LUNG CANCER

PRINCIPLES AND PRACTICE

LUNG CANCER

PRINCIPLES AND PRACTICE

SECOND EDITION

Editors

HARVEY I. PASS, MD

*Professor of Surgery and Oncology
Chief, Thoracic Oncology
Karmanos Cancer Institute
Wayne State University
Detroit, Michigan*

JAMES B. MITCHELL, PhD

*Branch Chief
Radiation Biology Branch
National Cancer Institute
Bethesda, Maryland*

DAVID H. JOHNSON, MD

*Cornelius A. Craig Professor of Medical & Surgical Oncology
Vanderbilt Ingram Cancer Center
Vanderbilt University School of Medicine
Nashville, Tennessee*

ANDREW T. TURRISI, MD

*Chairman
Department of Radiation Oncology
Medical University of South Carolina
Charleston, South Carolina*

JOHN D. MINNA, MD

*Chairman
Hamon Center for Therapeutic Oncology Research
University of Texas Southwestern Medical Center
Dallas, Texas*

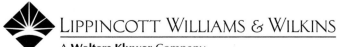

LIPPINCOTT WILLIAMS & WILKINS
A **Wolters Kluwer** Company

Philadelphia · Baltimore · New York · London
Buenos Aires · Hong Kong · Sydney · Tokyo

Developmental Editor: Tanya Lazar
Production Editor: Rakesh Rampertab
Manufacturing Manager: Colin J. Warnock
Cover Designer: Christine Jenny
Compositor: Maryland Composition Company Inc.
Printer: Courier Westford

© **2000 by LIPPINCOTT WILLIAMS & WILKINS**
530 Walnut Street
Philadelphia, PA 19106 USA
LWW.com

Printed in the USA

Library of Congress Cataloging-in-Publication Data

Lung cancer: principles and practice / Harvey I. Pass . . . [et al.].
    p.; cm.
    Includes bibliographical references and index.
    ISBN 0-7817-1791-4 (alk. paper)
    1. Lungs—Cancer. I. Pass, Harvey I.
    [DNLM: 1. Lung Neoplasms. WF 658 L9632 2000]
RC280.L8 L782 2000
616.99'424—dc21   99-051908

10 9 8 7 6 5 4 3 2 1

*This book is dedicated to our families. There are no substitutes
for their patience, encouragement, love, and support.*

*To
Helen, Ally, and Eric Pass*

Gloria Mitchell

Beverly and Mary-Michael Johnson

*Kathy, Richard, Casey, Harmon, Katie,
Carolyn, and, mostly, little Emilia Turrisi*

And the family of John Minna

*The inspiration for this endeavor came from
our patients, students, and residents,
as well as from our colleagues and mentors.
These sources of incredible wisdom and diversity
forced us to grapple with our limitations,
and help us to recognize how we can best utilize our strengths.*

CONTENTS

CONTRIBUTING AUTHORS

Amir Abolhoda, MD Instructor in Surgery/Department of Cardiothoracic Surgery, The University Hospital for Albert Einstein College of Medicine, 111 East 210 Street, Bronx, New York 10467-2490

Kathy S. Albain, MD Professor of Medicine, Division of Hematology/Oncology, Loyola University Medical Center, Cardinal Bernardin Cancer Center, Maywood, Illinois 60153

Joan Albanell, MD Attending Physician, Oncology Service, Hospital Universitari Vall d'Hebron, Barcelona, Spain

David L. Ball, MBBS, FRANZCR Head, Lung Unit, Division of Radiation Oncology, Peter MacCallum Cancer Institute, St. Andrews Place, East Melbourne, Victoria 3002, Australia

Frank A. Baciewicz, Jr, MD Associate Professor, Department of Cardiothoracic Surgery, Wayne State University, 3990 John R., #2162, Detroit, Michigan 48201

Steven A. Belinsky, PhD Senior Scientist, Department of Lung Cancer Program, Lovelace Respiratory Research Institute, PO Box 5890, Albuquerque, New Mexico 87185

Eric J. Bernhard, PhD Research Assistant Professor, Department of Radiation Oncology, University of Pennsylvania, 185 John Morgan Building, Philadelphia, Pennsylvania 19104-6072

Andrea Bezjak, MDCM, MSc, FRCPC Radiation Oncologist, Department of Radiation Oncology, Princess Margaret Hospital, University Health Network, 610 University Avenue, Toronto, Ontario M5G 2M9, Canada

Susan Blackwell, PA-C, MHS Senior Physician Assistant, Department of Medicine, Duke University Medical Center, Box 1-3198, Rm 25178, Morris Building, Duke University Medical Center, Erwin Road/Trent Drive, Durham, North Carolina 27710

James A. Bonner, MD Professor, Department of Radiation Oncology, University of Alabama, Birmingham, 619 South 19th Street, WTI-105, Birmingham, Alabama 35294

Robert F. Bonner, PhD Chief, Section of Medical Biophysics, Laboratory of Integrative and Medical Biophysics, National Institute of Child Health and Development, 13 South Drive, Bethesda, Maryland 20892-5772

Robert K. Bright, PhD Chief, Laboratory of Prostate Cancer Biology, Robert W. Franz Cancer Research Center, Providence Portland Medical Center, 4805 Northeast Glisan, 5F40, Portland, Oregon 97213

David P. Carbone, MD, PhD Professor of Medicine and Oncology, Division of Hermatology and Oncology, Vanderbilt-Ingram Cancer Center, 648 Medical Research Building II, Nashville, Tennessee 37232-6838

Murali Cherakuri, MD, Radiation Biology Branch, Division of Clinical Sciences, National Cancer Institute, Bethesda, Maryland 20892-1906

Pier Paolo Claudio, MD Department of Pathology, Anatomy and Cell Biology, Thomas Jefferson Medical College, 1020 Locust Street, Suite 226, Philadelphia, Pennsylvania 19107-6799

Keith Coffee, MD 648 Medical Research Center Building II, The Vanderbilt Cancer Center, Nashville, Tennessee 37232-6838

Andrew J. Coldman, PhD Head, Department of Cancer Control, British Columbia Cancer Agency, 600 West 10 Avenue, Vancouver, British Columbia, Canada, V5Z 4E6

John F. Conforti, DO Assistant Professor, Department of Pulmonary and Critical Care, Medicine, 2500 North State Street, Jackson, Mississippi 39216-4505

Denis A. Cortese, MD Chair, Board of Governors, Mayo Clinic Jacksonville, 4500 San Pablo Road, Jacksonville, Florida 32224

Douglas Coyle, MA, MSc Principal Investigator, Clinical Epidemiology Unit, Loeb Research Institute, 1053 Carling Avenue, Ottawa, Ontario 4E9, Canada

Jeffrey Crawford, MD Professor of Medicine, Box 3198, Rm. 25178, Morris Building, Duke University Medical Center, Erwin Road/Trent Drive, Durham, North Carolina 27710

Carlo M. Croce, PhD   Director, Kimmel Cancer Center, Thomas Jefferson University, BLSB Room 1050, 233 South 10th Street, Philadelphia, Pennslyvania 19107

Walter J. Curran, Jr, MD   Chairman, Department of Radiation Oncology, Kimmel Cancer Center at Thomas Jefferson, University Hospital, 111 South 11th Street, Philadelphia, Pennsylvania 19107-5097

Thomas A. D'Amico, MD   Assistant Professor, Department of Surgery, Duke University Medical Center, Box 3496, Durham, North Carolina 27710

Russell F. DeVore III, MD   Associate Professor, Department of Medicine, Vanderbilt University, 1956 TCV, Nashville, Tennessee 37232

Afshin Dowlati, MD   Fellow, Hematology/Oncology, Department of Medicine, Case Western Reserve University, 11100 Euclid Avenue, Cleveland, Ohio 44106

Ruth Louise Eakin, MRCPI, FRCR   Consultant, Department of Oncology, Northern Ireland Cancer Centre, Belfast, Nothern Ireland

Craig C. Earle, MD, FRCPC   Cancer Care Ontario Fellow, Center for Outcomes and Policy Research, Dana Farber Cancer Institute, Harvard Medical School, 25 Shattuck Street, Boston, Massachusettes 02115

Eric S. Edell, MD   Co-chair, Department of Pulmonary Critical Care, Mayo Clinic, 200 First Street Southwest, Rochester, Minnesota 55905

Michael R. Emmert-Buck, MD, PhD   Chief, Pathogenetics Unit, Laboratory of Pathology, National Cancer Institute, NIH, Bethesda, Maryland 20892

William K. Evans, MD, FRCPC   Chief Executive Officer, Ottawa Regional Cancer Centre, 501 Smyth Road, Ottawa, Ontario K1H 8L6, Canada

Eta Erdogan, MD   Department of Thoracic Surgery, Massachusetts General Hospital, Fruit Street, Boston, Massachusetts 02114

L. Penfield Faber, MD   Director, Section of General Thoracic Surgery, Department of Cardiovascular Thoracic Surgery, Rush-Presbyterian-St. Luke Medical Center, 1653 West Congress Parkway, Chicago, Illinois 60612

Ronald Feld, MD   Staff Physician, Department of Medical Oncology and Hematology, Princess Margaret Hospital, 610 University Avenue, Toronto, Ontario M5G 2M9, Canada

Mark K. Ferguson, MD   Professor, Department of Surgery, University of Chicago, 5841 South Maryland Avenue, Chicago, Illinois 60637

Frank V. Fossella, MD   Medical Director, Department of Thoracic Oncology, Multidisciplinary Center, M.D. Anderson Cancer Center, 1515 Holcombe Boulevard, Box 80, Houston, Texas 77030

Joseph M. Fugaro, MD   Resident in General Surgery, Karmanos Cancer Institute, Wayne State University, Detroit Medical Center, 110 East Warren Avenue, Detroit, Michigan 48201

Isaac R. Francis, MBBS   Department of Radiology, University of Michigan, 1500 East Medical Center Drive, Ann Arbor, Michigan 48109-0030

Adi F. Gazdar, MD   Professor of Pathology, Hamon Center for Oncology Research, University of Texas Southwestern Medical Center, 5323 Harry Hines Boulevard, Dallas, Texas 75235-8593

John Gillespie, MD   Research Fellow, Department of Pathogenetics Unit, Laboratory of Pathology, National Cancer Institute, 10 Center Drive, Building 10/Room 2C500, Bethesda, Maryland 20892

Robert J. Ginsberg, MD   Professor of Surgery, Cornell University Medical College, 525 East 68th Street, New York, New York 10021

Antonio Giordano, MD, PhD   Associate Professor, Department of Pathology, Anatomy, and Cell Biology, Thomas Jefferson Medical College, 1020 Locust Street, Philadelphia, Pennsylvania 19107

Mary V. Graham, MD   Director, Radiation Oncology, Philips County Regional Medical Center, 1000 West 10th Street, Rolla, Missouri 65401

Barry H. Gross, MD   Professor of Radiology, Department of Radiology, University of Michigan Medical Center, 1500 East Medical Center Drive, Ann Arbor, Michigan 48109-0030

Anjali K. Gupta, MD   Instructor, Department of Radiation Oncology, 2 Donner Building, The University of Pennsylvania, 3400 Spruce Street, Philadelphia, Pennsylvania 19104

Kenneth R. Hande, MD   Professor of Medicine and Pharmacology, Vanderbilt University School of Medicine, 1956 The Vanderbilt Clinic, Nashville, Tennessee 37232

Paul M. Harari, MD   Associate Professor, Department of Human Oncology, University of Wisconsin, 600 Highland Avenue, #K4/B100, Madison, Wisconsin 53792

William B. Harms, MD   Radiation Oncology Center, Washington University, Mallinckrodt Institute of Radiology, St. Louis, Missouri 63108

David H. Harpole, Jr, MD Associate Professor, Division of Thoracic Surgery, Duke University Medical Center, Trent Drive, #3617, Durham VA Medical Center, Durham, North Carolina 27710

Eleanor E.R. Harris, MD Department of Radiation Oncology, Hospital of the University of Pennsylvania, 3400 Spruce Street, Philadelphia, Pennsylvania 19104

Roy S. Herbst, MD, PhD Assistant Professor, Department of Thoracic/Head & Neck Medical Oncology, University of Texas M.D. Anderson Cancer Center, 1515 Holcombe Boulevard, Box 80, Houston, Texas 77030

Penelope Hopwood, MD, MSc, FRC Psych Honorary Consultant Psychiatrist, CRC Psychological Medicine Group, Christie Hospital NHS Trust, Wilmslow Road, Withington, Manchester M20 4BX, United Kingdom

Waun Ki Hong, MD Professor and Chairman, Department of Thoracic/Head & Neck Medical Oncology, University of Texas M.D. Anderson Cancer Center, 1515 Holcombe Boulevard, Box 80, Houston, Texas 77030

Kay Huebner, PhD Professor, Department of Microbiology Immunology, Thomas Jefferson University, Kimmel Cancer Institute, 233 South 10th Street, Room 1050, BLSB, Philadelphia, Pennsylvania 19107

Mark Iannettoni, MD Associate Professor of Surgery, Section of General Thoracic Surgery, University of Michigan, 1500 East Medical Center Drive, Ann Arbor, Michigan 48109-0344

Pasi A. Jänne, MD, PhD Clinical Fellow in Oncology, Lowe Center for Thoracic Oncology, Department of Adult Oncology, Dana Farber Cancer Institute, 44 Binney Street, Boston, Massachusettes 02115

Bruce Evans Johnson, MD Chief, Lowe Center for Thoracic Oncology, Dana Farber Cancer Institute, 44 Binney Street, Boston, Massachusettes 02115

David H. Johnson, MD Cornelius A. Craig Professor of Medical & Surgical Oncology, Vanderbilt Ingram Cancer Center, Vanderbilt University School of Medicine, Nashville, Tennessee 37232-5536

Gregory P. Kalemkerian, MD Associate Professor, Department of Internal Medicine, University of Michigan, 1500 East Medical Center Drive, Ann Arbor, Michigan 48109-0922

Harubumi Kato, MD Department of Surgery, Tokyo Medical College, 6-7-1, Nishishinjuku, Shinjuku-ku, Tokyo 160 Japan

Steven M. Keller, MD Chief, Division of Thoracic Surgery, Beth Israel Medical Center, First Avenue and 16th Street, New York, New York 10003

Fadlo R. Khuri, MD Assistant Professor of Medicine, Department of Thoracic/Head & Neck Medical Oncology, University of Texas M.D. Anderson Cancer Center, 1515 Holcombe Boulevard, Box 80, Houston, Texas 77030

Timothy J. Kinsella, MS, MD Director, Department of Radiation Oncology, University Hospitals of Cleveland Health System and Ireland Cancer Center, Lerner Tower, Room 6068, 11100 Euclid Avenue, Cleveland, Ohio 44106-6068

Ritsuko Komaki, MD Professor of Radiation Oncology, Department of Radiation Oncology, University of Texas M.D. Anderson Cancer, Center, 1515 Holcombe Boulevard, Box 97, Houston, Texas 77030

Michael Kraut, MD Associate Professor of Medicine, Department of Hematology/Oncology, Karmanos Cancer Institute, Harper Hospital, 3990 John R., Suite 5 Hudson, 110 E Warren Avenue, Detroit, Michigan 48201

John J. Kresl, MD, PhD Attending Staff Radiation Oncologist, Department of Radiation Oncology, St. Joseph's Hospital, 350 West Thomas Road, Phoenix, Arizona 85013

Samir Kubba, MD 648 Medical Research Building II, The Vanderbilt Cancer Center, Nashville, Tennessee 37232-6838

Stephen Lam, MD Professor of Medicine, British Columbia Cancer Center, 2775 Heather Street, Vancouver, British Columbia V5Z 2J5, Canada

Christine L. Lau, MD Resident in General and Thoracic Surgery, Duke University Medical Center, Durham, North Carolina 27710

Michael LeBlanc The Ontario Cancer Center, 500 Sherbourne Street, Toronto, Ontario M4X 1K9, Canada

John F. Lechner, PhD Professor, Department of Oncology and Pathology, Karmanos Cancer Institute, 110 East Warren Avenue, Detroit, Michigan 48201

Choon-Taek Lee, MD 688 Medical Research Building II, The Vanderbilt Cancer Center, Nashville, Tennessee 37232-6838

Rayman Lee, MD Department of Medicine, University of Texas Medical Branch, 301 University Boulevard, Galveston, Texas 77555

James Linder, MD   Professor, Department of Pathology and Microbiology, University of Nebraska College of Medicine, 986545 Nebraska Medical Center, Omaha, Nebraska 68198

Lance A. Liotta, MD, PhD   Chief, Laboratory of Pathology, National Cancer Institute, Bethesda, Maryland 20892

Fulvio Lonardo, MD   Assistant Professor of Pathology, Wayne State University, Harper Hospital and Karmanos Cancer Center, 110 East Warren Avenue, Detroit, Michigan 48201

Alvin M. Malkinson, PhD   Professor, Department of Pharmaceutical Sciences, University of Colorado, 4200 East 9th Street, Denver, Colorado 80262

Fernando J. Martinez, MD   Associate Professor, Department of Internal Medicine, University of Michigan, 1500 East Medical Center Drive, 3616, Taubman Center, Ann Arbor, Michigan 48109-0360

Douglas Mathisen, MD   Professor of Surgery, Chief, General & Thoracic Surgery, Massachusetts General Hospital, 32 Fruit Street, Blake Building, Room 1570, Boston, Massachusetts 02114

Bruce Mackay, MD, PhD   Department of Pathology, University of Texas M.D. Anderson Cancer Center, Houston, Texas 77030

W. Gillies McKenna, MD, PhD   Professor and Chair, Department of Radiation Oncology, University of Pennsylvania, 3400 Spruce Street, Philadelphia, Pennsylvania 19104

Minesh P. Mehta, MD   Associate Professor and Interim Chair, Department of Human Oncology, University of Wisconsin-Madison, 600 Highland Avenue, K4/312-3684, Madison, Wisconsin 53792

Mark R. Middleton, MA, MRCP   Lecturer, CRC Department of Medical Oncology, Christie Hospital NHS Trust, Wilmslow Road, Manchester, M20 9BX, United Kingdom

York E. Miller, MD   Staff Physician, Department of Medicine, University of Colorado Heath Sciences Center, 4200 East 9th Avenue, Denver, Colorado 80262

John D. Minna, MD   Chairman, Hamon Center for Therapeutic Oncology Research, University of Texas Southwestern Medical Center, 5323 Harry Hines Boulevard, Dallas, Texas 75235

James B. Mitchell, PhD   Branch Chief, Radiation Biology Branch, National Cancer Institute, Building 10, Room B3-B69, 9000 Rockville Pike, Bethesda, MD 20892

Mark Mostovych, MD   1820 Barrs Street, Suite #701, Jacksonville, Florida 32204

Clifton F. Mountain, MD   Clinical Professor of Surgery, Division of Cardiothoracic Surgery, University of California, San Diego, West Arbor Drive, San Diego, California 92103-8892

Mary J. Mulligan-Kehoe, PhD   Borwell 552 E, 1 Medical Center Drive, Dartmouth College, Lebanon, New Hampshire, 03756

Nevin Murray, MD, FRCPC   Department of Medical Oncology, British Columbia Cancer Agency, 600 West 10th Avenue, Vancouver, British Columbia V5Z 4E6, Canada

Ruth J. Muschel, MD   Department of Pathology and Laboratory Medicine, University of Pennsylvania, 3400 Spruce Street, Philadelphia, Pennsylvania 19104

Christopher Mutrie, BS   Columbia University, College of Physicians & Surgeons, 630 West 168th Street, New York, NY 10032

Jonathan C. Nesbitt, MD   Staff Surgeon Department of Cardiothoracic Surgery, St. Thomas Hospital, 4320 Harding Road, Nashville, Tennessee 37205

Yasuhiko Ohta, MD   Department of Surgery, Kanazawa University, School of Medicine, Takara-machi 13-1, Kanazawa, 920-8641, Japan

Herbert K. Oie, PhD   National Naval Medical Center, NCI/Naval Medical Oncology Branch, Building 8, Room 5105, Bethesda, Maryland 20892

Jemi Olak, MD   Associate Professor of Clinical Surgery, Lutheran General Hospital, 1700 Luther Lane, Park Ridge, Illinois 60068

Roberto Pacelli, MD   Radiotherapy Department, Medical School, University "Federico II", Naples, Italy

Robert Paine, II, MD   Associate Professor of Internal Medicine, Department of Internal Medicine, University of Michigan, Ann Arbor, Michigan 48109-0360

Harvey I. Pass, MD   Professor of Surgery and Oncology, Chief, Thoracic Oncology, Karmanos Cancer Institute, Wayne State University, 3990 John R, Suite 2102, Detroit, Michigan 48201

David G. Payne, MSc, MD   Department of Radiation Oncology, Princess Margaret Hospital, University Health Network, 610 University Avenue, Toronto, Ontario M5G 2M9, Canada

Thomas L. Petty, MD   Professor Of Medicine, Department of Medicine, University of Colorado, 4200 East 9th Avenue, Denver, Colorado 80218

Jennifer A. Pietenpol, PhD Associate Professor, Department of Biochemistry, Vanderbilt University School of Medicine, 652 Medical Research Building II, Nashville, Tennessee 37232

William Piccione, MD Associate Professor, Department of Cardiothoracic Surgery, Rush Medical Center, 1725 West Harrison Street, Suite 425, Chicago, Illinois 60612

Katherine M.W. Pisters, MD Associate Professor, Department of Thoracic/Head & Neck Medical, Oncology, University of Texas M.D. Anderson Cancer Center, 1515 Holcombe Boulevard, Box 80, Houston, Texas 77030

Jeffrey Port, MD Division of Thoracic Surgery, Department of Surgery, Memorial Sloan-Kettering Cancer Center, New York, New York 10021

William A. Pryor, PhD Director and Professor, Biodynamics Institute, Louisiana State University, 711 Choppin, Baton Rouge, Louisiana 70803

Leslie E. Quint, MD Professor of Radiology, Department of Radiology, University of Michigan Health Systems, 1500 East Medical Center Drive, Ann Arbor, Michigan 48109-0030

Angelo Russo, MD Radiation Biology Branch, National Cancer Institute, Building 10, Room B3-B69, National Institutes of Health, Bethesda, Maryland 20892

Uri Sagman The Ontario Cancer Institute, 500 Sherbourne Street, Toronto, Ontario M4X 1K9, Canada

Aravind B. Sankar, MD Department of Surgery, University of Texas Medical Branch, 301 University Boulevard, Galveston, Texas 77555-0534

Timothy E. Sawyer, MD Senior Associate Consultant, Department of Radiation Oncology, Mayo Clinic, 200 First Street Southwest, Rochester, Minnesota 55905

Joan H. Schiller, MD Professor, Department of Medicine/Medical Oncology Section, University of Wisconsin Hospital and Clinics, Room K4/636 CSC, 600 Highland Avenue, Madison, Wisconsin 53792

Ann G. Schwartz, PhD, MPH Associate Professor, Department of Epidemiology, Karmanos Cancer Institute, 110 East Warren Avenue, Detroit, Michigan 48201

David Schottenfeld, MD, MSc John G. Searle Professor of Epidemiology, Department of Epidemiology, University of Michigan, 109 Observatory Street, Ann Arbor, Michigan 48109-2029

Frances A. Shepherd, MD, FRCPC Senior Staff Physician, Department of Medical Oncology and Hematology, Princess Margaret Hospital, 610 University Avenue, Toronto, Ontario M5G 2M9, Canada

Deborah Shure, MD Director, Pulmonary and Critical Care Medicine, University of Mississippi Medical Center, 2500 North State Street, Jackson, Mississippi 39216

Nicole L. Simone, BS Laboratory of Pathology, National Cancer Institute, 900 Rockville Pike, Bethesda, Maryland 20892

Gabriella Sozzi, PhD Head of Molecular-Cytogenetic Unit, Department of Experimental Oncology, Instituto Nazionale Tumori, Via Venezian 1, 20133 Milano, Italy

Burton L. Speiser, MD, MS Director, Department of Radiation Oncology, St. Joseph's Medical Center, 350 West Thomas Road, Phoenix, Arizona 85013

Seth M. Steinberg, PhD Head, Biostatistics and Data Management Section, Division of Clinical Sciences, National Cancer Institute, 6116 Executive Boulevard, Room 702, MSC 8325, Bethesda, Maryland 20892-8325

Francis J. Sullivan, MB, MRCPI Medical Director, Maryland Regional Cancer Care, 2121 Medical Park Drive, Suite 4, Silver Springs, Maryland 20902

Suzanne T. Szak Department of Biochemistry, Vanderbilt University, Medical Research Building II, Room 652, Nashville, Tennessee 37232

Joseph R. Testa, PhD Director, Human Genetics Program, Population Science Division, Fox Chase Cancer Center, 7701 Burholme Avenue, Philadelphia, Pennsylvania 19111

Nicholas Thatcher, MD Chairman, Department of Lung Cancer Surgery, Christie Hospital NHS Trust, Wilmslow Road, Manchester, M20 4BX, United Kingdom

Ralph de la Torre, MD Assistant Professor of Cardiothoracic Surgery, Boston Medical Center, 88 East Newton, Boston, Massachusetts 02114

Alessandra Tosolini, BSc Research Assistant, Department of Population Science, Fox Chase Cancer Center, 7701 Burholme Avenue, Philadelphia, Pennsylvania 19111

Elizabeth L. Travis, PhD Professor, Division of Radiation Oncology, University of Texas M.D. Anderson Cancer Center, 1515 Holcombe Boulevard, Box 066, Houston, Texas 77030-4095

William D. Travis, MD Department of Pulmonary and Mediastinal Pathology, Building 54, Room M003B, Armed Forces Institute of Pathology, 6825 Northwest 16th Street, Washington, D.C. 20306-6000

Andrew T. Turrisi, MD Chairman, Department of Radiation Oncology, Medical University of South Carolina, 169 Ashley Avenue, Box 250318, Charleston, South Carolina 29425

Maria-Luisa Veronese, MD Postdoctoral Fellow, Division of Clinical Pharmacology, Thomas Jefferson University Hospital, 132 South 10th Street, Philadelphia, Pennsylvania 19107

Henry Wagner, Jr, MD Staff Physician, Department of Radiation Oncology, Moffitt Cancer Center, 12902 Magnolia Drive, Tampa, Florida 33612-9497

Richard L. Wahl, MD Professor, Department of Internal Medicine, B1G412 University Hospital, Ann Harbor, Michigan 48109-0028

William H. Warren, MD Professor, Department of Cardiovascular-Thoracic Surgery, Rush Medical Center, 1725 West Harrison Street, Suite 218, Chicago, Illinois 60612

Yoh Watanabe, MD Professor, Department of Surgery, Kanazawa University School of Medicine, 13-1 Takaramachi, Kanazawa 920-864, Japan

Ignacio I. Wistuba, MD Department of Pathology, Pontificia Universidad Catolica de Chile, Santiago, P.O. Box 114-D, Chile

Antoinette Wozniak, MD Associate Professor, Department of Medicine, Wayne State University, 3990 John R, Suite 5 Hudson, Detroit, Michigan 48201

Joseph B. Zwischenberger, MD Director of General Thoracic Surgery, ECMO Program, Division of Cardiothoracic Surgery, University of Texas Medical Branch, 301 University Boulevard, Galveston, Texas 77555-0528

PREFACE

It is now three years since we wrote that "lung cancer is the leading cause of cancer-related deaths in North America and Europe, and its incidence is rising elsewhere," ensuring an increasing number of lung cancer deaths worldwide. Unfortunately, we can substitute "remains the leading cause" for "is the leading cause." In 1997 alone, 178,100 new lung cancer patients were diagnosed in the United States. Lung cancer is rising at an exponential rate in women and in under-served populations. Children and young adults continue to smoke in alarming proportions. That's the bad news.

The encouraging news is that lung cancer and tobacco abuse are getting the attention necessary to actually open pocket books for related clinical and benchwork research. Advocacy groups for lung cancer, virtually unheard of in 1996, are taking a more proactive stance in the education of patients, families, and primary care physicians. An unprecedented resurgence in early detection, screening, and lung cancer prevention is gaining momentum, which could eventually translate into stage migration. New imaging techniques are being validated for increased sensitivity that may even change surgical staging practices. Aggressive multimodality therapy is moving into clinical trials for patients with earlier stages. Even the staging system (biologic staging) is different! Scientists are beginning to lay out an evolutionary molecular model of airway carcinogenesis. This model may predict or describe either the earliest event that could signal the development of lung cancer, or the event in the spectrum that is the latest, but reversible, so that it would be possible to indicate who will move on to neoplasia.

The task for all of us involved in the management of lung cancer is to look critically at past, present, and novel therapies for lung cancer. After this survey, we must assess the reasons for their failure, and study new therapies in ways that will delivers answers, hopefully at an unprecedented pace.

This, the second edition of *Lung Cancer: Principles and Practice,* retains the specifications that were made for its predecessor. It contains contributions from clinicians in *all* relevant disciplines—surgery, radiation oncology, medical oncology, pathology, and pulmonology. Also, it includes contributions from basic scientists working in the field. We have attempted to blend clinical reality with benchwork

dreams in a manner that assumed nothing regarding the reader's basic knowledge of lung cancer. Additionally, we have retained a similar format, starting with the biology of the disease. This concept extends to the clinical disciplines, with discussions of basic principles regarding surgery, radiotherapy, and chemotherapy. After the groundwork is laid, indepth discussions of innovative or aggressive treatments are outlined by authors who offer original detailed descriptions. This book alludes to the advantages, limits, and results of a multidisciplinary approach throughout, while making a concerted effort to unite concepts regarding this disease, such that the reader is armed with a greater understanding of the natural history, biology, and treatment options for lung cancer.

This second edition is meant to serve as a *comprehensive reference* for any individual interested in lung cancer; one that would appeal to scientists with very basic information of lung cancer, clinicians, and serve to broaden the knowledge base of medical students, primary care physicians, and cancer specialists.

Although the format may look similar, this edition has changed in accordance with the changes that occurred in the world of lung cancer. The book is bigger, and this reflects the increasing fund of clinical and benchwork knowledge that occurred since 1996. Newer aspects of the molecular genetics and biology of lung cancer are found in contributions concerning *FHIT,* telomerase, and *erbB*-2, as well as the intricacies of the cell cycle and angiogenesis. Lung cancer immunology and gene therapy are completely updated, and the newest elements of genetic susceptibility are included as a separate chapter. Technical changes, even in processing material for molecular evaluation are discussed, as is the use of these techniques in defining preneoplasia at the chromosomal/genetic level. Obviously, this requires that both biologic staging and morphologic/pathologic staging be discussed separately. There is a greater emphasis on screening and prevention for early disease, as well as the management of the elderly with lung cancer. The explosion of new cytotoxic agents for lung cancer and their interaction with radiation therapy is given a prominent role in this edition. Palliation is discussed again as a separate section, but a new discussion of cost-effectiveness of lung-cancer therapies reminds us of the economic realities of this problem.

The editors cannot emphasize enough the attention to detail and the cooperation shown by the contributing authors. All are experts who have made contributions to the study of lung cancer and the care of the lung cancer patient.

The editors would also like to express their gratitude to Lippincott Williams & Wilkins, specifically Stuart Freeman, who was always supportive of this effort, and Tanya Lazar, whose skillful coordination between contributors, editors, and Lippincott kept the project moving without incident.

Lung Cancer: Principles and Practice is intended to provide both the practitioner and the trainee with a reference source that will be useful in those moments of frustration in dealing with this disease. The editors' most profound wish is that the material presented will stimulate other investigators to join in the fight against lung cancer, so that future editions will describe therapies that will move the survival curves upward and towards the right.

Harvey I. Pass, MD
James B. Mitchell, PhD
David H. Johnson, MD
Andrew T. Turrisi, MD
John D. Minna, MD

LUNG CANCER

PRINCIPLES AND PRACTICE

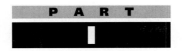

BIOLOGY OF LUNG CANCER

GENERAL CONCEPTS

1

GENERAL CONCEPTS OF MOLECULAR BIOLOGY RELATED TO LUNG CANCER

MARY J. MULLIGAN-KEHOE
ANGELO RUSSO

Molecular biology has assumed a preeminent role in biomedical research. The rapid ascension of molecular biology has occurred because it provides a solid framework for explaining and extending biological phenomena that were previously only observable. Certainly there continues to be a descriptive approach to biology, but more and more these descriptions are fashioned in molecular terms. Furthermore, molecular biology extends into so many fields of study because the methods employed are relatively straightforward, easily learned, and rapidly applied. Upon opening any biological or medical journal one quickly sees that molecular biology methods are being applied to all biological sciences. Minuscule quantities of potentially short-lived biomaterials can be amplified, isolated, studied, and subsequently perturbed and reevaluated. Within this chapter we emphasize the molecular biology of gene regulation and expression because we fundamentally believe that lung cancer occurs as a result of deregulation of normal gene expression. We also provide a compendium that defines and explains frequently used terms and illustrates the common methods employed by those who apply molecular biology to the study of lung cancer.

DNA STRUCTURE

Cellular function and structure are predetermined by the genetic profile of the cell. Although viruses are capable of archiving genetic information as ribonucleic acid (RNA), single-stranded (ss) deoxyribonucleic acid (DNA), or double-stranded (ds) DNA, prokaryotic (nonnucleated) and eukaryotic (nucleated) cells store genetic information within dsDNA.[1] Upon isolation and purification of DNA, one finds that it is formed from two purine nucleotides, adenine (A) and guanine (G), and two pyrimidine nucleotides, thymidine (T) and cytosine (C) (Figure 1.1).[2] Single-stranded DNA is a linear biopolymer resulting from covalent phosphate diester bonds between the deoxyribose sugars of the nucleotides. The hydrogen bonding between two ssDNA molecules results from individual As of one chain bonding with Ts of the other chain, likewise for the Gs with Cs (Figure 1.2). Consequently, in dsDNA the percentage of A always equals T, and likewise G equals C. Each nucleotide of the individual single strand inclines approximately at a right angle to the axis of the deoxyribose backbone. As the nucleotides project toward one another and wind about the axis of the backbone, they overlap to greater or lesser degrees, and as such there is an additional stability to the structure that results from Van der Waal's stacking forces. Approximately ten nucleotides form each 360-degree turn of the biopolymer. The hydrophilic phospho-sugars within the backbone establish major contact with the water environment of the cell, and the pendent nucleotides bind the two chains together and create a more hydrophobic interior. The macromolecular structure formed from such an arranged paired of ssDNA molecules, running in opposite directions, is a right-handed, antiparallel, double helix (Figure 1.3).[3-5] As is seen in Figure 1.3, in addition to the above structural characteristics, the double helix has a major and a minor groove.

One might assume that the double helix is a monotonous set of deoxyribonucleotides winding about a central axis, and the information stored within this string of nucleotidyl bases is but a simple alphabetic display which can be represented by a long piece of thin tape having an extensive display of doublets of As and Ts or Gs and Cs. This is not the case. The helix is conformationally flexible or polymorphic as a result of the local nucleotide sequences. The actual twist and bend of the helical structure may change as a function, for instance, of the A to T ratio. A homopolymer of A/T has a twist of approximately 36 degrees per base step or ten bases per turn of the helix, that is, the helix is overwound relative to an average of 34 degrees per base found in random-sequence DNA.[6] Moreover, if one considers the actual nucleotide sequence, for instance A:T pairs that are binding from the individual ssDNA through two

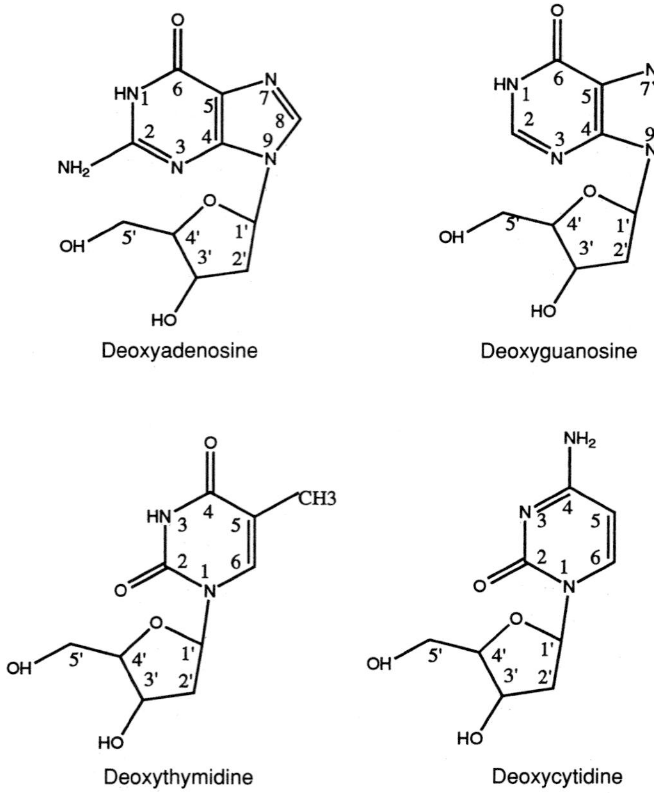

Deoxyadenosine

Deoxyguanosine

Deoxythymidine

Deoxycytidine

FIGURE 1.1. The four nucleotides that form DNA. Note the formal nomenclature for the deoxynucleotides. In common usage these are referred to as adenosine, guanosine, thymidine, and cytidine. These nucleotides are composed of nucleoside bases and deoxyribose sugars.

structure. If nucleotide sequences repeat at a frequency corresponding to the helical periodicity, that is, approximately every ten bases, it becomes even more apparent that local structure can function to exert bending forces on the helical structure.[7] The nucleotide sequences can and do influence the depth and width of the major or minor grooves, and the depth and width of the grooves may determine if or how effectively a protein binds DNA. Therefore a DNA-binding protein may not recognize just a linear sequence of bases, but local environment as well. This means that not only do nucleotides code for specific amino acids, but also that the sequence of nucleotides encodes local topological information that may have profound implications on DNA-protein interactions or intracellular conduction of transduced signals or may simply the ease by which DNA unwinds, which in itself may affect recombination or replication or transcription.

The double-helical DNA contains all the cell's genetic information, that is the genome. A bacterium's genome is composed of one linear dsDNA structure (chromosome) and is measured in the millions of nucleotides; whereas eukaryotic genomic dsDNA is composed, for the most part, of many individual chromosomes, each composed of 10^7 to greater than 10^8 nucleotides. In bacteria there are no DNA-binding histone complexes. The DNA is not compacted; it is spread generally throughout the central aspect of the cell in a structure which contains no nuclear membrane and is referred to as a nucleoid shape.[8] In contrast, eukaryotic chromosomal DNA is within a nuclear envelope and, for the most part, is highly compacted around histone protein complexes that are further compressed.[9] A consequence of this fundamental difference in storage of information is that bacteria are more readily able to access DNA either to dupli-

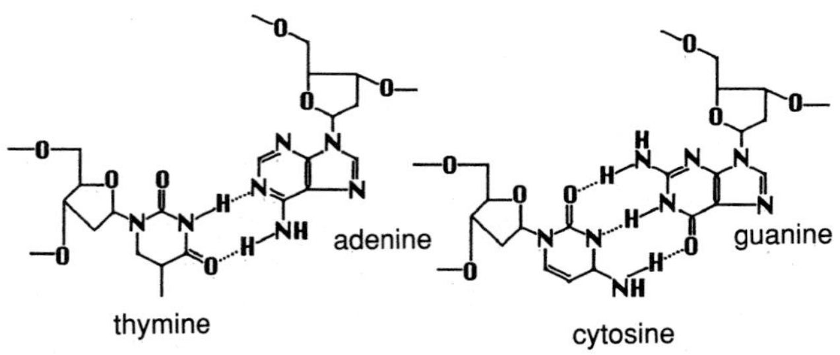

hydrogen bonds, then there is, when compared to G:C pairs that have three hydrogen bonds, a greater chance that the individual A and T will be slightly twisted relative to the right-angle plane of the axis of the helix (Figure 1.4). The result of A and T being potentially positioned slightly out of the plane is local distortion and/or stress in the helical

thymine   adenine

cytosine   guanine

FIGURE 1.2. The nucleotides are shown to demonstrate the hydrogen bonding between nucleotides. Note that adenine and thymine share two hydrogen bonds, whereas guanine and cytosine share three hydrogen bonds.

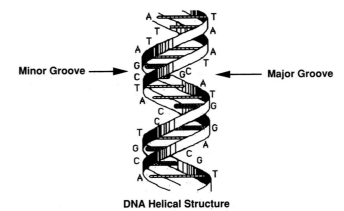

Minor Groove →   ← **Major Groove**

DNA Helical Structure

FIGURE 1.3. Double-stranded DNA is presented in its double helical form. The horizontal lines represent hydrogen bonding between the nucleotides within each single-stranded DNA molecule. The major and minor grooves of the helix are depicted with arrows.

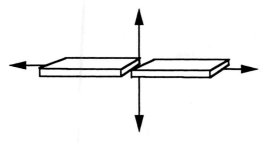

Parallel Base Pairing

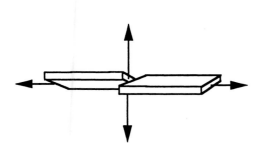

Propellar Twist Pairing

FIGURE 1.4. In **(A)** the nucleotide bases within DNA are represented schematically as two parallel bases. In **(B)** the bases are slightly twisted and consequently they are no longer parallel.

cate or to decode genetic information than are eukaryotes. The genome of a eukaryotic cell can therefore be viewed as an encrypted genetic archive made of sequences of linear arrayed nucleotides existing in a double helix, and the helix is further structured by virtue of bends and torsions and by winding around histone core protein complexes that are capable of assuming yet higher organizational structures.

TRANSCRIPTION

The array of nucleotides contains specific signals that allow proteins access to sites to start genomic duplication (origin of replication)[10,11] or gene transcription.[12–14] Transcription—copying DNA in an RNA form—of a gene is always started at the 5′ portion of the gene. In bacteria the nucleotide sequences containing information for gene transcription are streamlined. The nucleotide sequence coding for a specific gene product (a polypeptide or RNA) is composed of a promoter region followed immediately by a gene. In some cases the gene is transcribed as a single unit of RNA. In other cases the promoter is followed by a sequence that

results in transcription of multiple, juxtaposed, metabolically related genes.[15] The gene(s) in the DNA is transcribed into an exact complementary single strand of RNA that is usually translated into a polypeptide. This is the operon model of gene expression that is used by prokaryotes.[16,17] It is simple and exceedingly efficient. As messenger RNA (mRNA) destined to be translated into protein is being synthesized, it is immediately tethered to a ribosome,[18–21] wherein triplets of nucleotides (codons) of the mRNA sequences[22] are translated by aligning with a triplet nucleotide structure (anticodon) within an amino acid carrier molecule, transfer RNA (tRNA), which is positioned in the ribosomal structure. Rapidly thereafter the amino acid charged tRNA transfers its specific amino acid to a growing polypeptide chain. Each successive codon is translated by positioning another tRNA, until the stop codon is reached, whereupon the process of translating RNA into protein is completed. In the bacteria translation begins while the mRNA is being synthesized.[23] In fact, the amino terminal portion of a protein—that which corresponds to the 5′ segment of the gene—is frequently being synthesized while the 3′ segment of the gene is being transcribed. For bacteria, speed of gene expression is facilitated by such an efficient means of protein synthesis.

Prokaryote Transcription

In bacteria, a rather simple promoter sequence is the DNA determinant for the site of initiation of gene expression. The promoter is always in front (5′) of the gene. It usually has a TATA-box lying ten nucleotides 5′ of the start of transcription, that is, -10 nucleotides form the transcriptional initiation start site (Figure 1.5). Usually directly upstream of the TATA-box is the region where proteins can bind to DNA to either repress or stimulate synthesis.[24,25] Transcription begins when an open TATA-box or promoter element is recognized by one of a set of alternative protein transcriptional factors, σ, that binds to a multi-subunit RNA polymerase core enzyme (E)—composed of $\beta\beta'\alpha_2$—to form the transcriptional complex holoenzyme (Eσ).[26] The structure of $\beta\beta'\alpha_2$ is triangular, with $\beta\beta'$ forming the two sides and α_2 the base.[27,28] σ-factor fits in the middle of the triangle and makes contact with the TATA-box element. E without a σ-factor has the characteristics of nonspecific binding to DNA and has the capability of synthesizing long pieces of RNA from nicked DNA or single-stranded DNA. When a σ factor binds to the core enzyme it effects a conformational change in E.[29] With this conformational change, Eσ no longer binds DNA nonspecifically but rather recognizes specific promoter sites and initiates transcription from the start site, that is, σ changes E to an initiation-specific RNA polymerase. The σ-factor appears more than just to change the conformation of the

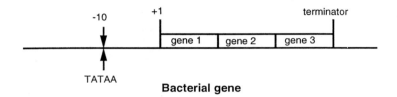

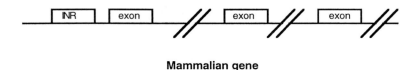

FIGURE 1.5. Contrast the construction of a bacterial gene containing three tandem genes with that of a mammalian gene which has an initiation element (INR), exons, and intervening introns.

core enzyme in order to allow it to bind the − 10 TATA-box site, it also allows the holoenzyme to interact with the DNA approximately two turns more 3′ or 5′ to the − 10 site, that is, in the vicinity of − 35 relative to the initiation origin. Once Eσ binds to the promoter region at the TATA-box, the closed complex is formed in which the RNA polymerase is bound to the DNA, but the DNA has not started to unwind. Since hydroxyl radicals are highly reactive species that will damage any exposed DNA, they have been used to demonstrate that in the closed-complex state, RNA polymerase protein complex protects the DNA from hydroxyl radical-induced base damage on one side of the helix by virtue of partially enwrapping the DNA. In the open complex it appears as if the DNA is completely enwrapped and both sides of it are protected.[30,31] This implies that in the closed complex, the initiation complex rests on only one side of the DNA, whereas in the open complex the DNA is surrounded by the initiation complex. As the DNA unwinds there is separation of the two strands to form a "bubble,"[32,33] and thereby to allow Eσ to align incoming ribonucleotides with the corresponding coding strand of DNA and to start synthesis of a complementary nucleotide polymer in an RNA format; that is, transcription begins. When the RNA polymerase complex proceeds past the initiation site—approximately ten nucleotides beyond the start site—the σ detaches from the core enzyme structure, and elongation of RNA commences and continues until, and beyond, the gene or operon terminus, whereupon E dissociates from the DNA, and the mRNA continues to be translated.[34–37] The selection of individual promoters to be transcribed is determined by the concentration of individual σ-factors which are in competition with one another. The σ^{70}-factor is the most abundant of the σ-factors in *Esche-*

richia coli (*E. coli*). In general, σ^{70} recognizes the most commonly employed promoter element in bacteria; the TATA-box sequence. As σ^{70} concentration decreases, there is greater utilization of other promoter-specific σ-factors, which in turn results in transcriptional selection of more specific genes.[38,39] In general, transcriptional regulation of housekeeping genes is controlled by the concentration of a specific σ. Most recently, another aspect of σ concentration regulation has been found in which anti-σ-factors bind specifically to specific σ-factors to regulate the available concentration of σ-factors available to initiate transcription.[40] In bacteria, once the mRNA is synthesized, its lifetime is measured in minutes, usually being degraded immediately after being translated. This is not necessarily the case for eukaryotic mRNA.

It should be recognized that a bacterium is a single-cell organism that sustains itself, for the most part, by multiplying at a faster rate than its competitors. Therefore, rapid doubling times demand ready access to the DNA for duplication and transcription. Regulation of transcription is essentially minimalistic, with on and off switches being controlled by accessibility to the promoter by the transcriptional complex containing RNA polymerase. Models of prokaryotic transcription envision the RNA polymerase complex being bound to dispersed DNA awaiting a signal to permit synthesis. Gram-negative *E. coli*'s cytoplasm is surrounded by an envelope composed of two membranes having an intermediate zone called the periplasmic space. The bacterium must therefore direct proteins to the cytoplasm, the inner or outer membrane, and the periplasmic space and react to its environment by quickly transducing messages directly to the DNA. Consequently, bacteria have trafficking signals (amino acid sequences that direct a protein to a specific site) and have specific pores for entry of substrates that will be metabolized by or interact with macromolecules. The bacterium must utilize nutrients efficiently and therefore be able to activate quickly a set of proteins that metabolize a specific substrate (gene arrangement in an operon facilitates such an existence) and subsequently suppress the synthesis of unnecessary proteins. It is the rule that repressed on/off promoters remain so until they are needed or until σ-factors are produced or activated as a result of adaptive stress. The entire life process in molecular biologic terms is efficiently fast because life depends on the ability to take advantage of the environment by multiplying and thereby replicating and producing proteins and other needed metabolic products faster than competing rivals.

Eukaryote Transcription

Although eukaryotes have comparable macromolecular structure to the bacterium, the higher eukaryotic cells for the most part are much more elaborate than bacteria by virtue of cellular structure and function. In eukaryotic cells, rapid multiplication is not usually the life-sustaining issue; controlled growth in concert with other cells is paramount. Deviation from concerted growth patterns results in unfavorable consequences. Stated differently, loss of regulatory control of any cell within a multicellular organism may have untoward effects, such as death of the cell or worse, and more threatening to the entire organism is development of cancer and subsequent death of the entire organism. Consequently, a universal theme in the molecular biology of higher eukaryotic cells is regulation that depends upon skillfully arranging elaborate networks to modulate an individual cellular function.

Chromatin Structure

For mammalian cells the important cellular function of transcribing information from DNA becomes much more complex than that described for prokaryotes. In fact, the entire genome is larger and more elaborate and more regulatory controls are manifest in both the DNA interacting proteins as well as, or maybe because of, the DNA structure itself. As noted above, the bacterial genome is, for the most part, set for rapid access and utility; whereas the mammalian genome, for the most part, is compacted into defined structures that may be bound to the nuclear membrane and other intranuclear matrix filamentous structure. Before a sequence of DNA (gene) can be transcribed, it must be exposed. The chromatin structure of eukaryotic cells is composed of a basic structure, the nucleosome.[41] Core nucleosomes contain approximately 146 base pairs wrapped twice around a core octameric histone protein complex (Figure 1.6). The core of the histone octamer is constructed from a central tetramer composed of two H3 and two H4 histones in con-

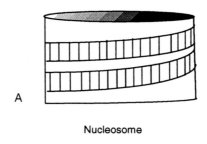

Nucleosome

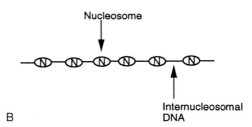

FIGURE 1.6. **A:** the core nucleosome, which is 7 nm in diameter, composed of a tetramer of histones with two loops of the DNA strand wrapped around the outermost aspect of the histone tetramer. **B:** the "beads on a string" arrangement of nucleosomal DNA.

tinuity on each side with two heterodimers of histone H2A and H2B. This fundamental nucleosomal structure has a 7-nm diameter and when viewed by electron microscopy has the appearance of beads that are linked to one another by threads of nonnucleosomal DNA. In higher eukaryotic cells the core nucleosomes can then associate with H1 histone, which can then result in a more elaborate compacted display in which the individual nucleosomes are wound together in a structure that results in further compression of the chromatin into a 30 nm structure. The 30 nm fibers can then be further organized into a more compact structure by interacting with nonhistone proteins to result in a highly compressed genome.[9,42–45] As would be expected from the nucleosomal structure, there would be limited access to an embedded mammalian gene within the highly compressed chromatin structure. Even in the state where the chromatin has been decompressed to the individual nucleosomal complex, the face of the DNA that is in contact with the internal histone octamer is not accessible to activator proteins. Stated differently, proteins that do interact with the nucleosomal DNA must do so by interacting with only the outer surface of the DNA. Initiation sites that are enwrapped within the nucleosome cannot be accessed by, nor accommodate a transcriptional complex. One can only conclude that the very structure of chromatin is acting in a regulatory sense as a suppressor. Experimental proof of chromatin repression is difficult, yet Straka and Horz were able to show just that.[46] In yeast, a lower eukaryotic cell which does not have H1 histone but does form nucleosomes, there is chromatin structure made of histones that are highly homologous to that in higher eukaryotes. Expression utilizing PHO5, a yeast gene that remains suppressed until there are low phosphate levels in the medium, is known to be highly responsive to the phosphate status of the environment. The activator response elements are structured in two upstream activating sites (UAS) which are the equivalent of enhancer elements in higher eukaryotes. *In vivo* basal expression of PHO5 is negligible until it is induced. The UAS and promoter elements are thought to be embedded in nucleosomal structure. A mutant having the H4 gene deleted from both chromosomes and a galactose conditional episomal (not part of the genomic DNA) copy of H4 was constructed. When galactose is the food source, H4 is induced in ample quantities; however, when glucose is substituted for galactose, H4 synthesis immediately stops. Glucose-fed cells do not assemble new nucleosomes as they go through the DNA replicative or synthesis phase (S-phase). As a result of not having new nucleosomes and therefore having PHO5 in a spread out or accessible state, PHO5 expression increased dramatically in the absence of any specific induction—a clear example that demonstrates that the nucleosomal structure functions as a suppressor element.

DNase I hypersensitivity assays[47] show that chromatin structure is loosened when there is active gene synthesis. Furthermore, data acquired from transfection experiments with the β-globin gene show that a DNA locus control region (LCR) that resides greater than 50 kilobases upstream of the transcriptional start site is the primary regulator that institutes relaxation of heterochromatin structure within the domain that contains the globin gene cluster and exposes the region to DNase hypersensitivity.[48,49] When the LCR is deleted, the domain becomes DNase I resistant and gene expression is down-regulated. The chromatin is tethered to the nuclear matrix attachment sites (MAR)[50] at both the 5'- and 3'-ends of the domain that contains the gene or gene cluster (Figure 1.7). These domains, moreover, may have certain DNA sequences which limit the effect of accession by activators or conformational changes that would result from LCR-like elements. In *Drosophila melanogaster,*

the heat shock genes are clustered in a domain that has demarcating sequences ranging in size from 200 to 350 bases called specialized chromatin structures[51–53] that function to limit the spreading of chromatin conformational changes to adjoining genes, that is, loosening and DNase hypersensitivity, that occur when a gene is activated.

Such observations demonstrate that unlike bacteria, mammalian cell promoter construction is not simply an "on/off" switch composed of a few tens of nucleotides positioned immediately before the gene to be synthesized. The very definition of promoter becomes one that has to encompass a sequence structure that may be composed of multiple different enhancer or repressor elements (nucleotide sequences that interact with protein or in some manner change the structure of the DNA) that can be vast distances in front of or behind or, for that matter, within the gene to be transcribed. There are specific sets of intranuclear proteins whose function is to acetylate histones within the nucleosomal structures. The acetylated histones allow greater access to DNA-binding proteins. In general, histone structure without acetylated groups results in compaction of DNA structure; whereas acetylated histones loosen up DNA structure for access by protein complexes to the DNA so that the myriad of events that are requires for transcription and replication and repair may occur.[54]

The picture that develops from such a paradigm of gene construction is one which shows that gene regulation begins by a set of commands that controls opening and shutting of entry to heterochromatin (Figure 1.8). Such a view would further allow one to appreciate that the complexity resulting from the presence of many regulatory elements built into the promoter can provide numerous places for concerted control of gene expression. If the repressor or enhancer proteins that bind to specific elements within the DNA or DNA sequences themselves acting as structural elements are thought of as keys that either lock or unlock embedded DNA sequences, then an expanded view of the eukaryotic promoter construction would be considered necessary to provide insight into how access to and transcription of the gene is selectively accomplished. Therefore, the potential of having to open heterochromatin in response to stimulatory signals in a eukaryote would be expected to be relatively slow, but speed is sacrificed for control. Furthermore, if a

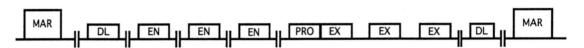

FIGURE 1.7. A portion of chromosomal DNA is represented by a line structure. The hashed marks denote varying lengths of DNA. The matrix attachment region (MAR) in a DNA sequence is associated with increased levels of AT and is also attached to the nuclear matrix. DL denotes a delimiting sequence that stops propagation of transcription; EN denotes enhancer elements; PRO is the core promoter; and EX is the abbreviation form of exon.

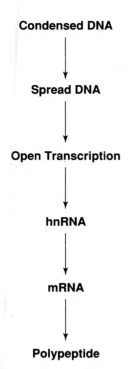

Condensed DNA

↓

Spread DNA

↓

Open Transcription

↓

hnRNA

↓

mRNA

↓

Polypeptide

FIGURE 1.8. Denotes the cascade of events that starts at condensed heterochromatin and ends with synthesis of the gene product: the polypeptide.

merases which, as a consequence of their order of elution from a chromatography column, are designated RNA polymerase I, II, and III. RNA polymerase I is responsible for the transcription of ribosomal preRNA 45S,[56] RNA polymerase III transcribes all tRNA and 5S RNA and like genes,[57] and RNA polymerase II transcribes, among other genes, all genes responsible for proteins that are made in the cell. The RNA polymerases can be distinguished biochemically on the basis of their inhibition by α-amanitin (RNA polymerase I is not sensitive, II is sensitive, and III may or may not be inhibitable, depending on the species). Type II genes are those genes that are transcribed by RNA polymerase II.

Promoter Region

Expression of type II genes is highly regulated at all levels, but the greatest degree of regulation occurs at the transcriptional level. It follows naturally that the construction of the promoter sequence and the enhancer or inhibitory elements associated with the promoter are of primary importance in regulation of gene expression. A core or minimal promoter may, then, be defined as one that does not contain binding sites for sequence specific factors; rather it contains elements that interact with general transcriptional factors (GTF) and transcriptional-associated factors that are required for basal transcription (Figure 1.9).[58–60] The core or minimal promoter in higher eukaryotes has at least one of two distinct elements that affect transcription: the initiation (Inr) element[61] which encompasses the site of transcriptional initiation and, at −30 relative to the start site, an AT-rich element of which the TATA box is the cognate or consensus sequence.[25,62,63] All promoters examined to date have at least one of these two elements. In referring to a promoter and its related gene, +1 is the start site for transcription, those nucleotides that follow the start site are—reading left to right—consecutively numbered +2, +3, . . . , +N, and those nucleotides that precede the initiation site are numbered from right to left, −1, −2, . . . , −N. There is no zero.

segment of DNA is opened or partially opened by a set of response elements, then, in a eukaryotic cell, DNA accessibility could be thought of as being preset by a cascade of DNA-interacting proteins, such as hypermobility group (HMG) proteins,[55] without there necessarily being an immediate gene expression response or, for that matter, expression at all unless subsequent signals are received.

Once the DNA is loosened, there is a requirement that different sets of proteins must interact with the DNA before transcription begins. Unlike in bacteria, eukaryotes do not utilize one RNA polymerase core enzyme complex for synthesis of all genes; rather there are three specific RNA poly-

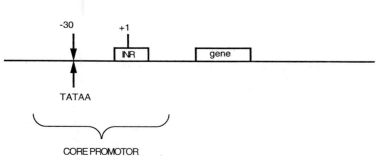

FIGURE 1.9. The core promoter is depicted by curled brackets. The horizontal line denotes double-stranded DNA having a TATAA box, transcriptional initiation element (INR), and a downstream gene.

Transcriptional Factors

There are at least seven general transcriptional factors (GTFs) which have been defined to date. They are named transcriptional factor TF, IIA, IIB, IID, IIE, IIF, IIH, and IIJ.[64] Of these, only TFIID interacts with DNA independent of the other factors. TFIID recognizes and binds most tightly to the TATAA consensus sequence −30 to −25 nucleotides relative to the start site (Figure 1.10). Within TFIID there is a TATA-binding protein (TBP) and at least seven other associated factors called TBP-associated factors

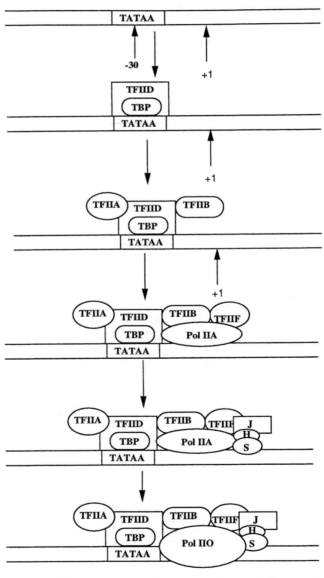

FIGURE 1.10. Demonstrates the cascade of transcriptional activation by the transcription factors (TF) for RNA polymerase II (Pol II). The TATAA box is −30 bp upstream from the transcription start site denoted by 0. TBP stands for TATA-binding protein. Pol IIA is the closed form of RNA polymerase II and Pol IIO is the open form of the RNA polymerase II.

(TAFs) having molecular weights of 250, 125, 95, 78, 50, and 30.[65–68] TBP, as would be expected from its name, is the subunit within TFIID that specifically binds the TATA-box element.[69] Moreover, TBP also participates in RNA polymerase I and III transcription.[70,71] Human recombinant TBP is a 38 kD protein whose crystal structure shows it to be a saddle-shaped protein.[72] Most sequence-specific transcriptional activator and inhibitor factors recognize elements by binding to nucleotides within the major groove of the DNA, but TBP binds within the minor groove and severely distorts and opens the minor groove.[73,74] The avidity of TBP is greatest for the consensus TATAA but it does bind to lesser degrees to other AT-rich sequences in the −30 to −25 area. The decrease in binding to sequences that diverge from the consensus sequence may be a means of regulation. TBP binds to a small sequence of bases in the vicinity of −30; however, the holo-TFIID rests on nucleotides from −30 to +10. Moreover, TBP does not have to interact directly with RNA polymerase for there to be basal transcription, yet there is evidence to support that TFIID does directly interact with the carboxy or C-terminal domain (CTD) of the largest subunit of RNA polymerase II to increase the frequency of initiation of transcription.[75] Furthermore, TBP is not affected by sequence-specific activator-dependent transcription, but TFIID, that is, TBP with its associated TAFs, has been shown to interact with such factors. This implies that activators can bind to the TAFs and thereby enhance transcription by nucleating the promoter with TFIID at the −30 site.[76,77] Furthermore, the TAFs, by associating with TBP, probably determine the binding efficiency by which TBP binds to AT-rich sequences that have diverged from the consensus sequence.[78]

Once TFIID associates with the TATA element, there is an ordered assembly of the other transcriptional factors. TFIIB associates with TFIID that has already associated with DNA to form the DB complex (TFIID-TFIIB complex).[79,80] TFIIB, like TBP, may be a sequence-binding cofactor that senses sequences immediately upstream of the TATA box and contributes to the evolving transcriptional complex.[81] TFIIB interacts with both RNA polymerase and TFIID and is probably responsible for the spacing between TFIID and RNA polymerase which allows for site-specific initiation of transcription. In addition to TFIIB directly interacting with TFIID, TFIIA associates with the DB complex to form the DAB complex.[82] Although there is controversy regarding the essential role of TFIIA in formation of the preinitiation complex, TFIIA does seems to function as an anti-inhibitor by preventing TFIID from being inhibited; consequently, TFIIA stimulates initiation of transcription.[83] TFIIB, in addition to its other function, may also interact with element-specific activators.[84] Once the DAB complex forms, then TFIIF (RAP30/74), along with RNA polymerase, associates with the DAB complex and binds to the DNA at the transcription initiation site (Inr).[85] Besides its role in binding to the DAB complex, RAP30/74 functions like bacterial σ, in that the heterodimer binds to RNA polymerase in solution and prevents nonspecific DNA binding by RNA polymerase II.[86,87] Unlike σ,[70] TFIIF does not directly bind to DNA; however, within the context of the preinitiation complex, TFIIF may bind to the Inr element. TFIIE then associates with the preinitiation complex to increase stability of the initiation complex by promoting binding of RNA polymerase to the Inr element.[88] Along with binding of TFIIE is the binding of TFIIH,[89] which promotes productive binding of the preinitiation complex. TFIIH is a complex transcriptional factor composed of at least five subunits (95–35 kD polypeptides)[90] that have, among other functions, ATPase, CTD kinase, and DNA helicase activity.[91] Each of these functional components are essential for RNA polymerase II to proceed beyond the initiation site. That is, ATPase activity is necessary for there to be energy for the RNA polymerase to activate. The CTD kinase activity is absolutely required for the RNA polymerase II to switch from the unphosphorylated (IIA)[92] and therefore nonelongating polymerase to the highly phosphorylated (IIO)[93] RNA polymerase II that elongates or proceeds with transcription. It is obvious that in order for there to be transcription from one of the strands of the double-stranded DNA, there is a requirement for helicase, that is, unwinding of the DNA. So once the DBPo1F complex is formed, then TFIIE associates with the complex, followed then by TFIIH, TFIIJ. TFIIS may be analogous to prokaryotic Nus A, which functions as an anti-terminator.[94] When transcribing RNA polymerase comes to a pause site, TFIIS, by functioning to remove several nucleotides from the 3'-end of the nascent RNA, allows for "relocation" or backward movement of the RNA polymerase by several nucleotides and then for RNA synthesis to recommence.[95–97] The human retroviruses HIV and HTLV express anti-terminators, TAT and TAX respectively, which promote transcriptional elongation early in transcription by specifically binding the transcribed RNA so that termination of transcription is aborted.[98] Both TAT and TAX either directly interact with the transcriptional complex through space because they bind elements on the RNA which are free of the RNA polymerase complex and, therefore, not associated with DNA, or they indirectly promote transcription by interacting through adaptor proteins. In either case, the sum effect of these viral proteins is, like TFIIS, continuation of transcriptional elongation. The preinitiation complex has an aggregate molecular weight of greater than 3.2 million dalton and is composed of greater than 32 proteins. All of this care is involved in setting up the core apparatus for RNA polymerase II to begin transcription. Purified pol II transcribes about 300 nucleotides per minute; whereas *in vivo* the pol II complex transcribes about 2,000 nucleotides per minute. The discordant rates probably result in part from the delay in movement of the initiation complex from the initiation start site. Yet the pol II complex, once moving, encounters multiple impediments to smooth and rapid elongation, for example, the nucleosome structures. There are families of elongation factors that modulate the rate of transcriptional progression. Factors such as TFIIF, ELL, SII, SIII, P-TEBf, FACT, and HSF1 have been shown to be involved in changing the rate of transcriptional elongation.[99,100] In fact, the B-C component of SIII has been shown to interact with von Hipple-Linau (VHL) tumor suppressor gene.[101]

As mentioned previously, bacterial RNA polymerase core enzyme is composed of four subunits. In the case of mammalian RNA polymerase II, there are at least ten subunits ranging in molecular mass from 10 to 240 kD.[102] The two largest subunits of RNA polymerase II that are thought to be involved in nucleotide and DNA binding have homology that persists from the β, β′ of *E. coli,* through yeast, into *Drosophila* and higher mammals.[103,104] The large subunit of RNA polymerase II has a unique heptad repeat unit, Tyr-Ser-Pro-Thr-Ser-Pro-Ser, which is not present in RNA polymerase I or III.[105,106] In mice and humans the heptad repeats 52 times.[102,107,108] Genetic deletion of more than half of the heptads from the large subunit is lethal. As stated above, the heptad phosphorylation or the transition from the RNA polymerase IIA to the phosphorylated IIO form is a potential regulatory point that serves to transform the preinitiation complex to the active transcriptional complex.

In yeast, the TATA box may be anywhere from − 40 to − 100 nucleotides upstream of the start site of transcription, and the orientation of the TATA sequence is strict. This is not the case for higher eukaryotes. In fact, in higher eukaryotes there are promoters that do not contain TATA boxes or AT-rich regions approximately − 30 to − 25 nucleotides upstream from the start site.[61,109–111] These TATA-less promoters are divided into two classes; those with GC-rich promoters which are associated with housekeeping genes,[112] and several upstream sequence-specific SP1 sites.[113] For the TATA-less promoters, the Inr element is a weak consensus sequence of A at the + 1 site and C at the − 1 site and T at + 3 with preferentially pyrimidine bases upstream and downstream of these sequence elements.[114] It is possible that the Inr sequence is recognized by a specific Inr-binding protein, and it is this protein which nucleates the ordered assembly of the transcriptional factors.[60] So even within these TATA-less promoters, the TFIID transcriptional factor containing the TBP is required for transcription; however, in this case the binding may be effected through adaptors or tethering factors which are probably one of an array of alternative TAFs that has been positioned by either the Inr-binding protein or sequence-specific activators (above).[84]

Regulatory Elements

The line between what is the promoter region and what is the enhancer region in eukaryotic genes is blurred. The trend is to consider the core promoter as the sequence just upstream and through the Inr sequence, and the rest of the elements that modulate transcription are referred to as the regulon or some such name that connotes transcriptional regulatory function. Since many genes can be regulated by proteins that interact with DNA upstream, within, and downstream of the transcriptional unit of the gene, description of regulatory elements will be restricted to the more common elements usually found upstream of the Inr element. By no means do we mean that the other elements are not important for efficient transcription of any individual gene. Moreover, specific regulatory elements within higher eukaryotes are not necessarily directionally dependent, nor is it uncommon to find that one element will be repeated several times or that multiple elements will be employed within a given regulatory region, that is, the regulatory elements are modular, and all of the elements can be coordinated as a functional unit. Eukaryotic-regulating proteins or enhancer-element-recognizing proteins must interact with a specific sequence within the extended promoter and additionally interact with other sequence-specific recognition proteins or the transcriptional factors themselves (Figure 1.11).[115] *In vitro* the activator molecules typically enhance transcription by two- to five-fold; however, *in vivo* the activators can enhance transcription by a thousandfold. In contrast to TBP, typically transcriptional activators recognize specific elements and bind to the nucleotides within the DNA sequence through the major groove. These regulatory proteins frequently consist of more than one protein subunit. The interplay of these regulatory proteins with one another and with DNA for the most part determines the

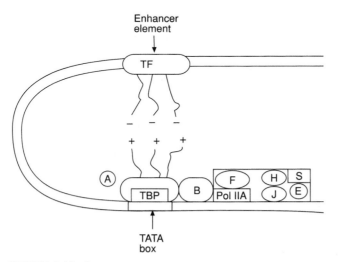

FIGURE 1.11. Demonstrates a negatively charged transcription factor (TF) binding to an enhancer element on double-stranded DNA that is forming a looped structure. The transcription factor may, by virtue of its charge and position, act in assisting the position of TFIID which is positively charged and contains the TATA-binding protein and is also binding with TFIIA (A) and TFIIB (B). F, H, J, E, and S denote TFIIF, H, J, E, and S. Pol IIA is the closed complex of RNA polymerase II.

tissue specificity and timing and frequency of gene transcription.

The CCAAT-box is an element that is frequently found in promoters approximately 75 bp upstream of the start site.[116] Multiple factors from different species bind the CCAAT element. Among those are the CCAAT-binding factor, CBF, which is a heterodimer,[117] CP1 functions in α-globin gene, CP2, which is γ-fibrinogen activating,[118] CDP, which may function to displace CCAAT-binding factors,[119] which is analogous in function to NF-E that downregulates fetal globin synthesis,[120] CCAAT transcription factor (CTF/NF-1),[121] CCAAT-enhancer binding factor (C/EBF),[122] and others.[123-127] The important thing to be learned from the CCAAT-binding factors is that given such an array of different binding proteins with possibly different preferences for the CCAAT element or mutations from the consensus sequence, regulation based on binding the same element may provide exquisite tissue and chronologic modulation of gene transcription.

The octamer element, ATTTGCAT, is another ubiquitous regulatory element which is usually bound by the Oct-1 factor and is an element module in promoters for the H2B histone,[128] U2 snRNA,[128] SV40 promoter,[129] γ-globulin, and major histocompatibility HLA-DQβ genes.[130] The octamer element in lymphoid tissues regulates γ-globulin synthesis and illustrates that a tissue-specific factor (Oct-2) recognizes the general octamer element, whereas Oct-1 does not function as a γ-globulin regulatory protein.[131] Here is a clear example of tissue-specific gene regulation by tissue regulatory factor expression.

The GC-rich Sp1 element has a consensus sequence of GGCGGG and is found within the six 21 bp repeat units of SV40 early promoter.[113,132-135] The Sp1 element is a frequently used motif within numerous genes, including the monocyte chemo-attractant protein-1,[136] TGF-β,[137] thymidylate syntase,[138] and apolipoprotein E,[139] among others. Sp1 is a heterodimeric structure composed of 105 and 95 kD subunits which seems to function as a single unit without subset subunit mixing to other factors.[140] Modulation of regulation from the Sp1 element is usually in concert with other regulatory factors or possibly, as discussed above for TBP, the degeneracy of the element away from the consensus sequence may be a means of altering affinity and therefore modulating enhancement.

Since higher eukaryotic cells must regulate protein expression in the context of the entire organism, it is not surprising that molecular communication between cells results in transcriptional modulation. To that end, it is not surprising that there are transcription factors that are responsive to hormones and to membrane receptor stimulation. The hormone response elements interact with the steroid/thyroid superfamily transcriptional factors, which include estrogen, androgen, glucocorticoid, mineralocorticoid, vitamin D, retinoic acid, thyroid, and other orphan receptors.[141-143] The action of the family of transcriptional factors is superficially reminiscent of bacterial activators and repressors in that the ligand (hormone) interacts with the intranuclear receptor, which subsequently results in a conformational change in the receptor that facilitates DNA binding and transcriptional activation or repression. The hormone receptors act as dimeric structures, either in a homo- or heterodimeric form.[144] Within this family there is a considerable degree of homology among the receptors.[145] In general members of this group of transcriptional factors share considerable functional homology. All of the steroid receptor proteins can be dissected into three functional domains.[146–148] The N-terminal domain is highly variable, activates gene-specific transcription, and binds other protein factors. Domain II functions in DNA binding, provides response-element recognition specificity and is highly conserved. Domain III, which is the C-terminal region of the receptor, actually contains two separate motifs: the hinge and the ligand-binding portion of the receptor. The hinge contains the nuclear localization signal, participates in transcriptional activation, and functions in dimer formation. Lastly, the steroid-binding region binds the specific activating ligand, interacts with heat-shock proteins, contributes to nuclear localization, and for the same receptor species is highly conserved. Domain-swapping experiments in which chimeric proteins between one specific DNA-binding domain of one receptor with that of the ligand-recognition domain of different class of hormone receptor show that the DNA and ligand domains act functionally in an independent manner. The consensus recognition sequence for the hormone androgen, glucocorticoid, progesterone, and mineralocorticoid receptors is GGTACANNNTGTTCT; the consensus sequence for the estrogen and thyroid receptor is GGTCA(N)xTGACC, where x is equal to zero for the estrogen response element and three for the thyroid response element; and the consensus element for retinoids is AGGTCA.[149–151] The mechanism by which the different hormone receptors compete for a common element may be mediated by concentration of the individual receptor within the cell, the interaction of composite elements within the promoter, changes of DNA structure, phosphorylation of the receptor, and/or the interaction of the hormone receptors with other proteins or tissue-specific nuclear factors.[152–159] Since phosphorylation can occur at multiple sites within the receptor and thereby change its structure, it would not be surprising that regulation of such transcriptional regulators could then be networked into other regulatory pathways such as tyrosine kinase, kinase A, and ultimately to signal transduction mediated from G-proteins.[160–164] Moreover, the steroid receptors are known to regulate the synthesis of nuclear protooncogenes and facilitate or inhibit the binding of other transcriptional activators.[165–168] In those cases where the receptor interacts with such protooncogenic regulatory elements, mutation of the hormone receptor could very well result in loss of coordinate cellular control.[169]

Insight into regulatory control is found when one considers the structural activation of the steroid hormone receptor.[170,171] These receptors do not exist intracellularly as monomeric or dimeric receptors; rather they are associated with a set of nonreceptor chaperone molecules that confer stability to the receptor such that they are held in a conformational state so that they may interact with the incoming ligand. The chaperone molecules are composed in part by heat-shock protein 94 and 70.[172–175] The heat-shock protein/receptor complex also associates with other proteins to form an aggregate species.[176] It is this aggregate species that functions to position the hormone receptor within the nucleus by associating with nuclear matrix proteins.[177] Such a display of positional control may imply that the topological position of segments of DNA within the nucleus is highly important and fixed by binding to specific proteins and potentially RNA molecules that match up with specific sequences of DNA. Furthermore, when the receptor reacts with its cognate steroid ligand, it may be released from some of the constraints of binding to the chaperone proteins and associate with another steroid receptor which allows binding to its respective response element within DNA. Since the aggregate is associated with nuclear matrix and DNA, then such changes in the aggregate structure can be translated into changes in chromatin structure or possibly into altering the bending patterns of DNA, which can then result in looping the composite enhancer region into a spatial position to associate with the transcriptional apparatus.[178,179] Once again, by considering the simple steroid-receptor transcriptional activator, we find that the eukaryotic cell has networked multiple regulatory paths to ensure exquisite control.

In higher eukaryotic cells, genes are structured differently from those found in bacteria. For one thing, they are not arranged in an operonic motif. That is, in higher eukaryotes one promoter corresponds to one gene rather than a cascade of genes as is found in bacteria. Moreover, eukaryotic genes are usually substantially larger than those found in bacteria. In a bacterium, a single gene coding for a fairly large polypeptide having a molecular weight of 100,000 dalton (100 kDa) would be considered unusually large. If one estimates that the average molecular weight of an amino acid is 100 Da, then the number of amino acids in a 100 kDa protein would be 1,000. Since three nucleotides code for one amino acid, the 100 kDa protein would correspond to a gene composed of 3,000 nucleotides. In mammals, as in prokaryotes, a single polypeptide is rarely larger than 100 kDa. However, when compared to the size of an average higher eukaryotic genes, the large 3-kbase prokaryotic gene would be considered small because in mammals it is not unusual to find genes spanning more than 100 kbases. For instance, the cystic fibrosis gene spans over 500 kbases, and the breast cancer gene, BCII, may span 1,000,000 bases—approximately one third the size of the genome of *E. coli*. The average size of a higher eukaryotic gene is 10 to 20 kD.[180]

The obvious conclusion is that gene structure in higher eukaryotic cells is much more elaborate than that found in prokaryotic cells. The gene has a dispersed structure. In mammalian cells most of the nucleotide sequences that are transcribed from a gene are not translated into protein. Intragenic, transcribed, but not necessarily translated, sequences within a gene are referred to as introns. The size and number of introns may vary depending on the gene but average between 6 to 8 introns per gene. Why would the cell invest so much energy into forming such long pieces of RNA only to have most of the nucleotide sequence degraded; and further, what are the advantages of having genetic material dispersed over so much of the DNA? The evolution of this mode of packaging eukaryotic genetic material probably reflects greater control of (a) transcription initiation—within introns cis-acting elements can reside, as well as elements for trans-acting proteins to activate or inhibit transcription, (b) genetic swapping of information,[181] and (c) development and specific tissue production of multiple isoforms of a particular protein at particular times during the life of the cell at the posttranscriptional level.

Posttranscriptional Processing Events

In prokaryotes, mRNA is translated as soon as transcription begins. This is not the case for eukaryotes.[180] Once transcription has occurred and the resultant RNA is synthesized, there is a vast array of events that occur. When RNA is synthesized, it is not in a suitable form to function as tRNA or rRNA or mRNA. Newly synthesized or nascent RNA is termed pre-messenger RNA or heterologous RNA (hnRNA). Pre-mRNA is single-stranded and corresponds to a one-to-one direct transcript of the original DNA representation of the gene. The RNA has a complex secondary structure that is not simply a linear array of nucleotides.[182] This secondary structure without doubt dictates how the pre-mRNA is processed and how other molecules within the nucleus interact with the nascent RNA. In such a state, hnRNA associates with intranuclear proteins and small nuclear RNA (snRNA). Introns and exons are present and there has been no RNA terminus processing, that is, no polyadenylation nor any modification of the 5′-bases. The panoply of processes that occur on hrRNA are referred to as posttranscriptional events.

The posttranscriptional processing events occur virtually immediately and simultaneously. For heuristic ease they will be discussed individually and as if these processes start at the 5′-end of hnRNA and end at the 3′-end. When the transcript is being made, the 5′-end begins to associate with proteins within the nuclear matrix. As discussed above in reference to transcriptional control, these proteins can impact on transcriptional elongation. But such proteins also begin to organize the growing RNA chain into a structure that lends itself to processing by specific modifying intranuclear complexes. With the exception of a few specialized

cases, such as the picornaviruses that contain as part of their RNA genome-specific sequences that code for precise ribosomal recognition sites, invariably, mRNAs are processed before translation.[183]

Methylated 5′ Cap

The original, start-site, transcribed nucleotide has a triphosphate group at the 5′-end. However, this nucleotide is never found in mRNA. The mRNA 5′-end is invariably processed or modified such that there is a special nucleotidyl structure composed of a 7-methylguanosine connected through an unusual triphosphate linkage to the first nucleotide of the pre-mRNA (Figure 1.12).[184] This results in a 5′ to 5′ bond between ^{7m}G and the penultimate nucleotide. The resulting ^{7m}GpppAp 5′-end in higher eukaryotes may then be further modified by secondary methylation at the 2′-hydroxyl group of the ribose, as well as potential nucleotide base methylation of adjoining nucleotides.[185,186] Methylation of the 2′-OH group of the penultimated nucleotide stabilizes against base catalyzed hydrolysis because there is no chance of anchiomeric assistance from the adjoining hydroxyl group to facilitate the cyclic diester intermediate that would proceed hydrolysis. These methylations are catalyzed by specific methylation enzymes that recognize the ^{7m}GpppAp of the 5′-end of mRNA.[187] What determines the methylation pattern is not known. The ^{7m}Gppp^{2m}Ap structure also ensures that there is no free 5′-OH group, and as such the mRNA molecule has a 3′ free hydroxyl group on both its 5′- and 3′-ends. Although mRNA stability may result from many factors, the absence of the free phosphorylated 5′-OH group protects the mRNA from 5′-OH-specific exoRNase catalyzed degradation and thereby the inverted linkage of 5′ to 5′ OHs stabilizes and preserves mRNAs.[188–192] The collectively modified 5′-end of mRNA is referred to as the cap structure. This structure associates with a cap-binding protein which is integral to initiation of translation—decoding the mRNA into protein—and possibly the associated CPB is important in transport of mRNA out of the nucleus and into the cytoplasm to be translated by ribosomes.[193–195] Further, the cap structure is crucial for binding and positioning pre-RNA into intranuclear complexes for further processing.[196]

Transcriptional Termination

In prokaryotes termination of transcription is controlled by either the presence of specific proteins or terminating cis-elements within the gene.[37,197] For the most part, this is not the case in eukaryotes wherein the emphasis has changed from specific transcription termination sites to a more vague transcriptional end point with subsequent exquisitely accurately regulated 3′-end processing.[198] The pre-mRNA may terminate either shortly or considerably downstream of the end of the mRNA. The control of where the transcriptional

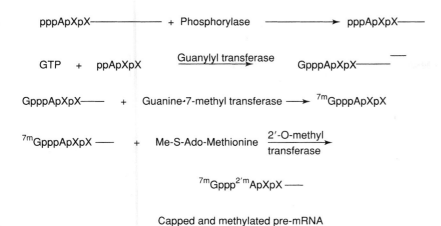

FIGURE 1.12. The capping and methylation of pre-mRNA goes through several steps. pppApXpX represents the 5′-end of pre-mRNA. GpppApXpX is the unusual 5′ to ′5 capped structure without methylation of the 7-nitrogen of guanosine. ^{7m}Gppp$^{2'm}$ApXpX is the fully methylated capped structure of pre-mRNA.

apparatus stops transcribing is not known; however, considerable effort has been expended in understanding the processes that define the 3′-terminus of mRNA.[199–201] Approximately 10 to 30 nucleotides upstream of the pre-mRNA is a hexameric element that has a consensus of AAUAAA and defines the subsequent 3′ cleavage site of pre-RNA.[202,203] Once 3′ endonucleolytic cleavage of pre-mRNA occurs, then between 200 and 250 As are added by poly(A) polymerase to form the poly(A) tail of mRNA (Figure 1.13).[24,204] But not all AAUAAA elements define the 3′ cleavage site. The AAUAAA element must be in the context of other regulatory elements that are downstream of the cleavage site. Two such downstream cognate sequences exist: the GU or U-rich sequences.[205,206] The enzyme that is responsible for polyadenylation has been isolated and purified.[207] Poly(A) polymerase must act in concert with other factors that determine 3′-end site selection and define endonucleolytic sites. There are several candidates for these factors such as cleavage and polyadenylation factor, CPF, and CF1.[208,209] As is seen in the selection of the exact isoform of diverse proteins such as dihydrofolate reductase, membrane or secreted IgM, α-amylase, and calcitonin and calcitonin gene-related peptide are subject to contextual constraints of cleavage site selection on the basis of tissue or cell

development (Figure 1.14).[210–212] For instance, selection of which of two mRNAs will be made from the same pre-mRNA that codes for the membrane bound or secreted IgM forms appears to depend on specific factors that are present as a function of the developmental maturity of the lymphocyte,[213,214] whereas the selection of synthesis of calcitonin versus calcitonin gene-related peptide appears to depend on the function of tissue specific factors, in that the calcitonin gene-related peptide is primarily synthesized in the hypothalamus, and calcitonin in the thyroid.[215,216] So not only do we find that the 3′-end of mRNA is a regulatory checkpoint, but also that polyadenylation can be dependent on the choice of intragenic exon selection that is defined by splice site selection.[217]

Spliceosomes

Since the ultimate mRNA is fashioned such that it will be efficiently utilized to translate genetic information into utilizable protein, it is not surprising that a major posttranscriptional regulatory checkpoint is compression of the dispersed pre-mRNA into RNA. The capped and poly(A) tailed prespliced RNA is composed in a modular fashion of exons and introns. The introns must be removed and the exons stitched together to result in a transcriptional unit that will be translated. The posttranscriptional process of removing introns and annealing the exons into a protein-coding RNA ready for translation is defined as splicing (Figure 1.15).[196,218–220] It is not surprising, considering the modular or motif nature of higher eukaryotic proteins, that exon sizes are fairly small and are usually less than 300 nucleotides.[221] This is not the case for introns, which can vary in size from approximately 60 to 100,000 nucleotides.[219,220] Since the initial pre-mRNA transcript for class II genes can be extremely large and composed of 50 or more introns of varying sizes, precise splicing must be maintained to ensure ultimate functional proteins.[219,221] There are three

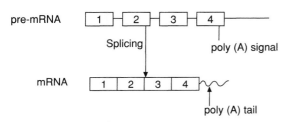

FIGURE 1.13. Demonstrates the pre-mRNA being processed by sequential splicing of exon 1, 2, 3, and 4. The polyadenylation signal is denoted at the terminal region of exon 4.

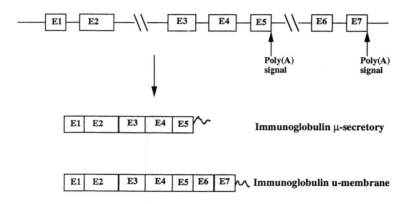

FIGURE 1.14. The selection of an immunoglobulin gene product for either secretion or membrane attachment depends on the use of one of two possible polyadenylation (poly[A]) elements within the immunoglobulin gene. When the first poly(A) site is selected, two exons are not incorporated into the gene product.

general classes of splicing reactions. The first two depend on autocatalytic splicing, which is highly dependent on the intron structure, whereas the third type of splicing, which is utilized for class II genes, depends on the pre-mRNA associating with an intranuclear structure referred to as the spliceosome complex.[220] The spliceosome is a 60S particle containing 5 small nuclear RNAs (snRNAs), U1, U2, U4, U5, and U6, as well as many small nuclear ribonuclear proteins (snRNP).[222–224] This spliceosome complex may form just after the capping modification has occurred; however, normally the complex forms on the capped and poly(A) tailed pre-mRNA. First U1 and U2 snRNP form with the

pre-RNA and then U4, U5, and U6 snRNP, as well as small ribonuclear (SR) proteins associated with the pre-spliceosome to form the catalytic spliceosome.[225–228] The splicing reaction requires the obvious presence of pre-mRNA, the spliceosome, and ATP.[229] When considering the great variability in the size and number of exons and introns of a transcribed gene, it becomes intuitive that mandatory cis-elements within the intron/exon contribute to the precise recognition by the splicing apparatus. There are cognate cis-elements at the 5'- and 3'-ends, as well as intraintronic sequences, that define the splicing junctions for removal of intron. As is seen in Figure 1.15, the sequence of events for

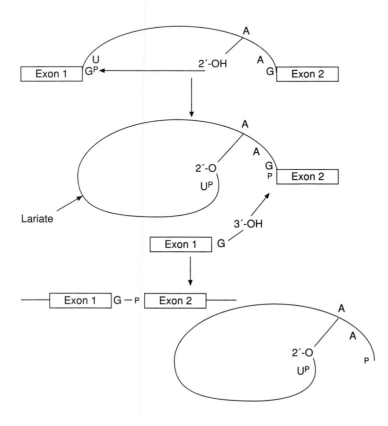

FIGURE 1.15. The splicing reaction is shown diagrammatically. The exons are represented as boxes, the intron as a single line between the two exons. The 2'-hydroxyl group of the adenosine (A) at the branch point is shown with the intron. The lariat structure which results from the branch 2'-hydroxyl group reacting with the phosphate ester between G and U at the 5'-end of the intron is indicated by an arrow. The resulting processed and spliced exons are joined together.

splicing proceeds first by cleavage at the 5′-end of the intron, followed by subsequent ligation of the 3′-end of the cleaved exon to the 5′-end of the exons with concomitant excision of the intron.[219,220] The first step of the splicing reaction involves a transesterification reaction in which the free 2′-hydroxyl group of an adenine at the branch point within the intron near the 3′-end of the intron reacts with the 5′-most guanosine within the intron to create a nucleotide that has phosphate esters on the 2′ and 3′ groups of the ribose sugar.[230,231] This creates the 5′ exon with a free hydroxyl group and a lariat structure composed of the intron and its connected 3′ exon. The second reaction, which appears *in vivo* to occur simultaneous with the first reaction, is the excision of the intron containing the lariat and ligation of the two exons. The U1 snRNP of the spliceosome interacts with pre-mRNA at the 5′ splice junction site of the intron.[232,233] The 5′ junction invariably contains a GU nucleotide; in a few cases GCs have replaced the GU.[234] The 5′ GU dinucleotide is positioned in a consensus sequence of AG*GU*AAGU that spans from the 3′-end of the exon into the 5′-end of the intron.[235] It has been shown that changing the G or the U can completely inactivate the splice junction.[236,237] Furthermore, alterations within the consensus sequence of the 5′ junction site may inactivate the primary junction site, decrease the rate of splicing, or activate alternative junction sites that may be either in the exon or intron.[237] These alternative or cryptic 5′ junctional sites invariable have a GU dinucleotide.[237,238] For instance, in β^E-thalassemia, a G to A mutation within the first exon of β-globin changes the nucleotide sequence in the vicinity of GU, and thereby activates an intra-exon cryptic 5′ junction site that results in aberrant mRNA.[238,239] Therefore, selection of the 5′ splice is a function of its closeness to the consensus sequence and conjoining sequences as well as of the distance from the 3′ junction site.[240]

The 3′ junction site contains a rather large consensus sequence that is composed of an invariant AG which resides immediately before the second exon and an upstream pyrimidine-rich tract with an intervening single purine or pyrimidine and then a pyrimidine just before the junction site AG. The consensus is therefore, a $(Py)_{11}$ NYAG-exon.[218,235] The 3′ pyrimidine-rich region interacts with the U5 snRNP as well as the U1 snRNP of the spliceosome.[241–243] The 3′ junction site and the pyrimidine-rich tract are an absolute requirement for the first endonucleolytic cleavage of the 5′ junctional site to occur.[244] The implication is that within the spliceosome, the recognition order probably is U1 followed by U2 and then U5 snRNP, or U1 in conjunction with U2 forms a complex with U5 and other snRNPs to conform to the 3′-end of the intron so that the branch point adenine which interacts with U2 can be positioned by the U1/U5/U4/U6/SR complex to react with the 5′ junctional site. Alternatively, there is a stepwise assembly of snRNPs that forms complexes with prespliced mRNA which results in rearrangement of the snRNPs to conform the pre-RNA

for splicing. In any case, U2 snRNP protects the branch point region from digestion by RNase.[245] Even though the branch point adenine is crucial for lariat formation and therefore intron excision, unlike yeast, in higher eukaryotes only a weak consensus sequence of UACUAAC exists.[231,246] What appears to be the case is that there is a strict requirement that the branch point of the lariat be 16 to 60 nucleotides upstream of the 3′ junction site.[218,219] Deletion of the original branch point adenine slows the splicing reaction and unmasks a cryptic branch point site.[247]

Alternate Splicing

It must be that in addition to the normally found snRNPs that make up the spliceosome, other nuclear proteins function in the splicing event. This becomes particularly obvious when one considers the mechanism by which cells regulate the splicing reaction such that alternative splicing events occur.[180,248] Alternative splicing provides to the cell a regulatory control to produce alternative proteins or isozymes without the need to store within the genome genes that code for each individual protein. To effect alternative splicing, the cell type must produce a nuclear protein that acts directly with the spliceosome to result in selection of alternative splice sites or, because the pre-mRNA has considerable secondary structure, the tissue-specific protein may interact with the pre-mRNA while it is forming to fold it in such a fashion that certain splice sites are not available to the spliceosome. It may be that the tissue-specific proteins may associate with the spliceosome such that certain intronic or exonic sequences are recognized as alternative splice sites. Whatever the underlying mechanism(s) of alternative splicing the end result is that in either the case of normal sequential splicing or of alternative splice, pre-RNA, once it has been capped and polyadenylated and spliced, is ready to be carried from the nucleus to the ribosome for translation.

TRANSLATION

During translation the mRNA carrying the genetic code is decoded into amino acids. Each amino acid is represented by at least one codon found as a triplet within the nucleotide sequence of mRNA. Translation in prokaryotes is a very rapid process, which occurs while transcription is still in progress. This is possible within a prokaryotic cell because both transcriptional and translational events are in the same cellular compartment. On the other hand, translation and transcription in eukaryotic cells are in separate cellular compartments. Moreover, because of posttranscriptional modifications and transport, there is a lag of a few hours between the two molecular events.[249,250]

Ribosome Structure

Ribosomes (ribonucleoprotein structures) provide the site for recognition between an mRNA codon and tRNA antico-

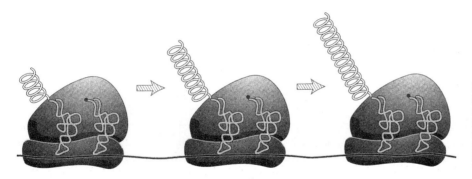

FIGURE 1.16. Polysomes are many ribosomes simultaneously translating the same molecule of RNA, resulting in synthesis of many polypeptides of different lengths from the same RNA molecule. (From Lewin B. *The assembly line for protein synthesis.* New York: Oxford University Press, 1990: 143, with permission.)

don with subsequent assembly of translated amino acids into polypeptides. Ribosomes attach to the 5′ end of mRNA, translating each nucleotide triplet into an amino acid as the triplets move in a 5′ to 3′ direction. A strand of mRNA can be simultaneously translated by more than one ribosome. Multiple ribosome constructs are referred to as a polysome. Polysomes contain variable numbers of ribosomes, each one synthesizing an individual polypeptide (Figure 1.16). There are generally a greater number of ribosomes per prokaryote mRNA molecule since the mRNA in these organisms is much longer than that found in eukaryotes. Bacteria can add approximately 15 amino acids to the growing polypeptide chain every second, therefore synthesizing a protein of about 300 amino acids in 20 seconds. Eukaryotic cells proceed at a slower rate, adding about two amino acids to the growing chain per second.[249]

A ribosome is composed of two subunits which can be dissociated from each other by reducing the Mg^{2+} concentration. The subunits can be isolated through zonal centrifugation in Mg^{2+}-sucrose gradient.[251,252] The sedimentation rate has been adopted as nomenclature for each subunit, with a higher S value indicating a greater rate of sedimentation and a larger mass.[253] Bacterial ribosomal subunits sediment at 30S (small subunit) and 50S (large subunit) forming a 70S reassociated ribosome. The small (30S) subunit is composed of 21 different proteins and 32 different proteins comprise the large 50S subunit. One of the small subunit proteins is identical to one found in the large subunit yielding a total of 52 different proteins within an intact prokaryote ribosome.[254] Eukaryotic cytoplasmic ribosomes are larger, sedimenting at 80S for the intact ribosome and 40S and 60S for the small and large subunits respectively. The ribosomal RNA has a molecular weight of 2,300 kD with an additional 1,700 to 1,800 kD of absorbed ribosomal proteins such as initiation factors, elongation factors, and enzymes.[255] Ribosomal proteins in both prokaryotes and eukaryotes have insoluble, basic properties.[256] The genes coding for ribosomal proteins are present 10 to 12 times in higher eukaryotic genomes, but there is only one copy of each ribosomal protein gene in prokaryotes.[257,258] *E. coli* rRNA genes are cotranscribed as a 16S-23s-5s linked

unit.[258] In higher eukaryotes the rRNA genes are linked as an 18s-5.8s-28s transcriptional unit while the 5s gene is transcribed separately by a different polymerase.[259–261] A comparison of rRNA sequences between bacteria and chloroplasts reveals 74% homology between the 16S subunits[262,263] and nearly 70% homology between the 23s subunits.[264,265] However, comparison of *E. coli* and eukaryote 16S rRNA shows no homology except within nucleotides 9–51 at the 3′-end of *E. coli* 16S rRNA. The region of homology is located just upstream from an 8 nucleotide region in *E. coli* 16S rRNA which is a necessary sequence in initiation of translation.[266–269]

Initiation Complex

An initiation complex must first be formed before a ribosome can begin the process of decoding mRNA triplets into amino acids. Formation of an initiation complex requires initiation factors to function as chaperones in bringing together the small ribosomal subunit, mRNA, an initiator tRNA, and the large ribosomal subunit (Figure 1.17). The translational process involves association of the proper amino acyl tRNA anticodon with a complementary mRNA codon. Each ribosome has two sites for tRNA binding; the A or entry site is occupied by the incoming amino acyl tRNA whose anticodon is the compliment of the mRNA codon, which is next in line to be translated. The adjacent P (donor) site is occupied by the growing polypeptide chain bound to peptidyl tRNA. When both the A and P sites are filled, a peptide bond is formed between the newly translated amino acid in the A site and the previously translated amino acid in the P site (Figure 1.18). These complexes of proteins and other initiation factors associated with a ribosome make up the active site for participation in one of the three stages of translation: (a) initiation; (b) elongation; and (c) termination. The following discussion will address the general mechanisms in each of these stages as well as the regulatory events and deviations which can occur in translation.[270,271]

Initiation of translation requires multiple steps to assemble a ribosomal initiation complex which can bind mRNA at or near a site containing an initiation codon (AUG). Formation of the initiation complex requires different initiation factors whose number and complexity of function increase from prokaryotic to eukaryotic translation. There are four main events in the initiation of translation: (a) dissociation of the small and large ribosomal subunits found in the free ribosome pool; (b) binding of the initiator tRNA to the small ribosomal subunit along with initiation factors to form a preinitiation complex; (c) binding of mRNA to the preinitiation complex to form an initiation complex with the small subunit; and (d) reassociation of the large and small subunits to form an 80S initiation complex.[272]

Initiation Complex in Prokaryotes

Assembly of the 30S preinitiation complex in prokaryotes requires three initiation factors (IF1, IF2, and IF3), GTP, 30S ribosomal subunits, initiator tRNA (formyl methionyl-tRNA), and mRNA. In order to form a preinitiation complex, the small ribosomal subunit (30S) must be available in the free ribosome pool. Normally 30S is found tightly coupled with 50S as a 70S ribosome, which must be dissociated in order to make 30S available.[273,274] Initiation factors IF1 and IF3 are part of the dissociation process. The IF1 association with the 70S ribosome increases the rate of dissociation of 30S from 50S.[275–277] Once the subunits

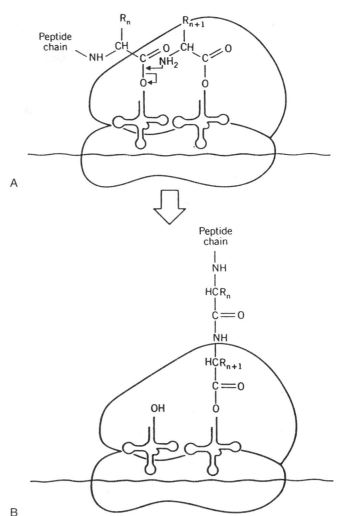

FIGURE 1.18. **A:** Each ribosome has two sites for tRNA binding. The entry (A) site is occupied by the incoming mRNA codon and the complimentary tRNA anticodon. The donor (P) site contains the elongation polypeptide bound to peptidyl tRNA. When both sites are filled, a peptide bond is formed between the two newly synthesized amino acids. **B:** The peptide chain with the most recently synthesized amino acid is translocated back to the A site.

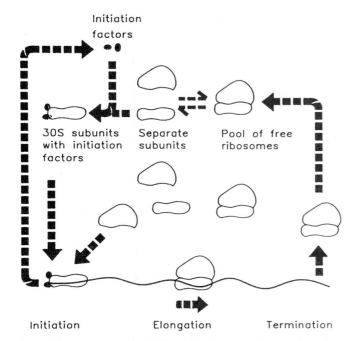

FIGURE 1.17. Formation of an initiation complex requires the dissociation of the ribosomal subunits in the "free pool" before the initiation factors, small ribosomal subunit, initiator tRNA, and mRNA can begin assembly of the initiation complex. (From Lewin B. *The assembly line for protein synthesis. Genes IV* New York: Oxford University Press, 1990:113, with permission.)

have separated from each other, IF3 complexes with 30S and prevents it from reassociating with 50S.[277–279] All three initiation factors, IF1, IF2, and IF3 then bind 30S subunits in the free pool, forming a 30S-IF1-IF2-IF3 complex. Each of the three initiation factors are capable of independently binding 30S; however, the stability of the binding is enhanced by the addition of one or more of the remaining initiation factors.[280–283] The binding sites on the 30S subunit for all three initiation factors are adjacent to or overlapping the 3′ end of 16S RNA.[284–287] IF2 is specifically needed for binding fMet-tRNA and chaperoning it to the 30S binding site. IF1 and GTP are present in complex formation. The presence of GTP reduces the number of molecules of IF2 needed to bind fMet-tRNA, and IF1 stabilizes the binding of IF2 to the 30S subunit.[280,281,288–290] IF3 is required for formation of the 30S-mRNA complex at the ribosomal binding site near the initiation codon. IF3 remains complexed with 30S until the large subunit joins the initiation complex at the site of initiation (Figure 1.19).[291,292] IF3 is present in exceedingly small amounts in bacterial cells, which makes it a determinant in how much 30S rRNA is available to initiate translation.[23]

The ribosomal binding site, found in prokaryotic mRNA, contains important sequences: (a) the Shine-Dalgarno sequence, AGGAGGU, which is the ribosome recognition site; and (b) the initiation codon AUG (or also GUG or UUG). In 1974, Shine and Dalgarno showed that a purine-rich sequence located upstream from the initiator methionine codon is complementary to the 3'-end of *E. coli* 16S rRNA.[293] Since then, approximately 150 additional bacterial and bacteriophage rRNA sequences have verified the presence of a Shine-Dalgarno sequence, which can be found preceding each cistron in a prokaryotic polycistronic message.[294–298] The efficiency with which the Shine-Dalgarno sequence binds the mRNA to initiate translation is contingent upon the number of nucleotides that form complementary base pairs with the 3' 16S rRNA nucleotide sequence. The stretch of complementary base pairing is usually three to nine continuous nucleotides.[294] However, the exact site within the 3' 16S rRNA where the Shine-Dalgarno sequence binds is dependent upon the degree of secondary structure present within that region, with the most favored sequence being CUCC found within the 3' pyrimidine-rich region (GAUCACCUCCUUA$_{OH}$3').[299] The advantage of this base pairing is that it brings the initiation codon into position for initiator tRNA binding.[288] The distance between the Shine-Dalgarno sequence and AUG is approximately seven nucleotides with 7 ± 2 being the ideal distance (Figure 1.20).[300–302]

AUG, the initiation triplet, codes for methionine which can be carried by two different tRNA molecules—one is the initiator methionine and the other is recognized in elongation. In bacteria and mitochondria, the initiator tRNA

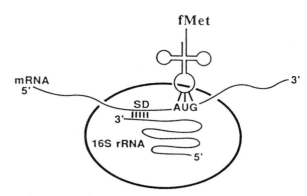

FIGURE 1.20. The Shine-Dalgarno (SD) sequence located upstream of the initiation codon is the motif recognized by ribosomes. The SD sequence forms complimentary base pairs with a 3' 16S rRNA. The number of nucleotides forming complementary bonds affects translation efficiency. (From Merrick WC. Eukaryotic mRNAs: strange solutions require unusual problems. In: Hill WE, Dahlberg A, Garrett RA, et al. *The ribosome: structure, function and evolution.* Washington, DC: American Society for Microbiology, 1990:292, with permission.)

is the formylated methionine, N-formyl-methionyl-tRNA, and it is the only amino acyl tRNA with which IF2 will interact (Figure 1.21).[303] The other methionine, whose function is to recognize an internal AUG codon, cannot be formylated. Formylated methionine (and eukaryotic initiator tRNAs) has the unique capability of bypassing the A site and entering directly into the P site of the ribosome to initiate protein synthesis. Once a growing polypeptide becomes 15 to 30 amino acids long, the formyl group at the NH2 terminus is removed. The function of the enzyme deformylase is to remove the formyl group and generate a normal NH2 terminus. The following set of reactions provides a summation of events in formation of an active 70S initiation complex.[270]

In contrast to the bacterial initiation of translation, the eukaryotic process is different, more complex, and requires many more factors to orchestrate the event. The main differences are that: (a) eukaryotes have larger ribosomes; (b) eukaryotes have more initiation factors (8 eIFs); (c) the Met-tRNA is not formylated; (d) most mRNA has a 5' cap structure; and (e) mRNA is monocistronic.

Initiation Complex in Eukaryotes

Eukaryotic mRNA has two distinguishing structures: the 5' cap and poly A tail, both of which are shown to be part of (although not necessary to) the translation process. It has been demonstrated that without a 5' cap, mRNA can be translated,[304,305] but the presence of the cap structure greatly enhances protein synthesis. The 5' cap structure, a methylated guanosine (position 7) that is connected to the first mRNA nucleotide by a 5' to 5' triphosphate bridge, functions to bring the 40S subunit of the ribosome to the

$$70S \xrightarrow{+ \text{ IF-3, IF-1}} 50S + [30S \cdot \text{IF-3} \cdot \text{IF-1}]$$

$$[30S \cdot \text{IF-3} \cdot \text{IF-1}] + \text{IF-2} \rightarrow [30S \cdot \text{IF-2} \cdot \text{IF-1} \cdot \text{IF-3}] \xrightarrow{+ \text{mRNA}}$$

$$[30S \cdot \text{mRNA} \cdot \text{IF-2} \cdot \text{IF-1} \cdot \text{IF-3}]$$

$$[30S \cdot \text{mRNA} \cdot \text{IF-2} \cdot \text{IF-1} \cdot \text{IF-3}] + \text{fMet-tRNA}_f \text{ GTP} \rightarrow$$

$$[30S \cdot \text{mRNA} \cdot \text{IF-2} \cdot \text{IF-1} \cdot \text{fMet-tRNA}_f \cdot \text{GTP}] + \text{IF-3}$$

30S · Initiation Complex

$$[30S \cdot \text{mRNA} \cdot \text{IF-2} \cdot \text{IF-1} \cdot \text{fMet-tRNA}_f \cdot \text{GTP}] + 50S \rightarrow$$

$$[\text{mRNA} \cdot 70S \cdot \text{fMet-tRNA}_f] + \text{IF-2} + \text{GDP} + \text{P}_i + \text{IF-1}$$

Active 70S Initiation Complex

FIGURE 1.19. The sequence of events and molecules involved with formation of an active 70S initiation complex.

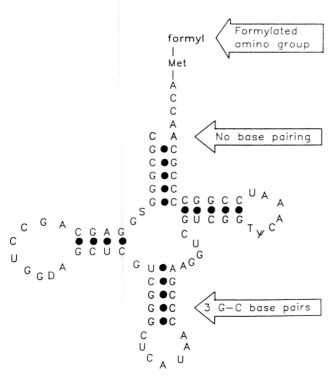

formyl
|
Met
|
A
C
C
A

Formylated amino group

No base pairing

3 G–C base pairs

FIGURE 1.21. The prokaryote initiator tRNA is formyl methionyl-t-RNA which has a formulated amino group making it structurally different from all other tRNAs. (From Lewin B. *The assembly line for protein synthesis.* New York: Oxford University Press, 1990: 113, with permission.)

mRNA to initiate translation. The four basic steps involved with the initiation of translation in eukaryotes are:

1. Dissociation of the 80S ribosome into two subunits: 40S and 60S;
2. Formation of a preinitiation complex consisting of methionyl-tRNA-40S-eIF2-GTP;
3. Formation of an initiation complex consisting of the preinitiation complex bound to mRNA;
4. Formation of an 80S initiation complex consisting of 40S and 60S subunits, initiator methionine, tRNA, and mRNA.

The initial step in eukaryotic translation is the formation of a complex containing GTP, eukaryotic initiation factor 2 (eIF2) and methionine-tRNA$_1$ (the initiator methionine in eukaryotes is not formylated). GTP binds to eIF2 to enhance the affinity of eIF2 for methionine-tRNA$_I$. Once the met-tRNA-eIF2-GTP complex is formed, it can then bind a free 40S ribosomal subunit found in the free ribosomal pool resulting in the formation of a 43S preinitiation complex.[306] The number of free 40S and 60S ribosomal subunits found in the free ribosomal pool is small since the formation of 80S is favored in the cellular milieu. The dissociation of the two subunits is maintained by eIF6 bind-

ing to the 60S subunit and eIF3 to 40S.[307–311] The 43S complex binds to the 5′ CAP region and moves along the mRNA until it reaches the AUG initiation codon. Here eIF5 triggers hydrolysis of GTP, which results in a conformational change in eIF2 and a reduced affinity for 40S; eIF2-GDP dissociates from the 43S; 40S forms an active 80S ribosome with 60S. eIF2 binds GDP with a 400-fold higher affinity than GTP,[312] resulting in a slow off rate of GDP. This would be a rate-limiting step in protein synthesis if it were not for the presence of another factor, guanine nucleotide exchange factor (GEF or eIF2B). GEF mediates the nucleotide exchange so that eIF2 now becomes GTP-bound, enabling this complex to be recycled in formation of another preinitiation complex. Protein synthesis begins when the 5′ cap structure is recognized by the initiation factor 4E(eIF4E) component of the eIF4F complex that also includes eIF4G. The 24-kD eIF4E, also known as the cap-binding protein, recognizes, binds to, and cross-links the 5′ cap structure.[313–315] The N-terminal domain of eIF4G functions as a bridge between eIF4E and eIF4A and its C-terminal domain interacts with eIF3 complexed to 40S-tRNA-GTP structure, thus creating a bridge between the cap structure and the 40S subunit.[316–320] After eIF4E has bound and cross-linked the 5′ cap structure, eIF4A and eIF4B become part of the initiation complex. eIF4A alone is a single-stranded RNA-dependent ATPase and belongs to a family of RNA helicase (unwinding) proteins. eIF4B has several functions, the most important of which is stimulation of ATP-dependent RNA helicase activity of eIF4A (Figure 1.22).[321–323] The coding region of eIF4B contains two sequence motifs, AFLGNL and KGFGYAEF, that are homologous with other RNA recognition motifs, suggesting that this factor acts as an mRNA cross-linking protein.[321–324] These two factors, eIF4A and eIF4B, are essential in melting the 5′ untranslated region (5′ UTR) of mRNA, making the initiation codon accessible to the ribosomes (Figure 1.23).

Initiation factor eIF4E is of considerable interest due to its important role in controlling the rate of initiation of translation as well as its role in the regulation of translation. For example, the promoter of the eIF4E gene has an E-box that c-Myc binds to activate transcription, thus increasing the level of eIF4A expression. Malignant transformation of cells overexpressing eIF4E has been demonstrated;[325,326] cells supplemented with growth factors, hormones, and mitogens can stimulate phosphorylation of eIF4E, and post-translational modifications such as phosphorylation have been shown to increase the initiation of translation by enhancing eIF4E affinity for the 5′ cap;[327–330] cellular inhibitory proteins, 4E-binding proteins, function as negative regulators of gene expression. They act as repressors of 5′ cap-binding by interfering with the association of eIF4E with the bridging factor eIF4G, thus inhibiting the formation of the initiation complex. The 4E-binding proteins contain an amino acid sequence homologous to the N-terminal domain

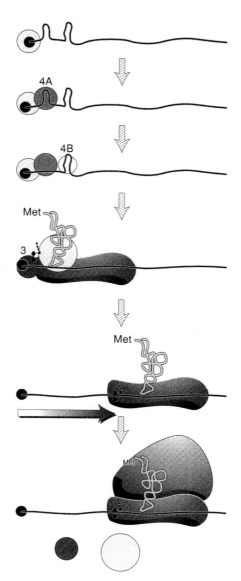

FIGURE 1.22. Eukaryotic initiation factors eIF-A and eIF-B function as helicase enzymes, unwinding the secondary structure of the mRNA in front of them as they move in a 5′ to 3′ direction. (From Lewin B. *The apparatus for protein localization.* New York: Oxford University Press, 1990:279, with permission.)

of eIF4G. This sequence in eIF4G normally associates with eIF4E.[317,331–333] The x-ray crystallography structure of eIF4E bound to 7-methyl-GDP has recently been reported,[334] thus giving additional insight into the interactions of this initiation factor with other factors and mRNA.

As might be expected, some viruses have an efficient alternative to the 5′ cap structure stimulation of translation. Positive-stranded picornoviruses (polio) have a 650 to 1,300 nucleotide long 5′ noncoding region (5′ NCR) containing many AUG codons and extensive secondary structure. This region is capable of efficiently initiating translation of the

viral mRNA. These regions are named internal ribosome entry sites (IRES) and are found in all picornoviruses, hepatitis A and C viruses mRNA.[335–337] IRES elements have been located in some cellular mRNAs, such as IgG heavy chain binding protein, Bip, fibroblast growth factor 2, *Drosophilia antennapedia* protein, and human eIF4G.[338–342]

It should be noted that there is evidence from experiments performed in amphibian oocytes and yeast indicating that the 3′ polyadenylation tail is involved in the stimulation of mRNA translation. These studies have shown that a poly(A) tail binding protein, Pab1p, is required for stimulation of translation and that it was capable of stimulating translation in the absence of eIF4E. It has also been shown that the poly(A) tail enhances the binding of the 40S subunit to mRNA as well as enhancing the joining of the 60S subunit to the initiation complex. Taken together, models of the poly(A) tail involvement in translation have been suggested, although many aspects remain unresolved.[343] At this juncture, the reader should make special note of these data and anticipate that this aspect of translation will be unraveled in the near future.

Unlike bacteria, eukaryotes do not have a specific ribosome-binding site on the mRNA to direct the initiation complex to the proper initiation codon. The precise mechanism by which eukaryotes locate the AUG initiator codon is still unknown; however, there are several hypotheses, all of which are variations of a "scanning" mechanism. The current hypothesis is that the 40S ribosomes bind mRNA at or near the 5′-end cap and move toward the interior of the mRNA sequence.[344–346] Recognition of the AUG initiator codon depends on the flanking sequences, with A/GNNAUGG providing the best context for binding of the initiation complex. If the first AUG is in this optimal context, then the 40S initiation complex will bind at that initiation codon without scanning the remainder of the mRNA. However, if the first AUG does not have the ideal flanking sequences, then the 40S will continue to scan the mRNA sequence until it locates another AUG, binds it and initiates translation at that codon.[347] In a few cases, some 40S subunits bind the first AUG flanked by nonoptimal sequences, while other ribosomes continue scanning and finally bind an AUG codon further downstream. Given these circumstances, two proteins would be synthesized from a single message. This is a highly unusual event in eukaryotes since they do not have bicistronic transcripts.[23] The ability of a mRNA to be actively involved in translation is determined by: (a) how accessible the 5′ capped mRNA is to the initiation complex; (b) how readily the 40S ribosomal subunit can scan the mRNA downstream from its entry point at the 5′ end; and (c) how easily the initiation complex can locate the AUG initiator codon in the optimal context.[272]

Ribosome "scanning" can be impeded by secondary structures in the mRNA. Extensive secondary structure, common to mRNA, can form stable stem-loop structures

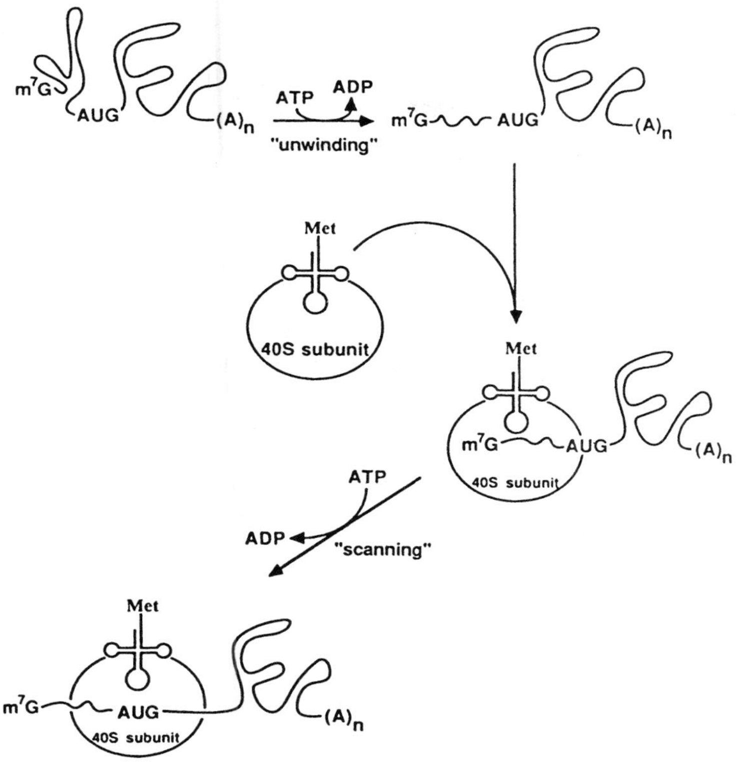

FIGURE 1.23. The initiation of translation in eukaryotes requires the formation of an initiation complex to initiate translation. This requires the functions of many enzymes performing their specific activity at the appropriate time. (From Merrick WC. Eukaryotic mRNAs: strange solutions require unusual problems. In: Hill WE, Dahlberg A, Garrett RA, et al. *The ribosome: structure, function and evolution*. Washington, DC: American Society for Microbiology, 1990:292, with permission.)

through complementary base pairing (Figure 1.24). If the stem-loop structure is so stable that it cannot be melted, then the 40S ribosome may not be able to pass the stem loop as it scans the mRNA. A stem loop at the 5′ CAP region can prevent the initiation complex from binding the mRNA at its normal site of entry.[345]

The formation of the initiation complex (joining of 60S to the preinitiation complex at the initiator codon) requires eIF5. This protein is a single polypeptide having ribosome-dependent GTPase activity. The function of this factor is to hydrolyze the GTP molecule bound to eIF2 prior to the addition of the 60S subunit. This hydrolysis reaction removes eIF2-GDP, eIF1 and eIF3 from the preinitiation complex so they can be recycled to continue their role in formation of new preinitiation complexes.[309,311,348–351]

Elongation

After the initiation complex is formed, the elongation step can begin. There are three major steps in the elongation that keep repeating themselves. They are: (a) binding of aminoacyl-tRNA to the ribosomal A site; (b) formation of a peptide bond; (c) translocation of the tRNAs and mRNA (Figure 1.25). There are elongation factors involved in the elongation steps. It should be noted that these factors are not a requirement, because the ribosome can carry out elongation without them.[352,353] However, catalysis of these steps by two GTP-dependent factors increases the speed and fidelity of protein synthesis.[354] These factors bind to specific components and are then released and recycled for use in the addition of the next amino acid in the nascent polypeptide chain.[355]

The process of elongation in prokaryotes and eukaryotes

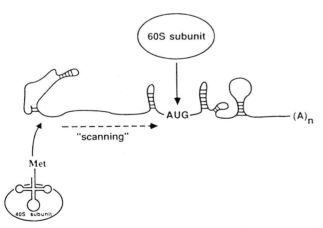

FIGURE 1.24. Ribosome scanning can be impeded by the secondary structure of mRNA, which can potentially prevent initiation at the correct AUG site. (From Merrick WC. Eukaryotic mRNAs: strange solutions require unusual problems. In: Hill WE, Dahlber A, Garrett RA, et al. *The ribosome: structure, function and evolution*. Washington, DC: American Society for Microbiology, 1990: 292, with permission.)

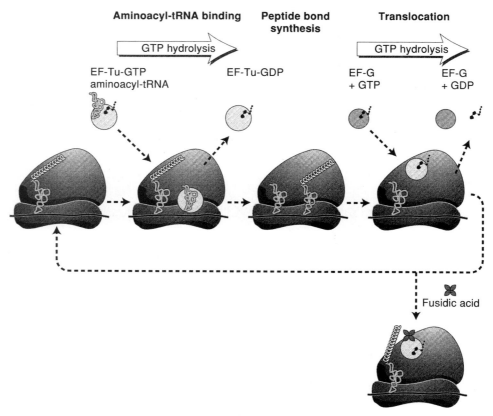

FIGURE 1.25. The four major elongation steps in prokaryotes require the functions of elongation factors. (From Lewin B. *The assembly line for protein synthesis.* New York: Oxford University Press, 1994:163, with permission.)

is similar. At this time the elongation process is under intense investigation. As more precise data obtained from more sophisticated technology are being accumulated, they more specifically define the interactions and functions of the elongation factors with the tRNA, mRNA, and ribosome subunits.

The initial step in elongation begins with an initiator tRNA in the P (peptidyl) site and the small ribosomal subunit and initiation factors that bind to the mRNA in a configuration that allow entry only into the P site of the ribosome. The aminoacyl (A) site is now available for introduction of an aminoacyl-tRNA having an anticodon complementary to the mRNA codon that will occupy the A site. The appropriate aminoacyl-tRNA is escorted to the A site by a GTP-bound elongation factor (EF-Tu in prokaryotes and eEF-1α in eukaryotes) introduced as an aminoacyl-tRNA-EF-Tu-GTP complex. The GTP undergoes hydrolysis and EF-Tu (eEF-1α) is released. Another factor is required to displace the GDP from the elongation factor. This factor, EF-Ts in bacteria and EF-1$\beta\gamma$ in eukaryotes, forms an intermediary with EF-Tu and is subsequently displaced by GTP as shown in the following diagram:

$$\text{EF-Tu-GDP} \rightarrow \text{EF-Tu-EF-Ts} \rightarrow \text{EF-Tu-GTP}$$

The EF-Tu-GDP complex is then available to undergo another cycle in chaperoning a tRNA to the A site. This can be a rate-limiting step in elongation just as it was in initiation, because a subsequent binding reaction cannot occur until the EF-GDP is released for recycling.

Release of the EF-Tu-GDP enables the aminoacyl-tRNA to bind to the A site. The anticodon regions of the tRNA in both sites interact with the small subunit of the ribosome, and likewise the acceptor regions of both tRNAs interact with the large ribosomal subunit. A peptide bond is formed when an α-amino group of aminoacyl-tRNA attacks the peptidyl-tRNA bond in a reaction catalyzed by peptidyl transferase. Following formation of the peptide bond, the nascent peptide chain translocates to the A site. At the time of translocation, another GTP-dependent elongation factor (EF-G in prokaryotes and EF-2 in eukaryotes) binds to the ribosomes and catalyzes the movement of the two tRNAs and mRNA by one codon. The deacylated aminoacyl-tRNA moves from the A site to the exit (E) site[356] and then dissociates from the ribosome.[354]

The GTP-dependent translocation step involving EF-G (eEF-2) is under intense debate. The previously viewed mechanism was that GTP-EF-G bound to the ribosome to induce translocation and ensure that translocation occurred in one direction.[357–359] This has been considered a rate-limiting step. Pre-steady-state experiments now show that GTP hydrolysis of EF-G occurs before translocation and increases the movement by more than 50-fold.[360] Recent evidence from experiments using directed hydroxyl radical probing and low-resolution electron microscope reconstruction to map the position of EF-G in the ribosome has led to the start of a new model which needs further verification. These studies indicate that the GTPase activity of EF-G triggered by the interaction of contacts in the G domain of EF-G with elements of 23S rRNA creates a conformational change in EF-G.[354,361] This conformational change would reposition domains in EF-G such that it contacts ribosomal elements, catalyzing the reaction for "unlocking"[358] of the tRNA-ribosome complex. The unlocking event would then allow relaxation of tRNA-binding contacts and movement of ribosomal substructures, followed by movement of tRNA and mRNA. As tRNA leaves the 30S A site, a domain of EF-G would occupy the site, thus preventing reversal of translocation while the ribosome is still in an unlocked state. This positional change of the EF-G domain would release it from the configurational state that enabled EF-G to catalyze unlocking of ribosome, thus reestablishing the locked position and release of EF-G. Such an event would explain the speed of translocation and diminish the likelihood of previous suggestions that this is a rate-limiting step in translation elongation.[354,360,361]

Once EF-Tu-GDP is released and a peptide bond is formed between the peptidyl-tRNA and the aminoacyl-tRNA, then the subsequent step—translocation—can occur. This step requires an elongation factor (EF-G in bacteria and EF-2 in eukaryotes), GTP, and the enzyme peptidyl transferase. The function of the elongation factor is to bind the ribosome while the polypeptide chain attached to tRNA in the P site is transferred to the aminoacyl tRNA in the A site (Figure 1.26). The elongation factor is then released from the ribosome by GTP hydrolysis, the polypeptide chain-tRNA moves to the P site, and the mRNA moves three nucleotides so that the next amino acid codon is in the empty A site. The cycle repeats itself.[362–364] This cyclical event continues until an in-frame termination codon—UAA, UGA, or UAG—enters the A site, signifying the end of the translatable sequence. However, in order to terminate protein synthesis: (a) the completed polypeptide must be released from peptidyl-tRNA; (b) the tRNA must be released from the ribosome; and (c) the ribosome must be dissociated from the mRNA.

Termination

An aminoacyl-tRNA with an anticodon for UAA, UGA, or UAG does not exist. Rather than the RNA-RNA interactions which normally occur in decoding, termination codons interact with protein factors for catalysis of the termi-

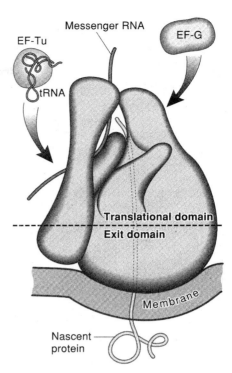

FIGURE 1.26. Bacterial elongation factor EF-Tu escorts the appropriate tRNA to the ribosome entry site A. EF-G binds the ribosome while translocation is occurring. (From Oakes MI, Scheinman A, Atha T, et al. Ribosome structure: three-dimensional locations of rRNA and proteins. In: Hill WE, Dahlberg A, Garrett RA, et al. *The ribosome: structure, function and evolution.* Washington DC: American Society for Microbiology, 1990:292, with permission.)

nation reaction. These proteins, called release factors, are found in both prokaryotes and eukaryotes. They recognize and decode the termination codons by an as-yet unknown mechanism.

Bacteria have two release factors (RF): (a) RF1 recognizes UAA and UAG; (b) RF2 recognizes UGA and UAA. *RF1* gene has a single reading frame which is directly translated into RF1 protein. *RF2* gene is in two open reading frames requiring a +1 frame shift for the entire RF protein to be synthesized. The first reading frame is terminated by an RF2-specific codon, UGA. It is postulated that RF2 is autoregulated. Evidence to support this idea was obtained from *in vitro* translation experiments in which addition of purified RF2 caused a significant decline in RF2 synthesis.[365] Other experiments using a *LacZ-RF2* fusion gene construct further demonstrated that RF2 frameshifting occurred 30% to 50% of the time.[366,367] The autoregulated mechanism would terminate protein synthesis at the first open reading frame termination codon when RF2 was in excess or unneeded. A frameshift would result in synthesis of both open reading frames yielding the RF2 protein when it was needed to terminate protein synthesis.[368,369]

The way RFs recognize termination codons remains unknown. However, there is evidence to support the idea: (a) that RFs bind directly to the termination codon; and (b) that rRNA is involved in this recognition mechanism. Competition experiments showed that repressor tRNA can compete with RF2 for binding to the termination codon, demonstrating that RF2 binds directly to the anticodon.[370] Other binding studies demonstrated that RF2 can bind termination codon UGA with a tenfold greater affinity than UAG in the presence of ribosomes, but does not bind UAG without ribosomes.[371] The RF2 in-frame UGA codon used when frameshifting occurs has a short sequence immediately upstream of UGA which interacts with the Shine-Dalgarno region of the 3' 16S rRNA.[367,372] This probably facilitates binding of RF2 to the appropriate termination codon just as it did for the AUG codon/tRNA in initiation.

Eukaryotic cells have only one release factor—eRF—which requires GTP for it to bind ribosomes. It is thought that eRF has a common recognition site for all three of the eukaryotic termination codons and that all three codons compete with each other to form the eRF-ribosome complex.[373] However, Brown and co-workers proposed a model for termination recognition in eukaryotes. They analyzed sequences surrounding the natural termination codon and found that UAA(A/G) is the codon and 3' nucleotide most preferred by eukaryotes. Based on this data they proposed a "tetranucleotide" termination signal which is recognized by RF rather than the trinucleotide. They further suggest that the total GC content of the mRNA would influence whether an A or G was selected in the fourth position.[374,375]

Stop codons do not always signal termination of protein synthesis. They can be read incorrectly by a normal or a suppressor tRNA and can incorporate an amino acid rather than terminate protein synthesis.

Regulation of Translation

When all of the tightly woven intricacies of translation are considered, it should not be a surprise that there are some regulatory mechanisms involved with the process. The regulatory differences between prokaryotes and eukaryotes are quite unalike. Prokaryotes have two basic regulatory mechanisms: (a) alteration in mRNA structure; and (b) repressor/activator proteins which bind to mRNA. Unlike prokaryotes, eukaryotes do not have mRNA-binding proteins, that is, repressor/activators that regulate translation. In eukaryotic cells, each protein is made in amounts proportional to the concentration of mRNA. For example, if the cell synthesizes more ribosomal proteins than the ribosomes can use, the ribosomal proteins are degraded. Many of the translational regulatory mechanisms in eukaryotes are reversible phosphorylation events with some examples of autoregulated translation.

E. coli and some bacteriophages have ribosomal proteins (rp) which regulate translation by binding mRNA and act-

ing as a repressor of protein synthesis. Most translational repressor proteins bind a specific nucleic acid site having a characteristic stem-loop structure. The unpaired loop region frequently constitutes the binding region in these structures.[376–378] Nomura suggested that initiation may be regulated via these secondary structure formations. He thought that sites on a repressor molecule which bind mRNA may be homologous with the sequences in rRNA which bind the ribosome binding site (RBS). If that was the case, the repressor protein may compete with rRNA for the RBS thereby inhibiting protein synthesis.[379] Specific examples of this are found in *E. coli* L1, L10, and S4 repressor proteins. All three bind to a hairpin loop located very near the ribosome-binding site. This brings the repressor protein in close proximity to the Shine-Dalgarno and initiation site, thus interfering with rRNA accessibility to the RBS. The binding sites for L1 and L10 repressor proteins are hairpin loops located very close to the ribosomal binding site.[380,381] The ribosome repressor S4 binds a GGGC sequence in a stem loop distal to the RBS. The GGGC forms complementary base pairs with sequences located immediately downstream from a GUG initiator codon. This type configuration, called a pseudoknot, puts S4 in close proximity to the initiation site, where it acts as an initiation repressor.[382]

Frameshifting is a translational event where the mRNA in the ribosome complex moves one nucleotide such that the pairing between the codon and anticodon in the P site is broken, allows pairing to occur with the nucleotide in the next codon, and in so doing has shifted the reading frame. A well-documented example is the +1 frameshift in translation of *E. coli* release factor 2 mRNA, as discussed earlier. Frameshift is also found in eukaryotes. For example, expression of the mammalian gene, ornithine decarboxylase (ODC), is needed for polyamine biosynthesis. When the ornithine decarboxylase antizyme protein binds to ODC, it targets ODC for ubiquitin-proteasome degradation. When the concentration of polyamines is high, it causes a frameshift in antizyme mRNA, resulting in more antizyme synthesis. More antizyme synthesis regulates the rate/degree of ODC degradation.[383–386] Further stimulation (2.5-fold) of the frameshift is provided by a 3' pseudoknot (stem loops whose sequence can pair with down- or upstream sequences) in the mRNA structure three nucleotides from the frameshift site.[386,387]

Frameshifting is a common regulatory event in expression of retroviral proteins. The common shift is a −1 at a heptanucleotide sequence that results in a gag-pol fusion protein rather than a gag or pol protein. This shift occurs at a particular stage in the life cycle of the virus.[388–394] Reversible phosphorylation is not an uncommon event in translational regulation in eukaryotes. Some steps in formation of the preinitiation complex are able to be regulated through reversible phosphorylation of initiation factors. The best-documented example is the phosphorylation of eIF2. As mentioned earlier, eIF2-GTP is bound to the 40S ribosomal subunit in the preinitiation complex. GTP hydrolysis causes a conformational change in eIF2, causing it to dissociate from 40S as an eIF2-GDP complex. Since eIF2 binds GDP with a 400-fold greater affinity than GTP,[312] it requires a guanine nucleotide exchange factor—GEF—to mediate the GDP to GTP exchange with eIF2. This is a rate-limiting step in protein synthesis because eIF2 must be bound to GTP in order for the factor to be recycled for a subsequent preinitiation complex formation. If an eIF2 alpha subunit becomes phosphorylated, then GEF has a 100-fold increased affinity for the phosphorylated eIF2, forming an eIF2(αP)-GDP-GEF complex. GEF is not an abundant protein and becomes less available. In fact, all of the available GEF can potentially become bound to eIF2(αP), stopping all new protein synthesis.[395] One example of eukaryotic autoregulation of translation is observed in alpha and beta tubulin. These proteins are the major constituents of tubulin, forming a heterodimer consisting of one alpha and one beta polypeptide. These heterodimers regulate the stability of tubulin mRNA.[396–399] Other requirements which are necessary for autoregulation are polysome-bound tubulin mRNA, free tubulin, and four specific amino-terminus β-tubulin amino acids. Translation of the first 13 nucleotides of β-tubulin mRNA (the first four amino acids are Met-Arg-Glu-Ile in β-tubulin) is necessary for autoregulated destabilization/degradation of polysome-bound tubulin mRNA.[400–402] Although the exact mechanism for this example of autoregulation remains unclear, it is known that continued elongation of the polypeptide being synthesized from the β-tubulin mRNA is a necessary step for autoregulated degradation of β-tubulin mRNA bound by polysomes.[403]

A second example of autoregulation of eukaryotic translation is found in the mRNA for ferritin and the transferrin receptor. In higher eukaryotes, iron uptake and detoxification are regulated by two proteins, ferritin and the transferrin receptor. Once in the cytoplasm (delivered via the receptor-mediated endocytosis), iron is either utilized or, if in excess, is sequestered in ferritin.[404–406] The expression of both proteins is highly regulated by the amount of iron present in the cell. The number of receptors increases with an iron deficiency, and conversely the number of receptors decreases with an abundance of iron. Ferritin is decreased proportionally to a decrease in iron and increases with an iron increase. Both of the proteins have a cis-acting iron responsive element, IRE,[407,408] whose location is variable. It can be found in either the 5′ untranslated regions (UTR) or 3′ untranslated regions (UTR) of mRNA. An IRE-binding protein[409,410] can repress translation if it binds the IRE located in the 5′ UTR. However, when this IRE-BP binds the IRE in the 3′ UTR of the transferrin receptor mRNA, it represses the degradation of mRNA. Therefore, this IRE-BP can regulate translation by: (a) increasing the amount of transferrin receptor synthesis, thereby repressing degradation of mRNA; (b) downregulating expression of transferrin

by binding the IRE in the 5′ UTR in the transferrin mRNA.[407,408] Deletion analysis studies showed that a 350 base pair region in the 5′ UTR is necessary and sufficient for these iron translational regulation mechanisms.[407]

There is a 680 nucleotide fragment in the 3′ UTR of the transferrin receptor that has been found to be necessary for iron-dependent regulation. Within the 680 nucleotide region are five stem loops whose structure resembles the secondary structure found in the 5′ UTR of the ferritin mRNA.[407,408] In fact the 3′ UTR containing the transferrin receptor IRE could be substituted for the 5′ UTR IRE in ferritin mRNA and regulate translation of ferritin mRNA.[409,410]

GCN4 is a transcriptional activating protein of yeast *Saccromyces cerevisiae*. It activates transcription of more than 30 genes in response to amino acid starvation. The expression of GCN4 itself is transcriptionally regulated by the amount of available amino acids. The GCN4 mRNA leader sequence has four upstream open reading frames (uORF) which inhibit translation of GCN4 when amino acids are abundant (nonstarvation). The uORFs are bound by negative regulatory proteins encoded by the GCD gene. Upon amino acid starvation, GCN2 and GCN3 gene products act as positive regulators by antagonizing the GCD protein's negative effect. The result is increased translation of GCN4 mRNA.[411] uORF3 and 4 in GCN4 mRNA inhibit GCN4 mRNA translation much better than uORF1 and 2. It has been demonstrated that uORF2 is more repressive than uORF1 because it is in closer proximity to the GCN4 AUG codon.[412,413] Hinnebusch's group showed that replacing the last codon and ten additional double-stranded nucleotides from uORF4 with the same nucleotides located in the uORF1 increased the repressor activity of uORF1 tenfold. It was proposed that this was due to the important relative distance of the termination codon of uORF1 to the AUG site in GCN4 mRNA.[414]

The general description and illustrations tend to give the reader the misconception that these beautifully designed and organized translational (like transcriptional) mechanisms are fail-proof (or nearly) systems. However, as in all replication, transcription, and translation reactions that function with precision, we hear ourselves frequently using the word "fidelitous." For a molecular biologist, fidelity means "exactness, as in a copy." How frequently can we expect to find error in the incorporation of the correct amino acid based on the genetic code? There is approximately one error for every 10,000 amino acids synthesized.[415]

The way in which the mRNA codon and tRNA anticodon interact has a major impact on fidelity and/or efficiency in incorporating the correct amino acid. These interactions can be less precise when: (a) the tRNA structure is altered through point mutation, modification of tRNA bases, or a point mutation in the tRNA gene; (b) changes occur in the mRNA sequence or the context of the codon.

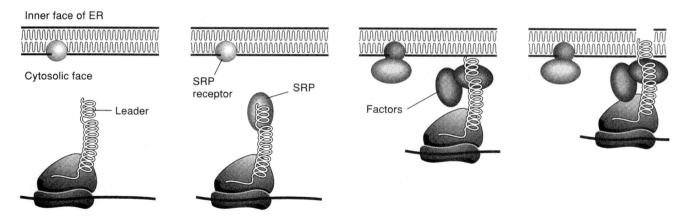

FIGURE 1.27. Proteins are synthesized on ribosomes located in the cytoplasm or bound to the endoplasmic reticulum. The proteins are then directed to the cellular compartment where they perform a specific function. (From Lewin B. *The apparatus for protein localization.* New York: Oxford University Press, 1990:279, with permission.)

Protein Modifications

Newly synthesized proteins must be directed to the compartment where they perform their function (Figure 1.27). Most soluble proteins are synthesized on free ribosomes in the cytosol, which is also where they are generally needed. Proteins that function as membrane or transported proteins are synthesized on the ribosomes attached to the surface of the ER. Protein sorting begins in the ER, and certain proteins are restricted to either smooth or rough endoplasmic reticulum. The newly synthesized protein is transported through a hydrophilic channel whose function is to translocate proteins for secretion as well as inserting membrane proteins into a lipid bilayer. The channel is part of a complex that has a defined function in transport of each specific protein by either a cotranslational or postranslational mechanism. In cotranslational translocation, the growing polypeptide chain is simultaneously being transported and synthesized, whereas a posttranslationally translocated protein is first synthesized, then transported.

Proteins that are co- or posttranslationally transported are synthesized with a short peptide on the amino terminus called a "signal peptide" in eukaryotes and a "leader sequence" in prokaryotes. In cotranslationally transported proteins, the newly synthesized signal peptide emerges from the ribosome and is recognized and bound by a signal recognition particle (SRP). The SRP then binds tightly to the ribosome, causing a pause (elongation arrest) in translation of the new protein. A complex made up of a ribosome, SRP, and a nascent protein with a signal sequence is needed for translocation or integration across/into ER membrane. The SRP interacts with the SRP membrane receptor. SRP is released from the complex, and the ribosome forms a junction with the ER membrane. This series of interactions tar-

gets the signal peptide to the ER membrane (Figure 1.28). Proteins that are posttranslationally translocated also have the same signal peptide, but the mechanism by which it functions in transport is still undefined.

The channel through which the proteins are trans-

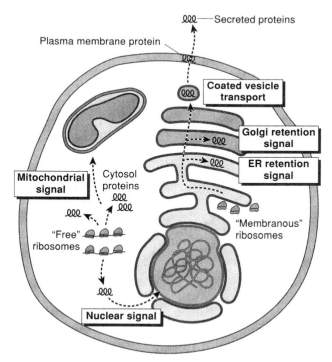

FIGURE 1.28. Signal peptides are sets of specific sequences on the amino terminus of the newly synthesized peptide. They function to transfer the protein to a membrane receptor. (From Lewin B. *The apparatus for protein localization.* New York: Oxford University Press, 1990:185, with permission.)

ported/translocated also requires a Sec61P complex (eukaryotes) or a SecYEG complex (prokaryotes), a ribosome if translocation is cotranslational, Sec62/63P complex and BIP protein in yeast, or Sec A in bacteria. The signal sequence of the translocating substrate induces the opening of the Sec61 channel in the lumenal direction. Sec61p and ribosome form a tight seal over the channel, allowing the translocating polypeptide to move in only one direction, from the ribosome through the pore and into the ER lumen. Furthermore, the positioning of the ribosome over the pore forms a tight seal[416–419] that prevents other molecules from crossing the membrane along with the polypeptide. The exact mechanism by which the channel opens/closes and/or the components required for formation of the channel remain unknown. Interestingly, the Sec61p complex can transport proteins from the ER to the cytoplasm. This reverse transport is termed "retrograde" transport.[420,421]

The inside of the channel must open in order for transmembrane sequences of integrated membrane proteins to become localized in the lipid bilayer. This is an even more complex situation because the transmembrane proteins must cross the membrane more than once, therefore requiring a much greater level of control in opening and closing of the channel and ribosome binding to the channel. The details of a model remain uncertain.[422]

Proteins translocated to the ER lumen undergo further modifications and sorting to provide them with direction to their destination. Posttranslational modifications are additions of side chain groups to a polypeptide chain that is forming bonds necessary for a protein to fold properly or to be held in a particular configuration or location (Figure 1.29). The endoplasmic reticulum lumen is the primary location for proteins undergoing folding and modification. This compartment ensures that only those proteins that are completely assembled with appropriate folding and modification will be allowed further transport in the secretory pathway. Those proteins that do not meet that criteria are selected out by the ER-associated protein degradation pathway. While proteins are undergoing the folding process, they have exposed hydrophobic regions which cause them to aggregate to bury the hydrophobic domains. Aggregation causes proteins to fall out of solution; therefore it takes longer for them to become properly folded and exit the endoplasmic reticulum lumen.[423] Other proteins are retained in the ER and selected for degradation despite the lack of an aberrant nature. The secretion of such proteins can be dependent upon the differentiated state of the cell, as seen with IgM[424–426] or the metabolic status of the cell.[427–429]

The ER serves as a "quality control" checkpoint making

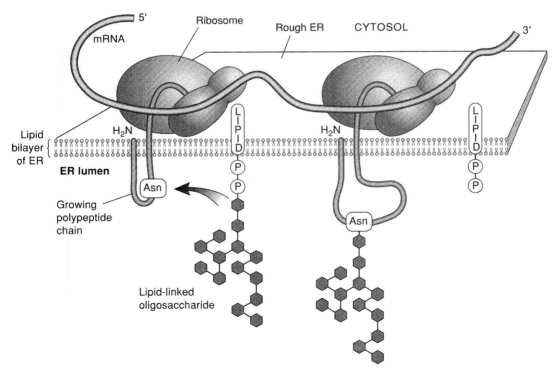

FIGURE 1.29. Posttranslational modifications of proteins are additions of side chain groups to newly synthesized peptide. These modifications are necessary for a protein to be properly folded. (From Alberts A, Bray D, Lewis J, et al. *Intracellular sorting and maintenance of cellular compartments.* New York: Garland Publishing Inc., 1989:405, with permission.)

certain that newly synthesized proteins are properly folded, processed, and assembled before they leave the ER. Those proteins that do not pass the criteria for further transport are selected for degradation by the endoplasmic reticulum-associated protein degradation pathway (ERAD). The ER lumen contains chaperone proteins that are involved with selection of proteins for the degradation process.[430-432] There is recent evidence to show that newly synthesized proteins transported to the ER and subsequently selected for degradation are transported back to the cytosol, where they are degraded by the proteasomes.[433-437] To exit the ER, the aberrant proteins utilize the Sec61p complex retrograde transport mechanism.

When the retrograde transported proteins reach the cytosol, they undergo a posttranslational modification that adds ubiquitin to the protein, marking it for degradation in the proteasome. A proteasome is where most eukaryotic cellular protein degradation occurs, and is part of an ATP-dependent pathway. Proteasomal degradation by means of the ubiquitin-proteasome pathway is a highly selective, highly regulated form of posttranslational modification. In this process, single or multiple ubiquitin molecules are conjugated to a protein. Following the ubiquitin conjugating process, the protein is degraded by a proteasome consisting of a 26S protease complex that contains a 20S protease catalytic core.[438-443] By itself, the 20S core functions as a proteasome, capable of degrading small peptides or proteins that are already denatured,[442,444] whereas the 26S complex is required for degradation of an intact protein structure.[443,445] When a ubiquitin-bound targeted protein is degraded, the ubiquitin(s) are released and reutilized. There is a three-step mechanism for ubiquitin modification of a protein that requires three enzymes—E1, E2, and E3. E1 is a ubiquitin-activating enzyme that catalyzes the ATP activation of a ubiquitin C-terminal Gly to a thiol ester intermediate. The ubiquitin intermediate is then transferred to a substrate (protein targeted for degradation) that is bound by E3, a ubiquitin-protein ligase. The transfer of the ubiquitin intermediate to the substrate requires E2, the ubiquitin-conjugating enzyme. In the transfer, an isopeptide bond is formed between the ubiquitin C-terminal Gly and an ϵ-amino group on a lysine residue in the targeted protein.[441]

There are specific examples of regulated protein degradation by the ubiquitin-proteasome pathway: tumor suppressor p53, IkB, yeast transcriptional factors AP-1, MATα2 (yeast) and GCN4 (yeast), cyclins that control eukaryotic cell cycle, Mos kinase involved in oocyte maturation, transmembrane proteins such as the T-cell receptor, platelet-derived growth factor receptor, and cystic fibrosis transmembrane conductance regulator.[439,442,445,446]

Although there is no clearly defined signal for ubiquitin-mediated degradation there are some reports of sequence motifs that have been shown to be involved with the selection of a protein for degradation by the ubiquitin pathway.[447-450]

Other posttranslational modifications also occur within the cytosol.[451] Many of the cytosolic modifications function to regulate specific protein activity and are often reversible (e.g., phosphorylation/dephosphorylation).

The addition of oligosaccharides to a protein is a posttranslational modification called glycosylation (Figure 1.30). Glycosylation was thought to occur in all eukaryotic proteins destined for secretion. However, there is substantial evidence that glycosylation of nuclear and cytoplasmic eukaryotic proteins at multiple sites by single o-linked N-acetylglucosamine (O-GlcNac) is abundant. In many of the proteins where this is found, this type of glycosylation is found to be reciprocal to phosphorylation and on sites similar to phosphorylation sites. This type of glycosylation occurs in response to cellular signals or cellular stages and may, therefore, play an important role in regulation. There is evidence that glycosylated proteins exist in the nuclear pore complex and are involved in nuclear transport;[452,453] every RNA polymerase transcription factor that has been examined,[454-458] as well as the C-terminal domain of the largest subunit of RNA polymerase II;[459,460] the transactivation domain of c-*myc* that binds retinoblastoma;[461,462] p53 tumor suppressor;[463] microtubule-associated protein tau;[464,465] a 67-kD multiply glycosolyated protein that protects initiation factor 2 (eIF2) from phosphorylation, thus enabling the initiation of protein synthesis to continue.[466,467] For recent reviews see 468–470.

Glycosylation does occur in all eukaryotic proteins destined for secretion. For these proteins the sugar moieties can be added in either the endoplasmic reticulum or the Golgi. A single oligosaccharide added to the NH2 group of asparagine in the endoplasmic reticulum (N-linked glycosylation) can also be linked to many other proteins. The entire glycosylation process involves cleaving parts of the oligosaccharide while it is still in the endoplasmic reticulum, followed by further modifications or additions as the process continues in the Golgi. Similarly, addition of an oligosaccharide to the $-$OH group of hydroxylysine, serine, or threonine (O-linked glycosylation) entails multiple enzyme-catalyzed reactions to add sugar groups to the protein.[471-474] These large, protruding oligosaccharide molecules are thought to provide protection from protease digestion.[475]

Prenylation is the addition of an isoprenyl to a cysteine by a thioester bond (Figure 1.31) which functions to maintain a protein at either the plasma or internal membranes.[476,477] There are two primary groups of prenylated proteins: those with a CAAX motif or those with a CC or CxC motif. The CAAX is most commonly found whereas the CC or CxC group consists mainly of Rab proteins that are GTP-binding proteins involved in intracellular membrane trafficking.[478] There are three enzymes that catalyzes the addition of isoprenoid to the cysteine of a CAAX motif protein. Farnesyl transferase transfers a farnesyl group from farnesyl diphosphate to the CAAX-cysteine, geranylgeranyl

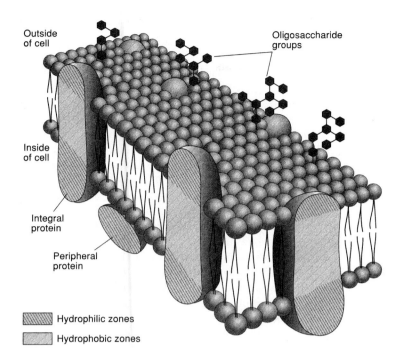

Outside
of cell

Oligosaccharide
groups

Inside
of cell

Integral
protein

Peripheral
protein

Hydrophilic zones

Hydrophobic zones

FIGURE 1.30. Glycosylation is the addition of sugar moieties to a protein. It is thought that these large sugar groups protect the protein from proteolytic degradation. (From Singer SJ, Nicolson GL. The fluid mosaic model of the structure of cell membranes. *Science* 1972:175, with permission.)

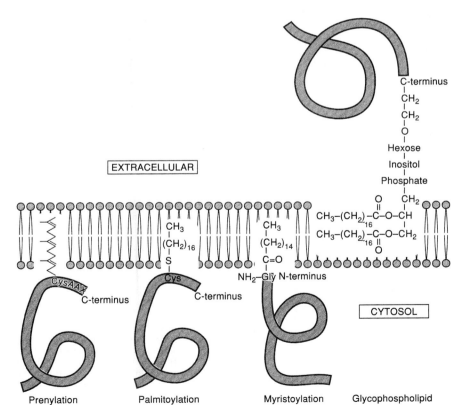

C-terminus
CH_2
CH_2
O
Hexose
Inositol
Phosphate

EXTRACELLULAR

CH_3
$(CH_2)_{16}$
S

CH_3
$(CH_2)_{14}$
C=O
NH_2–Gly N-terminus

CH_3–$(CH_2)_{16}$–C–O–CH
CH_3–$(CH_2)_{16}$–C–O–CH_2

CysAAX
C-terminus

Cys
C-terminus

CYTOSOL

Prenylation

Palmitoylation

Myristoylation

Glycophospholipid

FIGURE 1.31. Some posttranslational modifications hold a protein in a specific configuration at a particular cellular membrane. (From Lewin B. *Receptors and signal transduction: channels and ion uptake.* New York: Oxford University Press, 1994:319, with permission.)

transferase type I transfers a geranylgeranyl group from geranylgeranyl diphosphate to a CAAX-cysteine, geranylgeranyl transferase type II transfers geranylgeranyl groups from geranylgeranyl diphosphate to both cysteins in a CC- or CxC-containing protein. The X in the CAAX motif determines which isoprenoid will be added. A protein with a serine, methionine, or glutamine in the X position will have a farnesyl group transferred to cysteine and a leucine will signal a geranylgeranyl modification to the CAAX cysteine.[479,480] The CAAX- and CxC-motif proteins undergo a methylation of the terminal carboxyl on cysteine following prenylation.

Prenylated proteins are predominant in signal transduction cascades; for example, ras proteins undergo farnesylation of a cysteine at a carboxy CAAX that anchors it into the cytoplasmic side of the plasma membrane. This modification is necessary for H-, K-, and N-ras mutants to display transforming capabilities.[480–484] Studies show that not only is the prenylation important for membrane association, but the methylation step enhances[485] the affinity of the protein for the membrane.

Additional stability in a prenylated protein's association with a particular membrane can be provided by further post-translational modifications such as myristoylation or palmitoylation[486,487] Myristoylation is the formation of an irreversible covalent bond between 14-carbon unsaturated fatty acid and an amino group of a terminal glycine. An interesting example of this is found in the SRC oncogene (protein

kinase activity), which has a myristic acid fatty chain covalently linked to an amino-terminal glycine. This myristoylation keeps the Src protein in a configuration that enables it to transform normal cells into cancer cells. If this specific glycine is changed to an alanine so that myristic acid cannot form a bond, then the src protein functions normally as a protein kinase without transforming cells.[488] Palmitoylation entails the linkage of a 16-carbon-chain saturated fatty acid—palmitic acid—to a cysteine residue near either end of the protein. However, it has been shown through biophysical measurements that the 14-carbon myristate does not have sufficient binding energy to maintain the association of a protein with a lipid membrane, and consequently myristoylated proteins are found in the cytoplasm.[489,490] In situations where a myristoylated protein needs to associate with a membrane in a reversible manner, the reversibility of membrane association is regulated by another mechanism, such as guanine nucleotide binding or phosphorylation.[491–493] Palmitoylated proteins are almost always membrane-bound and are able to undergo a palmitoylated/depalmitoylated process due to the labile thioester bond between palmitate and cysteine residue in the modified protein.

A modified protein will remain in the endoplasmic reticulum if it contains a specific K(H)DEL sequence at the carboxy terminus;[494] membrane proteins have either a di-lysine or di-arginine close to the end of their cytoplasmic domain; the di-lysine motif binds COP1, a cytosolic coat

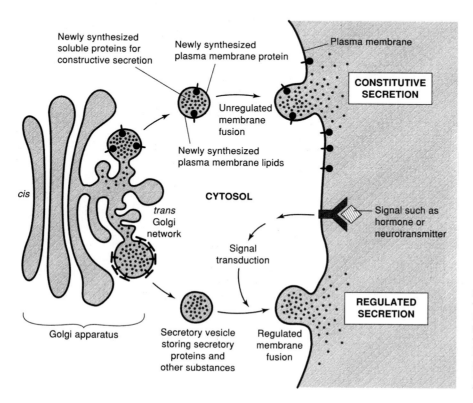

FIGURE 1.32. Proteins which have been transported through the endoplasmic reticulum and the Golgi are transported inside small vesicles which are "pinched off" from the Golgi membrane. (From Alberts A, Bray D, Lewis J, et al. *Intracellular sorting and maintenance of cellular compartments.* New York: Garland Publishing Inc., 1989: 405, with permission.)

protein complex that signals a retrieval of the protein from the Golgi back into the endoplasmic reticulum.[495,496] The ER must maintain certain proteins necessary for its function, such as proteins needed for translocation and vesicle transport, folding chaperoning, posttranslational modifications, maintenance of a calcium supply, and additional protein needed for ER function in a specific tissue type.

Protein Localization

A newly synthesized peptide which has successfully reached the membrane of the ER, crossed the membrane, folded properly, and has been modified as it moves through the ER and Golgi is now ready to be transported to its destination. Transportation is done in coated vesicles, which are pinched-off regions of the Golgi membrane. The "coat" that covers the vesicle is made up of protein which is identified for direction to the proper membrane (Figure 1.32). Once the coated vesicle has delivered the encapsulated protein to the appropriate site, it becomes uncoated and fuses with the targeted membrane, depositing the protein through the membrane. There are specific proteins and ATP associated with the uncoating and fusion process (Figure 1.33).[497–503]

CANCER DEFINED AS UNREGULATED TRANSCRIPTION/TRANSLATION

In studying the molecular biology of cancer, the most essential requirement is having access to nucleic acid, that is, DNA and RNA, as well as proteins and other macromolecular structures of the cell. Typically, cancer cells that are harvested from an animal contain many normal cellular components, such as matrix substituents, vessels, and a diverse group of infiltrating and circulating cells. Additionally, there may be heterogeneity within the cancer cells themselves. Therefore, any biomaterial taken from such specimens invariably contain mixtures from varying cell types. Relatively pure cellular preparations can be acquired from *in vivo* samples when flow cytometric techniques are used to separate dispersions of cancer cells gathered from *in vivo* specimens; however, the number of cells harvested is usually limited, and the separation techniques depend on the ready availability of technical expensive equipment and extended acquisition times.

As will be apparent in subsequent chapters, many of the cellular and molecular biologic studies dealing with cancer depend on there being homogenous populations of normal and cancerous cells. The methodology of tissue culture, wherein cells are grown *ex vivo* in a glass or plastic petri dish containing a buffered solution supplemented with fetal calf serum or defined medium containing added growth factors, provides a method of growing large numbers of a pure population of cells. When normal cells are removed

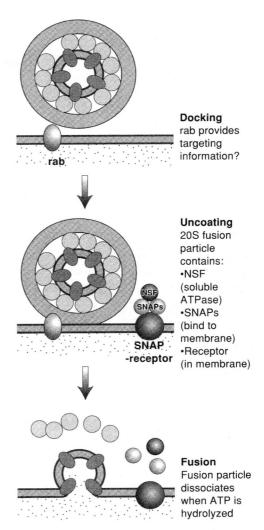

FIGURE 1.33. The coated vesicles which transport proteins deliver their contents to a specific cellular location in a complex with other proteins which are present during membrane fusion. (From Lewin B. *The apparatus for protein localization.* New York: Oxford University Press, 1994:279, with permission.)

directly from an animal and placed in tissue culture, they are referred to as a cell strain or primary culture. Cells within a primary culture grow for a while, usually less than 50 divisions, and then undergo a crisis wherein the vast majority, or all, the cells die. The reasons for and mechanisms by which cells within the primary culture die are not understood.[482,504] Rarely, a cellular clone—a population of cells derived from a single cell—will become immortalized. That is, the cells will continue to divide in tissue culture, and an established "normal" cell line will be formed. Immortalized cell lines rarely arise from human primary cultures but much more frequently result from murine primary cultures. Such cells do not have the characteristics of a malignant or cancerous cell; they are not transformed. The immortalized cells, not being malignant, have many of the characteristics of the primary culture. That is, they are still dependent on serum or growth factors and usually display cell-to-cell contact or density-dependent inhibition of their growth, and a need for attachment to a solid surface that is manifested by cytoskeletal organization that allows the cell to flatten and grow as a monolayer on the petri dish surface.[505] Frequently the immortalized cells do not have the normal chromosomal diploid number; rather they are aneuploid. In contrast, malignant cells have gone beyond the stage of immortalization and have transformed to a cell that is not contact inhibited, that is they tend to overgrow and pile up, have a tendency to assume a rounded structure and float in the tissue culture medium, have less or no dependency on serum factors, and, when injected into athymic or species-specific mice, grow as a tumor with the potential to metastasize—leave the initial site of implantation and grow in other sites within the animal.[506] Both primary and immortalized cells can be transformed to a malignant state. It is assumed that the immortalized cell with the capability of indefinite growth characteristic has assumed at least one characteristic that is different from a normal primary cell and, therefore, has progressed the path from normal to the transformed state. It is also assumed that by investigating the characteristics of malignant cells and comparing and contrasting those with normal cells, a molecular basis of cancer can be reached.

Usually multiple changes are required for a cell to become malignant. Normal cells can be made to undergo a malignant transformation by physical (x-ray), genetic (tumor viruses), or chemical (chemical carcinogens) means. Carcinogens can either initiate malignant transformation or promote transformation in a cell that has gone partially along the path toward malignancy. A means of studying carcinogenic promoters is provided by using immortalized 3T3 cells and exposing them to potential carcinogens, followed by noting phenotypic changes in the treated cells, that is, loss of contact inhibition or "focus" formation.[507,508]

The genetic events that result in malignant transformation after exposure to agents such as x-rays or chemicals in some cases are beginning to be understood. Assuredly, there are certain families, kindred, or individuals who have a genetic predisposition toward cancer. In several instances we know that individuals who genetically lack the ability to repair specific types of DNA damage resulting from ultraviolet light exposure (xeroderma pigmentosum) or ionizing radiation (ataxia telangiectasia) have a marked propensity for developing cancers.[509,510] Only most recently has additional insight into the mechanisms of malignant transformation been achieved by noting how certain viral infections produce cancers.[511]

In a number of instances a tumor-promoting virus such as an adenovirus or polyoma virus will infect a cell, undergo intracellular replication, and subsequently lyse the cell with release of the viral progeny. Those cell types that allow such

a process are not transformable and are said to be permissive. There are instances in which the tumor virus infects a nonpermissive cell type—the virus is unable to go further in its life cycle to replicate and lyse the host cell—yet the cell assumes a malignant phenotype until the viral genome is degraded or diluted out by host cell duplication. Afterwards the cell assumes a normal phenotype. An abortive transformation has occurred. However, in other cases the tumor virus does not replicate and lyse the cell, does not degrade or dilute out, but rather the viral genome integrates into the host genome as a provirus. In such a state, viral-origin mRNA is produced that is subsequently processed and translated into protein that results in malignant transformation. The gene that produces the protein that results in malignant transformation is referred to as an oncogene.[512–514]

One property of an oncogene is that the transformed cell is released from some aspect of cellular regulation. Frequently, the oncogene (viral oncogene or v-oncogene) has a normal cellular component (protooncogene or c-oncogene) that is highly regulated. In the transformed cell either the protooncogene brought in by the virus is mutated to a v-oncogene so that it is no longer regulated, or the c-oncogene is introduced into a cell that normally does not express that protooncogene, or a c-oncogene is dysregulated by being produced in greater quantity than normal. In each case, the result is that the cell, because of having been infected by a tumor virus, has acquired unregulated or new function. Nearly 100 oncogenes have been identified.[515,516]

Tumor-promoting viruses are either DNA or RNA tumor viruses. The major DNA tumor viruses carrying oncogenes are papovaviruses (polyoma and SV40 carrying T-antigen oncogene), herpes viruses, of which papilloma viruses are known to produce the E6 and E7 oncogenes, Epstein-Barn containing BNLF-1 oncogene, and adenoviruses having E1A and E1B oncogenes. Papovaviruses have small genomes containing only a few early genes (large T, small t, and possibly middle T antigen) and the late genes which result in viral coat protein. Of the papovaviruses, polyoma viruses have been identified that produce tumors in mice, SV40 in rhesus monkey, and BK and JC viruses in humans. SV40 large T antigen has been cloned into cells and shown to be capable of transforming them. Usually a normal cell has enough regulatory redundancy to overcome the effect of introducing only one oncogene. The fact that large T antigen as a single oncogene can malignantly transform a cell implies that large T antigen either must have multiple cellular functions or affects a major cellular switch that results in a cascade of events that leads to cancer. The most frequently seen transformations result from more than one oncogene, which implies that there is cooperativity among oncogenes. Such is the case with polyoma virus that produces three T antigens, of which large T antigen promotes indefinite growth and middle T antigen morphological transformation.[517,518]

Another class of tumor viruses is the retroviruses that have a RNA genome of approximately 10 kbases. These viruses can effect transformation by at least two means. The retrovirus may insert into the host genome in such a manner that the viral LTR (long terminal repeat) acts as a nonregulable promoter of a protooncogene. This is seen when a retrovirus inserts itself within the first intron of the nuclear transcriptional factor *myc*. *Myc* has three exons, of which in a normal cell only the latter two are translated. When a retrovirus containing a LTR promoter inserts into the first intron, exon 2 and 3 are transcribed in excess amounts. The consequence of such a genetic event is transformation of the cell. In the example of *myc*-mediated transformation, a LTR containing potential enhancers can also insert both upstream and downstream of the gene and result in excess gene expression.[519,520] Other protooncogenes that have been found to be activated by retroviral insertion include c-*raf*,[521] c-*mos*,[522] and c-*erbB*.[523]

A more common means by which retroviruses effect malignant transformation is by having an oncogene inserted within their genome (Figure 1.34). Frequently, the protooncogene that is carried by the retrovirus has major deletions (*fms, erbB, erbA, src, myb*) or mutations (*myc, H-ras, K-ras, sis*) within regions of the gene that are responsible for regulation of the protooncogene. As would be expected, the retroviral oncogenes usually have a great degree of homology with the corresponding protooncogenes. Moreover, the v-oncogenes are invariably derived from recombination between the viral genomic RNA and host RNA, rather than by capturing the original DNA-formatted protooncogene, which would be much larger because of the normal dispersed nature of eukaryotic genes.

The v-oncogenes can be divided into four major classes. The first class associated with growth factors is v-*sis*, which corresponds to the normal cellular *PDGFB* chain, v-*wnt1*, which is related to wingless, and v-*int2* and v-KS/*hst*, which have as a protooncogene counterpart FGF. The class II oncogenes are associated with cell receptors and include v-*kit*, which has as a cellular counterpart (c-*kit*) the steel receptor, v-*erb1* and 2(*neu*), which have the corresponding c-*erb1*

and 2(c-*neu*) coding for EGF receptor kinase and receptorlike kinase respectively, v-*mas*, which is related to c-*mas* or the angiotensin receptor, and v-*fms*, which has the corresponding protooncogene CSF-1 receptor kinase. The class III viral oncogenes are divided into subclasses that are either membrane-associated or intracellular transducers such as v-*gsp* and v-*gip*, which are related to G protein/signal transduction, v-*ras*, corresponding to c-*ras*, which is a GTP-binding protein, v-*src*, which is membrane-associated and related to the normal cellular tyrosine kinase c-*src*, or intracellular transducers such as v-*abl* and v-*fps* and v-*met* and v-*yes*, which are related to their corresponding c-oncogenes that function as tyrosine kinases.[481,488,524]

Other class III oncogenes that are associated with intracellular transducers are v-*raf* and v-*mos*, corresponding to the normal cellular protooncogene c-*raf* and c-*mos*, which are serine/threonine kinases, as well as the oncogenes that are associated with signaling, such as v-*crk* and v-*vav*, corresponding to c-*crk* (SH2/SH3 regulator with phospholipase C activity) and c-*vav* (SH2 regulator). The class IV oncogenes are nuclear transcription factors and include v-*jun*, v-*fos*, v-*myc*, v-*erbA*, v-*ski*, and v-*myb*.[525]

The most important lesson that the viral oncogene teaches us about cellular regulation is that excess or lack of control of a cellular function leading to stimulation of cell growth factor can result in cancer. We also learn from those viral oncogenes having cellular counterparts that oncogenesis generally requires the presence of more than one oncogene and that the oncogenes are invariably involved either in those processes that induce a cascade of events resulting in expression of multiple genes or where the oncogene itself is a nuclear transcription factor that promotes gene(s) expression. We also learn that protooncogenes that have acquired mutations resulting in changes in amino acid residues associated with regulatory regions within oncoproteins may result in malignant transformation. Additionally, we have examples wherein certain protooncogenes are expressed in excess quantities and as such produce cancer. Basically, studies elucidating the role of viral oncogenes provide information whereby we better understand how in nor-

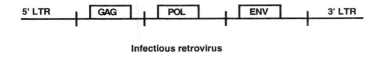

Infectious retrovirus

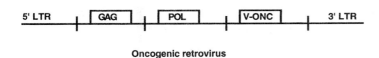

Oncogenic retrovirus

FIGURE 1.34. Retroviruses: the infectious retrovirus has a complete genome with *GAG, POL,* and *ENV* genes, flanked by LTRs. The oncogenic retrovirus has replaced the *ENV* gene with a viral oncogene through a recombination event.

mal cells alteration or mutations within a gene or DNA amplification or chromosomal translocations can result in the production of either an aberrant gene product or excess quantities of a gene product that then results in malignant transformation. Stated differently, the viral oncogene is a dominant mutation that results in overriding the corresponding normal allelic protooncogene.

Although oncogenes carry us a long way to understanding the mechanisms by which oncogenesis occurs, they do not present us with the possibility of understanding how loss of function of a gene may cause cancer. Such cases usually require that both allelic genes be lost, and as such represent the case whereby the normal function of the lost genes is tumor suppression. The RB and p53 protein represent such tumor-suppressor proteins.[526,527] Retinoblastoma, osteosarcomas, and small lung cancer result from the loss of or mutation within the RB gene from chromosome 13. Papilloma virus E7, adenovirus E1A, and SV40 large T antigen are known to bind to RB and as such may result in removing one of the constraints on the path toward malignant transformation. It is now known that RB is a nuclear phosphoprotein that functions to regulate the cell cycle. Like RB protein, p53 functions as a tumor suppressor, and like RB, p53 is a nuclear phosphoprotein that functions to retard progression of cells through the cell cycle.[528–530] p53 was originally found to be associated with SV40 large T-antigen. It is known from the Li-Fraumeni syndrome that mutation in p53 results in an array of tumor types. Many tumors are found to have increased levels of p53, but in each case such proteins are mutated and therefore do not function to restrain growth. Further, p53 probably exists as a tetrameric species that can lose function when just one of the proteins within the tetramer is aberrant. The loss of function of p53 results in unrestrained growth of the cell. Unrestrained growth may result in destabilizing DNA that may result in less efficient DNA repair with a concomitant increase in translocations and amplification that ultimately predisposes the normal cell to malignant transformation.

TECHNIQUES IN MOLECULAR BIOLOGY

Cloning Vectors

As stated at the beginning of the chapter, the techniques employed in molecular biology have allowed the elucidation of complex cellular biologic phenomena. Two aspects of bacterial metabolism are the foundational pins of molecular biologic research: (a) the existence of an array of restriction endonucleolytic enzymes, and (b) plasmids. Plasmids are small, circular pieces of DNA that exist in many types of bacteria and were initially found in bacteria that had acquired resistance to antibiotic treatment. That is, the plasmidal DNA that is not part of the bacteria chromosome (epichromosomal) was providing to the host bacterium a selective advantage by carrying a gene that detoxified a given

antibiotic. Plasmids possess an origin of replication that allows their replication independent of bacterial chromosomal reproduction. Although a bacterium may carry only a single copy of a plasmid, over the years plasmids have been engineered so that large copy numbers—many copies of the individual plasmid are found within an individual bacterium—can be accommodated. With their high copy number and ability to be transferred from one bacterium to another, plasmids are useful in producing recombinant DNA molecules, since foreign DNA can be inserted into plasmids without inactivating essential genes. Additionally, a eukaryotic gene can be placed under the control of an appropriate bacterial promoter within the plasmid to provide means of producing or expressing eukaryotic proteins within bacteria, that is, recombinant protein production.

While the vast majority of plasmids are derived from bacteria, there are a few plasmids found in lower eukaryotic cells. In yeast, plasmid 2μ exists as an independent epichromosomal replication element.[531] Many derivative plasmids containing the 2μ replication elements have been constructed for use in yeast molecular biologic studies. In mammalian cells, plasmids have been constructed based on viral genes that can persist as epichromosomal elements in high copy number. These plasmids use replication elements from bovine papilloma virus, Epstein-Barr virus and BK virus, among others, to provide replication capability.[532,533]

Restriction Endonucleases

The field of recombinant DNA technology for all practical purposes began with the description in 1970 of the first restriction endonuclease enzyme, HindIII. Restriction enzymes are part of the normal armamentarium of bacteria to ward off bacterial-specific viral (phage) infections. The host bacterium modifies its genome by methylating its DNA in a species-specific pattern. Restriction endonucleases often do not cut methylated base sequences. Incoming viral DNA, which does not have the appropriate methylation pattern, is susceptible to digestion and destruction, and therefore the virus's host range is constrained. Restriction endonucleases fall into three broad categories depending on their ability to cleave and methylate DNA.[534] Type I restriction endonuclease enzymes have three protein subunits that are responsible for recognition of the target DNA. Their function is methylation if the DNA is recognized as host DNA and cleavage of foreign DNA at a nonspecific site at least 1,000 bases away from the recognition site. Type III restriction endonucleases have two subunits, one of which is responsible for recognition and methylation, the other for cleavage. Type II restriction endonuclease enzymes, such as HindIII, are those most commonly used in molecular biological applications, because the recognition and cleavage activities are on a single protein separate from the methylation activity. There are a number of different restriction enzymes and as such they have offered a cornucopia of potential reagents for use by molecular biologists. Depending on the choice of the particular restriction endonuclease enzyme, one can cut DNA that contains many different specific sequences of bases, usually a four-to-six-base palindrome. The resulting restriction cut DNA usually has compatible ends that can be annealed together and, by subsequent use of ligating enzymes, can be covalently joined together. As an example, the enzyme HindIII recognizes the following sequence:

5′-AAGCTT-3′
3′-TTCGAA-5′

and cuts both strands to leave these compatible ends:

5′-A and AGCTT-3′
3′-TTCGA A-5′

The ends can reanneal to form the noncovalently bound sequence as follows:

5′-A*AGCTT-3′
3′-T TCGA*A-5′

The addition of a DNA ligase, such as that from bacteriophage T4, will repair the broken phosphate bond in each strand, resulting in a double-stranded DNA again, indistinguishable from the starting material. This technology gives us the ability to cut DNA at reproducible sites and relegate to similarly cut DNA from any other source having compatible ends.

Restriction nucleases have become useful tools in genetic linkage analysis. A short, specific DNA sequence having a specific restriction nuclease recognition site is selected based on the genetic defect one wishes to identify. The DNA from two different individuals (or normal versus tumor tissue from the same individual) is cut with specific restriction endonucleases which create DNA fragments. The fragments are then annealed with a specific probe and visualized on a Southern blot autoradiograph. Analysis of the fragment sizes could indicate differences in single base pair change, deletions, insertions, or rearrangements. This technique, which is a sensitive means of detecting specific mutations, is called restriction fragment length polymorphism (RFLP).[535,536]

The availability of Type II restriction endonucleases has greatly simplified the cloning of DNA. Genomic DNA is cut into manageable pieces by the application of one or more restriction enzymes, leaving restricted ends. An appropriate plasmid is cut with the same endonuclease, leaving compatible ends that can then be ligated. The two types of DNA are mixed together under conditions that favor annealing of the ends of the plasmid DNA with the cut pieces of genomic DNA, followed by treatment with DNA ligase to form covalently bound DNA. The result is genomic DNA incorporated into a circular plasmid. The recombinant DNA within the plasmid is then transfected into bacteria wherein the plasmid can be amplified into a source of vir-

tually unlimited quantities of a specific piece of exogenous genomic DNA.

DNA can be isolated from any eukaryotic cell, digested with appropriate restriction enzymes, and the collection of fragments cloned into plasmids. These plasmids can then be transfected into bacteria and amplified. The collection of DNA fragments, taken together, is called a library and represents the total genome divided into small, manageable pieces of DNA that can be individually isolated and amplified. The ability to clone DNA allows researchers to sort through an entire genome to find a particular gene of interest.

The most commonly used plasmid for DNA cloning has been pBR322 that was originally isolated from *E. coli* (Figure 1.35). Since pBR322 allows for only single copy plasmid per bacteria, other high copy number plasmids have been constructed, either as derivatives of pBR322 or from other sources. No matter the source of the plasmid, they all function in a fashion similar to pBR322. pBR322 is capable of accepting a piece of foreign DNA of up to 10 kbase pairs, approximately two and a half times its own size. The cloning of larger pieces of DNA causes the plasmid to become unstable, thereby slowing plasmid replication and causing the bacteria to delete the excess DNA. For these reasons other cloning systems have been developed which are more versatile than pBR322-like plasmids.

Phage λ is a virus or bacteriophage that infects *E. coli.* Its normal genome is approximately 50 kbase pairs packaged into a protein coat for infection. Packing of λ phage DNA can be accomplished *in vitro,* that is, outside a cell, by mixing the purified components of the phage together in a test tube. Normally λ phage DNA forms long, multigenomic strands that are cleaved by a phage enzyme into the appropriate sizes for assembly into the coat protein structure. The λ DNA sequence that is specifically cut is the *cos* site located

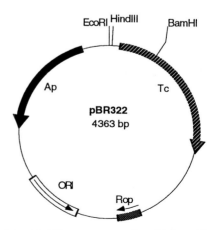

FIGURE 1.35. pBR322: a common plasmid found in *E. coli* and the basis for many artificial plasmids. Tc confers tetracycline resistance; Ap confers ampicillin resistance; ORI, origin of replication, allows the plasmid to be replicated epichromosomally.

at either end of the strands of the λ genome. Since λ has about 15 kbase pairs in the center of the genome that are not essential for replication, modified λ cloning vectors have been developed in which the nonessential sequences have been removed so that foreign DNA to be cloned can be inserted.[537] λ containing the foreign DNA is allowed to assemble into the infectious viral coat for use in transfecting *E. coli*. Each virally infected bacterium is carrying an individual λ containing one segment of foreign DNA, not more than 15 kbases, to be subsequently isolated for study (Figure 1.36).

Unfortunately, for some purposes even longer pieces of genomic DNA are required for study. For such studies segments of DNA of 35 to 45 kbase pairs in length can be cloned into λ phage using cosmid vectors. These cosmid plasmids containing a *cos* site, without any of the other phage genes, can be amplified in bacteria. When cleaved with appropriate restriction endonuclease enzymes and ligated to foreign DNA, the cosmid and foreign DNA form

long linear chains or concatemers separated by *cos* sites. The concatemers can be cut by λ protein A, which recognizes the *cos* sequence, and subsequently packaged into a viral coat for subsequent bacterial transfection. Within the bacterium the cosmid DNA circularizes because of the cohesive *cos* site sequences on either end of the recombinant λ. Besides containing the foreign DNA and *cos* sites, the cosmid contains an origin of replication for intrabacterial replication and a gene(s) for antibiotic selection. The consequence of such a construction is that bacteria that do not contain the transfected cosmid will be killed when exposed to a selected antibiotic; whereas the bacteria containing the cosmid will be replicated and the foreign DNA contained within the cosmid will be amplified.

Libraries

Although genomic libraries are important, when one wishes to study which genes are being expressed within a particular

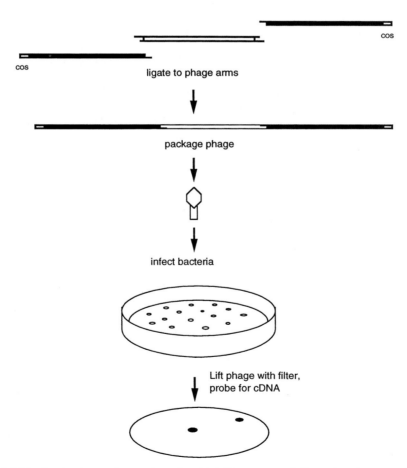

FIGURE 1.36. Production and screening of a cDNA library. cDNA is ligated to the arms of phage λ, which can self-assemble *in vitro*. The phage infect *E. coli*, which are plated on agar. When colonies appear, a filter is laid on top of the plate, then the filter is hybridized with a synthetic DNA probe.

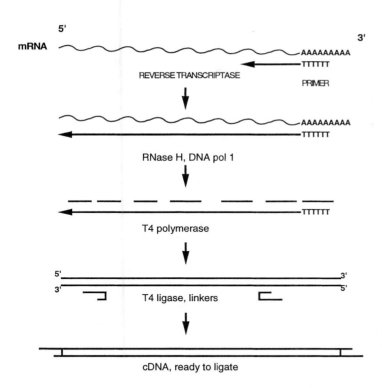

FIGURE 1.37. Production of cDNA from mRNA. Isolated mRNA contains a poly(A) tail which binds a synthetic poly(T) primer. Reverse transcriptase extends the primer, using the mRNA as the template. RNase H and DNA polymerase remove the RNA strand, leaving fragments of DNA. T4 polymerase fills the gaps, leaving double-stranded DNA. T4 ligase adds synthetic linkers containing restriction enzyme sites on the ends, ready to ligate into a cloning vector.

cell it becomes necessary to isolate mRNA. Libraries constructed from DNA retro transcribed from mRNA are called cDNA libraries.[538] To produce a cDNA library it is first necessary to reverse transcribe mRNA into DNA. Reverse transcriptase is an enzyme that uses RNA as a template to produce DNA. So once mRNA is isolated, DNA can be produced for packaging into a plasmid (Figure 1.37). Since most mRNA molecules contain poly(A) chains at their 3′-end, a short section of single-stranded synthetic poly(T) can be used to hybridize to the poly(A)-end of mRNA. The poly(T) then serves as a primer for reverse transcriptase, in the presence of the four deoxynucleotides A, T, G, C, because of its polymerase activity to produce a single strand of DNA complementary (cDNA) to the original mRNA. The resulting hybrid molecule is made of one strand of RNA and one of cDNA. The RNA can be removed by RNase H and the subsequent single-stranded DNA made into double-stranded DNA by DNA polymerase I. The resulting double-stranded DNA can be ligated into a plasmid or a cosmid to produce a cDNA library.

After a cDNA library has been made and amplified, it is necessary to screen the library to find the bacteria containing the cDNA of interest. The technique of filter hybridization allows tens of thousands of bacterial clones to be tested at the same time for the presence of an individual segment of DNA. Bacteria are spread on an agar plate and allowed to form colonies. Each colony is derived from a single bacterium that has been transfected, so all the bacteria in the colony carry the same piece of cloned DNA. However, each

colony on the plate contains a different piece of cloned DNA. A nitrocellulose filter is laid over the plate, whereupon some of the bacteria from each colony stick to the filter. The nitrocellulose filter is removed and treated to lyse the bacteria and remove proteins, RNA, and the remaining DNA is fixed to the filter. A probe is made consisting of a short piece of DNA complementary to the cDNA sequence of interest and either radioactive or light-emitting. The probe is allowed to hybridize to the filter, that is, to bind to complementary DNA by specific base pairing. After the hybridization has occurred, the excess probe is removed and the nitrocellulose filter is placed on photographic film. Those colonies retaining the probe will cause black spots on the film (Figure 1.36). When the film is developed, the original colony containing the cDNA of interest can be identified and the bacteria grown in large quantity to provide DNA for further study.

Expression libraries are used to isolate cDNA which codes for the expression of a particular protein. A cDNA library is made as described above, using expression vectors—plasmids which allow the inserted foreign DNA to be transcribed into RNA and translated into protein. The bacteria or yeast containing the plasmid library are plated on agar to form colonies and overlaid with a nitrocellulose filter to pick up a sample of each colony. The filter is incubated with antibody directed against the protein of interest, which binds to the colonies producing that protein. The antibody can then be visualized using standard histochemical techniques, identifying the colonies producing the recombinant protein, and these colonies can then be grown in culture, producing large quantities of the protein.

Transfection

For simple plasmids containing recombinant DNA that one wishes to amplify, one must be able to target or transfect the plasmid into the desired cell. Although viral transfection systems like λ phage are convenient because the virus infects the cells and delivers the recombinant DNA to the interior of the cell for subsequent amplification, the host range for transfection is limited to the range of cells that the virus can infect. Therefore, extensive effort has gone into devising chemical and mechanical techniques to facilitate transfection. Previously, the most commonly used method for introducing a plasmid into eukaryotic cells consisted of mixing the plasmid DNA in a phosphate buffer with calcium chloride that precipitates the DNA as the calcium salt. When the precipitated DNA is added to cultured cells, the DNA is taken up by endocytosis and some of the DNA is transported to the nucleus wherein genes encoded on the DNA can be transcribed. Although calcium phosphate transfections has been used extensively with a variety of fibroblast and epithelial cells, producing stable transfection rates in as high as 10% to 50% of the cases, other cells such as immunocytes are poorly transfected by calcium phosphate. In addition, calcium phosphate has been found to be toxic to many cell types at the concentration needed for transfections. Therefore, other transfection methods have been devised.

Among the other transfections methods, Polybrene (Abbott Laboratonica, Abbott Park, IL) has been used to facilitate retroviral transfection. Polybrene, being a poly-cation, binds to the negatively charged retroviral coat, thereby removing the negative charge and leaving a positively charged surface on the retrovirus that is then more efficiently bound to the negatively charged surface of the cell to be transfected. The Polybrene method has been extended to use with plasmidal DNA because the poly-cation is attracted to the negatively charged DNA and facilitates DNA adhering to the surface of the cell.[539] Then dimethylsulfoxide (DMSO) is added to the mix to make the cell membrane more permeable, thereby causing uptake of the membrane-bound DNA, of which some is transported into the nucleus to be subsequently expressed or integrated into the host genome. Polybrene/DMSO has been reported to produce stable transfectants at a frequency of 0.01% to 0.1%.

When lipids are mixed in an aqueous environment under the right conditions, they are capable of forming small vesicles composed of bilayers with negatively charged groups on both sides of the bilayered membrane and enclosing an aqueous center; that is, a liposome is formed. Liposomes are frequently used to entrap small-molecular-weight chemicals within the aqueous center and subsequently fuse the chemical-carrying liposome with the membrane of a cell. By such means, one can deliver into the cell small molecules and occasionally larger protein structures. Unfortunately, plasmid DNA is much larger than simple proteins, and as such simple liposomes, although exceedingly interesting as drug carrier systems, have had limited success as DNA delivery systems. To overcome the limitation of simple liposomes, cationic liposomes have been developed which are made from a synthetic positively charged lipid, *N*1-(2,3-dioleyloxy)propyl]-*N,N,N*-trimethylammonium and dioleoyl phosphatidyl ethanolamine.[540] The mixture is marketed under the trade name Lipofectin (Life Technologies, Gaithersburg, MD). When Lipofectin is mixed with polyanionic DNA or RNA, complexes form that capture the nucleic acid with high efficiency. Due to the cationic nature of Lipofectin, the liposomes bind with high avidity to the negatively charged surface of the cell and fuse with the membrane, thereby discharging DNA into the cell without being engulfed and subsequently lysosomally degraded. Lipofectin has been used to transfect DNA as large as 130 kbases, as well as to transfect mRNA directly into cells, a capability not found with the use of other transfection systems.

In a conceptual fashion similar to the Lipofectin polycationic molecule used for transfection, poly-*L*-lysine has been used as a DNA carrier molecule for transfection. Poly-*L*-lysine, being a positively charged polypeptide, is capable of complexing negatively charged DNA. If appropriate targeting molecules are covalently bound to the poly-*L*-lysine, the resulting DNA/polylysine complex can be targeted to specific cellular receptors for uptake. For example, asialogalactosyl-*poly-L*-lysine has been used to target DNA to a unique receptor on the surface of hepatic cells, resulting in successful *in vivo* transfection.[541] Transferrin-poly-*L*-lysine has also been used to transfect a variety of cells using the transferrin receptor. In both cases, however, most of the DNA is degraded after endocytosis in lysosomes, and the intracellularly remaining DNA is not targeted to the nucleus for expression.

Adenoviruses infect a wide variety of cell types and have the useful property of being endocytosed yet not lysosomally degraded. Spike proteins on the surface of the virus cause disruption of the endosome before being taken up by the lysosome organelle. Additionally, once inside the cell, adenoviruses are transported in their entirety into the nucleus. With such properties, it is not surprising that adenovirus constructs have been engineered to effect transfection. Among the adenovirus transfection systems, one consists of a genetically engineered antigen on the surface of the virus coupled to poly-*L*-lysine bound to an antibody that can target specific antigens on the surface of a cell.[542] Upon mixing DNA with the adenovirus particle/polylysine/antibody, a complex is formed that can be used to deliver DNA to the surface of the cell, which is subsequently endocytosed, disrupted within the cytoplasm, and targeted to the nucleus. Such a transfection system is attractive because there is no size limitation to the transfected DNA and the adenovirus does not need to be infective to result in efficient transfection. In fact, the chicken adenovirus CELO, which is completely noninfectious to mammalian cells, has been successfully used to transfect DNA into mammalian cells.[543]

In addition to the chemical means mentioned above, physical means have been developed to transfect DNA into cells. When cells are placed in a strong DC electrical field, pores appear in the cell membrane, allowing intracellular molecules to escape and extracellular molecules to enter.[544] This technique of introducing molecules into cells, called electroporation, has been used extensively to transfect DNA into many types of mammalian cells and numerous species of yeast, bacteria, and plants. Electroporation is now the most commonly employed method in the research laboratory to transfect DNA into cells. However, because of the requirement for electrical fields in the range of 500 per V cm in mammalian cells, electroporation can be used only *ex vivo* and with small numbers of cells. Unfortunately, the greatest transfection efficiencies are found under conditions causing 50% to 90% cell death; therefore electroporation, although an efficient laboratory tool, has limited use in clinical application.

Biolistics is a unique form of DNA transfection which uses accelerated gold microspheres to carry DNA into cells.[545] In this method, the DNA-coated microspheres are accelerated to high velocity by helium gas and then physically shot into cells. Biolistics has been used to transfect DNA into a wide variety of plant and animal cells and potentially can be used *in vivo*. Recently, biolistics transfection was used to transfect DNA for HIV gp120 into mouse muscle cells that had been surgically exposed for this purpose. The DNA transfected in this manner was shown to express glycoprotein, as demonstrated by the host developing an immune response to gp120.

After DNA has been transfected into a cell, it exists epichromosomally or separate from the host's chromosome. Genes within epichromosomal DNA can be expressed; however, the expression will be transient, lasting at best only a few weeks, the time in which the DNA is degraded. In mammalian cells, such epichromosomal DNA is inherently unstable because the foreign DNA is subject to degradation or dilution as the cell continues to divide but the plasmid does not. The exception to this in mammalian cells is EB virus or bovine papilloma virus vector constructs that can remain epichromosomal, as was discussed earlier. At a very low frequency, plasmids will recombine with chromosomal DNA to become integrated into the genome. Such intragenomic incorporated genes can be stably expressed for the life of the cell and are passed on to the daughter cells like any other chromosomal gene.

Because of the inherent limitation of most of the transfection methods discussed so far producing primarily transient transfectants, much effort has gone into identifying methods to effect efficient integrated transfection. To that end

numerous eukaryotic viral vectors have been studied. The most successful viral transfection systems to date have been those derived from retroviruses. Retroviruses have a relatively small genome (less than 10 kbases) made of RNA composed of a small number of genes, most of which can be removed and replaced. Most important, particularly for gene therapy, is that retroviruses efficiently integrate their genome into the host's genome, thereby effecting a permanent transfectant. A normal retrovirus consists of a protein capsid coat surrounding the diploid RNA genome and an envelope derived from the membrane of the cell in which the retrovirus was made. Protruding from the host-derived membrane envelope are envelope glycoproteins which are needed for binding to the target cell during the infectious phase of the life cycle of the virus. Once the retrovirus attaches to the specific receptors on the cell that is being infected, it is endocytosed. The envelope fuses with the endocytic vesicle, with subsequent release of the viral capsid into the cytoplasm. Once inside the cytoplasm, the host cell provides a tRNA molecule that is used by the reverse transcriptase to synthesize its genome in a circular DNA format. Once the DNA has been synthesized, then integrase, a viral protein found within the viral capsid structure, attaches to the virally derived DNA and also to the host genomic DNA. The viral genome, in the form of DNA, is then integrated into the host chromosome. From that point the integrated retroviral genome is a permanent part of the cell's genome, passed on to daughter cells like any other gene. After integration into the host genome, the virus makes full-length mRNA transcripts of its genome. The long terminal repeats (LTR) which are found on both the 5'- and 3'-end of the viral genome contain the viral promoter plus enhancer elements that vary as a function of the individual retroviral type. The mRNA copies of the viral genome can be either packaged as the genome of the daughter viruses or translated into protein.

Retroviruses are valuable vectors for transfecting DNA because the *gag, pol,* and *env* genes which code for the capsid proteins, reverse polymerase, and envelope proteins can be removed from the viral genome and replaced with foreign sequences without destroying the infectivity of the virus. Packaging cell lines have been engineered which do not produce infectious virions because they lack retroviral genomes with the *psi* packaging signal but yet are capable of producing all the proteins necessary to build a retrovirus.[546] When an appropriate genome is introduced into a packaging cell line, viruses are made which carry the altered genome and are made of the proteins from the packaging cell line. Such viruses are capable of infecting a new cell and integrating their genome into the host chromosome, but cannot produce progeny viruses because they lack the genes to produce the virion proteins.

Miller and Rosman have introduced a series of retroviral vectors that have been widely used both in the research laboratory and in clinical trials for gene therapy.[547] These so

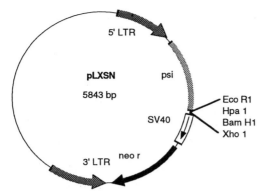

FIGURE 1.38. pLXSN: a retroviral expression vector. When transfected into an appropriate packaging cell line, pLXSN causes production of retrovirus particles containing the LTRs and everything between them as the genome. *psi* is the packaging region; 5′ LTR (long terminal repeat), acts as a promoter for a gene cloned into one of the restriction enzyme sites; SV40, a viral promoter, controls expression of the neo[r] gene; neo[r] is the neomycin phosphotransferase gene.

called pLN retroviral vectors have LTRs and a *psi* packaging region derived from murine retroviruses but lack *gag, pol,* and *env* genes (Figure 1.38). In their place is a promoter derived from either SV40 or cytomegalovirus that controls expression of a neomycin phosphotransferase gene, as well as space to insert a gene of interest. The viral sequences have been ligated into pBR322 so the recombinant DNA techniques described previously can be used to insert new genes into the viral genome. After the plasmid is transfected into a packaging cell line by electroporation or another methods, the cells begin producing replication-defective retroviruses that carry the engineered genome and are capable of infecting and integrating but cannot reproduce. A retroviral capsid can carry a genome of up to 10 kbases. Since as little as 2.5 kbases of the genome are necessary for efficient packaging and integration, retroviral vectors can theoretically carry inserted regions up to 7.5 kbases in length.

Retroviral transfection vectors have drawbacks resulting from inherent unique properties of their life cycle. Since the 3′ LTR has the same promoter and enhancer elements as the 5′ LTR, cellular genes downstream from the insertion site of the retroviral genome could theoretically be activated by the insertion of the virus upstream. If the virus were to insert upstream of a cellular protooncogene, the cell could become transformed into a malignant cell. Also, retroviruses have a very high recombination rate while in the RNA form and are, therefore, capable of incorporating genes expressed by the host cell into their genome. Early packaging cell lines were plagued by the problems of engineered viral genomes becoming replication-competent as a result of recombining with the mRNA transcription of the *gag, pol,* and *env* genes. Newer versions of packaging cell lines have much lower incidences of replication-competent revertants, but the in-

advertent production of such viruses and their possible introduction into patients while conducting gene therapy protocols remains a grave concern. In addition, it has been found that promoters inserted into the region between the two LTRs tend to be repressed or silenced. This problem can be circumvented by using an inserted promoter for the antibiotic resistance gene and using the 5′ LTR as the promoter for the gene of interest. Since very little enzyme is needed for inactivation of antibiotics, promoter repression is not a significant problem.

No matter which method is used to introduce DNA into a cell, the efficiency is not 100%. Therefore, it is often necessary to separate the transfected cells from those which are not transfected. This is easily accomplished by including a selectable marker in the transfected DNA. Commonly used selectable markers for eukaryotic cells are genes coding for resistance to the antibiotics hygromycin or the neomycin analogue G418 (geneticin). After transfection, the cells are given a brief period in culture to express the proteins coded for by the selection marker, for instance, neomycin phosphotransferase. Then G418 is added to the culture medium, and only those cells that carry the antibiotic resistance gene are able to inactivate G418 and grow in the presence of the drug.[548] The cells that were not successfully transfected are incapable of producing neomycin phosphotransferase, and are killed. This results in a pure population of cells that carry both the antibiotic resistance gene and the gene of interest.

Identification and Analysis of DNA

A wide variety of powerful techniques have been developed for the identification and analysis of DNA. The techniques allow the base sequence of the DNA to be determined accurately, the expression of mRNA from the DNA to be rapidly and accurately determined, the interaction of the particular DNA of interest with DNA-binding proteins to be determined, and the protein expressed from the genes to be studied and isolated. The simplest form of DNA analysis consists of digesting genomic DNA with restriction endonucleases and determining the size of the resulting fragments. With the development of the Southern blotting technique, the size of the fragment containing a particular DNA sequence could be determined readily.[549] A Southern blot is performed by digesting genomic DNA with one or more restriction enzymes to generate a large number of fragments of varying sizes (Figure 1.39). The fragments can be separated from each other on the basis of size by agar or polyacrylamide gel electrophoresis. Subsequently, the sized DNA can be transferred to a nylon or nitrocellulose filter by the application of an electric current or simply by buffers to carry the DNA out of the gel onto the filter. The filter can then be hybridized with a labeled probe that complements the DNA of interest. Southern blotting can be extremely useful for examining the large structure of DNA

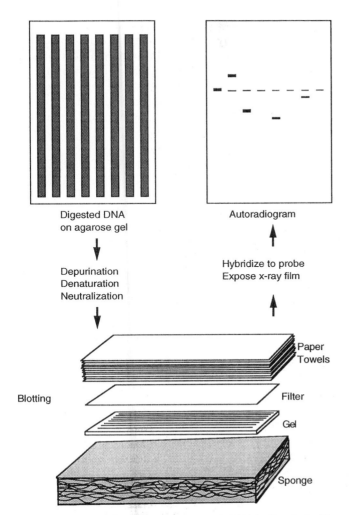

Digested DNA
on agarose gel

Autoradiogram

↓ Depurination
Denaturation
Neutralization

↑ Hybridize to probe
Expose x-ray film

Blotting

Paper
Towels

Filter

Gel

Sponge

FIGURE 1.39. Southern blotting: genomic DNA is digested with restriction endonucleases and electrophoresed in agarose to separate the fragments by size. The DNA is transferred to the filter by the flow of buffers from the sponge to the paper towels. The filter is hybridized to a radioactive probe specific for a particular DNA sequence. Bands appear on the autoradiograph where that sequence is found on the filter.

and for isolating specific fragments of DNA. Southern blots have also proven to be clinically useful in the diagnosis of malignancy, since the gene rearrangements found in a number of malignancies can be detected.

The basic methodology of Southern blotting, by which nucleic acids are separated on a gel by size and immobilized on filters for further analysis, has spawned a number of variations. A Northern blot is prepared and used essentially as is the Southern blot technique, except that RNA is run on the gel instead of DNA.[550] The filter is then hybridized with a probe to demonstrate the presence of a particular RNA species. Since the intensity of the signal from the probe is proportional to the amount of probe that is bound, a Northern blot can demonstrate the production, quantity, and base sequence of RNA isolated from cells.

Like DNA and RNA, proteins can also be separated by virtue of size or charge on polyacrylamide gels and subsequently transferred and probed. The technique is referred to as Western blotting.[551] Total cell lysates are separated by size (PAGE-gel) or charge (isoelectrically focused), or both (two-dimensional gels), then the proteins are transferred by electrical current to and immobilized on a nylon filter. The immobilized proteins can then be visualized with stains, or individual proteins can be localized by probing the filter with monoclonal antibodies that can be used with immunochemical stains.

Nuclease S1 Protection Assay

Nuclease S1 protection assays are used extensively to locate the termini of mRNA and/or the position of introns within hnRNA. The method is basically a modification of Southern and Northern blotting. The basic procedure involves hybridizing denatured DNA with mRNA. Those segments of DNA that do not hybridize to mRNA represent introns. Nuclease S1 is an enzyme which degrades ssDNA or RNA so that those segments of DNA that have not hybridized with mRNA will be digested, whereas those segments that have hybridized (exon) will be protected. Once the digestion has been completed, the protected fragments are separated by size on a gel and subsequently transferred to nitrocellulose and probed. As in Southern or Northern blotting, the DNA fragments are elucidative, thereby providing extremely valuable information regarding the length and concentration of the genomic DNA gene.[552–554]

Nuclear Run-On

Nuclear run-on experiments are used to determine the relative changes in nuclear transcription that results from introducing a foreign molecule into the cell (Figure 1.40). For several hours a cell population is treated with a foreign molecule, cells are harvested and lysed. Nuclei are isolated and incubated with the four nucleotides needed for RNA synthesis plus a trace of radiolabeled GTP. Following incorporation of the radiolabel into mRNA, the nuclei are pelleted. mRNA is isolated from the nuclei and hybridized to DNA that has been denatured and immobilized on a nitrocellulose filter. After exposing the washed filter to x-ray film, the film is developed and assessed to determine the amount of synthesis that has occurred as a result of stimulating the cells with the foreign molecule. Increases in nuclear transcription can then be quantitated by densitometric analysis. The procedure provides a ready means of analyzing those factors that affect transcription.[553,555–558]

Single-Stranded Conformation Polymorphism (SSCP)

Single-stranded conformation polymorphism (SSCP) is a method that will detect sequence changes as minor as a

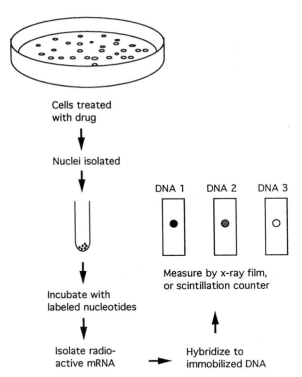

FIGURE 1.40. Nuclear run-on assay: cells are treated *in vitro* with a drug. The intact nuclei are isolated from the cells and incubated with radioactive nucleotides which incorporate into nascent RNA molecules in the nuclei. The mRNA is isolated and hybridized to cDNA of known sequence immobilized on filter strips. The mRNA which binds is measured in a scintillation counter.

single base difference.[559] The conformation of single-stranded DNA, under non-denaturing conditions, is dependent mainly on intrastrand interactions. Consequently, the mobility characteristics of the single-strand DNA in polyacrylamide gel electrophoresis will be based on its nucleotide sequence. In this technique, sample DNA, genomic or fragments amplified via polymerase chain reaction (PCR), is

denatured and evaluated on polyacrylamide gels under non-denaturing conditions. Electrophoretic mobility changes of the DNA bands have been found to be indicative of base sequence changes. Single base changes in DNA fragments up to 200 nucleotides long can be detected as mobility shifts.[560] The sensitivity of this technique allows one to analyze specific DNA sequences for mutations, especially when combined with PCR technology.

Antisense

Antisense technology provides a powerful tool which has uses in the research laboratory and potential applications in the clinic. In general, the object of the method is to prepare oligonucleotides that will specifically hybridize to RNA sequence as they are being made or processed into mRNA (Figure 1.41). The result of introducing either an antisense oligonucleotide or a plasmid which has a DNA fragment coding for RNA that will hybridize to mRNA is inhibition of translation of a selective mRNA. Although fraught with numerous technical difficulties, the method has the potential to produce a *de facto* mutation (selective decrease in a functional protein product) without resorting to mutation of DNA.[561–563]

DNA Sequencing

While DNA is composed of a combination of only four bases, it should be remembered that the genetic code is ultimately a language more powerful and expressive than any devised by humans. Within the sequence of bases is described the structure of all proteins, as well as information concerning when the proteins should be made and each step in their processing, distribution, and function. Through the action of the proteins encoded therein, the DNA contains all of the information for the all of the components of the cell or organism, including the lipids and carbohydrates that modify proteins as well as the individual synthesis of the

ANTISENSE TECHNOLOGY

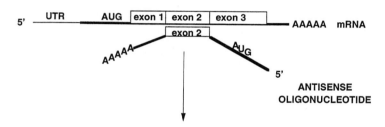

INHIBITION OF TRANSLATION OF EXON 2

FIGURE 1.41. Antisense technology: mRNA is normally single-stranded. A complementary piece of DNA or RNA which is capable of binding to a region of the mRNA will stop translation from that mRNA molecule.

DIDEOXY SEQUENCING TECHNIQUE

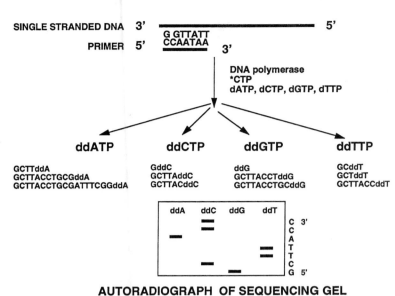

AUTORADIOGRAPH OF SEQUENCING GEL

FIGURE 1.42. Sanger dideoxy sequencing: four reactions are run in parallel. A single-stranded DNA template is hybridized to a synthetic primer. DNA polymerase extends the primer, incorporating a radioactive label in the process. Each of the reaction tubes contains one dideoxynucleotide, which terminates the reaction at that base. The radioactive strands are separated on a polyacrylamide gel which is exposed to x-ray film. The sequence is read from the film.

lipids and carbohydrates that are key structural parts of the cell and its matrix.

Although there are two primary means of determining DNA sequence, the Sanger method, utilizing the dideoxynucleotide sequencing technique, has now become the most common.[564] Before sequencing, the DNA is first denatured into single strands, then synthetic primers specific for one site on the DNA are allowed to hybridize (Figure 1.42). In the presence of the appropriate nucleotides, a DNA polymerase will extend the primer sequence to create a copy of the DNA. The sheer genius of Sanger's simple method is that it employs the addition of either the A or G or C or T dideoxynucleotide to the reaction mixture. When the dideoxynucleotide is added to the elongating end of the complementary strand, the chain elongation is terminated. Then, for instance, if the reaction contains all four normal bases and a trace of dideoxythymidine, a collection of terminated DNA chains is produced. Each of these terminated chains ends with a dideoxythymidine substituting for a potential thymidine nucleotide. The length at which the chain terminates corresponds to the location of a thymidine within the sequence. In practice four parallel reactions are run separately with one of the corresponding radioactive dideoxynucleotides of A, G, C, or T. After the reaction is stopped, all four reactions are run in juxtaposed wells of a polyacrylamide gel which separates the strands according to length of the chain. The gel is dried and exposed to x-ray film. The resulting developed film is imaged as four ladders of bands, each indicating a synthesized DNA strand which ends at one particular base in the sequence. The complete sequence can be literally read directly from the film by start-

ing at the bottom and observing the order of the chain length. For this technique, Sanger won his second Nobel prize in 1980. The Sanger sequencing technique has undergone many extensions and simplifications. The sequencing gel frequently yields the most reliable information when determined from a single strand of DNA, but single-stranded DNA is frequently difficult to obtain. Messing used an M13 bacteriophage as a cloning vector for insertion of DNA of interest.[565] To simplify the use of M13 for DNA sequencing, Messing inserted the M13 genome into a plasmid to create a phagemid. The phagemid contains all the sequences needed for replication and selection in bacteria and, in addition, carries a M13 phage genome that can be rescued by infecting the bacteria with a replication-defective helper phage. Upon infection of the helper phage, the phagemid begins rolling circle replication to produce single-stranded DNA copies of the phagemid that are packaged as infectious phage and extruded from the cell. The bacteriophage can be isolated and the single-stranded DNA isolated and purified for ready use in the Sanger sequence technique. The phagemid vectors have the advantage of being able to carry larger pieces of DNA without recombination or deletion seen in standard M13 phage. The pUC 119 phagemid, derived from pUC plasmid that was originally modified from BR322, is particularly useful for stably carrying large pieces of cloned DNA while still producing phage in high titer.

Reporter Genes

In addition to the expression vectors, discussed above, which are used to express proteins in bacteria, yeast, insects, and mammalian cells, some protein expression systems are designed to examine the regulatory elements controlling gene expression. These vectors use reporter genes to provide easy measurement of gene expression under different conditions. Three popular reporter genes are chloramphenicol acetyltransferase or *cat*, the firefly gene luciferase, and a bacterial gene β-galactosidase. Chloramphenicol acetyltransferase is a bacterial gene that inactivates the antibiotic chloramphenicol. The value of the *cat* reporter gene lies in the fact that there is no mammalian enzyme with a similar activity to confound measurement of expressed protein. The assay is performed by first expressing the *cat* gene within the cell, isolating the total protein lysate of the transfected cell, and finally, with the aid of scintillation counting of an organic extract of the protein lysate, one can determine the amount of radio-acetylchloramphenicol produced by transfer of radiolabeled acetate from acetyl CoA to chloramphenicol.

Luciferase is an enzyme which, when expressed and combined with luciferin and ATP, produces light.[566] The amount of expressed protein can be easily quantitated by a luminometer. Similarly, when the β-galactosidase gene is placed downstream of a promoter containing regulatory elements, those aspects of cellular function that up- or downregulate the expression of the gene can be followed simply by using visible spectroscopy, since the activity of β-galactosidase can be measured by the production of a blue precipitate from its substrate, X-Gal.[567] Additionally, the luciferase and β-galactosidase reporter gene methods have been extended to studying regulation of gene expression in viable cells, because whole intact cells can be used to measure light production or absorbance, respectively, in a dynamic manner.

DNA Amplification: Polymerase Chain Reaction (PCR)

Since the beginning of molecular biology, scientists have been plagued with the problem of generating sufficient amounts of specific pieces of DNA to carry on research efficiently. For example, many genes exist as only a few copies in the genome and are expressed at very low levels, generating few copies of mRNA. Such genes can be extremely difficult to clone using the techniques described earlier, yet no simple and direct way existed until recently to select and amplify a particular piece of DNA. Kary Mullis solved the problem in a simple and insightful manner, for which he received the Nobel prize in 1993.[568] It had been known that DNA could be produced enzymatically *in vitro* by emulating the process by which DNA is replicated *in vivo*. Short stretches of chemically synthesized DNA (primers) could be mixed with the DNA (template) one wished to amplify (Figure 1.43). The mixture is heated to cause the double-stranded DNA strands to separate, then cooled to allow the primers to anneal to the long strands of DNA. In the presence of the four deoxynucleotides and DNA polymerase, a matching strand of DNA would be

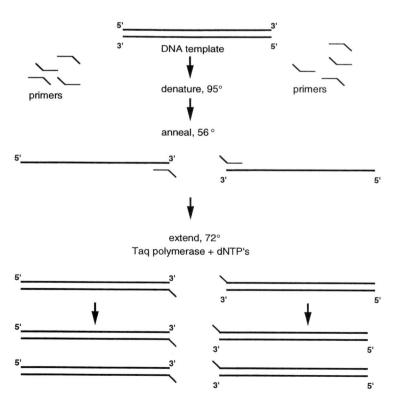

FIGURE 1.43. The polymerase chain reaction: the DNA template is mixed with synthetic primers complementary to regions flanking the DNA to be amplified. The template is denatured at 95°, then the primers are allowed to anneal to the template strands. *Taq* polymerase extends the primers into full-length strands of DNA. Each PCR cycle results in a doubling of the number of template molecules of DNA.

synthesized. Such a method would result in the production of only one strand of new DNA. Mullis made the key observation that if primers were made complementary to the regions flanking the DNA segment of interest, each cycle of the reaction would result in doubling the number of DNA strands available to use as template, thus causing the number of DNA strands to increase geometrically. Furthermore, the problem of heat inactivation of the polymerase could be avoided by using a heat-stable polymerase from *Thermus aquaticus,* a bacterium that thrives in the hot springs of Yellowstone Park.

In the short time since Mullis's insightful introduction of the polymerase chain reaction (PCR), the method has become an extremely powerful tool in any attempt to analyze DNA. Further, when the PCR is used following reverse transcription of mRNA, rare and scarce mRNA can be amplified by the RT-PCR technique. PCR is used extensively to search for genetic mutations, to match criminal suspects to evidence found at crime scenes, and in cancer diagnosis. The method has been elaborated on and extended to every aspect of molecular biology. Virtually every molecular biology laboratory now has at least one thermal cycler for use with PCR.

Transgenic and Knockout Technology

Most of the studies in molecular biology involve studying cells that are grown in tissue culture. However, no matter what cells are studied *in vitro,* the molecular biologist is ultimately presented with the fact that the cell types and systems that he has selected for use can bias his results and select for results that favor the initial assumptions of the researcher. When entire animals are used to investigate the importance of a particular gene product, we begin to understand a marvelous feature of the entire organism: there are many built in duplications. One method that is increasingly used in molecular biology is the creation of whole animals in which a foreign gene has been placed into the genome of embryonic cells (transgenic mice) or production of an animal in which a gene has been deleted or "knocked out." In the transgenic mouse technology, the role of overexpression can be studied. The mouse is the most commonly used animal to study expression of a foreign gene. The foreign gene or the gene construct having a promoter which allows for overexpression of a given gene is first placed into a single cell mouse embryo. The mouse embryo cells can be obtained by hormonally inducing ovulation, mating the mouse, and subsequently collecting fertilized embryo cells that can be manipulated for a short while in an *in vitro* environment. Once the fertilized cells are obtained, linearized DNA containing the gene of interest is microinjected into the embryo and subsequently incubated overnight. The transgenic embryonic cells are than introduced into the infundibulum of a pseudopregnant female mouse and, after the appropriate gestational period, live mice pups are obtained. The tails of the individual mice are then clipped and prepared for Southern blotting to determine if and which of the offspring contain the DNA insert. Then mRNA can be obtained to determine if gene expression is occurring. The most rapid and sensitive means of studying this for low-level expression is by RT-PCR. Alternatively, protein assay techniques (Western blotting) can be used. The techniques allow the study of oncogene expression and how that may affect tumor development.

For knockout mice technology, what is required is disruption of endogenous genes within the embryonic stem cells.[569] Since the stem cells have the potential to develop into a fully differentiated cell, mice can be produced that lack a particular gene product. The use of such models allows study of the importance of any gene and provides a clear means to study the manner by which the entire animal deals with a single mutation. The technique requires that homologous recombination occur between a transfected replacement vector and the endogenous gene of the stem cell. The insertion vector must contain between 3 and 10 bases of uninterrupted homologous sequence. Selection of the stem cell in which the gene has been knocked out is facilitated by the vector containing selectable markers such as neomycin phosphotransferase and herpes thymidylate kinase, whereupon the stem cell population is incubated with these selectable markers: G418 and gancyclovir. Although the selection marker greatly simplifies the task of determining which stem cells have undergone integration of insertion vector, it does not assure that there has been homologous recombination with resultant knockout. Therefore, DNA from clones of individual cells carrying the selection marker is further delineated by PCR to determine that there has been homologous recombination. Once this has been done, stem cells are injected into a blastocyst that has been implanted into a foster mother mouse. After gestation, the chimeric offspring are identified, which is frequently facilitated by hair color. These chimeras are bred with normal mice to determine if the germ line is chimeric. Then germ line chimeras are used to produce the homozygous knockout mice, in which the two copies of the target gene have been knocked out. The technique is extremely powerful in providing *in vivo* information regarding the importance of a particular gene in regulation of expression or suppression of tumor formation or development of disease.

MICROARRAY CHIP TECHNOLOGY

Biological experiments are frequently conducted in a manner that probes a single pathway or gene activation or event. The experimental consequence of such an approach is, for the most part, that a single assay or a small set of assays is used to probe the biological parameter that is being studied. With the most recent introduction of microarray technology to biology, it becomes distinctly possible that not only the face of the biological sciences will change, but likewise the manner in which experiments are thought of and executed will change.[570–572] Microarrays converge solid-state chemistry, transistor technology, laser optics, robotics, computer analysis, and biology to produce a new paradigm for the simultaneous study of multiple events. Although the technology will undoubtedly be applied to carbohydrate, protein, and lipid biochemistry, at the present time its main application is molecular biology. In particular, microarray technology is being applied to DNA sequencing, mutation analysis, and gene expression. When applied to gene expression, DNA chips or microarrays technology is an extremely powerful and informative tool.

At first glimpse, gene expression as assessed by microarrays appears to be an extension of membrane hybridization experiments. However, with the use of a glass template for affixing large number of DNA molecules to specific sites according to a predetermined XY coordinate system, the expression of thousands of genes can be selectively queried. The technique requires that an indexed expressed sequence tag (EST) be positioned precisely onto a solid matrix, usually a glass slide. The number of known sequences are ever increasing. A single chip can accommodate as many as 400,000 oligomers on a 1.6 cm^2 surface or up to 25,000 cloned DNA sequences on a 3.5 cm^2 surface.[571,572] Obviously such numbers cannot be positioned by hand, and so robotic technology is used to create slides with numerous precisely positioned ESTs, that is, DNA chips.

Within any given experiment, at any one time, steady-state mRNA is harvested and converted to cDNA (Figure 1.44). The cDNA is labeled with a specific fluorochrome, typically Cy3 or C5, and this sample is hybridized to the premade DNA chip. After rinsing, the individual XY coordinates are interrogated by laser light for the presence and extent of hybridized fluorochrome. In fact, two different expression sets can be studied at the same time by labeling one set of mRNA with Cy3 and the other with C5. Then the fluorescence from each set can be assessed simultaneously and a comparison generated between two different cell or tissue groups. Since there is a distinct chance of introducing intensity errors (particular when assaying different cells), sets of constitutively expressed housekeeping genes are used as internal standards. In that manner the entire data set can be normalized to the expression of housekeeping genes, and then the particular expressed gene and level of expression can be determined. Since thousands of genes can be queried simultaneously, the amount of data generated from any one experiment is frequently immense and, more important, the data are relational. Ultimately, one experiment will be compared with an array of other experiments. Therefore, there is an absolute requirement for bioinformatics to hold and catalogue results, as well as to provide ready access and easy querying sessions. A number of URLs are now being formed for compiling experiments in manner similar to that of Gene Bank. Likewise,

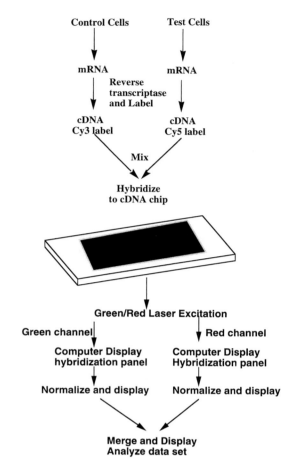

FIGURE 1.44. Diagram of a microchip array illustrating a typical experiment in which a set of control and test DNA are being compared to define transcriptional changes that result from a given test experiment. The cDNA is labeled, mixed, and hybridized to the oligonucleotides that have been precisely placed on the chip. Two different frequency lasers are used to excite the hybridized cDNA. Thereafter, emission from each x-y coordinate is collected, stored, and processed for further interrogation as to new or changes in transcribed genes.

URLs are becoming available to describe experimental conditions and results and availability of chips. Algorithms will be written to assist in processing and interrogating the large data sets. Such databases will permit perusal by investigators from anywhere. Patterns of up- and down-regulation of gene expression will undoubtedly emerge when comparing the results from similar and contrasting experiments.

Already DNA chips are being used to catalogue changes in enzyme profiles that result from exposure of cells to drugs. An example is an experiment when DNA chips were used to monitor differential expression of cytochrome 450 isoforms after exposure to phenobarbital. Increasingly, such studies will be done with regularity to assess detoxication and to repair enzymes that are modulated with respect to different antineoplastic drug exposure, as well as for profiling of expression sets of similar histochemical types of cancers.[573,574] Such studies will invariably increase understanding of the molecular events of and new targets for cancer.

At this time the DNA chips can "see" as little as three copies of mRNA per cell. Moreover, not only can the method determine new mRNA synthesis, but down-regulation of a particular gene(s) can be queried. With the vast amount of new data, it will not be long before interrelations between different molecular cascades will be routine. Ultimately, the technology promises to provide a format that will enable subtle questions to be asked in a virtual biology environment. The technology is new, the cost is expensive, improvements are occurring at rapid rate, and availability is limited. Moreover, the databases are still being formed. When the human genome project is finished, every gene will be followed by high levels of certainty. As some of the technical and expensive aspects of the techniques are addressed, interrogation by microarray chips of transcriptional and mutational events as they apply to fundamental and applied cancer research will begin in earnest. Once the gene expression format has been attended to, more and more will chip technology shift to translational protein chips. The future is indeed bright for molecular biology discovery.

GLOSSARY

alternative splicing: RNA that is spliced at alternate sites, yielding different but related RNAs coding for related proteins.

amber codon: a UAG triplet that signals termination of translation.

aminoacyl t-RNA: an aminoacyl ester of a tRNA carrying an amino acid.

amplification: synthesis of additional copies of chromosomal or extrachromosomal DNA.

annealing: complementary base pairing of two single strands of DNA.

anticoding strand: the strand of duplex DNA that serves as the template for synthesis of a complementary strand of RNA.

Chromosome: a large (long) molecule of double strand of DNA containing many genes.

cis-acting protein: a protein that activates a sequence of DNA within the same molecule of DNA from which the protein was expressed.

cis-acting: activation of a sequence of DNA within the same molecule; compare with **trans.**

clone: a large number of cells (molecules) that are all identical to the single parent from which they were derived.

cloning vector: DNA containing necessary fragments of DNA to replicate a foreign gene inserted in an appropriate position within the vector.

closed complex: the configuration of DNA while RNA polymerase is bound to DNA but before the DNA has started to unwind.

codon: three continuous nucleotides that code for an amino acid or termination signal.

constitutive genes: genes whose product is expressed at a steady level through RNA polymerase/promoter interactions without additional regulation.

core particle: a fragment of nucleosome-associated DNA consisting of a 146 base pair histone octamer resistant to nuclease digestion.

CAAT-box: a conserved DNA motif found upstream of initiation site in eukaryotic genes and recognized/bound by transcriptional factors.

cap: a posttranscriptional modification in which a GTP is added to the 5'-end of eukaryotic pre-mRNA through a 5' to 5' triphosphate bond.

cDNA: a single strand of DNA complementary to the coding strand of DNA.

chromatin: compacted molecules of DNA complexed with specific DNA-binding proteins.

degeneracy: a term used in reference to amino acids having more than one codon with the variation found in the third nucleotide.

deletion: removal of a sequence of DNA followed by rejoining of surrounding fragments.

denaturation: separation of double strands of DNA or RNA into single strands.

direct repeats: identical sequences of DNA found in two or more copies in the same orientation within the same molecule of DNA.

DNA polymerase: an enzyme that catalyzes the synthesis of a complementary strand of DNA.

DNAse I hypersensitive sites: regions of DNA that are sensitive to nuclease degradation by the enzyme DNase I.

downstream: denotes those sequences of nucleotides found further 3' in the DNA strand.

elongation factors: proteins whose functions are required at a specific step(s) in polypeptide elongation of protein synthesis.

end labeling: addition of a radioactive or chemically labeled molecule to one strand of DNA.

endonucleases: enzymes that cleave bonds within a strand of single-stranded or double-stranded DNA or RNA.

enhancer: a sequence motif that acts in cis to increase the level of transcription of DNA from a eukaryotic promoter. It can be located either upstream or downstream from the promoter.

episome: circularized DNA that replicates epichromosomally but is capable of integrating into bacterial genomic DNA.

eukaryotes: organisms that have compartmentalized their DNA within a nucleus.

exon: a coding region of a gene which becomes part of the mRNA.

exonucleases: enzymes that cleave in a systematic way either the 5′ or 3′ nucleotides from the end of a strand of DNA or RNA.

expression vector: a cloning vector containing the required regulatory elements which will enable a gene of interest (if properly inserted) to be translated into the correct protein.

frameshift mutation: an addition or deletion of nucleotide(s) which alters the reading frame for protein synthesis, resulting in an incorrect sequence of amino acids, hence an incorrect protein.

gene: a sequence of DNA that codes for a protein.

genetic code: a sequence of DNA or RNA triplet codons which correspond to an amino acid.

helper virus: when cells are coinfected with helper virus and defective virus, the helper virus provides those proteins whose functions are necessary for the defective virus to be an infectious particle.

heterochromatin: a highly condensed, nontranslated region of the genome.

heterogeneous nuclear RNA: nuclear RNA transcribed by RNA polymerase II which has not undergone splicing or posttranscriptional modifications.

histones: DNA-binding proteins in eukaryotes which form the nucleosome.

housekeeping genes: genes whose product is constitutively expressed because it is necessary for a basic cellular function.

hybridization: base pairing between complementary strands of RNA and DNA.

inducer: a molecule that binds to a specific regulator, resulting in initiation of transcription.

initiation factors: specific proteins that interact with each other, with ribosomes, and/or with mRNA to form a translation initiation complex.

integration: insertion and chemical bonding of extracellular DNA into genomic DNA.

intron: a noncoding region of DNA which is transcribed into RNA but removed by splicing of primary transcript into mRNA placing exons adjacent to each other.

inverted repeat: the same sequence of DNA represented more than once in the same molecule of DNA but in opposite orientation.

kilobase (kbase or kb):   or 1,000 base pairs of DNA or RNA.

lariat: a folded-over sequence of pre-RNA which forms a circular splicing intermediate resembling a loop of rope.

leader sequence: a nontranslated sequence located at either end or within the DNA sequence which directs translated proteins across membranes into a specific cellular compartment.

ligation: an enzymatic reaction requiring ligase and ATP to form a phosphodiester bond between two ends of nicked/cut double-stranded DNA.

lipid bilayer: the configuration of lipid membranes formed by phospholipids which align themselves so that the hydrophobic tail is in the interior milieu and the hydrophilic head is facing the exterior.

LTR: (long terminal repeat) sequences of DNA in a retroviral genome which are repeated at the 5′- and 3′-ends.

MAR: (matrix attachment site) an AT-rich region of DNA which attaches to the cellular matrix.

monocistronic: mRNA that codes for only one protein.

multicopy plasmids: plasmids that replicate themselves many times within a single cell per doubling.

mutation: any change in the nucleotide sequence of DNA.

negative regulators: molecules that can "turn off" transcription or translation.

nick translation: the enzymatic reaction which occurs when *E. coli* DNA polymerase I adds nucleotides to the free 3′ hydroxyl end of nicked double-stranded DNA.

Northern blotting: a technique that involves transfer of RNA to nitrocellulose filter for hybridization to a complementary strand of DNA.

nucleosome: the basic foundational chromatin structure in eukaryotic cells.

oncogenes: genes whose product can transform normal eukaryotic cells into a growth pattern resembling tumor cells.

open reading frame: a series of codons coding for amino acids.

operon: a group of bacterial genes expressed and regulated from same promoter and promoter elements.

origin: a sequence of DNA where replication begins.

packing ratio: the ratio of the length of DNA when stretched out to the length of the structure formed when it is condensed.

PCR: (polymerase chain reaction) technique that amplifies nucleic acids by using thermophilic DNA polymerase to synthesize complementary strands of DNA into many copies through multiple cycles of denaturing, annealing, and elongation temperatures.

periodicity: the number of base pairs of DNA in one turn of the double helix.

phage: (bacteriophage) virus that infects bacterial cells.

plasmid: a circular piece of DNA capable of replicating itself extrachromosomally.

point mutation: any change in a single base pair.

polyadenylation: posttranslational modification in eukaryotic cells involving addition of multiple polyadenylic acids.

polycistronic: a single prokaryotic mRNA containing the genetic code for more than one gene.

polysome: multiple ribosomes simultaneously translating a single mRNA.

primary transcript: RNA that has been transcribed and has not yet undergone splicing or posttranscriptional modification.

primer: a short sequence of single-stranded DNA or RNA with a free 3′ hydroxyl and complementary to one strand of DNA, therefore providing DNA polymerase a DNA synthesis start site.

prokaryote: an organism which does not have a nucleus.

promoter: a sequence motif found within DNA near the RNA polymerase transcriptional initiation site which forms a transcription complex when bound by transcriptional factors and RNA polymerase.

prophage: phage DNA covalently integrated into the host chromosome.

proteolytic enzyme: an enzyme that catalyzes hydrolysis of a peptide or protein.

protooncogenes: normal cellular genes from which oncogenes originate.

provirus: a viral genome covalently integrated into host genome.

reading frame: the alignment of bases in RNA to give a succession of triplets which are recognized as codons. Insertion or deletion of one or two bases will shift the reading frame; insertion or deletion of three bases will not.

regulatory gene: DNA whose gene product is a protein which functions in the regulation/control of nucleic acids or another protein.

repression: inhibition of transcription or translation when a repressor molecule binds to a specific region within the DNA or mRNA.

restriction enzyme: an endonuclease which cleaves DNA at a specific recognition sequence.

retrovirus: an RNA virus having the enzyme reverse transcriptase which transcribes the RNA into double-stranded DNA, enabling the viral genome to integrate into the host genome.

reverse transcription: synthesis of single-stranded DNA complementary to an RNA template by the enzyme reverse transcriptase.

RFLP: (restriction fragment length polymorphism) a technique used to detect nucleotide changes by comparing the sizes of restriction endonuclease cleaved genomic DNA fragments.

RNase: an enzyme which degrades RNA.

RNA polymerase: an enzyme which synthesizes RNA using a DNA template.

Shine-Dalgarno sequence: a 5 to 8 base pair purine-rich sequence located about 10 nucleotides upstream from the initiation codon which is complementary to 3′ sequences in 16S rRNA; the complementary base pairing strongly influences binding of 30S rRNA to mRNA.

sigma factor: the subunit of bacterial RNA polymerase which is necessary to initiate transcription.

signal transduction: a cellular reaction involving the binding of a ligand to a cell surface receptor which in turn transmits an intracellular signal initiating a cellular pathway/mechanism.

SSCP: (single-stranded conformation polymorphism) a technique that will detect single base changes in DNA through electrophoretic mobility shifts of denatured DNA on a polyacrylmaide gel.

Southern blotting: a technique for transferring DNA from an agarose gel to a nitrocellulose membrane, followed by probing the membrane with a labelled primer; hybridization is visualized on an autoradiograph.

snRNPs: small nuclear ribonucleoproteins.

splicing: the removal of introns followed by the joining together of exons in the primary RNA transcript.

splice junctions: sequences that are found in RNA at the boundary of an exon and intron.

start point: the triplet of DNA at which RNA polymerase initiates transcription.

stop codons: specific triplets (UAA, UAG, UGA) that code for termination of translation.

structural gene: any gene that codes for a protein which is not under cellular regulation.

suppression: a change that reverses the effects of a mutation without altering the original DNA sequence.

Tm: the melting temperature of double-stranded nucleic acids.

tandem repeats: many copies of the same repeated sequence next to each other.

TATA-box: a conserved, short T-A DNA motif in a fixed location which is part of the transcriptional complex.

termination codon: a triplet sequence coding for amino acid, signaling termination of protein synthesis; the termination codons are UAG, UAA, and UGA.

tertiary structure: the three-dimensional configuration of a biopolymer.

trans: sites located on two different molecules of DNA; compare with **cis.**

transcription: the enzymatic reaction that uses one strand of DNA as a template to make a complementary strand of RNA.

transduction: the transfer of genetic material from one cell to another with the use of a virus (usually phage).

transfection: introduction of new genetic material into cells.

transformation: the acquisition of new characteristics by a cell as the result of introduction of new genetic material or modification of endogenous genes.

translation: the process that translates the genetic information carried by the codons in mRNA into amino acids forming a polypeptide.

translocation: when a copy of a gene is found in a location within the genome different from the location where it was originally found.

transmembrane protein: a protein that protrudes through a lipid bilayer and is therefore exposed to an aqueous environment on both sides of the membrane.

transposon: a DNA sequence that moves to new location within the genome.

transposition: movement of transposon to a new location within the genome.

upstream: the nontranslated sequences of DNA found prior to the initiation site for transcription.

vector: a molecule or structure used to carry genetic information into a cell; a vector can be, for example, DNA plasmid or a virus.

REFERENCES

1. Avery OT, MacLeod CM, McCarty M. Studies on the chemical nature of the substance inducing formation of pneumococcal types. Induction of transformation by a deoxyribonucleic acid fraction isolated from a pneumococcal Type III. *J Exp Med* 1944;79:137.
2. Chargaff E. Chemical specificity of nucleic acids and mechanisms of their enzymative degradation. *Experientia* 1950;6:201.
3. Watson JD, Crick FH. A structure for deoxyribonucleic acid. *Nature* 1953;171:737.
4. Watson JD, Crick FH. Genetical implications of the structure of deoxyribonucleic acid. *Nature* 1953;171:964.
5. Watson JD, Crick FH. The structure of DNA. *Cold Spring Harb Symp Quant Biol* 1954;18:123.
6. Wang JC. Helical repeat of DNA in solution. *Proc Natl Acad Sci U S A* 1979;76:200.
7. Freeman LA, Garrard WT. DNA supercoiling in chromatin structure and gene expression. *Crit Rev Eukaryot Gene Expr* 1992;2:165.
8. Hobot JA, Villiger W, Escaig J, et al. Shape and fine structure of nucleoids observed on sections of ultrarapidly frozen and cryosubstituted bacteria. *J Bacteriol* 1985;162:960.
9. Sperling R, Wachtel EJ. The histones. *Adv Protein Chem* 1981; 34:1.
10. Kornberg A. Biological synthesis of deoxyribonucleic acid. *Science* 1960;131:1503.
11. Kornberg A. Aspects of DNA replication. *Cold Spring Harb Symp Quant Biol* 1979;43[Pt 1]:1.
12. Shenk T. Transcriptional control regions: nucleotide sequence requirements for initiation by RNA polymerase II and III. *Curr Top Microbiol Immunol* 1981;93:25.
13. Dynan WS, Tjian R. Control of eukaryotic messenger RNA synthesis by sequence-specific DNA-binding proteins. *Nature* 1985;316:774.
14. Fire A, Samuels M, Sharp PA. Interactions between RNA polymerase II, factors, and template leading to accurate transcription. *J Biol Chem* 1984;259:2509.
15. Schibler U, Sierra F. Alternative promoters in developmental gene expression. *Annu Rev Genet* 1987;21:237.
16. Jacob F, Monod F. Molecular and biological characterization of RNA. *J Mol Biol* 1961;3:318.
17. Matthews KS. DNA looping. *Microbiol Rev* 1992;56:123.
18. Hultin T. Incorporation *in vivo* of 15N-labelled glycine into liver fractions of newly hatched chicks. *Exp Cell Res* 1950;1: 376.
19. Hershey AD, Dixon J, Chase M. Nucleic acid economy in bacteria infected with bacteriophage T2. *J Gen Physiol* 1953;36:777.
20. Volkin E, Astrachan L. Phosphorous incorporation in *E. coli* ribonucleic acid after infection with bacteriophase T2. *Virology* 1956;2:149.
21. Tissiers A, Watson JD. Ribonucleoprotein particles from *E. coli Nature* 1958;182:778.
22. Nirenberg MW, Matthaei JH. The dependence of cell free protein synthesis in *E. coli* upon naturally occurring or synthetic polyribonucleotides. *Proc Natl Acad Sci* 1961;47:1588.
23. Kozak M. Comparison of initiation of protein synthesis in procaryotes, eucaryotes, and organelles. *Microbiol Rev* 1983;47:1.
24. Nevins JR. The pathway of eukaryotic mRNA formation. *Annu Rev Biochem* 1983;52:441.
25. Breathnach R, Chambon P. Organization and expression of eucaryotic split genes coding for proteins. *Annu Rev Biochem* 1981;50:349.
26. Helmann JD, Chamberlin MJ. Structure and function of bacterial sigma factors. *Annu Rev Biochem* 1988;57:839.
27. Darst SA, Kubalek EW, Kornberg RD. Three-dimensional structure of *Escherichia coli* RNA polymerase holoenzyme determined by electron crystallography. *Nature* 1989;340:730.
28. Heumann H, Lederer H, Baer G, et al. Spatial arrangement of DNA-dependent RNA polymerase of *Escherichia coli* and DNA in the specific complex. A neutron small-angle scattering study. *J Mol Biol* 1988;201:115.
29. Ishihama A. Role of the RNA polymerase alpha subunit in transcription activation. *Mol Microbiol* 1992;6:3283.
30. Buc H, McClure WR. Kinetics of open complex formation between *Escherichia coli* RNA polymerase and the lac UV5 promoter. Evidence for a sequential mechanism involving three steps. *Biochemistry* 1985;24:2712.
31. Straney DC, Crothers DM. Comparison of the open complexes formed by RNA polymerase at the *Escherichia coli* lac UV5 promoter. *J Mol Biol* 1987;193:279.
32. Schickor P, Metzger W, Werel W, et al. Topography of intermediates in transcription initiation of *E. coli*. *EMBO J* 1990;9: 2215.
33. Suh WC, Ross W, Record MTJ. Two open complexes and a requirement for Mg2+ to open the lambda PR transcription start site. *Science* 1993;259:358.
34. Roberts JW. Termination factor for RNA synthesis. *Nature* 1969;224:1168.
35. Platt T, Bear D. The role of RNA polymerase, Rho factor, and ribosomes. Beckwith J, Davies J, Gallant J, eds. New York: Cold Spring Harbor Laboratory Press, 1983;123.
36. Ryan T, Chamberlin MJ. Transcription analyses with heteroduplex trp attenuator templates indicate that the transcript stem and loop structure serves as the termination signal. *J Biol Chem* 1983;258:4690.
37. Platt T. Transcription termination and the regulation of gene expression. *Annu Rev Biochem* 1986;55:339.

38. McClure WR. Mechanism and control of transcription initiation in prokaryotes. *Annu Rev Biochem* 1985;54:171.

39. Reznikoff WS, Siegele DA, Cowing DW, et al. The regulation of transcription initiation in bacteria. *Annu Rev Genet* 1985;19:355.

40. Hughes KT, Mathee K. The anti-sigma factors. *Annu Rev Microbiol* 1988;52:231.

41. Paranjape SM, Kamakaka RT, Kadonaga JT. Role of chromatin structure in the regulation of transcription by RNA polymerase II. *Annu Rev Biochem* 1994;63:265.

42. Wolffe AP. Nucleosome positioning and modification: chromatin structures that potentiate transcription. *Trends Biochem Sci* 1994;19:240.

43. Wolffe AP. The transcription of chromatin templates. *Curr Opin Genet Dev* 1994;4:245.

44. Kornberg RD, Lorch Y. Chromatin structure and transcription. *Annu Rev Cell Biol* 1992;8:563.

45. Pederson DS, Thoma F, Simpson RT. Core particle, fiber, and transcriptionally active chromatin structure. *Annu Rev Cell Biol* 1986;2:117.

46. Straka C, Horz W. A functional role for nucleosomes in the repression of a yeast promoter. *EMBO J* 1991;10:361.

47. Weintraub H, Groudine M. Chromosomal subunits in active genes have an altered conformation. *Science* 1976;193:848.

48. Grosveld F, van Assendelft GB, Greaves DR, et al. Position-independent, high-level expression of the human beta-globin gene in transgenic mice. *Cell* 1987;51:975.

49. Forrester WC, Takegawa S, Papayannopoulou T, et al. Evidence for a locus activation region: the formation of developmentally stable hypersensitive sites in globin-expressing hybrids. *Nucleic Acids Res* 1987;15:10159.

50. Vemuri MC, Raju NN, Malhotra SK. Recent advances in nuclear matrix function. *Cytobios* 1993;76:117.

51. Kingston RE. Transcriptional regulation of heat shock genes. In: Cohen P, Foulkes JE, eds. The hormonal control regulation and gene transcription New York: Elsevier Science, 1991:377.

52. Wu C. The 5′ ends of *Drosophila* heat-shock genes in chromatin are hypersensitive to DNase I. *Nature* 1980;286:854.

53. Keene MA, Corces V, Lowenhaupt K, et al. DNase I hypersensitive sites in *Drosophila* chromatin occur at the 5′ ends of regions of transcription. *Proc Natl Acad Sci U S A* 1981;78:143.

54. Kadonaga JT. Eukaryotic transcription: an interlaced network of transcription factors and chromatin-modifying machines. *Cell* 1998;92:307.

55. Hess JL. Chromosomal translocations in benign tumors: the HMGI proteins. *Am J Clin Pathol* 1998;109:251.

56. Sollner-Webb B, Tower J. Transcription of cloned eukaryotic ribosomal RNA genes. *Annu Rev Biochem* 1986;55:801.

57. Geiduschek EP, Tocchini-Valentini GP. Transcription by RNA polymerase III. *Annu Rev Biochem* 1988;57:873.

58. Parvin JD, Timmers HT, Sharp PA. Promoter specificity of basal transcription factors. *Cell* 1992;68:1135.

59. Zawel L, Reinberg D. Advances in RNA polymerase II transcription. *Curr Opin Cell Biol* 1992;4:488.

60. Smale ST. Core promoter architecture for eukaryotic protein-coding genes. In: Conaway RC, Conaway JW, eds. Transcription: mechanisms and regulations. New York: Raven Press, 1994:63.

61. Smale ST, Baltimore D. The initiator as a transcription control element. *Cell* 1989;57:103.

62. Buratowski S, Hahn S, Sharp PA, et al. Function of a yeast TATA element-binding protein in a mammalian transcription system. *Nature* 1988;334:37.

63. Bucher P. Weight matrix descriptions of four eukaryotic RNA polymerase II promoter elements derived from 502 unrelated promoter sequences. *J Mol Biol* 1990;212:563.

64. Serizawa H, Conaway JW, Conaway RC. Transcription: mechanisms and regulation. New York: Raven Press, 1994:632.

65. Zhou Q, Lieberman PM, Boyer TG, et al. Holo-TFIID supports transcriptional stimulation by diverse activators and from a TATA-less promoter. *Genes Dev* 1992;6:1964.

66. Zhou Q, Boyer TG, Berk AJ. Factors (TAFs) required for activated transcription interact with TATA box-binding protein conserved core domain. *Genes Dev* 1993;7:180.

67. Hoey T, Weinzierl RO, Gill G, et al. Molecular cloning and functional analysis of *Drosophila* TAF110 reveal properties expected of coactivators. *Cell* 1993;72:247.

68. Ruppert S, Wang EH, Tjian R. Cloning and expression of human TAFII250: a TBP-associated factor implicated in cell-cycle regulation. *Nature* 1993;362:175.

69. Kao CC, Lieberman PM, Schmidt MC, et al. Cloning of a transcriptionally active human TATA binding factor. *Science* 1990;248:1646.

70. Lobo SM, Lister J, Sullivan ML, et al. The cloned RNA polymerase II transcription factor IID selects RNA polymerase III to transcribe the human U6 gene *in vitro*. *Genes Dev* 1991;5:1477.

71. Comai L, Tanese N, Tjian R. The TATA-binding protein and associated factors are integral components of the RNA polymerase I transcription factor, SL1. *Cell* 1992;68:965.

72. Nikolov DB, Hu SH, Lin J, et al. Crystal structure of TFIID TATA-box binding protein. *Nature* 1992;360:40.

73. Kim Y, Geiger JH, Hahn S, et al. Crystal structure of a yeast TBP/TATA-box complex. *Nature* 1993;365:512.

74. Kim JL, Nikolov DB, Burley SK. Co-crystal structure of TBP recognizing the minor groove of a TATA element [see comments]. *Nature* 1993;365:520.

75. Conaway RC, Bradsher JN, Conaway JW. Mechanism of assembly of the RNA polymerase II preinitiation complex. Evidence for a functional interaction between the carboxyl-terminal domain of the largest subunit of RNA polymerase II and a high molecular mass form of the TATA factor. *J Biol Chem* 1992;267:8464.

76. Pugh BF, Tjian R. Mechanism of transcriptional activation by Sp1: evidence for coactivators. *Cell* 1990;61:1187.

77. Goodrich JA, Hoey T, Thut CJ, et al. *Drosophila* TAFII40 interacts with both a VP16 activation domain and the basal transcription factor TFIIB. *Cell* 1993;75:519.

78. Goodrich JA, Tjian R. TBP-TAF complexes: selectivity factors for eukaryotic transcription. *Curr Opin Cell Biol* 1994;6:403.

79. Ha I, Lane WS, Reinberg D. Cloning of a human gene encoding the general transcription initiation factor IIB. *Nature* 1991;352:689.

80. Buratowski S, Hahn S, Guarente L, et al. Five intermediate complexes in transcription initiation by RNA polymerase II. *Cell* 1989;56:549.

81. Lagrange T, Kapanidis AN, Tang H, et al. New core promoter element in RNA polymerase II-dependent transcription: sequence-specific DNA binding by transcription factor IIB. *Genes Dev* 1998;12:34.

82. DeJong J, Roeder RG. A single cDNA, hTFIIA/alpha, encodes both the p35 and p19 subunits of human TFIIA. *Genes Dev* 1993;7:2220.

83. Inostroza JA, Mermelstein FH, Ha I, et al. Dr1, a TATA-binding protein-associated phosphoprotein and inhibitor of class II gene transcription. *Cell* 1992;70:477.

84. Roeder RG. The complexities of eukaryotic transcription initiation: regulation of preinitiation complex assembly. *Trends Biochem Sci* 1991;16:402.

85. Greenblatt J. RNA polymerase-associated transcription factors. *Trends Biochem Sci* 1991;16:408.

86. Killeen MT, Greenblatt JF. The general transcription factor

RAP30 binds to RNA polymerase II and prevents it from binding nonspecifically to DNA. *Mol Cell Biol* 1992;12:30.

87. McCracken S, Greenblatt J. Related RNA polymerase-binding regions in human RAP30/74 and *Escherichia coli* sigma 70 [published erratum appears in *Science* 1992;255(5049):1195]. *Science* 1991;253:900.

88. Peterson MG, Inostroza J, Maxon ME, et al. Structure and functional properties of human general transcription factor IIE. *Nature* 1991;354:369.

89. Gerard M, Fischer L, Moncollin V, et al. Purification and interaction properties of the human RNA polymerase B(II) general transcription factor BTF2. *J Biol Chem* 1991;266:20940.

90. Flores O, Lu H, Reinberg D. Factors involved in specific transcription by mammalian RNA polymerase II. Identification and characterization of factor IIH. *J Biol Chem* 1992;267:2786.

91. Schaeffer L, Roy R, Humbert S, et al. DNA repair helicase: a component of BTF2 (TFIIH) basic transcription factor. *Science* 1993;260:58.

92. Lu H, Flores O, Weinmann R, et al. The nonphosphorylated form of RNA polymerase II preferentially associates with the preinitiation complex. *Proc Natl Acad Sci U S A* 1991;88:10004.

93. Laybourn PJ, Dahmus ME. Phosphorylation of RNA polymerase IIA occurs subsequent to interaction with the promoter and before the initiation of transcription. *J Biol Chem* 1990;265:13165.

94. Reinberg D, Roeder RG. Factors involved in specific transcription by mammalian RNA polymerase II. Transcription factor IIS stimulates elongation of RNA chains. *J Biol Chem* 1987;262:3331.

95. Reines D. Elongation factor-dependent transcript shortening by template-engaged RNA polymerase II. *J Biol Chem* 1992;267:3795.

96. Reines D, Mote JJ. Elongation factor SII-dependent transcription by RNA polymerase II through a sequence-specific DNA-binding protein. *Proc Natl Acad Sci U S A* 1993;90:1917.

97. Donahue BA, Yin S, Taylor JS, et al. Transcript cleavage by RNA polymerase II arrested by a cyclobutane pyrimidine dimer in the DNA template. *Proc Natl Acad Sci U S A* 1994;91:8502.

98. Vaishnav YN, Wong-Staal F. The biochemistry of AIDS. *Annu Rev Biochem* 1991;60:577.

99. Reines D, Conaway JW, Conaway RC. The RNA polymerase II general elongation factors. *Trends Biochem Sci* 1996;21:351.

100. Shilatifard A. The RNA polymerase II general elongation complex. *Biol Chem* 1998;379:27.

101. Duan DR, Pause A, Burgess WH, et al. Inhibition of transcription elongation by the VHL tumor suppressor protein. *Science* 1995;269:1402.

102. Zawel L, Reinberg D. Initiation of transcription by RNA polymerase II: a multi-step process. *Prog Nucleic Acid Res Mol Biol* 1993;44:67.

103. Allison LA, Wong JK, Fitzpatrick VD, et al. The C-terminal domain of the largest subunit of RNA polymerase II of *Saccharomyces cerevisiae, Drosophila melanogaster,* and mammals: a conserved structure with an essential function. *Mol Cell Biol* 1988;8:321.

104. Allison LA, Moyle M, Shales M, et al. Extensive homology among the largest subunits of eukaryotic and prokaryotic RNA polymerases. *Cell* 1985;42:599.

105. Zehring WA, Lee JM, Weeks JR, et al. The C-terminal repeat domain of RNA polymerase II largest subunit is essential *in vivo* but is not required for accurate transcription initiation *in vitro. Proc Natl Acad Sci U S A* 1988;85:3698.

106. Bartolomei MS, Halden NF, Cullen CR, et al. Genetic analysis of the repetitive carboxyl-terminal domain of the largest subunit of mouse RNA polymerase II. *Mol Cell Biol* 1988;8:330.

107. Young RA. RNA polymerase II. *Annu Rev Biochem* 1991;60:689.

108. Thompson CM, Koleske AJ, Chao DM, et al. A multisubunit complex associated with the RNA polymerase II CTD and TATA-binding protein in yeast. *Cell* 1993;73:1361.

109. Grosschedl R, Birnstiel ML. Identification of regulatory sequences in the prelude sequences of an H2A histone gene by the study of specific deletion mutants *in vivo. Proc Natl Acad Sci U S A* 1980;77:1432.

110. Weis L, Reinberg D. Transcription by RNA polymerase II: initiator-directed formation of transcription-competent complexes. *FASEB J* 1992;6:3300.

111. Means AL, Farnham PJ. Transcription initiation from the dihydrofolate reductase promoter is positioned by HIP1 binding at the initiation site. *Mol Cell Biol* 1990;10:653.

112. Sehgal A, Patil N, Chao M. A constitutive promoter directs expression of the nerve growth factor receptor gene. *Mol Cell Biol* 1988;8:3160.

113. Dynan WS, Tjian R. The promoter-specific transcription factor Sp1 binds to upstream sequences in the SV40 early promoter. *Cell* 1983;35:79.

114. Javahery R, Khachi A, Lo K, et al. DNA sequence requirements for transcriptional initiator activity in mammalian cells. *Mol Cell Biol* 1994;14:116.

115. Wingender E. Transcription regulating proteins and their recognition sequences. *Crit Rev Eukaryot Gene Expr* 1990;1:11.

116. Maity SN, Golumbek PT, Karsenty G, et al. Selective activation of transcription by a novel CCAAT binding factor. *Science* 1988;241:582.

117. Hatamochi A, Golumbek PT, Van Schaftingen E, et al. A CCAAT DNA-binding factor consisting of two different components that are both required for DNA binding. *J Biol Chem* 1988;263:5940.

118. Chodosh LA, Baldwin AS, Carthew RW, et al. Human CCAAT-binding proteins have heterologous subunits. *Cell* 1988;53:11.

119. Barberis A, Superti-Furga G, Busslinger M. Mutually exclusive interaction of the CCAAT-binding factor and of a displacement protein with overlapping sequences of a histone gene promoter. *Cell* 1987;50:347.

120. Superti-Furga G, Barberis A, Schaffner G, et al. The −117 mutation in Greek HPFH affects the binding of three nuclear factors to the CCAAT region of the gamma-globin gene. *EMBO J* 1988;7:3099.

121. Jones KA, Yamamoto KR, Tjian R. Two distinct transcription factors bind to the HSV thymidine kinase promoter *in vitro. Cell* 1985;42:559.

122. Ray BK, Ray A. Expression of the gene encoding alpha 1-acid glycoprotein in rabbit liver under acute-phase conditions involves induction and activation of beta and delta CCAAT-enhancer-binding proteins. *Eur J Biochem* 1994;222:891.

123. Graves BJ, Johnson PF, McKnight SL. Homologous recognition of a promoter domain common to the MSV LTR and the HSV tk gene. *Cell* 1986;44:565.

124. Dorn A, Durand B, Marfing C, et al. Conserved major histocompatibility complex class II boxes—X and Y—are transcriptional control elements and specifically bind nuclear proteins. *Proc Natl Acad Sci U S A* 1987;84:6249.

125. Eilers A, Bouterfa H, Triebe S, et al. Role of a distal promoter element in the S-phase control of the human H1.2 histone gene transcription. *Eur J Biochem* 1994;223:567.

126. Wright KL, Vilen BJ, Itoh-Lindstrom Y, et al. CCAAT box binding protein NF-Y facilitates *in vivo* recruitment of upstream DNA binding transcription factors. *EMBO J* 1994;13:4042.

127. Dorn A, Bollekens J, Staub A, et al. A multiplicity of CCAAT box-binding proteins. *Cell* 1987;50:863.

128. Sive HL, Roeder RG. Interaction of a common factor with conserved promoter and enhancer sequences in histone H2B, immunoglobulin, and U2 small nuclear RNA (snRNA) genes. *Proc Natl Acad Sci U S A* 1986;83:6382.

129. Bohmann D, Keller W, Dale T, et al. A transcription factor which binds to the enhancers of SV40, immunoglobulin heavy chain and U2 snRNA genes. *Nature* 1987;325:268.

130. Miwa K, Strominger JL. The HLA-DQ beta gene upstream region contains an immunoglobulin-like octamer motif that binds cell-type specific nuclear factors. *Nucleic Acids Res* 1987; 15:8057.

131. Scheidereit C, Heguy A, Roeder RG. Identification and purification of a human lymphoid-specific octamer-binding protein (OTF-2) that activates transcription of an immunoglobulin promoter *in vitro*. *Cell* 1987;51:783.

132. Letovsky J, Dynan WS. Measurement of the binding of transcription factor Sp1 to a single GC box recognition sequence. *Nucleic Acids Res* 1989;17:2639.

133. Fromm M, Berg P. Deletion mapping of DNA regions required for SV40 early region promoter function *in vivo*. *J Mol Appl Genet* 1982;1:457.

134. Gidoni D, Kadonaga JT, Barrera-Saldana H, et al. Bidirectional SV40 transcription mediated by tandem Sp1 binding interactions. *Science* 1985;230:511.

135. Sun D, Hurley LH. Cooperative bending of the 21-base-pair repeats of the SV40 viral early promoter by human Sp1. *Biochemistry* 1994;33:9578.

136. Ueda A, Okuda K, Ohno S, et al. NF-kappa B and Sp1 regulate transcription of the human monocyte chemoattractant protein-1 gene. *J Immunol* 1994;153:2052.

137. Humphries DE, Bloom BB, Fine A, et al. Structure and expression of the promoter for the human type II transforming growth factor-beta receptor. *Biochem Biophys Res Commun* 1994;203:1020.

138. Kaneda S, Nalbantoglu J, Takeishi K, et al. Structural and functional analysis of the human thymidylate synthase gene. *J Biol Chem* 1990;265:20277.

139. Smith JD, Melian A, Leff T, et al. Expression of the human apolipoprotein E gene is regulated by multiple positive and negative elements. *J Biol Chem* 1988;263:8300.

140. Briggs MR, Kadonaga JT, Bell SP, et al. Purification and biochemical characterization of the promoter-specific transcription factor, Sp1. *Science* 1986;234:47.

141. Baniahmad A, Tsai MJ. Mechanisms of transcriptional activation by steroid hormone receptors. *J Cell Biochem* 1993;51:151.

142. Evans RM. The steroid and thyroid hormone receptor superfamily. *Science* 1988;240:889.

143. Fuller PJ. The steroid receptor superfamily: mechanisms of diversity. *FASEB J* 1991;5:3092.

144. Forman BM, Samuels HH. Dimerization among nuclear hormone receptors. *New Biol* 1990;2:587.

145. Carson-Jurica MA, Schrader WT, O'Malley BW. Steroid receptor family: structure and functions. *Endocr Rev* 1990;11:201.

146. Green S, Kumar V, Theulaz I, et al. The N-terminal DNA-binding "zinc finger" of the oestrogen and glucocorticoid receptors determines target gene specificity. *EMBO J* 1988;7:3037.

147. Mader S, Kumar V, de Verneuil H, et al. Three amino acids of the oestrogen receptor are essential to its ability to distinguish an oestrogen from a glucocorticoid-responsive element. *Nature* 1989;338:271.

148. Jensen EV. Overview of the nuclear receptor family. In: Parker MG, eds. Nuclear hormone receptors. New York: Academic Press, 1991;125.

149. Beato M. Transcriptional control by nuclear receptors. *FASEB J* 1991;5:2044.

150. Giguere V, Ong ES, Segui P, et al. Identification of a receptor for the morphogen retinoic acid. *Nature* 1987;330:624.

151. Mangelsdorf DJ, Borgmeyer U, Heyman RA, et al. Characterization of three RXR genes that mediate the action of 9-cis retinoic acid. *Genes Dev* 1992;6:329.

152. Gilbert DM, Losson R, Chambon P. Ligand dependence of estrogen receptor induced changes in chromatin structure. *Nucleic Acids Res* 1992;20:4525.

153. Pina B, Hache RJ, Arnemann J, et al. Hormonal induction of transfected genes depends on DNA topology. *Mol Cell Biol* 1990;10:625.

154. Schrader M, Muller KM, Nayeri S, et al. Vitamin D3-thyroid hormone receptor heterodimer polarity directs ligand sensitivity of transactivation. *Nature* 1994;370:382.

155. Schrader M, Carlberg C. Thyroid hormone and retinoic acid receptors form heterodimers with retinoid X receptors on direct repeats, palindromes, and inverted palindromes. *DNA Cell Biol* 1994;13:333.

156. Mader S, Leroy P, Chen JY, et al. Multiple parameters control the selectivity of nuclear receptors for their response elements. Selectivity and promiscuity in response element recognition by retinoic acid receptors and retinoid X receptors. *J Biol Chem* 1993;268:591.

157. Moudgil VK. Phosphorylation of steroid hormone receptors. *Biochim Biophys Acta* 1990;1055:243.

158. Auricchio F. Phosphorylation of steroid receptors. *J Steroid Biochem* 1989;32:613.

159. Weigel NL, Tash JS, Means AR, et al. Phosphorylation of hen progesterone receptor by cAMP-dependent protein kinase. *Biochem Biophys Res Commun* 1981;102:513.

160. Denton RR, Koszewski NJ, Notides AC. Estrogen receptor phosphorylation. Hormonal dependence and consequence on specific DNA binding. *J Biol Chem* 1992;267:7263.

161. Migliaccio A, Di Domenico M, Green S, et al. Phosphorylation on tyrosine of *in vitro* synthesized human estrogen receptor activates its hormone binding. *Mol Endocrinol* 1989;3:1061.

162. Nordeen SK, Moyer ML, Bona BJ. The coupling of multiple signal transduction pathways with steroid response mechanisms. *Endocrinology* 1994;134:1723.

163. Truss M, Beato M. Steroid hormone receptors: interaction with deoxyribonucleic acid and transcription factors. *Endocr Rev* 1993;14:459.

164. Tesarik J, Moos J, Mendoza C. Stimulation of protein tyrosine phosphorylation by a progesterone receptor on the cell surface of human sperm. *Endocrinology* 1993;133:328.

165. Rigaud G, Roux J, Pictet R, et al. *In vivo* footprinting of rat TAT gene: dynamic interplay between the glucocorticoid receptor and a liver-specific factor. *Cell* 1991;67:977.

166. Schule R, Muller M, Kaltschmidt C, et al. Many transcription factors interact synergistically with steroid receptors. *Science* 1988;242:1418.

167. Diamond MI, Miner JN, Yoshinaga SK, et al. Transcription factor interactions: selectors of positive or negative regulation from a single DNA element. *Science* 1990;249:1266.

168. Weisz A, Rosales R. Identification of an estrogen response element upstream of the human c-*fos* gene that binds the estrogen receptor and the AP-1 transcription factor. *Nucleic Acids Res* 1990;18:5097.

169. Fuqua SA, Chamness GC, McGuire WL. Estrogen receptor mutations in breast cancer. *J Cell Biochem* 1993;51:135.

170. Landers JP, Spelsberg TC. New concepts in steroid hormone action: transcription factors, proto-oncogenes, and the cascade model for steroid regulation of gene expression. *Crit Rev Eukaryot Gene Expr* 1992;2:19.

171. Rossini GP. The quaternary structures of untransformed steroid hormone receptors: an open issue. *J Theor Biol* 1994;166:339.

172. Pratt WB, Welsh MJ. Chaperone functions of the heat shock proteins associated with steroid receptors. *Semin Cell Biol* 1994; 5:83.

173. Bresnick EH, Dalman FC, Sanchez ER, et al. Evidence that the 90-kDa heat-shock protein is necessary for the steroid binding conformation of the L-cell glucocorticoid receptor. *J Biol Chem* 1989;264:4992.

174. Smith DF. Dynamics of heat-shock protein 90-progesterone receptor binding and the disactivation loop model for steroid receptor complexes. *Mol Endocrinol* 1993;7:1418.

175. Hutchison KA, Dittmar KD, Czar MJ, et al. Proof that hsp70 is required for assembly of the glucocorticoid receptor into a heterocomplex with hsp90. *J Biol Chem* 1994;269:5043.

176. Prendergast P, Onate SA, Christensen K, et al. Nuclear accessory factors enhance the binding of progesterone receptor to specific target DNA. *J Steroid Biochem Mol Biol* 1994;48:1.

177. Landers JP, Subramaniam M, Gosse B, et al. The ubiquitous nature of the progesterone receptor binding factor-1 (RBF-1) in avian tissues. *J Cell Biochem* 1994;55:241.

178. Onate SA, Prendergast P, Wagner JP, et al. The DNA-binding protein HMG-1 enhances progesterone receptor binding to its target DNA sequences. *Mol Cell Biol* 1994;14:3376.

179. Renoir JM, Pahl A, Keller U, et al. Immunological identification of a 50 kDa Mr FK506-binding immunophilin as a component of the non-DNA binding, hsp90 and hsp70 containing, hetero-oligomeric form of the chick oviduct progesterone receptor. *C R Acad Sci III* 1993;316:1410.

180. Leff SE, Rosenfeld MG, Evans RM. Complex transcriptional units: diversity in gene expression by alternative RNA processing. *Annu Rev Biochem* 1986;55:1091.

181. Lambowitz AM, Belfort M. Introns as mobile genetic elements. *Annu Rev Biochem* 1993;62:587.

182. Szekely M. The structure of mRNA. From DNA to protein: the transfer of genetic information. New York: John Wiley and Sons, 1980:149.

183. Sonenberg N. Poliovirus translation. *Curr Top Microbiol Immunol* 1990;161:23.

184. Shatkin AJ. Capping of eucaryotic mRNAs. *Cell* 1976;9:645.

185. Wei CM, Moss B. Methylated nucleotides block 5'-terminus of *vaccinia* virus messenger RNA. *Proc Natl Acad Sci U S A* 1975;72:318.

186. Perry RP, Kelley DE. Kinetics of formation of 5' terminal caps in mRNA. *Cell* 1976;8:433.

187. Moss B, Gershowitz A, Wei CM, et al. Formation of the guanylylated and methylated 5'-terminus of *vaccinia* virus mRNA. *Virology* 1976;72:341.

188. Peltz SW, Brewer G, Bernstein P, et al. Regulation of mRNA turnover in eukaryotic cells. *Crit Rev Eukaryot Gene Expr* 1991; 1:99.

189. Peltz SW, Brewer G, Kobs G, et al. Substrate specificity of the exonuclease activity that degrades H4 histone mRNA. *J Biol Chem* 1987;262:9382.

190. Stevens A, Maupin MK. A 5'–3' exoribonuclease of *Saccharomyces cerevisiae*: size and novel substrate specificity. *Arch Biochem Biophys* 1987;252:339.

191. Sachs AB. Messenger RNA degradation in eukaryotes. *Cell* 1993;74:413.

192. Rhoads RE. Regulation of eukaryotic protein synthesis by initiation factors. *J Biol Chem* 1993;268:3017.

193. Pantopoulos K, Johansson HE, Hentze MW. The role of the 5' untranslated region of eukaryotic messenger RNAs in translation and its investigation using antisense technologies. *Prog Nucleic Acid Res Mol Biol* 1994;48:181.

194. Hamm J, Mattaj IW. Monomethylated cap structures facilitate RNA export from the nucleus. *Cell* 1990;63:109.

195. Rose JK, Lodish HF. Translation *in vitro* of vesicular stomatitis virus mRNA lacking 5'-terminal 7-methylguanosine. *Nature* 1976;262:32.

196. Hodges D, Bernstein SI. Genetic and biochemical analysis of alternative RNA splicing. *Adv Genet* 1994;31:207.

197. Das A. Control of transcription termination by RNA-binding proteins. *Annu Rev Biochem* 1993;62:893.

198. Birnstiel ML, Busslinger M, Strub K. Transcription termination and 3' processing: the end is in site! *Cell* 1985;41:349.

199. Manley JL, Yu H, Ryner L. RNA sequence containing hexanucleotide AAUAAA directs efficient mRNA polyadenylation *in vitro*. *Mol Cell Biol* 1985;5:373.

200. Zarkower D, Stephenson P, Sheets M, Wickens M. The AAUAAA sequence is required both for cleavage and for polyadenylation of simian virus 40 pre-mRNA *in vitro*. *Mol Cell Biol* 1986; 6:2317.

201. Jacob ST, Terns MP, Hengst-Zhang JA, et al. Polyadenylation of mRNA and its control. *Crit Rev Eukaryot Gene Expr* 1990; 1:49.

202. Wahle E. The end of the message: 3'-end processing leading to polyadenylated messenger RNA. *BioEssays* 1992;14:113.

203. Fitzgerald M, Shenk T. The sequence 5'-AAUAAA-3‡ forms parts of the recognition site for polyadenylation of late SV40 mRNAs. *Cell* 1981;24:251.

204. Sheets MD, Wickens M. Two phases in the addition of a poly(A) tail. *Genes Dev* 1989;3:1401.

205. McDevitt MA, Hart RP, Wong WW, et al. Sequences capable of restoring poly(A) site function define two distinct downstream elements. *EMBO J* 1986;5:2907.

206. Gil A, Proudfoot NJ. Position-dependent sequence elements downstream of AAUAAA are required for efficient rabbit beta-globin mRNA 3' end formation. *Cell* 1987;49:399.

207. Wahle E. Purification and characterization of a mammalian polyadenylate polymerase involved in the 3' end processing of messenger RNA precursors. *J Biol Chem* 1991;266:3131.

208. Gilmartin GM, Nevins JR. Molecular analyses of two poly(A) site-processing factors that determine the recognition and efficiency of cleavage of the pre-mRNA. *Mol Cell Biol* 1991;11: 2432.

209. Christofori G, Keller W. 3' cleavage and polyadenylation of mRNA precursors *in vitro* requires a poly(A) polymerase, a cleavage factor, and a snRNP. *Cell* 1988;54:875.

210. Denome RM, Cole CN. Patterns of polyadenylation site selection in gene constructs containing multiple polyadenylation signals. *Mol Cell Biol* 1988;8:4829.

211. Hook AG, Kellems RE. Localization and sequence analysis of poly(A) sites generating multiple dihydrofolate reductase mRNAs. *J Biol Chem* 1988;263:2337.

212. Helfman DM, Cheley S, Kuismanen E, et al. Nonmuscle and muscle tropomyosin isoforms are expressed from a single gene by alternative RNA splicing and polyadenylation. *Mol Cell Biol* 1986;6:3582.

213. Alt FW, Bothwell AL, Knapp M, et al. Synthesis of secreted and membrane-bound immunoglobulin mu heavy chains is directed by mRNAs that differ at their 3' ends. *Cell* 1980;20:293.

214. Danner D, Leder P. Role of an RNA cleavage/poly(A) addition site in the production of membrane-bound and secreted IgM mRNA. *Proc Natl Acad Sci U S A* 1985;82:8658.

215. Amara SG, Jonas V, Rosenfeld MG, et al. Alternative RNA processing in calcitonin gene expression generates mRNAs encoding different polypeptide products. *Nature* 1982;298:240.

216. Bovenberg RA, Adema GJ, Jansz HS, et al. Model for tissue-specific calcitonin/CGRP-I RNA processing from *in vitro* experiments. *Nucleic Acids Res* 1988;16:7867.

217. Brady HA, Wold WS. Competition between splicing and polyadenylation reactions determines which adenovirus region E3 mRNAs are synthesized. *Mol Cell Biol* 1988;8:3291.

218. Padgett RA, Grabowski PJ, Konarska MM, et al. Splicing of messenger RNA precursors. *Annu Rev Biochem* 1986;55:1119.
219. Green MR. Pre-mRNA splicing. *Annu Rev Genet* 1986;20:671.
220. Sharp PA. Splicing of messenger RNA precursors [published erratum appears in *Science* 1987;237(4818):964]. *Science* 1987;235:766.
221. Naora H, Deacon NJ. Relationship between the total size of exons and introns in protein-coding genes of higher eukaryotes. *Proc Natl Acad Sci U S A* 1982;79:6196.
222. Busch H, Reddy R, Rothblum L, et al. SnRNAs, SnRNPs, and RNA processing. *Annu Rev Biochem* 1982;51:617.
223. Guthrie C, Patterson B. Spliceosomal snRNAs. *Annu Rev Genet* 1988;22:387.
224. Guthrie C. Messenger RNA splicing in yeast: clues to why the spliceosome is a ribonucleoprotein. *Science* 1991;253:157.
225. Krainer AR, Conway GC, Kozak D. Purification and characterization of pre-mRNA splicing factor SF2 from HeLa cells. *Genes Dev* 1990;4:1158.
226. Ge H, Manley JL. A protein factor, ASF, controls cell-specific alternative splicing of SV40 early pre-mRNA *in vitro. Cell* 1990;62:25.
227. Green MR. Biochemical mechanisms of constitutive and regulated pre-mRNA splicing. *Annu Rev Cell Biol* 1991;7:559.
228. Moore MJ, Query CC, Sharp PA. In the RNA World. New York: Cold Spring Harbor Laboratory Press, 1993:303.
229. Hardy SF, Grabowski PJ, Padgett RA, et al. Cofactor requirements of splicing of purified messenger RNA precursors. *Nature* 1984;308:375.
230. Padgett RA, Konarska MM, Grabowski PJ, et al. Lariat RNAs as intermediates and products in the splicing of messenger RNA precursors. *Science* 1984;225:898.
231. Ruskin B, Krainer AR, Maniatis T, et al. Excision of an intact intron as a novel lariat structure during pre-mRNA splicing *in vitro. Cell* 1984;38:317.
232. Mount SM, Pettersson I, Hinterberger M, et al. The U1 small nuclear RNA-protein complex selectively binds a 5′ splice site *in vitro. Cell* 1983;33:509.
233. Zhuang Y, Weiner AM. A compensatory base change in U1 snRNA suppresses a 5′ splice site mutation. *Cell* 1986;46:827.
234. King CR, Piatigorsky J. Alternative RNA splicing of the murine alpha A-crystallin gene: protein-coding information within an intron. *Cell* 1983;32:707.
235. Mount SM. A catalogue of splice junction sequences. *Nucleic Acids Res* 1982;10:459.
236. Montell C, Fisher EF, Caruthers MH, et al. Resolving the functions of overlapping viral genes by site-specific mutagenesis at a mRNA splice site. *Nature* 1982;295:380.
237. Wieringa B, Meyer F, Reiser J, et al. Unusual splice sites revealed by mutagenic inactivation of an authentic splice site of the rabbit beta-globin gene. *Nature* 1983;301:38.
238. Treisman R, Proudfoot NJ, Shander M, et al. A single-base change at a splice site in a beta 0-thalassemic gene causes abnormal RNA splicing. *Cell* 1982;29:903.
239. Orkin SH, Kazazian HHJ, Antonarakis SE, et al. Abnormal RNA processing due to the exon mutation of beta E-globin gene. *Nature* 1982;300:768.
240. Nelson KK, Green MR. Mechanism for cryptic splice site activation during pre-mRNA splicing. *Proc Natl Acad Sci U S A* 1990;87:6253.
241. Chabot B, Black DL, LeMaster DM, et al. The 3′ splice site of pre-messenger RNA is recognized by a small nuclear ribonucleoprotein. *Science* 1985;230:1344.
242. Seraphin B, Rosbash M. The yeast branchpoint sequence is not required for the formation of a stable U1 snRNA-pre-mRNA complex and is recognized in the absence of U2 snRNA. *EMBO J* 1991;10:1209.
243. Zillmann M, Rose SD, Berget SM. U1 small nuclear ribonucleoproteins are required early during spliceosome assembly. *Mol Cell Biol* 1987;7:2877.
244. Reed R, Maniatis T. Intron sequences involved in lariat formation during pre-mRNA splicing. *Cell* 1985;41:95.
245. Black DL, Chabot B, Steitz JA. U2 as well as U1 small nuclear ribonucleoproteins are involved in pre-messenger RNA splicing. *Cell* 1985;42:737.
246. Keller EB, Noon WA. Intron splicing: a conserved internal signal in introns of animal pre-mRNAs. *Proc Natl Acad Sci U S A* 1984;81:7417.
247. Ruskin B, Greene JM, Green MR. Cryptic branch point activation allows accurate *in vitro* splicing of human beta-globin intron mutants. *Cell* 1985;41:833.
248. Breitbart RE, Andreadis A, Nadal-Ginard B. Alternative splicing: a ubiquitous mechanism for the generation of multiple protein isoforms from single genes. *Annu Rev Biochem* 1987;56:467.
249. Higgins CF, Peltz SW, Jacobson A. Turnover of mRNA in prokaryotes and lower eukaryotes. *Curr Opin Genet Dev* 1992;2:739.
250. Lindahl L, Hinnebusch A. Diversity of mechanisms in the regulation of translation in prokaryotes and lower eukaryotes. *Curr Opin Genet Dev* 1992;2:720.
251. Chao FC. Dissociation of macromolecular ribonucleoprotein of yeast. *Arch Biochem Biophys* 1957;70:426.
252. Tissieres A, Watson JD. Ribonuleoprotein particles from *E. coli. Nature* 1957;182:778.
253. Noll M, Hapke B, Noll H. Structural dynamics of bacterial ribosomes. II. Preparation and characterization of ribosomes and subunits active in the translation of natural messenger RNA. *J Mol Biol* 1973;80:519.
254. Nierhaus KH. Structure, assembly, and function of ribosomes. *Curr Top Microbiol Immunol* 1982;97:81.
255. Spirin AS, Ajtkhozhin MA. Informosomes and polyribosome-associated proteins in eukaryotes. *Trends Biochem Sci* 1985;10:162.
256. Wool IG. The structure and function of eukaryotic ribosomes. *Annu Rev Biochem* 1979;48:719.
257. Monk RJ, Meyuhas O, Perry RP. Mammals have multiple genes for individual ribosomal proteins. *Cell* 1981;24:301.
258. Nomura M, Morgan EA. Genetics of bacterial ribosomes. *Annu Rev Genet* 1977;11:297.
259. Long EO, Dawid IB. Repeated genes in eukaryotes. *Annu Rev Biochem* 1980;49:727.
260. Perry RP. Processing of RNA. *Annu Rev Biochem* 1976;45:605.
261. Gegenheimer P, Apirion D. Processing of procaryotic ribonucleic acid. *Microbiol Rev* 1981;45:502.
262. Schwarz Z, Kossel H. The primary structure of 16s rDNA from Zea mays chloroplast is homologous to *E. coli* 16s rRNA. *Nature* 1980;283:739.
263. Tohdoh N, Sugiura M. The complete nucleotide sequence of 16S ribosomal RNA gene from tobacco chloroplasts. *Gene* 1982;17:213.
264. Edwards K, Kossel H. The rRNA operon from Zea mays chloroplasts: nucleotide sequence of 23S rDNA and its homology with *E. coli* 23S rDNA. *Nucleic Acids Res* 1981;9:2853.
265. Takaiwa F, Sugiura M. The complete nucleotide sequence of a 23S rRNA gene from tobacco chloroplasts. *Eur J Biochem* 1982;124:13.
266. Hagenbuchle O, Santer M, Steitz JA, et al. Conservation of the primary structure at the 3′ end of 18S rRNA from eucaryotic cells. *Cell* 1978;13:551.
267. Salim M, Maden BE. Nucleotide sequence of Xenopus laevis 18S ribosomal RNA inferred from gene sequence. *Nature* 1981;291:205.

268. Samols DR, Hagenbuchle O, Gage LP. Homology of the 3′ terminal sequences of the 18S rRNA of *Bombyx mori* and the 16S rRNA of *Escherichia coli*. *Nucleic Acids Res* 1979;7:1109.

269. Van Charldorp R, Van Knippenberg PH. Sequence, modified nucleotides and secondary structure at the 3′-end of small ribosomal subunit RNA. *Nucleic Acids Res* 1982;10:1149.

270. Maitra U, Stringer EA, Chaudhuri A. Initiation factors in protein biosynthesis. *Annu Rev Biochem* 1982;51:869.

271. Kozak M. Regulation of translation in eukaryotic systems. *Annu Rev Cell Biol* 1992;8:197.

272. Hershey JW. Translational control in mammalian cells. *Annu Rev Biochem* 1991;60:717.

273. Davis BD. Role of subunits in the ribosome cycle. *Nature* 1971;231:153.

274. Noll M, Hapke B, Schreier MH, et al. Structural dynamics of bacterial ribosomes. I. Characterization of vacant couples and their relation to complexed ribosomes. *J Mol Biol* 1973;75:281.

275. Naaktgeboren N, Roobol K, Voorma HO. The effect of initiation factor IF-1 on the dissociation of 70-S ribosomes of *Escherichia coli*. *Eur J Biochem* 1977;72:49.

276. Grunberg-Manago M, Dessen P, Pantaloni D, et al. Light-scattering studies showing the effect of initiation factors on the reversible dissociation of *Escherichia coli* ribosomes. *J Mol Biol* 1975;94:461.

277. Thibault J, Chestier A, Vidal D, et al. Interaction of the radioactive translation initiation factor IF3 with ribosomes. *Biochimie* 1972;54:829.

278. Sabol S, Ochoa S. Ribosomal binding of labelled initiation factor F3. *Nature New Biol* 1971;234:233.

279. Pon CL, Friedman SM, Gualerzi C. Studies on the interaction between ribosomes and 14 CH 3-F3 initiation factor. *Mol Gen Genet* 1972;116:192.

280. Lockwood AH, Sarkar P, Maitra U. Release of polypeptide chain initiation factor IF-2 during initiation complex formation. *Proc Natl Acad Sci U S A* 1972;69:3602.

281. Fakunding JL, Hershey JW. The interaction of radioactive initiation factor IF-2 with ribosomes during initiation of protein synthesis. *J Biol Chem* 1973;248:4206.

282. Vermeer C, Boon J, Talens A, et al. Binding of the initiation factor IF-3 to *Escherichia coli* ribosomes and MS2 RNA. *Eur J Biochem* 1973;40:283.

283. Vermeer C, Kievit RJ, Alphen WJ, et al. Recycling of the initiation factor IF-3 on 30 S ribosomal subunits of *E. coli*. *FEBS Lett* 1973;31:273.

284. Baan RA, Duijfjes JJ, van Leerdam E, et al. Specific *in situ* cleavage of 16S ribosomal RNA of *Escherichia coli* interferes with the function of initiation factor IF-1. *Proc Natl Acad Sci U S A* 1976;73:702.

285. Langberg S, Kahan L, Traut RR, et al. Binding of protein synthesis initiation factor IF1 to 30S ribosomal subunits: effects of other initiation factors and identification of proteins near the binding site. *J Mol Biol* 1977;117:307.

286. van Duin J, Kurland CG, Dondon J, et al. Near neighbors of IF3 bound to 30S ribosomal subunits. *FEBS Lett* 1975;59:287.

287. Czernilofsky AP, Kurland CG, Stoffler G. 30S ribosomal proteins associated with the 3′-terminus of 16S RNA. *FEBS Lett* 1975;58:281.

288. Dubnoff JS, Lockwood AH, Maitra U. Studies on the role of guanosine triphosphate in polypeptide chain initiation in *Escherichia coli*. *J Biol Chem* 1972;247:2884.

289. Mazumder R. Initiation factor 2-dependent ribosomal binding of N-formylmethionyl-transfer RNA without added guanosine triphosphate. *Proc Natl Acad Sci U S A* 1972;69:2770.

290. Hershey JW, Dewey KF, Thach RE. Purification and properties of initiation factor f-1. *Nature* 1969;222:944.

291. Jay G, Kaempfer R. Initiation of protein synthesis. Binding of messenger RNA. *J Biol Chem* 1975;250:5742.

292. Steitz JA. *Biological Regulation and Control.* New York, Plenum, 1978:349.

293. Shine J, Dalgarno L. The 3′-terminal sequence of *Escherichia coli* 16S ribosomal RNA: complementary to nonsense triplets and ribosome binding sites. *Proc Natl Acad Sci U S A* 1974;71:1342.

294. Steitz JA. RNA-RNA interactions during polypeptide chain initiation. In: Chambliss G, Craven GR, Davies J, et al., eds. Ribosomes: structure, function and genetics. Baltimore: University Park Press, 1980:479.

295. Gold L, Pribnow D, Schneider T, et al. Translational initiation in prokaryotes. *Annu Rev Microbiol* 1981;35:365.

296. Yanofsky C, Platt T, Crawford IP, et al. The complete nucleotide sequence of the tryptophan operon of *Escherichia coli*. *Nucleic Acids Res* 1981;9:6647.

297. Pauza CD, Karels MJ, Navre M, et al. Genes encoding *Escherichia coli* aspartate transcarbamoylase: the pyrB-pyrI operon. *Proc Natl Acad Sci U S A* 1982;79:4020.

298. Post LE, Nomura M. DNA sequences from the *str* operon of *Escherichia coli*. *J Biol Chem* 1980;255:4660.

299. Stroynowski I, van Cleemput M, Yanofsky C. Superattenuation in the tryptophan operon of Serratia marcescens. *Nature* 1982;298:38.

300. Stormo GD, Schneider TD, Gold LM. Characterization of translational initiation sites in *E. coli*. *Nucleic Acids Res* 1982;10:2971.

301. Gheysen D, Iserentant D, Derom C, et al. Systematic alteration of the nucleotide sequence preceding the translation initiation codon and the effects on bacterial expression of the cloned SV40 small-T antigen gene. *Gene* 1982;17:55.

302. Roberts TM, Bikel I, Yocum RR, et al. Synthesis of simian virus 40 T antigen in *Escherichia coli*. *Proc Natl Acad Sci U S A* 1979;76:5596.

303. Sundari RM, Pelka H, Schulman LH. Structural requirements of *Escherichia coli* formylmethionyl transfer ribonucleic acid for ribosome binding and initiation of protein synthesis. *J Biol Chem* 1977;252:3941.

304. Ohlmann T, Rau M, Morley SJ, et al. Proteolytic cleavage of initiation factor eIF-4 gamma in the reticulocyte lysate inhibits translation of capped mRNAs but enhances that of uncapped mRNAs. *Nucleic Acids Res* 1995;23:334.

305. Gunnery S, Mathews MB. Functional mRNA can be generated by RNA polymerase III. *Mol Cell Biol* 1995;15:3597.

306. Merrick WC. Mechanism and regulation of eukaryotic protein synthesis. *Microbiol Rev* 1992;56:291.

307. Raychaudhuri P, Stringer EA, Valenzuela DM, et al. Ribosomal subunit antiassociation activity in rabbit reticulocyte lysates. Evidence for a low molecular weight ribosomal subunit antiassociation protein factor (Mr = 25,000). *J Biol Chem* 1984;259:11930.

308. Russell DW, Spremulli LL. Purification and characterization of a ribosome dissociation factor (eukaryotic initiation factor 6) from wheat germ. *J Biol Chem* 1979;254:8796.

309. Peterson DT, Safer B, Merrick WC. Role of eukaryotic initiation factor 5 in the formation of 80 S initiation complexes. *J Biol Chem* 1979;254:7730.

310. Trachsel H, Erni B, Schreier MH, et al. Initiation of mammalian protein synthesis. II. The assembly of the initiation complex with purified initiation factors. *J Mol Biol* 1977;116:755.

311. Benne R, Hershey JW. The mechanism of action of protein synthesis initiation factors from rabbit reticulocytes. *J Biol Chem* 1978;253:3078.

312. Panniers R, Rowlands AG, Henshaw EC. The effect of Mg2 + and guanine nucleotide exchange factor on the binding of gua-

nine nucleotides to eukaryotic initiation factor 2. *J Biol Chem* 1988;263:5519.

313. Edery I, Pelletier J, Sonenberg J. Role of eukaryotic messenger RNA cap-binding protein in regulation of translation. In: Ilan J, ed. Translational regulation of gene expansion. New York: Plenum, 1987:335.

314. Rhoads RE, Hiremath LS, Rychlik W, et al. The messenger RNA cap binding protein. In: Smuckler EA, Clawson GA, eds. Nuclear envelope structure and RNA maturation. New York: Alan R. Liss, Inc., 1985:427.

315. Sonenberg N. Cap-binding proteins of eukaryotic messenger RNA: functions in initiation and control of translation. *Prog Nucleic Acid Res Mol Biol* 1988;35:173.

316. Lamphear BJ, Kirchweger R, Skern T, et al. Mapping of functional domains in eukaryotic protein synthesis initiation factor 4G (eIF4G) with picornaviral proteases. Implications for cap-dependent and cap-independent translational initiation. *J Biol Chem* 1995;270:21975.

317. Mader S, Lee H, Pause A, et al. The translation initiation factor eIF-4E binds to a common motif shared by the translation factor eIF-4 gamma and the translational repressors 4E-binding proteins. *Mol Cell Biol* 1995;15:4990.

318. Ohlmann T, Rau M, Pain VM, et al. The C-terminal domain of eukaryotic protein synthesis initiation factor (eIF) 4G is sufficient to support cap-independent translation in the absence of eIF4E. *EMBO J* 1996;15:1371.

319. Joshi B, Yan R, Rhoads RE. *In vitro* synthesis of human protein synthesis initiation factor 4 gamma and its localization on 43 and 48 S initiation complexes. *J Biol Chem* 1994;269:2048.

320. Jaramillo M, Dever TE, Merrick WC, et al. RNA unwinding in translation: assembly of helicase complex intermediates comprising eukaryotic initiation factors eIF-4F and eIF-4B. *Mol Cell Biol* 1991;11:5992.

321. Abramson RD, Dever TE, Merrick WC. Biochemical evidence supporting a mechanism for cap-independent and internal initiation of eukaryotic mRNA. *J Biol Chem* 1988;263:6016.

322. Lawson TG, Lee KA, Maimone MM, et al. Dissociation of double-stranded polynucleotide helical structures by eukaryotic initiation factors, as revealed by a novel assay. *Biochemistry* 1989; 28:4729.

323. Rozen F, Edery I, Meerovitch K, et al. Bidirectional RNA helicase activity of eucaryotic translation initiation factors 4A and 4F. *Mol Cell Biol* 1990;10:1134.

324. Milburn SC, Hershey JW, Davies MV, et al. Cloning and expression of eukaryotic initiation factor 4B cDNA: sequence determination identifies a common RNA recognition motif. *EMBO J* 1990;9:2783.

325. Jones RM, Branda J, Johnston KA, et al. An essential E box in the promoter of the gene encoding the mRNA cap-binding protein (eukaryotic initiation factor 4E) is a target for activation by c-myc. *Mol Cell Biol* 1996;16:4754.

326. Lazaris-Karatzas A, Montine KS, Sonenberg N. Malignant transformation by a eukaryotic initiation factor subunit that binds to mRNA 5′ cap. *Nature* 1990;345:544.

327. Joshi B, Cai AL, Keiper BD, et al. Phosphorylation of eukaryotic protein synthesis initiation factor 4E at Ser-209. *J Biol Chem* 1995;270:14597.

328. Whalen SG, Gingras AC, Amankwa L, et al. Phosphorylation of eIF-4E on serine 209 by protein kinase C is inhibited by the translational repressors, 4E-binding proteins. *J Biol Chem* 1996; 271:11831.

329. Joshi-Barve S, Rychlik W, Rhoads RE. Alteration of the major phosphorylation site of eukaryotic protein synthesis initiation factor 4E prevents its association with the 48 S initiation complex. *J Biol Chem* 1990;265:2979.

330. Sonenberg N. mRNA 5′ cap-binding protein eIF4E and control of cell growth. In: Hershey WB, Matthews M, Sonenberg N, eds. Translational Control. New York: Cold Spring Harbor Laboratory Press, 1996:245.

331. Pause A, Belsham GJ, Gingras AC, et al. Insulin-dependent stimulation of protein synthesis by phosphorylation of a regulator of 5′-cap function. *Nature* 1994;371:762.

332. Haghighat A, Mader S, Pause A, et al. Repression of cap-dependent translation by 4E-binding protein 1: competition with p220 for binding to eukaryotic initiation factor 4E. *EMBO J* 1995;14:5701.

333. Altmann M, Schmitz N, Berset C, et al. A novel inhibitor of cap-dependent translation initiation in yeast: p20 competes with eIF4G for binding to eIF4E. *EMBO J* 1997;16:1114.

334. Marcotrigiano J, Gingras AC, Burley SK. Cocrystal structure of the messenger RNA 5′ cap-binding protein (eIF4E) bound to 7-methyl-GDP. *Cell* 1997;89:951.

335. Jackson RJ, Kaminski A. Internal initiation of translation in eukaryotes: the picornavirus paradigm and beyond. *RNA* 1995; 1:985.

336. Tsukiyama-Kohara K, Iizuka N, Kohara M, et al. Internal ribosome entry site within hepatitis C virus RNA. *J Virol* 1992;66:1476.

337. Wang C, Sarnow P, Siddiqui A. Translation of human hepatitis C virus RNA in cultured cells is mediated by an internal ribosome-binding mechanism. *J Virol* 1993;67:3338.

338. Iizuka N, Chen C, Yang Q, et al. Cap-independent translation and internal initiation of translation in eukaryotic cellular mRNA molecules. *Curr Top Microbiol Immunol* 1995;203:155.

339. Macejak DG, Sarnow P. Internal initiation of translation mediated by the 5′ leader of a cellular mRNA. *Nature* 1991;353:90.

340. Oh SK, Scott MP, Sarnow P. Homeotic gene Antennapedia mRNA contains 5′-noncoding sequences that confer translational initiation by internal ribosome binding. *Genes Dev* 1992; 6:1643.

341. Vagner S, Gensac MC, Maret A, et al. Alternative translation of human fibroblast growth factor 2 mRNA occurs by internal entry of ribosomes. *Mol Cell Biol* 1995;15:35.

342. Gan W, Rhoads RE. Internal initiation of translation directed by the 5′-untranslated region of the mRNA for eIF4G, a factor involved in the picornavirus-induced switch from cap-dependent to internal initiation. *J Biol Chem* 1996;271:623.

343. Sachs AB and Sarrow P. Starting at the beginning, middle, and end: translation initiation in eukaryotes. *Cell* 1997;89:831.

344. Kozak M. How do eucaryotic ribosomes select initiation regions in messenger RNA? *Cell* 1978;15:1109.

345. Kozak M. Evaluation of the scanning model for initiation of protein synthesis in eucaryotes. *Cell* 1980;22:7.

346. Kozak M. Mechanism of mRNA recognition by eukaryotic ribosomes during initiation of protein synthesis. *Curr Top Microbiol Immunol* 1981;93:81.

347. Kozak M. Possible role of flanking nucleotides in recognition of the AUG initiator codon by eukaryotic ribosomes. *Nucleic Acids Res* 1981;9:5233.

348. Raychaudhuri P, Chaudhuri A, Maitra U. Formation and release of eukaryotic initiation factor 2 X GDP complex during eukaryotic ribosomal polypeptide chain initiation complex formation. *J Biol Chem* 1985;260:2140.

349. Brown-Luedi ML, Meyer LJ, Milburn SC, et al. Protein synthesis initiation factors from human HeLa cells and rabbit reticulocytes are similar: comparison of protein structure, activities, and immunochemical properties. *Biochemistry* 1982;21:4202.

350. Merrick WC, Kemper WM, Anderson WF. Purification and characterization of homogeneous initiation factor M2A from rabbit reticulocytes. *J Biol Chem* 1975;250:5556.

351. Schreier MH, Erni B, Staehelin T. Initiation of mammalian

protein synthesis. I. Purification and characterization of seven initiation factors. *J Mol Biol* 1977;116:727.

352. Pestka S. Studies on the formation of transfer ribonucleic acid-ribosome complexes. VI. Oligopeptide synthesis and translocation on ribosomes in the presence and absence of soluble transfer factors. *J Biol Chem* 1969;244:1533.

353. Gavrilova LP, Kostiashkina OE, Koteliansky VE, et al. Factor-free (non-enzymic) and factor-dependent systems of translation of polyuridylic acid by *Escherichia coli* ribosomes. *J Mol Biol* 1976;101:537.

354. Wilson KS, Noller HF. Molecular movement inside the translation engine. *Cell* 1998;92:337.

355. Ofengand J, Ciesiolka J, Denman R, et al. Structural and functional interactions of the tRNA-ribosome complex. Structure, function, and genetics of ribosomes. New York: Springer-Verlag, 1986:473.

356. Rheinberger HJ, Sternbach H, Nierhaus KH. Three tRNA binding sites on *Escherichia coli* ribosomes. *Proc Natl Acad Sci U S A* 1981;78:5310.

357. Inoue-Yokosawa N, Ishikawa C, Kaziro Y. The role of guanosine triphosphate in translocation reaction catalyzed by elongation factor G. *J Biol Chem* 1974;249:4321.

358. Spirin AS. Ribosomal translocation: facts and models. *Prog Nucleic Acid Res Mol Biol* 1985;32:75.

359. Kaziro Y. The role of guanosine 5′-triphosphate in polypeptide chain elongation. *Biochim Biophys Acta* 1978;505:95.

360. Rodnina MV, Savelsbergh A, Katunin VI, et al. Hydrolysis of GTP by elongation factor G drives tRNA movement on the ribosome. *Nature* 1997;385:37.

361. Stark H, Rodnina MV, Rinke-Appel J, et al. Visualization of elongation factor Tu on the *Escherichia coli* ribosome. *Nature* 1997;389:403.

362. Neirhaus KH, Rheinberger HJ, Geigenmuller U, et al. Three tRNA binding sites involved in the ribosomal elongation cycle. In: Hardesty B, Kramer G, eds. Structure, function, and genetics of ribosomes. New York: Springer-Verlag, 1986:454.

363. Watson JD. The synthesis of proteins upon ribosomes. *Bull Soc Chim Biol* 1964;46:1399.

364. Baranov VI, Ryabova LA. Is the three-site model for the ribosomal elongation cycle sound? *Biochimie* 1988;70:259.

365. Craigen WJ, Caskey CT. The function, structure and regulation of *E. coli* peptide chain release factors. *Biochimie* 1987;69:1031.

366. Craigen WJ, Caskey CT. Expression of peptide chain release factor 2 requires high-efficiency frameshift. *Nature* 1986;322:273.

367. Curran JF, Yarus M. Use of tRNA suppressors to probe regulation of *Escherichia coli* release factor 2. *J Mol Biol* 1988;203:75.

368. Poole ES, Brown CM, Tate WP. The identity of the base following the stop codon determines the efficiency of *in vivo* translational termination in *Escherichia coli*. *EMBO J* 1995;14:151.

369. Curran JF. Analysis of effects of tRNA:message stability on frameshift frequency at the *Escherichia coli* RF2 programmed frameshift site. *Nucleic Acids Res* 1993;21:1837.

370. Beaudet AL, Caskey CT. Release factor translation of RNA phage terminator codons. *Nature* 1970;227:38.

371. Lang A, Friemert C, Gassen HG. On the role of the termination factor RF-2 and the 16S RNA in protein synthesis. *Eur J Biochem* 1989;180:547.

372. Weiss RB, Dunn DM, Dahlberg AE, et al. Reading frame switch caused by base-pair formation between the 3′ end of 16s and the mRNA during elongation of protein synthesis in *Escherichia coli*. *EMBO J* 1988;7:1503.

373. Tate WP, Beaudet AL, Caskey CT. Influence of guanine nucleotides and elongation factors on interaction of release factors with the ribosome. *Proc Natl Acad Sci U S A* 1973;70:2350.

374. Cavener DR, Ray SC. Eukaryotic start and stop translation sites. *Nucleic Acids Res* 1991;19:3185.

375. Brown CM, Stockwell PA, Trotman CN, et al. Sequence analysis suggests that tetra-nucleotides signal the termination of protein synthesis in eukaryotes. *Nucleic Acids Res* 1990;18:6339.

376. Romaniuk PJ, Lowary P, Wu HN, et al. RNA binding site of R17 coat protein. *Biochemistry* 1987;26:1563.

377. Thomas MS, Nomura M. Translational regulation of the L11 ribosomal protein operon of *Escherichia coli*: mutations that define the target site for repression by L1. *Nucleic Acids Res* 1987;15:3085.

378. Freedman LP, Zengel JM, Archer RH, et al. Autogenous control of the S10 ribosomal protein operon of *Escherichia coli*: genetic dissection of transcriptional and posttranscriptional regulation. *Proc Natl Acad Sci U S A* 1987;84:6516.

379. Nomura M, Yates JL, Dean D, et al. Feedback regulation of ribosomal protein gene expression in *Escherichia coli*: structural homology of ribosomal RNA and ribosomal protein MRNA. *Proc Natl Acad Sci U S A* 1980;77:7084.

380. Kearney KR, Nomura M. Secondary structure of the autoregulatory mRNA binding site of ribosomal protein L1. *Mol Gen Genet* 1987;210:60.

381. Fiil NP, Friesen JD, Downing WL, et al. Post-transcriptional regulatory mutants in a ribosomal protein-RNA polymerase operon of *E. coli*. *Cell* 1980;19:837.

382. Deckman IC, Draper DE. S4-alpha mRNA translation regulation complex. II. Secondary structures of the RNA regulatory site in the presence and absence of S4. *J Mol Biol* 1987;196:323.

383. Hayashi S, Murakami Y. Rapid and regulated degradation of ornithine decarboxylase. *Biochem J* 1995;306:1.

384. Atkins JF, Lewis JB, Anderson CW, et al. Enhanced differential synthesis of proteins in a mammalian cell-free system by addition of polyamines. *J Biol Chem* 1975;250:5688.

385. Rom E, Kahana C. Polyamines regulate the expression of ornithine decarboxylase antizyme *in vitro* by inducing ribosomal frame-shifting [published erratum appears in *Proc Natl Acad Sci U S A* 1994;91(19):9195]. *Proc Natl Acad Sci U S A* 1994;91:3959.

386. Matsufuji S, Matsufuji T, Miyazaki Y, et al. Autoregulatory frameshifting in decoding mammalian ornithine decarboxylase antizyme. *Cell* 1995;80:51.

387. Matsufuji S, Matsufuji T, Wills NM, et al. Reading two bases twice: mammalian antizyme frameshifting in yeast. *EMBO J* 1996;15:1360.

388. Wickner RB. Yeast virology. *FASEB J* 1989;3:2257.

389. Atkins JF, Weiss RB, Gesteland RF. Ribosome gymnastics—degree of difficulty 9.5, style 10.0. *Cell* 1990;62:413.

390. Moore R, Dixon M, Smith R, et al. Complete nucleotide sequence of a milk-transmitted mouse mammary tumor virus: two frameshift suppression events are required for translation of gag and pol. *J Virol* 1987;61:480.

391. Jacks T, Townsley K, Varmus HE, et al. Two efficient ribosomal frameshifting events are required for synthesis of mouse mammary tumor virus gag-related polyproteins. *Proc Natl Acad Sci U S A* 1987;84:4298.

392. Parkin NT, Chamorro M, Varmus HE. Human immunodeficiency virus type 1 gag-pol frameshifting is dependent on downstream mRNA secondary structure: demonstration by expression *in vivo*. *J Virol* 1992;66:5147.

393. Jacks T, Power MD, Masiarz FR, et al. Characterization of ribosomal frameshifting in HIV-1 gag-pol expression. *Nature* 1988;331:280.

394. Wilson W, Braddock M, Adams SE, et al. HIV expression strategies: ribosomal frameshifting is directed by a short se-

quence in both mammalian and yeast systems. *Cell* 1988;55:1159.

395. Rowlands AG, Panniers R, Henshaw EC. The catalytic mechanism of guanine nucleotide exchange factor action and competitive inhibition by phosphorylated eukaryotic initiation factor 2. *J Biol Chem* 1988;263:5526.

396. Caron JM, Jones AL, Rall LB, et al. Autoregulation of tubulin synthesis in enucleated cells. *Nature* 1985;317:648.

397. Caron JM, Jones AL, Kirschner MW. Autoregulation of tubulin synthesis in hepatocytes and fibroblasts. *J Cell Biol* 1985;101:1763.

398. Pittenger MF, Cleveland DW. Retention of autoregulatory control of tubulin synthesis in cytoplasts: demonstration of a cytoplasmic mechanism that regulates the level of tubulin expression. *J Cell Biol* 1985;101:1941.

399. Lau JT, Pittenger MF, Havercroft JC, et al. Reconstruction of tubulin gene regulation in cultured mammalian cells. *Ann N Y Acad Sci* 1986;466:75.

400. Yen TJ, Machlin PS, Cleveland DW. Autoregulated instability of beta-tubulin mRNAs by recognition of the nascent amino terminus of beta-tubulin. *Nature* 1988;334:580.

401. Yen TJ, Gay DA, Pachter JS, et al. Autoregulated changes in stability of polyribosome-bound beta-tubulin mRNAs are specified by the first 13 translated nucleotides. *Mol Cell Biol* 1988;8:1224.

402. Pachter JS, Yen TJ, Cleveland DW. Autoregulation of tubulin expression is achieved through specific degradation of polysomal tubulin mRNAs. *Cell* 1987;51:283.

403. Gay DA, Sisodia SS, Cleveland DW. Autoregulatory control of beta-tubulin mRNA stability is linked to translation elongation. *Proc Natl Acad Sci U S A* 1989;86:5763.

404. Crichton RR, Charloteaux-Wauters M. Iron transport and storage. *Eur J Biochem* 1987;164:485.

405. Maxfield FR, Yamashiro DJ. In: Steer CJ, Hanover JA, eds. Intracellular trafficking of protein. New York, Cambridge University Press, 1991.

406. Theil EC. Ferritin: structure, gene regulation, and cellular function in animals, plants, and microorganisms. *Annu Rev Biochem* 1987;56:289.

407. Hentze MW, Caughman SW, Rouault TA, et al. Identification of the iron-responsive element for the translational regulation of human ferritin mRNA. *Science* 1987;238:1570.

408. Casey JL, Hentze MW, Koeller DM, et al. Iron-responsive elements: regulatory RNA sequences that control mRNA levels and translation. *Science* 1988;240:924.

409. Koeller DM, Casey JL, Hentze MW, et al. A cytosolic protein binds to structural elements within the iron regulatory region of the transferrin receptor mRNA. *Proc Natl Acad Sci U S A* 1989;86:3574.

410. Mullner EW, Neupert B, Kuhn LC. A specific mRNA binding factor regulates the iron-dependent stability of cytoplasmic transferrin receptor mRNA. *Cell* 1989;58:373.

411. Hinnebusch AG. Mechanisms of gene regulation in the general control of amino acid biosynthesis in *Saccharomyces cerevisiae*. *Microbiol Rev* 1988;52:248.

412. Miller PF, Hinnebusch AG. Sequences that surround the stop codons of upstream open reading frames in GCN4 mRNA determine their distinct functions in translational control. *Genes Dev* 1989;3:1217.

413. Williams NP, Mueller PP, Hinnebusch AG. The positive regulatory function of the 5′-proximal open reading frames in GCN4 mRNA can be mimicked by heterologous, short coding sequences. *Mol Cell Biol* 1988;8:3827.

414. Abastado JP, Miller PF, Jackson BM, et al. Suppression of ribosomal reinitiation at upstream open reading frames in amino acid-starved cells forms the basis for GCN4 translational control. *Mol Cell Biol* 1991;11:486.

415. Loftfield RB, Vanderjagt D. The frequency of errors in protein biosynthesis. *Biochem J* 1972;128:1353.

416. Corsi AK, Schekman R. Mechanism of polypeptide translocation into the endoplasmic reticulum. *J Biol Chem* 1996;271:30299.

417. Ito K. Protein translocation genetics. *Adv Cell Mol Biol Membr Organelles* 1995;4:35.

418. Matlack KE, Mothes W, Rapoport TA. Protein translocation tunnel vision. *Cell* 1998;92:381.

419. Oliver J, Jungnickel B, Gorlich D, et al. The Sec61 complex is essential for the insertion of proteins into the membrane of the endoplasmic reticulum. *FEBS Lett* 1995;362:126.

420. Pilon M, Schekman R, Romisch K. Sec61p mediates export of a misfolded secretory protein from the endoplasmic reticulum to the cytosol for degradation. *EMBO J* 1997;16:4540.

421. Wiertz EJ, Tortorella D, Bogyo M, et al. Sec61-mediated transfer of a membrane protein from the endoplasmic reticulum to the proteasome for destruction. *Nature* 1996;384:432.

422. Crowley KS, Reinhart GD, Johnson AE. The signal sequence moves through a ribosomal tunnel into a noncytoplasmic aqueous environment at the ER membrane early in translocation. *Cell* 1993;73:1101.

423. Lodish HF. Transport of secretory and membrane glycoproteins from the rough endoplasmic reticulum to the Golgi. A rate-limiting step in protein maturation and secretion. *J Biol Chem* 1988;263:2107.

424. Sidman C. B lymphocyte differentiation and the control of IgM mu chain expression. *Cell* 1981;23:379.

425. Dulis BH, Kloppel TM, Grey HM, et al. Regulation of catabolism of IgM heavy chains in a B lymphoma cell line. *J Biol Chem* 1982;257:4369.

426. Sitia R, Neuberger MS, Milstein C. Regulation of membrane IgM expression in secretory B cells: translational and post-translational events. *EMBO J* 1987;6:3969.

427. Borchardt RA, Davis RA. Intrahepatic assembly of very low density lipoproteins. Rate of transport out of the endoplasmic reticulum determines rate of secretion. *J Biol Chem* 1987;262:16394.

428. Davis RA, Thrift RN, Wu CC, et al. Apolipoprotein B is both integrated into and translocated across the endoplasmic reticulum membrane. Evidence for two functionally distinct pools. *J Biol Chem* 1990;265:10005.

429. Sato R, Imanaka T, Takatsuki A, et al. Degradation of newly synthesized apolipoprotein B-100 in a pre-Golgi compartment. *J Biol Chem* 1990;265:11880.

430. Bole DG, Hendershot LM, Kearney JF. Posttranslational association of immunoglobulin heavy chain binding protein with nascent heavy chains in nonsecreting and secreting hybridomas. *J Cell Biol* 1986;102:1558.

431. Flynn GC, Pohl J, Flocco MT, et al. Peptide-binding specificity of the molecular chaperone BiP. *Nature* 1991;353:726.

432. Kozutsumi Y, Segal M, Normington K, et al. The presence of malfolded proteins in the endoplasmic reticulum signals the induction of glucose-regulated proteins. *Nature* 1988;332:462.

433. Werner ED, Brodsky JL, McCracken AA. Proteasome-dependent endoplasmic reticulum-associated protein degradation: an unconventional route to a familiar fate. *Proc Natl Acad Sci U S A* 1996;93:13797.

434. Ogata M, Chaudhary VK, Pastan I, et al. Processing of *Pseudomonas* exotoxin by a cellular protease results in the generation of a 37,000-Da toxin fragment that is translocated to the cytosol. *J Biol Chem* 1990;265:20678.

435. Chaudhary VK, Jinno Y, FitzGerald D, et al. *Pseudomonas* exotoxin contains a specific sequence at the carboxyl terminus that

is required for cytotoxicity. *Proc Natl Acad Sci U S A* 1990;87: 308.

436. Sandvig K, Garred O, Prydz K, et al. Retrograde transport of endocytosed Shiga toxin to the endoplasmic reticulum. *Nature* 1992;358:510.

437. Simpson JC, Dascher C, Roberts LM, et al. Ricin cytotoxicity is sensitive to recycling between the endoplasmic reticulum and the Golgi complex. *J Biol Chem* 1995;270:20078.

438. Hilt W, Wolf DH. Proteasomes: destruction as a programme. *Trends Biochem Sci* 1996;21:96.

439. Weissman AM. Regulating protein degradation by ubiquitination. *Immunol Today* 1997;18:189.

440. Goldberg AL, Rock KL. Proteolysis, proteasomes and antigen presentation. *Nature* 1992;357:375.

441. Cienchanover A. The ubiquitin-proteasome proteolytic pathway. *Cell* 1994;79:13.

442. Hochstrasser M. Ubiquitin, proteasomes, and the regulation of intracellular protein degradation. *Curr Opin Cell Biol* 1995;7: 215.

443. Coux O, Tanaka K, Goldberg AL. Structure and functions of the 20S and 26S proteasomes. *Annu Rev Biochem* 1996;65:801.

444. Hochstrasser M. Ubiquitin and intracellular protein degradation. *Curr Opin Cell Biol* 1992;4:1024.

445. Jentsch S, Schlenker S. Selective protein degradation: a journey's end within the proteasome. *Cell* 1995;82:881.

446. Dick LR, Aldrich C, Jameson SC, et al. Proteolytic processing of ovalbumin and beta-galactosidase by the proteasome to a yield antigenic peptides. *J Immunol* 1994;152:3884.

447. Gottesman S, Maurizi MR. Regulation by proteolysis: energy-dependent proteases and their targets. *Microbiol Rev* 1992;56: 592.

448. Varshavsky A. The N-end rule. *Cell* 1992;69:725.

449. Kornitzer D, Raboy B, Kulka RG, et al. Regulated degradation of the transcription factor Gcn4. *EMBO J* 1994;13:6021.

450. Bachmair A, Varshavsky A. The degradation signal in a short-lived protein. *Cell* 1989;56:1019.

451. Aitken A. Identification of Protein Consensus Sequences. England: Ellis Horwood, 1990:35.

452. Forbes DJ. Structure and function of the nuclear pore complex. *Annu Rev Cell Biol* 1992;8:495.

453. Finlay DR, Newmeyer DD, Price TM, et al. Inhibition of *in vitro* nuclear transport by a lectin that binds to nuclear pores. *J Cell Biol* 1987;104:189.

454. Hart GW, Haltiwanger RS, Holt GD, et al. Glycosylation in the nucleus and cytoplasm. *Annu Rev Biochem* 1989;58:841.

455. Jackson SP, Tjian R. O-glycosylation of eukaryotic transcription factors: implications for mechanisms of transcriptional regulation. *Cell* 1988;55:125.

456. Scheffner M, Huibregtse JM, Vierstra RD, et al. The HPV-16 E6 and E6-AP complex functions as a ubiquitin-protein ligase in the ubiquitination of p53. *Cell* 1993;75:495.

457. Lichtsteiner S, Schibler U. A glycosylated liver-specific transcription factor stimulates transcription of the albumin gene. *Cell* 1989;57:1179.

458. Reason AJ, Morris HR, Panico M, et al. Localization of O-GlcNAc modification on the serum response transcription factor. *J Biol Chem* 1992;267:16911.

459. Kelly WG, Dahmus ME, Hart GW. RNA polymerase II is a glycoprotein. Modification of the COOH-terminal domain by O-GlcNAc. *J Biol Chem* 1993;268:10416.

460. Zawel L, Reinberg D. Common themes in assembly and function of eukaryotic transcription complexes. *Annu Rev Biochem* 1995;64:533.

461. Chou TY, Dang CV, Hart GW. Glycosylation of the c-myc transactivation domain. *Proc Natl Acad Sci U S A* 1995;92: 4417.

462. Chou TY, Hart GW, Dang CV. c-myc is glycosylated at threonine 58, a known phosphorylation site and a mutational hot spot in lymphomas. *J Biol Chem* 1995;270:18961.

463. Shaw P, Freeman J, Bovey R, et al. Regulation of specific DNA binding by p53: evidence for a role for O-glycosylation and charged residues at the carboxy-terminus. *Oncogene* 1996;12: 921.

464. Goedert M, Jakes R, Spillantini MG, et al. Tau protein in Alzheimer's disease. *Biochem Soc Trans* 1995;23:80.

465. Mandelkow EM, Mandelkow E. Tau as a marker for Alzheimer's disease. *Trends Biochem Sci* 1993;18:480.

466. Datta B, Chakrabarti D, Roy AL, et al. Roles of a 67-kDa polypeptide in reversal of protein synthesis inhibition in heme-deficient reticulocyte lysate. *Proc Natl Acad Sci U S A* 1988;85: 3324.

467. Datta B, Ray MK, Chakrabarti D, et al. Glycosylation of eukaryotic peptide chain initiation factor 2 (eIF-2)-associated 67-kDa polypeptide (p67) and its possible role in the inhibition of eIF-2 kinase-catalyzed phosphorylation of the eIF-2 alpha-subunit. *J Biol Chem* 1989;264:20620.

468. Hart GW, Greis KD, Dong LY, et al. O-linked N-acetylglucosamine: the yin-yang of Ser/Thr phosphorylation? Nuclear and cytoplasmic glycosylation. *Adv Exp Med Biol* 1995;376:115.

469. Hart GW, Kreppel LK, Comer FI, et al. O-GlcNAcylation of key nuclear and cytoskeletal proteins: reciprocity with O-phosphorylation and putative roles in protein multimerization. *Glycobiology* 1996;6:711.

470. Hart GW. Dynamic O-linked glycosylation of nuclear and cytoskeletal proteins. *Annu Rev Biochem* 1997;66:315.

471. Hart GW. Glycosylation. *Curr Opin Cell Biol* 1992;4:1017.

472. Warren CE. Glycosation. *Curr Opin Biotechnol* 1993;4:596.

473. Harding JJ, Crabbe JC. Post translational modification of proteins. New York: CRC Press, 1992.

474. Graves DJ, Martin BL, Wang JH. Co- and post-translational modification of proteins: chemical principles and biological effects. New York: Oxford University Press, 1994.

475. West CM. Current ideas on the significance of protein glycosylation. *Mol Cell Biochem* 1986;72:3.

476. Clarke S. Protein isoprenylation and methylation at carboxyl-terminal cysteine residues. *Annu Rev Biochem* 1992;61:355.

477. Schultz AM, Henderson LE, Oroszlan S. Fatty acylation of proteins. *Annu Rev Cell Biol* 1988;4:611.

478. Zhang FL, Casey PJ. Protein prenylation: molecular mechanisms and functional consequences. *Annu Rev Biochem* 1996; 65:241.

479. Volker C, Lane P, Kwee C, et al. A single activity carboxyl methylates both farnesyl and geranylgeranyl cysteine residues. *FEBS Lett* 1991;295:189.

480. Perez-Sala D, Gilbert BA, Tan EW, et al. Prenylated protein methyltransferases do not distinguish between farnesylated and geranylgeranylated substrates. *Biochem J* 1992;284:835.

481. Kohl NE, Mosser SD, deSolms SJ, et al. Selective inhibition of ras-dependent transformation by a farnesyltransferase inhibitor. *Science* 1993;260:1934.

482. Todaro GJ, Green H. Quantitative studies of the growth of mouse embryo cells in culture and their development into established lines. *J Cell Biol* 1963;17:299.

483. Gelb MH. Protein prenylation, et cetera: signal transduction in two dimensions. *Science* 1997;275:1750.

484. Casey PJ, Solski PA, Der CJ, et al. p21ras is modified by a farnesyl isoprenoid. *Proc Natl Acad Sci U S A* 1989;86:8323.

485. Parish CA, Smrcka AV, Rando RR. Functional significance of beta gamma-subunit carboxymethylation for the activation of phospholipase C and phosphoinositide 3-kinase. *Biochemistry* 1995;34:7722.

486. Hancock JF, Paterson H, Marshall CJ. A polybasic domain or

palmitoylation is required in addition to the CAAX motif to localize p21ras to the plasma membrane. *Cell* 1990;63:133.

487. Hancock JF, Magee AI, Childs JE, et al. All ras proteins are polyisoprenylated but only some are palmitoylated. *Cell* 1989; 57:1167.

488. Kamps MP, Buss JE, Sefton BM. Mutation of NH2-terminal glycine of p60src prevents both myristoylation and morphological transformation. *Proc Natl Acad Sci U S A* 1985;82:4625.

489. James G, Olson EN. Fatty acylated proteins as components of intracellular signaling pathways. *Biochemistry* 1990;29:2623.

490. Peitzsch RM, McLaughlin S. Binding of acylated peptides and fatty acids to phospholipid vesicles: pertinence to myristoylated proteins. *Biochemistry* 1993;32:10436.

491. Kahn RA, Yucel JK, Malhotra V. ARF signaling: a potential role for phospholipase D in membrane traffic. *Cell* 1993;75: 1045.

492. Aderem A. The MARCKS brothers: a family of protein kinase C substrates. *Cell* 1992;71:713.

493. Blackshear PJ. The MARCKS family of cellular protein kinase C substrates. *J Biol Chem* 1993;268:1501.

494. Munro S, Pelham HR. A c-terminal signal prevents secretion of luminal ER proteins. *Cell* 1987;48:899.

495. Teasdale RD, Jackson MR. Signal-mediated sorting of membrane proteins between the endoplasmic reticulum and the golgi apparatus. *Annu Rev Cell Dev Biol* 1996;12:27.

496. Bishop WR, Bell RM. Assembly of phospholipids into cellular membranes: biosynthesis, transmembrane movement and intracellular translocation. *Annu Rev Cell Biol* 1988;4:579.

497. Griffiths G, Simons K. The trans Golgi network: sorting at the exit site of the Golgi complex. *Science* 1986;234:438.

498. Orci L, Ravazzola M, Amherdt M, et al. The trans-most cisternae of the Golgi complex: a compartment for sorting of secretory and plasma membrane proteins. *Cell* 1987;51:1039.

499. Griffiths G, Pfeiffer S, Simons K, et al. Exit of newly synthesized membrane proteins from the trans cisterna of the Golgi complex to the plasma membrane. *J Cell Biol* 1985;101:949.

500. Dunphy WG, Rothman JE. Compartmental organization of the Golgi stack. *Cell* 1985;42:13.

501. Goldstein JL, Anderson RG, Brown MS. Coated pits, coated vesicles, and receptor-mediated endocytosis. *Nature* 1979;279: 679.

502. Burgess TL, Kelly RB. Constitutive and regulated secretion of proteins. *Annu Rev Cell Biol* 1987;3:243.

503. Pearse BM, Crowther RA. Structure and assembly of coated vesicles. *Annu Rev Biophys Biophys Chem* 1987;16:49.

504. Tsao MC, Walthall BJ, Ham RG. Clonal growth of normal human epidermal keratinocytes in a defined medium. *J Cell Physiol* 1982;110:219.

505. Burridge K, Fath K, Kelly T, et al. Focal adhesions: transmembrane junctions between the extracellular matrix and the cytoskeleton. *Annu Rev Cell Biol* 1988;4:487.

506. Christensen B, Kieler J, Vilien M, et al. A classification of human urothelial cells propagated *in vitro*. *Anticancer Res* 1984; 4:319.

507. Prescott DM, Flexer AS. *Cancer: the misguided cell* 1986:2.

508. Ritchie AC. The classification, morphology, and behaviour of tumours. In: Florey H, eds. General pathology. London: Lloyd-Luke, 1970:668.

509. McKinnon PJ. Ataxia-telangiectasia: an inherited disorder of ionizing-radiation sensitivity in man. Progress in the elucidation of the underlying biochemical defect. *Hum Genet* 1987;75:197.

510. Gatti RA, Boder E, Vinters HV, et al. Ataxia-telangiectasia: an interdisciplinary approach to pathogenesis. *Medicine* (Baltimore) 1991;70:99.

511. Hynes RO. Role of cell surface alterations in cell transformation. *Cell* 1974;1:147.

512. Weinberg RA. Oncogenes and the molecular origins of cancer. New York: Cold Spring Harbor Laboratory Press, 1989.

513. Bishop JM. Cellular oncogenes and retroviruses. *Ann Rev Biochem* 1983;52:301.

514. Levine AJ. Oncogenes of DNA tumor viruses. *Cancer Res* 1988; 48:493.

515. Hunter T. Cooperation between oncogenes. *Cell* 1991;64:249.

516. Klein G. *Cellular Oncogene Activation*. 1988.

517. Green M. Transformation and oncogenesis: DNA viruses. In: Fields BN, ed. Virology. New York: Reven Press, 1985:183.

518. Tooze J. Molecular biology of tumor viruses: DNA tumor viruses. New York: Cold Spring Harbor Laboratory Press, 1981.

519. Ratner L, Josephs SF, Wong-Staal F. Oncogenes: their role in neoplastic transformation. *Annu Rev Microbiol* 1985;39:419.

520. Dang CV. c-myc oncoprotein function. *Biochim Biophys Acta* 1991;1072:103.

521. Rapp UR. Role of Raf-1 serine/threonine protein kinase in growth factor signal transduction. *Oncogene* 1991;6:495.

522. Canaani E, Dreazen O, Klar A, et al. Activation of the c-mos oncogene in a mouse plasmacytoma by insertion of an endogenous intracisternal A-particle genome. *Proc Natl Acad Sci U S A* 1983;80:7118.

523. Graf T, Beug H. Role of the *v-erb*A and *v-erb*B oncogenes of avian erythroblastosis virus in erythroid cell transformation. *Cell* 1983;34:7.

524. James GL, Goldstein JL, Brown MS, et al. Benzodiazepine peptidomimetics: potent inhibitors of Ras farnesylation in animal cells. *Science* 1993;260:1937.

525. Lewin B. Oncogenic conversion by regulatory changes in transcription factors. *Cell* 1991;64:303.

526. Vogelstein B, Kinzler KW. p53 function and dysfunction. *Cell* 1992;70:523.

527. Lane DP, Benchimol S. p53: oncogene or anti-oncogene? *Genes Dev* 1990;4:1.

528. Wiman KG. The retinoblastoma gene: role in cell cycle control and cell differentiation. *FASEB J* 1993;7:841.

529. Clerico L, Mancuso T, Noonan D, et al. Oncosuppressor genes: mechanisms of inactivation for the retinoblastoma gene and p53. *Boll Soc Ital Biol Sper* 1993;69:725.

530. Weinberg RA. The retinoblastoma gene and gene product. *Cancer Surv* 1992;12:43.

531. Broach JR. Construction of high copy yeast vectors using 2-microns circle sequences. *Methods Enzymol* 1983;101:307.

532. Karin M, Cathala G, Nguyen-Huu MC. Expression and regulation of a human metallothionein gene carried on an autonomously replicating shuttle vector. *Proc Natl Acad Sci U S A* 1983;80:4040.

533. Oh SJ, Chittenden T, Levine AJ. Identification of cellular factors that bind specifically to the Epstein-Barr virus origin of DNA replication. *J Virol* 1991;65:514.

534. Brooks JE. Properties and uses of restriction endonucleases. *Methods Enzymol* 1987;152:113.

535. Botstein D, White RL, Skolnick M, et al. Construction of a genetic linkage map in man using restriction fragment length polymorphisms. *Am J Hum Genet* 1980;32:314.

536. White R, LaLouel JM. Chromosome mapping with DNA markers. *Sci Am* 1988;258:40.

537. Murray NE. Phage lambda and molecular cloning. In: Hendrix RW, Roberts J, Stahl F, et al., eds. Lambda II. Cold Spring Harbor, NY: CSH Laboratory, 1983:395.

538. Gubler U, Hoffman BJ. A simple and very effective method for generating cDNA libraries. *Gene* 1983;25:263.

539. Chaney WG, Howard DR, Pollard JW, et al. High-frequency transfection of CHO cells using polybrene. *Somat Cell Mol Genet* 1986;12:237.

540. Felgner PL, Gadek TR, Holm M, et al. Lipofection: a highly

efficient, lipid-mediated DNA-transfection procedure. *Proc Natl Acad Sci U S A* 1987;84:7413.

541. Wu GY, Wu CH. Receptor-mediated gene delivery and expression *in vivo*. *J Biol Chem* 1988;263:14621.

542. Curiel DT, Wagner E, Cotten M, et al. High-efficiency gene transfer mediated by adenovirus coupled to DNA-polylysine complexes. *Hum Gene Ther* 1992;3:147.

543. Cotten M, Wagner E, Zatloukal K, et al. Chicken adenovirus (CELO virus) particles augment receptor-mediated DNA delivery to mammalian cells and yield exceptional levels of stable transformants. *J Virol* 1993;67:3777.

544. Chernomordik L. Electropores in lipid bilayers and cell membranes. In: Chang D, Chassy B, Saunders J, Sowers A, eds. Guide to electroporation and electrofusion. New York: Academic Press, Inc., 1992:63.

545. Sanford JC, Smith FD, Russell JA. Optimizing the biolistic process for different biological applications. *Methods Enzymol* 1993;217:483.

546. Markowitz D, Goff S, Bank A. Construction and use of a safe and efficient amphotropic packaging cell line. *Virology* 1988; 167:400.

547. Miller A, Rosman G. Improved retroviral vectors for gene transfer and expression. *Biotechniques* 1989;7:980.

548. Southern PJ, Berg P. Transformation of mammalian cells to antibiotic resistance with a bacterial gene under control of the SV40 early region promoter. *J Mol Appl Genet* 1982;1:327.

549. Southern EN. Detection of specific sequences among DNA fragments separated by gel electrophoresis. *J Mol Biol* 1975;98: 503.

550. Krumlauf R. Northern blot analysis of gene expression. In: Murray EJ, eds. Methods in molecular biology. Clifton, NJ: The Humana Press, Inc., 1991:307.

551. Salinovich O, Montelaro RC. Reversible staining and peptide mapping of proteins transferred to nitrocellulose after separation by sodium dodecylsulfate-polyacrylamide gel electrophoresis. *Anal Biochem* 1986;156:341.

552. Berk AJ, Sharp PA. Sizing and mapping of early adenovirus mRNAs by gel electrophoresis of S1 endonuclease-digested hybrids. *Cell* 1977;12:721.

553. Favaloro J, Treisman R, Kamen R. Transcription maps of polyoma virus-specific RNA: analysis by two-dimensional nuclease S1 gel mapping. *Methods Enzymol* 1980;65:718.

554. Vogt VM. Purification and further properties of single-strand-specific nuclease from *Aspergillus oryzae*. *Eur J Biochem* 1973; 33:192.

555. Groudine M, Peretz M, Weintraub H. Transcriptional regulation of hemoglobin switching in chicken embryos. *Mol Cell Biol* 1981;1:281.

556. Chomczynski P, Sacchi N. Single-step method of RNA isolation by acid guanidinium thiocyanate-phenol-chloroform extraction. *Anal Biochem* 1987;162:156.

557. Pasco DS, Boyum KW, Merchant SN, et al. Transcriptional and post-transcriptional regulation of the genes encoding cytochromes P-450c and P-450d *in vivo* and in primary hepatocyte cultures. *J Biol Chem* 1988;263:8671.

558. Alwine JC, Kemp DJ, Stark GR. Method for detection of specific RNAs in agarose gels by transfer to diazobenzyloxymethyl-paper and hybridization with DNA probes. *Proc Natl Acad Sci U S A* 1977;74:5350.

559. Orita M, Iwahana H, Kanazawa H, et al. Detection of polymorphisms of human DNA by gel electrophoresis as single-strand conformation polymorphisms. *Proc Natl Acad Sci U S A* 1989; 86:2766.

560. Orita M, Suzuki Y, Sekiya T, et al. Rapid and sensitive detection of point mutations and DNA polymorphisms using the polymerase chain reaction. *Genomics* 1989;5:874.

561. Green PJ, Pines O, Inouye M. The role of antisense RNA in gene regulation. *Annu Rev Biochem* 1986;55:569.

562. Erickson RP, Izant JG. Gene regulation: biology of antisense RNA and DNA. 1992:1.

563. Nepveu A, Marcu KB. Intragenic pausing and anti-sense transcription within the murine c-myc locus. *EMBO J* 1986;5: 2859.

564. Sanger F, Nicklen S, Coulson AR. Dna sequencing with chain-terminating inhibitors. *Proc Natl Acad Sci U S A* 1977;74:5463.

565. Messing J. New M13 vectors for cloning. *Methods Enzymol* 1983;101:20.

566. Giguere V. Application of the firefly luciferase reporter gene. *Methods Mol Biol* 1991;7:237.

567. MacGregor GR, Nolan GP, Fiering S, et al. Use of *E. coli* lacZ as a reporter gene. *Methods Mol Biol* 1991;7:217.

568. Mullis K, Faloona F, Scharf S, et al. Specific enzymatic amplification of DNA *in vitro*: the polymerase chain reaction. *Cold Spring Harb Symp Quant Biol* 1986;51[Part 1]:263.

569. Thompson S, Clarke AR, Pow AM, et al. Germ line transmission and expression of a corrected HPRT gene produced by gene targeting in embryonic stem cells. *Cell* 1989;56:313.

570. Brown PO, Botstein D. Exploring the new world of the genome with DNA microarrays. *Nat Genet* 1999;21:33.

571. Gerhold D, Rushmore T, Caskey CT. DNA chips: promising toys have become powerful toys. *Trends Biochem Sci* 1999;24: 168.

572. Khan J, Bittner ML, Chen Y, et al. DNA microarray technology: the anticipated impact on the study of human disease. *Biochim Biophys Acta* 1999;1423:M17.

573. Moch H, Schraml P, Bubendorf L, et al. High-throughput tissue microarray analysis to evaluate genes uncovered by cDNA microarray screening in renal cell carcinoma. *Am J Pathol* 1999; 154:981.

574. Osin P, Shipley J, Lu YJ, et al. Experimental pathology and breast cancer genetics: new technologies. *Recent Results Cancer Res* 1998;152:35.

2

OVERVIEW OF CELL CYCLE AND APOPTOSIS

ANJALI K. GUPTA
ELEANOR E.R. HARRIS
ERIC J. BERNHARD
RUTH J. MUSCHEL
W. GILLIES McKENNA

Normally, cells respond to extracellular signals by either undergoing division or withdrawing into a resting state. Cancer, on the other hand, is characterized by uncontrolled cell proliferation. Cancers, including those of the lung, frequently have alterations in genes that directly regulate the cell cycle, thereby disrupting cell cycle controls. Molecular changes that have been demonstrated in lung cancer include activation of oncogenes such as *ras, myc, bcl*-2, and c-*erbB*-2, and loss of tumor suppressor genes such as *p53, RB*, and p16^{INK4A}. Most oncogenes and tumor suppressor genes function in signal transduction pathways that regulate cell proliferation. The activation of oncogenes provides persistent mitogenic stimulation, while inactivation of tumor suppressor genes removes the blocks to uncontrolled growth. Understanding the cell cycle and its control points has provided a better understanding of how a cell is transformed into cancer. More importantly, however, this knowledge will now point to new approaches for the treatment and prevention of cancer.

In this chapter, we will first review the cell cycle and its regulation. We will then review the signals that trigger apoptosis and the relationship between the cell cycle checkpoints and apoptosis. The molecular changes in oncogenes and genes for cell cycle control proteins that are found in lung cancers will then be reviewed. Finally, potential therapeutic options provided by our knowledge of cell cycle progression and apoptosis will be discussed.

THE CELL CYCLE

A normal cell exhibits a highly regulated system of proliferation and differentiation that responds to both extra- and intracellular signals. Cancer cells have escaped these regulatory constraints through mutations in genes controlling cell proliferation, such that they are able to grow and proliferate with little restriction. Understanding the mechanisms controlling the cell cycle in both normal cells and cancer cells may enable researchers to develop more specific anticancer therapies by targeting alterations in cell cycle control exhibited by the cancer cell. Normal cells may be in a state of quiescence (G0) where the cell remains metabolically active but is not progressing through the cell cycle towards division. Certain populations of quiescent cells are terminally differentiated and no longer have the ability to cycle or proliferate. In contrast, in response to growth stimuli, cells that are not terminally differentiated may enter the cell cycle, passing through the various phases: G1, the gap prior to replication; S, the DNA synthesis phase; G2, the gap after replication; and M, the mitotic phase leading to cell division (Figure 2.1).

G1 is the phase during which the cell prepares for DNA replication and division by accumulating the macromolecules, such as histones and enzymes, that are required for cell cycle transit. Cellular differentiation may be initiated in G1.[1] While the other cell cycle phases are of relatively constant duration among different cell types, G1 phase has the most variable duration—over a range of zero to several hours. Cells are required to pass a regulatory point to proceed from G1 to S. This commitment point has been defined most clearly in yeast cells, where it is called "Start." The comparable point in animal cells is called the restriction point, (R). Quiescent cells are considered to have withdrawn from the cell cycle into another state resembling G1 but distinct because they are unable to proceed directly into S phase. This noncycling state is called G0. Some cells can be stimulated to leave G0 and reenter the cell cycle. Withdrawal from or reentry into a cell cycle occurs before the restriction point in G1. After the restriction point, inhibitors will not reverse progression to S-phase.

The DNA synthesis phase (S-phase) results in the replication of the entire cellular DNA content and associated archi-

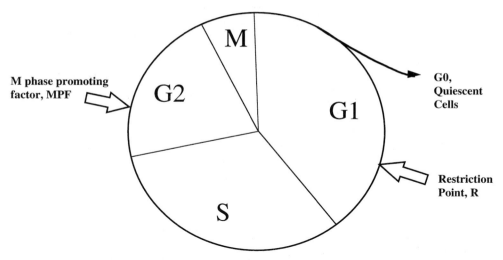

FIGURE 2.1. The cell cycle. The cell cycle consists of four phases—G1, S, G2, and M. Normal cells in G1 can go into a state of quiescence (G0) where they remain metabolically active but are not progressing towards division. Cells must pass the restriction point, R, to proceed from G1 to S.

tectural apparatus. The total content of DNA increases from a diploid value of 2 n to the fully replicated value of 4 n. Through specific, highly regulated patterns, multiple sites of bidirectional replication are initiated. S-phase is usually of constant duration within a given cell type. Initiation requires a change in the conformation of the DNA at replication sites. Upon initiation, clusters of replication units called replicons begin simultaneously, although different replicons initiate at different times in S-phase.[2] Individual genes have been shown to replicate at specific times within S-phase[2] with genes that are transcribed as part of S-phase replicating early on.[3]

After the completion of S-phase, the cell enters G2 phase, during which events lead to the commitment to and completion of mitosis. It is during this phase that replication errors and other DNA damage can be repaired. DNA damage may prolong G2 and prevent the progression into M-phase.[4,5] Under normal circumstances, G2 tends to be of constant duration. The coordination of the numerous processes required for cell division, including the ability to recognize the completion of synthesis, nuclear envelope dissolution, chromatin condensation, and organization of the cytoskeleton, are all initiated in G2 prior to entry into mitosis.

Mitosis itself is the process by which the cell equally divides its chromosome complement at cell division, and is composed of four stages. In prophase the replicated chromosomes condense while the microtubule assemblies rearrange, forming a centrosome which guides the movement of the chromosomes. The chromosomes are then positioned and oriented in association with the spindle fibers in prometaphase. These originate at the centrosome and are attached to kinetochores on the chromosome. Anaphase is characterized by the separation of the chromosomes and movement to opposite poles of the cell. This separation requires action of the spindle fibers. Finally, in telophase the nuclei are reformed around each group of chromosomes, after which they decondense. Once nuclear division is complete, cell division usually occurs.[6]

REGULATION OF THE CELL CYCLE

Identifying the factors that trigger the transitions between the cell cycle states (G1, S, G2, M) has been a major goal of cell cycle research. Initial work was done with cell fusion experiments where cells were synchronized at various stages of the cell cycle, then fused with nonsynchronized cells.[7,8] These studies revealed that S-phase nuclei contain a factor, S-phase promoting factor (SPF), capable of inducing G1 cells to enter S-phase. These studies also demonstrated that only cells in G1 are capable of initiating DNA synthesis. If S-phase nuclei were fused with G2 cells, no DNA replication occurred. In addition, late G2 or M-phase cells contain an M-phase promoting factor (MPF) capable of accelerating the onset of mitosis in early G2 cells.[9] Subsequent studies have identified the components of SPF and MPF, which are now known to be a complex of regulatory cyclin proteins and catalytic kinases known as cyclin-dependent kinases (CDK). In higher eukaryotes, more than ten CDK-related proteins have been discovered with numerous cyclin interactions.[10]

The activation of CDKs is tightly regulated by complex mechanisms to ensure proper timing and coordination of cell cycle events. This regulation is primarily posttranscriptional, and CDK levels remain fairly constant during the cell cycle.[11] Different kinases are active in different phases of the cell cycle (Figure 2.2). Their activity is controlled in

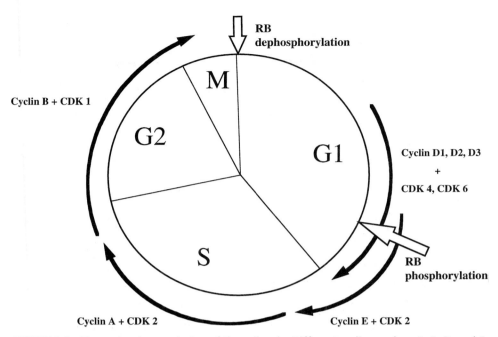

FIGURE 2.2. The molecular regulation of the cell cycle. Different cyclins, such as A, B, D, and E, complex with specific cyclin-dependent kinases (CDKs) during specific phases of the cell cycle. These cyclin/CDK complexes are held in an inactive state by physical interactions with CDK inhibitors such as p16, p21, and p27. Cyclin/CDK complexes phosphorylate key substrates, resulting in progression through the cell cycle at specific points.

part by the formation of complexes with cyclin proteins, so named because their expression varies throughout the cell cycle. The cyclins have homologous conserved domains, called cyclin boxes, responsible for CDK binding and activation. This binding is predicted to activate the partner CDK by altering the conformation of the N-terminal region, displacing a region called the T-loop that partially obscures the substrate binding site of the kinase. Complete activation of CDKs requires more than just cyclin binding; the CDK subunit must also be phosphorylated.[10,11] A CDK-activating kinase (CAK, also MO15 or CDK7) phosphorylates a conserved threonine residue which sits in the CDK substrate binding site (the T-loop).[10] Its phosphorylation seems to induce structural changes allowing the cyclin to bind the CDK protein and the complex to form.[12] Mutation of the threonine residue in the T-loop greatly reduces the kinase activity.[10]

Further regulation of the cyclin CDK complex is provided by controlled phosphorylation and dephosphorylation. Major CDKs involved in cell cycle control can be inhibited by phosphorylation of the CDK subunit at a conserved tyrosine (Tyr15) and the adjacent threonine (Thr14). For example, inhibitory phosphorylation contributes to the timing of mitosis in many organisms.[13,14] Prior to mitosis, CDK1-cyclin B complexes are held in an inactive state by phosphorylation at both these sites. At the end of G2, abrupt dephosphorylation triggers CDK1 activation and mitosis.[13,14] This phosphorylation is catalyzed by trans-

membrane kinases located in the endoplasmic reticulum of cells, Wee 1 and Myt 1.[15,16] Dephosphorylation of both sites is carried out by phosphatases of the Cdc25 family.[17] Inhibitory phosphorylation may control progression through early cell cycle stages as well. During S-phase, human CDK2 is extensively phosphorylated at both inhibitory sites,[18] and expression of a nonphosphorylated CDK2 mutant is lethal in human cells.[19]

Negative regulation of CDKs is also mediated by a family of inhibitory subunits called cyclin-dependent kinase inhibitors, or CKIs. The CKIs bind to the activating phosphorylation sites and inactivate CDK complexes. The CKIs are a diverse family of proteins including p21 (CIP1/WAF1), and p27 (KIP1), which associate with CDK2, and p16[INK4] and p15[INK4] (Figure 2.3), which act on CDKs 4 and 6.[20] The transcription of the CKIs is induced by p53, although p27 seems to be regulated posttranscriptionally.[21] Many human tumors demonstrate p16[INK4] rearrangements or deletions, while p16[INK4] expression is elevated in cells that are senescent.[22]

During the course of normal cell cycle progression, cyclin-CDK complexes are inactivated at specific times through degradation of the cyclin partner by regulated proteolysis.[10] The importance of cyclin degradation is most apparent in the control of the exit from mitosis, where destruction of mitotic cyclins is required for the onset of telophase, as well as for preparation for the next cell cycle.[23]

Cyclin degradation results from ubiquitin-dependent proteolysis[24] and requires a small sequence motif (the destruction box) near the N-terminus of mitotic cyclins.[24] Recent work has identified the key regulated component in mitotic cyclin destruction as a large multi-subunit complex known as the anaphase-promoting complex (APC), or cyclosome, which acts as an E3 enzyme to catalyze the transfer of ubiquitin in various mitotic substrates, including cyclins and putative inhibitors of anaphase.[25] The APC is thought to be activated by CDK1-cyclin B.[25] APC activity remains high in G1 and then declines concurrent to the appearance of G1 cyclins.[25] In yeast, APC activity was recently shown to require binding to an activating protein called Hct-1.[26] Binding of Hct-1 to the APC was regulated by CDK-mediated phosphorylation, and mitotic cyclins and CDK activity were in turn absent when Hct-1 was not phosphorylated. Thus Hct-1 in yeast (and the human CDK1 homologue[27]) appear to regulate mitotic cyclin degradation by APC.

The cell cycle phases are coordinated by the expression and/or activation of regulatory proteins, including complexes of cyclins and cyclin-dependent kinases. In the early G1-phase, D-type cyclins (D1, D2, and D3) and early CDKs (CDK4 and CDK6) accumulate. In addition, the protein levels of proliferating cell nuclear antigen (PCNA), a factor that stimulates the processing ability of DNA-polymerase-delta and associates with cyclin D-CDK4, increases.[28] High levels of CKIs (cyclin-dependent kinase inhibitors) decline on induction of cell cycle entry in mitogen-deprived (G0) cells.[29] The CKI binds to and inhibits G1-phase CDKs and cyclin/CDK complexes.[30,31] Free cyclin D-CDK4-PCNA complexes are activated through phosphorylation by CAK (cyclin-dependent kinase activating kinase).[29] The decline of CKIs, which results both from the down-regulation of CKI protein levels and from the stoichiometric titration of CKI to cyclin D-CDK4-PCNA complexes, also allows an enzymatic activation of CDK2.[29] Cyclin E synthesis follows cyclin D accumulation in G1. Cyclin E interacts with CDK2 in late G1 and at the beginning of S-phase to induce the initiation of DNA synthesis, and then it is rapidly degraded. After cyclin E is degraded, CDK2 binds cyclin A throughout the rest of S-phase.

Passage through G1 into S-phase is regulated by an elaborate feedback loop involving pRb, the retinoblastoma gene product, a growth-suppressing protein, and a family of related proteins, including p107, p130 and p300 (see also Chapter 7). pRb exerts most of its effect in early and mid-G1 by binding and sequestering E2F transcription factors[28] (Figure 2.3). Repression of transcription by pRb may also involve histone deacetylase recruitment and modification of chromatin structure.[32,33] pRb levels are relatively constant throughout the cell cycle, but its phosphorylation state varies.[34] Cyclin D- and E-dependent kinases have been implicated in the phosphorylation of Rb. It is known that loss of cyclin D-dependent kinase activity before the restriction point prevents many cultured cell lines from entering S-

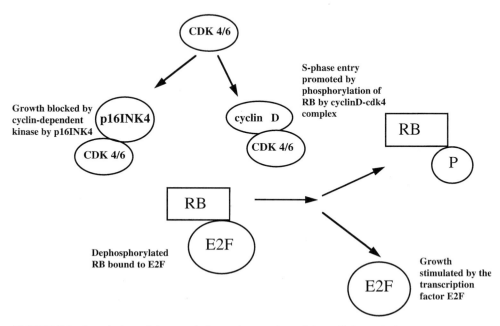

FIGURE 2.3. Regulation of the restriction point. Passing of the cell through the restriction point (R) is a key step in cell cycle progression. Cyclin D interacts with CDK 4 and 6 during G1, and phosphorylates RB. This releases the transcription factor E2F, allowing it to interact with nuclear targets to stimulate the synthesis of various proteins required for progression. Cyclin kinase inhibitors such as p16[INK4A] are able to bind to CDK 4/6 and thus prevent the binding of CDK 4/6 to cyclin D.

phase, but its absence later in the cell cycle is without effect.[35] Complete inactivation of pRb requires sequential phosphorylation first by cyclin D-CDK 4 or 6 complexes and subsequently by cyclin E-CDK2.[36,37] Also, cyclin D-dependent kinases are dispensable for passage through the restriction point in cultured cells that lack functional Rb, and in this setting, ectopic expression of INK4 proteins does not induce G1 phase arrest.[38] Thus INK4 proteins inhibit cyclin D-dependent kinases that, in turn, phosphorylate Rb. Conditions that cause pRb phosphorylation favor cell proliferation. Hypophosphorylated pRb can bind the transcription factor E2F, while phosphorylation leads to a loss of this association.[34]

E2F is actually a group of transcription factors which contain a consensus binding site specific for sequences in the promoters of a number of cell growth control genes, such as dihydrofolate reductase, PCNA, CDK1, cyclin E, cyclin A, c-*myc,* and TK.[39] One model of this negative feedback loop involves pRb sequestration of E2F in order to control the transcription of genes necessary for cell cycle progression. Upon phosphorylation, pRb releases E2F, leading to the induction of p16^{INK4}. This CKI binds to CDK4 and 6, preventing their binding cyclin D, which is subsequently degraded. This cascade of events mediates the transition into S-phase. Various growth inhibitory signals prevent pRb phosphorylation via CDK activity and thus block the cell cycle. Such signals include transforming growth factor β (TGF-β), cyclic AMP (cAMP) and contact inhibition. TGF-β can induce expression of the CKI, p15^{INK4B}, which also targets CDK4 and CDK6 and competes for binding with cyclin D. Cell proliferation by this pathway occurs only in cells with functional pRb. TGF-β also reduces CDK4 levels in some cells. Another CKI, p27, interacts with CDK2 in cells treated with TGF-β. DNA damage by radiation or other damaging agents blocks pRb phosphorylation through the CKI, p21, to maintain the pRb regulated cell block in order to complete DNA damage repair.[34]

The primary structures of pRb, p107 and p130, have several regions of highly conserved sequences that likely represent functional domains. The most strongly conserved regions correspond to binding sites. Both p107 and p130 contain a spacer region in common which is not found on pRb and is required for interaction with cyclin A and possibly cyclin E. These two proteins are phosphorylated, but the function of this change is not known. Both proteins can bind the same transcription factors which associate with pRb, including E2F. p130 is found in E2F complexes, primarily in G0, and is lost at the G1/S transition. At that time, E2F is found in complex with p107 instead. Both complexes associate with cyclin A and E complexes. Overexpression of p107 results in growth arrest in some cell lines, and this does not seem to relate to E2F binding. Overexpression of p130 results in arrest of cell proliferation in some tumor cell lines as well.[40] In general, the pRb family of proteins is thought to have similar, possibly overlapping, but not identical roles in the regulation of cell cycle. The

fourth protein, p300, has a bromodomain distinct from the other members of the family, implicating a role as a transcriptional co-activator. It also interacts with the TATA-binding protein, indicating a role in transcriptional regulation.[41]

After DNA replication is complete, the cell progresses into the G2-phase. At this time, the levels of cyclin B increase. This protein then forms a complex with CDK1, also known as CDC2, to form the M-phase promoting factor (MPF). Activation of MPF requires the phosphorylation of CDK1 on a threonine residue (Thr161) by CAK and dephosphorylation of a tyrosine residue (Tyr15) by CDC25 phosphatase. Activated MPF then initiates prophase and also induces the ubiquitin proteosome pathway that subsequently causes cyclin B destruction and the initiation of anaphase.[42] Finally, CDK1 is inactivated by the dephosphorylation of Thr161, and the cell cycle clock is reset.[43]

Cell proliferation often requires the presence of external growth factors, which usually influence the cell's commitment to division in G1. Growth factor stimulation of cell cycle entry is believed to be mediated by the upregulated transcription of the protooncogenes c-*fos*, c-*myb*, B-*myb*, and *ras*. Their gene products act as transcription factors that increase the expression of specific cell-cycle regulatory genes.[44] For example, stimulation of smooth muscle cells or fibroblasts results in a rapid induction of c-*fos*, which in turn increases cyclin D1, CDK4, and cyclin E mRNA expression.[45] Growth factors also increase levels of c-*myc*,[46] a protein crucial for the progression through both the G1- and the G2-phases of the cell cycle.[47] Like c-*fos*, c-*myc* induces early G1-phase cyclin accumulation and augments cyclin D- and cyclin E-associated kinase activities.[48,49] H-*ras* is a membrane-associated, guanine nucleotide-binding protein that couples growth regulatory signals from cell surface tyrosine kinase receptors to cytoplasmic second messenger pathways.[50] Abolition of *ras* activity, through the use of dominant negative mutants or neutralizing antibodies, inhibits entry of cells into S-phase,[51] while activation or constitutive overexpression of *ras* protein increases cyclin D levels and shortens G1-phase.[52] Furthermore, *myc* and *ras* proteins collaborate in activating cyclin E/CDK2 and E2F coincident with the loss of the CKI p27Kip1.[53]

A role for the tumor suppressor protein p53 in cell cycle regulation has also been suggested (see also Chapter 6).[54] It was recently proposed that p53 was induced by expression of oncogenic *ras* through the intermediary p19Arf.[55] p53 can act as a transcription factor to up-regulate the expression of a number of genes, including that for p21. Expression of p53 can arrest cells in the G1-phase in response to DNA damage and provides the primary mechanism of the antiproliferative effect in G1 of irradiation. This protective mechanism has been linked to p53-stimulated accumulation of p21.[54,56] p21 is able directly to block the ability of PCNA to increase the processing ability of DNA-polymerase-delta, thereby arresting DNA replication and allowing

DNA repair.[57] Alternatively, p53 can promote apoptosis, particularly in the presence of free E2F, providing another defense against the propagation of damaged DNA in cells that have progressed past the restriction point R.[58]

Many cells exhibit a G2 arrest following exposure to DNA-damaging agents, including ionizing radiation as well as drugs such a nitrogen mustard, cisplatinum, and etoposide. It has been hypothesized that this arrest may serve a protective function, perhaps allowing cells to repair damage before progressing through the cell cycle.[4] There is evidence correlating length of G2 delay following radiation to survival. In the budding yeast *S. cerevisiae,* a particular mutant, *rad9,* which fails to arrest G2 following radiation, displays much greater radiosensitivity that the wild type which does not arrest in G2.[5] It has been found that rat embryo fibroblasts transfected with H-*ras* and *myc* were significantly more radioresistant than cells transfected with *myc* alone (Do 1.68–2.17 versus 1.06–1.08) and that they also showed a greater duration of G2 delay following radiation.[59] No differences were found in the induction of rate of repair of DSBs between these lines.[60] In addition, drugs such as pentoxyfilline and caffeine, which shorten the length of the G2 arrest following radiation, increase radiosensitivity.[61,62]

Further study of the mechanism underlying G2 arrest has shown that synchronized HeLa cells irradiated with 10 Gy in S-phase remained in G2 phase for at least nine hours longer than control unirradiated cells.[63] Since it is known that cyclin B in complex with CDK1 is required for exit from G2 and entry into mitosis, the effect of radiation on cyclin B expression was studied. In these cells, a profound suppression of both cyclin B mRNA and protein expression was seen compared to unirradiated control cells which corresponded temporally to the G2 delay.[64] In addition, this suppression of cyclin B was seen with doses as low as 2 Gy.[64] HeLa cells irradiated in G2-phase at a time when cyclin B message expression was elevated with 10 Gy also remained in G2 much longer than control cells and showed a depression in cyclin B protein levels. In contrast, cyclin A expression was not suppressed following radiation; in fact, its level actually rose to a higher level than seen in unirradiated control cells.[64] Both caffeine and staurosporine, which reduce the length of G2 arrest following radiation, also reversed the suppression of cyclin B expression.[65]

However, cyclin B suppression is not the only regulator of G2/M progression. Studies by Kao and co-workers demonstrated that forcing increased expression of cyclin B1 after irradiation using a plasmid encoding cyclin B1 on a dexamethasone inducible promoter only partially reversed the G2 arrest.[66] Thus further controls exist that regulate the passage through G2/M after DNA damage. Phosphorylation of Thr14 and Tyr15 on CDK1 renders the cyclin B/CDK1 complex inactive. These residues must be dephosphorylated in order for the complex to become activated.[11] Paules and co-workers found that irradiation of normal human diploid fibroblasts with 3 Gy led to a rapid inhibition of entry into mitosis (G2 delay) which was accompanied by an accumulation of hyperphosphorylated CDK1.[67] Likewise, this effect has been seen during the G2 arrest in CHO cells[68] and in human lymphoma line[69] after treatment with etoposide and nitrogen mustard respectively.

APOPTOSIS

Apoptosis, or programmed cell death, is a genetically regulated form of cell death which, under normal circumstances, is involved in organogenesis, tissue homeostasis, and the editing of the immune system to remove autoreactive clones.[70,71] However, apoptosis is also linked to cellular proliferation and can be triggered by the loss of cell-cycle controls resulting from the activation of oncogenes that leads to cell transformation.[70] Thus apoptosis also serves as a protective mechanism against the development of tumors. Apoptosis can also be triggered in response to external stimuli, including hormonal or growth factor manipulations,[71] and in response to a number of toxic agents, including chemotherapeutic drugs and x-rays.[72] It is for these reasons that apoptosis has generated great interest among oncologists and cancer biologists, both because of the potential insights the study of apoptosis may yield into carcinogenesis, and in the hope of improving established treatments or developing new strategies for cancer treatment to maximize tumor cell apoptosis.

An apoptotic cell loses contact with its neighbors, decreases in size, and shows condensation of chromatin,[73] characteristics which allow for the identification of apoptotic cells in tissue. In apoptotic cells, the DNA is often degraded by nucleases at internucleosomal linker sites, yielding DNA fragments in multiples of 180 bp which can be detected as nucleosomal ladders after DNA extraction and agarose gel electrophoresis.[73] However, nucleosomal DNA cleavage is not universal,[73] and sometimes the DNA is degraded into larger fragments.[74] This enzymatic degradation of DNA forms the basis for one method of apoptosis detection, the TUNEL assay,[75] which relies on the labeling of enzymatically cleaved DNA fragments by the enzyme terminal deoxynucleotidyl-transferase. Apoptotic cell membrane proteins are cross-linked, making the membrane more rigid.[76] The altered membrane characteristics lead to phagocytosis of apoptotic cells by adjacent cells or macrophages. The removal of apoptotic cells by this means greatly reduces the inflammation that would otherwise occur with cell death and lysis.[71]

As discussed in the previous section, in response to DNA damage, cells greatly increase their transit time through the cell cycle, due primarily to arrests at G1 and G2. These arrests were described in the first paper accurately defining the phases of the cell cycle.[77] In this classic work Howard and Pelc described the G1, S, G2, and M components of the cell cycle and noted that both G1 and G2, but not S or M, were prolonged in irradiated cells. It was subsequently noted that all eukaryotic cells undergo a G2 delay after irradiation but that many tumor cells fail to arrest in G1.[78] Many of the genes that affect the G1 arrest also influence whether cells undergo apoptosis. For example, overexpression of *myc* leads to a bypass of the G1 arrest normally induced by serum starvation. However, accompanying the loss of the G1 checkpoint is the induction of apoptosis in response to serum withdrawal.[79] Similarly, p53 both functions in the regulation of the G1/S checkpoint,[80] and is a positive regulator of apoptosis. The loss of G1 arrest resulting from absent or mutated p53 does not necessarily lead to apoptosis however, since the proapoptotic function of p53 is also lost.[81] Induction of wild-type p53 expression will cause certain cells to undergo a G1 arrest, while in other cases wild-type p53 leads to apoptosis. For example, irradiated fibroblasts with wild-type p53 undergo a G1 arrest but do not undergo apoptosis over the first 72 hours after irradiation,[82,83] whereas thymocytes rapidly undergo apoptosis that is p53-dependent.[84] Since p53 mutations are among the most frequent lesions present in human tumor cells (seen in 50% of NSCLC and 80% of SCLC[85]), loss of this checkpoint may have a considerable impact on the survival of tumor cells during chemo- or radiotherapy. An important question under investigation is what the determinants are that regulate whether a cell will arrest in G1 or will instead undergo apoptosis. Kastan and co-workers have postulated that in one system, that of a cell line dependent upon IL-3, the absolute level of p21 (WAF1/CIP1) might contribute to this determination,[86] but while intriguing, there is as yet no general support of this observation (see also Chapters 6, 33).

Apoptosis has also been linked to the expression of oncogenes such as *bcl*-2. It has been shown that expression of bc1-2 can delay or even prevent apoptosis.[87,88] Conversely down-regulation of *bcl*-2 has been shown to promote apoptosis. *bcl*-2 is a membrane-associated protein that in the intact cell is largely found in the nuclear envelope, endoplasmic reticulum, and mitochondria.[89,90] It is a member of a family of genes including Bax, Bcl-X (which gives rise to protein products, Bcl-X$_L$ and Bcl-X$_S$) Mc1-1 and A1. It is also similar to the ced-9 gene of *C. elegans*,[91] and related in function and, to some extent, in sequence to a number of viral proteins such as p19-E1B of adenovirus, p30 of baculovirus and BHFR-1 of Epstein-Barr virus.[92,93] Some of the gene products of these genes function like Bcl-2 in preventing apoptosis (p19-E1B, Bcl-X$_L$,) others (Bax, Bcl-X$_S$) oppose *bcl*-2 action and hence promote apoptosis. It has been suggested that apoptosis is regulated not by *bcl*-2 alone but by the ratio of *bcl*-2 to Bax in the cells where both are found. Korsmeyer and co-workers have suggested that the *bcl*-2/Bax heterodimer constitutes a "preset rheostat within cells" determining the extent of apoptosis.[92] Another

bcl-2-binding protein, BAD, may act in a similar way to Bax.[93]

In normal tissues there is a counterbalance between cell proliferation and programmed cell death or apoptosis. A characteristic feature of many tumors is the loss of G1-specific regulators of proliferation.[94] However, if tumor cells are to continue to proliferate and to increase in cell number, then they must also lose the apoptotic response. Mutation of p53 appears to confer both deregulation of the G1/S checkpoint and diminished apoptosis. One example where p53 loss has been shown in tumor progression is during ultraviolet-light-induced skin carcinogenesis. Cells with DNA damage may die by apoptosis after irradiation due to induction of wild-type p53, but cells that have p53 mutations will continue to proliferate and actually establish sectors of skin bearing the mutation.[95] Zarbi and co-workers have described similar sectors of cells with *ras* mutations in the mammary glands of mice that give rise to tumors upon N-nitroso-N-methylurea exposure.[96] These mutations may also act to suppress apoptosis during mammary carcinogenesis, as *ras* can inhibit apoptosis in some settings.[83,97] These observations have led to the hypothesis that the loss of G1-specific regulation must be accompanied by suppression of apoptosis as a necessary step in carcinogenesis. Similar selection for p53 mutations may occur during severe hypoxia in tumors. Graeber and co-worker.[98] showed that cells with wild-type p53 undergo apoptosis at very low oxygen tensions, while cells with mutations in p53 do not, leading to a selection for cells with mutations in p53 under hypoxic conditions both *in vitro* and *in vivo*.

The loss of the G1 checkpoint in itself does not lead to the inability of cells to undergo apoptosis. Many tumor cells that have lost components of G1 regulation, including loss of G1 arrest after serum starvation or irradiation, can nonetheless be induced to undergo apoptosis after treatment with a variety of other stimuli, including radiation and some chemotherapeutic drugs.[83,99,100] The study of human tumor cells in tissue culture and oncogene transfection of cells allows modeling of some of these situations. We have studied oncogene-transfected rat embryo fibroblasts and found that *myc*-transfected rat embryo fibroblasts lack a radiation-induced G1 block, but are induced to undergo apoptosis by radiation or by serum withdrawal.[83] Co-transfection of *ras* with *myc* overrides the apoptotic effect of x-rays but not of serum withdrawal. *Ras* transfection does not restore the G1 checkpoint but greatly increases the radiation-induced G2 delay.[59] A similar situation is seen in HeLa cells, which are very resistant to radiation-induced apoptosis, lack a G1 checkpoint, but have a pronounced G2 checkpoint after x-rays.[78] Thus effects at the G1 checkpoint cannot be the sole determinants of apoptosis in tumor cells, and we have proposed the hypothesis that events controlling the G2 checkpoint also can impact on the induction of apoptosis similar to the effects at G1.[83] This checkpoint, however, will come into play only in those situations where a G2 checkpoint is induced.

Finally it should be noted that apoptosis is clearly independent of cell-cycle effects in some cases. Treatment of thymocytes with steroids occurs while the cells are in G0, and the resulting apoptosis is a p53-independent process.[70,84,101] There is also no evidence that apoptosis induced by hormone withdrawal from prostate or breast tissue is related to the cell cycle.[102,103]

MOLECULAR CHANGES IN LUNG CANCER

Lung cancer has been shown to be associated with molecular and genetic abnormalities, many of which affect cell cycle control and apoptosis. These include expression of oncogenes such as *ras, myc, bcl-2* and *c-erb*B-2, and loss of tumor suppressor genes like p53, RB, and p16[INK4A]. In the following section, we will examine each of these in detail and its association with lung cancer (see also Chapters 4, 5, 67).

RAS

The *ras* genes code for 21 kD proteins that are known as G proteins because they bind GDP or GTP (see also Chap-

ter 4). G proteins are members of signal transduction pathways which transmit signals from the cell's extracellular environment to the machinery that controls gene expression (Figure 2.4) thereby controlling cell proliferation and the cellular response to its environment. Signaling is initiated by growth factor binding to an extracellular receptor domain. This leads to guanine nucleotide exchange factors' (GEFs) recruitment to promote the formation of the active, GTP-bound form of *ras*.[104] GTPase activating proteins (GAPs) accelerate the intrinsic GTP hydrolytic activity of *ras* to promote the formation of the inactive, GDP-bound form of *ras*.[104] Activated *ras* interacts with several downstream signal transduction pathways, such as the raf, rac/rho, and PI3 kinase pathways,[105] thereby causing the signal to move to the nucleus. Mutations in *ras* at amino acids 12, 13, or 61 make *ras* consituitively active by making it nonresponsive to GAPs.[106] This causes a sustained signal to be transmitted through *ras* to the downstream effectors.

There are three forms of *ras:* H-*ras* (homologous to the Harvey murine sarcoma virus oncogene), K-*ras* (homologous to the Kirsten murine sarcoma virus oncogene) and N-*ras* (initially isolated from a neuroblastoma cell line). Activating mutations of *ras* can be seen in up to 30% of all human tumors. In addition, *ras* activity is up-regulated in many cancers by overexpression in the absence of activating

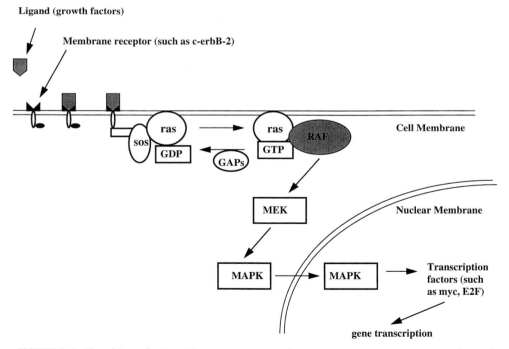

FIGURE 2.4. Signal transduction. Many oncogenes and tumor suppressor genes are members of the signal transduction pathway. In this model, a growth factor in the extracellular environment interacts with its receptor. This event is signaled to the nucleus via a G protein (ras) which leads to alterations in kinase activity. The activation of the kinase cascade results in the binding of a transcription factor to the regulatory sequence of a gene, which causes a change in its expression by alteration in mRNA transcription.

mutations.[107,108] *Ras* overexpression has been shown to impact on treatment of cancers as well. In a series of experiments by McKenna and co-workers with rat embryo fibroblast cells transfected with H-*ras* and *myc* or *myc* alone, it was noted that cell lines transfected with both oncogenes were significantly more radioresistant than if transfected with *myc* alone. The more resistant cell line also showed a greater G2 delay following irradiation.[59]

In lung cancer, K-*ras* has been shown to be mutated or overexpressed in 30% of adenocarcinomas, 30% of carcinoid tumors, 13% of large-cell carcinomas, and none of the squamous or small-cell carcinomas (see also Chapter 4).[109,110] K-*ras* overexpression has been shown to correlate with a worse prognosis in resectable cases.[111–113] A retrospective review of 244 patients with stage I non-small-cell lung cancer (NSCLC) treated surgically at the Brigham and Women's Hospital (Boston, MA) evaluated the effect of a number of molecular and clinical factors on cancer-free survival. They found K-*ras* mutations as an independent predictor of recurrence on multivariate analysis.[114] Although *ras* mutations have been shown to affect response to radiation and chemotherapy in cell culture,[115] no difference in response has been noted in patients with or without *ras* mutations in terms of treatment with chemotherapy.[116] Genetic changes including *ras* mutations can occur in bronchial epithelium well before the development of a tumor that can be clinically detected. In adenocarcinomas, point mutations of *ras* were detected in sputum samples of 11 out of 22 patients by the Point-EXACCT method one month to almost four years prior to the clinical diagnosis of lung cancer.[117] It is possible that screening of sputum samples in high-risk patients may potentially improve survival by leading to earlier diagnosis.

MYC

Three forms of *myc* have been described: c-*myc* is cellular, n-*myc* was originally isolated from neuroblastoma cell lines, and l-*myc* was isolated from small-cell lung cancer (SCLC). *myc* proteins are transcription factors that act via an amino-terminal transactivating domain and are involved in both cell proliferation and apoptosis.[118] Although they may be activated by truncation, *myc* genes are not usually mutated in carcinogenesis; instead they are activated by overexpression by either up-regulation or gene amplification.[119] In nontransformed cells, *myc* expression is linked to mitogenic stimuli and is a prerequisite for cell growth. *myc* expression has been shown to be both necessary and sufficient to cause G0 fibroblasts to enter the cell cycle.[120] Conversely, immortalized fibroblasts that constituitively express *myc* are unable to exit the cycle upon serum withdrawal and then undergo apoptosis.[119] The *myc* oncogene is an early-response gene whose expression rises rapidly at the G0-G1 transition and whose currently known functions are largely linked to G1 and early S. Unlike most early-response genes, however, *myc*

expression is sustained throughout the cell cycle. In addition to its proliferative function, *myc* can be shown to induce apoptosis in G0 and G1.[118]

In lung cancer, *myc* amplification is most commonly found in SCLC (see also Chapter 5). In NSCLC, *myc* amplification is rare (5% to 10%), and if it occurs, it is in adenocarcinomas without *ras* mutations.[121] *myc* amplification in SCLC is associated with the variant morphology. In classic SCLC (approximately 70% of small-cell lung cancers), the cells grow as tightly packed floating cellular aggregates with long doubling times and low colony-forming efficiencies. They also have a typical biochemical profile. The remaining 30% of small-cell lung cancers can be subdivided into the biochemical variant category that only have altered biochemical profile, or the morphological-variant category that have an altered biochemical profile with morphologic features of large-cell undifferentiated carcinoma. The morphological variant of SCLC is almost exclusively associated with *myc* gene amplification[122] Analysis of RNA expression shows that 80% to 90% of all SCLC overexpress *myc* as compared to normal lung tissue.[123] The overexpression of *myc* has been associated with poorer survival. In cell lines established from SCLC patients, 7 of 52 (11%) untreated patients had *myc* amplification, as compared to 16 of 44 (36%) patients who had relapsed after chemotherapy.[124] *myc* expression, however, has not been definitively shown to alter radiosensitivity.[125]

BCL-2

The *bcl-2* oncogene was discovered as a gene whose expression was increased by chromosomal translocations in B-cell malignancies.[126] During development, *bcl-2* is expressed in tissues from all three germ layers. In adults, however, it is expressed in tissues that are renewed from stem cells, have proliferative ability, or that are long lived.[127] In the past, the function of *bcl-2* was viewed like that of many other oncogenes as promoting proliferation or cooperating with other oncogenes in doing so. More recently, however, expression of *bcl-2* has been shown to delay or even prevent apoptosis.[87,88]

The expression of *bcl-2* in small-cell lung cancer is quite high at 75% to 80%.[128,129] It has not been associated with any particular histological subtype.[128] In NSCLC, *bcl-2* protein expression is found in 25% of squamous-cell carcinomas and 12% of adenocarcinomas.[130] The studies are inconclusive to whether *bcl-2* has any affect on prognosis. In one study, results in squamous-cell carcinoma were improved for patients that had *bcl-2* expression.[130] Other studies in squamous-cell carcinomas, however, have failed to show a difference in survival.[131,132]

c-erbB-2

(see also Chapter 4.) The stimulation for cells to grow without regulation can also occur through the expression of growth-factor receptors on the surface of the cell membrane. The c-*erbB*-1 protooncogene is known to encode for a tyrosine kinase growth factor receptor. The c-*erb*-B2 gene (also known as the *HER*-2/neu) encodes a protein originally isolated from rat neuroblastomas by virtue of structural similarities to EGF receptor.[133] In the rat neuroblastomas, a mutation in the transmembrane domain of neu resulted in constitutive receptor activation. c-*erb*-B2 is rarely mutated in human tumors, but is rather overexpressed or amplified.[134] The EGF and c-*erb*-B2 receptors have a glycosylated extracellular amino terminus where the ligand binds, a hydrophobic transmembrane region, and a kinase domain contained within the intracytoplasmic carboxy terminus. In the cytoplasmic domains of these receptors are several tyrosines that can become phosphorylated upon activation and thereafter bind to proteins that contain SH2 (*src* homology) domains. The SH2 domains mediate binding of these proteins to the phosphorylated tyrosine residues on the receptor.[134,135]

Gene amplification or overexpression of c-*erbB*-2 is rare in SCLC, whereas overexpression occurs in approximately 25% of NSCLC.[136,137] The highest expression levels are found in adenocarcinomas. c-erbB-2 overexpression, as documented by immunohistochemistry, has been shown to correlate with decreased survival in NSCLC[138] and to chemoresistance.[139] Since NSCLC has also been shown to produce EGF like substances, the possibility of an autocrine loop is raised such that a tumor cell expresses both a growth factor and its receptor.[140] An antibody against p185neu has been shown to inhibit proliferation of NSCLC cell lines.[141]

P53

(See also Chapter 6.) P53 mutations are the most common genetic changes in human cancer.[142] They are seen in more than 50% of NSCLC and 80% of SCLC.[85,143,144] Mutant p53 was first isolated as what was believed to be a dominant cooperating oncogene which behaved in many ways like *myc* or the E1A gene of adenovirus, in that it would cooperate with *ras* in transformation assays of 3T3 cells.[145] Subsequently it was realized that the form of p53 which was first isolated encoded a mutant, inactive, but long-lived form of the protein which displaced the wild-type but short-lived native form from its binding site and because of this acted as a dominant oncogene. p53 is now correctly thought of as a tumor suppressor gene. The action of p53 is complex. It binds to many important cellular proteins and is involved in the control of gene expression.[146] The last several years have seen an intense focus on its roles in cell-cycle delay in G1 phase and in apoptosis. It is now recognized that p53 can both regulate cell proliferation and induce apoptosis, depending on the circumstances and cellular background.[54,56]

The p53 gene is located at 17p13.1 and encodes a 53 kD nuclear protein.[85] Mutations in p53 in lung cancer are

of all types: missense, nonsense, splicing, and large deletions.[147] Missense mutations are associated with prolonged protein half-life and thus with increased steady-state protein level which can be detected via immunohistochemistry.[148] Immunohistochemical staining, however, misses about one third of mutations in p53 (mostly splicing and nonsense) and occasionally yields false positives.[148] Antibodies to p53 have been observed in lung cancer patients and appear to be correlated with the presence of a mutation in the tumor.[149] Antibodies to p53 may precede the development of clinical cancer.[150]

Abnormal expression of p53 has been shown to correlate with both better and worse prognosis. Early studies reported strong adverse prognostic impact,[151] but subsequent studies found either no association or even a survival advantage in patients with tumors bearing p53 mutations.[152] More recently, the multidrug-resistance-associated protein (MRP) expression in NSCLC was found to be correlated with p53 mutation, and this resulted in a worse prognosis.[153]

RB

(See also Chapter 7.) The RB gene is located on chromosome 13q14.11 and encodes for a 106 kD nuclear protein. It is phosphorylated in a cell-cycle-dependent manner, interacts with the transcription factor E2F, and is important in regulating cell cycle during G0/G1-phase.[34] When the cell enters late G1-phase to transition into S-phase, the RB protein becomes hyperphosphorylated.[34] RB protein, when hypophosphorylated, is complexed to E2F.[28] A crucial event in progression of the cell cycle is dissociation of the RB-E2F complex when RB becomes hyperphosphorylated. E2F is actually a group of transcription factors which contain a consensus binding site specific for sequences in the promoters of a number of cell-growth control genes, such as dihydrofolate reductase, PCNA, CDK1, cyclin E, cyclin A, c-*myc,* and TK.[39]

The RB gene is mutated or absent in more that 80% of SCLC and 40% of NSCLC.[154] In addition, disruptions of the RB pathway (RB, cyclin D1 and/or p16) can be seen in 90% of NSCLCs.[155] Thus the RB pathway plays an important role in tumorigenesis in lung cancer. Prognostically, however, no correlation has been found with alterations in RB and clinical outcome.[156] Like p53, it has been shown to be correlated to the multidrug-resistance gene and may be a marker for the assessment of sensitivity to some chemotherapeutic drugs.[157]

P16^{INK4a}

P16^{INK4A} is a cyclin-dependent kinase inhibitor which binds to CDK4 and 6, preventing their binding cyclin D.[34] As a result, RB is hypophosphorylated, and E2F is not released. P16^{INK4A} therefore functions as a tumor suppressor by contributing to the G1/S cell cycle checkpoint. Mutations in p16^{INK4A} are found in 50% of NSCLC and not reported in SCLC.[158] These mutations are frameshift, methylation, or homozygous deletion.[158] There is an inverse relationship between the presence of p16^{INK4A} mutations and RB expression in tumors.[159] Levels of p16^{INK4A} have not been shown to correlate with prognosis.

CLINICAL APPLICATIONS IN LUNG CANCER

Lung cancer is one of the most prevalent and lethal cancers. Despite recent advances in treatment, the long-term survival data show that only 10% of all patients are long-term survivors for NSCLC and 3% for SCLC.[160,161] To make an impact on the curability of lung cancer, we need to understand the biology of the disease and apply this to the development of novel diagnostic and therapeutic approaches. As outlined in the previous sections, numerous advances have been made recently in understanding the biology of lung cancer. These have led to potential techniques for diagnosing lung cancer at earlier stages, prognostic information to identify poor-risk patients, and various therapeutics under investigation such as gene therapy, antisense therapy, monoclonal antibody therapy, biologic response modifiers, and agents to enhance apoptosis.

Diagnosis of lung cancer at earlier stages can certainly make an impact on survival. Surgery in stage I/II disease can lead to five-year survival rates of 40% to 60%.[162] Development of *ras* mutations in bronchial epithelium can be detected in sputum samples as early as one month to four years prior to the clinical diagnosis of lung cancer.[117] p53 protein has also been found in sputum samples of patients with bronchial dysplasia.[163] Antibodies to p53 have been observed in lung cancer patients and appear to be correlated with the presence of a mutation in the tumor.[149] Antibodies to p53 may precede the development of clinical cancer.[150] Aberrant methylation of p16^{INK4A} has been found to be an early event in lung cancer, with its frequency increasing with disease progression from basal cell hyperplasia (17%) to squamous metaplasia (24%) to carcinoma *in situ* (50%).[164] With the application of these advancements in molecular biology techniques, it is possible that lung cancer could be detected in the preinvasive stages.

Mutations in *ras, myc,* and c-*erb*B-2 have been shown to correlate with a worse prognosis.[111–113,124,138] In addition, mutations of p53 and RB have been associated with the multidrug-resistance gene and may be markers for the assessment to some chemotherapeutic drugs.[153,157] It is plausible that assessing the bimolecular profile of the patient's tumor may assist in selecting the best therapy and prognostic category for patients to determine whether more aggressive treatment is warranted (see also Chapter 33).

With the various molecular changes seen in lung cancer, it can be hypothesized that replacing the defective gene/protein or decreasing the expression of the overexpressed ones may be a potential treatment. Studies have mostly focused on p53, c-*erb*B-2, and *ras*. Work on p53 done by Roth and co-workers has shown that administration of an adenoviral p53 vector to 21 patients with advanced non-small-cell lung cancer produced little toxicity and increased the sensitivity to cisplatinum in a phase I clinical trial.[165] A phase II clinical trial is being planned. In addition, a liposome-p53 complex delivered through the airway was effective in inhibiting lung tumor formation in transgenic mice with p53 deletions.[166] This may be a more direct way of getting p53 to the involved tissue (see also Chapters 6, 16).

Both K-*ras* and c-*erb*B-2 are overexpressed in lung tissue. One way to decrease their expression is by antisense therapy where a construct that binds to the active form is introduced into the cells. In nude mice, the introduction of a retroviral vector expressing antisense K-*ras* was reported to induce a marked reduction in tumor size and number of tumors with established tumor nodules created by intratracheal inoculation of human lung cancer cells.[167] With the overexpression of surface vectors such as c-*erb*B-2, toxins that specifically bind to the surface receptor have been tried. In mice with renal cell carcinoma, which also overexpresses c-*erb*B-2 as lung cancer does, systemic treatment with a recombinant c-*erb*B-2 receptor-specific tumor toxin reduced the number and size of pulmonary metastasis.[168]

We have been investigating molecular events that occur following ionizing radiation leading to DNA damage and repair, apoptosis, and cell cycle arrests.[59,60,63–66] We and others have studied the radiosensitizing effect of drugs such as caffeine[61] and pentoxyfylline[62] which alter G2 arrest. Unfortunately, these compounds are too toxic for clinical use in the doses that are required for radiosensitization. However, less toxic analogues are being developed.[169,170] *ras* has been implicated in the radioresistant phenotype,[171] and we have been investigating drugs that can inhibit its function so that tumors may become more radiosensitive. We have studied farnesyl transferase inhibitors that block *ras* processing that is required for its activity.[172] The treatment of tumor cells with FTI's has been shown to radiosensitize these tumors that express activated H- and K-*ras in vitro*.[100,173] Studies of their effect *in vivo* are underway.

REFERENCES

1. Pardee AB, Dubrow R, Hamlin JL, et al. Animal cell cycle. *Annu Rev Biochem* 1978;47:715.
2. Jackson DA, Pombo A. Replicon clusters are stable units of chromosome structure: evidence that nuclear organization contributes to the efficient activation and propagation of S phase in human cells. *J Cell Biol* 1998;140:1285.
3. Villarreal LP. Relationship of eukaryotic DNA replication to committed gene expression: general theory for gene control. *Microbiol Rev* 1991;55:512.
4. Tobey RA. Different drugs arrest cells at a number of distinct stages in G2. *Nature* 1975;254:245.
5. Weinert TA, Hartwell LH. The RAD9 gene controls the cell

cycle response to DNA damage in *Saccharomyces cerevesiae. Science* 1988;241:317.

6. McIntosh JR, Koonce MP. Mitosis. *Science* 1989;246:622.
7. Cross F, Roberts J, Weintraub H. Simple and complex cell cycles. *Annu Rev Cell Biol* 1989;5:341.
8. Rao PN, Johnson RT. Mammalian cell fusion: studies on the regulation of DNA synthesis and mitosis. *Nature* 1970;225:159.
9. Johnson RT, Rao PN. Mammalian cell fusion: induction of premature chromosome condensation in interphase nuclei. *Nature* 1970;226:717.
10. Morgan DO. Cyclin dependent kinases: engines, clocks, and microprocessors. *Annu Rev Cell Dev Biol* 1997;13:261.
11. Morgan DO. Principles of CDK regulation. *Nature* 1995;374:131.
12. Jeffrey PD, Russo AA, Polyak K, et al. Mechanism of CDK activation revealed by the structure of a cyclin A-CDK2 complex. *Nature* 1995;376:313.
13. Dunphy WG. The decision to enter mitosis. *Trends Cell Biol.* 1994;4:202.
14. Lew DJ, Kornbluth S. Regulatory roles of cyclin-dependent kinase phosphorylation in cell cycle control. *Curr Opin Cell Biol* 1996;8:795.
15. Booher R, Holman PS, Fattaey A. Human Myt1 is a cell cycle regulated Cdc2 inhibitory kinase. *J Biol Chem* 1997;272:22300.
16. Liu F, Stanton JJ, Wu Z, et al. The human Myt1 kinase preferentially phosphorylates Cdc2 on threonine 14 and localizes to the endoplasmic reticulum and Golgi complex. *Mol Cell Biol* 1997;17:571.
17. Galaktionov K, Chen X, Beach D. Cdc25 cell-cycle phosphatase as a target of c-*myc*. *Nature* 1996;382:511.
18. Gu Y, Rosenblatt J, Morgan DO. Cell cycle regulation of CDK2 activity by phosphorylation of Thr160 and Tyr15. *EMBO J* 1992;11:3995.
19. Jin P, Gu Y, Morgan DO. Role of inhibitory CDC2 phosphorylation in radiation-induced G2 arrest in human cells. *J Cell Biol* 1996;134:963.
20. Harper JW, Elledge SJ. Cdk inhibitors in development and cancer. *Curr Opin Genet Dev* 1996;6:56.
21. Morgan DO. Principles of CDK regulation. *Nature* 1995;374:131.
22. Noble JR, Rogan EM, Neumann AA, et al. Association of extended *in vitro* proliferative potential with loss of p16ink4 expression. *Oncogene* 1996;19:1259.
23. King RW, Deshaies RJ, Peters J-M, et al. How proteolysis drives the cell cycle. *Science* 1996;274:1652.
24. Chun KT, Mathias N, Goebl MG. Ubiquitin dependent proteolysis and cell cycle control in yeast. *Progress in Cell Cycle Res* 1996;2:115.
25. Page AM, Hieter P. The anaphase promoting complex. *Cancer Surveys* 1997;29:133.
26. Zachariae W, Schwab M, Nasmyth K, et al. Control of cyclin ubiquitination by CDK-regulated binding of Hct1 to the anaphase promoting complex. *Science* 1998;282:1721.
27. Fang G, Yu H, Kirschner MW. Direct binding of CDC20 protein family members activates the anaphase-promoting complex in mitosis and G1. *Mol Cell Biol* 1998;2:163.
28. Stillman B. Smart machines at the DNA replication fork. *Cell* 1994;78:725.
29. Sherr CJ. G1 phase progression: cycling on cue. *Cell* 1994;79:551.
30. Sherr CJ, Roberts JM. Inhibitors of mammalian G1 cyclin-dependent kinases. *Genes Dev* 1995;9:1149.
31. Hall M, Bates S, Peters G. Evidence for different modes of action of cyclin-dependent kinase inhibitors: p15 and p16 bind to kinases, p21 and p27 bind to cyclins. *Oncogene* 1995;19:1581.
32. Magnaghi-Jaulin L, Groisman R, Naguibneva I, et al. Retinoblastoma protein represses transcription by recruiting a histone deacetylase. *Nature* 1998;391:601.
33. Brehm A, Miska EA, McCance DJ, et al. Retinoblastoma protein recruits histone deacetylase to repress transcription. *Nature* 1998;391:597.
34. Weinberg RA. The retinoblastoma protein and cell cycle control. *Cell* 1995;81:323.
35. Baldin V, Lukas J, Marcote MJ, et al. Cyclin D1 is a nuclear protein required for cell cycle progression in G1. *Genes Dev* 1993;7:812.
36. Hatakeyama M, Brill JA, Fink GR, et al. Collaboration of G1 cyclins in the functional inactivation of the retinoblastoma protein. *Genes Dev* 1994;8:1759.
37. Lundberg AS, Weinberg RA. Functional inactivation of the retinoblastoma protein requires sequential modification by at least two distinct cyclin-cdk complexes. *Mol Cell Biol* 1998;18:753.
38. Lukas J, Bartkova J, Rohde M, et al. Cyclin D1 is dispensable for G1 control in retinoblastoma gene-deficient cells independent of CDK4 activity. *Mol Cell Biol* 1995;15:2600.
39. DeGregori J, Kowalik T, Nevins JR. Cellular targets for activation by the E2F1 transcription factor include DNA synthesis and G1/S regulatory genes. *Mol Cell Biol* 1995;15:4215.
40. Whyte P. The retinoblastoma protein and its relatives. *Sem in Cancer Biology* 1995;6:83.
41. Ludlow JW, Skuse GR. Viral oncoprotein binding to pRb, p107, p130 and p300. *Virus Res* 1995;35:113.
42. King RW, Jackson PK, Kirschner MW. Mitosis in transition. *Cell* 1994;79:563.
43. King RW, Deshaies RJ, Peters JM, et al. How proteolysis drives the cell cycle. *Science* 1996;274:1652.
44. Hunter T. Oncoprotein networks. *Cell* 1997;88:333.
45. Phuchareon J, Tokuhisa T. Deregulated c-Fos/AP-1 modulates expression of the cyclin and the cdk gene in splenic B cells stimulated with lipopolysaccharide. *Cancer Lett* 1995;92:203.
46. Kelly K, Cochran BH, Stiles CD, et al. Cell specific regulation of the c-*myc* gene by lymphocyte mitogenes and platelet derived growth factor. *Cell* 1983;35:603.
47. Shichiri M, Hanson KD, Sedivy JM. Effects of c-*myc* expression on proliferation, quiescence, and the G0 to G1 transition in nontransformed cells. *Cell Growth Differ* 1993;4:93.
48. Daksis JI, Lu RY, Facchini LM, et al. *Myc* induces cyclin D1 expression in the absence of *e novo* protein synthesis and links mitogen stimulated signal transduction to the cell cycle. *Oncogene* 1994;9:3635.
49. Steiner P, Philipp A, Lukas J, et al. Identification of a *myc* dependent step during the formation of active G1 cyclin-CDK complexes. *EMBO J* 1995;14:4814.
50. Avruch J, Zhang XF, Kyriakis JM. *Raf* meets *Ras:* completing the framework of a signal transduction pathway. *Trends Bioch Sci* 1994;19:279.
51. Dobrowlski S, Harter M, Stacey DW. Cellular *ras* activity is required for passage through multiple points of the G0/G1 phase in BALB/c 3T3 cells. *Mol Cell Biol* 1994;14:5441.
52. Liu JJ, Chao JR, Jiang MC Ng Sy, et al. *Ras* transformation results in as elevated level of cyclin D1 and acceleration of G1 progression in NIH 3T3 cells. *Mol Cell Biol* 1995;15:3654.
53. Leone G, DeGregori J, Sears R, et al. *Mac* and *Ras* collaborate in inducing accumulation of active cyclin E/CDK2 and E2F. *Nature* 1997;387:422.
54. Levine AJ. p53, the cellular gatekeeper for growth and division. *Cell* 1997;88:323.
55. Palmero I, Pantoja C, Serrano M. p19ARF links the tumor suppressor p53 to *ras*. *Nature* 1998;395:125.

56. el-Deiry WS, Tokino T, Velculescu VE, et al. WAF1, a potential mediator of p53 tumor suppression. *Cell* 1993;75:817.

57. Waga S, Hannon GJ, Beach D, et al. The p21 inhibitor of cyclin dependent kinases controls DNA replication by interaction with PCNA. *Nature* 1994;369:574.

58. Lowe SW, Schmitt EM, Smith SW, et al. p53 is required for radiation induced apoptosis in mouse thymocytes. *Nature* 1993; 362:847.

59. McKenna WG, Iliakis G, Weiss MC, et al. Increased G2 delay in radiation-resistant cells obtained by transformation of primary rat embryo cells with the oncogenes H-*ras* and v-*myc*. *Radiat Res* 1991;125:283.

60. Iliakis G, Metzger L, Muschel RJ, et al. Induction and repair of DNA double strand breaks in radiation-resistant cells obtained by transformation of primary rat embryo cells with the oncogenes H-*ras* and V-*myc*. *Cancer Res* 1990;50:6575.

61. Busse PM, Bose SK, Jones RW, et al. The action of caffeine on X-irradiated HeLa cells. Enhancement of X-ray induced killing during G2 arrest. *Radiat Res* 1978;76:292.

62. Kim SH, Khil MS, Ryu S, et al. Enhancement of radiation response on human carcinoma cells in culture by pentoxyfylline. *Int J Radiat Oncol Biol Phys* 1993;25:61.

63. Muschel RJ, Zhang HB, Iliakis G, et al. Cyclin B expression in HeLa cells during the G2 block induced by ionizing radiation. *Cancer Res* 1991;51:5113.

64. Muschel RJ, Zhang HB, McKenna WG. Differential effect of ionizing radiation on the expression of cyclin A and cyclin B in HeLa cells. *Cancer Res* 1993;53:1128.

65. Bernhard EJ, Maity A, Muschel RJ, et al. Increased expression of cyclin B1 mRNA coincides with diminished G2-phase arrest in irradiated HeLa cells treated with staurosporine or caffeine. *Radiat Res* 1994;140:393.

66. Kao GD, McKenna WG, Maity A, et al. Cyclin B1 availability is a rate limiting component of the radiation induced G2 delay in HeLa cells. *Cancer Res* 1997;57:753.

67. Paules RS, Levedakow EN, Wilson SJ, et al. Defective G2 checkpoint function in cells from individuals with familial cancer syndromes. *Cancer Res* 1995;55:1763.

68. Lock RB. Inhibition of p34CDC2 kinase activation, p34CDC2 tyrosine dephosphorylation, and mitotic progression in chinese hamster ovary cells exposed to etoposide. *Cancer Res* 1992;52: 1817.

69. O'Connor PM, Ferris DK, Pagano M, et al. G2 delay induced by nitrogen mustard in human cells affect cyclin A/Cdk2 and cyclin B1/Cdc2-kinase complexes differently. *J Biol Chem* 1993; 268:8298.

70. Clarke AR, Purdie CA, Harrison DJ, et al. Thymocyte apoptosis induced by p53-dependent and independent pathways. *Nature* 1993;362:849.

71. Kerr JFK, Wyllie AH, Currie AH. Apoptosis, a basic biological phenomenon with wider implications in tissue kinetics. *Br J Cancer* 1972;26:239.

72. D'Amico AV, McKenna WG. Apoptosis and a reinvestigation of the biologic basis for cancer therapy. *Radiother Oncol* 1994; 33:3.

73. Arends MJ, Morris RG, Wyllie AH. Apoptosis. The role of the endonuclease. *Am J Pathol* 1990;136:593.

74. Walker PR, Sikorska M. Endonuclease activities, chromatin structure, and DNA degradation in apoptosis. *Biochem Cell Biol* 1994;72:615.

75. Whiteside G, Munglani R. TUNEL, hoechst and immunohisto-chemistry triple-labelling: an improved method for detection of apoptosis in tissue sections—an update. *Brain Res Protoc* 1998; 1:52.

76. Dive C, Gregory CD, Phipps DJ, et al. Analysis and discrimination of necrosis and apoptosis (programmed cell death) by mul-

77. tiparameter flow cytometry. *Biochemica et Biophysica Acta* 1992; 1133:275.

77. Howard A, Pelc SR. Synthesis of deoxyribonucleic acid in normal and irradiated cells and its relation to chromosome breakage. *Heredity [Suppl.]* 1953;6:261.

78. Yamada M, Puck TT. Action of radiation on mammalian cells, IV. Reversible mitrotic lag in the S3 HeLa cell produced by low doses of X-rays. *Proc Nat Acad Sci USA* 1961;47:1181.

79. Evan GI, Gilbert CS, Littlewood TD, et al. Induction of apoptosis in fibroblasts by c-*myc* protein. *Cell* 1992;69:119.

80. Kastan MB, Onyekwere O, Sidransky D, et al. Participation of p53 protein in the cellular response to DNA damage. *Cancer Res* 1991;511:6304.

81. Hermeking H, Eick D. Mediation of c-*myc*-induced apoptosis by p53. *Science* 1994;265:2091.

82. Di Leonardo A, Linke SP, Clarkin K, et al. DNA damage triggers a prolongued p53-dependent G1 arrest and long-term induction of Cip-1 in normal human fibroblasts. *Genes Dev* 1994; 8:2540.

83. McKenna WG, Bernhard EJ, Markiewicz DA, et al. Regulation of radiation induced apoptosis in oncogene transfected fibroblasts: influence of H-*ras* on the G2 delay. *Oncogene* 1996;12: 237.

84. Lowe SW, Schmitt EM, Smith SW, et al. p53 is required for radiation-induced apoptosis in mouse thymocytes. *Nature* 1993; 362:847.

85. Sidransky D, Hollstein M. Clinical implications of the p53 gene. *Annu Rev Med* 1996;47:285.

86. Canman CE, Gilmer TM, Coutts SB, et al. Growth factor modulation of p53 mediated growth arrest versus apoptosis. *Genes Dev* 1995;9:600.

87. Sentman CL, Shutter JR, Hockenbery D, et al. *Bcl*-2 inhibits multiple forms of apoptosis but not negative selection in thymocytes. *Cell* 1991;67:879.

88. Vanhaesebroek B, Reed JC, De Valck D, et al. Effect of *bcl*-2 proto-oncogene expression on cellular sensitivity to tumor necrosis factor-mediated cytotoxicity. *Oncogene* 1993;8:1075.

89. Akao Y, Otsuki Y, Kataoka S, et al. Multiple subcellular localization of *bcl*-2: detection in nuclear outer membrane, endoplasmic reticulum membrane, and mitochondrial membranes. *Cancer Res* 1994;54:2468.

90. de Jong D, Prins FA, Mason DY, et al. Subcellular localization of the *bcl*-2 protein in malignant and normal lymphoid cells. *Cancer Res* 1994;54:256.

91. Craig RW. The *bcl*-2 gene family. *Sem Cancer Biol* 1995;6:35.

92. Oltvai ZN, Milliman CL, Korsmeyer SJ. *Bcl*-2 heterodimerizes *in vivo* with a conserved homolog, bax, that accelerates programmed cell death. *Cell* 1993;74:609.

93. Williams GT, Smith CA. Molecular regulation of apoptosis: genetic controls on cell death. *Cell* 1993;74:777.

94. Hartwell LH, Kastan MB. Cell cycle control and cancer. *Science* 1994;266:1821.

95. Zeigler A, Jonason AS, Leffell DJ, et al. Sunburn and p53 in the onset of skin cancer. *Nature* 1994;372:773.

96. Cha RS, Thilly WG, Zarbl H. N-nitroso-N-methylurea-induced rat mammary tumors arise from cells with preexisting oncogenic H-*ras*-1 gene mutations. *Proc Natl Acad Sci USA* 1994;91:3749.

97. Nooter K, Boersma AWM, Oostrum RG, et al. Constitutive expression of the c-H-*ras* oncogene inhibits doxorubicin-induced apoptosis and promotes cell survival in a rhabdomyosarcoma cell line. *British J of Cancer* 1995;71:556.

98. Graeber TG, Osmanian C, Jacks T, et al. Hypoxia-mediated selection of cells with diminished apoptotic potential in solid tumors. *Nature* 1996;379:88.

99. Lock RB, Galperina OV, Feldhoff RC, et al. Concentration-

dependent differences in the mechanism by which caffeine potentiates etoposide cytotoxicity in Hela cells. *Cancer Res* 1994; 54:4933.

100. Bernhard EJ, Muschel RJ, Bakanauskas VJ, et al. Reducing the radiation-induced G2 delay causes HeLa cells to undergo apoptosis instead of mitotic death. *Int J Radiant Biol* 1996;69: 575.

101. Donehower LA, Harvey M, Slagle BL, et al. Mice deficient for p53 are developmentally normal but susceptible to spontaneous tumours. *Nature* 1992;356:215.

102. Berges RR, Furuya Y, Remington L, et al. Cell proliferation, DNA repair, and p53 function are not required for programmed death of prostatic glandular cells induced by androgen ablation. *Proc Natl Acad Sci USA* 1993;90:8910.

103. Kyprianou N, English HF, Davidson NE, et al. Programmed cell death during regression of the MCF-7 human breast cancer following estrogen ablation. *Cancer Res* 1991;51:162.

104. Bourne H, Sanders D, McCormick F. The GTPase superfamily: conserved structure and molecular mechanism. *Nature* 1991; 349:117.

105. Lim L, Manser E, Leung T, et al. Regulation of phosphorylation pathways by p21 GTPases: the p21 *ras*-related rho family and its role in phosphorylation signalling pathways. *Eur J Biochem* 1996;242:171.

106. Bos JL. *Ras* oncogenes in human cancer: a review. *Cancer Res* 1989;49:4682.

107. Ben-Levy R, Paterson HF, Marshall CJ, et al. A single autophosphorylation site confers oncogenicity to the neu/*erb*B-2 receptor and enables coupling to the MAP kinase pathway. *EMBO J* 1994;13:3302.

108. DeClue JE, Papgeorge AG, Fletcher JA, et al. Abnormal regulation of mammalian p21*ras* contributes to malignant tumor growth in von Recklinghausen (type 1) neurofibromatosis. *Cell* 1992;69:265.

109. Sagawa M, Saito Y, Fujimura S, et al. K-*ras* point mutation occurs in the early stage of carcinogenesis in lung cancer. *Br J Cancer* 1998;77:720.

110. Mitsudomi T, Viallet J, Mulshine JL, et al. Mutations of *ras* genes distinguish a subset non-small-cell lung cancer cell lines from small-cell lung cancer cell lines. *Oncogene* 1991;6:1353.

111. Harada M, Dosaka-Akita H, Miyamoto H, et al. Prognostic significance of the expression of *ras* oncogene product in non-small-cell lung cancer. *Cancer* 1992;69:72.

112. Sugio K, Ishida T, Yokoyama T, et al. *Ras* gene mutations as a prognostic marker in adenocarcinoma of the human lung without lymph node metastasis. *Cancer* 1992;52:2903.

113. Rossell R, Li S, Skacel Z. Prognositc impact of mutated K-*ras* gene in surgically resected non-small-cell lung cancer patients. *Oncogene* 1993;8:2407.

114. Kwiatkowski DJ, Harpole DH, Godleski J, et al. Molecular pathologic substaging in 244 stage I non-small-cell lung cancer patients: clinical implications. *J Clin Oncol* 1998;16:2468.

115. Sklar MD. Increased resistance to cis-diamminedichloroplatinum (II) in NIH3T3 cells transformed by *ras* oncogenes. *Cancer Res* 1988;48:793.

116. Rodhenhuis S, Boerrigter L, Top B, et al. Mutational activation of the K-*ras* oncogene and the effect of chemotherapy in advanced adenocarcinoma of the lung: a prospective study. *J of Clin Oncol* 1997;15:285.

117. Somers VA, Pietersen AM, Theunissen PH, et al. Detection of K-*ras* point mutations in sputum from patients with adenocarcinoma of the lung by point-EXACCT. *J Clin Oncol* 1998;16: 3061.

118. Evan GI, Littlewood TD. The role of c-*myc* in cell growth. *Curr Opin Genet Dev* 1993;3:44.

119. Wong AJ, Ruppert JM, Eggleston J, et al. Gene amplification of c-*myl* and n-*myc* in small-cell carcinoma of the lung. *Science* 1986;233:461.

120. Eilers M, Schirm S, Bishop JM. The *myc* protein activates transcription of the alpha-prothymosin gene. *EMBO J* 1991;10: 133.

121. Slebos RJ, Evers SG, Wagenaar SS, et al. Cellular protooncogenes are infrequently amplified in untreated non-small-cell lung cancer. *Br J Cancer* 1989;59:76.

122. Gazdar AF, Carney DN, Nau MM, et al. Characterization of variant subclasses of cell lines derived from small-cell lung cancer having distinctive biochemical, morphological, and growth properties. *Cancer Res* 1985;45:2924.

123. Takahashi T, Obata Y, Sekido Y, et al. Expression and amplification of *myc* gene family in small-cell lung cancer and its relation to biological characteristics. *Cancer Res* 1989;49:2863.

124. Johnson BE, Russell E, Simmons AM, et al. *Myc* family DNA amplification in 126 tumor cell lines from patients with small-cell lung cancer. *J Cell Biochem* 1996;24:210.

125. Rygaard K, Slebos RJ, Spang-Thomsen M. Radiosensitivity of small-cell lung cancer xenografts compared with activity of c-*myc*, n-*myc*, l-*myc*, c-*raf*-1, and k-*ras* protooncogenes. *Int J Cancer* 1991;49:279.

126. Reed JC, Kitada S, Takayama S, et al. Regulation of chemoresistance by the *bcl*-2 oncoprotein in non-Hodgkin's lymphoma and lymphocytic leukemia cell lines. *Annals Oncol* 1994;[Suppl. 1]:61.

127. Novack DV, Korsmeyer SJ. *Bcl*-2 protein expression during murine development. *Am J Pathol* 1994;145:61.

128. Stefanaki K, Rontogiannis D, Vamvouka C, et al. Immunohistochemical detection of *bcl*-2, p53, mdm2, and p21/waf1 proteins in small cell lung carcinomas. *Anticancer Res* 1998;18(3A): 1689.

129. Kaiser U, Schilli M, Haag U, et al. Expression of *Bcl*2 protein in small cell lung cancer. *Lung Cancer* 1996;15:31.

130. Pezzella F, Turley H, Kuzu I, et al. *Bcl*-2 protein in non-small-cell lung carcinoma. *NEJM* 1993;329:690.

131. Anton RC, Brown RW, Younes M, et al. Absence of prognostic significance of *bcl*-2 immunopositivity in non-small-cell lung cancer: analysis of 427 cases. *Hum Pathol* 1997;28:1079.

132. Silvestrini R, Costa A, Lequaglie C, et al. *Bcl*-2 protein and prognosis in patients with potentially curable non-small-cell lung cancer. *Virchows Archiv* 1998;432:441.

133. Schechter AL, Stern DF, Vaidyanathan L, et al. The neu oncogene: an *erb*-B related gene encoding a 185,000 Mr tumour antigen. *Nature* 1984;312:513.

134. Ullrich A, Schlessinger J. Signal transduction by receptors with tyrosine kinase activity. *Cell* 1990;61:203.

135. Aaronson S. Growth factors and cancer. *Science* 1991;254:1146.

136. Knyazev PG, Imyanitov EN, Chernitca OI, et al. Amplification of the ERBB2 (HER2/NEW) oncogene in different neoplasms of patients from USSR. *Oncology* 1992;49:162.

137. Weiner DB, Nordberg J, Robinson R, et al. Expression of the new gene-encoded protein (P185neu) in human non-small-cell carcinoma of the lung. *Cancer Res* 1990;50:421.

138. Kern JA, Schwartz DA, Nordberg JE, et al. p185neu expression in human lung adenocarcinomas predicts shortened survival. *Cancer Res* 1990;50:5184.

139. Tsai CM, Chang KT, Wu LH, et al. Correlations between intrinsic chemoresistance and HER-2/new gene expression, p53 gene mutations, and cell proliferation characteristics in non-small-cell lung cancer cell lines. *Cancer Res* 1996;56:206.

140. Carbone DP. The biology of lung cancer. *Seminars in Oncology* 1997;24:388.

141. Kern J, Filderman A. Oncogenes and growth factors in human lung cancer. *Clin Chest Med* 1993;14:31.

142. Hollstein M, Sidransky D, Vogelstein B, et al. p53 mutations in human cancers. *Science* 1991;253:49.

143. Chiba I, Takahashi T, Nau MM, et al. Mutations in the p53 gene are frequent in primary, resected non-small-cell lung cancer. *Oncogene* 1990;5:1603.

144. D'Amico D, Carbone D, Mitsudomi T, et al. High frequency of somatically acquired p53 mutations in small cell lung cancer cell lines and tumors. *Oncogene* 1992;7:339.

145. Parada LF, Land H, Weinberg RA, et al. Cooperation between gene encoding p53 tumor antigen and *ras* in cellular transformation. *Nature* 1984;312:649.

146. Miyashita T, Krajewski S, Krajewska M, et al. Tumor supressor p53 is a regulator of *bcl*-2 and *bax* gene expression *in vitro* and *in vivo*. *Oncogene* 1994;9:1799.

147. Caron de Fromental C, Soussi T. The p53 tumor suppressor gene: a model for investigating human mutagenesis. *Genes Chromosomes Cancer* 1992;4:1.

148. Bodner SM, Minna J, Jensen SM, et al. Expression of mutant p53 proteins in lung cancer correlates with the class of p53 gene mutations. *Oncogene* 1992;7:743.

149. Winter SF, Minna JD, Johnson BE, et al. Development of antibodies against p53 in lung cancer patients appears to be dependent on the type of p53 mutations. *Cancer Res* 1992;52:4168.

150. Lubin R, Zalcman G, Bouchet L, et al. Serum p53 antibodies as early markers of lung cancer. *Nature Med* 1995;1:701.

151. Quinlan DC, Davidson AG, Summers CL, et al. Accumulation of p53 protein correlates with a poor prognosis in human lung cancer. *Cancer Res* 1992;52:4828.

152. Lee JS, Yoon A, Kalapurakal SK, et al. Expression of p53 oncoprotein in non-small-cell lung cancer: a favorable prognostic factor. *J Clin Oncol* 1995;13:1893.

153. Oshika Y, Nakamura M, Tokunaga T, et al. Mulitdrug resistance-associated protein and mutant p53 protein expression in non-small-cell lung cancer. *Mod Pathol* 1998;11:1059.

154. Shimizu E, Zhao M, Shinohara A, et al. Differential expressions of cyclin A and the retinoblastoma gene product in histological subtypes of lung cancer cell lines. *J Cancer Res Clin Oncol* 1997;123:533.

155. Tenaka H, Fujii Y, Hirabayashi H, et al. Disruption of the RB pathway and cell-proliferative activity in non-small-cell lung cancers. *Int J Cancer* 1998;79:111.

156. Volm M, Koomagi R, Rittgen W. Clinical implications of cyclin-dependent kinases, RB and E2F1 in squamous-cell lung carcinoma. *Int J Cancer* 1998;79:294.

157. Yamamot Y, Shimizu E, Masuda N, et al. RB protein status and chemosensitivity in non-small-cell lung cancers. *Oncol Rep* 1998;5:447.

158. Gazzeri S, Gouyer V, Vour'ch C, et al. Mechanisms of p16ink4A inactivation in non-small-cell lung cancers. *Oncogene* 1998;16:497.

159. Fujishita T, Mizushima Y, Kashii T, et al. Coincidental alterations of p16INK4A/CDKN2 and other genes in human lung cancer cell lines. *Anticancer Res* 1998;18:1537.

160. Parker S, Tong T, Bolden S. Cancer statistics 1997. *CA Cancer J Clin* 1997;47:5.

161. Skarin A. Analysis of long term survivors with small cell lung cancer. *Chest* 1993;103:440.

162. al-Kattan K, Sepsas E, Townsend ER, et al. Factors affecting long term survival following resection for lung cancer. *Thorax* 1996;12:1266.

163. Mitsudomi T, Lam S, Shirakusa T, et al. Detection and sequencing of p53 gene mutations in bronchial biopsy samples in patients with lung cancer. *Chest* 1993;104:362.

164. Belinsky SA, Nikula KJ, Palmisano WA, et al. Aberrant methylation of p16(INK4a) is an early event in lung cancer and a potential biomarker for early diagnosis. *Proc Natl Acad Sci USA* 1998;95:11891.

165. Roth JA, Swisher SG, Merritt JA, et al. Gene therapy for non-small-cell lung cancer: a preliminary report of a phase I trial of adenoviral p53 gene replacement. *Semin Oncol* 1998;3:33.

166. Zou Y, Zong G, Ling YH, et al. Effective treatment of early endobronchial cancer with regional administration of liposome-p53 complexes. *J Natl Cancer Inst* 1998;90:1130.

167. Georges RN, Mukhopadhyay T, Zhang Y, et al. Prevention of orthotopic human lung cancer growth by intratracheal instillation of a retroviral antisense K-*ras* construct. *Cancer Res* 1993;53:1743.

168. Maurer-Gebhard M, Schmidt M, Azemar M, et al. Systemic treatment with a recombinant *erb*B-2 recetor-specific tumor toxin efficiently reduces pulmonary metastases inmice injected with genetically modified carcinoma cells. *Cancer Res* 1998;58:2661.

169. Husain A, Rosales N, Schwartz GK, et al. Lisofylline sensitizes p53 mutant human ovarian carcinoma cells to the cytotoxic effects of cis-diamminedichloroplatinum (II). *Gynec Onc* 1998;70:17.

170. Wong JS, Ara G, Keyes SR, et al. Lisofylline as a modifier of radiation therapy. *Oncol Res* 1996;8:513.

171. McKenna WG, Weiss MC, Endlich B, et al. Synergistic effect of the v-*myc* oncogene with H-*ras* of radioresistance. *Cancer Res* 1990;50:97.

172. Kohl NE, Mosser SD, DeSolms SJ, et al. Selective inhibition of *ras* dependent transformation by a farnesyltransferase inhibitor. *Science* 1993;260:1934.

173. Bernhard EJ, McKenna WG, Hamilton AD, et al. Inhibiting *ras* prenylation increases the radiosensitivity of human tumor cell lines with activating mutations of *ras* oncogene. *Cancer Res* 1998;58:1754.

3

CIGARETTE SMOKE DAMAGE TO DNA AND OTHER BIOMOLECULES

WILLIAM A. PRYOR

The oxidants in smoke, including both free radicals and nonradical oxidants, are responsible for the biological damage caused by smoke, including damage to DNA,[1-13] proteins,[8] and lipids.[14-17]

Cigarette smoke is operationally divided into two phases: a particulate phase ("tar"), and gas-phase smoke. The two phases are separated using a filter, typically a Cambridge filter made of glass fibers that retains more than 99.9% of the particles 0.1 μm or larger. The principal compounds in gas-phase smoke and tar are shown in (Table 3.1). Gas-phase smoke and tar contain very different types of free radicals and oxidants.

GAS PHASE SMOKE

Gas-phase cigarette smoke contains high concentrations of both oxy-radicals and nitrogen oxides (which also are free radicals), particularly nitric oxide.[18] The organic radicals produced by the flame itself are too short-lived to reach the lung. The organic radicals in gas-phase smoke are formed by the slow oxidation of nitric oxide, $\cdot$NO, to nitrogen dioxide, $\cdot NO_2$ (Reaction 1). Nitrogen dioxide, which is more reactive toward organic compounds than is $\cdot$NO, then adds to isoprene and other reactive olefins in the smoke to produce carbon-centered radicals, as shown in Reaction 2. The carbon-centered radicals then react with dioxygen to form peroxyl radicals (Reaction 3), and these species can cause lipid peroxidation and other types of biological oxidations.[2,19-22] The peroxyl radicals also can react with nitric oxide to form esters of peroxynitrite (Reaction 4).[7,22]

$$\cdot NO + \tfrac{1}{2}O_2 \text{—slow} \rightarrow \cdot NO_2 \quad [1]$$

$$\cdot NO + \text{isoprene} \rightarrow R\cdot \text{ (carbon-centered radicals)} \quad [2]$$

$$R\cdot + O_2 \rightarrow ROO\cdot \quad [3]$$

$$ROO\cdot + \cdot NO \rightarrow ROO\text{-}NO \text{ (peroxynitrite esters)} \quad [4]$$

The radicals in gas-phase smoke are very short lived and react within a fraction of a second on entering the lung.[2,19] When smoke is absorbed by models of the lung lining fluid, these species produce a complex mixture of reactive oxygen species (ROS), such as hydrogen peroxide, peroxyl and alkoxyl radicals, and reactive nitrogen species (RNS), including peroxynitrite, peroxynitrate, and their esters, as shown above.[2,7,20,22] The oxidants in gas-phase smoke initiate lipid peroxidation.[14-17] They also oxidize the principal human anti-proteinase, α-1-proteinase inhibitor; in this case, it is H_2O_2 that is the principal oxidant.[8,23]

AQUEOUS CIGARETTE TAR (ACT) EXTRACTS AND DNA DAMAGE

In contrast to the short-lived radicals in the gas phase, cigarette tar contains high concentrations (more than 10^{17} radicals per gram) of extremely stable radicals. These stable radicals can be directly observed by EPR methods, either directly on the filter or in organic[24] or aqueous solutions.[7-13] At least four different radicals have been identified in tar, based on their EPR characteristics;[24] the most interesting is a low-molecular-weight semiquinone (QH$\cdot$) that is in equilibrium with quinones (Q) and polyphenols (QH$_2$).[2,19] The principal polyphenols in aqueous cigarette tar (ACT) extracts are hydroquinone and catechol.[6,11,25-27]

The tar-radical system is readily water-soluble and can be extracted into aqueous solutions; the EPR spectra of ACT solutions contain a broad signal with a G value of 2.0035 that is typical of organic semiquinones.[7,28] (The G value of a radical can be used to characterize its chemical type.)

Since the tar radical is water-soluble, the aqueous fluids bathing the lung will contain this long-lived radical; for this reason, we have concentrated our studies on the biological damage that this tar radical can produce.[2,3,7-13,19,24] ACT solutions nick plasmid DNA,[29] producing nicks of a type that are not easily repairable.[4] Thus error-prone mechanisms may be involved in the repair of the tar-radical–induced nicks, and these erroneous repairs could lead to muta-

TABLE 3.1. CONSTITUENTS IN TAR AND GAS-PHASE (MAINSTREAM) SMOKE[26]

Tar	mg/Cigarette	Gas-Phase Smoke	mg/Cigarette
Nicotine	1.6	NO	0.3
Polyphenols	0.6	Ethylene	0.2
Aldehydes	0.5	Isoprene	0.4
Nitrosamines	1.5	Methanol	0.2
PAH	0.004	Acetaldehyde	0.9

tions. The tar-radical system can also penetrate rat thymus cells, reach the nucleus, and bind to and nick the nuclear DNA.[7,10–13] Thus the radical system is sufficiently stable to be able to diffuse through the lung lining fluid, reach and penetrate cells and subcellular organelles, and thus reach nuclear DNA.

The first interaction of the tar-radical system with DNA appears to be an association of the semiquinone radical with DNA; this association is probably a complexation of the quinones, polyphenols and semiquinones with DNA, and this complex also probably binds metal ions.[10–12] We demonstrated this binding by isolating DNA from intact rat alveolar macrophage (RAM) cells that had been exposed to ACT extracts and showing that the tar radical EPR signal becomes incorporated into the DNA. After binding, DNA nicks are observed, and the nicking follows saturation kinetics, suggesting that the binding occurs to certain sites on the DNA chain that then become saturated.[7,10,13,30] The EPR properties and the DNA-damaging effects of main-

stream and sidestream tar solutions are comparable to those of aged catechol solutions, as shown in (Table 3.2).[27]

Based on these nicking and binding studies, we have proposed a model in which the tar radical first binds to and then nicks DNA.[3,13] This model is shown in (Figure 3.1).

FRACTIONATION OF ACT SOLUTIONS

Fractionation of ACT extracts by Sephadex chromatography allows the isolation and identification of those fractions that contain the $Q/QH_2/QH\cdot$ system. These fractions absorb dioxygen and undergo autoxidation to produce superoxide and hydrogen peroxide, as shown in Reactions 5 to 7.

$$QH_2 + O_2 \rightarrow QH\cdot + O_2\cdot^- + H^+ \qquad [5]$$

$$QH\cdot + O_2 \rightarrow Q + O_2\cdot^- + H^+ \qquad [6]$$

$$2O_2\cdot^- + 2H^+ \rightarrow H_2O_2 \cdot + O_2 \qquad [7]$$

Cigarette tar binds metals such as iron, and either this tar-bound iron or iron present in the biological mileau causes the iron-catalyzed production of hydroxyl radicals, as shown in Reaction 8 (the Fenton reaction).

$$H_2O_2 + Fe^{2+} \rightarrow HO\cdot + O_2 + HO^- \qquad [8]$$

We find that the DNA-nicking activity of the tar is virtually exclusively possessed by the fractions that contain the

TABLE 3.2. COMPARISON OF DNA DAMAGE, HYDROGEN PEROXIDE PRODUCTION, AND THE EFFECTS OF INHIBITORS FOR TAR EXTRACTS FROM MAINSTREAM AND SIDESTREAM SMOKE AND AGED CATECHOL SOLUTIONS

Parameter	Mainstream Cigarette Tar	Sidestream# Cigarette Tar	Aged Catechol Solutions
Number of cigarettes, or cigarette equivalents (for aged catechol) needed to cause maximum DNA damage	0.24 cigarettes	1.0 cigarettes	0.34 cigarette equivalents
H_2O_2 production/g tar**	25–60 μmol/mg	1–5 μmol/mg	2.5–4 μmol/mg
Protection by catalase, %	83 ± 12	96 ± 4	18 ± 14*
Protection by boiled catalase, %			2
Protection by superoxide dismutase, %	38	24 ± 12	10 ± 13
Protection by boiled SOD, %	35	25	16
Protection by 200 mM GSH, %	85 ± 7	87 ± 3	84 ± 4
Protection by 20 mM DTPA, %	28 ± 5	42 ± 8	not tested
Protection by 1 mM deferoxamine, %	27 ± 9	not tested	29 ± 17

* Catechol is an effective inhibitor of catalase, thus no protection is observed. (Keilin D, Hartree EF. Catalase, peroxidase, metmyoglobin as catalysts of coupled peroxidatic reactions. *Biochem J* 1955;60:310, with permission Ogura Y, Tonomura Y, Hino S, et al. Studies on the reaction between catalase molecule and various inhibitory substances, I. *J Biochem Tokyo* 1950;37:153, with permission.)
** The ACT solution was dried and the tar weighed; this is H_2O_2 production calculated on a per gram of tar basis.
# Sidestream smoke rises from the cigarette into the environment between puffs; it is the principal component of environmental tobacco smoke (ETS).
(From Pryor WA, Stone K, Zhang L-Y, et al. Fractionation of aqueous cigarette tar extracts: fractions that contain the tar radical cause DNA damage. *Chem Res Toxicol* 1998;11:441, with permission.)

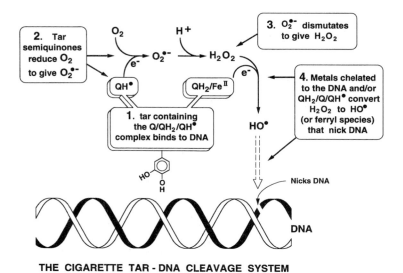

THE CIGARETTE TAR - DNA CLEAVAGE SYSTEM

FIGURE 3.1. Model of the tar radical binding to and nicking DNA. **1:** Aqueous extracts of cigarette tar contain a semiquinone/hydroquinone/quinone radical in a low-molecular-weight polymeric matrix that binds to DNA. **2:** The semiquinone radicals reduce dioxygen to form superoxide. **3:** Superoxide then dismutates to form hydrogen peroxide. (Hydrogen peroxide may also diffuse into the nucleus from other loci in the cell.) **4:** Metals chelated to the tar react with hydrogen peroxide to form hydroxyl radical (or ferryl) species that nick DNA. (From Pryor WA. Cigarette smoke and the involvement of free radical reaction in chemical carcinogenesis *Br J Cancer* 1987;55[Suppl. VIII]:19; Pryor WA, Stone K. Oxidants in cigarette smoke: radicals, hydrogen peroxide, peroxyritrate, and peroxynitrite. In: Diana J, Pryos W, eds. *Tobacco smoking and nutrition: influence of nutrition on tobacco associated health risks.* Annals of the New York Academy of Sciences, Vol. 686, New York: New York Academy of Sciences, 1993: 12; Pryor WA. Cigarette smoke radicals and the role of free radicals in chemical calcinogenicity. *Environ Health Perspect* 1997;105:875, with permission.)

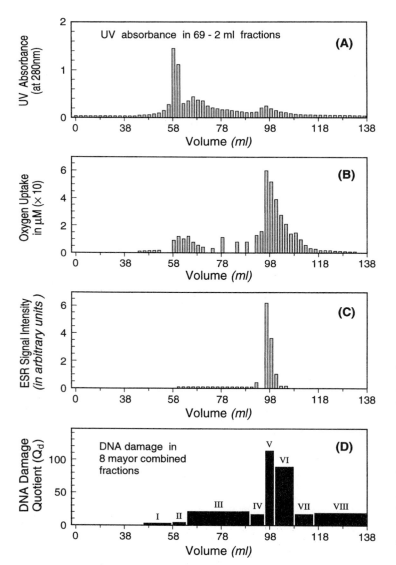

FIGURE 3.2. The separation of ACT solutions by Sephadex chromatography, showing that the DNA nicking activity is primarily in the fractions that contain the tar radical. **A:** Absorbance at 280 nm for 78 fractions of ACT subjected to Sephadex chromatography. **B:** Hydrogen peroxide production (determined indirectly as the uptake of dioxygen) for all 78 fractions. **C:** The EPR signal intensity of the stable free radical signal for all 78 fractions. The EPR signal intensity was estimated by the height of the highest peak. EPR parameters were: microwave power, 10 mW; modulation amplitude, 0.63 G; time constant, 0.2 s; receiver gain, 2 × 104; scan time, 200 s. **D:** The 78 ACT fractions were consolidated (based on their UV spectra) into eight major fractions, and these eight fractions were assayed for DNA-damaging activity in rat thymocytes (Qd, DNA damage quotient). (From Pryor WA. Cigarette smoke radicals and the role of free radicals in chemical carcinogenicity. *Environ Health Perspect* 1997;105:875; Pryor WA, Stone 15, Zhang L-Y, et al. Fractionation of aqueous cigarette tar extracts: fractions that contain the tar radical cause DNA damage. *Chem Res Toxicol* 1998;11:441, with permission.)

$Q/QH_2/QH\cdot$ system[11,13,27] (Figure 3.2). We believe it is the hydroxyl radical, produced in the close vicinity of the DNA strand by the Fenton reaction (Reaction 4), that is responsible for the DNA nicks that ACT solutions cause.[13,29,31]

ACT solutions also contain large amounts of nicotine and nitrosamines. To test if the $Q/QH_2/QH\cdot$ system is the agent in cigarette tar that causes DNA damage, and to dissociate the toxicity of nicotine from the effects of the tar-radical system, we developed a simplified model to study the tar radical. Aged solutions of catechol form a radical that has a similar G value, 2.0035, to the radical observed in ACT.[2,7] Fresh solutions of catechol do not nick DNA;[32–34] however, catechol autoxidizes to give semiquinone radicals. We have used autoxidized solutions of catechol as a simplified model for ACT; these solutions contain a radical similar to that in ACT solutions, yet any unreacted (unoxidized) material would have no effect. Aged solutions of catechol, like tar extracts, nick DNA in rat thymocytes. (Thymocytes are a frequently used cell type in the DNA nicking assay.[35])

These aged catechol solutions, like the ACT solutions, contain a semiquinone radical that becomes associated with double-stranded DNA in RAM and then causes nicking with saturation kinetics.[10,13,27] In addition, using radiolabeled catechol, we have shown that this tarlike $Q/QH_2/QH\cdot$ system binds to DNA and in about the expected amounts based on nicking data (unpublished work by Dr. M.G. Salgo). The similarity of aged catechol solutions and the cigarette tar radical extracts leave little doubt that it is the $Q/QH_2/QH\cdot$ system in tar that is responsible for the nicking observed.

PRODUCTION OF HYDROGEN PEROXIDE AND RADICALS FROM TAR EXTRACTS

It is our hypothesis that superoxide and hydrogen peroxide result from the reduction of dioxygen by the semiquinone radicals in aqueous tar solutions and in aged catechol solutions (see Reactions 5 to 7). Superoxide and hydroxyl radicals have both been observed in aqueous tar extracts by EPR methods.[11] We detect hydrogen peroxide in ACT extracts from both mainstream and sidestream smoke and also from aged catechol solutions, as summarized in Table 3.2.[7,11,27] (Sidestream smoke rises into the environment between puffs.) Hydrogen peroxide can be reduced to the hydroxyl radical by metals such as iron (reaction 8), and iron is present in tar extracts. The hydroxyl radical is known to be able to nick DNA. In addition, superoxide can lead to the liberation of iron from ferritin.[6]

DNA NICKING AND SCAVENGERS

Cigarette tar extracts from both mainstream and sidestream smoke nick DNA in rat thymocytes, and aged catechol solu-

tions also cause DNA nicking. This nicking appears to follow saturation kinetics in all three cases. To investigate the mechanism of DNA nicking by smoke extracts and aged catechol solutions, we studied the effects of catalase, superoxide dismutase, glutathione, deferoxamine, and diethylamine pentaacetic acid (DTPA). Catalase protected DNA against damage by both mainstream and sidestream tar extracts. Catechol did not protect DNA against nicking, probably because catechol is an effective inhibitor of catalase. Superoxide dismutase (SOD) did not protect against DNA damage. Deferoxamine and DTPA are divalent metal ion chelators and neither had a very dramatic effect. Our model of tar causing DNA nicking involves the presence of metals; however, the metals probably are tightly complexed to the cigarette tar or to the DNA, and thus unaffected by chelators in solution. Table 3.2 summarizes our results for these inhibitor studies.

CONCLUDING REMARKS

The oxidants in gas-phase smoke and in cigarette tar are quite different, but both appear to be involved in the damage to biomolecules that cigarette smoke causes. The oxidants in gas-phase smoke are shorter lived and more transient, but those in tar are long lived and can be expected to be a part of the aqueous fluid that bathes a smoker's lungs. In particular, we have shown that the tar radical, a semiquinone radical that reduces dioxygen to form superoxide, hydrogen peroxide, and ultimately the hydroxyl radical, can penetrate cells and cause DNA damage.

ACKNOWLEDGMENT

Our cigarette-smoking research has been supported in part by NIH.

REFERENCES

1. Kodama M, Kaneko M, Aida M, et al. Free radical chemistry of cigarette smoke and its implication in human cancer. *Anticancer Res* 1997;17:433.
2. Church DF, Pryor WA. Free-radical chemistry of cigarette smoke and its toxicological implications. *Environ Health Perspect* 1985; 64:111.
3. Pryor WA. Cigarette smoke and the involvement of free radical reactions in chemical carcinogenesis. *Br J Cancer* 1987;55[Suppl. VIII]:19.
4. Borish ET, Pryor WA, Venugopal S, et al. DNA synthesis is blocked by cigarette tar-induced DNA single-strand breaks. *Carcinogenesis* 1987;8:1517.
5. Church DF, Burkey TJ, Pryor WA. Preparation of human lung tissue from cigarette smokers for analysis by electron spin resonance spectroscopy. *Methods Enzymol* 1990;186:665.
6. Moreno JJ, Foroozesh M, Church DF, et al. Release of iron from

ferritin by aqueous extracts of cigarette smoke. *Chem Res Toxicol* 1992;5:116.

7. Pryor WA, Stone K. Oxidants in cigarette smoke: radicals, hydrogen peroxide, peroxynitrate, and peroxynitrite. In: Diana J, Pryor WA, eds. *Tobacco smoking and nutrition: influence of nutrition on tobacco associated health risks,* Annals of the New York Academy of Sciences, Vol. 686. New York: New York Academy of Sciences, 1993:12.

8. Evans MD, Pryor WA. An invited review: cigarette smoking, emphysema and damage to alpha-1-proteinase inhibitor. *Am J Physiol (Lung Cell Mol Physiol 10)* 1994;266:L593.

9. Bermúdez E, Stone K, Carter KM, et al. Environmental tobacco smoke is just as damaging to DNA as mainstream smoke. *Environ Health Perspect* 1994;102:870.

10. Stone K, Bermúdez E, Pryor WA. Aqueous extracts of cigarette tar containing the tar free radical cause DNA nicks in mammalian cells. *Environ Health Perspect* 1994;102:173.

11. Stone K, Bermúdez E, Zang L-Y. The ESR properties, DNA nicking and DNA association of aged solutions of catechol versus aqueous extracts of tar from cigarette smoke. *Arch Biochem Biophys* 1995;319:196.

12. Zang L-Y, Stone K, Pryor WA. Detection of free radicals in aqueous extracts of cigarette tar by electron spin resonance. *Free Radic Biol Med* 1995;19:161.

13. Pryor WA. Cigarette smoke radicals and the role of free radicals in chemical carcinogenicity. *Environ Health Perspect* 1997;105:875.

14. Frei B, Forte TM, Ames BN, et al. Gas phase oxidants of cigarette smoke induce lipid peroxidation and changes in lipoprotein properties in human blood plasma. Protective effects of ascorbic acid. *Biochem J* 1991;277:133.

15. Churg A, Cherukupalli K. Cigarette smoke causes rapid lipid peroxidation of rat tracheal epithelium. *Int J Exp Path* 1993;74:127.

16. Lapenna D, Mezzetti A, De Gioia S, et al. Plasma copper and lipid peroxidation in cigarette smokers. *Free Radic Biol Med* 1995;19:849.

17. Ueyama K, Yokode M, Arai H, et al. Cholesterol efflux effect of high-density lipoprotein is impaired by whole cigarette smoke extracts through lipid peroxidation. *Free Radic Biol Med* 1998;24:182.

18. Cueto R, Church DF, Pryor WA. Quantitative fourier transform infrared analysis of gas phase cigarette smoke and other gas mixtures. *Anal Lett* 1989;22:751.

19. Pryor WA, Prier DG, Church DF. Electron-spin resonance study of mainstream and sidestream cigarette smoke: nature of the free radicals in gas-phase smoke and in cigarette tar. *Environ Health Perspect* 1983;47:345.

20. Pryor WA, Tamura M, Church DF. ESR spin trapping study of the radicals produced in NOx/olefin reactions: a mechanism for the production of the apparently long-lived radicals in gas-phase cigarette smoke. *J Am Chem Soc* 1984;106:5073.

21. Pryor WA, Dooley MM, Church DF. Mechanisms of cigarette smoke toxicity: the inactivation of human alpha-1-proteinase inhibitor by nitric oxide/isoprene mixtures in air. *Chem Biol Interact* 1985;54:171.

22. Pryor WA, Dooley MM, Church DF. The inactivation of alpha-1-proteinase inhibitor by gas-phase cigarette smoke: protection by antioxidants and reducing species. *Chem Biol Interact* 1986;57:271.

23. Pryor WA. The free radical chemistry of cigarette smoke and the inactivation of alpha-1-proteinase inhibitor. In: Taylor JC, Mittman C, eds. *Pulmonary emphysema and proteolysis: 1986.* Orlando, FL: Academic Press, 1987:369.

24. Pryor WA, Hales BJ, Premovic PI, et al. The radicals in cigarette tar: their nature and suggested physiological implications. *Science* 1983;220:425.

25. Wynder EL, Hoffmann D. *Tobacco and tobacco smoke: studies in experimental carcinogenesis.* New York: Academic Press, 1967.

26. Guerin MR. Chemical composition of cigarette smoke. In: Gori GB, Bock FG, eds. *The Banbury report 3; a safe cigarette?* Cold Spring Harbor, NY: Cold Spring Harbor Laboratory, 1980:191.

27. Pryor WA, Stone K, Zhang L-Y, et al. Fractionation of aqueous cigarette tar extracts: fractions that contain the tar radical cause DNA damage. *Chem Res Toxicol* 1998;11:441.

28. Sealy RC, Felix CC, Hyde JS, et al. Structure and reactivity of melanins: influence of free radicals and metal ions. In: Pryor WA, ed. *Free radicals in biology,* Vol. 4. New York, NY: Academic Press, Inc., 1980:209.

29. Borish ET, Cosgrove JP, Church DF, et al. Cigarette tar causes single-strand breaks in DNA. *Biochem Biophys Res Commun* 1985;133:780.

30. Borish ET, Cosgrove JP, Church DF, et al. Cigarette smoke, free radicals, and biological damage. In: Rotilio G, ed. *Superoxide and superoxide dismutase in chemistry, biology, and medicine.* Amsterdam, Netherlands: Elsevier, 1986:467.

31. Cosgrove JP, Borish ET, Church DF, et al. The metal-mediated formation of hydroxyl radical by aqueous extracts of cigarette tar. *Biochem Biophys Res Commun* 1985;132:390.

32. Leanderson P, Tagesson C. Cigarette smoke-induced DNA damage in cultured human lung cells: role of hydroxyl radicals and endonuclease activation. *Chem Biol Interact* 1992;81:197.

33. Lewis JG, Stewart W, Adams DO. Role of oxygen radicals in induction of DNA damage by metabolites of benzene. *Cancer Res* 1988;48:4762.

34. Walles SAS. Mechanisms of DNA damage induced in rat hepatocytes by quinones. *Cancer Lett* 1992;63:47.

35. McLean JR, McWilliams RS, Kaplan JG, et al. Rapid detection of DNA strand breaks in human peripheral blood cells and animal organs following treatment with physical and chemical agents. In: Bora KC, ed. *Progress in mutation research,* Vol. 3. Amsterdam: Elsevier/North-Holland Biomedical Press, 1982:137.

36. Keilin D, Hartree EF. Catalase, peroxidase, metmyoglobin as catalysts of coupled peroxidatic reactions. *Biochem J* 1955;60:310.

37. Ogura Y, Tonomura Y, Hino S, et al. Studies on the reaction between catalase molecule and various inhibitory substances, I. *J Biochem Tokyo* 1950;37:153.

MOLECULAR GENETICS

4

RAS AND *ERBB 2*

JOHN F. LECHNER
JOSEPH M. FUGARO

Malignant transformation of a normal lung epithelial cell is the culmination of multiple genetic aberrations,[1,2] and two that are frequently associated with human lung cancer are *ras* and *erb*-B2. This chapter overviews these two oncogenes, their mechanisms of action, and their effect upon clinical outcome.

(Genes are denoted in italics and protein products are written in capital letters.)

RAS ONCOGENES

The family of *RAS* genes of H-*RAS,* K-*RAS,* and N-*RAS* is differentiated by their homology to different sarcoma oncogenes. Each of these codes for a 188 amino acid, 21 kD (p21) guanine-binding protein that is localized to the inner side of the plasma membrane. Such location and composition enable *RAS* proteins to "transduce" an appropriate signal from the extracellular milieu to the cell nucleus, thereby affecting gene transcription and directing cellular response to external stimuli. *RAS* constitutes the α subunit of a complex that also includes a receptor, an effector, and a $\beta\gamma$ dimer (see Figure 4.1). Most *RAS* protein within a cell exists in an inactive state with bound guanosine diphosphate (GDP). The $\beta\gamma$ subunit connects the α subunit to the receptor. When a signal ligand binds to the receptor, there is a conformational change in the guanine-binding site on the α molecule that promotes the exchange of guanosine triphosphate (GTP) for GDP. This action also moves the α molecule from the $\beta\gamma$ subunit to the effector molecule. The effector for *RAS* is a tyrosine kinase that can phosphorylate amino acid residues of proteins such as RAF1, one of the mitogen-activated protein kinases (MAPK).[3]

An example of *RAS* signal transduction is the epidermal growth factor receptor (EGFR) and *ERB* B2 heterodimer receptor, as shown in Figure 4.1. When TGF-α binds to this receptor complex, *RAS* is activated, subsequently inducing nuclear transcription factors that enhance cellular proliferation. In the process, the receptor is phosphorylated and the associated tyrosine kinase activates the Src homologous protein complex (SHC) that promotes dimerization of two other tyrosine kinases, Son of Sevenless (SOS) and growth factor response binding protein (GRB2). The newly formed dimer binds and activates RAS by producing a conformational change that enables *RAS* to bind GTP.[4] Thus, *RAS* acts as a "switch" that initiates a cascade of protein activations, beginning with RAF1, to transmit a signal from the cell membrane to the nuclear transcription machinery. Ultimately, the *RAS* signal transduction pathway activates nuclear protooncogenes that can form leucine zippers or helix-loop-helix transcription factors such as *MYC, FOS,* and *JUN.* These latter factors influence many cellular activities including transcription, translation, cytoskeletal organization, Golgi trafficking, vesicle formation, and cell-cell interactions. The effector will remain active until the α subunit's GTPase dephosphorylates the bound GTP to GDP.

RAS Oncogenes and Lung Cancer

One can imagine that if *RAS* became constitutively activated, there would be an exaggeration of the downstream effects, especially cell division. In keeping with this supposition, researchers have found two general mechanisms for aberrant *RAS* activation. The first is point mutations that cause irreversible binding of GTP. The most common mutations are within codons 12, 13, or 61, although Japanese and Chinese studies have also implicated codons 59 and 63.[5] While mutational activations of *HRAS* and *NRAS* are rare events in human lung cancer, several laboratories have reported a frequent association with *KRAS.*[6] For example, Richardson's study of 52 lung cancer patients revealed a prevalence of 15% to 20% of all non–small cell lung cancers (NSCLC), with the most common subtype being adenocarcinoma. In this study as well as others, the incidence of *KRAS* mutations for adenocarcinoma tumor tissue is approximately 30%.[2] Similar mutations are rarely detected in small cell lung cancer (CLC). Richardson noted that 85% of the lung cancer specimens that had *KRAS* mutations showed point mutations on codon 12, and nearly 70% of these were G-to-T transversions that change a glycine codon (GGT) to valine (GGT) or cysteine (TGT).[7]

In an attempt to establish a link between carcinogen

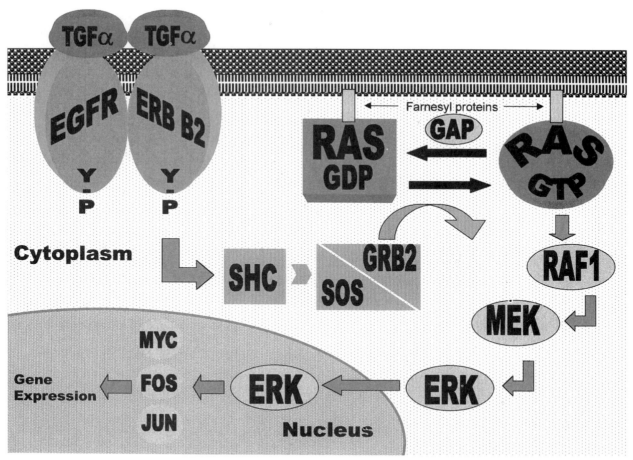

FIGURE 4.1. *Ras* signaling transduction pathway. *Ras* functions as a switch to relay extracellular ligand-stimulated signals from the inner cell membrane surface through the cytoplasm, and to the nucleus. The pathway places *RAS* downstream from a receptor tyrosine kinase, such as the epidermal growth factor receptor (EGFR)/*ERB* B2 heterodimer, and upstream of multiple serine/threonine kinases. A signal can be carried from outside the cell to the cell nucleus, where activated extracellular signal-regulated kinase (ERK) can be transported across the nuclear membrane and activate transcription factors known as *MYC, JUN,* and *FOS*. Tumor growth factor alpha (TGF-α), Src homology complex (SHC), Son of Sevenless (SOS), growth factor response binding protein (GRB2), GTPase activating protein (GAP), guanosine diphosphate (GDP), guanosine triphosphate (GTP), MAPK/ERK kinase (MEK). (From Vojtek AB, Der CJ. Increasing complexity of the Ras signaling pathway. *J Biol Chem* 1998;273:19925, with permission.) (See Color Figure 4.1.)

exposure and *RAS* mutations, Prahalad and associates examined the mutational spectra of *RAS* exposed to benzopyrene, one of the carcinogenic ingredients of tobacco smoke.[8] The predominant mutations found in chemically induced murine lung tumors were transversion mutations in codons 12 and 61. Cells which acquired mutations in both *p53* and *KRAS* lost the G1 arrest phase of the cell cycle.[9] These cells are unchecked and grow with progressive cellular dysregulation, leading to overt neoplasia.

The second model of *RAS*-mediated oncogenesis involves protein overexpression. Theoretically, the affected pulmonary epithelial cells could produce enough *RAS* protein that some *RAS* could bind GTP without the "activation" of the SHC/GRB2/SOS complex. Anti-H-*RAS*-specific antibodies

have been shown to improve sensitivity of tumor tissue screening to 80% in adenocarcinomas and 40% in squamous carcinomas.[10] A tenfold increase in transcription of H-*RAS* is sufficient to confer a functionally active amount of GTP-bound *RAS* in a cell,[11] and since signal-transducing protein dysfunctions downstream from *HRAS* should produce similar oncologic phenotypes, overexpression can initiate malignancy. However, the importance of H-*RAS* activation in human lung cancer by overexpression is controversial because the observed levels may be insufficient, based upon *in vitro* studies with human and murine cells.[12] Yet overexpression of *HRAS* detected by immunohistochemistry has been reported to be a highly frequent character of lung squamous cell carcinomas.[13]

RAS as a Biomarker of Early Detection of Lung Cancer

Recently studies to identify individuals at high risk for lung cancer have assessed cells from sputum,[14] bronchial alveolar lavage (BAL)[15] or endobronchial biopsies[16] for *KRAS* mutations. The Johns Hopkins Lung Project utilized sputum samples to retrospectively assess for an incidence of *KRAS* mutations. From 15 patients who later developed adenocarcinoma of the lung, eight sputum samples showed *KRAS* mutations in codon 12. The sputum PCR analysis was positive as early as four months prior to clinical diagnosis and reverted following curative resection in all cases. Lehman and colleagues[15] used BAL specimens from patients who have already been surgically treated for NSCLC. Using a ligase chain reaction, these researchers were able to detect *KRAS* mutation in five out of 12 patients in spite of a background of 99% normal airway DNA. Clements and associates evaluated bronchoscopic biopsies of patients with varied histological diagnoses of lung cancer. The biopsies were paired samples of endobronchial lesions and distant airway sites. The patients' airway epithelium exhibited cellular changes ranging from histologically normal to metaplastic to frankly malignant. The samples were then assayed for K-*RAS* mutations. In only 50% of the eight patients with adenocarcinoma, *KRAS* mutations were present at the site of the lesion. Meanwhile, two of the nine patients with histologic inflammatory changes showed evidence of *KRAS* mutations. Clinical experimentation shows that while *KRAS* mutations can predict the presence of carcinogen-insulted bronchial epithelium, this molecular marker is not ubiquitous in neoplasms, nor is it activated only in oncologic states.[17] Therefore, a positive *RAS* assay may correlate to DNA damage without necessarily conferring malignant potential.

Prognostic Impact of RAS

Many researchers suggest that K-*RAS* mutations portend a poor clinical prognosis for patients with adenocarcinoma.[13,18,19] See Figure 4.2 as an example of this relationship. Clinicians have attributed the increased mortality to therapeutic resistance. However, this largely retrospective observation was not supported when Rodenhuis performed a prospective study on late-stage (inoperable) cancers.[20] The study showed that *KRAS* mutations had no correlation with late-stage cancer survival or chemosensitivity. This conclusion was confirmed by a later Japanese study.[21] Furthermore, Tsai and associates used an *in vitro* model to refute the contention that cancers with *KRAS* mutations have increased resistance to chemotherapy and radiotherapy.[22] The prognostic impact of *RAS* may be more relevant to patients without lymphatic involvement. A Japanese study of 115 surgical patients without lymph-node metastasis showed a significant survival advantage in stage I and stage IIIA can-

cers without *KRAS* mutations (see Figure 4.3).[23] Therefore, the survival advantage of patients without K-*RAS* mutations is seemingly limited to premetastatic stages of lung cancer.

Therapy

The well-described details of *RAS* protein (p21) biochemistry have prompted many to generate antitumor therapy through inhibiting the activity of this protein. Several pharmacologic approaches to this end have been proposed to interfere with the effective cellular activity of p21. To date, there are five approaches to *RAS* inhibition in antitumor therapy: antisense exposure; ribozymes that block expression of the protein; GTPase activating proteins (GAP) stimulation to dephosphorylate activated *RAS;* signal transduction interference; and blocking membrane localization of *RAS*.

Experiments with antisense oligonucleotides have also shown that it is possible to inhibit selectively the expression of mutated *RAS* with little interference upon the wild-type *RAS* gene expression. Employing antisense oligonucleotide methylphosphates, concentrations in the range of 100 μM have been required to achieve selective inhibition of mutated *KRAS* mRNA. Using phosphorylated oligonucleotides of optimal size (17 nucleotides), somewhat lower concentrations may be effective, but it is not clear whether it will be possible to create the conditions under which it is possible *in vivo*. In a preclinical study of gene therapy to cause complete inactivation of the mutated gene transcript, a retrovirus that transduces an anti-K-*RAS* antisense construct has been instilled intratracheally in mice.[24] This treatment prevented outgrowth of orthotopically implanted human lung cancer cells, and human trials are anticipated. An alternative approach could be gene therapy in which DNA coding for ribozymes that specifically cleave mutated *KRAS* mRNA is introduced. Ribozymes directed against mutant *HRAS* have been shown to inhibit colony formation and induce reversion of cell morphology to a more normal appearing phenotype.[25]

The GAP proteins (see Figure 4.1) for *RAS* are novel and responsible for stimulation of the GTPase activity associated with the α subunit of a protein. *KRAS* mutations are thought to decrease the sensitivity of *RAS* to GAP, and leave *RAS* in a GTP-bound, activated state. These suppositions have been borne out in *in vitro* studies.[26,27] Therefore, the generation of an engineered *RAS* GAP may serve to stimulate GTPase activity even in oncogenic *RAS*.

As previously mentioned, activated *RAS* undergoes a conformational change to promote GTP binding. If the signal cascade were interrupted directly or indirectly, the increased *RAS* signal would not reach the cell nucleus. Accordingly, some researchers have suggested a GTP analog to bind the activated *RAS* and inhibit RAF1 phosphorylation (see Figure 4.1).[25] Others suggest blocking signal transduction from the MEK (MAP/ERK kinase) and MAP kinases of the cascade.[28,29] However, MEK and RAF1 mutants do not trans-

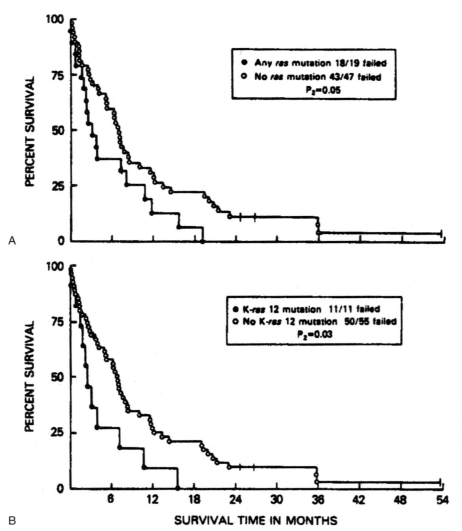

FIGURE 4.2. Comparison of survival with RAS mutations. Survival is significantly elevated in patient populations without RAS mutation in evaluating the time from tissue acquisition with respect to **(A)** any RAS mutations, and **(B)** K-*RAS* codon 12 mutation. (From Mitsudomi T, Steinberg SM, Oie HK, et al. *Ras* gene mutations in non–small cell lung cancers are associated with shortened survival irrespective of treatment intent. *Cancer Res* 1991;51:4999, with permission.)

form lung cells nor are they found in lung cancer cells except in exceedingly rare cases. Thus, successful applications of these approaches appear remote.

A particularly interesting target for pharmacologic interventions may be the enzyme farnesylprotein transferase, which is responsible for farnesylation of p21.[30] Farnesylation is a requirement for membrane attachment of the molecule. The enzyme can be inhibited *in vitro* by small peptides that compete with *RAS* protein; however, the toxicity to normal tissues might be significant. Lastly, data from *in vitro* studies employing plasmids containing antisense *KRAS* constructs suggest that blocking K-*RAS* mRNA translation may result in inhibited growth and in decreased tumorigenicity.

RAS is only one of many proteins that are responsible for signal transduction and cell fate determination. This protein has a historical role in molecular oncology in that it represents the first direct link of genetics to malignancy.

However, other researchers have confirmed that RAS mutation or *RAS* overexpression is not alone sufficient to transform normal epithelial cells.[31] Therefore this pathway requires further clarification of mechanism and utility as an oncogenic focus.

ERBB-2

Ligand binding is used to categorize the first three of the four members of the *ERB* B gene family of receptor tyrosine kinases. The first group includes epidermal growth factor (*EGF*), transforming growth factor-α (TGF-α), and amphiregulin; these all recognize the original member of this family, *EGF* receptor (*EGFR*). In the second group are the ligands betacellulin (BTC), heparin-binding EGF-like growth factor, and epiregulin; these bind to both *EGFR* and HER4. Neuregulin-3 (NRG3) is the only known member

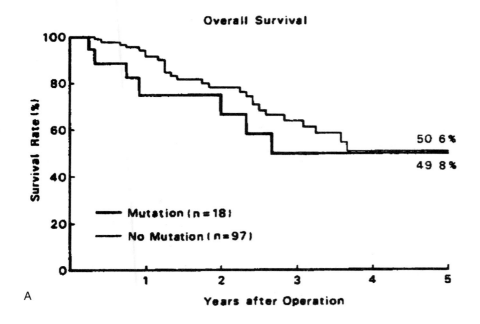

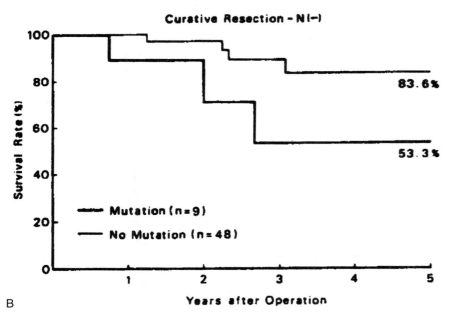

FIGURE 4.3. Comparison of nonmetastatic survival with RAS mutations. The Kaplan Meier survival curves after surgery for adenocarcinoma of the lung with respect to presence or absence of RAS mutations. Overall survival is unaffected by presence of RAS mutations **(A)** p = 0.1513 by generalized Wilcoxon test. However, absence of RAS mutation in patients without lymph node metastasis following curative resection had a significant impact upon survival **(B)** p = 0.212 by generalized Wilcoxon test. The numbers of patients with stage I and stage IIIA disease were 44 and 4 in the RAS negative group, and 8 and 1 in the RAS positive group respectively. (From Sugio K, Ishida T, Yokoyama H, et al. *Ras* gene mutations as a prognostic marker in adenocarcinoma of the human lung without lymph node metastasis. *Cancer Res* 1992;52:2903, with permission.)

of the third category; it has specificity only for *erbB-4*. The last group of ligands are the heregulin differentiation factors HRGβ1, sensory and motor neuron-derived factor (SMDF), and neuregulin-2 (NRG2); they all bind to *erbB-3* and *erbB-4*. The last member of the family, *erbB-2* (also designated as HER2 or p185^neu) is a 185 kD glycoprotein. The molecule has a glycosylated amino-terminal extracellular region containing the ligand binding site, a hydrophobic transmembrane region, a cytoplasmic carboxyl terminal domain containing the kinase activity, and presumed regulatory sites. However, it does not directly bind any known

ligand. Instead, it heterodimerizes with the three other family members, and enhances ligand-binding affinity and reduces the rate of dissociation. These heterodimers also amplify the elicited signal through activation of the *erbB-2* intracellular kinase domain and auto-cross-phosphorylation. The phosphorylated tyrosine residues in the receptor's cytoplasmic tail, in turn, serve as high-affinity binding sites for cytosolic substrates containing SRC-homology 2 (SH2) domains, for example, GRBs. Depending on the heterodimerization partner, the signal then traverses the *RAS*, P13K, or CDC42 cascades to the nucleus.[32–38] These signal cascades culminate in the nucleus, where they regulate transcription. Elevated expression of *ERB* B family members has been reported in a variety of human cancers. With respect to lung tissue, normal epithelial cells, carcinoids, and NSCLC cells are either negative, or minimally positive for expression of *erbB-2* to 4.[39–43] In contrast, *erbB-2* is highly expressed in 30% to 90% of SCLC tumors. However, contrary to the common gene amplification mechanism seen in most other cancers,[32] lung tumors overexpress this receptor by a mechanism that remains to be delineated.[2] *erbB-3* is also frequently overexpressed in NSCLC tumors, and information on the potential importance of elevated expression of *erbB-4* in NSCLC lung carcinogenesis has been intimated.[44–46]

The mechanism(s) whereby excess *erbB-2,* and possibly *erbB-3* and *erbB-4,* contribute to lung carcinogenesis is unclear. However, recent observations by Gerwin and co-workers[46–49] have shown, using an *in vitro* model system, that excess autocrine expression of the ligand TGF-α can be involved. By transfecting Beas2B human airway epithelial cells with a constitutively expressing *erbB-2* construct, these investigators found that conversion of the cells to tumorigenicity was directly associated with excessive autocrine expression of TGF-α.[48] They have shown elevation of MAPK activity in tumorigenic cells (see Figure 4.1), and signaling pathway depression of cells transfecting with a TGF-α antisense construct. The antisense-expressing cells also lost the tumorigenic phenotype. These studies indicate that overexpressed *erbB-2* implements TGF-α manifested tumorigenicity. More recent work supports this supposition by showing that excess *erbB-2* forces constitutive heterodimerization with EGFR and constitutively activates transcription of the signal transducer and activator of transcription (STAT).[49] Thus these workers propose that although overexpression of *erbB-2* alone is insufficient to convey the tumorigenic phenotype, it is necessary for tumorigenicity to arise through the TGF-α signal transduction pathway.

Gerwin and associates also report that TGF-α antisense reduces the steady-state levels of *erbB-3* and *erbB-4.* Thus a possible role of excess constitutive *erbB-2/erbB-3* and *erbB-2/erbB-4* dimers cannot be ruled out as also having a role in producing tumorigenicity. In keeping with this latter suggestion is the recent report by al Moustafa and colleagues.[43] These investigators showed that *erbB-2, erbB-3* and *erbB-4* are all constitutively activated in lung cancer cell lines. Lastly, Funayama and co-workers[45] reported that overexpression of *erbB-3* is frequently seen in squamous cell carcinomas, and its level of expression in metastatic nodules was higher than in the primary tumor.

By immunohistochemistry, Sozzi and colleagues[50] detected overexpression of *erbB-2* in three of 13 normal bronchial specimens from patients with a second primary lung tumor, suggesting that receptor overexpression is an early genetic change in the evolution of a NSCLC. However, four large studies[51–54] comprised of approximately 400 NSCLC specimens used different antibodies from those used by Sozzi and colleagues, and failed to detect *erbB-2* overexpression in nontumor lung epithelial cells. Reconciliation of these disparate results, as well as the prognostic interpretations described below, can be attributed to fact that these investigators used different antibodies and antigen retrieval techniques. Furthermore, not all studies deemed the specimens positive by scoring only the cells that specifically exhibited membrane staining. Another possible reason is illustrated by Tesfaigzi and colleagues.[55] These investigators studied rats exposed to a single intratracheal dose of the noncarcinogen endotoxin. Using immunohistochemical staining and Western blotting, they characterized a wave of hyperplasia followed by epithelium remodeling in the lungs of these animals. Interestingly, the hyperplastic cells exhibited a transient and marked expression of both *EGFR* and *erbB-2.* Therefore, the results of Sozzi and co-workers[50] may reflect a background of subclinical infections or smoking-associated epithelium wound repair.

Prognostic Associations of *erbB-2*

Kern and colleagues[52] were the first to report a statistical association of shorter survival time for adenocarcinoma and *erbB-2* overexpression. Subsequently, data from 119 adenocarcinomas and 84 squamous cell tumors showed that detectable *erbB-2* expression was statistically associated with shorter five-year survival, larger tumor size, and higher stage.[53] In addition, a study of 120 NSCLC tumors found that the frequency of overexpression was statistically higher in adenocarcinomas than in squamous cancers (81% versus 44%). However, expression was more frequent in clinical stages II and III than in stage I, regardless of histology. *erbB-2* expression was also positively correlated with lymph node metastasis in a cohort of 50 squamous lung carcinomas but not in a group of 32 lung adenocarcinomas.[54] Together these earlier studies supported a prognostic significance for *erbB-2* expression in NSCLC.

Subsequent studies have supported and refuted the correlation between *erbB-2* overexpression and shortened survival. Yu and colleagues[56] found significant relationships between *erbB-2* overexpression, a higher incidence of earlier recurrence, and an overall survival for 69 patients diagnosed with adenocarcinoma, but not for 47 with squamous tumors. A study by Hsieh and co-workers[57] of 42 stage I adenocarcinoma patients also showed that patients with *erbB-2* overexpression had a significantly higher incidence of early tumor recurrence and a lower overall survival expectation. Nemunaitis and colleagues[11] arrived at the same conclusion from studying 103 adenocarcinoma and large cell cancer patients. Most recently, D'Amico and colleagues[58] studied 408 stage I NSCLC patients and found that *erbB-2* overexpression equated with a "hazard ratio" of 1.43. Sloman and co-workers[59] and Guddo and co-workers[60] also reported that shorter survival correlated with *erbB-2* expression. Lastly, Diez and colleagues[61] have suggested that the risk of recurrence is directly related to the amount of *erbB-2* activity, and that for every increase of 100 units there is a 30% increase in risk. Interestingly, Yu and colleagues[62] have reported that high *erbB-3* expression is also associated with shortened survival, but the significance is associated only with advanced disease.

In contrast to the above reports, other studies, such as Pastorino and co-workers[63] failed to find any prognostic relationship between *erbB-2* overexpression and disease outcome. However, because of highly stringent scoring criteria, only 4% of their tumors were scored as positive; thus their small numbers precluded reliable inferences. On the other hand, Giatromanolaki and co-workers[64] examined *erbB-2* as a prognostic marker for 176 early-stage NSCLC patients and failed to find any significant relationship between survival of either adenocarcinomas or squamous carcinomas and survival. Likewise, Greatens and colleagues[65] studied 101 consecutive patients with primarily stage I or II NSCLC and failed to find any significant prognostic survival value for *erbB-2* overexpression. Interestingly, both Giatromanolaki and colleagues and Greatens and colleagues suggest that differences between their results and those studies that revealed a correlation could be due to chance, population differences, or interobserver variability. Finally, Fontanini and co-workers[66] reported a study of 195 patients; no significant correlation was found for either *erbB-2* or *erbB-3*.

ERBB-2 as a Target for Antitumor Therapy

Although an association between overexpression of *erbB-2* and adverse prognosis has not been firmly established, unlike *RAS*, *erbB-2* overexpression has been associated with enhancement of the metastatic properties and chemoresistance of lung cancer cells. The metastatic relationship was uncovered through transfection of the pSV2*erbB-2* plasmid DNA into low-expressing lung NSCLC cells.[62] Three independent clones were isolated that exhibited varying degrees of *erbB-2* expression. The untransfected, antisense transfected, and low-expressing cells exhibited minimal motility and ability to invade Matrigel, and produced few sites of pulmonary and extrapulmonary metastasis when injected into nude mice. In marked contrast, the two high-expressing clones were highly mobile and invasive, and produced multiple sites of metastasis.[22,67] With respect to chemoresistance, Tsai and colleagues[22] have shown that introduction of an *erbB-2* construct into lung cancer cells made them more resistant to doxorubicin, cisplatin, mitomycin, and etoposide. Interestingly, Tsai and associates[67,68] have also reported lung cell lines that are intrinsically high expressers of *erbB-2* lung cells lines are more chemoresistant. Importantly, chemoresistance was attenuated if the chemotherapeutic agent was combined with tyrosine kinase inhibitors that preferentially inhibited *erbB-2* kinase.[68,69]

The above studies all support the assertion that overexpression of *erbB-2* is involved in lung carcinogenesis and,

therefore, it is a potential target for mechanism-directed chemoprevention modalities. Support for this hypothesis came when lung tumor cells constitutively expressing *erbB-2* antisense RNA exhibited a reduced level of anchorage-independent growth, and fewer sites inoculated subcutaneously with the cells developed tumors.[70] Further, studies with anti-*erbB-2* antibodies have shown that cell growth is inhibited if the antibodies are incorporated into the culture medium.[71] In addition, mice with orthotopically implanted lung tumor cells developed smaller tumors if they received five weeks of injections of recombinant anti-*erbB-2* antibodies coupled with *Pseudomonas* endotoxin.[72] As a consequence of these encouraging results, a phase I trials for Herceptin anti-*erbB-2* antibodies is in progress.[73-75]

Finally, serum levels of *erbB-2* protein have been shown to correlate with extensive clinical cancer, and to be reduced after surgery.[76] Also, Brandt-Rauf and co-workers[77] showed that significant increases in the level of receptor protein in serum could be detected up to 60 months before clinical diagnosis, supporting the conclusion of Sozzi and colleagues[50] that the extracellular portion of the protein may be a useful biomarker of early disease.

REFERENCES

1. Braithwaite KR, Rabbitts PH. Multistep evolution of lung cancer. *Semin Cancer Biol* 1999;9:255.
2. Sekido Y, Fong KM, Minna JD. Progress in understanding the molecular pathogenesis of human lung cancer. *Biochim Biophys Acta* 1998;1378:F21.
3. Mora-Garcia P, Sakamoto KM. Cell signaling defects and human disease. *Mol Genet Metab* 1999;66:143.
4. Vojtek AB, Der CJ. Increasing complexity of the Ras signaling pathway. *J Biol Chem* 1998;273:19925.
5. Wang YC, Lee HS, Chen SK, et al. Analysis of K-ras gene mutations in lung carcinomas: correlation with gender, histological subtypes, and clinical outcome. *J Cancer Res Clin Oncol* 1998; 124:517.
6. Rodenhuis S, Boerrigter L, Top B, et al. Mutational activation of the K-ras oncogene and the effect of chemotherapy in advanced adenocarcinoma of the lung: a prospective study. *J Clin Oncol* 1997;15:285.
7. Richardson G, Johnson B. The biology of lung cancer. *Semin Oncol* 1993;20:105.
8. Prahalad AK, Ross JA, Nelson GB, et al. Dibenzo[a,l]pyrene-induced DNA adduction, tumorigenicity, and Ki-ras oncogene mutations in strain A/J mouse lung. *Carcinogenesis* 1997;18:1955.
9. Greenblatt MS, Bennett WP, Hollstein M, et al. Mutations in the p53 tumor suppressor gene: clues to cancer etiology and molecular pathogenesis. *Cancer Res* 1994;54:4855.
10. Kim YC, Park KO, Kern JA, et al. The interactive effect of Ras, HER2, P53 and Bcl-2 expression in predicting the survival of non–small cell lung cancer patients. *Lung Cancer* 1998;22:181.
11. Nemunaitis J, Klemow S, Tong A, et al. Prognostic value of K-ras mutations, ras oncoprotein, and c-ERB B-2 oncoprotein expression in adenocarcinoma of the lung. *Am J Clin Oncol* 1998; 21:155.
12. O'Brien W, Stenman G, Sager R. Suppression of tumor growth by senescence in virally transformed human fibroblasts. *Proc Natl Acad Sci U S A* 1986;83:8659.

13. Rosell R, Li S, Skacel Z, et al. Prognostic impact of mutated K-ras gene in surgically resected non–small cell lung cancer patients. *Oncogene* 1993;8:2407.

14. Mao L, Hruban R, Boyle J, et al. Detection of oncogene mutations in sputum precedes diagnosis of lung cancer. *Cancer Res* 1994;54:1634.

15. Lehman TA, Scott F, Seddon M, et al. Detection of K-ras oncogene mutations by polymerase chain reaction-based ligase chain reaction. *Anal Biochem* 1996;239:153.

16. Clements N, Nelson M, Wymer J, et al. Analysis of K-ras gene mutations in malignant and non-malignant endobronchial tissue obtained by fiberoptic bronchoscopy. *Am J Respir Crit Care Med* 1995;152:1374.

17. Yakubovskaya MS, Spiegelman V, Luo FC, et al. High frequency of K-ras mutations in normal appearing lung tissues and sputum of patients with lung cancer. *Int J Cancer* 1995;63:810.

18. Slebos RJC, Kibbelaar RE, Dalesio O, et al. K-ras oncogene activation as a prognostic marker in adenocarcinoma of the lung. *NEJM* 1991;323:561.

19. Mitsudomi T, Steinberg SM, Oie HK, et al. Ras gene mutations in non–small cell lung cancers are associated with shortened survival irrespective of treatment intent. *Cancer Res* 1991;51:4999.

20. Rodenhuis S, Boerrigter L, Top B, et al. Mutational activation of the K-ras oncogene and the effect of chemotherapy in advanced adenocarcinoma of the lung: a prospective study. *J Clin Oncol* 1997;15:285.

21. Fukuyama Y, Mitsudomi T, Sugio K, et al. K-ras and p53 mutations are an independent unfavourable prognostic indicator in patients with non–small cell lung cancer. *Br J Cancer* 1997;75:1125.

22. Tsai C-M, Chang KT, Perng RP, et al. Correlation of intrinsic chemoresistance of non–small cell lung cancer cell lines with HER-2/neu gene expression but not with ras gene mutations. *J Natl Cancer Inst* 1993;85:897.

23. Sugio K, Ishida T, Yokoyama H, et al. Ras gene mutations as a prognostic marker in adenocarcinoma of the human lung without lymph node metastasis. *Cancer Res* 1992;52:2903.

24. Georges RN, Mukbopadhyay T, Zhang Y, et al. Prevention of orthotopic human lung cancer growth by intratracheal instillation of a retroviral antisense K-ras construct. *Cancer Res* 1993;53:1743.

25. Cox AD, Der CJ. Farnesyltransferase inhibitors and cancer treatment: targeting simply Ras? *Biochim Biophys Acta* 1997;1333:F51.

26. Zhang K, DeClue JE, Vass WC, et al. Suppression of c-ras transformation by GTPase-activating protein. *Nature* 1990;346:754.

27. Huang DC, Marshall CJ, Hancock JF. Plasma membrane-targeted ras GTPase-activating protein is a potent suppressor of p21ras function. *Mol Cell Biol* 1993;13:2420.

28. Miwa W, Yasuda J, Yashima K, et al. Absence of activating mutations of the RAF1 protooncogene in human lung cancer. *Biol Chem Hoppe Seyler* 1994;375:705.

29. Bansal A, Ramirez RD, Minna JD. Mutation analysis of the coding sequences of MEK-1 and MEK-2 genes in human lung cancer cell lines. *Oncogene* 1997;14:231.

30. Gibbs JB, Oliff A. The potential of farnesyltransferase inhibitors as cancer chemotherapeutics. *Annu Rev Pharmacol Toxicol* 1997;37:143.

31. Hahn WC, Counter CM, Lundberg AS, et al. Creation of human tumour cells with defined genetic elements. *Nature* 1999;400:464.

32. Ross JS, Fletcher JA. The HER-2/neu oncogene: prognostic factor, predictive factor and target for therapy. *Seminars Cancer Biol* 1999;9:125.

33. Sundaresan S, Roberts PE, King KL, et al. Biological response to ERB B ligands in nontransformed cell lines correlates with a specific pattern of receptor expression. *Endocrinology* 1998;139:4756.

34. Adam L, Vadlamudi R, Kandapaka SB, et al. Heregulin regulates cytoskeletal reorganization and cell migration through p21-activated kinase-1 via phosphatidylinositol-3 kinase. *J Biol Chem* 1998;273:28238.

35. Crovello CS, Lai C, Cantley LC, et al. Differential signalizing by the epidermal growth factor-like growth factors neuregulin-1 and neuregulin-2. *J Biol Chem* 1998;273:26954.

36. Olayioye MA, Graus-Porta D, Beerli RR, et al. ERB B-1 and ERB B-2 acquire distinct signaling properties dependent upon their dimerization partner. *Mol Cell Biol* 1998:5042.

37. Tzahar E, Pinkas-Kramarski R, Moyer JD, et al. Bivalence of EGF-like ligands drives the ERB B signaling network. *EMBO J* 1997;16:4938.

38. Fiddes RJ, Campbell DH, Janes PW, et al. Analysis of Grb7 recruitment by heregulin-activated ERB B receptors reveals a novel target selectivity for ERB B3. *J Biol Chem* 1998;273:7717.

39. Press MF, Cordon-Cardo C, Slamon DJ. Expression of the HER2/neu proto-oncogene in normal human adult and fetal tissues. *Oncogene* 1990;5:953.

40. Schneider PM, Hung M-C, Chiocca SM, et al. Differential expression of the c-ERB B-2 gene in human small cell and non–small cell lung cancer. *Cancer Res* 1989;49:4968.

41. Wilkinson N, Hasleton PS, Wilkes S, et al. Lack of C-ERB B-2 protein expression in pulmonary carcinoid tumors. *Clin Pathol* 1991;44:343.

42. Rachwal WJ, Bongiorno PF, Orringer MB, et al. Expression and activation of ERB B-2 and epidermal growth factor receptor in lung adenocarcinomas. *Br J Cancer* 1995;72:56.

43. al Moustafa AE, Alaoui-Jamali M, Paterson J, et al. Expression of p185ERB B-2, p160ERB B-3, P180ERB B-4 and heregulin alpha in human normal bronchial epithelial and lung cancer cell lines. *Anticancer Res* 1999;19:481.

44. Eunhee S, Haarclerode D, Gondo M, et al. High c-ERB B-3 protein expression is associated with shorter survival in advanced non–small cell lung carcinomas. *Mol Pathol* 1997;10:142.

45. Funayama T, Nakanishi T, Takahashi S, et al. Overexpression of c-ERB B3 in various stages of squamous cell carcinomas. *Oncology* 1998;55:161.

46. Fernandes AM, Hamburger AW, German BI. Production of EGF related ligands in tumorigenic and benign human lung epithelial cells. *Cancer Lett* 1999;142:55.

47. Noguchi M, Murakami M, Bennett W, et al. Biological consequences of overexpression of a transfected c-ERB B-2 gene in immortalized human bronchial epithelial cells. *Cancer Res* 1993;53:2035.

48. Hamburger AW, Fernandes A, Murakami M, et al. The role of transforming growth factor alpha production and ERB B-2 overexpression in induction of tumorigenicity of lung epithelial cells. *Br J Cancer* 1998;77:1066.

49. Fernandes AM, Hamburger AW, Gerwin BI. Dominance of ERB B-1 heterodimers in lung epithelial cells overexpression ERB B-2: Both ERB B-1 and ERB B-2 contribute significantly to tumorigenicity. *Am J Respir Mol Biol* 1999;21:701.

50. Sozzi G, Iflozzo M, Tagliabue E, et al. Cytogenetic abnormalities and overexpression of receptors for growth factors in normal bronchial epithelium and tumor samples of lung cancer patients. *Cancer Res* 1991;51:400.

51. Weiner DB, Nordberg J, Robimon R, et al. Expression of the neu gene-encoded protein (P185) in human non–small cell carcinomas of the lung. *Cancer Res* 1990;50:42.

52. Kern JA, Schwartz DA, Nordberg JE, et al. p185neu expression in human lung adenocarcinomas predicts shortened survival. *Cancer Res* 1990;50:5184.

53. Tateishi M, Ishida T, Mitsudomi T, et al. Prognostic value of

cERB B-2 protein expression in human lung adenocarcinoma and squamous cell carcinoma. *Eur J Cancer* 1991;27:1372.

54. Shi D, He G, Cao S, et al. Overexpression of the c-ERB B-2/neu-encoded p185 protein in primary lung cancer. *Mol Carcinog* 1992;5:213.

55. Tesfaigzi J, Johnson NF, Lechner JF. Induction of EGF receptor and ERB B-2 during endotoxin-induced alveolar type II cell proliferation in the rat lung. *Int J Exp Path* 1996;77:143.

56. Yu C-J, Shun C-T, Yang P-C, et al. Sialomucin expression is associated with ERB B-2 oncoprotein overexpression, early recurrence, and cancer death in non–small cell lung cancer. *Am J Respir Crit Care Med* 1997;155:1419.

57. Hsieh C-C, Chow K-C, Fahn H-J, et al. Prognostic significance of HER-2/neu overexpression in stage I adenocarcinoma of lung. *Ann Thorac Surg* 1998;66:1159.

58. D'Amico TA, Massey M, Herndon II JE, et al. A biologic risk model for stage I lung cancer: immunohistochemical analysis of 408 patients with the use of ten molecular markers. *J Thorac Cardiovasc Surg* 1999;117:736.

59. Sloman A, D'Amico F, Yousem SA. Immunohistochemical markers of prolonged survival in small cell carcinomas of the lung. *Arch Pathol Lab Med* 1996;120:465.

60. Guddo F, Giatromanolaki A, Koukourakis MI, et al. MUC1 (episialin) expression in non–small cell lung cancer is independent of EGFR and c-ERB B-2 expression and correlates with poor survival in node positive patients. *J Clin Pathol* 1998;51:667.

61. Diez M, Pollan M, Maestro M, et al. Prediction of recurrence by quantification of p185neu protein in non–small cell lung cancer. *Br J Cancer* 1997;75:684.

62. Yu D, Wang S-S, Dulski KM, et al. C-ERB B-2/neu overexpression enhances metastatic potential of human lung cancer cells by induction of metastasis-associated properties. *Cancer Res* 1994; 54:3260.

63. Pastorino U, Andreola S, Tagliabue E, et al. Immunohistochemical markers in stage I lung cancer: Relevance to prognosis. *J Clin Oncol* 1977;15:2858.

64. Giatromanolaki A, Gorgoulis V, Chetty R, et al. C-ERB B-2 oncoprotein expression in operable non–small cell lung cancer. *Anticancer Res* 1996;16:987.

65. Greatens TM, Niehans GA, Rubins JB, et al. Do molecular markers predict survival in non–small cell lung cancer? *Am J Respir Crit Care Med* 1998;157:1093.

66. Fontanini G, DeLaurentiis M, Vignati S, et al. Evaluation of epidermal growth factor-related growth factors and receptors and of neoanginogenesis in completely resected stage I-IIIA non–small cell lung cancer: amphiregulin and microvessel count are independent prognostic indicators of survival. *Clin Cancer Res* 1998;4:241.

67. Tsai C-M, Yu D, Chang K-T, et al. Enhanced chemoresistance by elevation of p185^{neu} levels in HER-2/neu-transfected human lung cancer cells. *J Natl Cancer Inst* 1995;87:682.

68. Tsai, C-M, Levitzki A, Wu LH, et al. Enhancement of chemoresistance by AG825 in high-p185^{neu} expressing non–small cell lung cancer cells. *Cancer Res* 1996;56:1068.

69. Tsai C-M, Chang K-T, Chen JY, et al. Correlations between intrinsic chemoresistance and HER-2/neu gene expression, p53 gene mutations, and cell proliferation characteristics in non–small cell lung cancer cell lines. *Cancer Res* 1996;56:206.

70. Nenard CP, Malandrin MS, Rigo CN, et al. Inhibition of tumorigenicity in lung adenocarcinoma cells by c-ERB B-2 antisense expression. *Int J Cancer* 1997;72:631.

71. Kern JA, Torney L, Weiner D, et al. Inhibition of human lung cancer cell line growth by an anti-p185HER2 antibody. *Am J Respir Cell Mol Biol* 1993;9:448.

72. Skrepnik N, Araya JC, Qian Z, et al. Effects of anti-ERB B2 (HER-2/neu) recombinant oneotoxin AR209 on human non–small cell lung carcinoma growth orthotopically in athymic nude mice. *Clin Cancer Res* 1996;2:1851.

73. O'Rourke DM, Greene MI. Immunologic approaches to inhibiting cell-surface residing oncoproteins in human tumors. *Immunol Res* 1998;17:179.

74. Goldenberg MM. Trastuzumab, a recombinant DNA-derived humanized monoclonal antibody, a novel agent for the treatment of metastatic breast cancer. *Clin Ther* 1999;21:309.

75. Trastuzmab plus chemotherapy in treating patients with advanced non–small cell lung cancer. Eastern Cooperative Oncology Group: protocol E-2598.

76. Osaki T, Mitsudomi T, Oyama T, et al. Serum level and tissue expression of c-ERB B-2 protein in lung adenocarcinoma. *Chest* 1995;108:157.

77. Brandt-Rauf P, Luo J-C, Carney WP, et al. Detection of increased amounts of the extracellular domain of the cERB B-2 oncoprotein in serum during pulmonary carcinogenesis in humans. *Int J Cancer* 1994;56:383.

5

THE ROLE OF *MYC, JUN,* AND *FOS* ONCOGENES

PASI A. JÄNNE
BRUCE EVAN JOHNSON

The *MYC, JUN,* and *FOS* families of protooncogenes all share sequence homology with retroviruses, code for nuclear binding proteins with short half-lives, and share common structures. These proteins all contain a basic region of amino acids followed by a leucine zipper which allows the protein to dimerize with other proteins and bind to DNA. The protein products of these gene families localize to the nucleus and regulate gene transcription. The functions and characteristics of the *MYC* and *JUN* and families genes have been recently reviewed.[1–10] Structural DNA, mRNA expression and protein studies have implicated them in the pathogenesis and progression of lung cancer. The following chapter provides information about the normal structure and function of each of these protooncogenes and focuses on the evidence for the *MYC, JUN,* and *FOS* families' playing a role in the development and maintenance of lung cancer. The readers are referred to other reviews for more detailed information about the function of *JUN* in other animal and human tumor systems.[1–3,5–9]

MYC FAMILY PROTOONCOGENES

MYC Family Gene Structure

The *MYC* family genes studied in lung cancer include *MYC, NMYC,* and *LMYC.* The studies of the human *MYC* gene were prompted by the studies of the RNA tumor virus v-*myc*. The v-*myc* gene was first identified in an avian RNA tumor virus, MC29, which caused leukemias, carcinomas, and sarcomas in chickens.[11] This virus carried incomplete retroviral gene sequences along with the transforming gene, v-*myc*. v-*myc* shared a greater than 99% nucleotide sequence and amino acid homology with the normal second and third exon of the chicken *MYC* gene. This suggested that the retrovirus MC29 had picked up sequences of the chicken *MYC* gene by inaccurate recombination of retroviral gene sequences.[11] The human *MYC* gene was able to be cloned from normal DNA because of the close sequence homology

between the previously cloned murine *MYC* gene and the human *MYC* gene.[12]

The human *MYC* gene is a 3 exon gene spanning approximately 5 kbases located on chromosome 8q24 Figure 5.1. mRNA transcription originates from at least two different promoters separated by 150 nucleotides in the first exon and gives rise to mRNA of 2.2 and 2.4 kbases.[12–15] *MYC* protein translation starts in exons 1 or 2 to give rise to phosphoproteins of 439 and 453 amino acids with an apparent molecular weight of 64,000 and 67,000 D and a half-life of approximately 30 minutes.[12,16,17]

The *NMYC* gene was initially identified in neuroblastomas and neuroblastoma cell lines because of DNA amplification of sequences homologous to the MC38 avian retrovirus v-*myc* but different from the human *MYC* gene.[18] A fragment of the *NMYC* gene was also subsequently cloned from DNA fragments isolated from a homogeneously staining region (HSR) in a neuroblastoma cell line.[19] Hybridization of this radiolabeled fragment to DNA isolated from neuroblastoma cell lines showed intense signals representative of DNA amplification.

The human *NMYC* gene is a 3 exon gene spanning approximately 6.5 kbases located on chromosome 2p25.[1,20–23] mRNA transcription gives rise to a predominant mRNA of 3.1 kbases.[19,24,25] The *NMYC* protein is translated from exons 2 and 3 to give rise to phosphoproteins of 453 and 456 amino acids with apparent molecular weights of 65,000 and 67,000 D and half-lives of 30 minutes.[1,26–29]

The human *LMYC* gene was initially identified in small cell lung cancer cell lines and tumors because of DNA amplification of sequences homologous to but different from the human *MYC* and *NMYC* gene.[18] The human *LMYC* gene is a 3 exon gene spanning approximately 6.5 kbases located on chromosome 1p32.[30,31] Transcription of the *LMYC* gene gives rise to 3.6 and 3.9 kbase mRNAs but alternative processing in small cell lung cancer cells can give rise to smaller forms of the *LMYC* mRNA which will be described later.[1,29,30] The *LMYC* protein is normally trans-

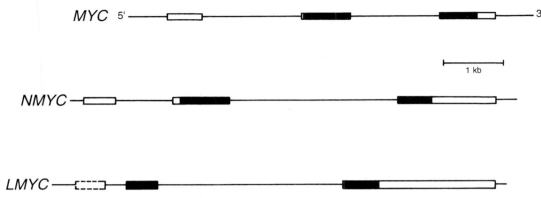

FIGURE 5.1. Gene structure of the *MYC* family genes: This diagramatically depicts the structure of the *MYC* family genes (*MYC, NMYC,* and *LMYC*). The boxes represent the exons and the lines between represent the introns. The black portions of the boxes represent exon domains that correspond to the protein-coding signals.

lated from exons 2 and 3 and produces a phosphoprotein of 364 amino acids with an apparent molecular weight of 60,000 to 66,000 D and a half-life of 45 to 120 minutes.[30,32,33]

The *MYC* family genes share a similar structure and a close sequence homology, and have similar functions in biological assays. *MYC, NMYC,* and *LMYC* all have 3 exons with 2 introns. The predominant areas of sequence homology are contained within exons 2 and 3. The first exons of the *MYC* family genes are not closely related and do not typically code for protein. Translation initiation typically takes place within the second exon in all three genes and the major protein coding regions lie within exons 2 and 3 (Figure 5.1).

There are five areas of close sequence homology in the second and third exons of *MYC, NMYC,* and *LMYC* Figure 5.2. The area of sequence homology in the carboxy-terminal is contained in the 85 amino acids of the *MYC* family proteins. This region contains a basic region, helix-loop-helix structure, the leucine zipper.[34] The basic region contains a high proportion of basic amino acids and binds to the DNA; the helix-loop-helix has two amphipathic helices of 12 and 13 amino acids separated by a loop structure, a leucine zipper characterized by a leucine or hydrophobic amino acid every 7 amino acids for four repeats in the carboxy-terminal amino acids.[35] This helix-loop-helix and leucine zipper structure allows proteins to form homo- or heterodimers which allow the basic portion of the molecule to contact the DNA and regulate gene transcription. The amino-terminus contains the transactivation domain and the highly conserved *MYC*-box (Mb I and Mb II) domains.[6] The Mb I domain is located at amino acids 45 to 63, while the Mb II domain is at amino acids 129 to 141 of the human *MYC* protein.[6] The Mb domains are evolutionarily conserved, show a greater than 90% homology between the *MYC* family members, and are sites of protein interactions, diagrama-

tically depicted in Figure 5.2.[4,36] In addition, the Mb II domain is essential for *MYG*-mediated cell transformation in a rat embryo fibroblast assay.[37] Thus the *MYC* family of genes has the ability to participate in diverse functions, including protein-protein interactions, binding of DNA sequences, and modulation of gene transcription.

Molecular Mechanisms of *MYC* Action

The *MYC* family of genes contains two highly conserved dimerization motifs: the helix-loop-helix domain, and the leucine zipper domain. *MYC* proteins do not homodimerize, and it was subsequently discovered that *MYC* forms heterodimers with another BR-HLH-Zip protein known as MAX (see Figure 5.2). All of the biologic activities of *MYC* occur as a heterodimer with MAX. *MYC, NMYC,* and *LMYC* all heterodimerize with MAX.[6] These heterodimers bind DNA at sequence-specific sites known as the E-box with the consensus sequence of CAC(G/A)TG, and activate transcription. The E-box elements are found in *MYC* target genes and are located in promoter regions, the first or second introns, and even in protein coding sequences.[4] In addition to heterodimerizing with *MYC*, MAX can homodimerize or bind to a multitude of other BR-HLH-Zip proteins, including MAD, MAD 3, MAD 4, MXI, and MNT.[3] These complexes can compete with *MYC*-MAX heterodimers at the E-box sites and act as transcriptional repressors. This provides a complex network of regulation and allows for transcriptional activation or repression depending on the intracellular stoichiometry of the *MYC* binding partners.

The *MYC* family of proteins also binds with various other proteins through highly conserved motifs (Figure 5.2). In addition to MAX, *MYC* can form complexes through the BR-HLH-Zip domain with the transcription factors YY-1, AP-2, and MIZ-1. In general, the binding of *MYC* to these proteins leads to repression of transcription either by inhib-

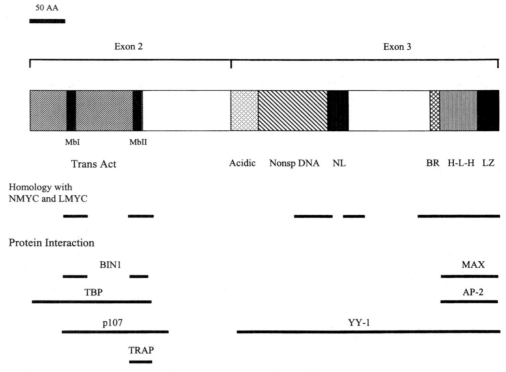

FIGURE 5.2. Functional domains of the *MYC* protein and the location of protein-binding sites: This diagramatically represents the functional domains of the *MYC* protein. The portions of the *MYC* protein encoded by exon 2 and 3 are represent by the brackets above the bar. The letters below the bar represent abbreviations for the functional domains of the *MYC* protein. The initial diagonal region represents the transactivation domain (Trans Act), the black dots represent the acidic domain (Acidic), the next diagonal lines represent the nonspecific DNA-binding domain (Nonsp DNA), the white dots represent the nuclear localization domain (NL), the crosshatched lines represent the basic region (BR), the dark dots represent the helix-loop-helix domain (H-L-H), and the dark diagonal lines represent the leucine zipper (LZ). The black boxed areas represent the *MYC*-binding domains (Mb I and Mb II). The dark lines below the bar represent the areas of close sequence homology between the other two *MYC* family proteins. The dark lines below represent the regions where *MYC* interacts with various proteins, and the specific proteins are listed on the right-hand column: TBP (TATA-binding protein), BIN-1 (box-dependent *MYC*-interacting protein-1), and TRAP (transformation associated protein).

iting the native transcriptional activation of the binding partners (YY-1 and MIZ-1) or by interfering with *MYC*-MAX transcriptional activation (AP-2).[4] The amino-terminus of *MYC* can combine with proteins including TRAP (transformation associated protein), the p107 tumor supressor, BIN-1, TBP (TATA-binding protein), and α-tubulin (see Figure 5.2). These interactions can regulate *MYC* function by different mechanisms and can occur in the presence of MAX. TRAP binding to the Mb II region appears to be required for *MYC*-mediated transformation.[43] The Rb family member p107 interacts with *MYC* at Mb I, and its binding inhibits the transactivation activity of *MYC*.[4] BIN 1 association with *MYC* occurs via the Mb I and Mb II domains. BIN 1 inhibits *MYC*-mediated transformation of primary rat embryo fibroblats.[38] BIN 1 expression is frequently reduced or absent in various tumor cell lines (including half of lung cancer cell lines examined) and in some

primary tumors.[38] Thus BIN 1 potentially functions as a tumor suppressor gene. These various protein interactions underscore the diverse functions of *MYC* and specifically its role as a transcriptional activator and repressor.

The Biology of the *MYC* Family of Genes

The *MYC* proteins are important regulators of cell proliferation. The regulation of *MYC* expression is crucial for normal cellular proliferation. Deregulated expression characterized by constitutive, inappropriate, or nonphysiologic expression is seen in a variety of tumor cells and primary tumors.[4,6] The majority of this type of expression occurs via gene amplification, increased mRNA expression, or chromosomal translocations. The *MYC* genes also play key roles in differentiation and apoptosis.[6,39] The expression of *MYC* is tightly regulated in normal tissues and is controlled at multiple levels by signal transduction pathways.[36] Several potential targets of *MYC* activation and repression have been identified. These include genes coding for enzymes regulating the production of essential molecules for DNA synthesis, proteins involved in RNA structure and metabolism, proteins involved in cell cycle control, and those with no known function.[4] *MYC* protein mediation of these downstream events by either direct or indirect mechanisms is presently under investigation.[40] Thus, the *MYC* family of genes is involved in many diverse biologic functions. The various roles of *MYC* and their relationship to the pathogenesis of human lung cancer have not yet been thoroughly investigated.

MYC Family mRNA Expression Studies in Developing and Adult Mouse and Human Tissues

The pattern of *MYC* family mRNA expression has been studied by Northern blot analyses and *in situ* hybridization in normal tissues of mice during fetal development through adulthood, in human embryos, and in nonneoplastic lung tissue.[41–44] *myc*, N-*myc*, and L-*myc* are expressed in murine tissues during development. By *in situ* hybridization, N-*myc* is expressed in both the embryonic ectoderm and extraembryonic ectoderm. As development proceeds, N-*myc* expression becomes more restricted and is abundantly expressed in the developing nervous system.[45] This includes expression in both the developing central nervous system and in the cranial and spinal ganglia of the developing peripheral nervous system.[45] N-*myc* is also expressed in the developing gut, kidney, and lung. Its expression is located in the luminal areas of the developing lung; these will later go on to form bronchioles. N-*myc* expression is low or undetectable in most adult tissues.[41] Thus N-*myc* may play a role in early differentiation as its level of expression decreases with development. Also expressed in early development during active cellular proliferation is *myc*. The levels of *myc* expression in general are much lower than of N-*myc*. It is expressed in the majority of tissues but during early development is predominately found in the extraembryonic tissues. *myc* expression is also found in the mesenchymal cells of the developing gut and lung, and in the developing liver. *myc* continues to be expressed in adult mice in various tissues including the lung.[33,37,38] The expression of L-*myc* in development is more limited than that of *myc* or N-*myc*. In early developing embryos, L-*myc* is expressed at high levels in the neuroectoderm of the brain and neural tube.[46] By day 12 of mouse development, L-*myc* is expressed at the highest levels in the CNS, nasal epithelium, metanephric kidney, and the developing lung. Newborn mice express high levels of L-*myc* in the brain, kidney, and lung.[46] Thus L-*myc* may also play a role in differentiation. From these studies, it also appears that L-*myc* is expressed in cells that express either c-*myc* or

N-*myc*, whereas this observation does not hold for the other *myc* gene family members.

In situ hybridization studies of human embryos studied three to ten weeks after conception showed abundant *MYC* mRNA expression in more than 20% of the cells of the lung.[47] *NMYC* and *LMYC* mRNA expression was not studied. The human adult nonneoplastic lung has also been studied in patients whose lung cancer has been resected. *In situ* hybridization showed detectable *MYC* mRNA expression in all samples of nonneoplastic cells studied.[48] The expression was most detectable in the basal cell layer of the bronchial epithelium, type II alveolar cells, and endothelial cells. *NMYC* and *LMYC* mRNA expression was not detected in the adult nonneoplastic tissues.

The studies of mRNA expression from the *MYC* family genes in the lungs of mice and humans show that *MYC* is expressed during fetal development and in the adult lung. The various family members may be important for different functions in developing and adult lung tissues.

Functional Studies of *MYC* Family Genes

The role of the *MYC* gene family in multistage carcinogenesis initially proposed by Land and colleagues was defined in a rat embryo fibroblast system.[49] Transfection of an activated *HRAS*1 gene into the rat embryo fibroblasts allowed the formation of cells with an altered cellular morphology or foci which formed colonies in soft agarose but did not form tumors in athymic nude mice. Established cancer cell lines will typically grow and form tumors in athymic nude mice. The cells transfected with the activated *H-RAS*1 and a *MYC* gene provided an establishment function in the rat embryo fibroblasts which allowed the cells to continue growing and form tumors in athymic nude mice.[31,50–52] *NMYC* and *LMYC* complement the *RAS* family in this assay as well. However, the transforming activity of *LMYC* is only 1% to 10% of that of *MYC*.[52,53] This appears to be due to amino acid differences in the transactivation domains of these two proteins.[54] The transforming ability of *NMYC* is also less than that of *MYC* but stronger than *LMYC*.[53] Further proof of the role of *MYC* in carcinogenesis has been obtained from studies performed in mice. Transgenic mice have been used to study the role of *MYC* in tumorigenesis and its effects on proliferation and differentiation.[55] Using tissue-specific promoters, high levels of *MYC* expression have been obtained in tissues such as the mammary gland, the lymphoid system, the liver, the pancreas, the heart, and the lens. Tumorigenesis was observed in the mammary gland, lymphoid system, liver, and pancreas, while hyperplasia was seen in the heart. The neoplastic phenotypes and the effects on differentiation and proliferation vary depending on the *MYC* family member used. For example, mice overexpressing L-*MYC* in the lens (using α A crystal promoter) show abnormalities in differentiation, while mice with *MYC* overexpression have abnormal lens cell proliferation.[56] The onset of tumor formation is accelerated in double transgenic mice containing cytoplasmic oncogenes, including *HRAS* and *PIM*1.[31,55] These studies confirm the oncogenic role of *MYC* family genes and have allowed further study into the role of the *MYC* family members in differentiation and proliferation. These studies have not specifically addressed *MYC* overexpression in the lung.

The role of the *MYC* family members in normal development has been studied using mice lacking the normal *MYC* family members. Mice deficient in all of the *MYC* family members have been generated using homologous recombination techniques. Mice homozygously deficient in *myc* die early in development, usually by day 10.5.[57] The homozygous mice show a generalized delay in development, with pathologic abnormalities including cardiac enlargement, pericardial effusion, and neural tube defects.[57] N-*myc* homozygously deficient mice die between day 10.5 and 12.5 of development.[45,58] The homozygous mice exhibit multiple developmental abnormalities, mostly in tissues where N-*myc* is normally expressed. The developing lungs from these mice demonstrate nonbranching of the trachea and bronchi with a hypoplastic epithelium. Similar findings of organ hypoplasia are seen in the developing of gut and genitourinary system, suggesting a role for N-*myc* in regulating cellular proliferation. In marked contrast, mice deficient in L-*myc* develop normally into adulthood and have no detectable phenotypic consequences.[46] It is possible that one of the other family members compensates for the lack of L-*myc*. As mentioned above, L-*myc* is often coexpressed with either N-*myc* or c-*myc*, whereas this is not the case for the other two family members.

These studies demonstrate that genes of the *MYC* family share some similar functions but that they also have unique roles in normal development.

MYC Family DNA Structural Abnormalities in Lung Cancer

DNA Amplification

A rodent cell line selected *in vitro* for resistance to methotrexate developed gene amplification of dihydrofolate reductase, the target enzyme for methotrexate.[59,60] This increased the amount of dihydrofolate reductase enzymatic activity and allowed the cells to escape the growth inhibition caused by methotrexate. The amplified gene encoding dihydrofolate reductase localized to homogeneously staining regions and double minute chromosomes. This association of gene amplification with double minute chromosomes and homogenous staining region led to the discovery of oncogene amplification in human cancers. The initial discovery of *MYC* DNA amplification in human cancer was initially identified in a leukemia cell line which had double minute chromosomes, HL-60, and a colon cancer cell line (COLO 320) which had both homogeneously staining regions and

double minute chromosomes.[61,62] A radiolabeled fragment of the chicken *MYC* gene DNA hybridized intensely to the DNA from the HL-60 cell line and a radiolabeled fragment of v-*myc* hybridized to the DNA from COLO 320, representing DNA amplification. *In situ* hybridization studies of metaphase spreads from COLO 320 showed a radiolabeled *MYC* fragment hybridized to the homogeneously staining region on the X chromosome. Therefore *MYC* DNA amplification and high levels of expression were present in these human cancer cell lines and localized to a marker associated with gene amplification, a homogeneously staining region in a different location (the X chromosome) from the normal locus on chromosome 8q24.

Double minute chromosomes and homogeneously staining regions had been identified by karyotypic analyses of small cell lung cancer (SCLC) cell lines.[63,64] The screening of these cell lines with DNA fragments from oncogenes and protooncogenes identified DNA amplification of the *MYC* gene in a subset of SCLC cell lines.[65,66] Amplification of all three members of the *MYC* family has been identified in lung cancer cell lines.[24,65,67] These cell lines with amplified *MYC* family DNA contain 4 to 135 copies of the *MYC* family genes.[68–71] The size of the DNA segment amplified in the SCLC cell line NCI-N417 has been estimated at 120 and 130 bases of DNA and NCI-H82 at 300 bases.[71,72] The amplified *MYC* DNA in this SCLC cell line, NCI-N417, has been localized to a homogeneously staining region on chromosome 1.[71] Therefore, in both COLO 320 and NCI-N417 the amplified *MYC* gene is localized to chromosomal loci different from its location in normal cells.

DNA Rearrangement

Additional signals have been detected in lung cancer cell lines that have *MYC* family DNA amplification which represent rearrangements of the DNA.[24,67] Rearrangements of the *LMYC* gene in SCLC with *LMYC* DNA amplification have been extensively investigated. The initial studies involved immunoprecipitation of the *LMYC* protein in two SCLC cell lines which showed proteins of 72 to 77 kD, 10 kD larger than expected for *LMYC* proteins from other lung cancer cell lines.[58] Subsequent investigations of the DNA and mRNA from SCLC cell lines with *LMYC* DNA amplification identified a gene RLF, which stands for Rearranged L-*myc* Fusion.[73,74] The RLF gene is approximately 500 bases 5′ from the LMYC gene on chromosome 1p32 (Figure 5.3). The RLF/L-*MYC* locus undergoes an intrachromosomal rearrangement and RLF is brought into proximity to the L-*MYC* gene in some SCLCs with L-*MYC* DNA amplification.[73] The mechanism involved in the generation of this fusion transcript is complex and can occur at different breakpoints sites 5′ of *LMYC*.[73] These breakpoints appear to cluster in regions containing highly repetitive DNA sequences.[75]

The mRNA studies show that the first exon of the RLF

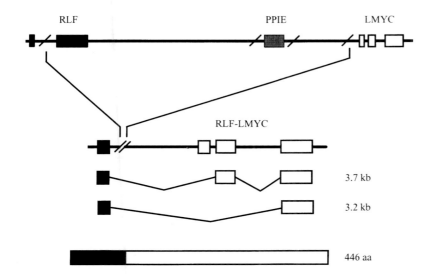

100 kb

RLF   PPIE   LMYC

RLF-LMYC

3.7 kb

3.2 kb

446 aa

FIGURE 5.3. Chromosomal rearrangement of *RLF* and *L-MYC:* The bracket at the top represents distance covered by 100 kbases of DNA on the uppermost diagram, representing the normal configuration of the *RLF* gene and the *LMYC* gene. The black boxes represent the hypothetical exons of the *RLF* gene, but the exon-intron structure beyond the first exon and intron have not yet been reported. The open boxes represent the three exons of the L-*MYC* gene. The PPIE is located in between *RLF* and *L-MYC:* its exact position is not known. (From Kim JO, Nau MM, Allikian KA, et al. Co-amplification of a novel cyclophilin-like gene [PPIE] with L-*myc* in small cell lung cancer cell lines. *Oncogene* 1998;17:1019, with permission). The diagonal lines connecting the exons represent the mRNA splicing which brings the exons together. Kb represents kilobases, and aa represents amino acids. (From Vastrik I, Makela TP, Keskinen PJ, et al. *myc, max,* and a novel *rlf*-L-*myc* fusion protein in small-cell lung cancer. In: Harris CC, ed. *Multistage Carcinogenesis.* Boca Raton: CRC Press, 1992:307, with permission.)

gene is spliced to the second or third exon of the *LMYC* gene, giving rise to novel mRNAs of 3.7 and 3.2 bases (Figure 5.3).[58,60] The 3.7 base mRNA gives rise to a protein with 466 amino acids—79 from RLF exon 1, 3 from previously untranslated sequences in exon 2, and 364 amino acids from the *LMYC* coding sequences. These rearrangements give rise to the fusion proteins which have only been observed in SCLC cell lines and tumors and which have DNA amplification of *LMYC*. These rearrangements have not been observed in 99 cell lung cancer (NSCLC) tumors studied.[74] The fusion protein formed by RLF and *LMYC* appears to take place in a subset of SCLC cell lines with *LMYC* DNA amplification and therefore is present in less than 10% of the SCLC cell lines studied.

The normal RLF gene encodes for a 1914 amino acid protein containing six zinc finger motifs and a leucine zipper.[76] Thus its function appears to be that of a transcription factor, and the spacing of the zinc fingers suggests that it is related to the transcription factor Zn-15. Zn-15 is a transcription factor involved in the transcriptional activation of the growth hormone gene. However, there are large regions without homology between these two proteins. RLF expression has been analyzed by Northern and RNAse protection analyses. It is widely expressed in human fetal and adult tissues, including the fetal lung but not in the adult lung.[76] The RLF-*LMYC* fusion product contains only the first 79 amino acids of the normal RLF gene, and this does not include the zinc finger motifs. In a transformation assay of primary rat embryo fibroblasts, the RLF-L-*MYC* fusion protein had a similar transforming capacity as the normal L-*MYC* gene.[76] Attempts to create transgenic mice using this fusion gene (under the normal RLF promoter) failed

to create mice expressing the chimeric transcript.[77] When this construct was introduced into embryonic stem (ES) cells, the cells failed to develop into proper embryoid bodies. Taken together, these experiments suggest that the deregulation of the normal L-*MYC* expression brought about by the RLF promoter is critical to the phenotypic findings and not a novel function associated with the RFL/*LMYC* fusion product. The significance of this for SCLC is unknown. The phenotype of SCLC cells lines with *LMYC* amplification compared with those additionally containing the RLF-*LMYC* fusion appears to be similar with respect to doubling times, cloning efficiency in soft agar, and *in vitro* and *in vivo* morphology.[69,78]

A second rearrangement product from the same locus has also been identified. This involves a novel cyclophilin-like gene named PPIE (pedtidyl-prolyl *cis-trans* isomerase E) and shows 83% amino acid identity with the central conserved region of cyclophilin A.[78] In a subset of SCLC cell lines that have *LMYC* amplification, 64% (7 of 11 cell lines) showed amplification of PPIE, whereas RLF amplification was seen in 36% (4 of 11) of the cell lines. Consistent with the higher rate of PPIE amplification, it appears that the PPIE gene lies in between RLF and *LMYC* on chromosome 1. One of amplified cell lines, NCI-H378, shows a PPIE fusion product with exon 2 of *LMYC* in the antisense orientation.[78] The function of this chimeric transcript (if any) is not know and to date has not been identified in primary lung cancers.

Other rearrangements of the *MYC* family genes have been in SCLC cell lines[24,65,67,79–82] and tumors[24,83–85] as well as NSCLC tumors.[84–87] The rearrangements can appear or disappear after the cells are placed in culture.[82,83]

Several of the cell lines with rearrangements of the *MYC* family genes give rise to a different-sized mRNA.[24,65] Most rearrangements of the *MYC* gene family take place with gene amplification and are present in both the lung cancer cell line and the lung cancer from which it arises, although there are examples where the rearrangement takes place in cell culture or in xenografts. These rearrangements can bring a novel segment of DNA near the *MYC* family locus, but relatively few of these rearrangements have been well characterized.

MYC DNA Amplification and Phenotype of Small Cell Lung Cancer Cell Lines

Some experimental evidence shows that increased amounts of *MYC* gene product are associated with increased growth in multiple tumor systems.[1,29] There is less evidence that increased amounts of *NMYC* and *LMYC* gene product are associated with growth.[1,29]

The definition of classic and variant subclasses of SCLC cell lines was proposed in 1985 using biochemical, morphologic, and growth properties.[69,88] The majority of cell lines (classic subclass) grew as tightly packed floating aggregates in cell culture media (NCI-H209 Figure 5.4) and formed intermediate histology when injected into athymic nude mice.[89] They grew with long doubling times and low colony-forming efficiencies in soft agarose. The classic SCLC cell lines had markers of neuroendocrine differentiation.

The cell lines had enzymatic L-dopa decarboxylase activity (an enzyme in the pathway to form dopaminergic amines), bombesinlike immunoreactivity, neuron-specific enolase, and the brain isoenzyme of creatine kinase.

In contrast, the variant cell lines grew as loosely attached floating aggregates (Figure 5.4; NCI-N417) and formed small cell/large cell morphology when injected into athymic nude mice.[89] The variant cell lines had shorter doubling times and higher cloning efficiencies in soft agarose than classic cell lines. The variant SCLC cell lines retained the brain isozyme of creatine kinase but had lower concentrations of neuron-specific enolase and L-dopa decarboxylase.

The original description of *MYC* family DNA amplification in lung cancer cell lines showed the five SCLC cell lines with greater than 20-fold *MYC* DNA amplification were all in the variant subclass of SCLC cell lines.[65] Subsequent studies showed that amplification of the *MYC* gene was associated with the shorter doubling times and higher cloning efficiencies in soft agarose.[69] The variant cell lines NCI-N417 and NCI-H82 were also found to be relatively resistant to low doses of radiation, NCI-H146 had intermediate sensitivity, and NCI-H249, NCI-H187, NCI-H209, and NCI-H69 were all sensitive to low doses of radiation.[90] NCI-N417 and NCI-H82 had greater than 20-fold *MYC* family DNA amplification, NCI-H146 did not have DNA amplification but did have abundant expression of the *MYC* gene, and NCI-H249, NCI-H187, and NCI-H209 did not have detectable *MYC* expression.

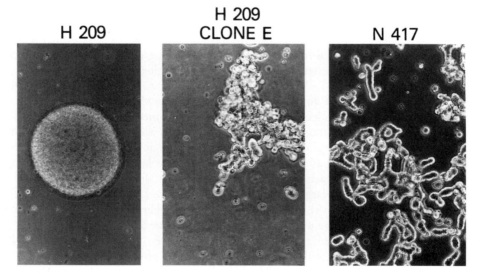

H 209

H 209 CLONE E

N 417

FIGURE 5.4. Cellular morphology of small cell lung cancer cell lines and a transfected clone: Small cell lung cancer cell lines NCI-H209 and NCI-H209 transfected with six copies of the normal *MYC* gene, and NCI-N417 growing in log phase. The cells have been photographed using a phase contrast Nikon photomicroscope (100 × magnification). (From Johnson BE, Battey JF, Linnoila I, et al. Changes in the phenotype of human small cell lung cancer cell lines after transfection and expression of the c-*myc*. *J Clin Invest* 1986;78:525 by copyright permission of the Society of Clinical Investigation.)

Other authors have commented on the association with the variant phenotype and *MYC* family amplification and expression. H22, H24, H86, GLC16, GLC 19, and SCLC-SK2 have high degrees of *MYC* DNA amplification but do not have a variant phenotype.[70,81,91] Although it appears that there is a link between *MYC* DNA amplification and the variant phenotype, numerous convincing examples of classic phenotype with *MYC* DNA amplification have been published.[70,81,91] In addition, cell lines with variant characteristics have been reported with *NMYC*[24] DNA amplification and *LMYC* DNA amplification.[81] We await additional information about additional potential etiologies for the variant phenotype in other cell lines.

Further support for the *MYC* gene playing a role in the increased growth of SCLC cells came from transfection studies. The normal human *MYC* gene with its own promoter, 5 kbases of upstream regulatory sequences, and a selectable marker were transfected into a tumor cell line (NCI-H209) which did not express detectable *MYC* mRNA.[15] One to six copies of the gene were introduced into a clone of NCI-H209 and different amounts of the mature form of *MYC* mRNA were expressed in the transfected clones (Figure 5.4). The amounts of *MYC* mRNA expressed in clones A to C and E were similar to the amount expressed in NCI-H146, the cell line which did not have *MYC* DNA amplification but did express abundant *MYC* mRNA. There was no detectable *MYC* mRNA in clone D because the third exon of the *MYC* gene was deleted. The amount of *MYC* mRNA in all the clones was less than the amount expressed by the cell line with *MYC* DNA amplification, NCI-N417.

The clone with the most abundant expression of *MYC* mRNA (clone E) used the first promoter (P1) in preference to P2, similar to Burkitt lymphoma cell lines which have a *MYC* gene translocated into the immunoglobin locus.[12] Therefore, in both these system where the *MYC* gene is placed into an altered location in the genome by transfection or translocation in Burkitt's lymphoma, the promoter utilization is changed.

The morphology of the original clone, NCI-H209, formed the typical tightly packed floating aggregates typical of a classic subclass cell line while NCI-N417 formed loosely attached floating aggregates typical of a variant cell line (Figure 5.4). The *MYC*-transfected clone E of NCI-H209 changed to loosely attached floating aggregates and formed small cell/large cell morphology when injected into athymic nude mice. The NCI-H209 clone E cells had a shorter doubling time and greater cloning efficiency but no difference in L-dopa decarboxylase enzymatic activity and bombesinlike immunoreactivity than the original clone. Therefore *MYC* transfection with increased gene expression is associated with a change in morphology and increased growth characteristics but not detectable change in biochemical characteristics. We were unable to examine these transfected clones for changes in the sensitivity to radiation because of the low cloning efficiency in soft agarose of the original clone, NCI-H209.

Retinoic acid studies have also provided evidence for the *MYC* gene playing a role in the increased growth of rate of SCLC cells.[92,94] The variant cell lines NCI-H82 and NCI-H417 have *MYC* DNA amplification and high levels of *MYC* mRNA expression. The addition of retinoic acid dramatically reduces *MYC* mRNA expression, which is associated with development of typical features of classic SCLC cells. In addition, NCI-H82 and NCI-H417 have a reduction in the growth rate of the cells and cloning efficiency in soft agarose and development of a classic morphology in cell culture after addition of retinoic acid.[92,94] However, retinoic acid treatment of these cell lines did not result in an increase in L-dopa decarboxylase activity, a feature of classic SCLC lines.[92] L-*MYC* expression increased dramatically in NCI-H82 cells treated with retinoic acid.[94] The mechanism by which retinoic acid induces *LMYC* expression is by an increase in *LMYC* transcriptional initiation.[95] This can be observed at a retinoic acid concentration of 1 μm; a concentration that is easily achievable in the plasma of patients undergoing treatment with retinoic acid. The mechanism by which the addition of retinoic acid leads to an increase in *LMYC* transcriptional initiation is presently undefined. The mechanism of *MYC* down-regulation appears to involve an increase in transcript attenuation at the exon 1 intron 1 boundary.[95] Transcript attenuation is a transcriptional regulatory mechanism reducing the elongation of mRNA molecules at the exon 1/intron 1 boundary of the *MYC* gene.[96] Thus these experiments demonstrate that the addition of retinoic acid to NCI-H82 SCLC cell lines leads them to assume a classic SCLC cell morphology and decreases their growth rate and cloning efficiency, which are accompanied by an increase in *LMYC* and a decrease in *MYC* gene expression.

The findings from these cell culture studies have been applied to a clinical study. A phase II clinical trial incorporated retinoic acid (all-*trans*-retinoic acid) with cisplatin and etoposide for previously untreated patients with extensive stage small cell lung carcinoma.[97] Retinoic acid was given at 150 mg per m^2 and was begun on day 1 of treatment and continued for one year. Of the 22 evaluable patients, 59% discontinued retinoic acid due to toxicity. These included mucocutaneous reactions, headaches, anorexia, fatigue, nausea/emesis, myalgias, and confusion.[97] The overall response rate was 45%, with a median survival of 10.9 months. Presently the combination of retinoic acid with combination chemotherapy is not effective enough and too toxic for routine use. Newer synthetic retinoids which have less toxicity and are more potent inhibitors of SCLC cell growth in culture than retinoic acid are presently being evaluated.[98]

MYC FAMILY AMPLIFICATION, mRNA EXPRESSION, AND PROTEIN STUDIES IN HUMAN LUNG CANCER

The *MYC* family genes have been studied in a large number of tumor cell lines and tumors. Tables 5.1–5.5 list the studies done of lung cancer cell lines and lung cancers. If a lung cancer or lung cancer cell line is reported in more than one publication, the cell line in the table is listed with the article in which it first appeared and is not included when studied in subsequent publications.

MYC Family DNA Amplification and Expression in Small Cell Lung Cancer Cell Lines

MYC family DNA amplification and expression have been studied in 185 and 73 SCLC cell lines and xenografts respectively. Approximately 40% of tumor cell lines established from patients with SCLC have *MYC* family DNA amplification (Table 5.1). *MYC* and *LMYC* DNA amplification are present in 15% and 18% respectively of the tumor cell lines, while N-*MYC* is present in 7%. Three cell lines have been described that have amplification of more than one member of the *MYC* family of genes. These include Lu-135 (*MYC* and *LMYC*), DMS-273 (*MYC* and *LMYC*), and NCI-H2552 (*LMYC* and *NMYC*).[80,99,100]

TABLE 5.1. MYC FAMILY DNA AMPLIFICATION IN SMALL CELL LUNG CANCER CELL LINES

Investigators	*MYC*	N-*MYC*	L-*MYC*
Little, et al.[65]	5/11	ND	ND
Saksela, et al.[66]	2/4	0/4	ND
Gazdar, et al.[69]	4/8	ND	ND
Nau, et al.[67]	ND	ND	4/7
Nau, et al.[24]	ND	5/11	ND
Bepler, et al.[82]	1/1	0/1	0/1
Graziano, et al.[140]	0/1	1/1	ND
Keifer, et al.[70]	3/4	0/4	ND
Waters, et al.[141]	0/9	3/9	3/9
Yokota, et al.[80]	1/4	0/4	1/4
Kok, et al.[91]	0/1	1/1	0/1
Takahashi, et al.[81]	2/13	0/13	4/13
*Gazzeri, et al.[142]	0/14	1/14	6/14
*Gazzeri, et al.[83]	4/11	0/11	0/11
Brennan, et al.[106]	2/60	1/62	1/61
Makela, et al.[143]	ND	ND	4/4
**Rygaard, et al.[99]	1/13	0/13	3/13
Johnson, et al.[100]	2/27	2/27	4/27
Gasperi-Campani, et al.[144]	0/1	0/1	0/1
Total	27/182 (15%)	13/176 (7%)	30/166 (18%)

* These studies were performed on human lung xenografts grown in athymic nuce mice.
** These studies were performed on cell lines and on xenografts grown in athymic nude mice.

TABLE 5.2. MYC FAMILY mRNA EXPRESSION IN SMALL CELL LUNG CANCER CELL LINES

Investigators	MYC	N-*MYC*	L-*MYC*
Little, et al.[65]	8/8	ND	ND
Saksela, et al.[66]	3/4	ND	ND
Nau, et al.[67]	ND	ND	4/7
Nau, et al.[24]	ND	4/9	ND
Bepler, et al.[82]	1/1	0/1	0/1
Graziano, et al.[140]	0/1	1/1	ND
Keifer, et al.[70]	4/4	4/4	ND
Kok, et al.[91]	0/1	1/1	0/1
Takahashi, et al.[81]	5/13	0/13	6/13
*Gazzeri, et al.[142]	2/14	1/14	7/14
*Gazzeri, et al.[83]	5/11	6/11	0/11
**Rygaard, et al.[99]	8/13	1/13	7/13
Arvelo, et al.[145]	0/3	0/3	1/3
Total	36/73 (49%)	18/70 (26%)	25/63 (39%)

* These studies were performed on human lung xenografts grown in athymic nude mice.
** These studies were performed on cell lines and on xenografts grown in athymic nude mice.

Four different reports describe *MYC* family DNA amplification in 16 tumor cell lines established from seven patients with SCLC at different times during their clinical course.[70,81,91,99] In three of these studies, the *MYC* family DNA amplification status appears to be consistent in five of the patients.[70,81,99] In the tumor cell lines established from the individual patients, the same *MYC* family gene

TABLE 5.3. MYC FAMILY DNA AMPLIFICATION AND EXPRESSION IN TUMORS FROM PATIENTS WITH SMALL CELL LUNG CANCER

Investigators	*MYC*	N-*MYC*	L-*MYC*
Amplification			
Wong, et al.[68]	2/45	3/45	ND
Heighway, et al.[146]	0/3	ND	ND
Johnson, et al.[139]	0/38	4/38	2/38
Yokota, et al.[80]	0/17	1/17	3/17
Shiraishi, et al.[87]	1/8	0/8	2/6
Kok, et al.[91]	0/1	1/1	0/1
Takahashi, et al.[81]	2/23	0/23	3/23
Noguchi, et al.[105]	1/47	5/47	5/47
*Gazzeri, et al.[83]	2/11	0/11	0/11
Gazzeri, et al.[84]	5/29	1/29	6/29
Total	12/219 (5%)	15/219 (7%)	21/174 (12%)
Expression			
Takahashi, et al.[81]	1/6	0/6	4/6
*Gazzeri, et al.[83]	1/5	0/5	0/5
Gazzeri, et al.[84]	8/29	1/29	9/29
Total	10/40 (25%)	1/40 (3%)	13/40 (33%)

* These studies were performed on human lung xenografts grown in athymic nude mice.

TABLE 5.4. MYC FAMILY DNA AMPLIFICATION AND EXPRESSION OF NON–SMALL CELL LUNG CANCER CELL LINES

Reference	*MYC*	*N-MYC*	*L-MYC*
Amplification			
Little, et al.[65]	1/5	ND	ND
Saksela, et al.[66]	0/2	0/2	ND
Nau, et al.[67]	0/1	ND	ND
Nau, et al.[24]	ND	0/2	ND
*Gazzeri, et al.[142]	5/7	0/7	0/5
*Gazzeri, et al.[83]	0/11	1/11	1/11
Sekido, et al.[73]	ND	ND	0/9
Total	6/26 (23%)	1/22 (5%)	1/25 (4%)
Expression			
Saksela, et al.[66]	1/2	ND	ND
Nau, et al.[24]	ND	0/1	ND
*Gazzeri, et al.[142]	5/5	0/5	0/5
*Gazzeri, et al.[83]	6/11	1/11	3/11
Total	12/18 (67%)	1/17 (6%)	3/16 (19%)

* These studies were performed on human lung xenografts grown in athymic nude mice.

was amplified in each series of cell lines. *MYC* was amplified in five cell lines from two patients, LMYC in four cell lines from two patients, and none in four cell lines from two patients. An exception to this observation has been reported.[91] Hole and colleagues have described a series of three cell lines established from a single patient with SCLC at presentation, at recurrence after nine cycles of chemotherapy, and after a subsequent course of radiotherapy. The tumor cell lines established prior to the initiation of treat-

TABLE 5.5. MYC FAMILY DNA AMPLIFICATION AND EXPRESSION IN TUMORS FROM PATIENTS WITH NON—SMALL CELL LUNG CANCER

Reference	*MYC*	*N-MYC*	*L-MYC*
Amplification			
Heighway, et al.[146]	0/22	ND	ND
Cline, et al.[147]	3/27	0/27	ND
Yokota, et al.[80]	3/36	0/36	0/36
Shiraishi, et al.[87]	13/129	0/129	4/102
Hajj, et al.[148]	1/54	0/54	0/54
Gazzeri, et al.[83]	1/11	0/11	0/11
Total	21/279 (8%)	0/257 (0%)	4/203 (3%)
Expression			
Gazzeri, et al.[84]	33/69	ND	ND
Total	33/69 (33%)		

ment had *NMYC* DNA amplification, while the two cell lines established after the patients recurred had *MYC* DNA amplification. This is the single example where tumor cell lines established from the same patient at different times during treatment course had a different *MYC* family gene amplified.

MYC family mRNA expression in SCLC cell lines have been studied by Northern blot analyses, nuclear run-off studies, S1 nuclease analyses, and *in situ* hybridization.[12,15,25,10] An S1 nuclease analysis (Figure 5.5) using an antisense *MYC* probe encompassing the first exon showed that the SCLC cell lines NCI-H82, NCI-H146, and NCI-N417 use both promoters (P1 and P2) within the first exon.[15,101] The second promoter is preferentially used, as has been typical of normal cells.[12,101] *In situ* hybridization of the cytospins and xenografts of SCLC cell lines with DNA amplification of *MYC* (NCI-N417, NCI-H82), *NMYC* (NCI-H526), and L-*MYC* (NCI-H378) showed cell lines which had easily detectable *MYC* family mRNA expression.[102] *MYC* family mRNA expression is detected more commonly than *MYC* family DNA amplification in SCLC cell lines and xenografts. *MYC* mRNA expression is present in approximately half, and *NMYC* and *LMYC* mRNA expression is present in 26% and 39% respectively (Table 5.2). Multiple cell lines have been described that have detectable mRNA expression of more than one *MYC* family member.[99] The mRNA expression of the *MYC* family genes is two to four times as common as DNA amplification of the genes. Therefore SCLC cell lines and xenografts commonly have increased mRNA expression of the *MYC* family genes without evidence of DNA amplification.

The regulation of *MYC* family mRNA expression has been studied in a subset of SCLC cell lines.[101,103] The DNase I sensitivity patterns and methylation patterns of the *MYC* gene in the SCLC cell lines NCI-H82 and NCI-H378 have been investigated. Chromosomal regions undergoing active transcription tend to be sensitive to DNase I treatment and are hypomethylated in the CpG (cytosine-guainine) dinucleotides, while chromosomal regions that are quiescent are not sensitive to DNase treatment and are hypermethylated. NCI-H82 has 40 to 50-fold *MYC* DNA amplification and abundant expression, while NCI-H378 has a single copy of the *MYC* gene and undetectable mRNA expression. The DNase hypersensitivity sites were identical in the two cell lines, and the hypomethylation and partial methylation patterns in the *MYC* gene locus were very similar. Therefore these structural chromatin patterns did not appear to be the mechanism of altered *MYC* gene expression.

In addition to an increase in *MYC* family mRNA expression caused by amplification, attenuation of mRNA expression takes place within the first intron in *MYC* and *LMYC*, which reduces the amount of steady-state mature mRNA.[103] Attenuation blocks the transcription of a gene after it is initiated. This attenuation takes place in tumor cell lines

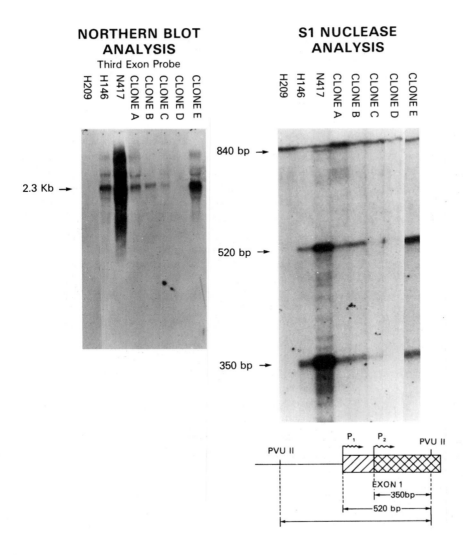

FIGURE 5.5. Northern blot and S1 nuclease analysis of small cell lung cancer cell lines and transfected clones: Cells grown from a clone of NCL-H209 were transfected with the normal human *MYC* gene with a selectable marker, individual clones were grown, and RNA was isolated. Northern blots were prepared and S1 nuclease analyses done as described in reference 15. NCI-H209, NCI-H146, and NCI-N417 represent SCLC cell lines, and clones A to E represent different clones transfected with the human *MYC* gene. Clones A to C have one intact *MYC* gene, clone D has deleted the *MYC* gene, and clone E has six copies of the *MYC* gene. The Northern blot was hybridized with a Cla-Eco R1 third exon fragment of the human *MYC* gene, and the signal at 2.3 kilobases (Kb) represents the mRNA. The S1 nuclease analysis shows a first exon probe hybridized to the mRNA, and the single strands of mRNA and antisense probe are digested away with S1 nuclease. The signal at 840 base pairs (bp) represents undigested probe, the signal at 520 bp represents the mRNA initiated at the first promoter, and the signal at 350 base pairs represents the mRNA initiated at the second promoter. (From Johnson BE, Battey JF, Linnoila I, et al. Changes in the phenotype of human small cell lung cancer cell lines after transfection and expression of the c-myc. *J Clin Invest* 1986;78: 525, by copyright permission of the Society of Clinical Investigation.)

which do and do not have amplification of the same *MYC* family gene. The loss of this attenuation in intron 1 of the *MYC* gene (NCI-H146) and *LMYC* (NCI-H432) is associated with increased mRNA expression of these genes. Increased expression of *NMYC* is associated with increased promoter function and gene amplification.

Antisense mRNA expression of the *NMYC* gene has been shown to play a potential role in the regulation of the *NMYC* gene.[25] Antisense mRNA expression refers to the transcription of the DNA strand complimentary to the strand coding for the *NMYC* gene product. Antisense *NMYC* mRNA initiates within the first intron and transcribes through the first exon in NCI-H249. Most of this antisense *NMYC* mRNA exists as a complex with the first exon and intron of sense *NMYC* mRNA, suggesting that this duplex could control mRNA processing and thereby regulate the production of the *NMYC* gene product.

Eleven tumor cell lines from nine patients have been studied for their mechanisms of increased *MYC* family

mRNA expression in the absence of DNA amplification. The mechanism for increased *MYC* family mRNA expression in the absence of amplification has not been established in the vast majority of tumor cell lines. However, mechanisms that increase *MYC* family mRNA expression other than gene amplification are likely to be important because the majority of lung cancers and lung cancer tumor cell lines with *MYC* family mRNA expression do not have *MYC* family DNA amplification of the corresponding gene.

Variability in processing of mRNA can also give rise multiple forms of the mRNA, leading to altered protein products in SCLC (Figure 5.6).[30] The *LMYC* gene can give rise to two different long forms of mature mRNA, which can either retain the first intron sequences (3.9 kbase mRNA) or process them out (3.6 kbase mRNA). The presence or absence of the first intron *LMYC* sequences has been demonstrated in mRNA extracted from normal human testis as well.[104] This shows alternative *LMYC* mRNA processing can take place in both normal tissue as well as tumor tissue.

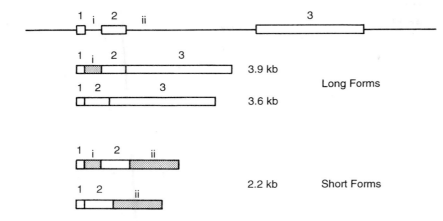

FIGURE 5.6. mRNA processing of the *LMYC* gene: The upper diagram depicts the genomic structure of L-*MYC*. The open boxes represent the three exons and the two lines between the boxes are the two introns. The four boxes below the genomic structure represent the portions of the introns and exons included in the mRNAs in both the long and short forms of mRNA. (From Kaye F, Battey J, Nau M, et al. Structure and expression of the human L-*myc* gene reveal a complex pattern of alternative mRNA processing. *Mol Cell Biol* 1988;8:186, with permission.)

The *LMYC* gene can also give rise to two different short forms of mature mRNA when the RNA polymerase continues reading into the second intron and uses one of several potential polyadenylation signals to terminate transcription in the second intron. These short forms can either retain the first intron or process it out (2.2 kbase mRNA). These four different forms are present in two different SCLC cell lines. The predicted amino acid sequence of these short forms will be different because they do not contain the protein coding sequences contained in the absent third exon. Antibodies generated by immunizing rabbits detected only proteins predicted to be translated from the long forms of mRNA.[32] In contrast, antibodies directed against homologous sequences present in all three *MYC* genes identified proteins the size predicted from the short forms of mRNA as well as the long forms.[33] The presence of proteins translated from the short forms of mRNA remains unresolved and their potential role remains undefined.

MYC FAMILY DNA AMPLIFICATION AND EXPRESSION IN SMALL CELL LUNG CANCER TUMORS

MYC family DNA amplification and expression have been studied in 219 and 40 tumors respectively from patients with SCLC (Table 5.3). Approximately 22% of the tumors from patients with SCLC have *MYC* family DNA amplification. *MYC* family DNA amplification is less common in tumors than in tumor cell lines and xenografts. *MYC* DNA amplification is about one third as common in tumors as in tumor cell lines (5% versus 15%), *NMYC* DNA is similar (8% in both), *LMYC* DNA amplification is two thirds as common in the tumors as in the tumor cell lines (12% versus 18%). No tumor from a SCLC patient has DNA amplification of more than one *MYC* family gene.

Two studies showed that the *MYC* family DNA copy number was similar in multiple sites of metastatic disease

from 26 different patients with SCLC.[68,81] Wong and associates reported on four patients where all ten metastatic lesions had amplified copies of the *MYC* family genes two patients with *MYC* and two with N-*MYC* DNA amplification).[68] In addition, 17 patients' original tumors did not have *MYC* family DNA amplification, nor did their 41 metastatic lesions. Takahashi and co-workers reported on five SCLC patients' 11 simultaneous tumor samples.[81] One patient's tumor samples had *MYC*, one had *LMYC*, and three had no *MYC* family DNA amplification. In addition, one patient with SCLC had *MYC* DNA amplification in the tumor before treatment and at postmortem examination.

In contrast, two other reports have described different *MYC* family DNA copy numbers in different sites from the same SCLC patient. Yokota and colleagues reported on a patient with SCLC where they studied the primary tumor and four different sites of metastases.[80] The primary tumor, pulmonary hilar lymph node, and pleural metastasis all had about 100-fold amplification of *NMYC*, while a liver metastasis and para-aortic lymph node did not have *NMYC* DNA amplification. Noguchi and co-workers were able to study tumors from 47 patients with SCLC.[105] Eleven patients had *MYC* family DNA amplification in their primary tumor. Nine of the 11 had similar degrees of *MYC* family DNA amplification in the metastatic sites as in the primary tumor site. One of the other two patients had *NMYC* DNA amplification in part of the primary tumor and three metastatic sites, while a different part of the primary tumor and three metastatic sites did not have *NMYC* DNA amplification. The other patient had *LMYC* DNA amplification in metastatic lymph nodes present at postmortem examination but not present in the primary lesion which had been resected prior to the patient death. No investigators found DNA amplification of multiple members of the *MYC* family DNA in the same sample.

MYC family mRNA expression is detected more commonly than *MYC* family DNA amplification in tumors obtained from patients with SCLC (Table 5.3). *MYC* and

LMYC mRNA expression is present in approximately one fourth to one third respectively, and N-*MYC* mRNA expression is detectable in only a single tumor. The mRNA expression of the *MYC* and *LMYC* is three to four times as common as DNA amplification of the genes, while N*MYC* expression is less common. Therefore SCLC cell lines and xenografts commonly have increased mRNA expression of the *MYC* family genes without evidence of DNA amplification. The incidence of *MYC* family DNA amplification and mRNA expression is less common in the tumor than in the tumor cell lines.

MYC Family DNA Amplification in Tumors, Tumor Cell Lines, and Xenografts from the Same Patient with Small Cell Lung Cancer

The *MYC* family copy number is nearly always similar in the tumors and the tumor cell lines plus the athymic nude mouse xenografts established from tumors obtained from patients with SCLC. One report showed that the *MYC* family DNA copy number was similar in tumors and tumor cell lines from 16 patients with SCLC.[106] Figure 5.7 shows examples of *NMYC* DNA amplification in tumors and tumor cell lines from the same individuals but having a single copy in the normal tissue. The intense signals in NCI-H720, the tumor from patient 1, NCI-H526 and the tumor from patient 2, NCI-H526 and the tumor from patient 2, NCI-H689 and the tumor from patient 3, and the tumor from patient 4 show *NMYC* DNA amplification. The normal tissues from all these patients show a less intense 1.9 base signal, representing a single copy of the gene, which shows that the amplification takes place only in the cancer and not in the patients' normal tissue. The single exception was in a patient where the tumor DNA had degraded so the DNA copy number of the tumor could not be accurately determined.

Yokota and associates reported that the cell line Lu-135 was amplified for both *MYC* and *LMYC*.[80] The tumor from which Lu-135 was established had *LMYC* DNA amplification but did not have *MYC* DNA amplification. Dr. Yokota also reported on a second tumor cell line, Lu-139, which had *MYC* DNA amplification while the original tumor did not. Takahashi and colleagues reported on two patients with SCLC who had both their tumors and tumor cell lines studied.[81] One had *MYC* DNA amplification in two tumor samples as well as two tumor cell lines established from these tumor specimens. The other patient with SCLC did not have *MYC* family DNA amplification in either the two tumor cell lines or the tumors. Kok and colleagues reported on the *MYC* family DNA amplification status of a tumor and tumor cell line established from the same patient prior to starting his therapy.[91] The supraclavicular lymph node and the tumor cell line established from it, GLC-14, had *MYC* DNA amplification. In contrast, the tumor cell lines

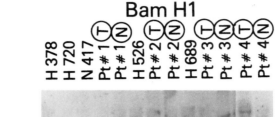

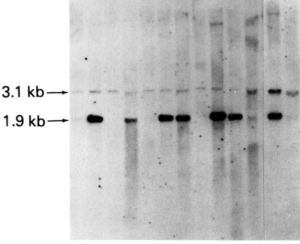

FIGURE 5.7. N-*MYC* DNA amplification in patients' tumors and tumor cell lines: Southern blot of 10 micrograms of DNA digested with the Bam H1 restriction endonuclease from SCLC tumors, normal tissues, and tumor cell lines hybridized to N-*MYC* exon 2 fragment. The tumor for each patient is designated T and the normal tissue is designated N. SCLC cell line NCI-H526 was derived from a tumor from patient number 2, and NCI-H689 was derived from a tumor from patient number 3. The signals that appear at 1.9 kb represent the signal from the fragment N-*MYC*. The signal at 3.1 kilobases represents gastrin-releasing peptide gene, present in a single copy. (From Johnson BE, Makuch RW, Simmons AD, et al. *myc* family DNA amplification in small cell lung cancer patients' tumors and corresponding cell lines. *Cancer Res* 1988;48:5163, with permission.)

established from tumors after treatment, GLC-16 and GLC-19, had *MYC* DNA amplification and the tumors were not available for study.

The *MYC* family DNA copy number was also examined in tumors and xenografts from 13 patients with SCLC. Four of the 13 patients with SCLC had *MYC* family DNA amplification (two *MYC*, one N-*MYC*, and one L-*MYC*) in both their tumors and xenografts. Two patients had *MYC* DNA amplification in their xenografts but not in the primary cancer. All primary cancers and xenografts which had *MYC* family DNA amplification had abundant expression of that *MYC* family gene.[93]

There is evidence that *MYC* DNA amplification occurs more commonly in tumor cell lines and xenografts than in tumors (Tables 5.3 and 5.4). This is likely to be caused by a combination of *MYC* gene amplification which takes after cells are placed in culture[80] or in xenografts,[83,85] and the tumor cell lines are more likely to grow if they have *MYC*

DNA amplification. These two reasons likely explain the more than three fold higher incidence of *MYC* family DNA amplification in tumor cell lines and xenografts (15%) than in the tumors taken directly from patients (4%). The incidence of *NMYC* and *LMYC* DNA amplification in tumors, tumor cell lines, and xenografts is similar.

MYC Family DNA Amplification in Tumors from Patients with Small Cell Lung Cancer: Clinical Status and Course

MYC family DNA amplification and expression in tumors and tumor cell lines from patients with SCLC have also been associated with chemotherapy treatment and shortened survival.[105–107] However, all three studies are retrospective, and two studied the tumors or tumor cell lines obtained after the patients died[105] or had relapsed after initial treatment.[106]

Brennan reported on *MYC* family DNA amplification in tumors and tumor cell lines obtained from patients either before or after chemotherapy treatment.[106] *MYC* family DNA amplification was detected in 19 out of 67 (28%) of the specimens (35 tumor cell lines and 32 tumors) from patients previously treated with chemotherapy. Seven specimens from previously treated patients had *MYC,* seven had *NMYC,* and five had *LMYC* DNA amplification. This was significantly more than the incidence of *MYC* family DNA amplification detect in the specimens obtained from patients prior to the initiation of treatment (3 of 40; p = 0.01) where one had N-*MYC* and two had L-*MYC* DNA amplification. Other authors have not directly analyzed the effect of chemotherapy treatment on the incidence of *MYC* family DNA amplification, so information from other groups is not available (Table 5.1).

Noguchi and his colleagues obtained tumor samples from 47 patients with SCLC who underwent postmortem examination.[105] Dot blot hybridization of the DNA extracted from paraffin-embedded tissue was used to determine the DNA copy number of the *MYC* family genes. One patient had *MYC,* five patients had *NMYC,* and five had *LMYC* DNA amplification in their tumor sample. If the five patients whose tumor had *MYC* family DNA amplification of ten or less (two with *NMYC* and three with *LMYC*) were removed from the analysis, the patients with *MYC* family DNA amplification of ten copies or greater lived a shorter time than patients without *MYC* family DNA amplification (p = 0.06). This study's shortcomings include that the studies were done on the tumors from patients with SCLC after they had died of their cancer, they were done after the patients had been treated with chemotherapy, and their data were extensively analyzed before arriving at a survival difference.

The other study evaluated 69 tumor cell lines established from patients with SCLC,[106] with a recent update including additional 27 cell lines.[100] Fifty-two were established from patients who had not been previously treated with chemotherapy, while 44 were established from patients previously treated with chemotherapy. The survival of the patients who had tumor cell lines established prior to the start of chemotherapy was much shorter than patients whose tumor cell lines were established after the start of therapy, so the two groups were analyzed separately. Eight of the 44 tumor cell lines established from patients previously treated with chemotherapy had *MYC* DNA amplification. The patients whose tumor cell lines had *MYC* DNA amplification lived a shorter time (median of 25 weeks) than the patients whose tumor cell lines did not (median of 54 weeks) Figure 5.8. There was no association between *NMYC* or *LMYC* DNA amplification in the patients' tumor cell lines and patient outcome. However, this study's shortcomings include that the studies were done on tumor cell lines instead of the tumors from patients with small cell lung cancer, they were done on a small subset of the entire patient group (44 out of 306), and they were done after the patients had been treated with chemotherapy.

A single small study has examined *MYC* family mRNA expression and patient outcome.[107] Fifteen patients with SCLC who underwent mediastinal biopsies were selected. The seven patients whose formalin-fixed, paraffin-embedded mediastinal biopsies had abundant expression of *NMYC* mRNA by *in situ* hybridization were less likely to have a complete response and lived a shorter time than the eight patients whose tumors did not have detectable *NMYC* mRNA. The shortcomings of this study were that the other *MYC* family genes were not evaluated, only a small number of patients were examined, and there were potential patient selection factors.

Despite the defects in these three studies, *in vitro* evidence shows *MYC* amplification and expression being associated with growth of SCLC, and there is prospective data showing that DNA amplification of N-*MYC* in pretreatment specimens of childhood neuroblastoma is associated with shortened survival.[108]

MYC Family DNA Amplification and Expression in Non–Small Cell Lung Cancer Cell Lines

The information of *MYC* family DNA amplification and expression in tumor cell lines and xenografts established from patients with NSCLC is much less extensive than that from patients with SCLC. *MYC* family DNA amplification and expression has been studied in 26 and 18 NSCLC cell lines and xenografts respectively. Less than one third of tumor cell lines established from patients with NSCLC have *MYC* family DNA amplification (Table 5.4). *MYC* DNA amplification is present in 23% while *NMYC* and *LMYC* are present in a single cell line.

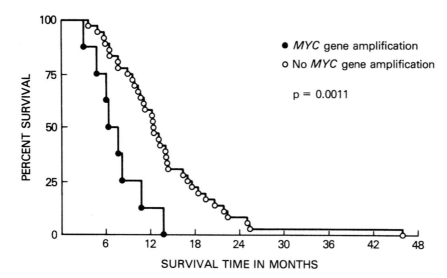

FIGURE 5.8. Survival from the initiation of chemotherapy of small cell lung cancer patients whose cell lines established at relapse had *MYC* DNA amplification compared with patients whose cell lines did not. Patients whose cell lines had DNA amplification of *MYC* lived a shorter time compared to those patients without *MYC* amplification (p = 0.0011). (From Johnson BE, Russell E, Simmons AM, et al. MYC family DNA amplification in 126 tumor cell lines from patients with small cell lung cancer. *J Cell Biochem Suppl* 1996;24:210, with permission.)

MYC family mRNA expression is detected more commonly than *MYC* family DNA amplification in tumor cell lines and xenografts obtained from patients with NSCLC (Table 5.4). *MYC* and *LMYC* mRNA expression is present in approximately two thirds to one fourth respectively and N-*MYC* mRNA expression is detectable in only a single tumor. The mRNA expression of the *MYC* and *LMYC* is three to four times as common as DNA amplification of the genes, while *NMYC* expression is less common. Therefore, NSCLC cell lines and xenografts commonly have increased mRNA expression of the *MYC* family genes without evidence of DNA amplification.

MYC Family DNA Amplification and Expression in Non–Small Cell Lung Cancer Tumors

MYC family DNA amplification and expression have been studied in 279 and 69 tumors from patients with NSCLC. Approximately 10% of the tumors from patients with NSCLC had *MYC* family DNA amplification (Table 5.5). *MYC* and *LMYC* DNA amplification was present in the tumors in 8% and 3% respectively. None of the tumors from 257 patients with non–small cell lung cancer had *NMYC* DNA amplification. In addition, no tumor from a patient with NSCLC patient had DNA amplification of more than one *MYC* family gene.

MYC mRNA expression was detected more commonly than *MYC* DNA amplification in tumors from patients with NSCLC. *MYC* mRNA expression was present in one third and *NMYC* and *LMYC* mRNA expression were so uncommon that they were not examined in the following refer-

ence.[84] *MYC* mRNA expression was four times as common as DNA amplification of the genes.

MYC Proteins in Patients with Non–Small Cell Lung Cancer

The presence of *MYC* protein has been studied by flow cytometry and immunohistochemistry on clinical samples of surgically resected NSCLC. Two studies examined 30 NSCLCs for the presence of the *MYC* protein in the surgically resected cancers.[109,110] Fifteen NSCLCs were surgically resected, frozen, cell suspensions prepared, and incubated with a murine monoclonal antibody directed against the *MYC* protein. The cells stained with the antibody were passed through a cell sorter, and the percentage of cells staining with the murine monoclonal antibody was determined. Of the 15 (67%) NSCLCs seven adenocarcinomas and three squamous cell carcinomas, ten had abundant *MYC* protein detected.[109] Another study examined 15 frozen sections of NSCLCs with antibodies directed against *MYC*.[110] Six of the 15 (40%) had protein detectable by immunuhistochemistry. Three of these six also had foci of squamous metaplasia, and the *MYC* protein was detectable in all three of these foci.

Two different reports from the same institution showed the percentage of NSCLC with *MYC* protein detectable by immunohistochemistry of paraffin-embedded tissues and its relationship to clinical outcomes.[110,111] About one half of patients (48% to 57%) had detectable *MYC* protein in their NSCLC. The authors showed a statistically significant association between the presence of *MYC* protein in the surgically resected NSCLC and the presence of metastases in a univariate analysis.[111] These studies show the presence of the *MYC* protein in approximately half of NSCLCs, which is similar to the percentage of NSCLC cell lines and tumors expressing *MYC* mRNA. However, *MYC* DNA amplification, mRNA expression, and protein have been studied in very few NSCLC cell lines and tumors, so the studies are only correlative to date.

Gene Therapy with *MYC* in Lung Cancer

The *MYC* family of genes appears to have a prominent role in the pathogenesis and progression of SCLC. These genes are attractive targets for gene therapy. One approach is to inhibit *MYC* mRNA by using antisense oligonucleotides. This technology has been used successfully to inhibit *MYC* expression in hematopoetic cell lines, colon cancer cell lines, and neuroblastoma cell lines. Studies using *LMYC* antisense constructs have been performed using the SCLC cell line NCI-H209.[112] The antisense oligonucleotide was used at a concentration of 10 μM and was shown to inhibit cell growth *in vitro* in a sequence and dose-dependant manner (range 1.6 to 10 μM). The levels of *LMYC* protein were also shown to be decreased (to ~30% of control) in the treated cells. This antisense inhibition was *LMYC*-specific, as the construct was unable to inhibit the growth of cell line NCI-H82, which is known to contain an amplification of *MYC*.[112] Antisense studies using c-*myc* have also been performed in SCLC cell line GLC$_4$ and its two drug-resistant (*in vitro* acquired) subclones to cisplatin (GLC$_4$-cDDP) and adriamycin (GLC$_4$-Adr).[113] These studies have been performed using both purified antisense oligonucleotides and using a plasmid construct containing a dexamethasone-inducible expression system.[113,114] These studies resulted showed aon ~30% growth reduction in the GLC$_4$ cell lines tested. In addition, increased cisplatin sensitivity (12% more cell kill at IC25 and 16% more cell kill at IC50) was observed in the cisplatin-resistant subclone (GLC$_4$-cDDP) after treatment with antisense *MYC* but not in the native cell line.[114] In NSCLC cell lines, *MYC* antisense oligonucleotides have been used with NSCLC cell lines A427, A549, and SKMES-1. This also resulted in a 20% to 40% reduction in cell proliferation in these cell lines.[115]

A second gene therapeutic approach is to take advantage of the *MYC* family overexpression in SCLC cells. Kumagai and colleagues constructed a plasmid containing an E-box element upstream of a herpes simplex virus (HSV) thymidine kinase (TK) promoter and structural gene.[116] Using a chloramphenicol acetyltransferase system, they could demonstrate that any *MYC* gene family member could activate the TK promoter. When this construct was transfected into cells and the cells were treated with gancyclovir, a significant increase in gancyclovir sensitivity could be demonstrated due to the presence of this construct. The increase varied depending on which *MYC* family member was overexpressed and was 33-fold for *MYC* (cell line OC-10), 500-fold for *LMYC* (cell line OS-2-R), and 22-fold for *NMYC* (cell line OS1).[116] Similar findings were seen *in vivo* when

these tumor cells were placed into nude mice that were subsequently treated with gancyclovir. Complete tumor regression was seen in 7 of 10 (OC-10 cells) and 5 of 10 mice (OS2-R cells). Interestingly, mice with tumors containing a mixture of the TK construct transfected cells (with OS2-R cells) and parental cells showed greater inhibition of growth after gancyclovir administration than would be expected on the basis of the transfected cells alone. This suggested that the nontransfected cells were also being effected, a process known as the bystander effect.

The data presented above using a cell culture systems and mice are encouraging but preliminary and far from being applied as effective treatment options for patients with lung cancer. One of the main problems is delivery of the DNA (oligonucleotides or constructs) to the tumor(s) in adequate concentrations to achieve the effect observed *in vitro*. A proposed mechanism to improve the delivery problem has been the use of lipid-packaging systems. *In vitro*, incorporation of *LMYC* antisense oligonucleotides into cationic virosomes resulted in decrease in *LMYC* protein expression (32% of control) and an inhibition in thymidine incorporation (by 60% to 70%) in NCI-H209 cells using only picamolar concentrations of the oligonucelotide.[117] This may be a more efficient system to try in patients. However, as mentioned above, not all SCLC tumors overexpress *MYC* family genes, and thus patient's tumors would have to be intially analyzed to identify appropriate targets for treatment. Our knowledge of the *MYC* family of proteins and their interacting partners has grown significantly in the last few years. These binding partners also provide new targets of therapeutic intervention but have not yet been used *in vitro* in lung cancer.

JUN AND *FOS* FAMILY PROTOONCOGENES

The AP-1 (activating protein-1) family of transcription factors is composed of *JUN*, *FOS*, and *ATF* (activating transcription factor) proteins. These transcription factors form homo- and heterodimers and bind DNA at (TGACTCA or TGACGTCA) sequence-specific sites to activate transcription. These genes belong to a group of immediate early genes and are induced by a variety of mitogens including growth factors, serum, and phorbol esters. The information available on the *JUN* and *FOS* family of protooncogenes in lung cancer is sparse. Therefore the information given in this review will be brief, and readers are referred to the more complete reviews for mechanism of *JUN* and *FOS* family function.[7-10]

The human family of *JUN* protooncogenes is comprised of *JUN*, *JUNB*, and *JUND*. These human protooncogenes share sequence homology with the oncogene contained in the avian sarcoma virus 17 (ASV 17.[118] This avian retrovirus was isolated from a sarcoma in an adult chicken, and the retrovirus can transform chicken embryo fibroblasts into neoplastic cells. *JUN, JUNB,* and *JUND* human sequences have cloned. *JUN* and *JUNB* are approximately 2 to 3 kbases long and do not have any introns in their gene structure.[119,120] These genes code for predominant mRNAs of 2.0 to 2.7 kbases with a predicted number of amino acids in the *Jun* proteins of 331 and 347 amino acids. An incomplete human *JUNB* cDNA sequence has also been reported.[121]

The human family of FOS protooncogenes is comprised of the related genes *FOS, FOS-B,* and *FRA*1 and *FRA*2. These human protooncogenes share sequence homology with the oncogene contained in the FBJ murine osteosarcoma virus.[122] This murine retrovirus was isolated from a spontaneous sarcoma in a mouse, and the retrovirus can transform fibroblasts into neoplastic cells. Human genomic *FOS* sequences show that *FOS* has four exons contained within approximately 3.5 kbases of DNA.[123] The *FOS* gene codes for an mRNAs of 2.2 kbases with a predicted protein sequence of 380 amino acids. The cDNA sequences for the murine-related gene *FOS-B,*[124] and human *FRA*1 and *FRA*2 have been reported.[125] Although *FOS-B, FRA*1, and *FRA*2 have been have been identified in other systems, their specific role in lung cancer remains undefined.

The *JUN* and *FOS* family genes all code for a basic region of amino acids followed by a leucine zipper similar to those described within the *MYC* family genes, but they do not have the helix-loop-helix structure present in the *MYC* family genes.[8] The *JUN* proteins dimerize with themselves or with *FOS* proteins to form an activation protein complex (AP-1).[126,127,128] This AP-1 complex recognizes and binds to the consensus DNA sequence TGAGTCAG upstream from a number of genes, including collagenase and metallotheonein II, which stimulates their mRNA expression. The mRNA expression of these two genes increases rapidly following addition of exogenous growth factors or nonspecific stimulation by adding serum to serum-starved cells.[7,8,9] In addition, *JUN* is regulated posttranscriptionally by phosphorylation at serine and threonine residues, whereas *FOS* is primarily regulated by a transcriptional mechanism.[10] These genes are involved in various biologic mechanisms including cell proliferation, differentiation, and apoptosis.[129]

JUN and *FOS* Expression in NSCLC Cell Lines, Primary Tumors from Patients, and Clinical Course

The published information available on the *JUN* and *FOS* genes in lung cancer is somewhat conflicting. *JUN* and *FOS* mRNA expression increases within 30 minutes in primary bronchial epithelial cells and in the SCLC cell line NCI-H345 in response to exogenously added growth factors or serum.[130] Serum stimulation of SCLC cell line NCI-H345 is accompanied by an increase in *FOS* and *JUN* mRNA expression (analyzed by Northern), whereas there is no increase in NCI-H82 cells. This cell line also contains an amplified *MYC* gene (25 copies), whereas NCI-H345 cells

have a single copy of the *MYC* gene. The association of *MYC* amplification with the expression of *FOS* and *JUN* following serum stimulation is undefined. In the NSCLC cell line NCI-H125 there is low baseline mRNA expression of both *FOS* and *JUN*. Their expression increases rapidly following serum stimulation (*JUN* more than *FOS*) followed by a down-regulation of *FOS* expression.[52,96] Another NSCLC line (A549) also shows increase in *JUN* and *FOS* mRNA expression, but the level of *FOS* expression is greater (11-fold) than *JUN* (nine fold) in these cell lines. These cell lines also show increase in *FOS* and *JUN* mRNA expression comparable to that seen with serum following stimulation with TGF-β, insulin, and IGF-1.[96] This increase in expression is accompanied by an increase in AP-1 transcriptional activity. Lee and colleagues described the level of *FOS* and *JUN* expression as being higher in normal bronchial epithelial cells (HBE) than in tumorigenic HBE cells (these cell lines have been immortalized and developed in nude mice).[132] This is accompanied by a decrease in AP-1 transcriptional activity and has also been observed in NSCLC cell lines Chago K1 and SKMES-1.[131] This decrease in AP-1 transcriptional activity appears to be due in part to suppression of *FOS* transcription.[132] The mRNA expression of the *FOS* and *JUN* family members has also been studied. *JUNB* and *JUND* MRNA expression (by Northern analysis) was detected in ten of ten NSCLC cell lines studied while *FRA*1 mRNA expression was high in two of ten cell lines (NCI-H1299 and NCI-H441) and minimal in four of ten cell lines.[133]

The expression of *JUN* appears to occur early in the process of lung carcinogenesis.[133] *JUN* is not detectable in normal bronchial epithelium but is found by immunohistochemistry in bronchial hyperplasias (two of three specimens), squamous metaplasias (five of five specimens), bronchial dysplasias (three of three positive), and carcinomas *in situ* (four of five positive). In NSCLC tumor specimens, *JUN* was detected by immunohistochemistry in 31% of specimens including squamous cell carcinomas, adenocarcinomas, and large cell carcinomas. There was no statistically significant difference in expression between the various histologic subtypes. However, Levin and colleagues have found that *FOS* and *JUN* were expressed at high levels in normal tissues and that the expression was much lower in the adjacent malignant tissues (in 72% of cases) in the same specimen.[134] This was confirmed both by RNA expression studies and using immunohistochemistry with four different histologic subtypes of NSCLC.

The clinical significance of *JUN* or *FOS* expression in human lung tumors is presently under investigation. *JUN* protein has been detected in 31% to 51% of the tumors, and *FOS* protein was detected in 42% to 60% of the NSCLC cancers.[110,111,133] In a xenograft model, tumors (squamous cell carcinomas) overexpressing *FOS* or *JUN* grew better in athymic nude mice compared to those without overexpression.[135] Analysis of patients with squamous cell carcinoma showed that *FOS* expression in the tumor specimen (as assayed by immunohistochemistry) was a significant negative prognostic factor independent of lymph node involvement.[133,136,137] Patients whose tumors were positive for either *FOS* (60% of tumors) or *JUN* (49% of tumors) had significantly shorter median survivals. These studies were retrospective and nature and need to be confirmed prospectively and in additional patient populations. Szabo and colleagues report no association between *JUN* protein expression in NSCLC and survival.[133] However, this study included four different histologic subtypes of NSCLC.

FUTURE STUDIES OF THE *MYC, JUN,* and *FOS* FAMILIES IN LUNG CANCER

Over the last few years, a great deal has been learned about the *MYC* family of genes and their dimerization partners. In addition, the role of the *MYC* family of genes in normal development (including lung development) has been elucidated. The role of the various *MYC*-binding proteins in lung cancer (if any) remains to be defined. The lung cancer cell lines and tumors have been extensively characterized for *MYC* family mRNA expression and protein production. There are numerous examples of increased expression and protein production of various members of the *MYC* family in different lung cancers and lung cancer cell lines. This will offer fertile territory for investigation into the interaction of MAX, MAD, and MXI1 gene products within a class of human cancers known for its abnormalities with this family of genes. In addition, these dimerization partners may be appropriate for gene therapeutic interventions.

Extensive work will need to be done on the *JUN* and *FOS* family of protooncogenes to understand their role within lung cancer. We already know that the genes are expressed in bronchial epithelial cells and lung cancer cell lines, though there appear to be discrepancies regarding their expression in primary lung cancers. The role of *FOS* and *JUN* in the generation and maintenance of lung cancer is yet to be elucidated. Future studies of these nuclear oncogenes will be needed to understand better their role in lung cancer.

SUMMARY

The extensive studies on the *MYC* family protooncogenes in lung cancer have shown that *MYC* plays a prominent role in the growth in lung cancer. *MYC* mRNA expression is present in the normal developing and mature adult lung. The majority of lung cancers express one or more *MYC* family mRNAs, while a minority of lung cancers have *MYC* family DNA amplification. The *MYC* gene appears to be more closely linked with more rapid growth than *NMYC* and *LYMC*, because it is more active in establishing perma-

nent cell lines in the rat embryo fibroblast system, is more closely linked with the variant SCLC phenotype and appears to select for increased chance of growth in xenografts and cell culture. Amplification of the *MYC* gene is associated with more rapid growth of SCLC as measured by doubling times and increased cloning efficiency in soft agarose. Transfection of the *MYC* gene into a SCLC cell line that does not express *MYC* mRNA changes its morphology into a variantlike cell line and increases its growth rate. Retinoic acids decrease the amount of *MYC* mRNA expression and the growth rate of SCLC cell lines. In addition *MYC* family DNA amplification in SCLC is associated with shortened patient survival. Therefore, the *MYC* gene appear to be active in the development of the phenotype of lung cancer cells *in vitro* and *in vivo* in patients with lung cancer.

The *JUN* and *FOS* nuclear protooncogenes are in their very early stages of study in lung cancer and additional studies are needed to define their role.

REFERENCES

1. Marcu KB, Bossone SA, Patel AJ. *myc* function and regulation. *Ann Rev Biochem* 1992;61:809.
2. Prins J, De Vries EG, Mulder NH. The *myc* family of oncogenes and their presence and importance in small cell lung carcinoma and other tumour types. *Anticancer Res* 1993;13:1373.
3. Bouchard C, Staller P, Eilers M. Control of cell proliferation by Myc. *Trends Cell Biol* 1998;8:202.
4. Facchini LM, Penn LZ. The molecular role of Myc in growth and transformation: recent discoveries lead to new insights. *Faseb J* 1998;12:633.
5. Hoffman B, Liebermann DA. The proto-oncogene c-*myc* and apoptosis. *Oncogene* 1998;17:3351.
6. Henriksson M, Luscher B. Proteins of the Myc network: essential regulators of cell growth and differentiation. *Adv Cancer Res* 1996;68:109.
7. Vogt PK, Bos TJ. *jun*: oncogene and transcription factor. *Adv Cancer Res* 1990;55:1.
8. Angel P, Karin M. The role of Jun, Fos, and the AP-1 complex in cell-proliferation and transformation. *Biochem Biophys Acta* 1991;1072:129.
9. Distel RJ, Spiegelman BM. Protooncogene c-*fos* as a transcription factor. *Adv Cancer Res* 1990;55:37.
10. Karin M, Liu Z, Zandi E. AP-1 function and regulation. *Curr Opin Cell Biol* 1997;9:240.
11. Watson DK, Reddy EP, Duesberg PH, et al. Nucleotide sequence analysis of chicken c-*myc* gene reveals homologous and unique coding regions by comparinson with the transforming gene of avian myelocytomatosis virus MC29, *gag-myc. Proc Natl Acad Sci U S A* 1983;80:2146.
12. Battey J, Moulding C, Taub R, et al. The human c-*myc* oncogene: structural consequences of translocation into the IgH locus in Burkitt lymphoma. *Cell* 1983;34:779.
13. Taub R, Kirsch I, Morton C, et al. Translocation of the c-*myc* gene into the immunoglobulin heavy chain locus in human Burkitt lymphoma and murine plasmacytoma cells. *Proc Natl Acad Sci U S A* 1982;79:7837.
14. Dalia-Favera R, Bregal M, Erikson J, et al. The human c-*myc* oncogene is located on the region of chromosome 8 that is translocated in Burkitt lymphoma cells. *Proc Natl Acad Sci U S A* 1982;79:7824.

15. Johnson BE, Battey JF, Linnoila I, et al. Changes in the phenotype of human small cell lung cancer cell lines after transfection and expression of the c-*myc*. *J Clin Invest* 1986;78:525.

16. Hann SR, Eisenman RN. Proteins encoded by the human c-*myc* oncogene: differential expression in neoplastic cells. *Mol Cell Biol* 1984;4:2486.

17. Ramsay G, Evan GI, Bishop JM. The protein encoded by the human proto-oncogene c-*myc*. *Proc Natl Acad Sci U S A* 1984; 81:7742.

18. Schwab M, Alitalo K, Klempaauer KH, et al. Amplified DNA with limited homology to *myc* cellular oncogene is shared by human neuroblastoma cell lines and a neuroblastoma tumour. *Nature* 1983;305:245.

19. Kohl NE, Kanda N, Schreck RR, et al. Transposition and amplification of oncogene-related sequences in human neuroblastomas. *Cell* 1983;35:359.

20. Stanton LW, Schwab M, Bishop JM. Nucleotide sequence of the human N-*myc* gene. *Proc Natl Acad Sci U S A* 1986;83: 1772.

21. Kohl NE, Legouy E, DePinho RA, et al. Human N-*myc* is closely related in organization and nucleotide sequence to c-*myc*. *Nature* 1986;319:73.

22. Kanda N, Schreck R, Alt F, et al. Isolation of amplified DNA sequences from IMR-32 human neuroblastoma cells: facilitation by fluorescence-activated flow sorting of metaphase chromosomes. *Proc Natl Acad Sci U S A* 1983;80:4069.

23. Schwab M, Varmus HE, Bishop JM, et al. Chromosome localization in normal human cells and neuroblastomas of a gene related to c-*myc*. *Nature* 1984;308:288.

24. Nau MM, Brooks BJ, Jr., Carney DN, et al. Human small-cell lung cancers show amplification and expression of the N-*myc* gene. *Proc Natl Acad Sci U S A* 1986;83:1092.

25. Krystal GW, Armstrong BC, Battey JF. N-*myc* mRNA forms an RNA-RNA duplex with endogenous transcripts. *Mol Cell Biol* 1990;10:4180.

26. Makela TP, Saksela K, Alitalo K. Two N-*myc* polypeptides with distinct amino terminal encoded by the second and third exons of the gene. *Mol Cell Biol* 1989;9:1545.

27. Ramsay G, Stanton L, Schwab M, et al. Human proto-oncogene N-*myc* encodes nuclear proteins that bind DNA. *Mol Cell Biol* 1986;6:4450.

28. Chodesh LA, Olesen J, Hahn S, et al. A yeast and a human CCAAT-binding protein have heterologous subunits that are functionally interchangeable. *Cell* 1988;53:25.

29. Prins J, De Vries EGE, Mulder NH. The *myc* family of oncogenes and their presence and importance in small-cell lung carcinoma and other tumour types. *Anticancer Res* 1993;13:1373.

30. Kaye F, Battey J, Nau M, et al. Structure and expression of the human L-*myc* gene reveal a complex pattern of alternative mRNA processing. *Mol Cell Biol* 1988;8:186.

31. DePinho RA, Hatton KS, Tesfaye A, et al. The human *myc* gene family: structure and activity of L-*myc* and an L-*myc* pseudogene. *Genes and Dev* 1987;1:1311.

32. De Greve J, Battey J, Fedorko J, et al. The human L-*myc* gene encodes multiple nuclear phosphoproteins from alternatively processed mRNAs. *Mol Cell Biol* 1988;8:4381.

33. Ikegaki N, Minna J, Kennett RH. The human L-*myc* gene is expressed as two forms of protein in small cell lung carcinoma cell lines: detection by monoclonal antibodies specific to two *myc* homology box sequences. *EMBO J* 1989;8:1793.

34. Blackwood EM, Eisenman RN. Max: A helix-loop-helix zipper protein that forms a sequence-specific DNA-binding complex with *myc*. *Science* 1991;251:1211.

35. Murre C, McCaw PS, Baltimore D. A new DNA binding and dimerization motif in immunoglobulin enhancer binding, daughterless, MyoD, and *myc* proteins. *Cell* 1989;56:777.

36. Lemaitre JM, Buckle RS, Mechali M. c-*myc* in the control of cell proliferation and embryonic development. *Adv Cancer Res* 1996;70:95.

37. Brough DE, Hofmann TJ, Ellwood KB, et al. An essential domain of the c-*myc* protein interacts with a nuclear factor that is also required for E1A-mediated transformation. *Mol Cell Biol* 1995;15:1536.

38. Sakamuro D, Elliott KJ, Wechsier-Reya R, et al. BIN1 is a novel MYC-interacting protein with features of a tumour suppressor. *Nat Genet* 1996;14:69.

39. Evan GI, Wyllie AH, Gilbert CS, et al. Induction of apoptosis in fibroblasts by c-*myc* protein. *Cell* 1992;69:119.

40. Grandori C, Eisenman RN. Myc target genes. *Trends Biochem Sci* 1997;22:177.

41. Zimmerman KA, Yancopoulos GD, Collum RG, et al. Differential expression of *myc* family genes during murine development. *Nature* 1986;319:780.

42. Mugrauer G, Alt F, Ekblom P. N-*myc* proto-oncogene expression in the developing organogenesis in the developing mouse as revealed by *in situ* hybridization. *J Cell Biol* 1988;107:1325.

43. Schmid P, Schulz WA, Hameister H. Dynamic expression pattern of the *myc* protooncogene in midgestation mouse embryos. *Science* 1989;243:226.

44. Hirning U, Schmid P, Schultz WA, et al. A comparative analysis of N-*myc* and c-*myc* expression and cellular proliferation in mouse organogenesis. *Mech Dev* 1991;33:119.

45. Stanton BR, Perkins AS, Tessarollo L, et al. Loss of N-*myc* function results in embryonic lethality and failure of the epithelial component of the embryo to develop. *Genes Dev* 1992;6: 2235.

46. Hatton KS, Mahon K, Chin L, et al. Expression and activity of L-*myc* in normal mouse development. *Mol Cell Biol* 1996; 16:1794.

47. Pfeifer-Ohlsson S, Rydnert J, Goustin AS, et al. Cell-type-specific pattern of *myc* protooncogene expression in developing human embryos. *Proc Natl Acad Sci U S A* 1985;82:5050.

48. Broers JLV, Viallet J, Jensen SM, et al. Expression of c-*myc* in progenitor cells of the bronchopulmonary epithelium and in a large number of non-small cell lung cancers. *Am J Respir Cell Mol Biol* 1993;9:33.

49. Land H, Parada LF, Weinberg RA. Tumorigenic conversion of primary embryo fibroblasts requires at least two cooperating oncogenes. *Nature* 1983;304:596.

50. Schwab M, Varmus HE, Bishop JM. Human N-*myc* gene contributes to neoplastic transformation of mammalian cells in culture. *Nature* 1985;316:160.

51. Yancopoulos GD, Nisen PD, Tesfaye A, et al. N-*myc* can cooperate with *ras* to transform normal cells in culture. *Proc Natl Acad Sci U S A* 1985;82:5455.

52. Birrer MJ, Segal S, DeGreve JS, et al. L-*myc* cooperates with *ras* to transform primary rat embryo fibroblasts. *Mol Cell Biol* 1988;8:2668.

53. Mukherjee B, Morgenbesser SD, DePinho RA. Myc family oncoproteins function through a common pathway to transform normal cells in culture: cross-interference by Max and transacting dominant mutants. *Genes Dev* 1992;6:1480.

54. Barrett J, Birrer MJ, Kato GJ, et al. Activation domains of L-*myc* and c-*myc* determine their transforming potencies in rat embryo cells. *Mol Cell Biol* 1992;12:3130.

55. Morgenbesser SD, DePinho RA. Use of transgenic mice to study *myc* family gene function in normal mammalian development and in cancer. *Semin Cancer Biol* 1994;5:21.

56. Morgenbesser SD, Schreiber-Agus N, Bidder M, et al. Contrasting roles for c-*myc* and L-*myc* in the regulation of cellular growth and differentiation *in vivo*. *EMBO J* 1995;14:743.

57. Davis AC, Wims M, Spotts GD, et al. A null c-*myc* mutation

causes lethality before 10.5 days of gestation in homozygotes and reduced fertility in heterozygous female mice. *Genes Dev* 1993;7:671.

58. Charron J, Malynn BA, Fisher P, et al. Embryonic lethality in mice homozygous for a targeted disruption of the N-*myc* gene. *Genes Dev* 1992;6:2248.

59. Nunberg JH, Kaufman RJ, Schimke RT, et al. Amplified dihydrofolate reductase genes are localized to a homogenously staining region of a single chromosome in a methotrexate-resistant Chinese hamster ovary cancer cell line. *Proc Natl Acad Sci U S A* 1978;75:5553.

60. Kaufman RJ, Brown RC, Schimke RT. Amplified dihydrofolate reductase genes in unstably methotrexate resistant cells are associated with double minute chromosomes. *Proc Natl Acad Sci U S A* 1979;76:5669.

61. Collins S, Groudine M. Amplification of endogenous *myc*-related DNA sequences in a human myeloid leukaemia cell line. *Nature* 1982;298:679.

62. Alitalo K, Bishop JM, Smith DH, et al. Nucleotide sequence to the v-*myc* oncogene of avian retrovirus MC29. *Proc Natl Acad Sci U S A* 1983;80:100.

63. Whang-Peng J, Knutsen T, Gazdar A, et al. Nonrandom structural and numerical chromosome changes in non-small-cell lung cancer. *Genes Chromosom Cancer* 1981;3:168.

64. Wurster-Hill DH, Cannizzaro LA, Pettengill OS, et al. Cytogenetics of small cell carcinoma of the lung. *Cancer Genet Cytogenet* 1984;13:303.

65. Little CD, Nau MM, Carney DN, et al. Amplification and expression of the c-*myc* oncogene in human lung cancer cell lines. *Nature* 1983;306:194.

66. Saksela K, Bergh J, Lehto VP, et al. Amplification of the c-*myc* oncogene in a subpopulation of human small cell lung cancer. *Cancer Res* 1985;45:1823.

67. Nau MM, Brooks BJ, Battey J, et al. L-*myc*, a new *myc*-related gene amplified and expressed in human small cell lung cancer. *Nature* 1985;318:69.

68. Wong AJ, Ruppert JM, Eggleston J, et al. Gene amplification of c-*myc* and N-*myc* in small cell carinoma of the lung. *Science* 1986;233:461.

69. Gazdar AF, Carney DN, Nae MM, et al. Characterization of variant subclasses of small cell ung cancer cell lines having classic and variant features. *Cancer Res* 1985;45:2924.

70. Kiefer PE, Bepler G, Kubasch M, et al. Amplification and expression of protooncogenes in human small cell lung cancer cell lines. *Cancer Res* 1987;47:6236.

71. Feo S, Di Liegro C, Jones T, et al. The DNA region around the c-*myc* gene and its amplification in tumour cell lines. *Oncogene* 1994;9:955.

72. Kinzier KW, Zehnbauer BA, Brodeur GM, et al. Amplification units containing human N-*myc* and c-*myc* genes. *Proc Natl Acad Sci U S A* 1986;83:1031.

73. Sekido Y, Takahashi T, Makela TP, et al. Complex intrachromosomal rearrangement in the process of amplification of the L-*myc* gene in small-cell lung cancer. *Mol Cell Biol* 1992;12:1747.

74. Makela TP, Kere J, Winqvist R, et al. Intrachromosomal rearrangements fusing L-*myc* and *rif* in small-cell lung cancer. *Mol Cell Biol* 1991;11:4015.

75. Makela TP, Saksela K, Alitalo K. Amplification and rearrangement of L-*myc* in human small-cell lung cancer. *Mutat Res* 1992;276:307.

76. Makela TP, Hellsten E, Vesa J, et al. The rearranged L-*myc* fusion gene (RLF) encodes a Zn-15 related zinc finger protein. *Oncogene* 1995;11:2699.

77. MacLean-Hunter S, Makela TP, Grzeschiczek A, et al. Expression of a *rif*/L-*myc* minigene inhibits differentiation of embryonic stem cells and embroid body formation. *Oncogene* 1994; 9:3509.

78. Kim JO, Nau MM, Allikian KA, et al. Co-amplification of a novel cyclophilin-like gene (PPIE) with L-*myc* in small cell lung cancer cell lines. *Oncogene* 1998;17:1019.

79. Gazdar AF, Carney DN, Nau MM, et al. Characterization of variant subclasses of cell lines derived from small cell lung cancer having distinctive biochemical, morphological, and growth properties. *Cancer Res* 1985;45:2924.

80. Yokota J, Wada M, Yoshida T, et al. Heterogeneity of lung cancer cells with respect to the amplification and rearrangement of *myc* family oncogenes. *Oncogene* 1988;2:607.

81. Takahashi T, Obata Y, Sekido Y, et al. Expression and amplification of *myc* gene family in small cell lung cancer and its relation to biological characteristics. *Cancer Res* 1989;49:2683.

82. Bepler G, Jaques G, Havemann K, et al. Characterization of two cell lines with distinct phenotypes established from a patient with small cell lung cancer. *Cancer Res* 1987;47:1883.

83. Gazzeri S, Brambilla E, Jacrot M, et al. Activation of *myc* gene family in human lung carcinomas and during heterotransplantation into nude mice. *Cancer Res* 1991;51:2566.

84. Gazzeri S, Brambilla E, Caron de Fromentel C, et al. p53 genetic abnormalities and *myc* activation in human lung carcinoma. *Int J Cancer* 1994;58:24.

85. Gemma A, Nakajima T, Shiraishi M, et al. *myc* family gene abnormality in lung cancers and its relation to xenotranplantability. *Cancer Res* 1988;48:6025.

86. Yoshimoto K, Shiraishi M, Hirohashi S, et al. Rearrangement of the c-*myc* gene in two giant cell carcinomas of the lung. *Jpn J Cancer Res* 1986;77:731.

87. Shiraishi M, Noguchi M, Shimosato Y, et al. Amplification of protooncogenes in surgical specimens of human lung carcinomas. *Cancer Res* 1989;49:6474.

88. Carney DN, Gazdar AF, Bepler G, et al. Establishment and identification of small cell lung cancer cell lines having classic and variant features. *Cancer Res* 1985;45:2913.

89. Hirsch FR, Matthews MJ, Aisner S, et al. Histopathologic classification of small cell lung cancer changing concepts and terminology. *Cancer* 1988;62:973.

90. Carney DN, Mitchell JB, Kinselia TJ. *In vitro* radiation and chemosensitivity of established human small cell lung cancer and its large cell morphologic variants. *Cancer Res* 1983;43:2806.

91. Kok K, Osinga J, Schotanus DC, et al. Amplification and expression of different *myc*-family genes in a tumor specimen and 3 cell lines derived from one small-cell lung cancer patient during longitudinal follow-up. *Int J Cancer* 1989;44:75.

92. Doyle LA, Giangiulo D, Hussain A, et al. Differentiation of human variant small cell lung cancer cell lines to a classic morphology by retinoic acid. *Cancer Res* 1989;49:6745.

93. Johnson BE, Makuch RW, Simmons AD, et al. MYC family amplification in small cell lung cancer patients' tumors and corresponding cell lines. *Cancer Res* 1988;48:5163.

94. Kalemkerian GP, Jasti RK, Celano P, et al. All-*trans*-retinoic acid alters *myc* gene expression and inhibits *in vitro* progression in small cell lung cancer. *Cell Growth Differ* 1994;5:55.

95. Ou X, Campau S, Slusher R, et al. Mechanism of all-*trans*-retinoic acid-mediated L-*myc* gene regulation in small cell lung cancer. *Oncogene* 1996;13:1893.

96. Sabichi AL, Birrer MJ. Regulation of nuclear oncogenes expressed in lung cancer cell lines. *J Cell Biochem Suppl* 1996;24:218.

97. Kalemkerian GP, Jiroutek M, Ettinger DS, et al. A phase II study of all-*trans*-retinoic acid plus cisplatin and etoposide in patients with extensive stage small cell lung carcinoma: an Eastern Cooperative Oncology Group Study. *Cancer* 1998;83:1102.

98. Kalemkerian GP, Slusher R, Ramalingam S, et al. Growth inhibition and induction of apoptosis by fenretinide in small-cell lung cancer cell lines. *J Natl Cancer Inst* 1995;87:1674.

99. Rygaard K, Vindelov LL, Spang-Thomsen M. Expression of *myc* family oncoproteins in small-cell lung-cancer cell lines and xenografts. *Int J Cancer* 1993;54:144.

100. Johnson BE, Russell E, Simmons AM, et al. MYC family DNA amplification in 126 tumor cell lines from patients with small cell lung cancer. *J Cell Biochem Suppl* 1996;24:210.

101. Seifter EJ, Sausville EA, Battey J. Comparison of amplified and unamplified c-*myc* gene structure and expression in human small cell lung carcinoma cell lines. *Cancer Res* 1986;46:2050.

102. Gu J, Linnoila RI, Seibel NL, et al. A study of *myc*-related gene expression in small cell lung cancer by *in situ* hybridization. *Am J Pathol* 1988;132:13.

103. Krystal G, Birrer M, Way J, et al. Multiple mechanisms for transcriptional regulation of the *myc* gene family in small-cell lung cancer. *Mol Cell Biol* 1988;8:3373.

104. Saksela K, Makela TP, Alitalo K. Oncogene expression in small-cell lung cancer cell lines and and testicular germ-cell tumor: activation of the N-*myc* gene and decreased RB mRNA. *Int J Cancer* 1989;44:182.

105. Noguchi M, Hirohashi S, Hara F, et al. Heterogenous amplification of *myc* family oncogenes in small cell lung carcinoma. *Cancer* 1990;66:2053.

106. Brennan J, O'Connor T, Makuch RW, et al. *myc* family DNA amplification in 107 tumor and tumor cell lines from patients with small cell lung cancer treated with different combination chemotherapy regimens. *Cancer Res* 1991;51:1708.

107. Funa K, Steinholtz L, Nou E, et al. Increased expression of N-*myc* in human small cell lung cancer biopsies predicts lack of response to chemotherapy and poor prognosis. *Am J Clin Pathol* 1987;88:216.

108. Seeger RC, Brodeur GM, Sather H, et al. Association of multiple copies of the N-*myc* oncogene with rapid progression of neuroblastomas. *N Engl J Med* 1985;313:1111.

109. Morkve O, Halvorsen OJ, Stangeland L, et al. Quantitation of biological markers (*p53, c-myc*, Ki-67, and DNA ploidy) by multiparameter flow cytometry in non-small cell lung cancer. *Int J Cancer* 1992;52:851.

110. Volm M, Efferth T, Mattern J. Oncoprotein (c-*myc*, c-*erb*B1, c-*erb*B2, c-*fos*) and suppressor gene product (*p53*) expression in squamous cell carcinomas of the lung. Clinical and biological correlations. *Anticancer Res* 1992;12:11.

111. Volm M, Drings P, Wodrich W, et al. Expression of oncoproteins in primary human non-small cell lung cancer and the incidence of metastases. *Clin Exp Metastasis* 1993;11:325.

112. Dosaka-Akita H, Akie K, Hiroumi H, et al. Inhibition of proliferation by L-*myc* antisense DNA for the translational initiation site in human small cell lung cancer. *Cancer Res* 1995;55:1559.

113. Van Waardenburg RC, Meijer C, Burger H, et al. Effects of an inducible anti-sense c-*myc* gene transfer in a drug-resistant human small-cell-lung-carcinoma cell line. *Int J Cancer* 1997;73:544.

114. Van Waardenburg RC, Prins J, Meijer C, et al. Effects of c-*myc* oncogene modulation on drug resistance in human small cell lung carcinoma cell lines. *Anticancer Res* 1996;16:1963.

115. Robinson LA, Smith LJ, Fontaine MP, et al. c-*myc* antisense oligodeoxyribonucleotides inhibit proliferation of non-small cell lung cancer. *Ann Thorac Surg* 1995;60:1583.

116. Kumagai T, Tanio Y, Osaki T, et al. Eradication of Myc-overexpressing small cell lung cancer cells transfected with herpes simplex virus thymidine kinase gene containing Myc-Max response elements. *Cancer Res* 1996;56:354.

117. Waelti ER, Gluck R. Delivery to cancer cells of antisense L-*myc* oligonucleotides incorporated in fusogenic, cationic-lipid-reconstituted influenza-virus envelopes (cationic virosomes). *Int J Cancer* 1998;77:728.

118. Maki Y, Bos TJ, Davis C, et al. Avian sarcoma virus 17 carries the *jun* oncogene. *Proc Natl Acad Sci U S A* 1987;84:2848.

119. Hattori K, Angel P, Le Beau MM, et al. Structure and chromosomal localization of the functional intronless human *JUN* protooncogene. *Proc Natl Acad Sci U S A* 1988;85:9148.

120. Schutte J, Viallet J, Nau M, et al. *jun*-B inhibits and c-*fos* stimulates the transforming and transactivating activities of c-*jun*. *Cell* 1989;59:987.

121. Nomura N, Ide M, Sasamoto S, et al. Isolation of human cDNA clones of *jun*-related genes, *jun*-B and *jun*-D. *Nucleic Acids Res* 1990;18:3047.

122. Curran T, Peter G, Van Beveren C, et al. FBJ murine osterosarcoma virus: identification and molecular cloning of biologically active proviral DNA. *J Virol* 1982;44:674.

123. Van Straaten F, Muller R, Curran T, et al. Complete nucleotide sequence of a human c-oncogene: Deduced amino acid sequence of the human c-*fos* gene. *Proc Natl Acad Sci U S A* 1983;80:3183.

124. Zerial M, Toschi L, Ryseck RP, et al. The product of a novel growth factor activated gene, *fos* B, interacts with *JUN* proteins enhancing their DNA binding activity. *EMBO J* 1989;8:805.

125. Matsui M, Tokuhara M, Konuma Y, et al. Isolation of human *fos*-related genes and their expression during monocyte-macrophage differentiation. *Oncogene* 1990;5:249.

126. Angel P, Imagawa M, Chiu R, et al. Phorbol ester-inducible genes contain a common *cis* element recognized by a TPA-modulated *trans*-acting factor. *Cell* 1987;49:729.

127. Lee W, Mitchell P, Tjian R. Purified transcription factor AP-1 interacts with TPA-inducible enhancer elements. *Cell* 1987;49:741.

128. Angel P, Allegretto EA, Okino ST, et al. Oncogene *jun* encodes a sequence specific *trans*-activator similar to AP-1. *Nature* 1988;332:166.

129. Karin M. The regulation of AP-1 activity by mitogen-activated protein kinases. *Philos Trans R Soc Lond B Biol Sci* 1996;351:127.

130. Birrer MJ, Alani R, Cuttitta F, et al. Early events in the neoplastic transformation of respiratory epithelium. *J Natl Cancer Inst Monogr* 1992;13:31.

131. Lee HY, Dawson MI, Claret FX, et al. Evidence of a retinoid signaling alteration involving the activator protein 1 complex in tumorigenic human bronchial epithelial cells and non-small cell lung cancer cells. *Cell Growth Differ* 1997;8:283.

132. Lee HY, Chaudhary J, Walsh GL, et al. Suppression of c-*fos* gene transcription with malignant transformation of human bronchial epithelial cells. *Oncogene* 1998;16:3039.

133. Szabo E, Riffe ME, Steinberg SM, et al. Altered c*JUN* expression: an early event in human lung carcinogenesis. *Cancer Res* 1996;56:305.

134. Levin WJ, Press MF, Gaynor RB, et al. Expression patterns of immediate early transcription factors in human non-small cell lung cancer. The Lung Cancer Study Group. *Oncogene* 1995;11:1261.

135. Volm M, Mattern J. Correlation between successful heterotransplantation of lung tumors in nude mice, poor prognosis of patients and expression of Fos, Jun, ErbB1, and Ras. *Anticancer Res* 1993;13:2021.

136. Volm M, Drings P, Wodrich W. Prognostic significance of the expression of c-*fos*, c-*jun* and c-*erb*B-1 oncogene products in human squamous cell lung carcinomas. *J Cancer Res Clin Oncol* 1993;119:507.

137. Volm M, Rittgen W, Drings P. Prognostic value of *ERB*B-1, VEGF, cyclin A, *FOS*, *JUN* and *MYC* in patients with squa-

mous cell lung carcinomas [published erratum appears in *Br J Cancer* 1998;77(7):1198]. *Br J Cancer* 1998;77:663.

138. Vastrik I, Makela TP, Koskinen PJ, et al. *myc, max,* and a novel *rif*-L-*myc* fusion protein in small-cell lung cancer. In: Harris CC, ed. *Multistage Carcinogenesis.* Boca Raton: CRC Press, 1992:307.

139. Johnson BE, Makuch RW, Simmons AD, et al. *myc* family DNA amplification in small cell lung cancer patients' tumors and corresponding cell lines. *Cancer Res* 1988;48:5163.

140. Graziano SL, Cowan BY, Carney DN, et al. Small cell lung cancer cell line derived from a primary tumor with a characteristic deletion of 3p. *Cancer Res* 1987;47:2148.

141. Waters JJ, Ibson JM, Twentyman PR, et al. Cytogenetic abnormalities in human small cell lung carcinoma: cell lines characterized for *myc* gene amplification. *Cancer Genet Cytogenet* 1988; 30:213.

142. Gazzeri S, Brambilla E, Chauvin C, et al. Analysis of activation of the *myc* family oncogene and of its stability over time in xenografted lung carcinomas. *Cancer Res* 1990;50:1566.

143. Makela TP, Shiraishi M, Borrello MG, et al. Rearrangement and co-amplification of L-*myc* and *rif* in primary lung cancer. *Oncogene* 1992;7:405.

144. Gasperi-Campani A, Roncuzzi L, Zoli W, et al. Chromosomal alterations, biological features and *in vitro* chemosensitivity of SCLC-R1, a new cell line from human metastatic small cell lung carcinoma. *Eur J Cancer* 1998;34:724.

145. Arvelo F, Poupon MF, Le Chevalier T. Establishment and characterization of five human small cell lung cancer cell lines from early tumor xenografts. *Anticancer Res* 1994;14:1893.

146. Heighway J, Hasleton PS. c-Kl-*ras* amplification in human lung cancer. *Br J Cancer* 1986;53:285.

147. Cline MJ, Battifora H. Abnormalities of protooncogenes in non-small cell lung cancer: correlations with tumor type and clinical characteristics. *Cancer* 1987;60:2669.

148. Hajj C, Akoum R, Bradley E, et al. DNA alterations at protooncogene loci and their clinical significance in operable non-small cell lung cancer. *Cancer* 1990;66:733.

6

P53

SUZANNE T. SZAK
JENNIFER A. PIETENPOL
DAVID P. CARBONE

Cancers arise by a multi-step process in which cells become malignant by multiple genetic alterations affecting cell growth, differentiation, and survival. To suppress tumor formation, multicellular organisms have evolved mechanisms to protect against the uncontrolled growth of cells. One such mechanism involves the tumor suppressor gene *p53*.

p53 is a tumor suppressor that is activated in cells that have undergone stress, such as exposure to genotoxic agents or oncogene activation (Figure 6.1). Once active, p53 initiates either cell cycle arrest or programmed cell death (apoptosis). It does so, in part, by binding to specific DNA sequences that control the expression of genes whose products govern cell growth and cell death. The timepoint in the genesis of a tumor at which p53 mutation occurs depends on the tumor type and can vary from an early event to a late step in tumor progression. Relatively early mutation of p53 appears to occur in cells that are chronically exposed to DNA-damaging agents and inflammation. The differences in the timing of p53 loss during tumor progression among different tumor types suggest that the tumor suppressor is active under specific conditions, and only then does tumor progression select for cells that have lost normal p53 activity. This selection then requires the inactivation of p53 for continued tumor growth because restoring p53 function to these tumor cells results in either growth arrest or death. Loss or mutation of the *p53* gene occurs often in lung cancers.

Research on p53 over the past decade has demonstrated that p53 is a protein toward which many signals are directed and from which many signaling cascades emanate. This chapter focuses on the p53 protein, outlines the biochemical signals that are upstream and downstream of p53, and discusses its clinical relevance to human lung cancer. Understanding the signaling pathways that regulate and are regulated by p53 have allowed, and will continue to provide, increased understanding of the clinical behavior of lung cancer and opportunities for clinical intervention in lung cancer cells lacking functional p53.

P53 STRUCTURE AND FUNCTION

The p53 protein can be divided into three functional domains (Figure 6.2). Each individual domain plays a critical role in p53 function. The amino terminus (amino acids 1–100) of the protein contains an acidic transactivation domain. Proteins that bind this domain either stimulate or inhibit the ability of p53 to regulate transcription of genes. When basal transcription factors (TF) such as TFIID[1] or the TFIIH complex[2] are recruited to this domain, transcription of p53 downstream target genes is activated. In addition to its role in transcription, TFIIH is required for transcription-coupled DNA repair, which has led to the speculation that p53 may have a role in DNA repair.[3–9] The transcriptional co-activator p300 also binds p53 at its amino-terminus.[10] This interaction is proposed to be necessary for p53-mediated G1/S arrest and apoptosis[10] and has been shown to result in p53 acetylation *in vitro*.[11] Inhibitors of p53-mediated transcription, such as murine double minute 2 (MDM2)[12,13] and the 55 kDa adenoviral protein E1B, have been shown to bind to the amino-terminal domain of p53 and are hypothesized to block access of the basal transcriptional machinery to p53. The crystal structure of the amino-terminus of p53 bound to the MDM2 protein has been solved. It reveals that the hydrophobic amino acids that constitute an amphipathic helix in the amino-terminus of p53 are involved in MDM2 binding.[14] A proline-rich subdomain in the amino-terminus of p53 has also been shown to be critical for the growth-suppressive effects of p53 but unnecessary for transcriptional activation.[15]

The central domain of p53 is required for sequence-specific DNA binding.[16] A majority of tumor-derived p53 mutations reside in this domain, underscoring the importance of p53 DNA-binding activity in tumor suppression.[17] The mutations predominantly occur in the four regions of the central domain that are highly conserved across many species. In lung cancer, p53 codons 157, 248, and 273 are often found mutated,[18,19] abrogating the ability of p53 to bind DNA. When the crystal structure of a complex containing the central domain of p53 and a cognate DNA-binding site was solved,[16] it provided great insight into how tumor-derived mutations inactivate p53 function. The structure of the core domain revealed a β sandwich motif that acts as a scaffold for two large loops and a loop-sheet-helix configuration. These latter motifs are required for the

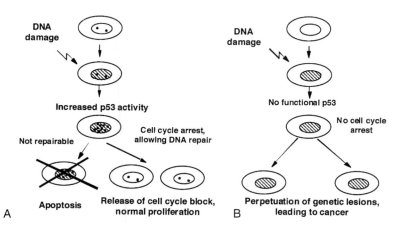

FIGURE 6.1. Schematic of p53 tumor suppression. **A:** p53 levels in normal cells are very low. After DNA damage, the levels and activity of p53 protein increase. If DNA damage is extensive, p53 activity is thought to result in apoptosis. Otherwise, p53 mediates cell cycle arrest, allowing time for the damage to be repaired before the cell resumes cycling. **B:** if p53 is absent or mutant in a cell, it is unable to mediate cell cycle arrest or apoptosis after DNA damage. Thus any mutations resulting from the DNA damage are perpetuated.

interaction of p53 with DNA. The two large loops involved in DNA binding are connected by a stretch of amino acids that includes a cysteine and histidine; together, these two amino acids coordinate a zinc ion, which is required for p53 activity.[20] Mutations in p53 either destroy the structural integrity of the central domain or alter the amino acids that directly contact the DNA. In addition to binding DNA in a sequence-specific manner, p53 can interact with insertion/deletion mismatches (IDLs). An intact central domain is required for complex formation with IDLs because tumor-derived mutants lack this activity.

The carboxyl-terminus (amino acids 293–393) of p53 is basic and appears to be the site of numerous posttranslational modifications that regulate p53 activity, including

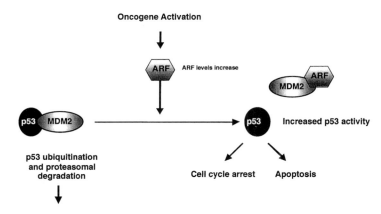

FIGURE 6.2. Schematic representation of the p53 protein. The protein has 393 amino acids. Five regions, shown in gray, are evolutionarily conserved in sequence content. Amino acids 1–60 constitute the transactivation domain. Conserved region 1 within this domain is the site at which the MDM2 protein binds p53. The center of the protein, from amino acid 100 to 300, is the DNA-binding domain and contains four conserved sequences. The basic C-terminal regulatory domain of p53 is encompassed by amino acids 363–393 and is represented by the checkered region in the diagram. The hatched area shows the location of the tetramerization domain within the C-terminus (amino acids 323–356). Circles in the diagram represent sites of posttranslational modifications. Seven amino acids in the amino-terminus can be phosphorylated. Of note, the ATM kinase and DNA-dependent protein kinase (DNA PK) phosphorylate Serine 15 of p53 after DNA damage. DNA PK has also been shown to phosphorylate Serine 37. Serine 33 can be phosphorylated by cdk-activating kinase (CAK). Following phosphorylation of Serine 15, p53 is thought to be acetylated by p300 (Lysines 373 and 382) and/or pCAF (Lysine 320). In addition to acetylated amino acids, the carboxyl-terminus may be phosphorylated by casein kinase II (CKII), protein kinase C (PK-C), and cdk complexes (CDK).

phosphorylation, acetylation, and glycosylation.[11,21–24] The carboxyl-terminus of p53 also reportedly binds nonspecifically to both short, single-stranded DNA, RNA and double-stranded DNA containing nucleotide loops.[8,25–27] Many functional motifs are encompassed within the carboxyl-terminus, such as the nuclear localization signal and an amphipathic helix involved in oligomerization;[28] p53 is thought to be transcriptionally active when it is in a homodimeric or homotetrameric form.[29] A crystal structure of the oligomerization domain of p53 has been solved.[30–32] Solution of this structure predicts a tetramer or dimer of a dimer. Each p53 monomer has a large hydrophobic area composed of both β strands and α helices that is buried upon tetramerization of the protein. The oligomerization capability of p53 is the basis for the dominant-negative effect of mutant p53 proteins; oligomerization of mutant p53 with wild-type p53 inhibits DNA-binding ability and thus transcriptional activation of the wild-type protein.[33]

The biochemical analyses of p53 that defined the transactivation and sequence-specific DNA-binding domains have led to the classification of p53 as a transcription factor that can regulate the expression of other gene products. These downstream target genes of p53 are thought to mediate its apoptotic and cell cycle effects. As targets, these genes have consensus p53 DNA-binding sites in their promoters, and the level of gene product increases after p53 activation. In addition to its role as a transcriptional activator, p53 can act as a transcriptional repressor. This repressor function is thought to be mediated by p53 binding to the basal transcriptional machinery, sequestering it from certain promoters.[34,35] Expression of several genes has been reported to be down-regulated by p53. These genes include bcl2, topoisomerase IIα, MAP4, Wee1, proliferating cell nuclear antigen (PCNA), c-fos, β-actin, and hsp70.[36–41]

P53 TUMOR SUPPRESSION

What are the tumor-suppressive functions of p53 and how are they regulated? Initially, it was observed that the wild-type but not the mutant form of p53 blocks cells at the G1 phase of the cell cycle.[42,43] Recent studies have confirmed that an important role of p53 is to regulate cell proliferation and survival following DNA damage and perhaps during disruption of normal differentiation pathways,[44,45] p53 levels and/or activity increase in cells that have activated oncogenes[46–48] or cells exposed to genotoxic agents.[49,50] Whether the increased level of p53 protein,[49,50] posttranslational modification,[23,51] or both are responsible for transcriptional activation of downstream genes is not well understood. The increase in p53 protein level is thought to be caused by metabolic stabilization of the protein and is associated with the transcriptional induction of specific genes, cell cycle arrest, or in some cases, apoptosis. However, the mechanisms involved in regulating p53 levels and bio-

chemical activity in normal and damaged cells is still not completely known.

P53 AND CONTROL OF THE CELL CYCLE

The G1/S cell cycle arrest mediated by p53 is governed by one of its target genes, p21$^{Waf1/Cip1}$ (see also Chapter 2).[52,53] The p21$^{Wof1/Cip1}$ protein is a cell cycle inhibitor.[54,55] One way in which p21$^{Wof1/Cip1}$ exerts its effect is by binding to and inhibiting cyclin/cdk complexes; the kinase activity of these complexes is essential for the coordinated transitions between cell cycle phases.[56–59] The enzymatic activity of cyclin/cdk complexes is suppressed by p21$^{Waf1/Cip1}$ binding, and thus the cell cycle arrests. A second way in which p21$^{Waf1/Cip1}$ can inhibit DNA replication (the S-phase of the cell cycle) is to bind and block the function of proliferating cell nuclear antigen (PCNA), a DNA polymerase processivity factor.[60] GADD45, another gene transcriptionally activated in a p53-dependent manner after DNA damage,[61] also binds PCNA, preventing the onset of S-phase.[62] Similar to p21,$^{Waf1/Cip1}$ however, the role of PCNA in DNA nucleotide excision repair is unaffected when bound to GADD45.[63–65]

In addition to monitoring the G1/S cell cycle checkpoint, p53 may also play a role in regulating the G2/M transition. The cdc25C phosphatase is essential for activating the cyclin/cdk complex that stimulates transition of a cell from the G2 phase of the cell cycle into mitosis (M); however, it is inactivated when bound to a 14-3-3 protein family member.[66,67] After DNA damage, when p53 is activated, the transcription of the 14-3-3σ gene has been shown to be upregulated.[68] However, the relevance of this observation is unclear because the 14-3-3σ isoform is not detectable in any cell type after irradiation, and its binding to cdc25C has not been demonstrated. Nevertheless, overexpression of p53 in the absence of DNA damage causes accumulation of cells in the G2/M phase of the cell cycle.[69,70] In the absence of either p53 or p21, the G2 arrest following DNA damage cannot be sustained, and the cell advances into mitosis.[71]

Integral to cell cycle regulation is the proper coordination of mitotic exit and subsequent S-phase entry. Intact checkpoint pathways are needed to prevent the S-phase entry of cells that have failed to properly segregate their chromosomes during mitosis. Recent studies have demonstrated that after treatment with microtubule inhibitors (MTIs), cells may undergo an aberrant mitotic exit, reenter G1 with a 4N DNA content, and enter S-phase, a process known as endoreduplication that results in polyploid cells. Although how mitotic slippage occurs is not understood, studies have shown that cells with deficient spindle checkpoint function endoreduplicate after treatment with drugs that inhibit microtubule dynamics.[72] Furthermore, cells lacking the gene products involved in G1/S checkpoint function, including p53,[73–75] pRb[73,76] or p21,[75–77] endoreduplicate if aberrant mitotic exit occurs after MTI treatment. These studies suggest that, in addition to playing a role in checkpoint function after DNA damage, p53 also functions to prevent inappropriate S-phase entry after an aberrant mitotic exit and thus is critical to proper coordination of S-phase and mitosis. Moreover, Stewart et al. have shown that epithelial tumor cells with defective p53 signaling pathways have enhanced sensitivity to Taxol and vincristine-induced apoptosis.[78]

Insulinlike growth factor binding protein 3 (IGF1-BP3) has been shown to be upregulated by p53 after inducible expression of p53 as well as after treatment of cells with genotoxic agents.[79] IGF-BP3 is secreted from cells and blocks the mitogenic action of the growth factor insulinlike growth factor 1 (IGF1). These observations suggest that p53 may play a role in cell cycle regulation by paracrine or autocrine growth factors.

P53 AND APOPTOSIS

Several studies have shown that p53 transcriptional activity is necessary for the growth-suppressive effects of p53;[29,80] however, the importance of p53 transcriptional activity for promoting apoptosis is debatable (see also Chapter 2). Genes upregulated by p53 that mediate the apoptotic effects of p53 are less well characterized than those involved in cell cycle arrest. Nevertheless, several genes involved in apoptosis have been found to be upregulated in a p53-dependent fashion, suggesting that the role of p53 in initiating programmed cell death is that of a transcription factor.

p53-induced genes (PIGs) were found to be differentially expressed in cells undergoing p53-dependent apoptosis.[81] PIGs are hypothesized to be involved in the generation of intracellular reactive oxygen species that are thought to trigger a cascade of biochemical events culminating in the release of proteins from the mitochondria and initiating apoptosis. Bax, a member of the bcl-2 family of proteins that has a proapoptotic effect when overexpressed in cells, is upregulated by activated p53 in some cells and may therefore have a role in p53-mediated apoptosis.[82]

However, p53-dependent apoptosis may not require the transcriptional upregulation of these genes. Some studies have demonstrated p53-dependent apoptosis in the absence of new RNA or protein synthesis,[83] or in the presence of MDM2, an inhibitor of p53 transcriptional activity.[84] Thus the p53-directed signaling to the initiators or effectors of apoptosis is currently unclear. Cell fate, whether cell cycle arrest or apoptosis, is likely to be dictated not only by p53 but also by a combination of other genetic alterations present in the cell and other stimulated signaling pathways.[85]

INHIBITORS OF P53 ACTIVITY

The fact that normal cells express p53 without adverse effects implies that the tumor-suppressive functions of the protein are tightly regulated. In normal, nonstressed cells, the level of p53 protein is low because of its short half-life. After a stress event, the levels of p53 increase resulting from a posttranslational modification that prolongs its half-life. The rapid turnover of wild-type p53 *in vivo* may be caused by degradation by the ubiquitin proteolytic system, and the stability of the protein observed after DNA damage is likely caused by an inhibition of this process.[86,87]

A cellular protein proposed to play an integral role in p53 half-life is MDM2. MDM2 is transcriptionally activated by p53.[88] In turn, the MDM2 protein binds to the transactivation domain of p53, terminating its action as a transcription factor.[89] Additionally, MDM2 can target p53 for ubiquitin-mediated proteolysis.[90,91] In effect, an autoregulatory feedback loop is created. The MDM2 protein is oncogenic, and although the gene is often amplified in tumors, this is not usually the case in lung cancer.[92] The oncogenic phenotype observed with MDM2 overexpression is believed to be through its binding to p53 protein. The importance of MDM2 in regulating the apoptotic and growth arrest functions of p53 is suggested by the MDM2$^{-/-}$ mouse model; these animals die as embryos, but the double p53$^{-/-}$, MDM2$^{-/-}$ knockout mice are viable.[93,94]

Cells with mutant p53 also exhibit high p53 levels; this overexpression is probably caused by loss of the p53/MDM2 biofeedback loop. The increased half-life of mutant p53 protein allows the detection of mutant p53-containing cells by immunohistochemistry. The latter has been used as a prognostic tool in lung cancer. The high levels of mutant p53 in cells may also result from selective binding of p53 mutants by heat-shock protein 70.[95]

Viruses have evolved mechanisms to hijack the growth control of a host cell. One of the ways in which many DNA viruses exert their oncogenic effects is through the inactivation of p53. Indeed, much p53 biology was pioneered in virology studies. The E1B 55 kDa protein expressed by adenovirus binds, and therefore blocks, the transactivation domain of p53. SV40 large T antigen associates with the central domain of p53, inhibiting its DNA-binding ability. In fact, SV40 induces mesotheliomas in hamsters, and 60% of human mesotheliomas contain and express SV40 sequences.[96] Whether SV40 contributes to the development of human mesothelioma is not known and requires further investigation. Lastly, the human papilloma virus type 16 (HPV-16) partially exerts its tumorigenic action through its E6 protein that, together with the E6-associated protein (E6-AP), binds and inactivates the p53 tumor-suppressor protein[97,98] by targeting it for degradation through the ubiquitin proteolytic system.[98,99]

STIMULATORS OF P53 ACTIVITY

Hyperproliferative signals in cells resulting from aberrant or excessive activity of oncogenes can elevate p53 levels and/or activity. For example, overexpression of c-myc[46] or Ras[48,100] can activate apoptosis and growth arrest, respectively, in a p53-dependent manner; however, the absence of functional p53 under these conditions results in cell transformation. In the case of oncogene activation, signaling to p53 is mediated by the p19[ARF] tumor suppressor, an alternative reading frame of the INK4A locus[101] (Figure 6.3). p19[ARF] can bind MDM2, preventing both the MDM2-mediated degradation of p53 and inhibition of p53 transactivation.[102–106] p19[ARF] is not required in DNA damage signaling pathways involving p53.

p53 is also activated in hypoxic conditions.[107,108] The lack of oxygen resulting from restricted blood supply at the core of many tumors represents a stress event that can activate p53. In such a milieu, p53 causes the cell to undergo apoptosis. However, if the cells at the core of the tumor are mutant for p53, these cells do not die but rather adopt a selective growth advantage in such an environment over cells with intact p53.[108] The stress sensor stimulated in hypoxic conditions, which activates p53, is probably an altered cellular redox environment; both REF1[109] and HIF1-α proteins regulated by hypoxia have been shown to stimulate p53 transcriptional activity.

Radio- and chemotherapy manifest pleiotropic effects, but the DNA damage they induce is a potent activator of p53.[60] In fact, merely introducing nucleases or a damaged DNA template into cells induces a p53-dependent cell cycle arrest.[110,111] A cell can acquire DNA damage in many ways. Each form of genotoxic insult triggers an independent pathway to p53 activation even though the end result is the same. For example, phosphorylation of p53 on the amino acid serine 15 and acetylation at lysine 382 occur after cells are treated with ionizing or ultraviolet radiation.[23] The kinase responsible for the serine-15 phosphorylation after ionizing radiation is either ATM or DNA-dependent protein kinase (DNA-PK), whereas the activity of these kinases is not necessary for this site-specific phosphorylation after ultraviolet radiation. The acetylation of p53 may be regulated by phosphorylation of its amino-terminus by either the ATM kinase or DNA-PK.[23,112–114] Finally, serine 392 is phosphorylated after ultraviolet, but not ionizing, radiation.[115] Generally, these posttranslational modifications of p53 following a cellular stress event activate p53 for DNA binding.[11,114,116,117]

P53 MUTATIONS ARE COMMON IN LUNG CANCERS

p53 mutations in lung cancer were first described in 1989.[118] Since then many authors have analyzed hundreds of lung cancer tumors and cell lines for somatically acquired abnormalities of p53.[119] In non–small cell lung cancer (NSCLC), most series report that 50% to 60% of tumors have identifiable mutations,[120,121] and in small cell lung cancer (SCLC) the frequency is 90% or greater.[122,123] In contrast to *ras,* where the mutations occur overwhelmingly in a single codon, the mutations in p53 are distributed throughout the open reading frame (see Figure 6.4). The majority of mutations are substitutions of one amino acid residue for another at a single codon, but frame shifts, insertions, deletions, and splicing mutations have been re-

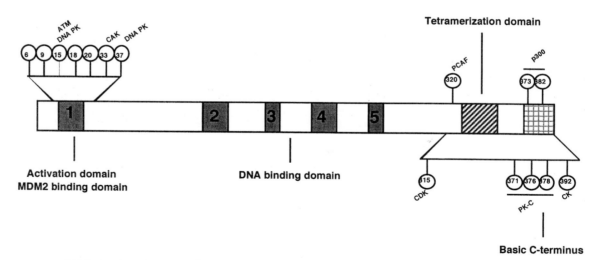

FIGURE 6.3. Schematic of molecular interactions after oncogene activation. In normal cells, MDM2 binds p53, targeting it for degradation. With oncogene activation, levels of the ARF protein increase. ARF protein is thought to bind MDM2, freeing p53 to trigger either cell cycle arrest or apoptosis in the cell.

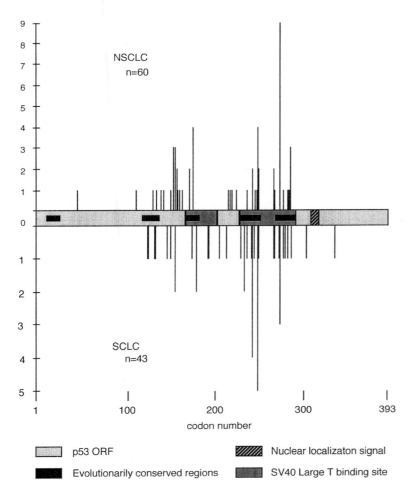

FIGURE 6.4. Histogram showing the distribution of mutations in the p53 open reading frame (ORF) from non–small cell lung cancer and small cell lung cancer. The vertical axis represents the number of mutations at a given codon, and the horizontal axis represents codons in the p53 open reading frame. Above the bar are data from non-small cell lung cancer, and below the bar are those from small cell lung cancer. (From Mitsudomi T, Steinberg SM, Nau MM, et al. p53 gene mutations in non-small cell lung cancer cell lines and their correlation with the presence of *ras* mutations and clinical features. *Oncogene* 1992;7:171, and D'Amico D, Carbone D, Mitsudomi T, et al. High frequency of somatically acquired p53 mutations in small cell lung cancer cell lines and tumors. *Oncogene* 1992;7:339, with permission.)

ported.[124] p53 consists of 11 exons, divided into 3 functional regions as discussed previously. The majority of mutations are found in the central region, composed of exons 5 through 8. Although apparent "hotspot" codons exist, at which multiple tumors have been found to have mutations (e.g., codon 248 and 273 in Figure 6.4), this condition is still the minority of cases. Mutations at these "hotspot" codons result in several different amino acid substitutions as well.

Cigarette smoke is the greatest risk factor for lung cancer, accounting for approximately 85% of cases, and contains polycyclic aromatic hydrocarbons and nitrosamines.[125] These compounds are metabolically hydrolyzed, resulting in the formation of benzo[a]pyrene, a potent carcinogen and mutagen that can form adducts on DNA that manifest as G-to-T transitions in DNA (see also Chapter 3). In smokers with lung cancer, codons 157, 158, 179, 248, 249, and 273 of the p53 gene are the most commonly mutated.[19] Interestingly, benzo[a]pyrene diol epoxide (BPDE), when added to cells in culture, preferentially forms covalent adducts to the guanine residues at codons 157, 248, and 273,

precisely the hotspot mutations observed in smokers with lung cancer.[18] Also interestingly, the mutation spectrum observed in colon cancer, a tumor not strongly associated with polycyclic aromatic hydrocarbons, is predominantly G to A, and the hotspots differ, with colon cancer having a strong predominance at codon 175. The mutational spectrum of the p53 gene in nonsmokers with lung cancer differs from that observed in smokers as well. For nonsmokers, codons 179 and 249 are hotspots for mutations, and nonsmokers generally have fewer G-to-T transitions and more G-to-C transversions.[19] These observations suggest that exposure to certain mutagens can lead to specific mutations in the p53 gene.

At least two known homologues to p53 are present in the human genome, but abnormalities in the known p53 homologues are uncommon in human tumors. A few mutations have been observed in one of them, known as p73, in cell lines containing mutant p53.[126] A recent report has also found a single, apparently functionally significant mutation in 80 tumors examined for abnormalities in a new p53 homologue, p51A/TAp63 gamma.[127]

INHERITED LESIONS OF P53 AND LUNG CANCER

Inherited lesions of p53 lead to the Li-Fraumeni syndrome, and affected individuals have a greatly increased risk of brain and breast tumors, as well as soft tissue sarcomas. Lung cancer is also found in these families, although it is such a common malignancy that increased predisposition is not apparent. Transgenic mice that have a mutant p53 expressed in every cell in their bodies develop a high incidence of tumors,[128] as do mice that have a homozygous deletion of p53,[129] although both are viable. Neither of these strains of mice exhibit a high incidence of lung cancer. Among known Li-Fraumeni families few cases of lung cancer are reported, with a recent series reporting 81 breast cancers, 25 brain tumors, 19 bone tumors, 18 sarcomas, and only 8 lung cancers in 91 families.[130]

A known polymorphism at codon 72 in p53 (Arg versus Pro) has been associated with alterations in lung cancer risk,[131] with the Pro/Pro genotype associated with increased risk. Nonsmoker lung cancer patients had a significant excess of Arg/Arg homozygotes in another study.[132] Several studies have recently looked at whether apparent familial clustering of lung cancer cases might be associated with otherwise unrecognized inherited mutations of p53. In a study of 64 lung cancer patients with early-onset tumors or affected first-degree relatives, one family was found to have an inherited mutation at codon 235, and no increased frequency of the codon 72 Pro/Pro genotype was observed.[133] In another study, of 1,068 families of patients with lung cancer, only 4 had more than three relatives affected. Two successive generations were affected in 36 families, and one family had Li-Fraumeni syndrome.[134] Thus although p53 mutations are common in lung cancer, having an inherited p53 mutation does not seem to dramatically increase the lung cancer risk, relative to other cancer types. This correlation is likely to be caused by the relatively late role of p53 in lung cancer carcinogenesis.

P53 IN PRENEOPLASIA

p53 overexpression has been observed in preneoplastic epithelium adjacent to overt lung cancers (see also Chapter 23).[135,136] Most studies indicate that in the development of squamous cell lung cancer, loss of heterozygosity at 17p (suggesting loss of wild-type p53 function) occurs at the transition of preneoplasia to carcinoma *in situ*.[137] With the advent of polymerase chain reaction-based detection of mutations in p53, it has become possible to analyze ever-decreasing amounts of tissue for abnormalities in oncogenes possibly allowing molecular early detection of lung cancer. Sidransky et al. have detected oncogene mutations in pulmonary cytological specimens.[138,139] Unfortunately, these assays require prior knowledge of the precise location of the mutation, which eliminates most of its usefulness as a screening procedure for p53, unless complex banks of oligonucleotide probes are used. However, molecular detection of residual disease at surgical margins would be feasible with this approach. A recent study of the lungs of a smoker without lung cancer showed a single mutant p53 gene present at seven of ten sites sampled from widely dispersed areas of both lungs.[140] This finding suggested to the authors that a single progenitor bronchial epithelial cell clone harboring a p53 mutation had spread to distant sites within the bronchial tree. If this phenomenon is common, then sputum, or perhaps even something as simple as a buccal wash, could be used to detect occult genetic damage leading to upper aerodigestive malignancies in presymptomatic populations. Studies of allele loss, gene mutation, and other genetic abnormalities in preneoplastic tissues are underway toward that end.

PROGNOSTIC SIGNIFICANCE OF P53 MUTATIONS IN LUNG CANCER

The prognostic significance of p53 mutations in lung cancer is controversial, and the answer may depend on the precise technique used to assay for it and the patient population selected. In SCLC, such a study would be difficult because as almost all SCLC have p53 mutations. In NSCLC, however, many groups have studied this problem. Horio et al. analyzed resected Japanese lung cancer cases and found adverse prognostic significance, especially in early-stage tumors.[141] Other groups have evaluated the prognostic significance of p53 abnormalities as measured by immunohistochemical analysis. An early report found a highly significant adverse effect on survival,[142] and another report the same year found no effect whatsoever,[143] using similar numbers of patients from the United States and England, respectively. In fact, another group found that extremely high p53 protein expression was associated with a favorable prognosis.[144] One study to evaluate both gene mutations and immunostaining on the same group of patients found no prognostic significance to mutations in the gene, but a modest adverse prognosis to p53 overexpression.[145]

Recently, several large studies have been published (see also Chapter 33). D'Amico et al. published on 408 consecutive resected stage I NSCLC patients and showed a modest adverse prognostic impact of p53 overexpression (RR1.68, p = 0.004.[146] An even larger study of 515 resected stage I NSCLC showed no difference in survival for p53 positive immunostaining,[147] but rather that the pathologic T-stage was the only important factor. In summary, the isolated impact of having a mutant p53 or p53 overexpression on time to recurrence or overall survival in lung cancer is unclear and probably not clinically significant.

P53 STATUS AS A PREDICTOR OF CLINICAL RESPONSE TO CHEMOTHERAPY AND RADIATION

The previous studies evaluated stage I patients treated with surgery alone for overall survival. When stage I lung cancer recurs, the second-line treatment modalities vary widely, and time to death is often short. In addition, the general efficacy of therapy in this setting is limited. Thus if p53 had an effect on whether patients responded to radiation or chemotherapy, it might not be detected unless it is specifically evaluated. Several studies have attempted to evaluate this relationship.

Stage III NSCLC is often given initial chemotherapy or chemoradiation therapy, and several studies have evaluated these tumors for p53 status in relation to response. In one study, 52 patients with stage IIIA NSCLC were evaluated for p53 expression and response to cisplatin-based induction chemotherapy. High levels of p53 expression were found to be predictive for lack of pathologic response at the time of surgery.[148] Interestingly, no correlation existed with clinical response assessed radiographically. Other studies have found positive immunostaining to be predictive of resistance.[149] In one of these studies a cohort of stage III patients were analyzed for both p53 mutations and immunohistochemistry,[150] and a normal p53 genotype was found to be highly predictive of response to chemotherapy ($p < 0.001$). No association of response was found with immunohistochemistry, but surprisingly, no association was found between genotype and immunohistochemistry. Because most studies find at least a good correlation between mutations and immunostaining,[145] the immunostain results of this study are questionable.

Response to radiation therapy has also been analyzed. In a group of 34 NSCLC patients with recurrent disease treated with radiation therapy alone, p53 gene sequence abnormalities significantly predicted resistance to treatment (15% response vs. 62% response).[151] When stage III patients are treated with radiation alone, a significant correlation has been observed between lack of p53 immunostain positivity and both response and survival.[152]

Thus the response of clinical lung cancers to chemotherapy or radiation appears worse in the presence of a mutation in p53; however, larger prospective studies specifically addressing this issue are needed to confirm these data. If confirmed, p53 status could potentially be used to select the subset of lung cancers most likely to benefit from nonsurgical interventions and to allow those patients with a small potential benefit to avoid the toxicity of treatment.

ANTI-P53 IMMUNE RESPONSES IN LUNG CANCER PATIENTS

Lung cancer patients sometimes spontaneously make antibodies in their serum that react specifically with p53.[153] We found that 13% of lung cancer patients (but none of the controls) had such naturally occurring antibodies. All patients with antibodies had missense mutations of p53 in their tumors and had detectable levels of protein by ELISA.[153] None of these antibodies were mutant-specific on Western blot, indicating that they are detecting a conformational epitope rather than the actual altered amino acid sequence. Subsequent studies have confirmed these findings, including a recent study of 188 resected NSCLC patients, 38 of whom had detectable anti-p53 antibodies.[154] No relationship existed between antibodies and survival in the subset of 171 patients resected with curative intent. Other studies have evaluated the correlation of anti-p53 antibodies with survival and reported that it was a favorable predictor of survival after radiation therapy[155] or an adverse prognostic factor in the subset of tumors overexpressing p53.[156] Antibodies are consistently reported to be more prevalent in large cell and squamous cell than in adenocarcinomas.[157] In SCLC, a study of 170 patients reported an incidence of 16% and no prognostic impact.[158]

The development of antibodies to p53 when tumors express mutant p53 suggests that antigen presentation to the humoral immune system may indeed depend on the presence of particular protein abnormalities commonly associated with cancer. Antibodies to other proteins such as HuD in lung cancer patients lead to the autoimmune paraneoplastic syndromes,[159] but no such syndrome has been identified for p53. Antibody development has even been reported to be detectable before the development of clinically apparent cancer,[160] but its low frequency limits its usefulness as a screening marker. Correlation with the ability to bind to hsp70 has been described in cases of breast cancer,[161] implicating hsp70 in the antigenic presentation of p53 to the humoral immune system. The significance of these antibodies in a host antitumor immune response and their association with outcome is unknown.

Antibodies can only detect surface proteins in intact cells, but the cellular immune system, and MHC class I-restricted cytotoxic T lymphocytes in particular, can readily detect single amino acid missense substitutions in intracellular and even intranuclear proteins.[162] It has recently been shown that mutant p53-specific cytotoxic T lymphocytes (CTL) can be generated by mutant oncopeptide vaccination, and that these CTL can kill tumor cells that endogenously present the intact mutant p53.[163–166] Effective p53-specific immunity can also be induced using a recombinant adenovirus to overexpress wild-type p53 in dendritic cells.[167] We have also recently shown that we can detect these responses in cancer patients and induce them with peptide vaccination.[168] The therapeutic potential of these p53-specific CTL remains to be determined (see also Chapter 16).

THERAPEUTIC POTENTIAL FOR *P53* GENE THERAPY AND P53-TARGETED SMALL MOLECULES

As discussed previously, expression of wild-type p53 has been shown to result in growth arrest or death of lung cancer cell lines. For example, the H358 lung cancer cell line contains a homozygous deletion of the *p53* gene and thus expresses no p53 protein at all. When expression vectors containing mutant p53 were transfected into this cell line, many stable transfectants that expressed the mutant protein were observed. However, when wild-type p53 was transfected, many fewer clones were isolated, and none of those expressed the normal p53 protein.[169] In contrast, in another tumor expressing a dominant mutant p53, decreased numbers of colonies were found, but stable co-expression was observed. This finding suggests that despite the multiple genetic abnormalities associated with lung cancer, expression of normal p53 protein can inhibit tumor cell growth. Both retroviruses and adenoviruses have been used in animal models[170,171] and humans[172,173] to deliver wild-type p53 for therapy, and these applications are discussed in more detail elsewhere in this book.

Another interesting potential therapeutic approach was suggested by the fact that a subset of p53 mutations are "conditionally mutant." For example, the temperature-sensitive mutation Val-135, which is biochemically mutant at 37.5°C but wild-type at 32.5°C.[174] Similar mutants have been found in human lung cancer.[175] Subsequently, certain antibodies were shown to cause this conformational shift, and the activity of p53 was found to be regulated by phosphorylation as described previously. These facts suggest, at least in a subset of mutant p53 molecules expressed in tumors, that it may be possible to switch p53 from a mutant to a wild-type conformation pharmacologically with therapeutic intent. These strategies are currently under investigation.

CONCLUSION

p53 is often mutated in the process of lung tumor development, and recent studies are beginning to clarify its role in normal and tumor cell physiology. Knowledge of these lesions in clinical samples is beginning to be used for genetic counseling, early and more accurate diagnoses, prognoses, and detection of residual disease. Therapeutic strategies or drugs that can directly affect mutant p53 function may ultimately allow more effective and more tumor-specific treatments of lung cancer patients.

REFERENCES

1. Truant R, Xiao H, Ingles CJ, et al. Direct interaction between the transcriptional activation domain of human p53 and the TATA box-binding protein. *J Biol Chem* 1993;268:2284.
2. Xiao H, Pearson A, Coulombe B, et al. Binding of basal transcription factor TFIIH to the acidic activation domains of VP16 and p53. *Mol Cell Biol* 1994;14:7013.
3. Smith ML, Chen I-T, Zhan Q, et al. Involvement of the p53 tumor suppressor in repair of u.v.-type DNA damage. *Oncogene* 1995;10:1053.
4. Abramova NA, Russell J, Botchan M, et al. Interaction between replication protein A and p53 is disrupted after UV damage in a DNA repair-dependent manner. *Proc Natl Acad Sci USA* 1997; 94:7186.
5. Nishino H, Knoll A, Buettner VL, et al. p53 wild-type and p53 nullizygous Big Blue transgenic mice have similar frequencies and patterns of observed mutation in liver, spleen and brain. *Oncogene* 1995;11:263.
6. Wang XW, Yeh H, Schaeffer L, et al. p53 modulation of TFIIH-associated nucleotide excision repair activity. *Nature Genet* 1995;10:188.
7. Ford JM, Hanawalt PC. Li-Fraumeni syndrome fibroblasts homozygous for p53 mutations are deficient in global DNA repair but exhibit normal transcription-coupled repair and enhanced UV resistance. *Proc Natl Acad Sci USA* 1995;92:8876.
8. Szak ST, Pietenpol JA. High affinity insertion/deletion lesion binding by p53—evidence for a role of the p53 central domain. *J Biol Chem* 1999;274:3904.
9. Leveillard T, Andera L, Bissonnette N, et al. Functional interactions between p53 and the TFIIH complex are affected by tumour-associated mutations. *Embo J* 1996;15:1615.
10. Avantaggiati ML, Ogryzko V, Gardner K, et al. Recruitment of p300/CBP in p53-dependent signal pathways. *Cell* 1997;89: 1175.
11. Gu W, Roeder RG. Activation of p53 sequence-specific DNA binding by acetylation of the p53 C-terminal domain. *Cell* 1997;90:595.
12. Momand J, Zamvetti G, Olson DC, et al. The mdm-2 oncogene product forms a complex with the p53 protein and inhibits p53 mediated transactivation. *Cell* 1992;69:1237.
13. Oliner JD, Pietenpol JA, Thiagalingam S, et al. Oncoprotein MDM2 conceals the activation domain of tumour suppressor p53. *Nature* 1993;362:857.
14. Kussie PH, Gorina S, Marechal V, et al. Structure of the MDM2 oncoprotein bound to the p53 tumor suppressor transactivation domain. *Science* 1996;274:948.
15. Walker KK, Levine AJ. Identification of a novel p53 functional domain that is necessary for efficient growth suppression. *Proc Natl Acad Sci USA* 1996;93:15335.
16. Cho Y, Gorina S, Jeffrey PD, et al. Crystal structure of a p53 tumor suppressor-DNA complex: understanding tumorigenic mutations. *Science* 1994;265:346.
17. Nigro JM, Baker SJ, Preisinger AC, et al. Mutations in the p53 gene occur in diverse human tumour types. *Nature* 1989;342: 705.
18. Denissenko MF, Pao A, Tang MS, et al. Preferential formation of benzo[*a*]pyrene adducts at lung cancer mutational hotspots in *P53*. *Science* 1996;274:430.
19. Hernandez-Boussard TM, Hainaut P. A specific spectrum of p53 mutations in lung cancer from smokers: review of mutations compiled in the IARC p53 database. *Environ Health Perspect* 1998;106:385.
20. Rainwater R, Parks D, Anderson ME, et al. Role of cysteine residues in regulation of p53 function. *Mol Cell Biol* 1995;15: 3892.

21. Hupp TR, Meek DW, Midgley CA, et al. Regulation of the specific DNA binding function of p53. *Cell* 1992;71:875.

22. Jayaraman L, Prives C. Activation of p53 sequence-specific DNA binding by short single strands of DNA requires the p53 C-terminus. *Cell* 1995;81:1021.

23. Sakaguchi K, Herrera JE, Saito S, et al. DNA damage activates p53 through a phosphorylation-acetylation cascade. *Genes and Deve* 1998;12:2831.

24. Shaw P, Freeman J, Bovey R, et al. Regulation of specific DNA binding by p53: evidence for a role for O-glycosylation and charged residues at the carboxy-terminus. *Oncogene* 1996;12: 921.

25. Reed M, Woelker B, Wang P, et al. The C-terminal domain of p53 recognizes DNA damaged by ionizing radiation. *Proc Natl Acad Sci USA* 1995;92:9455.

26. Wang Y, Reed M, Wang P, et al. p53 domains: identification and characterization of two autonomous DNA-binding regions. *Genes Dev* 1993;7:2575.

27. Lee S, Elenbaas B, Levine A, et al. p53 and its 14 kDa C-terminal domain recognize primary DNA damage in the form of insertion/deletion mismatches. *Cell* 1995;81:1013.

28. Sturzbecher HW, Brian R, Addison C, et al. *Oncogene* 1992; 7:1513.

29. Pietenpol JA, Tokino T, El-Deiry WS, et al. Sequence-specific transcriptional activation is essential for growth suppression by p53. *Proc Natl Acad Sci USA* 1994;91:1998.

30. Jeffrey PD, Gorina S, Pavletich NP. Crystal structure of the tetramerization domain of the p53 tumor suppressor at 1.7 angstroms. *Science* 1995;267:1498.

31. Clore GM, Ernst J, Clubb R, et al. Refined solution structure of the oligomerization domain of the tumour suppressor p53. *Nature Struct Biol* 1995;2:321.

32. Clore GM, Omichinski JG, Sakaguchi K, et al. High-resolution structure of the oligomerization domain of p53 by multidimensional NMR. *Science* 1994;265:386.

33. Kuerbitz SJ, Plunkett BS, Walsh WV, et al. Wild-type p53 is a cell cycle checkpoint determinant following irradiation. *Proc Natl Acad Sci USA* 1992;89:7491.

34. Seto E, Usheva A, Zambetti GP, et al. Wild-type p53 binds to the TATA-binding protein and represses transcription. *Proc Natl Acad Sci USA* 1992;89:12028.

35. Mack DH, Vartikar J, Pipas JM, et al. Specific repression of TATA-mediated but not initiator-mediated transcription by wild-type p53. *Nature* 1993;363:281.

36. Wang QJ, Zambetti GP, Suttle DP. Inhibition of DNA topo-isomerase IIα gene expression by the p53 tumor suppressor. *Mol Cell Biol* 1997;17:389.

37. Subler MA, Martin DW, Deb S. Modulation of cellular and viral promoters by mutant human p53 proteins found in tumor cells. *J Virol* 1992;66:4757.

38. Murphy M, Hinman A, Levine AJ. Wild-type p53 negatively regulates expression of a microtubule-associated protein. *Genes Dev* 1996;10:2971.

39. Leach SD, Scatena CD, Keefer CJ, et al. Negative regulation of Wee1 expression and Cdc2 phosphorylation during p53-mediated growth arrest and apoptosis. *Cancer Res* 1998;58: 3231.

40. Ginsberg D, Mechta F, Yaniv M, et al. Wild-type p53 can down-modulate the activity of various promoters. *Proc Natl Acad Sci USA* 1991;88:9979.

41. Miyashita T, Harigai M, Hanada M, et al. Identification of a p53-dependent negative response element in the *bcl*-2 gene. *Cancer Res* 1994;54:3131.

42. Diller L, Kassel J, Nelson CE, et al. p53 functions as a cell cycle control protein in osteosarcomas. *Mol Cell Biol* 1990;10:5772.

43. Baker SJ, Markowitz S, Fearon ER, et al. Suppression of human colorectal carcinoma cell growth by wild-type p53. *Science* 1990; 249:912.

44. Giaccia AJ, Kastan MB. The complexity of p53 modulation: emerging patterns from divergent signals. *Genes Dev* 1998;12: 2973.

45. Ko LJ, Prives C. p53: puzzle and paradigm. *Genes Dev* 1996; 10:1054.

46. Hermeking H, Eick D. Mediation of c-myc-induced apoptosis by p53. *Science* 1994;265:2091.

47. Jacks T, Weinberg RA. Cell-cycle control and its watchman. *Nature* 1996;381:643.

48. Serrano M, Lin AW, McCurrach ME, et al. Oncogenic *ras* provokes premature cell senescence associated with accumulation of p53 and p16^{INK4a}. *Cell* 1997;88:593.

49. Maltzman W, Czyzyk L. UV irradiation stimulates levels of p53 cellular tumor antigen in nontransformed mouse cells. *Mol Cell Biol* 1984;4:1689.

50. Kastan MB, Onyekwere O, Sidransky D, et al. Participation of p53 protein in the cellular response to DNA damage. *Cancer Res* 1991;51:6304.

51. Weinberg WC, Azzoli CG, Chapman K, et al. p53-mediated transcriptional activity increases in differentiating epidermal keratinocytes in association with decreased p53 protein. *Oncogene* 1995;10:2271.

52. El-Deiry WS, Tokino T, Velculescu VE, et al. *WAF1,* a potential mediator of p53 tumor suppression. *Cell* 1993;75:817.

53. El-Deiry WS, Harper JW, O'Connor PM, et al. *WAF1/CIP1* is induced in *p53*-mediated G$_1$ arrest and apoptosis. *Cancer Res* 1994;54:1169.

54. Brugarolas J, Chandrasekaran C, Gordon JI, et al. Radiation-induced cell cycle arrest compromised by p21 deficiency. *Nature* 1995;377:552.

55. Waldman T, Kinzler KW, Vogelstein B. p21 is necessary for the p53-mediated G$_1$ arrest in human cancer cells. *Cancer Res* 1995;55:5187.

56. Harper JW, Adami GR, Wei N, et al. The p21 Cdk-interacting protein Cip1 is a potent inhibitor of G1 cyclin-dependent kinases. *Cell* 1993;75:805.

57. Xiong Y, Hannon GJ, Zhang H, et al. p21 is a universal inhibitor of cyclin kinases. *Nature* 1993;366:701.

58. Gu Y, Turck CW, Morgan DO. Inhibition of CDK2 activity *in vivo* by an associated 20K regulatory subunit. *Nature* 1993; 366:707.

59. Deng CX, Zhang PM, Harper JW, et al. Mice lacking p21 CIP1/WAF1 undergo normal development, but are defective in G1 checkpoint control. *Cell* 1995;82:675.

60. Prelich G, Tan CK, Kostura M, et al. Functional identity of proliferating cell nuclear antigen and a DNA polymerase-delta auxiliary protein. *Nature* 1987;326:517.

61. Kastan MB, Zhan Q, El-Deiry WS, et al. A mammalian cell cycle checkpoint pathway utilizing p53 and GADD45 is defective in ataxia-telangiectasia. *Cell* 1992;71:587.

62. Smith ML, Chen I-T, Zhan Q, et al. Interaction of the p53-regulated protein Gadd45 with proliferating cell nuclear antigen. *Science* 1994;266:1376.

63. Kazantsev A, Sancar A. Does the p53 up-regulated Gadd45 protein have a role in excision repair? *Science* 1995;270:1003.

64. Kearsey JM, Shivji MKK, Hall PA, et al. Does the p53 up-regulated Gadd45 protein have a role in excision repair? *Science* 1995;270:1004.

65. Li R, Waga S, Hannon GJ, et al. Differential effects by the p21 CDK inhibitor on PCNA-dependent DNA replication and repair. *Nature* 1994;371:534.

66. Sanchez Y, Wong S, Thoma RS, et al. Conservation of the Chk1 checkpoint pathway in mammals: linkage of DNA damage to Cdk regulation through Cdc25C. *Science* 1997;277:1497.

67. Peng C-Y, Graves PR, Thoma RS, et al. Mitotic and G$_2$ checkpoint control: regulation of 14-3-3 protein binding by phosphorylation of Cdc25c on Serine-216. *Science* 1997;277:1501.

68. Hermeking H, Lengauer C, Polyak K, et al. 14-3-3σ is a p53-regulated inhibitor of G2/M progression. *Mole Cell Biol* 1998; 1:3.

69. Agarwal ML, Agarwal A, Taylor WR, et al. p53 controls both the G$_2$/M and the G$_1$ cell cycle checkpoints and mediates reversible growth arrest in human fibroblasts. *Proc Natl Acad Sci USA* 1995;92:8493.

70. Stewart N, Hicks GG, Paraskevas F, et al. Evidence for a second cell cycle block at G2/M by p53. *Oncogene* 1995;10:109.

71. Bunz F, Dutriaux A, Lengauer C, et al. Requirement for p53 and p21 to sustain G$_2$ arrest after DNA damage. *Science* 1998; 282:1497.

72. Sorger PK, Dobles M, Tournebize R, et al. Coupling cell division and cell death to microtubule dynamics. *Curr Opin Cell Biol* 1997;9:807.

73. Di Leonardo A, Khan SH, Linke SP, et al. DNA rereplication in the presence of mitotic spindle inhibitors in human and mouse fibroblasts lacking either p53 or pRb function. *Cancer Res* 1997;57:1013.

74. Cross SM, Sanchez CA, Morgan CA, et al. A p53-dependent mouse spindle checkpoint. *Science* 1995;267:1353.

75. Lanni JS, Jacks TS. Characterization of the p53-dependent postmitotic checkpoint following spindle disruption. *Mol Cell Biol* 1998;18:1055.

76. Khan SH, Wahl GM. p53 and pRb prevent rereplication in response to microtubule inhibitors by mediating a reversible G$_1$ arrest. *Cancer Res* 1998;58:396.

77. Stewart ZA, Leach SD, Pietenpol JA. p21 Waf1/Cip1 inhibition of cyclin E/Cdk2 activity prevents endoreduplication after mitotic spindle disruption. *Mol Cell Biol* 1999;19:205.

78. Stewart ZA, Mays D, Pietenpol JA. Defective G1/S cell cycle checkpoint function sensitizes cells to microtubule inhibitor-induced apoptosis. *Cancer Res* 1999;59:3831.

79. Buckbinder L, Talbott R, Velasco-Miguel S, et al. Induction of the growth inhibitor IGF-binding protein 3 by p53. *Nature* 1995;377:646.

80. Crook T, Marston NJ, Sara EA, et al. Transcriptional activation by p53 correlates with suppression of growth but not transformation. *Cell* 1994;79:817.

81. Polyak K, Xia Y, Zweier JL, et al. A model for p53-induced apoptosis. *Nature* 1997;389:300.

82. Miyashita T, Reed JC. Tumor suppressor p53 is a direct transcriptional activator of the human *bax* gene. *Cell* 1995;80:293.

83. Caelles C, Helmberg A, Karin M. p53-dependent apoptosis in the absence of transcriptional activation of p53-target genes. *Nature* 1994;370:220.

84. Haupt Y, Barak Y, Oren M. Cell type-specific inhibition of p53-mediated apoptosis by mdm2. *Embo J* 1996;15:1596.

85. Pan H, Yin C, Dyson NJ, et al. Key roles for E2F1 in signaling p53-dependent apoptosis and in cell division within developing tumors. *Mole Cell Biol* 1998;2:283.

86. Maki CG, Huibregtse JM, Howley PM. *In vivo* ubiquitination and proteasome-mediated degradation of p53. *Cancer Res* 1996; 56:2649.

87. Maki CG, Howley PM. Ubiquitination of p53 and p21 is differentially affected by ionizing and UV radiation. *Mol Cell Biol* 1997;17:355.

88. Barak Y, Juven T, Haffner R, et al. *mdm2* expression is induced by wild type p53 activity. *Embo J* 1993;12:461.

89. Wu X, Bayle JH, Olson D, et al. The p53-mdm-2 autoregulatory feedback loop. *Genes Dev* 1993;7:1126.

90. Haupt Y, Maya R, Kazaz A, et al. Mdm2 promotes the rapid degradation of p53. *Nature* 1997;387:296.

91. Kubbutat MHG, Jones SN, Vousden KH. Regulation of p53 stability by Mdm2. *Nature* 1997;387:299.

92. Marchetti A, Buttitta F, Pellegrini S, et al. mdm2 gene amplification and overexpression in non-small cell lung carcinomas with accumulation of the p53 protein in the absence of p53 gene mutations. *Diag Mol Pathol* 1995;4:93.

93. Jones SN, Roe AE, Donehowes LA, et al. Rescue of embryonic lethality in Mdm2-deficient mice by absence of p53. *Nature* 1995;378:206.

94. Luna RMD, Wagner DS, Lozano G. Rescue of early embryonic lethality in *mdm2*-deficient mice by deletion of *p53*. *Nature* 1995;378:203.

95. Hainaut P, Milner J. Interaction of heat-shock protein 70 with p53 translated in vitro: evidence for interaction with dimeric p53 and for a role in the regulation of p53 conformation. *Embo J* 1992;11:3513.

96. Carbone M, Rizzo P, Grimley PM, et al. Similan virus-40 large-T antigen bind p53 in human mesotheliomas. *Nature Med* 1997;8:908.

97. Werness BA, Levine AJ, Howley PM. Association of human papillomavirus types 16 and 18 E6 proteins with p53. *Science* 1990;248:76.

98. Scheffner M, Werness BA, Hulbregtse JM, et al. The E6 oncoprotein encoded by human papillomavirus types 16 and 18 promotes the degradation of p53. *Cell* 1990;63:1129.

99. Huibregtse JM, Scheffner M, Howley PM. Cloning and expression of the cDNA for E6-AP, a protein that mediates the interaction of the human papillomavirus E6 oncoprotein with p53. *Mol Cell Biol* 1993;13:775.

100. Palmero I, Pantoja C, Serrano M. p19 ARF links the tumour suppressor p53 to Ras. *Nature* 1998;395:125.

101. De Stanchina E, McCurrach ME, Zindy F, et al. E1A signaling to p53 involves the p19 ARF tumor suppressor. *Genes Dev* 1998; 12:2434.

102. Kamijo T, Weber JD, Zambetti G, et al. Functional and physical interactions of the ARF tumor suppressor with p53 and Mdm2. *Proc Natl Acad Sci USA* 1998;95:8292.

103. Pomerantz J, Schreiber-Agus N, Liegeois NJ, et al. The *Ink4a* tumor suppressor gene product, p19 Arf, interacts with MDM2 and neutralizes MDM2's inhibition of p53. *Cell* 1998;92:713.

104. Bates S, Phillips AC, Clark PA, et al. p14 ARF links the tumour suppressors RB and p53. *Nature* 1998;395:124.

105. Zhang YP, Xiong Y, Yarbrough WG. ARF promotes MDM2 degradation and stabilizes p53: *ARF-INK4a* locus deletion impairs both the Rb and p53 tumor suppression pathways. *Cell* 1998;92:725.

106. Stott F, Bates SA, James M, et al. The alternative product from the human CDKN2A locus, p14 ARF, participates in a regulatory feedback loop with p53 and mdm2. *Embo J* 1998;17:5001.

107. Graeber TG, Peterson JF, Tsai M, et al. Hypoxia induces accumulation of p53 protein, but activation of a G1-phase checkpoint by low-oxygen conditions is independent of p53 status. *Mol Cell Biol* 1994;14:6264.

108. Graeber TG, Osmanian C, Jacks T, et al. Hypoxia-mediated selection of cells with diminished apoptotic potential in solid tumours. *Nature* 1996;379:88.

109. Jayaraman L, Murthy KGK, Zhu C, et al. Identification of redox/repair protein Ref-1 as a potent activator of p53. *Genes Dev* 1997;11:558.

110. Nelson WG, Kastan MB. DNA strand breaks: the DNA template alterations that trigger p53-dependent DNA damage response pathways. *Mol Cell Biol* 1994;14:1815.

111. Huang L, Clarkin K, Wahl GM. Sensitivity and selectivity of the DNA damage sensor responsible for activating p53-dependent G arrest. *Proc Natl Acad Sci USA* 1996;93:4827.

112. Banin S, Moyal L, Shieh SY, et al. Enhanced phosphorylation

of p53 by ATN in response to DNA damage. *Science* 1998;
281:1674.

113. Canman CE, Lim DS, Cimprich KA, et al. Activation of the
ATM kinase by ionizing radiation and phosphorylation of p53.
Science 1998;281:1677.

114. Shieh SY, Ikeda M, Taya Y, et al. DNA damage-induced phosphorylation of p53 alleviates inhibition by MDM2. *Cell* 1997;
91:325.

115. Kapoor M, Lozano G. Functional activation of p53 via phosphorylation following DNA damage by UV but not gamma
radiation. *Proc Natl Acad Sci USA* 1998;95:2834.

116. Hupp TR, Lane DP. Allosteric activation of latent p53 tetra-
mers. *Curr Biol* 1994;1994:865.

117. Wang Y, Prives C. Increased and altered DNA binding of
human p53 by S and G2/M but not G1 cyclin-dependent kinases. *Nature* 1995;376:88.

118. Takahashi T, Nau MM, Chiba I, et al. p53: a frequent target
for genetic abnormalities in lung cancer. *Science* 1989;246:491.

119. Soussi T, Caron de Fromentel C, May P. Structural aspects of
the p53 protein in relation to gene evolution. *Oncogene* 1990;
5:945.

120. Chiba I, Takahashi T, Nau MM, et al. Mutations in the p53
gene are frequent in primary, resected non-small cell lung cancer. *Oncogene* 1990;5:1603.

121. Mitsudomi T, Steinberg SM, Nau MM, et al. p53 gene mutations in non-small-cell lung cancer cell lines and their correlation
with the presence of *ras* mutations and clinical features. *Oncogene* 1992;7:171.

122. Sameshima Y, Matsuno Y, Hirohashi S, et al. Alterations of the
p53 gene are common and critical events for the maintenance
of malignant phenotypes in small-cell lung carcinoma. *Oncogene*
1992;7:451.

123. D'Amico D, Carbone D, Mitsudomi T, et al. High frequency
of somatically acquired p53 mutations in small cell lung cancer
cell lines and tumors. *Oncogene* 1992;7:339.

124. Takahashi T, D'Amico D, Chiba I, et al. Identification of intronic point mutations as an alternative mechanism for p53
inactivation in lung cancer. *J Clin Invest* 1990;86:363.

125. Hecht SS, Carmella SG, Murphy SE, et al. Carcinogen biomarkers related to smoking and upper aerodigestive tract cancer.
J Cell Biochem 1993;17F:27.

126. Yoshikawa H, Nagashima M, Khan MA, et al. Mutational analysis of p73 and p53 in human cancer cell lines. *Oncogene* 1999;
18:3415.

127. Sunahara M, Shishikura T, Takahashi M, et al. Mutational
analysis of p51A/TAp63gamma, a p53 homolog, in non-small
cell lung cancer and breast cancer. *Oncogene* 1999;18:3761.

128. Lavigueur A, Maltby V, Mock D, et al. High incidence of lung,
bone, and lymphoid tumors in transgenic mice overexpressing
mutant alleles of the p53 oncogene. *Mol Cell Biol* 1989;9:3982.

129. Donehower LA, Harvey M, Slagle BL, et al. Mice deficient for
p53 are developmentally normal but susceptible to spontaneous
tumours. *Nature* 1992;356:215.

130. Kleihues P, Schauble B, zur Hausen A, et al. Tumors associated
with p53 germline mutations: a synopsis of 91 families. *Am J
Pathol* 1997;150:1.

131. Jin X, Wu X, Roth JA, et al. Higher lung cancer risk for younger
African-Americans with the Pro/Pro p53 genotype. *Carcinogenesis* 1995;16:2205.

132. Murata M, Tagawa M, Kimura M, et al. Analysis of a germ
line polymorphism of the p53 gene in lung cancer patients;
discrete results with smoking history. *Carcinogenesis* 1996;17:
261.

133. Auer H, Warncke K, Nowak D, et al. Variations of p53 in
cultured fibroblasts of patients with lung cancer who have a
presumed genetic predisposition. *Am J Clin Oncol* 1999;22:278.

134. Tomizawa Y, Adachi J, Kohno T, et al. Identification and characterization of families with aggregation of lung cancer. *Jpn J
Clin Oncol* 1998;28:192.

135. Bennett WP, Colby TV, Travis WD, et al. p53 protein accumulates frequently in early bronchial neoplasia. *Cancer Res* 1993;
53:4817.

136. Rusch V, Klimstra D, Linkov I, et al. Aberrant expression of
p53 or the epidermal growth factor receptor is frequent in early
bronchial neoplasia and coexpression precedes squamous cell
carcinoma development. *Cancer Res* 1995;55:1365.

137. Wistuba, II, Lam S, Behrens C, et al. Molecular damage in the
bronchial epithelium of current and former smokers. *J Natl
Cancer Inst* 1997;89:1366.

138. Sidransky D, Tokino T, Hamilton SR, et al. Identification of
ras oncogene mutations in the stool of patients with curable
colorectal tumors. *Science* 1992;256:102.

139. Sidransky D, Von Eschenbach A, Tsai YC, et al. Identification
of p53 gene mutations in bladder cancers and urine samples.
Science 1991;252:706.

140. Franklin WA, Gazdar AF, Haney J, et al. Widely dispersed p53
mutation in respiratory epithelium. A novel mechanism for field
carcinogenesis [published erratum appears in *J Clin Invest* 1997
Nov 15;100(10):2639]. *J Clin Invest* 1997;100:2133.

141. Horio Y, Takahashi T, Kuroishi T, et al. Prognostic significance
of p53 mutations and 3p deletions in primary resected non-
small cell lung cancer. *Cancer Res* 1993;53:1.

142. Quinlan DC, Davidson AG, Summers CL, et al. Accumulation
of p53 protein correlates with a poor prognosis in human lung
cancer. *Cancer Res* 1992;52:4828.

143. McLaren R, Kuzu I, Dunnill M, et al. The relationship of p53
immunostaining to survival in carcinoma of the lung. *Br J Cancer* 1992;66:735.

144. Mrkve O, Halvorsen OJ, Skjaerven R, et al. Prognostic significance of p53 protein expression and DNA ploidy in surgically
treated non-small cell lung carcinomas. *Anticancer Res* 1993;13:
571.

145. Carbone D. p53 immunostaining is imperfectly correlated with
gene mutations in non-small cell lung cancer. *Proceed Am Soc
Clin Oncol* 1993;abstract.

146. D'Amico TA, Massey M, Herndon JE, 2nd, et al. A biologic risk
model for stage I lung cancer: immunohistochemical analysis of
408 patients with the use of ten molecular markers. *J Thorac
Cardiovasc Surg* 1999;117:736.

147. Pastorino U, Andreola S, Tagliabue E, et al. Immunocytochemical markers in stage I lung cancer: relevance to prognosis. *J Clin
Oncol* 1997;15:2858.

148. Rusch V, Klimstra D, Venkatraman E, et al. Aberrant p53
expression predicts clinical resistance to cisplatin-based chemotherapy in locally advanced non-small cell lung cancer. *Cancer
Res* 1995;55:5038.

149. Kawasaki M, Nakanishi Y, Kuwano K, et al. Immunohistochemically detected p53 and P-glycoprotein predict the response
to chemotherapy in lung cancer. *Eur J Cancer* 1998;34:1352.

150. Kandioler-Eckersberger D, Kappel S, Mittlbock M, et al. The
TP53 genotype but not immunohistochemical result is predictive of response to cisplatin-based neoadjuvant therapy in stage
III non-small cell lung cancer. *J Thorac Cardiovasc Surg* 1999;
117:744.

151. Matsuzoe D, Hideshima T, Kimura A, et al. p53 mutations
predict non-small cell lung carcinoma response to radiotherapy.
Cancer Lett 1999;135:189.

152. Langendijk JA, Thunnissen FB, Lamers RJ, et al. The prognostic
significance of accumulation of p53 protein in stage III non-
small cell lung cancer treated by radiotherapy. *Radiother Oncol*
1995;36:218.

153. Winter SF, Minna JD, Johnson BE, et al. Development of

antibodies against p53 in lung cancer patients appears to be dependent on the type of p53 mutation. *Cancer Research* 1992; 52:4168.

154. Mitsudomi T, Suzuki S, Yatabe Y, et al. Clinical implications of p53 autoantibodies in the sera of patients with non-small-cell lung cancer. *J Natl Cancer Inst* 1998;90:1563.

155. Bergqvist M, Brattstrom D, Larsson A, et al. P53 auto-antibodies in non-small cell lung cancer patients can predict increased life expectancy after radiotherapy. *Anticancer Res* 1998;18:1999.

156. Komiya T, Hirashima T, Takada M, et al. Prognostic significance of serum p53 antibodies in squamous cell carcinoma of the lung. *Anticancer Res* 1997;17:3721.

157. Segawa Y, Kageyama M, Suzuki S, et al. Measurement and evaluation of serum anti-p53 antibody levels in patients with lung cancer at its initial presentation: a prospective study. *Br J Cancer* 1998;78:667.

158. Rosenfeld MR, Malats N, Schramm L, et al. Serum anti-p53 antibodies and prognosis of patients with small-cell lung cancer. *J Natl Canc Inst* 1997;89:381.

159. Dalmau JO, Posner JB. Paraneoplastic syndromes. *Arch Neurol* 1999;56:405.

160. Trivers GE, Cawley HL, DeBenedetti VM, et al. Anti-p53 antibodies in sera of workers occupationally exposed to vinyl chloride. *J Natl Cancer Inst* 1995;87:1400.

161. Davidoff AM, Iglehart JD, Marks JR. Immune response to p53 is dependent upon p53/HSP70 complexes in breast cancers. *Proc Natl Acad Sci USA* 1992;89:3439.

162. Germain R, Margolis D. The biochemistry and cell biology of antigen processing and presentation. *Ann Rev Immunol* 1993; 11:403.

163. Yanuck M, Carbone DP, Pendleton CD, et al. A mutant p53 tumor suppressor protein is a target for peptide-induced CD8 + cytotoxic T cells. *Cancer Res* 1993;53:3257.

164. Gabrilovich DI, Nadaf S, Cunningham T, et al. Cytotoxic T-lymphocytes (CTL) specific for mutant p53-peptides in peripheral blood of patients with cancer: support for specific immune intervention. *9th Internatl Cong Immunol* 1995:A3964.

165. Gabrilovich DI, Cunningham HT, Carbone DP. IL-12 and mutant p53 peptide-pulsed dendritic cells for the specific immunotherapy of cancer. *J Immunotherapy* 1997;19:414.

166. McCarty TM, Yu Z, Liu X, et al. An HLA-restricted, p53 specific immune response from HLA transgenic p53 knockout mice. *Ann Surg Oncol* 1998;5:93.

167. Ishida T, Stipanov M, Chada S, et al. Dendritic cells transduced with wild type p53 gene elicit potent antitumor immune responses. *J Clin Exp Immunol* 1999;117:224.

168. Carbone DP, Kelley M, Smith MC, et al. Results of NCI T93-0148: detection of immunologic responses and vaccination against tumor specific mutant ras and p53 peptides in patients with cancer. *Proc ASCO* 1999.

169. Takahashi T, Carbone D, Takahashi T, et al. Wild-type but not mutant p53 suppresses the growth of human lung cancer cells bearing multiple genetic lesions. *Cancer Res* 1992;52:2340.

170. Fujiwara T, Cai DW, Georges RN, et al. Therapeutic effect of a retroviral wild-type p53 expression vector in an orthotopic lung cancer model. *J Natl Cancer Inst* 1994;86:1458.

171. Zhang WW, Fang X, Mazur W, et al. High-efficiency gene transfer and high-level expression of wild-type p53 in human lung cancer cells mediated by recombinant adenovirus. *Cancer Gene Ther* 1994;1:5.

172. Swisher SG, Roth JA, Nemunaitis J, et al. Adenovirus-mediated p53 gene transfer in advanced non-small-cell lung cancer. *J Natl Cancer Inst* 1999;91:763.

173. Roth JA. Therapy of human lung cancer with a retrovirus carrying wild-type p53. *Nature Medicine* 1996;2:985.

174. Ginsberg D, Michael-Michalovitz D, Ginsberg D, et al. Induction of growth arrest by a temperature-sensitive p53 mutant is correlated with increased nuclear localization and decreased stability of the protein. *Mol Cell Biol* 1991;11:582.

175. Medcalf EA, Takahashi T, Chiba I, et al. Temperature-sensitive mutants of p53 associated with human carcinoma of the lung. *Oncogene* 1992;7:71.

7

RB1 AND *RB2*

PIER PAOLO CLAUDIO
ANTONIO GIORDANO

GENETIC BASIS OF CANCER

Cancer is a genetic disease that results from multiple genomic changes. These changes ultimately lead to the deregulation of the cell cycle machinery and to autonomous cell proliferation. Neoplastic transformation involves four sets of genes: (a) oncogenes; (b) tumor-suppressor genes; (c) mutator genes; and (d) apoptotic genes. In the hematopoietic system, the first step in oncogenesis is the activation of an oncogene, which may then be followed by the activation of an additional oncogene and/or the loss of function of a tumor-suppressor gene. The activation of oncogenes may play a predominant role in the formation of sarcomas as well. Tumors of both the hematopoietic system and soft tissues exhibit a karyotype close to normal. On the other hand, carcinomas, the most prevalent forms of cancer, are predominantly caused by the loss of function of tumor-suppressor genes with multiple sites of loss of heterozygosity (LOH), and they have dramatic alterations in the karyotype.[1]

The discovery of tumor-suppressor genes revolutionized the field of cancer research and of cell cycle molecular biology. According to Knudson's "two-hit" hypothesis,[2] the development of several human cancers is thought to involve LOH of putative tumor-suppressor genes, several of which are not yet identified. Many forms of malignancies have been linked to mutations in the retinoblastoma-susceptibility gene (*RB*), the first tumor-suppressor gene identified. RB provides a link among the cell cycle machinery, the G1/S cyclins, and cyclin-dependent kinases (Cdks), and the transcription of genes necessary for entry into S-phase. Another tumor suppressor, p53, is found mutated in more than 50% of human tumors.[3] Both tumor-suppressor genes, *RB* and *p53,* are negative regulators of the cell cycle and are involved in growth arrest. p53 is also implicated in the recognition and repair of DNA damage, as well as in the induction of programmed cell death, apoptosis. Recently, it has become increasingly clear that these two proteins interact with each other through various pathways in order to exert their effects on cellular events.

THE CELL CYCLE CLOCK

The mammalian cell cycle machinery involves the formation, activation, inactivation, and degradation of sequential complexes of cyclins with Cdks. This process is governed by positive and negative feedback regulations at various critical transition points to ensure that the necessary molecular events occur in each phase of the cell cycle prior to progression to the next stage. Uncoupling of this intricately controlled regulatory process often results in cellular transformation and oncogenesis.

Disruptions in the cell cycle machinery are implicated in the development of certain cancers. Cyclins are cell cycle regulators first identified in marine embryos and named for their cyclical accumulation and degradation at each stage of the cell cycle.

In humans the overexpression of certain G1 cyclins is associated with oncogenesis. Hepatitis B viral integration into the cyclin A gene is found in some cases of hepatocellular carcinoma.[4] Elevated levels of cyclin A are also correlated with hematologic malignancies.[5] Gene derangement and aberrant expression of cyclins are reported in breast, esophageal, and skin malignancies.[6–8] The candidate oncogene, PRAD1, found to be overexpressed and rearranged in parathyroid tumors, actually encodes for the cyclin D1.[9] Certain colorectal cancer cell lines have amplifications of cyclin D2 and cyclin E.[10] Unregulated, persistent expression of cyclins D1 and D3 are found in various human tumor cell lines,[11] and an overabundance of cyclin D3 expression is detected in subsets of breast tumors and lymphomas.[12] The transforming protein E1A, from a DNA oncovirus, associates with cyclin A in adenovirus-transformed cells.[13,14] This association is the first evidence for the linkage between the cell cycle and the process of neoplastic transformation. The binding of E1A may promote cellular proliferation by disrupting the normal interaction between cyclin A and the E2F/DRTF1 transcription factor.[15] DNA oncoviruses, via their oncoproteins targeting key regulatory and proliferative proteins of the cell cycle, serve as valuable tools in the attempt to elucidate the complex mechanisms governing the cell cycle machinery.

It is well established that p34[cdc2] protein kinase plays an important role in the regulation of the cell division cycle. In fission yeast, cdc2 function is required at two points of the cell division cycle: prior to the initiation of DNA replication and at the time of initiation of mitosis. In *Xenopus* the cdc2 gene product has been identified as a component of M-phase promoting factor (MPF), a factor that causes an interphase cell to enter mitosis; other components include the product of the Suc1 gene and p62, homologous to the human cyclin B gene. The MPF complex also acts as a histone H1 kinase that is maximally active at mitotic metaphase. In mammalian cells the cdc2 kinase is required for mitosis and for the transition from G1 to S-phase (DNA replication).[16] At least two complexes of mammalian p34[cdc2] have been identified, the p62 (cyclin B)-p34[cdc2] complex and the p60 (cyclin A)-p34[cdc2] complex.[13,17] The p60 (cyclin A)-p34[cdc2] complex also displays a cell cycle–dependent histone H1 kinase activity, but it shifts the timing of maximal activity to interphase.[13] Another complex has been identified between p50 (cyclin E) and Cdk2, a member of the extended cdc2-related protein family.[18] These three complexes (cyclin B–Cdc2; cyclin A–Cdc2; cyclin E–Cdk2) display a cell cycle–dependent histone H1 kinase activity that has different timings of activation during the cell division cycle.[13,17,18]

G1-Phase

Throughout the G1 phase of the cell cycle, growth factors exhibit their effects by binding to specific surface receptors. This process leads to the activation of signaling cascades that control the transcription of immediate and delayed early-response genes. Even within cells that ultimately undergo divergent long-term responses, many of the same intracellular signaling molecules exhibit uniform activation. Withdrawal of growth factors in mammalian cells leads to arrest of the cells in early G1 into what is known as the G0-phase. In order for cells to reenter the cell cycle from quiescence, the Cdk complexes in the cells must be activated (Figure 7.1). Activation of the Cdk complexes requires the aggregation of cyclins and Cdk subunits, the derangement of inhibitory molecules such as p15, p16, p21, and p27[19–23] from the Cdk complexes, and phosphorylation by the Cdk-activating kinase (CAK).[24–26] The cyclins involved in G1 of mammalian cells include cyclins C, D, and E. In yeast these cyclins are encoded by CLN genes whose protein products regulate cdc2 activity at START, the point at which a cell commits to DNA replication.[27] Neither cyclin A nor B is available prior to S-phase. Throughout the cell cycle, cyclin C levels do not oscillate very much, exhibiting only a slight increase in early G1. However, this invariability is not the case for cyclin E, which has periodic expression and peaks at the G1/S transition, suggesting a possible role for it in the regulation of S-phase entry.[18,28]

There are three D-type cyclins, which vary in their rela-

tive levels among cell types.[29] Following serum addition to quiescent cells, D-type cyclins are induced. Subsequent induction and maintenance of D-type cyclin mRNAs depend on the presence of growth factors.[30,31] The D-type cyclins pose a possible link among cell cycle, signal transduction, and oncogenesis because the overexpression of cyclin D1 has been found in some tumors. The D-type cyclins have been shown to associate with four members of the Cdk protein family, Cdk2, 4, 5, and 6; however, the major catalytic partners of the D-type cyclins are Cdk4 and Cdk6.[31,32] Similar to all nascent cyclin–Cdk complexes, those containing cyclin D become activated only when phosphorylated by Cdk-activating kinase (CAK). In mammalian cells CAK has recently been shown to complex with cyclin H (thus termed Cdk7) and then to phosphorylate and activate Cdk2, Cdc2, and Cdk4 complexes.[24,25] Depletion of CAK from the cell lysates prevents the activation of cyclin–D-Cdk4 complexes.[25] This reaction demonstrates that the CAK protein is a necessary component of the Cdk4-activation kinase.

The three D-type cyclins may not be functionally equivalent because cyclin D1 forms a much less stable complex with pRb than either cyclins D2 or D3.[32–34] Unlike cyclin E or A, the D-type cyclins share the sequence Leu-X-Cys-X-Glu (LXCXE) near their amino-termini with the DNA viral oncoproteins, which bind pRb and pRb-related p107. Point mutations within this region disrupt the ability of D-type cyclins to bind to pRb and to p107 *in vitro;* thus, D-type cyclins can be more effectively complexed by oncoprotein-derived peptides containing the LXCXE residues.[34,35] Additional evidence of the possible functional divergence among the D-type cyclins comes from the observation that the overexpression of cyclins D2 and D3 in hematopoietic cell lines inhibits differentiation of granulocytes; however, overexpression of cyclin D1, which is not a normal constituent of these cells, does not affect their differentiation.[32] The effects of the D-type cyclins are cell type specific because in some cell types their overexpression results in an enhanced capacity of the cells to enter S-phase and lowers the cells' requirements for growth factors.[36,37]

Microinjection of antisense plasmids or antibodies of cyclin D1 during mid-G1 into quiescent fibroblasts is inhibitory to cell cycle progression upon serum stimulation, but it is ineffectual when administered near the G1/S boundary.[38] This relationship indicates a functional role for the D-type cyclins occurring after the G0/G1 transition. Recent studies have pointed to the possible necessity of down-regulation of cyclin D1 levels and/or their removal from the nucleus at the end of G1, which more precisely delineates the timing of the functional activity of the D-type cyclins. This conjecture originates from the findings that as cells enter S-phase, cyclin D1 vanishes from the nucleus and the total concentration of the protein markedly decreases.[38] This notion is also supported by the observation that the ectopic expression of cyclin D1 arrests fibroblasts prior to entering S-

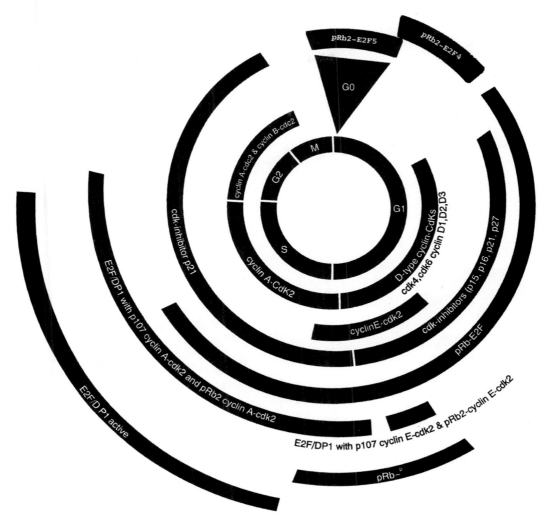

FIGURE 7.1. Schematic diagram of the cell cycle clock. (From "neoplastic transformation: onco-genes, tumor suppressors, cyclins, and cyclin-dependent kinases" by Candace M. Howard and Antonio Giordano in *Hormones and Cancer* 1996, Birkhäuser Boston, with permission).

phase and prevents their repair of damaged DNA.[39] When pRb becomes hyperphosphorylated by Cdk4, complexes between pRb and cyclin D2 and D3 become destabilized. However, this disruption may be overridden by the expression of a kinase-defective Cdk4 mutant instead of the wild type, and stable ternary complexes are formed once again.[33] This resolution suggests that the D-type cyclins may serve as multifunctional regulators by also targeting Cdk4 and other partners to specific substrates.

The D-type cyclins as well as their Cdk partners associate with proliferating cell nuclear antigen (PCNA), the auxiliary subunit of DNA polymerase delta, and with a 21 kD protein, p21.[40] As a subunit of DNA polymerase delta, PCNA is involved in DNA replication and excision repair.[41,42] The D-type cyclins, along with cyclins E and A, are implicated in the regulation of DNA replication. PCNA is not a phos-

phoprotein; however, other proteins present at replication origins are Cdk substrates.[43] The polypeptide p16, a Cdk inhibitor, binds Cdk4, resulting in destabilization of cyclin D complex formation and thus halting Cdk4 activity. The presence of p16 prevents the phosphorylation of pRb by the Cdk4–cyclin D complex that prevents the stimulation of releasing factors that would otherwise turn on DNA transcription and/or replication. This autoregulatory loop (as depicted in Figure 7.2) then comes full circle as the inactivation of pRb leads to the enhanced expression of p16 as cells approach S-phase.

Current evidence indicates that the D-type cyclins serve primarily as stimulants for the progression through the G1 stage of the cell cycle instead of as promoters of the G1/S transition. This concept is supported by the timing of D-type cyclins accumulation in relation to cyclin E. In cells

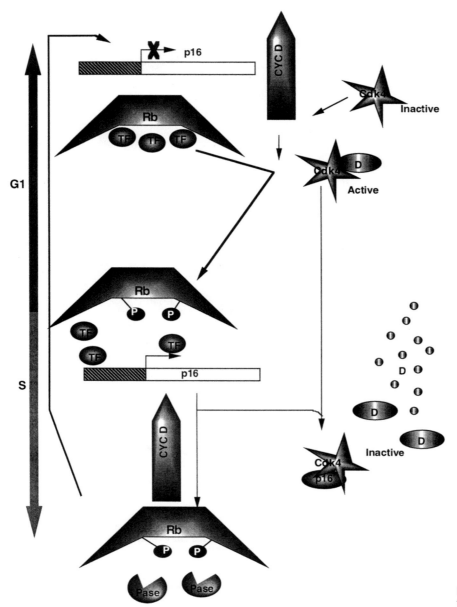

FIGURE 7.2. A schematic representation of the pRb regulatory loop.

of nonlymphoid origin, prior to the arrival of cyclin E, both cyclin D1 and Cdk4 amass in mid-G1. Cyclin D2 and its associated kinases, Cdk4 and Cdk6, accumulate early in G1 in stimulated human T lymphocytes.[30,44–47]

Cyclin D3 follows D1 and D2 in its appearance.[44,48,49] Most important, removal of growth factors from macrophages in S-phase results in a rapid decrease in cyclin D1–Cdk4 complexes; however, the cells are still capable of the completion of S-phase and division.[30] The importance of the timing of the microinjection of antisense constructs or antibodies to cyclin D1 early in G1 in order to elicit an inhibitory effect, as mentioned earlier, also lends further credence to the notion that the D-type cyclins are stimulants

for the progression through the G1 phase, rather than promoters of the G1/S transition.

The G1/S Transition

The rate-limiting factor involved in the G1/S transition is hypothesized to be cyclin E (Figure 7.1). Cyclin E associates primarily with Cdk2.[18] Currently, the precise mechanisms involved in the inactivation of cyclin E are unclear. The short half-life of the protein is thought to be mediated by its PEST sequences[28,50] because the removal of such sequences from yeast G1 cyclins increases their half-life.[51] In human foreskin fibroblasts and in Rat-1 cells the stable, ectopic overexpression of human cyclin E has been found to shorten their G1 interval, to decrease cell size, and to reduce their serum dependence for accomplishing the transition from G1 to S-phase without altering the generation time. Thus the shortened G1 interval is accompanied by lengthened S and G2 phases. The reduction in cell size suggests that the cell size may depend more on G1 cyclin levels than on the length of the cell cycle. Stepwise withdrawal of serum from the cells slowed the rate of decline in their S-phase fraction and created a less profound lengthening of their G1 interval. The generation times of the cyclin E overexpressors and the control group increase in parallel, and both growth arrest in 0.1% serum.[52,53] This finding means that cyclin E does not induce cell transformation and further, that overexpression of cyclin E retains the requirement for serum-dependent signals to continue cellular proliferation. Thus this study demonstrates that cyclin synthesis in mammalian cells is rate limiting for the G1/S transition. Possible oncogenic properties for cyclin E have been uncovered by the discovery of cyclin E overexpression in breast cancer resulting from a gene rearrangement.[54]

S-phase

Entry into S-phase does not depend on the presence of cyclins A or B.[55] The initiation of DNA replication, conversely, depends on the presence of functional cyclin A,[56] and a disruption of cyclin A function may upset the normal timely sequential relationship between the S and M phases.[57] Both cyclins A and B are first synthesized after the start of S-phase, and the synthesis and destruction of cyclin A occurs prior to that of cyclin B.[14,58] In humans, cyclin A localizes to the nucleus in interphase and is first detected near the G1/S transition, whereas cyclin B accumulates in the cytoplasm and does not enter the nucleus until just before the breakdown of the nuclear membrane.[14]

Progression through S-phase depends on the presence of cyclin A as shown by studies where the functional knockout of cyclin A–associated kinase activity, either by expression of plasmids encoding antisense cyclin A mRNA or by injection of anti–cyclin A antibodies, halts mammalian fibroblasts progression into S-phase.[56,59,60] The localization of the Cdk2–cyclin A complex to DNA replication foci by immunofluorescence,[61] and the demonstration of its ability to phosphorylate the p34 subunit of the DNA single-strand-binding protein, RPA p34,[62] illustrates the direct involvement of the Cdk2–cyclin A complex in DNA replication. A model has been proposed that implicates the cyclin A–Cdk2 complex and RPA p34 in playing an integral role in the DNA re-replication block that limits DNA synthesis to only one round of replication.[61] In this model, RPA p34, which is bound to DNA in G1-phase, is dissociated from the DNA and is translocated to the cytoplasm following phosphorylation by cyclin A–Cdk2. Within the cytoplasm, phosphatases may act on p34. As the activity of the cyclin A–Cdk2

complexes decreases in early G2, hypophosphorylated RPA p34 may regain its ability to bind DNA and signal the cell that the DNA has replicated and inhibits further DNA synthesis until the activation of Cdk2–cyclin A complexes in the next cycle, thus preventing endoreduplication.

Cyclin A–Cdk2 as well as cyclin E–Cdk2 associated subunits are able to form higher order complexes with pRb, p107 (Rb-related), and the transcription factor E2F. Such dynamic associations infer that Cdk2 may be functioning on a secondary level as a temporal regulator of gene transcription during the G1 and S phases of the cell cycle,[63] depending on which complexes it forms.

Mitosis

Cyclin B bound to p34^{cdc2} is linked to entry of the cell into the mitotic phase; however, the complex is present throughout the S and G2 phases (Figure 7.2). Hyperphosphorylation of the cyclin B–Cdc2 complex at Thr-14 and Tyr-15 within the p34^{cdc2} ATP-binding site inactivates the kinase to allow normal progression of the cell through the S and G2 phases. Dephosphorylation of the previously mentioned residues by the appropriate phosphatases and phosphorylation of the p34^{cdc2} at Thr-161 (thought to stabilize cyclin B binding) lead to activation of the p34^{cdc2} kinase and stimulate entry into mitosis.[64] Recent evidence, however, shows that the Thr-161 phosphorylation of p34^{cdc2} kinase has no effect on cyclin B binding ability, leaving the biologic significance of this event undefined.[65] This process does exhibit negative regulation in some systems. Unreplicated DNA in *Xenopus* egg extracts blocks the activation of the cyclin B–cdc2 complex by preventing the removal of the phosphates from the inhibitory sites in cdc2 (Tyr-15 and Thr-14). The inhibition of the cdc2 kinase occurs by the activation of the Wee1-Mik-1–related protein kinases that phosphorylate these residues.[66] Following successful DNA replication and progression past the G2/M transition, the cell divides and is able to exit mitosis by the abrupt degradation of cyclin B through ubiquitin mediation in anaphase. This process releases the p34^{cdc2} as a monomer, which is subsequently inactivated.[64]

CDK INHIBITORS

One of the most exciting findings in the area of the cell cycle and its connection to tumorigenesis has been the isolation of a family of small cyclin–Cdk inhibitor proteins. This discovery has uncovered an additional layer of regulation to the cell cycle machinery.

p27^{KIP1}

Cells are arrested in late G1 by inhibitors, transforming growth factor beta (TGF-β) prior to the phosphorylation of the retinoblastoma protein.[67] TGF-β inhibits the expression of Cdk4 in G1 while having no such effect on cyclin D; however, this inhibition blocks the activation of the cyclin D–Cdk4 complex Figure 7.3[68] Because overexpression of Cdk4 in TGF-β–responsive cells negates the TGF-β block of the cell cycle, this relationship suggests that the inhibition of Cdk4 expression is an important event in TGF-β–mediated cell cycle arrest. TGF-β has no effect on the expression levels of cyclin E or Cdk2; however, active cyclin E–Cdk2 complexes fail to form in cells treated with TGF-β.[69]

The TGF-β–mediated cell cycle arrest involves the indirect induction of an inhibitor of cyclin–Cdk complexes, p27[KIP1], which has recently been cloned.[20,22] The majority of p27 found in cycling cells is juxtaposed in the cyclin D–Cdk4 complexes (Figure 7.1).[68] TGF-β does not induce the transcription of p27.[20] Rather, by repressing the synthesis of Cdk4, TGF-β reduces the number of cyclin D–Cdk4 complexes, which then possibly frees p27 to inhibit other Cdks. The inactive form of cyclin E–Cdk2 in TGF-β–treated cells is found to complex with p27.[20,69]

Newly formed complexes of cyclin E–Cdk2 are activated by phosphorylation of Cdk2 on the residue Thr-160 by the activation enzyme CAK; however, the association of p27 to these new cyclin E–Cdk2 complexes effectively inhibits CAK and thus blocks the activation of the new complexes.[21] Both events, the decrease in the number of the cyclin D–Cdk4 complexes and the inactivation of the cyclin E–Cdk2 complexes, block the phosphorylation of not only pRb but also other regulatory factors by cyclin–Cdks that are necessary events for the transition of cells into S-phase.

The G1-specific cyclin–CDK inhibitor, p27[Kip1], is subject to various levels of translational and postranslational regulation, which include phosphorylation, noncovalent sequestration, and the ubiquitin-proteasome pathway. In S-phase, the abundance of p27 is regulated predominantly by specific proteolysis of the protein by the ubiquitin-proteasome pathway.[70] While in quiescent cells (G0), the accumulation of p27 is caused by an increase in the synthesis rate of p27 resulting from an enhancement in the amount of p27 mRNA associated in polyribosomes.[71] The complexity of the regulation of p27 increases considering that p27 also serves as a substrate for the cyclin E–Cdk2 kinase, whose activity p27 inhibits.[72] A kinetic model has been proposed where the binding of ATP to the Cdk determines whether p27 acts as a negative regulator of the cyclin–Cdk complex (low ATP concentrations, $<50~\mu M$) or as a substrate (higher ATP concentrations >1 mM).[72] Cyclin E–Cdk2 specifically phosphorylates p27 on threonine-187, which is a conserved C-terminal Cdk target site (TPKK).[72–74] Mutational analysis has shown that the selective degradation of p27 by the proteasome pathway depends on the association of p27 with active cyclin E–Cdk2 and subsequent phosphorylation by Cdk2 on the TPKK site.[74]

Because p27 is targeted by the adenovirus E1A oncoprotein,[75] the human papillomavirus E7 oncoprotein dissociates p27 from cyclin–Cdk complexes,[76] p27-deficient mice develop tumors of the pituitary gland with 100% penetrance,[77,78] and overexpression of p27 using a recombinant adenoviral vector triggers apoptosis in several different human cancer cell lines;[79] p27 is thought to be involved in

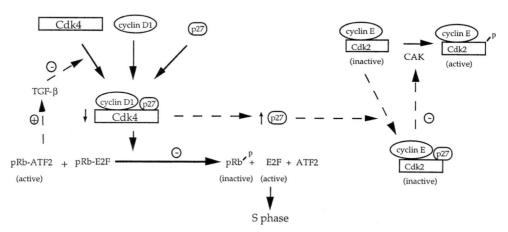

FIGURE 7.3. A model of the actions of the growth inhibitor transforming factor (TGF-β). TGF-β inhibits the expression of Cdk4 in the G1-phase of the cell cycle, leading to a decrease in the number of cyclin D–Cdk4 complexes. Because the majority of the Cdk-inhibitor p27 in cycling cells is found juxtaposed in the cyclin D–Cdk4 complexes, this results in an indirect induction of p27. The association of p27 with newly formed cyclin E–Cdk2 complexes inhibits their activation by CAK. The suppression and inhibition of cyclin D–Cdk4 and cyclin E–Cdk2 prevents the phosphorylation of pRb and the release of the E2F transcription factor required for the progression into S-phase. pRb is also able to bind and enhance the transcription factor ATF-2, which is thought to be involved in the expression of TGF-β, thus serving as a positive feedback loop for the G1 growth arrest.

neoplastic transformation. However, studies examining the genomic structure of p27 in cancer cell lines and primary human tumors have either failed to find abnormalities in the p27^{Kip1} gene in a variety of cancers[80] or have found p27 mutations to be rare.[81] The scarcity of p27 mutations found to date does not necessarily mean that this cell cycle regulatory protein is not involved in tumorigenesis, especially considering the complex levels of regulation of this protein. In fact, enhanced ubiquitin-proteasome–mediated degradation of p27 is found in aggressive colorectal carcinomas[82] and in NSCLC, where p27 is an independent prognostic factor correlating with the overall survival time of the patients.[83] In essence, functional inactivation of p27 is associated with tumorigenesis.

p21

Other mammalian Cdk inhibitors in addition to p27 have also been found, including p21, p16, p15, and p18 to name a few. In fact, p21 is the first Cdk inhibitor to be isolated, discovered simultaneously by several laboratories using various approaches, and has been termed Cip1, p21, p20^{CAP1}, Waf1, and Sdi1.[84–88] The importance of p21 presently seems to lie in three areas: (a) the p21 gene is transcriptionally regulated by the tumor suppressor protein p53;[87] (b) p21 is a Cdk inhibitor,[84,86] and (c) p21 may block the entry of senescent cells into the cell cycle.[88] In fact, p21 inactivation in normal diploid human fibroblasts by two sequential rounds of targeted homologous recombination renders cells capable of bypassing senescence. Cells lacking p21 fail to arrest the cell cycle in response to DNA damage at the checkpoint between the prereplicative phase of growth and the phase of chromosome replication; however, their apoptotic response and genomic stability are intact.[89] Interestingly, p21 induction during initiation of terminal differentiation occurs in a p53-independent manner.[90] This independence hints to a more universal function for p21 in differentiation as well as growth control. The Cdk inhibitors p21 and p27 share 44% identity in their amino-terminal regions, and *in vitro* p27 is able to inhibit the same gamut of Cdks as p21.[21] Normal fibroblasts exhibit a wide range of cyclin–Cdk complexes associated with p21. Strong associations occur with cyclin D–Cdk4 and cyclin E–Cdk2 complexes in the G1/S transition, as well as to the cyclin A–Cdk2 complex during mitosis.[40,84,85,91] However, cyclin B–Cdc2 forms only a weak partnership with p21 in M phase.[40] The strength of association of the cyclin–Cdk complexes with p21 is directly proportional to the ability of p21 to inhibit their functions *in vitro*. In addition to exerting negative control of the G1/S-phase transition, p21 may play a role at the onset of mitosis. In nontransformed fibroblasts, near the G2/M-phase boundary, p21 transiently reaccumulates in the nucleus, concurrent with the nuclear translocation of cyclin B1, and associates with a fraction of cyclin A–Cdk and cyclin B1–Cdk2 complexes in normal fibro-

blasts. Premitotic nuclear accumulation of cyclin B1 is reduced or not detectable in cells that are nullizygous for p21 (p21 − / −), cells such as fibroblasts transformed by the viral human papillomavirus type 16 E6 oncoprotein, which functionally inactivates p53, or tumor-derived cells with low p21 levels. Such cells exhibit accelerated entry into mitosis with concomitant higher levels of cyclin A- and cyclin B-associated kinase activities. This correlation suggests that p21 may aid the execution of late cell cycle checkpoint controls by promoting a transient interlude late in G2.[92]

In response to DNA damage, the expression levels of p53 dramatically increase, which leads to the transcriptional induction of DNA damage inducible genes. Within the promoter of the p21 gene are two consensus p53-binding sites.[87] Exposure of cells to DNA-damaging agents enhances transcription of p21, leading to the agglomeration of p21 in cyclin E–Cdk2 immune complexes. This reaction culminates in decreased kinase activity that is thought to mediate the G1 arrest of the cell cycle.[93,94] This scenario only occurs if the cells have wild-type p53 (and fails with mutant p53), thus supporting the hypothesis that p21 is the primary mediator of p53-dependent G1 arrest. Ectopic overexpression of p21 alone in normal fibroblasts is also able to elicit growth arrest.[84,88] Basal levels of p21 may also depend on the functional activity of p53 because p21 is absent from the Cdk complexes of various transformed cell lines lacking an active p53.[40,87,93] To date p21 mutants have not yet been identified in human cancers, thus leading medical researchers to look for additional p53-inducible genes involved in growth regulation.

In addition to serving in DNA-damage checkpoint regulation by causing G1 arrest through the inhibition of Cdks, the p21 protein has also been implemented in the cells proofreading system during cellular replication to improve fidelity. PCNA enhances processivity of DNA polymerase delta (pol D) by forming a homotrimer that holds the complex of pol D with its replication factor C (RFC) to the DNA template to allow synthesis of both the leading and lagging strands of DNA. *In vitro* studies show that p21 can effectively associate with PCNA and block pol D–dependent DNA replication, which may be overcome only by the addition of PCNA.[95,96] p21 may be serving important functions in this manner. p21 may be acting to reduce the processivity of the lagging strand, which is desirable because the rate-limiting step here is the dissociation of the DNA polymerase at the end of the Okazaki fragment. By inhibiting the elongation step of polymerization.[96] p21 is effectively slowing the replicative process to allow for the proofreading mechanisms of the replicative machinery to correct any errors in replication. The *in vivo* verification of these results is still pending. Whether p21 is able to affect other functions of PCNA is not currently known. This relationship is of interest because PCNA is also involved in excision repair. Here, one may again hypothesize a role for p21 in decreasing the processivity of the DNA polymerase repair complex because this activity would be beneficial in filling the excision repair gaps. If this correlation is the case, eukaryotes would have another similarity with bacteria because bacteria alter the processivity of polymerase III by interactions with proteins, where eukaryotes were thought before to augment processivity only by the implementation of three different DNA polymerases. This new model calls for a higher order of regulation of processivity of DNA polymerase than once thought.

p16[INK4]

The Cdk inhibitor p16, also known as Multiple Tumor Suppressor 1 (MTS1), is implicated as a tumor-suppressor gene directly linked to the cell cycle.[97] In certain transformed cells lacking the normal components of the Cdk4 complexes, such as the D-type cyclins, PCNA, and sometimes p21,[40] Cdk6 is found in association with p16. Complex formation of p16 with Cdk4 is thought to block or upset the D-type cyclin association.[23] This dissociation contrasts with the inhibitory mechanisms employed by the Cdk inhibitors, p21 and p27. p16 is the first Cdk inhibitor where structural homologues such as MTS2 (p15) have been indicated.[97] Also, p16 seems to have a higher selectivity than the other two Cdk inhibitors because p16 appears to specifically inhibit the D-type Cdks, Cdk4 and Cdk6. These unique characteristics of p16 suggest that this protein may play a specialized and important role in growth regulation. In addition, the human p16 gene maps to chromosome 9p21 (MTS1 locus), a region that is often deleted in gliomas and melanomas.[97,98] MTS1 is found homozygously deleted in cell lines derived from tumors of lung, breast, brain, bone, skin, bladder, kidney, ovary, and lymphocytes. In addition, nonsense, missense, or frameshift mutations are found in at least one copy of the gene in melanoma cell lines.[97] However, only 10% to 20% of primary tumors demonstrate an alteration in the locus.[97,99]

Direct evidence of the inhibitory ability of p16 on cell growth has been provided. Ectopic expression of p16 effectively blocks entry into S-phase of cells induced to proliferate by the H-*ras* oncogene and suppresses cellular transformation by oncogenic H-*ras* and *Myc*.[100] As an inhibitor of G1 Cdks (Cdk4/6), p16 serves as an upstream regulator of the tumor-suppressor pRb as they cooperate through feedback mechanisms to regulate cell cycle progression.[101,102] Essentially, pRb becomes hyperphosphorylated by the D-type cyclin-associated kinases in late G1 and subsequently releases several active transcription factors that induce transcription of p16. As p16 expression reaches threshold levels, the kinase activity of Cdk4/6 is inhibited. Phosphatases then return pRb to its active hypophosphorylated form, allowing pRb to sequester the transcription factors and thereby down-regulate the p16 promoter to a basal transcription level (Figure 7.2).[101] Supporting this model, cells that are nullizygous for the RB gene (RB −/−) overexpress the p16

gene, which disrupts the formation of complexes between Cdk4/6 and the D-type cyclins[102] such that no cyclin D–Cdk complexes are detectable.[103] The dependence on endogenous wild-type pRb for ectopic expression of p16 or p16-related proteins p15 and p18, homologues of the cyclin D–Cdk 4 inhibitor p16 that form binary complexes *in vitro* and *in vivo* with Cdk4/6, to suppress cell growth also supports the idea that p16 and pRb are involved in the same pathway.[23,104]

p15[INK4b/MTS2]

The TGF-β pathway also involves the induction of a Cdk-inhibitor, p15[INK4b/MTS2], a p16 homologue that also maps to the 9p21 locus. TGF-β transactivates p15, which inhibits the D-type–Cdk complexes (Cdk4/Cdk6).[105] This reaction releases additional p27 to inhibit other Cdks and thus promotes cell cycle arrest. The p15[INK4b/MTS2] gene is homozygously deleted in 20% of primary advanced head and neck squamous cell carcinomas.[106] Deletion of the p16/p15 locus (9p21) is common in NSCLC.[107] In multiple myeloma, a high incidence of p16 and p15 alterations occur solely by hypermethylation of the 5′ CpG islands, such that these alterations are the most common genetic abnormalities in this disease. Hypermethylation of p16/p15 is associated with blastic disease, whereas concomitant hypermethylation of both genes is related to development of plasmacytoma.[108] Additionally, codeletion of p16 and p15 in pancreatic tumors is found often.[109]

TUMOR SUPPRESSORS

The Retinoblastoma Protein (RB1)

The genetic characteristics and the epidemiologic studies of Knudson concerning familial and nonfamilial retinoblastoma led to the "Knudson Two-hit Hypothesis." This hypothesis laid the groundwork for the discovery of tumor-suppressor genes and for a revolutionary new way of thinking about oncogenesis. Knudson concluded that the familial form of retinoblastoma results when an individual inherits a mutant (nonfunctional) allele from the affected parent, and the childhood tumor manifests when the wild-type (normal) allele of the same gene is functionally "knocked out" by a somatic event, resulting in LOH. The nonfamilial form of retinoblastoma requires two separate somatic mutations of both alleles of the gene and thus accounts for the sporadic nature of this form of retinoblastoma and its appearance later in life.[2] Subsequent studies confirmed that all retinoblastomas carry mutations in both alleles of the same gene. Prior to this finding oncogenesis was thought to evolve by dominantly acting oncogenes, which could only occur by somatic mutations because the dominant oncogenic phenotype would result in the gestational death of the embryo if it were acquired from the germline. So, for the first time, a recessive mutation conferring an inherited increased risk of neoplasia could be envisioned. The finding of deletions on chromosome 13q14 in both familial and sporadic retinoblastomas[110,111] supported the Knudson hypothesis and lead to the eventual cloning of the first tumor-suppressor gene, the retinoblastoma gene, RB.[112-114]

The retinoblastoma gene encodes a 105 kDa protein product, pRb. The nuclear phosphoprotein, pRb, serves as a negative regulator of cell cycle progression, at least in some specific cell types. RB transcripts are present in all normal tissues examined.[114] In cell lines that lack a functional pRb protein, the restoration of pRb function, by either microinjection of the protein in early to mid-G1 or by transfection of the cDNA, arrests cell growth in the G1-phase of the cell cycle.[115-117] This inhibition of cell growth by pRb depends on the sequences necessary for the interaction of pRb with the transcription factor E2F, as well as a number of oncoproteins from human DNA viruses such as E1A, T antigen, and E7 (from adenovirus, simian virus 40 [SV40], and human papillomavirus, respectively).[118-121] Binding of pRb to this set of associated proteins occurs at a specific "pocket region" in pRb.

The "pocket region" of RB is also a common site of mutation in many human tumors, and it has been found altered or deleted in nearly all RB mutants from the tumors thus far examined.[111,122] Inactivation of RB function involves various genetic lesions, including large-scale deletions and splicing mutations resulting in the deletion of an exon.[123,124] Smaller deletions in the promoter region of RB and point mutations have also been found.[125,126] Genetic mutations in RB have been demonstrated in several human tumors such as osteosarcomas, bladder carcinomas, prostate carcinomas, breast carcinomas, small cell lung carcinomas, cervical carcinomas, and leukemias.[127]

pRb and the Cell Cycle

Posttranscriptional regulation of pRb involves changes in the phosphorylation state of pRb throughout the cell cycle.[128,129] During the G0 and G1 phases of the cell cycle, pRb is found in a hypophosphorylated form, which becomes increasingly phosphorylated on serine and threonine residues as the cell cycle progresses. The cell cycle–dependent phosphorylation of pRb may occur in several steps. In primary human T lymphocytes, pRb probably undergoes phosphorylation at discrete residues during three phases of the cell cycle: late G1, S-phase, and again, in G2/M.[128] All phosphorylations of pRb are on serine-threonine residues; to date, no evidence exists for phosphorylation on tyrosine residues in pRb.[129,130] As the cells emerge from mitosis and enter into the G1-phase again, or become senescent in G0, pRb is dephosphorylated back to its hypophosphorylated form, possibly by pp1 phosphatase.[131] The viral oncoproteins and the transcription factor E2F bind specifically to hypophosphorylated pRb.[118-121] Microinjection studies

show that hypophosphorylated pRb is the physiologically active form;[115] it exhibits the growth-suppressive function that can be inactivated in G1 by phosphorylation or by dimerization with viral oncoproteins to allow DNA replication.

The specific kinase(s) responsible for the *in vivo* phosphorylation of pRb is/are currently not known. Several Cdks have been found in association with pRb *in vivo* in a region similar to "the pocket." The A, B, D, and E Cdks as well as the recently discovered Cdc2-related kinase PITALRE (now known as Cdk9),[132] phosphorylate pRb *in vitro*.[68,84,116,133-135] Considering the timing of phosphorylation of pRb, as well as the peak activity intervals of the Cdks and their interactive abilities, it seems plausible that pRb is phosphorylated by the D-type–dependent kinases in early G1, cyclin E–Cdk2 at the G1/S transition, and by the cyclin A–Cdc2 complex at the G2/M transition. After completion of the cell cycle, cells generated by the mitotic process again display hypophosphorylated pRb caused by specific phosphatase activities. The Cdk inhibitors further guarantee the stringent timing of the activity of the Cdk complexes on pRb.[136] Because Interleukin 2 is stimulatory and TGF-β is inhibitory to cyclin E–Cdk2 activity, this offers one possible route by which exogenous growth-regulatory signals influence pRb and the cell cycle machinery.[20,69]

Phosphorylation of pRb by the D-type–dependent kinases may play a key role in overriding the G1 cell cycle arrest of pRb. Microinjection of cyclin D antibodies into RB +/+ cells but not into the RB −/− tumor cell line, SAOS-2 (human osteosarcoma), blocks entry into S-phase.[38] This reaction suggests that pRb may indeed be the key substrate for the D cyclins. Several cell lines harboring mutated, or pRb inactivated, by the expression of the oncoprotein SV40 large T antigen, exhibit an enhanced expression of the specific cyclin D–Cdk4 kinase inhibitor, p16.[23] Additionally, cell lines, which fail to express functional p16, are resistant to the growth-suppressive effects of ectopic pRb expression.[117] This resistance reflects the cooperative effort and codependence of p16 and pRb in regulating cell cycle progression, as shown in Figure 7.2.

pRb Cellular Targets

Functioning as a transcriptional regulator through the modulation of the activity of several transcription factors, pRb exerts its growth-suppressive effects. pRb binds directly to the transcription factor ATF-2 and enhances its activity.[137] ATF-2 is thought to be involved in the expression of TGF-β. In this example, pRb may actually upregulate the expression of TGF-β and thereby lead to growth suppression through the expression of this growth inhibitor. As discussed previously, TGF-β would in turn disrupt and inactivate the cyclin D–Cdk4 complexes, leading to the release of the Cdk inhibitor p27 and the effective inhibition of cyclin E–Cdk2 (Figure 7.3). This process would prevent the phosphorylation of pRb and thus serve as a positive feedback loop to block progression into S-phase.

The transcription factor E2F, first identified as a DNA-binding protein required for E1A-mediated induction of the adenovirus E2 promoter, binds to hypophosphorylated pRb in the "pocket region" during the G0 and G1 phases of the cell cycle.[15,63,118,138,139] E2F binding sites are located in the promoters of multiple growth-promoting and growth-responsive genes such as c-*myc*, c-*myb*, dihydrofolate reductase (DHFR), thymidine kinase (TK), thymidine synthetase, DNA polymerase alpha, RB, the gene for the Rb-related protein p107, cyclin A, cyclin D1, cdc2, and E2F-1 itself.[15,140,141] The heterodimer of pRb-E2F is thought to sequester the active form of E2F and in effect block the transactivation of genes, whose products are necessary for DNA synthesis.[63,141] The inhibition of transactivation potential of E2F-1 by pRb may occur by targeting a repressor domain to the transcription complex or by physically blocking the interaction of E2F-1 with a separate component of the transcription complex.[142] Association with the viral oncoproteins or the phosphorylation of pRb releases E2F in its functional form, which is then able to promote the transcription of genes required for S-phase entry and completion. The adenovirus early region 1 transforming proteins not only liberate the active form of E2F but also stabilize the protein by inhibiting targeted proteolysis of the transcription factor.[143]

Recently, four E2F-related proteins (E2F-2, E2F-3, E2F-4, and E2F-5) have been isolated and shown to share homologous domains with E2F;[144–147] thus confirming the speculation that an E2F family may exist. E2F binds as a heterodimer to DNA with dimerization partner-1 (DP1) (Figure 7.1).[148,149] DP1 is actually the patriarch of a family of DP genes with their own protooncogenic properties that are able to dimerize with E2F family members.[150–152] Besides the sequestering of E2F by pRb, the activity of the E2F/DP1 heterodimer is further regulated during the cell cycle by phosphorylation of DP1. As the phosphorylation level of DP1 increases, the DNA-binding activity of E2F/DP1 decreases proportionally.[153] Because a cyclin A–binding domain is located in the amino-terminus of E2F-1, cyclin A–Cdk2 is the most likely candidate for the late S-phase phosphorylation of DP1.[154] Moreover, cyclin A–Cdk2 interacts with E2F-1 directly both *in vivo* and *in vitro* and phosphorylates E2F-1, thereby inhibiting the DNA-binding activity of the E2F-1/DP-1 complex.[155] The regulation of transcriptional activity is made even more complex considering the involvement of the Rb-family proteins, p107 and pRb2/p130. The Rb-family is capable of association with the E2F family. This interaction seems to be temporally modulated and varies among family members. Several sources of data suggest that pRb and p107 associate with distinct E2F species. The *in vivo* results demonstrate that E2F-1, E2F-2, E2F-3, and E2F-4 all form complexes with pRb, but E2Fs one through three do not interact with

p107.[156] E2F4 and E2F5 were both cloned by their ability to interact with pRb2/p130. E2F4 undergoes complex formation *in vivo* with pRb2/p130 during G0 and G1, then later associates with p107 and pRb in late G1 and S phases as the levels of these regulators increase.[145–147,157] The vast majority of endogenous E2F activity stems from E2F-4. In fact, during G1 E2F-4 accounts for almost all of the free activity. During S-phase an equal mixture of E2F-4 and E2F-1 constitutes the free E2F activity.[157]

Another important feature of the interaction between pRb and E2F-dependent gene repression is that pRb protects E2F-1 from proteolytic degradation by the ubiquitin-proteasome pathway.[143,158,159] Furthermore, the antagonistic effect of pRb on E2F activity not only blocks transcription of growth-promoting genes but also may be the mechanism by which pRb protects against apoptosis in differentiating cells. Overexpression of E2F-1 induces apoptosis following entry of the cells into S-phase in cells with a wild-type p53 gene, but it favors proliferation in cells null for p53 (p53 −/−).[160,161] Coexpression of pRb with E2F-1 blocks the induction of apoptosis by E2F-1.[160] Additionally, studies involving homozygous disruption of the E2F-1 gene indicate that E2F plays a physiologic role in normal development, more than likely by the induction of apoptosis in a specific set of developing cells. This conclusion comes from the finding that at an early stage of development, mice null for the E2F1 gene show defects in cell types in which apoptosis plays a significant role in their terminal differentiation, such as epithelial cells of the testis and other exocrine glands and T-cells. Later in life these animals develop widespread tumors.[162,163] The stochastic levels of pRb and E2F-1 may prove to be critical not only in regulating cell cycle progression but also in determining cell fate and cellular specialization. Because terminal differentiation invariably involves permanent withdrawal from the cell cycle,[164] and because apoptosis is a constant phenomena in differentiating cells,[165] key proteins regulating such events would be predicted to be multifunctional in nature.

pRb and Cellular Differentiation

In addition to the role of pRb as a checkpoint regulator of the cell cycle, the protein is also implicated in cellular differentiation through complex formation and subsequent modulation of various tissue-specific transcription factors. The retinoblastoma protein is implicated in playing an integral role in adipogenesis, myogenesis, and hematopoiesis.[166] Members of the MyoD bHLH transcription factor family associate with pRb, and the binding of pRb to MyoD is thought to induce activation of muscle-specific genes. In fact, cell lines that lack a functional pRb are unable to undergo myogenic conversion. This ability points to a possible role of pRb in the myogenic activation of MyoD.[167] Similarly, in murine fibroblasts pRb activates CCAAT/enhancer-binding proteins (C/EBPs), a family of transcription factors crucial for adipocyte differentiation. The C/EBP zinc finger transcription factor and pRb form a complex in the E2F pocket-binding domain of pRb. Furthermore, conversion of fibroblasts to adipocytes by C/EBP transfection requires the presence of a functional retinoblastoma protein.[168] Furthermore, an intact retinoblastoma susceptibility protein family binding domain in SV40 large T-antigen is necessary for deletion mutants of this oncoprotein to block adipocyte differentiation.[169] This requirement further demonstrates that the Rb-family proteins are important in regulating adipocyte differentiation. Evidence directly links pRb with several other transcription factors that are involved in the withdrawal from the cell cycle and the induction of differentiation,[167,170] such as the brahma-related gene 1 (BRG1).

Perhaps the most convincing evidence for the importance of pRb in cellular differentiation and specialization stems from the studies of RB knockout mice. Homogeneous germline disruptions of the RB gene (RB −/−) are lethal mutations, with the mice dying *in utero* by the fourteenth day of gestation and manifesting gross defects in the development of the hematopoietic and central nervous systems.

The heterozygous mice (RB +/−) mature normally until 9 months of age when they develop thyroid and intermediate lobe pituitary tumors. Surprisingly, they show no indication of retinoblastoma.[171,172] The fact that the vast majority of cell division cycles in the RB −/− embryos occur without the presence of pRb suggests that other proteins, possibly the Rb-family members, can complement pRb function, or perhaps the cell can elicit a different signal transduction pathway to regulate the activities of proliferation. These results also point to pRb involvement in neurogenesis and hematopoiesis. The link between pRb and hematopoiesis is supported by recent transcriptional studies indicating that the RB gene plays an erythroid- and stage-specific functional role in normal human adult hematopoiesis, particularly at the level of late erythroid hematopoietic progenitor cells.[173]

Rb-Family

The "pocket region" of pRb is shared by two additional E1A-associated proteins, which has led to the identification of two members of the Rb-family, p107, and pRb2/p130.[117,174,175] All three Rb-family members (also known as pocket proteins) localize primarily to the nuclear compartment of the cell.[114,174,176] A schematic picture of pRb, p107, and pRb2/p130 is shown in Figure 7.4 highlighting the zones of high homology among the family members.

Essentially, the structures consist of (a) the N-terminal portion; (b) the pocket structure subdivided into domain A, spacer, and domain B; and (c) the C-terminal portion, also called domain C. The pocket functional domains A and B are the most conserved and are responsible for most of the interactions involving both endogenous proteins and viral oncoproteins. Amino acid comparisons of the three protein sequences of the Rb-family suggest a closer relationship of pRb2/p130 to p107.[175] Beyond the high structural homology, phylogenetic studies show that pRb is specific to vertebrates; however, p107 and pRb2/p130, which form their own subfamily defined by their homologous spacer region, are common to plants, insects, and vertebrates.[177,178]

Similar to pRb, ectopic expression of p107 and pRb2/p130 is able to suppress the growth of the osteosarcoma cell line SAOS-2.[116,117,121,179] Recent functional studies of p107 and pRb2/p130 indicate that although the Rb-family members may be able to complement each other, the proteins are not fully functionally redundant. Unlike pRb, both p107 and pRb2/p130 form stable complexes with cyclin A, cyclin E and Cdk2 *in vitro* and *in vivo*.[180–184]

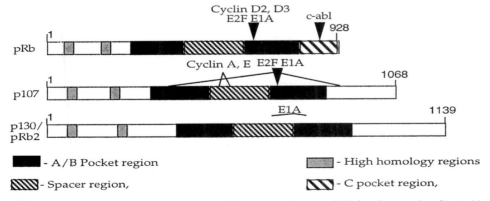

FIGURE 7.4. A schematic representation of the retinoblastoma (RB) family proteins. (From M. Paggi, Baldi A, Bonnetto F, et al., in "Retinoblastoma protein family in cell cycle and cancer," *J Cell Biochem* 1996;62:419, with permission.)

Both p107 and pRb2/p130 undergo cell cycle–dependent phosphorylation similar to pRb. As with pRb, p107 phosphorylation is cell cycle regulated with a high level of hyperphosphorylated p107 present during S-phase and at the G2/M transition.[185] The major complex responsible for p107 phosphorylation is the cyclin D1–Cdk4 complex.[182,186,187] As far as pRb2/p130 is concerned, it displays evident cell cycle changes in phosphorylation, coupled to an extensive microheterogeneity in SDS-PAGE migration pattern.[176,183,188] From a functional point of view, cyclins A, D-type, and E overexpression rescue pRb2/p130-mediated growth arrest in SAOS-2 human osteosarcoma cells.[183] This rescue may result from the cyclins targeting pRb2/p130 for phosphorylation and subsequent inactivation, and/or pRb2/p130 may negatively modulate cdk activity.

Additionally, pRb, p107, and pRb2/p130 all form complexes with specific E2F family members, as detailed previously.[118,145,146,156,185,189] However, the temporal order of complex formation appears to vary. For example, the binding of p107 to E2F is first detected at the G1-S boundary and remains stable throughout S-phase.[185,189] On the other hand, pRb-E2F complexes are found in the G1-phase and then dissociate in late G1.[118,119] The main form of E2F detected in the G0 to G1 phases in primary mouse fibroblasts is E2F bound to pRb2/p130, which is then replaced by p107-E2F complexes in late G1.[188] Therefore, pRb2/p130 is the major negative modulator of E2F activity in quiescent cells.

Similar to the case for pRb and E2F-1, p107 and pRb2/p130 through complex formation with E2F-4 stabilize the protein and protect E2F-4 from targeted proteolysis by the ubiquitin-proteasome pathway. Stabilization of the p107- and pRb2/p130-E2F4 complexes is thought to contribute to maintaining a state of active transcriptional repression in quiescent cells.[143] Unlike E2F-1, E2F-2, or E2F-3, which are constitutively nuclear, E2F-4 and E2F-5 lack a nuclear localization signal. The subcellular localization of E2F-4 is regulated in a cell cycle–dependent manner with high nuclear/cytoplasmic ratios in G0 and early G1, with a progressive increase in cytoplasmic E2F-4 as the cells proceed toward S-phase.[190] Co-transfection studies indicate that cellular compartmentalization of E2F-4 and E2F-5 becomes nuclear by complex formation with p107, pRb2/p130, DP-2, and/or DP-3δ.[190–192] E2F-4 nuclear accumulation induced by pRb2/p130 and p107 correlates with cell growth arrest, whereas overexpression of E2F-4 with DP-3δ stimulates reentry into the cell cycle in previously quiescent cells. This E2F-4/DP-3δ reactivation of the cell cycle, however, is efficiently counteracted by overexpression of either p107 or pRb2/p130.[192]

Genetic analysis of mice homozygously deleted for each of the retinoblastoma family members, as well as combined deletions of the p107 and RB genes and targeted disruptions of the RB2/p130 and p107 genes, further demonstrates that the Rb-family proteins have unique but partly overlapping functions that are required for the proper development and maintenance of vertebrate organisms.[171,172,193–195] The expression patterns of the Rb-family members during early development of wild-type mice correlates well with the tissue-specific damage elicited by the absence of different sets of the Rb-family proteins.[196] Moreover, deletion of different members of the Rb-family results in altered expression patterns of E2F-regulated genes in mouse embryonic fibroblasts (MEF) prepared from embryos of the knockout mice.[197] Severe deregulation of E2F-dependent transcription occurs in RB −/− and p107 −/−; RB2/p130 −/− double mutants, resulting in improper expression of S-phase–promoting and cell cycle–responsive genes such as p107 and pRb in RB2/p130 −/− MEFs, cyclin E in RB −/− MEFs, and cyclin A, b-myb, and E2F-1 in p107 −/−; RB2/p130 −/− MEFs.[197] This expression clearly demonstrates differences among the Rb-family in the transcriptional regulation of distinct genes.

Each of the retinoblastoma family proteins elicit cell cycle growth arrest in a unique manner. The E1A mutant pm928 that binds p107, but fails to bind pRb and pRb2/p130, is able to initiate DNA synthesis, but the transformation property of the oncoprotein is abrogated.[134,198,199] This condition implies that pRb2/p130 and pRb may elicit repression of cell cycle progression at similar checkpoints. Growth suppression by pRb requires an intact E1A oncoprotein-binding domain, whereas p107 does not.[116,117] p107 contains two functional domains that are able to block cell cycle progression independently in a cell type–specific manner. One domain, like pRb, corresponds to the sequences necessary for association with the transcription factor E2F. The interaction domain for cyclin A and cyclin E complexes forms the other. Only the cyclin-binding domain is an active growth suppressor in the cervical carcinoma cell line C33A, which is sensitive to p107-but resistant to pRb-mediated growth suppression.[200] This relationship illustrates an important functional difference between pRb and p107. Additionally, p107 and pRb2/p130, similar to the p21 family of Cdk inhibitors, can inhibit the phosphorylation of target substrates by cyclin A–Cdk2 and cyclin E–Cdk2 complexes through a structurally and functionally conserved kinase inhibitory domain in their N-terminal region. This domain also serves as an independent growth-suppressive domain.[201–203] The interactions between p21 and p107 with cyclin–Cdk2 complexes are mutually exclusive. p53-mediated induction of p21 levels in response to DNA damage leads to the dissociation of p107–cyclin–Cdk2 complexes to form p21–cyclin–Cdk2 complexes.[202] Furthermore, p107-E2F complexes dissociate upon activation of the p107-bound cyclin–Cdk kinases.[202] Together, these results suggest that different families of proteins, in a mutually exclusive manner in response to certain signals, can affect cdk activity, thereby regulating macromolecular assembly. Intriguingly, a unique domain of pRb2/p130 within the spacer region also acts as an inhibitor of Cdk2 kinase activity separate from that of p107. Increased expression of pRb2/p130 during various cellular processes correlates with decreased kinase activity of Cdk2. This correlation demonstrates that pRb2/p130 may act not only to bind and modify E2F activity but also to inhibit Cdk2 kinase activity in concert with p21 in a manner different from p107.[201]

Most interestingly, the T98G human glioblastoma cell line, which is resistant to the suppression effect of both pRb and p107,[117] demonstrates a drastic reduction in cellular proliferation upon overexpression of pRb2/p130.[179] This reaction suggests that pRb2/p130 may function in a completely different pathway than that of p107 or pRb, and that certain mutation(s) within the T98G cells predisposes them to be sensitive to the effects of pRb2/p130 but not to those of p107 or pRb. An alternate explanation may be that the three proteins may share functional properties, whereas pRb2/p130 has an additional property that p107 and pRb2 are unable to complement in this particular cell line.

In addition to these differences, no evidence supports the notion that p107 is normally a tumor suppressor. To date no examples of naturally occurring mutations of p107 have been found, despite the testing of several hundred human tumor samples and cell lines. In addition, p107 maps to chromosome 20q.11.2, a region not commonly found to be cytogenetically altered in human neoplasms.[174] Furthermore, the expression of p107 in cell lines derived

from retinoblastoma tumors implies that p107 is unable to complement the lack of pRb and to suppress tumor formation.[204] However, pRb2/p130 maps to human chromosome 16q12.2,[205] an area in which deletions have been found in several human neoplasms, including breast, ovarian, hepatic, and prostatic cancers.[205]

The introduction of wild-type pRb2/p130 in HONE-1 cells, a cell line of human nasopharyngeal carcinoma (NPC) that endogenously expresses a genetically altered form of pRb2/p130 at a very low level, causes a significant reduction in cell proliferation and a change in morphology.[179] The HONE-1 cell line expresses the RB gene product with normal size and abundance, and no point mutation has been detected in the common sites for RB mutations.[206] NPC shows no detectable retinoblastoma-susceptibility gene alterations.[206] These recent findings hint to a possible involvement of pRb2/p130 in nasopharyngeal carcinogenesis in the face of a functionally intact RB gene. NPC is a rare disease in most parts of the world; however, the disease has a racial and geographic distribution. The people of Southern China are among those that deviate from the low-risk profile so much that NPC is the most common cancer in the city of Guangzhow (Canton) and constitutes 32% of all cancer.[207,208] Furthermore, immunohistochemical studies indicate that lack of pRb2/p130 expression plays a role in the formation and/or progression of lung (Tables 7.1, 7.2, 7.3)[209,210] and endometrial cancer (Table 7.4 and Figure 7.5).[211] Serving as an independent prognostic factor, the expression level of pRb2/p130 is able to predict patient outcome and to identify groups of patients at a greater risk of

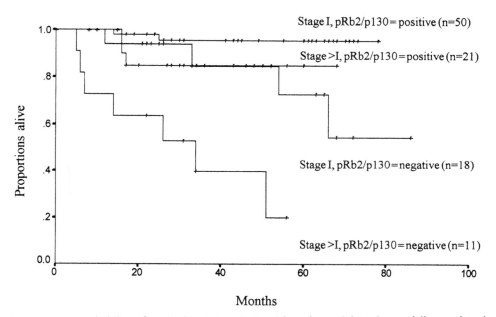

FIGURE 7.5. Probability of survival in 100 patients with endometrial carcinoma (all stages) and pRb2/p130 positive or -negative tumors. (From T. Susini, Baldi F, Howard CM, et al. "Expression of the retinoblastoma-related gene Rb2/p130 correlates with clinical outcome in endometrial cancer," *J Clin Oncol* 1998;16:1091, with permission.)

TABLE 7.1. RB-FAMILY PROTEINS AND PCNA EXPRESSION IN LUNG CANCER

Type	Grading	pRb/p105	p107	pRb2/p130	PCNA	Type	Grading	pRb/p105	p107	pRb2/p130	PCNA
squamous	3	3	2	0	2	adenocarcinoma	3	2	2	0	3
squamous	2	3	1	3	3	adenocarcinoma	1	2	1	2	1
squamous	1	3	1	3	2	adenocarcinoma	2	1	2	1	3
squamous	1	3	1	3	2	adenocarcinoma	2	2	1	1	1
squamous	2	2	1	2	2	adenocarcinoma	2	1	2	0	3
squamous	2	2	1	3	2	adenocarcinoma	2	2	1	1	1
squamous	3	3	1	1	2	adenocarcinoma	1	2	1	2	1
squamous	2	2	1	3	2	adenocarcinoma	3	2	2	0	3
squamous	2	2	1	1	2	adenocarcinoma	1	2	1	2	1
squamous	2	1	1	3	2	adenocarcinoma	3	2	2	0	3
squamous	2	2	1	3	2	adenocarcinoma	2	1	2	1	3
squamous	1	3	1	3	2	adenocarcinoma	2	2	1	0	1
squamous	3	1	1	1	3	bronchioloalveolar		2	1	3	3
squamous	1	3	1	3	2	bronchioloalveolar		3	1	3	2
squamous	3	3	2	0	2	bronchioloalveolar		2	1	3	2
squamous	2	2	1	2	2	bronchioloalveolar		2	1	3	2
squamous	2	2	1	3	2	bronchioloalveolar		3	1	3	2
squamous	2	2	1	1	2	bronchioloalveolar		2	1	3	3
squamous	1	3	1	3	2	bronchioloalveolar		3	1	3	2
squamous	3	1	1	1	3	bronchioloalveolar		2	1	3	3
squamous	2	2	1	3	2	bronchioloalveolar		2	1	3	2
squamous	3	3	1	2	2	small cell		0	0	1	2
squamous	2	3	1	3	3	small cell		1	1	0	3
squamous	2	1	1	3	1	small cell		0	0	0	3
squamous	2	2	1	3	2	small cell		0	1	1	2
squamous	1	3	1	3	2	small cell		1	1	1	2
squamous	3	3	2	1	2	small cell		0	0	0	3
squamous	2	3	1	3	3	carcinoid		1	1	0	1
squamous	1	3	1	3	2	carcinoid		2	1	0	1
squamous	1	3	1	3	2	carcinoid		1	1	0	1
squamous	2	2	1	2	2	carcinoid		1	1	1	1
squamous	2	2	1	3	2	carcinoid		1	1	0	1
squamous	3	3	1	3	2	carcinoid		2	1	0	1
squamous	2	2	1	3	2	carcinoid		1	1	0	1
squamous	2	2	1	0	2	carcinoid		2	1	0	1
squamous	2	1	1	3	2	carcinoid		1	1	1	1
squamous	2	2	1	3	2	lymphoepithelioma		3	2	3	3
squamous	1	3	1	3	2	carcinosarcoma		3	2	3	3
squamous	3	0	1	1	3						

dying from the cancer.[211] Morever, certain human tumor cell lines of nasopharyngeal and lung cancer harbor genetic mutations in the RB2/p130 gene.[179,212–214] This finding suggests a role for the RB2/p130 gene as a tumor-suppressor gene in human cancer.

TABLE 7.2. EXPRESSION PATTERN OF Rb-FAMILY MEMBERS AND PCNA IN LUNG CANCER

Expression	pRb/p105	p107	pRb2/p130	PCNA
High	23 (30%)	—	36 (47%)	19 (25%)
Medium	33 (43%)	10 (13%)	7 (9%)	42 (54%)
Low	16 (21%)	64 (83%)	16 (21%)	16 (21%)
Undetectable	5 (7%)	3 (4%)	18 (23%)	—

High = 60% to 100% of positive cells; Medium = 30% to 60% of positive cells; Low = 1% to 30% of positive cells; Undetectable = 0% of positive cells.

RB1 AND RB2 IN LUNG CANCER

Lung cancer is one of the leading causes of death related to cancer in the world. The high mortality rates for lung cancer may in part result from the absence of standard clinical procedures for diagnosis of early tumoral stages, in contrast to the screening modalities available for breast, prostate, and colon cancers.[215] Early studies indicated that several distinct chromosomal loci (3p, 9p, 13q, 17p, and others) are implicated in the pathogenesis of lung cancer, suggesting that sequential genetic events may occur during the initiation and progression of lung carcinogenesis.[216–218] PRb/p105 (RB1) maps to the chromosomal locus 13q and pRb2/p130 (RB2) on 16q.[114,205] Recently, frequent allelic losses on chromosomes 2q, 18q, and 22q have been reported in advanced NSCLC.[219] Additionally, frequent novel genetic alterations such as increased DNA copy number at 5p, 1q24,

TABLE 7.3. Rb2 PERCENTAGE OF EXPRESSION IN LUNG CANCER

Score[a]	Tumors			
	Squamous	Adenocarcinoma	SCLC[b]	Carcinoid
1	23 (19.5%)	8 (25%)	4 (100%)	
2	55 (46.6%)	18 (56.3%)		
3	40 (33.9%)	6 (18.7%)		4 (100%)

[a] 1, 0% to 10% of positive cells; 2, 10% to 50% of positive cells; 3, 50% to 100% of positive cells.
[b] SCLC, small cell lung cancer.

and Xq26 and decreased DNA copy number at 22q12.1–13.1, 10q26, and 16p11.2 have been identified in NSCLC.[220,221]

In all normal cells, two types of genes—oncogenes and anti-oncogenes (also known as tumor-suppressor genes—are expressed and control cell proliferation and differentiation. Cell growth is stimulated by oncogenes and inhibited by anti-oncogenes. Neoplastic transformation involves loss of growth control caused by defective gene expression either by overexpression of a normal growth-promoting protein or by expression of an abnormal mutated protein that may result in a gain or loss of function. Several oncogenes, such as *c-myc*, *N-myc*, and *L-myc*, have been identified as potential initiators of lung cancerogenes.[222] On the other hand, loss of anti-oncogene function has also been described in lung cancer. Mutations or deletions of the *RB* gene have been reported in non–small cell carcinomas in greater than 90% of the cases.[223] Likewise, mutations of other tumor-suppressor genes such as p53 have been reported with frequencies as high as 50% in NSCLC and 70% to 80% in SCLC.[222,223] Moreover, by immunohistochemistry the expression of *p53*, *pRb/p105*, *Ras*, and *Bcl-2* have been investigated in a panel of 65 samples of preneoplastic lesions of the bronchial epithelium. The frequency of p53-positive and pRb-negative microscopic fields was directly related to the morphologic grading of the lesions. One of the main patterns found to be correlated with the severity of histopathologic features was characterized by combined p53 hyperexpression and pRb hypoexpression.[224]

Lung cancer arises from a series of morphologic changes

that take several years to progress from a normal epithelium to an invasive cancer. During the progression from hyperplasia through metaplasia, to dysplasia, to carcinoma *in situ,* to invasive and finally to metastatic cancer, multiple molecular changes have been noted. The molecular changes include activation of dominant oncogenes as well as loss of recessive growth-regulatory genes or anti-oncogenes.[225] Interestingly, some authors correlated the prognostic significance of the loss of Rb protein either alone, or in combination with *Ras* or p53 mutations in patients with NSCLC. Individuals with the theoretically best pattern of protein expression in their tumors versus those with the theoretically worst pattern of gene expression (i.e., Rb+/*Ras*− versus Rb−/*Ras*+ and Rb+/p53− versus Rb−/p53+) showed a longer period of survival. The correlation between Rb and *Ras* proved to be a better prognostic factor than that of the Rb and p53 status in NSCLCs. In patients affected by squamous cell carcinoma, neither Rb/*Ras* nor Rb/p53 status was a significant prognostic factor in this cohort.[226]

RB2/p130 is the latest member of the Rb-family of proteins to be identified.[175,181,184] Immunohistochemic studies of the expression patterns of the Rb family members (pRb/p105, p107, and pRb2/p130) in 235 specimens of lung cancer indicate that pRb2/p130 may play an important role in the pathogenesis and progression of certain lung cancers (Tables 7.1, 7.2, and 7.3).[209,210] The same studies have suggested that *RB2/p130* protein expression inversely correlates with the histological grading and with PCNA expression in different lung cancer histotypes (Tables 7.1, 7.2, and 7.3).[209,210] The characterization of the genomic structure of the *RB2/p130* gene[227] allowed for mutational screening. Different authors reported that the majority of point mutations in the *RB/p105* gene are located in the C-terminal region.[228] Very little is known about the presence of mutations in human cancers in the *RB2/p130* gene instead. In two very recent studies, the *RB2/p130* gene has been found to be mutated in the carboxyl-terminus region in more than 80% of the human lung tumors analyzed, as well as in primary human lymphomas and NPCs by single-strand conformation polymorphism (SSCP) analysis and direct DNA sequence analysis (Figure 7.6).[213,214] Interestingly, the vast majority of those lung tumors were adenocarcinomas spanning from poorly to moderately differentiated.

TABLE 7.4. FIVE-YEAR SURVIVAL RATES BY TYPE OF TREATMENT AND pRb2/p130 STATUS IN ENDOMETRIAL CANCER

Adjuvant Treatment	No. of Cases	pRb2/p130 (%)		P Value
		Positive	Negative	
None	57	97.4%	68.5%	<.01
Radiotherapy	37	86.8%	50.3%	<.05
Chemotherapy	6	66.6%	0	<.01

Exon 21

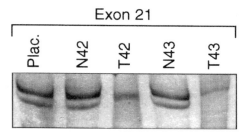

FIGURE 7.6. Representative example of single-strand conformation polymorphyism analysis of exon 21 of the *RB2/p130* gene in primary lung tumors compared to the normal genomic DNA extracted from peripheral blood of the corresponding patient, indicating that the mutations found in the tumors were somatic. (From P.P. Claudio, et al. "Mutations in the retinoblastoma-related gene RB2/p130 in lung tumors and suppression of tumor growth *in vivo* by retroviral-mediated gene transfer," *Cancer Res,* [*in press*], 1999.)

As a model to study carcinogenesis, mice are among the most suitable. Mice develop lung tumors with a similar histology and molecular features to peripheral adenocarcinomas in humans. Additionally, mice are an easy and firmly established model to grow tumors *in vivo* and to study different delivery systems suitable for human gene therapy. The advantage of this model system is that events early in tumorigenesis can be studied at the molecular level. Decreased expression of p15, p16, Rb, cyclin D1, Apc, Mcc, and Gjal occur during tumor formation in both rodents and humans.[229]

Gene therapy models in different types of cancers using viral vectors to deliver either a functional p53 or pRb have been attempted.[230–237] In a recent study, using a tetracycline-regulated gene expression system to control the expression of *RB2/p130* in JC virus-induced hamster brain tumor cells, it was demonstrated for the first time that *RB2/p130* could be used to inhibit the growth of such tumors *in vivo*. Induced expression of pRb2/p130 in this *in vivo* study brought about a 3.2 fold or 69% reduction in tumor mass in *nude* mice.[238]

The effects of expressing pRb2/p130 *in vivo* in a lung adenocarcinoma cell line were also analyzed using a retroviral delivery approach.[213] Retroviruses are among the most efficient vector systems for transducing genes into mammalian cells, and they have been successfully used to deliver therapeutic genes into humans.[232,239] The requirement for host cells to actively divide to allow viral genes to integrate into the host genome[240] may be advantageous for cancer gene therapy. This requirement would limit exogenous gene delivery to rapidly proliferating cancer cells while sparing delivery to other nonproliferating cells within the effected organ.

It has been recently shown that *in vivo* retroviral transduction of the *RB2/p130* gene in established tumors, derived from injection of the lung adenocarcinoma cell line

H23 grown subcutaneously in *nude* mice, greatly reduced the tumor mass. The average tumor weight of the excised tumors transduced with *RB2/p130* was over 12 fold smaller compared to those transduced with retroviruses carrying the puromycin (*Pac*) resistance alone or the *Lac-Z* gene.[213]

Functional inactivation of tumor-suppressor gene products by way of interaction with viral oncoproteins of DNA tumor viruses represent another mechanism of tumorigenesis. Such a scenario has been proposed for the oncoprotein of simian virus 40, the SV40 large T antigen (Tag) that targets and inactivates cell cycle regulatory proteins such as the Rb-family and p53, leading to transformation of human cell lines *in vitro*, and producing tumors *in vivo* in rodent models.[241–243] Even though mesotheliomas are among the most aggressive human cancers, alterations of important cell cycle "controllers," such as the Rb-family genes, have never been reported in these tumors. However, SV40-like sequences have been detected in 86% of archival specimens of mesothelioma; furthermore, SV40 Tag was isolated from frozen biopsies of human mesothelioma that retained its ability to bind each of the Rb-family proteins: pRb/p105, p107, and pRb2/p130.[242] This finding raises the question of whether the tumorigenic potential of SV40 Tag in some human mesotheliomas may stem from its ability to interact with and thereby inactivate several tumor- and/or growth-suppressive proteins.

The absence of mutations in Rb-family proteins and the unusually high level of expression of pRb, pRb2/p130, and p107 in the mesothelioma specimens may be explained by the physical association of these proteins with SV40 Tag, which should lead to their functional inactivation. All members of the Rb gene family share the ability to interact physically with certain oncoproteins of DNA tumor viruses. These viral oncoproteins compete with the E2F family of transcription factors for binding to the Rb-family proteins.[244] Release of the E2F family members from the pocket structure leads to the induction of genes needed to proceed through the cell cycle. The finding that p53, a well-characterized tumor-suppressor gene, is also a target of SV40 Tag,[241,245] further supports the model of viral transformation via the binding of the viral oncoproteins to a specific region of cell growth-suppressor genes.

A paradigm is forming that the removal or inactivation of functional tumor-suppressor proteins such as pRb/p105 or pRb2/p130 by way of tumor viral oncoproteins, as is the case in SV40 large T antigen–associated mesothelioma,[242,245] or by way of genetic alteration as is the case in lung cancer,[124,213,215,217,218,222,223,225,246] may be a critical event in the malignant transformation of a cell.

Considering the impact of lung cancer in terms of morbidity and mortality on the Western world,[247] it is possible to suggest that *RB1* (pRb/p105) and/or *RB2* (pRb2/p130) in combination with *p53, Ras,* and other cell cycle regulatory genes, may serve as valuable tools in establishing the molecular diagnosis and/or prognosis of lung cancer. Additionally, identification of mutations within these tumor-suppressor loci in lung cancer could have possible implications on guiding and designing standard as well as novel therapeutic regimes.

CONCLUSION

The prototypic tumor-suppressor gene *RB* is mutated in several human tumors, and numerous studies are now beginning to identify their role in cancer development, as well as in normal cell physiology. In cell lines that lack a functional pRb protein, the restoration of protein function suppresses the cells' neoplastic properties.[115,116] These data have led to the exploration of the possibility of replacement of the wild-type *RB* gene as a clinical treatment for human cancers.[231–233,235–237,248–251]

The fact that transforming oncoproteins such as SV40 Tag must maintain an intact Rb-family binding domain (LXCXE domain; L = Leucine, X = any amino acid, C = Cystein, B = Glutamine) to transform *RB* −/− cells indicates that p107 and/or pRb2/p130 are also strategically important targets for SV40 Tag-mediated transformation and implicates them as putative tumor-suppressor genes.[252] In support of an involvement of the *RB2/p130* gene in human cancer as a tumor-suppressor gene, it maps to human chromosome 16q12.2, an area in which deletions have been found in several human neoplasias including breast, ovarian, hepatic, and prostatic cancers.[205] Intriguingly, differential expression of pRb2/p130 in human endometrial cancer, where the expression level of pRb2/p130 inversely correlates with tumor grade and prognosis, has been detected.[211] These findings have significant clinical implications involving prognosis and implementation of therapeutic strategies. Immunohistochemic data examining the expression of the Rb-family proteins in 235 patient samples of lung carcinoma suggest an independent role for the reduction or loss of pRb2/p130 expression in the formation and/or progression of lung carcinoma Tables 7.1, 7.2, and 7.3.[209,210] Additionally, different groups have detected mutations in the *RB2/p130* gene in human cell lines of small cell and adenocarcinoma[212] as well as patient tumor specimens.[213] This finding suggests that functional inactivation of one or more of the Rb-family genes by genomic mutation or by transforming oncoprotein may provide the cell with a growth advantage resulting in tumor formation.

Additionally, it has recently beer shown that the induction of pRb2/p130 expression is growth suppressive to tumor formation *in vivo.*[213,238] This data predicts that *RB2/p130* gene therapy may serve as a beneficial therapeutic alternative for cancer and lays the foundation for exploring this avenue of research in addition to other gene therapeutic models that are under current investigation.[253]

In summary, pRb2/p130 is proving to be a complex multifunctional protein that is directly linked to the cell cycle machinery by its Cdk-inhibitory activity. Furthermore, the fact that induction of pRb2/p130 expression or overexpression by retrovirally delivered pRb2/p130 inhibits tumor growth *in vivo,*[213,238] along with the mapping of the *RB2/p130* locus to a region altered in several human neoplasms,[205] immunohistochemic data indicating an independent role for pRb2/p130 in the development and/or progression of human lung (Tables 7.1, 7.2, and 7.3)[209,210] and endometrial cancer (Table 7.4 and Figure 7.5),[211] and the identification of mutations in the *RB2/p130* gene in human tumor cell lines[212] and primary tumors,[213,214] strongly supports the hypothesis that *RB2/p130* is a tumor-suppressor gene as well as RB1/p105.

REFERENCES

1. Rabbitts TH. Chromosomal translocations in human cancer. *Nature* 1994;372:143.
2. Knudson AG, Jr. Mutation and cancer: statistical study of retinoblastoma. *Proc Natl Acad Sci USA* 1971;68:820.
3. Bienz-Tadmor B, Zakut-Houri R, Libresco S, et al. The 5' region of the p53 gene: evolutionary conservation and evidence for a negative regulatory element. *Embo J* 1985;4:3209.
4. Wang J, Chenivesse X, Henglein B, et al. Hepatitis B virus integration in a cyclin A gene in a hepatocellular carcinoma. *Nature* 1990;343:555.
5. Paterlini P, Suberville AM, Zindy F, et al. Cyclin A expression in human hematological malignancies: a new marker of cell proliferation. *Cancer Res* 1993;53:235.
6. Keyomarsi K, Pardee AB. Redundant cyclin overexpression and gene amplification in breast cancer cells. *Proc Natl Acad Sci USA* 1993;90:1112.
7. Jiang W, Kahn SM, Tomita N, et al. Amplification and expression of the human cyclin D gene in esophageal cancer. *Cancer Res* 1992;52:2980.
8. Bianchi AB, Fischer SM, Robles AI, et al. Overexpression of cyclin D1 in mouse skin carcinogenesis. *Oncogene* 1993;8:1127.
9. Motokura T, Bloom T, Kim HG, et al. A novel cyclin encoded by a bcl1-linked candidate oncogene [see comments]. *Nature* 1991;350:512.
10. Leach FS, Elledge SJ, Sherr CJ, et al. Amplification of cyclin genes in colorectal carcinomas. *Cancer Res* 1993;53:1986.
11. Juan G, Gong J, Traganos F, et al. Unscheduled expression of cyclins D1 and D3 in human tumour cell lines. *Cell Prolif* 1996;29:259.
12. Bartkova J, Zemanova M, Bartek J. Abundance and subcellular localisation of cyclin D3 in human tumours. *Int J Cancer* 1996;65:323.
13. Giordano A, Whyte P, Harlow E, et al. A 60 kd cdc2-associated polypeptide complexes with the E1A proteins in adenovirus-infected cells. *Cell* 1989;58:981.
14. Pines J, Hunter T. Human cyclin A is adenovirus E1A-associated protein p60 and behaves differently from cyclin B. *Nature* 1990;346:760.
15. Chellappan SP. The E2F transcription factor: role in cell cycle regulation and differentiation. *Mol Cell Diff* 1994:201.
16. King RW, Jackson PK, Kirschner MW. Mitosis in transition [see comments]. *Cell* 1994;79:563.
17. Draetta G, Beach D. Activation of cdc2 protein kinase during mitosis in human cells: cell cycle-dependent phosphorylation and subunit rearrangement. *Cell* 1988;54:17.
18. Koff A, Giordano A, Desai D, et al. Formation and activation

of a cyclin E-cdk2 complex during the G1 phase of the human cell cycle. *Science* 1992;257:1689.

19. Kato JY, Matsuoka M, Polyak K, et al. Cyclic AMP-induced G1 phase arrest mediated by an inhibitor (p27Kip1) of cyclin-dependent kinase 4 activation. *Cell* 1994;79:487.

20. Polyak K, Kato JY, Solomon MJ, et al. p27Kip1, a cyclin-Cdk inhibitor, links transforming growth factor-beta and contact inhibition to cell cycle arrest. *Genes Dev* 1994;8:9.

21. Polyak K, Lee MH, Erdjument-Bromage H, et al. Cloning of p27Kip1, a cyclin-dependent kinase inhibitor and a potential mediator of extracellular antimitogenic signals. *Cell* 1994;78:59.

22. Toyoshima H, Hunter T. p27, a novel inhibitor of G1 cyclin-Cdk protein kinase activity, is related to p21. *Cell* 1994;78:67.

23. Serrano M, Hannon GJ, Beach D. A new regulatory motif in cell-cycle control causing specific inhibition of cyclin D/CDK4 [see comments]. *Nature* 1993;366:704.

24. Fisher RP, Morgan DO. A novel cyclin associates with MO15/CDK7 to form the CDK-activating kinase. *Cell* 1994;78:713.

25. Matsuoka M, Kato JY, Fisher RP, et al. Activation of cyclin-dependent kinase 4 (cdk4) by mouse MO15-associated kinase. *Mol Cell Biol* 1994;14:7265.

26. Kato JY, Matsuoka M, Strom DK, et al. Regulation of cyclin D-dependent kinase 4 (cdk4) by cdk4-activating kinase. *Mol Cell Biol* 1994;14:2713.

27. Hunter T, Pines J. Cyclins and cancer. *Cell* 1991;66:1071.

28. Koff A, Cross F, Fisher A, et al. Human cyclin E, a new cyclin that interacts with two members of the CDC2 gene family. *Cell* 1991;66:1217.

29. Draetta GF. Mammalian G1 cyclins. *Curr Opin Cell Biol* 1994;6:842.

30. Matsushime H, Roussel MF, Ashmun RA, et al. Colony-stimulating factor 1 regulates novel cyclins during the G1 phase of the cell cycle. *Cell* 1991;65:701.

31. Matsushime H, Roussel MF, Sherr CJ. Novel mammalian cyclins (CYL genes) expressed during G1. *Cold Spring Harb Symp Quant Biol* 1991;56:69.

32. Kato JY, Sherr CJ. Inhibition of granulocyte differentiation by G1 cyclins D2 and D3 but not D1. *Proc Natl Acad Sci USA* 1993;90:11513.

33. Kato J, Matsushime H, Hiebert SW, et al. Direct binding of cyclin D to the retinoblastoma gene product (pRb) and pRb phosphorylation by the cyclin D-dependent kinase CDK4. *Genes Dev* 1993;7:331.

34. Ewen ME, Sluss HK, Sherr CJ, et al. Functional interactions of the retinoblastoma protein with mammalian D-type cyclins. *Cell* 1993;73:487.

35. Dowdy SF, Hinds PW, Louie K, et al. Physical interaction of the retinoblastoma protein with human D cyclins. *Cell* 1993;73:499.

36. Quelle DE, Ashmun RA, Shurtleff SA, et al. Overexpression of mouse D-type cyclins accelerates G1 phase in rodent fibroblasts. *Genes Dev* 1993;7:1559.

37. Musgrove EA, Lee CS, Buckley MF, et al. Cyclin D1 induction in breast cancer cells shortens G1 and is sufficient for cells arrested in G1 to complete the cell cycle. *Proc Natl Acad Sci USA* 1994;91:8022.

38. Baldin V, Lukas J, Marcote MJ, et al. Cyclin D1 is a nuclear protein required for cell cycle progression in G1. *Genes Dev* 1993;7:812.

39. Pagano M, Theodoras AM, Tam SW, et al. Cyclin D1-mediated inhibition of repair and replicative DNA synthesis in human fibroblasts. *Genes Dev* 1994;8:1627.

40. Xiong Y, Zhang H, Beach D. D type cyclins associate with multiple protein kinases and the DNA replication and repair factor PCNA. *Cell* 1992;71:505.

41. Prelich G, Stillman B. Coordinated leading and lagging strand synthesis during SV40 DNA replication in vitro requires PCNA. *Cell* 1988;53:117.

42. Shivji KK, Kenny MK, Wood RD. Proliferating cell nuclear antigen is required for DNA excision repair. *Cell* 1992;69:367.

43. Heichman KA, Roberts JM. Rules to replicate by [see comments]. *Cell* 1994;79:557.

44. Meyerson M, Harlow E. Identification of G1 kinase activity for cdk6, a novel cyclin D partner. *Mol Cell Biol* 1994;14:2077.

45. Sewing A, Burger C, Brusselbach S, et al. Human cyclin D1 encodes a labile nuclear protein whose synthesis is directly induced by growth factors and suppressed by cyclic AMP. *J Cell Sci* 1993;104:545.

46. Ajchenbaum F, Ando K, DeCaprio JA, et al. Independent regulation of human D-type cyclin gene expression during G1 phase in primary human T lymphocytes. *J Biol Chem* 1993;268:4113.

47. Surmacz E, Reiss K, Sell C, et al. Cyclin D1 messenger RNA is inducible by platelet-derived growth factor in cultured fibroblasts. *Cancer Res* 1992;52:4522.

48. Tam SW, Theodoras AM, Shay JW, et al. Differential expression and regulation of Cyclin D1 protein in normal and tumor human cells: association with Cdk4 is required for Cyclin D1 function in G1 progression. *Oncogene* 1994;9:2663.

49. Musgrove EA, Hamilton JA, Lee CS, et al. Growth factor, steroid, and steroid antagonist regulation of cyclin gene expression associated with changes in T-47D human breast cancer cell cycle progression. *Mol Cell Biol* 1993;13:3577.

50. Lew DJ, Dulic V, Reed SI. Isolation of three novel human cyclins by rescue of G1 cyclin (Cln) function in yeast. *Cell* 1991;66:1197.

51. Nash R, Tokiwa G, Anand S, et al. The WHI1+ gene of Saccharomyces cerevisiae tethers cell division to cell size and is a cyclin homolog. *Embo J* 1988;7:4335.

52. Ohtsubo M, Roberts JM. Cyclin-dependent regulation of G1 in mammalian fibroblasts. *Science* 1993;259:1908.

53. Resnitzky D, Gossen M, Bujard H, et al. Acceleration of the G1/S phase transition by expression of cyclins D1 and E with an inducible system. *Mol Cell Biol* 1994;14:1669.

54. Keyomarsi K, O'Leary N, Molnar G, et al. Cyclin E, a potential prognostic marker for breast cancer. *Cancer Res* 1994;54:380.

55. Fang F, Newport JW. Evidence that the G1-S and G2-M transitions are controlled by different cdc2 proteins in higher eukaryotes. *Cell* 1991;66:731.

56. Girard F, Strausfeld U, Fernandez A, et al. Cyclin A is required for the onset of DNA replication in mammalian fibroblasts. *Cell* 1991;67:1169.

57. Walker DH, Maller JL. Role for cyclin A in the dependence of mitosis on completion of DNA replication. *Nature* 1991;354:314.

58. Minshull J, Golsteyn R, Hill CS et al. The A- and B-type cyclin associated cdc2 kinases in Xenopus turn on and off at different times in the cell cycle. *Embo J* 1990;9:2865.

59. Pagano M, Pepperkok R, Verde F, et al. Cyclin A is required at two points in the human cell cycle. *Embo J* 1992;11:961.

60. Pagano M, Draetta G, Jansen-Durr P. Association of cdk2 kinase with the transcription factor E2F during S phase. *Science* 1992;255:1144.

61. Cardoso MC, Leonhardt H, Nadal-Ginard B. Reversal of terminal differentiation and control of DNA replication: cyclin A and Cdk2 specifically localize at subnuclear sites of DNA replication. *Cell* 1993;74:979.

62. Pan ZQ, Amin AA, Gibbs E, et al. Phosphorylation of the p34 subunit of human single-stranded-DNA-binding protein in cyclin A-activated G1 extracts is catalyzed by cdk-cyclin A

complex and DNA-dependent protein kinase. *Proc Natl Acad Sci USA* 1994;91:8343.

63. Nevins JR. E2F: a link between the Rb tumor suppressor protein and viral oncoproteins. *Science* 1992;258:424.

64. Hartwell LH, Weinert TA. Checkpoints: controls that ensure the order of cell cycle events. *Science* 1989;246:629.

65. Desai D, Wessling HC, Fisher RP, et al. Effects of phosphorylation by CAK on cyclin binding by CDC2 and CDK2. *Mol Cell Biol* 1995;15:345.

66. Smythe C, Newport JW. Coupling of mitosis to the completion of S phase in Xenopus occurs via modulation of the tyrosine kinase that phosphorylates p34cdc2. *Cell* 1992;68:787.

67. Laiho M, DeCaprio JA, Ludlow JW, et al. Growth inhibition by TGF-beta linked to suppression of retinoblastoma protein phosphorylation. *Cell* 1990;62:175.

68. Ewen ME, Sluss HK, Whitehouse LL, et al. TGF beta inhibition of Cdk4 synthesis is linked to cell cycle arrest. *Cell* 1993;74:1009.

69. Koff A, Ohtsuki M, Polyak K, et al. Negative regulation of G1 in mammalian cells: inhibition of cyclin E-dependent kinase by TGF-beta. *Science* 1993;260:536.

70. Pagano M, Tam SW, Theodoras AM, et al. Role of the ubiquitin-proteasome pathway in regulating abundance of the cyclin-dependent kinase inhibitor p27 [see comments]. *Science* 1995;269:682.

71. Millard SS, Yan JS, Nguyen H, et al. Enhanced ribosomal association of p27(Kip1) mRNA is a mechanism contributing to accumulation during growth arrest. *J Biol Chem* 1997;272:7093.

72. Sheaff RJ, Groudine M, Gordon M, et al. Cyclin E-CDK2 is a regulator of p27Kip1. *Genes Dev* 1997;11:1464.

73. Morisaki H, Fujimoto A, Ando A, et al. Cell cycle-dependent phosphorylation of p27 cyclin-dependent kinase (Cdk) inhibitor by cyclin E/Cdk2. *Biochem Biophys Res Commun* 1997;240:386.

74. Vlach J, Hennecke S, Amati B. Phosphorylation-dependent degradation of the cyclin-dependent kinase inhibitor p27. *Embo J* 1997;16:5334.

75. Mal A, Poon RY, Howe PH, et al. Inactivation of p27Kip1 by the viral E1A oncoprotein in TGFbeta-treated cells. *Nature* 1996;380:262.

76. Zerfass-Thome K, Zwerschke W, Mannhardt B, et al. Inactivation of the cdk inhibitor p27KIP1 by the human papillomavirus type 16 E7 oncoprotein. *Oncogene* 1996;13:2323.

77. Fero ML, Rivkin M, Tasch M, et al. A syndrome of multiorgan hyperplasia with features of gigantism, tumorigenesis, and female sterility in p27(Kip1)-deficient mice. *Cell* 1996;85:733.

78. Kiyokawa H, Kineman RD, Manova-Todorova KO, et al. Enhanced growth of mice lacking the cyclin-dependent kinase inhibitor function of p27(Kip1). *Cell* 1996;85:721.

79. Katayose Y, Kim M, Rakkar AN, et al. Promoting apoptosis: a novel activity associated with the cyclin-dependent kinase inhibitor p27. *Cancer Res* 1997;57:5441.

80. Kawamata N, Morosetti R, Miller CW, et al. Molecular analysis of the cyclin-dependent kinase inhibitor gene p27/Kip1 in human malignancies. *Cancer Res* 1995;55:2266.

81. Spirin KS, Simpson JF, Takeuchi S, et al. p27/Kip1 mutation found in breast cancer. *Cancer Res* 1996;56:2400.

82. Loda M, Cukor B, Tam SW, et al. Increased proteasome-dependent degradation of the cyclin-dependent kinase inhibitor p27 in aggressive colorectal carcinomas [see comments]. *Nat Med* 1997;3:231.

83. Esposito V, Baldi A, De Luca A, et al. Prognostic role of the cyclin-dependent kinase inhibitor p27 in non-small cell lung cancer. *Cancer Res* 1997;57:3381.

84. Harper JW, Adami GR, Wei N, et al. The p21 Cdk-interacting protein Cip1 is a potent inhibitor of G1 cyclin-dependent kinases. *Cell* 1993;75:805.

85. Xiong Y, Hannon GJ, Zhang H, et al. p21 is a universal inhibitor of cyclin kinases [see comments]. *Nature* 1993;366:701.

86. Gu Y, Turck CW, Morgan DO. Inhibition of CDK2 activity in vivo by an associated 20K regulatory subunit. *Nature* 1993;366:707.

87. el-Deiry WS, Tokino T, Velculescu VE, et al. WAF1, a potential mediator of p53 tumor suppression. *Cell* 1993;75:817.

88. Noda A, Ning Y, Venable SF, et al. Cloning of senescent cell-derived inhibitors of DNA synthesis using an expression screen. *Exp Cell Res* 1994;211:90.

89. Brown JP, Wei W, Sedivy JM. Bypass of senescence after disruption of p21CIP1/WAF1 gene in normal diploid human fibroblasts. *Science* 1997;277:831.

90. Jiang H, Lin J, Su ZZ, et al. Induction of differentiation in human promyelocytic HL-60 leukemia cells activates p21, WAF1/CIP1, expression in the absence of p53. *Oncogene* 1994;9:3397.

91. Xiong Y, Zhang H, Beach D. Subunit rearrangement of the cyclin-dependent kinases is associated with cellular transformation. *Genes Dev* 1993;7:1572.

92. Dulic V, Stein GH, Far DF, et al. Nuclear accumulation of p21Cip1 at the onset of mitosis: a role at the G2/M-phase transition. *Mol Cell Biol* 1998;18:546.

93. el-Deiry WS, Harper JW, O'Connor PM, et al. WAF1/CIP1 is induced in p53-mediated G1 arrest and apoptosis. *Cancer Res* 1994;54:1169.

94. Dulic V, Kaufmann WK, Wilson SJ, et al. p53-dependent inhibition of cyclin-dependent kinase activities in human fibroblasts during radiation-induced G1 arrest. *Cell* 1994;76:1013.

95. Waga S, Hannon GJ, Beach D, et al. The p21 inhibitor of cyclin-dependent kinases controls DNA replication by interaction with PCNA [see comments]. *Nature* 1994;369:574.

96. Flores-Rozas H, Kelman Z, Dean FB, et al. Cdk-interacting protein 1 directly binds with proliferating cell nuclear antigen and inhibits DNA replication catalyzed by the DNA polymerase delta holoenzyme. *Proc Natl Acad Sci USA* 1994;91:8655.

97. Kamb A, Gruis NA, Weaver-Feldhaus J, et al. A cell cycle regulator potentially involved in genesis of many tumor types [see comments]. *Science* 1994;264:436.

98. Nobori T, Miura K, Wu DJ, et al. Deletions of the cyclin-dependent kinase-4 inhibitor gene in multiple human cancers. *Nature* 1994;368:753.

99. Spruck CH, 3rd, Gonzalez-Zulueta M, Shibata A, et al. p16 gene in uncultured tumours [letter] [see comments]. *Nature* 1994;370:183.

100. Serrano M, Gomez-Lahoz E, DePinho RA, et al. Inhibition of ras-induced proliferation and cellular transformation by p16INK4. *Science* 1995;267:249.

101. Li Y, Nichols MA, Shay JW, et al. Transcriptional repression of the D-type cyclin-dependent kinase inhibitor p16 by the retinoblastoma susceptibility gene product pRb. *Cancer Res* 1994;54:6078.

102. Parry D, Bates S, Mann DJ, et al. Lack of cyclin D-Cdk complexes in Rb-negative cells correlates with high levels of p16INK4/MTS1 tumour suppressor gene product. *Embo J* 1995;14:503.

103. Bates S, Parry D, Bonetta L, et al. Absence of cyclin D/cdk complexes in cells lacking functional retinoblastoma protein. *Oncogene* 1994;9:1633.

104. Guan KL, Jenkins CW, Li Y, et al. Growth suppression by p18, a p16INK4/MTS1- and p14INK4B/MTS2-related CDK6 inhibitor, correlates with wild-type pRb function. *Genes Dev* 1994;8:2939.

105. Sherr CJ. G1 phase progression: cycling on cue [see comments]. *Cell* 1994;79:551.

106. Gonzalez MV, Pello MF, Lopez-Larrea C, et al. Deletion and methylation of the tumour suppressor gene p16/CDKN2 in primary head and neck squamous cell carcinoma. *J Clin Pathol* 1997;50:509.

107. Xiao S, Li D, Corson JM, et al. Codeletion of p15 and p16 genes in primary non-small cell lung carcinoma. *Cancer Res* 1995;55:2968.

108. Ng MH, Chung YF, Lo KW, et al. Frequent hypermethylation of p16 and p15 genes in multiple myeloma. *Blood* 1997;89:2500.

109. Naumann M, Savitskaia N, Eilert C, et al. Frequent codeletion of p16/MTS1 and p15/MTS2 and genetic alterations in p16/MTS1 in pancreatic tumors. *Gastroenterology* 1996;110:1215.

110. Cavenee WK, Hansen MF, Nordenskjold M, et al. Genetic origin of mutations predisposing to retinoblastoma. *Science* 1985;228:501.

111. Knudson AG, Jr. The genetics of childhood cancer. *Cancer* 1984;35:1022.

112. Friend SH, Bernards R, Rogelj S, et al. A human DNA segment with properties of the gene that predisposes to retinoblastoma and osteosarcoma. *Nature* 1986;323:643.

113. Fung YK, Murphree AL, T'Ang A, et al. Structural evidence for the authenticity of the human retinoblastoma gene. *Science* 1987;236:1657.

114. Lee WH, Bookstein R, Hong F, et al. Human retinoblastoma susceptibility gene: cloning, identification, and sequence. *Science* 1987;235:1394.

115. Goodrich DW, Wang NP, Qian YW, et al. The retinoblastoma gene product regulates progression through the G1 phase of the cell cycle. *Cell* 1991;67:293.

116. Hinds PW, Mittnacht S, Dulic V, et al. Regulation of retinoblastoma protein functions by ectopic expression of human cyclins. *Cell* 1992;70:993.

117. Zhu L, van den Heuvel S, Helin K, et al. Inhibition of cell proliferation by p107, a relative of the retinoblastoma protein. *Genes Dev* 1993;7:1111.

118. Chellappan SP, Hiebert S, Mudryj M, et al. The E2F transcription factor is a cellular target for the RB protein. *Cell* 1991;65:1053.

119. Hiebert SW, Chellappan SP, Horowitz JM, et al. The interaction of RB with E2F coincides with an inhibition of the transcriptional activity of E2F. *Genes Dev* 1992;6:177.

120. Qian Y, Luckey C, Horton L, et al. Biological function of the retinoblastoma protein requires distinct domains for hyperphosphorylation and transcription factor binding. *Mol Cell Biol* 1992;12:5363.

121. Qin XQ, Chittenden T, Livingston DM, et al. Identification of a growth suppression domain within the retinoblastoma gene product. *Genes Dev* 1992;6:953.

122. Weinberg RA. Tumor suppressor genes. *Science* 1991;254:1138.

123. Horowitz JM, Yandell DW, Park SH, et al. Point mutational inactivation of the retinoblastoma antioncogene. *Science* 1989;243:937.

124. Kaye FJ, Kratzke RA, Gerster JL, et al. A single amino acid substitution results in a retinoblastoma protein defective in phosphorylation and oncoprotein binding. *Proc Natl Acad Sci USA* 1990;87:6922.

125. Bookstein R, Shew JY, Chen PL, et al. Suppression of tumorigenicity of human prostate carcinoma cells by replacing a mutated RB gene. *Science* 1990;247:712.

126. Bookstein R, Rio P, Madreperla SA, et al. Promoter deletion and loss of retinoblastoma gene expression in human prostate carcinoma. *Proc Natl Acad Sci USA* 1990;87:7762.

127. Horowitz JM, Park SH, Bogenmann E, et al. Frequent inactivation of the retinoblastoma anti-oncogene is restricted to a subset of human tumor cells. *Proc Natl Acad Sci USA* 1990;87:2775.

128. DeCaprio JA, Furukawa Y, Ajchenbaum F, et al. The retinoblastoma-susceptibility gene product becomes phosphorylated in multiple stages during cell cycle entry and progression. *Proc Natl Acad Sci USA* 1992;89:1795.

129. Chen PL, Scully P, Shew JY, et al. Phosphorylation of the retinoblastoma gene product is modulated during the cell cycle and cellular differentiation. *Cell* 1989;58:1193.

130. Ludlow JW, DeCaprio JA, Huang CM, et al. SV40 large T antigen binds preferentially to an underphosphorylated member of the retinoblastoma susceptibility gene product family. *Cell* 1989;56:57.

131. Durfee T, Becherer K, Chen PL, et al. The retinoblastoma protein associates with the protein phosphatase type 1 catalytic subunit. *Genes Dev* 1993;7:555.

132. Wei P, Garber ME, Fang SM, et al. A novel CDK9-associated C-type cyclin interacts directly with HIV-1 Tat and mediates its high-affinity, loop-specific binding to TAR RNA. *Cell* 1998;92:451.

133. Bandara LR, Adamczewski JP, Hunt T, et al. Cyclin A and the retinoblastoma gene product complex with a common transcription factor. *Nature* 1991;352:249.

134. Giordano A, Lee JH, Scheppler JA, et al. Cell cycle regulation of histone H1 kinase activity associated with the adenoviral protein E1A. *Science* 1991;253:1271.

135. Grana X, De Luca A, Sang N, et al. PITALRE, a nuclear CDC2-related protein kinase that phosphorylates the retinoblastoma protein in vitro. *Proc Natl Acad Sci USA* 1994;91:3834.

136. MacLachlan TK, Sang N, Giordano A. Cyclins, cyclin-dependent kinases and cdk inhibitors: implications in cell cycle control and cancer. *Crit Rev Eukaryot Gene Expr* 1995;5:127.

137. Kim SJ, Wagner S, Liu F, et al. Retinoblastoma gene product activates expression of the human TGF-beta 2 gene through transcription factor ATF-2. *Nature* 1992;358:331.

138. Bandara LR, La Thangue NB. Adenovirus E1a prevents the retinoblastoma gene product from complexing with a cellular transcription factor. *Nature* 1991;351:494.

139. Raychaudhuri P, Bagchi S, Devoto SH, et al. Domains of the adenovirus E1A protein required for oncogenic activity are also required for dissociation of E2F transcription factor complexes. *Genes Dev* 1991;5:1200.

140. Zhu L, Xie E, Chang LS. Differential roles of two tandem E2F sites in repression of the human p107 promoter by retinoblastoma and p107 proteins. *Mol Cell Biol* 1995;15:3552.

141. Sala A, Nicolaides NC, Engelhard A, et al. Correlation between E2F-1 requirement in the S phase and E2F-1 transactivation of cell cycle-related genes in human cells. *Cancer Res* 1994;54:1402.

142. Slansky JE, Farnham PJ. Introduction to the E2F family: protein structure and gene regulation. *Curr Top Microbiol Immunol* 1996;208:1.

143. Hateboer G, Kerkhoven RM, Shvarts A, et al. Degradation of E2F by the ubiquitin-proteasome pathway: regulation by retinoblastoma family proteins and adenovirus transforming proteins. *Genes Dev* 1996;10:2960.

144. Ivey-Hoyle M, Conroy R, Huber HE, et al. Cloning and characterization of E2F-2, a novel protein with the biochemical properties of transcription factor E2F. *Mol Cell Biol* 1993;13:7802.

145. Hijmans EM, Voorhoeve PM, Beijersbergen RL, et al. E2F-5, a new E2F family member that interacts with p130 in vivo. *Mol Cell Biol* 1995;15:3082.

146. Beijersbergen RL, Kerkhoven RM, Zhu L, et al. E2F-4, a new member of the E2F gene family, has oncogenic activity and associates with p107 in vivo. *Genes Dev* 1994;8:2680.

147. Ginsberg D, Vairo G, Chittenden T, et al. E2F-4, a new member of the E2F transcription factor family, interacts with p107. *Genes Dev* 1994;8:2665.

148. Huber HE, Edwards G, Goodhart PJ, et al. Transcription factor E2F binds DNA as a heterodimer. *Proc Natl Acad Sci USA* 1993;90:3525.

149. Bandara LR, Buck VM, Zamanian M, et al. Functional synergy between DP-1 and E2F-1 in the cell cycle-regulating transcription factor DRTF1/E2F. *Embo J* 1993;12:4317.

150. Ormondroyd E, de la Luna S, La Thangue NB. A new member of the DP family, DP-3, with distinct protein products suggests a regulatory role for alternative splicing in the cell cycle transcription factor DRTF1/E2F. *Oncogene* 1995;11:1437.

151. Jooss K, Lam EW, Bybee A, et al. Protooncogenic properties of the DP family of proteins. *Oncogene* 1995;10:1529.

152. Rogers KT, Higgins PD, Milla MM, et al. DP-2, a heterodimeric partner of E2F: identification and characterization of DP-2 proteins expressed in vivo. *Proc Natl Acad Sci USA* 1996;93:7594.

153. Bandara LR, Lam EW, Sorensen TS, et al. DP-1: a cell cycle-regulated and phosphorylated component of transcription factor DRTF1/E2F which is functionally important for recognition by pRb and the adenovirus E4 orf 6/7 protein. *Embo J* 1994;13:3104.

154. Krek W, Ewen ME, Shirodkar S, et al. Negative regulation of the growth-promoting transcription factor E2F-1 by a stably bound cyclin A-dependent protein kinase. *Cell* 1994;78:161.

155. Xu HJ, Quinlan DC, Davidson AG, et al. Altered retinoblastoma protein expression and prognosis in early-stage non-small-cell lung carcinoma. *J Natl Cancer Inst* 1994;86:695.

156. Chittenden T, Livingston DM, DeCaprio JA. Cell cycle analysis of E2F in primary human T cells reveals novel E2F complexes and biochemically distinct forms of free E2F. *Mol Cell Biol* 1993;13:3975.

157. Moberg K, Starz MA, Lees JA. E2F-4 switches from p130 to p107 and pRB in response to cell cycle reentry. *Mol Cell Biol* 1996;16:1436.

158. Hofmann F, Martelli F, Livingston DM, et al. The retinoblastoma gene product protects E2F-1 from degradation by the ubiquitin-proteasome pathway. *Genes Dev* 1996;10:2949.

159. Campanero MR, Flemington EK. Regulation of E2F through ubiquitin-proteasome-dependent degradation: stabilization by the pRB tumor suppressor protein. *Proc Natl Acad Sci USA* 1997;94:2221.

160. Qin XQ, Livingston DM, Kaelin WG, Jr., et al. Deregulated transcription factor E2F-1 expression leads to S-phase entry and p53-mediated apoptosis. *Proc Natl Acad Sci USA* 1994;91:10918.

161. Shan B, Lee WH. Deregulated expression of E2F-1 induces S-phase entry and leads to apoptosis. *Mol Cell Biol* 1994;14:8166.

162. Field SJ, Tsai FY, Kuo F, et al. E2F-1 functions in mice to promote apoptosis and suppress proliferation. *Cell* 1996;85:549.

163. Yamasaki L, Jacks T, Bronson R, et al. Tumor induction and tissue atrophy in mice lacking E2F-1. *Cell* 1996;85:537.

164. Nadal-Ginard B. Commitment, fusion and biochemical differentiation of a myogenic cell line in the absence of DNA synthesis. *Cell* 1978;15:855.

165. Jacobson MD, Weil M, Raff MC. Programmed cell death in animal development. *Cell* 1997;88:347.

166. Condorelli G, Giordano A. Synergistic role of E1A-binding proteins and tissue-specific transcription factors in differentiation. *J Cell Biochem* 1997;67:423.

167. Gu W, Schneider JW, Condorelli G, et al. Interaction of myogenic factors and the retinoblastoma protein mediates muscle cell commitment and differentiation. *Cell* 1993;72:309.

168. Chen PL, Riley DJ, Chen Y, et al. Retinoblastoma protein positively regulates terminal adipocyte differentiation through direct interaction with C/EBPs. *Genes Dev* 1996;10:2794.

169. Higgins C, Chatterjee S, Cherington V. The block of adipocyte differentiation by a C-terminally truncated, but not by full-length, simian virus 40 large tumor antigen is dependent on an intact retinoblastoma susceptibility protein family binding domain. *J Virol* 1996;70:745.

170. Dunaief JL, Strober BE, Guha S, et al. The retinoblastoma protein and BRG1 form a complex and cooperate to induce cell cycle arrest. *Cell* 1994;79:119.

171. Lee EY, Chang CY, Hu N, et al. Mice deficient for Rb are nonviable and show defects in neurogenesis and haematopoiesis [see comments]. *Nature* 1992;359:288.

172. Clarke AR, Maandag ER, van Roon M, et al. Requirement for a functional Rb-1 gene in murine development [see comments]. *Nature* 1992;359:328.

173. Condorelli GL, Testa U, Valtieri M, et al. Modulation of retinoblastoma gene in normal adult hematopoiesis: peak expression and functional role in advanced erythroid differentiation. *Proc Natl Acad Sci USA* 1995;92:4808.

174. Ewen ME, Xing YG, Lawrence JB, et al. Molecular cloning, chromosomal mapping, and expression of the cDNA for p107, a retinoblastoma gene product-related protein. *Cell* 1991;66:1155.

175. Mayol X, Grana X, Baldi A, et al. Cloning of a new member of the retinoblastoma gene family (pRb2) which binds to the E1A transforming domain. *Oncogene* 1993;8:2561.

176. Baldi A, De Luca A, Claudio PP, et al. The RB2/p130 gene product is a nuclear protein whose phosphorylation is cell cycle regulated. *J Cell Biochem* 1995;59:402.

177. Cobrinik D. Regulatory interactions among E2Fs and cell cycle control proteins. *Curr Top Microbiol Immunol* 1996;208:31.

178. Wang JY. Retinoblastoma protein in growth suppression and death protection. *Curr Opin Genet Dev* 1997;7:39.

179. Claudio PP, Howard CM, Baldi A, et al. p130/pRb2 has growth suppressive properties similar to yet distinctive from those of retinoblastoma family members pRb and p107. *Cancer Res* 1994;54:5556.

180. Ewen ME, Faha B, Harlow E, et al. Interaction of p107 with cyclin A independent of complex formation with viral oncoproteins. *Science* 1992;255:85.

181. Li Y, Graham C, Lacy S, et al. The adenovirus E1A-associated 130-kD protein is encoded by a member of the retinoblastoma gene family and physically interacts with cyclins A and E. *Genes Dev* 1993;7:2366.

182. Faha B, Ewen ME, Tsai LH, et al. Interaction between human cyclin A and adenovirus E1A-associated p107 protein. *Science* 1992;255:87.

183. Claudio PP, De Luca A, Howard CM, et al. Functional analysis of pRb2/p130 interaction with cyclins. *Cancer Res* 1996;56:2003.

184. Hannon GJ, Demetrick D, Beach D. Isolation of the Rb-related p130 through its interaction with CDK2 and cyclins. *Genes Dev* 1993;7:2378.

185. Shirodkar S, Ewen M, DeCaprio JA, et al. The transcription factor E2F interacts with the retinoblastoma product and a p107-cyclin A complex in a cell cycle-regulated manner. *Cell* 1992;68:157.

186. Beijersbergen RL, Carlee L, Kerkhoven RM, et al. Regulation of the retinoblastoma protein-related p107 by G1 cyclin complexes. *Genes Dev* 1995;9:1340.

187. Lees E, Faha B, Dulic V, et al. Cyclin E/cdk2 and cyclin A/cdk2 kinases associate with p107 and E2F in a temporally distinct manner. *Genes Dev* 1992;6:1874.

188. Cobrinik D, Whyte P, Peeper DS, et al. Cell cycle-specific asso-

ciation of E2F with the p130 E1A-binding protein. *Genes Dev* 1993;7:2392.

189. Cao L, Faha B, Dembski M, et al. Independent binding of the retinoblastoma protein and p107 to the transcription factor E2F. *Nature* 1992;355:176.

190. Lindeman GJ, Gaubatz S, Livingston DM, et al. The subcellular localization of E2F-4 is cell-cycle dependent. *Proc Natl Acad Sci USA* 1997;94:5095.

191. Magae J, Wu CL, Illenye S, et al. Nuclear localization of DP and E2F transcription factors by heterodimeric partners and retinoblastoma protein family members. *J Cell Sci* 1996;109:1717.

192. Puri PL, Cimino L, Fulco M, et al. Regulation of E2F4 mitogenic activity during terminal differentiation by its heterodimerization partners for nuclear translocation. *Cancer Res* 1998;58:1325.

193. Jacks T, Fazeli A, Schmitt EM, et al. Effects of an Rb mutation in the mouse [see comments]. *Nature* 1992;359:295.

194. Lee MH, Williams BO, Mulligan G, et al. Targeted disruption of p107: functional overlap between p107 and Rb. *Genes Dev* 1996;10:1621.

195. Cobrinik D, Lee MH, Hannon G, et al. Shared role of the pRB-related p130 and p107 proteins in limb development. *Genes Dev* 1996;10:1633.

196. Jiang Z, Zacksenhaus E, Gallie BL, et al. The retinoblastoma gene family is differentially expressed during embryogenesis. *Oncogene* 1997;14:1789.

197. Hurford RK, Jr., Cobrinik D, Lee MH, et al. pRB and p107/p130 are required for the regulated expression of different sets of E2F responsive genes. *Genes Dev* 1997;11:1447.

198. Giordano A, McCall C, Whyte P, et al. Human cyclin A and the retinoblastoma protein interact with similar but distinguishable sequences in the adenovirus E1A gene product. *Oncogene* 1991;6:481.

199. Moran E. DNA tumor virus transforming proteins and the cell cycle. *Curr Opin Genet Dev* 1993;3:63.

200. Zhu L, Enders G, Lees JA, et al. The pRB-related protein p107 contains two growth suppression domains: independent interactions with E2F and cyclin/cdk complexes. *Embo J* 1995;14:1904.

201. De Luca A, MacLachlan TK, Bagella L, et al. A unique domain of pRb2/p130 acts as an inhibitor of Cdk2 kinase activity. *J Biol Chem* 1997;272:20971.

202. Zhu L, Harlow E, Dynlacht BD. p107 uses a p21CIP1-related domain to bind cyclin/cdk2 and regulate interactions with E2F. *Genes Dev* 1995;9:1740–52.

203. Woo MS, Sanchez I, Dynlacht BD. p130 and p107 use a conserved domain to inhibit cellular cyclin- dependent kinase activity. *Mol Cell Biol* 1997;17:3566.

204. Ewen ME, Ludlow JW, Marsilio E, et al. An N-terminal transformation-governing sequence of SV40 large T antigen contributes to the binding of both p110Rb and a second cellular protein, p120. *Cell* 1989;58:257.

205. Yeung RS, Bell DW, Testa JR, et al. The retinoblastoma-related gene, RB2, maps to human chromosome 16q12 and rat chromosome 19. *Oncogene* 1993;8:3465.

206. Sun Y, Hegamyer G, Colburn NH. Nasopharyngeal carcinoma shows no detectable retinoblastoma susceptibility gene alterations. *Oncogene* 1993;8:791.

207. Yan L, Xi Z, Drettner B. Epidemiological studies of nasopharyngeal cancer in the Guangzhou area, China. Preliminary report. *Acta Otolaryngol* (Stockh) 1989;107:424.

208. Mascolo A, Levin S, Giordano A. A molecular biological approach to the study of nasopharyngeal cancer in Chinese Garment workers. *Ramazzini Newsletter* 1992;2:54.

209. Baldi A, Esposito V, De Luca A, et al. Differential expression of the retinoblastoma gene family members, Rb/p105, p107 and pRb2/p130, in lung cancer. *Clin Cancer Res* 1996;7:1239–1245.

210. Baldi A, Esposito V, De Luca A, et al. Differential expression of Rb2/p130 and p107 in normal human tissues and in primary lung cancer. *Clin Cancer Res* 1997;3:1691.

211. Susini T, Baldi F, Howard CM, et al. Expression of the retinoblastoma-related gene Rb2/p130 correlates with clinical outcome in endometrial cancer. *J Clin Oncol* 1998;16:1085.

212. Helin K, Holm K, Niebuhr A, et al. Loss of the retinoblastoma protein-related p130 protein in small cell lung carcinoma. *Proc Natl Acad Sci USA* 1997;94:6933.

213. Howard CM, Claudio PP, Gallia GL, et al. Retinoblastoma-related protein pRb2/p130 and suppression of tumor growth in vivo. *JNCI* 90:1451.

214. Cinti C, Claudio PP, Howard CM, et al. Genetic alterations disrupting the nuclear localization of the retinoblastoma related gene *RB2/p130* in human cell lines and primary tumors (*in press*, 1998).

215. Wiest JS, Franklin WA, Drabkin H, Genetic markers for early detection of lung cancer and outcome measures for response to chemoprevention. *J Cell Biochem Suppl* 1997;29:64.

216. Todd S, Franklin WA, Varella-Garcia M, et al. Homozygous deletions of human chromosome 3p in lung tumors. *Cancer Res* 1997;57:1344.

217. Wiest JS, Franklin WA, Otstot JT, et al. Identification of a novel region of homozygous deletion on chromosome 9p in squamous cell carcinoma of the lung: the location of a putative tumor suppressor gene. *Cancer Res* 1997;57:1.

218. Shimizu E, Sone S. Tumor suppressor genes in human lung cancer. *J Med Invest* 1997;44:15.

219. Shiseki M, Kohno T, Nishikawa R, et al. Frequent allelic losses on chromosomes 2q, 18q, and 22q in advanced non-small cell lung carcinoma. *Cancer Res* 1994;54:5643.

220. Levin NA, Brzoska PM, Warnock ML, et al. Identification of novel regions of altered DNA copy number in small cell lung tumors. *Genes Chromosomes Cancer* 1995;13:175.

221. Levin NA, Brzoska P, Gupta N, et al. Identification of frequent novel genetic alterations in small cell lung carcinoma. *Cancer Res* 1994;54:5086.

222. Demoly P, Pujol JL, Godard P, et al. [Oncogenes and anti-oncogenes in lung cancer]. *Presse Med* 1994;23:291.

223. Salgia R, Skarin AT. Molecular abnormalities in lung cancer. *J Clin Oncol* 1998;16:1207.

224. Ferron PE, Bagni I, Guidoboni M, et al. Combined and sequential expression of p53, Rb, Ras and Bcl-2 in bronchial preneoplastic lesions. *Tumori* 1997;83:587.

225. Gazdar AF. The molecular and cellular basis of human lung cancer. *Anticancer Res* 1994;14:261.

226. Dosaka-Akita H, Hu SX, Fujino M, et al. Altered retinoblastoma protein expression in nonsmall cell lung cancer: its synergistic effects with altered ras and p53 protein status on prognosis. *Cancer* 1997;79:1329.

227. Baldi A, Boccia V, Claudio PP, et al. Genomic structure of the human retinoblastoma-related Rb2/p130 gene. *Proc Natl Acad Sci USA* 1996;93:4629.

228. Yandell DW, Campbell TA, Dayton SH, et al. Oncogenic point mutations in the human retinoblastoma gene: their application to genetic counseling [see comments]. *N Engl J Med* 1989;321:1689.

229. Malkinson AM. Molecular comparison of human and mouse pulmonary adenocarcinomas. *Exp Lung Res* 1998;24:541.

230. Dunst J. [Gene therapy with wild-type p53 in lung tumors]. *Strahlenther Onkol* 1997;173:431.

231. Carbone DP, Minna JD. In vivo gene therapy of human lung

cancer using wild-type p53 delivered by retrovirus [editorial; comment]. *J Natl Cancer Inst* 1994;86:1437.

232. Roth JA, Nguyen D, Lawrence DD, et al. Retrovirus-mediated wild-type p53 gene transfer to tumors of patients with lung cancer [see comments]. *Nat Med* 1996;2:985.

233. Roth JA, Swisher SG, Merritt JA, et al. Gene therapy for non-small cell lung cancer: a preliminary report of a phase I trial of adenoviral p53 gene replacement. *Semin Oncol* 1998;25:33.

234. Nguyen DM, Wiehle SA, Koch PE, et al. Delivery of the p53 tumor suppressor gene into lung cancer cells by an adenovirus/DNA complex. *Cancer Gene Ther* 1997;4:191.

235. Nguyen DM, Spitz FR, Yen N, et al. Gene therapy for lung cancer: enhancement of tumor suppression by a combination of sequential systemic cisplatin and adenovirus-mediated p53 gene transfer. *J Thorac Cardiovasc Surg* 1996;112:1372; discussion 1376.

236. Riley DJ, Nikitin AY, Lee WH. Adenovirus-mediated retinoblastoma gene therapy suppresses spontaneous pituitary melanotroph tumors in Rb+/− mice. *Nat Med* 1996;2:1316.

237. Fueyo J, Gomez-Manzano C, Yung WK, et al. Suppression of human glioma growth by adenovirus-mediated Rb gene transfer [see comments]. *Neurology* 1998;50:1307.

238. Howard CM, Claudio PP, Gallia GL, et al. Retinoblastoma-related protein pRb2/p130 and suppression of tumor growth in vivo [In Process Citation]. *J Natl Cancer Inst* 1998;90:1451.

239. Miller AD. Progress toward human gene therapy. *Blood* 1990; 76:271.

240. Miller DG, Adam MA, Miller AD. Gene transfer by retrovirus vectors occurs only in cells that are actively replicating at the time of infection [published erratum appears in *Mol Cell Biol* 1992 Jan;12(1):433]. *Mol Cell Biol* 1990;10:4239.

241. Carbone M, Rizzo P, Grimley PM, et al. Simian virus-40 large-T antigen binds p53 in human mesotheliomas [see comments]. *Nat Med* 1997;3:908.

242. De Luca A, Baldi A, Esposito V, et al. The retinoblastoma gene family pRb/p105, p107, pRb2/p130 and simian virus-40 large

T-antigen in human mesotheliomas [see comments]. *Nat Med* 1997;3:913.

243. Pass H, Rizzo P, Donington J, et al. Further validation of SV40-like DNA in human pleural mesotheliomas [In Process Citation]. *Dev Biol Stand* 1998;94:143.

244. Fattaey AR, Harlow E, Helin K. Independent regions of adenovirus E1A are required for binding to and dissociation of E2F-protein complexes. *Mol Cell Biol* 1993;13:7267.

245. Vousden KH. Regulation of the cell cycle by viral oncoproteins. *Sem Cancer Biol* 1995;6:109.

246. Anderson M, Sladon S, Michels R, et al. Examination of p53 alterations and cytokeratin expression in sputa collected from patients prior to histological diagnosis of squamous cell carcinoma. *J Cell Biochem Suppl* 1996;25:185.

247. Carney DN. Lung cancer biology. *Curr Opin Oncol* 1991;3: 288.

248. Santoso JT, Tang DC, Lane SB, et al. Adenovirus-based p53 gene therapy in ovarian cancer [see comments]. *Gynecol Oncol* 1995;59:171.

249. Fujiwara T, Grimm EA, Mukhopadhyay T, et al. A retroviral wild-type p53 expression vector penetrates human lung cancer spheroids and inhibits growth by inducing apoptosis. *Cancer Res* 1993;53:4129.

250. Sumegi J, Uzvolgyi E, Klein G. Expression of the RB gene under the control of MuLV-LTR suppresses tumorigenicity of WERI-Rb-27 retinoblastoma cells in immunodefective mice. *Cell Growth Differ* 1990;1:247.

251. Lefebvre D, Gala JL, Heusterspreute M, et al. Introduction of a normal retinoblastoma (Rb) gene into Rb-deficient lymphoblastoid cells delays tumorigenicity in immunodefective mice. *Leuk Res* 1998;22:905.

252. Zalvide J, DeCaprio JA. Role of pRb-related proteins in simian virus 40 large-T-antigen-mediated transformation. *Mol Cell Biol* 1995;15:5800.

253. Romano G, Claudio PP, Kaiser HE, et al. Recent advances, prospects and problems in designing new strategies for oligonucleotide and gene delivery in therapy. *In Vivo* 1998;12:59.

8

THE ROLE OF THE *FHIT* GENE IN THE PATHOGENESIS OF LUNG CANCER

MARIA-LUISA VERONESE
GABRIELLA SOZZI
KAY HUEBNER
CARLO M. CROCE

Lung cancer is a major cause of mortality worldwide, and despite progress in early detection and treatment, the overall survival rate has not improved significantly during the past two decades.[1] A direct association between lung cancer and smoking is well known, being first observed 55 years ago by Ochsner and DeBakey[2] and subsequently confirmed by epidemiologic studies.[3,4] Lung tumors that develop in nonsmokers account for only 5% to 10% of all lung cancers.[5,6] Although the relationship between carcinogen exposure and tumorigenesis has long been recognized, the molecular events resulting in lung cancer have been defined only recently. Lung cancer, similar to other cancers, results from the sequential accumulation of specific genetic changes. These changes involve deletions of the short arm of chromosome 3 (3p), inactivation of tumor-suppressor genes *TP53*, *CDKN2*, and *RB*, deregulated expression of *EGER* and *HER2/neu* oncogenes, and alteration in expression of proteins involved in apoptosis control, such as Bcl2, as well as point mutations in *KRAS2* and amplification of *myc* oncogene family members (see also Chapters 4, 5, 6, 7, 23).[7] Definition of the genetic alterations and the associated alterations in biologic behavior of lung cancer will undoubtedly aid in the design of novel therapies, as well as in early diagnosis and prevention of the disease.

Evidence linking exposure to carcinogens in cigarette smoke and specific genetic alterations of the bronchial tissue is accumulating. In particular, deletions of loci on the short arm of chromosome 3, which have been recognized as early events in lung tumor development, seem to be preferential targets of tobacco smoke carcinogens.[8,9] We have shown that the *FHIT* gene at chromosome 3p14.2 plays a critical and early role in lung carcinogenesis.[10] Interestingly, this gene that spans more than 1.5 Mb of DNA contains the most inducible of the constitutive fragile sites of the human genome, *FRA3B*, a common target of rearrangements in lung carcinogenesis.

In this chapter we examine the importance of the 3p14.2 region and the *FRA3B* fragile site in lung cancer. We summarize previous studies on the cloning and characterization of the *FHIT* gene and the investigation of the Fhit protein and its biologic function. We also describe the biallelic alterations of the *FHIT/FRA3B* locus in human cancers, methods to detect these alterations, and our theories about the mechanisms involved in deletion. Finally, we discuss the role of *FHIT* in lung tumors and the clinical implications of its loss of function.

THE GENE

The Short Arm of Chromosome 3 and the FRA3B

Chromosomal deletions and loss of heterozygosity (LOH) involving the short arm of chromosome 3 (3p) are often detected in carcinomas of the lung, head and neck, kidney, stomach, breast, cervix, and ovary.[11–17] At least four distinct regions—3pl12, 3p14, 3p21, and 3p24–25—have been identified by LOH studies, suggesting the presence of tumor-suppressor genes involved in the pathogenesis of several epithelial neoplasia in these regions. The von Hippel-Lindau gene (*VHL*) at chromosome 3p25 was isolated several years ago.[18] This gene is responsible for some familial kidney carcinomas, is inactivated in a large fraction of sporadic renal cancers, but does not seem to be involved in lung cancer.[19] A gene at chromosome band 3p14.2 has been sought for many years because this region is the site of a balanced chromosome translocation, t(3;8)(p14.2;q24), associated with familial clear cell renal carcinoma.[20] This translocation is also known to be close to an interesting genetic landmark, *FRA3B*, the most inducible of the constitutive or common human chromosomal fragile sites.[21,22]

Fragile sites are specific chromosome regions that reveal specific cytogenetically detectable gaps or breaks when cells are exposed to certain chemicals, for example inhibitors of

DNA synthesis such as aphidicolin, and are divided into two classes, common and rare.[23,24] Common fragile sites are highly conserved during evolution, are induced by agents that perturb DNA replication, and have been implicated in interchromosomal and intrachromosomal rearrangements, deletions and translocations in hybrid cells, and plasmid and viral integration.[25-28] Expression of fragile sites can also trigger gene overexpression, suggesting their possible role in oncogenic amplification during tumorigenesis.[29] The coincident chromosome location of common fragile sites, characteristic cancer breakpoints, and genes involved in tumor development has suggested that fragile sites could be involved in specific chromosomal rearrangements in malignant diseases, or harbor oncogenes or tumor-suppressor genes that are altered in the process of carcinogenesis.

Interestingly, *FRA3B*, the most inducible constitutive fragile site, located at 3p14.2 and is expressed after exposure of cultured cells to diverse carcinogens, including benzo[*a*]pyrene diol epoxide, the ultimate carcinogen of benzo[*a*]pyrene, a major constituent of tobacco smoke.[28] In addition, homozygous deletions within the *FRA3B* in primary lung cancers have been shown to correlate with exposure to cigarette carcinogens and asbestos.[9] Understanding the structure of the *FRA3B* could provide clues to the mechanism of fragility. We sequenced approximately 800 kb of the 3p14.2 region containing the *FRA3B* locus and precisely located the homozygous deletion breakpoints of numerous cancer cell lines, including those derived from lung cancers.[22,30,31] The *FRA3B* locus has a low content of Alu repeats and is abundant in LINE repeats over 1 kb in length, mostly of the L1 subtype; most of the deletion endpoints in tumor-derived cell lines involve L1 repeats greater than 1 kb in length or long terminal repeats (LTRs).[22,30,31]

This finding suggests that homologous recombination between L1 sequences or LTRs can result in internal deletions within the *FHIT* gene in response to carcinogen-induced double-strand breaks at the *FRA3B* fragile region. The breakpoints are induced by agents such as aphidicolin, an inhibitor of DNA polymerase α and δ apparently occurring in regions of the highest DNA flexibility, confirming a relationship between fragility and DNA flexibility, as suggested by Mishmar et al.[32,33] Thus double-strand breaks occurring in regions of high flexibility, which could result in cell death, may be rescued by homologous recombination involving LINE 1 elements or LTRs, leading to deletion of the intervening DNA sequences.

Cloning and Characterization of the *FHIT* Gene

The definition of the region of hemi- and homozygous loss at 3p14.2 within YAC clone 850A6, telomeric to the t(3; 8) translocation, in cancer-derived cell lines, facilitated the cloning of the *FHIT* gene, a portion of which was included in the homozygously deleted region.[34,35] We constructed a cosmid contig covering this common deleted region, the t(3;8) translocation and the *FRA3B* region, and identified and cloned the *FHIT* gene. Individual cosmids were used in exon-trapping experiments, and primer extension was used to obtain a 5' extended product from the initial trapped *FHIT* exon 5. A full-length cDNA was characterized and the genomic structure determined. The 1.1-kb *FHIT* cDNA consists of 10 small exons and is distributed over a genomic locus of greater than one megabase. The protein coding region begins in exon 5 and ends in exon 9 (Figure 8.1).

We characterized deletions in numerous cancer-derived cell lines and observed that homozygous deletions can occur in several discontinuous segments within the *FRA3B/FHIT* locus and often involve loss of specific *FHIT* exons (Figure 8.2).[36] The common deleted region originally defined in tumor-derived cell lines often involves exon 5.[35,36] The first three 5' exons of the gene are centromeric to the t(3;8) break, an observation that is consistent with the involvement of *FHIT* in the development of familial clear cell renal carcinoma because one copy of the gene is disrupted by the translocation.[35] Further characterization of the complex homozygous deletions revealed that they are often the result of overlap of independent deletions of the two *FRA3B/FHIT* alleles.[22,36] For example, a stomach carcinoma–derived cell line, AGS, exhibited three separate regions of homozygous deletions, including exon 3, a portion of intron 4, and exon 5.[36] The Kato III cell line showed independent biallelic deletions resulting in absence of Fhit protein, and the Siha cervical carcinoma cell line exhibited a small homozygous deletion in intron 4, also the result of overlap of biallelic deletions.[36,30,31] Figure 8.2 illustrates portions of *FHIT* alleles missing within the gene in some cancer-derived cell lines.

Northern blot analysis indicated that *FHIT* is expressed at variable levels in all normal human tissues tested, as a 1.1-kb mRNA. The highest levels have been detected in epithelial tissues. Initial studies of primary gastrointestinal tumors, compared to their normal counterparts, using reverse transcription-polymerase chain reaction (RT-PCR) showed a mixture of apparently normal size transcripts and aberrant transcripts in the tumor tissues, with complete absence of the full-length product in some tumors.[35] Sequence analysis of these short abnormal transcripts revealed that regions between exons 4 and 9 were missing, whereas mRNA from matched normal tissue did not exhibit alteration. Several studies later reported presence of similar aberrant transcripts in mRNA from some normal cells, such as white blood cells, raising the question of the cancer-specificity of the alterations initially detected.[37,38] Such transcripts in normal cells are, however, faint and not reproducible, suggesting that such transcripts in normal cells are artifacts. Numerous experiments have shown consistent, reproducible, and abundant aberrant *FHIT* transcripts in cancer cells, supporting the original observation that detection of abnor-

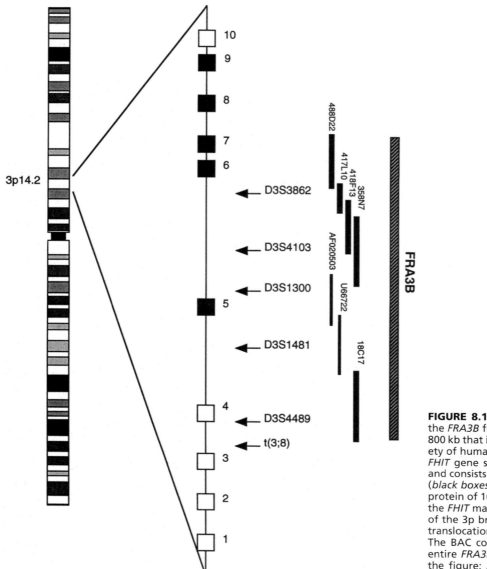

FIGURE 8.1. The *FHIT* gene at 3p14.2 contains the *FRA3B* fragile site, a region of approximately 800 kb that is often involved in deletions in a variety of human cancers, including lung cancer. The *FHIT* gene spans well over 1 Megabase of DNA and consists of 10 exons, of which five are coding (*black boxes*). It encodes a mRNA of 1.1 kb and a protein of 16.8 kD. The position of 3p markers on the *FHIT* map is described, as well as the position of the 3p break involved in the t(3;8)(p14.2;q24) translocation in a family with renal cell carcinoma. The BAC contig we have used to sequence the entire *FRA3B* region is described on the right of the figure; AF020503 and U66722 are Genbank accession numbers for published sequences.

mal *FHIT* RT-PCR products indicates the presence of *FHIT* genomic alterations.

The genetic alterations to the *FHIT* gene, usually involving independent deletions within both alleles, rather than point mutations, are probably the result of the particular location of the *FRA3B* fragile region within the *FHIT* gene, rendering it more susceptible to deletions than point mutations. When antibodies recognizing the Fhit protein became available, we demonstrated a good correlation between DNA and RNA alterations and the absence of the expression of the Fhit protein in tumors.[36] Initial studies in gastric cancer cell lines showed that absence of *FHIT* mRNA by Northern blot analysis and presence of aberrant RT-PCR products were associated with absence of Fhit protein.[39]

Immunohistochemic analysis showed absence of Fhit protein in gastric carcinomas and strong *FHIT* expression in the normal epithelial cells within the same tissue sections.[39]

Similar results have been reported in lung cancer, breast cancer, cervical cancer, pancreatic cancer, and clear renal cell carcinoma.[40–44] Of particular interest is the finding that Fhit protein was absent in low-grade, low-stage clear cell renal carcinomas, whereas higher grade and stage tumors displayed a mixture of Fhit-positive and -negative cancer cells.[44] These results suggest that the *FHIT* gene plays a role during the early steps of tumor development in the low-grade renal carcinomas and is associated with progression in the high-grade tumors. Subsequent studies in lung cancers showed Fhit inactivation in preneoplastic lesions,[10] in line

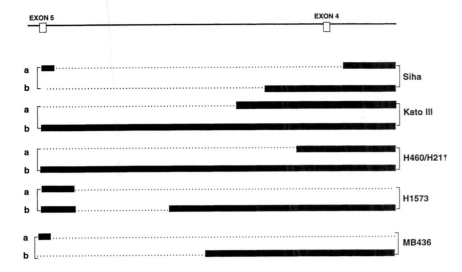

FIGURE 8.2. Biallelic *FHIT* deletions involving the *FRA3B* fragile site in human tumor-derived cell lines. Five cell lines derived from cervical cancer (Siha), gastric cancer (Kato III), lung cancer (H460/H211, H1573), and breast cancer (MB436) were studied for alterations of the *FHIT* gene. The DNA junctions associated with the deletions were sequenced by inverted PCR as described by Mimori et al. (From Mimori K, Druck T, Inoue H, et al. Cancer specific chromosome alterations in the constitutive fragile region. *FRA3B. Proc Natl Acad Sci USA* 1999;96:7456, with permission.) As shown in the figure, the region between intron 3 and exon 5 is involved in deletions in these cell lines. In the gastric cancer cell line, Kato III, the deletion in the allele b occurred past exon 5. In the lung carcinoma H460/H211, the deletion of the allele b is outside the region shown. The black bars represent the undeleted portions of alleles.

with the observation that loss at 3p14/*FHIT* is the earliest LOH event observed in preneoplastic lung lesions,[45,46] and showing that complete Fhit loss is a very early event in the development of lung cancer.

THE PROTEIN

The Fhit Protein and the HIT Family

The *FHIT* gene encodes a polypeptide of 16.8 kD that consists of 147 amino acids that show 52% identity and 69% similarity to a core region of 109 amino acids of the diadenosine 5′, 5′′′-P1,P4-tetraphosphate (Ap$_4$A) hydrolase from the fission yeast *Schizosaccaromyces pombe*.[35,47,48] This latter enzyme catalyzes the *in vitro* hydrolysis of dinucleoside polyphosphates, with Ap$_4$A as the preferred substrate. Both the Fhit protein and the *S. pombe* Ap$_4$A are members of the Histidine Triad (HIT) protein family. HIT proteins are characterized by four conserved histidines, three of which form a histidine triad sequence that, together with a distinct protein fold, binds nucleotides (Figure 8.3).[48,49] Although *FHIT* also cleaves Ap$_4$A efficiently, biochemical studies and site-directed mutagenesis analysis demonstrated that the Fhit protein could be classified as an Ap$_3$A hydrolase on the basis of its *in vitro* enzymatic activity and that all three conserved histidines are required for full activity (Figure 8.3).[50] Structural analysis and sequence comparison linked Fhit to Hint (triad nucleotide-binding protein) proteins, whose most conserved residues mediate nucleotide binding.[51,52] The HIT motif forms part of the phosphate-binding loop of Hint proteins. Thus Fhit is a member of the HIT family involved in nucleotide metabolism. Interestingly, Fhit substrates, Ap$_4$A and Ap$_3$A, accumulate in human cultured cells as a consequence of toxic stress or interferon induction, suggesting a possible involvement of Fhit in signaling responses to cellular stress.[53,54]

Biologic Function of Fhit

As mentioned previously, Fhit is a mammalian member of the HIT family of proteins. Insight into the enzymatic function of Fhit came from its similarity to the yeast enzyme, Ap$_4$A hydrolase, and our data have shown that Fhit has Ap$_3$A hydrolase activity.[50] However, the *in vitro* enzymatic activity of Fhit did not suggest a biologic function for Fhit. Because established cancer cell lines can be positive or negative for Fhit expression, and because Fhit-negative cell lines and their Fhit-positive DNA transfectants grow well *in vitro*, Fhit expression did not seem to alter the ability to grow in culture.[55] This experiment is not conclusive, however, because the Fhit-expressing clones are selected for constitutive Fhit expression. In addition, the pattern of Fhit expression did not correlate with any phase of the cell cycle.

To analyze Fhit biologic function, several cancer cell lines, including lung, kidney, and gastric, were transfected with *FHIT* cDNA.[55] The number of colonies obtained after transfection with the *FHIT* vector was lower compared to transfection with the empty vector, and only a few of the selected colonies expressed Fhit, suggesting that overexpression *FHIT* was selected against. The lung cancer clones expressing exogenous Fhit exhibited a longer doubling time in liquid medium than the parental Fhit-negative H460 cells and formed fewer colonies in soft agar. The Fhit-expressing gastric (MKN74*FHIT* and AGS*FHIT*) and kidney (RC48*FHIT*) cancer clones did not show changes in the *in vitro* growth pattern compared to the negative parental cells. *In vivo* experiments conducted by inoculating Fhit-expressing clones of each cell line, as well as empty-vector transfected clones, into nude mice showed that the expression of Fhit in the clones suppressed their tumorigenicity *in vivo*.[55] Thus the expression of Fhit strongly affects the ability of cells to form tumors *in vivo*.

Evidence is also accumulating that binding to diadenos-

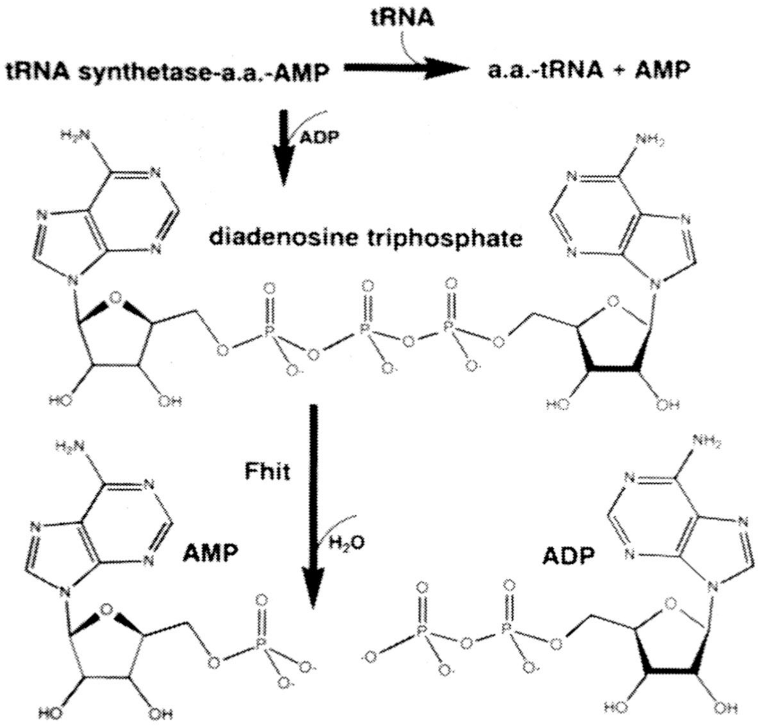

FIGURE 8.3. Fhit encodes an Ap_3A hydrolase. Diadenosine triphosphate (Ap_3A) is a product of the tryptophan tRNA synthetase. Ap_3A is cleaved by Fhit into AMP and ADP. As mentioned in the text, Ap_3A is found to be elevated in a variety of human cancers.

ine triphosphate regulates the activity of Fhit. In particular, transfectants with a mutant form of Fhit that binds diadenosine polyphosphates well but does not cleave them are unable to form tumors in nude mice or to form tumors of reduced size.[50,55,56] This finding indicates that Fhit binding with a dinucleotide polyphosphate is important for tumor-suppressor activity and that the Fhit-Ap_3A complex may send the tumor-suppression signal. Similarly, activated Ras p21, a nucleotide-binding protein, exerts its tumorigenic action by decreasing guanosine triphosphatase (GTPase) activity.[57] Because the GTP-bound form of Ras stimulates cell division, oncogenic-activating mutations of Ras lead to cellular transformation. X-ray crystallography provided an attractive model of the structural consequences of *Fhit*-substrate binding, reminiscent of the conformational change of GTP-bound Ras, which results in activation of mitogenic effectors.[56] Two diadenosine polyphosphate substrates fill the positively charged cleft of the Fhit dimer in its empty form and convert it to a bulging electronegative surface. It is possible that the tumor-suppressing effectors of Fhit recognize this change in protein appearance, interact with the Fhit-substrate complex, and are activated.

Fhit and Apoptosis

To gain insight into the biologic mechanisms underlying Fhit overexpression in lung cancer cells, we studied H460/*FHIT* clones overexpressing Fhit for proliferation, apoptosis, and cell cycle profiles.[58]

We focused on the lung cancer cell line H460 and on H460/*FHIT* clones transfected with a *FHIT*-FLAG expression vector under control of a CMV promoter. Endogenous wild-type *FHIT* mRNA transcript and protein are undetectable in the H460 cells. Only a few stable Fhit-expressing clones were isolated after transfection of H460 cells with pRC-CMV/*FHIT,* suggesting that constitutive overexpression negatively affects cell growth. In contrast, in 293 adenovirus 5 transformed human kidney cells, which express endogenous Fhit, enforced Fhit overexpression does not affect cell growth, as reflected in the high yield of rescued colonies and the high number of Fhit expressors among them.[55] Analysis of apoptosis by *in situ* TUNEL assay (TdT mediated dUTP Nick End Labelling) revealed a high rate of apoptosis-induced DNA strand breaks in stable H460/*FHIT* clones. *In situ* results were confirmed by FACS can analysis, which showed an apoptotic rate of 44% to 47% compared to a 15% level in the control H460 cells. No significant changes in Bcl2, BclX, and Bax protein expression levels were observed in the transfected clones as compared to the control H460 cells, whereas a two-fold increase in Bak protein levels was noted.[58] An increased level of $p21^{waf}$ protein, paralleled by an upregulation of $p21^{waf}$ transcripts, was also found in Fhit-expressing clones compared to H460 parental cells. No differences in p53 levels were observed in the same cells, suggesting a p53-independent effect.[58]

These data suggest that the observed growth-inhibitory effect in Fhit-expressing H460 cells could be related to apoptosis and cell cycle arrest, and link the tumor-suppressor activity of Fhit to a proapoptotic function. Interestingly, it has been reported that apoptosis in human cultured cells is associated with a decrease of free Ap_3A levels,[59] suggesting that Fhit, through binding with Ap_3A, is involved in induction of apoptosis.

A recent paper from J. Roth's group strengthens the observation of Fhit involvement in apoptosis, with relevant *in vitro* and *in vivo* experiments.[60] In this study an adenovirus-*FHIT* vector was used to study the effect of Fhit expression in several cancer cell lines, including H460, and normal human bronchial epithelial cells. Transient overexpression of exogenous Fhit resulted in cell growth inhibition of tumor cell lines, associated with induction of apoptosis and alteration of cell cycle processes. Moreover, the tumorigenicity of the highly tumorigenic H1299 lung cancer cells transduced by Ad-*FHIT* was eliminated *in vivo*. Together, these results suggest that the *FHIT* gene functions as a tumor-suppressor gene.

ROLE IN CANCER

Detection of *FHIT* Gene Alterations

The characterization and sequencing of the *FHIT* gene and the *FRA3B* fragile region facilitated the detection of *FHIT* rearrangements in primary cancers and cancer-derived cell lines.[30,31,35] Alterations at the *FHIT* locus are characterized by deletions, including homozygous deletions, of coding exons, intronic deletions, deletions involving one coding exon in one allele and another coding exon on the other allele, multiple discontinuous regions of deletion in some cell lines, and deletions affecting the 5' untranslated exons, such as exons 3 and 4.[22,36] The effect of all these alterations is the loss or severe reduction of expression of Fhit protein.[22,36] The pattern of alterations characteristic of the *FHIT* gene in cancer cells is different from that of other tumor-suppressor genes, and for this reason the involvement of *FHIT* in human cancer has been slow to be accepted, that is, since *FHIT* is not p53.

Analysis of the levels of *FHIT* transcripts in cases with complex deletions within the *FHIT* gene presents a challenge; *FHIT* mRNA is not abundant and its detection requires poly A^+ RNA, which is usually not available from primary cancers. Therefore, *FHIT* expression has often been studied by RT-PCR. Cancer-derived cell lines and primary tumors exhibited different sized transcripts, ranging from apparent normal to short products, or absence of products.[36] Short abnormal transcripts were often detected in cell lines with defined deletions, consistent with the suggestion that aberrant products reflect DNA lesions.[22,36] Several

laboratories observed similar short *FHIT* products in normal cells and normal *FHIT* transcripts in cancer cells and argued against the tumor-specificity or relevance to tumor development of these abnormalities.[37,38] Such aberrant transcripts in normal tissues are, however, not consistent from one experiment to another and may be artifacts of the amplification process. Extensive analysis of many tumors revealed that abnormal *FHIT* transcripts are consistently detected and much more common in cancer tissues, indicating that although the RT-PCR assay has pitfalls and must be interpreted with caution, aberrant *FHIT* amplification products often indicate DNA damage.

The availability of antiserum against the Fhit protein allowed the demonstration of the abundant expression of Fhit protein in normal epithelial tissues and its absence in tumors.[39-44] Western blot analysis showed that cancer cell lines with *FHIT* DNA deletions or aberrant transcripts lacked Fhit protein; cancer cell lines with no *FHIT* DNA or RNA alterations expressed normal Fhit protein; and cancer cell lines with a mixture of normal and aberrant *FHIT* products exhibited reduced levels of Fhit expression.[36] Even more exciting were the results of immunohistochemic analysis of cytologic preparations from cancer cell lines and tumor sections. Nine of eleven lung cancer–derived cell lines, 73% of primary small cell lung cancer (SCLC) tested, lacked Fhit protein expression, and near concordance was observed between RNA alteration and protein expression.[40] Similar results were obtained by analyzing cervical cancers.[42] Seventy percent of cervical carcinomas showed reduction or lack of Fhit expression, whereas the normal cervical tissue in the same section showed normal Fhit expression. Again, a correlation existed between Fhit expression and DNA or RNA alterations.

Thus immunohistochemic methods are useful in determining the relevance of Fhit in tumorigenesis and are the best way to assess the level of Fhit involvement in a clinical setting.

FHIT Abnormalities in Human Cancer

The *FHIT* gene is inactivated in a wide range of solid tumors, including breast cancer, head and neck cancer, gastrointestinal and esophageal cancer, renal cancer, cervical cancer, and lung cancer. Analysis of numerous cell lines derived from tumors of the gastrointestinal tract, as well as from other sites, demonstrated a correlation of DNA lesions at the *FHIT* locus with aberrant RT-PCR products and altered *FHIT* protein.[36] The most common type of alterations were deletions and/or rearrangements within the gene. In addition, the same study showed that Fhit protein may be reduced or absent, even in absence of detectable DNA or RNA alterations, suggesting the usefulness of Western blot analysis and immunohistochemistry in assessing the level of Fhit involvement.

Baffa et al.[39] analyzed 32 primary adenocarcinomas of

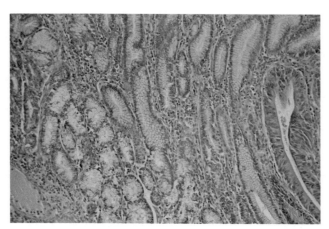

FIGURE 8.4. Immunohistochemistry of a gastric adenocarcinoma for expression of Fhit protein. As shown in the figure, the normal gastric epithelial cells stain strongly positive for Fhit, whereas the adenocarcinoma cells are completely negative (From Croce C, Sozzi G, Huebner K. Role of FHIT in human cancer. *J Clin Oncol* 1999;17:1618, with permission.) (See Color Figure 8.4.)

the stomach and 8 gastric cancer–derived cell lines using RT-PCR, Southern analysis, Western blot analysis, and immunohistochemistry. Four of the eight cell lines and eighteen of the primary gastric cancers (56%) showed deletions or rearrangements within the *FHIT* gene, together with absence of the wild-type transcript and Fhit protein (Figure 8.4). Although not statistically significant, there was a trend toward a higher frequency of Fhit immunonegativity in intestinal-type carcinoma (76%), which is thought to develop from carcinogenic exposure, compared with the diffuse-type adenocarcinoma (50%). Thus results of this study were consistent with the hypothesis that abnormal *FHIT* transcripts result from carcinogen-mediated DNA damage leading ultimately to Fhit inactivation. Another study involving 40 matched normal and gastric cancer tissues using PCR single-strand conformation polymorphism (SSCP) and sequencing revealed the presence of a missense mutation in exon 6 in a signet ring cell adenocarcinoma.[61]

The discovery that the t(3;8) chromosome translocation was associated with hereditary renal cancer in a large three-generation family was the first suggestion that the 3p14.2 region could be involved in kidney cancer. The *FHIT* gene is interrupted by this translocation and is likely to play a role in renal tumor development. An extensive analysis of renal cell carcinomas of different subtypes showed a variable spectrum of Fhit expression from the almost 100% strongly positive oncocytomas through mostly positive papillary renal carcinomas to the predominantly negative clear cell carcinomas.[44] Loss of *FHIT* protein in clear cell renal carcinomas agrees with previous studies showing LOH of markers within the *FHIT* gene in more than 80% of this subtype of kidney tumor.[62]

A high frequency of LOH at 3p14 was demonstrated in head and neck cancers,[63,64] which have been recognized to

be associated with tobacco and alcohol use,[63,64] and interestingly, in oral dysplastic lesions at the precancerous stage.[65,66] Virgilio et al.[67] analyzed 26 head and neck cancer–derived cell lines for *FHIT* alterations by Southern blot analysis, RT-PCR, and interphase fluorescence *in situ* hybridization (FISH). Homozygous deletions within the *FHIT* gene were observed in three cell lines, aberrant transcripts were detected in 55% of them, and FISH analysis revealed the presence of more than one cellular population lacking portions of *FHIT* alleles in 65% of cell lines. Mao et al.[68] reported LOH at 3p14.2 in 81% of 16 head and neck cancer cell lines and abnormal *FHIT* expression in 45%.

Interstitial deletions of the short arm of chromosome 3 have been repeatedly detected in breast carcinomas by LOH and cytogenetics, and the minimal common deleted segment was 3p14.[69–71] Similar deletions were also found in hyperproliferative breast disease and *in situ* ductal carcinoma, suggesting that 3p alterations are probably early events in breast carcinogenesis.[72,73] Analysis of a series of breast cancer cell lines and primary tumors revealed *FHIT* alterations, mainly consisting in aberrant transcripts, in approximately 30% of cases.[74] Involvement of *FHIT* in breast tumor development was confirmed by analysis of three benign proliferative breast disease samples with cytogenetic rearrangements of chromosome 3p14.[75] The level of *FHIT* expression was either reduced or absent by RT-PCR analysis in samples with atypical hyperplasia, consistent with the hypothesis of a role for the *FHIT* gene in the early steps of tumorigenesis. Another study tested the level of Fhit protein expression in a group of 29 primary breast tumors in the normal and tumor epithelia of the same patients and in a second group of 156 primary breast carcinomas.[41] This analysis found that more than 60% of the breast cancers displayed reduced or absent Fhit protein and that Fhit inactivation was associated with a poorly differentiated phenotype.[41]

Greenspan et al. analyzed 7 cervical carcinoma cell lines and 35 primary cervical carcinoma by RT-PCR, Northern blot analysis, and immunohistochemistry.[42] Six of seven cell lines and 68% of primary tumors exhibited aberrant *FHIT* transcripts, and the same cases displayed markedly reduced Fhit protein by immunohistochemic analysis. Conversely, nonneoplastic squamous and glandular epithelium revealed strong Fhit positivity.

Finally, a study analyzing 19 pancreatic cancer cell lines and 21 primary tumors by RT-PCR, Western blot analysis, and immunohistochemistry found that 42% of the cell lines and 62% of the primary cancers displayed *FHIT* inactivation.[76]

In summary, these studies provide strong evidence that the *FHIT* gene is involved in a variety of epithelial tumors and that abnormalities in this gene are among the most common genetic changes occurring in human cancers; these studies also represent the first molecular evidence linking the instability of fragile sites to cancer. Of particular interest is the finding of *FHIT* alterations in the earliest stage of tumorigenesis and their association with carcinogen-induced tissue damage.

FHIT Alterations in Lung Cancer

Analysis of primary lung tumors for abnormalities of *FHIT* expression by RT-PCR showed that 80% of SCLCS and 42% of non–small cell lung cancers (NSCLCS) exhibited aberrant transcripts.[77] The absence of *FHIT* exons 4 or 5 through 8 was the most common abnormality detected by sequencing these altered transcripts.

Eleven lung cancer cell lines were studied by Southern blot analysis, RT-PCR, Western blot analysis, and immunohistochemistry.[40] Southern blot analysis using cDNA and specific cosmid probes covering large intronic regions of *FHIT* revealed deletions or rearrangements involving exon 3, exon 4, intron 5, and a more distal region surrounding exon 6 in three cell lines. One cell line showed a homozygous deletion in intron 5. RT-PCR analysis showed complete absence of *FHIT* transcripts in three cell lines and a mixture of abnormal transcripts lacking exons 3 or 4 through 8 or 9 in two cell lines. Both normal-size and aberrant transcripts were present in six cell lines, and only two showed the wild-type transcript only. Western blot analysis revealed that indeed 9 of the 11 lung cell lines did not produce Fhit protein and immunocytochemistry displayed a clear cytoplasmic immunostaining in the two cell lines expressing Fhit. These data confirmed that immunohistochemistry is the simplest assay to investigate the involvement of the *FHIT* gene in lung tumors. Indeed, absence or reduction of Fhit protein expression was observed in cancer cell lines and tumors for which DNA or RNA alterations were not detected.

We have investigated 474 NSCLCs for the expression of Fhit by immunohistochemistry and found that 73% of tumors were negative (Table 8.1; Figure 8.5), as were approximately 85% of dysplastic lesions (Table 8.2).[10] Fhit inactivation was significantly more common than p53 (46%), Egfr (50%), and Bcl2 (19%) overexpression, and

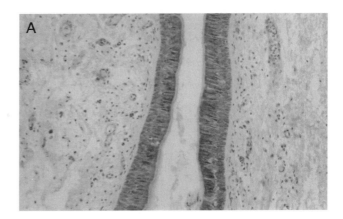
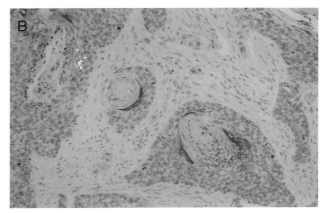
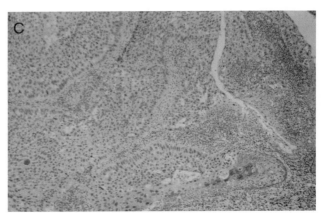

FIGURE 8.5. Loss of Fhit expression in human non–small cell lung carcinoma (hNSCLC). As shown in **(A)**, all cells of the normal bronchus stain positively with the anti-Fhit antibody. On the contrary, NSCLCs are negative for Fhit expression **(B,C)**. (From Croce C, Sozzi G, Huebner K. Role of FHIT in human cancer. *J Clin Oncol* 1999; 17:1618; Sozzi G, Pastorino U, Moiraghi L, et al. *Cancer Res* 1998; 58:5032, with permission.) (See Color Figure 8.5.)

TABLE 8.1. LOSS OF Fhit EXPRESSION IN DIFFERENT HISTOLOGIC TYPES OF NON–SMALL CELL LUNG CANCER

	Fhit Reactivity		Total	% Fhit negative	P-value
	+	−			
Squamous cell carcinoma	31	202	233	87	<0.01
Adenocarcinoma	84	112	196	57	<0.01
Large cell carcinoma	31	14	45	69	<0.01

was an independent biological marker. Notably, absence of Fhit protein was not related to p53 overexpression, thus indicating that Fhit and p53 inactivation represent independent biological pathways in lung cancer.

In the same study, a larger fraction of squamous-type

TABLE 8.2. LOSS OF Fhit EXPRESSION IN BRONCHIAL DYSPLASIA

	Fhit Expression			
	+	−	Total	% Fhit Negative
Dysplasia	3	17	20	85
Carcinoma *in situ*	0	25	25	100

carcinomas were Fhit negative compared with adenocarcinomas (87% versus 57%), whereas the other histotypes (large cell carcinoma, mucoepidermoid carcinoma) displayed an intermediate value (69%). Interestingly, adenocarcinomas had a strong association between the pattern of Fhit expression and the level of cell differentiation; positive immunostaining was shown in the more differentiated cells and weaker protein expression in the less differentiated areas of the tumor. Of relevance is the loss of Fhit expression in the earliest stages of the neoplastic process, indicating that Fhit loss is a very early event in lung carcinogenesis, as illustrated in the cartoon shown in Figure 8.6. This finding

is particularly important because the highest frequency of Fhit loss of expression is observed in the squamous type of lung cancer, which is associated with bronchial dysplastic lesions. In fact, positive Fhit immunostaining was observed in 326 hyperplastic bronchial mucosa and in 78 squamous metaplasia lesions; however, in several cases of incomplete metaplasia, Fhit immunostaining was weaker then in normal bronchus. Modulation of Fhit expression was observed in the bronchial lesions of increasing grade, occurring in 34 patients. A progressive loss of Fhit protein expression occurred in moderate and severe dysplasia lesions, whereas the mild dysplasia analyzed showed positive immunoreactivity. Negative immunostaining was observed in all of the 25 (100%) *carcinoma in situ* (CIS) lesions. Overall, 85% of dysplastic lesions and 93% of all the precancerous lesions analyzed showed negative Fhit immunostaining.

Of interest, p53 overexpression and loss of Fhit protein expression were concordant in these lesions. However, the frequency of Fhit-negative, high-grade preinvasive lesions (dysplasia and CIS) was significantly higher than that of p53 overexpression (93% versus 55%) and reflected that observed in tumors of the squamous type. Thus the level

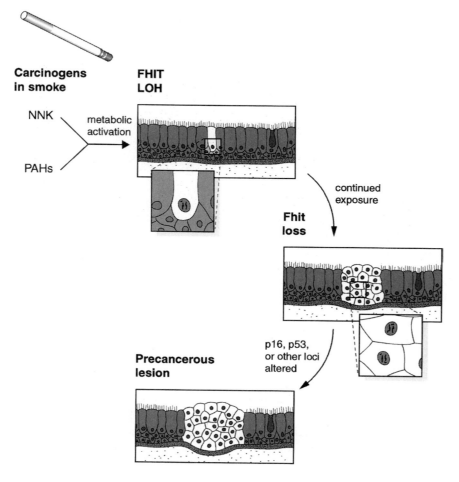

FIGURE 8.6. Tobacco smoking causes loss of function of the *FHIT* gene. Carcinogens present in tobacco smoke cause deletion in a *FHIT* allele. Continued exposure causes deletion in the second allele, leading to loss of Fhit expression. *FHIT* alterations and then mutations in p16, *p53,* and other loci cause precancerous lesions (bronchial dysplasia), some of which will later evolve into frank carcinomas. (From Huebrev K, Sozzi G, Brenner C, et al. *FHIT* loss in lung cancer: diagnostic and therapeutic implication. *Adv Oncology* 1999;15:3, with permission.) (See Color Figure 8.6.)

TABLE 8.3. SMOKING AND LOSS OF Fhit EXPRESSION

	Fhit Expression		Total	% Fhit Negative	P-value
	+	−			
Nonsmokers	14	9	23	39	<0.01
Smokers	115	336	451	75	<0.01

of sensitivity of Fhit immunostaining is higher than that achieved by p53 immunoreactivity in precancerous lesions. These findings reinforce the hypothesis that Fhit may act as a "gatekeeper" in the lung carcinogenetic process, and the similar temporal sequence of Fhit and p53 alterations in lung carcinogenesis points to a role for both pathways in lung carcinogenesis.

We also found that loss of Fhit expression was significantly more common in tumors occurring in smokers (75%) than in those of nonsmokers (39%), which was also true in the subset of adenocarcinoma patients (Table 8.3). These results, together with other evidence discussed in the next section, indicate that Fhit alterations preferentially occurred in the tumors of heavy smokers and were not correlated with p53 mutations. Fhit expression did not seem to correlate with prognosis of squamous tumors, consistent with the role of Fhit in the initiation of the tumorigenic process rather than in the progression to invasive and metastatic disease.

Tomizawa et al.[78] also found that Fhit loss correlated with the squamous cell subtype of lung cancer and smoking history but indicated poorer prognosis for patients with stage I NSCLC. This study also concluded that Fhit protein expression could be a marker of aggressiveness in stage I NSCLC. Although differing in several aspects, these two studies agree on important points: A larger proportion of squamous lung cancers showed Fhit inactivation; loss of Fhit protein expression was associated with a less differentiated morphology, especially in adenocarcinomas, and the *FHIT* gene is a preferential target of tobacco carcinogens.

A very recent study (Tseng JE, Proceedings AACR 1999, abstract #1228, page 184) investigated whether loss of Fhit expression is associated with prognosis in stage I NSCLC. Fhit levels were determined by immunohistochemistry in 86 specimens; 52% of NSCLC samples lacked Fhit immunostaining and 48% showed at least moderate staining. Loss or reduced staining was observed in multiple areas of preneoplastic lesions and even normal-appearing bronchial epithelium. However, Fhit expression status was not associated with disease-free survival or overall survival. The lack of association between Fhit expression and prognosis in NSCLC in this study may reflect the occurrence of alterations in the *FHIT* gene at an early stage in lung carcinogenesis.

The common loss of Fhit in early-stage NSCLC and preneoplastic lesions suggests a role for Fhit in initiation of lung cancer and indicates that assessment of Fhit protein could be an important aspect of screening programs (see also Chapter 23).

FHIT/FRA3B Alterations and Smoking Habits

We undertook molecular analysis of microsatellite alterations within the *FHIT* gene and *FRA3B* in lung tumors from heavy smokers and in tumors developed in never-smokers to seek genetic damage attributable to tobacco smoking.[8] LOH affecting at least one locus of the *FHIT* gene was observed in 41 out of 51 tumors in the smokers group (80%) but in only 9 out of 40 tumors in the nonsmokers (22%) (p = 0.0001). These findings suggest that the *FHIT* gene is a preferential target of carcinogens in tobacco smoke and indicate the possibility of using LOH at *FHIT* and *FRA3B* as early molecular indicators of damage related to tobacco smoke in screening high-risk individuals, such as those belonging to the heavy smokers category. Accordingly, Nelson et al.[9] observed homozygous deletions of *FHIT* exons in 13 of 30 (43%) microdissected primary lung cancers. These authors also observed an association of *FHIT* exon deletion with smoking duration and asbestos exposure.

Lung cancer is directly linked to smoking, and genetic changes similar to those observed in tumors can be detected in the normal bronchial epithelium of smokers or previous smokers. The association between LOH at 3p14.2 alleles and smoking history was investigated by many authors, and common agreement exists that deletions at the *FHIT*/*FRA3B* locus are early and common events in lung carcinogenesis and are associated with smoking history.[8,45,46] Mao et al.[45] analyzed DNA microdissected from bronchial biopsies from 54 current and former smokers for LOH at three different loci within or near candidate lung tumor–suppressor genes (3p14, 9p21, and 17p13). Overall LOH tended to be more common in current smokers than in former smokers (82% versus 62%), but the difference was not statistically significant, indicating that cigarette smoke induces genetic alterations in the bronchial tissue that persist after smoking cessation. Current smokers, however, showed a higher frequency of loss at the 3p14 locus than former smokers, a finding that was attributed to reversal of squamous metaplasia following smoking cessation.

In a similar study, Wistuba et al.[46] obtained multiple biopsies from current smokers, former smokers, and nonsmokers without cancer. Fifteen microsatellite markers were used to assess LOH at five chromosomal arms. Eighty-six percent of subjects with a history of smoking demonstrated LOH in at least one biopsy specimen, whereas none of the nonsmokers showed genetic alterations. In addition, LOH at 3p and 9p was more common than LOH at other chromosomal loci.[46]

Overall, these studies highlight the linkage between tobacco smoking and genetic alterations that initiate the process of carcinogenesis in the bronchial epithelium, and are followed by the accumulation of additional mutations during the neoplastic process leading to invasive and metastatic cancer. The studies also agree that deletions at chromosome 3p14.2 are common and early events in the carcinogenesis, being detected in precancerous lesions, and that *FHIT* is a preferential molecular target of carcinogens contained in tobacco smoke. Consistent with this finding is the low frequency (20%) of LOH at 3p14.2 in lung tumors from subjects who had never smoked.[5,6] Thus the discovery that *FHIT* inactivation is an important determinant in lung tumorigenesis and represents an early step during the neoplastic process provides the basis for molecular approaches in screening, diagnosis, prognosis, and, possibly, treatment.

Diagnostic and Therapeutic Implications

As mentioned previously, lung cancer is the leading cause of cancer-death among men and women worldwide, and smoking is the single biggest risk factor. Because the diagnosis is often reached when lung cancer is at advanced stages, efforts to significantly decrease mortality, including new therapeutic approaches and early diagnosis, have been relatively unsuccessful. So far sputum cytology or screening by radiography, as means of early detection, have proved unsatisfactory.[79]

The studies discussed previously have clearly shown that, similarly to other epithelial tumors, lung cancer evolves throught a multi-step process over time. The occurrence of these sequential genetic changes, which we are beginning to characterize and understand, can provide the basis for novel molecular diagnostic approaches.

Thus although alterations of almost every chromosome can be observed in lung cancers, deletions at chromosome 3p are commonly detected in both SCLC and NSCLC and in the earliest preneoplastic lesions of the bronchial epithelium.[10,77,78] As the malignant transformation progresses, mutations of p53, p16 inactivation, and mutations and deregulated expression of Ras, Egfr, Her2/neu, Bcl2, and Myc oncoproteins can be demonstrated.[7] In addition, LOH at multiple chromosomal loci and microsatellite instability occur at various frequencies in NSCLC and may serve as clonal markers for cancer detection.[7] The possibility of using such genetic markers for early detection of lung cancer has been suggested primarily for tissue biopsies[45,46,80,81] and exfoliated cells in sputum and bronchoalveolar lavage.[82–85] Assessment of the level of Fhit protein in biopsy or cytologic specimens from smokers and former smokers could be included in screening programs to identify high-risk patients and to provide markers for prevention regimens.

Of particular interest is the presence of genetic alterations, mostly involving LOH at 3p14.2, in the respiratory mucosa of smokers, even in the absence of recognizable preneoplastic lesions. These changes gradually accumulate with duration of smoking and persist after smoking cessation, suggesting that the risk of developing lung cancer never returns to that of nonsmokers.

Despite pronouncements to the contrary,[86–88] evidence is accumulating that the *FHIT* gene is a critical determinant in lung tumorigenesis and that it could be a long-awaited link between chromosomal fragile sites and cancer. The characterization of the *FHIT/FRA3B* locus is therefore likely to provide important means for the screening, diagnosis, and prognosis of lung cancer.

Because *FRA3B* is constitutively fragile, it might be supposed that this locus would be equally vulnerable to carcinogens in all individuals. However, polymorphisms that could confer increased fragility and susceptibility to lung cancer in certain subjects may be present within the *FRA3B* locus. The complete sequence of *FRA3B* may allow for definition and eventual screening of individuals for cancer risk. Moreover, knowing that a specific genetic alteration defines a true cancer risk factor and that it is easily detectable, could reinforce smoking cessation programs by providing a powerful screening tool.

Recent studies have demonstrated the possibility of detecting genetic alterations in plasma or serum DNA from patients with various cancers. In a recent study,[89] we looked for microsatellite alterations at the *FHIT/FRA3B* locus and other genomic loci in circulating plasma DNA of 87 stage I–III NSCLC and 14 controls. Sixty-one percent of the NSCLC patients showing allele shift and LOH in tumor samples also displayed a microsatellite change in plasma, irrespective of tumor size and stage, suggesting that circulating tumor DNA is present in early phases of lung tumor development.

Of interest, plasma DNA abnormalities were detectable in 43% of pathologic stage I and in 45% of cases with tumors up to 2 cm of maximum diameter. These findings highlight new prospects for early tumor detection by noninvasive screening procedures based on the analysis of genetic changes in plasma.

Finally, a long-term goal of research strategies in lung cancer is to directly modify lung cancer cells in order to restore the function of an altered gene product that suppresses the malignant phenotype. Candidate genes for replacement are those that are commonly altered in human cancers, inactivated in early phases of carcinogenesis, and/or involved in relevant cellular biochemic and biologic pathways. If we could identify the earliest genetic changes that initiate the process of malignant transformation, we might be able to detect these changes in premalignant lesions and develop novel therapeutic approaches to eliminate premalignant cells. The overall high frequency and precocity of Fhit loss in lung carcinogenesis and its role in controlling apoptosis prompt FHIT gene replacement as a gene therapy approach for early lesions accompanying lung carcinogenesis.

ACKNOWLEDGMENTS

We thank Yuri Pekarsky and Eric Martin for technical assistance in the preparation of the figures. M.L. Veronese was supported by NIH Training Grant 5T32 GM08562.

REFERENCES

1. Ginsberg RJ, Vokes EE, Raben A. Non-small cell lung cancer. In: DeVita VT, Hellman S, Rosenberg SA, eds. *Cancer: principles & practice of oncology,* 5th ed. Philadelphia: Lippincott-Raven, 1997; 858.
2. Ochsner A, DeBakey M. Carcinoma of the lung. *Archives of Surgery* 1941;42:209.
3. Parkin DM, Pisani P, Lopez AD, et al. At least one in seven cases of cancer is caused by smoking. Global estimates for 1985. *Int J Cancer* 1994;5904:494.
4. Shopland DR, Eyre HJ, Pechacek TF. Smoking attributable cancer mortality in 1991: is lung cancer now the leading cause of death among smokers in the United States? *J Natl Cancer Inst* 1991;83:1142.
5. Brownson RC, Loy TS, Ingram E, et al. Lung cancer in nonsmoking women. *Cancer* 1995;75:29.
6. Marchetti A, Pellegrini S, Sozzi G, et al. Genetic analysis of lung tumors of non-smoking subjects: p53 gene mutations are constantly associated with loss of heterozygosity at the *FHIT* locus. *British J Cancer* 1998;78:73.
7. Minna JD, Sekido Y, Fong KM, et al. Cancer of the lung. In: DeVita VT, Hellman S, Rosenberg SA, eds. *Cancer: principles & practice of oncology,* 5th ed. Philadelphia: Lippincott-Raven 1997; 849.
8. Sozzi G, Sard L, De Gregorio L, et al. Association between cigarette smoking and *FHIT* gene alterations in lung cancer. *Cancer Res* 1997;57:2121.
9. Nelson HH, Wiencke JK, Gunn L, et al. Chromosome 3p14 alterations in lung cancer: evidence that *FHIT* exon deletion is a target of tobacco carcinogens and asbestos. *Cancer Res* 1998; 58:1804.
10. Sozzi G, Pastorino U, Moiraghi L, et al. Loss of *FHIT* function in lung cancer and preinvasive bronchial lesions. *Cancer Res* 1998; 58:5032.
11. Devilee P, Van den Broek M, Kuipers-Dijkshoorn N, et al. At least four different chromosomal regions are involved in loss of heterozygosity in human breast carcinoma. *Genomics* 1989;5:554.
12. Hibi K, Takahashi T, Yamakawa K, et al. Three distinct regions involved in 3p deletion in human lung cancer. *Oncogene* 1992; 7:445.
13. Lothe RA, Fossa SD, Stenwig AE, et al. Loss of 3p or 11p alleles is associated with testicular cancer tumors. *Genomics* 1989;5:134.
14. Ogawa O, Kakehi Y, Ogawa K, et al. Allelic loss at chromosome 3p characterizes clear cell phenotype of renal cell carcinoma. *Cancer Res* 1991;51:949.
15. Yang-Feng TL, Han H, Chen KC, et al. Allelic loss in ovarian cancer. *Int J Cancer* 1993;54:546.
16. Kohno T, Takayama H, Hamaguchi M, et al. Deletion mapping of chromosome 3p in human uterine cervical cancer. *Oncogene* 1993;8:1825.
17. Maestro R, Gasparotto D, Vukosavljevic T, et al. Three discrete regions of deletion at 3p in head and neck cancers. *Cancer Res* 1993;53:5775.
18. Latif F, Tory K, Gnarra J, et al. Identification of the von Hippel-Lindau disease tumor suppressor gene. *Science* 1993;260:1317.
19. Kaelin WG, Maher ER. The VHL tumor-suppressor gene paradigm. *Trends Genet* 1998;14:423.
20. Cohen AJ, Li FP, Berg S, et al. Hereditary renal-cell carcinoma associated with a chromosomal translocation. *New Engl J Med* 1979;301:592.
21. Glover TW, Coyle-Morris JF, Frederick PL, et al. Translocation t(3;8)(p14.2;q24.1) in renal cell carcinoma affects expression of the common fragile site at 3p14 (*FRA3B*) in lymphocytes. *Cancer Genet Cytogenet* 1988;31:69.
22. Huebner K, Garrison PN, Barnes LD, et al. The role of the *FHIT/FRA3B* locus in cancer. *Ann Rev Genet* 1998;32:7.
23. Sutherland GR. Chromosomal fragile sites. *Genet Anal Tech & Appl* 1991;8:161.
24. Sutherland GR, Richards RI. The molecular basis of fragile sites in human chromosomes. *Curr Opin Genet Develop* 1995;5:323.
25. Schmid M, Ott G, Haaf T, et al. Evolutionary conservation of fragile sites induced by 5-azacytidine and 5-azadeoxycytidine in man, gorilla, and chimpanzee. *Hum Genet* 1985;71:342.
26. Yunis JJ, Soreng AL. Constitutive fragile sites and cancer. *Science* 1984;226:1199.
27. Le Beau MM. Chromosomal fragile sites and cancer-specific rearrangements. *Blood* 1986;67:849.
28. Yunis JJ, Soreng AL, Bowe AE. Fragile sites are targets of diverse mutagens and carcinogens. *Oncogene* 1987;1:59.
29. Coquelle A, Pipiras E, Toledo F, et al. Expression of fragile sites triggers intrachromosomal mammalian gene amplification and sets boundaries to early amplicons. *Cell* 1997;89:215.
30. Inoue H, Ishii H, Alder H, et al. Sequence of the *FRA3B* common fragile region: implications for the mechanism of *FHIT* deletion. *Proc Natl Acad Sci USA* 1997;94:14584.
31. Mimori K, Druck T, Inoue H, et al. Cancer specific chromosome alterations in the constitutive fragile region, *FRA3B*. *Proc Natl Acad Sci USA* 1999;96:7456.
32. Mishmar D, Rahat A, Scherer SW, et al. Molecular characterization of a common fragile site (FRA7H) on human chromosome 7 by the cloning of a simian virus 40 integration site. *Proc Natl Acad Sci USA* 1998;95:8141.
33. Mishmar D. Common fragile sites: G-band characteristics within an R-band. *Am J Hum Genet* 1999;64:908.
34. Kastury K, Baffa R, Druck T, et al. Potential gastrointestinal tumor suppressor locus at the 3p14.2 FRA3B site identified by homozygous deletions in tumor cell lines. *Cancer Res* 1996;56: 978.
35. Ohta M, Inoue H, Cotticelli MG, et al. The *FHIT* gene, spanning the chromosome 3p14.2 fragile site and renal carcinoma-associated t(3;8) breakpoint, is abnormal in digestive tract cancers. *Cell* 1996;84:587.
36. Druck T, Hadaczek P, Fu T-B, et al. Structure and expression of the human *FHIT* gene in normal and tumor cells. *Cancer Res* 1997;57:504.
37. Gayther SA, Barski P, Batley SJ, et al. Aberrant splicing of the *TSG101* and *FHIT* genes occurs frequently in multiple malignancies and in normal tissues and mimics alterations previously described in tumors. *Oncogene* 1997;15:119.
38. Panagopoulos I, Thelin S, Mertens F, et al. Variable *FHIT* transcripts in non-neoplastic tissues. *Genes Chromosomes Cancer* 1997; 19:215.
39. Baffa R, Veronese ML, Santoro R, et al. Loss of *FHIT* expression in gastric carcinoma. *Cancer Res* 1998;58:4708.
40. Sozzi G, Tornielli S, Tagliabue E, et al. Absence of *FHIT* protein in primary lung tumors and cell lines with *FHIT* gene abnormalities. *Cancer Res* 1997;57:5207.
41. Campiglio M, Pekarsky Y, Menard S, et al. *FHIT* loss of function in human primary breast cancer correlates with advanced stage of the disease. *Cancer Res* (in press, 1999).
42. Greenspan DL, Connolly DC, Wu R, et al. Loss of *FHIT* expression in cervical carcinoma cell lines and primary tumors. *Cancer Res* 1997;57:4692.

43. Simon B, Bartsch D, Barth P, et al. Frequent abnormalities of the putative tumor suppressor gene *FHIT* at 3p14.2 in pancreatic carcinoma cell lines. *Cancer Res* 1998;58:1583.

44. Hadaczek P, Kovatich A, Gronwald J, et al. Loss or reduction of *FHIT* expression in renal neoplasias: correlation with histogenic class. *Hu Path* 1999;11:1276.

45. Mao L, Lee JS, Kurie JM, et al. Clonal genetic alterations in the lungs of current and former smokers. *J Natl Cancer Inst* 1997; 89:857.

46. Wistuba II, Lam S, Behrens C, et al. Molecular damage in the bronchial epithelium of current and former smokers. *J Natl Cancer Inst* 1997;89:1366.

47. Robinson AK, de la Pena CE, Barnes LD. Isolation and characterization of diadenosine tetraphosphate (Ap4A) hydrolase from Schizosaccharomyces pombe. *Biochim Biophys Acta* 1993;1161: 139.

48. Huang Y, Garrison PN, Barnes LD. Cloning of the Schizosaccharomyces pombe gene encoding diadenosine 5′,5′′′-P1,P4-tetraphosphate (Ap4A) asymmetrical hydrolase: sequence similarity with the histidine triad (HIT) protein family. *Biochem J* 1995; 312:925.

49. Seraphin B. The HIT protein family: a new family of proteins present in prokaryote yeast and mammals. *DNA Seq* 1992;3:177.

50. Barnes LD, Garrison PN, Siprashvill Z, et al. *FHIT*, a putative tumor suppressor in humans, is a dinucleoside 5′,5′′′-P^1,P^3-triphosphate hydrolase. *Biochemistry* 1996;35:11529.

51. Gilmour J, Liang N, Lowenstein JM. Isolation, cloning and characterization of a low-molecular-mass purine nucleoside- and nucleotide-binding protein. *Biochem J* 1997;326:471.

52. Brenner C, Garrison P, Gilmour J, et al. Crystal structures of HINT demonstrate that histidine triad proteins are GalT-related nucleotide-binding proteins. *Nature Struct Biol* 1997;4:231.

53. Vartanian A, Narovlyansky A, Amchenkova A, et al. Interferons induce accumulation of diadenosine triphosphate (Ap3A) in human cultured cells. *FEBS Letters* 1996;381:32.

54. Segal E, Le Pecq JB. Relationship between cellular diadenosine 5′,5′′′-P1,P4-tetraphosphate level, cell density, cell growth stimulation and toxic stresses. *Exp Cell Res* 1986;167:119.

55. Siprashvili Z, Sozzi G, Barnes LD, et al. Replacement of *FHIT* in cancer cells suppresses tumorigenicity. *Proc Natl Acad Sci USA* 1997;94:13771.

56. Pace HC, Garrison PN, Barnes LD, et al. Genetic, biochemical and crystallographic definition of a substrate analog complex with the fragile histidine triad protein as the active signaling form of *FHIT*. *Proc Natl Acad Sci USA* 1998;95:5484.

57. Huebner K, Sozzi G, Brenner C, et al. *FHIT* loss in lung cancer: diagnostic and therapeutic implications. *Adv Oncology* 1999;15: 3.

58. Sard L, Accornero P, Tornielli S, et al. The tumor suppressor gene *FHIT* is involved in the regulation of apoptosis and in cell cycle control. *Proc Natl Acad Sci USA* 1999;15:8489.

59. Kisselev LL, Justesen J, Wolfson AD, et al. Diadenosine oligophosphates (Ap(n)A), a novel class of signalling molecules? *FEBS Letters* 1998;427:157.

60. Ji L, Fang B, Yen N, et al. Induction of apoptosis, inhibition of tumorigenicity, and suppression of tumor growth by adenovirus vector-mediated *FHIT* gene overexpression *in vitro* and *in vivo*. *Cancer Res* 1999;59:3333.

61. Gemma A, Hagiwara K, Ke Y, et al. *FHIT* mutations in human primary gastric cancer. *Cancer Res* 1997;57:1435.

62. Hadaczeck P, Siprashvili Z, Markiewski M, et al. Absence or reduction of *FHIT* expression in most clear cell renal carcinomas. *Cancer Res* 1998;58:2946.

63. Nawroz H, van der Riet P, Hruban RH, et al. Allelotype of head and neck squamous cell carcinoma. *Cancer Res* 1994;54:1152.

64. Ishwad CS, Ferrell RE, Rossie KN, et al. Loss of heterozygosity of the short arm of chromosomes 3 and 9 in oral cancer. *Int J Cancer* 1996;69:1.

65. Roz L, Wu CL, Porter S, et al. Allelic imbalance on chromosome 3p in oral dysplastic lesions: an early event in oral carcinogenesis. *Cancer Res* 1996;56:1228.

66. Mao L, Lee JS, Fan YH, et al. Frequent microsatellite alterations at chromosomes 9p21 and 3p14 in oral premalignant lesions and their value in cancer risk assessment. *Nature Med* 1996;2: 682.

67. Virgilio L, Shuster M, Gollin SM, et al. (1996). *FHIT* gene alterations in head and neck squamous cell carcinomas. *Proc Natl Acad Sci USA* 1996;93:9770.

68. Mao L, Fan YH, Lotan R, et al. Frequent abnormalities of *FHIT*, a candidate tumor suppressor gene, in head and neck cancer cell lines. *Cancer Res* 1996;56:5128.

69. Pandis N, Jin Y, Limon J, et al. Interstitial deletion of the short arm of chromosome 3 as a primary chromosome abnormality in carcinomas of the breast. *Genes Chrom Cancer* 1993;6:151.

70. Buchhagen DL, Qiu L, Etkind P. Homozygous deletion, rearrangement and hypermethylation implicate chromosome region 3p14.3-3p21.3 in sporadic breast-cancer development. *Int J Cancer* 1994;57:473.

71. Pandis N, Jin Y, Gorunova L, et al. Chromosome analysis of 97 primary breast carcinomas: identification of eight karyotypic subgroups. *Genes Chrom Cancer* 1995;12:173.

72. Dietrich CU, Pandis N, Teixeira MR, et al. Chromosome abnormalities in benign hyperproliferative disorders of epithelial and stromal breast tissue. *Int J Cancer* 1995;60:49.

73. Teixeira MR, Pandis N, Bardi G, et al. Karyotypic comparisons of multiple tumorous and macroscopically normal surrounding tissue samples from patients with breast cancer. *Cancer Res* 1996; 56:855.

74. Negrini M, Monaco C, Vorechovsky I, et al. The *FHIT* gene at 3p14.2 is abnormal in breast carcinomas. *Cancer Res* 1996;56: 3173.

75. Panagopoulos I, Pandis N, Thelin S, et al. (1996). The *FHIT* and PTPRG genes are deleted in benign proliferative breast disease associated with familial breast cancer and cytogenetic rearrangements of chromosome band 3p14. *Cancer Res* 1996;56:4871.

76. Sorio C, Baron A, Orlandini S, et al. The *FHIT* gene is expressed in pancreatic ductular cells and is altered in pancreatic cancer. *Cancer Res* 1999;59:1308.

77. Sozzi G, Veronese ML, Negrini M, et al. The *FHIT* gene at 3p14.2 is abnormal in lung cancer. *Cell* 1996;85:17.

78. Tomizawa Y, Nakajima T, Kohno T, et al. Clinico-pathological significance of *FHIT* protein expression in stage I non-small cell lung carcinoma. *Cancer Res* 1998;58:5478.

79. Roland M, Rudd RM. Genetics and pulmonary medicine: somatic mutations in the development of lung cancer. *Thorax* 1998; 53:979.

80. Sozzi G, Miozzo M, Donghi R, et al. Deletions of 17p and p53 mutations in preneoplastic lesions of the lung. *Cancer Res* 1992; 52:6079.

81. Thiberville L, Payne P, Vielkinds J, et al. Evidence of cumulative gene losses with progression of premalignant epithelial lesions to carcinoma of the bronchus. *Cancer Res* 1995;55:5133.

82. Mao L, Hruban RH, Boyle JO, et al. Detection of oncogene mutations in sputum precedes diagnosis of lung cancer. *Cancer Res* 1994;54:1634.

83. Miozzo M, Sozzi G, Musso K, et al. Microsatellite alterations in bronchial and sputum specimens of lung cancer patients. *Cancer Res* 1996;56:2285.

84. Mills NE, Fishman CL, Scholes J, et al. Detection of K-ras oncogene mutations in bronchoalveolar lavage fluid for lung cancer diagnosis. *J Natl Cancer Inst* 1995;87:1056.

85. Somers VA, Pietersen AM, Theunissen PH, et al. Detection of

K-ras point mutations in sputum from patients with adenocarcinoma of the lung by point-EXACCT. *J Clin Oncol* 1998;16:3061.

86. Li Mao. Tumor suppressor genes: does *FHIT* fit? *J Natl Cancer Inst* 1998;90:412.

87. Le Beau M, Drabkin H, Glover TW, et al. An *FHIT* tumor suppressor gene? *Genes Chromo Cancer* 1998;21:281.

88. Fong KM, Biesterveld EJ, Virmani A, et al. *FHIT* and FRA3B 3p14.2 allele loss are common in lung cancer and preneoplastic bronchial lesions and are associated with cancer-related *FHIT* cDNA splicing aberrations. *Cancer Res* 1997;57:2256.

89. Sozzi G, Musso K, Ratcliffe C, et al. Microsatellite alterations in plasma DNA of non small cell lung cancer patients: a prospect for early diagnosis. *Clin Cancer Res* 1999;5:2689.

9

TELOMERASE IN LUNG CANCER

FULVIO LONARDO
JOAN ALBANELL

A distinguishing biological feature of tumor cells is their ability to undergo unlimited cell divisions. The discovery that the enzyme telomerase plays a crucial role in immortalization has constituted a major advance in the biology of cell transformation and has offered insights into the pathogenesis of lung cancer. Further, it has highlighted the clinical relevance of telomerase activity as an important molecular marker of lung cancer and a potential target of therapy.

BIOLOGY OF TELOMERES AND TELOMERASE

Structure

Telomeres are DNA-protein complexes located at the end of linear chromosomes, made up of multiple repeats of the oligomeric sequence 5'-TTAGGG-3' which can be up to 15 kbases long[1] and are associated with specialized nucleoproteins.[2] In the absence of telomerase activity, telomeres shorten with each cell division (end-replication problem). Telomerase is an RNA-dependent DNA polymerase (reverse transcriptase) specialized in the synthesis of telomeric repeats, an activity which cannot be carried out by conventional DNA polymerases.[3–5] Telomerase is composed of an RNA component and multiple associated proteins.[2] It is a unique polymerase in that its integral RNA component provides its own template for the synthesis of oligomeric repeats. Studies in *Tetrahymena* show that, in addition to acting as a template, this RNA component is endowed with regulatory functions, affecting the affinity of RNA binding to the catalytic protein and the fidelity of transcription.[6,7] Cloned constituents of human telomerase include an RNA component named hTR[8] and two associated proteins: hTERT (also named TP2 or hEST2),[9,10] endowed with polymerase activity,[11] and a telomerase-associated protein with unknown function, named TP1.[12] The presence of homology between the TP2 component, the yeast homologue EST2, retroviral reverse transcriptases, and transposons,[5,13] in regions that are crucial for its polymerase activity,[11] points to a common evolutionary origin of these molecules. Reconstitution studies *in vitro* have shown that the minimal core complex still capable of telomerase activity

is constituted by the RNA and the TP2 reverse transcriptase components.[14]

Tissue Expression

The availability of molecular probes has allowed the study at the cellular level of correlations between expression of telomerase constituents, proliferation, and differentiation, in both normal and neoplastic tissues. This availability has also allowed the study of how expression of single telomerase components affects telomerase activity by allowing a comparison between cellular expression of telomerase components through *in situ* hybridization and immunohistochemistry and telomerase enzymatic activity assessed by the TRAP assay (see *infra*). Thus Yashima and colleagues[15] have found that, by *in situ* hybridization, hTR expression is predominantly found in proliferating, undifferentiated tissue during embryogenesis. In contrast, differentiation is accompanied in most tissues by decreased or absent expression. In adult tissues, expression is restricted to actively dividing cells of gonads, lymphoid tissue, and epithelia. These include primary and secondary spermatocytes; ovarian follicular cells and oocytes; follicular center cells of lymphoid follicles; basal cells of respiratory epithelia and of keratinized and nonkeratinized squamous epithelia, including the skin; and intestinal crypt cells. In the normal lung, hTR is expressed in the basal cells of bronchi and in bronchioles.[15,16] An exception is provided by the presence of weak positivity for hTR in differentiated, nonproliferating ganglion cells in normal tissue, ganglioneuroblastomas, and ganglioneuromas.[17] These studies show a general correlation between hTR expression, telomerase activity, and proliferative potential in normal tissues. Studies on the cellular localization of hTR in histologically preneoplastic lesions of the cervix, bronchi, and breast (see *infra*) also point to a direct correlation between hTR expression and proliferation. In addition, they highlight an indirect correlation with differentiation. Thus cervical dysplastic lesions, while showing a cellular redistribution of hTR positivity, also reveal that the lowest levels of positivity are found in the superficial, differentiated component of the dysplastic epithelium.[18] Studies on germ cell tumors also point out an inverse correlation between differentiation and hTR expression. Differentiated tissue within ovarian germ cell tumors and mature testicular teratomas lacks detectable hTR expression by *in situ* hybridization.[19] In contrast, germ cell cancers and immature teratomas show telomerase activity.[20] Such an inverse correlation between telomerase activity and differentiation in germ cell tumors is supported by *in vitro* and *in vivo* studies.[20,21]

Use of reverse transcripture chain reaction (RT-PCR) has shown that hTR is also present in somatic tissues, although at much lower levels than in cancers and gonads.[8] Analyses of the tissue distribution of hTR conducted by Northern blot (NB) have generally revealed a wider tissue distribution than those conducted by *in situ* hybridization. Thus Feng and co-workers found by NB that hTR was expressed in tissues such as brain and lung that are respectively negative or positive only in a small cell population. *In situ* hybridization, although less sensitive, offers the advantage of precisely localizing subsets of cells positive for hTR. Furthermore, a correlation exists between the presence of hTR and telomerase activity[16,22] when this is detected by the latter technique but not by NB.[23]

The chromosomal site where the gene for hTR resides has been mapped to chromosome 3q26.3. Interestingly, this region is frequently overexpressed in head and neck squamous cell carcinomas,[24,25] raising the prospect that increased levels of hTR found in tumors may be secondary to gene amplification.

These data highlight that telomerase activation is usually accompanied by upregulation of hTR levels. However, data exist supporting the view that control of levels of the hTERT component is the key element in regulating telomerase activity. Thus, immortalization is accompanied by upregulation of this component, and differentiation by its down-regulation;[10] and introduction of this component extends the recipient's cell life span.[26] Further evidence of an important role of this component in carcinogenesis is suggested by the frequent amplification of the 5p chromosome in approximately 70% of non–small cell lung carcinomas (NSCLC),[27,28] where the EST2 gene resides at 5p.33. A comparative analysis by RT-PCR of all three components of human telomerase components in renal cell carcinomas reveals that the expression of hTERT is a critical determinant of telomerase activity in this cancer. Here, TP1 and hTR mRNA were constitutively expressed both in tumor and in normal tissue. In contrast, the expression of hTERT was found to be limited to cancer and correlated with telomerase activity.[29] Recently, the finding by immunohistochemistry of hTERT protein in colonic crypt cells, known to represent the proliferative component of this epithelium, further confirms the important role of this component in regulating telomerase activity.[30]

Another mechanism of regulation of telomerase activity may be operating through telomerase inhibitors.[8,23] An inhibitor of telomerase activity has been demonstrated to reside on the short arm of chromosome 3 at 3p.21.2–3p21.3.[24,31] This region frequently undergoes loss of heterozygosity in NSCLC[32] and has tumor suppressive ability *in vitro*,[33,34] thus raising the prospect that it may act as a tumor suppressor gene *in vivo*. This hypothesis awaits further confirmation by a detailed mapping of the genes involved in the deletion.

The TRAP Assay

Telomerase activity was originally detected by the visualization of the direct enzymatic products generated by cell extracts in the presence of a synthetic primer and labeled nucleotides. The subsequent introduction of a different method of cell lysis (detergent-mediated lysis versus hypotonic shock) and, most important, of a polymerase chain reaction (PCR) step in the technique greatly enhanced the sensitivity of the telomeric repeat amplification protocol (TRAP) assay.[35] The oligomeres generated in the reaction, instead of being immediately separated and visualized by electrophoresis, are first used as templates in a PCR reaction, which allows their exponential amplification. The typical TRAP product appears as a "ladder" composed of multiple bands of increasing length, each differing from the other by 6bp, spanning the entire length of the gel. Telomerase activity is quantified by measuring the intensity of the generated bands, normalized for background activity. This modified technique is reported to be able to detect 10^{-4} telomerase-positive cells in a mixed cell population. The high sensitivity of the TRAP assay, in conjunction with the differential expression of telomerase activity in normal versus cancer tissue, constitutes the premises for its potential clinical use as a marker of cancer, as discussed later. Recently, the development of an *in situ* version of this assay has been reported in the Japanese literature.[36]

Function

Telomeres have multiple functions. Telomere integrity is crucial for maintenance of chromosomal stability, and for preventing chromosome fusions, translocations, and non-disjunctions.[37] Telomere shortening constitutes an end point of oxidative stress, thus controlling ageing. Genetically transmitted human diseases characterized by early aging, such ataxia telangiectasia, and Down's syndrome, have all been described as showing accelerated telomeric attrition and a reduced proliferative life span.[24] A large body of evidence, briefly reviewed here, further highlights that telomerase activity can control the cell's life span, and its deregulation constitutes a key event in cell transformation.

In vivo, differentiated cells do not proliferate and are constantly replaced by new cells. Examples of replicating cells include bone marrow stem cells, neck cells of the intestinal crypts, and basal cells of squamous epithelia. The extended proliferative potential of these cells allows for the generation of differentiated elements able to carry out specialized biological functions but incapable of division. It has long been known that *in vitro,* primary cell lines undergo senescence after a limited, set number of cell passages.[38] In contrast, immortal cell lines have an unlimited proliferative potential. Advances in our knowledge of the interactions between telomerase, telomeres, and cell proliferation have shed new light on the molecular basis of this process. Namely, a host of data suggest that telomere length constitute the cell's clock to monitor the number of cell divisions it has gone through and that there is a correlation between telomere length, telomerase activity, and proliferative potential.

A progressive shortening of telomeric ends takes place with each cell division in mortal cells lacking telomerase activity, with a loss of approximately 50 bp per division for cultured human fibroblasts, until a critical telomere length is reached. When cells reach this point (named Mortality Stage 1) they stop proliferating and undergo senescence.[39] Senescence is characterized by the inability of the cell to express transcription factors crucial in allowing progression into G1, such as c-*fos* and members of the E2F family, in addition to overexpression of the cyclin-dependent kinase inhibitors p21 and p16.[37] Whereas this model implies a link between telomere length, transcription factors, and kinase inhibitors in controlling cell cycle progression, the molecular details of this mechanism are unknown. It has been hypothesized that a short telomere may trigger a DNA damage response through a "sensor" molecule, and *p53* is a candidate for this role.[40] Alternatively, a short telomere may directly bind transcription factors or indirectly repress the transcription of regulatory genes as a consequence of tridimensional changes in the DNA structure.[37]

Oncogene activation or tumor-suppressor gene inactivation allows somatic cells to bypass cell senescence, extending their life span. In particular, *p53* and Rb are thought to have a crucial role in controlling this checkpoint.[41] With continuing cell divisions, telomeres become progressively shorter, until a critical length is reached and cells undergo a second crisis (Mortality Stage 2). Further proliferation and cell survival at this stage are critically dependent on the presence of telomerase activity, which appear spontaneously *in vitro* in rare tumor clones which become immortal.[1,39]

Activated lymphocytes are an exception among normal cells in that they express telomerase activity.[42,43] This has important clinical bearings, limiting the role of telomerase as a molecular marker of cancer (see *infra*).[44] As for its biological relevance in the context of the presented model, it has been shown that lymphocytes lose telomeric DNA with cell proliferation, in spite of the presence of this telomerase activity.[43] These data highlight that low-level telomerase activity present in rare somatic cells is not sufficient to overcome the end-replication problem.

In contrast to mortal cells, germ cells and a great majority of spontaneously immortalized human cancer cell lines and

human tumor specimens exhibit telomerase activity at a level sufficient to stabilize telomerase,[45,46] and have unlimited proliferative potential.

These data prompt a model envisioning progressive telomere shortening as a crucial factor determining cell senescence. This process is counterbalanced by telomerase activity which, by stabilizing telomere length, allows cells to undergo unlimited cell divisions. In tune with this model, telomerase activity is found in immortal cell lines but not in mortal ones *in vitro. In vivo,* it is restricted to cells with unlimited life span, including gonads, tumors cells,[39,46] and renovating cell subsets within differentiated epithelia.[15,39,47] This proposed association between unlimited life span and telomerase activity has been further confirmed by several *in vitro* data. The reverse transcriptase component of human telomerase has the ability to expand the recipient's cell life span when introduced in telomerase-negative retinal pigment and foreskin fibroblasts,[26] and its message is upregulated during immortalization.[10] Furthermore, transfection of the immortal HeLa cell line with an antisense to the RNA component of telomerase results in loss of telomeric DNA and cell death.[8]

However, it should be stressed that the control of senescence is multifactorial. Thus four sets of genes acting as complementation groups were revealed by cell hybrids to control senescence.[37] Further, inactivation of crucial tumor-suppressor genes such as *p53*[40] and Rb is crucial in allowing continuing cell proliferation and transformation, despite critically short telomeres.[37] Particularly, it has been proposed that *p53* may act as a "sensor" of telomere length. According to this model, *p53* deficiency allows cancer cells to escape the growth arrest that telomere shortening induces in normal cells by upregulation of wt *p53*.[40] Unrestricted cell proliferation can occur in rare cases in the face of absent telomerase activity by alternative mechanisms of telomere lengthening.[48]

Studies show that papilloma virus's E6 and E7 and SV40 constitute a convenient experimental model for the study of the molecular pathways of immortalization and have shed further light on this mechanism. It was previously assumed that papilloma virus–mediated immortalization depended entirely on the combined inactivation carried out by E6 and E7 of *p53*[49] and Rb.[50] In contrast, it has recently been demonstrated that the minimal requirement for immortalization of human keratinocytes or mammary epithelial cells is constituted by the combination of telomerase activation carried out by E6 and E7-induced Rb/p16 inactivation, and that *p53* inactivation is dispensable.[51] Further highlighting the multifactorial nature of cell transformation, cells transfected with the enzymatic component of telomerase hTERT have extended life span but are nontumorigenic.[52,53] In contrast, it has been shown that the transformed phenotype can be reproduced by the transfection of an activated *RAS* and a large T in addition to hTERT.[54]

These data highlight that acquisition of telomerase activity may constitute an obligatory step for the acquisition of an unlimited life span, but cooperation with other molecules is required to achieve immortalization and cell transformation. The molecular details of the interrelationships between telomerase activation and deregulation of other cell cycle–controlling molecules remain largely uncharacterized.

TELOMERASE IN LUNG CANCER

Telomerase in the Pathogenesis of Lung Cancer

The noninvasive lesions associated with the development of lung carcinoma are well characterized for squamous cell carcinoma both at the morphological[55] and at the molecular level (reviewed in Colby[56]). Increasing molecular alterations have been described as occurring in these lesions, paralleling their increasing histological grades. These include alterations in cyclins D1 and E,[57] EGFR, and *p53*,[58] and loss of heterozygosity at loci at chromosomes 3p, 9p-21 and 5q.[56,59] Only one study has addressed the timing, within this histological continuum, of telomerase deregulation. Yashima and colleagues studied the cellular distribution of the RNA component of human telomerase (hTR) in normal, preneoplastic, and invasive carcinoma. They found a correlation between hTR positivity as detected by *in situ* hybridization, and telomerase activity as detected by the TRAP assay. In normal lung, hTR expression is restricted to small bronchioles (23%) and the basal cells of bronchi (26%).[16] In contrast, virtually all preneoplastic lesions show deregulated expression (20 out of 22). This is two-fold. First, a cellular redistribution of hTR is present. Thus, while positive only in the basal layer in normal bronchial mucosa and in the basal and parabasal layer in hyperplastic lesions, in dysplasia it becomes expressed throughout the entire thickness of the epithelium. A similar redistribution is also observed in cervical dysplasia.[18] This phenomenon reproduces the redistribution of epidismal growth factor receptor (EGFR) positivity observed in bronchial dysplasia by immunohistochemistry.[58] Second, low-level telomerase activity appeared in dysplasia. This was severalfold lower than that detected in invasive carcinoma; however carcinoma *in situ* (CIS) in the vicinity of invasive carcinoma had telomerase levels comparable to those of invasive carcinoma. Similar results were obtained in studies of preneoplastic lesions of the breast[22] and cervix uteri.[18]

Overall, these data highlight that increasing histological grades are associated with increasing telomerase activity and hTR expression in histological models of preneoplasia (see also Chapter 23). Because in these sites, including the bronchus, increasing proliferative rates are associated with increasing histological grades,[59] these data also highlight an association between telomerase activity and proliferative rate. The positivity of the basal bronchial layer in normal and hyperplastic conditions for hTR is further in tune with this association, because this cell type is believed to play a crucial role in the turnover of the bronchial mucosa.[60] An intriguing association is also evident in this cell type between telomerase positivity and positivity for EGFR.[58] Interestingly, the basal cells of the skin, which are assumed to play the same role in the epithelium, are also reported to be positive for telomerase activity.[47]

These observations seem further to indicate out that progression to invasive carcinoma is marked by a progressive increase in the *level* of telomerase activity rather than by its *acquisition*. Were this model confirmed, it would justify the employment of telomerase inhibitors as prevention agents to arrest the progression of preinvasive bronchial lesions to overt cancer in patients with bronchial dysplasia. This group of patients is rarely detected clinically yet comprises the target of early lung cancer detection screening programs.[61]

The view that invasive adenocarcinomas arise from noninvasive proliferative lesions of small bronchioles and alveoli, termed atypical alveolar hyperplasia (AAH) (see also Chapter 26) is substantiated by a large body of experimental and morphological evidence (reviewed in Colby[56]). Only one study has studied telomerase activation in these lesions. Yashima and colleagues found that, although 23% of small bronchioles were positive for telomerase, the six samples of AAH examined were all negative. Yet overt invasive adenocarcinomas (*infra*) frequently express telomerase activity. Furthermore, AAH lesions of different nuclear grades exist, and the occurrence of molecular alterations such as *p53* accumulation has previously been shown to increase with nuclear grades in these lesions for *p53*.[62] However, the nuclear grade of the lesions analyzed was not commented on in this small series. Thus further studies are needed to address the timing of telomerase activation in the pathogenesis of lung adenocarcinoma.

Telomerase in Invasive Lung Cancer

The data from the three major studies performed so far on telomerase in lung cancer are provided in Table 9.1. The incidence of telomerase positivity in NSCLC in these series ranges from 80%[63,64] to 85% [84 of 99],[65] compared with a range of positive expression in normal tissue of 0%[65] to 7.7%.[64] Only Hiyama and associates have also analyzed small cell carcinomas (SSC)[63] finding telomerase activity in all 11 cases examined. No significant differences in telomerase activity have been found in these series between squamous cell carcinomas, adenocarcinomas, and large cell undifferentiated carcinomas. In these series, the bronchioloalveolar carcinomas category has been incorporated with adenocarcinomas or within a third miscellaneous group.[64] However, in view of the distinctive clinical and pathological features of this histological type,[66] it would be intriguing to find out if its incidence of telomerase positivity is different from that of ordinary adenocarcinoma. A positive correlation between high telomerase activity and high pathological (TNM) stage has been reported in the only study

TABLE 9.1. REPORTED DISTRIBUTION OF TELOMERASE POSITIVITY IN RESECTED LUNG CANCER

Author	Cases Analyzed	Overall Positivity	Adenocarcinoma	Squamous Cell Carcinoma	Other Histotypes
Wu et al.	100	80%	80% (n = 54)	79% (n = 44)	83% (n = 12)[¶]
Hiyama et al.	136	80%	70% (n = 65)	88% (n = 52)	85% (n = 19)[†]
Albanell et al.	99	85%	86% (n = 56)	83% (n = 36)	86% (n = 7)[‡]

[¶] Includes: large cell carcinomas, bronchiololaveolar carcinoma; poorly differentiated carcinomas NOS.
[†] Includes adenosquamous (4/5 positive), large cell (1/2 positive), carcinoid (1/1 positive) and Small Cell Carcinomas (11/11 positive).
[‡] Includes only large cell carcinoma (n = 7).

analyzing the association between telomerase and clinical-pathological features in lung cancer (Figure 9.1).[65] This study confirms the association between telomerase activity and stage which has also been repeated in gastric[67] and breast cancer[68] and leukemias[69] but not in renal cell carcinoma,[70] highlighting the importance of telomerase as a molecular cancer marker in these malignancies.

A positive correlation has also been found between high telomerase activity and proliferative rate, determined by immunohistochemical stain for Ki-67, a nuclear antigen expressed only in proliferating cells.[71] This latter finding is in agreement with the demonstrated role of telomerase in the control of cell proliferation. However, though associated with proliferation, as discussed before, the expression of telomerase is likely to reflect immortality and therefore to constitute a more meaningful parameter than the proliferative rate as assessed by traditional pathological markers.

No associations were found by Albanell and associates[65] between the level of telomerase activity and tumor histological grade or the amount of lymphocytes infiltrating the tumor. This latter analysis was prompted by the reported positivity of activated lymphocytes for telomerase,[42] a finding that, as discussed later, hinders the use of this test in molecular staging.[72]

Albanell and associates[65] found that telomere lengths were not significantly different in groups with low, moderate, and high telomerase activity and were not associated with pathological stage. Furthermore, in 34 cases, telomere restriction fragments (TRFs) were determined in both tumor samples and adjacent normal tissue, revealing mean TRFs reduced in the tumor in 18% of cases and elongated in 6%. Peak TRFs were similar in tumor and normal tissue in 68% of cases, reduced in 24%, and elongated in 9% of cases. These data are in agreement with others, showing that many tumors have mean telomerase length similar to those of adjacent normal tissue.[68,70,73,74] They are also in agreement with *in vitro* data showing that in tumor-derived cell lines there is no association between telomerase activity and telomere length.[63]. Thus, telomere length alone is unlikely to be a predictor of cell immortality.[75]

Though these data point out that telomerase activity is associated with tumor progression, not much is known about the specific molecular deregulation underlying such

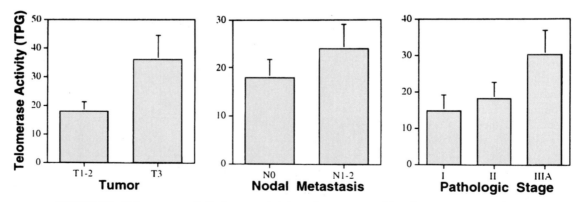

FIGURE 9.1. Telomerase activity (average total product generated [TPG] +/− standard error of the mean [SEM]) was associated with tumor size and extension of the primary lesion (left pane, two-sided P = 0.03), the presence of lymph node metastasis (middle panel, two-sided P = 0.05), and pathologic TNM stage (right panel, two-sided P = 0.01) in non–small cell lung cancer. (From Albanell J, Lonardo F, Rusch V, et al. High telomerase activity in primary lung cancers: association with increased cell proliferation rates and advanced stage. *J Natl Cancer Inst* 1997;89:1609, with permission.)

process. Interestingly, a statistically significant association between *p53* positivity and presence of telomerase activity has also been found in NSCLC.[64] Further correlative studies are needed to define whether telomerase activation is significantly associated with deregulation of other cell cycle–controlling molecules and their nature.

TRAP Assay as a Molecular Test of Lung Cancer?

The widespread positivity of telomerase in human tumors, including lung cancer, and its infrequent positivity in nonneoplastic tissues have prompted investigations on its value as a molecular marker of cancer. These studies have addressed the value of positive telomerase activity in cytological specimens as a diagnostic test of cancer, as well as in lymph node tissue in patients with known cancer, for the purpose of molecular staging. The first line of investigation has been pursued in several organ systems, including the upper and lower aerodigestive system. Califano and colleagues[76] have studied oral rinses from 44 patients with head and neck SCC and found telomerase activity in 14 of them, in contrast to 1 of 22 rinses from control patients without cancer. Both primary tumor and oral rinses were analyzed in 19 cases. A positive telomerase activity in the primary tumor was detected in 17 of 19 samples. Among these 17 telomerase-positive cases, activity was detected in both tumor and oral rinses in seven cases and only in the primary tumor in ten cases; no case showed telomerase activity only in oral rinses.[76] Thus, in this setting, the utility of telomerase as a cancer marker is severely hindered by its low sensitivity.

Three studies have addressed the role of detection of telomerase activity in cytological specimens in the diagnosis of lung cancer. The combined results, showing telomerase activity in benign versus neoplastic cases, are shown in Table 9.2. The reported rates of telomerase positivity in bronchioalveolar lavage fluids from cancer patients ranged from 44% (14 of 34),[77] to 82% (29 of 37),[78] (18 of 22),[79] with an overall positive percentage of 65% (61 of 93). In contrast, a study of the incidence of *KRAS*, *p53* mutations, and microsatellite alterations and methylations of the p16 gene in

bronchoalveolar lavage fluid from patients with lung cancer yielded a sensitivity of only 53% in the diagnosis of cancer.[72] The positivity for telomerase activity detected in cytological specimens from nonneoplastic pulmonary disease was of seven of 128 in the series by Hiyama and colleagues including four of 106 bronchoalveolar lavage fluids, which contained a large number of lymphocytes.[77] Among 21 combined specimens from normal and inflammatory conditions, positive telomerase was found in two cases of sarcoidosis, two cases of tuberculosis, and two normal samples by Arai and associates.[78] Yahata and colleagues[79] found no telomerase positivity in seven normal specimens and only one low-level positivity in 12 nonneoplastic conditions. Two studies compared the sensitivity of telomerase with that of cytology in the detection of lung cancer. Arai and associates[78] found that the TRAP assay detected 29 of 37 clinically proven cancers, versus 24 of 37 for cytology. In the series of Yahata and colleagues[79] telomerase activity detected 18 of 22 cancer cases, cytological examination nine of 22. Interestingly, Yahata and colleagues[79] have combined a traditional TRAP assay with a recently modified *in situ* version of the assay. They found that the sensitivity of the assay significantly improved when both assays were combined.

These results are particularly intriguing in view of the limited sensitivity of cytology alone[61] and of currently available molecular markers[72] in the detection of lung cancer in cytology specimens. In particular they highlight the possibility that telomerase activity may complement currently available screening tests in the diagnostic workup of suspected lung cancer, a possibility that needs further testing in large clinical cohorts.

Only one study has addressed the role of detection of telomerase activity in the molecular staging of lung cancer. These authors found positivity in eight of nine histologically positive and 26 of 48 histologically negative nodes, including three of four lymph nodes found to contain cancer cells by the *p53* plaque assay hybridization. In comparison, assessment of *p53* mutations by plaque hybridization revealed positivity in three of three histologically positive and three of 27 histologically negative nodes. Assessment of *KRAS* mutations revealed positivity in all six histologically positive nodes and in one of 21 histologically negative nodes. It is unlikely that all telomerase-positive, histologically negative lymph nodes harbor metastases, because these patients remained recurrence-free.[44] Furthermore, normal lymph nodes have been shown to contain telomerase activity.[42] These data thus show that the assessment of telomerase activity, while representing a promising molecular marker in the detection of suspected lung cancer, is of little utility in the molecular staging of NSCLC.

SUMMARY

The acquisition of telomerase activity represents a key event in the biology of immortalization *in vitro* and tumorigenesis

TABLE 9.2. DISTRIBUTION OF TELOMERASE POSITIVITY IN BRONCHOALVEOLAR LAVAGE FLUID*

Nonneoplastic	Neoplastic
14/161 (9%)	62/93 (65%)

* Combined data from Hiyama K, Ishioka S, Shay JW, et al. Telomerase activity as a novel marker of lung cancer and immune-mediated associated lung disease. *Int J Mol Med* 1998;3:545. Arai T, Yasuda Y, Takaya T, et al. Application of telomerase activity for the screening of primary lung cancer in bronchoalveolar lavage fluid. *Oncol Rep* 1998;5:405. Yahata N, Okyashiki K, Okyashiki JK, et al. Telomerase activity in lung cancer cells obtained from bronchial washings. *J Natl Cancer Inst* 1998;90:684, with permission.

in vivo, including the progression of preneoplastic bronchial lesions. Telomerase activity is an important molecular marker of lung cancer because it is present very rarely in the nonneoplastic lung, while appearing in more than or equal to 80% of NSCLC, where it correlates with tumor pathological stage and proliferative rate. Its assessment may thus help identify lung cancer patients with unfavorable pathological features and, in addition, potentially may assist the clinician in the diagnostic workup of suspected lung cancer. Furthermore, its ubiquitous role in carcinogenesis and its differential expression in normal and tumor cells make it an attractive target for novel therapeutic and/or chemopreventive intervention in overt and/or preinvasive lung cancer.

REFERENCES

1. Rhyu MS. Telomeres, telomerase and immortality. *J Natl Cancer Inst* 1995;87:884.
2. Muniyappa K, Kironmai KM. Telomerase structure, replication and length maintenance. *Crit Rev Mol Biol* 1998;33:297.
3. Lingner J, Cech TR. Telomerase and chromosomal end maintenance. *Curr Opin Genet Dev* 1998;8:226.
4. Cech Tr, Lingner J. Telomerase and the chromosome end replication problem. *Ciba Found Symp* 1997;211:20.
5. Cech TR, Nakamura TM, Lingner J. Telomerase is a true reverse transcriptase. A review. *Biochemistry* 1997;62:1202.
6. Licht JD, Collins K. Telomerase RNA function in recombinant *Tetrahymena* telomerase. *Genes Dev* 1999;13:1116.
7. Autexier C, Greide CW. Mutational analysis of the *Tetrahymena* telomerase RNA: identification of residues affecting telomerase activity *in vitro. Nucleic Acids Res* 1998;26:787.
8. Feng J, Funk WD, Wang SS, et al. The RNA component of telomerase. *Science* 1995;269:1236.
9. Nakamura TM, Morin GB, Chapman KB, et al. Telomerase catalytic subunit homologs from fission yeast and human. *Science* 1997;277:955.
10. Meyerson M, Counter CM, Eaton EN, et al. hEST2, the putative human telomerase catalytic subunit gene, is up-regulated in tumor cells and during immortalization. *Cell* 1997;90:785.
11. Harrington L, Zhou W, McPhail T, et al. Human telomerase contains evolutionary conserved catalytic and structural subunits. *Genes Dev* 1997;11:3109.
12. Harrington L, McPhail T, Mar V, et al. A mammalian telomerase associated protein. *Science* 1997;275:973.
13. Pardue ML, Danilevskaya ON, Traverse KL, et al. Evolutionary links between telomerase and transposable elements. *Genetica* 1997;100:73.
14. Beattie TL, Zhou W, Robinson MO, et al. Reconstitution of human telomerase activity *in vitro. Curr Biol* 1998;8:177.
15. Yashima K, Maitra A, Rogers BB, et al. Expression of the RNA component of telomerase during human development and differentiation. *Cell Growth Differ* 1998;9:805.
16. Yashima K, Litzky LA, Kaiser L, et al. Telomerase expression in respiratory epithelium during the multistage pathogenesis of lung carcinoma. *Cancer Res* 1997;57:2373.
17. Maitra A, Yashima K, Rathi A, et al. The RNA component of telomerase as a marker of biological potential and clinical outcome in childhood neuroblastic tumors. *Cancer* 1999;85:741.
18. Yashima K, Ashfaq H, Nowak J, et al. Telomerase activity and expression of its RNA component in cervical lesions. *Cancer* 1998;82:1319.
19. Soder AI, Going JJ, Kaye SB, et al. Tumor specific regulation of telomerase RNA gene expression visualized by *in situ* hybridization. *Oncogene* 1998;16:979.
20. Albanell J, Bosl GJ, Engelhardt M, et al. Telomerase activity in germ cell cancers and mature teratomas. *J Natl Cancer Inst* 1999; 91:1321.
21. Albanell J, Han W, Mellado B, et al. Telomerase activity is repressed during differentiation of maturation sensitive but not resistant human tumor cell lines. *Cancer Res* 1996;56:1503.
22. Yashima K, Milchgrub S, Gollahon LS, et al. Telomerase enzyme activity and RNA expression during the multistage pathogenesis of breast carcinoma. *Clin Cancer Res* 1998;4:229.
23. Avilion A, Piatyszek M, Gupta J, et al. Human telomerase activity in immortal cell lines and human tumor tissues. *Cancer Res* 1996; 56:645.
24. Parkinson EK, Newbold RF, Keith WN. The genetic basis of human keratinocyte immortalisation in squamous cell carcinoma development: the role of telomerase reactivation. *Eur J Cancer* 1997;33:727.
25. Speicher MR, Howe C, Crotty P et al. Comparative genomic hybridization detects novel deletions and amplifications in head and neck squamous cell carcinomas. *Cancer Res* 1995;55:1010.
26. Bodnar AG, Ouelette M, Frolkis M, et al. Extension of life span by introduction of telomerase into normal cells. *Science* 1998; 279:349.
27. Balsara BR, Sonoda G, duManoir S, et al. Comparative genomic hybridization analysis detects frequent, often high level, overrepresentation of DNA sequences at 3p, 5p, 7p and 8q in human non–small cell lung carcinoma. *Cancer Res* 1997;57:2116.
28. Peterson I, Bujard M, Petersen S, et al. Patterns of chromosomal imbalances in adenocarcinoma and squamous cell carcinoma of the lung. *Cancer Res* 1997;57:2321.
29. Kanaya T, Kyo S, Takakura M, et al. hTERT is a critical determinant of telomerase activity in renal-cell carcinoma: *Int J Cancer* 1998;78:539.
30. Tahara H, Yasui W, Fujimoto E, et al. Immunohistochemical detection of human telomerase catalytic component, hTERT, in human colorectal tumor and non-tumor tissue. *Oncogene* 1999; 18:1561.
31. Ohmura H, Tahara H, Suzuki M. Restoration of the cellular senescene program and repression of telomerase by chromosome 3. *Jpn J Cancer Res* 1995;86:899.
32. Kok K, Osinga J, Carritt B, et al. Deletion of a DNA sequence at the chromosomal region 3p21 in all major types of lung cancer. *Nature* 1987;330,578.
33. Killary McNeill A, Wolf ME, et al. Definition of a tumor suppressor locus within human chromosome 3p21-p22. *Proc Natl Acad Sci U S A* 1992;89:10877.
34. Daly MC, Xiang RH, Buchhagen D, et al. A homozygous deletion on chromosome 3 in a small cell lung cancer cell line correlates with a region of tumor suppressor activity. *Oncogene* 1993; 8:1721.
35. Kim NW, Piatyszek MA, Prowse KR, et al. Specific association of human telomerase activity with immortal cells and cancer. *Science* 1994;266:2011.
36. Okyashiki K, Yahata N, Okyashiki JK. Development of an *in situ* assay detecting telomerase activity in cells. *Nippon Rinsho* 1998;56:1159.
37. Campisi J. The biology of replicative senescene. *Eur J Cancer* 1997;33:703.
38. Hayflick L. The limited *in vitro* lifetime of human diploid cell strains. *Exp Cell Res* 1965;37:614.
39. Holt SE, Wright WE, Shay JW. Multiple pathways for the regulation of telomerase activity: *Eur J Cancer* 1997;33:761.
40. Chin L, Artandi SE, Shen Q et al. p53 deficiency rescues the

adverse effects of telomere loss and cooperates with telomere dysfunction to accelerate carcinogenesis. *Cell* 199;97:527.

41. Wynford TD. Proliferative lifespan checkpoints: cell-type specificity and influence on tumor biology. *Eur J Cancer* 1997;33:716.

42. Norrback KF, Dahlenborg K, Carlsson R, et al. Telomerase activation in normal B lymphocytes and non-Hodgkin's lymphomas. *Blood* 1996;88:222.

43. Engelhardt M, Kumar, Albanell J, et al. Telomerase regulation, cell cycle and telomere stability in primitive hematopoietic cells. *Blood* 1997;90:182.

44. Ahrendt SA, Yang SC, Wu L, et al. Comparison of oncogene mutation detection and telomerase activity for the molecular staging of non small cell lung cancer. *Clin Cancer Res* 1997;3:1207.

45. Kim NW. Clinical implications of telomerase in cancer. *Eur J Cancer* 1997;33:781.

46. Shay JW, Bacchetti S. A survey of telomerase activity in human cancer. *Eur J Cancer* 1997;33:787.

47. Harle-Bachor C, Boukamp P. Telomerase activity in the regenerative basal layer of the epidermis in human skin and immortal and carcinoma derived skin keratinocytes. *Proc Natl Acad Sci U S A* 1996;93:647.

48. Bryan TM, Reddel RR. Telomere dynamics and telomerase activity in *in vitro* immortalized human cells *Eur J Cancer* 1997;33:767.

49. Scheffner M, Werness BA, Huibregtse JM, et al. The E6 oncoprotein encoded by human papillomavirus types 16 and 18 promotes the degradation of *p53*. *Cell* 1990;63:1129.

50. Dyson N, Howley PM, Münger K, et al. The human papilloma virus-16 E7 oncoprotein is able to bind to the retinoblastoma gene product. *Science* 1989;243:934.

51. Kiyono T, Foster SA, Koop JI, et al. Both Rb/p16INK4A inactivation and telomerase activity are required to immortalize epithelial cells. *Nature* 1998;396:84.

52. Morales CP, et al. Absence of cancer-related changes in human fibroblasts immortalized with telomerase. *Nat Genet* 1999;21:115.

53. Jiang XR, et al. Telomerase expression in human somatic cells does not induce changes associated with a transformed phenotype. *Nat Genet* 1999;21:111.

54. Hahn WC, Counter CM, Lundberg AS, et al. Creation of human tumor cells with defined genetic elements *Nature* 1999;400:464.

55. Auerbach O, Brewster GJ, Forman JB, et al. Changes in the bronchial epithelium in relation to smoking and cancer of the lung. *N Engl J Med* 1957;256:97.

56. Colby TV, Wistuba II, Gazdar A. Precursors to pulmonary neoplasia. *Adv Anat Pathol* 1998;5:205.

57. Lonardo F, Rusch V, Langenfeld J, et al. Aberrant expression of cylins D1 and E is frequent in preneoplastic bronchial lesions and precedes the development of squamous cell carcinoma. *Cancer Res* 1999;59:2470.

58. Rusch V, Klimstra D, Linkov I, et al. Aberrant expression of p53 or EGFR is frequent in early bronchial preneoplasia and coexpression precedes development of squamous cell carcinoma. *Cancer Res* 1995;55:1365.

59. Thiberville L, Payne P, Vielkinds J, et al. Evidence of cumulative genetic losses with progression of premalignant epithelial lesions to carcinoma of the bronchus. *Cancer Res* 1995;55:5133.

60. Emura M. Stem cells of the respiratory epithelium and their *in vitro* cultivation. *In Vitro Cell Dev Biol Anim* 1997;33:3.

61. Eddy DM. Screening for lung cancer. *Ann Intern Med* 1989;111:232.

62. Kitamura H, Kameda Y, Nakamura N, et al. Atypical adenomatous hyperplasia and bronchioloalveolar lung carcinoma. Analysis by morphometry and the expression of p53 and carcino-embryogenic antigen. *Am J Surg Pathol* 1996;20:553.

63. Hiyama K, Hiyama E, Ishioka S. Telomerase activity in small-cell and non–small cell lung cancers. *J Natl Cancer Inst* 1995;87:895.

64. Wu X, Kemp B, Honn SE, et al. Associations among telomerase activity, p53 protein overexpression, and genetic instability in lung cancer. *Br J Cancer* 1999;80:453.

65. Albanell J, Lonardo F, Rusch V, et al. High telomerase activity in primary lung cancers: association with increased cell proliferation rates and advanced stage. *J Natl Cancer Inst* 1997;89:1609.

66. Colby TV, Koss MN, Travis WD. Tumors of the respiratory tract. In: Rosai J, ed. *Atlas of Tumor Pathology,* 3rd series. Armed Forces Institute of Pathology, Washington, DC 1995:91.

67. Hiyama E, Yokohama, Tatsumoto N, et al. Telomerase activity in gastric cancer. *Cancer Res* 1995;55:3258.

68. Hiyama E, Gollahon L, Kataoka T, et al. Telomerase activity in human breast tumors. *J Natl Cancer Inst* 1996;88:116.

69. Counter CM, Gupta J, Harley CB, et al. Telomerase activity in normal leukocytes and in hematological malignancies. *Blood* 1995;85:2315.

70. Hiyama E, Yokohama T, Hiyama K, et al. Alterations of telomeric repeat length in adult and childhood solid neoplasias. *Int J Oncol* 1995;6:13.

71. Cattoretti G, Becker MH, Key G, et al. Monoclonal antibodies against recombinant parts of the Ki-67 antigen detect proliferating cells in microwave processed, formalin fixed paraffin sections. *J Pathol* 1992;168:357.

72. Ahrendt SA, Chow JT, Xu LH, et al. Molecular detection of tumor cells in broncholaveolar lavage fluid from patients with early stage lung cancer. *J Natl Cancer Inst* 1999;91:332.

73. Hiyama E, Hiyama K, Yokohama T, et al. Correlating telomerase activity levels with human neuroblastoma outcome. *Nat Med* 1995;1:249.

74. Bacchetti S, Counter CM. Telomeres and telomerase in human cancer. *Int J Oncol* 1995;7:423.

75. Hiyama E, Gollahon L, Kataoka T, et al. Telomerase activity in human tumors. *J Natl Cancer Inst* 1996;88:116.

76. Califano J, Ahrendt SA, Meininger G, et al. Detection of telomerase activity in oral rinses from head and neck squamous cell carcinoma patients. *Cancer Res* 1996;56:5720.

77. Hiyama K, Ishioka S, Shay JW, et al. Telomerase activity as a novel marker of lung cancer and immune-mediated associated lung diseases. *Int J Mol Med* 1998;3:545.

78. Arai T, Yasuda Y, Takaya T, et al. Application of telomerase activity for the screening of primary lung cancer in bronchoalveolar lavage fluid. *Oncol Rep* 1998;5:405.

79. Yahata N, Okyashiki K, Okyashiki JK, et al. Telomerase activity in lung cancer cells obtained from bronchial washings. *J Natl Cancer Inst* 1998;90:684.

HOST-TUMOR INTERACTIONS

10

GROWTH FACTORS

GREGORY P. KALEMKERIAN

Various growth factors and growth factor receptors have been implicated in the pathogenesis and progression of both small cell (SCLC) and non–small cell (NSCLC) lung cancer. Many of these factors and receptors are preferentially expressed by either SCLC or NSCLC cells, and their effects on proliferation are similarly cell-type specific. Growth factors generally act through interactions with specific membrane-associated receptors, resulting in the activation of intracellular signal transduction pathways that carry mitogenic signals to the nucleus where cell cycle activation leads to cellular division. These pathways are also involved in the transmission of survival signals that can maintain malignant clones by interfering with appropriate apoptotic, or cell death, signals. Therefore, the dysregulation of the expression or function of specific growth factors, receptors, or signal transduction mediators can result in uncontrolled proliferation and malignant transformation. Although most growth factors induce proliferation, several growth-inhibitory factors have also been identified. The production of autocrine growth factors by lung cancer cells plays an important role in the establishment and survival of primary tumors and metastatic deposits. Proof of an autocrine growth pathway requires the demonstration of growth factor production, specific receptor expression, and growth factor–mediated proliferation within a homogenous cell population. Growth factors secreted by tumor cells or associated stromal cells can also act in a paracrine fashion by interacting with specific receptors on neighboring cancer cells. Recent advances in our understanding of the specific pathways through which growth factors affect the survival and proliferation of cancer cells has allowed the development of novel, tumor-specific therapeutic strategies.

GROWTH FACTORS IMPLICATED IN SMALL CELL LUNG CANCER

SCLC cell lines (see also Chapter 18) can be categorized into two phenotypic subsets: classic and variant. The majority of SCLC cells exhibit a classic phenotype with a high degree of neuroendocrine differentiation. Variant cell lines are less differentiated and tend to have shorter doubling times and

greater treatment resistance. In light of the neuroendocrine nature of SCLC, it is not surprising that a wide variety of neuropeptides and neuropeptide receptors are expressed by SCLC cell lines and tumors. Several of these neuropeptides have mitogenic potential and have been shown to be important mediators of SCLC proliferation (Table 10.1).

Bombesinlike Peptides

Gastrin-releasing peptide (GRP) is the 27-amino acid mammalian homologue of the 14-amino acid amphibian neuropeptide bombesin. The C-terminal region of these peptides is a highly conserved receptor-binding domain that allows interaction with a family of G-protein-coupled, membrane-associated receptors. Thus far, three mammalian bombesinlike peptide receptors have been identified: GRP receptor (GRP-R), neuromedin B receptor (NMB-R), and bombesin receptor subtype-3 (BRS-3). Significant GRP expression has been reported in bronchial neuroendocrine cells and fetal, but not adult, lung preparations.[1,2] A role for inappropriate GRP expression in lung carcinogenesis was suggested by studies demonstrating that high levels of bombesinlike immunoreactivity (BLI) are present in bronchoalveolar lavage fluid from smokers,[3] and that bombesin and GRP can induce the proliferation of normal human bronchial epithelial cells and classic SCLC xenografts in nude mice.[4–6]

Initial reports of BLI in SCLC cells led to the finding that most SCLC cell lines and tumors produce and secrete GRP, and that those lacking BLI generally exhibit a variant phenotype.[7–9] The expression of GRP in SCLC cells is not constitutive, but is regulated by numerous factors, including several proteins found in nuclear extracts of classic, but not variant, SCLC cells that interact with cis-acting regulatory elements in the 5′ flanking region of the GRP gene.[10,11] In addition, somatostatin down-regulates BLI in SCLC cells,[12] whereas retinoic acid,[13] vasoactive intestinal peptide,[14] and corticotophin-releasing factor[15] induce the expression of GRP. The complexity of the GRP signaling system was underscored by the finding that extensive alternate splicing and posttranslational processing of GRP mRNA result in the expression of multiple GRP gene-associated proteins in SCLC cells.[16–18]

TABLE 10.1. GROWTH FACTORS AND RECEPTORS IMPLICATED IN SMALL CELL LUNG CANCER

Stimulatory Factors/Receptors
Gastrin-releasing peptide/GRP receptor
Neuromedin B/NMB receptor
Vasopressin/V$_1$ receptors
Bradykinin/B$_2$ receptor
Gastrin/CCK-B/gastrin receptor
Cholecystokinin/CCK-B/gastrin receptor
Neurotensin/NT receptor
Galanin/Galanin receptor
Insulinlike growth factor I/IGF-I receptor
Stem cell factor/SCF receptor (c-*kit*)
Transferrin/TF receptor
Interleukin-3/IL-3 receptor
Testosterone/Androgen receptor
Nicotine/Nicotinic acetylcholine receptor

Inhibitory Factors/Receptors
Transforming growth factor β_1/TGFβ-RII receptor
Opioids-endorphins/Opioid receptors
Somatostatin/SST receptors
Physalaemin

Bifunctional Factors/Receptors
Vasoactive intestinal peptide/VIP receptor
Nerve growth factor/NGF receptors

protein complexes then activate phospholipase C-β (PLC), which cleaves phosphotidyl inositol 4,5-biphosphate (PIP$_2$) into inositol 1,4,5-triphosphate (IP$_3$) and 1,2-diacylglycerol (DAG).[21,22] IP$_3$ induces intracellular calcium ion mobilization, whereas DAG activates protein kinase C (PKC).[23,24] Mitogen-activated protein kinase (MAPK) pathways, including the c-jun amino-terminal kinase (JNK) and extracellular signal-regulated kinase (ERK) pathways, are activated by both PKC-dependent and -independent mechanisms, culminating in the transcriptional activation of early-response genes (c-*fos*, c-*jun*, c-*myc*), DNA synthesis, and mitosis.[25,26] Neuropeptide receptors have also been shown to activate arachidonic acid signaling pathways, leading to an accumulation of cyclic AMP (cAMP). Further evidence of GRP's role as an autocrine growth factor in SCLC comes from studies in which the monoclonal antibody 2A11, with specificity for the C-terminus of bombesin, blocked GRP:GRP-R binding, inhibited clonal growth of SCLC cells *in vitro,* and induced the regression of human SCLC xenografts in nude mice.[27] The expression of neuromedin B and its receptor, NMB-R, has been identified in some SCLC and NSCLC cells, and exogenous neuromedin B induces clonal proliferation in classic SCLC cell lines.[28,29]

Although only a few NSCLC specimens have been reported to express GRP or BLI,[30–32] most NSCLCs do express either GRP-R or NMB-R,[33,34] and activation of these receptors by bombesin can induce intracellular calcium ion shifts and PKC translocation.[35] However, despite a few reports suggesting that GRP can stimulate the growth of NSCLC cells, most studies have failed to demonstrate any

High-affinity GRP-R and NMB-R have been identified on most SCLC cells, whereas BRS-3 is expressed by a smaller subset of tumors.[19,20] In SCLC cells, the binding of bombesin or GRP to these receptors activates several G-proteins that initiate the second messenger cascade by hydrolyzing guanine nucleotides (Figure 10.1). Activated G-

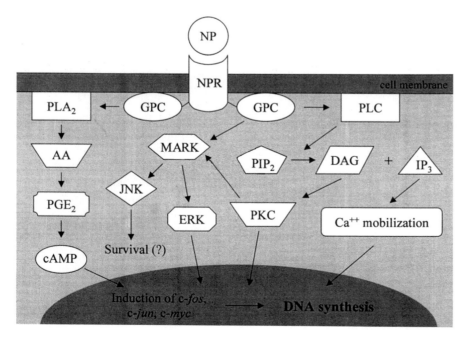

FIGURE 10.1. Schematic representation of neuropeptide-mediated signal transduction pathways. *NP*, neuropeptide growth factor; *NPR*, neuropeptide receptor; *GPC*, G-protein complex; *PLC*, phospholipase C; *PIP$_2$*, phosphotidylinositol 4,5-bisphosphate; *DAG*, 1,2-diacylglycerol; *IP$_3$*, inositol 1,4,5-triphosphate; *PKC*, protein kinase C; *MAPK*, mitogen-activated protein kinase; *JNK*, c-jun amino-terminal kinase; *ERK*, extracellular signal-regulated kinase; *PLA$_2$*, phospholipase A$_2$; *AA*, arachidonic acid; *PGF$_2$*, prostaglandin E$_2$; *cAMP*, cyclic adenosine monophosphate. (From Woll PJ. Growth factors and lung cancer. In: Pass HI, Mitchell JB, Johnson DH, Turrisi AT, eds. *Lung cancer: principles and practice,* 1/e, Philadelphia: Lippincott-Raven, 1996:123, with permission.)

GRP or bombesin-mediated mitogenic effects in NSCLC.[26,36]

GRP has been evaluated as a clinical tumor marker for SCLC, with several trials reporting elevated plasma pro-GRP or GRP concentrations in more than 70% of patients with SCLC, but not in those with NSCLC.[37–39] In addition, high levels of cerebrospinal fluid GRP were noted in 75% of SCLC patients with carcinomatous meningitis.[40] However, most studies have found that low sensitivity and specificity severely limit the clinical utility of plasma GRP levels in patients with SCLC.[41,42]

Although many other neuropeptides induce biochemical evidence of signal transduction pathway activation, such as mobilization of intracellular calcium ion stores, relatively few have been shown to enhance the proliferation of SCLC cells.[43,44] Among this latter group are vasopressin, bradykinin, cholecystokinin, gastrin, neurotensin, and galanin.

Vasopressin

Vasopressin, a hypothalamic nonapeptide, is a regulator of blood pressure and the adrenal axis, and is the major antidiuretic hormone (ADH) in humans. These physiologic functions are mediated through a family of vasopressin-specific receptors, V_{1a}, V_{1b}, and V_2, which are all expressed by most classic and variant SCLC cell lines.[45] Activation of the V_{1a} receptor results in an increase in cytosolic calcium ion concentrations and activation of PKC and phospholipases C, D, and A_2, whereas the V_2 receptor acts through cAMP-coupled increases in protein kinase A (PKA). Vasopressin is produced by 67% of SCLC tumors, but not by NSCLC, and is responsible for the syndrome of inappropriate ADH secretion, which causes paraneoplastic hyponatremia in 11% of SCLC patients.[46,47] (see also Chapter 29.) Vasopressin enhances the clonal growth of classic SCLC cell lines, an effect that can be antagonized by synthetic substance P analogues, suggesting that it is an autocrine mediator of SCLC proliferation.[48–50]

Bradykinin

Bradykinin is a nonapeptide that regulates diverse physiologic processes, including coagulation and nociceptive neurotransmission. Although few lung tumors produce bradykinin, normal lung tissue and many lung cancers do express B_2 bradykinin receptors.[51,52] Activation of B_2 receptors by bradykinin in both SCLC and NSCLC cells results in cytosolic calcium ion flux and stimulation of growth through a $PKC\alpha$ pathway.[48,53,54] In light of these findings, long-acting, N-terminally-linked bradykinin antagonist dimers containing the novel amino acid, indanylglycine, were developed and shown to inhibit the growth of SCLC cells *in vitro* and in xenograft models through the induction of apoptosis.[55] It has been suggested that the anti-SCLC activity of these bradykinin antagonist dimers and of substance P analogues is caused by discordant signaling. Specifically,

these compounds activate or inhibit specific G-proteins, resulting in the activation of JNK pathways without activating PLC or PKC, a signal transduction pattern that can stimulate apoptotic pathways. Additionally, the activity of bradykinin antagonist dimers is synergistic with that of standard chemotherapeutic agents, even in SCLC cells exhibiting a multidrug-resistance phenotype.[56]

Gastrin and Cholecystokinin

Both gastrin and cholecystokinin (CCK) mediate their biologic activity through an identical C-terminal pentapeptide sequence that binds to CCK-B/gastrin receptors and, to a lesser extent, CCK-A receptors. Pro-gastrin is produced and processed by both SCLCs and NSCLCs,[57] but pre-pro-CCK and carboxyamidated bioactive CCK are expressed only by SCLC cells.[58] CCK-B/gastrin receptors are present on most SCLC cells, but are rarely expressed by NSCLC, and only a few lung tumors have been reported to express CCK-A receptors.[59,60] The concurrent expression of gastrin and CCK-B/gastrin receptors in many SCLCs has raised the possibility that they may be components of an autocrine loop. Both gastrin and CCK induce intracellular calcium ion shifts and stimulate proliferation of SCLC cells that possess CCK-B/gastrin receptors,[61] and several CCK analogues have been reported to antagonize CCK-B/gastrin receptor-mediated signal transduction events in SCLC cells.[62,63] CCK also enhances clonal growth through activation of CCK-A receptors in some SCLC cell lines.[64]

Vasoactive Intestinal Peptide

Vasoactive intestinal peptide (VIP) is a 28-amino acid neuropeptide that binds to a transmembrane receptor and activates both G-protein- and cAMP-mediated signal transduction pathways. Expression of VIP occurs in approximately 50% of lung cancers and is a rare cause of paraneoplastic watery diarrhea.[65] The VIP receptor is expressed in normal lung alveoli, as well as by SCLC and NSCLC cell lines.[66] In NSCLC cell lines, VIP stimulates proliferation,[67,68] and a hybrid peptide consisting of the N-terminus of neurotensin fused to the C-terminus of VIP has been shown to antagonize VIP-mediated induction of cAMP and inhibit the growth of NSCLC cells and xenografts.[69] In SCLC cells, VIP induces the secretion of GRP and has been reported to have both growth-stimulatory and -inhibitory potential, the latter of which is potentiated by an antibombesin monoclonal antibody.[70–72]

Neurotensin

Neurotensin is a 13-amino acid neuropeptide that is expressed and processed by most classic SCLC cells, but not by variant SCLC or NSCLC cells.[73,74] Both neurotensin and the bioactive C-terminal fragment, NT(8–13), bind with high affinity to classic SCLC cells, resulting in the release of calcium from intracellular stores, PKC-dependent activation of ERK pathways, and enhancement of proliferation, suggesting an autocrine growth-stimulatory pathway.[48,75–77]

Galanin

Galanin is a 29-amino acid polypeptide that is widely distributed in neurons and has diverse physiologic functions. In classic SCLC cells, galanin-mediated stimulation of clonal proliferation is associated with increases in intracellular calcium ion concentrations and inositol phosphatase activity, as well as activation of ERK pathways in a PKC-dependent manner.[48,77,78]

Tachykinins

The tachykinins are a group of neuropeptides that mediate a diverse range of biologic activities, including pulmonary inflammation and the proliferation of mesenchymal and epithelial cells. Tachykinin receptors, such as the NK1 receptor, have been identified in human bronchial epithelium and are linked to G-proteins that activate PLC signaling pathways.[79] Mammalian tachykinins, including substance P and the neurokinins, induce calcium ion mobilization in SCLC cells, but have little effect on DNA synthesis or proliferation.[80,81] A peptide with immunologic and biologic homology to the amphibian tachykinin, physalaemin, has been infrequently identified in human SCLC,[82] and picomolar concentrations of physalaemin have been reported to inhibit the growth of both classic and variant SCLC cells.[80]

Therapeutic Strategies Targeting Neuropeptide Pathways

The profound influence of GRP and other neuropeptides on SCLC proliferation has led to a variety of therapeutic strategies targeting relevant growth factor pathways. Thus far, the most extensively studied approaches involve receptor-specific and broad-spectrum neuropeptide antagonists.[83] Numerous peptide analogues of bombesin and GRP have been synthesized and evaluated for anticancer activity in SCLC cells. Among these compounds, short-chain peptides with homology to the C-terminal region of bombesin and GRP, especially those containing reduced peptide bonds, appear to possess the greatest antitumor activity.[84,85] These analogues interact specifically with GRP-R, competitively blocking bombesin/GRP binding and inhibiting bombesin/GRP-mediated calcium ion mobilization and PIP$_2$ turnover in classic SCLC cells.[86,87] Receptor-specific antagonists also down-regulate the expression of GRP-R and epidermal growth (EGF-R) block DNA synthesis, and inhibit basal and bombesin/GRP-mediated proliferation in a cytostatic manner in some SCLC cell lines and xeno-

grafts.[88–90] However, receptor-specific neuropeptide antagonists are inactive against NSCLC cell lines and SCLC cells lacking expression of bombesin/GRP receptors.[88,90]

Because the growth and survival of SCLC depends on the combined actions of a variety of neuropeptide growth factors, substantial effort has been directed toward the design of broad-spectrum neuropeptide antagonists. In this light, a variety of substance P peptide analogues have been developed and evaluated for activity in SCLC. These substance P antagonists inhibit neuropeptide-mediated calcium ion mobilization, protein tyrosine kinase activation, and DNA synthesis in SCLC cell lines.[91,92] In addition, these compounds inhibit the growth induced by multiple neuropeptides, including bombesin/GRP vasopressin, bradykinin, cholecystokinin and others, in SCLC cell lines and xenografts.[83,93–95] Broad-spectrum substance P analogues are generally more potent inhibitors of SCLC growth than receptor-specific neuropeptide antagonists, despite being less potent inhibitors of neuropeptide binding and receptor activation.[83] In addition, the activity of substance P analogues does not consistently depend on the expression of neuropeptide receptors by the target cell, suggesting that these compounds may inhibit basal and neuropeptide-stimulated SCLC growth through unpredicted mechanisms.[81,96] The activity of full-length analogues, such as [D-Arg^1, D-Phe^5, D-Trp^{7,9}, Leu^{11}] substance P (antagonist D), depends on relatively high antagonist concentrations, a finding that has hampered clinical development. In contrast, some short-chain analogues, such as [Arg^6, D-Trp^{7,9}, N-MePhe^8] substance P(6–11) (antagonist G) and [D-MePhe^6, D-Trp^{7,9}, $\psi^{10,11}$, Leu^{11}] substance P(6-11) (NY3460), inhibit SCLC growth *in vitro* and *in vivo* at low micromolar concentrations.[50,97,98] The activity of antagonist G is additive with that of the tyrosine kinase inhibitor, tyrphostin,[99] and NY3460 has recently been shown to be a potent inducer of apoptosis in some SCLC cell lines.[100] Preclinical evaluation of the metabolism, pharmacokinetics, and toxicity of antagonist G yielded favorable results, and a phase I–II clinical trial is currently underway.[101]

Another therapeutic strategy aimed at interrupting autocrine growth loops in SCLC involves murine monoclonal antibody 2A11 directed against the C-terminal region of GRP. This antibody blocks bombesin-mediated PLC activation and PIP$_2$ turnover,[87] and inhibits the growth of SCLC cells and xenografts that express at least one bombesin-family receptor.[102] Recently, Kelley and colleagues reported a clinical trial in which monoclonal antibody 2A11 induced a complete response in a patient with relapsed SCLC.[103] An alternate immunotherapeutic strategy involves the fusion of a GRP analogue with a monoclonal antibody directed against the Fc$_1$RI or Fc$_1$RIII cytotoxic trigger molecules on immunologic effector cells. This immunoconjugate binds to SCLC cells that express GRP-R and attracts cytokine-activated monocytes and NK cells that mediate the lysis of the targeted SCLC cells *in vitro*.[104]

A similar approach utilizes an immunoconjugate in which the active domains of diphtheria toxin are fused to either GRP (DAB$_{389}$-GRP) or substance P (DAB$_{389}$-SP). Exposure to nanomolar concentrations of DAB$_{389}$-GRP or DAB$_{389}$-SP results in the inhibition of both protein synthesis and proliferation in SCLC cells expressing GRP-R or NMB-R.[105]

Second-messenger molecules can also serve as effective targets for the disruption of autocrine growth factor pathways. The recognition of the importance of protein phosphorylation in neuropeptide-mediated proliferative signal transduction pathways has led to studies evaluating the antitumor activity of kinase inhibitors. Several tyrosine kinase inhibitors, including the tyrphostins and genestein, inhibit basal and neuropeptide-mediated SCLC growth at low-micromolar levels, with the induction of p53- and bcl-2-independent apoptosis (see also Chapter 6) at higher concentrations.[92,99] The serine/threonine kinase, p70^{s6k}, is constitutively active in classic SCLC cells and is involved in neuropeptide-mediated mitogenesis. Rapamycin, an immunosuppressant that inhibits p70^{s6k} phosphorylation and activation, induces the dephosphorylation of p70^{s6k} and inhibits basal and galanin-stimulated proliferation in classic SCLC cells.[106]

Neutral endopeptidase (CD10/NEP, CALLA, EC 3.4.24.11) is a cell surface metalloproteinase that regulates growth factor–mediated proliferation by hydrolyzing and inactivating many neuropeptides, including GRP, neurotensin, and bradykinin. A possible role for CD10/NEP in lung carcinogenesis has been suggested by the finding that cigarette smoke not only induces neuropeptide production but also inhibits CD10/NEP expression, leading to a dramatic increase in the concentration of neuropeptide growth factors in the bronchial epithelium of smokers. In addition, although CD10/NEP is highly expressed by normal airway epithelial cells, CD10/NEP mRNA and protein levels are low or absent in most SCLC and NSCLC tumors and cell lines.[107,108] In cultured NSCLC and human bronchial epithelial cells, the expression of CD10/NEP is inversely related to that of proliferating cell nuclear antigen (PCNA),[109] and the inhibition of CD10/NEP activity potentiates neuropeptide-induced signaling and cellular growth.[107,110] *In vitro* studies have shown that recombinant CD10/NEP inhibits neuropeptide-mediated calcium ion mobilization, DNA synthesis, and proliferation in most SCLC and NSCLC cells, but that this activity requires prolonged exposure to high concentrations of CD10/NEP.[107,108,110] *In vivo*, high doses (10 mg/kg/day) of CD10/NEP administered intraperitoneally reversibly slowed the development of subcutaneous classic and variant SCLC xenografts in nude mice, but had no effect on large, established xenografts.[108]

Somatostatin

The somatostatins physiologically inhibit the secretion of many amine and peptide hormones and growth factors. As such, they can act as growth-inhibitory factors for a variety of normal and malignant cell types that rely on autocrine growth factors. The activity of somatostatin is mediated through specific membrane-associated receptors, SST-R1 and SST-R2, that are expressed by a variety of cancers. These receptors are linked to G-protein signaling pathways that inhibit cAMP production and calcium ion influx and activate tyrosine phosphatases, thereby interfering with a range of proliferative signaling pathways.[111] Somatostatin expression has been detected in approximately 25% of SCLC cell lines and tumors, but is rare in NSCLC,[112–114] and 15% of patients with SCLC have elevated plasma levels of somatostatin.[115] In addition, functional somatostatin receptors have been identified on most SCLC, but few NSCLC, cell lines and tumors.[116–118] Somatostatin inhibits VIP-induced autocrine growth factor release in classic SCLC cells,[119] but has no effect on the growth of Lewis lung carcinoma cells with an NSCLC phenotype.[120] In light of the short half-life of natural somatostatins, several long-acting analogues with somatostatin agonist activity have been developed (e.g., octreotide, BIM 23014C, RC-160). These analogues inhibit the proliferation of some SCLC and NSCLC cells and xenografts in a cytostatic manner that is additive with cisplatin.[121–123] Mechanistically, somatostatin agonists have been reported to inhibit growth factor–stimulated MAPK activation and to down-regulate EGF-R and IGF-I-R expression.[90,124] However, their anticancer activity does not correlate with the expression of known somatostatin receptors, or with the inhibition of calcium ion influx or cAMP production.[90,121,124] Clinical trials of octreotide have reported only one partial response in a total of 22 patients with SCLC.[121,125] Although the antitumor activity of somatostatin analogues has been disappointing, they have been effective in blocking hormone secretion and alleviating paraneoplastic syndromes associated with a variety of neuroendocrine tumors. The presence of somatostatin receptors in most SCLC tumors has also led to interest in the use of radiolabeled analogues for detection and staging; however, the clinical utility of such imaging studies is severely limited by low sensitivity in detecting metastatic foci.[126,127]

Nerve Growth Factor

High-affinity receptors for nerve growth factor (NGF) have been identified in a subset of SCLC cells but not in NSCLC.[128,129] However, the biologic effects of NGF on SCLC remain unclear. One study found that NGF stimulated *in vitro* growth of several SCLC cell lines in a specific manner that was inhibited by anti-NGF antibodies and the tyrosine kinase inhibitor, genestein,[129] but a conflicting report suggested that NGF inhibited basal and nicotine-mediated SCLC proliferation and tumorigenicity.[130]

GROWTH FACTORS IMPLICATED IN NON–SMALL CELL LUNG CANCER

The factors and receptors involved in the regulation of NSCLC proliferation have also been identified as growth mediators in many other epithelial tumors (Table 10.2). The frequent dysregulation of these pathways in NSCLC and other malignancies suggests that they are important determinants of neoplastic growth and rational targets for novel anticancer strategies.

Epidermal Growth Factor Receptor and Its Ligands

EGF-R, a transmembrane receptor with tyrosine kinase activity encoded by the c-*erbB*-1 oncogene, can be activated by several ligands, including EGF, transforming growth factor α (TGFα), and amphiregulin. Both EGF and TGFα induce mitogenic signals through EGF-R, whereas amphiregulin is a bifunctional growth factor with both stimulatory and inhibitory potential. Normal lung tissue and many NSCLC tumors express EGF-R, TGFα, and amphiregulin, but most studies have failed to demonstrate significant expression of EGF-R or its ligands in SCLC.[131–134] Rusch and colleagues reported overexpression of EGF-R and TGFα relative to normal bronchial epithelium in 45% and 61% of NSCLC tumors, respectively, with co-overexpression in 38%.[135] In contrast, amphiregulin was underexpressed in 63% of tumors, with simultaneous EGF-R overexpression and amphiregulin underexpression in only 21%. Although EGF was not detected in any tumors in this study, another report noted overexpression of EGF in 50% of lung adenocarcinomas.[136] Studies demonstrating that the growth of NSCLC cell lines is enhanced by EGF or TGFα and inhibited by monoclonal antibodies directed against EGF-R or TGFα suggest that these molecules participate in auto-

crine or paracrine loops in NSCLC.[137–139] Treatment of NSCLC cell lines with exogenous EGF results in rapid autophosphoylation of EGF-R followed by activation of MAPK pathways, including the ERK and JNK pathways, with subsequent enhancement of proliferation.[140,141] Inhibition of JNK pathways with specific antisense oligonucleotides blocked EGF-induced growth, whereas inhibition of ERK activity had no effect on proliferation, suggesting separable MAPK signaling pathway functions.[141]

A role for TGFα in lung carcinogenesis has been suggested by reports that TGFα enhances tumorigenicity in lung epithelial cells expressing EGF-R and p185[HER2].[142] In addition, increased expression of TGFα has been associated with malignant transformation of SV-40 immortalized human bronchial epithelial cells (BEAS-2B) induced by tobacco-specific N-nitrosamines or cigarette smoke condensate.[143] Although some reports have noted an association between EGF-R expression and drug resistance, lymph node metastases, and shortened survival,[144,145] most studies have failed to demonstrate any prognostic significance for the expression of EGF-R or its ligands,[135,146,147] suggesting that these factors modulate local tumor growth without affecting tumor progression or metastatic potential. However, in lung adenocarcinomas the expression of TGFα or EGF appeared to portend a poorer prognosis in patients whose tumors also expressed EGF-R, but not in those with EGF-R-negative tumors.[136] In a recent study of 195 patients who underwent resection of a stage I–III NSCLC, multivariate analysis revealed that lymph node involvement, high microvessel counts and overexpression of amphiregulin correlated with poor prognosis, whereas overexpression of EGF-R, TGFα, and p185[HER2] did not.[148]

EGF-R-mediated proliferative pathways have become popular targets for experimental therapeutic interventions in NSCLC. A variety of anti-EGF-R monoclonal antibodies have been shown to block the binding of TGFα or EGF to EGF-R, and to inhibit EGF-R activation and the proliferation of NSCLC cell lines and xenografts.[138,149] The growth-inhibitory activity of anti-EGF-R monoclonal antibodies can be augmented by combining them with GM3, an anti-tyrosine kinase ganglioside that further suppresses the activation of EGF-R.[150] Clinical trials have found that anti-EGF-R monoclonal antibodies localize to EGF-R-expressing lung tumors, down-regulate EGF-R tyrosine kinase activity *in vivo,* and have minimal toxicity.[151–153] Anti-TGFα monoclonal antibodies also inhibit the proliferation of NSCLC cell lines.[154] In addition, the experimental anticancer agent, suramin, can interfere with the binding of EGF or TGFα to EGF-R and can inhibit growth factor–induced DNA synthesis and proliferation in NSCLC cells.[139,155] TGFα-PE40, a recombinant fusion protein consisting of TGFα and a 40kD cytotoxic fragment of *Pseudomonas* exotoxin A that was designed to target EGF-R-expressing tumor cells, partially inhibited the growth of NSCLC colonies and xenografts, and its cytotoxicity was

TABLE 10.2. GROWTH FACTORS AND RECEPTORS IMPLICATED IN NON-SMALL CELL LUNG CANCER

Stimulatory Factors/Receptors
Epidermal growth factor/EGF receptor (c-*erbB*-1)
Transforming growth factor α/EGF receptor (c-*erbB*-1)
Platelet-derived growth factor/PDGF receptor
Insulin-like growth factors I & II/IGF-I receptor
Parathyroid hormone-related peptide
Vasoactive intestinal peptide/VIP receptor
Transferrin/TF receptor
p185[HER2] (*HER2/neu*)

Inhibitory Factors/Receptors
Transforming growth factor β_1/TGFβ-RII receptor
Interleukin-6/IL-6 receptor
Tumor necrosis factor α/TNFα receptor

Bifunctional Factor/Receptor
Amphiregulin/EGF receptor (c-*erbB*-1)

associated with the expression of EGF-R.[156,157] An EGF-R deletion-mutant with unique peptide sequences, EGF-R type III, has been identified in up to 16% of NSCLCs, but not in normal lung tissue, suggesting that it may serve as a tumor-specific therapeutic target.[158,159] Strategies targeting the signal transduction pathways downstream of EGF-R are also being developed. Genestein, a naturally occurring tyrosine kinase inhibitor, abrogates EGF-induced receptor phosphorylation and MAPK activation and induces apoptosis in NSCLC cells.[140] Finally, the high level of expression of EGF-R in NSCLC cells has been exploited to develop an efficient gene therapy delivery system in which the gene of interest is fused to EGF. This EGF-DNA conjugate specifically targets EGF-R-expressing cells, resulting in efficient heterologous expression of the delivered gene.[160]

HER2/neu

The *HER2/neu* (c-*erbB*-2) oncogene encodes p185[HER2], a transmembrane growth factor receptor with tyrosine kinase activity that shares significant sequence homology with EGF-R (see also Chapter 4). Overexpression of p185[HER2] occurs in 25% to 60% of NSCLC tumors and cell lines but not in SCLC.[161,162] However, unlike the case in breast cancer and other tumors where gene amplification is the primary mode of *HER2/neu* dysregulation, gene amplification is rare event in NSCLC.[163,164] Studies with transgenic mice and immortalized human bronchial epithelial cells have suggested that although overexpression of p185[HER2] appears to be involved in the development of neoplastic lung lesions, it is not sufficient for malignant transformation.[165,166] Transfection experiments have also shown that p185[HER2] overexpression results in increased invasiveness and metastatic potential in NSCLC cells.[167]

P185[HER2] has become a common target for novel therapeutic strategies because of reports that have identified an association between *HER2/neu* overexpression and advanced-stage disease or shortened survival in patients with NSCLC.[162,168] High levels of p185[HER2] expression also appear to correlate with chemoresistance, and the treatment of p185[HER2]-overexpressing NSCLC cells with the tyrosine kinase inhibitors tyrphostin AG825 and emodin suppressed p185[HER2] activation and increased sensitivity to cisplatin, etoposide, and doxorubicin.[169–171] Similarly, the inhibition of p185[HER2] expression through the transfection of a *HER2/neu* antisense-containing vector suppressed growth and tumorigenicity of *HER2/neu*-expressing NSCLC cells.[172] A murine monoclonal anti-p185[HER2] antibody conjugated to gelonin, a potent ribosomal inhibitor, was also found to be a potent selective inhibitor of p185[HER2]-positive NSCLC cell growth.[173] The significant clinical activity of Herceptin a humanized monoclonal antibody targeting p185[HER2], as a single agent and in combination with chemotherapy in patients with breast cancer, has led to substantial interest in applying this approach to patients with NSCLC.[174,175]

Platelet-Derived Growth Factor

Platelet-derived growth factor (PDGF) is a chemotactic and growth factor for normal mesenchymal and endothelial cells. Most NSCLC cell lines and tumors express the PDGF A and B subunits, whereas SCLC cells do not.[176,177] The available data on PDGF-receptors (PDGF-R) in lung tumors is less clear, with conflicting reports of frequent or rare expression in NSCLC.[177–179] Most studies agree that coexpression of PDGF and PDGF-R is uncommon in lung cancer and that PDGF does not appear to mediate an autocrine proliferative effect. However, PDGF-R is highly expressed in stromal and endothelial cells within and around lung tumors, suggesting that tumor-derived PDGF may act in a paracrine manner to stimulate the development of tumor stroma and/or angiogenesis.[178]

Parathyroid Hormone-Related Protein

A large percentage of squamous cell carcinomas of the lung produce parathyroid hormone-related protein (PTHrP), which is responsible for the clinical syndrome of paraneoplastic humoral hypercalcemia.[180,181] The expression of PTHrP is enhanced by TGFα and is associated with increased proliferation in some squamous cell lung cancer cell lines, suggesting an autocrine pathway.[182] PTHrP may also act as an autocrine regulator of differentiation in bronchioloalveolar carcinoma cells.[183]

OTHER GROWTH FACTORS IMPLICATED IN LUNG CANCER

Insulinlike Growth Factors

Although insulin is essential for the serum-free propagation of SCLC and NSCLC cells in culture, it is probably not an important mediator of lung cancer growth in humans. The insulinlike growth factors, IGF-I and IGF-II, are polypeptides that share structural homology with insulin and mediate embryonic development, growth, and differentiation primarily through interactions with a high-affinity IGF-I-R membrane-associated receptor with tyrosine kinase activity.[184] A second receptor, IGF-II/M-6-PR, binds both IGF-I and IGF-II with a low affinity, but appears to lack intracellular signaling activity. The biologic activity of the IGFs is regulated by interactions with at least six IGF-binding proteins, IGF-BP1–6. The IGFs are predominantly produced in the liver and exert physiologic autocrine and paracrine effects in most organs, including the lung. Secretion of a precursor-form of IGF-II by some tumors is a rare cause of paraneoplastic hypoglycemia. A role for the IGF pathways in carcinogenesis is supported by the finding that the overexpression of IGF-I-R induces IGF-dependent cellular transformation.[185]

Nearly all lung cancer cell lines and tumors express both types of IGF receptors,[186–189] and IGF-I-R mediates the invasiveness and metastatic potential of Lewis lung carcinoma cells.[190] Although IGF-I is expressed by most SCLC and NSCLC cell lines and tumors, few lung cancer cells actually secrete IGF-I.[191–193] In contrast, IGF-I is secreted by lung fibroblasts and can stimulate the proliferation of both SCLC and NSCLC cells *in vitro,* suggesting that IGF-I affects lung cancer growth in a paracrine, rather than an autocrine, manner.[189,192,194,195] IGF-II, which is expressed and secreted by most SCLC and NSCLC cell lines,[191,196] preferentially binds the active IGF-I-R instead of IGF-II/M-6-PR[197] and is a more potent mitogen than IGF-I in NSCLC cells,[198] suggesting that IGF-II participates in an autocrine growth pathway in NSCLC. In addition to its effects on tumor cell growth, recent studies have noted that IGF-II also promotes the proliferation of vascular endothelial cells.[199] The potential pathophysiologic role of the IGFs in SCLC is less clear because both IGF-I and IGF-II preferentially bind to membrane-associated IGF-BP2, rather than IGF-I-R, without inducing proliferation in SCLC cells.[198] The IGF-BPs are differentially expressed by SCLC and NSCLC cell lines, but conflicting reports on individual IGF-BP expression and our lack of understanding of their specific functions make it difficult to explain their possible role in lung cancer.[191,198,200,201] Studies evaluating the potential use of IGFs or IGF-BPs as tumor markers have found that although plasma levels of IGF-I are not elevated in patients with lung cancer, 93% of patients with SCLC or NSCLC have elevated plasma concentrations of IGF-BP.[202]

The apparent importance of the IGF-I-R signaling pathway in lung cancer led to the development of an IGF-I-R-antisense-containing adenoviral vector that inhibits the proliferation of NSCLC cells and improves survival in mice with human NSCLC xenografts.[203] Other potential therapeutic approaches targeting the IGF pathway that have been shown to inhibit the growth of NSCLC cells include αIR-3, a monoclonal antibody specific for IGF-I-R,[204] and distamycin A derivatives that block the binding of IGF to IGF-I-R.[205]

Transforming Growth Factor β

The transforming growth factor β (TGFβ) family consists of several growth factors and receptors with pleiotropic effects on growth and differentiation in normal and malignant cells. The TGFβ-receptors (TGFβ-RI, -RII, and -RIII) are serine/threonine kinases that induce p21[WAFI] expression and cell cycle arrest. In normal tracheobronchial epithelial cells, TGFβ inhibits growth and regulates normal mucoepithelial differentiation.[206] The dysregulation of TGFβ pathways has been implicated in the pathogenesis of lung cancer,

and the role of TGFβ as an autocrine tumor suppressor is supported by the finding that the development of urethane-induced pulmonary adenomas in A/J mice is preceded by the down-regulation of TGFβ-RII expression.[207] In addition, transgenic mice expressing a dominant-negative mutant TGFβ-RII exhibit a higher frequency of lung and breast tumors after carcinogen exposure than nonengineered controls.[208] Most SCLC and NSCLC cell lines and tumors express TGFβ, primarily as TGFβ.[209–211] TGFβ[1] inhibits the growth of SCLC and NSCLC cells and xenografts,[212,213] and can enhance the cytotoxicity of DNA-damaging agents, such as gamma irradiation and cisplatin.[214] TGFβ[1] also increases the motility and invasiveness of NSCLC cells *in vitro*[215] and suppresses IL-2-dependent T-lymphocyte proliferation,[216] suggesting a role for TGFβ in lung cancer progression and immunosuppression, respectively. Although many lung cancers express TGFβ-receptors,[209,210] TGFβ-RII expression is often suppressed, and resistance to the growth-inhibitory effects of TGFβ is associated with the loss of TGFβ-RII expression.[213,217,218] It has been suggested that TGFβ may be a useful prognostic factor in lung cancer because patients with NSCLC whose tumors express high levels of TGFβ or have concordant expression of TGFβ and p21[WAFI] (i.e., both high or low) appear to have better survival rates than patients with low TGFβ or discordant expression.[219,220]

Opioids and Nicotine

The discovery of opioid and nicotine responsive signaling pathways in lung cancer cells led to important insights into the potential role of the dysregulation of growth factor pathways by tobacco carcinogens in the development of lung cancer. Both SCLC and NSCLC cells express natural opioids, including β-endorphin and enkephalin, along with high-affinity δ, κ, and μ opioid receptors.[221,222] Proopiomelanocortin, the precursor of β-endorphin, is produced by one-third of SCLCs and two-thirds of pulmonary carcinoids.[223] Opioid agonists act as negative regulators of lung cancer growth, and exposure to nicotine abrogates the tumor-suppressive activity of autocrine opioids.[222] In some SCLC cells, β-endorphin enhances proliferation through activation of atypical opioid signaling pathways.[224]

Pulmonary neuroendocrine cells and tumors, including SCLC, express neuronal-type nicotinic acetylcholine receptors (nAChR) that regulate cation flux directly and through interactions with voltage-sensitive calcium channels.[225,226] These receptors can be activated by nicotine or nicotine-derived N-nitrosamines, such as NNK, resulting in increased proliferation of normal and malignant neuroendocrine cells, suggesting that chronic nicotine exposure may play a role in the promotion of pulmonary neoplasms.[227–229] In a Syrian hamster model, the mitogenic effect of nicotine plus elevated pCO_2 on pulmonary neuroendocrine cells was blocked by nAChR antagonists,[230] and the combination of nicotine or NNK and chronic hyperoxia, which induces emphysematous lung injury, resulted in neuroendocrine lung tumors.[231] In SCLC cells, nicotine has been shown to alter the balance between cellular proliferation and death by activating MAPK and PKC growth-stimulatory pathways and by inducing the expression of bcl-2, an inhibitor of apoptosis.[232,233] In addition, nicotine-mediated proliferation in SCLC cells is associated with increased expression of serotonin, a neuropeptide that stimulates SCLC growth through an autocrine mechanism, suggesting that both nicotinic and serotonergic receptors are potential targets for therapeutic or chemopreventive interventions.[234]

Hepatocyte Growth Factor

Hepatocyte growth factor (HGF), the ligand for the receptor product of the *c-met* protooncogene, is a physiologic mediator of angiogenesis, cellular motility, and invasion. HGF is expressed by normal bronchial epithelial cells and most NSCLC tumors but is rarely produced by SCLC cells.[235–237] C-*met* is expressed in nearly all SCLC and NSCLC cell lines and tumors, but overexpression relative to normal bronchial epithelium has been demonstrated in only 25% to 50% of NSCLC specimens.[235–238] Conflicting studies have reported that HGF can either enhance or inhibit the proliferation of NSCLC and SCLC cells, with growth stimulation occurring through calcium-independent pathways.[239–242] In contrast, HGF consistently potentiates the *in vitro* motility and invasiveness of lung cancer cells and normal bronchial epithelial cells,[239,241] suggesting that the HGF-c-*met* pathway may mediate lung cancer progression rather than proliferation. In support of this concept, high levels of HGF and c-*met* expression have been identified as negative prognostic factors in patients with resected early-stage NSCLC.[243]

Sex-Steroid Hormones and Receptors

The finding that women with lung cancer have better stage-specific survival than men has led to the study of sex-steroid hormones and their receptors in lung cancer. Androgen-receptor (AR) expression has been reported in most NSCLC and a few SCLC cell lines, and testosterone can stimulate the growth of AR-expressing SCLC cells.[244,245] Progesterone receptors are expressed in many NSCLC samples, but not in SCLC.[245–247] Although most NSCLC cell lines and tumors exhibit estrogen-receptor (ER) immunoreactivity,[248,249] recent studies have shown that this reaction is primarily caused by the expression of p29 ER-related protein or type II estrogen-binding sites, and that very few NSCLCs actually express ER.[246,247,250] Nevertheless, tamoxifen, an anti-estrogen, inhibits the growth of NSCLC cells in culture,[251] and

the intensity of p29 expression is directly associated with poor survival in women, but not men, with NSCLC.[250]

Transferrin

Iron is required for cellular proliferation, and transferrin—a glycoprotein that transports iron through interactions with transferrin receptors—is an essential factor for the *in vitro* growth of both SCLC and NSCLC cells in serum-free media.[252,253] Transferrin is produced by normal lung cells in culture and can act in a paracrine fashion to support tumor cell growth.[254] The expression of transferrin receptors, which are found in more than 75% of NSCLC tumors, is associated with increased mitotic activity and poor prognosis.[255,256] In addition, transferrin has autocrine growth-stimulatory activity in SCLC cell lines that express both transferrin and transferrin receptors.[257,258]

CYTOKINES IMPLICATED IN LUNG CANCER
Hematopoietic Growth Factors

The hematopoietic growth factors were initially characterized based on their ability to stimulate the growth and differentiation of specific subsets of hematopoietic progenitor cells. Subsequently, these factors have also been found to influence the biologic properties of some normal and malignant epithelial cells. The expression of granulocyte colony-stimulating factor (G-CSF) and its receptor have been reported in a small subset of SCLC and NSCLC cell lines and tumors.[259,260] In contrast, granulocyte-macrophage colony-stimulating factor (GM-CSF) is produced by both normal bronchial epithelial cells and about one-half of NSCLC tumors and cell lines, and several NSCLC and SCLC cell lines express GM-CSF receptors.[261,262] Exposure to G-CSF or GM-CSF enhanced *in vitro* proliferation in at least 10 lung cancer cell lines, mostly of the small cell phenotype.[259,262–265] However, these cytokines are not likely important activators of lung cancer cell proliferation because the growth of most SCLC and NSCLC cell lines is not affected by exposure to G-CSF or GM-CSF.[261,266–268] Interestingly, both GM-CSF and interleukin-3 (IL-3) stimulated the growth of one SCLC cell line *in vitro,* but they failed to affect the growth of these cells in an *in vivo* xenograft model.[269] Despite the concerns raised by some of these studies, numerous clinical trials have not revealed any adverse consequences resulting from the use of G-CSF or GM-CSF in patients with SCLC.

Cytokines can influence cellular properties other than proliferation. GM-CSF has been shown to enhance the *in vitro* invasiveness and *in vivo* metastatic potential of murine Lewis lung carcinoma cells through activation of PKA pathways.[270] In addition, GM-CSF increases the production of matrix metalloproteinases in human squamous cell lung carcinoma cells, and both GM-CSF and G-CSF can enhance the *in vitro* invasiveness of human NSCLC cells.[261,271] Macrophage-CSF (M-CSF, CSF-1) and its receptor, CSF-1R, the product of the *c-fms* oncogene, mediate normal macrophage invasiveness. In NSCLC cells expressing CSF-1R, M-CSF increases basement membrane invasiveness *in vitro*.[272] However, the expression of heterologous M-CSF in human squamous and SCLC cell lines decreased hematogenous and lymphatic metastases in *in vivo* xenograft models,[273] and treatment of mice bearing subcutaneous Lewis lung carcinoma transplants with M-CSF results in fewer pulmonary metastases.[274] The effect of M-CSF on metastasis may be immune-mediated, as suggested by a study in which the pretreatment of mice with irradiated Lewis lung cancer cells that were engineered to express heterologous M-CSF resulted in the inhibition of tumor formation after subsequent injection of untreated Lewis lung cancer cells.[275]

Lymphokines

The proliferation of most lung cancer cell lines appears to be unaffected by interleukins (IL-1, IL-2, IL-3, IL-4, IL-6) and interferons (IFNα, IFNβ, IFNγ).[266,267,276] However, IL-3 can stimulate the growth of some SCLC cell lines that express IL-3 receptors, and it can partially inhibit the cytotoxic effects of cisplatin and doxorubicin.[267,277] In addition, IL-6 inhibits and anti-IL-6 antibodies enhance the proliferation of some NSCLC cells that express IL-6 and IL-6 receptors, suggesting an autocrine growth-inhibitory loop.[278] The finding that NSCLC cells are less sensitive to the inhibitory effects of IL-6 than are normal bronchial epithelial cells also suggests that escape from autocrine IL-6 control may be involved in lung carcinogenesis. Finally, TNFα and IL-1β, which are induced by retinoic acid, can inhibit the growth of lung cancer cells *in vitro*, and the inhibitory activity of TNFα can be potentiated by IFNγ.[266,279]

Stem Cell Factor and c-*Kit*

Stem cell factor (SCF), a growth and differentiation factor that affects multiple hematopoietic lineages, and its receptor, the product of the *c-kit* oncogene, are coexpressed by at least 70% of SCLC cell lines and tumors[235,280,281] and constitute an autocrine loop that can cooperate with other growth factor pathways in SCLC.[282] In contrast, *c-kit* is not expressed by normal bronchial epithelial cells,[281,283] and only 15% of NSCLC tumors coexpress SCF and *c-kit*.[284] SCF mediates both proliferation and chemotaxis in SCLC cells that express *c-kit*, suggesting that the *c-kit* pathway is a rational therapeutic target.[284,285] Antisense oligonucleotides targeting *c-kit* and SCF inhibited the growth of NSCLC cells that coexpress *c-kit* and SCF.[286] In addition, infection of SCLC cells that express *c-kit* with a *c-kit* antisense-containing adenoviral vector significantly inhibited cellular proliferation.[287] Krystal and colleagues demonstrated that

AG1296, a tyrosine kinase inhibitor that is relatively selective for *c-kit*, induced apoptosis in SCLC cells that coexpress *c-kit* and SCF.[288] These investigators also reported that activation of kit by SCF enhanced the activity of lck, a src-family tyrosine kinase, and that treatment of SCLC cells with PP1, a lck-selective inhibitor of src-family kinases, antagonized SCF-mediated proliferation and inhibition of apoptosis.[289]

CONCLUSION

Recent advances in our understanding of the signaling pathways that regulate the survival and proliferation of both small cell and non–small cell lung cancer have allowed the development of a wide variety of therapeutic strategies designed to specifically target various components of these pathways, including growth factors, growth factor receptors, and second messenger molecules (Table 10.3). Although the ultimate clinical utility of these approaches has yet to be determined, future advances in the prevention and therapy of cancer will depend on further research aimed at expanding our knowledge of the cellular and molecular determinants of the malignant phenotype.

TABLE 10.3. THERAPEUTIC STRATEGIES EXPLOITING GROWTH FACTOR PATHWAYS IN LUNG CANCER

Growth Factor–Targeted
Anti-growth factor (*GRP, TGFα*) monoclonal antibodies
Anti-growth factor (*SCF*) antisense oligonucleotides
Neutral endopeptidase
Inhibitory growth factors (*TGFβ, SST analogues*)

Receptor-Targeted
Receptor-selective neuropeptide antagonists (*GRP/ bombesin analogues, bradykinin antagonist dimers CCK analogues*)
Broad-spectrum neuropeptide antagonists (*substance P analogues*)
Anti-receptor (*IGF-I-R, EGF-R, p185^{HER2}*) monoclonal antibodies (*Herceptin*)
Anti-receptor (*c-kit, IGF-I-R, p185^{HER2}*) antisense oligonucleotides/gene therapy
Immunoconjugates (*GRP analogue: anti-FC, RI/III monoclonal antibody*)
Growth factor: toxin fusion proteins (*GRP: diphtheria toxin, TGFα: Ps. exotoxin A*)
Receptor-selective tyrosine kinase inhibitors (*anti-c-kit, anti-EGF-R, anti-p185^{HER2}*)
Growth factor: receptor (*IGF: IGF-I-R*) binding inhibitors (*distamycin A derivatives*)
Growth factor (*EGF*): DNA conjugate gene therapy delivery system

Signal Transduction Pathway–Targeted
Tyrosine kinase inhibitors (*tyrphostins, genestein, PP1*)
Serine/threonine kinase inhibitors (*rapamycin*)

(parentheses) indicate examples under preclinical or clinical development

REFERENCES

1. Wharton J, Polak JM, Bloom SR, et al. Bombesin-like immunoreactivity in the lung. *Nature* 1978;273:769.
2. Yamaguchi K, Abe K, Kameya T, et al. Production and molecular size heterogeneity of immunoreactive gastrin-releasing peptide in fetal and adult lungs and primary lung tumors. *Cancer Res* 1983;43:3932.
3. Aguayo SM, Kane MA, King TE, et al. Increased levels of bombesin-like peptides in the lower respiratory tract of asymptomatic cigarette smokers. *J Clin Invest* 1989;84:1105.
4. Willey JC, Lechner JF, Harris CC. Bombesin and the C-terminal tetradecapeptide of gastrin-releasing peptide are growth factors for normal human bronchial epithelial cells. *Exp Cell Res* 1984;153:245.
5. Siegfried JM, Guentert PJ, Gaither AL. Effects of bombesin and gastrin-releasing peptide on human bronchial epithelial cells from a series of donors: individual variation and modulation by bombesin analogs. *Anatomical Record* 1993;236:241.
6. Alexander RW, Upp JR, Poston GJ, et al. Effects of bombesin on growth of human small cell lung carcinoma in vivo. *Cancer Res* 1988;48:1439.
7. Moody TW, Pert CB, Gazdar AF, et al. High levels of intracellular bombesin characterize human small-cell lung carcinoma. *Science* 1981;214:1246.
8. Erisman MD, Linnoila RI, Hernandez O, et al. Human lung small-cell carcinoma contains bombesin. *Proc Natl Acad Sci USA* 1985;79:2379.
9. Sausville EA, Lebacq-Verheyden AM, Spindel ER, et al. Expression of the gastrin-releasing peptide gene in human small cell lung cancer. *J Biol Chem* 1986;261:2451.
10. Aguayo SM, Miller Y, Boose D, et al. Nonconstitutive expression of the gastrin-releasing peptide autocrine growth system in human small cell lung carcinoma NCI-H345 cells. *Cell Growth Differ* 1996;7:563.
11. Nagalla SR, Spindel ER. Functional analysis of the 5′-flanking region of the human gastrin-releasing peptide gene in small cell lung carcinoma cell lines. *Cancer Res* 1994;54:4461.
12. Kee KA, Finan TM, Korman LY, et al. Somatostatin inhibits the secretion of bombesin-like peptides from small cell lung cancer cells. *Peptides* 1988;9(suppl):257.
13. Ravi RK, Scott FM, Cuttitta F, et al. Induction of gastrin releasing peptide by all-trans retinoic acid in small cell lung cancer cells. *Oncol Rep* 1998;5:497.
14. Korman LY, Carney DN, Citron ML, et al. Secretin/vasoactive intestinal peptide-stimulated secretion of bombesin/gastrin releasing peptide from human small cell carcinoma of the lung. *Cancer Res* 1986;46:1214.
15. Moody TW, Zia F, Venugopal R, et al. Corticotropin-releasing factor stimulates cyclic AMP, arachidonic acid release and growth of lung cancer cells. *Peptides* 1994;15:281.
16. Spindel ER, Chin WW, Price J, et al. Cloning and characterization of cDNAs encoding human gastrin-releasing peptide. *Proc Natl Acad Sci USA* 1984;81:5699.
17. Lebacq-Verheyden AM, Kasprzyk PG, Raum MG, et al. Post-translational processing of endogenous and baculovirus-expressed human gastrin-releasing peptide precursor. *Mol Cell Biol* 1988;8:3129.
18. Reeve JR Jr, Cuttitta F, Vigna SR, et al. Multiple gastrin-releasing peptide gene-associated peptides are produced by a human small cell lung cancer line. *J Biol Chem* 1989;264:1928.
19. Moody TW, Carney DN, Cuttitta F, et al. High affinity receptors for bombesin/GRP-like peptides on human small cell lung cancer. *Life Sci* 1985;37:105.
20. Corjay MH, Dobrzanski DJ, Way JM, et al. Two distinct bombesin receptor subtypes are expressed and functional in human lung carcinoma cells. *J Biol Chem* 1991;266:18771.
21. Trepel JB, Moyer JD, Heikkila R, et al. Modulation of bombesin-induced phosphatidylinositol hydrolysis in a small-cell lung cancer cell line. *Biochem J* 1988;255:403.
22. Kado-Fong H, Malfroy B. Effects of bombesin on human small cell lung cancer cells: evidence for a subset of bombesin non-responsive cell lines. *J Cell Biochem* 1989;40:431.
23. Heikkila R, Trepel JB, Cuttitta F, et al. Bombesin-related peptides induce calcium mobilization in a subset of human small cell lung cancer cell lines. *J Biol Chem* 1987;262:16456.
24. Sausville EA, Moyer JD, Heikkila R, et al. A correlation of bombesin-responsiveness with myc-family gene expression in small cell lung carcinoma cell lines. *Ann N Y Acad Sci* 1988;547:310.
25. Draoui M, Chung P, Park M, et al. Bombesin stimulates c-fos and c-jun mRNAs in small cell lung cancer cells. *Peptides* 1995;16:289.
26. Carney DN, Cuttitta F, Moody TW, et al. Selective stimulation of small cell lung cancer clonal growth by bombesin and gastrin-releasing peptide. *Cancer Res* 1987;47:821.
27. Cuttitta F, Carney DN, Mulshine J, et al. Bombesin-like peptides can function as autocrine growth factors in human small-cell lung cancer. *Nature* 1985;316:823.
28. Cardona C, Rabbitts PH, Spindel ER, et al. Production of neuromedin B and neuromedin B gene expression in human lung tumor cell lines. *Cancer Res* 1991;51:5205.
29. Moody TW, Staley J, Zia F, et al. Neuromedin B binds with high affinity, elevates cytosolic calcium and stimulates the growth of small-cell lung cancer cell lines. *J Pharmacol Exper Therap* 1992;263:311.
30. Siegfried JM, Han YH, DeMichele MA, et al. Production of gastrin-releasing peptide by a non-small cell lung carcinoma cell line adapted to serum-free and growth factor-free conditions. *J Biol Chem* 1994;269:8596.
31. Kiriakogani-Psaropoulou P, Malamou-Mitsi V, Martinopoulou U, et al. The value of neuroendocrine markers in non-small cell lung cancer: a comparative immunohistopathologic study. *Lung Cancer* 1994;11:353.
32. Hamid QA, Corrin B, Dewar A, et al. Expression of gastrin-releasing peptide gene in large cell undifferentiated carcinoma of the lung. *J Pathol* 1990;161:145.
33. Toi-Scott M, Jones CL, Kane MA. Clinical correlates of bombesin-like peptide receptor subtype expression in human lung cancer cells. *Lung Cancer* 1996;15:341.
34. Fathi Z, Way JW, Corjay MH, et al. Bombesin receptor structure and expression in human lung carcinoma cell lines. *J Cell Biochem* 1996;24(suppl):237.
35. Moody TW, Zia F, Venugopal R, et al. GRP receptors are present in non-small cell lung cancer cells. *J Cell Biochem* 1996;24(suppl):247.
36. Weber S, Zuckerman JE, Bostwick DG, et al. Gastrin releasing peptide is a selective mitogen for small cell lung carcinoma in vitro. *J Clin Invest* 1985;75:306.
37. Maruno K, Yamaguchi K, Abe K, et al. Immunoreactive gastrin-releasing peptide as a specific tumor marker in patients with small cell lung carcinoma. *Cancer Res* 1989;49:629.
38. Holst JJ, Hansen M, Bork E, et al. Elevated plasma concentrations of C-flanking gastrin-releasing peptide in small-cell lung cancer. *J Clin Oncol* 1989;7:1831.
39. Miyake Y, Kodama T, Yamaguchi K. Pro-gastrin-releasing peptide (31–98) is a specific tumor marker in patients with small cell lung carcinoma. *Cancer Res* 1994;54:2136.
40. Pedersen AG, Becker KL, Bach F, et al. Cerebrospinal fluid bombesin and calcitonin in patients with central nervous system

metastases from small-cell lung cancer. *J Clin Oncol* 1986;4:1620.

41. Pert CB, Schumacher UK. Plasma bombesin concentrations in patients with extensive small cell carcinoma of the lung. *Lancet* 1982;1:509.

42. Wood SM, Wood JR, Ghatei MA, et al. Is bombesin a tumour marker for small-cell carcinoma? *Lancet* 1982;1:690.

43. Woll PJ, Rozengurt E. Multiple neuropeptides mobilise calcium in small cell lung cancer: effects of vasopressin, bradykinin, cholecystokinin, galanin and neurotensin. *Biochem Biophys Res Commun* 1989;164:66.

44. Bunn PA, Dienhart DG, Chan D, et al. Neuropeptide stimulation of calcium flux in human lung cancer cells: delineation of alternative pathways. *Proc Natl Acad Sci USA* 1990;87:2162.

45. North WG, Fay MJ, Longo KA, et al. Expression of all known vasopressin receptor subtypes by small cell tumors implies a multifaceted role for this neuropeptide. *Cancer Res* 1998;58:1866.

46. Friedmann AS, Malott KA, Memoli VA, et al. Products of vasopressin gene expression in small-cell carcinoma of the lung. *Br J Cancer* 1994;69:260.

47. Friedmann AS, Memoli VA, North WG. Vasopressin and oxytocin production by non-neuroendocrine lung carcinomas: an apparent low incidence of gene expression. *Cancer Lett* 1993;75:79.

48. Sethi T, Rozengurt E. Multiple neuropeptides stimulate clonal growth of small cell lung cancer: effects of bradykinin, vasopressin, cholecystokinin, galanin and neurotensin. *Cancer Res* 1991;51:3621.

49. Fay MJ, Friedmann AS, Yu XM, et al. Vasopressin and vasopressin-receptor immunoreactivity in small-cell lung carcinoma cell lines: disruption in the activation cascade of V_{1a} receptors in variant SCCL. *Cancer Lett* 1994;82:167.

50. Woll PJ, Rozengurt E. A neuropeptide antagonist that inhibits the growth of small cell lung cancer in vitro. *Cancer Res* 1990;50:3968.

51. DiMattei P. Occurrence of bradykinin in human pulmonary carcinoma. *Biochem Pharmacol* 1967;16:909.

52. Trifilieff A, Lach E, Dumont P, et al. Bradykinin binding sites in healthy and carcinomatous human lung. *Br J Pharmacol* 1994;111:1228.

53. Levesque L, Dean NM, Sasmor H, et al. Antisense oligonucleotides targeting human protein kinase C-α inhibit phorbol ester-induced reduction of bradykinin-evoked calcium mobilization in A549 cells. *Mol Pharmacol* 1997;51:209.

54. Bunn PA, Chan D, Dienhart DG, et al. Neuropeptide signal transduction in lung cancer: clinical implications of bradykinin sensitivity and overall heterogeneity. *Cancer Res* 1992;52:24.

55. Stewart JM, Gera L, Chan DC, et al. Potent, long-acting, orally-active bradykinin antagonists for a wide range of applications. *Immunopharmacol* 1997;36:167.

56. Bunn PA, Chan D, Johnson G, et al. Anti-growth factor therapy for lung cancer. *Lung Cancer* 1997;18(suppl 2):10.

57. Rehfeld JF, Bardram L, Hilsted L. Gastrin in human bronchogenic carcinomas: constant expression but variable processing of progastrin. *Cancer Res* 1989;49:2840.

58. Geijer T, Folkesson R, Rehfeld JF, et al. Expression of the cholecystokinin gene in a human (small-cell) lung carcinoma cell-line. *FEBS Lett* 1990;270:30.

59. Reubi JC, Schaer JC, Waser B. Cholecystokinin(CCK)-A and CCK-B/gastrin receptors in human tumors. *Cancer Res* 1997;57:1377.

60. Matsumori Y, Katakami N, Ito M, et al. Cholecystokinin-B/gastrin receptor: a novel molecular probe for human small cell lung cancer. *Cancer Res* 1995;55:276.

61. Sethi T, Rozengurt E. Gastrin stimulates Ca^{2+} mobilization and clonal growth in small cell lung cancer cells. *Cancer Res* 1992;52:6031.

62. Staley J, Jensen RT, Moody TW. CCK antagonists interact with CCK-B receptors on human small cell lung cancer cells. *Peptides* 1990;11:1033.

63. Witte DG, Nazdan AM, Martinez J, et al. Characterization of the novel CCK analogs JMV-180, JMV-320, and JMV-332 in H345 cells. *Peptides* 1992;13:1227.

64. Sethi T, Herget T, Wu SV, et al. CCKA and CCKB receptors are expressed in small cell lung cancer lines and mediate Ca^{2+} mobilization and clonal growth. *Cancer Res* 1993;53:5208.

65. Davidson A, Moody TW, Gozes I. Regulation of VIP gene expression in general-human lung cancer cells in particular. *J Mol Neurosci* 1996;7:99.

66. Shaffer MM, Carney DN, Korman LY, et al. High affinity binding of VIP to human lung cancer cell lines. *Peptides* 1987;8:1101.

67. Scholar EM, Paul S. Stimulation of tumor cell growth by vasoactive intestinal peptide. *Cancer* 1991;67:1561.

68. Moody TW, Zia F, Draoui M, et al. A vasoactive intestinal peptide antagonist inhibits non-small cell lung cancer growth. *Proc Natl Acad Sci USA* 1993;90:4345.

69. Moody TW, Leyton J, Coelho T, et al. (Stearyl, norleucine 17)VIP hybrid antagonizes VIP receptors on non-small cell lung cancer cells. *Life Sci* 1997;61:1657.

70. Moody TW, Zia F, Makheja A. Pituitary adenylate cyclase activating polypeptide receptors are present on small cell lung cancer cells. *Peptides* 1993;14:241.

71. Korman LY, Carney DN, Citron ML, et al. Secretin/vasoactive intestinal peptide-stimulated secretion of bombesin/gastrin releasing peptide from human small cell carcinoma of the lung. *Cancer Res* 1986;46:1214.

72. Maruno K, Said SI. Small-cell lung carcinoma: inhibition of proliferation by vasoactive intestinal peptide and helodermin and enhancement of inhibition by anti-bombesin antibody. *Life Sci* 1993;52:PL267.

73. Goedert M, Reeve JG, Emson PC, et al. Neurotensin in human small cell lung carcinoma. *Br J Cancer* 1984;50:179.

74. Moody TW, Carney DN, Korman LY, et al. Neurotensin is produced by and secreted from classic small cell lung cancer cells. *Life Sci* 1985;36:1727.

75. Davis TP, Crowell S, McInturff B, et al. Neurotensin may function as a regulatory peptide in small cell lung cancer. *Peptides* 1991;12:17.

76. Allen AE, Carney DN, Moody TW. Neurotensin binds with high affinity to small cell lung cancer cells. *Peptides* 1988;9 suppl 1:57.

77. Seufferlein T, Rozengurt E. Galanin, neurotensin, and phorbol esters rapidly stimulate activation of mitogen-activated protein kinase in small cell lung cancer cells. *Cancer Res* 1996;56:5758.

78. Sethi T, Rozengurt E. Galanin stimulates Ca^{2+} mobilization, inositol phosphate accumulation, and clonal growth in small cell lung cancer cells. *Cancer Res* 1991;51:1674.

79. Naline E, Molimard M, Regoli D, et al. Evidence for functional tachykinin NK1 receptors on human isolated small bronchi. *Am J Physiol* 1996;271:L763.

80. Bepler G, Carney DN, Gazdar AF, et al. *In vitro* growth inhibition of human small cell lung cancer by physalaemin. *Cancer Res* 1987;47:2371.

81. Takuwa N, Takuwa Y, Ohue Y, et al. Stimulation of calcium mobilization but not proliferation by bombesin and tachykinin neuropeptides in human small cell lung cancer cells. *Cancer Res* 1990;50:240.

82. Lazarus LH, DiAugustine RP, Jahnke GD, et al. Physalaemin: an amphibian tachykinin in human lung small-cell carcinoma. *Science* 1983;219:79.

83. Bunn PA, Chan D, Stewart J, et al. Effects of neuropeptide analogues on calcium flux and proliferation in lung cancer cell lines. *Cancer Res* 1994;54:3602.

84. Coy DH, Jensen RT, Jiang NY, et al. Systematic development of bombesin/gastrin-releasing peptide antagonists. *J Natl Cancer Inst Monogr* 1992;13:133.

85. Mahmoud S, Staley J, Taylor J, et al. [Psi[13,14]] bombesin analogues inhibit growth of small cell lung cancer in vitro and in vivo. *Cancer Res* 1991;51:1798.

86. Moody TW, Venugopal R, Zia F, et al. BW2258U89: a GRP receptor antagonist which inhibits small cell lung cancer growth. *Life Sci* 1995;56:521.

87. Sharoni Y, Viallet J, Trepel JB, et al. Effect of guanine and adenine nucleotides on bombesin-stimulated phospholipase C activity in membranes from Swiss 3T3 and small cell lung carcinoma cells. *Cancer Res* 1990;50:5257.

88. Thomas F, Arvelo F, Antoine E, et al. Antitumoral activity of bombesin analogues on small cell lung cancer xenografts: relationship with bombesin receptor expression. *Cancer Res* 1992;52:4872.

89. Halmos G, Schally AV. Reduction in receptors for bombesin and epidermal growth factor in xenografts of human small-cell lung cancer after treatment with bombesin antagonist RC-3095. *Proc Natl Acad Sci USA* 1997;94:956.

90. Pinski J, Schally AV, Halmos G, et al. Effects of somatostatin analogue RC-160 and bombesin/gastrin-releasing peptide antagonists on the growth of human small-cell and non-small cell lung carcinomas in nude mice. *Br J Cancer* 1994;70:886.

91. Bepler G, Zeymer U, Mahmoud S, et al. Substance P analogues function as bombesin receptor antagonists and inhibit small cell lung cancer clonal growth. *Peptides* 1988;9:1367.

92. Tallett A, Chilvers ER, Hannah S, et al. Inhibition of neuropeptide-stimulated tyrosine phosphorylation and tyrosine kinase activity stimulates apoptosis in small cell lung cancer cells. *Cancer Res* 1996;56:4255.

93. Seckl MJ, Higgins T, Widmer F, et al. [D-Arg[1],D-Trp[5,7,9],Leu[11]]substance P: a novel potent inhibitor of signal transduction and growth *in vitro* and *in vivo* in small cell lung cancer cells. *Cancer Res* 1997;57:51.

94. Everard MJ, Macauley VM, Miller JL, et al. In vitro effects of substance P analogue [D-Arg[1], D-Phe[5], D-Trp[7,9], Leu[11]]substance P on human tumour and normal cell growth. *Br J Cancer* 1992;65:388.

95. Woll PJ, Rozengurt E. [D-Arg[1],D-Phe[5],D-Trp[7,9],Leup[11]]substance P, a potent bombesin antagonist in murine Swiss 3T3 cells, inhibits the growth of human small cell lung cancer cells in vitro. *Proc Natl Acad Sci USA* 1988;85:1859.

96. Layton JE, Scanlon DB, Soveny C, et al. Effects of bombesin antagonists on the growth of small cell lung cancer cells in vitro. *Cancer Res* 1988;48:4783.

97. Langdon S, Sethi T, Ritchie A, et al. Broad spectrum neuropeptide antagonists inhibit the growth of small cell lung cancer *in vivo*. *Cancer Res* 1992;52:4554.

98. Orosz A, Schrett J, Nagy J, et al. New short-chain analogs of a substance P antagonist inhibit proliferation of human small-cell lung cancer cells *in vitro* and *in vivo*. *Int J Cancer* 1995;60:82.

99. Seckl MJ, Rozengurt E. Effect of tyrphostin combined with a substance P related antagonist on small cell lung cancer cell growth *in vitro*. *Eur J Cancer* 1996;32A:342.

100. Rosati R, Adil MR, Ali MA, et al. Induction of apoptosis by a short-chain neuropeptide analog in small cell lung cancer. *Peptides* 1998;19:1519.

101. Jones DA, Cummings J, Langdon SP, et al. Preclinical studies on the broad-spectrum meuropeptide growth factor antagonist G. *Gen Pharmac* 1997;28:183.

102. Yang HK, Scott FM, Trepel JB, et al. Correlation of expression of bombesin-like peptides and receptors with growth inhibition by an anti-bombesin antibody in small-cell lung cancer cell lines. *Lung Cancer* 1998;21:165.

103. Kelley MJ, Linnoila RI, Avis IL, et al. Antitumor activity of a monoclonal antibody directed against gastrin-releasing peptide in patients with small-cell lung cancer. *Chest* 1997;112:256.

104. Chen J, Zhou JH, Mokotoff M, et al. Lysis of small cell carcinoma of the lung cells by cytokine-activated monocytes and natural killer cells in the presence of bispecific immunoconjugates containing a gastrin-releasing peptide analog or a GRP antagonist. *J Hematotherapy* 1995;4:369.

105. VanderSpek JC, Sutherland JA, Zeng H, et al. Inhibition of protein synthesis in small cell lung cancer cells induced by the diphtheria toxin-related fusion protein DAB$_{389}$ GRP. *Cancer Res* 1997;57:290.

106. Seufferlein T, Rozengurt E. Rapamycin inhibits constitutive p70^{s6k} phosphorylation, cell proliferation and colony formation in small cell lung cancer cells. *Cancer Res* 1996;56:3895.

107. Cohen AJ, Bunn PA, Franklin W, et al. Neutral endopeptidase: variable expression in human lung, inactivation in lung cancer and modulation of peptide-induced calcium flux. *Cancer Res* 1996;56:831.

108. Bunn PA, Helfrich BA, Brenner DG, et al. Effects of recombinant neutral endopeptidase (EC 3.4.24.11) on the growth of lung cancer cell lines *in vitro* and *in vivo*. *Clin Cancer Res* 1998;4:2849.

109. Ganju RK, Sunday M, Tsarwhas DG, et al. CD10/NEP in non-small cell lung carcinomas: relationship to cellular proliferation. *J Clin Invest* 1994;94:1784.

110. Shipp MA, Tarr GE, Chen CY, et al. CD10/neutral endopeptidase 24.11 hydrolyzes bombesin-like peptides and regulates the growth of small cell carcinomas of the lung. *Proc Natl Acad Sci USA* 1991;88:10662.

111. O'Byrne KJ, Carney DN. Somatostatin and the lung. *Lung Cancer* 1993;10:151.

112. Szabo M, Berelowitz M, Pettengill OS, et al. Ectopic production of somatostatin-like immuno-and bioactivity by cultured human pulmonary small cell carcinoma. *J Clin Endocrin Metabol* 1980;51:978.

113. Kasurinen J, Syrjanen KJ. Peptide hormone immunoreactivity and prognosis in small-cell carcinoma of the lung. *Respiration* 1986;49:61.

114. Bepler G, Rotsch M, Jaques G, et al. Peptides and growth factors in small cell lung cancer: production, binding sites and growth effects. *J Cancer Res Clin Oncol* 1988;114:235.

115. Roos BA, Lindall AW, Ells J, et al. Increased plasma and tumor somatostatin-like immunoreactivity in medullary thyroid carcinoma and small cell lung cancer. *J Clin Endocri Metabol* 1981;52:187.

116. Sagman U, Mullen JB, Kovacs K, et al. Identification of somatostatin receptors in human small cell lung carcinoma. *Cancer* 1990;66:2129.

117. Reubi JC, Waser B, Sheppard M, et al. Somatostatin receptors are present in small-cell but not in non-small-cell lung carcinomas: relationship to EGF-receptors. *Int J Cancer* 1990;45:269.

118. O'Byrne KJ, Halmos G, Pinski J, et al. Somatostatin receptor expression in lung cancer. *Eur J Cancer* 1994;30A:1682.

119. Kee KA, Finan TM, Korman LY, et al. Somatostatin inhibits the secretion of bombesin-like peptides from small cell lung cancer cells. *Peptides* 1988;9 suppl 1:257.

120. Lenzhofer R, Cerni C, Frohlich I, et al. Failure of somatostatin to influence experimental tumor cell growth *in vivo* and *in vitro*. *Experientia* 1981;37:1015.

121. Macauley VM, Smith IE, Everard MJ, et al. Experimental and

clinical studies with somatostatin analogue octreotide in small cell lung cancer. *Br J Cancer* 1991;64:451.

122. Bogden AE, Taylor JE, Moreau JP, et al. Response of human lung tumor xenografts to treatment with a somatostatin analogue (Somatuline). *Cancer Res* 1990;50:4360.

123. Taylor JE, Moreau JP, Baptiste L, et al. Octapeptide analogues of somatostatin inhibit the clonal growth and vasoactive intestinal peptide-stimulated cyclic AMP formation in human small cell lung cancer cells. *Peptides* 1991;12:839.

124. Cattaneo MG, Amoroso D, Gussoni G, et al. A somatostatin analogue inhibits MAP kinase activation and cell proliferation in human neuroblastoma and in human small cell lung carcinoma cell lines. *FEBS Lett* 1996;397:164.

125. Anthony L, Johnson D, Hande K, et al. Somatostatin analogue phase I trials in neuroendocrine neoplasms. *Acta Oncol* 1993; 32:217.

126. Berenger N, Moretti JL, Boaziz C, et al. Somatostatin receptor imaging in small cell lung cancer. *Eur J Cancer* 1996;32A:1429.

127. Reisinger I, Bohuskavitzki KH, Brenner W, et al. Somatostatin receptor scintigraphy in small-cell lung cancer: results of a multicenter study. *J Nucl Med* 1998;39:224.

128. Sherwin SA, Minna JD, Gazdar AF, et al. Expression of epidermal and nerve growth factor receptors and soft agar growth factor production by human lung cancer cells. *Cancer Res* 1981; 41:3538.

129. Olemann E, Sreter L, Schuller I, et al. Nerve growth factor stimulates clonal growth of human lung cancer cell lines and a human glioblastoma cell line expressing high-affinity nerve growth factor binding sites involving tyrosine kinase signaling. *Cancer Res* 1995;55:2219.

130. Missale C, Codignola A, Sigala S, et al. Nerve growth factor abrogates the tumorigenicity of human small cell lung cancer cell lines. *Proc Natl Acad Sci USA* 1998;95:5366.

131. Cerny T, Barnes DM, Hasleton P, et al. Expression of epidermal growth factor receptor in human lung tumors. *Brit J Cancer* 1986;54:265.

132. Liu C, Tsao MS. *In vitro* and *in vivo* expressions of transforming growth factor α and tyrosine kinase receptors in human non-small-cell lung carcinomas. *Am J Pathol* 1993;142:1155.

133. Gamou S, Hunts J, Harigai H, et al. Molecular evidenced for the lack of epidermal growth factor gene expression in small cell lung carcinoma cells. *Cancer Res* 1987;47:2668.

134. Haeder M, Rotsch M, Bepler G, et al. Epidermal growth factor receptor expression in human lung cancer cell lines. *Cancer Res* 1988;48:1132.

135. Rusch V, Baselga J, Cordon-Cardo C, et al. Differential expression of the epidermal growth factor receptor and its ligands in primary non-small cell lung cancers and adjacent benign lung. *Cancer Res* 1993;53:2379.

136. Tateishi M, Ishida T, Mitsudomi T, et al. Immunohistochemical evidence of autocrine growth factors in adenocarcinoma of the human lung. *Cancer Res* 1990;50:7077.

137. Rabiasz GJ, Langdon SP, Bartlett JM, et al. Growth control by epidermal growth factor and transforming growth factor-α in human lung squamous carcinoma cells. *Br J Cancer* 1992;66: 254.

138. Lee M, Draoui M, Zia F, et al. Epidermal growth factor receptor monoclonal antibodies inhibit the growth of lung cancer cell lines. *J Natl Cancer Inst Monogr* 1992;13:117.

139. Putnam EA, Yen N, Gallick GE, et al. Autocrine growth stimulation by transforming growth factor α in human non-small cell lung cancer. *Surg Oncol* 1992;1:49.

140. Lei W, Mayotte JE, Levitt ML. EGF-dependent and independent programmed cell death pathways in NCI-H596 nonsmall cell lung cancer cells. *Biochem Biophys Res Comm* 1998;245: 939.

141. Bost F, McKay R, Dean N, et al. The JUN kinase/stress-activated protein kinase pathway is required for epidermal growth factor stimulation of growth of human A549 lung carcinoma cells. *J Biol Chem* 1997;272:33422.

142. Hamburger AW, Fernandes A, Murakami M, et al. The role of transforming growth factor α production and ErbB-2 overexpression in induction of tumorigenicity of lung epithelial cells. *Brit J Cancer* 1998;77:1066.

143. Klein-Szanto AJ, Iizasa T, Momiki S, et al. A tobacco-specific N-nitrosamine or cigarette smoke condensate causes neoplastic transformation of xenotransplanted human bronchial epithelial cells. *Proc Natl Acad Sci USA* 1992;89:6693.

144. Volm M, Efferth T, Mattern J. Oncoprotein (c-myc, c-erbB1, c-erbB2, c-fos) and suppressor gene product (p53) expression in squamous cell carcinomas of the lung: clinical and biological correlations. *Anticancer Res* 1992;12:11.

145. Fontanini G, Vignati S, Bigini D, et al. Epidermal growth factor receptor expression in non-small cell lung carcinomas correlates with metastatic involvement of hilar and mediastinal lymph nodes in the squamous subtype. *Eur J Cancer* 1995;31A:178.

146. Pfeiffer P, Clausen PP, Andersen K, et al. Lack of prognostic significance of epidermal growth factor receptor and the oncoprotein p185[HER2] in patients with systematically untreated non-small-cell lung cancer: an immunohistochemical study on cryosections. *Brit J Cancer* 1996;74:86.

147. Pastorino U, Andreola S, Tagliabue E, et al. Immunocytochemical markers in stage I lung cancer: relevance to prognosis. *J Clin Oncol* 1997;15:2858.

148. Fontanini G, DeLaurentis M, Vignati S, et al. Evaluation of epidermal growth factor-related growth factors and receptors and of neoangiogenesis in completely resected stage I-IIIA non-small-cell lung cancer: amphiregulin and microvessel count are independent prognostic indicators of survival. *Clin Cancer Res* 1998;4:241.

149. Dean C, Modjtahedi H, Eccles S, et al. Immunotherapy with antibodies to the EGF receptor. *Int J Cancer* 1994;8(suppl): 103.

150. Suarez Pestana E, Greiser U, Sanchez B, et al. Growth inhibition of human lung adenocarcinoma cell by antibodies against epidermal growth factor receptor and by ganglioside GM3: involvement of receptor-directed protein tyrosine phosphatase(s). *Brit J Cancer* 1997;75:213.

151. Divgi CR, Welt S, Kris M, et al. Phase I and imaging trial of indium[111]-labeled anti-epidermal growth factor receptor monoclonal antibody 225 in patients with squamous cell lung carcinoma. *J Natl Cancer Inst* 1991;83:97.

152. Perez-Soler R, Donato NJ, Shin DM, et al. Tumor epidermal growth factor receptor studies in patients with non-small cell lung cancer or head and neck cancer treated with monoclonal antibody RC 83852. *J Clin Oncol* 1994;12:730.

153. Modjtahedi H, Hickish T, Nicolson M, et al. Phase I trial and tumor localisation of the anti-EGFR monoclonal antibody ICR62 in head and neck and lung cancer. *Brit J Cancer* 1996; 73:228.

154. Imanishi K, Yamaguchi K, Kuranami M, et al. Inhibition of growth of human lung adenocarcinoma cell lines by anti-transforming growth factor-α monoclonal antibody. *J Natl Cancer Inst* 1989;81:220.

155. Fujiuchi S, Ohsaki Y, Kikuchi K. Suramin inhibits the growth of non-small-cell lung cancer cells that express the epidermal growth factor receptor. *Oncology* 1997;54:134.

156. Kirk J, Carmichael J, Stratford IJ, et al. Selective toxicity of TGFα-PE40 to EGFR-positive cell lines: selective protection of low-EGFR-expressing cell lines by EGF. *Brit J Cancer* 1994; 69:988.

157. Draoui M, Siegall CB, FitzGerald D, et al. TGFα-PE40 inhibits non-small cell lung cancer growth. *Life Sci* 1994;54:445.

158. Garcia de Palazzo IE, Adams GP, Sundareshan P, et al. Expression of mutated epidermal growth factor receptor by non-small cell lung carcinomas. *Cancer Res* 1993;53:3217.

159. Wikstrand CJ, Hale LP, Batra SK, et al. Monoclonal antibodies against EGFRvIII are tumor specific and react with breast and lung carcinomas and malignant gliomas. *Cancer Res* 1995;55:3140.

160. Cristiano RJ, Roth JA. Epidermal growth factor mediated DNA delivery into lung cancer cells via the epidermal growth factor receptor. *Cancer Gene Ther* 1996;3:4.

161. Kern JA, Schwartz DA, Nordberg JE, et al. p185^{aeu} expression in human lung adenocarcinomas predicts shortened survival. *Cancer Res* 1990;50:5184.

162. Shi D, He G, Cao S, et al. Overexpression of the c-erbB-2/neu-encoded p185 protein in primary lung cancer. *Mol Carcinog* 1992;5:213.

163. Kern JA, Robinson RA, Gazdar A, et al. Mechanisms of p185^{HER2} expression in human non-small cell lung cancer cell lines. *Am J Respir Cell Mol Biol* 1992;6:359.

164. Schneider PM, Hung MC, Chiocca SM, et al. Differential expression of the c-erbB-2 gene in human small cell and non-small cell lung cancer. *Cancer Res* 1989;49:4968.

165. Noguchi M, Murakami M, Bennett W, et al. Biological consequences of overexpression of a transfected c-erbB-2 gene in immortalized human bronchial epithelial cells. *Cancer Res* 1993;53:2035.

166. Stocklin E, Botteri F, Groner B. An activated allele of the c-erbB-2 oncogene impairs kidney and lung function and causes early death in transgenic mice. *J Cell Biol* 1993;122:199.

167. Yu D, Wang SS, Dulski KM, et al. C-erbB-2/neu overexpression enhances metastatic potential of human lung cancer cells by induction of metastasis-associated properties. *Cancer Res* 1994;54:3260.

168. Kern JA, Slebos RJ, Top B, et al. C-erbB-2 expression and codon 12 K-ras mutations both predict shortened survival for patients with pulmonary adenocarcinomas. *J Clin Invest* 1994;93:516.

169. Tsai CM, Chang KT, Wu LH, et al. Correlations between intrinsic chemoresistance and HER2/neu gene expression, p53 gene mutations and cell proliferation characteristics in non-small-cell lung cancer cell lines. *Cancer Res* 1996;56:206.

170. Tsai CM, Levitzki A, Wu LH, et al. Enhancement of chemosensitivity by tyrphostin AG825 in high-p185 expressing non-small cell lung cancer cells. *Cancer Res* 1996;56:1068.

171. Zhang L, Hung MC. Sensitization of HER2/neu-overexpressing non-small cell lung cancer cells to chemotherapeutic drugs by tyrosine kinase inhibitor emodin. *Oncogene* 1996;12:571.

172. Casalini P, Menard S, Malandrin SM, et al: Inhibition of tumorigenicity in lung adenocarcinoma cells by c-erbB-2 antisense expression. *Int J Cancer* 1997;72:631.

173. Snider JM, Bushnell LJ, Chen LC, et al. C-erbB-2/p185-directed therapy in human lung adenocarcinoma. *Ann Thorac Surg* 1996;62:1454.

174. Slamon D, Leyland-Jones B, Shak S, et al. Addition of Herceptin to first line chemotherapy for HER2 overexpressing metastatic breast cancer markedly increases anticancer activity [abstract]. *Proc Am Soc Clin Oncol* 1998;17:98a.

175. Cobleigh MA, Vogel CL, Tripathy D, et al. Efficacy and safety of Herceptin as a single agent in 222 women with HER2 overexpression who relapsed following chemotherapy for metastatic breast cancer [abstract]. *Proc Am Soc Clin Oncol* 1998;17:97a.

176. Soderdahl G, Betsholtz C, Johansson A, et al. Differential expression of platelet-derived growth factor and transforming growth factor genes in small-and non-small-cell human lung carcinoma lines. *Int J Cancer* 1988;41:636.

177. Antoniades HN, Galanopoulos T, Neville-Golden J, et al. Malignant epithelial cells in primary human lung carcinomas coexpress *in vivo* platelet-derived growth factor (PDGF) and PDGF receptor mRNA and their protein products. *Proc Natl Acad Sci USA* 1992;89:3942.

178. Vignaud JM, Marie B, Klein N, et al. The role of platelet-derived growth factor production by tumor-associated macrophages in tumor stroma formation in lung cancer. *Cancer Res* 1994;54:5455.

179. Forsberg K, Bergh J, Westermark B. Expression of functional PDGF β receptors in a human large-cell lung carcinoma cell line. *Int J Cancer* 1993;53:556.

180. Moseley JM, Kubota M, Diefenbach-Jagger H, et al. Parathyroid hormone-related protein purified from a human lung cancer cell line. *Proc Natl Acad Sci USA* 1987;84:5048.

181. Kitazawa S, Fukase M, Kitazawa R, et al. Immunohistologic evaluation of parathyroid hormone-related protein in human lung cancer and normal tissue with newly developed monoclonal antibody. *Cancer* 1991;67:984.

182. Burton PBJ, Knight DE. Parathyroid hormone-related peptide can regulate the growth of human lung cancer cells and may form part of an autocrine TGF-α loop. *FEBS Lett* 1992;305:228.

183. Hastings RH, Summers-torres D, Cheung TC, et al. Parathyroid hormone-related protein, an autocrine regulatory factor in alveolar epithelial cells. *Am J Physiol* 1996;270,L353.

184. LeRoith D. Insulin-like growth factors. *N Engl J Med* 1997;336:633.

185. LeRoith D, Baserga R, Helman L, et al. Insulin-like growth factors and cancer. *Ann Int Med* 1995;122:54.

186. Nakanishi Y, Mulshine JL, Kasprzyk PG, et al. Insulin-like growth factor-I can mediate autocrine proliferation of human small cell lung cancer cell lines in vitro. *J Clin Invest* 1988;82:354.

187. Macaulay VM, Everard MJ, Teale D, et al. Autocrine function for insulin-like growth factor 1 in human small cell lung cancer cell lines and fresh tumor cells. *Cancer Res* 1990;50:2511.

188. Kaiser U, Schardt C, Brandscheidt D, et al. Expression of insulin-like growth factor receptors I and II in normal human lung and in lung cancer. *J Cancer Res Clin Oncol* 1993;119:665.

189. Favoni RE, deCupis A, Ravera F, et al. Expression and function of the insulin-like growth factor I system in human non-small-cell lung cancer and normal lung cell lines. *Int J Cancer* 1994;56:858.

190. Long L, Rubin R, Brodt P. Enhanced invasion and liver colonization by lung carcinoma cells overexpression the type I insulin-like growth factor receptor. *Exp Cell Res* 1998;238:116.

191. Reeve JG, Brinkman A, Hughes S, et al. Expression of insulin-like growth factor and IGF-binding protein genes in human lung tumor cell lines. *J Natl Cancer Inst* 1992;84:628.

192. Ankrapp DP, Bevan DR. Insulin-like growth factor I and human lung fibroblast-derived insulin-like growth factor I stimulate the proliferation of human lung carcinoma cells *in vitro*. *Cancer Res* 1993;53:3399.

193. Shigematsu K, Kataoka Y, Kamio T, et al. Partial characterization of insulin-like growth factor I in primary human lung cancers using immunohistochemical and receptor autoradiographic techniques. *Cancer Res* 1990;50:2481.

194. Minuto F, Del Monte P, Barreca A, et al. Evidence for autocrine mitogenic stimulation by somatomedin-C/insulin-like growth factor I on an established human lung cancer cell line. *Cancer Res* 1988;48:3716.

195. Siegfried JM, Owens SE. Response of primary human lung

carcinomas to autocrine growth factors produced by a lung carcinoma cell line. *Cancer Res* 1988;48:4976.

196. Quinn KA, Treston AM, Unsworth EJ, et al. Insulin-like growth factor expression in human cancer cell lines. *J Biol Chem* 1996;271:11477.

197. Schardt C, Rotsch M, Erbil C, et al. Characterization of insulin-like growth factor II receptors in human small cell lung cancer cell lines. *Exp Cell Res* 1993;204:22.

198. Reeve JG, Morgan J, Schwander J, et al. Role for membrane and secreted insulin-like growth factor-binding protein-2 in the regulation of insulin-like growth factor action in lung cancer. *Cancer Res* 1993;53:4680.

199. Hagiwara K, Kobayashi T, Tobita M, et al. Isolation of a cDNA for a growth factor of vascular endothelial cells from human lung cancer cells: its identity with insulin-like growth factor II. *Jap J Cancer Res* 1995;86:202.

200. Kiefer P, Jaques G, Schöneberger J, et al. Insulin-like growth factor binding protein expression in human small cell lung cancer cell lines. *Exp Cell Res* 1991;192:414.

201. Jaques G, Kiefer P, Schöneberger HJ, et al. Differential expression of insulin-like growth factor binding proteins in human non-small cell lung cancer cell lines. *Eur J Cancer* 1992;28A:1899.

202. Reeve JG, Payne JA, Bleehen NM. Production of immunoreactive insulin-like growth factor-I and IGF-I binding proteins by human lung tumours. *Br J Cancer* 1990;61:727.

203. Lee CT, Wu S, Gabrilovich D, et al. Antitumor effects of an adenovirus expressing antisense insulin-like growth factor I receptor on human lung cancer cell lines. *Cancer Res* 1996;56:3038.

204. Zia F, Jacobs S, Kull F, et al. Monoclonal antibody αIR-3 inhibits non-small cell lung cancer growth *in vitro* and *in vivo*. *J Cell Biochem* 1996;24:269.

205. De Cupis A, Ciomei M, Pirani P, et al. Anti-insulin-like growth factor-I activity of a novel polysulphonated distamycin A derivative in human lung cancer cell lines. *Br J Pharmacol* 1997;120:537.

206. Jetten AM, Vollberg TM, Nervi C, et al. Positive and negative regulation of proliferation and differentiation in tracheobronchial epithelial cells. *Am Rev Respir Dis* 1990;142:S36.

207. Jakowlew SB, Moody TW, You L, et al. Reduction in transforming growth factor β type II receptor in mouse lung carcinogenesis. *Mol Carcinogen* 1998;22:46.

208. Böttinger EP, Jakubezak JL, Haines DC, et al. Transgenic mice overexpressing a dominant-negative mutant type II transforming growth factor β receptor show enhanced tumorigenesis in the mammary gland and lung in response to the carcinogen 7,12-dimethylbenz-[a]-anthracene. *Cancer Res* 1997;57:5564.

209. Damstrup L, Rygaard K, Spang-Thomsen, et al. Expression of transforming growth factor β receptors and expression of TGFβ_2, TGFβ_2, and TGFβ_3 in human small cell lung cancer cell lines. *Br J Cancer* 1993;67:1015.

210. Jakowlew SB, Mathias A, Chung P, et al. Expression of transforming growth factor β ligand and receptor messenger RNAs in lung cancer cell lines. *Cell Growth Differ* 1995;64:465.

211. Colasante A, Mascetra N, Brunetti M, et al. Transforming growth factor β_1 interleukin-8 and interleukin-1 in non-small cell lung tumors. *Am J Respir Crit Care Med* 1997;156:968.

212. Twardzik DR, Ranchalis JE, McPherson JM, et al. Inhibition and promotion of differentiated-like phenotype of a human lung carcinoma in athymic mice by natural and recombinant forms of transforming growth factor β. *J Natl Cancer Inst* 1989;81:1182.

213. Norgaard P, Damstrup L, Rygaard K, et al. Growth suppression by transforming growth factor β_1 of human small-cell lung

cancer cell lines is associated with expression of the type II receptor. *Br J Cancer* 1994;69:802.

214. Raynal S, Nocentini S, Croisy A, et al. Transforming growth factor β_1 enhances the lethal effects of DNA-damaging agents in a human lung cancer cell line. *Int J Cancer* 1997;72:356.

215. Mooradian DL, McCarthy JB, Komanduri KV, et al. Effects of transforming growth factor β_1 on human pulmonary adenocarcinoma cell adhesion, motility and invasion *in vitro*. *J Natl Cancer Inst* 1992;84:523.

216. Fischer JR, Darjes H, Lahm H, et al. Constitutive secretion of bioactive transforming growth factor β_1 by small cell lung cancer cell lines. *Eur J Cancer* 1994;30A:2125.

217. DeJonge RR, Garrigue-Antar L, Vellucci VF, et al. Frequent inactivation of the transforming growth factor β type II receptor in small-cell lung carcinoma cells. *Oncogene Res* 1997;9:89.

218. Norgaard P, Spang-Thomsen M, Poulsen HS. Expression and autoregulation of transforming growth factor beta receptor mRNA in small-cell lung cancer cell lines. *Br J Cancer* 1996;73:1037.

219. Inoue T, Ishida T, Takenoyama M, et al. The relationship between the immunodetection of transforming growth factor-beta in lung adenocarcinoma and longer survival rates. *Surg Oncol* 1995;4:51.

220. Bennett WP, El-Deiry WS, Rush WL, et al. p21$^{\text{wafl/cipl}}$ and transforming growth factor β1 protein expression correlate with survival in non-small cell lung cancer. *Clin Cancer Res* 1998;4:1499.

221. Roth KA, Barchas JD. Small cell carcinoma cell lines contain opioid peptides and receptors. *Cancer* 1986;57:769.

222. Maneckjee R, Minna JD. Opioid and nicotine receptors affect growth regulation of human lung cancer cell lines. *Proc Natl Acad Sci USA* 1990;87:3294.

223. Black M, Carey FA, Farquharson MA, et al. Expression of the pro-opiomelanocortin gene in lung neuroendocrine tumours: *in situ* hybridization and immunohistochemical studies. *J Pathol* 1993;169:329.

224. Melzig MF, Nylander I, Vlaskivska M, et al. β-endorphin stimulates proliferation of small cell lung carcinoma cells *in vitro* via nonopioid binding sites. *Exp Cell Res* 1995;219:471.

225. Sciamanna MA, Griesmann GE, Williams CL, et al. Nicotinic acetylcholine receptors of muscle and neuronal (α7) types coexpressed in a small cell lung carcinoma. *J Neurochem* 1997;69:2302.

226. Tarroni P, Rubboli F, Chini B, et al. Neuronal-type nicotinic receptors in human neuroblastoma and small-cell lung carcinoma cell lines. *FEBS Lett* 1992;312:66.

227. Quik M, Chan J, Patrick J. α-bungarotoxin blocks the nicotinic receptor mediated increase in cell number in a neuroendocrine cell line. *Brain Res* 1994;655:161.

228. Codignola A, Tarroni P, Cattaneo MG, et al. Serotonin release and cell proliferation are under the control of α-bungarotoxin-sensitive nicotinic receptors in small-cell lung carcinoma cell lines. *FEBS Lett* 1994;342:286.

229. Schuller HM. Nitrosamine-induced lung carcinogenesis and Ca^{2+}/calmodulin antagonists. *Cancer Res* 1992;52:2723s.

230. Schuller HM, Miller MS, Park PG, et al. Promoting mechanisms of CO$_2$ on neuroendocrine cell proliferation mediated by nicotinic receptor stimulation: significance for lung cancer risk in individuals with chronic lung disease. *Chest* 1996;109:20S.

231. Schuller HM, McGavin MD, Orloff M, et al. Simultaneous exposure to nicotine and hyperoxia causes tumors in hamsters. *Lab Invest* 1995;73:448.

232. Cattaneo MG, D'atri F, Vicentini LM. Mechanisms of mitogen-activated protein kinase activation by nicotine in small-cell lung carcinoma cells. *Biochem J* 1997;328:499.

233. Heusch WL, Maneckjee R. Signaling pathways involved in nicotine regulation of apoptosis of human lung cancer cells. *Carcinogenesis* 1998;19:551.

234. Cattaneo MG, Codignola A, Vicentini LM, et al. Nicotine stimulates a serotonergic autocrine loop in human small-cell lung carcinoma. *Cancer Res* 1993;53:5566.

235. Rygaard K, Nakamura T, Spang-Thomsen M. Expression of the proto-oncogenes c-met and c-kit and their ligands hepatocyte growth factor/scatter factor and stem cell factor, in SCLC cell lines and xenografts. *Br J Cancer* 1993;67:37.

236. Olivero M, Rizzo M, Madeddu R, et al. Overexpression and activation of hepatocyte growth factor/scatter factor in human non-small cell lung carcinomas. *Br J Cancer* 1996;74:1862.

237. Harvey P, Warn A, Newman P, et al. Immunoreactivity for hepatocyte growth factor/scatter factor and its receptor, met, in human lung carcinomas and malignant mesotheliomas. *J Pathol* 1996;180:389.

238. Tsao MS, Liu N, Chen JR, et al. Differential expression of met/hepatocyte growth factor receptor in subtypes of non-small cell lung cancers. *Lung Cancer* 1998;20:1.

239. Rygaard K, Spang-Thomsen M. Hepatocyte growth factor/scatter factor is an inhibitor of growth and a migration factor in some small cell lung cancer cell lines expressing the corresponding receptor [Abstract]. *Proc Am Assoc Cancer Res* 1993;34:519.

240. Seckl MJ, Seufferlein T, Rozengurt E. Lysophosphatidic acid-depleted serum, hepatocyte growth factor and stem cell growth factor stimulate colony growth of small cell lung cancer cells through a calcium-independent pathway. *Cancer Res* 1994;54: 6143.

241. Yi S, Chen JR, Viallet J, et al. Paracrine effects of hepatocyte growth factor/scatter factor on non-small-cell lung carcinoma cell lines. *Br J Cancer* 1998;77:2162.

242. Tsao MS, Zhu H, Giaid A, et al. Hepatocyte growth factor/scatter factor is an autocrine factor for human normal bronchial epithelial and lung carcinoma cells. *Cell Growth Differ* 1993;4:571.

243. Siegfried JM, Weissfeld LA, Singh-Kaw P, et al. Association of immunoreactive hepatocyte growth factor with poor survival in resectable non-small cell lung cancer. *Cancer Res* 1997;57:433.

244. Maasberg M, Rotsch M, Jaques G, et al. Androgen receptors, androgen-dependent proliferation, and 5 α-reductase activity of small-cell lung cancer cell lines. *Int J Cancer* 1989;43:685.

245. Kaiser U, Hofmann J, Schilli M, et al. Steroid-hormone receptors in cell lines and tumor biopsies of human lung cancer. *Int J Cancer* 1996;67:357.

246. Cagle PT, Mody DR, Schwartz MR. Estrogen and progesterone receptors in bronchogenic carcinoma. *Cancer Res* 1990;50:6632.

247. Su JM, Hsu HK, Chang H, et al. Expression of estrogen and progesterone receptors in non-small-cell lung cancer: immunohistochemical study. *Anticancer Res* 1996;16:3803.

248. Beattie CW, Hansen NW, Thomas PA. Steroid receptors in human lung cancer. *Cancer Res* 1985;45:4206.

249. Canver CC, Memoli VA, Vanderveer PL, et al. Sex hormone receptors in non-small-cell lung cancer in human beings. *J Thorac Cardiovasc Surg* 1994;108:153.

250. Vargas SO, Leslie KO, Vasek PM, et al. Estrogen-receptor-related protein p29 in primary non-small cell lung carcinoma: pathologic and prognostic correlations. *Cancer* 1998;82:1495.

251. Caltagirone S, Ranelletti FO, Rinelli A, et al. Interaction with type II estrogen binding sites and antiproliferative activity of tamoxifen and quercetin in human non-small-cell lung cancer. *Am J Respir Cell Mol Biol* 1997;17:51.

252. Simms E, Gazdar AF, Abrams PG, et al. Growth of human small cell carcinoma of the lung in serum-free growth factor-supplemented medium. *Cancer Res* 1980;40:4356.

253. Brower M, Carney D, Oie HK, et al. Growth of cell lines and clinical specimens of human non-small cell lung cancer in a serum-free defined medium. *Cancer Res* 1986;46:798.

254. Cavanaugh PG, Nicolson GL. Lung-derived growth factor that stimulates the growth of lung-metastasizing tumor cells: identification as transferrin. *J Cell Biochem* 1991;47:261.

255. Kondo K, Noguchi M, Mukai K, et al. Transferrin receptor expression in adenocarcinoma of the lung as a histologic indicator of prognosis. *Chest* 1990;97:1367.

256. Whitney JF, Clark JM, Griffin TW, et al. Transferrin receptor expression in nonsmall cell lung cancer: histopathologic and clinical correlates. *Cancer* 1995;76:20.

257. Nakanishi Y, Cuttitta F, Kasprzyk PG, et al. Growth factor effects on small cell lung cancer cells using a colorimetric assay: can a transferrin-like factor mediate autocrine growth? *Exp Cell Biol* 1988;56:74.

258. Vostrejs M, Moran PL, Seligman PA. Transferrin synthesis by small cell lung cancer cells acts as an autocrine regulator of cellular proliferation. *J Clin Invest* 1988;82:331.

259. Avalos BR, Gasson JC, Hedvat C, et al. Human granulocyte colony-stimulating factor: biologic activities and receptor characterization on hematopoietic cells and small cell lung cancer cell lines. *Blood* 1990;75:851.

260. Nakamura M, Oshika Y, Abe Y, et al. Gene expression of granulocyte colony stimulating factor in non-small-cell lung cancer. *Anticancer Res* 1997;17:573.

261. Tsuruta N, Yatsunami J, Takayama K, et al. Granulocyte-macrophage-colony stimulating factor stimulates tumor invasiveness in squamous cell lung carcinoma. *Cancer* 1998;82: 2173.

262. Baldwin GC, Gasson JC, Kaufman SE, et al. Nonhematopoietic tumor cells express functional GM-CSF receptors. *Blood* 1989; 73:1033.

263. Ruff MR, Farrar WL, Pert CB. Interferon gamma and granulocyte/macrophage colony-stimulating factor inhibit growth and induce antigens characteristic of myeloid differention in small-cell lung cancer cell lines. *Proc Natl Acad Sci USA* 1986;83:6613.

264. Inoue M, Minami M, Fujii Y, et al. Granulocyte colony-stimulating factor and interleukin-6-producing lung cancer cell line LCAM. *J Surg Oncol* 1997;64:347.

265. Foulke RS, Marshall MH, Trotta PP, et al. In vitro assessment of the effects of granulocyte-macrophage colony-stimulating factor on primary human tumors and derived lines. *Cancer Res* 1990;50:6264.

266. Munker M, Munker R, Saxton RE, et al. Effect of recombinant monokines, lymphokines, and other agents on clonal proliferation of human lung cancer cell lines. *Cancer Res* 1987;47:4081.

267. Vellenga E, Biesma B, Meyer C, et al. The effects of five hematopoietic growth factors on human small cell lung carcinoma cell lines: interleukin 3 enhances the proliferation in one of the eleven cell lines. *Cancer Res* 1991;51:73.

268. Twentyman PR, Wright KA. Failure of GM-CSF to influence the growth of small cell and non-small cell lung cancer cell lines in vitro. *Eur J Cancer* 1991;27:6.

269. Berdel WE, Zafferani M, Senekowitsch R, et al. Effect of interleukin-3 and granulocyte-macrophage colony-stimulating factor on growth of xenotransplanted human tumor cell lines in nude mice. *Eur J Cancer* 1992;28:377.

270. Young MR, Lozano Y, Djordjevic A, et al. Granulocyte-macrophage colony-stimulating factor stimulates the metastatic properties of Lewis lung carcinoma cells through a protein kinase A signal-transduction pathway. *Int J Cancer* 1993;53:667.

271. Pei XH, Nakanishi Y, Takayama K, et al. Granulocyte-colony stimulating factor promotes invasion by human lung cancer cell lines in vitro. *Clin Exp Metastsis* 1996;14:351.

272. Filderman AE, Bruckner A, Kacinski BM, et al. Macrophage colony-stimulating factor (CSF-1) enhances invasiveness in CSF-1 receptor-positive carcinoma cell lines. *Cancer Res* 1992; 52:3661.

273. Yano S, Nishioka Y, Nokihara H, et al. Macrophage colony-stimulating factor gene transduction into human lung cancer cells differentially regulates metastasis formation in various organ nicroenvironments of natural killer cell-depleted SCID mice. *Cancer Res* 1997;57:784.

274. Lu L, Shen RN, Lin ZH, et al. Anti-tumor effects of recombinant human macrophage colony-stimulating factor alone or in combination with local irradiation in mice inoculated with Lewis lung carcinoma cells. *Int J Cancer* 1991;47:143.

275. Morita T, Ikeda K, Douzono M, et al. Tumor vaccination with macrophage colony-stimulating factor-producing Lewis lung carcinoma in mice. *Blood* 1996;88:955.

276. Nachbaur D, Denz H, Zwierzina H, et al. Stimulation of colony formation of various human carcinoma cell lines by rhGM-CSF and rhIL-3. *Cancer Lett* 1990;50:197.

277. Pedrazzoli P, Bacciocchi G, Bergamaschi G, et al. Effects of granulocyte-macrophage colony-stimulatin factor and interleukin-3 on small cell lung cancer cells. *Cancer Invest* 1994;12: 283.

278. Takizawa H, Ohtoshi T, Ohta K, et al. Growth inhibition of human lung cancer cell lines by interleukin-6 *in vitro:* a possible role in tumor growth via an autocrine mechanism. *Cancer Res* 1993;53:4175.

279. Ross HJ. The antiproliferative effect of trans-retinoic acid is associated with selective induction of interleukin-1β, a cytokine that directly inhibits growth of lung cancer cells. *Oncol Res* 1996; 8:171.

280. Hibi K, Takahashi T, Sekido Y, et al. Coexpression of the stem cell factor and the c-kit genes in small-cell lung cancer. *Oncogene* 1991;6:2291.

281. Matsuda R, Takahashi T, Nakamura S, et al. Expression of the c-kit protein in human solid tumors and in corresponding fetal and adult normal tissues. *Am J Path* 1993;142:339.

282. Krystal GW, Hines SJ, Organ CP. Autocrine growth of small cell lung cancer mediated by coexpression of c-*kit* and stem cell factor. *Cancer Res* 1996;56:370.

283. Hida T, Ueda R, Sekido Y, et al. Ectopic expression of c-*kit* in small cell lung cancer. *Int J Cancer* 1994;8:108.

284. Pietsch T, Nicotra MR, Fraioli R, et al. Expression of the c-*kit* receptor and its ligand SCF in non-small cell lung carcinomas. *Int J Cancer* 1998;75:171.

285. Sekido Y, Takahashi T, Ueda R, et al. Recombinant human stem cell factor mediates chemotaxis of small-cell lung cancer cell lines aberrantly expressing the c-kit protooncogene. *Cancer Res* 1993;53:1709.

286. DiPaola RS, Kuczynski WI, Onodera K, et al. Evidence for a functional kit receptor in melanoma, breast and lung carcinoma cells. *Cancer Gene Ther* 1997;4:176.

287. Yamanishi Y, Maeda H, Hiyama K, et al. Specific growth inhibition of small-cell lung cancer cells by adenovirus vector expressing antisense c-*kit* transcripts. *Jap J Cancer Res* 1996;87:534.

288. Krystal GW, Carlson P, Litz J. Induction of apoptosis and inhibition of small cell lung cancer growth by the quinoxaline tyrphostins. *Cancer Res* 1997;57:2203.

289. Krystal GW, DeBerry CS, Linnekin D, et al. J. Lck associates with and is activated by kit in a small cell lung cancer cell line: inhibition of SCF-mediated growth by the src family kinase inhibitor PP1. *Cancer Res* 1998;58:4660.

11

CURRENT CONCEPTS OF ANGIOGENESIS RELATED TO PRIMARY LUNG CANCER

YASUHIKO OHTA
YOH WATANABE

As a route for nutrients, oxygen, and metastasis, blood vessels are an integral component of malignant solid tumors. Angiogenesis is the phenomenon of the development of new blood vessels from preexisting blood vessels (Figure 11.1). Development of metastases includes many steps, among which are angiogenesis and growth of tumor cells in the primary site, followed by invasion, intravasation, transport, arrest, attachment, and extravasation. The same series of steps, including angiogenesis and growth, should occur at the metastatic site. Theoretical simulations have led us to believe that tumors with rich vascularization are likely to have faster growth and higher risk of distant metastasis compared to those with poor vascularization. Tumor angiogenesis is of particular interest not only as a promising prognostic indicator but also as a target for possible innovative therapeutic interventions against tumor growth and metastasis. Folkman has been foremost in the concept that tumor growth is angiogenesis-dependent and that the acquisition of an angiogenic phenotype clearly has a decisive meaning in the development of tumor cells.[1,2] His hypotheses were first substantiated when he proved that tumors grown in isolated perfused organs without proliferating blood vessels were limited to 1 to 2 mm^3, but expanded rapidly after vascularization in an *in vivo* model system.[3]

Among the many reported angiogenesis-associated factors, vascular endothelial growth factor (VEGF) is the most powerful endothelial cell-specific mitogen that is associated with tumor neovascularization. This novel angiogenic stimulator has a peculiar background in that it was originally detected as a vascular permeability factor in malignant ascites fluid in 1983[4] To date, two definite VEGF receptors, kinase insert domain-containing receptor (KDR)/Flk-1 and fms-like tyrosine kinase 1(flt-1), have been identified in its signal transduction pathways.[5–8] Several factors that are related to the regulation of VEGF expression have also been identified. Transforming growth factor (TGF)-β, epidermal growth factor (EGF), platelet-derived growth factor (PDGF), and basic fibroblast growth factor (bFGF), which are all angiogenesis stimulators, appear to be major stimulants of VEGF expression.[9,10] Recent studies have also revealed a connection between mutant *p53*, mutations in the H-*ras* or K-*ras* oncogene, and *Src* oncogene and the stimulation of VEGF expression in tumor angiogenesis.[11–14] These results suggest that VEGF participates in the key role of tumor angiogenesis. In this chapter, we highlight VEGF/vascular permeability factor expression in primary lung cancer, outlining clinical implications that are just being realized. The areas that are covered include (a) intratumoral microvessel density and its clinical implications in primary lung cancer, (b) tumor angiogenesis and VEGF expression in lung cancer, (c) the association of VEGF expression with metastasis, (d) assessment of lymphatic vessel density in tumor tissue and its association with VEGF family expressions, (e) other angiogenesis-associated agents that appear to take part in the progression of lung cancer, and (f) inhibition of angiogenesis for cancer treatment.

NEOVASCULARIZATION ASSESSED BY INTRATUMORAL MICROVESSEL DENSITY IN PRIMARY LUNG CANCER—ITS CLINICAL IMPLICATIONS

In primary lung cancer, Macchiarini et al. first observed a relationship between neovascularization of tumors in early stages and metastasis in 1992.[15] In this study, neovascularization was assessed by counting microvessels by using anti-Factor VIII (FVIII) immunohistochemistry in the most vascularized "hotspot" area. In 1994, Yamazaki and colleagues found that microvessel density similarly assessed by FVIII was positively correlated to the relapse of patients with lung adenocarcinoma after resection. These authors also suggested that intratumoral microvessel counts were associated with the aggressiveness of the tumor.[16] Since then, many reports have assessed the impact of intratumoral microvessel density on the prognosis in primary lung cancer, and some researchers have found that intratumoral vascularity has a close relationship to poor prognosis in the assessment of

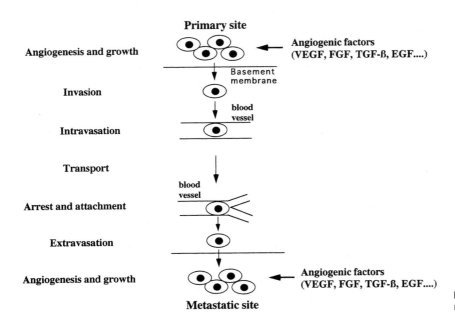

FIGURE 11.1. Schematic sequential steps of the metastatic cascade.

overall survival or disease-free intervals.[17-22] However, not all studies agree with the concept of microvessel density as prognostic in lung cancer.[23-25] This inconsistency may partly be a result of the lack of homogeneity of experimental methods and/or conditions, heterogeneity of angiogenesis in samples used, and the character of markers mostly used for the detection of endothelial cells that recognize both blood and lymphatic vessels.

Harpole et al. studied 275 consecutive non–small cell lung cancer (NSCLC) patients with stage I disease using anti-FVIII immunohistochemistry and found an increased positive correlation between microvessel density and poor outcome of the patients.[18] Giatromanolaki et al. studied 134 NSCLC patients with stage I–II diseases using both anti-FVIII and anti-CD31 antibodies, also revealing a positive correlation with poor prognosis.[20] Duarte et al. also found a significant association between vascularization assessed by anti-FVIII antibody and cancer-related mortality rate in 106 patients with stage I NSCLC.[22] Ohta, using 104 randomly selected stage I NSCLC patients with or without recurrence for a follow-up period of at least 5 years, reported that the mean microvessel density in tumors with recurrence was significantly greater than that in tumors without recurrence (18.2 ± 10.5 versus 8.5 ± 5.0, $p < 0.0001$).[26] Vascularity may be able to reduce the risk of recurrence of lung cancer with curative resections in early stages. The limitations of FVIII analysis are well described. FVIII antigen is not necessarily expressed in all endothelial cells and is actually consumed by the endothelium of newly formed capillaries. In addition, the endothelial cells from microvessels are inferior to those from macrovessels in the expression of Weibel-Palade bodies, which store factor VIII antigen.[27]

Research using other antibodies has confirmed a similar significant association between intratumoral microvessel density and prognosis. For example, using anti-CD34 monoclonal antibody (which has a higher specificity compared to anti-FVIII), Fontanini reported that microvessel count was an independent prognostic indicator among 195 patients with stage I–IIIA NSCLC.[21] Conventional wisdom, therefore, implies that direct counting of microvessels, which is mainly based on immunohistochemical staining for endothelial cells, will define the risk of recurrence and outcomes for lung cancer patients who undergo potentially curative operations.

TUMOR ANGIOGENESIS AND VEGF EXPRESSION IN PRIMARY LUNG CANCER

Molecular cloning has found four VEGF alternative spliced transcripts from the single VEGF gene on chromosome 6p21.3; that is, VEGF121, 165, 189, and 206. Although the longer forms, designated as VEGF189 and 206, are mostly cell-associated and have vascular permeation ability, VEGF121 and 165, which are translated from shorter transcripts, are efficiently secreted and promote mitogenesis of endothelial cells.[28] A positive correlation between VEGF expression and microvessel density has already been observed in a variety of tumors.[23,29-31] Michenko and colleagues have found that VEGF is associated with the mechanisms underlying the induction of angiogenesis by hypoxia.[32] According to the study, which used primary cultured vascular cells, the number of both endothelial cells and pericytes increased significantly under hypoxic conditions, along with an increase of mRNAs coding for the secretory forms of VEGF (VEGF121 and 165). VEGF receptors

KDR and flt-1 were found to be constitutively expressed in endothelial cells, but only flt-1 mRNA was expressed in pericytes under hypoxic conditions.[33] Secretory forms of VEGF seem to be involved in tumor angiogenesis not only through autocrine mechanisms but also through paracrine systems. As a tumor increases in size with resulting ischemic change, angiogenic mechanisms may be influenced.

The significance of each spliced variant of VEGF is not yet clear. Using the quantitative reverse transcription-PCR (RT-PCR) method, we previously examined the VEGF mRNA expressions in primary lung cancer tissues.[34] Human lung cancer cell lines (PC-6, PC-10, QG-56, and QG-96) all had secretory forms of VEGF mRNA, and large amounts of the secretory forms of VEGF mRNAs were also found in resected lung cancer tissues independent of histologic subtypes (71.4% in total). VEGF121 mRNA expression levels also correlated with patient outcomes. Although the sample scale was small, VEGF121 gene expression levels were associated with poor prognosis in patients in the early stages of lung cancer. In patients who underwent a curative operation at stage I of the disease (n = 17), the median survival of the VEGF high-expression group was 8 months, and that of the VEGF low-expression group was 151 months. The 3- and 5-year survival rates of the high-expression group were 50.0% and 16.7%, respectively, and those of the low-expression group were 90.9% and 77.9%, respectively. Further, among eight cases of long-term survival beyond 5 years, seven cases had low or no VEGF121 mRNA expression. In contrast, among 18 cases with VEGF121 mRNA overexpression, 17 cases died because of recurrence. These data imply that gene expressions of the secretory forms of VEGF mainly pertain to cancer cells and have an important role in lung cancer progression.

According to the results of another study using 90 randomly selected primary lung cancer patients without distant metastasis,[35] the percentage of positive cases for each spliced variant in tumors (T) and surrounding normal lung tissue samples (N) was 84.3% in T and 66.7% in N for VEGF121, 76.5% in T and 56.9% in N for VEGF165, and 47.1% in T and 7.8% in N for VEGF189. Among the four alternatively spliced variants, although VEGF121 and 165 were the dominant types in both lung cancer tissue and surrounding normal lung tissue, VEGF189 appeared to be dominant only in tumor tissue. The mean relative intensities of VEGF121 mRNA expression (VEGF121/β-actin) in tumor (T) (20.2 ± 5.2) was significantly higher than that in normal (N) (3.5 ± 1.1, p = 0.0024). In addition, if tumors were classified as high or low VEGF121 expression group relative to the mean value of densitometry index in N, the percentage of high-expression cases was 65.0% in T, whereas only 10.9% in N. These results reveal that the secretory form of VEGF, VEGF121, is overexpressed in lung cancer tissue compared to surrounding normal lung tissue. Moreover, overexpression of VEGF is found in adjacent normal lung tissue in advanced stages, including pleural involvement.[35]

The association of VEGF with pleural dissemination, however, needs further definition.

If VEGF is involved in tumor angiogenesis through both autocrine and paracrine systems, then the expression in normal lung tissue may participate in the mitogenic activity in tumor angiogenesis. Although the meaning and significance of each alternatively spliced variant of VEGF remains unclear, the majority of studies support the importance of VEGF121 isoform for the progression of lung cancer. Regarding the role of VEGF121 in tumorigenesis, it has been found that transfection of this isoform into a human breast carcinoma cell line promotes tumor growth and angiogenic response.[36] Although VEGF189 expression is not as high as that of VEGF121, its specific expression in tumors suggests that VEGT 189 may be involved in tumor progression. The specific upregulation of the VEGF189 isoform in confluent cultures compared to sparse monolayers has been found in colon cancer cell lines,[37] implying a potential role for the isoform in cellular interaction.[38,39] In colon cancer patients, VEGF189 isoform has also been found to be correlated with liver metastasis.[40]

Lung alveoli (together with adrenal cortex, renal glomeruli, and cardiac myocytes) are rich in VEGF expression.[41] This particular condition may promote malignant development in patients with lung cancer. Strong VEGF expression in tumors seems to predict a poor outcome in lung cancer patients.[23,34,42–44] VEGF expression levels have been assessed chiefly by the immunohistochemistry using antibodies that recognize multiple VEGF spliced variants at a time. In 1995, Mattern et al., in a study of 204 patients with primary NSCLC, demonstrated a trend that patients with VEGF-positive tumors had worse prognoses than those with VEGF-negative tumors.[23] They also reported that the proliferating cell nuclear antigen (PCNA) labeling index significantly increased with increasing VEGF expression, but that no association existed between PCNA labeling index and tumor vascularity. These findings imply that VEGF may participate in tumor progression and development through at least two separate mechanisms; that is, as a growth factor for tumor cells and as a mitogen for vascular endothelial cells.[45] Data have also demonstrated that VEGF expression, based on immunohistochemic staining methods, was an independent prognostic indicator in lung cancer patients.[43,44]

Limited data exist regarding serum VEGF protein levels in lung cancer patients, and high VEGF expression levels in serum have been associated with poor outcomes in these patients.[46] Recent studies have also shown that serum VEGF is produced by megakaryocytes and platelets *in vitro*, and its concentrations are correlated with platelet counts.[47,48]

ASSOCIATION OF VEGF EXPRESSION WITH LYMPH NODE METASTASIS

Two routes are involved in the development of lymph node metastasis. An anatomic route involves the blood circulation to the lymphatic hilum, in which tumor cells in the blood can be transported and arrested in the lymph nodes. An increasing number of tumor cells in the blood may result in a high frequency of nodal involvement, and tumor angiogenesis may be involved in nodal metastasis via this medium. The second route involves a direct invasion of tumor cells into lymphatic vessels. In tumors with an increase in newly formed lymphatic vessels, both preexisting lymphatic and neolymphatic vessels may be the route for lymph node metastasis. If the neolymphatics develop from preexisting lymphatic endothelium as do blood vessels, the number of preexisting lymphatics should affect the lymphatic density. Although this neolymphatic route is hypothetical, it implies that tumor angiogenesis as well as lymphangiogenesis may be involved in lymph node metastasis formation. The study on neovascularization of lymphatics in tumors has just begun to be explored and no conclusive data have been reported. Consistent with this hypothesis, however, are previous data that indicate a relationship between microvessel density and lymph node metastasis, using antibodies that recognize both blood and lymphatic microvessels.[49,50] This area of study is controversial, however, with minimal data supporting the mechanism.[16,23]

A correlation between VEGF expression and lymph node metastasis in primary lung cancer has been documented.[35] Primary lung cancer tissue and surrounding normal lung from 90 patients without distant metastasis had the intensity of VEGF mRNA expression levels calculated by the sum of the relative intensities of both the tumor tissue and corresponding adjacent normal lung tissue using quantitative RT-PCR analysis. A trend to higher VEGF mRNA expression levels occurred in patients with nodal metastasis (23.2 ± 39.9, n = 35) than in those patients without nodal

metastasis (8.8 ± 17.9, n = 55) (p = 0.051). When stratified by nodal status, the VEGF expression levels had a tendency to increase with the progression of nodal status [N1, 12.0 ± 14.9 (n = 7); N2, 21.2 ± 36.2 (n = 21), and N3, 40.5 ± 66.1 (n = 7)]. Moreover, VEGF expression could be detected in lymph nodes. Ten lymph nodes (four nodes positive and six nodes negative), together with the corresponding primary lung tumors and surrounding normal lung tissue, were simultaneously examined. To obtain an exact diagnosis of nodal micrometastasis, keratin 19 mRNA expression was also investigated by using the RT-PCR technique along with histologic examination. VEGF expression levels in metastatic lymph nodes were conspicuously higher than those in the primary site, and all the expression levels from nodes without metastases were lower than those of the primary tumors (Figure 11.2). These results suggest that tumor cells with high VEGF expression may metastasize selectively to nodes. VEGF expression within lymph nodes, although a small sample scale renders the meaning inconclusive, may imply the existence of another function of VEGF for the development of nodal metastasis independent of the proliferation of endothelial cells. In fact, Gabrilovich and colleagues recently reported a potential role for VEGF in allowing tumor cells to avoid the induction of an immune response.[51]

ASSESSMENT OF LYMPHANGIOGENESIS AND ITS CONNECTION WITH VEGF FAMILY

Partly because of the difficulties in making exact distinctions between blood and lymphatic microvessels and because of the lack of suitable *in vivo* or *in vitro* model systems for the

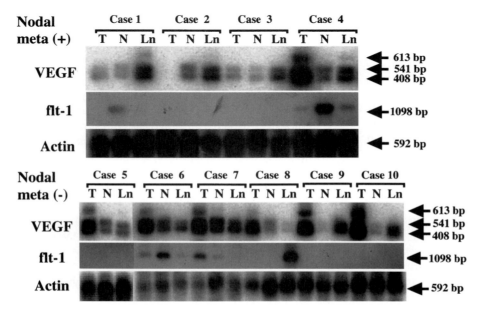

FIGURE 11.2. RT-PCR analysis of VEGF mRNAs in lymph nodes (*Ln*), correspondent lung cancer tissue (*T*), and adjacent normal lung tissue (*N*). Among the 10 lymph node samples, 4 from node-positive patients were metastatic (samples 1–4) and 6 from node-negative patients were nonmetastatic (samples 5–10). This assessment of lymph node metastasis was done by histopathologic examination using enzyme-histochemistry staining and the RT-PCR method for the detection of keratin 19 mRNA as a sensitive assay for the micrometastasis. Other receptors (flt-4 and KDR) could not be found in this study. (From Ohta Y, Watanabe Y, Murakami, et al. Vascular endothelial growth factor and lymph node metastasis in primary lung cancer. *Br J Cancer* 1997;76:1041, with permission.)

study of lymphatic endothelial cells, little information is available about the phenomenon of "lymphangiogenesis" in tumors; that is, the neovascularization of lymphatic vessels in tumors. As previously detailed, this phenomenon is not well documented, and its existence is controversial. In human primary cutaneous melanoma, de Waal et al. recently reported the lack of lymphangiogenesis in tumors even in the presence of extensive hemangiogenesis based on the results of a differential immunohistochemic double-staining method.[52] It was concluded from this study that hemangiogenesis might indirectly enhance lymphatic invasion as the driving force behind tumor expansion. Despite the infrequent observation of lymphatics inside the tumor, the expanding cutaneous melanoma tumor mass appeared to facilitate entrapping of lymphatics in tumors and the invasion of tumor cells into lymphatics at the site of the subepidermal lymphatic plexus. Other reports have suggested the existence of the specific pathways involved in the formation of lymphatics separately from those of hemangiogenesis.[53–56] Among the VEGF family members, the function of VEGF type C (VEGF-C) appears to extend to the lymphatic systems, where it serves as a ligand for fms-like tyrosine kinase 4 (flt–4).[53,54]

The correlation between VEGF-C expression levels and microlymphatic vessel density in malignant pleural mesothelioma has been recently examined.[57] An attempt was made to discriminate lymphatics from blood vessels using an enzyme-histochemistry assay for 5′-nucleotidase (5′-NA).[58] The activity of the enzyme is higher in lymphatic endothelial cells compared to that in blood capillary endothelial cells, and as such is used to discriminate lymphatics from capillary endothelial cells after adequate inhibition of its activity.[59–62] Among 54 malignant pleural mesotheliomas, significant positive correlations were found between VEGF-C and flt-4 gene expression levels that were assessed by semiquantitative RT-PCR analysis ($p = 0.0018$, $r = 0.67$). Further, the association between microlymphatic vessel density and VEGF-C expression levels was especially strong ($p < 0.0001$, $r = 0.63$). The correlation of microlymphatic vessel density with flt-4 expression levels was also confirmed ($p = 0.0164$, $r = 0.64$). The microlymphatic vessel density, however, within mesothelioma tumor tissue had no impact on nodal metastasis. Instead, the expression of VEGF had a tendency to be greater in node-positive than in node-negative patients, suggesting its association with nodal metastasis independent of the number of lymphatics in malignant pleural mesothelioma tumors. In addition, flt-4, which was originally described in lymphatic endothelium,[63,64] was highly expressed in malignant pleural mesothelioma tissues, in human malignant mesothelioma cell lines, and in normal pleural tissue samples. Although the role of flt-4 in mesothelioma is not well known, flt-4 expression was confirmed in normal mesothelial cells.[65] These results suggest a possibility that VEGF-C has some role for the autocrine growth of mesothelioma cells.

VEGF-C is actually expressed in a variety of human tumors,[66] and its family members encompass VEGF-B,[67] VEGF-C,[63,68] and VEGF-D.[69,70] The significance of these VEGF-associated factors as novel stimulators for vascular endothelial cells and/or lymphatic ones needs to be further studied to elucidate their connections with proliferation of lymphatic endothelium and lymph node metastasis.

The relationship between microlymphatic vessel density in tumors and the capacity of tumors to develop lymph node metastasis has been studied using the microlymphatic vessel density (MLD) method in SCID mice injected subcutaneously with various human tumor cells (PC-14, DLD-1, OST, and MNNG/HOS). Subcutaneous regional lymph nodes and lungs were dissected when the primary tumor volume reached 2 cm[3]. As a result, lymph node metastases were detected in mice injected with PC-14, and primary PC-14 tumors had high MLD (15.3—7.6). Tumors with no lymph node metastasis had low MLD (DLD-1, 0 and MNNG/HOS, 0) except for OST (13.5—6.0). Moreover, an interesting contrast was found between PC-14 and MHHG/HOS tumors in that, while PC-14 tumors developed lymph node metastasis, all MNNG/HOS tumors developed lung metastasis, paralleling the contrast of the relatively high MLD in PC-14 tumors to low MLD in MNNG/HOS tumors. DLD-1 developed no lymph node metastasis or lung metastasis, and this cell line had low MLD. On the other hand, OST tumors developed no lymph node metastasis despite relatively high MLD. These findings suggest that high microlymphatic vessel density is not necessarily associated with nodal involvement, although some tumors appear to have a tendency to develop lymph node metastasis when they are rich with lymphatic vessels.

OTHER ANGIOGENESIS-ASSOCIATED AGENTS THAT ARE RELATED TO THE PROGRESSION OF LUNG CANCER

Of the nine fibroblast growth factors (FGFs), FGF-2 (bFGF) is the leading candidate for being a stimulator of angiogenesis. The functions of FGF-2 include vascular endothelial and smooth muscle cell proliferation, capillary tube formation, and chemotaxis of endothelial cells. A recent study also suggests an antiapoptotic effect of FGF-2 via induction of Mdm-2 with the subsequent inhibition of p53 function and via down-regulation of bcl-2.[72,73] In NSCLC the potential role of bcl-2 in suppressing tumor angiogenesis has been reported.[74] There have been suggestions of an association between FGF-2 and VEGF;[75–78] however, clinical investigations using resected tumor specimens have not necessarily disclosed a significant association between them.[31,34] The significance of bFGF as a prognostic indicator still needs to be defined in lung cancer. In breast carcinoma, low expression of bFGF is reportedly associated with a poor prognosis.[79] In lung cancer, one report found a significant correlation between bFGF expression and patient survival,[80] whereas another did not.[81]

Platelet-derived endothelial cell growth factor (PD-ECGF)/thymidine phosphorylase is also an angiogenesis stimulant and promotes tumor cell growth.[82,83] PD-ECGF expression has been observed in a variety of human tumors, including NSCLC cell lines.[84,85] In NSCLC patients, tumors with PD-ECGF overexpression have reportedly been associated with poor prognosis.[86,87]

Interleukin 8 (IL-8) is one of the most studied chemokines that stimulate angiogenesis. The production of IL-8 has been confirmed in NSCLC cell lines and in resected NSCLC specimens alike, and it appears to act as a promoter of human NSCLC tumor growth through angiogenesis activation.[88,89] A study using human glioma cell lines suggested that the paracrine control of tumor angiogenesis by IL-8 was independent of that by VEGF/bFGF.[90]

Thrombospondin (TSP) is a matricellular glycoprotein that is secreted by a variety of cells, including tumor cells.[91,92] Among the five structurally different members (TSP-1–5) of the TSP family, TSP-1 and -2 have a molecular architecture similar to angiogenesis inhibitors. Recent data suggest that TSP-1 may also function as an angiogenesis stimulator.[93,94] For example, a domain analysis has revealed that TSP-1 possesses binding sites for $\alpha v \beta 3$ integrin and TGF-β, which are both proangiogenic.[93,95,96] In addition, the role of TSP-1 seems to be multifunctional and to be associated with adhesion, chemotaxis, and proliferation of endothelial cells.[93] Further, recent studies have also suggested that *p53* can down-regulate TSP-1 expression,[97] raising the possibility that inactivation of *p53* may induce transcriptional activation of TSP-1 in affected tumors. In primary lung cancer, although little information is available on the role and clinical implications of TSP, a recent study suggested an inhibitory role of TSP-2 in angiogenesis and progression of NSCLC.[98]

INHIBITION OF ANGIOGENESIS FOR CANCER TREATMENT (Table 11.1)

Candidates for Antiangiogenic Cancer Treatment

Antiangiogenic therapy is being used as a new anticancer "dormancy therapy" to promote stabilization or shrinkage of disease. The process of new blood vessel generation is divided into multiple major steps; that is, (a) proliferation of endothelial cells, (b) resolution of the extracellular matrix, and (c) migration of endothelial cells.[99] Several antiangiogenic agents or drugs are expected to be feasible for cancer therapy that targets these angiogenic steps (Figure 11.3). For inhibition of the first step, neutralization antibodies to angiogenic factors (VEGF, bFGF), antiangiogenic agents [fumagillin analogues (TNP-470/AGM-1470), interleukin-12, suramin, linomide, minocycline, tamoxifen, thalido-

mide, interferons, platelet-factor 4(PF4), pentosan polysulphate, genestein, etc.], and angiogenesis-inhibitory factors (angiostatin, endostatin, thrombospondin, etc.), are representative agents so far.[100] For the second and third steps, metalloproteinase inhibitors, antibody to $\alpha v \beta 3$ integrin, and linomide are also potential candidates.[100] Some of these agents (e.g., linomide, PF4, pentosan polysulphate, neutralization antibodies to VEGF, metalloproteinase inhibitors, fumagillin analogues, interleukin-12, thalidomide, and so on) are already in clinical trials.[100,101]

Inhibition of Angiogenesis for Cancer Treatment by Targeting VEGF and its Receptors

VEGF itself may be a potential molecular target for the treatment of lung cancer. Using *in vivo* model systems, inhibition of VEGF function has successfully controlled tumor growth, dissemination, and distant metastasis by a variety of anti-VEGF agents such as neutralizing anti-VEGF antibodies, anti-sense VEGF cDNA, and soluble VEGF receptor.[102–108] Kim first demonstrated the effectiveness of a monoclonal antibody against tumor cells having VEGF expression in 1993.[102] Human sarcoma cells injected into nude mice were inhibited by the administration of anti-VEGF antibody A.4.6.1. The monoclonal antibody had no direct inhibitory effect on tumor cell growth *in vitro*, suggesting the importance of the inhibition of paracrine VEGF mechanisms from both host and tumor cells in order to control tumor angiogenesis and tumor progression. In addition to antibody cocktails that recognize all VEGF-spliced isoforms, those antibodies to VEGF121 secretory form alone can also inhibit tumor growth and metastasis. Asano found that a neutralizing monoclonal antibody to VEGF121 could inhibit the growth and formation of spontaneous lung metastasis of human sarcoma HT-1080 cells subcutaneously inoculated into nude mice.[109]

Targeting of VEGF receptors also serves as a possible therapeutic intervention to inhibit tumor angiogenesis and tumor growth.[110,111] A clinical investigation of colon cancer found that upregulation of VEGFR-2 (KDR) was associated with metastasis[31] and that inhibition of angiogenesis by blocking VEGFR-2 (KDR) prevents tumor cell invasion.[111] These results suggest a mutually close relationship between VEGF and tumor invasion, and that anti-VEGF therapy may have a direct therapeutic influence against cancer invasion or metastasis together with antiangiogenic effects for tumor angiogenesis.

The timing of the antiangiogenesis therapy may be important, as suggested by Yoshiji.[112] No growth inhibition of human breast carcinoma T-47D cells was observed when anti-VEGF treatment was started for tumors that had reached a certain size (820 mm^3) despite the observation of significant inhibitory effects for smaller tumors. This correlation suggests that VEGF may not be the crucial an-

TABLE 11.1. THE EFFECT OF ANTIANGIOGENIC AGENTS ON LYMPH NODE METASTASIS

Authors	Journal	Antiangiogenic Agent	Animal	Cell Line	LN Metastasis
1. Kurebayashi et al. (1994)	*Breast Cancer*	AGM-1470	Nude mouse	MKL-4	Inhibit
2. Futami et al. (1994)	*Proc Am Assoc Cancer Res*	AGM-1470	Rat	AS653HM	Inhibit
3. McLeskey et al. (1996)	*Br J Cancer*	AGM-1470	Mouse	MCF-7	No effect
4. Mu et al. (1996)	*Jpn J Cancer Res*	FR118487	Nude mouse	OV-HM	Inhibit
5. Singh et al. (1996)	*Breast Cancer Res Treat*	TNP-470	Rat	KPL-1	Inhibit
6. Hori et al. (1997)	*Br J Cancer*	AGM-1470	Rat	LY80	Promote
7. Ohta et al. (1997)	*Br J Cancer*	TNP-470	Nude mouse	HT1080	Inhibit

giogenic factor for larger tumors or that angiogenic factors may alternatively be changed and superseded by other factors after the suppression of VEGF. If VEGF is essential at the initial phase of tumor development and angiogenesis, the practical usage of anti-VEGF treatment may then be most expected for the control of micrometastasis.

The Effect of Antiangiogenic Drugs on Tumor Growth, Distant Metastasis, and Lymph Node Metastasis

Antitumor or antimetastatic activity with antiangiogenic therapies have been documented in a variety of metastatic model systems using various antiangiogenic drugs. Most of the experimental studies have reported inhibitory effects for bloodborne distant metastases, such as liver and lung metastases, and few comments have been made on possible thera-

peutic effects for lymph node metastasis. Because nodal involvement is one of the most important factors influencing the survival of surgical patients with primary lung cancer, the effects of antiangiogenic drugs on lymph node metastasis need to be clarified.

Ohta assessed the inhibitory action of a semisynthetic analogue of fumagillin, TNP-470/AGM-1470, on lymph node metastasis in a metastatic model system using athymic nude mice.[113] In this study, lymph node metastases were detected by PCR and Southern blotting for human β-globin-related sequence. After mice were injected subcutaneously with human fibrosarcoma HT-1080 cells, various amounts of the antiangiogenic agent (10, 30, and 100 mg/kg) were injected subcutaneously every other day beginning seven days after tumor inoculation. Five weeks after tumor inoculation, DNA was extracted from axillary and inguinal lymph nodes. Antitumor effects on the primary

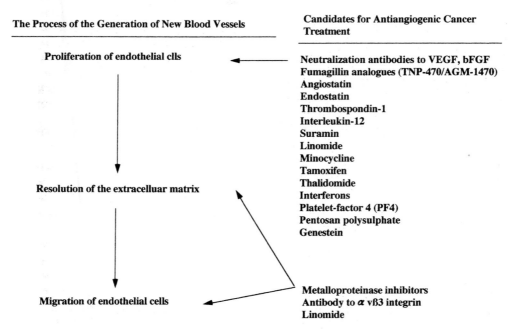

FIGURE 11.3. Candidates for antiangiogenic cancer treatment.

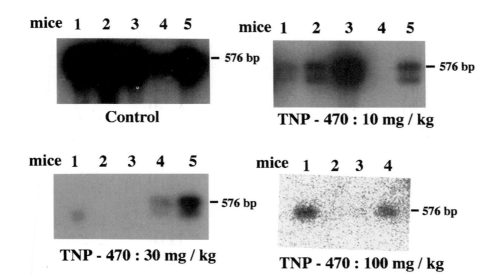

FIGURE 11.4. Effects of TNP-470 (10, 30, and 100 mg/kg) on lymph node metastasis of HT-1080 cells. TNP-470 was subcutaneously injected every other day from 1 week after tumor inoculation on mice. Mouse lymph nodes were then dissected at 5 weeks after tumor inoculation. Following extraction of DNA from dissected lymph nodes, specific detection of human β-globin gene in metastasized human tumor cells in nude mice (576 bp) was performed by the PCR technique and analized by Southern blotting. (From Ohta Y, Watanabe Y, Tabata T, et al. Inhibition of lymph node metastasis by an anti-angiogenic agent, TNP-470. *Br J Cancer* 1997;75:512, with permission.)

sites were seen only in the 100 mg/kg treatment group. Lymph node metastases were detected in all mice in the no treatment group, and the incidence of lymph node metastasis in treated mice was 2/4 mice (100 mg/kg), 2/5 mice (30 mg/kg), and 4/5 mice (10 mg/kg). Further, the inhibition ratios of lymph node metastasis were 82.3% in 10 mg/kg, 97.2% in 30 mg/kg, and 97.5% in 100 mg/kg, respectively, implying that antiangiogenic treatment can be useful in inhibiting nodal metastasis (Figure 11.4). In the literature, Mu has also observed an almost complete inhibition of metastasis to lymph nodes in mice with murine ovarian carcinoma cells by administering an angiogenesis-inhibitory fumagillin analog, FR118487.[114] A similar inhibitory action of TNP-470/AGM-1470 against lymph node metastasis in breast cancer cell lines and rat fibrosarcoma cell line has also been reported.[115,116] Other studies have reported variable results on lymph node metastasis with antiangiogenic agents.[117,118]

The fumagillin analogues have been shown to inhibit *distant metastasis* and tumor growth via inhibition of tumor angiogenesis.[119,123] TNP-470/AGM-1470 inhibits the growth of human umbilical vein endothelial (HUVE) cells in a biphasic manner, cytostatic and cytotoxic.[123] Exposure to TNP-470 arrests HUVE cells in G0/G1 phases, and this cytostatic inhibition may be the mechanism for the antigiogenic activity.[124–126] In addition, other studies have suggested a variable effect of the agent on the host immune system, involving B-cell proliferation in the presence of T-cells.[127,128]

Safety of Antiangiogenic Drugs for Cancer Treatment in Practical Usage

In *in vivo* experimental model systems, the treatment by a combination of antiangiogenic drugs has been found to be more effective compared to that by only a single agent. In addition, a combination therapy using both antiangiogenic agents and cytotoxic anticancer drugs has also been shown to have a greater effect than that using only cytotoxic anticancer drugs.[129–131] These results offer implications about the practical usage of the antiangiogenic agents for cancer treatment to achieve optimal therapeutic effects.

Most angiogenesis inhibitors appear to have less toxicity and no drug resistance, making for an advantageous contrast to conventional cytotoxic anticancer drugs. These merits give credence to the permanent or long-term administration of these drugs to sustain the stabilization of the cancer or to continue to inhibit the development of metastasis. So far, although drug-induced side effects should be carefully investigated in a long period of dosage, no major side effects have been reported from results of phase I clinical studies using antiangiogenic agents for cancer treatment. Reversible neurologic side effects have been reported to be the dose-limiting toxicity[132] of fumagillin analogue TNP-470. Among 18 patients in the phase I trial[132] with recurring or metastatic squamous cell carcinoma of the cervix, one patient had a complete response and three patients had stable disease. A phase I clinical trial using orally administered pentosan polysulphate in patients with advanced cancers revealed no major side effects.[133]

Antiangiogenic Therapy and Micrometastasis

Via the biomolecular or immunohistochemical techniques for the detection of the specific biologic marker for cancer cells, such as cytokeratin fragments, it has been found that tumor cells are present in some distant organs such as bone marrow, peripheral blood circulation, and lymph nodes in a significant proportion of various cancer patients, including lung cancer, even if any distant metastasis cannot be detected by conventional clinical examinations.[134–142] Importantly, a recent study also showed worse postoperative outcomes of such patients and their trend toward recurrence after curative operations.[134,139–142] These findings suggest a necessity to take some steps for patients with micrometastasis before the manifestation of the occult disease. In patients with NSCLC, the percentage of the patients with micrometastasis of bone marrow has been reported to be 21.9% to 59.7% in total.[139–141] If stratified by pathologic stages, its rates were reported to be 29% in stage I or II and 46% in stage III.[140] For lymph node micrometastasis, 63.0% of NSCLC patients were revealed to have micrometastasis despite negative studies based on the conventional examination using hematoxylin and eosin stained slides.[138,142] Folkman previously proposed an interesting theory that is related to the clinical patterns of metastasis.[143] According to the theory, the duration of metastatic disease-free interval after operation depends on "the switch to the angiogenic phenotype as a net balance of positive and negative regulators of blood vessel growth." The antiangiogenic therapy may theoretically improve the survival of the patients with micrometastasis after curative resection of the primary site by keeping the micrometastatic cells in the dormant state. Exploitation of this strategy will require the proper selection of patients and greater assessment to determine the phenotype of cancer cells with potential metastatic ability as a function of short or long periods after operation.

REFERENCES

1. Folkman J. Tumor angiogenesis: therapeutic implications. *N Engl J Med* 1971;285:1182.
2. Folkman J. What is the evidence that tumors are angiogenesis dependent? *J Natl Cancer Inst* 1990;82:4.
3. Folkman J, Cole P, Zimmerman S. Tumor behavior in isolated perfused organs: in vitro growth and metastasis of biopsy material in rabbit thyroid and canine intestinal segment. *Ann Surg* 1966;164:491.
4. Senger DR, Galli SJ, Dvorak AM, et al. Tumor cells secrete a vascular permeability factor that promotes accumulation of ascites fluid. *Science* 1983;219:983.
5. Millauer B, Wizigmann Voos S, et al. High affinity VEGF binding and developmental expression suggest Flk-1 as a major regulator of vasculogenesis and angiogenesis. *Cell* 1993;72:835.
6. Oelrichs RB, Reid HH, Bernard O, et al. NYK/FLK-1: a putative receptor protein tyrosine kinase isolated from E10 embryonic neuroepithelium is expressed in endothelial cells of the developing embryo. *Oncogene* 1993;8:11.
7. Terman BI, Dougher-Vermazen M, Carrion, ME, et al. Identification of the KDR tyrosine kinase as a receptor for vascular endothelial cell growth factor. *Biochem Biophys Res Commun* 1993;187:1579.
8. De Vries C, Escobedo JA, Ueno H, et al. The fms-like tyrosine kinase, a receptor for vascular endothelial growth factor. *Science* 1992;255:989.
9. Dolecki GJ, Connolly DT. Effect of a variety of cytokines and inducing agents on vascular permeability factor mRNA levels in U937 cells. *Biochem Biophys Res Commun* 1991;180:572.
10. Tsai J, Goldman CK, Gillespie GY. Vascular endothelial growth factor in human glioma cell lines: induced secretion by EGF, PDGF-BB, and bFGF. *J Neurosurg* 1995;82:864.
11. Keiser A, Weich HA, Brandner G, et al. Mutant p53 potentiates protein kinase-C induction of vascular endothelial growth factor expression. *Oncogene* 1994;9:963.
12. Rak J, Mitsuhashi Y, Bayko L, et al. Mutant ras oncogenes upregulate VEGF/VPF expression: implications for induction and inhibition of tumor angiogenesis. *Cancer Res* 1995;55:4575.
13. Grugel S, Finkenzeller G, Weindel K, et al. Both v-Ha-Ras and v-Raf stimulate expression of the vascular endothelial growth factor in NIH 3T3 cells. *J Biol Chem* 1995;270:25915.
14. Mukhopadhyay D, Tsiokas L, Sukhatme VP. Wild-type p53 and v-Src exert opposing influences on human vascular endothelial growth factor gene expression. *Cancer Res* 1995;55:6161.
15. Macchiarini P, Fontanini G, Hardin MJ, et al. Relation of neovascularisation to metastasis of non-small-cell lung cancer. *Lancet* 1992;340:145.
16. Yamazaki K, Abe S, Takekawa H, et al. Tumor angiogenesis in human lung adenocarcinoma. *Cancer* 1994;74:2245.
17. Fontanini G, Bigini D, Vignati S, et al. Microvessel count predicts metastatic disease and survival in non-small cell lung cancer. *J Pathol* 1995;177:57.
18. Harpole DH, Richards WG, Herndon II JE, et al. Angiogenesis and molecular biologic substaging in patients with stage I non-small cell lung cancer. *Ann Thorac Surg* 1996;61:1470.
19. Giatromanolaki A, Koukourakis M, O'Byrne K, et al. Prognostic value of angiogenesis in operable non-small cell lung cancer. *J Pathol* 1996;179:80.
20. Giatromanolaki A, Koukourakis M, Theodossiou D, et al. Comparative evaluation of angiogenesis assessment with anti-factor-VIII and anti-CD31 immunostaining in non-small cell lung cancer. *Clin Cancer Res* 1997;3:2485.
21. Fontanini G, Laurentiis MD, Vignati S, et al. Evaluation of epidermal growth factor-related growth factors and receptors and of neoangiogenesis in completely resected stage I-IIIA non-small-cell lung cancer: amphiregulin and microvessel count are independent prognostic indicators of survival. *Clin Cancer Res* 1998;4:241.
22. Duarte IG, Bufkin BL, Pennington MF, et al. Angiogenesis as a predictor of survival after surgical resection for stage I non-small-cell lung cancer. *J Thorac Cardiovasc Surg* 1998;115:652.
23. Mattern J, Koomägi R, Volm M. Vascular endothelial growth factor expression and angiogenesis in non-small cell lung carcinomas. *Int J Oncol* 1995;6:1059.
24. Pezzella F, Bacco AD, Andreola S, et al. Angiogenesis in primary lung cancer and lung secondaries. *Eur J Cancer* 1996;32A:2494.
25. Chandrachud LM, Pendleton N, Chisholm DM, et al. Relationship between vascularity, age and survival in non-small-cell lung cancer. *Br J Cancer* 1997;76:1367.
26. Ohta Y, Tomita Y, Oda M, et al. Tumor angiogenesis and recurrence in stage I non-small cell lung cancer. *Ann Thorac Surg* 1999;68:1034.
27. Querrec AL, Duval D, Tobelem G. Tumor angiogenesis. *Bailliere Clin Haematol* 1993;6:711.
28. Ferrara N, Houck K, Jakeman L, et al. Molecular and biological properties of the vascular endothelial growth factor family of proteins. *Endocr Rev* 1992;13:18.
29. Toi M, Hoshina S, Takayanagi T, et al. Association of vascular endothelial growth factor expression with tumor angiogenesis and with early relapse in primary breast cancer. *Jpn J Cancer Res* 1994;85:1045.
30. Samoto K, Ikezaki K, Ono M, et al. Expression of vascular endothelial growth factor and its possible relation with neovascularization in human brain tumors. *Cancer Res* 1995;55:1189.
31. Takahashi Y, Kitadai Y, Bucana CD, et al. Expression of vascular

endothelial growth factor and its receptor, KDR, correlates with vascularity metastasis, and proliferation of human colon cancer. *Cancer Res* 1995;55:3964.

32. Michenko A, Bauer T, Salceda S, et al. Hypoxic stimulation of vascular endothelial growth factor expression in vitro and in vivo. *Lab Invest* 1994;71:370.

33. Nomura M, Yamagishi S, Harada S, et al. Possible participation of autocrine and paracrine vascular endothelial growth factors in hypoxia-induced proliferation of endothelial cells and pericytes. *J Biol Chem* 1995;270:28316.

34. Ohta Y, Endo Y, Tanaka M, et al. Significance of vascular endothelial growth factor messenger RNA expression in primary lung cancer. *Clin Cancer Res* 1996;2:1411.

35. Ohta Y, Watanabe Y, Murakami S, et al. Vascular endothelial growth factor and lymph node metastasis in primary lung cancer. *Br J Cancer* 1997;76:1041.

36. Zhang H-T, Craft P, Scott PAE, et al. Enhancement of tumor growth and vascular density by transfection of vascular endothelial cell growth factor into MCF-7 human breast carcinoma cells. *J Natl Cancer Inst* 1995;87:213.

37. Koura AN, Wenbiano L, Kitadai Y, et al. Regulation of vascular endothelial growth factor expression in human colon carcinoma cells by cell density. *Cancer Res* 1996;56:3891.

38. Ferrara N, Houck KA, Jakeman LB, et al. The vascular endothelial growth factor family of polypeptides. *J Cell Biochem* 1991; 47:211.

39. Houck KA, Ferrara N, Winer J, et al. The vascular endothelial growth family: identification of a fourth molecular species and characterization of alternate splicing of RNA. *Mol Endocrinol* 1991;5:1806.

40. Tokunaga T, Oshika Y, Abe Y, et al. Vascular endothelial growth factor (VEGF) mRNA isoform expression pattern is correlated with liver metastasis and poor prognosis in colon cancer. *Br J Cancer* 1998;77:998.

41. Berse B, Brown LF, Water LVD, et al. Vascular permeability factor (vascular endothelial growth factor) gene is expressed differentially in normal tissues, macrophages, and tumors. *Mol Biol Cell* 1992;3:221.

42. Volm M, Koomagi R, Mattern J. Prognostic value of vascular endothelial growth factor and its receptor Flt-1 in squamous cell lung carcinoma. *Int J Cancer* 1997;74:64.

43. Fontanini G, Vignati S, Boldrini L, et al. Vascular endothelial growth factor is associated with neovascularization and influences progression of non-small cell lung carcinoma. *Clin Cancer Res* 1997;3:861.

44. Volm M, Rittgen W, Drings P. Prognostic value of ERBB-1, VEGF, cyclin A, FOS, JUN and MYC in patients with squamous cell lung carcinomas. *Br J Cancer* 1998;77:663.

45. Mattern J, Koomagi R, Volm M. Association of vascular endothelial growth factor expression with intratumoral microvessel density and tumour cell proliferation in human epidermoid lung carcinoma. *Br J Cancer* 1996;73:931.

46. Salven P, Ruotsalainen T, Mattson K, et al. High pre-treatment serum level of vascular endothelial growth factor (VEGF) is associated with poor outcome in small-cell lung cancer. *Int J Cancer* 1998;79:144.

47. Mohle R, Green D, Moore MA, et al. Constitutive production and thrombin-induced release of vascular endothelial growth factor by human megakaryocytes and platelets. *Proc Natl Acad Sci USA* 1997;94:663.

48. Verheul HMW, Hoekman K, Bakker SL, et al. Platelet: transporter of vascular endothelial growth factor. *Clin Cancer Res* 1997;3:2187.

49. Bosari S, Lee AKC, Dlellis RA, et al. Microvessel quantitation and prognosis in invasive breast carcinoma. *Hum Pathol* 1992; 23:755.

50. Weidner N, Folkman J, Pozza F, et al. Tumor angiogenesis: a new significant and independent prognostic indicator in early-stage breast carcinoma. *J Natl Cancer Inst* 1992;84:1875.

51. Gabrilovich DI, Chen HI, Girgis KR, et al. Production of vascular endothelial growth factor by human tumors inhibits the functional maturation of dendritic cells. *Nature Med* 1996;2:1096.

52. de Waal RMW, van Altena MC, Erhard H, et al. Lack of lymphangiogenesis in human primary cutaneous melanoma. *Am J Pathol* 1997;150:1951.

53. Kukk E, Lymboussaki A, Taira S, et al. VEGF-C receptor binding and pattern of expression with VEGFR-3 suggests a role in lymphatic vascular development. *Development* 1996;122:3829.

54. Jeltsch M, Kaipainen A, Joukov V, et al. Hyperplasia of lymphatic vessels in VEGF-C transgenic mice. *Science* 1997;276: 1423.

55. Wilting J, Birkenhager R, Eichmann A, et al. VEGF121 induces proliferation of vascular endothelial cells and expression of flk-1 without affecting lymphatic vessels of chorioallantoic membrane. *Dev Biol* 1996;176:76.

56. Oh SJ, Jeltsch MM, Birkenhager R, et al. VEGF and VEGF-C: specific induction of angiogenesis and lymphangiogenesis in the differentiated avian chorioallantoic membrane. *Dev Biol* 1997;188:96.

57. Ohta Y, Shridhar V, Bright RK, et al. VEGF and VEGF type C play an important role in angiogenesis and lymph angiogenesis in human malignant mesothelioma tumors. *Br J Cancer* 1999;81:54.

58. Wachstein M, Meisel E. The histochemical distribution of 5-nucleotidase and unspecific alkaline phosphatase in the testicle of various species and in two human seminomas. *J Histochem* 1954;2:137.

59. Vetter W. Alkaline phosphatasen in mastzellen, blut-und lymphagefäßen der rattenzunge. 5'-nucleotidase-, unspezifische alkalische phosphatase- und polyphosphatase-(ATP'ase) aktivität unter besonderer berücksichtigung des pH. *Z Anat Entwicklungsgesch* 1970;130:153.

60. Turner RR, Beckstead JH, Warnke RA, et al. Endothelial cell phenotypic diversity. In situ demonstration of immunologic and enzymatic heterogeneity that correlates with specific morphologic subtypes. *Am J Clin Pathol* 1987;87:569.

61. Airas L, Niemela J, Salmi M, et al. Differential regulation and function of CD73, a glycosyl-phosphatidylinositol-linked 70-kD adhesion molecule, on lymphocytes and endothelial cells. *J Cell Biol* 1997;136:421.

62. Ji RC, Kato S. Enzyme-histochemical study on postnatal development of rat stomach lymphatic vessels. *Microvasc Res* 1997; 54:1.

63. Joukov V, Pajusola K, Kaipainen A, et al. A novel vascular endothelial growth factor, VEGF-C, is a ligand for the FLT-4(VEGFR-3) and KDR (VEGFR-2) receptor tyrosine kinases. *Embo J* 1996;15:290.

64. Kaipainen A, Korhonen J, Mustonen T, et al. Expression of the fms-like tyrosine kinase 4 gene becomes restricted to lymphatic endothelium during development. *Proc Natl Acad Sci USA* 1995;92:3566.

65. Hewett PW, Murray JC. Coexpression of flt-1, flt-4 and KDR in freshly isolated and cultured human endothelial cells. *Biochem Biophys Res Commun* 1996;221:697.

66. Salven P, Lymboussaki A, Heikkilä P, et al. Vascular endothelial growth factors VEGF-B and VEGF-C are expressed in human tumors. *Am J Pathol* 1998;153:103.

67. Olofsson B, Pajusola K, Kaipainen A, et al. Vascular endothelial growth factor B, a novel growth factor for endothelial cells. *Proc Natl Acad Sci USA* 1996;93:2576.

68. Lee J, Gray A, Yuan J, et al. Vascular endothelial growth factor-

related protein: A ligand and specific activator of the tyrosine kinase receptor Flt4. *Proc Natl Acad Sci USA* 1996;93:1988.

69. Yamada Y, Nezu J, Shimane M, et al. Molecular cloning of a novel vascular endothelial growth factor, VEGF-D. *Genomics* 1997;42:483.

70. Achen MG, Jeltsch M, Kukk E, et al. Vascular endothelial growth factor D (VEGF-D) is a ligand for the tyrosine kinases VEGF receptor 2 (Flk1) and VEGF receptor 3 (Flt4). *Proc Natl Acad Sci USA* 1998;95:548.

71. Ohta Y, Tanaka M, Endo Y, et al. Relationship between microlymphatic vessel density within tumors and lymph node metastasis. *Oncology Rep* 1997;4:889.

72. Shaulian E, Resnitzky D, Shifman O, et al. Induction of Mdm2 and enhancement of cell survival by bFGF. *Oncogene* 1997;15:2717.

73. Wang Q, Maloof P, Wang H, et al. Basic fibroblast growth factor down regulates Bcl-2 and promotes apoptosis in MCF-7 human breast cancer cells. *Exp Cell Res* 1998;238:177.

74. Koukourakis MI, Giatromanolaki A, O'Byrne KJ, et al. Potential role of bcl-2 as a suppressor of tumour angiogenesis in non-small-cell lung cancer. *Int J Cancer* 1997;74:565.

75. Pepper MS, Ferrara N, Orci L, et al. Potent synergism between vascular endothelial growth factor and basic fibroblast growth factor in the induction of angiogenesis in vitro. *Biochem Biophys Res Commun* 1992;189:824.

76. Goto F, Goto K, Weindel K, et al. Synergistic effects of vascular endothelial growth factor and basic fibroblast growth factor on the proliferation on cord formation of bovine capillary endothelial cells within collagen gels. *Lab Invest* 1993;69:508.

77. Brogi E, Wu T, Namiki A, et al. Indirect angiogenic cytokines upregulate VEGF and bFGF gene expression in vascular smooth muscle cells, whereas hypoxia upregulates VEGF expression only. *Circulation* 1994;90:649.

78. Stavri GT, Zachary IC, Baskerville PA, et al. Basic fibroblast growth factor upregulates the expression of vascular endothelial growth factor in vascular smooth muscle cells. Synergistic interaction with hypoxia. *Circulation* 1995;92:11.

79. Colomer R, Aparicio J, Montero S, et al. Low levels of basic fibroblast growth factor (bFGF) are associated with a poor prognosis in human breast carcinoma. *Br J Cancer* 1997;76:1215.

80. Takanami I, Tanaka F, Hashizume T, et al. The basic fibroblast growth factor and its receptor in pulmonary adenocarcinomas: an investigation of their expression as prognostic markers. *Eur J Cancer* 1996;32A:1509.

81. Volm M, Koomagi R, Mattern J, et al. Prognostic value of basic fibroblast growth factor and its receptor (FGFR-1) in patients with non-small cell lung cancer. *Eur J Cancer* 1997;33:691.

82. Moghaddam A, Bicknell R. Expression of platelet-derived endothelial cell growth factor in Escherichia coli and confirmation of its thymidine phosphorylase activity. *Biochemistry* 1992;31:12141.

83. Moghaddam A, Zhang HT, Fan TPD, et al. Thymidine phosphorylase is angiogenic and promotes tumor growth. *Proc Natl Acad Sci USA* 1995;92:998.

84. Yoshimura A, Kuwazuru Y, Furukawa T, et al. Purification and tissue distribution of human thymidine phosphorylase; high expression in lymphocytes, reticulocytes and tumors. *Biochim Biophys Acta* 1990;1034:107.

85. Heldin NE, Usuki K, Bergh J, et al. Differential expression of platelet-derived endothelial cell growth factor/thymidine phosphorylase in human lung carcinoma cell lines. *Br J Cancer* 1993;68:708.

86. Koukourakis MI, Giatromanolaki A, O'Byrne KJ. Platelet-derived endothelial cell growth factor expression correlates with tumor angiogenesis and prognosis in non-small-cell lung cancer. *Br J Cancer* 1997;75:477.

87. Koukourakis MI, Giatromanolaki A, Kakolyris S, et al. Different patterns of stromal and cancer cell thymidine phosphorylase reactivity in non-small-cell lung cancer: impact on tumour neoangiogenesis and survival. *Br J Cancer* 1998;77:1696.

88. Yatsunami J, Tsuruta N, Ogata K, et al. Interleukin-8 participates in angiogenesis in non-small cell, but not small cell carcinoma of the lung. *Cancer Lett* 1997;120:101.

89. Arenberg DA, Kunkel SL, Polverini PJ, et al. Inhibition of interleukin-8 reduces tumorigenesis of human non-small cell lung cancer in SCID mice. *J Clin Invest* 1996;97:2792.

90. Wakabayashi Y, Shono T, Isono M, et al. Dual pathways to tubular morphogenesis of vascular endothelial cells by human glioma cells: vascular endothelial growth factor/basic fibroblast growth factor and interleukin-8. *Jpn J Cancer Res* 1995;86:1189.

91. Varani J, Rister BL, Hughes LA, et al. Characterization of thrombospondin synthesis, secretion and cell surface expression by human tumor cells. *Clin Exp Metastasis* 1989;7:265.

92. Castle V, Varani J, Fligiel S, et al. Antisense-mediated reduction in thrombospondin reverses the malignant phenotype of a human squamous carcinoma. *J Clin Invest* 1991;87:1883.

93. Nicosia RF, Tuszynski GP. Matrix-bound thrombospondin promotes angiogenesis in vitro. *J Cell Biol* 1994;124:183.

94. Bornstein P. Diversity of function is inherent in matricellular proteins: an appraisal of thrombospondin 1. *J Cell Biol* 1995;130:503.

95. Gao AG, Lindberg FP, Dimitry JM, et al. Thrombospondin modulates alpha V beta 3 function through integrin associated protein. *J Cell Biol* 1996;135:533.

96. Dawson DW, Pearce SF, Zhong R, et al. CD36 mediates the in vitro inhibitory effects of thrombospondin-1 on endothelial cells. *J Cell Biol* 1997;138:707.

97. Dameron KM, Volpert OV, Tainsky MA, et al. Control of angiogenesis in fibroblast by p53 regulation of thrombospondin-1. *Science* 1994;265:1582.

98. Oshika Y, Masuda K, Tokunaga T, et al. Thrombospondin 2 gene expression is correlated with decreased vascularity in non-small cell lung cancer. *Clin Cancer Res* 1998;4:1785.

99. Denijn M, Ruiter DJ. The possible role of angiogenesis in the metastatic potential of human melanoma: clinicopathological aspects. *Melanoma Res* 1993;3:5.

100. Gasparini G. Angiogenesis research up to 1996. A commentary on the state of art and suggestions for future studies. *Eur J Cancer* 1996;32A:2379.

101. Folkman J. Clinical applications of research on angiogenesis. *New Engl J Med* 1995;333:1757.

102. Kim KJ, Li B, Winer J, et al. Inhibition of vascular endothelial growth factor-induced angiogenesis suppresses tumour growth in vivo. *Nature* 1993;362:841.

103. Warren RS, Yuan H, Matli MR, et al. Regulation by vascular endothelial growth factor of human colon cancer tumorigenesis in a mouse model of experimental liver metastasis. *J Clin Invest* 1995;95:1789.

104. Borgström P, Hillan KJ, Spiramarao P, et al. Complete inhibition of angiogenesis and growth of microtumors by anti-vascular endothelial growth factor neutralizing antibody: novel concepts of angiostatic therapy from intravital videomicroscopy. *Cancer Res* 1996;56:4032.

105. Melnyk O, Shuman MA, Kim KJ. Vascular endothelial growth factor promotes tumor dissemination by a mechanism distinct from its effect on primary tumor growth. *Cancer Res* 1996;56:921.

106. Presta LG, Chen H, O'Connor SJ, et al. Humanization of an anti-vascular endothelial growth factor monoclonal antibody for the therapy of solid tumors and other disorders. *Cancer Res* 1997;57:4593.

107. Saleh M, Stacker SA, Wilks AF. Inhibition of growth of C6

glioma cells in vivo by expression of antisense vascular endothelial growth factor sequence. *Cancer Res* 1996;56:393.

108. Lin P, Sankar S, Shan S, et al. Inhibition of tumor growth by targeting tumor endothelium using a soluble vascular endothelial growth factor receptor. *Cell Growth Differ* 1998;9:49.

109. Asano M, Yukita A, Matsumoto T, et al. Inhibition of tumor growth and metastasis by an immunoneutralizing monoclonal antibody to human vascular endothelial growth factor/vascular permeability factor$_2$. *Cancer Res* 1995;55:5296.

110. Strawn LM, McMahon G, App H, et al. Flk-1 as a target for tumor growth inhibition. *Cancer Res* 1996;56:3540.

111. Skobe M, Rockwell P, Goldstein N, et al. Halting angiogenesis suppresses carcinoma cell invasion. *Nature Med* 1997;3:1222.

112. Yoshiji H, Harris SR, Thorgeirsson UP. Vascular endothelial growth factor is essential for initial but not continued in vivo growth of human breast carcinoma cells. *Cancer Res* 1997;57:3924.

113. Ohta Y, Watanabe Y, Tabata T, et al. Inhibition of lymph node metastasis by an anti-angiogenic agent, TNP-470. *Br J Cancer* 1997;75:512.

114. Mu J, Abe Y, Tsutsui T, et al. Inhibition of growth and metastasis of ovarian carcinoma by administering a drug capable of interfering with vascular endothelial growth factor activity. *Jpn J Cancer Res* 1996;87:963.

115. Singh Y, Shikata N, Kiyozuka Y, et al. Inhibition of tumor growth and metastasis by angiogenesis inhibitor TNP-470 on breast cancer cell lines in vitro and in vivo. *Breast Cancer Res Treat* 1997;45:15.

116. Futami H, Iseki H, Tamaguchi K. Inhibition of lymphatic metastasis of rat fibrosarcoma by an angiogenesis inhibitor, AGM-1470. *Proc Am Assoc Cancer Res* 1994;35:184.

117. Hori K, Li H-C, Saito S, et al. Increased growth and incidence of lymph node metastases due to the angiogenesis inhibitor AGM-1470. *Br J Cancer* 1997;75:1730.

118. McLeskey SW, Zhang L, Trock BJ, et al. Effects of AGM-1470 and pentosan polysulphate on tumorigenicity and metastasis of FGF-transfected MCF-7 cells. *Br J Cancer* 1996;73:1053.

119. Ingber D, Fujita T, Kishimoto S, et al. Synthetic analogues of fumagillin that inhibit angiogenesis and suppress tumor growth. *Nature* 1990;348:555.

120. Yamaoka M, Yamamoto T, Masaki T, et al. Inhibition of tumor growth and metastasis of rodent tumors by the angiogenesis inhibitor O-(chloroacetyl-carbamoyl) fumagillol (TNP-470; AGM-1470). *Cancer Res* 1993;53:4262.

121. Yanase T, Tamura M, Fujita K, et al. Inhibitory effect of angiogenesis inhibitor TNP-470 on tumor growth and metastasis of human cell lines in vivo and in vitro. *Cancer Res* 1993;53:2566.

122. Tanaka H, Taniguchi H, Mugitani T, et al. Intra-arterial administration of the angiogenesis inhibitor TNP-470 blocks liver metastasis in a rabbit model. *Br J Cancer* 1995;72:650.

123. Sasaki A, Alcalde RE, Nishiyama A, et al. Angiogenesis inhibitor TNP-470 inhibits human breast cancer osteolytic bone metastasis in nude mice through the reduction of bone resorption. *Cancer Res* 1998;58:462.

124. Kusaka M, Sudo K, Matsutani E, et al. Cytostatic inhibition of endothelial cell growth by the angiogenesis inhibitor TNP-470 (AGM-1470). *Br J Cancer* 1994;69:212.

125. Hori A, Ikeyama S, Sudo K. Suppression of cyclin D1 mRNA expression by the angiogenesis inhibitor TNP-470 (AGM-1470) in vascular endothelial cells. *Biochem Biophys Res Commun* 1994;204:1067.

126. Antoine N, Greimers R, De Roanne C, et al. AGM-1470, a potent angiogenesis inhibitor, prevents the entry of normal but not transformed endothelial cells into the G1 phase of the cell cycle. *Cancer Res* 1994;54:2073.

127. Antoine N, Daukandt M, Heinen E, et al. In vitro and in vivo stimulation of the murine immune system by AGM-1470, a potent angiogenesis inhibitor. *Am J Pathol* 1996;148:393.

128. Antoine N, Daukandt M, Locigno R, et al. The potent angioinhibin AGM-1470 stimulates normal but human tumoral lymphocytes. *Tumori* 1996;82:27.

129. Parangi S, O'Reilly M, Christofori G, et al. Antiangiogenic therapy of transgenic mice impairs de-novo tumor-growth. *Proc Natl Acad Sci USA* 1996;93:2002.

130. Teicher BA, Holden SA, Ara G, et al. Potentiation of cytotoxic cancer therapies by TNP-470 alone and with other anti-angiogenic agents. *Int J Cancer* 1994;57:920.

131. Herbst RS, Takeuchi H, Teicher BA. Paclitaxel/carboplatin administration along with antiangiogenic therapy in non-small-cell lung and breast carcinoma models. *Cancer Chemother Pharmacol* 1998;41:497.

132. Kudelka AP, Levy T, Verschraegen CF, et al. A phase I study of TNP-470 administered to patients with advanced squamous cell cancer of the cervix. *Clin Cancer Res* 1997;3:1501.

133. Marshall JL, Wellstein A, Rae J, et al. Phase I trial of orally administered pentosan polysulfate in patients with advanced cancer. *Clin Cancer Res* 1997;3:2347.

134. Redding WH, Coombes RC, Monaghan P, et al. Detection of micrometastases in patients with primary breast cancer. *Lancet* 1983;Dec 3:1271.

135. Lindemann F, Schlimok G, Dirschedl P, et al. Prognostic significance of micrometastatic tumour cells in bone marrow of colorectal cancer patients. *Lancet* 1992;340:685.

136. Moreno JG, Croce CM, Fischer R, et al. Detection of hematogenous micrometastasis in patients with prostate cancer. *Cancer Res* 1992;52:6110.

137. Pantel K, Schlimok G, Braun S, et al. Differential expression of proliferation-associated molecules in individual micrometastatic carcinoma cells. *J Natl Cancer Inst* 1993;85:1419.

138. Chen Z-L, Perez S, Holmes EC, et al. Frequency and distribution of occult micrometastases in lymph nodes of patients with non-small-cell lung carcinoma. *J Natl Cancer Inst* 1993;85:493.

139. Pantel K, Izbichi JR, Angstwurm M, et al. Immunocytological detection of bone marrow micrometastasis in operable non-small cell lung cancer. *Cancer Res* 1993;53:1027.

140. Cote RJ, Beattie EJ, Chaiwun B, et al. Detection of occult bone marrow micrometastases in patients with operable lung carcinoma. *Ann Surg* 1995;222:415.

141. Pantel K, Izbicki J, Passlick B, et al. Frequency and prognostic significance of isolated tumour cells in bone marrow of patients with non-small-cell lung cancer without overt metastases. *Lancet* 1996;347:649.

142. Izbicki JR, Passlick B, Hosch SB, et al. Mode of spread in the early phase of lymphatic metastasis in non-small-cell lung cancer: significance of nodal micrometastasis. *J Thorac Cardiovasc Surg* 1996;112:623.

143. Folkman J. Angiogenesis in cancer, vascular, rheumatoid and other disease. *Nature Med* 1995;1:27.

BASICS OF THERAPEUTICS

12

RADIATION BIOLOGY

ROBERTO PACELLI
FRANCIS J. SULLIVAN
MURALI CHERAKURI
JAMES B. MITCHELL

The study of the effects of ionizing radiation on biologic tissue has contributed greatly to the management of cancer patients. Techniques first developed and described by radiation biologists have elucidated much important information in the understanding of basic cellular biology and the response of biologic tissues to therapeutic agents. Lung cancer is an enormous therapeutic challenge to the clinician. The following chapter is intended as a summary of key radiation biologic contributions to our understanding and management of this disease. By no means is it intended to be an exhaustive treatise on this important topic. Many fine textbooks and reviews fulfill this need. These texts have been liberally referenced as appropriate throughout the chapter. The reader requiring a more detailed review is encouraged to review these texts.

THE CHEMISTRY OF RADIATION BIOLOGY

Introduction

The transfer of energy from radiation to an absorbing medium can cause either excitation or ionization of the component molecules. If the energy of the incident radiation is sufficient to eject an electron from the outer orbital of an atom or molecule, then the incident radiation is defined as ionizing radiation. Ionizing radiation releases energy sufficient to exceed bond energies of many chemical bonds (5 eV) and thereby break them. Radiation that causes excitation without ionization has wavelengths in the UV/visible region.

Both electromagnetic radiation and particulate radiation such as alpha-particles, protons, and neutrons can cause ionization. X-rays that are produced extranuclearly and gamma-rays that are produced intranuclearly are two forms of electromagnetic radiation that possess sufficient energy to cause ionization of atoms or molecules. Electromagnetic radiation and particulate radiation, which have high energies, are slowed down in the absorbing medium by interacting with the electrons of the component molecules with

characteristic dependence on linear energy transfer (LET). LET is defined as the energy lost from the charged particle per unit length of the absorbing medium it traverses and has units of KeV/μm (kilo electron Volts/micrometer). Generally, particulate radiations have higher LET. However, for a given type of radiation, LET is inversely proportional to the energy of the radiation. LET values for typically used radiation are Cobalt 60 gamma-rays: 0.2; 150 MeV protons: 0.5; 250 kV x-rays: 2.0; 10 MeV protons: 4.7; and 2.5 MeV alpha-particles: 166.

Photons of ionizing radiation are absorbed by two processes depending on their energies and the chemical composition of the absorbing material. At high photon energy, characteristic of therapeutic radiation, the *Compton scattering process* is important. In this process, the x-ray photon interacts with and ejects an electron whose binding energy is negligible compared to the photon energy. On collision, part of the photon energy is given as kinetic energy to the ejected electron. The x-ray photon with the diminished energy continues, deflected from its original path, to cause subsequent ionization. After the initial collision, in place of an original x-ray photon, an ejected electron and a scattered photon of diminished energy appear. In the second process, the *photoelectric process,* the x-ray photon interacts with a strongly bound orbital electron and transfers all of its energy to it. Part of its energy is utilized to overcome the binding energy of the electron to release it from the orbital, and the remaining energy is converted to the kinetic energy of the ejected electron. In diagnostic radiology, where lower energy x-rays are used, the photoelectric process dominates. The absorption of the radiation through Compton scattering is independent of the atomic number of the component molecules of the absorbing material, whereas the energy absorption by the photoelectric process is proportional to the cube of the atomic number of the absorbing material. Hence, in diagnostic radiology (low-energy x-rays), the photoelectric process predominates, and a greater extent of the energy is absorbed by the bone that contains atoms with high atomic number (e.g., calcium). This reaction provides the sharp contrast between bone and soft tissue necessary for diagnostic evaluation. In the case of high-energy therapeutic radiation, the absorbed dose is the same in the bone, muscle, and soft tissue. However, in both cases, the energy of the photon is converted into the kinetic energy of the fast electron, leading to ionization events.

Direct and Indirect Effects

Particulate radiation such as alpha-particles, neutrons, and protons, which have high LET values, cause direct ionization by disturbing the atomic structure of molecules of the absorbing material, thereby causing chemical and subsequent biologic changes. On the other hand, when x-rays are absorbed in biologic material, they can directly ionize a critical site (direct effect) or interact with other molecules to produce reactive radicals, which can subsequently damage critical biologic molecules (indirect effect). The chemical nature of the free radicals produced by indirect effects depends on the abundance of chemical species in the absorbing material.

Because 80% of biologic matter is composed of water, the effect of radiation on water molecules is important in understanding the indirect effects causing damage to critical molecules, which eventually lead to biologic damage. The two major effects of radiation on water molecules are excitation and ionization and are described below.

$$H_2O \rightarrow H_2O^{+\cdot} + e^- \text{ (ionization)} \quad [1]$$
$$H_2O \rightarrow H_2O^* \text{ (excitation)} \quad [2]$$

The electron e^- becomes solvated by the surrounding water molecules and is called the solvated electron (eq. 3), which can also produce H-atoms (eq. 4).

$$e^- + (H_2O)_n \rightarrow e_{ag}^- \quad [3]$$
$$e_{aq}^- + H^+ \rightarrow H\cdot \quad [4]$$

The H_2O^+ produced by ionization (eq. 1) is strongly acidic and loses a proton to the surrounding water molecules to give the hydroxyl radical $\cdot OH$.

$$H_2O^{+\cdot} + H_2O \rightarrow \cdot OH + -OH \quad [5]$$

The water molecule in the excited state (H_2O^*) can also homolyze to produce H-atoms and $\cdot OH$ radicals.

$$H_2O^* \rightarrow H\cdot + \cdot OH \quad [6]$$

The H-atoms and OH radicals should be distinguished from the protons (H +) and the hydroxide ion (− OH). H^+ and ^-OH both have their outer orbital electrons completely paired up without any free electrons, unlike for H-atoms and $\cdot OH$ radicals.

All these free-radical species react with each other within the spur (regions of high local concentrations of ionization products) or diffuse into the bulk of the solution. Solvated electrons (e_{aq}^-) can react with protons to produce H-atoms.

Recombination reactions of all the water radiolysis products in the spur are described below.

$$H\cdot + H\cdot \rightarrow H_2 \quad [7]$$
$$e_{aq}^- + e_{aq}^- \rightarrow H_2 + 2 \, ^-OH \quad [8]$$
$$\cdot OH + \cdot OH \rightarrow H_2O_2 \quad [9]$$

The primary radicals can also be converted to water in the spurs

$$H\cdot + \cdot OH \rightarrow H_2O \quad [10]$$
$$e_{aq}^- + \cdot OH \rightarrow \, ^-OH \quad [11]$$

The initial ionizing events leading to primary lesions are completed in less than 10^{-10} sec. The transfer of energy from the primary species to cause lesions on biologically important molecules such as DNA and to cause genetic or metabolic alterations is completed in less than 10^{-6} sec (1 μsec). All the above recombination reactions that occur in the spur after the initial ionizing event are practically diffusion controlled and hence are very efficient. However, considerable quantities of the radicals formed escape the spur and can be intercepted by critical biologic targets or radical scavengers. The scavenging efficiency of a given radical depends on the rate constant of reaction of the scavenger with the radical and the scavenger concentration. All the primary radical species produced by ionizing radiation are highly reactive and abstract H-atoms or add to various target molecules, causing chemical modification.

The radiochemical yields are expressed in terms of G-values. G-value is defined as the number of molecules damaged or formed per 100 eV of absorbed energy. The G-values for the various products of water radiolysis produced by 250 kV x-radiation are as follows: $e_{aq}^- = 2.63$; $\cdot OH = 2.72$; $\cdot H = 0.55$; $H_2 = 0.45$; $H_2O_2 = 0.68$. The concentration of individual species produced by 10 Gy radiation can be derived by multiplying the G-value with 1 $\times$ 10^- 1. The concentration of $\cdot OH$ radicals produced by irradiating water to a radiation dose of 1 Gy is 2.72 $\times$ $10 \rightarrow$ M.

The formation of single-strand breaks in the DNA of cells is a linear function of the dose of irradiation of the DNA solutions. For double-stranded 10^6 dalton DNA, the efficiency of single-strand breaks is 0.2–0.3 breaks/100 Gy, whereas for isolated chromatin particles, the value is 0.5–1.5 $\times$ 10^{-2}.[1,2] Are these ages or rations example, 1.5 $\times$ 10^{-2} or 1.5 $\times$ 10^{-2}. The dependence of double-strand breaks in double-stranded DNA and isolated chromatin depends on the radiation dose in a complex manner. At a dose of 100 Gy, the yield of double-strand breaks in a 10^6 dalton DNA molecule is 3–9 $\times$ 10^{-2}. The same value for chromatin is 0.6–1.7 $\times$ 10^{-4}.[3] As discussed later, a total body dose of 4.5 Gy may be lethal to a human, despite efficient chemical DNA repair mechanisms, whereas much larger doses are required for detectable DNA damage in isolated DNA and chromatin *in vitro*.

Cellular Targets in Radiation Biology

DNA is considered to be a critical target for damage induced by ionizing radiation either by direct or indirect processes.[4] However, in therapeutic radiology utilizing high-energy x-rays, damage mediated by H·, e_{aq}^- and ·OH radicals (indirect effects) are important. The rates of reactions of H·, e_{aq}^-, and ·OH radicals with free nucleic acid bases and ribose have been determined, which give information about the relative efficiencies of attack by the primary species. Based on the rate constants, the site of attack of e_{aq}^- is exclusively the *base components* of various monomeric nucleic acid compounds. H-atom also attacks heterocyclic bases rather than the sugar moiety. Approximately 20% of the ·OH radicals react with the sugar moiety. Because the product of reaction among the primary radical species with DNA is still a radical, it must further react before converting into a stable and chemically modified state. This process can occur via radical reactions in three mechanisms: (a) unimolecularly, (b) bimolecularly with other radicals, and (c) bimolecularly with another molecule. For the *in vivo* situation, the radical-molecule reaction (c), particularly with oxygen or a drug, is the relevant pathway.

DNA adducts of OH radicals are considered to be the most damaging. The damage has been found to be DNA-DNA cross-links, base damage, sugar damage leading to DNA single-strand breaks, as well as base release. Model studies of irradiated aqueous aerobic solutions of DNA have revealed (a) unaltered bases and their radiation-induced oxidation products that are released by the rupture of the N-glycosidic bond and (b) altered bases attached to DNA. The main site of OH radical attack on pyrimidines is the 5, 6 double bond leading to ring saturation. In the case of purines, OH radical attack has been suggested to mediate scission of the bond between C-8 and N-9 atoms in the imidazole ring. In the case of halogenated pyrimidines (e.g., 5-bromouracil), a uracilyl radical is formed by splitting the C-Br bond, presumably by both direct effects as well as by reaction with solvated electrons. This radical is highly reactive and can abstract an H-atom from neighboring sugar moiety. This process induces a DNA strand break as well as a uracil moiety into the DNA.

Although 20% of the OH radicals react with the sugar moiety, scission of the sugar-phosphate bond (leading to strand breaks) and release of unaltered bases can be induced by sugar radicals. It has also been proposed that radicals on base moiety can lead to strand breaks by radical transfer to sugar moiety.

Radiation Repair and Sensitization

In addition to enzymatic repair of DNA lesions caused by radiation, chemical repair can be accomplished by reducing agents, the most abundant being *reduced glutathione* as

shown in the simplified model. If TH is the critical radiobiologic target

$$TH + (x\text{-rays}) \rightarrow T\cdot + H^+ \text{ (radical formation)} \quad [12]$$

The radical site on the target can be fixed by O_2 or chemical radiosensitizers, leading to subsequent base modification or strand breaks.

$$T\cdot + O_2 \rightarrow TOO\cdot \text{ (damage fixation)} \quad [13]$$
$$T\cdot + S \rightarrow TS \quad [14]$$
$$(S = \text{sensitizer, e.g., nitric oxide or nitroxides})$$

However, glutathione can compete with the damage fixation reaction by chemical restitution by donating an H-atom.

$$T\cdot + GSH \rightarrow TH + GS\cdot \quad [15]$$

The GS· radical is an extremely weak oxidant and may not mediate further damage and forms disulfides

$$GS\cdot + GS\cdot \rightarrow GSSG$$

Lipid Peroxidation

Cellular membranes can also be damaged by radiation-induced lipid peroxidation. The initiating event is the radiation-induced formation of a radical on the membrane lipid. The radical formation can be caused by H-atom abstraction by ·OH radicals among other radiation-induced reactive intermediates.

$$RH + \cdot OH \rightarrow R\cdot + H_2O \quad [16]$$

Reaction of the radical species (R·) with oxygen produces the *lipid peroxyl* radical

$$R\cdot + O_2 \rightarrow ROO\cdot \quad [17]$$

The lipid peroxyl radicals are very unstable and form lipid hydroperoxides by reaction with other lipids by abstracting an H-atom.

$$ROO\cdot + RH \rightarrow ROOH + R\cdot \quad [18]$$

Reaction (16) is the initiating reaction in the lipid peroxidation process. After this reaction, a chain reaction is set up in the system in the presence of dissolved oxygen (reactions 17 and 18). Thus a significant amount of damage can be induced through a single initiating reaction through the process of lipid peroxidation and may also contribute to radiation-induced cytotoxicity by inducing membrane damage. The lipid peroxidation *can be inhibited by the use of antioxidants* that scavenge the initiating radical species such as ·OH radicals or by terminating the chain reaction by acting as radical acceptors. Natural antioxidants such as vitamin E are purported to terminate chain reactions by terminating reactions 17 and 18.

Importance of Free Radicals in Biology and Medicine

Generation of free radicals in biologic systems in the normal course of metabolism and abnormal states has gained increasing attention in recent years to explain several aspects of human disease processes, such as inflammation, mutagenesis, carcinogenesis and cancer, atherosclerosis and postischemic reperfusion injury of cardiac tissue, Alzheimer's disease, and Parkinson's disease.[5] In addition, free-radical intermediates in the metabolism or activation of anticancer drugs are being recognized (Adriamycin, Mitomycin C, Streptonigrin, Neocarzinostatin, etc.). In most of the cases where radicals are generated naturally by biochemical processes in the normal metabolic pathways, or in the presence of xenobiotic agents capable of generating free radicals by enzymatic processes, the radical species are similar in chemical nature and reactivity to those generated by radiolysis. Of more direct relevance to lung cancer, some of the detrimental effects of cigarette smoke have been attributed to free-radical damage, (see also Chapter 3).

CELL DEATH AND VIABILITY

Biologic tissue must possess the ability to either repair or reproduce itself in order to maintain function and the health of the organism throughout natural life span. A tumor owes part of its malignant potential to the ability of cells to reproduce in an uncontrolled way and thus grow and invade local tissues and even metastasize throughout the body. One of the most important consequences of exposing biologic tissue (and its component cells) to ionizing radiation is the loss of the cell's ability to reproduce and thus the ultimate death of the cell. Cell death is the main cause of the early and late toxic effects of radiation on normal tissues and the reason that radiation may be used to sterilize human tumors.

Such cell death must be defined. It is to be distinguished from the intuitive concept we have of death: that is, complete, instantaneous, and irreversible loss of *all* function. Although super-high doses of radiation (in the region of several hundred gray [Gy]) certainly cause such a death to occur as surely as though the cell were physically crushed, lower radiation doses (several hundred centigray [cGy]) exert no such obvious effect. In fact, the vast majority of such irradiated cells appear morphologically normal and continue to perform complex biologic functions including protein and DNA synthesis. They may even be able to pass through a limited number of mitoses and give rise to some progeny. However, in terms of the continued health of that biologic tissue, a proportion of these cells lose their ability to sustain indefinite reproduction and die at the next or subsequent mitosis, or give rise to progeny incapable of reproduction. The cell's ability to sustain indefinite reproduction and to produce "clones" of itself is referred to as its *clonogenic* potential. For many tissues, the greater the proportion of clonogenic cells damaged by ionizing radiation, the greater the perturbation on the function of that tissue. In normal tissue as well as tumors, a variable proportion of cells are clonogenic; their number is decreased by ionizing radiation. Thus both normal tissues and tumors may be damaged by radiation. In studying these biologic effects, therefore, it is particularly important to be able to determine a cell's sensitivity to loss of reproductive or clonogenic potential. Several methods have been devised to assess cell viability *in vitro* and *in vivo*. These tools are potent not only in radiation biology but also in studying the effects of other cytotoxic agents such as chemotherapy. Before examining these tools individually, the concept of the *survival curve* is explored.

IDEALIZED RADIATION DOSE-RESPONSE CURVES AND MODELING

A single cell that has retained its clonogenic viability is capable of reproducing multiple clones of itself, which may be visualized as discrete colonies in tissue culture flasks or petri dishes. This type of assay, first described by Puck and Marcus in 1956[4] provides *in vitro* evidence of clonogenic viability. Samples of normal tissues as well as tumors can be disaggregated physically and with proteolytic enzymes such as trypsin into single-cell suspensions. These cells may be seeded into culture flasks under aseptic conditions at 37°C with medium appropriate to support growth for 1 to 2 weeks. Viable cells attach to the plate and grow to form colonies that may be stained and counted. The number of single cells seeded may be counted using an automated cell counter, and therefore the *plating efficiency (PE)* for each cell suspension may be calculated. Typically, only 50% to 90% of the cells form colonies (PE = 50% to 90%) even in the absence of any cytotoxic agents. Some loss inevitably occurs due to handling or failure to accurately determine the exact numbers of cells seeded or colonies counted. Plating efficiencies may therefore be compared, in the absence of any cytotoxic agent (controls) and in the presence of various doses of the cytotoxic agent to be tested. For example, a population of such clonogenic cells may be divided into several samples, and each sample maybe exposed to increasingly larger doses of radiation. The numbers of colonies formed in each plate is expressed as a percentage of the control plate (surviving fraction, SF), and survival curves generated. To increase accuracy, samples are plated in triplicate, and results are expressed as mean values with appropriate standard deviations.

Conventionally, the results are plotted on semiogarithmic coordinates, with the doses of the test agent expressed linearly on the ordinate (x-axis), and the logarithm of the SF on the abscissa (y-axis). A smooth curve is drawn between the experimental points, allowing for the uncertainty of each

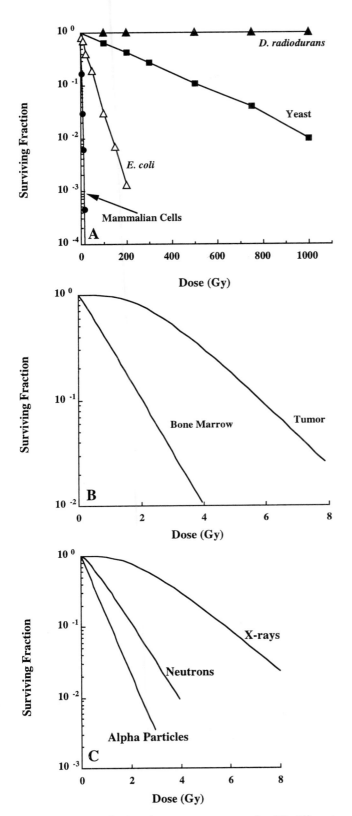

FIGURE 12.1. Radiation dose response curves for **(A)** different species, **(B)** typical human bone marrow and tumor, and **(C)** different types of radiation of varying LET.

point. The shape and slope of the curve then become important characteristics defining the response of these cells and by inference, the biologic tissues from which they derive, to the cytotoxic agent tested. Radiation survival curves may vary according to the biologic system studied (e.g., bacteria, yeast, mammalian cells), the inherent x-ray sensitivity of different mammalian cell types, and the type of radiation (e.g., x-rays, neutrons, α particles) as shown in Figure 12.1. Figure 12.1A illustrates the vast range of sensitivities among different biologic species. In particular, note how sensitive mammalian cells are when compared to other species. Figure 12.1B shows that in humans, a significant difference in radiation sensitivity may exist between normal tissue and malignant cells. This difference may be exploited for therapeutic gain, and at times may be a potential problem in terms of normal tissue toxicity. For example, bone marrow toxicity may be a significant problem when irradiation fields encompass a large quantity of bone marrow. An inability to repair the effects of densely ionizing radiation (α particles) when compared to sparsely ionizing radiation (x-rays) is illustrated in the differential response of mammalian cells to these types of radiation in Figure 12.1C.

Various mathematical functions may be used to represent these survival curves, and biophysical models have been proposed to account for their shape and characteristics. Mathematical modeling can provide values of the SF over the range of radiation doses studied. Less accurately perhaps, these mathematical models suggest biophysical theories as to how the cell might be killed. For example, surviving fractions that fall exponentially with increasing dose suggest a "single-hit, single-target" theory, where each particle traversing a cell may produce a lethal event. The total number of lethal events therefore increases in direct proportion to the dose. Although these models can provide useful guidelines in predicting biologic responses, none is precise enough to be truly representative of the complex response of living tissues to radiation. It is worthwhile, however, to examine "reference" radiation survival curves utilizing X- or γ-rays given over a short time under well-oxygenated conditions. *Exponential* ("straight") survival curves, as well as survival curves with *initial shoulders* ("curved") are described, and three of the many mathematical models used to predict responses in this dose range are outlined.

Exponential Survival Curves

The relationship between the surviving fraction (SF) and the radiation dose (D) is given by the mathematical equation

$$SF = e^{-\alpha D}$$

where α is a constant and e is the base of the natural logarithm

We now define a specific dose, the mean lethal dose (D_0), which reduces the SF to 37% of the initial cell number.

Thus when $D_0 = 1/\alpha$

$$SF = e^{-D/D0}$$

$$\log SF = -\alpha(D)$$

This equation is now in the form of a general equation [y = m(x)], describing a line with a slope m. On semilogarithmic coordinates, this plots a "straight" line with slope

$$m = -\alpha \text{ or } -1/D_0$$

Thus D_0 becomes an important comparative number when evaluating radiation sensitivity of cells or tissues. D_0 is the dose (on an exponential curve, or portion of a curve) that reduces the surviving fraction of the cells to 37% of the number present prior to irradiation. Further, because D_0 is inversely related to α ($D_0 = 1/\alpha$), the slope of the line ($-\alpha$) provides a visual demonstration of the sensitivity of the tissues irradiated. The steeper the slope, the more sensitive the tissue, and the smaller the D_0. It now becomes possible to compare at a glance the radiation sensitivity of cell populations or tissues that fit an exponential modeling curve when irradiated. Furthermore, because no shoulder (or flat portion) is present on this curve, no dose exists, however small, which will not bring about some cell kill. This distinction from survival curves with initial flatter portions or "shoulder" as described below is important.

Survival Curves with an Initial Shoulder

Mammalian cells irradiated with x- or γ-rays generally show some curvature or "shoulder" in the initial (or low-dose) segment of the survival curve. Often, although not invaria-

bly, at higher radiation doses the curve becomes straight with a constant exponential slope downwards as shown in Figure 12.2A. Because the initial curved portion cannot be described by a line equation with a single slope, as is true of the exponential lines, the concept of a mean lethal dose (D^0) cannot be used to define radiation sensitivity at low doses in mammalian survival curves. This concept is particularly important because daily doses of radiation used in the clinic (150 to 200 cGy) often fall in this low-dose region of the curve. Two other parameters, the *extrapolation number* (ñ) and the *quasi-threshold dose (D_q)* are used to characterize the width of the initial shoulder. These parameters become important when attempting to characterize the sensitivity of mammalian cells to the radiation dose fraction sizes used in cancer treatment. Extrapolation of the terminal "straight" portion of the mammalian curve back to the point at which it intersects the abscissa, defines ñ. Thus when ñ is large (10.0 to 15.0), the survival curve has a broad shoulder, and when ñ is small (1.2 to 2.0) the shoulder is narrow. The dose point at which the same extrapolated line intersects the dose axis at SF = 1 defines the quasi-threshold dose (D_q). The quasi-threshold dose may be thought of as that dose below which no measurable effect of the radiation on cell killing occurs. Both parameters define the size of the initial shoulder and may define the cell's ability to repair sublethal radiation damage (see following). The three parameters $D\rightarrow$, D_q and ñ are linked together by the equation:

$$\log_e (ñ) = D_q/D_0$$

Doses at or around the D_q on the curved portion of the curve are interesting in that each incremental increase in

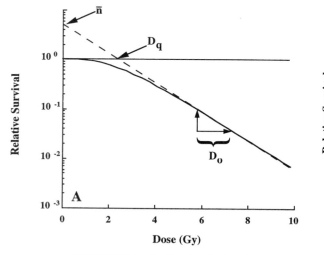

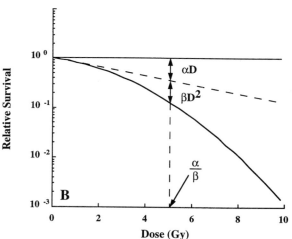

FIGURE 12.2. Idealized radiation dose-response curves. **A:** exhibits survival parameters based on the multitarget, single-hit model. The terms extrapolation number (ñ), quasi-threshold dose (D_q), and mean lethal dose (D_0) are defined in the text. **B:** shows a survival curve based on the linear-quadratic model. Note how the curve has an initial slope and lacks a terminal "straight" or exponential portion. The α/β ratio, or the dose at which the linear and quadratic components of cell killing are equal in this example, is ~5Gy.

dose produces a proportionally larger (as opposed to equivalent) effect on cell kill. This response suggests that cell death may be resulting from an accumulation of effects on critical targets, where individual "hits" are ineffectual or sublethal but become lethal when added together. Alternatively, the cell may be less efficient at repairing sublethal damage when it accumulates. Several mathematical models have been proposed to fit such "shouldered" survival curves. Three of the more popular models are further described.

Single-Hit Multitarget Model

In this model, as opposed to a single critical target, the cell is theorized to have multiple (n) targets, all of which must be inactivated before the cell is killed. The cell surviving fraction (SF) in this model is given by the equation:

$$SF = 1 - (1 - e^{-D/D0})^n$$

Thus when n = 1, as in the single-hit model, the equation solves to $SF = e^{-D/D0}$ as shown previously. Furthermore, as the dose (D) gets larger, then SF tends toward $n(e^{-D/D0})$, which is an exponential line with slope $-1/D_0$ intercepting the ordinate at the extrapolation point (ñ). Note also that this curve starts out with zero initial slope, which infers zero mortality from small radiation doses. This property does not with most experimental results and is further discussed in following sections.

Quadratic Model

Cell death in this model is caused by the addition of two independent "hits" on a single critical target, from two separate radiation-induced particles. The mean number of lethal events is proportional to the square of the dose, so the SF is given by the equation:

$$SF = e^{-\beta D^2}$$

Here β is a constant relating to the probability of a dose of radiation producing a sublethal event. Note that this equation also plots a line with zero initial slope. Thus the "single-hit multitarget" and "quadratic" models are probably not accurate when dealing with the response of mammalian cells to small doses of radiation. One further model is described to address this important point.

Linear-Quadratic Model

This model assumes that cell killing was two components. One component is proportional to the given dose (D), and the second is proportional to the square of the given dose (D^2). The equation that plots this survival curve is

$$SF = -e^{\alpha D - \beta D^2}$$

Here α and β are constants of proportionality. The components of cell kill proportional to the dose and square of the dose are equal when

$$\alpha D = \beta D^2$$
$$D = \alpha/\beta$$

Expressing this relationship in words, the linear and quadratic components of cell killing are equal at a dose equal to the α/β ratio. Such a curve is shown in Figure 12.2B. It has an initial slope (α), so it is perhaps a better predictor of the response of mammalian cells to low doses of radiation. However, such a curve continuously curves downward with increasing dose, which does not correlate well with the exponential ("straight") response to larger radiation doses in actual experiments.

Thus no single mathematical model accurately fits experimentally observed cell survival across a broad range of radiation doses. The linear-quadratic model is a useful representation of the data, however, because it has only two adjustable parameters and is accurate in the range of doses used in daily standard fractionated radiation therapy.[6] This model is often used when predicting the biologic effect of altering radiation-dose fractionation schemes and comparing them to standard (180–200 cGy per day) treatment regimens. The coefficients α and β relate to the two modes of cell killing, and the α/β ratio thus gives an indication about the relative importance of each. When α is large relative to β, the α/β ratio is high and the survival curve slopes steeply and near exponentially. Early-reacting normal tissues and tumors tend to have high α/β ratios. When β is large relative to α, the curve starts out with a shallow slope and a broad shoulder. This response is typical of late-reacting normal tissues. α/β ratio is a dose expressed in Gy; α is expressed in Gy^{-1} and β in Gy^{-2}.

Predictive Assays

In vitro assays of radiosensitivity are important tools in radiobiology with the potential to guide clinical practice. If *in vitro* assays of radiosensitivity truly reflect *in vivo* radiosensitivity, then such assays may prove to be of considerable help in predicting those patients who are potentially curable with radiation, and those perhaps requiring more aggressive multimodality treatment. Several candidate factors, including hypoxia, clonogenic cell number, and intrinsic tumor cell radiosensitivity, have all been tested as potential predictive assays in this context. One assay, the fraction of cells surviving a dose of 2 Gy (SF 2Gy) has recently received much attention. The observation was originally made by Fertil and Malaise[7] and Deacon et al.[8] that the radiosensitivity of cell lines derived from human tumors was characteristic of tumor type, and that tumors more difficult to cure in the clinic produced cell lines that are more resistant to low doses of radiation *in vitro*. The technique involves disaggregating tumor cells enzymatically, attaching cells as single-cell suspensions to tissue culture plates, irradiating the cells typically over dose ranges of 0.5 to 6.0 Gy, incubating the irradiated cells in culture medium for up to 2 weeks, then assaying for surviving fraction. The data derived are typically fitted to the linear-quadratic modeling described previously and survival curves are generated. From these curves, the SF 2 Gy may be derived. Several preliminary reports are now available comparing clinical local control with SF 2Gy, and in at least some instances, a correlation is emerging. This assay has problems, however,[10] and as yet no consensus has been reached as to whether it will prove clinically useful enough to be routinely used.

REPAIR OF RADIATION DAMAGE

If cells could successfully repair all radiation damage, then ionizing radiation would produce no lasting biologic effect. Fortunately for the radiation oncologist, absolutely radioresistant cells do not exist. Biologic tissues clearly possess a differential ability to accumulate and repair radiation damage. Irradiated cells can be shown to behave differently *in vivo* versus *in vitro*. Malignant cells often fail to adequately repair accumulated radiation damage that is effectively repaired by normal tissue. An understanding of radiation damage and repair is helpful in exploiting the differential response of normal tissues and tumor cells, and thus the effective use of radiation in the treatment of cancer. Two operationally defined terms, *sublethal damage repair* (SLDR) and *potentially lethal damage repair* (PLDR) have been coined to account for the observation that cells can survive radiation under certain conditions. Although these terms were originally defined in an abstract way, without reference to the molecular or subcellular entities experiencing the actual radiation damage, a wealth of experimental data now exists to support the concepts, and perhaps to allow for the design of therapeutic strategies in the treatment of cancer.[11]

Potentially Lethal Damage Repair

It was found that by altering a cell's environment following radiation, a proportion of the radiation injury could be obviated. This phenomenon was observed both in normal tissues and tumors, and it suggested that a component of radiation damage is repairable under certain environmental conditions and irreparable in others. *In vitro,* allowing cells to remain in a density-inhibited state (plateau phase) for several hours postirradiation, or incubating them in a balanced salt solution instead of culture medium, leads to improved survival indicative of PLDR. Similar conditions may be mimicked *in vivo*. For example, mouse thyroid or mammary cells may be irradiated *in situ*, then transplanted into a fat pad for survival assay. If the transplant is delayed several hours, then enhanced survival is seen, which is thought to be caused by PLDR.[12] The hypothesis underlying such observations is that a *porportion of radiation damage may be repaired if cells are somehow prevented from attempting the complex process of mitosis and cell division for a period following the radiation.* This theory may then be of relevance to both normal tissues and tumors.

Normal tissues are often in a resting (nondividing) state akin to plateau-phase cell cultures *in vitro*. Tumors under certain conditions (e.g., nutritional impairment, hypoxia, etc.) may be unable to cycle a proportion of their cells through mitosis and thus create PLDR efficiently. The exact relevance of PLDR in the clinic is uncertain. No good evidence supports a differential in PLDR between normal and malignant tissue, so it is difficult to define a method to exploit this phenomenon in the clinic.[12] It is noteworthy that the *quality* of the radiation is important in PLDR. It has been shown that PLDR does not occur following densely ionizing (high-LET) irradiation, such as neutrons, but can be shown in the same cells irradiated with sparsely ionizing (low-LET) irradiation, such as ^{50}Co γ-rays.[13] The relevance of this finding in terms of the mechanism of such repair is unknown.

Sublethal Damage Repair

As discussed previously, the survival curve for mammalian cells irradiated *in vitro* has a characteristic shape (Figure 12.2A). The initial portion of the curve is shallower, sweeping downward in a continuously curving "shoulder" of varying magnitude and extent. The terminal portion has a steeper slope and falls "exponentially." The general interpretation of the initial shoulder region is that a proportion of the radiation damage is being repaired and therefore not producing lethality. After sufficient radiation damage has been accumulated, each additional dose causes exponential cell kill. Although these lower radiation doses are not producing exponential cell kill, they are causing "sublethal" damage, which the cell appears capable of repairing under appropriate conditions. The association between the initial shoulder on the survival curve and SLDR has been well established.[14] Bacterial cells genetically deficient in repair enzymes, such as (rec-) *E. coli*, have exponentially falling survival curves with no shoulder (Figure 12.1A). Herein lies one of the most important observations in radiobiology: Mammalian cells exposed to smaller doses of radiation (i.e., in the initial "shoulder" region) can repair proportion of the radiation damage ("sublethal damage") given sufficient time and nutrients. *A proportion of the cells irradiated,* however, will sustain lethal damage and will not survive. Adding a second small dose of radiation reproduces exactly the same initial curve, and kill the same proportion of the remaining cells (Figure 12.3). The survival curve for multifractionated irradiation can be generated by joining these curves as shown. Theoretically, this curve approaches an exponential decline, with a uniform albeit *shallower* slope than seen with acute single-dose exposures. The broader the shoulder, the greater the capacity for repair. In general, the

Radiation Biology **221**

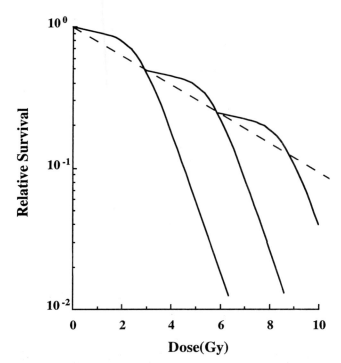

FIGURE 12.3. Theoretical survival curves illustrating the effect of repeated administration of 3 Gy doses of radiation to a population of mammalian cells. Because of the cells' capacity to repair sublethal damage caused by these doses, a proportion of the cells survive each time, giving rise to the shoulder. The net effect of such fractionation yields an exponentially falling curve (*dotted line*) much shallower than when single doses are used (*solid lines*). Thus the "sparing" effect of radiation dose fractionation.

survival curves of late-reacting normal tissues have such "shoulders." Thus multifractionated radiation schedules, using small doses per fraction, tend to spare late reactions in normal tissues.

Evidence for this important phenomenon was first provided in the classic studies of Elkind and Sutton.[15] In a series of experiments comparing the lethality of a large single dose of radiation with the same total dose, split into two smaller fractions and separated by a time interval (fractionated irradiation), it was shown that the split dose produced *less* lethality.[16] The interval between the two fractions allows SLDR. The half-time for this repair has been estimated at 0.5 to 1.5 hours depending on the cells studied.[14] The *fading-time* has been defined as the time taken for this repair to decay to an undetectable level (e.g., less than 5%). Thus one can calculate that in acute-reacting cells, including most tumors, where SLDR is less developed (e.g., less than 20%), the fading-time would be three to four hours for acute effects. In late-reacting normal tissues, where sublethal damage repair may be significant (50%), the fading-time may be on the order of 5 to 6 hours for late effects. As a direct consequence of these observations, clinical studies using altered radiation-dose fractionation (e.g., hyperfractionation)

have usually incorporated a time interval of at least 6 hours between fractions to avoid severe late normal tissue reactions.[17] Such studies involving patients with head and neck cancers,[18] as well as small cell lung cancer (SCLC)[19] have generally shown equivalent to improved local control rates with acceptable long-term toxicities. Just as has been observed in the case of PLDR, sublethal damage is significant for low-LET radiation, including x-rays, but is insignificant following neutron-beam irradiation.[12]

Dose-Rate Effect

The sparing effect of fractionating a radiation dose over time has been explained by the SLDR in those cells whose survival curve is characterized by an initial "shoulder" (e.g., late-reacting normal mammalian tissues). As shown previously, it is a feature of low-LET irradiation (i.e., X- and γ-rays) and is not seen for high-LET irradiation (i.e., neutrons, α-particles, etc.). Stated a different way, a given single dose of radiation tends to spare normal tissues if it is protracted over time. Dose fractionation is one example of protracting the treatment time to spare such tissue. A second example is provided *by slowing the rate* at which a single continuous dose is given. This process is referred to as the *dose-rate effect*. This effect has been demonstrated *in vitro* as well as *in vivo* and is an important radiobiologic tenet underlying effective administration of radiation in the clinic. Reducing the dose-rate at which certain cell lines are irradiated *in vitro* shows a progressive sparing effect, most marked between 1 to 100 cGy/min as shown in Figure 12.4.[20–22] Tremendous variability exists among differing cell lines irradiated at varying dose-rates *in vitro*, depending on their ability to accumulate and create SLDR.[12] Furthermore, little if any additional effect is seen at rates above 100 cGy/min. However, over a range of dose rates between 0.3 to 1.6 cGy/min, a paradoxical "inverse" dose-rate effect is observed (Figure 12.4); the survival curve becomes steeper once again as cell-cycle effects increase the radiation sensitivity and outweigh the effect of SLDR.[21] Of course, similar to fractionating radiation doses, little benefit would be gained in altering dose-rates in the clinic, if the lower dose-rates also spared tumor cells. Fortunately, data suggest that tumor cells do not show the same response to altered dose-rates as to normal tissue.[12] The EMT6 mammary sarcoma and the KHT sarcoma in the mouse show much less sparing effect to reduced dose-rates than normal tissues.[23,24] Thus we may begin to exploit the differential response of normal and malignant cells to varying radiation dose-rate.

The dose-rate effect has proven to be important in the response of both normal lung and lung tumors to radiation. Clinical and experimental studies have clearly shown a marked sparing effect in the lung as a result of fractionating radiation doses.[25–27] *In vivo* assays in the mouse model showed a sparing effect of low dose-rate irradiation in terms of the development of radiation pneumonitis.[28] Histologic

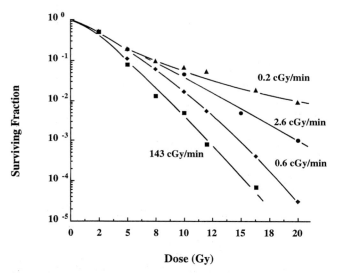

FIGURE 12.4. Radiation dose-response curves for human S3 HeLa cells exposed to varying dose-rates of continuous radiation. Note that as the dose-rate is lowered, a greater proportion of the cells survive. Note also the paradoxic increased killing at 0.6 cGy/min, which is caused by cell cycle blockade. At this dose-rate, the cells are selectively blocked at G2/M, a more radiosensitive phase of the cell cycle. (From Mitchell JB, Bedford JS, Bailey SM. Dose-rate effects in mammalian cells in culture III. Comparison of cell killing and cell proliferation during continuous irradiation for six different cell lines. *Radiat Res* 1979;79:537, with permission.)

comparison of radiation reactions in the lungs of mini-pigs exposed to 750 cGy total body irradiation revealed a quantitative effect on the lungs with higher dose-rates (25 cGy/min) when compared to lower dose-rates (5 cGy/min).[29] Radiation pneumonitis in humans has been shown to correlate not only with absolute dose within the lung[30] but also with dose rate.[31] Experience with wide-field irradiation, including hemibody and total body irradiation, estimates that a dose of 930 cGy at 50 cGy/min is equivalent to 1,100 cGy at 10 cGy/min. Protocols using total-body irradiation for marrow transplant have sought to avoid lung toxicity by limiting the dose-rate to the lungs to the region of 10 cGy/min.[32]

Limited data exist on radiation dose-rate effects in lung carcinoma cells in culture. When clonogenic survival alone is used as an end point, sparing effect of dose-rate reduction may be expressed as a dose-reduction factor (DRF).[33,34] This factor is defined as the ratio of doses required to reduce clonogenic survival (for example to 1%), at low and high dose-rates. A series of four lung cancer lines so studied showed DRFs ranging from 1.19 to 1.57. No clear correlation between the overall radiation sensitivity of these lines and the DRF could be seen.[34] However, the more radiosensitive SCLC lines showed significantly more residual DNA damage (double-strand breaks), suggesting a failure of these cells to produce SLDR even at low dose-rates, whereas the more resistant non–small cell lung cancer (NSCLC) lines showed significantly less residual DNA damage, in keeping with efficient repair at low dose-rates. Lung carcinoma lines in culture exhibit a marked heterogeneity in response to varying dose rates, as shown in Figure 12.5.[35] Although NSCLC lines (NCI-H460 and A549) show increased survival at low dose-rates, the SCLC line (NCI-H69) shows no such variation in response.

These findings suggest a possible strategy for improving the therapeutic outcome in SCLC. A reduced dose-rate (1 to 5 cGy/min) in SCLC would effect cell killing equivalent to standard/high dose-rate irradiation (100 to 200 cGy/min), with less toxicity to normal tissue (e.g., lung and esophagus). This strategy has been recently brought to clinical trial at the National Cancer Institute (NCI), and early tumor responses are encouraging, with a suggestion of less acute toxicity. Should tumor response rates be equivalent to standard radiation responses, with less acute toxicity, this might allow for the possibility of escalating the total radiation dose and/or treating greater tumor volumes.

RESPONSE OF NORMAL TISSUES TO RADIATION

The differential response of normal tissue and tumors underlies the successful use of ionizing radiation in treating cancer patients. In order to predict the likelihood of sterilizing a tumor and protecting the surrounding normal tissues, we must have some method of assaying radiation effects *in vivo* as well as *in vitro*. Here the biologic end points of relevance are altered structure or loss of function of a tissue or organ. When considering the radiotolerance of tissue, the critical targets may be thought of as functional subunits, and the tolerance of the tissue is related to the number as well as the radiosensitivity of such units. Biologic tissue consists of a heterogenous population of living cells, interacting in a complex fashion. Clinical effects of radiation are not predictable solely on the basis of cell kill but on a host of interrelated variables that may be difficult to accurately quantitate. It is recognized, however, that death of critical cells or functional subunits may contribute significantly to loss of function of the tissue or organ. Thus clonogenic assays that can quantitate cell death *in vivo* may predict functional impairment within tissue. This process is particularly dramatic in tissues consisting of cells that are proliferating rapidly as part of their normal function (e.g., bone marrow, gastrointestinal mucosa, testis, skin, hair follicles). Clonogenic assays can be used to construct dose-response curves reflecting the radiosensitivity of such tissues. The dose required to see a measurable effect on the function of such a tissue is termed the *threshold dose* and may be quite low, depending on the intrinsic radiosensitivity of the individual cells.

A second strategy for estimating radiation effects in tis-

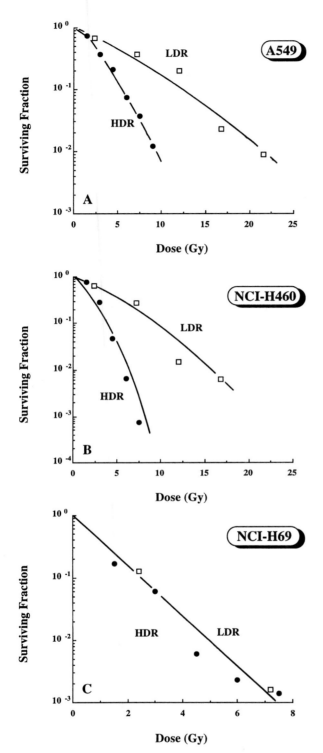

FIGURE 12.5. Radiation dose-response curves for three human tumor cell lines as a function of dose-rate (HDR = 100 cGy/min, LDR = 1 cGy/min). **A:** A549, adenocarcinoma. **B:** NCI-H460, adeno-carcinoma. **C:** NCI-H69, small cell. The non–small cell lines have shouldered survival curves and exhibit a dose-rate sparing effect, whereas small cell carcinoma has an exponential curve, and survival is unaffected by altering dose-rate. (From Sullivan FJ, Carmichel J, Glatstein E et al. Radiation biology of lung cancer. *J Cell Biochem* 1996;24:152, with permission.)

sues relies on loss of observed function (including death of the animal) with increasing radiation dose. Such assays have been described for normal lung, skin, and spinal cord tissues among others. The following sections discuss the tolerance of various organs and biologic systems to irradiation. The concept of radiotolerance needs to be further defined. Individual variability makes medicine an inexact "science." Nothing better exemplifies this concept than the tolerance of human tissue to ionizing radiation. Extrapolating *in vitro* and animal data to humans is a risky business. Nonetheless, this process and the collective (and often empiric) observations of clinicians in the practice of radiotherapy, guide us in treating patients. Ideally, one would like to know the tolerance of the whole body and each organ system (e.g., respiratory, gastrointestinal, neurologic, etc.) to both single doses as well as fractionated irradiation. In practice, these data are not completely available. For some situations, the only available information is the dose of irradiation that is known to kill 50% of animals tested. Such lethal dose (LD_{50}) data are available from a variety of sources for different animal models as well as organ systems.[36] The most widely utilized measure of radiotolerance in the human is the tolerance dose (TD) system described by Rubin et al.[37] This system assesses a percentage risk of a complication occurring within a given time interval after treatment. The $TD_{5/5}$ represents a 5% risk of severe complication within 5 years. This percentage is usually taken as the minimal tolerance dose. The $TD_{50/5}$ represents a 50% chance of severe reaction within 5 years. These doses are limited in that they make no allowance for patient age, nutritional status, or the presence of other important factors such as prior surgery, chemotherapy, or irradiation. Recent attempts have been made to review accepted normal tissue tolerance levels with respect to the influence of volumes irradiated.[38] It should be borne in mind that these doses are only guidelines and may be overridden in certain clinical situations. For example, it may be perfectly reasonable to expose a patient to a higher than usually considered acceptable risk of radiation injury if the clinical situation warrants intervention, if no reasonable alternative is available and if the patient is fully informed and accepts such risk. In general, however, clinicians prefer not to exceed quoted doses, especially in an environment dominated by fear of litigation. These data are provided, together with experimental models where available, and clinical information for each body system.

Cell Death in Tissue: Necrosis and Apoptosis

The classic observation by Kerr et al. in the early 1970s of a distinct mode of cell death, distinguishable histologically and in other ways from necrosis, paved the way for a fascinating series of observations concerning a genetically programmed cell death.[39] *Apoptosis,* or *programmed cell death*

TABLE 12.1. FEATURES OF CELLULAR NECROSIS

- Early plasma membrane changes leading to a loss of K^+, influx of Ca^{++} and Na^+
- Acidosis
- Osmotic shock caused by uptake of water
- Blebbing of the cell surface
- Clumping of chromatin and nuclear pyknosis

These changes are accompanied by:
- Activation of mitochondrial phospholipase
- A loss of oxidative phosphorylation
- A drop in ATP production and a loss of synthetic and homeostatic capability
- Random DNA degradation by lysosomal enzymes

(PCD) has since been reported as a consequence of a bewildering variety of stimuli and may be important in several disease states.[40,41] *Cellular necrosis* is a consequence of environmental insults such as hypoxia, toxins, complement attack, hyperthermia, viral lysis, and so on, and follows a relatively well-defined morphologic and biochemical path (Table 12.1). Apoptosis, on the other hand, shows morphologic features quite distinct from necrosis. The original description by Kerr was "shrinking necrosis" (Table 12.2).

Although the final pathway of both processes has similarities, the triggering events are very distinct. PCD is a highly active process requiring energy (ATP) and signaling factors including calcium[42] essential for the activation of specific endonucleases.[43] A burst of cellular protein and RNA synthetic activity always precedes PCD, and inhibition of endonuclease activity, such as by protein inhibitors (actinomycin-D, cycloheximide), blocks apoptosis. This process is not true of necrosis, which is accompanied by a loss of protein synthesis and a decline in oxidative phosphorylation that is not affected by actinomycin D.

Apoptosis has been shown following irradiation in several systems.[44-47] The intriguing phenomenon of interphase death in lymphocytes following irradiation suggested a role for apoptosis.[48-50] The rapidity of onset of this mode of death (6 to 7 hours)[44] offers perhaps a more appealing explanation for the well-known ability of radiation to induce measurable and rapid shrinkage in certain tumors,[51] and

TABLE 12.2. FEATURES OF APOPTOSIS

- Cell-to-cell contact breaks down early
- Loss of cellular features such as microvilli and desmosomes
- Distinct margination and blebbing of chromatin
- Chromatolysis involving the activation of endonuclease, the chromatin is cleaved into nonfunctional fragments of *180 to 190 base pair DNA* (laddering)
- The cell ruptures into several membrane-bound spheres (apoptotic bodies) and is phagocytosed by neighboring cells or macrophages

early acute reactions in normal tissues, than mitotic-linked death. Attempts are currently underway to link apoptosis in the causation of acute radiation effects in the clinic.

"Acute" and "Late" Radiation Reactions

The effects of ionizing radiation on biologic tissues can be usefully considered in two categories. Those occurring during or immediately following the course of radiation are considered "acute" or "early," whereas those occurring months to years after completing therapy are termed "chronic" or "late." The exact chronology of these events is not strictly defined, and some authors have preferred the terms "acute," "subacute," "chronic," and "late," depending on the time of observation.[52,53] We will define "acute/subacute" effects as those occurring during and up to 6 months, and "late" effects as those occurring from 6 months to several years from treatment. These terms are important not only in understanding the pathophysiology of radiation effects, but also in counseling patients receiving radiation therapy in the clinic.

Acute Effects

As noted previously, reproductive cell death is thought to be the most important consequence of radiating biologic tissue. The *threshold dose* is that which kills a sufficiently large proportion of the cells so that a measurable effect may be observed in the tissue. Actively cycling cells are particularly sensitive to the effects of ionizing radiation and undergo mitotic-linked death when attempting reproduction. It follows, therefore, that tissues composed predominantly of actively cycling cells (e.g., bone marrow, gastrointestinal mucosa, skin, and rapidly growing tumors) are most susceptible to cell kill, and furthermore manifest a measurable radiation effect relatively quickly after doses in excess of the threshold dose.[54] Such tissues in which active cell division is required to maintain the function of the organ are often referred to as *acutes reacting tissues*. It is further true that loss of a cell destined to undergo differentiation along multiple lines, such as a pluripotent stem cell in the bone marrow, also results in loss of all potential progeny, and therefore exerts a greater biologic effect than loss of a relatively well-differentiated cell, such as a late normoblast or mature myelocyte.[14] The radiation sensitivity of each tissue thus depends to a great extent on the number and cell cycle kinetics of these target or stem cells.

Nonetheless, measurable effects of radiation can sometimes be encountered in a matter of hours, too fast to be easily explained by cells attempting to undergo mitosis. The link between apoptosis (PCD) and radiation has been recently established as described previously. The rapidity of apoptotic cell death (hours) is a more appealing explanation for rapid onset "acute" radiation reactions and may well be an important component of such events. This correlation has not as yet been definitively shown. In addition to actual cell death, it should further be borne in mind that the body's reaction to acute injury of any kind, including inflammatory response, hyperemia, edema, release of chemotactic, and other factors, also underlies the acute radiation reaction.[55] Such effects are important in the body's homeostasis and repair of radiation injury to normal tissues. In practice, virtually all patients undergoing therapeutic irradiation experience acute symptoms caused by radiation injury to normal tissues in the irradiated field. These symptoms range in severity from insignificant to severe and at times life-threatening. Acute reactions are usually rapidly repaired and completely reversible. The vast majority resolve within 4 to 6 weeks of completing the course of therapy. These effects are further elaborated by individual body system in following sections.

Late Effects

In contradistinction to acute radiation effects, "late" effects differ in time course and natural history from acute reactions. The onset is usually several months following completion of therapy, and they are generally irreversible. The degree to which a late side effect of radiation is clinically important is highly variable. Although patients treated with modern radiation technique almost invariably experience self-limiting acute effects that are clinically apparent, the occurrence of clinically significant late effects is far less common. The occurrence of an acute reaction is not necessarily predictive of subsequent late reactions. The pathologic hallmarks are *fibrosis, atrophy, vascular damage,* and less frequently *necrosis.* Although the exact cause of late effects is debatable, it seems likely that a combination of *direct* cytotoxicity on tissue stem cells, allied to *indirect effects* from damage to microenvironmental supporting tissues (e.g., vascular and lymphatic systems) is important.

Tissues particularly at risk for late reactions are generally those with slow cellular renewal and long cell cycle times. Reduction in the number of stem cells[56] and loss of reproductive ability in those remaining have both been implicated in the genesis of late reactions. The slower proliferation rate and longer cell cycle times (months to years) account for the delayed onset and gradual manifestation of these effects. For example, it has been shown that the turnover time of normal tissue endothelium in the mouse is estimated to be 20 to 2,000 times longer (47 to 23,000 days) than tumor cells derived from the same animal (2.4 to 13 days).[57] In addition, loss of vascular endothelial and other supporting stromal cells along with growth and regulatory factors may also play a role.[58] Although the latent interval between radiation and late effects shortens with increasing total radiation dose,[59] the severity of these effects worsens with increasing radiation dose-fraction size. It has been suggested that stem cells in late-reacting tissues may have a better capacity

to repair damage from smaller fraction of radiation, possibly related to the prolonged cell cycle times, than early-reacting stem cells.[58]

The following sections detail the response of those normal tissues most often irradiated in the radiation management of lung cancer. The skin, gastrointestinal tract, and bone marrow are early-reacting tissues, whereas the spinal cord and lung are late-reacting.

Skin

Skin is a complex structure comprising an epidermis and dermis. The epidermis contains keratinocytes, dendritic cells, melanocytes, Langerhans cells, and hair follicles. It is regenerated from proliferative units in the basal layer. The epidermis is a rapidly proliferating (acute-reacting) body tissue. The dermis is a dense connective tissue containing fibroblasts, sebaceous glands, and lymphovascular channels, which play a major role in the radiation response. It is considered a slowly proliferating (late-reacting) tissue. Thus the full spectrum of normal tissue reactions, both acute and chronic, are easily seen in the skin and are a common feature of clinical radiotherapy.

Clinical Features. The acute and chronic skin reactions are listed in Table 12.3. The hallmark of acute damage is *erythema,* which appears in three phases.[58] Erythema is the result of keratinocyte damage in the epidermis and dilatation of superficial blood vessels in the dermis. The phases are early (within 24 hours of a single dose of 4.5 to 5.0 Gy) lasting 2 to 3 days; main erythematous reaction (appearing within 8 days of a single 8 to 10 Gy dose) peaking within 8 days; and a third phase, which sometimes develops 6 to 7 weeks following a course of irradiation and lasts 2 to 3 weeks. Marked erythema is seen to conform exactly to the irradiated portal. Intermediate doses of irradiation (10 to 12 Gy single dose) produce *dry desquamation* within 1 month. High (15 Gy single-dose) or tumoricidal fractionated doses kill all basal cells and expose the underlying der-

TABLE 12.3. CLINICAL FEATURES OF RADIATION SKIN INJURY

Acute	Chronic
• Erythema	• Atrophy
-early phase	• Thickening/fibrosis
-main phase	• Telangiectasia
-postirradiation phase	• Sebaceous gland dysfunction
• Dry desquamation	• Impaired sweating and
• Moist desquamation	temperature control
• Bulla formation	• Altered pigmentation
• Altered pigmentation	• Altered hair growth and color
• Altered hair growth	• Necrosis
and color	• Carcinogenesis
• Impaired wound healing	• Impaired wound healing

mis. Serous weeping from the exposed dermis is termed *moist desquamation.* Very high doses of irradiation result in epidermal necrosis with separation of the epidermis from the dermis and bulla formation. Melanocytes are located in the basal layer of the epidermis at a 1:10 ratio to the keratinocytes and produce melanin, which pigments human skin and hair.[60] Stimulation of the melanocytes after irradiation may produce increased melanin, which may be deposited in the dermis and appear as increased *pigmentation.* Higher doses may kill melanocytes and cause depigmentation. Altered pigmentation is a feature of both acute and chronic radiation injury.[61] Actively growing hair follicles are particularly radiosensitive. It has been estimated that as many as 86% of scalp follicles are in the anagen phase at any point in time,[61] thus hair loss and pigment change is a feature of radiation skin injury. The extent of loss and subsequent recovery is a function of radiation dose. Permanent *alopecia* may result from high doses. Added insult from chemotherapy may also affect recovery. Late radiation changes produce atrophy, hyperkeratosis, fibrosis, telangiectasia, and marked reduction in resistance to subsequent injury (infection, surgery, chemotherapy, etc.). Reduction in dermal fibroblasts, and cross-linking of collagen result in loss of elasticity.[58] Altered sweat gland function is particularly important in patients receiving total electron skin therapy for diseases such as mycosis fungoides. Increased risk of *carcinogenesis* is most marked in children and patients receiving low doses of radiation (2 to 10 Gy). Low doses are thought more likely to induce mutations, whereas high doses sterilize irradiated skin. The Radiation Therapy Oncology Group (RTOG) and European Organization for Research and Treatment of Cancer (EORTC) have defined clinical grading criteria for skin injury due to radiation.[62] These grading systems are useful for ensuring uniformity in reporting radiation toxicities.

Radiobiologic Features. Since the earliest observation of radiation-induced skin changes by Freund in 1897, an im-

mense amount of radiation biology has been learned by the study of various skin model systems. Both clonogenic and functional assays have been described, and much important time dose fractionation (TDF) information has been applied to radiation treatment strategies. The following section outlines the model systems used and lists the basic radiobiologic information derived.

Clonogenic Assays. Classic studies by Withers provided *in vivo* clonogenic data for radiation reactions in mouse skin.[63–65] Data deriving from these experiments are shown in Table 12.4.

Functional Assays. Classic observations by Strandqvist[66] on 280 patients undergoing skin irradiation at various TDF schedules attempted to define isoeffect curves for the irradiation of human skin. Further work by Ellis[67,68] and Fowler et al.[69–71] brought to light the importance of number of fractions used as well as the overall treatment time. The observation of acute and long-term effects on the skin of rodents as well as pigs has provided invaluable information regarding skin tolerance and the effects of fractionation. Pig skin is remarkably similar to human skin in many respects. Fowler derived a scale of acute reactions to irradiation.[69] The acute and long-term reactions were found to correlate well with those observable in humans. The expense of the pig model led to the development of similar models in rodents, and scales of acute and long-term reactions have proven reproducible in these studies.[36]

Gastrointestinal Tract

The vast majority of patients irradiated for lung cancer receive an obligatory radiation dose to the esophagus. The anatomic proximity of this organ to the lung and mediastinum make this treatment unavoidable. Anatomically, the entire length of the gastrointestinal (GI) tract shares common generalized structural features. From superficial to deep, the major subdivisions are mucosa, submucosa, mus-

TABLE 12.4. SKIN: BASIC RADIOBIOLOGIC PARAMETERS

- Single dose $D_0 = 1.35$ Gy (mouse skin) Range tested 8 to 25 Gy [Withers]
- Quasi-threshold dose $D_q = 3.5$ Gy (mouse skin)
- Rate of loss of basal (stem) cells = 2.6% +/− 0.2% per day (pig skin) following single and fractionated doses [Bernstein]
- Repopulation: Usually at 1 week postirradiation. Following modest dose, from the hair follicles and high dose from the edge of the irradiated area.
- α/β ratios (X-ray): α/β (Gy) [Tubiana]

Acute desquamation	9.4 to 21
Epilation (anagen)	7.7
Epilation (telogen)	5.5
Late effects	3.0

cularis mucosae, muscularis propria, subserosa, and serosa (in part only). The mucosa of the esophagus is lined with nonkeratinizing stratified squamous epithelium. The mucosa and submucosa are surrounded by the muscularis propria, composed of striated muscle in the superior portion and smooth muscle inferiorly. The esophagus does not uniformly have a surrounding serosa.[72] The major acute reactions in the gut are typically a result of the effects of irradiation on the superficial layers (mucosa and submucosa). The late effects of irradiating the gut tend to produce full-thickness effects.

Clinical Features. *Acute radiation esophagitis* is a common accompaniment of radiation treatment in lung cancer. The epithelium of the esophagus is a moderately radiosensitive acute-reacting tissue. Large single doses are seldom if ever administered to the esophagus in clinical practice, so relatively little information exists on the acute reaction to such doses in the human. In a rat model, doses of 30 Gy produced submucosal edema at 4 days, necrosis of the basal epithelium at 6 days, intraluminal sloughing at 10 days, and re-epithelialization beginning at 14 days and complete at 20 days.[73] Even fractionated radiation produces mucosal injury. Symptoms include dysphagia and odynophagia, usually beginning in the second to third week of therapy. Symptoms generally increase in severity throughout the treatment course and subside within 1 to 2 weeks after completing therapy. The severity varies from mild, responsive to simple analgesics, to severe, requiring narcotic analgesia and parenteral support. The radiation tolerance of the esophagus is generally accepted as 60 to 65 Gy in 6 to 7 weeks at standard fractionation.[72] The late effects of radiation damage in the GI tract develop at 12 to 24 months following treatment. Gut mobility is reduced, and wall thickening, induration, and fibrosis occur. Ulceration may lead to perforation. Mesenteric thickening and fibrous adhesions are common, and subacute/acute bowel obstruction may occur. The likelihood of adhesions is increased by prior surgery and chemotherapy. The incidence of late complications to the small bowel increases after fractionated doses in excess of 40 to 45 Gy to large volumes. Smaller volumes of small bowel will likely tolerate doses of 45 to 55 Gy. The radiation tolerance of the colon and rectum is greater, and doses of 55 to 70 Gy are generally tolerated to small-volume fields.[58]

Radiobiologic Features. Both clonogenic and functional assays have been described for the GI tract, reflecting measures of both acute and late radiation gut injury.

Clonogenic Assays. Normal jejunal mucosa include villi and crypts. Stem cells divide rapidly, repopulate the crypts, and differentiate as they move up through the villi, to be eventually sloughed off into the lumen. They can be used as the basis for a clonogenic assay. Irradiating mouse jejunum initially denudes crypts (sensitive stem cells) and leaves villi (resistant differentiated cells) unscathed. Eventually the villi also disappear because of a lack of replacement cells from the irradiated crypts. Graded doses of total-body irradiation in mice (11 to 16 Gy) sterilize varying proportions of the crypt stem cells. Three to four days later the mice are sacrificed, and histologic sections of the jejuni are made to count the number of regenerating crypts per circumference.[36] Such assays like the one described by Withers[74,75] can yield information on gut radiation response as shown in Table 12.5. The late effects of radiation on the esophagus include a reduction in the number of capillaries, submucosal fibrosis and stricture of the lumen.

Functional Assays. Acute esophageal radiation reactions have been studied *in vivo*.[36] Thoracic irradiation in air-breathing mice denudes the esophagus in 6 to 10 days and kills a proportion of the treated animals by 28 days. Those animals surviving at 28 days eventually go on to die from radiation pneumonitis. The early deaths are attributed to radiation esophagitis, and thus $LD_{50/28}$ may be calculated reflecting acute radiation esophagitis (Table 12.5). Such experiments provide useful information on the effects of different types of radiation and fractionation, as well as chemosensitization data, but are not useful for determining dose-response information.

Lung

The radiation response of normal lung is critically important in considering the radiation biology and management of

TABLE 12.5. GASTROINTESTINAL: BASIC RADIOBIOLOGIC PARAMETERS

• Single dose	D_0 = 1.2 to 1.3 Gy (mouse gut) Range tested 9 to 16 Gy)
• Quasi-threshold dose	D_q = 4.0 to 4.5 Gy (mouse gut)
• α/β ratio (X-rays)	
	α/β Gy [Tubiana]
Acute effects (jejunum)	7.1 Gy
Late effects (bowel)	3.0 to 5.0 Gy
Functional Assays:	
• *In vivo* esophageal toxicity	$LD_{60/28}$ = 27 Gy

lung cancer, and this subject is also discussed in detail in Chapter 13. The lungs are generally considered among the late-reacting tissues, but both "acute" as well as "late" clinical reactions are well described following irradiation. In addition, the lungs are susceptible to damage from certain chemotherapeutic agents (bleomycin, cyclophosphamide, nitrogen mustard, procarbazine, etc.), and such effects must also be considered in the treatment of lung cancer patients.

Anatomy.   The lung consists of two physiologically distinct sections with separate functions in respiration.[76] The *respiratory tract,* which conducts air from the trachea to the terminal bronchioles, and the *acinar units,* containing the alveoli that actually perform the gas exchange. At least five cell types occupy the alveoli: epithelial cell (type 1 and 2 pneumocytes), endothelial cells, macrophages, and interstitial cells. Type 2 pneumocytes are a proliferating population of cells that produce, store, and secrete surfactant. They are the progenitors of type 1, membranous pneumocytes. After radiation, the type 2 pneumocytes, which are relatively radiosensitive, swell and release surfactant into the interstitial spaces and alveoli. This reaction is a marker for early radiation injury in the lung.

Clinical Features.   Two clinical syndromes, histologically distinct and chronologically separate, are described following irradiation of the lung. *Radiation pneumonitis* occurs 1 to 3 months following a course of radiation and is characterized by either asymptomatic pulmonic infiltrates on radiographic evaluation or a clinical syndrome of cough, fever, and shortness of breath.[58] The infiltrate on chest x-ray (or CT scan) characteristically corresponds to the radiotherapy treatment portal. The syndrome is generally self-limiting, but may require treatment with corticosteroids, and in severe cases, intensive ventilatory support.[77] If steroids are used, they must be cautiously withdrawn to avoid recrudescence of the syndrome. Pathophysiologically, damage to type 2 pneumocytes is believed to cause loss of surfactant, alveolar collapse, and interstitial edema.[76] *Pulmonary fibrosis* occurs as an inevitable consequence of the acute pulmonary reaction to radiation, whether or not the patient has shown evidence of acute radiation pneumonitis. The onset is generally 6 to 12 months after irradiation, and it is irreversible. Alveolar wall sclerosis, obliterative vasculitis, interstitial fibrosis, lung volume loss, and pleural thickening have been described.[77] Arterial hypoxia and a restrictive defect may be seen on pulmonary function testing. The functional impact of these reactions on the patient is largely related to the amount of lung irradiated, the total dose used, and the dose per fraction.

Radiobiologic Features.   The lack of clear evidence as to the nature of the critical target cells following irradiation, coupled with the slow cell cycle times of those implicated (type 2 pneumocytes cell cycle time of 1 to 2 months[58]),

means that no reliable clonogenic assay can assess lung radiosensitivity *in vitro.*[76] Thus we must rely on *in vivo* functional or histological end points for such assessments.

Functional Assays of Lung Radiation Response.   The ultimate test of function of a vital organ after radiation is survival. LD_{50} estimates have been described by Phillips et al.[25] Animals surviving the first wave of death (80 to 180 days) exhibited a second phase of damage at 6 to 12 months. This phase is thought to relate to radiation fibrosis. Dyspnea, manifested by increased breathing rate, can also be quantitated in animals to assess lung damage.[78] Airtight total-body plethysmography allows for a noninvasive test that can be sequentially applied to a single animal at intervals post irradiation.[76] Respiratory rate climbs rapidly with doses exceeding 11 Gy in association with radiation pneumonitis at 14 to 24 weeks and fibrosis at 52 weeks.[36] Other functional end points, such as arterial blood gas analysis, have also been described in this context. Most experimental systems involve whole lung irradiation, and as such are not totally representative of the more common partial lung irradiation used in the clinic. Table 12.6 summarizes the quantitative data derived from these and other assays, as well as from clinical observation of the occurrence of lung damage following partial or whole lung irradiation. Although differing estimates of lung tolerance are quoted depending on the author and system used, the figures quoted in Table 12.6 are useful guidelines in the clinic.

Heart
Portions of the heart often receive substantial doses of radiation that are unavoidable with current techniques. In the radiation management of the lymphomas, especially Hodgkin's disease, and certain carcinomas, including lung and breast, this radiation effect may be clinically relevant and at times life-threatening. Both acute and late effects are seen, and all anatomic structures of the heart are vulnerable. The radiotolerance of the heart is not clearly defined. Furthermore, as techniques assessing cardiac function have become more sensitive, it appears that probably no radiation dose to the heart is not accompanied by some measurable decrement in function. A useful rule of thumb in the clinic is that 60% of the volume of the heart appears to tolerate 40 Gy at standard fractionation, whereas 40% of the heart generally tolerates doses up to 60 Gy. This statement is empiric and imprecise. It must also be remembered that preexisting cardiac conditions are common and may be important in altering the radiotolerance. Similarly, chemotherapeutic agents (e.g., anthracycline drugs) may greatly affect cardiac function in this context.

Acute pericarditis may appear a few weeks to several years following radiation. Features include fever, tachycardia, substernal pain, and a friction rub. Pericardial effusion and even tamponade may occur, with radiographic and electrocardiographic changes typical of these syndromes. Approxi-

TABLE 12.6. LUNG: RADIOBIOLOGIC PARAMETERS AND TOLERANCE DATA

Single dose:
• Estimated D_0 = 0.6 Gy

Species	Treated Volume	Dose Tolerated
• Mouse	Whole lung	12 to 13 Gy ($LD_{50/160}$)
• Man	Whole lung	6 Gy (threshold dose)
• Man	Whole lung	8 Gy ($TD_{10/5}$)
• Man	Whole lung	10 Gy ($TD_{50/5}$)
Fractionated doses*:		
• Mouse	Whole lung	47 Gy ($LD_{50/160}$)
• Man	Whole lung	22 to 24 Gy ($TD_{5/5}$)
• Man	Whole lung	26.4 to 28.8 Gy ($TD_{50/5}$)
• Man	Partial lung	45–50Gy (volume dependent)

* 200 cGy/day five days a week.
** From Tubiana M, Dutreix J, Wambersic A. Effects on normal tissues. In: *Introduction to radiobiology.* Tubiana M, Dutreix J, Wambersic A, eds. London: Taylor & Francis, 1990;126, with permission.

mately one-half of the cases are self-limiting, whereas the remainder progress to chronic pericarditis of varying clinical significance. Most patients will have received doses in the 40 to 50 Gy range in 4 to 6 weeks to substantial portions of the heart. The incidence of significant pericarditis rises with doses in excess of 50 Gy in 5 weeks.[79] Chronic pericarditis occurs from 6 months to several years following radiation. The clinical syndrome comprises chronic restrictive changes with associated cardiac fibrosis and effusion. Clinical features are those of constrictive pericarditis, effusion, and ultimately progressive cardiac failure. Antecedent history of acute pericarditis is only elicited in approximately 50% of patients.

Myocardial dysfunction occurs because of vascular damage and progressive fibrosis and thickening of the myocardium. Coronary artery stenosis and occlusion is a particularly significant component of radiation injury to the heart. With mature follow-up now available from earlier studies using radiation therapy in diseases such as Hodgkin's disease and breast cancer, comes the realization of the importance of cardiac toxicity caused by radiation in clinical practice. Early trials of chest wall radiation in patients with breast cancer actually revealed a decrement in survival on the irradiated arm. It is now appreciated that this outcome was caused by excess cardiac deaths. Important causative factors included poor choice of radiation fields (internal mammary node groups), lower energy equipment, and higher daily doses (>2.5 Gy). With attention to proper technique, cardiac injury is no longer being encountered, and more recent trials are beginning to show a trend toward improved survival.[80] Likewise, long-term follow-up of patients treated with radiation for Hodgkin's disease are now also showing markedly increased rates of various cardiac injuries including myocardial infarctions.[81] Factors implicated again include higher total doses and dose per fractions used. The recent development of sophisticated cardiac pacemaker devices, and the

frequent coexistence of lung cancer in patients fitted with them has highlighted the occurrence of pacemaker malfunction caused by ionizing radiation. Guidelines are now being drawn to avoid clinical problems in such patients.[82] Careful attention to these factors is therefore warranted in the radiation management of the lung cancer patient.

Hematopoietic Tissues

The sensitivity of hematopoietic tissues is perhaps the single most important factor limiting the dose of cytotoxic therapies in the clinic. The requirement for rapid reproduction of the cellular elements in blood to maintain homeostasis (gas exchange, immune protection, and coagulation) calls for a prodigious clonogenic output and therefore renders this tissue especially sensitive to ionizing radiation and myelotoxic chemotherapies. An exhaustive discussion on this topic is beyond the scope of this chapter, but key points are highlighted as they apply to the management of lung cancer patients.

Anatomy and Physiologic Features. The bone marrow may thus be regarded as a single organ with structural organization for hematopoiesis.[58] Given the quantitative importance of radiation volume in terms of toxicity, the location of active marrow within the adult skeleton becomes a key issue (Figure 12.6).[83]

Clinical Features. When functional bone marrow is included in the radiation portal, an inevitable loss of stem cells occurs. The greater the volume of marrow, the greater the loss. Clinical effects are thus most easily observed following total-body irradiation (TBI). However, limited-field irradiation can cause measurable marrow toxicity, especially when significant amounts of the axial skeleton and pelvis are irradiated (Figure 12.6). Prior or concomitant myelotoxic chemotherapies can also aggravate the situation. Changes in peripheral blood counts may not mirror cytotoxic damage in time or extent because compensatory mechanisms may

Marrow Distribution (adult)

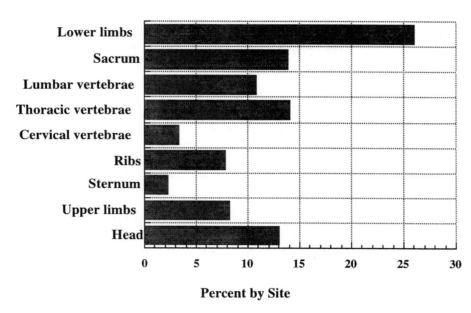

FIGURE 12.6. A graphic representation of the distribution of active bone marrow in the adult skeleton. Note that more than 80% of active marrow in health is in the axial skeleton, with approximately 30% in the vertebral bodies. (From Ellis, Thames HD, Withers HR, Peters LJ, et al. Changes in early and late radiation responses with altered dose fractionation: implications for dose-survival relationships. *Int J Radiat Oncol Biol Phys* 1982;8:219, with permission.)

mask the marrow toxicity, and the life cycle of mature cellular elements in the blood may be sufficiently long (e.g., red cell = 120 ± 30 days) so as to obscure the effect on the marrow. As always, *stem cells are most sensitive to radiation, whereas the more mature and differentiated cells are relatively resistant.* Following a TBI dose of 30 cGy, peripheral lymphocyte counts fall in humans.[58] Doses of 3 to 8 Gy cause profound lymphopenia, followed by granulocytopenia, thrombocytopenia, and anemia. The nadir in counts occurs at 2 to 3 weeks, and death occurs in a proportion of cases. A measure of bone marrow toxicity from radiation is the $LD_{50/30}$ for animals and $LD_{50/60}$ for humans. This measure is the dose that kills 50% of those irradiated at 30 days (animals) and 60 days (humans). The $LD_{50/60}$ for humans is variously quoted at 3 to 4 Gy.[38] Death occurs as a consequence of infection or bleeding. The higher the dose, the deeper and more prolonged the nadir.[58] It should be stressed that with modern medical support, including empiric broad-spectrum antibiotics, transfusions, and marrow "rescue," patients may survive whole-body doses up to 8 Gy. Above 10 Gy the patient will likely die from gastrointestinal toxicity. Following *partial marrow* irradiation, compensatory hyperplasia in the unirradiated marrow usually maintains peripheral blood counts. With doses greater than 30 Gy, hemopoiesis rarely returns to normal in the irradiated volume. However, if substantial portions of the marrow are irradiated, regeneration occurs to a greater extent within the irradiated field, probably because of intense humoral stimulation needed to recover.[58] Typically, when hypoplasia occurs following partial-marrow irradiation, platelet counts are the slowest to recover.

Radiobiologic Features. Clonogenic assays are available to assess the radiation sensitivity of bone marrow *in vivo.* The classic work of Till and McCulloch using supralethally irradiated mice (9 to 11 Gy), in whom marrow is infused following increasing exposure to radiation, has yielded much valuable information on the radiosensitivity of hematopoietic tissue.[84] The spleen is assayed for the number of colonies, each representing a pluripotent stem cell surviving the test irradiation dose. These and other studies have confirmed that hematopoietic tissue is an acute-reacting and relatively radiosensitive tissue (Table 12.7).

Central Nervous System
The proximity of the spinal cord to the lung and mediastinal nodes makes it virtually impossible to avoid obligatory irradiation of this critical structure. The tolerance of the cord

---

TABLE 12.7. HEMATOPOIETIC TISSUE: BASIC RADIOBIOLOGIC PARAMETERS*

General:
n = 1.2 to 1.5 (small shoulder)
D_0 = 0.9 Gy
α/β ratio = 20 Gy (high)

Lymphocytes:
n = 1.0 to 1.2
D_0 = 0.8 to 1.0 Gy

---

* From Tubiana M, Dutreix J, Wambersic A. Effects on normal tissues. In: *Introduction to radiobiology.* Tubiana M, Dutreix J, Wambersic A, eds. London: Taylor & Francis, 1990;126, with permission.

is therefore of paramount importance in the radiation management of the lung cancer patient. Nervous system tissue is a classic example of late-reacting tissue, and although acute toxicities can occur, the major concern is avoidance of a catastrophic late sequela—myelopathy.

Anatomy. Neurons are terminally differentiated cells that do not undergo cell division. As such, they are relatively resistant to radiation. However, important stromal support tissue, including Schwann cells, oligodendrocytes, and vascular endothelium, are susceptible. Damage to Schwann cells and oligodendrocytes is thought to cause loss of the myelin sheath, a protective support tissue. Demyelinization is implicated in the early radiation injury to the cord.

Clinical Features. Although a long-held belief states that the tolerance of the spinal cord varies according to the anatomic segment irradiated, objective evidence supports this belief.[85,86] The factors associated with the development of cord injury are principally dose (total and fraction size[87]) and volume. When greater than 10 cm of cord is irradiated, most clinicians do not exceed total doses of 45 to 50 Gy at standard fractionation (1.8 to 2.0 Gy/day). It is also important to realize that other factors, such as concomitant chemotherapy, may also reduce the tolerance of the cord to radiation.[88] *Early reversible myelopathic syndromes* may appear within a few weeks following cord doses of 50 to 60 Gy. *Lhermitte's syndrome* is characterized by an acute episode of demyelination, with symptoms of "electric shock" or "tingling" in the spine, aggravated by tilting the head (the "barber's chair sign"). This syndrome is generally self-limiting and is not associated with the inevitable development of permanent myelopathy. *Late radiation injury* to the spinal cord is a potentially catastrophic event that can usually be avoided by adhering to doses and fractionation schedules considered "safe." The most common cause of late radiation injury in clinical practice is overdosage at the junction of two abutting radiation fields. The onset is 6 months to 4 years from the end of treatment. The incidence is hard to determine because irradiated patients often do not survive their cancer long enough to be at risk for such damage. Although dose and fractionation are clearly extremely important, the occurrence of myelopathy with doses considered within "tolerance," indicates that other factors must be involved. Demyelination and atrophy of the cord is visible on MRI scanning, and histologic evidence of absent glial cells, necrosis, infarcts, and hyaline degeneration may be seen microscopically.[58] Clinically, a Brown-Sequart syndrome evolves and is generally irreversible.

Radiobiologic Features. Just as is true in the case of the late-reacting tissues of the lung, no useful clonogenic assays can detect the slowly dividing normal tissues of the central nervous system (CNS). However, several useful animal models provide information on tolerance of the spinal cord

and the effects of fractionation. The rat model with atrophy and dysfunction of the hind limbs has been used to study different fractionation schedules and the effects of reirradiation.[89,90] The potential protective effects of hyperbaric oxygen have been assessed in the mouse.[91] Other models utilize the guinea pig[92,93] rhesus monkey,[94] and the dog.[95]

MODIFICATION OF RADIOSENSITIVITY
Biological Aspects

In 1961 Terasima and Tolmach showed that cells vary in their radiosensitivity as a function of their position in the cell cycle.[96] In general, the ordering of radiosensitivies from the most resistant to the most sensitive response with respect to phases in the cell cycle are as follows: late S, early S, early G1, late G1, G2, M.[97] The difference in radiosensitivity from a cell in late S-phase versus mitosis is on the order of 2.5 to 3.0 fold. It is impressive that the same cell would vary so much in radiosensitivity as it simply traverses the cell cycle. Little is known as to why this happens. Possible explanations may be differential repair capacities, inability to appropriately arrest in critical phases of the cell cycle for repair, or changes in the biophysical nature of DNA as cells progress through the cell cycle. Presently this area of research is fruitful now that several molecules (in particular, the cyclins) have been discovered that are important in controlling movement through the cell cycle.[98–100]

Considerable radiosensitization could be achieved in a population of cells if they could somehow be synchronized into radiosensitive phases of the cell cycle such as G2, M, or the interface of G1 and S-phase. Radiation exposure (either acute exposures or continuous low dose-rate irradiation) has long been known to impose cell cycle blocks, in particular, in the radiosensitive G2-phase of the cell cycle.[21,101] Recent information identifies increased levels of mitotic cyclins as key biochemical events initiating mitosis. In HeLa cells, cyclin B mRNA and protein levels have been shown to increase in G2 and to decrease after division is completed. Cyclin B protein binds to cdc2, resulting in histone kinase activity, which is necessary for the initiation of mitosis. Radiation has been shown to alter levels of cyclin B and thus may interfere with the progression of cells from G2 to mitosis.[102] Indeed, continuous irradiation at low dose-rate has been shown to become much more efficient with respect to cell killing once cells are blocked in G2.[21]

Likewise, several drugs impose cell cycle blocks and have been used as radiation sensitizers.[103] Two examples are hydroxyurea (HU), evaluated many years ago, and more recently, paclitaxel (taxol). HU blocks cells at the G1/S-phase interface, is cytotoxic to cells in S-phase, and inhibits radiation damage repair.[104] If HU is exposed to cells for a time equivalent to the total cell cycle time, then cells in S-phase are killed and cells that were in G2, M, and G1 are synchronized at the G1/S-phase interface. When HU is removed, this cohort of cells moves synchronously through the cell cycle, and the cells become more radiosensitive as they move into G2 and M. This observation has been shown for *in vitro* cell cultures,[105–107] but it has been more difficult to demonstrate *in vivo*. Nonetheless, HU has been extensively evaluated in the clinic as a potential radiation-sensitizing drug.[108–118]

Paclitaxel binds to microtubules, possibly at a site on *β*-tubulin,[119] and interferes with normal microtubule structure and function. The effects of paclitaxel on nuclear microtubules probably account for most of the cytotoxicity manifested by the drug. Nuclear microtubules become shortened and form numerous abnormal spindle asters as paclitaxel-treated cells enter mitosis.[120] Normally, only two spindle asters appear in cells during mitosis, and these cells facilitate the separation of chromosomes before cell division. The abnormal microtubule asters that arise in mitotic cells following paclitaxel exposure do not contribute to cellular division. Indeed, paclitaxel markedly prolongs the duration of mitosis.[121] In order for paclitaxel to exert cytotoxicity, cells must be moving through the cell cycle because cells in plateau phase are resistant to paclitaxel (Figure 12.7A).[122] Long-term treatment of cells with relatively low concentrations of paclitaxel results in radiosensitization of log-phase cells, but no radiosensitization is observed for cells exposed to paclitaxel and subsequently irradiated (Figure 12.7B).[123] This radiosensitization is most likely caused by the paclitaxel-mediated G2/M block in the cell cycle.[123–125] In clinical trials, paclitaxel alone has exhibited activity against several malignancies, including ovarian,[126] breast,[127] head and neck,[128] and NSCLC carcinomas.[129] Combination of paclitaxel with radiation may have utility in lung cancer treatment given paclitaxel's activity alone in lung cancer and its ability to block cells in radiosensitive phases of the cell cycle.

Physical Aspects

The response of cells and tissues depends on the type of radiation used.[130,131] Examples of different types of radiation include x-rays, electrons, protons, neutrons, *α*-particles, and heavy-charged ions (e.g., C, Ne, Ar). As a photon or charged particle moves through cells or tissue, it transfers its energy randomly. The average energy lost per unit of track length of the photon or charged particle is referred to as LET. The radiation response of cells and tissues depends on the LET. In general, as the LET increases, the effectiveness of radiation increases and the dependence on oxygen (see following) decreases.[53,132] For example, cell killing for a given dose of radiation is greater for neutrons and *α*-particles (LETs, 2-10, and 100-200 kev/*μ*, respectively) than for x-rays (LET, 1 kev/*μ*) (Figure 12.1C). The use of high LET for cancer treatment carries several potential advantages over conventional x-ray treatment, including improved dose distribution, enhanced radiosensitization of hypoxic cells, and less radiation damage repair.[53] Despite these

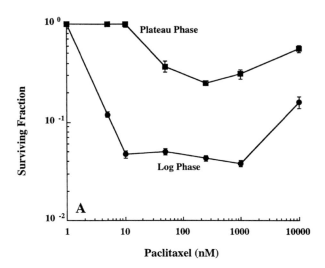

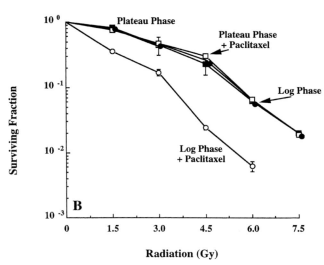

FIGURE 12.7. Cytotoxicity of paclitaxel (taxol) in V79 cells. **A:** illustrates the cell cycle specificity of paclitaxel. Because paclitaxel interferes with microtubule function during mitosis, actively cycling cells are much more sensitive. **B:** shows that paclitaxel sensitizes log-phase (cycling) but not plateau-phase (resting) cells to radiation. (From Liebmann JE, Cook JA, Fisher J, et al. Cytotoxic studies of paclitaxel (Taxol) in human tumour cell lines. *Br J Cancer* 1993;68:1104, with permission.)

potential advantages, the use of high LET has not become a mainstay in clinical radiotherapy. Some problems reside in unacceptable normal tissue toxicities observed with high-LET treatments and simply the cost and complexity involved in maintaining such sophisticated equipment.

Chemical Aspects

The inherent radiosensitivity of cells and tissues can be influenced by several chemical approaches and manipulations, which is important for at least two reasons. First, modifying the radiosensitivity by specific agents of known mechanisms of action can provide information about how radiation damage is registered and repaired. Second, selective modification of radiosensitivity, for example, in tumor as opposed to normal tissue, could provide therapeutic possibilities. In radiation oncology the major goal is to develop a treatment that affords a therapeutic gain; that is, enhanced tumor response without increased damage to surrounding normal tissue. It is well established that, for most tumors, increasing the radiation dose results in improved local control.[133–137] Ideally, the use of *tissue-specific radiation sensitizers or protectors* could result in an effective increase in the tumor radiation dose. For example, if a tumor-specific radiation sensitizer enhanced the effectiveness of radiation by a factor of 1.5, a delivered dose of 10 Gy would actually be equivalent to 15 Gy. Likewise, a specific radiation protector of normal tissue would allow for more radiation dose to be delivered to the tumor without enhancing normal tissue damage. Much research has gone into the development of both radiation sensitizers and protectors as a means of improving the local control of tumors by radiation, and examples of major classes are discussed in following sections.

RADIATION SENSITIZERS

Oxygen

Perhaps the most efficient radiation sensitizer is molecular oxygen. Oxygen has long been known to enhance the effectiveness of radiation (x-rays) in killing cells in culture by a factor of 2 to 3 compared to when irradiation is conducted under oxygen-free conditions.[138] In other words, if cells are irradiated in an hypoxic (<0.5% oxygen) as opposed to aerobic (~20% oxygen) environment, they are two to three times more resistant to the cytotoxic effects of radiation. When comparing the radiosensitivity of cells in aerobic versus hypoxic conditions, radiobiologists use the term oxygen enhancement ratio (OER), thus the OER for mammalian cells exposed to x-rays is 2.0 to 3.0. As discussed previously, it has been postulated that radiation produces carbon-centered radicals (most likely in the cellular DNA) that can react with molecular oxygen (a diradical molecule) to yield a lesion that is toxic and if not repaired results in death of the cell.[139] Under hypoxic conditions very few, if any, oxygen-related lesions are formed, and hence less cell killing results.

A major research effort has been directed toward the potential problem of the presence of viable hypoxic cells within tumors. In 1955 Thomlinson and Gray published a landmark study, which hypothesized that the presence of hypoxic cells in tumors may limit the effectiveness of radiation therapy.[140] This theory was based on the observation that tumor biopsy material taken from lung cancer patients contained distinct regions of viable tumor always near or surrounding blood capillaries. With increasing distances from the capillaries, regions of necrosis were noted. These observations prompted Thomlinson and Gray to make a

series of calculations regarding the maximum distance oxygen could diffuse through actively metabolizing tissue. The distance obtained from their calculations was between 150 to 200 μM. Actual measurements of their biopsy material revealed that viable tumor cells extended approximately 150 to 200 μM from the capillaries; beyond this distance, evidence for necrosis was apparent. Thus Thomlinson and Gray hypothesized that a gradient of oxygen concentrations may exist as a function of distance from capillaries and that tumor cells located at 150 to 200 μM, although still viable, are in an environment of extremely low oxygen concentrations. Such cells would be considered resistant to radiation, and thus their presence could limit the effectiveness of radiation cancer treatment. Considerable creditability was given to this hypothesis from the findings of Powers and Tolmach,[141] who showed quantitatively using a rodent tumor model that viable radiobiologically hypoxic cells exist *in vivo*. The experiments of Powers and Tolmach are not amenable to the study of hypoxic cell presence in human tumors, and thus scientists have assumed their presence in human tumors and sought means to eliminate them.

Only recently has technology been available to determine if, in fact, hypoxic cells are present in human tumors. When oxygen electrodes are directly inserted into tumors and many readings are taken as the electrode is tracked through the tissue, regions within the tumor have been recorded as having low oxygen levels (<10 mm Hg). The presence of hypoxia has been demonstrated in various tumor types, including head and neck carcinomas[142] breast carcinoma,[143] malignant brain tumors,[144] and cervical cancer.[145] Regional hypoxia has also been observed using noninvasive positron emission tomography of [18F]fluoromisonidazole for prostate and SCLC.[146] As more experience is gained with *in situ* oxygen measurements of tumors, it may be possible to select patients prior to therapy whose tumor has a significant hypoxic fraction and use approaches targeted at this radioresistant compartment.

To address the problem of hypoxic cells in tumors, radiobiologists and radiotherapists for the past 30 years have actively pursued various approaches to sensitize hypoxic cells to radiation. The goal of this research is to identify an approach that will reduce the OER from ~3.0 to 1.0; that is, hypoxic cells will have the same response to radiation as aerobic cells. Use of high LET radiation (i.e., neutrons) has been proposed because hypoxic cells exhibit less radioresistance under hypoxia to neutrons (OER = 1.7) than to x-rays.[138] The use of neutrons in clinical radiotherapy has not yielded significant improvement in tumor response, and because of the cost of constructing and maintaining a clinical neutron facility, this option is not likely to be explored extensively. The use of hyperbaric oxygen has been evaluated both experimentally and clinically. The idea here is to force oxygen into hypoxic regions of tumors using hyperbaric oxygen (100%). This approach has shown some degree of hypoxic radiosensitization in rodent tumors,[141] but the results in the clinic have not been impressive, primarily because of low patient accrual because of the problems associated with multiple treatments (~20 to 30) at hyperbaric oxygen levels.

Another approach that has received more attention is the development of chemicals that would not be metabolized like oxygen but could diffuse into hypoxic regions in tumors and sensitize hypoxic cells to radiation.[147] A class of compounds known as *nitroimidazoles* was identified to have such characteristics.[147] These compounds were shown not to radiosensitize aerobic cells; however, at concentrations of ~1mM, hypoxic cells were radiosensitized (OER = 1.6). The mechanism of hypoxic cell radiosensitization by nitroimidazoles is unknown; however, it is hypothesized that they have similar electron affinity to that of oxygen, and under hypoxic conditions can react with carbon-centered free radicals produced by radiation, and hence like oxygen "fix" the damage on important biological molecules crucial for survival. Two nitroimadazoles have been introduced into clinical radiotherapy trials; misonidazole and SR-2508. Clinical evaluation of misonidazole was complicated by dose-limiting normal tissue toxicities, namely, peripheral neuropathy.[148] SR-2508 was synthesized specifically to circumvent this problem; however, clinical trials to date have not shown it to be an effective sensitizer.[149,150]

More recently, a new approach at radiosensitizing hypoxic cells has been identified. Nitric oxide (NO) has been unexpectedly found to be an important bioregulatory molecule synthesized throughout the animal kingdom.[151–154] NO has a wide variety of physiological functions, including cardiovascular effects, neurotransmission, smooth muscle relaxation, bronchodilation, and immunologic potentiation.[153,154] The use of NO gas in animals (or humans) as a hypoxic cell radiosensitizer is problematic because breathing high concentrations of NO gas can damage lung tissue, and pharmacologic delivery of adequate concentrations of gaseous NO to distant solid tumor sites is not possible. Recently, a series of compounds called NONOates [$(R_1R_2NN(O)(NO))$], which are amine derivatives of dimeric NO, have been shown to release NO in a predictable manner at physiologic conditions.[155] As shown in Figure 12.8, NO released from NONOates radiosensitize hypoxic cells.[156,157] Such agents may have utility in the treatment of lung cancer.

The view that the presence of hypoxic cells in human tumors may limit the effectiveness of radiation treatment is not uniformly agreed upon in the radiation community. The reason for this disagreement resides in the manner in which radiation is delivered to tumors and the phenomenon of tumor reoxygenation. Using a rodent tumor model, van Putten and Kallman demonstrated that following a multifraction course of radiation treatment, the hypoxic fraction remaining at the end of radiation treatment was the same as the hypoxic fraction before treatment.[158] From these

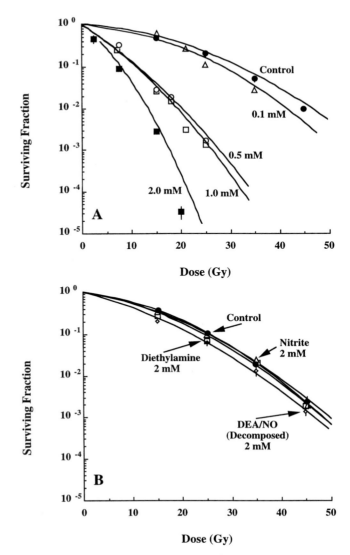

FIGURE 12.8. Radiation dose-response for Chinese hamster V79 cells exposed to radiation under hypoxic conditions in the absence or presence of **(A)** varying concentrations of the nitric oxide–releasing agent DEA/NO, or **(B)** 2 mM of nitrite, diethylamine, or decomposed DEA/NO. This study suggests that active nitric oxide is responsible for the sensitizing effect. (From Mitchell JB, Wink DA, DeGraff W, et al. Hypoxic mammalian cell radiosensitization by nitric oxide. *Cancer Res* 1993;53:5845, with permission.)

studies, van Putten and Kallman concluded that reoxygenation of hypoxic regions must have occurred during the fractionated course of radiation treatment. If no reoxygenation of hypoxic cells had occurred, then the proportion of hypoxic cells would have increased by the end of the fractionated radiation treatment. The fact that the hypoxic proportion remained the same during (and at the end of) treatment was interpreted to mean that for each radiation dose, aerobic cells were killed and the oxygen used by these cells was now diverted to reaerate hypoxic cells. The time course for reoxygenation in experimental tumor models varies widely among experimental rodent tumors ranging from 6 to 24 hours.[138] Thus with repeated daily exposures of radiation, reoxygenation of hypoxic regions should occur, along with killing of aerobic cells, with the net result after 20 to 30 radiation fractions being eradication of the tumor mass. If this correlation were true, then fractionated radiation therapy would not be greatly influenced by the presence of hypoxic cells. Technologic advances in the area of tumor oxygen measurements in human tumors allow for evaluation of the role of tumor hypoxia response and whether tumor reoxygenation during fractionated treatment adequately eliminates this potential problem.

Chemotherapy

As mentioned previously and covered in more detail in Chapter 15, the combination of chemotherapy and radiation may offer potential advantages with respect to tumor radiosensitization. Yet another practical aspect of combined modality therapy often arises in the clinical setting, involving whether chemotherapy-resistant cells are also radiation-resistant or vice versa, or whether previous treatment with one modality produces resistance to a different modality. These concerns have been partially addressed in cell culture studies, and considerable controversy exists. In general, chemotherapy-resistant cells are not radioresistant,[85,159–162] however, in some instances this is not the case.[163,164]

Does radiation treatment result in altered sensitivity to chemotherapy? Some *in vitro* reports indicate that prior radiation exposure increased drug resistance.[165–168] Hill et al. has reported that multiple fractions of radiation were able to induce the multidrug-resistant (MDR) phenotype in Chinese hamster ovary cells.[169] After radiation, these cells showed increased resistance to the vinca alkaloids, VP-16, adriamycin, and cisplatin; this resistance was reversed by the use of verapamil. Interestingly, these cells did not show amplification of the p-170 gene or of the p-170 mRNA; however, the cells did show an increased expression of the p-170 protein. The drug resistance induced using the radiation treatments was not as high as drug resistance produced by continuous low-dose exposure to colchicine. It should be noted that these interesting *in vitro* observations suggest that radiation could lead to changes in inherent cellular sensitivities (as a result of genomic alterations) to subsequent chemotherapy, but other possibilities certainly exist. For example, radiation treatment could alter the tumor vascular supply, tumor bed, and other physiological determinants that could compromise the delivery of the drug to the clonogenic tumor cells in the tumor. Careful work at both the cellular and tissue level will be required to work out these complexities; nonetheless, combined modality therapy remains an important research area in the laboratory and the clinic.

RADIATION PROTECTORS

As detailed previously, the successful treatment of human lung cancer with radiation is often limited by normal tissue complications. The anatomic location of lung tumors place several vital normal tissues at risk for radiation damage. If normal tissue could be protected selectively as opposed to tumor, more radiation dose could be delivered to the tumor with the expectation of greater tumor control with no or little additional damage to normal tissue. At the surface this task seems formidable; however, if blood flow is compromised to the tumor (this would be true if tumor hypoxia exists), a "window" of opportunity might open to deliver a radioprotector to normal tissues (well perfused) before appreciable quantities reach and the tumor. Alternatively, if a radioprotector could be developed such that it could be inactivated by tumor as opposed to normal tissues by virtue of differential metabolism, advantages might be expected.

Radioprotectors are classified in several categories. Some radioprotectors protect by *scavenging radiation-induced free radicals* and/or *donating reducing equivalents to oxidized molecules*. Others protect by *altering physiologic functions* that interfere with the effects of radiation, such as agents that cause vasoconstriction and hypoxia. This class of protectors actually reduces blood flow to normal tissues, such as bone marrow, rendering the tissue hypoxic. Because hypoxic cells are less responsive to the effects of radiation, the net result is radioprotection. Lastly, some radioprotectors act by *enhancing the recovery and/or repair of normal tissues*. Examples of these protectors include cytokines and hemopoietic growth factors.

Aminothiol Radioprotective Agents

The search for radioprotectors began in the 1940s when Patt et al. found that sulfhydryl compounds afforded protection against whole-body irradiation in rodents.[170] The dose modifying factor (DMF) for these experiments was −1.7. Subsequently, Bacq et al. found that cysteamine also protected animals from whole-body radiation.[171] The mechanism(s) by which these sulfhydryl compounds protect appears to involve their ability to scavenge radiation-induced free radicals and/or to donate reducing equivalents to oxidized molecules, although more recent studies suggest that induction of bone marrow hypoxia could also account for some of the protection.[172] These discoveries prompted the U.S. Army to sponsor the synthesis and screening of compounds to identify relatively nontoxic and potentially more effective radioprotectors.[173] From this massive screening effort, a thiophosphate compound, S-2-(3-aminopropyl-amino) ethylphosphorothioic acid (WR-2721), emerged. WR-2721 showed substantial and selective protection of normal tissues in murine models.[174–177] Yuhas et al. showed that WR2721 could protect normal tissues but did not protect tumor.[176] Subsequent studies established the basis for this observation to be slower penetration of WR2721 into tumor tissue than normal tissues.[177] Phase I studies of WR2721 defined the maximally tolerated dose under different treatment schemes.[178–180] Recent clinical trials has shown that WR2721 (amifostine) has been quite effective in protecting against radiation-induced normal tissue toxicities without reducing antitumor efficacy in NSCLC[181] and head and neck cancer.[182]

Nitroxides as Radiation Protectors

Recently, a new class of radioprotectors, the nitroxides, has been described.[183–185] Nitroxides are stable free-radical compounds that afford radioprotection both *in vitro*[183] and *in vivo*.[184] Tempol protected V79 cells against radiation in a dose-dependent fashion (Figure 12.9A), whereas, the reduced form of Tempol (Tempol-H), the hydroxylamine, did not provide aerobic radioprotection (Figure 12.9B). Likewise, although Tempol was rapidly reduced to the hydroxylamine (inactive radioprotector) *in vivo* (Figure 12.10A), significant radioprotection was observed in animals (DMF = 1.3) if irradiation was conducted within 10 minutes after drug administration. Figure 12.10B shows that the same concentration of Tempol administered to tumor-bearing mice receiving local tumor irradiation did not influence tumor response.[186] To identify a mechanism for the apparent differential protection of the hematopoietic system (Figure 10A) and tumor tissue, pharmacologic studies were carried out. The percentage of oxidized compound (nitroxide) was approximately 2-fold greater in the bone marrow compartment, compared to RIF-1 tumor at the time of irradiation. Greater bioreduction of Tempol occurred in the RIF-1 tumor. Such a result may provide at least a partial explanation for the absence of tumor radioprotection because it previously had been demonstrated that the oxidized form of Tempol is the active radioprotector. These preliminary data imply that a potential difference exists between normal and tumor tissues with respect to bioreduction.

CELLULAR PROPERTIES OF HUMAN LUNG CANCER CELLS AND THEIR RESPONSE TO RADIATION

The clinical variability in response among the different histologies of lung cancer to cytotoxic agents probably has many causes. One approach toward unraveling this complex issue has involved a systematic study of inherent properties of tumor cells that might be important in governing response to a particular treatment modality. Studies have focused on three main areas: (a) the human tumor stem-cell assay; (b) established permanent *in vitro* human tumor cell lines; and (c) xenografts of human tumors grown in athymic nude mice.

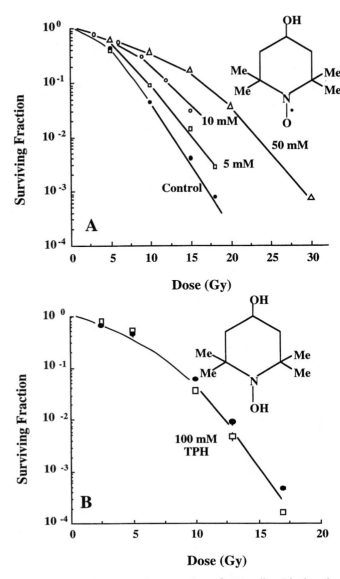

FIGURE 12.9. *In vitro* radioprotection of V79 cells with the nitroxide Tempol. **A:** Increasing concentrations of Tempol provide increasing aerobic radioprotection in a clonogenic assay. **B:** The reduced form of Tempol (Tempol-H) provides no radioprotection. (From Mitchell JB, DeGraff W, Kaufman D, et al. Inhibition of oxygen-dependent radiation-induced damage by the nitroxide superoxide dismutase mimic, Tempol. *Arch Biochem Biophys* 1991;289:62, with permission.)

Human Tumor Stem-Cell Assay

This process involves the disaggregation to a single-cell suspension of tumor cells obtained at biopsy, exposure to cytotoxic substances, and assessment of cloning or colony-forming capacity in medium made semisolid by the addition of

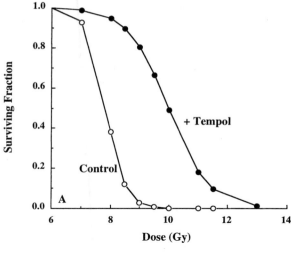

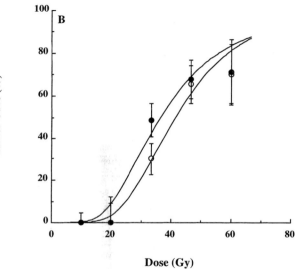

FIGURE 12.10. A: An LD$_{50/30}$ curve of whole-body radiation in C3H mice. Tempol injected intraperitoneally protects them against whole-body radiation. Data adapted from Hahn, et al. Tempol, a stable free radical, is a novel murine radiation protector. *Cancer Res* 1992;52:1750, with permission. **B:** Radiation tumor-control curves for animals treated in the absence or presence of Tempol. Closed circles: Tempol-treated mice; open circles: PBS-treated mice. No statistical difference existed between the two curves (p = 0.54). The calculated TCD$_{50/30}$ values for Tempol-treated and PBS-treated mice were 36.7 and 41.8 Gy, respectively. No statistical difference existed between these values (p = 0.32). The error bars represent one standard error above and below the value shown. (From Hahn SM, Sullivan FJ, DeLuca AM, et al. Evaluation of tempol radioprotection in a murine tumor model. *Free Radic Biol Med* 1997;22:1211, with permission.)

agarose.[187] This study allows the potential of tailoring patient therapy based on the sensitivity of their own cells *in vitro*. Unfortunately, at present, major problems with the assay limit its usefulness. These problems include long assay times, the low yield of growth from tumor biopsy specimens, difficulty in obtaining true single-cell suspensions

from solid tumors, and low cloning efficiencies, ranging from 0.001% to 0.1%.[188,189] A further disadvantage is the admixture of both normal and tumor cells in most specimens.[190] Improved culture media, as well as techniques to circumvent these issues, is required before this assay will become clinically useful.

Radiation Sensitivity of Lung Cancer Cell Lines

As noted previously, the use of cell lines to establish radiation sensitivity dates back to the classic work of Theodore Puck, who used the cervical carcinoma cell line (HeLa) to report the first mammalian x-ray survival curve.[4] Over the past decade or more, numerous investigators have reported on the *in vitro* radiation response of human tumor cell lines for various malignant conditions.[191–200] In the same time period, it has been estimated that more than 1,000 continuous human cell lines have been established from lung cancer biopsy specimens.[201] The major advantages of using established human cell lines for such assays include the availability of large numbers of cells to perform survival, biochemic, cytogenetic, and molecular studies, as well as reproducibility and generally acceptable cloning efficiencies.[198] NSCLC cells generally adhere to culture flasks and plate in monolayers and thus lend themselves easily to clonogenic assay.[202] In contrast, SCLC lines have been more difficult to establish and tend to aggregate and float in culture, making clonogenic assays more difficult.[203,204] Furthermore, SCLCs tend to clone inefficiently, especially newly established classic lines from untreated patients. Thus other assays, including dye exclusion techniques,[205] tritiated thymidine uptake,[206] radiolabeled glucose utilization,[207] and automated image analysis of crystal violet-stained cells,[208] have been evaluated as alternatives to the classic clonogenic assays. A semiautomated colorimetric assay has proven a reliable nonclonogenic alternative, allowing for rapid sensitivity screening of lung cancer cells to cytotoxic agents including chemotherapy[209] and radiation.[210] Such studies have confirmed a heterogeneity of *in vitro* response, which parallels the behavior of these diseases in the clinic. To illustrate this property, the radiation survival curves for established cell lines of six different histologic types of lung cancer are shown in Figure 12.11A. The most striking feature observed among these curves is the variation in the initial shoulder as well as the terminal slope of the different lines, indicative of a differential cell survival. The mean surviving fraction at 2 Gy, thought to be a reliable indicator of radiation sensitivity, is displayed in Figure 12.11B and demonstrates the heterogeneous response among the differing histologies. A summary of the radiation survival curve parameters for selected lines evaluated from the NCI lung cancer cell panel,[211] as well as the work of other investigators, confirms this heterogeneity and suggests that the response of lung cancer cell lines can be considered in three groups. Group 1 includes "clas-

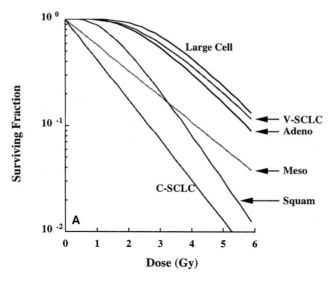

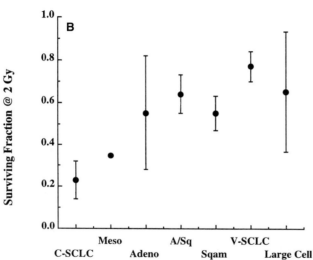

FIGURE 12.11. A: Radiation dose-response curves for six different types of human lung cancer cell lines. In this assay, small cell carcinoma is the most radiosensitive, a finding often reproduced in the clinic. **B:** Mean surviving fraction at 2 Gy for seven different types of human lung cancer cell lines, confirming the relative sensitivity of small cell *in vitro*. (From Carmichael J, DeGraff WG, Gamson J, et al. Radiation sensitivity of human lung cancer cell lines. *Eur J Cancer Clin Oncol* 1989;25:527, with permission.)

Therefore, the question may be asked: Is the intrinsic radiation-sensitivity values ($\bar{n}$, D_0, SF 2Gy) of these cell lines generally predictive of clinical responsiveness or curability? Weichselbaum and his colleagues in studies of cell lines from various malignancies found little or no correlation,[192] whereas the data from the studies of lung cancer lines appear predictive.[198,199,211] Classic SCLC is definitely responsive to radiation treatment in the clinic, although it is rarely cured because of its capacity for systemic spread.[212] Variant SCLC and NSCLC are clinically less responsive to radiation. Cell lines from responsive SCLC patients are characterized by low $\bar{n}$ values (1.0 to 3.3) and low SF 2 Gy values, whereas cell lines from variant SCLC or NCSLC tend to have larger $\bar{n}$ values (5.6 to 14) and higher SF 2 Gy values. A large shoulder on the survival curve (or high $\bar{n}$ value) implies a considerable capacity for SLDR, and thus a greater cell survival. Additionally, for a clinically relevant radiation dose of 2 Gy, the surviving fraction is usually greater for those cell lines having a higher $\bar{n}$ value.[211] The absence of a shoulder on the SCLC cell lines has important dose-rate implications discussed previously.

Xenografts

Almost 100 years ago, Livingood described a spontaneously occurring papillary mouse tumor in a mouse lung.[213] Chemically and transgenically induced primary lung tumors in mice share many of the morphologic, histologic, and biochemic features of human NSCLC.[214] For example, when a *ras* oncogene is transfected into SV-40 transformed human bronchial epithelial cells, and injected into a nu/nu mouse, adenocarcinoma of the lung results.[215] These models therefore offer the ability to study premalignant lung lesions, as well as models of lung tumor progression. *In vitro* clonogenic assays of human heterotransplants have been developed with cloning efficiencies ranging from 0.3% to 35%[216] Reasonable correlations have been reported between *in vivo* tumor responses to chemotherapy and observed responses in the clinic.[217] More recently, xenograft models have been utilized in the assessment of novel therapeutic strategies, including radiolabeled monoclonal antibody treatments in SCLC.[218] This approach has been relatively underutilized, and further work is warranted.[214]

MOLECULAR ASPECTS OF RADIATION SENSITIVITY AND RESISTANCE

Human lung cancer is a complex disease resulting from a series of inherited and somatically occurring defects in several critical genes. The genetic changes include mutations, deletions, and amplification of genes coding for proteins involved in fundamental regulatory functions such as signal transduction, nuclear transcription, cell cycle regulation, and apoptosis. Although such genetic alterations are funda-

sic" SCLC lines with D_0s in the range of 0.51 to 1.4 Gy and extrapolation numbers ($\bar{n}$) in the 1 to 3.3 range. These lines were clearly the most radiosensitive. Both NSCLC and "variant" SCLC lines could be considered as belonging to Group 2, with D_0s of 0.8 to 0.91 Gy and rather large $\bar{n}$ values of 5.6 to 14.0. Group 3 consists of the adenocarcinoma lines, with D_0s in the 0.97 to 1.3 Gy and $\bar{n}$ of 1.3 to 3.0. Somewhat surprisingly, mesothelioma cell lines tested appeared radiosensitive with low $\bar{n}$ in the 1.0 to 1.8 range and D_0 1.3 to 1.86 Gy, whereas the clinical experience with this tumor would suggest a more radioresistant response.

mental to many aspects of lung carcinogenesis and may provide the basis for a rational approach to primary and secondary prevention, many attempts have been made to relate molecular features to prognosis and/or to response to radiotherapy and chemotherapy. Can specific genetic alterations be shown to be associated with radiation resistance? The data are not consistent on this question. This section intends to briefly review the major molecular biologic advances in lung cancer made during the last few years and relate such information to clinical oncology. Particular effort is made to interweave these advances with our understanding of radiation biology.

p53

p53 gene mutation is the most common genetic alteration found in human cancers (see also Chapter 6).[219] *p53* is a tumor-suppressor gene linked to control of gene expression, cell cycle arrest at G1 by activation of p21 (an inhibitor of cyclin-dependent kinases) and GADD45 (an effector of growth arrest and DNA repair), and control of cell proliferation and apoptosis.[220] In lung cancer, *p53* is mutated in up to 80% of SCLC and 50% of NSCLC.[221] Fujino et al. showed p53 alterations to correlate with poorer prognosis in surgically resected NSCLC patients.[222] Moreover, their study demonstrated that the *p53* status was a strong predictor of survival in p21-ras negative patients. In fact, patients with altered expression of *p53* had a 43% five-year survival rate as compared to 87% in those patients without *p53* mutation.

A correlation between *p53* status of the tumor and response to gamma radiation or adriamycin *in vivo* has been demonstrated. It was found that the loss of *p53* function in tumors growing in immunocompromised mice was associated with resistance to both ionizing radiation and adriamycin treatment.[223] The loss of *p53* function probably suppresses the apoptotic signals that are activated chemically or physically by antineoplastic agents. Consistent with this view, Chang et al. have shown that transfection of a normal *p53* gene into cell lines with *p53* mutations restores the normal G1 checkpoint and the apoptotic pathway and sensitizes the cells to radiation.[224] However, it is not clear at present exactly how *p53* influences radiosensitivity. No relationship has been found between radiosensitivity and *p53* status among 24 head and neck cancer cell lines.[225] Likewise, abrogation of *p53* function by HPV16 E6 gene does not influence radiosensitivity.[226] More recently, a relationship between the ataxia telangiectasia (AT) gene product and *p53* activation in response to ionizing radiation has been shown.[227] The relationship between AT and *p53* suggests a potential mechanism underlying the exquisite susceptibility of AT patients to ionizing radiation and provides yet another instance of the importance of *p53* in determining the radiosensitivity of a cell.

Ras

Ras (K-*ras*, homologous to Kirsten murine sarcoma virus oncogene; H-*ras*, homologous to Harvey murine sarcoma virus oncogene; and N-*ras* isolated from a neuroblastoma cell line) codes for a 21 kilodalton protein (p21) with high homology to G-proteins that function in signal transduction and cell proliferation (see also Chapter 4). Point mutation at codon 12, 13, or 61 of the *ras* gene confers transforming potential to p21.[221] Although virtually absent in SCLC, mutated *ras* genes are found in approximately 20% of *in vivo* NSCLC tumors and NSCLC-derived cell lines. *Ras* mutations are more commonly found in adenocarcinoma (~30%) than in squamous and large cell carcinoma (~10%). A negative prognostic correlation in surgically resected NSCLC patients has been found for ras gene mutation or overexpression.[228] As noted previously, combining information about *p53* and *ras* status is helpful in more accurately defining the subset of patients at risk and possibly, in the future, defining the best choice of treatment modality.[222]

When mutated *ras* genes were transfected in murine fibroblast cell line NIH3T3, resistance to ionizing radiation was conferred. The implication of this acquired radiation resistance is that *ras* has an important function in the response to the physicochemical insult of ionizing radiation.[229] McKenna and colleagues, using a primary rat embryo cell (REC) model, suggested that transfection of H-*ras* oncogene alone conferred little alteration in radiation resistance, whereas the presence of a co-transfected cooperating oncogene (v-*myc*) induced a dramatic increase in radioresistance.[230–232] It was further suggested that increased radioresistance may be caused partly by cell cycle perturbation. The transfected cells had a more prolonged G_2 than sensitive cell lines.[233] A similar finding was reported by Su and Little when human fetal fibroblast cells were transfected with activated *ras* oncogene and or simian virus 40 T-antigen.[234] However, these results need to be interpreted with caution because transfection of REC and human cell lines with nononcogenic DNA sequences alone (pSV2neo, encoding only for neomycin resistance) and subjecting them to subsequent clonal selection, can also yield clones with increased resistance to radiation.[235] Likewise, considerable heterogeneity in radiation response exists among different clones of the NIH 3T3 cells as used by Sklar, such that when *ras*, *raf*, and *myc* genes were transfected, no clear modification of radiation sensitivity was attained when compared to the nontransfected parent lines.[236] Harris et al. used a temperature-sensitive rat kidney epithelial cell containing k-*ras* and found *increased* radiosensitivity with *ras* activation.[237] More recently, human tumor cell lines with mutations in H- or K-*ras* genes were radiosensitized after treatment with prenyltransferase inhibitors that prevent posttranslational modification of *ras*, required for its activity.[238] The use of prenyltransferase inhibitors in radiation oncology is presently undergoing phase I clinical trials.

ErbB 2

erbB 2 gene encodes a transmembrane glycoprotein receptor having homology with the epidermal growth factor receptor (see also Chapter 4). *ErbB 2* has a constitutive tyrosine kinase activity that is pivotal in the protein's function in growth regulation.[239] *ErbB 2* has been shown to confer the transformed phenotype to murine fibroblasts NIH3T3 *in vitro*,[240] and overexpression of *erbB 2* has been shown in lung cancer.[241] Immunohistochemic expression of *erbB 2* was detected in approximately 50% of lung adenocarcinomas.[242] As in the case with p53, *erbB 2* expression along with K-*ras* mutation has been associated with a poorer prognosis in lung adenocarcinoma patients.[243] Although *erbB 2* has not yet been defined as a treatment determinant in lung cancer, in early-stage breast cancer it has been shown that the presence of the *erbB 2* oncogene, p53 status, and the number of positive lymph nodes correlate with response to adjuvant chemotherapy and radiotherapy.[244]

Myc

Myc, a phosphoprotein with transcriptional regulatory activity, is involved in the control of development and growth of the normal cell (see also Chapter 5). C-Myc, of cellular origin and homologous to the *v-myc* oncogene of the avian myelocytic leukemia virus, has been found to be overexpressed in several neoplasms. Although overexpression of myc family genes: c-*myc*, n-*myc* (from neuroblastoma), and l-*myc* (from lung), has been found in approximately 20% of SCLC, being more common in pretreated patients, it is an uncommon finding in NSCLC. The presence of myc has been associated with more aggressive malignant behavior and poorer prognosis.[245] Transfection of c-*myc* into a human melanoma cell line has been shown to confer increased sensitivity to ionizing radiation. Interestingly, the opposite effect was found when myc was co-transfected with ras in the same cell line.[246]

Retinoblastoma

Retinoblastoma (RB) tumor suppressor gene product is a nuclear protein that in the dephosphorylated form acts negatively on cell cycle progression and holds the cell in the G_0-G1 phase (see also Chapters 2, 7). In a normal cell, Rb is phosphorylated by a complex cyclin D1-CDK4 (cyclin-dependent kinase 4) to allow the progression of the cell cycle to mitosis. This mechanism is complemented by p16, a product of cdkn2 gene, that inhibits the phosphorylation of RB by the complex cyclin/CDK. P16 expression is upregulated by the phosphorylated form of RB, the result of which is a feedback-type control. RB, cyclin D1, and p16 constitute the RB pathway. Alteration of any part of the pathway seems to play an important role in NSCLC tumorigenesis. In fact, loss of Rb was found in 42 of 101

(41.6%) NSCLC specimens, and disturbances in expression of at least one of the three components of the Rb pathway were found in 91 of 101 (90%) NSCLC specimens.[247] In other studies, altered *RB* gene has been found in 32% of NSCLC patients and 13% of SCLC primary tumors.[248] The absence of the Rb mRNA transcript was common in SCLC specimen and cell line.[249]

Correlation between expression of Rb and sensitivity to carboplatin and VP-16 has been shown in NSCLC cell lines.[250] In this study, the cell lines having higher expression of *RB* gene were more sensitive to the antineoplastic drugs. Interestingly, an inverse correlation was found for radiosensitivity in an *in vitro* study on non-Hodgkin's lymphoma cell line and in a clinical study on patients with bladder cancer. Both of the latter studies, in fact, show a negative correlation of Rb expression with response to radiation. Rb overexpression appeared to be associated with more resistance to ionizing radiation in an *in vitro* model.[251] Consistent with this study, a better response rate to radiotherapy was found in patients whose tumors were immunohistochemically negative for Rb protein.[252]

BCL2

BCL2 gene is an oncogene that was first identified in follicular lymphoma in which a translocation resulted in overexpression.[253] The BCL2 protein is an inhibitor of programmed cell death or apoptosis.[254] BCL2 overexpression is very common in SCLC (~75%)[255] and is found in approximately 25% of NSCLC, where it has been proposed as prognostic factor.[256] However, a study of 427 NSCLC cases showed BCL2 expression not to be an independent prognostic factor.[257] A recent study suggests that BCL2 expression may be a favorable prognostic indicator in some subgroups of patients, such as those having stage IIIa disease.[258] *In vitro* studies have associated BCL2 overexpression with radiation resistance.[259] Transgenic mice ubiquitously overexpressing BCL2 are more resistant to the lethal bone marrow effects of ionizing radiation, and lymphocytes that survive radiation in wild-type mice show higher levels of BCL2 expression.[260]

The evolving paradigm regarding tumorigenesis and ultimate treatment offers a vision of genetic determinism. However, at this time, our molecular biology knowledge is not yet at the level to provide general deterministic views with regard to therapeutic decisions. What may be required is a genetic determination of an array of expressed mRNAs, which will hopefully enable a better understanding of the complex relationship of a particular oncogene or tumors suppressor gene to other expressed genes within an individual tumor. Certainly, our technology is moving in that direction. It is assumed that as our knowledge grows, the role of oncogenes and tumor-suppressor genes in the context of tumor physiology will not only affect tomorrow's radiotherapy decisions, but will also define how to weave radiobiologic principles with molecular biology to arrive at optimal, curative therapy.

SUMMARY

This chapter has summarized the major areas of radiobiology as they relate to lung cancer. Future advances in the management of this disease will likely emerge from continued basic and applied research. Particularly exciting are the recent advances in molecular biology and their application to the understanding of the pathogenesis and treatment of lung cancer. Radiation continues to be one of the most active agents in the management of this disease. As the field of radiation biology incorporates novel molecular techniques, further advances will likely ensue.

REFERENCES

1. Frey R, Hagen U. Oxygen effect on gamma-irradiated DNA. *Radiat Environ Biophys* 1974;11:125.
2. Ward JF, Kuo I. Radiation damage to DNA in aqueous solution: a comparison of the response of the single-stranded form with that of the double-stranded form. *Radiat Res* 1978;75:278.
3. Mee LK. Radiation chemistry of biopolymers. In: Farhataziz, Rodgers MAJ, eds. *Radiation chemistry principles and applications.* New York: VCH Publishers, 1987:477.
4. Puck TT, Markus PI. Action of x-rays on mammalian cells. *J Exp Med* 1956;103:653.
5. Halliwell B, Gutteridge JMC. *Free radicals in biology and medicine.* Oxford, Oxford University Press, 1989.
6. Fowler JF. Dose response curves for organ function or cell survival. *Brit J Radiol* 1983;56:497.
7. Fertil B, Malaise EP. Intrinsic radiosensitivity of human cell lines is correlated with radioresponsiveness of human tumors: analysis of 101 published survival curves. *Int J Radiat Oncol Biol Phys* 1985;11:1699.
8. Deacon J, Peckham MJ, Steel GG. The radioresponsiveness of human tumours and the initial slope of the cell survival curve. *Radiother Oncol* 1984;2:317.
9. Brock WA, Baker FL, Wike JL, et al. Cellular radiosensitivity of primary head and neck squamous cell carcinomas and local tumor control. *Int J Radiat Oncol Biol Phys* 1990;18:1283.
10. Peters LJ, Brock WA. Cellular radiosensitivity as predictors of treatment outcome: where do we stand? *Int J Radiat Oncol Biol Phys* 1993;25:147.
11. Bedford JS. Sublethal damage, potentially lethal damage, and chromosomal aberrations in mammalian cells exposed to ionizing radiations. *Int J Radiat Oncol Biol Phys* 1991;21:1457.
12. Hall EJ. *Repair of radiation damage and the dose-rate effect.* Philadelphia: JB Lippincott, 1994:107.
13. Shipley WU, Stanley JA, Courtenay VD, et al. Repair of radiation damage in Lewis lung carcinoma cells following in situ treatment with fast neutrons and gamma-rays. *Cancer Res* 1975; 35:932.
14. Tubiana M, Dutreix J, Wambersie A. *Cellular effects of ionizing radiation. Cell survival curves.* London: Taylor and Francis, 1990:86.
15. Elkind MM, Sutton H. X-ray damage and recovery in mammalian cells in culture. *Nature* 1959;184:1293.
16. Elkind MM, Sutten-Gilbert H, Moses WB, et al. Radiation response of mammalian cells in culture V. Temperature dependence of the repair of x-ray damage in surviving cells (aerobic and hypoxic). *Radiat Res* 1965;25:359.
17. Fowler JF. Intervals between multiple fractions per day. *Acta Oncologica* 1988;27:181.
18. Gardner KE, Parsons JT, Mendenhall WM, et al. Time-dose relationships for local tumor control and complications following irradiation of squamous cell carcinoma of the base of tongue. *Int J Radiat Oncol Biol Phys* 1987;13:507.
19. Turrisi AT, Glover DJ, Mason BA. A preliminary report: concurrent twice-daily radiotherapy plus platinum-etoposide chemotherapy for limited small cell cancer. *Int J Radiat Oncol Biol Phys* 1988;15:183.
20. Bedford JS, Hall EJ. Survival of HeLa cells cultured in vitro and exposed to protracted gamma irradiation. *Int J Radiat Biol* 1963;7:337.
21. Mitchell JB, Bedford JS, Bailey SM. Dose-rate effects in mammalian cells in culture III. Comparison of cell killing and cell proliferation during continuous irradiation for six different cell lines. *Radiat Res* 1979;79:537.
22. Bedford JS, Mitchell JB, Fox MH. Variations in responses of several mammalian cell lines to low dose-rate irradiation. In: Meyn RE, Withers HR, eds. *Radiation biology in cancer research.* New York: Raven Press, 1980:251.
23. Hill RP, Bush RS. The effect of continuous or fractionated irradiation on a murine sarcoma. *Br J Radiol* 1973;46:167.
24. Fu KK, Phillips TL, Kane LJ, et al. Tumor and normal tissue response to irradiation in vivo: variation with decreasing dose rates. *Radiology* 1975;114:709.
25. Phillips TL, Margolis L. Radiation pathology and the clinical response of the lung and esophagus. In: Vaeth JM, ed. *Frontiers in radiation therapy and oncology.* Basel, Karger, 1972:254.
26. Wara WM, Phillips TL, Margolis LW, et al. Radiation pneumonitis: a new approach to the derivation of time-dose factors. *Cancer* 1973;32:547.
27. Field SB, Hornsey S, Kutsutani Y. Effects of fractionated irradiation on mouse lung and a phenomenon of slow repair. *Br J Radiol* 1976;49:700.
28. Down JD, Easton DF, Steel GG. Repair in the mouse lung during low dose-rate irradiation. *Radiother Oncol* 1986;6:29.
29. Proietti A, Murer B, Muretto P, et al. Effetti biologici della irradiazione corporea totale in dose unica somministrata con diverso dose-rate. *Minerva Med* 1991;82:723.
30. Van Dyk J, Keane TJ, Kan S, et al. Radiation pneumonitis following large single dose irradiation: a re-evaluation based on absolute dose to lung. *Int J Radiat Oncol Biol Phys* 1981;7:461.
31. Phillips TL. Pulmonary section-cardiorespiratory workshop. *Cancer Clin Trials* 1981;4:45.
32. Barrett AJ, Depledge MH, Powles RL. Interstitial pneumonitis following bone marrow transplantation after low dose rate total body irradiation. *Int J Radiat Oncol Biol Phys* 1983;9:1029.
33. Steel GG, Deacon JM, Duchesne GM, et al. The dose-rate effect in human tumour cells. *Radiother Oncol* 1987;9:299.
34. Cassoni AM, McMillian TJ, Peacock JH, et al. Differences in the level of DNA double-strand breaks in human tumour cell lines. Following low dose-rate irradiation. *Eur J Cancer* 1992; 28A:1610.
35. Sullivan FJ, Carmichael J, Glatstein E, et al. Radiation biology of lung cancer. *J Cell Biochem* 1996;24:152.
36. Hall EJ. Dose-response relationships for normal tissues. In: Hall EJ, ed. *Radiobiology for the radiologist.* 4th ed. Philadelphia: JB Lippincott, 1994:45.
37. Rubin P, Cooper R, Phillips TL. Radiation biology and radiation pathology syllabus (set RT 1: radiation oncology), Chicago, American College of Radiology, 1975.
38. Emami B, Lyman J, Brown A, et al. Tolerance of normal tissue

to therapeutic irradiation. *Int J Radiat Oncol Biol Phys* 1991; 21:109.

39. Kerr JF, Wyllie AH, Currie AR. Apoptosis: a basic biological phenomenon with wide-ranging implications in tissue kinetics. *Br J Cancer* 1972;26:239.

40. Alnemri ES, Fernandes TF, Haldar S, et al. Involvement of BCL-2 in glucocorticoid induced apoptosis of human pre-B-leukemias. *Cancer Res* 1992;32:491.

41. Shaw P, Bovey R, Tardy S, et al. Induction of apoptosis by wild-type p53 in a human colon tumor-derived cell line. *Proc Natl Acad Sci USA* 1992;89:4495.

42. Whitfield JF. Calcium signals and cancer. *Crit Rev Oncogen* 1992;3:55.

43. Arends MJ, Morris RG, Wyllie AH. Apoptosis. The role of the endonuclease. *Am J Pathol* 1990;136:593.

44. Sellins KS, Cohen JJ. Gene induction by gamma-irradiation leads to DNA fragmentation in lymphocytes. *J Immunol* 1987; 139:3199.

45. Ijiri K. Cell death (apoptosis) in mouse intestine after continuous irradiation with gamma rays and with beta rays from tritiated water. *Radiat Res* 1989;118:180.

46. Stephens LC, Ang KK, Schultheiss TE, et al. Apoptosis in irradiated murine tumors. *Radiat Res* 1991;127:308.

47. Warters RL. Radiation-induced apoptosis in a murine T-cell hybridoma. *Cancer Res* 1992;52:883.

48. Okada S. Radiation induced death. In: Altman G, Gerber G, Okada S, eds. *Radiation biochemistry*. New York: Academic Press, 1970:247.

49. Duvall E. Death and the cell. *Immunol Today* 1986;7:115.

50. Yamada T, Ohyama H. Radiation-induced interphase death of rat thymocytes is internally programmed (apoptosis). *Int J Radiat Biol* 1988;53:65.

51. Stephens LC, Hunter NR, Ang KK, et al. Development of apoptosis in irradiated murine tumors as a function of time and dose. *Radiat Res* 1993;135:75.

52. Rubin P, Casarett GW. *Clinical radiation pathology*. Philadelphia: WB Saunders, 1968.

53. Hall EJ, Cox JD. Physical and biologic basis of radiation therapy. In: Moss WT, Cox JD, eds. *Radiation oncology. Rationale, technique, results.* 6th ed. St. Louis: Mosby, 1989:1.

54. Michalowski A. Effects of radiation on normal tissues: hypothetical mechanisms and limitations of in situ assays of clonogenicity. *Radiat Environ Biophys* 1981;19:157.

55. Frindel E, Croizat H, Vassort F. Stimulating factors liberated by treated bone marrow: in vitro effect on CFU kinetics. *Exp Hematol* 1976;4:56.

56. Williams MV. The cellular basis of renal injury by radiation. *Br J Cancer Suppl* 1986;7:257.

57. Hobson B, Denekamp J. Endothelial proliferation in tumours and normal tissues: continuous labelling studies. *Br J Cancer* 1984;49:405.

58. Tubiana M, Dutreix J, Wambersie A. Effects on normal tissues. In: Tubiana M, Dutreix J, Wambersie A, eds. *Introduction to radiobiology*. London: Taylor & Francis, 1990:126.

59. Wheldon TE, Michalowski AS. Alternative models for the proliferative structure of normal tissues and their response to irradiation. *Br J Cancer* 1986;53 [Suppl. VII]:155.

60. Lever WF, Schaumburg-Lever G. *Histology of the skin,* 3rd ed. Philadelphia: JB Lippincott, 1990:9.

61. Bernstein EF, Sullivan FJ, Mitchell JB, et al. Biology of chronic radiation effect on tissues and wound healing. In: Granick MS, Salomon MP, Larson DL, eds. Philadelphia: WB Saunders, 1993:435.

62. Winchester DP, Cox JD. Standards for breast-conservation treatment. *CA Cancer J Clin* 1992;42:134.

63. Withers HR. The dose-response relationship for epithelial cells of skin. *Radiology* 1966;86:1110.

64. Withers HR. Recovery and repopulation in vivo by mouse skin epithelial cells during fractionated irradiation. *Radiat Res* 1967; 32:227.

65. Withers HR. The dose-survival relationship for irradiation of epithelial cells of mouse skin. *Br J Radiol* 1967;40:187.

66. Strandqvist M. Studien uber die kumulative Wirkung der Rontgenstrahlen bie Frakionierung. *Acta Radiol (Stockh)* 1944;55:1.

67. Ellis F. Dose time and fractionation: a clinical hypothesis. *Clin Radiol* 1969;20:1.

68. Ellis F. Nominal standard dose and the ret. *Br J Radiol* 1971; 44:101.

69. Fowler JF, Morgan RL, Sylvester JA, et al. Experiments with fractionated x-ray treatment of the skin of pigs. I. Fractionation up to 28 days. *Br J Radiol* 1963;36:188.

70. Fowler JF, Denekamp J, Page AL, et al. Fractionation with x-rays and neutrons in mice: response of skin and C3H mammary tumours. *Brit J Radiol* 1972;45:237.

71. Hegazy MA, Fowler JF. Cell population kinetics and desquamation skin reactions in plucked and unplucked mouse skin. II. Irradiated skin. *Cell Tissue Kinet* 1973;6:587.

72. Stevens KR. The esophagus. In: Moss WT, Cox JD, eds. *Radiation oncology. Rationale, technique, results,* 6th ed. St. Louis: Mosby, 1989:351.

73. Jennings FL, Arden A. Acute radiation effects in the esophagus. *AMA Arch Pathol* 1960;69:407.

74. Withers HR. Regeneration of intestinal mucosa after irradiation. *Cancer* 1971;28:75.

75. Thames HDJ, Withers R, Mason KA, et al. Dose-survival characteristics of mouse jejunal crypt cells. *Int J Radiat Oncol Biol Phys* 1981;7:1591.

76. Travis EL. Relative radiosensitivity of the human lung. *Adv Rad Biol* 1987;12:205.

77. Cox JD. The lung and thymus. In: Moss WT, Cox JD, eds. *Radiation oncology. Rationale, technique, results,* 6th ed. St. Louis: Mosby, 1989:285.

78. Travis EL, Down JD, Holmes SJ, et al. Radiation pneumonitis and fibrosis in mouse lung assayed by respiratory frequency and histology. *Radiat Res* 1980;84:133.

79. Byhardt RW, Moss WT. The heart and blood vessels. In: Moss WT, Cox JD, eds. *Radiation oncology. Rationale, technique, results,* 6th ed. St. Louis: Mosby, 1989:277.

80. Cuzick J, Stewart H, Rutqvist L, et al. Cause-specific mortality in long-term survivors of breast cancer who participated in trials of radiotherapy. *J Clin Oncol* 1994;12:447.

81. Cosset JM, Henry-Amar M, Pellae-Cosset B, et al. Pericarditis and myocardial infarctions after Hodgkin's disease therapy. *Int J Radiat Oncol Biol Phys* 1991;21:447.

82. Marbach JR, Sontag MR, Dyk JV, et al. Management of radiation oncology patients with implanted cardiac pacemakers: report of AAPM Task Group No. 34. *Medical Phys* 1994;21:85.

83. Ellis RE. The distribution of active bone marrow in the adult. *Phys Med Biol* 1961;5:255.

84. Till JE, McCullock EA. A direct measurement of the radiation sensitivity of normal mouse bone marrow cells. *Radiat Res* 1961; 14:213.

85. Marcus RB, Million RR. The incidence of myelitis after irradiation of the cervical spinal cord. *Int J Radiat Oncol Biol Phys* 1990;19:3.

86. Schultheiss TE. Spinal cord radiation "tolerance": Doctrine versus data. *Int J Radiat Oncol Biol Phys* 1990;19:219.

87. Jeremic B, Djuric L, Mijatovic L. Incidence of radiation myelitis of the cervical spinal cord at doses of 5500 cGy or greater. *Cancer* 1991;68:2138.

88. Bloss JD, DiSaia PJ, Mannel RS, et al. Radiation myelitis: a

complication of concurrent cisplatin and 5-fluorouracil chemotherapy with extended field radiotherapy for carcinoma of the uterine cervix. *Gynecol Oncol* 1991;43:305.

89. Wong CS, Minkin S, Hill RP. Re-irradiation tolerance of rat spinal cord to fractionated X-ray doses. *Radiother Oncol* 1993; 28:197.

90. Wong CS, Minkin S, Hill RP. Effect of small doses per fraction in rat spinal cord: influence of initial vs. final top-up doses. *Radiother Oncol* 1993;28:52.

91. Feldmeier JJ, Lange JD, Cox SD, et al. Hyperbaric oxygen as prophylaxis or treatment for radiation myelitis. *Undersea Hyperb Med* 1993;20:249.

92. Mason KA, Withers HR, Chiang CS. Late effects of radiation on the lumbar spinal cord of guinea pigs: re-treatment tolerance. *Int J Radiat Oncol Biol Phys* 1993;26:643.

93. van der Kogel AJ. Retreatment tolerance of the spinal cord [editorial]. *Int J Radiat Oncol Biol Phys* 1993;26:715.

94. Ang KK, Price RE, Stephens LC, et al. The tolerance of primate spinal cord to re-irradiation. *Int J Radiat Oncol Biol Phys* 1993; 25:459.

95. Powers BE, Beck ER, Gillette EL, et al. Pathology of radiation injury to the canine spinal cord. *Int J Radiat Oncol Biol Phys* 1992;23:539.

96. Terasima T, Tolmach LJ. Changes in x-ray sensitivity of HeLa cells during the division cycle. *Nature* 1961;190:1210.

97. Sinclair WK. Cyclic x-ray responses in mammalian cells in vitro. *Radiat Res* 1968;33:620.

98. Murray AW. Cell biology. Cyclins in meiosis and mitosis. *Nature* 1987;326:542.

99. Hanley-Hyde J. Cyclins in the cell cycle: an overview. *Curr Top Microbiol Immunol* 1992;182:461.

100. Sherr CJ. Mammalian G1 cyclins. *Cell* 1993;73:1059.

101. Mitchell JB, Bedford JS, Bailey SM. Dose-rate effects on the cell cycle and survival of S3 HeLa and V79 cells. *Radiat Res* 1979;79:520.

102. Muschel RJ, Zhang HB, Iliakis G, et al. Cyclin B expression in HeLa cells during the G2 block induced by ionizing radiation. *Cancer Res* 1991;51:5113.

103. Hill BT, Bellamy AS. *Antitumor drug-radiation interactions*. Boca Raton, FL: CRC Press, 1990.

104. Yarbro JW. Mechanism of action of hydroxyurea. *Semin Oncol* 1992;19:1.

105. Sinclair WK. The combined lethal effect of hydroxyurea and x-rays on Chinese hamster cells in vitro. ANL-7409. *ANL Rep* 1967;3.

106. Sinclair WK. The combined effect of hydroxyurea and x-rays on Chinese hamster cells in vitro. *Cancer Res* 1968;28:198.

107. Sinclair WK. Protection by cysteamine of cells sensitized by hydroxyurea to x radiation. ANL-7635. *ANL Rep* 1969;233.

108. Richards GJJ, Chambers RG. Hydroxyurea: a radiosensitizer in the treatment of neoplasms of the head and neck. *Am J Roentgenol Radium Ther Nucl Med* 1969;105:555.

109. Richards GJJ, Chambers RG. Hydroxyurea in the treatment of neoplasms of the head and neck. A resurvey. *Am J Surg* 1973; 126:513.

110. Piver MS, Barlow JJ, Vongtama V, et al. Hydroxyurea and radiation therapy in advanced cervical cancer. *Am J Obstet Gynecol* 1974;120:969.

111. Scheer AC, Wilson RF, Kalisher L. Combined radiotherapy and hydroxyurea in the management of lung cancer. *Clin Radiol* 1974;25:415.

112. Landgren RC, Hussey DH, Barkley HTJ, et al. Split-course irradiation compared to split-course irradiation plus hydroxyurea in inoperable bronchogenic carcinoma—a randomized study of 53 patients. *Cancer* 1974;34:1598.

113. Bhalla K, Birkhofer M, Bhalla M, et al. A phase I study of a combination of allopurinol, 5-fluorouracil and leucovorin followed by hydroxyurea in patients with advanced gastrointestinal and breast cancer. *Am J Clin Oncol* 1991;14:509.

114. Vokes EE, Haraf DJ, Panje WR, et al. Hydroxyurea with concomitant radiotherapy for locally advanced head and neck cancer. *Semin Oncol* 1992;19:53.

115. Levin VA. The place of hydroxyurea in the treatment of primary brain tumors. *Semin Oncol* 1992;19:34.

116. Vokes EE, Dolan ME, Krishnasamy S, et al. 5-Fluorouracil, hydroxyurea and escalating doses of iododeoxyuridine with concomitant radiotherapy for malignant gliomas: a clinical and pharmacologic analysis. *Ann Oncol* 1993;4:591.

117. Blumenreich MS, Kellihan MJ, Joseph UG, et al. Long-term intravenous hydroxyurea infusions in patients with advanced cancer. A phase I trial. *Cancer* 1993;71:2828.

118. Stehman FB, Bundy BN, Thomas G, et al. Hydroxyurea versus misonidazole with radiation in cervical carcinoma: long-term follow-up of a Gynecologic Oncology Group trial. *J Clin Oncol* 1993;11:1523.

119. Rao S, Horwitz SB, Ringel I. Direct photoaffinity labeling of tubulin with taxol. *J Natl Cancer Inst* 1992;84:785.

120. Rowinsky EK, Donehower RC, Jones RJ, et al. Microtubule changes and cytotoxicity in leukemic cell lines treated with taxol. *Cancer Res* 1988;48:4093.

121. Liebmann J, Cook J, Lipschultz C, et al. The Influence of Cremophor EL on the cell cycle effects of paclitaxel (taxol) in human tumor cell lines. *Cancer Chemother Pharmacol* 1994;33:331.

122. Liebmann JE, Cook JA, Lipschultz C, et al. Cytotoxic studies of paclitaxel (Taxol®) in human tumour cell lines. *Br J Cancer* 1993;68:1104.

123. Liebmann JE, Cook JA, Fisher J, et al. In vitro studes of paclitaxel (Taxol®) as a radiation sensitizer in human tumor cells. *J Natl Cancer Inst* 1994;86:441.

124. Cook JA, DeGraff W, Teague D, et al. Radiation sensitization of Chinese hamster V79 cells by paclitaxel. *Radiat Oncol Invest* 1993;1:103.

125. Liebmann JE, Cook JA, Fisher J, et al. Changes in radiation survival curve parameters in human tumor and rodent cells exposed to paclitaxel (Taxol®). *Int J Radiat Oncol Biol Phys* 1994; 29:559.

126. McGuire WP, Rowinsky EK, Rosenshein NB, et al. Taxol: a unique antineoplastic agent with significant activity in advanced ovarian epithelial neoplasms. *Ann Intern Med* 1989;111:273.

127. Holmes FA, Walters RS, Theriault RL, et al. Phase II trial of taxol, an active drug in the treatment of metastatic breast cancer. *J Natl Cancer Inst* 1991;83:1797.

128. Forastiere AA. Use of paclitaxel (Taxol) in squamous cell carcinoma of the head and neck. *Semin Oncol* 1993;20:56.

129. Chang A, Kim K, Glick J, et al. Phase II study of taxol in patients with stage IV non-small cell lung cancer (NSCLC): The Eastern Cooperative Oncology Group (ECOG) results. *Proc Am Soc Clin Oncol* 1992;11:293.

130. Withers HR. Biological basis for high-LET radiotherapy. *Radiology* 1973;108:131.

131. Withers HR. Biologic basis of radiotherapy. In: Perez CA, Brady LW, eds. *Principles and practice of radiation oncology*. Philadelphia: JB Lippincott, 1992:64.

132. Hall EJ. Linear energy transfer and relative biological effectiveness. In: Hall EJ, ed. *Radiobiology for the radiologist*. Philadelphia: JB Lippincott, 1994:153.

133. Fletcher GH, Shukovsky LJ. Isoeffect exponents for the production of dose-response curves in squamous cell carcinomas treated between 4 to 8 weeks. *J Radiol Electrol Med Nucl* 1976;57:825.

134. GH F. The evolution of the basic concepts underlying the practice of radiotherapy from 1949 to 1977. *Radiology* 1978;127: 3.

135. Walker M, Strike TA, Sheline GE. An analysis of dose effect relationship in the radiotherapy of malignant gliomas. *Int J Radiat Oncol Biol Phys* 1979;5:1725.

136. Perez CA, Stanley K, Rubin P, et al. A prospective randomized study of various irradiation doses and fractionation schedules in the treatment of inoperable non-oat cell carcinoma of the lung. Preliminary report by the Radiation Therapy Oncology Group. *Cancer* 1980;45:2744.

137. Parsons JT. Time-dose-volume relations in radiation therapy. In: Million RR, Cassisi NJ, eds. *Management of head and neck cancer: a multidisciplinary approach*. Philadelphia: JB Lippincott, 1994:203.

138. Hall EJ. The oxygen effect and reoxygenation. In: Hall EJ, ed. *Radiobiology for the radiologist*. Philadelphia: JB Lippincott 1994:133.

139. von Sonntag C. *The chemical basis of radiation biology,* London: Taylor and Francis, 1987.

140. Thomlinson RH, Gray LH. The histological structure of some human lung cancers and the possible implications for radiotherapy. *Br J Cancer* 1955;9:539.

141. Powers WE, Tolmach LJ. A multicomponent x ray survival curve for mouse lymphosarcoma cells irradiated in vivo. *Nature* 1963;197:710.

142. Gatenby RA, Kessler HB, Rosenblum JS, et al. Oxygen distribution in squamous cell carcinoma metastases and its relationship to outcome of radiation therapy. *Int J Radiat Oncol Biol Phys* 1988;14:831.

143. Vaupel P, Schlenger K, Knoop C, et al. Oxygenation of human tumors: evaluation of tissue oxygen distribution in breast cancers by computerized O2 tension measurements. *Cancer Res* 1991;51:3316.

144. Rampling R, Cruickshank G, Lewis AD, et al. Direct measurement of pO2 distribution and bioreductive enzymes in human malignant brain tumors. *Int J Radiat Oncol Biol Phys* 1994;29:427.

145. Hockel M, Schlenger K, Aral B, et al. Association between tumor hypoxia and malignant progression in advanced cancer of the uterine cervix. *Cancer Res* 1996;56:4509.

146. Rasey JS, Koh WJ, Evans ML, et al. Quantifying regional hypoxia in human tumors with positron emmision tomography of [18F]fluoromisonidazole: a pretherapy study of 37 patients. *Int J Radiat Oncol Biol Phys* 1996;36:417.

147. Adams GE, Flockhart IR, Smithen CE, et al. Electron-affinic sensitization. VII. A correlation between structures, one-electron reduction potentials, and efficiencies of nitroimidazoles as hypoxic cell radiosensitizers. *Radiat Res* 1976;67:9.

148. Phillips TL, Wasserman T. Promise of radiosensitizers and radioprotectors in the treatment of human cancer. *Cancer Treat Rep* 1984;68:291.

149. Lawton CA, Coleman CN, Buzydlowski JW, et al. Results of a phase II trial of external beam radiation with etanidazole (SR 2508) for the treatment of locally advanced prostate cancer (RTOG Protocol 90-20). *Int J Radiat Oncol Biol Phys* 1996;36:673.

150. Eschwege F, Sancho-Garnier H, Chassagne D, et al. Results of a European radomized trial of Etanidazole combined with radiotherapy in head and neck carcinomas. *Int J Radiat Oncol Biol Phys* 1997;39:275.

151. Marletta MA. Nitric oxide: biochemistry of formation and biological significance. *Trends Biochem Sci* 1989;14:488.

152. Furchgott RF, Vanhoutee PM. Endolthelium-derived relaxing and contracting factors. *FASEB* 1989;3:2007.

153. Moncada S, Palmer RMJ, Higgs EA. Nitric oxide: physiology, pathophysiology, and pharmacology. *Pharmacol Rev* 1991;43:109.

154. Feldman PL, Griffith OW, Stuehr DJ. The surprising life of nitric oxide. *Chem Engineering News* 1992;December 20:26.

155. Maragos CM, Morley D, Wink DA, et al. Complexes of NO with nucleophiles as agents for the controlled biological release of nitric oxide. Vasorelaxant effects. *J Med Chem* 1991;34:3242.

156. Mitchell JB, Wink DA, DeGraff W, et al. Hypoxic mammalian cell radiosensitization by nitric oxide. *Cancer Res* 1993;53:5845.

157. Mitchell JB, Cook JA, Krishna MC, et al. Radiation sensitization by nitric oxide releasing agents. *Br J Cancer* 1996;74:S181.

158. van Putten LM, Kallman RF. Oxygenation status of a transplantable tumor during fractionated radiotherapy. *J Natl Cancer Inst* 1968;40:441.

159. Belli JA, Harris JR. Adriamycin resistance and radiation response. *Int J Radiat Oncol Biol Phys* 1979;5:1231.

160. Wallner K, Li GC. Adriamycin resistance, heat resistance, and radiation response in Chinese hamster fibroblasts. *Int J Radiat Oncol Biol Phys* 1986;12:829.

161. Wallner KE, Li GC. Effect of cisplatin resistance on cellular radiation response. *Int J Radiat Oncol Biol Phys* 1987;13:587.

162. Mitchell JB, Gamson J, Russo A, et al. Chinese hamster pleiotropic multidrug-resistant cells are not radioresistant. *NCI Monogr* 1988;6:187.

163. Louie KG, Behrens BC, Kinsella TJ, et al. Radiation survival parameters of antineoplastic drug-sensitive and -resistant human ovarian cancer cell lines and their modification by buthionine sulfoximine. *Cancer Res* 1985;45:2110.

164. Lehnert S, Greene D, Batist G. Radiation response of drug-resistant variants of a human breast cancer cell line. *Radiat Res* 1989;118:568.

165. Hopwood LE, Moulder JE. Radiation induction of drug resistance in RIF-1 tumors and tumor cells. *Radiat Res* 1989;120:251.

166. Sharma RC, Schimke RT. Enhancement of the frequency of methotrexate resistance by gamma radiation in Chinese hamster ovary and mouse 3T6 cells. *Cancer Res* 1989;49:3861.

167. Osmak M, Perovic S. Multiple fractions of gamma rays induced resistance to cis-dichloro-diammineplatinum (II) and methotrexate in human HeLa cells. *Int J Radiat Oncol Biol Phys* 1989;16:1537.

168. Habraken Y, Laval F. Enhancement of 1,3-bis(2-chloroethyl)-1-nitrosourea resistance by γ-irradiation or drug pretreatment in rat hepatoma cells. *Cancer Res* 1991;51:1217.

169. Hill BT, Deuchars K, Hosking LK, et al. Overexpression of P-glycoprotein in mammalian tumor cell lines after fractionated X irradiation in vitro. *J Natl Cancer Inst* 1990;82:607.

170. Patt HM, Tyree EB, Staube RL, et al. Cysteine protection against X-irradiation. *Science* 1949;110:213.

171. Bacq ZM, Dechamps G, Fischer P, et al. Protection against X-rays and therapy of radiation sickness with β-mercaptoethylamine. *Science* 1953;117:633.

172. Allalunis-Turner MJ, Walden TL, Sawich C. Induction of marrow hypoxia by radioprotective agents. *Radiat Res* 1989;118:581.

173. Sweeny TR. *A survey of compounds from the antiradiation drug development program of the U.S. Army Medical Research and Development Command*. Washington, D.C.: Walter Reed Institute of Research, 1979.

174. Utley JF, Marlowe JF, Waddell WJ. Distribution of 35 S-labelled WR-2721 in normal and malignant tissues of the mouse. *Radiat Res* 1976;68:284.

175. Washburn LC, Carlton JE, Hayes RL. Distribution of WR-2721 in normal and malignant tissues of mice and rats bearing solid tumors: dependence on tumor type, drug dose and species. *Radiat Res* 1974;59:475.

176. Yuhas JM, Storer VB. Differential chemoprotection of normal and malignant tissues. *J Natl Cancer Inst* 1969;42:331.

177. Yuhas JM. Active versus passive absorption kinetics as the basis for selective protection of normal tissues by S-2-(3-aminopropylamino) ethylphosphorthioic acid. *Cancer Res* 1980;40:1519.

178. Kligerman MM, Shaw MT, Slavik M, et al. Phase I clinical studies with WR-2721. *Cancer Clin Trials* 1980;3:217.

179. Kligerman MM, Turrisi AT, Urtasun RC, et al. Final report on phase I trial of WR-2721 before protracted fractionated radiation therapy. *Int J Radiat Oncol Biol Phys* 1988;14:1119.

180. Turrisi AT, Glover DJ, Hurwitz S, et al. The final report of the phase I trial of single dose WR-2721, S-2-(3-aminopropylamino) ethylphosphorothioic acid. *Cancer Treat Rep* 1986; 70:1389.

181. Mehta MP. Protection of normal tissues from the cytotoxic effects of radiation therapy: focus on amifostine. *Semin Radiat Oncol* 1998;8:14.

182. Buntzel J, Kuttner K, Frohlich D, et al. Selective cytoprotection with amifostine in concurrent radiochemotherapy for head and neck cancer. *Ann Oncol* 1998;9:505.

183. Mitchell JB, DeGraff W, Kaufman D, et al. Inhibition of oxygen-dependent radiation-induced damage by the nitroxide superoxide dismutase mimic, Tempol. *Arch Biochem Biophys* 1991;289:62.

184. Hahn SM, Tochner Z, Krishna CM, et al. Tempol, a stable free radical, is a novel murine radiation protector. *Cancer Res* 1992;52:1750.

185. Goffman T, Cuscela D, Glass J, et al. Topical application of nitroxide protects radiation induced alopecia in guinea pigs. *Int J Radiat Oncol Biol Phys* 1992;22:803.

186. Hahn SM, Sullivan FJ, DeLuca AM, et al. Evaluation of tempol radioprotection in a murine tumor model. *Free Radic Biol Med* 1997;22:1211.

187. Salmon SE. *Cloning of human tumor stem cells.* New York: Alan R Liss, 1980.

188. Rupinak HT, Hill BT. The poor cloning ability in agar of human tumour cells. *Cell Biol Int Rep* 1980;4:479.

189. Selby P, Buick RN, Tannock T. A critical appraisal of the "human tumor stem-cell assay" *N Eng J Med* 1983;308:129.

190. Ioachim HL, Dorsett BH, Paluch E. The immune response at the tumor site in lung carcinoma. *Cancer* 1976;38:2296.

191. Barranco SC, Romsdahl MM, Humphrey RM. The radiation response of human malignant melanoma cells grown in vitro. *Cancer Res* 1971;31:830.

192. Weichselbaum RR, Epstein J, Little JB, et al. In vitro cellular radiosensitivity of human malignant tumors. *Eur J Cancer* 1976; 12:47.

193. Gerweck LE, Kornblith PL, Burlette P, et al. Radiation sensitivity of cultured human glioblastoma cells. *Radiology* 1977;27: 231.

194. Ohara H, Okamato T. A new in vitro cell line established from human oat cell carcinoma of the lung. *Cancer Res* 1977;37: 3088.

195. Weichselbaum RR, Nove J, Little JB. Radiation response of human tumor cells in vitro. *Rad Biol Can Res* 1980;345.

196. Weichselbaum RR, Greenberger JS, Schmidt A, et al. In vitro radiosensitivity of human leukemia cell lines. *Radiology* 1981; 139:485.

197. Fertil B, Malaise EP. Inherent cellular radiosensitivity as a basic concept for human tumor radiotherapy. *Int J Radiat Oncol Biol Phys* 1981;1:621.

198. Carney DN, Mitchell JB, Kinsella TJ. In vitro radiation and chemotherapy sensitivity of established cell lines of human small cell lung cancer and its large cell morphological variants. *Cancer Res* 1983;43:2806.

199. Morstyn G, Russo A, Carney DN, et al. Heterogeneity in the radiation survival curves and biochemical properties of human lung cancer cell lines. *J Natl Cancer Inst* 1984;73:801.

200. Brodin O, Lennartsson L, Nilsson S. Single-dose and fractionated irradiation of four human lung cancer cell lines in vitro. *Acta Oncologica* 1991;30:967.

201. Moody TW, Cuttitta F. Growth factor and peptide receptors in small cell lung cancer. *Life Sciences* 1993;52:1161.

202. Bergh J, Nilsson K, Ekman R, et al. Establishment and characterization of cell lines from human small cell and large cell carcinomas of the lung. *Acta Pathol Microbiol Scand* 1985;93: 133.

203. Gazdar AF, Carney DN, Russell EK, et al. Establishment of continuous, clonable cultures of small-cell carcinoma of lung which have amine precursor uptake and decarboxylation cell properties. *Cancer Res* 1980;40:3502.

204. Carney DN, Gazdar AF, Bepler G, et al. Establishment and identification of small cell lung cancer cell lines having classic and variant features. *Cancer Res* 1985;45:2913.

205. Weisenthal LM, Marsden JA, Dill PL, et al. A novel dye exclusion method for testing in vitro chemosensitivity of human tumors. *Cancer Res* 1983;43:749.

206. Twentyman PR, Walls GA, Wright KA. The response of tumor cells to radiation and cytotoxic drugs-a comparison of clonogenic and isotope uptake assays. *Brit J Cancer* 1984;50:625.

207. Van Hoff DD, Forseth B, Warfel LE. Use of a radiometric system to screen for antineoplastic agents: correlation with a human tumor cloning system. *Cancer Res* 1985;45:4032.

208. Fraser LB, Spitzer G, Ajani JA, et al. Drug and radiation sensitivity measurements of successful primary mono-layer culturing of human tumor cells using cell-adhesive matrix and supplemented medium. *Cancer Res* 1986;46:1263.

209. Carmichael J, DeGraff WG, Gazdar AF, et al. Evaluation of tetrazolium-based semiautomated colorimetric assay: assessment of chemosensitivity testing. *Cancer Res* 1987;47:936.

210. Carmichael J, DeGraff WG, Gazdar AF, et al. Evaluation of a tetrazolium-based semiautomated colorimetric assay: assessment of radiosensitivity. *Cancer Res* 1987;47:943.

211. Carmichael J, DeGraff WG, Gamson J, et al. Radiation sensitivity of human lung cancer cell lines. *Eur J Cancer Clin Oncol* 1989;25:527.

212. Matthews MJ, Kanhouwa S, Pickren J. Frequency of residual and metastatic tumor in patients undergoing curative surgical resection for lung cancer. *Cancer Chemother Rep* 1973;4:63.

213. Livingood LE. Tumors in the mouse. *Johns Hopkins Bull* 1896; 66/67:177.

214. Malkinson AM. Primary lung tumors in mice: An experimentally manipulable model of human adenocarcinoma. *Cancer Res [Suppl]* 1992;52:2670s.

215. Amstad P, Reddel RR, Pfeifer A, et al. Neoplastic transformation of a human bronchial epithelial cell line by a recombinant retrovirus encoding viral Harvey ras. *Mol Carcinog* 1988;1:151.

216. Smith IE, Courtenay VD, Mills J, et al. In vitro radiation response of cells from four human tumors propagated in immune suppressed mice. *Cancer Res* 1978;38:390.

217. Steel GG, Peckham MJ. Human tumor xenografts: a critical appraisal. *Br J Cancer* 1980;41 [suppl. 4]:133.

218. Hosono M, Endo K, Hosono MN, et al. Treatment of small-cell lung cancer xenografts with iodine-131-anti-neural cell adhesion molecule monoclonal antibody and evaluation of absorbed dose in tissue. *J Nuc Med* 1994;35:296.

219. Hollstein M, Sidransky D, Vogelstein B, et al. p53 mutations in human cancers. *Science* 1991;253:49.

220. Blank KR, Rudoltz MS, Kao GD, et al. The molecular regulation of apoptosis and implications for radiation oncology. *Int J Radiat Biol* 1997;71:455.

221. Salgia R, Skarin AT. Molecular abnormalities in lung cancer. *J Clin Oncol* 1998;16:1207.

222. Fujino M, Dosaka-Akita H, Harada M, et al. Prognostic signifi-

cance of p53 and ras p21 expression in nonsmall cell lung cancer. *Cancer* 1995;76:2457.

223. Lowe SW, Bodis S, McClatchey A, et al. p53 status and the efficacy of cancer therapy in vivo. *Science* 1994;266:807.

224. Chang EH, Jang YJ, Hao Z, et al. Restoration of the G1 checkpoint and the apoptotic pathway mediated by wild-type p53 sensitizes squamous cell carcinoma of the head and neck to radiotherapy. *Arch Otolaryngol Head Neck Surg* 1997;123:507.

225. Brachman DG, Beckett M, Graves D, et al. p53 mutation does not correlate with radiosensitivity in 24 head and neck cancer cell lines. *Cancer Res* 1993;53:3667.

226. Yu Y, Li CY, Little JB. Abrogation of p53 function by HPV16 E6 gene delays apoptosis and enhances mutagenesis but does not alter radiosensitivity in TK6 human lymphoblast cells. *Oncogene* 1997;14:1661.

227. Canman CE, Lim DS, Cimprich KA, et al. Activation of the ATM kinase by ionizing radiation and phosphorylation of p53. *Science* 1998;281:1677.

228. Harada M, Dosaka-Akita H, Miyamoto H, et al. Prognostic significance of the expression of ras oncogene in non-small cell lung cancer. *Cancer* 1992;69:72.

229. Sklar M. The ras oncogenes increase the intrinsic resistance of NIH 3T3 cells to ionizing radiation. *Science* 1988;239:645.

230. McKenna WG, Weiss MC, Endlich B, et al. Synergistic effect of the v-myc oncogene with H-ras on radioresistance. *Cancer Res* 1990;50:97.

231. McKenna WG, Weiss MC, Bakanauskas VJ, et al. The role of the H-ras oncogene in radiation resistance and metastasis. *Int J Radiat Oncol Biol Phys* 1990;18:849.

232. Iliakis G, Metzger L, Muschel RJ, et al. Induction and repair of DNA double strand breaks in radiation-resistant cells obtained by transformation of primary rat embryo cells with the oncogenes H-ras and v-myc. *Cancer Res* 1990;50:6575.

233. McKenna WG, Iliakis G, Weiss MC, et al. Increased G_2 delay in radiation-resistant cells obtained by transformation of primary rat embryo cells with the oncogenes H-ras and v-myc. *Radiat Res* 1991;125:283.

234. Su L-N, Little JB. Prolonged cell cycle delay in radioresistant human cell lines transfected with activated ras oncogene and/or Simian Virus 40 T-antigen. *Radiat Res* 1993;133:73.

235. Pardo FS, Bristow RG, Taghian A, et al. Role of transfection and clonal selection in mediating radioresistance. *Proc Natl Acad Sci USA* 1991;88:10652.

236. Kasid UN, Weichselbaum RR, Brennan T, et al. Sensitivities of NIH/3T3-derived clonal cell lines to ionizing radiation: Significance for gene transfer studies. *Cancer Res* 1989;49:3396.

237. Harris J, Chambers A, Tam A. Some ras-transformed cells have increased radiosensitivity and decreased repair of sublethal radiation damage. *Somatic Cell Mol Genet* 1990;16:39.

238. Bernhard EJ, McKenna WG, Hamilton AD, et al. Inhibiting Ras prenylation increases the radiosensitivity of human tumor cell lines with activating mutations of ras oncogenes. *Cancer Res* 1998;58:1754.

239. Coussens L, Yang-Feng TL, Liao YC, et al. Tyrosine kinase receptor with extensive homology to EGF receptor shares chromosomal location with neu oncogene. *Science* 1985;230:1132.

240. Di Fiore PP, Pierce JH, Kraus MH, et al. ErbB-2 is a potent oncogene when overexpressed in NIH3T3 cells. *Science* 1987;237:178.

241. Shi D, He G, Cao S, et al. Overexpression of the c-erbB-2/neu-encoded p185 protein in primary lung cancer. *Mol Carcinogen* 1992;5:213.

242. Nemunaitis J, Klemow S, Tong A, et al. Prognostic value of K-ras mutations, ras oncoprotein, and c-erb B-2 oncoprotein expression in adenocarcinoma of the lung. *Am J Clin Oncol* 1998;21:155.

243. Kern JA, Slebos RJ, Top B, et al. C-erbB-2 expression and codon 12 K-ras mutations both predict shortened survival for patients with pulmonary adenocarcinomas. *J Clin Invest* 1994;93:516.

244. Burke HB, Hoang A, Iglehart JD, et al. Predicting response to adjuvant and radiation therapy in patients with early stage breast carcinoma. *Cancer* 1998;82:874.

245. Schiller JH. Lung cancer: therapeutic modalities and cytoprotection. *Lung* 1998;176:145.

246. Pomp J, Ouwerkerk IJM, Hermans J, et al. The influence of oncogenes NRAS and MYC on the radiation sensitivity of cells of a human melanoma cell line. *Radiat Res* 1996;146:374.

247. Tanaka H, Fujii Y, Hirabayashi H, et al. Disruption of the RB pathway and cell-proliferative activity in non-small-cell lung cancers. *Int J Cancer* 1998;79:111.

248. Reissmann PT, Koga H, Figlin RA, et al. Inactivation of retinoblastoma susceptibility gene in non-small-cell lung cancer. The Lung Cancer Study Group. *Oncogene* 1993;8:1913.

249. Harbour JW, Lai SL, Whang-Peng J, et al. Abnormalities in structure and expression of the human retinoblastoma gene in SCLC. *Science* 1988;241:353.

250. Yamamoto Y, Shimizu E, Masuda N, et al. RB protein status and chemosensitivity in non-small cell lung cancers. *Oncol Rep* 1997;5:447.

251. Ishii H, Igarashi T, Saito T, et al. Retinoblastoma protein expressed in human non-hodgkin's lymphoma cells generates resistance against radiation-induced apoptosis. *Am J Hematol* 1997;55:46.

252. Pollack A, Czerniak B, Zagars GK, et al. Retinoblastoma protein expression and radiation response in muscle-invasive bladder cancer. *Int J Radiat Oncol Biol Phys* 1997;39:687.

253. Cleary ML, Smith SD, Sklar J. Cloning and structural analysis of cDNAs for bcl-2 and a hybrid bcl-2/immunoglobin transcript resulting from the t(14;18) translocation. *Cell* 1986;47:19.

254. Korsmeyer SJ. Regulators of cell death. *Trends Genet* 1995;11:101.

255. Stefanaki K, Rontogiannis D, Yamvouka C, et al. Immunohistochemical detection of bcl2, p53, mdm2 and p21/waf1 proteins in small-cell lung carcinomas. *Anticancer Res* 1998;18:1689.

256. Pezzella F, Turley H, Kuzu I, et al. bcl-2 protein in non-small-cell lung carcinoma. *N Engl J Med* 1993;329:690.

257. Anton RC, Brown RW, Younes M, et al. Absence of prognostic significance of bcl-2 immunopositivity in non-small cell lung cancer: analysis of 427 cases. *Hum Pathol* 1997;28:1079.

258. Silvestrini R, Costa A, Lequaglie C, et al. Bcl-2 protein and prognosis in patients with potentially curable non-small-cell lung cancer. *Vichows Arch* 1998;432:441.

259. Gilbert MS, Saad AH, Rupnow BA, et al. Association of BCL-2 with membrane hyperpolarization and radioresistance. *J Cell Physiol* 1996;168:114.

260. Domen J, Gandy KL, Weissman IL. Systemic overexpression of BCL-2 in the hematopoetic system protects transgenic mice from the consequences of lethal irradiation. *Blood* 1998;91:2272.

13

TREATMENT-RELATED LUNG DAMAGE

ELIZABETH L. TRAVIS
RITSUKO KOMAKI

Radiation therapy is an integral part of the treatment and management of lung cancer. More than 50% of patients with lung cancer receive radiation at some point during the management of their disease. Because these patients generally require the treatment of a large volume of lung to high doses, definitive radiotherapy of lung cancer requires the use of total doses that result in late sequelae. These late sequelae were observed as early as the 1920s, less than two decades after the discovery of x-ray.[1] The two phases of lung damage—radiation pneumonitis and radiation fibrosis—were first described in 1925 by Evans and Leucutia, who divided the damage into these now well-recognized sequelae of lung irradiation.[2] Although almost a century of studies in patients and experimental models has provided a wealth of information on these two potentially fatal complications, we remain unable totally to circumvent these untoward reactions. Both pneumonitis and fibrosis continue to limit the effective use of radiation in the treatment of malignant tumors of the lung.

Despite the fact that only three years have passed since the first edition of this book was published, significant advances have been made in understanding the genetic regulation and molecular basis of radiation-induced lung damage. In addition, the radiation dose-volume effect in mouse lung has been clearly defined, with substantiation of the experimental findings by clinical studies. As 3D conformal therapy has become the norm for treating lung cancer, new methods of estimating the risk of pulmonary injury from dose-volume histograms and normal tissue complication probability models have been developed. The goal of this chapter is to update the information specifically in these areas as well as to present new data regarding the development of quantitative and easily accessible markers of lung damage and predictive assays of pulmonary radiosensitivity.

In this chapter all the data, unless otherwise stated, will be from studies on normal nondiseased lungs, although preexisting lung disease in patients may have a significant impact on the effects of radiation or drugs on response.

DAMAGE VERSUS MORBIDITY

Damage and morbidity are terms which are frequently interchanged but, although related, they actually reflect different concepts. In clinical practice, the radiation oncologist accepts some structural lung damage, either pneumonitis or fibrosis, because of the large functional reserve of this tissue. Functionally, the whole organ does not fail if some part of it is destroyed. Morbidity is a clinical term that describes how an individual patient feels and/or how well a specific organ functions. The morbidity of treatment is determined by many factors, including the damage incurred by the tissue, the impact of this damage on organ function, and the impact of both of the above on the patient's well-being and lifestyle. Because of the functional reserve of the lung, structural damage is not necessarily reflected in clinical morbidity as assessed by whole-lung function.

The dissociation between damage and morbidity in the lung reflect the organization of those anatomical units responsible for lung function.[3] Morbidity is a reflection of two parameters: (a) the survival of sufficient numbers of cells to maintain tissue function, and (b) the organization of these cells into units that carry out tissue function. The spatial relationship between these functional subunits differs between tissues and is a critical determinant of the relationship between damage and any resultant morbidity. Anatomically, the lung is a system of branching ducts and accompanying blood vessels that ultimately terminate in the alveoli, the site of gas exchange. The functional subunit in the lung is most likely the acinus, which is structurally well defined, beginning at the ramification of the terminal bronchiole to the respiratory bronchioles and terminating in the alveolar sac, each of which bears numerous alveoli. Each acinus is a self-contained entity independent of its neighbor. It is suggested that the destruction of one acinus will have no measurable effect on lung function in a normal healthy lung and that functional damage, particularly total lung function, will be manifested only when a critical number of these units are destroyed. A useful analogy is a strand of Christmas tree lights arranged in parallel. When one burns out (damage), none of the others are affected and the overall effect is not diminished, that is, the damage is below the threshold of the human eye to distinguish it (no morbidity). However, when sufficient numbers of lights burn out such that this is noticeable (the threshold for damage in the human eye is now exceeded), the overall effect is diminished (morbidity occurs).

Many assays are available to quantify radiation-induced morbidity and damage in the lungs of experimental animals and in patients. In humans, regional pulmonary function tests or radiographic evidence of pneumonitis and fibrosis can be quantified, providing a scoring system for damage.[4-13] In rats and mice, the experimental animals most commonly used to study radiation and drug-induced lung injury, measurements of regional lung function are difficult and pulmonary function tests most often assess total lung function, a measure of morbidity.[14-18] Whereas in patients structural damage can be quantified by noninvasive methods, for example CT scans, assessment of such damage in small experimental animals is most often performed on autopsy specimens. In this chapter, clear distinctions will be made between damage and morbidity and the assessment of each.

RADIATION-INDUCED LUNG DAMAGE

Pathophysiology of Radiation-Induced Lung Injury

Radiation damage in the human lung has four well-described clinical phases: a phase of acute injury termed radiation pneumonitis, a subacute phase, a chronic phase characterized by lung fibrosis, and a late phase (Figure 13.1).[19-23] Two of these phases of damage are clearly separated in time; pneumonitis occurs from three to six months after the beginning of treatment, while fibrosis occurs from one year onward. Both pneumonitis and fibrosis have been well defined histopathologically under controlled conditions in animals. However, because animals can be studied at predetermined times after irradiation, an earlier phase of damage that is asymptomatic has been defined—the latent phase.[19,22,24] Thus radiation lung injury consists of distinct phases characterized by differences in time of expression after irradiation and distinct histologic and/or molecular changes.

Latent Phase

The weeks to months preceding the overt appearance of radiation pneumonitis is referred to as the "latent" period because no overt histopathologic, radiographic, or clinical signs and symptoms of radiation damage can be observed. In most cases, overt pulmonary reactions are not expressed either clinically or histologically in human and animal models for the first three months after irradiation, regardless of the volume of lung irradiated, although in humans, dam-

age may be expressed as early as two months after initiation treatment. Although no changes can be observed at the light microscopic level during this "latent" time, electron microscopy reveals degranulation and loss of Type II cells with attendant loss of surfactant, loss of basal laminar proteoglycans resulting in swelling of the basement membrane, and transudation of proteins into the alveolar spaces indicating increased capillary permeability and suggesting a loss of endothelial cells within the first month after whole-lung irradiation.[20,22,23] Endothelial cells themselves become vacuolated and pleomorphic and may slough, leading to denudation of the basement membrane and changes in capillary permeability.[25] Although these changes are dose-related and diffuse throughout the lung, they are not in themselves sufficiently severe to result in death during this time. Deaths do not occur before there is overt histologic damage.

It had been generally accepted that a series of biochemical events was occurring during this latent phase that ultimately culminated in the overt expression of damage in the next phase of lung injury, pneumonitis, although none had been identified. The advent of new molecular techniques and tools has shown that dramatic changes do occur during this period and, depending on the dose, may resolve or may progress to the next phase of radiation pneumonitis, which produces overt signs and symptoms. These molecular changes in the lung will be discussed later in this chapter.

"Classical" Pneumonitis

Structural changes in the lung appear within the first six months after irradiation of all or part of the lung of humans or experimental animals, resulting in diffuse alveolar damage.[1,19,22,24] Although this phase of damage occurs relatively long after lung irradiation, histologically it is an acute effect which is characterized by a prominent inflammatory cell infiltrate consisting of macrophages, lymphocytes, and mononuclear cells in the air sacs and in the pulmonary interstitium, the latter of which is normally devoid of cells.[3,19-24] The neutrophil is not a dominant cell in this inflammatory cell infiltrate in animal models. Although loosening and widening of the interstitium indicates interstitial edema, only after high doses is edema observed in the air spaces. When the whole of both lungs is irradiated in humans or experimental animals, the damage is diffuse and, if sufficiently severe, can be fatal.

This acute phase of damage in the lung is generally referred to as pneumonitis, a term that usually refers to an inflammatory reaction in the lung caused by local growth of bacteria, fungi, or parasites. In such situations, the cellular infiltrate contains polymorphonuclear leukocytes, a cell type rarely found in the "sterile" inflammatory infiltrate in the irradiated lungs of experimental animals. When present, these cells are indicative of a superimposed infection and the cause of death is unclear, that is, radiation or infection or both. Perhaps a more appropriate term for this phase of

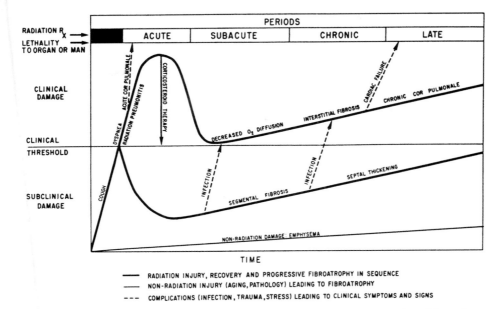

FIGURE 13.1. The clinical course of radiation induced pulmonary damage consists of four phases, each having distinct pathologic and clinical signs and symptoms. These changes are dependent on dose, as depicted in the upper curve (high dose) and the lower curve (low dose). The changes in the acute phase after high doses are those generally associated with radiation pneumonitis, while those occurring during the chronic and late phase are associated with pulmonary fibrosis. After low doses, the pathologic changes are subtle, consisting mostly of interstitial fibrosis which is usually not sufficiently severe to cause clinical symptoms. (From Rubin P and Casarett GW, eds, *clinical radiation pathology*, W.B. Saunders Company, 1968; 459, with permission.)

diffuse alveolar damage following lung irradiation is "alveolitis," which pathologically refers to an inflammatory reaction not caused by a microorganism.[26] Although an inflammatory cell infiltrate in the interstitium and the air sacs is a prominent component of radiation alveolitis, the relative contribution of these inflammatory events versus direct tissue injury from radiation in the pathogenesis of this syndrome is unclear.

In mice, pneumonitis begins at three months after radiation is administered and persists for up to six months, with the majority of deaths occurring between four and five months. The latent time for the appearance of damage is dose-dependent, appearing sooner after high doses than after low doses. To account for the dose-dependent difference in latent time and to include all responders in the assay, the standard time for scoring deaths from pneumonitis is between three and seven months in animal experiments. Techniques used to quantify this phase of lung damage in experimental animals include functional assays such as breathing rate[14,15,18] and CO uptake,[16] CT scans,[17] quantitative morphometry,[24,27] and of course, lethality from the syndrome.[3] These assays provide steep dose-response curves from which estimates of effect dose for a given severity of injury can be obtained. Generally, the Effect Dose 50 (ED50) or lethal dose that kills 50% of the population (LD50) is used. Estimates of the LD50 for radiation pneu-

monitis occurring between three and six months after whole-lung irradiation in mice range from 9 to greater than 16 Gy in mice, depending on the mouse strain. In the clinic, the use of large single doses to the upper-half body or the whole body has provided dose-response data for radiation pneumonitis in humans. Using incidence of pneumonitis[28–31] or computed tomographic (CT) scans[9,32] to quantify the increase in lung density in patients, the shape of the resultant dose-response curves for lung damage in humans is similar to those for mice. The ED50 for pneumonitis in humans, 9 to 10 Gy, is within the range of LD50s for pneumonitis measured for different mouse strains, although on the low end of the range. Although treatment of lung cancer can involve irradiation of large volumes of lung, rarely is the whole lung irradiated, and thus fatal pneumonitis occurs infrequently. However it is estimated that at least 5% to 15% of irradiated patients will develop clinical signs of pneumonitis, with an even higher proportion, 50%, showing lung changes consistent with pneumonitis on computed tomographic scans.

The diffuse alveolitis described above had been considered characteristic of the acute phase of radiation-induced lung damage in humans and animals, but histopathologic differences between mouse pneumonitis and human pneumonitis could not be explained. For example, a characteristic histologic finding in irradiated human lung is the presence of hyaline membranes. Unlike in mice, which do not develop fibrosis during the pneumonitis phase, focal areas of fibrosis have been reported in patients within the first month or two after lung irradiation, the time generally associated with the infiltrative, exudative lesions of radiation pneumonitis. These discrepancies between mice and humans have been partially resolved by the recent studies of Sharplin and Franko[27] that showed that the pathologic lesion of the acute phase was dependent on the strain of mouse used. For example, mice of the C3H and CBA strains showed a classical diffuse alveolitis (pneumonitis) with no evidence of fibrosis, while the C57B16 strain exhibited protein-rich edema, hyaline membranes, and focal fibrosis, with few of the changes characteristic of pneumonitis (Figure 13.2). These data indicate that the choice of mouse strain is critical in studies of radiation lung damage; mouse strains used to study pneumonitis would be different from those chosen to study fibrosis.

Intermediate Phase

If the dose is low or if less than a critical volume of lung is irradiated, the acute pneumonitis phase resolves. Although little data on this phase are available in patients, it has been characterized in irradiated mouse lung.[24] In those mice that survive the acute pneumonitis phase, lung function, as measured by breathing rate, improves. The lungs are not totally normal however, and foci of foamy macrophages are the dominant finding in the air spaces, along with hyperplasia of Type II epithelial cells. However no deaths occur during this phase of damage. Thus this phase appears to be one of resolution of the early exudative alveolitis.

Radiation Fibrosis

In contrast to the acute alveolitis, the chronic effects of radiation in humans are observed from months to years later, even though biochemical and histologic changes occur months earlier. Pulmonary fibrosis develops insidiously and may stabilize after one or two years. Although numerous studies have attempted to elucidate the mechanism(s) leading to pulmonary fibrosis, the pathogenesis of this late lung response remains elusive and controversial.

Pulmonary fibrosis is the end stage of a complex process of abnormal repair of damage that may be preceded by an inflammatory response dominated by macrophages and lymphocytes. It is generally accepted that radiation-induced lung fibrosis is the repair process that follows radiation pneumonitis, or radiation alveolitis. Fibrosis of the pulmonary parenchyma may occur as a diffuse or focal lesion, but the designation of pulmonary fibrosis is usually reserved for diffuse or widespread multifocal collagen deposition involving the peripheral airspaces. Although frequently referred to as interstitial fibrosis, collagenous thickening of alveolar walls is often a consequence of incorporation of organizing intra-alveolar exudate into the interstitium and subsequent reepithelialization, leading to a revision of alveolar architecture. In fact, it is frequently suggested that severe exudative alveolitis of long-standing duration results in a generalized fibrotic thickening of the alveolar septa.[26,33] Loss of pulmonary function results from focal microcollapse of alveoli and

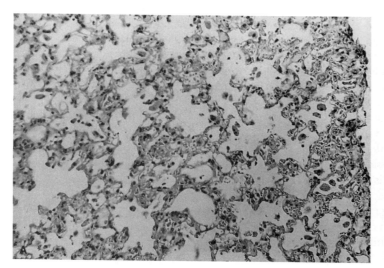
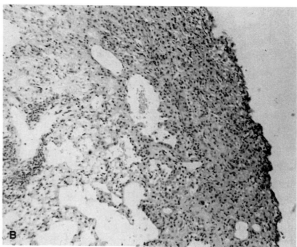

FIGURE 13.2. Characteristic changes in the lungs of C3Hf/Kam (**A**) mice and C57/BL6 (**B**) mice after equivalent single doses of radiation or cobalt-60 gamma rays to the whole thorax. The C3H mouse was sacrificed at 3.5 months because of overt signs of severe respiratory distress; the C57 mouse was sacrificed at 5 months. The lungs of the C3H mouse show a classic radiation alveolitis (pneumonitis), while the lungs of the C57 mouse show collapsed atelectatic alveoli with collagen superimposed—alveolitis is not a feature.

apposition of alveolar walls, leading to irreversible remodeling of pulmonary architecture.

Although data from lung irradiation studies in mice indicate that pneumonitis and fibrosis are directly related,[24,34–36] other data, also in murine models, show that these two sequelae of lung irradiation can be dissociated from each other, and radiation-induced lung fibrosis can and does occur without a preceding inflammatory event.[37–39] These studies suggest that this phase of injury may result from different pathogenic mechanisms.

The exact form of lung fibrosis that occurs after lung irradiation has been shown to be dependent on the strain of mouse. In the initial studies of radiation-induced lung damage, mice were terminated at seven months after irradiation, when the pneumonitis phase of damage ended. However, in later studies, mice surviving at seven months were followed for periods of up to a year after thoracic irradiation. When sacrificed, a diffuse thickening of the alveolar septa was observed in these mice that was characterized by collagen deposition.[37,38] The air spaces were clear, and patent and pulmonary architecture was preserved, although the lung was stiff. Recently, Sharplin and Franko[27,40] reported that radiation-induced lung fibrosis in mice is not always manifested as a diffuse thickening of the alveolar septa, but that some strains exhibit atelectasis accompanied by collagen deposition in the collapsed area, resulting in a focal contracted scar. In this form of lung fibrosis, alveolar architecture is obliterated. We too have found a difference in the fibrotic lesions in irradiated mouse lung, with the C57B1/6J mice exhibiting collapsed atelectatic alveoli with superimposed collagen, while the C3H strain shows a more diffuse fibrosis of the alveolar walls and small stellate scars surrounded by patent alveoli.[41] Unlike in the C57B1 mice, where the collagen appears in organized bundles, making it easily distinguishable on light microscopy with collagen-specific stains, the initial deposition of the collagen as fine, wispy fibrils in the alveolar wall of the C3H mouse make this type of fibrosis more difficult to resolve with the light microscope. In addition to distinct histological features, these two forms of fibrosis are distinguished further by the time they appear in the two strains after irradiation. Fibrosis in the C57 strain occurs within the first six months after irradiation, the period during which only pneumonitis is found in the C3H strain. In the latter strain, fibrosis of the alveolar walls does not occur until nine months (or later) after irradiation.

The suggestion from these mouse studies that radiation-induced pulmonary fibrosis may not have a uniform pathogenesis is consistent with the suggestion that there may be three different pathways to lung fibrosis which may be dependent on the toxic agent: *luminal fibrosis,* in which granulation tissue buds into the air spaces; *mural fibrosis,* in which exudate is incorporated into the alveolar walls; and *atelectatic induration,* which involves partial or complete collapse of alveoli and permanent apposition of alveolar walls followed

by fibrous tissue proliferation and collagen deposition in the area.[26] Franko and colleagues have suggested from breeding studies in inbred strains of mice that radiation-induced lung fibrosis results from two independent pathways which may involve different genes.[42] Further support for the hypothesis that multiple mechanisms lead to pulmonary fibrosis comes from the colon, in which it has been shown that two distinct types of fibrosis occur after irradiation, possibly as a result of two distinct mechanisms.[43]

Most studies in mice irradiated the whole lung, which is not the standard procedure for treating lung cancer with radiation, where a limited volume of lung is irradiated. Thus the question remains of the relevance of these data from experimental animal models to the treatment of lung cancer in humans with radiation. For example, hemithoracic irradiation in mice and rats does not produce the mortality and morbidity of whole-lung irradiation, due to hypertrophy of the contralateral lung, but the mechanisms of collapse and fibrosis of the irradiated lung may differ from those that occur after whole-lung irradiation. In the kidney, a paired organ like the lung, it was found that nephrectomy one day after bilateral kidney irradiation induces a proliferative response in the remaining irradiated kidney that results in a partial restoration of kidney function compared to that in irradiated nonnephrectomized mice.[44] Although it is important to be aware of these differences between animal experiments with radiation and treatment of humans for lung cancer, the clinical data indicate that similar-appearing damage occurs in humans and in mice after lung irradiation, supporting the use of these animal models for mechanistic studies. Most importantly, the studies in mice that defined a strain dependence for the form and severity of radiation-induced lung fibrosis suggest that this late sequelae of lung irradiation may be genetically regulated. Identifying, mapping, and cloning the gene(s) for radiation-induced lung fibrosis could provide a means to identify "sensitive" individuals in the population before treatment commenced.

The characteristic findings in each of these four phases of lung damage are summarized in Table 13.1.

Sporadic Radiation Pneumonitis

In humans, anecdotal reports of pneumonitis occurring outside the irradiated area have been reported for a number of years.[45–48] Since one of the characteristic features of classical radiation pneumonitis is that the damage is confined to the irradiated area, it has been suggested that the clinical and radiologic picture of radiation damage outside the irradiated field represents a hypersensitivity pneumonitis. First suggested by Holt in 1964,[49] this syndrome has been given little attention for two reasons: it occurs rarely, and in most of these cases, the contralateral lung received some dose, although the actual quantity was unknown. Three factors suggest that this clinical syndrome may be different from the classical form of radiation induced lung damage: (a) it

TABLE 13.1. PRINCIPAL HISTOPATHOLOGIC ABNORMALITIES AFTER IRRADIATION OF THE THORAX IN ANIMALS*

Site	Immediate and Early (0–2 mo)	Intermediate (2–9 mo)	Late (9+ mo)
Capillaries	2 h: Endothelial cell changes, increased capillary permeability	Marked capillary abnormalities with widespread obstruction due to platelets fibrin and collagen	Loss of many capillaries, regeneration of new capillaries
	2–7 d: Marked endothelial cell changes and separation from basement membrane and sloughing producing obstruction of lumen	Regeneration of capillaries; reduced capillary permeability	Reduced capillary permeability
	1+ mo: Many capillaries swollen and obstructed		
Type 1 pneumocytes	Degenerative changes or normal	Decreased number	Further decrease in number
Type 2 pneomocytes	Very early degenerative changes becoming more marked with time or normal	Large increase in size and number, abnormal appearance	Return to normal size and number
Basement membrane	Early swelling, indistinct, later very irregular	Folded and thickened	Folded and thickened
Interstitial space	Edema and debris, infiltrated with inflammatory cells and basophils; slight increase in connective tissue	Infiltrated with mononuclear cells, mast cells; inflammatory cells, and connective tissue	Few inflammatory cells; large increase in collagen
Alveolar space	Fibrin, hemorrhages, and debris. Increased number of alveolar macrophages	Becomes smaller	Small or absent, distortion of architecture
Bronchial epithelium	Early transient inflammatory reaction; cillary paralysis, increase in goblet cells or normal	Epithelial proliferation	—

* Mouse strain dependent.
From Gross NJ. Pulmonary effects of radiation therapy. *Ann Intern Med* 1977;86:81, with permission.

affects 10% to 15% of patients; (b) symptoms frequently resolve without sequelae; and (c) it frequently develops earlier than classical pneumonitis, that is within two to six weeks after the completion of therapy. In an extensive study of four breast cancer patients who developed bilateral changes after radiation confined solely to one lung, Gibson and colleagues[50] found that bronchoalveolar lavage (BAL) of the irradiated and nonirradiated lung showed a marked lymphocytosis in both the irradiated and nonirradiated lungs. Gallium scan confirmed these BAL findings, showing increased gallium uptake in both irradiated and nonirradiated lungs. In all four patients prompt symptomatic improvement was seen after corticosteroid administration. Based on these data, these authors concluded that the finding of abnormalities in both the irradiated and nonirradiated fields equally was not consistent with simple direct radiation-induced damage but implied an immunologically mediated mechanism such as a hypersensitivity pneumonitis.

More recently, Morgan and Breit have challenged the idea that bilateral radiation pneumonitis after unilateral lung irradiation is a relatively infrequent occurrence in the practice of radiotherapy.[51] These authors contend that the extreme dyspnea experienced by patients with radiation-induced pneumonitis appears out of proportion to the volume of lung irradiated and cannot be explained on the basis of localized tissue destruction. In a prospective study of 17 breast cancer patients, BAL analysis and gallium scans showed a diffuse lymphocytosis, increased gallium scan uptake, and decreased alveolar volume and vital capacity in both the irradiated and nonirradiated lung. Further analysis of the lymphocyte infiltrate in a patient with clinical radiation pneumonitis showed that these cells were almost exclusively recently activated CD4+ helper T-cells, cells that have been implicated in hypersensitivity pneumonitis after other insults. In a further analysis of these patients plus an additional five patients studied only after they developed clinical features of pneumonitis, these authors found no statistically significant difference between BAL findings on the irradiated and unirradiated sides of the chest either pretreatment or posttreatment and with or without clinical pneumonitis. Although bilateral lymphocytosis was found in 75% of the study population (13 of the 17 patients), only two (10%) of these patients developed clinical features of radiation-induced pneumonitis. Symptoms resolved spontaneously in the other 65% (11) patients. The remaining 25% did not develop subclinical or clinical symptoms. On the basis of these findings, these authors suggest that bilateral involvement of both lungs after irradiation of one lung represents an immune-mediated hypersensitivity pneumonitis which leads to the clinical picture of radiation pneumonitis in only 10% of the irradiated population. Because this syndrome appears to be due to an entirely different pathogenetic mechanism from classical radiation pneumonitis, these authors suggest that this form of radiation-induced lung damage be distinguished from the classical form and be called "sporadic radiation pneumonitis." What distinguishes this type of lung damage from the classical type is that it occurs in an unpredictable manner and involves unirradiated portions of the lung.

At this time, an animal model for sporadic radiation pneumonitis has not been identified. However, in a study of CT changes after irradiation of only the right lung of rats, Geist and Trott observed fluctuations in the radiological density in the shielded left lung of the irradiated rats that were greater than those observed in control rats and parallel to those occurring in the irradiated right lung, similar to the sporadic pneumonitis in humans.[52] In contrast to these data, it has been reported that irradiation of one lung of rabbits resulted in a decrease in the number of alveolar macrophages in only the irradiated lung. The number of alveolar macrophages in the contralateral unirradiated lung was not decreased.[53]

Pathogenesis of Radiation-Induced Lung Damage

Target Cells. It has been hypothesized that killing and depletion of a critical "target" cell by radiation in the lung is the initiating event leading, after a "latent" period, to the late sequelae of pneumonitis and fibrosis.[54] In addition, it has been generally accepted that the expression of radiation damage requires cell division. In tissues like the lung, therefore, in which damage is not overtly expressed for months after treatment is completed, the long latent time was thought to be due to a slowly proliferating target cell population. For these reasons, a major research focus has been to identify the target cell(s) for radiation-induced lung damage, with the intention of protecting this cell from radiation damage and thereby preventing or, at least minimizing, the severity of radiation-induced pneumonitis and fibrosis while not compromising tumor cell kill and tumor control. The two most likely target cells were thought to be the Type II cell[19,55–58] and the vascular endothelial cell.[19,59–63] The

Type II cell was shown to divide more frequently than other types of lung parenchymal cells; it is responsible for synthesizing, storing, and secreting surfactant, the surface active material that prevents alveolar collapse. The vascular endothelial cell also was a reasonable target cell candidate because it too was believed to divide more quickly than other cell types in the lung. Furthermore, edema is a consistent finding in the interstitium and air spaces after lung irradiation, indicating vascular leakage, which in turn implies radiation-induced killing and depletion of vascular endothelial cells.

Type II Cells as the Target. The first evidence that supported the hypothesis that Type II cells were the target cells for radiation pneumonitis was published in 1982 by Shapiro and associates.[58] These investigators showed that local irradiation of both lungs of mice with a range of single doses of x-rays produced dose-dependent changes in phospholipids in lung lavage fluid and in lung tissue as early as 24 hours after irradiation. These changes persisted for the first four weeks after irradiation, indicating that changes in the function of Type II cells occurred long before tissue damage was manifested at the light microscopic level. Although the relationship of these early events to the later incidence of pneumonitis and fibrosis was unclear, these data were the first demonstration that the latent period was not really quiet or latent at all. These investigators then sought to identify biochemical markers of surfactant that could be assessed in patients early during a course of radiotherapy prior to the onset of clinical and pathologic pneumonitis, with the aim of identifying patients at a high risk of developing severe radiation pneumonitis.[57] Their finding in rabbits that surfactant apoprotein in the serum was an accurate predictor and marker for radiation pneumonitis has led to a clinical trial in lung cancer patients. Blood is collected before treatment, weekly during treatment, and one week after treatment, and surfactant apoprotein is quantitated in the serum. These data will be compared with the incidence and severity of radiation pneumonitis and fibrosis assayed by CT scans every three months after treatment and by chest radiograph at one year.

Endothelial Cells as the Target. The suggestion that vascular damage was the underlying mechanism of radiation pneumonitis and fibrosis was based primarily on the hypothesis that the lung cell most likely to divide soon after irradiation was the capillary endothelial cell. The parenchymal cells, most importantly the Type II cells, were believed to be more slowly dividing than the endothelial cell. This hypothesis was substantiated by the pathologic findings in humans and experimental models that pneumonitis after irradiation was characterized by edema in the air spaces and interstitium, and an inflammatory cell infiltrate. Among the many studies aimed at elucidating the role of the vasculature in radiation-induced lung damage, Ward and colleagues[64-66] performed comprehensive studies that correlated changes in four parameters of endothelial function, angiotensin-converting enzyme activity, plasminogen activator activity, and prostacyclin and thromboxane production, with histopathologic and ultrastructural changes in rat lungs irradiated with the same doses, as well as changes in one vascular functional assay—arterial perfusion. These studies showed that dose-dependent changes occurred in all endothelial functional parameters and that these functional changes agreed well with pathologic changes in the lungs of these rats. These data suggest that changes in vasculature do occur after lung irradiation, but they do not necessarily implicate the endothelial cell as the target cell.

MOLECULAR BASIS OF RADIATION-INDUCED LUNG DAMAGE

It is obvious that changes in both the pulmonary parenchyma and pulmonary vasculature contribute to radiation pneumonitis and fibrosis, and that these sequelae of lung irradiation arise from a dynamic interaction between different cell types, the major players including both the Type II pneumocyte and the endothelial cell, as well as the fibroblast, macrophages, and lymphocytes, as shown in Figure 13.3.[67,68] However, the concept that one or more target cells are solely responsible for radiation-induced pneumonitis and pulmonary fibrosis has been replaced by the paradigm that it is not only cells but the messages that these cells produce that determine the final outcome. It is now well established that radiation is one of many insults that cause the release of trophic factors that subsequently act

through a variety of pathways to produce the end pathologic stage of radiation pneumonitis and fibrosis.[69-71] These messages are delivered via diffusion of soluble mediators over short distances, which may have been secreted by one population of cells and then act locally upon another population, referred to as paracrine stimulation, or upon the same population, known as autocrine stimulation, or which may involve membrane-associated molecules activating receptors on adjacent target cells, referred to as juxtacrine stimulation. These soluble mediators, or cytokines or growth factors, are currently recognized as playing an important part in stimulating cells to overproduce those extracellular matrix components that characterize fibrosis[69-74] Following their initial contact with the cell surface, these molecules are postulated to activate intracellular signaling pathways, which in turn lead to activation of a pleiotropic genetic program characteristic of the fibrotic response. This activation is thought to bring about changes in the expression of specific genes that determine the phenotype of cells involved in the healing of lung injury.

Perhaps the cytokine most frequently associated with lung fibrosis after a number of toxic insults, including radiation, is TGF-β.[73-76] TGF-β has been shown to be an important mediator of tissue damage in a variety of pathologies in which excessive collagen production is a characteristic feature. TGF-β has been shown to stimulate lymphocyte and fibroblast recruitment to the site of damage, to promote fibroblast proliferation, and to stimulate the production of collagen and fibronectin, the net effect being a net increase in extra cellular matrix material which replaces the normal architecture of the tissue. In addition, TGF-β increases the production of Type I plasminogen activator inhibitor, while

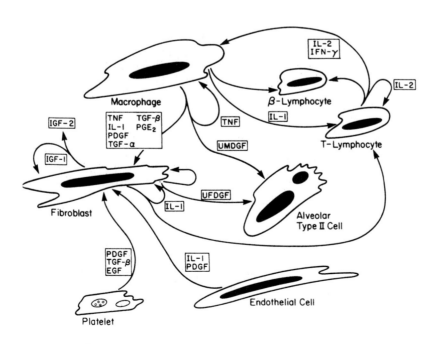

FIGURE 13.3. Diagram of hypothesized interaction of different lung target cells and cytokines and growth factors in the development of alveolitis and fibrosis. IGF, insulinlike growth factor; TNF, tumor necrosis factor; TGF, transforming growth factor; IL, interleukin; PDGF, platelet derived growth factor, EGF, epidermal growth factor; PGE, prostaglandin E2; UMDGF, UFDGF. (From King RJ, Jones MB, Minoo P. Regulation of lung cell proliferation by polypeptide growth factors. *Am J Physiol* 1989;257:23, with permission.)

simultaneously decreasing the production of plasminogen activators, resulting not only in an increase in the production of connective tissue but a decrease in its breakdown, leading ultimately to maturation of this excess connective tissue and scar formation.

Recently, Finkelstein and co-workers[71] have studied the latent period to determine whether changes in early expression of collagen precursors or cytokines, particularly TGF-β, known to be involved in the fibrotic process were expressed before damage was manifested histologically. These investigators used two single doses of radiation to the whole thorax of C57B1/6 mice, a strain known to be sensitive to the fibrogenic effects of lung radiation. The lowest dose used, 5 Gy, is well below the threshold known to induce clinical symptoms and pathologic changes of radiation pneumonitis and fibrosis, while the second higher dose of 12.5 Gy is closer to the reported LD50 for radiation-induced lung damage in this strain, although this dose itself does not cause any deaths from lung damage. The data showed that all three forms of TGF-β mRNA, that is, TGF-β1, β2, and β3, were increased in the lungs of C57B1/6 mice at 14 days, but a consistent dose response relationship was not found. For example, the increase in TGF-β1 was similar after both doses at 14 days; for TGF-β2, an increase was observed only after the higher dose of 12.5 Gy; whereas TGF-β3 was increased only after the lower dose of 12 Gy. Despite these inconsistencies, these data show clearly that after radiation doses that cause no clinical signs nor pathologic changes of radiation lung damage and before the onset of overt lung damage, alterations in expression of at least this fibrogenic cytokine occur which may ultimately lead to the development of chronic fibrosis.

However, just as there is not one target cell that, when depleted, leads to the complex pathologic process known as radiation pneumonitis and fibrosis, it is equally unlikely that the overexpression of only one cytokine initiates and promulgates the fibrogenic process in the lung. It is more likely that the damage, repair, and restructuring of the lung after irradiation as well as other toxic insults is the result of a cytokine network orchestrated by a few key cytokines, such as TNFα and TGF-β. Thus it may be the balance of a few positive profibrogenic cytokines and negative antifibrogenic cytokines generated from the interaction of a number of cytokines constituting these networks that may finally determine the outcome of lung injury and inflammation. Unfortunately, it is not easy to dissect out the role of any of these cytokines in lung damage and repair. However, one approach to determining the role of various cytokines in lung fibrosis is to take advantage of known differences in susceptibility to radiation-induced fibrosis in different inbred mouse strains.

Johnston and colleagues,[77] using the fibrosis-prone C57B1/6 strain and the fibrosis-resistant C3H/HeJ strain, showed that the elevation of mRNA levels of a number of chemokines known to play a role in the recruitment of inflammatory cells to sites of pulmonary damage was not different between the two strains when assessed at eight weeks after irradiation. However, by 26 weeks postirradiation, messages encoding transcripts produced predominantly by macrophages and lymphocytes were elevated only in the fibrosis-prone strain. These data indicate that lymphocytic recruitment and activation are key components of radiation-induced fibrosis, but their role in the pathogeny of this process remains unclear. Thus, despite abundant evidence that expression of a multitude of cytokines is elevated in radiation-induced pneumonitis and lung fibrosis, their actual *in vivo* role and the mechanism of their upregulation remain to be determined. Regardless of our lack of understanding of how these factors mediate damage and repair in the lung, it is now clear that the latent phase preceding the overt expression of radiation damage in the lung is not a quiescent time, but that molecular changes are occurring that may ultimately result in the later clinical and histopathologic picture of pneumonitis and fibrosis. The events that lead to the overt expression of radiation-induced lung damage involve a number of complex cellular and molecular processes, which explains why the nature of both the inflammatory responses and the triggering mechanism that induces the fibrotic response in the lung remain poorly understood.

Table 13.2 summarizes the proposed changes in target cells and growth factors after lung irradiation.

Time, Dose, and Volume Considerations

Fractionation. The sparing effects of fractionating dose in radiotherapy has been known since the experiments performed on rams' testicles in the 1920s and 1930s. Assuming that the testes were a model of a rapidly growing tumor and the skin of the scrotum was representative of normal tissues, it was found that the ram could not be sterilized by a single dose of radiation without causing extensive damage to the skin, while spreading the dose out over a period of weeks resulted in sterilization without producing unacceptable skin reactions. The basis of fractionation lies in the understanding that dose fractionation spares normal tissue reactions by allowing repair of sublethal damage and repopulation of target cells during treatment while increasing tumor cell kill by allowing reoxygenation and reassortment of cells into more sensitive parts of the cell cycle.[78–82] For years, the standard fractionation regimen was doses per fraction of 1.8 to 2.0 Gy over treatment times of four to six weeks. Modification of this conventional treatment schedule by increasing the dose per fraction in the treatment of lung cancer resulted in unacceptable sequelae in tissues such as the spinal cord. However, it was not until the early 1980s that we began to understand the basis for the differences in fractionation sensitivity of normal tissues.

Lung is a *late-responding normal tissue;* that is, damage is not manifested until weeks to months after completion

TABLE 13.2. TARGET CELLS AND GROWTH FACTORS ASSOCIATED WITH RADIATION-INDUCED PNEUMONITIS AND FIBROSIS

Pathophysiologic Target Cells	Biochemical Marker	Growth Factors	Lesion or Event
Type II pneumocyte	Surfactant released into alveolus	TGF-α TGF-β	Acute pneumonitis
Capillary endothelial cell	Surfactant protein enters into blood serum through altered permeability	FGF IL-1 PDGF	Acute pneumonitis and/or fibrosis
Macrophage	Surfactant persists for days or weeks due to decrease in macrophages essential to its removal	IL-1 PDGF TGF-α TGF-β	May protect against pneumonitis, increase septal fibrosis
Septal fibrocyte	Procollagen III appears preceding fibrosis buildup; also, metaloprotease appears, as does elastase and collagenese		

TGF, transforming growth factor; FGF, fibroblast growth factor; IL, interleukin; PDGF, platelet-derived growth factor.
From Rubin P. Finkelstein J, Shapiro D. Molecular biology mechanisms in the radiation induction of pulmonary injury syndromes: interrelationship between the alveolar macrophage and the septal fibroblast. *Int J Radiat Oncol Biol Phys* 1992;24:93, with permission.

of a standard course of radiotherapy, in contrast to tissues such as intestinal mucosa, which manifests damage during and shortly after the completion of a course of treatment and is an *acutely responding normal tissue*. An analysis of experimental data for a variety of both acutely and late-responding normal tissues by Thames and associates[83] demonstrated a clear and consistent difference between fractionation effects in these two categories of tissues. By plotting the total dose for an isoeffect specific to a variety of tissues versus the dose per fraction, it was found that the total dose for a given effect in any late-responding normal tissue increased more rapidly as the dose per fraction was decreased than did the total dose for an effect in any acutely responding normal tissue. This pattern was observed consistently in all acutely and late-responding tissues analyzed and suggests that late-responding tissues such as the lung are more sensitive to changes in dose per fraction than are acutely responding tissues. These data imply that decreasing the dose per fraction should spare late-responding tissues such as the lung more than acutely responding tissues as well as the tumor, if tumors respond like acutely responding normal tissues. It has been suggested that the difference in fractionation response for acutely and late-responding normal tissues is due to differences in the repair capacity or shoulder shape of the underlying dose-response curves for these two classes of tissues, that is, the dose-response curve for the late-responding tissues is curvier than that for acutely responding tissues.[83] One way of defining these differences is by the α/β ratio, which derives from the linear quadratic model of cell killing.[83–87] Briefly, this model assumes that there are two components of cell killing by radiation; one that is proportional to dose, and the second that is proportional to dose.[2] The α/β ratio then is the dose at which the linear and quadratic contributions to cell killing are equal. For late-responding tissues such as the lung, the dose-response curve bends at lower doses than for acutely responding tissues, and therefore the dose at which the α and β contribution to cell killing is equal is lower in late-responding than acutely responding tissues. In general, the α/β ratio is below 5 Gy for late-responding normal tissues and greater than 5 Gy for acutely responding normal tissues. For the lung, the α/β is about 3 Gy.[81,88–91] In clinical radiotherapy, then, significant sparing of normal lung damage can be gained by decreasing the size of the dose per fraction.

A second factor in the sparing of normal tissues is repopulation of surviving cells during treatment. However, the late response of the lung, that is, weeks to months after completion of treatment, suggests that repopulation does not occur during a conventional four-to-six week treatment schedule. Although retreatment studies in the lung suggest that this may not be totally correct and that repopulation may occur within the first four weeks after irradiation,[92] it remains a general axiom that conventional fractionation schedules extending for six weeks do not allow triggering of proliferation and subsequent repopulation in the lung, a late-responding tissue. Thus, in terms of clinical radiotherapy, prolonging overall treatment time will have little, if any, sparing effect on the lung.

It can be stated, then, that in the lung the size of the dose per fraction is the dominant factor in determining lung damage, while overall treatment time will have little influence. What is more important is that prolonging treatment time may decrease tumor response because of accelerated repopulation of surviving and proliferating tumor cells during treatment.[93–95]

These radiobiological findings have been translated into the clinical treatment of lung cancer using fractionation protocols that vary from the conventional protocols by reducing the size of the dose and giving more than one fraction per day, while keeping the overall treatment time the same as in traditional schedules. To compensate for the loss of cell killing in the tumor by the reduction in dose per fraction, higher total doses are given. Thus the goal is to hold the lung damage constant by the reduced dose per fraction, but simultaneously increase tumor control by giving a higher total dose. The fractionation schedule most commonly used in the treatment of lung cancer, termed hyperfractionation, gives two doses of 1.2 Gy per day. In initial clinical trials, the total doses given ranged from 60 Gy, the same total dose given in conventional schedules using one fraction of 2 Gy per fraction, to 69.6 Gy.[96,97] The risk of both acute and late effects was found to be acceptable, and there was a dose response for survival, with survival significantly improved in patients receiving the highest total dose. In a second trial, total doses were escalated to a maximum of 79.2 Gy, but this increase in total dose did not result in a significant survival advantage, although lung toxicity was still acceptable. Further clinical trials are underway to test this hyperfractionation protocol against conventional protocols using 2 Gy per fraction alone or combined with systemic radiotherapy.

Volume of Lung Irradiated. It is well accepted by the radiation oncologists that in addition to fractionation, an effective technique to reduce morbidity is to reduce the volume of normal lung irradiated. The advent of 3D treatment planning and conformal radiation therapy allow the use of more than the traditional two to four opposing treatment fields, making it possible to tailor the treatment plan to the individual patient and tumor. However, the dose distributions in these nontraditional plans may be very different from those used in standard two or three field treatments. For example, some plans may deliver a small dose to a larger volume of lung than in opposed fields, making it difficult for the radiotherapist to extrapolate from experience to predict the probability of incurring morbidity. In addition, the lung is a paired organ and has a large functional reserve, thus it is expected that it would exhibit a threshold volume, that is, a subvolume below which irradiation causes no detectable injury, even at very high doses.[3,98,99] However, since most experimental studies had been performed using whole-lung irradiation, neither the threshold volume nor the relationship of volume of lung irradiated, dose, and morbidity were defined.

In the past few years, with the impetus of conformal therapy and questions from radiotherapists regarding the volume response of the lung, experimental studies have been initiated in a number of labs to address these questions. Most of the data for partial lung irradiation have been obtained from hemithoracic irradiation studies in mice and rats. In these studies, single-dose irradiation of only one lung led to dose-dependent increases in one functional assay—breathing rate—but not in lethality (Travis, unpublished observations). The initial increase in breathing rate was followed by a decrease that was suggested to be coincident with compensatory hypertrophy of the unirradiated lung and/or the formation of new alveoli that increased the surface area of the lung. Both breathing rate and lethality are assays of total lung function, both the irradiated half and the unirradiated half, and show clearly that the lung has a large functional reserve. Other studies using blood flow changes in hemithoracic irradiated mice and rats showed that vascular changes in the irradiated lung were similar to those after whole-lung irradiation.[59] Thus this assay of regional function showed no difference after whole- versus partial-lung irradiation.

A series of experiments in mouse lung designed to define the relationship of dose and volume to damage assessed histopathologically and morbidity assessed by two tests of total lung function—breathing rate and lethality—has been reported recently.[100,101] In these studies, a range of lung volumes, from 20% to 100%, were irradiated. In addition, matched volumes were irradiated in the base or in the apex of the lung to test the hypothesis that the functional subunits were randomly and homogeneously distributed. Figure 13.4 shows the proportion of dead mice after irradiation of two of the matched volumes in the apex and base of the lung, 50% and 75%. Figure 13.5 shows breathing rate and lethality as a function of the percentage volume of lung irradiated in the apex or the base of the lung. It is clear from these data that for any given volume, the base of the lung is more sensitive than the same volume in the apex, that is, the isoeffect doses for both breathing rate and lethality are lower for all irradiated volumes in the base than in the apex.

Although the underlying mechanism of this spatial heterogeneity in the response of the mouse lung to radiation is unknown, Travis and co-workers[101] suggested that there is a heterogeneous distribution of target cells or functional subunits in the lung, which is due to the anatomy of the tracheobronchial tree. The alveoli are concentrated in the periphery of the lung, whereas the mid region of the lung is most occupied by conducting airways, which are not involved in gas exchange. Thus the base of the lung is more sensitive because there is a higher concentration of alveoli and fewer conducting airways in this region, whereas a large portion of the mid region of the lung is occupied by large branching bronchi and bronchioles. Boersma[102] suggested that these regional differences in the incidence of pneumonitis could be accounted for by differences in functionality of cells in the base and apex, rather than to a difference in density. Khan and co-workers[103] ascribe these regional differences in the incidence of radiation pneumonitis to differences in the amount of DNA damage sustained by the cells in the apex and the base, that is, the cells in the base sustain more DNA damage than those in the apex when either region is irradiated. Interestingly, this differential in DNA damage between cells isolated from the apex or base of the lung disappears when the whole lung is irradiated.

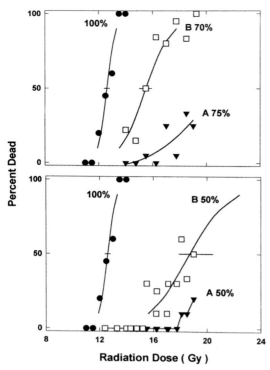

FIGURE 13.4. Dose-response curves of lethality after irradiation of two partial volumes of the lungs of C3H mice. 70% to 75% (**top**) or 50% (**bottom**), located in the apex (**A**) or base (**B**) of the lung. The dose-response curve for whole lung is shown for comparison. These data show a clear volume effect. The lethal dose that kills 50% of the population (LD50) for irradiation of 50% in either the base or apex is higher than the irradiation of the larger volume of 75% in these same two sites. In addition, these data show that the LD50 is dependent on the site of the lung irradiated. The isoeffect dose is less for both volumes irradiated in the base than in the apex, suggesting that the base is more sensitive than the apex. These data indicate that the volume effect is dependent not only on the volume of lung irradiated but also on the site of the lung irradiated.

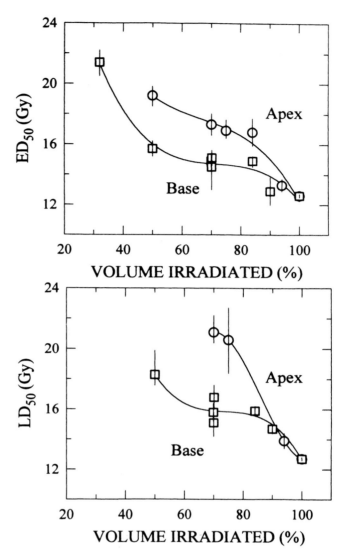

FIGURE 13.5. Breathing rate (ED 50, **top**) and lethality (LD 50, **bottom**) for radiation pneumonitis, plotted as a function of partial volume irradiated in the apex of base of the lung. The curves are second-order regression fits to the data. The curve for irradiation of a range of volumes in the base is consistently displaced below that for irradiation of the same volumes in the apex, that is, the isoeffect doses for both breathing rate and lethality are lower for all volumes irradiated in the base than in the apex. These data show clearly that the base is more sensitive than the same volume in the apex for the induction of radiation pneumonitis. (From Travis EL, Liao Z-X, Tucker SL. Spatial heterogeneity of the volume effect for radiation pneumonitis in mouse lung. *Int J Radiat Oncol Biol Phys* 1997;38:1050, with permission.)

Regardless of the mechanism underlying these regional differences, it is clear that the morbidity of lung irradiation will be related not only to the volume of lung irradiated but to the location of the irradiated subvolume within the lung. Based on these data, then, greater morbidity would be expected when the irradiation portal includes the base than when the apex is included. Also, when using conformal therapy, the data suggest that the volume irradiated in the base be kept as minimal as possible.

Regardless of the mechanism of the heterogeneity of the lung's response to partial-volume irradiation, these data impact on the use of nonconventional treatment techniques such as 3D conformal radiotherapy and more recently, intensity modulated radiotherapy (IRMT) in the treatment of lung cancer. Both of these latter techniques treat larger volumes of normal lung than conventional treatment techniques, although the normal lung would get a smaller dose. However, the question of whether a lot to a little (conven-

tional treatment) is better or worse than a little to a lot (3D and IMRT), has not been answered. Using the mouse data, Tucker and associates[104] calculated the incidence of pneumonitis for subvolumes of the lung irradiated with a fixed dose. As shown in Figure 13.6, the complication rate varies over the entire range of possible responses, from a 100% incidence after irradiation of the base, to a 0% incidence after irradiation of the mid-lung, with an intermediate incidence after irradiation of the apex. These data indicate that relatively small changes in the location of the irradiated subvolume in lung may correspond to significantly greater changes in the incidence of pneumonitis than moderate changes in either the dose or the size of the irradiated subvolume. Using the mouse data, Tucker and associates found, using a constant integrated dose of 12.7 Gy, that the risk of pneumonitis varied enormously depending on the site of the irradiated subvolume (Figure 13.7), whereas for both the apex and the mid-region of mouse lung, a little to a lot was found to be worse that a lot to a little, provided that the integrated dose, that is, the product of volume and dose, was kept constant. However, a quite different picture emerges for the base, where irradiation of 50% to 70% of the lung is predicted to be worse than irradiation of either larger or smaller subvolumes, again provided that the integrated dose is kept constant. After volumes larger than 70%, the decrease in the probability of pneumonitis occurs because the increase in the number of cells irradiated is more than offset by the decrease in dose required to maintain the constant integrated dose. In terms of the threshold volume, that is, that volume below which radiation causes no detectable injury even at very high doses, the predicted size of this volume depends on the region of lung irradiated and ranges from 10% in the base to 30% to 40% in the apex.

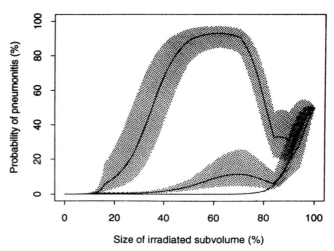

FIGURE 13.7. Predicted incidence of pneumonitis in mouse lung as a function of irradiated volume where the integrated dose (dose × volume) is kept fixed at 12.7 Gy, equal to the whole-lung LD50. The upper, middle, and lower curves represent volumes in the base, apex, or mid-region of the lung respectively. Stippled regions around the curves represent the 95% confidence limits. It is clear that whether a lot to a little is better than a little to a lot is critically dependent on the location of the irradiated subvolume. In the base, the risk of pneumonitis is highest after irradiation of an intermediate subvolume with an intermediate dose, whereas in the apex, a little to a lot is generally worse than a lot to a little. (From Tucker SL, Liao Z-X, Travis EL. Estimation of the spatial distribution of target cells for radiation pneumonitis in mouse lung. *Int J Radiat Oncol Biol Phys* 1997;38:1062, with permission.)

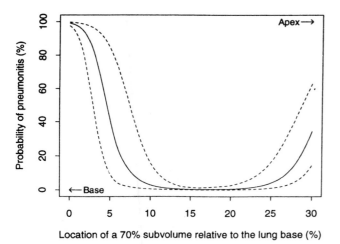

FIGURE 13.6. Effect of subvolume location on response calculated using estimates of cell density in different subvolumes of the lung. The solid curve shows the predicted incidence of pneumonitis in mice after irradiation of a subvolume of fixed size (70%) with a fixed dose (22 Gy), plotted as a function of the location in the lung of the irradiated subvolume. The complication rate varies over the entire range, from a 100% incidence rate after irradiation of the base to a 0% incidence after irradiation of the mid-lung to an intermediate incidence after irradiation of the apex. Dashed curves represent the 95% confidence band around the predicted curve, based on the uncertainty in the estimated cell density parameters. (From Tucker SL, Liao Z-X, Travis EL. Estimation of the spatial distribution of target cells for radiation pneumonitis in mouse lung. *Int J Radiat Oncol Biol Phys* 1997; 38:1062, with permission.)

Interestingly, a recent clinical study[105] found that the risk of pneumonitis in patients varied with the location of the irradiated site, exactly as had been observed in mouse lung. In a study of 60 patients treated with radiation and chemotherapy given either sequentially or concurrently for lung cancer, the site of irradiation in the lung was evaluated by dividing the whole lung into three-by-three areas, that is the right and left lung were divided into three equal areas from upper to lower lung field. When the risk of pneumonitis was analyzed by irradiated site, it was found that when the lower lung field was included in the radiation site, the incidence of pneumonitis was 70%, compared with 20% for other sites (p less than 0.01). Multivariate analysis revealed a significant relationship between radiation site and the risk of pneumonitis (p = 0.0096). These data are consistent with the data from the mouse studies, both of which show that irradiated site, the base of the lung, is a treatment factor significantly associated with a higher risk of pneumonitis following CRT.

In contrast to the data from lung function tests, no volume effect was found for damage in the studies of Liao and colleagues.[100] A characteristic pneumonitis was found in all mice regardless of the volume of lung irradiated. These data illustrate the necessity to define whether damage or morbidity is being assessed in both clinical and animal studies, as different answers may be obtained. In addition, these data indicate that tests of total lung function that reflect a summation of the function in the irradiated volume and the function of normal lung in the unirradiated volume will give a different answer from regional lung function tests that assess damage only in the irradiated area.

Quantifying Dose-Volume Relationship in Patients

Approximately 50% to 90% of patients who receive lung irradiation will have radiographic or pulmonary function abnormalities following treatment; however, the significance of these changes in terms of morbidity varies from minimal to severe, depending on the volume of lung irradiated. A comprehensive study of radiation pneumonitis after partial volume fractionated irradiation in patients was conducted by Mah and associates.[30] The end point was an increase in lung density within the irradiated volume on CT in the posttreatment period. The estimated single dose equivalent, ED50, was 10 ± 4 ED units, at the low end of the dose range for pneumonitis in various mouse strains (Figure 13.8). However, no information was obtained for the effect of these changes on pulmonary function. More

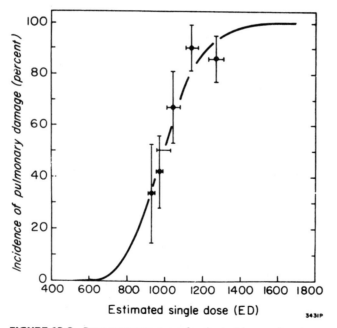

FIGURE 13.8. Dose-response curve for the incidence of acute radiation pneumonitis after fractionated radiotherapy of the whole lung in humans. The solid curve is the best fit sigmoid to the data points as determined by probit regression. An ED50 of 1,000 ED units with a standard error of 40 ED units is predicted. Vertical error bars are the standard deviation of the points. (From Mah K, Van Dyk J, Keane T, et al. Acute radiation-induced pulmonary damage: a clinical study on the response to fractionated radiation therapy. *Int J Radiat Oncol Biol Phys* 1987;13:179, with permission.)

recent studies by Boersma[4,6] and Marks and colleagues[11] in which changes in regional lung function were quantified showed that the dose-effect curves for both functional parameters studied—perfusion and ventilation (Figure 13.9)—were less steep than the dose-effect curve for structural changes as measured by density changes on CT published previously by Mah et al.[9,32] The lack of correlation between CT changes as a measure of structural damage and tests of regional lung function was more clearly observed in one study by Boersma[4] in which all assays were performed in the same patients. These data suggest that lung density may be a different biological end point from perfusion and ventilation, the former representing the late phase of fibrosis, while the functional assays measure the ability of the irradiated lung within that area to perform gas exchange.

Numerous studies in the literature describe changes in local lung function using a number of assays, such as those described above and others such as SPECT scanning. However, what is critical in 3D conformal treatment in which both dose and volume are changing is the effect of these changes in regional function and structure on whole-lung function. In other words, as the volume of normal lung irradiated increases, should the dose be decreased, and if so, by how much? Clearly, the correlation of clinical symptoms or changes in whole-lung function is heavily dependent on the volume of functioning lung remaining. What is well accepted is that there is a clear separation between whole organ and regional organ tolerance. The impact of changes in regional lung function and structure on whole-lung function will depend on the dose-volume histogram (DVH).

The most convenient way of expressing this type of information is a DVH which is then used to develop mathematical models that attempt to predict normal tissue complication probability (NTCP). Although NTCP models are useful tools in the treatment planning process, the absolute values of the predicted complication rates must be verified clinically. Because verification of the complication rates predicted from NTCP models requires a large number of patients, Kwa and co-workers,[106] in a large, five-center study of 540 patients, asked the question whether a parameter such as mean lung dose could predict the probability of radiation pneumonitis using doses calculated from 3D treatments. These authors have reported that the mean lung dose, NTD mean, is a useful predictor of the risk of radiation pneumonitis. This parameter is relatively easy to calculate from the 3D dose distribution and is far simpler than NTCP calculation. In addition, there was a good correlation between the mean biological dose, NTDmean, and the mean physical dose, Dmean, both of which have a clear meaning. Thus, until more complex predictive models can be proven to be superior, these authors suggest that calculation of simpler parameters such as the NTDmean may prove more useful for predicting the risk of lung complications when treatment volume is changed.

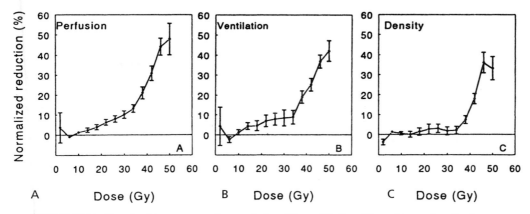

FIGURE 13.9. Dose-incidence curves for perfusion **(A)**, ventilation **(B)**, and lung-density changes **(C)** greater than 20%, indicating the fraction of patients with average local changes greater than 20%. The solid lines are logistic fits to the data points; the error bars on the points indicate the 68% confidence limits. (From Boersma LJ, Damen EMF, de Boer RW, et al. Dose-effect relations for local functional and structural changes of the lung after irradiation for malignant lymphoma. *Radiother Oncol* 1994;32:206, with permission.)

Intervention in the Pathogenesis of Radiation Pneumonitis and Fibrosis

Although changes in dose-fractionation schedules and information on the effect of irradiated volume on the incidence and severity of radiation pneumonitis and fibrosis have led to advances in the treatment of lung cancer, the challenge is to identify agents that either protect against lung damage or specifically intervene in the pathogenesis of pneumonitis or fibrosis. Although it has been generally thought that interventional techniques would not work, recent studies on the events occurring during the latent period could prove useful in designing compounds that specifically intervene in these events.

Much information has been obtained at the cellular and molecular level on the biology of connective tissue formation and the pathophysiology of connective tissue diseases. The knowledge that pharmacologic interventions can be specifically targeted at varying strategic points in the life cycle of fibroproliferative processes has broadened considerably the realm of therapeutic modalities that might be investigated to control these processes. Numerous approaches designed to control collagen deposition remain untested in the lung. It would be useful to develop delivery methods that exploit the unique aspects of the lung to overcome the toxicity associated with collagen inhibitors. Collagen degradation, use of steroidal and nonsteroidal anti-inflammatory drugs, and cyclic nucleotides offer opportunities to control the accumulation of extracellular matrix in the lung.

Cytokines. Studies of the events occurring during the "latent phase" of radiation lung injury have shown that a number of these molecules and growth factors are activated during this time, some of which may be exploited interventionally.

Basic Fibroblast Growth Factor (BFGF). A cytokine suggested to be useful in protecting against radiation pneumonitis in mice is the growth factor basic fibroblast growth factor, βFGF. Fuks and co-workers[107–109] have shown that this cytokine protects against radiation-induced apoptosis in bovine arterial endothelial cells *in vitro*[108,109] as well as against apoptosis in endothelial cells in irradiated lungs of mice.[107] βFGF also protected mice against the lethal effects of radiation pneumonitis.[107] However, neither the time of death nor the histological changes observed were consistent with classical radiation pneumonitis. Hemorrhage and edema in the air spaces was a consistent finding at eight to ten weeks, when the mice were sacrificed because they were moribund. In a separate study giving βFGF after radiation doses to the whole lung that induce a classical pneumonitis, no protection with βFGF was found.[110] Although the reason for the discrepancy between these two studies is not clear, it is possible that the higher doses used by Fuks and co-workers[107] produced "sporadic pneumonitis" whereas the lower doses used in the study by Tee[110] induced a classical pneumonitis. Despite these unresolved differences, these studies do indicate the potential for intervening in these reactions. These studies also indicate our incomplete understanding of the events that occur after chest irradiation.

Interferon γ (IFN-γ). The rationale for the use of this cytokine in modulating radiation pneumonitis is that IFN-γ has been shown to reduce the severity of bleomycin-induced fibrosis in mouse lung[111] and to inhibit acute inflammation.[112,113] Thus, if radiation-induced fibrosis is a sequelae of an acute inflammatory response, that is, pneumonitis, then IFN-γ could potentially reduce the severity of lung fibrosis after irradiation. In a study in rats, Rosiello and colleagues[114] showed that IFN-γ markedly reduced the neutrophil influx and protein leak into the alveoli after irradiation of rat lung with a single dose of 15 GY, suggesting that prophylactic administration of IFN-γ could reduce the severity of radiation pneumonitis in humans. However, long-term follow-up of these animals showed that although IFN-γ reduced early inflammatory events in irradiated lungs, the tissue response at 35 days, the end of the study, showed that the number of cells and exudate in the irradiated lungs of the IFN-γ-treated rats was not different from that in rats only irradiated. Thus it is unclear whether IFN-γ could be useful in modulating either radiation pneumonitis or fibrosis.

Noncytokine Protection. Because radiation damage in the lung is manifested as an alveolitis followed by focal scarring with an attendant increase in collagen, many studies have focused on identifying drugs active against either one or both of these lesions. One of the first drugs to be used clinically was the steroid prednisolone. It was hypothesized to modify radiation pneumonitis by reducing the inflammatory and exudative portion of lung injury, and both animal and human studies showed that prednisolone did protect against the early phase of pneumonitis. However, when drug administration was terminated, the alveolitis reappeared and in mice the LD50 for pneumonitis was not changed.

A second approach of these early studies was to attempt to intervene in the fibrotic process with collagen antagonists. Perhaps the most widely tested was D-penicillamine, a compound shown in experimental studies significantly to inhibit collagen accumulation in rat lung for up to one year after irradiation.[115,116] This biochemical effect was translated into significant improvement in pulmonary function. Although shown to be effective in rats at a concentration that produced no deleterious side effects, D-penicillamine was not widely tested in the clinic, perhaps because its effectiveness required continuous administration.

As more data became available on the different cell types involved in radiation pneumonitis, it became possible rationally to test drugs known to reduce cell killing in these different populations. To determine the role of endothelial dysfunction in the pathogenesis of radiation-induced pneumonitis and fibrosis, Ward and colleagues[64-66] quantitated markers of endothelial activity—angiotensin converting enzyme (ACE) and plasminogen activator—and correlated these changes with pulmonary perfusion scans and morphologic changes. A time- and dose-dependent decrease in ACE was observed after irradiation of either the whole thorax or hemithorax that was in good agreement with pulmonary perfusion scans. Based on these data, these investigators then sought agents which would protect the endothelial cell, the presumed target, against radiation-induced cell killing.[117-119] The most promising drug is one that is commonly used in the management of hypertension and congestive heart failure by millions of people—captopril.[120,121] This drug contains a free thiol and is an orally active com-

petitive inhibitor of ACE, the enzyme that metabolizes angiotensin 1 to the vasoconstrictor angiotensin 2 and inactivates the bradykinins. In preclinical studies, captopril has been shown to ameliorate endothelial dysfunction after irradiation and to reduce radiation-induced lung fibrosis in rats.[119,122] Further support for the use of captopril against radiation-induced lung fibrosis is that it reduces age-related and radiation-induced cardiac fibrosis in rats[123] and, in patients, decreases morbidity and mortality from left ventricular dysfunction after myocardial infarction.[124] Captopril has been shown to be effective also in experimental radiation nephropathy by reducing proteinuria, preserving kidney function, and enhancing survival in rats.[125-127] These promising preclinical studies, coupled with the clinical use of the drug for hypertension, have prompted a clinical trial of captopril in lung cancer patients treated with radiation. Although the mechanism of its protective effect is unknown, studies *in vitro* suggest that captopril acts by inhibiting proliferation of lung fibroblasts.[128]

GENETIC REGULATION OF RADIATION- AND DRUG-INDUCED PNEUMONITIS AND FIBROSIS

A body of data has emerged in this area since the first edition of this book. Clinically, it has been well recognized that there are individual differences in the severity of treatment-related complications, including the severity of radiation-induced pneumonitis and fibrosis after definitive radiotherapy for lung cancer. A recent study by Gears and colleagues[129] of a group of 56 patients with limited small cell lung cancer who were treated with chemoradiotherapy demonstrated patient-to-patient heterogeneity, suggesting that the risk of lung fibrosis is strongly affected by inherent factors that vary among individuals. Although this heterogeneity could be due to a number of factors, mouse studies indicate that at least part of this response may be regulated by genetic factors.

Twenty years ago Steel and co-workers[130] reported an anomalous finding after irradiation of the whole thorax of C57B1 mice. Using a dose range designed to capture the LD50 for radiation pneumonitis previously reported in other mouse strains, they found that the survival time of this inbred strain of mice was significantly prolonged beyond the standard 80 to 180 days reported for radiation pneumonitis in other mouse strains. However the LD50 for radiation pneumonitis was similar in this strain to that reported in other inbred strains, leading them to conclude that the C57B1/6J strain was not more "resistant" to radiation-induced lung damage, but that the survival time was simply prolonged. However, subsequent studies by Down and co-workers[131,132] in a number of inbred mouse strains showed that the incidence of radiation pneumonitis and fibrosis was strain-dependent. Although strain-dependent differences could be due to a number of factors, certainly one possibility is that there is a genetic basis to this strain dependence. Down and co-workers conducted studies on the F_1 hybrid of a cross of a sensitive and resistant parent, but no clear-cut genetic dominance for the fibrosing phenotype was found.[132] However, in an in-depth survey of the incidence of radiation pneumonitis and fibrosis in nine inbred mouse strains, Sharplin and Franko[40] showed that the strains could be categorized as fibrosing, nonfibrosing, or intermediate, based on quantitative histological data. Further studies by these authors showed that the crossbreeding of strains with different proneness to fibrosis produced hybrids with the same sensitivity of the least fibrotic parent; the F_1 hybrid of a fibrosing and a nonfibrosing strain was uniformly nonfibrosing while a cross of an intermediate with a fibrosing strain produced a hybrid intermediate in its proneness to fibrosis,[133] suggesting that sensitivity to radiation-induced fibrosis is an autosomal recessive trait.

Although the data indicate that radiation-induced fibrosis is under polygenic control, the availability of mapping technologies, a genetic map of the mouse genome, and the existence of over 3000 markers polymorphic for the fibrosis-prone C57BL/6J and the fibrosis-resistant C3H/HeJ inbred strains allow the undertaking of a search for those genes that regulate radiation-induced fibrosis in these two mouse strains. In breeding studies using the C57B1/6J and the C3Hf/Kam inbred strains of mice to produce F_2 progeny which were individually genotyped and phenotyped by quantifying fibrosis in the lungs of each mouse, Haston and colleagues[41] have reported one loci on chromosome 17 that segregates with the fibrosing phenotype. This loci, which is within the region containing the major histocompatibility locus (MHC), has also shown by these same authors to be linked to bleomycin-induced lung fibrosis.[134] This same loci has been shown to be linked to susceptibility to ozone-induced lung damage in mice.[135] These data suggest that at least one genetic factor regulating pulmonary fibrosis may be universal and independent of the etiologic, although other loci have been shown to be insult-dependent.

The genetic regulation of pathologic processes in the lung is not without precedent. It is well known that pulmonary inflammation is controlled by genes in the H-2 complex.[136–138] Mice with an H-2^k loci are high responders (i.e., C3H mice), and those with an H-2^b loci are low responders (i.e., C57B1 mice).[136,138,139] In the studies of Sharplin and Franko[40] and Down and associates,[132] pneumonitis was found to be strain-dependent and related to the H-2 loci, that is an inflammatory cell infiltrate was not a feature of pneumonitis in the highly fibrogenic C57B1 strain, while conversely, an inflammatory cell infiltrate was the most prominent characteristic of the pneumonitis phase in the weakly fibrogenic C3H strain. Although these observations refute the hypothesis that immune-inflammatory processes usually precede fibrosis, they clearly indicate that pneumonitis after irradiation of mouse lung is genetically

regulated. However, the strain sensitivity to radiation pneumonitis is exactly opposite that for radiation-induced fibrosis, that is, the C57B1 are highly fibrogenic and the C3H are weakly fibrogenic.

In Sharplin's and Franko's study,[40] lung fibrosis was defined as collagen deposition in the interstitium and air spaces, resulting in contracture and collapse of the alveoli, an obliteration of normal lung architecture, and an attendant loss of pulmonary function resulting in the death of the mouse. The designation of "highly fibrogenic" was based on the number of acini obstructed by this contracted scar; in their studies only the C57 strains met these criteria. Another form of fibrosis characterized by collagen deposited only in the interstitium, a process that maintains alveolar structure, was largely ignored because it was suggested that this lesion alone would not produce sufficient functional impairment to cause death. The strains exhibiting this lesion, that is, CBA and C3H, were considered weakly fibrogenic. Thus the genetic regulation that controls the contracted fibrotic process described by Sharplin and Franko[40] may not be identical to that controlling interstitial fibrosis although there may be overlaps. Contrary to Sharplin's and Franko's suggestion that interstitial fibrosis is not a lethal event, it has been shown previously that interstitial fibrosis in the lung[15,24] and colon[43] can and does cause the demise of both CBA[132] and C3H[15] mice. Thus these lesions may represent two types of fibrosis regulated by different genes or sets of genes. In further studies using a number of inbred strains, Franko and colleagues[42] have also suggested that radiation can elicit two independent mechanisms for the development of fibrosis in mouse lung, one of which is controlled by two autosomal recessive determinants which act additively, the other of which is regulated independently by two additional genes, one of which is X-linked. Thus it is clear that radiation-induced pulmonary fibrosis is genetically regulated at least in part, but the genetics underlying this pathologic process appear to be complex.

Of the nine strains studied by Sharplin and Franko, all the C57B1 strains were found to be high responders, while both the C3H and CBA mice were identified as low responders. Similar strain variations in pulmonary fibrosis after a number of other insults have been reported. Particularly interesting are the data obtained after treatment with bleomycin, another DNA-damaging agent often used to induce lung fibrosis in model systems. The most striking finding after bleomycin treatment is that C57B1 mice were high responders[140–142] while the C3H strain was weakly fibrogenic,[143] findings remarkably similar to that observed after radiation. These data suggest that genetic factors related to susceptibility to lung fibrosis may operate independently of the etiologic agent.

CONCLUSIONS AND FUTURE DIRECTIONS

Although intervention in the process that results in radiation-induced fibrosis is certainly one way of decreasing the morbidity of thoracic irradiation for lung cancer, this approach would be reactive rather than proactive, and would not necessarily allow for higher tumor control by increasing tumor dose. The ultimate goal is to identify individuals who are at a higher risk of developing treatment-related pneumonitis and fibrosis before treatment begins. Clinically, a wide variation exists in the severity of lung fibrosis exhibited by individual patients treated similarly. These and data in other normal tissues demonstrate that variations in radiosensitivity exist in the same normal tissue cell type from different individuals. However, "tolerance" doses of both drugs and radiation are determined empirically from population averages and may reflect the sensitivity of a genetically determined minority. These data imply then that a majority of patients could be treated with higher doses of either modality without exceeding their individual tolerance to the treatment. One approach to increasing tumor control while maintaining an acceptable level of lung morbidity is to be able to identify those sensitive individuals before treatment begins. Although studies in humans and mice suggest that radiation sensitivity is genetically regulated, none of the genes have been identified. Nonetheless, predictive assays are being developed to individual patients at risk of developing severe late radiation effects, including lung fibrosis.[144-146]

Radiation-Sensitivity Testing of Cultured Fibroblasts from Patients: Correlation with Tissue Fibrosis

It is now well documented that variations in radiosensitivity can be demonstrated in the same normal tissue cell type from different individuals, suggesting that radiosensitivity is genetically regulated. Data from patients with ataxia telangiectasia (AT) have established not only that these individuals are highly sensitive to ionizing radiation, but that in survival assays, fibroblasts isolated and cultured from AT patients are more radiosensitive by several logs than fibroblasts from unaffected individuals.[147-150] Even in the normal population, a wide range of radiosensitivities is known to exist. If normal tissue radiosensitivity has a genetic component, then the radiosensitivity of cultured cells isolated from individuals should reflect the genetics of the individual. A number of studies have been performed to determine the relationship between fibroblast radiosensitivity as measured by the function of cells surviving a dose of 2Gy (SF 2Gy) (see also Chapter 12) and late tissue damage in patients.[150-152] Although early studies reported variable results, more recent data suggest that fibroblast radiosensitivity may be a useful predictor of late radiation damage in vasculoconnective tissues. However, the majority of these studies have been performed using skin fibroblasts cultured from breast cancer patients. Fibroblast radiosensitivity as measured by SF2 was compared with both acute and late end points, and although the data do not demonstrate a clear relationship between fibroblast radiosensitivity and chronic skin damage, these data appeared to be promising.[150]

In the case of patients with lung cancer, there are two issues that must be resolved experimentally. First, is there a correlation between lung fibrosis and survival of cultured lung fibroblasts? Also, since it would be difficult to obtain biopsies of normal lung from patients with lung cancer before treatment, the second issue is whether the radiosensitivity of fibroblasts isolated from another tissue, for example skin, from the patient will have a similar radiosensitivity as lung fibroblasts. Both of these questions have been investigated using two inbred strains of mice with documented differences in radiation induced lung fibrosis.

Dileto and Travis[153] determined the radiosensitivity of fibroblasts cultured from the lung and skin of the fibrosis-prone C57B1/6 strain and the fibrosis-resistant C3Hf/Kam strains of mice. In these mouse models, lung fibroblast radiosensitivity was not different as measured by SF2, despite a more than 20-fold difference in fibrosis scores—5.1% and 0.2% in the fibrosis-prone and fibrosis-resistant strains respectively. Similar SF2 values were obtained for skin fibroblasts from the two strains, indicating that the radiosensitivity of fibroblasts isolated from lung and skin of the same strain is the same. These data indicate that the *in vitro* radiosensitivity of lung fibroblasts as assayed by survival at 2 Gy does not correlate with the development of lung fibrosis, at least in the two strains of mice used in the studies of Dileto.[153]

Thus the usefulness of the fibroblast radiosensitivity as measured by SF2 for predicting lung fibrosis remains unclear.

Transforming Growth Factor β

A second approach to identifying "at risk" patients would be to identify the expression of cytokines, growth factors or other factors during treatment that correlate with the later incidence of pneumonitis or fibrosis. The underlying rationale of this approach is to identify and intervene in the early expression of gene products that may participate in the pathogenesis of pneumonitis or fibrosis. The goal would be to define factors that could be monitored regularly and routinely during treatment. The requirement of such a test would be that these factors be easily accessible for multiple sampling.

Transforming growth factor β is a ubiquitous cytokine present in a number of organs undergoing fibrosis.[154-156] TGF-β also has been implicated in the causation of chronic pulmonary fibrosis in rats and mice exposed to bleomycin and cyclophosphamide[141,157-161] and in the development of hepatic fibrosis in irradiated rats.[162] For this reason, it has been suggested that plasma levels of TGF-β may be increased before the onset of fibrosis. Recently, Anscher and colleagues measured the circulating levels of TGF-β in breast cancer patients undergoing bone marrow transplantation[162] and correlated these values with the later incidence of pulmonary fibrosis and hepatic venoocclusive disease, both of which are significant side effects of this treatment. TGF-β was determined initially after induction chemotherapy but before the administration of high-dose chemotherapy and subsequently after high-dose chemotherapy and transplantation. Hepatic venoocclusive disease and lung fibrosis were observed clinically between one to three weeks and 40 to 75 days after transplantation respectively. Analysis of the TGF-β levels after induction chemotherapy with the later incidence of liver and pulmonary fibrosis in individual patients showed that plasma levels of TGF-β had a positive predictive value of more than 90% for the development of fibrosis in either of these organs in a given patient. Although plasma levels of TGF-β were not determined before any treatment, and thus its usefulness in selecting patients more likely to develop lung fibrosis before treatment begins is unknown, these data suggest that routine monitoring of plasma TGF-β in individual patients undergoing radiation or chemotherapy for lung cancer could be useful as a predictor of lung fibrosis. More recently, Anscher and colleagues[163] investigated in a prospective study the usefulness of TGF-β1 as a predictive marker for the development of radiation-induced lung damage. In this study, 73 lung cancer patients were treated with curative intent; all treatment parameters were similar in this patient cohort. TGF-β1 levels were measured before, weekly during treatment, and at each follow-up to six months after the completion of radiotherapy, when the study was ended. The end point was the development of radiation pneumonitis at six months after treatment, which was defined by National Cancer Institute common toxicity criteria. Only 15 (21%) of these patients developed symptomatic pneumonitis. In this study, a normal plasma TGF-β1 level by the end of radiotherapy was more common in patients who did not develop pneumonitis (Figure 13.10). A return of TGF-β1 plasma levels to normal accurately identified patients who would not develop pneumonitis with a positive predictive value of 90%, indicating that the level of this cytokine may be useful in identifying patients at low risk for the development of radiation pneumonitis. These patients could then be considered for dose escalation.

Such studies provide the impetus to search for other early markers of radiation- and drug-induced lung damage in the hope of preventing these potentially fatal complications.

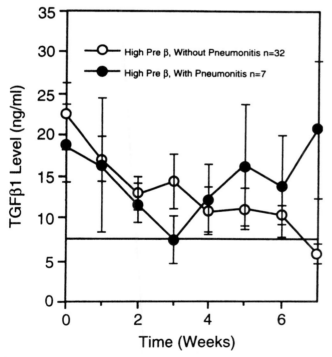

FIGURE 13.10. Plasma TGF-β-levels as a function of time for patients with an elevated pretreatment plasma TGF-β level who did not (*open symbols*) or did (*closed symbols*) develop radiation pneumonitis. Although both groups experienced a reduction in TGF-β levels during treatment, in one group this decrease was transient, and the TGF-β levels returned to high levels. This group had a significantly higher risk of developing pneumonitis than those patients whose TGF-β levels remained within control values. (From Anscher MS, Kong F-M, Andrews K, et al. Plasma transforming growth factor β1 as a predictor of radiation pneumonitis. *Int J Radiat Oncol Biol Phys* 1998;41:1032, with permission.)

REFERENCES

1. Groover TA, Christie AC, Merritt EA. Observations on the use of the copper filter in the roentgen treatment of deep-seated malignancies. *South Med J* 1922;15:440.
2. Evans WA, Leucutia T. Intrathoracic changes induced by heavy radiation. *AJR Am J Roentgenol* 1925;13:203.
3. Travis EL. Lung morbidity of radiotherapy. In: Plowman PN, McElwain TJ, Meadows AT, eds. *Complications of cancer management.* Oxford: Butterworth-Heineman, Ltd., 1991:232.
4. Boersma LJ, Damen EMF, de Boer RW, et al. Dose-effect relations for local functional and structural changes of the lung after irradiation for malignant lymphoma. *Radiother Oncol* 1994;32:201.
5. Mah K, Keane TJ, Van Dyk J, et al. Quantitative effect of combined chemotherapy and fractionated radiotherapy on the incidence of radiation-induced lung damage: A prospective clinical study. *Int J Radiat Oncol Biol Phys* 1994;28:563.
6. Boersma LJ, Damen EMF, de Boer RW, et al. A new method to determine the dose-effect relations for local lung function changes using correlated SPECT and CT data. *Radiother Oncol* 1993;29:110.
7. Choi NC, Kanarek DJ, Kazemi H. Physiologic changes in pulmonary function after thoracic radiotherapy for patients with lung cancer and a role of regional pulmonary function studies in predicting post-radiotherapy pulmonary function before radiotherapy. *Cancer Treat Symp* 1985;2:119.
8. Damen EMF, Muller SH, Boersma LJ, et al. Quantifying local lung perfusion and ventilation using correlated SPECT and CT data. *J Nucl Med* 1994;35:784.
9. Mah K, Van Dyk J. Quantitative measurement of changes in human lung density following irradiation. *Radiother Oncol* 1988;11:169.

10. Marks LB, Spencer DP, Bentel GC, et al. The utility of SPECT lung perfusion scans in minimizing and assessing the physiologic consequences of thoracic irradiation. *Int J Radiat Oncol Biol Phys* 1993;23:659.

11. Marks LB, Munley MT, Spencer DP, et al. Quantification of radiation-induced regional lung injury with perfusion imaging. *Int J Radiat Oncol Biol, Phys* 1997;38:399.

12. Kwa SLS, Theuws JCM, van Herk M, et al. Automatic three-dimensional matching of CT-SPECT and CT-CT to localize lung damage after radiotherapy. *J Nucl Med* 1998;39:1074.

13. Hebert ME, Lowe VJ, Hoffman JM, et al. Positron emission tomography in the pretreatment evaluation and follow-up of non–small cell lung cancer patients treated with radiotherapy: preliminary findings. *Am J Clin Oncol* 1996;19:416.

14. Travis EL, Vojnovic B, Davies EE, et al. A plethysmographic method for measuring lung function in locally irradiated mouse lung. *Br J Radiol* 1979;52:67.

15. Travis EL, Down JD, Holmes SJ, et al. Radiation pneumonitis and fibrosis in mouse lung assayed by respiratory frequency and histology. *Radiat Res* 1980;84:133.

16. Depledge MH, Collis CH, Barrett A. The technique for measuring carbon monoxide uptake in mice. *Int J Radiat Oncol Biol Phys* 1981;7:485.

17. Nicholas D, Down JD. The assessment of early and late radiation injury to the mouse lung using X-ray computerised tomography. *Radiother Oncol* 1985;4:253.

18. Lockhart SP, Hill D, King S, et al. A semi-automated method for breathing rate measurement in the mouse. *Radiother Oncol* 1991;22:68.

19. Rubin P, Casarett GW. *Clinical radiation pathology.* vol. II. Philadelphia: W.B. Saunders Company, 1968:1057.

20. Nonn RA, Gross NJ. Effects of radiation on the lung. *Curr Opin Pulmonary Med* 1996;2:390.

21. Marks LB. The pulmonary effects of thoracic irradiation. *Oncology* 1994;8:89.

22. McDonald S, Rubin P, Phillips TL, et al. Injury to the lung from cancer therapy: clinical syndromes, measurable endpoints, and potential scoring systems. *Int J Radiat Oncol Biol Phys* 1995; 31:1187.

23. Rosiello RA, Merrill WW. Radiation-induced lung injury. *Clin Chest Med* 1990;11:65.

24. Travis EL. The sequence of histological changes in mouse lungs after total lung irradiation. *Int J Radiat Oncol Biol Phys* 1980; 6:345.

25. Penney DP, Siemann DW, Rubin P, et al. Morphologic changes reflecting early and late effects of irradiation of the distal lung of the mouse: a review. *Scanning Electron Microsc* 1982;I:413.

26. Burkhardt A, Cottier H. Cellular events in alveolitis and the evolution of pulmonary fibrosis. B, cell pathology including molecular pathology *Virchows Arch* 1989;58:1.

27. Sharplin J, Franko AJ. Quantitative histological study of strain-dependent differences in the effects of irradiation on mouse lung during the early phase. *Radiat Res* 1989;119:1.

28. Van Dyk J, Keane TJ, Kan S, et al. Radiation pneumonitis following large single dose irradiation: A re-evaluation based on absolute dose to lung. *Int J Radiat Oncol Biol Phys* 1981;7:461.

29. Prato FS, Kurdyak R, Saibil EA, et al. The incidence of radiation pneumonitis as a result of single fraction upper half body irradiation. *Cancer* 1976;39:71.

30. Mah K, Van Dyk J, Keane T, et al. Acute radiation-induced pulmonary damage: a clinical study on the response to fractionated radiation therapy. *Int J Radiat Oncol Biol Phys* 1987;13: 179.

31. Van Dyk J, Mah K, Keane TJ. Radiation-induced lung damage: dose-time-fractionation considerations. *Radiother Oncol* 1989; 14:55.

32. Mah K, Poon PY, Van Dyk J, et al. Assessment of acute radiation-induced pulmonary changes using computed tomography. *J Comput Assist Tomog* 1986;10:736.

33. Bachofen M, Weibel ER. Alterations of the gas exchange apparatus in adult respiratory insufficiency associated with septicemia. *Am Rev Respir Dis* 1977;116:589.

34. Travis EL, Down JD, Holmes SJ, et al. Radiation pneumonitis and fibrosis in mouse lung assayed by respiratory frequency and histology. *Year Book of Cancer* 1982;364.

35. Ullrich RL, Casarett GW. Interrelationship between the early inflammatory response and subsequent fibrosis after radiation exposure. *Radiat Res* 1977;72:107.

36. Franko AJ, Sharplin J. Development of fibrosis after lung irradiation in relation to inflammation and lung function in a mouse strain prone to fibrosis. *Rad Res* 1994;140:347.

37. Travis EL, Down JD. Repair in mouse lung after split doses of X-rays. *Radiat Res* 1981;87:166.

38. Travis EL, Meistrich ML, Finch-Neimeyer MV, et al. Late functional and biochemical changes in mouse lung after irradiation: differential effects of WR-2721. *Radiat Res* 1985;103:219.

39. Pickrell JA, Diel JH, Slauson DO, et al. Radiation-induced pulmonary fibrosis resolves spontaneously if dense scars are not formed. *Exp Mol Pathol* 1983;38:22.

40. Sharplin J, Franko AJ. A quantitative histological study of strain-dependent differences in the effects of irradiation on mouse lung during the intermediate and late phases. *Radiat Res* 1989; 119:15.

41. Haston CK, Travis EL. Murine susceptibility to radiation-induced pulmonary fibrosis is influenced by a genetic factor implicated in susceptibility to bleomycin-induced pulmonary fibrosis. *Cancer Res* 1997;57:5286.

42. Franko AJ, Sharplin J, Ward WF, et al. Evidence for two patterns of inheritance of sensitivity to induction of lung fibrosis in mice by radiation, one of which involves two genes. *Radiat Res* 1996;146:68.

43. Followill DS, Kester D, Travis EL. Histological changes in mouse colon after single and split dose irradiation. *Radiat Res* 1993;136:280.

44. Liao ZX, Travis EL. Unilateral nephrectomy 24 hours fafter bilateral kidney irradiation reduces damage to function and structure of remaining kidney. *Radiat Res* 1994;139:290.

45. Cohen Y, Gellei B, Robinson E. Bilateral radiation pneumonitis after unilateral lung and mediastinal irradiation. *Radiol Clin Biol* 1974;43:465.

46. Bennett DE, Million RR, Ackerman LV. Bilateral radiation pneumonitis, a complication of the radiotherapy of bronchogenic carcinoma. *Cancer* 1969;23:1001.

47. Smith JC. Radiation pneumonitis: case report bilateral reaction after unilateral irradiation. *Am Rev Respir Dis* 1964;89:264.

48. Goldman AL, Enquist R. Hyperacute radiation pneumonitis. *Chest* 1975;67:613.

49. Holt JAG. The acute radiation pneumonitis syndrome. *J Collegiate Radiol Australasia* 1964;8:40.

50. Gibson PG, Bryant DH, Morgan GW, et al. Radiation-induced lung injury: a hypersensitivity pneumonitis? *Ann Intern Med* 1988;109:288.

51. Morgan GW, Breit SN. Radiation and the lung: a re-evaluation of the mechanisms mediating pulmonary injury. *Int J Radiat Oncol Biol Phys* 1995;31:361.

52. Geist BJ, Trott K-R. Radiographic and function changes after partial lung irradiation in the rat. *Strahlenther Onkol* 1992;168: 168.

53. Penney DP, Rubin P. Specific early fine structural changes in the lung following irradiation. *Int J Radiat Oncol Biol Phys* 1977; 2:1123.

54. Travis EL, Tucker SL. The relationship between functional as-

says of radiation response in the lung and target cell depletion. *Br J Cancer* 1986;53:304.

55. Rubin P, Shapiro DL, Finklestein JN, et al. The early release of surfactant following lung irradiation of alveolar type II cells. *Int J Radiat Oncol Biol Phys* 1980;6:75.

56. Rubin P, Siemann DW, Shapiro DL, et al. Surfactant release as an early measure of radiation pneumonitis. *Int J Radiat Oncol Biol Phys* 1983;9:1669.

57. Rubin P, McDonald S, Maasilta P, et al. Serum markers for prediction of pulmonary radiation syndromes. Part I: surfactant apoprotein. *Int J Radiat Oncol Biol Phys* 1989;17:553.

58. Shapiro DL, Finkelstein JN, Penney DP, et al. Sequential effects of irradiation on the pulmonary surfactant system. *Int J Radiat Oncol Biol Phys* 1982;8:879.

59. Peterson LM, Evans ML, Graham MM, et al. Vascular response to radiation injury in the rat lung. *Radiat Res* 1992;129:139.

60. Law MP, Ahier RG. Vascular and epithelial damage in the lung of the mouse after X rays or neutrons. *Radiat Res* 1989;117:128.

61. Law MP. Radiation induced vascular injury and its relation to late effects in normal tissues. *Adv Radiat Biol* 1981;9:37.

62. Gross NJ. Experimental radiation pneumonitis. IV. Leakage of circulatory proteins onto the alveolar surface. *J Lab Clin Med* 1980;95:19.

63. Hopewell JW. The importance of vascular damage in the development of late radiation effects in normal tissues. In: Meyn RE, Withers HR, eds. *Radiation biology in cancer research*. New York: Raven Press, 1980:449.

64. Ts'ao C-H, Ward WF, Port CD. Radiation injury in rat lung I. Prostacyclin (PGI_2) production, arterial perfusion, and ultrastructure. *Radiat Res* 1983;96:284.

65. Ward WF, Solliday NH, Molteni A, et al. Radiation injury in rat lung II. Angiotensin-converting enzyme activity. *Radiat Res* 1983;96:294.

66. Ts'ao C-H, Ward WF, Port CD. Radiation injury in rat lung III. Plasminogen activator and fibrinolytic inhibitor activities. *Radiat Res* 1983;96:301.

67. King RJ, Jones MB, Minoo P. Regulation of lung cell proliferation by polypeptide growth factors. *Am J Physiol* 1989;257:23.

68. Rubin P, Finkelstein J, Shapiro D. Molecular biology mechanisms in the radiation induction of pulmonary injury syndromes: interrelationship between the aveolar macrophage and the septal fibroblast. *Int J Radiat Oncol Biol Phys* 1992;24:93.

69. Rubin P, Johnston CJ, Williams JP, et al. A perpetual cascade of cytokines postirradiation leads to pulmonary fibrosis. *Int J Radiat Oncol Biol Phys* 1995;33:99.

70. Martinet Y, Menard O, Vaillant P, et al. Cytokines in human lung fibrosis. *Arch Toxicol* 1996;S18:127.

71. Finkelstein JN, Johnston CJ, Baggs R, et al. Early alterations in extracellular matrix and transforming growth factor β gene expression in mouse lung indicative of late radiation fibrosis. *Int J Radiat Oncol Biol Phys* 1994;28:621.

72. Finkelstein JN, Horowitz S, Sinkin RA, et al.: Cellular and molecular responses to lung injury in relation to induction of tissue repair and fibrosis. *Clin Perinatol* 1992;19:603.

73. McDonald S, Rubin P, Constine L, et al. Biochemical markers as predictors for pulmonary effects of radiation. *Radiat Oncol Invest* 1995;3:56.

74. Franklin TJ. Therapeutic approaches to organ fibrosis. *Int J Biochem Cell Biol* 1997;29:79.

75. Grande JP. Role of transforming growth factor-β in tissue injury and repair. *Proc Soc Exp Biol Med* 1997;214:27.

76. Anscher MS, Kong F-M, Marks LB, et al. Changes in plasma transforming growth factor beta during radiotherapy and the risk of symptomatic radiation-induced pneumonitis. *Int J Radiat Oncol Biol Phys* 1997;37:253.

77. Johnston CJ, Wright TW, Rubin P, et al. Alterations in the expression of chemokine mRNA levels in fibrosis-resistant and sensitive mice after thoracic irradiation. *Exp Lung Res* 1998;24:321.

78. Fowler JR. 40 years of radiobiology: Its impact on radiotherapy. *Phys Med Biol* 1984;29:97.

79. Withers HR, Peters LJ, Kogelnik HD. The pathobiology of late effects of irradiation. In: Meyn RE, Withers HR, eds. *Radiation biology in cancer research*. New York: Raven Press, 1980:439.

80. Travis EL, Parkins CS, Down JD, et al. Repair in mouse lung between multiple small doses of x-rays. *Rad Res* 1983;94:326.

81. Travis EL, Thames HD, Jr., Watkins TL, et al. The kinetics of repair in mouse lung after fractionated radiation. *Int J Radiat Biol* 1987;52:903.

82. Withers HR, Thames HD, Jr., Peters LJ. Dose fractionation and volume effects in normal tissue and tumors. *Cancer Treat Symp* 1984;1:75.

83. Thames HD, Withers HR, Peters LJ, et al. Changes in early and late radiation responses with altered dose fractionation: implications for dose-survival relationships. *Int J Radiat Oncol Biol Phys* 1982;8:219.

84. Douglas BG, Fowler JF. The effect of multiple small doses of x-rays on skin reactions in the mouse and a basic interpretation. *Radiat Res* 1976;66:401.

85. Fowler JF. The linear quadratic formula and progress in fractionated radiotherapy. *Br J Radiol* 1989;62:679.

86. Peters LJ, Withers HR, Thames HD. Radiobiological bases for multiple daily fractionation. In: Kaercher KH, Kogelnik HD, Reinartz G, eds. *Progress in radio-oncology* II. New York: Raven Press, 1982.

87. Withers HR, Thames HD, Peters LJ, et al. Normal tissue radioresistance in clinical radiotherapy. In: Fletcher GH, Nervi C, Withers HR, eds. *Biological bases and clinical implications of tumor radioresistance*. New York: Masson, 1983:139.

88. Vegesna V, Withers HR, Thames HD, et al. Multifraction radiation response of mouse lung. *Int J Radiat Biol* 1985;47:413.

89. Parkins CS, Fowler JR. Repair in mouse lung after multifraction X-rays and neutrons: extension to 40 fractions. *Br J Radiol* 1985;58:1097.

90. Parkins CS, Fowler JF, Maughan RL, et al. Repair in mouse lung for up to 20 fractions of X-rays or neutrons. *Br J Radiol* 1985;58:225.

91. Down JD, Easton DF, Steel GG. Repair in the mouse lung during low dose-rate irradiation. *Radiother Oncol* 1986;6:29.

92. Terry NHA, Tucker SL, Travis EL. Residual radiation damage in murine lung assessed by pneumonitis. *Int J Radiat Oncol Biol Phys* 1988;14:929.

93. Withers HR, Taylor JM, Maciejewski B. The hazard of accelerated tumor clonogen repopulation during radiotherapy. *Acta Oncol* 1988;27:131.

94. Withers HR, Maciejewski B, Taylor JM, et al. Accelerated repopulation in head and neck cancer. *Front Radiat Ther Oncol* 1988;22:105.

95. Maciejewski B, Withers HR, Taylor JM, et al. Hliniak A. Dose fractionation and regeneration in radiotherapy for cancer of the oral cavity and oropharynx: tumor dose-response and repopulation. *Int J Radiat Oncol Biol Phys* 1989;16:831.

96. Komaki R, Pajak TF, Byhardt RW, et al. Analysis of early and late deaths on RTOG non–small cell carcinoma of the lung trials: comparison with CALGB 8433. *Lung Cancer* 1993;10:189.

97. Cox JD, Azarnia N, Byhardt RW, et al. A randomized phase I/II trial of hyperfractionated radiation therapy with total doses of 60.0 Gy to 79.2 Gy: possible survival benefit with ±69.6 Gy in favorable patients with radiation therapy oncology group

stage III non-small-cell lung carcinoma: report of radiation therapy oncology group 83–11. *J Clin Oncol* 1990;8:1543.

98. Withers HR, Thames HD, Jr. Dose fractionation and volume effects in normal tissue and tumors. *Am J Clin Oncol* 1988;11:313.

99. Withers HR, Taylor JMG, Maciejewski B. Treatment volume and tissue tolerance. *Int J Radiat Oncol Biol Phys* 1988;14:751.

100. Liao Z-X, Travis EL, Tucker SL. Damage and morbidity from pneumonitis after irradiation of partial volumes of mouse lung. *Int J Radiat Oncol Biol Phys* 1995;32:1359.

101. Travis EL, Liao Z-X, Tucker SL. Spatial heterogeneity of the volume effect for radiation pneumonitis in mouse lung. *Int J Radiat Oncol Biol Phys* 1997;38:1045.

102. Boersma LJ, Theuws JCM, Kwa SLS, et al. Regional variation in functional subunit density in the lung: regarding Liao *et al.* IJROBP 32(5):1359–1370;1995. *Int J Radiat Oncol Biol Phys* 1996;34:1187.

103. Khan MA, Hill RP, Van Dyk J. Partial volume rat lung irradiation: an evaluation of early DNA damage. *Int J Radiat Oncol Biol Phys* 1998;40:467.

104. Tucker SL, Liao Z-X, Travis EL. Estimation of the spatial distribution of target cells in mouse lung. *Int J Radiat Oncol Biol Phys* 1997;38:1055.

105. Yamada M, Kudoh S, Hirata K, et al. Risk factors of pneumonitis following chemoradiotherapy for lung cancer. *Eur J Cancer* 1998;34:71.

106. Kwa SLS, Lebesque JV, Theuws JCM, et al. Radiation pneumonitis as a function of mean lung dose: an analysis of pooled data on 540 patients. *Int J Radiat Oncol Biol Phys* 1998;42:1.

107. Fuks Z, Persaud RS, Alfieri A, et al. Basic fibroblast growth factor protects endothelial cells against radiation-induced programmed cell death *in vitro* and *in vivo*. *Cancer Res* 1994;54:2582.

108. Haimovitz-Friedman A, Vladavsky I, Chaudhuri A, et al. Autocrine effects of fibroblast growth factor in repair of radiation damage in endothelial cells. *Cancer Res* 1991;51:2552.

109. Haimovitz-Friedman A, Balaban N, McLoughlin M, et al. Protein kinase C mediates basic fibroblast growth factor protection of endothelial cells against radiation-induced apoptosis. *Cancer Res* 1994;54:2591.

110. Tee PG, Travis EL. Basic fibroblast growth factor does not protect against classical radiation pneumonitis in two strains of mice. *Cancer Res* 1995;55:298.

111. Giri SN, Hyde DM, Marafino BJJ. Ameliorating effect of murine interferon gamma on bleomycin-induced lung collagen fibrosis in mice. *Biochem Med Metabol Biol* 1986;36:194.

112. Granstein RD, Deak MR, Jacques SL, et al. The systemic administration of gamma interferon inhibits collagen synthewis and acute inflammation in a murine skin wounding model. *J Invest Dermatol* 1989;93:18.

113. Granstein RD, Flotte TJ, Amento EP. Interferons and collagen production. *J Invest Dermatol* 1990;95:75S.

114. Rosiello RA, Merrill WW, Rockwell S, et al. Radiation pneymonitis: bronchoalveolar lavage assessment and modulation by a recombinant cytokine. *Am Rev Respir Dis* 1993;148:1671.

115. Ward WF, Shih-Hoellwarth A, Tuttle RD. Collagen accumulation in the irradiated rat lung: modification by D-penicillamine. *Radiology* 1983;146:533.

116. Ward WF, Molteni A, Ts'ao C-H, et al. Radiation injury in rat lung IV. Modification by D-penicillamine. *Radiat Res* 1983;98:397.

117. Ward WF, Kim YT, Molteni A, et al. Radiation-induced pulmonary endothelial dysfunction in rats: modification by an inhibitor of angiotensin converting enzyme. *Int J Radiat Oncol Biol Phys* 1988;15:135.

118. Ward WF, Molteni A, Ts'ao C, et al. Radiation pneumotoxicity in rats: modification by inhibitors of angiotensin converting enzyme. *Int J Radiat Oncol Biol Phys* 1992;22:623.

119. Ward WF, Lin PO, Wong PS, et al. Radiation pneumonitis in rats and its modification by the angiotensin-converting enzyme inhibitor captopril evaluated by high-resolution computed tomography. *Radiat Res* 1993;135:81.

120. Gavras I, Gavras H. The use of ACE inhibitors in hypertension. In: Kostis JB, DeFelice EA, eds. *Angiotensin converting enzyme inhibitors.* New York: Liss, 1987:93.

121. Franciosa JA. The use of ACE inhibitors in congestive heart failure. In: Kostis JB, DeFelice EA, eds. *Angiotensin converting enzyme inhibitors.* New York: Liss, 1987;123.

122. Ward WF, Molteni A, Ts'ao C, et al. Captopril reduces collagen and mast cell accumulation in irradiated rat lung. *Int J Radiat Oncol Biol Phys* 1990;19:1405.

123. Yarom R, Harper IS, Wynchank S, et al. Effect of captopril on changes in rats' hearts induced by long-term irradiation. *Radiat Res* 1993;133:187.

124. Rossi MA, Peres LC. Effect of captopril on the prevention and regression of myocardial cell hypertrophy and interstitial fibrosis in pressure overload cardiac hypertrophy. *Am Heart J* 1992;124:700.

125. Cohen EP, Fish BL, Moulder JE. Treatment of radiation nephropathy with captopril. *Radiat Res* 1992;132:346.

126. Moulder JE, Fish BL, Cohen EP. Treatment of radiation nephropathy with ACE inhibitors. *Int J Radiat Oncol Biol Phys* 1993;27:93.

127. Moulder JE, Cohen EP, Fish BL, et al. Prophylaxis of bone marrow transplant nephropathy with captopril, an inhibitor of angiotensin-converting enzyme. *Radiat Res* 1993;136:404.

128. Nguyen L, Ward WF, Ts'ao C-H, et al. Captopril inhibits proliferation of human lung fibroblasts in culture: a potential antifibrotic mechanism. *Proc Soc Exp Biol Med* 1994;205:80–84.

129. Geara FB, Komaki R, Tucker SL, et al. Factors influencing the development of lung fibrosis after chemoradiation for small cell carcinoma of the lung: evidence for inherent interindividual variation. *Int J Radiat Oncol Biol Phys* 1998;41:279.

130. Steel GG, Adams K, Peckham MJ. Lung damage in C57B1 mice following thoracic irradiation: enhancement by chemotherapy. *Br J Radiol* 1979;52:741.

131. Down JD, Steel GG. The expression of early and late damage after thoracic irradiation: a comparison between CBA and C57B1 mice. *Radiat Res* 1983;96:603.

132. Down JD, Nicholas D, Steel GG. Lung damage after hemithoracic irradiation: Dependence on mouse strain. *Radiother Oncol* 1986;6:43.

133. Franko AJ, Sharplin J, Ward WF, et al. The genetic basis of strain-dependent differences in the early phase of radiation injury in mouse lung. *Radiat Res* 1991;126:349.

134. Haston CK, Amos CI, King TM, et al. Inheritance of susceptibility to bleomycin-induced pulmonary fibrosis in the mouse. *Cancer Res* 1996;56:2596.

135. Kleeberger SR, Levitt RC, Zhang L-Y, et al. Linkage analysis of susceptibility to ozone-induced lung inflammation in inbred mice [Letter]. *Nat Genet* 1997;17:475.

136. Rossi GA, Hunninghake GW, Kawanami O, et al. Motheaten mice. An animal model with an inherited form of interstitial lung disease. *Am Rev Respir Dis* 1985;131:150.

137. Vaz NM, Vaz EM, Levine BB. Relationship between histocompatibility (H-2) genotype and immune responsiveness to low dose of ovalbumin in the mouse. *J Immunol* 1970;104:1572.

138. Wilson BD, Sternick JL, Yoshizawa Y, et al. Experimental murine hypersensitivity pneumonitis: multigenic control and influence by genes within the *I-B* subregion of the *H-2* complex. *J Immunol* 1982;129:2160.

139. Allen EM, Moore VL, Stevens JO. Strain variation in BCG-induced chronic pulmonary inflammation in mice I. Basic model and possible genetic control by non-H-2 genes. *J Immunol* 1977;119:343.

140. Schrier DJ, Kunkel RG, Phan SH. The role of strain variation in murine bleomycin-induced pulmonary fibrosis. *Am Rev Respir Dis* 1983;127:63.

141. Hoyt DG, Lazo JS. Alterations in pulmonary mRNA encoding procollagens, fibronectin and transforming growth factor-β precede bleomycin-induced pulmonary fibrosis in mice. *J Pharmacol Exp Ther* 1988;246:765.

142. Hoyt DG, Lazo JS. Bleomycin and cyclophosphamide increase pulmonary type IV procollagen mRNA in mice. *Am J Physiol* 1990;259:L47.

143. Mori H, Kawada K, Zhang P, et al. Bleomycin-induced pulmonary fibrosis in genetically mast cell-deficient WBB6F$_1$-W/W^V mice and mechanism of the suppressive effect of tranilast, an antiallergic drug inhibiting mediator release from mast cells, on fibrosis. *Int Arch Allergy Appl Immunol* 1991;95:195.

144. Peters LJ, Brock WA, Chapman JD, et al. Response predictors in radiotherapy: a review of research into radiobiologically based assays. *Br J Radiol* 1988;22S:96.

145. Peters LJ, Brock WA, Travis EL. Radiation biology at clinically relevant fractions. In: DeVita VT, Hellman S, Rosenberg SA, eds. *Important advances in oncology.* Philadelphia: J.B. Lippincott Company, 1990:65.

146. Peters LJ. Inherent radiosensitivity of tumor and normal tissue cells as a predictor of human tumor response. *Radiother Oncol* 1990;17:177.

147. Deschavanne PJ, Debieu D, Fertil B, et al. Re-evaluation of *in vitro* radiosensitivity of human fibroblasts of different genetic origins. *Int J Radiat Biol* 1986;50:279.

148. Cole J, Arlett CF, Green MHL, et al. Comparative human cellular radiosensitivity: II. The survival following gamma-irradiation of unstimulated (G$_0$) T-lymphocytes, T-lymphocyte lines, lymphoblastoid cell lines and fibroblasts from normal donors, from ataxia-telangiectasia patients and from ataxia-telangiectasia heterozygotes. *Int J Radiat Biol* 1988;54:929.

149. Woods WG, Byrne TD, Tae HK. Sensitivity of cultured cells to gamma radiation in a patient exhibiting marked *in vivo* radiation sensitivity. *Cancer* 1988;62:2341.

150. Brock WA, Tucker SL, Geara FB, et al. Fibroblast radiosensitivity versus acute and late normal skin responses in patients treated for breast cancer. *Int J Radiat Oncol Biol Phys* 1995;32:1371.

151. Geara FB, Peters LJ, Ang KK, et al. Radiosensitivity measurement of keratinocytes and fibroblasts from radiotherapy patients. *Int J Radiat Oncol Biol Phys* 1992;24:287.

152. Geara FB, Peters LJ, Ang KK, et al. Prospective comparison of *in vitro* normal cell radiosensitivity and normal tissue reactions in radiotherapy patients. *Int J Radiat Oncol Biol Phys* 1993;27:1173.

153. Dileto CL, Travis EL. Fibroblast radiosensitivity in vitro and lung fibrosis: comparison between a fibrosing and non-fibrosing mouse strain. *Radiat Res* 1996;146:61.

154. Border WA, Noble NA. Transforming growth factor β in tissue fibrosis. *N Engl J Med* 1994;331:1286.

155. Beck LS, DeGuzman L, Lee WP, et al. One systemic administration of transforming growth factor-β1 reverses age- or glucocorticoid-impaired wound healing. *J Clin Invest* 1993;92:2841.

156. Anscher MS, Peters WP, Reisenbichler H, et al. Transforming growth factor β as a predictor of liver and lung fibrosis after autologous bone marrow transplantation for advanced breast cancer. *N Engl J Med* 1993;328:1592.

157. Kelly J, Kobacs EJ, Nicholson K, et al. Transforming growth factor-β production by lung macrophages and fibroblasts. *Chest* 1991;[99 Suppl]:85S.

158. Khalil N, Bereznay O, Sporn M, et al. Macrophage production of transforming growth factor beta and fibroblast collagen synthesis in chronic pulmonary inflammation. *J Exp Med* 1989;170:727.

159. Raghow R, Irish P, Kang AH. Coordinate regulation of transforming growth factor β gene expression and cell proliferation in hamster lungs undergoing bleomycin-induced pulmonary fibrosis. *J Clin Invest* 1989;84:1836.

160. Phan SH, Giharaee-Kermani M, Wolber F, et al. Stimulation of rat endothelial cell transforming growth factor-β production by bleomycin. *J Clin Invest* 1991;87:148.

161. Hoyt DG, Lazo JS. Early increases in pulmonary mRNA encoding procollagens transforming growth factor-β in mice sensitive to cyclophosphamide-induced pulmonary fibrosis. *J Pharmacol Exp Ther* 1989;249:38.

162. Anscher MS, Crocker IR, Jirtle RL. Transforming growth factor-β1 expression in irradiated liver. *Radiat Res* 1990;122:77.

163. Anscher MS, Kong F-M Andrews K, et al. Plasma transforming growth factor β1 as a predictor of radiation pneumonitis. *Int J Radiat Oncol Biol Phys* 1998;41:1029.

14

CHEMOTHERAPY

KENNETH R. HANDE

Combination chemotherapy has been the cornerstone of treatment for patients with small cell lung cancer (SCLC) for nearly three decades.[1] More recently, chemotherapy has also become the standard of care for patients with stage III and IV non–small cell lung cancer (NSCLC).[2,3] Since over two thirds of NSCLC patients present with stages III or IV disease, chemotherapy is now being considered for most of the 170,000 patients diagnosed with lung cancer in the United States.[4] Despite the beneficial effects of drug treatment in producing tumor regressions, improving symptoms, and prolonging life, the use of chemotherapy is not appropriate for every patient. Cancer chemotherapy has a narrow therapeutic window, with the potential for producing life-threatening toxicity. Clinicians recommending chemotherapy for their patients must understand the goals of treatment and the potential for toxicity. This chapter outlines the general principles of cancer chemotherapy, including the pharmacology and toxicity of specific agents used for the treatment of lung cancer.

BIOLOGIC PRINCIPLES

Lung cancers commonly have several characteristics which limit the effectiveness of cancer chemotherapy. These factors include: (a) large tumor volume; (b) the presence of nondividing cells within the tumor; (c) cancer cells with different apoptotic pathways; and (d) the presence of drug-resistant tumor cells. The importance of these factors in treatment will be discussed in the following sections.

Cancer Biology

A 1 cm diameter tumor (rarely are lung cancers detected this early) contains 10^9 cells. A lethal tumor burden is only 3 logs higher (10^{12} cells). Chemotherapy generally kills a specific fraction of malignant cells.[5,6] The fractional cell kill (e.g., 90%, 99%, or 99.99% cell kill) depends on the sensitivity of cells to the antineoplastic drug and upon the dose of drug administered. The model of fractional cell kill leads to two important principles regarding chemotherapy. First, because of the large number of cells present at diagno-

sis (e.g. 10^{11}), multiple courses of treatment are required for therapy even if a drug or a combination of drugs produces a 99.9% cell kill (i.e., kills 999 of every 1,000 cells present). One treatment with a 99.9% cell kill will reduce a tumor population from 10^{11} to 10^8 cells. At least four treatments are, therefore, necessary to eliminate the final cancer cell, assuming there is no tumor cell growth during the treatment period. In fact, because of toxicity to normal tissues and time needed for normal tissue recovery, cancer chemotherapy is usually given on an intermittent basis. During the period between treatment cycles, tumor regrowth occurs. Thus most curative treatment regimens required multiple courses of chemotherapy, the number depending on the tumor mass at the time of diagnosis and upon the sensitivity of the tumor to the drugs.

A second concept from this model is that recurrent disease following "complete remission" (disappearance of all detectable disease) can be explained by the inability to detect fewer than 10^6 to 10^8 tumor cells in the body, even by the most sensitive test available. Chemotherapy that kills several logs of tumor cells (e.g., from 10^{11} to 10^4) eliminates all evidence of cancer and prolongs survival, but the cancer will recur at a later time. An example of the fractional kill concept with repeated cycles of chemotherapy is shown in Figure 14.1.

The cell cycle also plays an important role in designing cancer chemotherapy (see also Chapter 2). Two phases of a cell cycle can be directly observed and monitored: the S-phase and the M-phase. During S-phase (DNA synthesis), DNA replication occurs. During M-phase (mitosis), cellular division into two daughter cells is seen.[6] G_1 (gap-1) is the time from the end of mitosis to the start of the next S-phase. G_2 is the time between the completion of S and the start of M. Cells that have ceased to proliferate for prolonged periods have entered a G_0 phase (or resting phase) of the cell cycle (Figure 14.2). Most lung cancers exhibit a Gompertzian model of cell growth. With Gompertzian kinetics, the growth fraction decreases with time. In a Gompertzian model, large tumor masses have smaller growth fractions with more cells in G_0 phase. Some drugs (alkylating agents or platinum drugs) cause cytotoxicity when exposed to can-

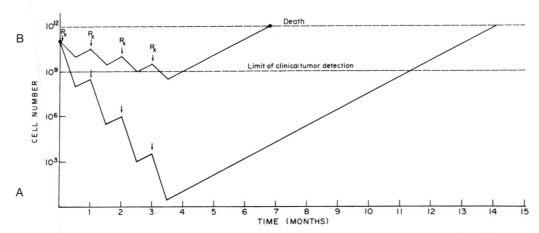

FIGURE 14.1. Schematic representation of clinical course of two patients with small cell lung cancer. Both patients A and B are diagnosed with an average-sized tumor mass (10^{11} cells). Both patients are treated with etoposide and cisplatin every four weeks for four cycles of chemotherapy. One course of therapy for patient A results in a three-log tumor cell kill (99.9%). Patient B's therapy results in only a one-log tumor cell kill (90%). Tumor growth occurs while waiting for normal tissue recovery before initiation of the next treatment. Four months into therapy, patient A has no clinically detectable disease (a CR) while patent B has had only a partial response. Patient A has a long disease-free survival, whereas patient B has a minimal survival advantage.

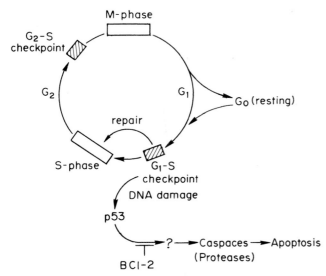

FIGURE 14.2. The cell cycle is marked by two observable events, the S- and M-phases. During S-phase, DNA synthesis occurs. In the M-phase (for mitosis) cells divide. G_1 and G_2 (for gap) are times between completion of M and start of S and the completion of S and beginning of M, respectively. During G_1 and G_2, the cell prepares for the S- and M-phases of the cell cycle. Cells may temporarily cease to divide and enter a resting or G_0 phase of the cell cycle. The G_1-S checkpoint is a critical phase in the cell cycle when directions for entering S-phase or committing to apoptosis (programmed cell death) are given. Cells can be damaged by chemotherapeutic drugs or growth factor deprivation. If the damage is sublethal, it may be repaired, and the cell proceeds into the S-phase. If significant DNA damage is present, the process of programmed cell death will be initiated. However, critical factors such as p53 and p21 gene products may be required for the cell to undergo apoptosis.

cer cells in any phase of the cell cycle. Other antineoplastic agents are phase-specific; that is, they are cytotoxic primarily in a selected phase of the cell cycle. Vinorelbine, for example, induces metaphase arrest (M-phase) by blocking formation of the microtubules forming the spindle apparatus. Cells in G_0 are not killed by antineoplastic chemotherapy. Larger masses are, therefore, more resistant to chemotherapy.

Antineoplastic Drug Action and Apoptosis

Antineoplastic drugs have a variety of initial targets. However, all antineoplastic agents cause a disruption in some normal cellular process which is so significant as to require the cell either to repair quickly the damage or to initiate the process of apoptosis or programmed cell death. All antineoplastic agents result in cell death through initiation of apoptosis. Apoptosis is the normal physiologic process of cellular suicide which occurs in all living organisms to eliminate unwanted, functionally abnormal, or harmful cells (see also Chapter 2). In apoptosis, in contrast with cellular necrosis, the cell shrinks and condenses, fragmenting into multiple membrane-bound bodies (apoptotic bodies) which are engulfed by surrounding cells without inflammation or damage to the surrounding tissues. Biochemically, apoptosis is characterized by fragmentation of nuclear DNA, as demonstrated by a typical DNA ladder pattern on agarose gel electrophoresis.[7] Several typical events of early cell cycle traverse are associated with apoptosis, for example, upregulation of proto oncogenes, such as c-*myc*, *ras*, c-*fos*, c-*jun*, *cdc*-2, and phosphorylation of the protein product of the tumor suppressor retinoblastoma gene.[8] There are different cellular thresholds, or set points, for apoptosis induction and subsequent signaling. Cell types vary in their susceptibility to activating the apoptotic pathway.

There are two general categories of apoptosis: primed apoptosis and unprimed apoptosis.[9] Primed apoptosis is found in most cell types of hematopoietic lineages, where all effector molecules are expressed in the cell. In this situation, the apoptosis program can be executed directly without the requirement of active gene transcription. In unprimed apoptosis, active gene transcription is required, and the process occurs more slowly than primed apoptosis. Cells successfully progress through one round of the cell cycle but die in the subsequent cycle.

The apoptotic process can be divided into four stages.[10] The first involves the interaction between the environment and the cell to provoke a cellular response (e.g., radiation, cytotoxic drugs, growth factor withdrawal, etc.). The second stage involves detection of an apoptotic signal and transduction of that signal to downstream events. The third stage is the effector arm of the apoptotic pathway, which involves a family of cysteine proteases (now called caspases) and endonucleases, as well as other positive and negative regulators of apoptosis. Recent evidence indicates that most signal transduction pathways converge at a common effector. The final stage, corpse disposal, is the phagocytosis and digestion of apoptotic cells by neighboring cells or macrophages.

Apoptosis is closely related to the proliferation status of a cell. Overexpression and activation of genes and proteins related to increased proliferative and cell cycle progression lowers the threshold for apoptosis. While apoptosis can occur during any phase of the cell cycle, sensitivity of proliferating cells to various death stimuli is usually cell cycle–phase specific.[11] Apoptosis induced by various DNA damaging agents can be affected by the presence or absence of the G_1 checkpoint, which is regulated by p53. p53, a tetrameric, sequence-specific DNA-binding phosphoprotein, is the product of a tumor suppressor gene whose mutation represents a genetic lesion found in 50% to 55% of all cancers.[12] With p53 present, the cell cycle is generally halted at the G_1-S checkpoint. At this point, cells determine whether to continue into the S-phase or initiate the process of apoptosis (Figure 14.2).[13] Passage into the S-phase requires activation of a series of enzymes called cyclin-dependent kinases (CDKs) which activate another group of enzymes (the cyclins) required for DNA synthesis.[14] If cellular repair occurs, cyclins are activated. If damage is extensive and/or if repair is unsuccessful, the cell is directed toward the apoptotic pathway. The critical factors needed for apoptosis are currently under investigation, but some important components have been recognized. At times, loss of functional p53 inhibits the induction of apoptosis by anticancer drugs and radiation, and correlates with poor response to chemotherapy.[15] However, p53-independent pathways do exist. Over expression of antiapoptotic genes can render cancer cells resistant to drug effects. *BCL2* and

$BCLX_1$ have the capacity to block apoptosis induction by a wide spectrum of chemotherapeutic drugs.[16] (See Figure 17.) It is clear that antineoplastic agents provide the initial trigger for initiating the pathway to programmed cell death. However, factors other than the initial interaction between a cytotoxic drug and its effector are important in determining whether tumor cell kill occurs.

Resistance to Anticancer Drugs

In the treatment of lung cancer, an initial tumor response with the subsequent growth of cells resistance to chemotherapy is a common clinical occurrence. Cancer cells can become resistant to an antineoplastic agent in many ways (Figure 14.3). In order for a drug to be active, it must: (a) be taken up into a cancer cell, and (b) be converted into an active metabolite. It must make its way within the cell to its target without being (c) metabolically inactivated, (d) chemically inactivated, or (e) excreted from the cell. Once it interacts with its cellular target, the cell must not be able to (f) alter the target or (g) repair the damage to the target. Finally, (h) mechanisms for apoptosis must be in place, as discussed in the preceding section. Examples of drug resistance caused by all of the mechanisms listed above have been described.

Cancer cell, may become simultaneously resistant to several types of chemotherapeutic drugs. Cells expressing the multidrug resistance (MDR) gene produce a glycoprotein

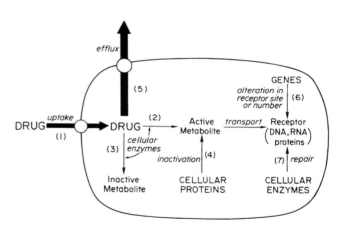

FIGURE 14.3. Potential pathways for antineoplastic drug disposition within tumor cells. In order for a drug to be effective, the drug, or its active metabolite, must reach its target site within the cell. Potential steps in the drug reaching its receptor include: (*1*) uptake into a cell through a particular transport protein; (*2*) enzymatic conversion of the drug to its active metabolite; (*3*) enzymatic conversion of the drug to an inactive metabolite; (*4*) binding of an active metabolite by a cellular protein or thiol, thereby inactivating drug; (*5*) excretion of the drug from the cell via an efflux transport pump; (*6*) alteration in the genetic makeup of the cell, changing the drug receptor site or number; (*7*) changes in the ability of a cell to repair damage of a drug at its receptor. All steps have been shown to be altered in various drug-resistant tumor cell lines.

of 170 kD weight known as p-glycoprotein or p170.[18] P-glycoprotein is a cell membrane protein that transports several antineoplastic agents across the cell membrane. Most p-glycoprotein transported agents are hydrophobic. These include the vinca alkaloids, epipodophyllotoxins, anthracyclines, actinomycin, and taxanes. Cells in which the MDR gene is activated develop simultaneous resistance to all of these antineoplastic agents. The presence of p-glycoprotein on tumor cells has been correlated with poor prognosis in SCLC.[19] Because of the potential role of MDR in tumor resistance, efforts have been directed at blocking this transporter. A number of agents, including analogs of verapamil and cyclosporine, are inhibitors of MDR. Clinical trials of combinations of these inhibitors with anticancer drugs have been undertaken. Other resistant cell lines have been identified which do not overexpress p-glycoprotein, but display a similar cross-resistance pattern. Some of these lines express a different transport protein called (MRP) multidrug resistance-associated protein.[20] MRP, like p-glycoprotein, is a member of the ATP binding cassette gene superfamily. However, MRP is structurally dissimilar to p-glycoprotein, with different inhibitors. The clinical significance of MRP is under study but, like p-glycoprotein, its presence in tumor cells may be a prognostic factor.

In summary, tumor cells can develop resistance to one or several antineoplastic drugs by numerous mechanisms. Resistance develops as a result of random mutational changes in a population of cancer cells. Mutations to a resistant phenotype are estimated to occur when a mass reaches 10^4 to 10^6 tumor cells, a size smaller than clinically detectable.[20] This suggests that drug-resistant populations will be present in the majority of tumors. It leads to the rationale for: (a) early treatment of cancers to avoid multiple resistant populations, and (b) use of multiple agents with differing mechanisms of action.

Toxicity

Antineoplastic agents have the potential for life-threatening toxicity. The therapeutic window for drugs used to treat lung cancer is narrow. Doses of drug needed to achieve tumor cell kill commonly result in toxicity to normal tissues. Chemotherapeutic agents may cause a variety of toxicities. Myelosuppression and nausea are the most common toxicities seen. Nausea and vomiting, although generally self-limited and not life-threatening, are often considered most distressing by patients. The emetogenic potential of antineoplastic agents varies from drug-to-drug and is dose-dependent.[21] Serotonin receptors, located within the vagal and splanchnic nerves of the gastrointestinal system, are critical in the initiation of nausea by chemotherapeutic agents.[22] The development of specific type 3 serotonin (5-hydroxytryptamine or $5HT_3$) receptor blockers, such as ondansetron and granisetron, has resulted in major improvement in control of acute chemotherapy-induced emesis.[23]

TABLE 14.1. EMETOGENIC POTENTIAL OF ANTINEOPLASTIC DRUGS USED FOR TREATMENT OF LUNG CANCER

High	
Cisplatin	Cyclophosphamide (>1.5 g/m²)

Moderate	
Carboplatin	Ifosfamide
Cyclophosphamide	Nitrosoureas
Doxorubicin	

Mild	
Docetaxel	Irinotecan
Etoposide	Paclitaxel
Gemcitabine	Topotecan
	Vinca Alkaloids

The emetogenic potential of chemotherapeutic agents used in lung cancer therapy is indicated in Table 14.1.

Myelosuppression is the most common dose-limiting toxicity encountered with antineoplastic agents. The suppression of specific hematopoietic cell lines is determined by the kinetics of the cell line in the peripheral compartment. Anemia occurs as a late effect because red blood cells have a long half-life (120 days). Thrombocytopenia occurs in an intermediate time frame shortly following granulocyte suppression. The white blood count (WBC) usually drops five to 14 days following drug administration, with recovery in three to ten days.

The range of toxicities associated with antineoplastic agents is great (Table 14.2). Oral,[24] renal,[25] neurologic,[26] hepatic,[27] pulmonary,[28] cardiac,[29] and cutaneous[30] toxicities from anticancer drugs are all seen. Many antineoplastic agents have teratogenic and mutagenic potential. Alkylating agents are the most damaging to testicular and ovarian function. Damage is dependent on drug dose, age of patient (the older being more likely to have toxicity), and sex (males greater than females).[31] Second malignancies (primarily acute leukemia) have been associated with alkylating agents, epipodophyllotoxins, nitrosoureas, and anthracycline.[32,33] Physicians need to be familiar with the toxicities of the drugs they are using and have support facilities adequate to care for patients developing treatment-related toxicity.

GENERAL PRINCIPLES OF LUNG CANCER CHEMOTHERAPY

A physician treating patients with cytotoxic chemotherapy must be certain of the diagnosis (histology is nearly always required). The physician and patient must understand the goals of treatment (cure versus palliation). Optimal therapy requires familiarity with individual to be treated, knowledge

TABLE 14.2. TOXICITIES OF ANTINEOPLASTIC AGENTS USED FOR TREATMENT OF LUNG CANCER

Bone Marrow	Nausea/ Vomiting	Mucositis	Alopecia	Neurologic	Diarrhea	Vesicant	Pulmonary	Renal	Cardiac	Hypersensitivity
Carboplatin	Carboplatin	Cyclophos- phamide	Carboplatin	Doxorubicin	Doxorubicin	Doxorubicin	Cyclophos- phamide	Carboplatin	Cyclophos- phamide	Docetaxel
Cisplatin	Cisplatin	Doxorubicin	Cisplatin	Irinotecan	Irinotecan	Vinblastine		Cisplatin	Doxorubicin	Etoposide
Cyclophos- phamide	Cyclophos- phamide	Etoposide	Docetaxel	Topotecan	Topotecan	Vincristine		Ifosfamide		Paclitaxel
Docetaxel	phamide	Ifosfamide	Ifosfamide			Vinorelbine				Teniposide
Doxorubicin	Doxorubicin	Irinotecan	Irinotecan							
Etoposide	Etoposide	Paclitaxel	Paclitaxel							
Gemcitabine	Fluorouracil	Vinblastine	Vinblastine							
Ifosfamide	Gemcitabine	Vincristine	Vincristine							
Irinotecan	Ifosfamide		Vinorelbine							
Paclitaxel	Irinotecan									
Teniposide										

of the drugs to be used, and the availability of appropriate laboratory and hospital support services. The physician should discuss with the patient the natural history of the cancer, the goals, and the toxicities of treatment. If cure is the goal, the patient and physician may be willing to tolerate more severe toxicity. The patient must be a partner in such decisions. In many cases, several options may be reasonable, and an informed patient can direct the physician as to whether intensive, potentially toxic therapy should be tried for a relatively small chance of cure.[34,35]

Combination chemotherapy (use of several drugs) is usually employed and multiple cycles of drugs administered to achieve adequate tumor cell kill without life-threatening toxicity or the development of tumor cell resistance. Patient selection factors are important in planning treatment. Age alone is not a reason to exclude patients from chemotherapy.[36,37] However, age-related changes in organ function, including reduced marrow reserve and decreased renal function, are commonly seen and may increase the risk of toxicity. The performance status of a patient usually correlates with response to chemotherapy. The nutritional state of a patient is important. Malnourished patients with hypoalbuminemia have increased toxicity when highly protein-bound drugs are used.[38] Appropriate dosing guidelines for obese patients are not available.[39] Doses based on actual body weight appear appropriate when the goal for therapy is cure,[40] whereas doses based on ideal body weight, with potential escalations later, are reasonable when palliation is the intent. Altered organ function may eliminate the oppor-

tunity to use certain drugs (e.g., doxorubicin in patients with heart failure or bleomycin in patients with severe pulmonary compromise). Drug doses should be modified for decreases in blood counts (Table 14.3) and also for changes in renal and hepatic function (Table 14.4). The patient must be carefully followed for toxicity and response to chemotherapy. It is common to reevaluate patients after two to three cycles of chemotherapy to determine treatment effectiveness. If a response is seen, therapy is usually continued for a set number of courses or two cycles past a complete response. If tumor progression is noted, therapy should be discontinued. For patients with stable disease, an assessment of drug toxicity is important. If therapy is tolerable, a decision to continue treatment is reasonable, with the understanding that disease progression will eventually occur.

PHARMACOLOGY OF CHEMOTHERAPEUTIC AGENTS USED IN THE TREATMENT OF LUNG CANCER

Many antineoplastic agents have been evaluated for treatment of lung cancer. A comprehensive review of all these

TABLE 14.3. GENERALIZED DOSE ADJUSTMENT GUIDELINES FOR HEMATOLOGIC TOXICITY

	100% Dose	75% Dose	50% Dose	Omit
Granulocyte	<2000	1500–1999	1000–1499	<1000
WBC	>3500	3000–3500	2500–2999	<2500
Platelet	>100,000	75–100,000	50–75,000	<50,000

TABLE 14.4. DRUGS COMMONLY USED IN TREATMENT OF LUNG CANCER WHICH REQUIRE DOSE ALTERATIONS FOR ORGAN TOXICITY

Nephrotoxicity	Hepatic Toxicity
Carboplatin	Doxorubicin
Cisplatin*	Docetaxel*
Cyclophosphamide (if CrCl <20 ml/min)	Irinotecan
Etoposide	Paclitaxel*
Ifosfamide	Vincristine*
Methotrexate*	Vinblastine*
Nitrosoureas*	Vinorelbine*
Topotecan	

* Major dose adjustment

drugs is beyond the scope of this chapter. Instead, this section will focus on the agents most commonly used for the therapy of small cell and non–small cell lung cancer. For each class of drugs, the mechanism of drug action, pharmacology, including route of drug elimination, and toxicities will be reviewed.

Alkylating Agents (Cyclophosphamide and Ifosfamide)

Cyclophosphamide and ifosfamide are members of a family of antineoplastic agents whose mechanism of action involves attachment of an alkyl group to DNA. Cyclophosphamide has been used for decades for treatment of both small cell and non–small cell lung cancer. Ifosfamide, an analog of cyclophosphamide, has also demonstrated activity in both diseases.[41,42] Although other alkylating agents are occasionally used for treatment of lung cancers, cyclophosphamide and ifosfamide are the primary agents employed, and their pharmacology will be emphasized.

Mechanism of Action. Alkylating agents covalently bind alkyl groups (one or more saturated carbon atoms) to cellular molecules, including DNA, RNA, and proteins. Alkylating agents form reactive carbonyl groups which attack at electron-rich sites on adenine or guanine in the DNA molecule.[43] The active metabolites of cyclophosphamide and ifosfamide contain two reactive nitrochlorethyl groups, allowing reaction with two strands of DNA, forming cross-linkage (Figure 14.4). Alkylation occurs at the N-7 position of guanine. Alkylating agents are cell cycle nonspecific. Spacing between the nitrochlorethyl groups in cyclophosphamide is slightly different from ifosfamide and may result in different cross-linkage sites.

Thiols are nucleophilic targets within the cell which can bind alkylating agents before they reach their DNA target. Increasing the concentration of thiols decreases antineoplastic drug activity and/or toxicity. Buthione sulfonamide (BSO) decreases synthesis of glutathione (a naturally occurring thiol) and increases drug cytotoxicity.[44] The radioprotective agent amifostine (WR2721) provides an exogenous nucleophilic thiol that can decrease alkylating agent toxicity.[45]

Pharmacology. Cyclophosphamide and ifosfamide require activation via the hepatic cytochrome P450 system to produce 4-hydroxy derivatives which are taken up in tumor tissue and undergo further metabolism to form an active mustard metabolite (Figure 14.5). Drugs inducing or inhibiting the microsomal enzyme system, such as phenobarbital, can alter the plasma kinetics of cyclophosphamide and its metabolites. However, these kinetic changes do not appear to have any effects on the toxicity of this drug.[46] Ifosfamide, a structural analog of cyclophosphamide, has a slightly different metabolite pathway from cyclophosphamide. Less drug is converted to a mustard (activated), so higher drug doses are required.[47] Only a small amount of the dichlorethyl metabolite (Figure 14.5) is formed when cyclophosphamide is administered, but this metabolite is generated to a significant extent following ifosfamide administration. The dichlorethyl metabolite likely accounts for the CNS toxicity seen with ifosfamide.[48] The excretion of reactive acrolein and dichlorethyl metabolites into the bladder following use of either cyclophosphamide or ifosfamide can result in cystitis. Mercaptoethane sulfonate (MESNA) is administered in equivalent doses to all patients receiving ifosfamide and to patients receiving high-dose cyclophosphamide to prevent cystitis by binding these reactive metabolites.[49] In plasma, MESNA circulates in an inactive dimesna form, so that antineoplastic activity of the alkylating agent is not affected.

Toxicity. Marrow suppression occurs in all hematopoietic cells with alkylating agent use. However, a relative platelet and stem cell sparing effect occurs with cyclophosphamide.[50] Nausea and vomiting are frequent with high doses of alkylating agents but decrease with low-dose oral regimens. Pulmonary fibrosis can be seen.[51] Bladder toxicity occurs with ifosfamide and cyclophosphamide. Renal toxicity has been reported with ifosfamide.[52] As previously mentioned, ifosfamide is associated with CNS toxicity (somno-

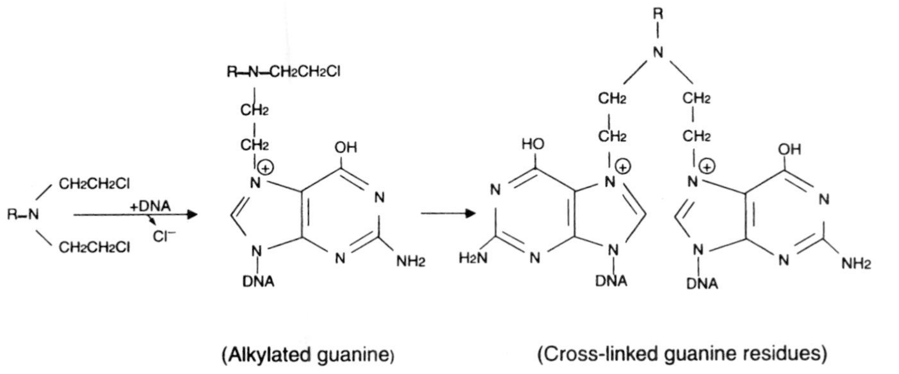

FIGURE 14.4. Mechanism of action of alkylating agents on DNA. Alkylating agents (in this case those with two nitrochlorethyl groups) form reactive intermediates which bind to two guanine molecules, resulting in cross-linkage of DNA strands.

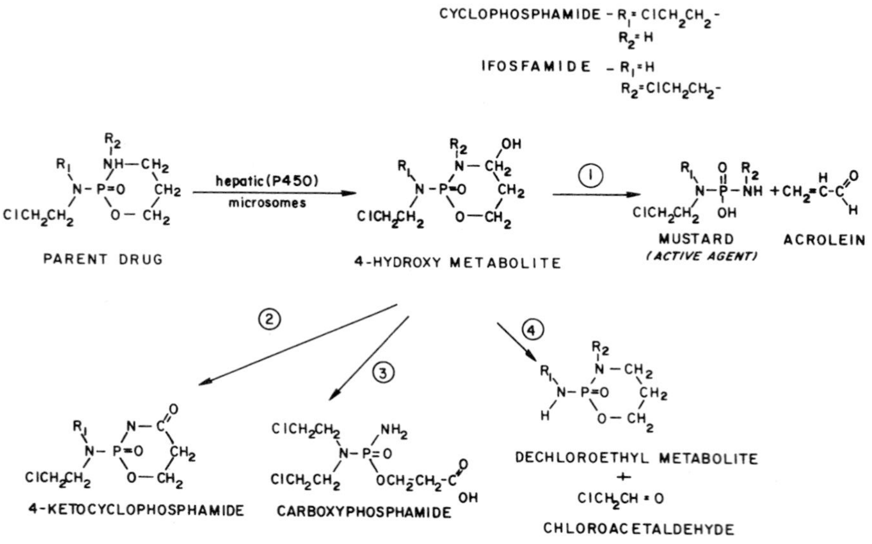

CYCLOPHOSPHAMIDE - R_1 = $ClCH_2CH_2$-
R_2 = H

IFOSFAMIDE - R_1 = H
R_2 = $ClCH_2CH_2$-

PARENT DRUG → hepatic (P450) microsomes → **4-HYDROXY METABOLITE** → ① → **MUSTARD** *(ACTIVE AGENT)* + **ACROLEIN**

② ③ **4-KETOCYCLOPHOSPHAMIDE**   **CARBOXYPHOSPHAMIDE**

④ **DECHLOROETHYL METABOLITE** + **CHLOROACETALDEHYDE**

FIGURE 14.5. Metabolism of cyclophosphamide and ifosfamide: these drugs can be metabolized to the active agents (mustards) or to inactive metabolites. Because of the minor structural differences, the rate of formation of different metabolites is different between cyclophosphamide and ifosfamide. Less ifosfamide is converted to active metabolite. The dichloro metabolite is formed to a greater extent with ifosfamide.

lence, confusion), particularly at high doses in patients with low serum albumin (less than 3g per dl) or high serum creatinine (more than 1.5 mg per dl).[53] Cyclophosphamide and ifosfamide, like all alkylating agents, are teratogenic and carcinogenic. Gonadal atrophy and permanent loss of reproductive function can occur.[54]

Platinum Analogs (Cisplatin, Carboplatin)

Mechanisms of Action. Cisplatin, carboplatin, and the investigational agent oxalloplatin are heavy-metal complexes that induce tumor cell kill by cross-linking DNA strands in a manner analogous to the alkylating agents. Reactive aquated platinum intermediates are formed within cells that directly and covalently bind to DNA, leading to DNA cross-links[55] (Figure 14.6). Cisplatin is more reactive in water than carboplatin. Chloride-containing solutions are required to stabilize cisplatin. The difference in aqueous stability between the various platinum analogs results in differences in each agent's pharmacokinetics and toxicity.

Pharmacology. Cisplatin and carboplatin are the only two platinum analogs currently used for treatment of lung cancer. Their pharmacology differs significantly. Cisplatin more rapidly forms reactive intermediates in plasma. Over 90% of cisplatin is protein-bound and inactivated within two to four hours.[56] Thus protein-binding represents the major route of drug elimination. Only the free (unbound) platinum species are cytotoxic.[57] Carboplatin is less reactive, with only 20% to 40% of total platinum protein-bound at two hours following drug administration. Renal excretion is the primary route of carboplatinum elimination (70% of total carboplatin clearance). Carboplatin clearance is highly correlated with creatinine clearance.[58] Carboplatinum doses

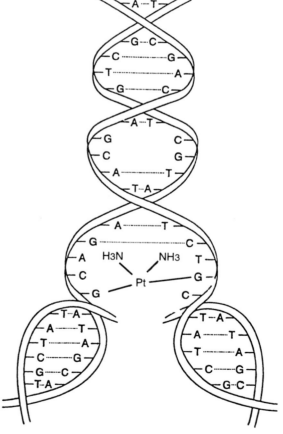

FIGURE 14.6. A schematic representation of cellular DNA showing covalently bonded cross-links from a cisplatin inhibiting the progress of DNA replication.

should be calculated based on an individual patient's creatinine clearance[59] rather than based on body weight or body surface area (BSA).[60]

Toxicity. The toxicity profiles of cisplatin and carboplatin differ.[61] Myelosuppression is rare with cisplatin, although moderate anemia is common. Nausea and vomiting are common cisplatin toxicities, but the frequency of emesis can be reduced with pretreatment use of dexamethasone (Decadron) and serotonin antagonists.[62] Nephrotoxicity, represented by azotemia and electrolyte disturbances (primarily hypokalemenia and hypomagnesemia), is dose-related. Although pre- and posttreatment hydration (with chloride-containing solutions) and diuresis reduce the incidence and severity of cisplatin nephrotoxicity, moderate and permanent reductions in GFR may still occur.[63] Neurotoxicity from cisplatin is cumulatively dose-related and usually begins as a "stocking-glove" type peripheral neuropathy. Hearing loss, cortical blindness, and seizures have also been reported. The toxicity profile of carboplatin is different from that of cisplatin, with dose-limiting myelosuppression (primarily thrombocytopenia) being the major toxicity, following carboplatin administration.[64] The renal, neurologic, and oto-toxicities noted with cisplatin are infrequent occurrences after carboplatin administration.[65] Dose reductions of carboplatin must be made in patients with impaired renal function. Several formulas are available for calculating dose adjustments, based on creatinine clearance and desired nadir platelet count.[59,60]

MICROTUBULAR INHIBITORS (Vincristine, Vinblastine, Vinorelbine, Paclitaxel, Docetaxel)

Several drugs initiate apoptosis through interactions with microtubulin, the protein used to form the mitotic spindle apparatus. The vinca alkaloids block the formation of microtubulin, while the taxanes increase assembly and stability of microtubulin.

Vinca Alkaloids (Vinblastine, Vincristine, and Vinorelbine)

Mechanism of Action. Several vinca alkaloids have been synthesized and evaluated preclinically. Three, vinblastine, vincristine and vinorelbine, are clinically available. All bind to tubulin and inhibit the formation of microtubulin, a protein that is essential for maintenance of cellular shape and for formation of the mitotic spindle.[66] Cells treated with vinca alkaloids are arrested in metaphase. Differences in activity and toxicity of the vinca alkaloids result from variations in their pharmacokinetic properties, differential effects on various tubulin isoforms, and upon differences in tissue penetration and cellular retention.[67] Resistance results

from the presence of p-glycoprotein or reduced tubulin-binding within tumor cells.

Pharmacology. All vincas are rapidly taken up into cells. However, the individual agents differ in their cellular retention (vinblastine greater than vincristine). All vincas are extensively bound to tissues and to protein.[68] Their terminal half-lives are long (20 to 60 hours). The vinca alkaloids are metabolized by the liver and excreted into the bile. Doses need to be reduced for hepatic dysfunction but not for renal insufficiency. Specific dose-reduction guidelines for hepatic function impairment are not available.

Toxicity. Vincristine causes little myelosuppression. Neurotoxicity occurs frequently and is dose-limiting.[69] It commonly presents as a symmetric, distal, sensory-motor neuropathy. Loss of deep tendon reflexes in the lower extremities and paresthesias of the fingers and toes are common early findings. Foot-drop or wrist-drop, neuropathies of cranial nerves, constipation, cramps, and paralytic ileus have been reported. The dose-limiting toxicity of vinblastine is hematopoietic.[70] The onset of myelosuppression occurs earlier with this agent than with other antineoplastics. Severe neurotoxic symptoms are unusual with vinblastine, but use of the drug is associated with myalgias and an autonomic neuropathy manifested by orthostatic hypotension or paralytic ileus. Vinorelbine shows toxicities similar to other vincas. Its dose-limiting toxicity is myelosuppression. Although the incidence of grade 3 to 4 neutropenia is high (60%), only 7% of patients develop neutropenia fever. Non-hematologic toxicity from vinorelbine is generally mild in severity. Constipation (30%), neuropathy (20%, severe in less than 1%) and nausea (grade 3 to 4 in 2%) are seen.[71] Vinca alkaloids are *vesicants* and need to be given with care.

Taxanes (Paclitaxel and Docetaxel)

Mechanism of Action. Paclitaxel and docetaxel bind to a unique site on microtubulin, resulting in increased microtubulin assembly and stabilization.[72] The bundling of microtubules induced by the taxanes blocks cells in metaphase and induces apoptosis. The taxanes have activity against most lung cancers.[73] They are also potent radiation sensitizers. Although both taxanes bind to the same site on the β subunit of tubulin, docetaxel produces microtubules of larger size. Docetaxel is also more avidly taken up by cells and is two to three times more potent than paclitaxel.[74] Paclitaxel and docetaxel are not cross-resistant.

Pharmacology. Paclitaxel is primarily cleared from the body by hepatic metabolism via cytochrome P450 2C8 and 3A4 enzymes.[75] This route of elimination can be saturated

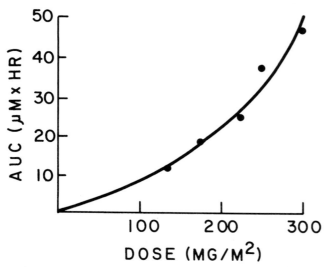

FIGURE 14.7. Plot of the area under the concentration time curve (AUC) of paclitaxel plotted against the dose of drug given as a three-hour infusion.

so that nonlinear kinetics are noted (Figure 14.7).[76] A 30% increase in drug dose (from 135 to 175 mg per m²) results in an increased plasma drug concentration of 75%.[77] Docetaxel is also metabolized by the hepatic microsomal enzyme system (predominantly CYP3A4). In contrast to paclitaxel, docetaxel exhibits linear kinetics. It has been postulated that the vehicle in which paclitaxel is dissolved (Cremophor EL) accounts for nonlinear paclitaxel kinetics by inhibiting hepatic drug excretion.[78] Drugs that inhibit CYP3A or CYP2C8 may inhibit the clearance of the taxanes.[79] Several drug interactions have been identified when paclitaxel is used. If cisplatin is given before paclitaxel, delayed paclitaxel clearance is noted, with increased neutropenia. In contrast, the combined use of carboplatin and paclitaxel results in decreased thrombocytopenia. Anticonvulsants and steroids increase paclitaxel clearance.[79] No drug interactions have been clearly demonstrated with docetaxel. Because of their extensive hepatic metabolism, dose reductions of both paclitaxel and docetaxel are needed in patients with hyperbilirubinemia.

Toxicity. Myelosuppression is the principle toxicity of both paclitaxel and docetaxel. Longer infusion of paclitaxel produces greater neutropenia than shorter infusions.[74] Hypersensitivity reactions (dyspnea, urticaria, and hypotension) were seen in 25% of patients initially treated with paclitaxel.[80] With prophylactic use of decadron and antihistamines, these reactions are uncommon (1%). Paclitaxel induces a peripheral neuropathy. Nausea and vomiting are uncommon but alopecia is seen. Docetaxel induces edema formation and an erythematous maculopapular rash in up to 60% of patients.[81] A syndrome of cumulative fluid reten-

tion (pleural effusions, edema) is also an effect unique to docetaxel, occurring in half of patients at cumulative doses of 400 mg per m.² Fluid retention can be treated with prophylactic steroid therapy. A dose-related syndrome of myalgias and arthralgias is seen 24 to 72 hours after paclitaxel but not with docetaxel. The combined use of paclitaxel and doxorubicin results in an increased rate of congestive heart failure.[82]

Topoisomerase Inhibitors (Etoposide, Doxorubicin, Irinotecan, and Topotecan)
Mechanism of Action. Topoisomerase II (topo II) normally functions within the cell to carry out necessary breakage-reunion reactions of mammalian DNA.[83] Etoposide, an epipodophyllotoxin, and doxorubicin, an anthracycline, bind with topo II and DNA to form a stabilized cleavable complex inhibiting the enzyme's ability to relegate cleaved DNA (Figure 14.8).[84,85] Irinotecan (CPT-11) and topotecan are anticancer agents that inhibit the activity of topoisomerase I, a separate enzyme also important in maintaining DNA structure. Topoisomerase I functions in a manner similar to topo II to help unwind supercoiled DNA.[86] Unlike topo II, topo I is expressed at relatively constant levels throughout the cell cycle.[87] It is hoped that topoisomerase I inhibitors may therefore be more active in tumors with low growth fractions. Topo I results in single-strand DNA breaks, while topo II can cause double-stranded breaks. The

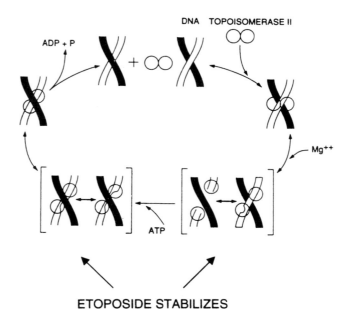

FIGURE 14.8. The catalytic cycle of topoisomerase II. Dimeric topoisomerase II binds to DNA. In the presence of magnesium and ATP, an intact DNA helix can pass through a temporary break in DNA with subsequent relegation. Etoposide and doxorubicin block the cycle at the stage of DNA cleavage.

activity of topoisomerase inhibitors appears to be schedule-dependent.[88]

Pharmacology. While the four topoisomerase agents have similar mechanisms of action, the pharmacology and toxicities of these agents differ significantly.

Etoposide can be given by both intravenous and oral routes. Oral bioavailability ranges from 40% to 70%, with significant interpatient variability.[89] Bioavailability decreases at doses greater than 300 mg. Etoposide is highly protein-bound. One third of drug is excreted intact into the urine, and 40% undergoes hepatic metabolism. Obstructive jaundice does not alter the clearance of etoposide.[90] Etoposide is poorly soluble in water and can precipitate in solution if not adequately diluted. It must be given as a one-hour infusion to avoid hypersensitivity reactions. Etoposide phosphate (Etopophos) is a water-soluble prodrug of etoposide which can be given as a rapid intravenous infusion.[91]

Doxorubicin (Adriamycin) is metabolized in the liver to its alcohol metabolite (doxorubincinol) and excreted into the bile.[92] Dose reductions in patients with hepatic function impairment are recommended. Specific guidelines as to appropriate dosing schedules are lacking.[93] Urinary excretion of doxorubicin is minimal. Use of paclitaxel prior to doxorubicin decreases doxorubicin clearance and increases its toxicity.[94]

Irinotecan is a prodrug that is rapidly converted through carboxylesterases to the active metabolite SN38 (7-ethyl-10 hydroxycamptothecin) (Figure 14.9). Both irinotecan and SN38 exist in open and closed lactone ring forms in the plasma, with the closed form being active.[95] SN38 is inactivated via glucuronidation. Irinotecan and metabolites are primarily cleared by biliary excretion. Renal excretion ac-

counts for 10% to 35% of drug clearance. Formal recommendations for dosing in patients with renal or hepatic function impairment have not been made, but patients with hyperbilirubinemia appear to at increased risk of myelosuppressive toxicity.[96] Decreased ability to conjugate SN38 may correlate with gastrointestinal toxicity.[97]

Topotecan also exists in open and closed lactone ring forms. Elimination of topotecan is primarily through the kidneys (30% to 65% of drug).[98] Dose reductions are recommended for patients with renal insufficiency (creatinine clearance less than 20 ml per min: no treatment; 20 to 40 ml per min: 50% dose reduction).[99] No dosing changes appear needed for patients with liver function impairment, although the number of patient studied is small.[100]

Toxicities. Common etoposide toxicities include bone marrow suppression, mild nausea, and hair loss.[101,102] Myelosuppression is the dose-limiting toxicity. At doses of 100 mg per m^2 per day for 3 days, 8% of patients develop a WBC nadir below 1000 per mm.^{3} An allergic reaction to drug administration, manifested by hypertension, wheezing, fever, and dyspnea, may occur when etoposide is given over periods shorter than one hour. This reaction may be related to the solvents needed to solubilize etoposide. Development of acute nonlymphocytic leukemia (ANNL) in patients treated with either etoposide or teniposide has been reported by several centers.[103,104] The leukemia is associated with cytogenetic abnormalities involving chromosome 11 (11q23). The six-year risk of developing leukemia in patients receiving high cumulative etoposide doses appears to be roughly 3%. Common *doxorubicin* toxicities include bone marrow suppression, mucositis, alopecia, and cardiac toxicity.[105,106] Myelosuppression and mucositis follow an acute course, with the maximum toxicity occurring seven to ten days after drug administration. The cardiac toxicity

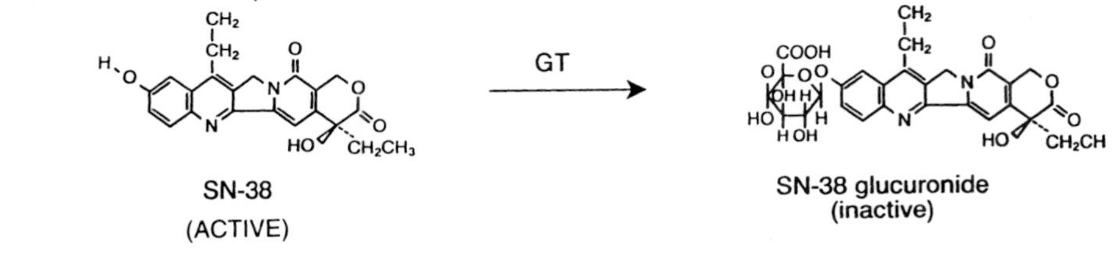

FIGURE 14.9. Metabolism of irinotecan. Parent drug is converted to an active metabolite (SN-38) through action of carboxylesterase enzymes. Hepatic metabolism via the hepatic cytochrome system (CYP3A4) or glucuronosyltransferase (GT) converts drug to inactive metabolites.

induced by anthracycline antibiotics can be manifested in both acute and chronic forms.[106] The mechanism of myocardial toxicity is thought to be drug-induced oxidative damage caused by free-radical generation. The risk of developing congestive heart failure is greater with increasing cumulative drug dose, increasing age, underlying cardiac disease, high peak plasma concentrations, and previous or concurrent cardiac irradiation.[107] High peak plasma drug concentrations induce greater free-radical formation. Therefore lower, more frequent drug doses result in less potential for development of heart failure. For doxorubicin, the most commonly used total dose limit is 550 mg per m.[2,108] At this cumulative dose, the risk of clinical cardiac toxicity is 3% to 7%. Heart failure can occur months to years after discontinuing treatment.[109] Dexrazoxane (Zinecard, ICRF-187) is an iron chelator that blocks the generation of free radicals from anthracyclines. It has been shown to prevent cardiac toxicity without altering antitumor activity.[110] Extravasation of the anthracycline antibiotics can lead to severe local tissue damage, which can progress over weeks to months. Administration of doxorubicin can result in recall of radiation-associated tissue damage, such as skin erythema, mucositis, and esophagitis.

Diarrhea and myelosuppression are the primary toxicities associated with *irinotecan* use. Administration of drug on an every three-week schedule produces more myelosuppression, while weekly treatment results in greater diarrhea.[111] Although neutropenia is common with irinotecan, other hematologic toxicities are generally mild, with only a minority of patients developing significant (grade 3 to 4) thrombocytopenia (4%) or anemia (16%). Irinotecan is associated with two forms of diarrhea. The first type occurs during or just after the infusion of irinotecan and has a cholinergic mechanism. The use of atropine at the onset of this diarrhea is effective. The second type of diarrhea begins three to five days after the infusion of irinotecan and may be moderate to severe in 20% of patients. Aggressive treatment with antimotility agents at the onset of the diarrhea (loperamide given at a dose of 4 mg at the time of first loose stool, then 2 mg every two hours until no bowel movements for 12 hours) may obviate the severity of the diarrhea.[112] If the diarrhea is not treated early, it usually runs a 5 to 7-day course. The mechanism for development of diarrhea is unknown but may be secondary to the biliary excretion of the active metabolite SN-38.[97] In addition to dose-limiting myelosuppression and diarrhea, other toxicities reported with irinotecan include alopecia, transaminasemia, and malaise.[95] The dose-limiting toxicities of topotecan are neutropenia and thrombocytopenia, usually short-lived (less than seven days). Heavily pretreated patients have more severe myelosuppression and may need a dose reduction.[113] Nausea is mild. Diarrhea is uncommon except after oral drug use.[114] Other nonhematologic toxicity includes mucositis, alopecia, skin rash, and fever, all mild.[98]

Antimetabolites (Gemcitabine)

Most antimetabolite antineoplastic agents are ineffective in the treatment of lung cancer. The primary exception is gemcitabine [2'-deoxy-2', 2'-difluorocytidine monohydrochoride; dFdC] which has shown significant activity in the treatment of NSCLC.

Mechanism of Action. Gemcitabine is an analog of deoxycytidine (Figure 14.10). It is a prodrug which is taken up into the cell and phosphoylated to gemcitabine di- and triphosphates, which are the active metabolites.[115] When gemcitabine triphosphate is incorporated into the DNA chain, DNA polymerase can add only a single additional nucleotide, after which chain elongation is terminated. Importantly, gemcitabine triphosphate in the nonterminal position DNA chain prevents detection and "repair" by proofreading exonucleases.[116] Additional effects of gemcitabine di- and triphosphates include inhibition of ribonucleotide reductase depleting deoxyribonucleotide pools available for DNA repair.[117]

Pharmacology. Plasma concentrations of gemcitabine generally reach a plateau 15 minutes after a 30-minute infusion. There is a linear relationship between the steady-state concentration of gemcitabine and dose up to 1,000 mg per m.[2118] Plasma protein-binding is negligible. Gemcitabine is inactivated by several aytidine deaminase in organs (blood, aytidine deaminase in liver, kidneys) so that its half-life is short (32–94 minutes).[119] Almost all administered drug is excreted in the urine as the inactive metabolite 2 deoxy-2, 2-difluorouridine.[120] No dose adjustments are needed for liver or hepatic insufficiency. Gemcitabine undergoes intracellular metabolism to the mono-, di- and triphosphate moieties; these metabolites are not found in plasma or urine.

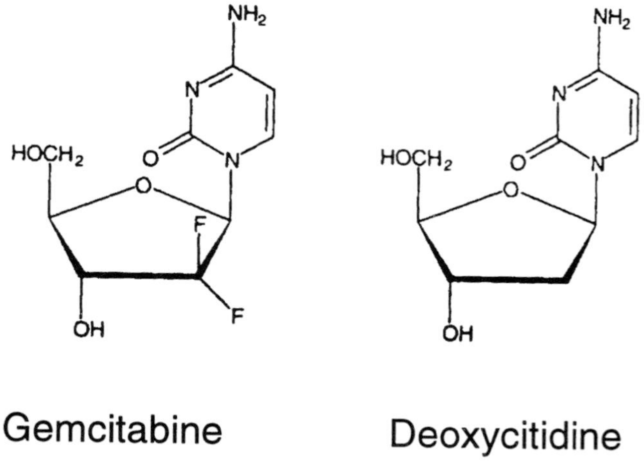

Gemcitabine   Deoxycitidine

FIGURE 14.10. Chemical structures of gemcitabine and deoxycytidine.

Toxicity. The primary toxicity of gemcitabine is myelosuppression. At an average dose of 1000 mg per m^2 given weekly for 3 weeks each month, 4% of patients have grade 4 neutropenia and 2% grade 4 thrombocytopenia.[118,119] Elevation in hepatic transaninases and alkaline phosphatase is frequently seen (10% of patients), but usually is transient and modest. Nausea and vomiting (all grades) are seen in many patients (70%), but are severe in only occasional patients (grade 3: 13%; grade 4: 1%).[120] Other reported toxicities include fever, rash, dyspnea, and hematuria.[121,122] Gemcitabine is not a vesicant.

REFERENCES

1. Aisner J, Alberto P, Bitran J, et al. Role of chemotherapy in small cell lung cancer: a consensus report of the international association for the study of lung cancer workshop. *Cancer Treat Rep* 1983;67:37.
2. Bunn PA, Kelly K. New chemotherapeutic agents prolong survival and improve quality of life in non—small cell lung cancer: a review of the literature and future direction. *Clin Cancer Res* 1998;5:1087.
3. Clinical practice guidelines for the treatment of unresectable non—small cell lung cancer. *J Clin Oncol* 1997;15:2996.
4. Landis SH, Murray T, Bolden S, Wingo PA. Cancer statistics 1998. *CA Canc J Clin* 1998;48:6.
5. DeVita VT. Principles of chemotherapy. In: DeVita VT, Hellman S, Rosenberg SA, ed. *Cancer: principles and practice of oncology,* 4th ed. Philadelphia: JB Lippincott, 1993;276.
6. Tannock IF. Tumor growth and cell kinetics. In: Tannock IF, Hill RP, ed. *The Basic science of oncology.* New York: Pergamon Press, 1987;140.
7. Han nun VA. Apoptosis and the dilemma of cancer chemotherapy. *Blood* 1997;89:1845–1853.
8. Pandey S, Wang E. Cells on route to apoptosis are characterized by the upregulation of c-*fos*, c-*myc*, c-*jun*, *cdcz* and RB phosphorylation resembling events of early cell traverse. *J Cell Biochem* 1995;58:135.
9. Wyllie AH, Arends MJ, Morris RG, et al. The apoptosis endonuclease and its regulation. *Sem Immunol* 1992;4:389.
10. Au JS, Panchal N, Li D, et al. Apoptosis: a new pharmacodynamic endpoint. *Pharmaceut Res* 1997;14:1659.
11. King KL, Cidlowski JA. Cell cycle and apoptosis: common pathways to life and death. *J Cell Biochem* 1995;58:175.
12. Hollstein M, Sidransky D, Vogelstein B, et al. P53 mutations in human cancer. *Science* 1991;253:49.
13. Martin SJ, Green DR. Apoptosis as a goal of cancer therapy. *Curr Opin Oncol* 1994;6:521.
14. Meikrantz W, Schlegel R. Apoptosis and the cell cycle. *J Cell Biochem* 1995;58:160.
15. Shimamura A, Fisher DE. P53 in life and death. *Clin Canc Res* 1996;2:435.
16. Miyashita T, Reed JC. Bcl-2 oncoprotein blocks chemotherapy-induced apoptosis in a human leukemia cell line. *Blood* 1993;81:151.
17. Walton MI, Whysong D, O'Conner PM, et al. Constitutive expression of human Bcl-2 modulates nitrogen mustard and camptothecin induced apoptosis. *Cancer Res* 1993;53:1853.
18. Gottesmann MM. How cancer cells evade chemotherapy: Sixteenth Richard and Hinda Rosenthal Foundation award lecture. *Cancer Res* 1993;53:747.
19. Holzmayer TA, Hilsenbeck S, VanHoff DD, et al. Clinical correlates of MDR1 (P-glycoprotein) gene expression in ovarian and small cell lung carcinomas. *J Natl Cancer Inst* 1992;84: 1486.
20. Goldie JH. Scientific basis for adjuvant and primary (neoadjuvant) chemotherapy. *Semin Oncol* 1987;14:1.
21. Hesketh PJ, Kris MG, Grunberg SM, et al. Proposal for classifying the emetogenicity of cancer chemotherapy. *J Clin Oncol* 1997;15:103.
22. Tyers MB. 5-HT$_3$ receptors. *Ann NY Acad Sci* 1990;600:194.
23. Grunberg SM, Hesketh PJ. Control of chemotherapy induced emesis. *N Engl J Med* 1993;329:1790.
24. Carl W. Oral complications of local and systemic cancer treatment. *Curr Opin Oncol* 1995;7:320.
25. Kintzel PE, Dorr RT. Anticancer drug renal toxicity and elimination: dosing guidelines for altered renal function. *Cancer Treat Rev* 1995;21:33.
26. Tuxen MK, Hansen SW. Neurotoxicity secondary to antineoplastic drugs. *Cancer Treat Rev* 1994;20:191.
27. Perry MC. Chemotherapeutic agents and hepatotoxicity. *Semin Oncol* 1992;19[Suppl]:551.
28. Kreisman H, Wolkove N. Pulmonary toxicity of antineoplastic therapy. *Semin Oncol* 1992;19[Suppl]:508.
29. Hochster H, Wasserheit C, Speyer J. Cardiotoxicity and cardioprotection during chemotherapy. *Curr Opin Oncol* 1995;7:304.
30. Adrian RM, Hood AF, Skarin AT. Mucocutaneous reaction to antineoplastic agents. *CA J Clin* 1980;30:143.
31. McInnes S, Schilsky RL. Infertility following cancer chemotherapy. In: Chabner BA, Longo DL, eds. *Cancer chemotherapy and biotherapy.* Philadelphia: Lippincott-Raven 1996;31.
32. Tucker MA, Coleman CN, Cox RS, et al. Risk of second cancers after treatment of Hodgkin's disease. *N Engl J Med* 1988;318: 76.
33. Pui CH, Ribaerio RC, Hancock ML, et al. Acute myeloid leukemia in children treated with epipodophyllotoxins for acute lymphoblastic leukemia. *N Engl J Med* 1991;325:1682.
34. Richards MA, Ramirez LF, Degner LF, et al. Offering choice of treatment to patients with cancers. *Eur J Cancer* 1995;31A: 112.
35. Samet J, Hunt WB, Key C, et al. Choice of cancer therapy varies with age of the patient. *JAMA* 1986;255:3385.
36. Einhorn LH. Approaches to drug therapy in older cancer patients. *Oncology* 1996;6[Suppl]:69.
37. Leslie WT. Chemotherapy in older cancer patients. *Oncology* 1992;6[Suppl]:74.
38. Stewart CF, Pieper JA, Arburk SG, et al. Altered protein binding of etoposide in patients with cancer. *Clin Pharmacol Ther* 1989; 45:49.
39. Baker SD, Growchow LB, Donehower RB. Should anticancer drug doses be adjusted in the obese patient? *J Natl Cancer Inst* 1995;87:333.
40. Georgiadis MS, Steinberg SM, Hankins LA, et al. Obesity and therapy related toxicity in patients treated for small cell lung cancer. *J Natl Cancer Inst* 1995;87:361.
41. Johnson DH. Ifosfamide in non-small cell lung cancer. *Semin Oncol* 1996;23[Suppl]:7.
42. Ettinger DB. Ifosfamide in the treatment of small cell lung cancer. *Semin Oncol* 1996;23[Suppl]:2.
43. Tew KD, Colvin M, Chabner BA. Alkylating agents. In: Chabner BA, Longo DL, ed. *Cancer chemotherapy and biotherapy.* Philadelphia: Lippincott-Raven 1996;297.
44. O'Dwyer, Hamilton TC, Young RC, et al. Depletion of glutathione in normal and malignant human cells in vivo by butathione sulfonamide: clinical and biochemical results. *J Natl Cancer Inst* 1992;84:264.
45. Glover D, Glick JH, Weiler C, et al. WR2721 protects against

the hematologic toxicity of cyclophosphamide: a controlled phase II trial. *J Clin Oncol* 1986;4:584.

46. Moore MJ. Clinical pharmacokinetics of cyclophosphamide. *Clin Pharmacokinet* 1991;20:194.

47. Colvin M. The comparative pharmacology of cyclophosphamide and ifosfamide. *Semin Oncol* 1982;9[Suppl]:2.

48. Sarosy G. Ifosfamide—pharmacologic overview. *Semin Oncol* 1989;16:2.

49. Shaw IC, Graham MI. Mesna—a short overview. *Cancer Treat Rev* 1987;14:67.

50. Fleming RA. An overview of cyclophosphamide and ifosfamide pharmacology. *Pharmacotherapy* 1997;17[Suppl]:146S.

51. Twohig KJ, Matthay RA. Pulmonary effects of cytotoxic agents other than bleomycin. *Clin Chest Med* 1990;11:31.

52. Skinner R, Sharkey IM, Pearson ADJ, et al. Ifosfamide, mesna and nephrotoxicity in children. *J Clin Oncol* 1993;11:173.

53. Meanwell CA, Blake AE, Kelly KA, et al. Prediction of ifosfamide/mesna associated encephalopathy. *Eur J Cancer Clin Oncol* 1986;22:815.

54. Sherins RJ, Devita VT. Effect of drug treatment for lymphoma on male reproductive capacity. *Ann Intern Med* 1973;79:216.

55. Dabholkar M, Reed E. Cisplatin. *Cancer Chemother Biol Response Modif* 1996;16:88.

56. Himmelstein KJ, Patton FT, Belt RJ, et al. Clinical kinetics of intact cisplatin and some related species. *Clin Pharmacol Ther* 1984;29:658.

57. Chu G. Cellular responses to cisplatin. The roles of DNA binding proteins and DNA repair. *J Biol Chem* 1994;269:787.

58. Egorin MJ, Van Echo DA, Olman EA, et al. Prospective validation of a pharmacologically based dosing scheme for cis-diamine-dichloroplatinum analog, diamminecyclobutane dicarboxylato-platinum. *Cancer Res* 1985;45:6502.

59. Calvert AH, Newell DR, Gimbrell LA, et al. Carboplatin dosage: prospective evaluation of a simple formula based on renal function. *J Clin Oncol* 1989;7:1748.

60. Hande KR. Pharmacologic-based dosing of carboplatin: a better method. *J Clin Oncol* 1993;11:2295.

61. Murry DJ. Comparative clinical pharmacology of cisplatin and carboplatin. *Pharmacotherapy* 1997;17:1405.

62. Perez EA. Review of the preclinical pharmacology and comparative efficacy of 5-hydroxytryptamine-3-receptor antagonists for chemotherapy induced emesis. *J Clin Oncol* 1995;13:1036.

63. Blachley JD, Hill JB. Renal and electrolyte disturbances associated with cisplatin. *Ann Intern Med* 1981;95:628.

64. Pinzani V, Bressolle F, Haug IJ, et al. Cisplatin-induced renal toxicity and toxicity-modulating strategies: a review. *Cancer Chemother Pharmacol* 1994;35:1.

65. McKeage MJ. Comparative adverse effect profiles of platinum drugs. *Drug Saf* 1995;13:228.

66. Correia JJ. Effects of antimitotic agents on tubulin-nucleotide interactions. *Pharmacol Ther* 1991;52:127.

67. Jones AL, Smith IE. Navelbine and the anthrapyrazoles. *Hematol Oncol Clin North Am* 1994;8:141.

68. Zhou XJ, Rahmani R. Preclinical and clinical pharmacology of vinca alkaloids. *Drugs* 1992;44[Suppl4]:1.

69. Legha SS. Vincristine neurotoxicity: Pathophysiology and management. *Med Toxicol* 1986;1:421.

70. Rowinsky EK, Donehower RC. The clinical pharmacology and use of antimicrotubule agents in cancer chemotherapeutics. *Pharmacol Ther* 1991;52:35.

71. Hohneker JA. A summary of vinorelbine (Novelbine) *Sem Oncol* 1995;22[Suppl 5]:80.

72. Schiff PH, Horwitz SB. Taxol stabilizes microtubules in mouse fibroblast cells. *Proc Natl Acad Sci U S A* 1980;77:1561.

73. Rowinsky EK, Cazenave LA, Donehower RC. Taxol: A novel investigational antimicrotubule agent. *J Natl Cancer Inst* 1990; 82:1247.

74. Eisenhauer EA, Vermorken JB. The taxoids: comparative clinical pharmacology and therapeutic potential. *Drugs* 1998;55:5.

75. Cresteil T, Monsarrat B, Alvinerie P, et al. Taxol metabolism by human liver microsomes: identification of cytochrome P450 isoenzymes involved in its biotransformation. *Cancer Res* 1994; 54:386.

76. Gianni L, Kearns CM, Giani A, et al. Nonlinear pharmacokinetics and metabolism of paclitaxel and its pharmacokinetic/pharmacodynamic relationships in humans. *J Clin Oncol* 1995;13:180.

77. Kearns CM. Pharmacokinetics of the taxanes. *Pharmacotherapy* 1997;17[Suppl]:105.

78. Sparreboom A, vanTellinger O, Noorjen WJ, et al. Non-linear pharmacokinetics of paclitaxel results from the pharmaceutical vehicle cremophor EL. *Cancer Res* 1996;56:2112.

79. Baker SD. Drug interactions with the taxanes. *Pharmacotherapy* 1997;17[Suppl]:126.

80. Rowinski EK, Eisenhauer EA, Chaudry V, et al. Clinical toxicities encountered with paclitaxel. *Semin Oncol* 1993;20[Suppl 3]:1.

81. Cortes JE, Pazdur R. Docetaxel. *J Clin Oncol* 1995;13:2643.

82. Gianni L, Munzone E, Capri G, et al. Paclitaxel by 3-hour infusion in combination with bolus doxorubicin in women with untreated metastatic breast cancer: high antitumor efficacy and cardiac effects in a dose-finding and sequence-finding study. *J Clin Oncol* 1995;13:2688.

83. Osheroff N, Zechiedrich EL, Gale KC. Catalytic function of DNA topoisomerase II. *Bioassays* 1991;12:269.

84. Liu LF. DNA topoisomerase poisons as antitumor drugs. *Ann Rev Biochem* 1989;58:351.

85. Walker PR, Smith C, Youdale T, et al. Topoisomerase II-reactive chemotherapeutic drugs induce apoptosis in thymocytes. *Cancer Res* 1991;51:1078.

86. Giovanella BC, Stehlin JS, Wall ME, et al. DNA topoisomerase I-targeted chemotherapy of human colon cancer in xenografts. *Science* 1989;246:1046.

87. Slichenmyer WJ, Rowinsky EK, Donehower RC, et al. The current status of camptothecin analogues as antitumor agents. *J Natl Cancer Inst* 1993;85:271.

88. Hande KR. The importance of drug scheduling in cancer chemotherapy: etoposide as an example. *Stem Cells* 1996;14:18.

89. Hande KR, Krozely MG, Greco FA, et al. Bioavailability of low-dose oral etoposide. *J Clin Oncol* 1993;11:374.

90. Hande KR, Wolff SN, Greco FA, et al. Etoposide kinetics in patient with obstructive jaundice. *J Clin Oncol* 1990;8:1101.

91. Thompson DS, Greco FA, Miller AA, et al. A phase I study of etoposide phosphate administered as a daily 30-minute infusion for five days. *Clin Pharmacol Ther* 1995;57:499.

92. Speth PAJ, vanHoesel QG, Haanen C. Clinical pharmacokinetics of doxorubicin. *Clin Pharmacokinet* 1988;15:15.

93. Brenner DE, Wiernik PH, Wesley M, et al. Acute doxorubicin toxicity: relationship to pretreatment liver function, response and pharmacokinetics in patients with acute non-lymphocytic leukemia. *Cancer* 1984;53:1042.

94. Holmes FA, Madden T, Newman RA, et al. Sequence-dependent alteration of doxorubicin pharmacokinetics by paclitaxel in a Phase I study of paclitaxel and doxorubicin in patients with metastatic breast cancer. *J Clin Oncol* 1996;14:2713.

95. Burris HA, Fields SM. Topoisomerase I inhibitors. *Hematol Oncol Clin North Am* 1996;8:333.

96. Chabot CG, Abigerges D, Catimel G, et al. Population pharmacokinetics and pharmacodynamics of irinotecan (CPT-11) and active metabolite SN-38 during phase I trials. *Ann Oncol* 1995; 6:141.

97. Gupta E, Lestingi TM, Mick R, et al. Metabolic fate of irinotecan in humans: correlation of glucuronidation with diarrhea. *Cancer Res* 1994;54:3723.

98. Takimoto CH, Arbuck SG. Clinical status and optimal use of topotecan. *Oncology* 1997;11:1635.

99. O'Reilly S, Rowinsky E, Slichenmyer W, et al. Phase I and pharmacologic studies of topotecan in patients with impaired renal function. *J Clin Oncol* 1996;14:3062.

100. O'Reilly S, Rowinsky E, Slichenmyer W, et al. Phase I and pharmacologic studies of topotecan in patients with impaired hepatic function. *J Nat Cancer Inst* 1996;88:817.

101. O'Dwyer PJ, Leyland-Jones B, Alonso MT, et al. Etoposide (VP-16-213). Current status of an active anticancer drug. *N Engl J Med* 1985;312:692.

102. Hande KR. Clinical applications of anticancer drugs targeted to topoisomerase II. *Biochem et Biophysica Acta* 1998;1400:173.

103. Rui CH, Riberiro RC, Hancock ML, et al. Acute myeloid leukemia in children treated with epipodophyllotoxins for acute lymphoblastic leukemia. *N Engl J Med* 1991;325:1682.

104. Nichols CR, Breeded ES, Loehrer PJ, et al. Secondary leukemia associated with a conventional dose of etoposide: review of serial germ cell tumor protocols. *J Natl Cancer Inst* 1993;85:36.

105. Young RC, Ozols RF, Myers CE. The anthracycline antineoplastic drugs. *N Engl J Med* 1981;305:139.

106. Doroshow JH. Anthracyclines and anthracendiones, in: Chabner BA, Long DL, eds. *Cancer chemotherapy and biotherapy: principles and practice.* Lippincott-Raven, Philadelphia: 1996;409.

107. Von Hoff DD, Layard MW, Basa P, et al. Risk factors for doxorubicin-induced congestive heart failure. *Ann Intern Med* 1979;91:710.

108. Shan K, Lincott AM, Young JB. Anthracycline-induced cardiotoxicity. *Ann Intern Med* 1996;125:47.

109. Steinherz LJ, Steinherz PG, Tan CD, et al. Cardiac toxicity 4 to 20 years after completing anthracycline therapy. *JAMA* 1991;266:1672.

110. Swain SM, Whaley FS, Gerber MD, et al. Cardioprotection with dexrazoxane for doxorubicin-containing therapy in advanced breast cancer. *J Clin Oncol* 1992;15:1318.

111. Eckardt J, Eckardt G, Villanona-Calero M, et al. New anticancer agents in clinical development. *Oncology* 1995;9:1191.

112. Abigerges D, Chabot GG, Armand JP, et al. Phase I and pharmacokinetic studies of the camptothecin analog irinotecan administered every 3 weeks in cancer patients. *J Clin Oncol* 1995;13:210.

113. Saltz L, Sirott M, Young C, et al. Phase I and pharmacology study of topotecan given for 5 consecutive days to patients with advanced solid tumors with an attempt at dose intensification using recombinant granulocyte colony stimulating factor. *J Natl Cancer Inst* 1993;85:1499.

114. Creemers GJ, Gerrits CH, Eckardt JR, et al. Phase I and pharmacologic study of oral topotecan administered twice daily for 21 days to adult patients with solid tumors. *J Clin Oncol* 1997;15:1087.

115. Huang P, Plunkett W. Fludarabine- and gemcitabine-induced apoptosis: incorporation of analogs into DNA is a critical event. *Cancer Chemother Pharmacol* 1995;36:181.

116. Plunkett W, Huang P, Xu Y-Z, et al. Gemcitabine: metabolism, mechanisms of action, and self-potentiation. *Semin Oncol* 1995;22[suppl 11]:3.

117. Stonnicolo AM, Allerheiligen SRB, Pearce HL. Preclinical pharmacologic and Phase I studies of gemcitabine. *Sem Oncol* 1997;24(7):52.

118. Noble S, Goa KL. Gemcitabine: a review of its pharmacology and clinical potential in non–small cell lung cancer and pancreatic cancer. *Drugs* 1997;54:447.

119. Eli Lilly and Company. Gemzar® (gemcitabine HCl) for injection. US prescribing information. Eli Lilly and Company (Indianapolis).

120. Abbruzzese JL, Grunewald R, Weeks EA, et al. A phase I clinical, plasma, and cellular pharmacology study of gemcitabine. *J Clin Oncol* 1991;9:491.

121. Abratt RP, Bezwoda WR, Falkson G, et al. Efficacy and safety profile of gemcitabine in non–small cell lung cancer: a phase II study. *J Clin Oncol* 1994;12:1535.

122. Carmichael J, Possinger K, Phillip P, et al. Advanced breast cancer: a phase II trial with gemcitabine. *J Clin Oncol* 1995;13:2731.

15

CHEMOTHERAPY–RADIATION INTERACTION

AFSHIN DOWLATI
RUTH LOUISE EAKIN
TIMOTHY J. KINSELLA

Combinations of chemotherapy and radiotherapy have been used and investigated in the treatment of human cancers for more than 30 years. During this time, clinical and laboratory investigations have become increasingly complex because the understanding of interactions and mechanisms have improved. Basic clinical observations have been critically important; for example, when local treatment such as radiotherapy was given successfully for apparently localized intrathoracic disease, systemic relapse was still seen to occur in a significant proportion of patients despite the maintenance of local control. Likewise, chemotherapy, which produced good responses in metastatic disease, particularly in the lymphomas, could not prevent relapse in sites of initial bulk disease. The potential advantages of combining modalities were obvious from early days.

The main context in which to consider chemotherapy–radiotherapy interactions in non–small cell lung cancer (NSCLC) is in locally advanced stage III disease, where until the last decade, radiation therapy and surgery have played the major roles. In contrast, chemotherapy has been the cornerstone of treatment for small cell lung cancer (SCLC) with the issues of thoracic radiotherapy and prophylactic cranial irradiation in limited-stage disease becoming increasingly important over the last two decades.

Radiation therapy has developed markedly over the last century, and optimal fractionation schedules continue to be sought, alongside the improvements in its technical and conformal application. Chemotherapy has, over the last 40 years, mushroomed in its complexity of combinations and integration of new compounds. The outlook for patients with SCLC has changed considerably in recent decades because of well-structured clinical trials designed to reveal the optimal combinations of chemoradiation, and is one of the many examples of progress in this field to date. On the other hand, progress in the treatment of NSCLC has made more modest gains. Local control has been hard to improve, and impacts of systemic therapy on survival have only been modest in comparison. Despite this progress treatment results in both major types of lung cancer are still poor overall,

although recent developments do allow significant optimism. Progress is being made, and with improved understandings of combined modality therapy at the molecular, cellular, and clinical levels, not only can clinical trial protocols be better designed, but of course, better outcomes, can also be realized for patients with small cell and non–small cell lung carcinomas.

BASIC CONCEPTS

When radiation therapy and chemotherapy are combined, the therapeutic result can be improved over single modality treatment by one or more theoretical means. They can contribute independently of each other (spatial cooperation); they can improve primary tumor response without increasing toxicity beyond tolerance; or they can decrease normal tissue toxicities without changing tumor response, thereby allowing increased doses or the addition of other anticancer agents. Two key considerations in any combination of radiotherapy and chemotherapy are doses and timing, relative to each other. If radiotherapy is given first, tumor bulk is likely to shrink, which would theoretically allow better drug distribution. It is also recognized clinically that chemotherapy is better able to achieve a sustainable response when small bulk of disease is present; however, giving radiotherapy first delays systemic therapy and may allow metastases to grow, making them subsequently less likely to be eliminated by chemotherapy. If chemotherapy is given first, it will theoretically tackle micrometastases at the earliest possible opportunity, thereby giving the best chance of elimination. However, delaying definitive management of the primary tumor can also be detrimental. Whatever way these many possible interactions are viewed, it is vital to be clear about definitions.

Definition of Terms

Having clear definitions is fundamental to the discussion of any complex interaction.[1] Terms that have been used previously in the context of chemoradiation include *synergy*, to describe an additive effect. This term does not clarify whether the synergistic combination resulted in an effect that was equal to the sum of the individual chemotherapy and radiotherapy effects, or whether it was in fact equivalent to slightly more or slightly less than the sum. The term synergy is often used to mean an effect greater than the sum of the individual effects. In addition, it is necessary to try and differentiate the *sensitization* of one modality by the other, from the simple cooperation of geographically remote effects of each modality.

Therapeutic Ratio and Dose Effects

Radiotherapy and chemotherapy *in vivo* unfortunately cannot treat cancer cells exclusively but will inevitably affect normal cells and tissues. During a course of radiotherapy, the target volume and beam arrangements are designed to maximize dose to tumor, while keeping dose to surrounding normal tissues as low as possible. Typically, for lung cancers, the dose-limiting factor is normal tissue tolerances to the adjacent normal lung, esophagus, and less commonly heart. Similarly with chemotherapy, the ability of normal tissues, principally bone marrow, to recover in relation to the rate of tumor regrowth again determines maximum tolerated doses. With certain drugs, such as the platinum analogs, there may be enhanced acute normal tissue toxicities, such as esophageal mucositis, when used concomitantly with thoracic irradiation. The *therapeutic ratio* is therefore defined as the ratio of effect(s) of any given intervention on tumor tissue to its effect(s) on normal tissues. Manipulation of treatment strategies is aimed at improving the therapeutic ratio. It should also be noted that a combination of treatments, in some circumstances, can improve therapeutic outcome without necessarily improving the therapeutic ratio.

In terms of combined modality therapy (CMT), the therapeutic ratio can be calculated using the concept of *dose-effect factor* (DEF).[2] The DEF is the ratio of radiation dose required for a given effect to the radiation dose required with chemotherapy to cause the same effect, and can be applied to effect on both tumor or on normal tissues. Thus the therapeutic ratio can be improved by either an increase in DEF for tumor with no change in DEF for normal tissue, or by no change in DEF for tumor and a decrease in DEF for normal tissue.

Spatial Cooperation

The concept of *spatial cooperation* was first described by Steel and Peckham,[3] and relates to situations where the effects of chemotherapy and radiotherapy are thought to be anatomically independent. Ideally, their combined toxicity is also independent, but in reality this does not always follow. An example of spatial cooperation is seen in SCLC, where prophylactic cranial irradiation is used to treat a common site of spread that chemotherapy does not reach because of the blood–brain barrier. In this type of beneficial combination, a physical interaction between the two modalities is not required to obtain an overall therapeutic benefit.

Enhancement

Enhancement is a global term for an increased cell-killing effect and should be used when it is not possible to be more precise. If the effect of combined chemoradiation is equal to the sum of the individual effects, then it is considered to be *additive*. If the combined effect is greater than the sum, then it is *supraadditive*. If it is less than the sum, but greater than the more effective single modality, then it is *subadditive*. If one of the two agents does not have an effect on its own, then it causes a *sensitizing* effect. Enhancement is seen to occur with intrathoracic radiotherapy plus combination chemotherapy, again in the CMT of SCLC and to a lesser extent, in the current combined modality treatment of NSCLC.

Diminution

In contrast, *diminution* implies reduction of overall effect. When the combined effect is less than that seen with the more effective single modality, then it constitutes *inhibition*. When it is not as effective as the less active single modality, then it is *antagonism*. When one of the agents is not active against the disease by itself, such as ethylol, then *protection* is used to describe the combined effect as it relates to a reduction of normal tissue toxicity, such as esophagitis.

How to accurately quantify these different combinations of effects remains difficult, although Steel and Peckham have described the important concept of isobologram analysis, in which "envelopes of additivity" are constructed.[3] These, however, only apply when the unimodal dose-response curves are close to linear. There are many known variables, such as the radiation fractionation, the time interval for combined modality therapy, and tumor cell kinetics, which unfortunately make this method not universally applicable.

Mechanisms of Interaction

Cellular damage by radiation is thought to be caused by direct photon "hits" on cellular DNA, and indirectly by free radical formation causing subsequent DNA damage. It is plausible that cytotoxic chemicals could interfere with the radiation reaction at this level by perhaps stabilizing free radicals, by enzyme inhibition, or by physically altering the molecular target for effective cell kill by radiation. The cell survival curves of megavoltage radiation for different cell lines are all remarkably similar, with a shoulder at the low-dose range and a log-linear exponential progression at higher doses. At lower doses, greater potential exists for DNA repair, or sublethal damage repair (SLDR), and the intrinsic repair capacity of the specific cellular DNA irradiated determines the initial slope of the curve. Chemotherapy may, by whatever means, cause inhibition of SLDR, or potentially lethal damage repair (PLDR), and in fact this action is predominantly implicated. These functionally defined repair processes are thought to represent the repair of single- and double-stranded DNA breaks, which occur in the first few hours after irradiation. Radiation could, of course, also inhibit the cellular repair processes activated following chemotherapy-induced damage. A more complete understanding of radiation damage and repair pathways, as currently understood, is reviewed recently (see also Chapters 12, 13).[4]

Other important radiobiologic components of fractionated radiation therapy include the phenomena of repopulation, redistribution, and reoxygenation. *Repopulation* results from continued cell division, and in some experimental tumor models it has been shown to accelerate after 2 to 3 weeks of treatment. *Redistribution* occurs because of varying sensitivity of cells in relation to the cell cycle, which can lead to recruitment of more cells out of the resting (Go) phase and thus a buildup of cells in any one part of the cell cycle. For example, one of the known actions of hydroxyurea is a G1/S-phase block, which could conceivably cause accumulation of cells by redistribution into a radiosensitive part of the cell cycle, thus enhancing the overall killing effect. By this mechanism, reduction of accelerated proliferation might also be induced, causing an enhanced radiation effect.

The mechanisms of *reoxygenation* are not clearly understood, but are probably caused in part by cell loss and improved vascular supply to acutely or chronically hypoxic cells. Chemotherapy could alter the proportion of oxygenated cells in the radiotherapy portal, thereby altering its effectiveness. Likewise, radiotherapy almost certainly causes improved blood supply and drug delivery to an area, if given prior to chemotherapy.

Whatever way the combination of drug(s) and radiation interact at a molecular or cellular level, clear evidence exists that bulk of tumor tissue plays an important role. This correlation is in part related to reoxygenation but also to improved blood supply, revascularisation, and drug delivery.

These concepts are some of the mechanisms that form the theoretical basis of interaction. Many other factors further complicate and influence these mechanisms to varying degrees, such as the specific chemotherapy drug or combination of drugs, drug doses, drug dose scheduling, radiotherapy fractionation scheme, radiation dose-per-fraction, overall radiation dose, radiation dose rate, and timing of chemoradiotherapy. In addition, the key to benefiting patients lies in the difference between what happens in normal tissues compared to tumor tissues. Dose-responses and timing are discussed in the next two sections.

Dose-Response Relationships

Much work has been done on dose-response for radiation and chemotherapy drugs, both on different tumor types and on different normal tissues. Underlying this work is the definition of cell survival, which is that the cell is able to retain its proliferative capacity for approximately five or six cell divisions; that is, clonogenic survival.

Radiotherapy Dose-Response

Survival curves for radiotherapy are similar in shape for different tissues and tumors. The shoulder, as discussed previously, is in the lower dose range and is thought to represent the ability of the cells to repair sublethal damage. When radiotherapy is fractionated, this phenomenon helps to increase the therapeutic ratio because of the intrinsic difference in SLDR capacity of tumor and normal tissue. Several representative mathematical models have been proposed over the years, the most widely and currently accepted being the linear-quadratic (LQ) model. This model allows for the theory of ionizing radiation either causing a single, lethal, chromosomal double-stranded break (alpha or linear interaction), or causing a sublethal, single-stranded break, in which case more than one is required to produce cell death (beta or quadratic component). On experimentally plotting survival curves for all the different normal tissues, it became apparent that there were basically two quite different types of normal tissue responders—early and late. The early-responding tissues, such as skin, bone marrow, and gastrointestinal mucosa, were noted to be tissues with a rapid cell turnover, and late-responding tissues, such as central nervous system, kidney, or lung, were noted to have a slow normal cell turnover rate. Tumor tissue was seen to act more like acute-responding normal tissues. The effects of increasing dose to tumor and to different types of normal tissue must be appreciated if the potential therapeutic effects of combined modality therapy are to be optimized.

Dose-response to radiotherapy is well documented clinically. One of the interesting questions often asked is in relation to how much more benefit could potentially be achieved by increasing the dose any further than is already achieved at standard dose. The standard dose represents the highest or most effective dose that can currently be given within the context of acceptable normal tissue toxicities. The only ways of further escalating the radiation dose to tumor, relative to normal tissues, would be by using more technical/conformal-based approaches, or by applying *in vivo* modulators (such as radioprotectors/radiosensitizers), both of which have their potential advantages and disadvantages. A recent Radiation Therapy Oncology Group (RTOG) study of hyperfractionated radiotherapy compared dose levels in NSCLC, and was able to indicate a dose above which no additional benefit was achieved.[5] Once a maximum radiation dose-tumor response relationship is established, then alternative approaches must be pursued.

The total radiation dose and radiobiologic dose must also be considered. For example, a total dose of 52.4Gy given over 20 daily fractions (262cGy per fraction) is considered to be radiobiologically equivalent to a total dose of 64Gy given over 32 daily fractions (200cGy per fraction), in terms of tumor cell kill. In this comparison, the higher dose per fraction regimen can cause worse late-normal tissue toxicities, even though the total dose is lower. The current development of altered fractionation schedules is based on radiobiologic data (both laboratory and clinical) suggesting ways of increasing the differential between tumor and normal tissue responses. In a *hyperfractionated* schedule, the total number of fractions is increased without altering overall treatment time, thereby allowing for an increased total dose but necessitating a reduced dose per fraction because of enhanced toxicity. In an *accelerated fractionation* schedule, the overall treatment time is shortened, with total dose, number of fractions, and dose per fraction being unchanged or slightly reduced. These factors are important when considering the addition of chemotherapy.

Chemotherapy Dose-Response

Survival curves for chemotherapy agents vary widely for different tissues.[6] They also vary depending on dose of drug, whether single or combination therapy is used, and whether a single administration or multiple administrations are given. If multiple administrations are given, the interval time and individual drug doses, plus any interaction, all participate in affecting overall response. In addition, the pharmacokinetic properties of individual drugs are extremely important in determining bioavailability, which is often further altered at the tumor site by factors such as heterogeneous tumor blood flow. Sanctuary sites, such as the central nervous system, and drug resistance are other reasons for chemotherapy failure, which simply increasing dose will not overcome.

An abundance of evidence supports the theory that increasing the dose results in increases in tumor response. However, two distinct categories of dose-escalation characteristics have been recognized: A dose-response survival curve, which levels off in the higher range (e.g., vinca alkaloids and methotrexate) and the classical log-linear dose-response curve, which continues indefinitely (e.g., alkylating agents). In recent years, the limiting factor for the latter (i.e., bone marrow toxicity) has been partially breached by the development of peripheral blood stem cell transplantation. It is now the other dose-limiting toxicities, such as gastrointestinal, pulmonary, or neurological toxicities, that continue to produce the barriers to any further dose escalation.

Mechanisms of Cell Death

As can be implicated by the preceding definition of cell survival (i.e., clonogenic or reproductive survival) the converse definition applies to the process of mitotic cell death (i.e., cells that are unable to sustain proliferation beyond one or a few cell divisions). This reaction occurs as a direct result of injury, whether through radiation, cytotoxic chemicals, heat, or other physical insults. DNA degradation occurs late, after cytoplasm and membrane breakdown. In contrast, programmed cell death or apoptosis is a normal physiological two-phase process involving the formation of microscopically recognizable apoptotic bodies, and occurs regularly *in vivo*. Characteristically, DNA degradation occurs first, followed by degeneration of the rest of the cell and subsequent loss of membrane integrity. This process is responsible for such natural events as tissue involution during embryonic development, or as part of the renewal process during regeneration of the gastrointestinal tract lining, and has been identified within tumors as well. Less than 20 years ago, radiation-induced apoptosis was also described, although it is thought to represent only a fraction of all radiation-induced cell death. It has nonetheless become an important line of investigation because the genes and proteins associated with controlling apoptosis become obvious potential targets for therapy.[4]

Timing of Radiation and Chemotherapy

In CMT, clearly the decision about sequencing is a key aspect to achieving optimal therapeutic benefit. Experimentally, the effectiveness can vary dramatically with timing of chemotherapy administration relative to irradiation, as has been illustrated by the varying times of maximum and minimum cell kill in intestinal crypt cells.[2] Hill and colleagues have also demonstrated that initial *in vitro* exposure of mammalian tumor cell lines to fractionated radiotherapy significantly alters their drug-response patterns, but prior exposure to chemotherapy does not generally alter radiation response.[7] The individual variation of different drugs might well prove to be of value, as will be discussed later when considering resistance and strategies.

Sequencing can be considered to fall into three major categories, as follows:

Neoadjuvant (Remote or Sequential)

The term *neoadjuvant* is used to describe upfront chemotherapy, prior to definitive management of the primary site by radiotherapy (or surgery). Advantages of this approach include the earliest possible treatment of micrometastases at a time when metastatic burden is lowest, and causing reduction of primary tumor size with possible elimination of radioresistant subclones. On the other hand, delaying definitive management of the primary site may allow chemotherapy-resistant clones to metastasize, which would otherwise have been dealt with by radiotherapy (or surgery) before becoming able to spread. This method may also increase proliferation of the primary tumor, thereby causing enhancement of its growth during fractionated radiotherapy.

Remote refers to a common practice in the community setting, where a planned break occurs between modalities to allow for normal tissue recovery. In these circumstances, both modalities can be given in full, independent of dose, making the most of the individual dose-response relationships and taking advantage of spatial cooperation. However, any interaction or possible benefit from enhancement at the primary site is minimized. In *sequential* treatments, radiotherapy is started within a few days of completion of chemotherapy. Although this method improves direct interaction at the primary site, it clearly also increases toxicity, which may ultimately prove to be a limiting factor in this neoadjuvant approach.

Concurrent (Including Alternating)

Simultaneous administration of chemotherapy during a course of fractionated radiation therapy has undoubtedly proven itself to be the optimal combination to date in certain situations, most notably in the management of various gastrointestinal cancers, where the important advantage over resection is organ preservation. In other circumstances, maximization of primary tumor response by this method often asks too high a price in terms of toxicity, and is therefore not the current standard of practice. Given the theoretical advantages, alternating protocols are under investigation in an attempt to make the toxicity acceptable. This approach gives chemotherapy (e.g., weekly), and allows gaps in the radiotherapy delivery, perhaps treating one week on, one week off. This type of strategy permits the use of full dose in each modality without undue delay for either, thereby reducing the potential for resistance to either modality.

Adjuvant (Remote or Sequential)

When chemotherapy is given after definitive treatment of the primary site by radiotherapy (or surgery), it is termed *adjuvant*. In this setting, the advantages are that treatment of the primary site is not delayed and that the ability of the local tumor to metastasize is potentially restricted, if not eliminated. The size of the primary tumor mass is reduced, allowing a better chance of complete response to chemotherapy.[8] In remote sequencing, chemotherapy can still tackle micrometastases, but in sequential treatment it does so immediately after radiation therapy. Sequential adjuvant treatment carries the same problems of increasing toxicity as sequential neoadjuvant therapy.

Drug Resistance

When a single chemotherapy drug is administered repeatedly or in a prolonged fashion, such as continuous infusion, a change in cellular response can occur in tumor cells. This change is entirely directed toward resisting the drug and its effects. The likelihood of these drug-resistant cells being present in any particular tumor may be related to the mass of the tumor, implying that smaller tumors are less likely to harbor these drug-resistant cells. Many mechanisms have been identified, and undoubtedly a combination of these mechanisms comes into play in any given situation. The development of drug resistance has clear implications for treatment failure, and consequently for new ways of trying to enhance the efficacy of current combinations. When designing protocols for chemoradiation strategies, overcoming intrinsic and/or acquired resistance is a key consideration.

Mechanisms

These mechanisms are summarized in part, in Table 15.1, and can be considered at a cellular/intrinsic level, or on an anatomic/pharmacokinetic basis. Although resistance can occur because of the latter, the development of intrinsic resistance has provoked much study since it was first recognized. This intrinsic resistance is acquired through self-adaptation of the cell and can be responsible for resistance to other chemotherapy compounds (i.e., cross-resistance). When this happens, it is termed *multidrug resistance* (MDR) and is believed to be responsible for the majority of clinical treatment failures that occur because of drug resistance.

Multidrug Resistance

MDR refers to the situation when resistance developed because of repeated exposure to one drug and extends to structurally and functionally different classes of drugs. Cross-resistance has been found to be associated, in most cases, with the overexpression of P-glycoprotein, which is an integral part of the cell membrane drug efflux mechanism. The MDR-I gene has been shown to encode for P-glycoprotein. MDR is also associated with inhibition of the spindle cell poisons, including drugs affecting functions of topoisomerase I and topoisomerase II (See also Chapter 14). These mechanisms have been shown to be quite different from P-glycoprotein-mediated MDR. In addition, MDR has been identified with the mechanism of increased activity of the enzymes that metabolize the drugs, such as glutathione. Several different ways of preventing or reversing these actions have been investigated, but none so far has proven to be clinically useful.[9]

Strategies for Chemoradiation

The best way to integrate these two modalities is the subject of increasing study, both in the laboratory and in the clinic.

TABLE 15.1. SOME MECHANISMS AND PATHWAYS OF DRUG RESISTANCE

Mechanism		Enzymes and/or Proteins Involved	Specific Drugs Involved (examples)
Cellular level			
Membrane properties	Decreased uptake; Increased drug efflux	P-glycoprotein; Lipidperoxidases; Glutathione	Alkylating agents, Vinca alkaloids, Methotrexate, Nitrogen mustard
Altered drug metabolism	Reduced conversion of prodrugs to active moiety; enhanced degradation	Kinases	5-FU, Doxorubicin, Cytosine arabinoside, Bleomycin, 6-MP, Cytosine arabinoside
Drug targets	Physical or chemical alteration; increased level of target enzyme	Dihydrofolate reductase; Topoisomerase II	5-FU, methotrexate
DNA	Increased repair capacity	Guanine alkyl transferase; mismatch repair proteins	Cisplatin, Cyclophosphamide, Mitomycin C, Melphalan, Nitrogen mustard, Nitrosureas
Noncellular level			
Sanctuary sites	Unable to cross blood–brain barrier or into testes	—	Most, except Nitrosureas
Macroscopic effects	Poor vascularization; Reduced oxygenation; Altered pH; Cell cycle distribution	—	All
In vivo factors	Absorption; Renal excretion	—	All

Different types of tumors are known to have different intrinsic levels of radiosensitivity and chemosensitivity.[10] Even within one tumor histology, such as SCLC, a heterogeneous population of cells and tissues often exists. In addition, it is important to remember that even similar groups of patients, with similar types and stages of disease, still have their differences, particularly in how they tolerate aggressive CMT. Nonetheless, it is feasible to construct models, based on factors such as likelihood of resistance and tumor burden, to help in trying to predict the best combination of modalities, doses, and timing that might prove to be superior. These theoretical strategies are important to develop, but they still need to undergo thorough testing in accurately defined conditions. Only by the results of carefully controlled randomized clinical trials will their place in clinical practice be properly defined.

Targeting tumor cells as early as possible in their growth is undoubtedly optimal. The more bulk that exists, the longer it takes to eliminate all the cells, as per the log-cell kill theory. In terms of overcoming drug resistance, it also seems logical to apply different chemotherapy agents as soon as possible so that cells becoming quickly resistant to one type of drug will be targeted by another one to which they have not developed resistance. As has been discussed earlier, good evidence supports the fact that the degree of response and resistance to chemotherapy can be related directly to tumor mass. It, therefore, follows that treating with radiation and combination chemotherapy simultaneously, if tox-

icity is acceptable, should prove to be superior. However, in order to make it tolerable, dose reductions are often necessary, thereby negating any potential benefit.

One way of trying to deal with this problem is to combine agents and modalities with nonoverlapping toxicities. Several reports have hinted that when compared with neoadjuvant or adjuvant chemotherapy relative to radiotherapy, concurrent treatment has been better in terms of tumor responses, although not reaching statistical significance.[11] In this light, the approach of alternating modalities is under investigation, and Goldie has proposed the use of non–cross-resistant drugs in an alternating rather than sequential fashion as one possible strategy.[12] The additional concept of quantitative symmetry of these drugs is analyzed in detail by Day, which is where the efficacy of individual drugs is taken into account, and delivery in terms of dose and timing is adjusted to compensate.[13] The possible advantages of alternating strategies include being able to maintain the chemotherapy schedule with non–cross-resistant drugs given as early as possible and delivering significant total doses of radiotherapy between drug administration.[14]

Non–Small Cell Lung Cancer

Until this decade, the relative effectiveness of chemotherapy at all, in this disease, was debated. In 1995, a metaanalysis reported a statistically significant survival benefit for chemotherapy, and interest has since grown exponentially (See also

Chapter 50.).[15] Several randomized studies have now shown significant improvement with chemoradiotherapy in locally advanced stage III disease (see also Chapter 52), prompting many questions about optimizing the overall combination.[16,17]

In attempting to define the best strategy, it is important to recognize the problems that need to be addressed. The importance of achieving local control in this disease cannot be underestimated.[18] The increasing use of conformal radiation techniques invites not only dose-escalation (overall or radiobiologic) but also improved tolerability of CMT. The optimal fractionation schedule, in itself, is currently a major research topic, and the CHART regimen (Continuous Hyperfractionated Accelerated Radiotherapy) from Mount Vernon reported an improvement in two-year survival from 20% to 30% in locally advanced NSCLC.[19]

Given the persistently high rate of metastatic relapse, neoadjuvant chemotherapy has been a focus for many studies. Although phase II trials consistently showed better responses than in the palliative setting, they failed to be convincing on the matter of any improvement of local or distant control rates.[20-22] Likewise, studies of adjuvant chemotherapy have been unimpressive to date. However, several phase III randomized trials using CMT have been encouraging, although the radiation techniques and doses were, in retrospect, less than current optimal standards.[16,17,23,24] In Trovo's recent overview, summaries of randomized trials comparing radiotherapy alone to combined chemoradiotherapy are presented.[25] Careful analysis reveals that although some evidence supports superiority of CMT, it is not overwhelming.

The progression to investigation of combination chemotherapy with radiation, including new chemotherapy agents, is reviewed by Vokes.[26] Paclitaxel and carboplatin have been of particular interest[27-29] but so has the combining of these agents with more advanced radiation techniques.[30-32] Alternating radiotherapy and chemotherapy in phase II trials has also been reported, from GOTHA (Groupe d'Oncologie Thoracique Alpine), suggesting feasibility and a possible gain in long-term survival,[33] but as yet no mature or substantial phase III data supports these kinds of combinations as optimal. A recently reported cancer and leukemia Group B/Eastern Cooperative Oncology Group (CALGB/ECOG) study did not confirm any significant benefit with concurrent daily carboplatin, given at a dose of 100mg/m^2/week.[34]

The newer drugs, such as the taxanes, navelbine, and gemcitabine, are now being incorporated into protocols, along with biologic response modifiers.[35] Likewise, the pharmacokinetics of combining topoisomerase inhibitors with radiation is under investigation.[36] How to combine these agents effectively with improved radiotherapy fractionation and technology will continue to provide much subject for study well into the next century. The potential for significant improvement in this hitherto relatively unresponsive disease is now very real.

Small Cell Lung Cancer

The benefits of chemotherapy in this essentially systemic disease is not disputed, instead the integration of radiation—how, when, and where—raises most of the questions. Trials incorporating thoracic radiotherapy and predominantly cyclophosphamide-doxorubicin–based chemotherapy, were initiated more than 20 years ago, and the survival benefit attributable to thoracic radiation was confirmed in a subsequent metaanalysis.[37] Since that time, platinum-based regimens and more intensive chemotherapy have become widely used (see also Chapter 53). Nonetheless, the question of radiotherapy timing remains controversial, and until recently was given predominantly as postchemotherapy consolidation.[38] The appropriate target volume (i.e., whether supraclavicular nodal areas should be included) and the correct total dose/dose-fractionation schedule are also unclear. These issues remain to be resolved. Turrisi summarizes some of the randomized trials of chemoradiation in SCLC, dividing them into sequential, alternating, and concurrent.[39] The benefit of thoracic radiotherapy becomes evident, but again, the optimal sequencing, and other factors, remain uncertain.

In 1996, Johnson et al. from the National Cancer Institute (NCI), reported a phase II trial treating patients with limited-stage SCLC with concurrent etoposide, cisplatin, and hyperfractionated thoracic radiotherapy (1.5Gy twice per day to total 45Gy), followed by cyclophosphamide, doxorubicin, and vincristine.[40] Out of fifty-four patients, nine were alive and disease free at a median time of 4 years (2 to 7 years). Thirty-eight patients had progression of their disease at a median of 1.2 years, and interestingly, one-third of these patients developed and subsequently died of isolated central nervous system (CNS) relapse. Their calculated actuarial survival rates were 43% at 1 year and 19% at 2 years. In contrast, a Southwest Oncology Group phase II study published in 1998 looked at concurrent chemoradiation incorporating prolonged oral etoposide and prophylactic cranial irradiation (PCI), and found this combination to be toxic.[41] Only 50% of patients (28/56) completed chemotherapy as per protocol, with 93% (52/56) completing radiotherapy. Eleven patients (20%) discontinued treatment because of toxicity and two patients died from treatment. Possibly because of poor tolerability, complete response rates were not significantly different from previous studies. The European Organization for Research and Treatment of Cancer evaluated alternating versus sequential treatment modalities in a phase III randomized study but failed to confirm any clinical advantage for either arm.[42] At least two studies have assessed the effects of maintenance chemotherapy after induction with either CMT, or chemotherapy alone, and neither found any advantage.[43,44]

The other main area of controversy is in the use of PCI. Many conflicting studies have been reported, often with heterogeneous patient, tumor, or radiation-dosing factors, making interpretation all the more difficult. Currently, PCI is recommended for good performance status limited-stage patients who achieve a complete response to chemotherapy (see also Chapter 56).[45,46]

Future strategies for SCLC therapy will almost certainly focus also on the growing pool of genetic information, either for patient selection, or as part of treatment in combined therapy protocols.

SPECIFIC CHEMOTHERAPEUTIC AGENTS USED IN CHEMORADIATION

This section concentrates on radiation–chemotherapy interactions of individual agents. More detail on individual drugs can be found in chapters 14, 42, 50–52, 53, 54, and 57.

Nucleoside Analogues

Drugs that affect nucleoside and nucleotide metabolism are among the most effective and most widely used agents to sensitize tumor cells to radiation treatment. Some of the older agents include the fluoropyrimidines (5-fluorouracil), thymidine analogues, and hydroxyurea. Newer agents in this category include gemcitabine (difluorodeoxycytidine) and fludarabine.

Hydroxyurea

Mechanisms of Action
Although hydroxyurea is not a nucleoside analogue, its primary mechanism of action is related to its inhibition of ribonuleotide reductase, a key enzyme for the conversion of ribonucleotides to deoxyribonucleotides.[47] Its role in the treatment of hematologic malignancies and myeloproliferative disorders is well established.[48]

Preclinical Data with Radiation
The mechanism of hydroxyurea radiosensitization has been attributed to the inhibition of DNA synthesis resulting from the inhibition of ribonucleotide reductase.[49] Exposure prior to radiation blocks cells at the G1/S phase border, although it is uncertain if this redistribution alone causes increased radiation sensitivity. Another mechanism may be through inhibition of DNA repair, as illustrated by radiosensitization when hydroxyurea is given during or after radiation treatment.[50] There seems to be no differential effect on tumor cells compared to normal cells, although more rapidly dividing cells may be more sensitive to its effect. More recent investigations are focusing on the role of ribonucleotide reductase rather than disruption of cell cycle kinetics.[51] Hydroxyurea may also modulate fluoropyrimidine-mediated radiosensitization of tumor cells. Hydroxyurea depletes intracellular deoxyuridine monophosphate pools, thus in-

creasing the ability of FdUMP to bind with thymidylate synthase. Synergism between these two drugs has been demonstrated in preclinical models.[52] Finally, hydroxyurea may have a role as a biochemical modulator of IdUrd radiosensitization in tumor cells.[53] Exposure to low doses of hydroxyurea with IdUrd prior to radiation has been shown to enhance IdUrd-DNA incorporation and radiosensitization in the human bladder cell line 647V.

Clinical Experience
The use of hydroxyurea as a radiosensitizer has been evaluated in cancer of the head and neck,[54] malignant glioma,[55] and cervical cancer.[56] Its role in cancer of the head and neck as well as gliomas is difficult to appreciate given the fact that hydroxyurea was part of a multidrug regimen in these trials. Positive results have been demonstrated in cervical cancer when hydroxyurea is given with radiation compared to radiation alone.[57] In lung cancer, several studies demonstrated the feasibility of such an approach, but overall it has had little impact on the natural course of this disease. Vokes has used hydroxyurea along with 5-FU and radiation with or without cisplatin in locally advanced NSCLC.[58,59] The role of hydroxyurea is unclear in this setting because cisplatin and 5-FU alone have also been shown to be clinically effective radiosensitizers.

Gemcitabine

Mechanisms of Action
Gemcitabine (2′, 2′-difluoro-2′-deoxycytidine) is an analog of deoxycytidine that, unlike cytarabine, has demonstrated effectiveness as a single agent against solid tumors, including pancreatic cancer, lung cancer, and breast cancer. Gemcitabine exhibits cell-cycle specificity by affecting cells undergoing DNA synthesis (S-phase) and by blocking the progression of the cells through the G1/S-phase boundary.[60] Gemcitabine is metabolized intracellularly by deoxycytidine kinase to the active forms of diphosphate and triphosphate nucleosides. Gemcitabine diphosphate inhibits ribonucleotide reductase, which catalyzes reactions and generates deoxynucleoside triphosphates for DNA synthesis. The reduction of intracellular concentration of deoxycytidine triphosphate facilitates the incorporation of gemcitabine triphosphate into DNA. Further chain elongation is terminated after gemcitabine triphosphate and one additional nucleotide are incorporated into the growing DNA strands. Gemcitabine is rapidly metabolized to an inactive uridine derivative by cytidine deaminase. However, in comparison with ara-C, gemcitabine has greater membrane permeability and enzyme affinity, as well as considerably longer intracellular retention.

Preclinical Data with Radiation
Shewach et al. first reported on preclinical investigations of gemcitabine as a radiation sensitizer in human colon carci-

noma cells (HT-29).[61] Maximal radiation sensitization was observed when cells were irradiated immediately following gemcitabine exposure instead of before or during drug treatment. Radiation sensitization was found to be dose and time dependent. Exposures of 10 nmol/l for 24 hours or 30 nmol/l for 16 hours both produced a radiation enhancement ratio of approximately 2. Radiosensitization of gemcitabine has also been investigated on pancreatic cell lines.[62] Radiation enhancement ratios of 1.7 to 1.8 have been obtained. Sensitization occurred when gemcitabine depleted the dATP pools below the level of 1 nmol/l. The previous data thus suggest that radiation sensitization is achieved at very low gemcitabine plasma concentrations, which are not by themselves cytotoxic.

Conditions to obtain radiosensitization can be achieved either by a long (24-hour) exposure to a low concentration of gemcitabine (10 nmol/l) or by a brief (2-hour) treatment with higher but clinically relevant concentrations (100 nmol/l to 3 μmol/l).[63] Under the latter conditions, sensitization can be detected 4 hours after treatment and last for up to 2 days. The mechanism by which gemcitabine radiosensitizes tumor cells is unclear. Studies indicate that the observed radiosensitization is not associated with either an increase in the radiation-induced DNA double-strand breaks or with a slowing of DNA double-strand break repair.[64] This finding suggests that radiosensitization by gemcitabine is unlike that produced by the fluoropyrimidines and the thymidine analogs. However, radiosensitization is associated with the depletion of deoxyadenosine triphosphate pools, suggesting that inhibition of ribonucleotide reductase may be relevant.[61,62]

Clinical Experience
A phase I study in head and neck cancer used a starting dose of 300 mg/m² week of gemcitabine, along with standard dose radiation (70 Gy in 2-Gy fractions).[65] Gemcitabine was found to be a potent radiation enhancer, leading to marked increase in normal tissue toxicities within the radiation field. In addition, long-term sequelae were noted. Three patients required gastric tubes 5 months after radiation therapy. As a result, doses of gemcitabine in this study were decreased from an initial dose of 300 mg/m²/week to 150 mg/m²/week. However, the observed clinical activity was very encouraging. A phase I trial evaluating the role of gemcitabine as a radiation sensitizer in lung cancer is in progress.[66] The CALGB is conducting a phase II trial evaluating cisplatin and gemcitabine in combination as induction chemotherapy and as radiation enhancers in locally advanced NSCLC.[67]

5-Fluorouracil (5-FU)

Mechanisms of Action
Fluorouracil (5-FU) is a synthetic analog of the naturally occurring pyrimidine, uracil. Several active metabolites of 5-FU have pharmacologic effects on the synthesis and function of cellular DNA and RNA. Inhibition of thymidylate synthase (TS) by 5-fluorodeoxyuridine monophosphate (FdUMP) is believed to be the primary mechanism of anticancer efficacy of 5-FU. Other active metabolites include 5-fluorouridine triphosphate (FUTP) and 5-fluorodeoxyuridine triphosphate (FdUTP). FUTP is misincorporated into RNA and may affect several aspects of RNA stability and function. Similarly, FdUTP can be misincorporated into DNA. Fluorodeoxyuridine nucleotides that have been misincorporated into DNA are recognized and cleaved by a glycosylase, yielding apyrimidinic sites in the DNA double helix and leading to DNA strand breaks.

Preclinical Data with Radiation
Recent laboratory investigations point to biochemical events at the G1/S-phase interface as potentially important determinants of fluoropyrimidine radiosensitization. Our group has shown that the use of minimally cytotoxic doses of fluoropyrimidines prior to irradiation results in an immediate inhibition of TS followed by a later (within several hours) expansion of an early S-phase tumor cell population that correlates temporally with enhanced *in vitro* radiosensitivity.[64] The enhanced radiosensitivity of the early S-phase tumor cell population is not seen using cell synchronization techniques alone. Instead, the period of radiosensitization is best correlated with the time course of an altered dTTP/dATP radio resulting from TS inhibition.[64] It is speculated that an accelerated release of cells from the G1/S checkpoint occurs as a consequence of the nucleoside pool imbalance prior to complete repair of radiation damage. The relationships of the proposed molecular sensors at the G1/S checkpoint (e.g., p53, cyclin-dependent kinases) responsible for ionizing radiation repair and these biochemical perturbations resulting from TS inhibition are currently being studied.

Clinical Experience
Positive trials of combined 5-FU and radiation have been reported for head and neck, esophageal, pancreatic, rectal, and anal cancers. Use of 5-FU in lung cancer has been limited. Multiple trials have been reported; all combined with other chemotherapy agents. Cisplatin, 5-FU, and etoposide have been used as induction neoadjuvant therapy prior to surgery in three different trials.[68] 5-FU has also been combined with hydroxyurea, cisplatin and interferon, and radiation for advanced chest malignancies.[58] In one study, radiation was given with or without a five-day continuous infusion of 5-FU in locally advanced NSCLC. This study demonstrated that the combined therapy arm resulted in a significantly higher response rate but also more toxicity.

Fludarabine

Mechanisms of Action
Fludarabine phosphate (2-fluoro-ara-AMP) is a synthetic analog of the naturally occurring purine nucleotide, deoxy-

adenosine monophosphate, and is a fluorinated nucleotide analog of the antiviral agent vidarabine. Following intravenous infusion, fludarabine phosphate is rapidly dephosphorylated to 2-fluoro-ara-A; intracellularly, 2-fluoro-ara-A is rephosphorylated to the active triphosphate, 2-fluoro-ara-ATP. This triphosphate metabolite is an inhibitor of several key enzymes in deoxyribonucleotide metabolism and DNA synthesis, including ribonucleotide reductase, DNA polymerase alpha, and DNA primase, resulting in impaired DNA synthesis and repair.[69] Fludarabine has clinical activity against hematologic cancers such as chronic lymphocytic leukemia and follicular non-Hodgkin's lymphoma.

Preclinical Data with Radiation

Kim et al.[70] have demonstrated that treatment with fludarabine and radiation substantially increased the control rate of Meth-A fibrosarcomas in BALB/c mice compared to radiation treatment alone. Investigators at M.D. Anderson Cancer Center have shown that the administration of fludarabine at a dose of 800 mg/kg 1 hour prior to radiation treatment lengthened regrowth delay over a range of conditions, but particularly if irradiation was performed 24 hours after drug treatment.[71-73] Subsequent studies suggested that this delay in radiosensitization reflected a fludarabine-induced loss of radioresistant S-phase cells (through apoptosis) and partial synchronization of cells into G2/M 24 hours later.

Clinical Experience

No clinical trials of fludarabine and radiation have been reported to date.

Plant Derivatives

Paclitaxel

Mechanisms of Action

The FDA approved the production of semisynthetic paclitaxel in 1995, and this form has replaced the original, which was derived from the bark of *Taxus brevifolia*. Its unique mechanism of action as a promotor of microtubule assembly distinguishes paclitaxel from the vinca alkaloids and other tubulin-interacting drugs. All aspects of tubulin polymerization are enhanced at concentrations as low as 0.05 μmol/l. By stabilizing the microtubule and preventing its disassembly, paclitaxel causes tubulin-microtubule disequilibrium, which eventually leads to cell death.

Preclinical Data with Radiation

In one study, human lung carcinoma cells (SW1573) were given five daily treatments with 3 Gy of x-rays during the continuous presence of 5 nM of taxol.[74] This study demonstrated that taxol, continuously present at low concentration with little cytotoxicity, causes a progressive reduction of the surviving cell population in combination with fractionated radiation, mainly by inhibiting the repopulation of surviving cells between the dose fractions. Other studies have demonstrated that 1 to 10 nmol/L appears to be the optimal paclitaxel concentrations (when given as a continuous infusion) for direct cytotoxicity and radiosensitization *in vitro*.[75] Preclinical data also suggests that low-dose daily infusions of paclitaxel for as long as possible during a course of radiotherapy are more likely to result in radiosensitization and prolonged cytotoxicity than high infusions given once a week.[76] In this study, A375 melanoma and S549 lung carcinoma cell lines were used. The minimum concentration of paclitaxel for measurable radiosensitization was 3nM for both cell lines. A minimum of 18 hours incubation with the drug was necessary for measurable effects, and radiosensitizing effects were soon lost after the removal of paclitaxel. Pharmacokinetic calculations predict that 15 mg/m^2 paclitaxel given as a 1-hour infusion 5 days per week for 3 weeks during radiotherapy should achieve both cytotoxicity and radiosensitization. The presumed mechanism of action of paclitaxel as a radiosensitizer has been that this drug blocks cells at the radiosensitive G2-M interface.[77] This reaction is independent of the p53 mutations in lung cancer. Although p53 mutations have been associated with radioresistance in the case of NSCLC, p53 mutations do not predict response to paclitaxel/radiation in this disease.[78]

Clinical Experience

Of the newer drugs, paclitaxel combined with radiation has been the most studied in lung cancer. A continuous exposure to paclitaxel in the preclinical setting has demonstrated superior radiosensitizing effects, which has been studied in a phase I trial. Rosenthal et al. gave escalating doses of continuous-infusion paclitaxel over 7 weeks concurrently with radiation.[79] Dose-limiting toxicity was not achieved at the time of the report at a dose of 6.5 mg/m^2/day. In a phase I trial of continuous (120 hours) infusions of paclitaxel along with radiation in malignant mesothelioma and NSCLC, the MTD was 105 mg/m^2 repeated every 3 weeks.[80] Twice weekly paclitaxel has also been investigated with radiation.[81] The MTD of paclitaxel was 35 mg/m^2 given twice weekly as a 1-hour infusion for 6 weeks along with the radiation. The MTD of paclitaxel given as a weekly 3-hour infusion along with radiation has been shown to be 55 to 60 mg/m^2 week.[82] Pharmacokinetic data with weekly paclitaxel dosing of 100 to 250 mg/m^2 has been shown to yield plasma concentrations that remain above the putative radiosensitizing threshold of 0.01 μmol/L for 4.5 to 10.7 days.[83] Combinations of paclitaxel along with carboplatin and radiation have also been studied.[84-85]

Taxotere

Mechanisms of Action

Docetaxel is a semisynthetic derivative of 10-deacetyl baccatin, a precursor of paclitaxel. It is extracted from the needles of the European yew, *Taxus baccata,* an abundantly available and renewable source. Its mechanism of action is similar to that of paclitaxel, promoting microtubule assembly and stabilization, arresting cells in the M-phase of the cell cycle. In a head-to-head *in vitro* comparison against a variety of human tumors, docetaxel was more cytotoxic than paclitaxel (1.3- to 12-fold). In addition, cross-resistance between these two agents is incomplete.

Preclinical Data with Radiation

Although docetaxel has been shown to have additive effects when combined with radiation, controversy exists as to whether this combination is synergistic. An *in vitro* study by Choy et al.[86] found that both paclitaxel and docetaxel have radiosensitizing effects on the human leukemic cell line (HL-60). When these cells were treated with either drug, up to 70% of the cells were blocked in the G2/M-phase as determined by flow cytometry. The radiosensitizing effects were measured by calculating the dose of radiotherapy required to reduce survival to 25% of baseline, to determine the sensitizer enhancement ratio (SER). The SER was found to be 1.5 to 2.0 when a low concentration of docetaxel (0.3 μM) was used. The synergistic effect was hypothesized to occur because of the drug's ability to block the cells in G2/M. In contrast, a more recent study by Hennequin et al.[87] found no *in vitro* synergism with the combination of docetaxel and radiation using Hela cell lines. In another *in vitro* study, Watanabe et al.[88] also found no synergistic effects with docetaxel and radiation. In this study, lung cancer cell lines, RERF-LCMS (adenocarcinoma) and RERF-LCMA (small cell carcinoma) were exposed to docetaxel for 1 hour. Cells were irradiated for various periods, before and after the 1-hour drug exposure. The combination effects of radiation and drug were analyzed using an isobologram. Results from this study demonstrated that docetaxel with radiation had an additive effect on lung cancer cell lines, but no synergistic effects were noted. Finally, docetaxel has been shown to potentiate the radiation response of the murine mammary carcinoma MCa-4, with the proposed mechanisms being through an increase in radiosensitive mitotic cells (inducing arrest in the G2/M cell-cycle phase) and enhanced apoptosis.[89]

Clinical Experience

A phase I trial of concomitant docetaxel and radiation in locally advanced NSCLC has been conducted. Except for severe dysphagia at docetaxel doses above 30 mg/m^2 given on days 1, 6, 16, and 21 of radiation, this regimen was well tolerated.[90] A phase I/II of accelerated radiotherapy and weekly docetaxel in locally advanced NSCLC has also been conducted. Doses up to 30 mg/m^2 given weekly were well tolerated with an overall response of 73%.[91]

Vinorelbine

Mechanisms of Action

Vinorelbine is a unique semisynthetic vinca alkaloid derived from the leaves of the periwinkle plant. It differs from the natural vinca alkaloids by an eight-as opposed to a nine-member catharanthine ring. This unique structure may be responsible for its greater microtubule specificity and antitumor activity. It is a classic antitubulin in that it causes mitotic arrest of cells by inhibiting tubulin assembly. Vinorelbine causes less neurotoxicity than other vinca alkaloids.

Preclinical Data with Radiation

The activity of this combination *in vitro* was evaluated in the human NSCLC cell line NCI-H460.[92] When cells were exposed to navelbine for 24 hours and then irradiated, the drug potentiated radiation in a dose-dependent manner, with the ratio of fractional survival ranging from 1.7-fold at 1 Gy to 5.5-fold at 6 Gy. When treatment sequence was reversed (i.e., radiation followed by drug exposure), similar survival ratios were obtained at navelbine concentrations that were 10-fold lower. In this cell line, radiation produced a block in the G2/M-phase of the cell cycle with a maximum (60% to 70%) by 10 hours. The best potentiation was seen when irradiated cells were exposed to navelbine after they had plateaued in the G2/M-phase of the cycle. Navelbine given early after radiation, when only 10% to 30% of the cells were in G2/M, produced survival ratios similar to radiation alone. These studies show that navelbine acts as a radiosensitizer, and that the potentiation is cell cycle dependent, with a maximal effect being obtained when the cells have reached the G2/M-phase of the cycle.[92]

Clinical Experience

Patients with advanced chest malignancies that required radiation were enrolled in a phase I study of standard chest radiation and concurrent chemotherapy with cisplatin 100 mg/m^2 every 3 weeks and vinorelbine starting at 20 mg/m^2/week.[93] This regimen was feasible, and the recommended phase II dose was cisplatin 80 mg/m^2 every 3 weeks and vinorelbine 15 mg/m^2 on days 1 and 8 of the 3-week schedule. Esophagitis was the dose-limiting toxicity, and neutropenia occurred at higher doses. The CALGB is currently conducting a phase II trial of this regimen in unresectable stage III NSCLC.

Etoposide

Mechanisms of Action

Etoposide is a derivative of podophyllotoxin, itself extracted from the American mandrake or *Podophyllum peltatum.* The major mechanism of action is through interference with DNA synthesis by interaction with the enzyme topoisomerase II. This enzyme is responsible for "untangling" daughter chromosomes during mitosis. During this process, it causes transient DNA strand breaks. These breaks are then resealed by this same enzyme. The resealing is inhibited by etoposide, leading to permanent DNA strand breakage.

Preclinical Data with Radiation

Etoposide inhibits replication of DNA but does not stimulate repair.[94] *In vitro* studies have indicated an enhanced cell killing with radiation combined with etoposide. Rapidly repairable radiation-induced DNA damage is fixed into lethal lesions by etoposide. Cells arrested in G2-phase by radiation are hypersensitive to etoposide. Apoptosis, a result of the expression of the p53 gene, can be induced by radiation or etoposide in the presence of the gene but not in cells that lack both copies.[95] Giocanti et al.[96] described a decrease in the shoulder of the cell survival curve. Some increase in resistance of cell lines to etoposide has been reported after fractionated radiation. *In vivo* studies using the C3H mammary tumor model suggest that the major enhancement of radiation response is in hypoxic cells.[97]

Clinical Experience

Because etoposide is almost always employed with other chemotherapy agents for lung cancer, it is difficult to discern the effect related to radiosensitization with etoposide. Lau et al. have demonstrated improved survival with concurrent carboplatin/etoposide with radiation in poor-risk patients with locally advanced NSCLC.[98] However, radiosensitization may be caused by the platinum alone as demonstrated in a randomized trial with platinum and radiation alone.

Vincristine and Vinblastine

Mechanisms of Action

These agents are generally considered to cause mitotic inhibition with arrest at metaphase. This effect is caused by binding of the drug to a pair of sites on each subunit of tubulin, which results in blockage of assembly of microtubules during S-phase. Depolymerized tubulin proteins do not allow assembly of the mitotic spindle, and cell division is thus halted in metaphase.

Preclinical Data with Radiation

Little evidence exists of interaction of these drugs with radiation. In *in vivo* animal experiments, the LAF1 mouse exhibited an MTD of 9 mg/m.[2] There was no effect on the sublethal dose enhancement factor for lung, esophagus, or kidney. In the intestinal crypt cells, vincristine showed a DEF of 1.1 and yielded little cell kill for intestinal crypt cells. There was no effect on repair of ionizing radiation damage.

Clinical Experience

No trials of these agents combined with radiation have been performed in NSCLC. In SCLC, the CAV regimen, containing vincristine, has been used along with radiation.

Topoisomerase I Inhibitors

Mechanisms of Action

Topoisomerases are DNA enzymes that control the topology of the supercoiled DNA double helix during the transcription and replication of cellular genetic material. Topoisomerase I initiates the cleavage of a strand of the DNA molecule, whereas topoisomerase II cleaves both DNA strands. These actions guarantee the subsequent replicative process of the DNA. A partial or complete inhibition of this DNA replicative mechanism results in the accumulation and stability of cleavable complexes and subsequent cell death. Although this process is widely accepted as the main mechanism by which topoisomerase I inhibitors produce their antitumor effect, the mechanism by which this class of drugs achieves any selective toxicity in cancer cells is not fully understood.

Camptothecin and 9-aminocamptothecin

Preclinical Data with Radiation

Studies indicate that the addition of topoisomerase I inhibitors shortly after irradiation causes conversion of single-strand breaks to double-strand breaks, resulting in synergistic lethality to cultured log-phase or quiescent human tumor cells. Dramatic enhancement of the response of a human melanoma cell line (U1-Mel) has been seen with camptothecin.[99] 9-amino-camptothecin also enhanced the cytotoxicity of radiation in a schedule-dependent manner in U1-Mel tumor cells.[100] This study also indicated that an intact stereospecific interaction between camptothecin derivatives and DNA topoisomerase I is essential in the induction of radiosensitization.

Clinical Experience

There is no experience with the drugs in combination with radiation for lung cancer as yet.

Topotecan

Preclinical Data with Radiation

Preclinical evidence indicates that topotecan may inhibit DNA repair following sublethal doses of ionizing radiation. Enhanced cytotoxicity was noted when topotecan was present during the first 30 minutes after single or multiple doses of irradiation.[101–103] The effect of topotecan on ionizing radiation-induced cytotoxicity has been studied in NSCLC H460 cell lines (containing high levels of topoisomerase I levels) and in glioblastoma multiforme cell lines (containing low topoisomerase I levels).[104] In this study, topotecan had a superadditive effect to radiation in the glioblastoma multiforme cell lines but not in the H460 cell line, suggesting that a potential clinical interaction exists for topoisomerase I inhibitors in combination with radiation for tumors expressing low topoisomerase I levels. Several studies were conducted to examine the effect of varying doses and time sequences of topotecan administration with respect to the administration of irradiation. Radiation sensitization appeared to depend on the drug concentration, the administration time, and exposure time.[101-103] Boscia et al.[105] demonstrated that radiation sensitization of topotecan was improved when daily administration of topotecan was followed by daily fractionated radiation as compared to a single dose of the drug with a single dose of irradiation.

Clinical Experience
A dose escalation clinical study with topotecan and concurrent radiation in patients with inoperable NSCLC has been conducted.[106] The MTD of topotecan was 0.5 mg/m^2 when given on days 1 to 5 and days 22 to 26 during a 6-week course (60 Gy) of external beam radiotherapy. Higher doses of topotecan were associated with high hematologic and gastrointestinal toxicity.

Irinotecan

Preclinical Data with Radiation
The ability of CPT-11 to increase tumor radiation-response *in vivo* using human lung tumor xenogratfs has been investigated.[107] Combinations of CPT-11 and radiation resulted in greater tumor regression compared to either modality alone. In flow cytometry studies, the proportion of cells in G2/M-phase, the most radiosensitive phase, increased after 1-hour exposure to the lowest dose of SN-38 (0.5 ng/ml), the active metabolite for CPT-11. The interaction of SN-38 and radiation *in vitro* in monolayer cultures and multicellular spheroids of HT-29 human colon adenocarcinoma cells has been studied.[108] SN-38 at a concentration of 2.5 μg/ml, which by itself was not cytotoxic, greatly increased the lethal effects of radiation in spheroids. Exposure to SN-38 following irradiation inhibited the PLDR. This reaction suggests that the mechanism of the radiosensitization by SN-38 is caused by PLDR repair inhibition.

Clinical Experience
A phase I/II study of concurrent chemoradiotherapy with CPT-11 and cisplatin was conducted to determine the maximum tolerated dose and efficacy of this regimen in patients with advanced NSCLC.[109] This trial had to be discontinued because of severe diarrhea and leukopenia causing chemotherapy delays as well as early termination of radiation. A trial of irinotecan alone with radiation is ongoing.

Platinum Analogs

Mechanisms of Action
The mechanism of cytotoxicity of the platinum analogs is similar to alkylating agents, and these drugs are therefore considered to be nonclassical alkylators. In the relatively high chloride concentrations of plasma, the cisplatin complex is deionized and able to pass through cell membranes. In the presence of low intracellular chloride concentrations, the chloride ligands of the complex are displaced by water and produce the positively charged platinum compound, which is toxic and probably the active form of the drug. The *cis* isomer forms intrastrand and interstrand cross-links between guanine-guanine pairs of DNA and inhibits DNA synthesis. Cisplatin to a lesser extent binds to protein and RNA, ultimately inhibiting RNA synthesis. Carboplatin is a cytotoxic platinum complex that, similar to cisplatin, reacts with nucleophilic sites on DNA.

Cisplatin

Preclinical Data with Radiation
Cisplatin is one of the drugs that has been most extensively studied for its interaction with radiation. A recent review published by Wheeler and Spencer[110] reported that cisplatin enhances the cytotoxicity of ionizing radiation in several studies using human tumor cell lines in both cell culture and tumor-bearing animals. The drug appears to cause supraadditive effects when given simultaneously with radiation. It also appears to inhibit the repair of sublethal damage. It is a hypoxic cell sensitizer at high doses, although it is unlikely that clinical doses achieve significant hypoxic cell sensitization. Some data suggest that at low doses per fraction, a DEF of 2.3 can be seen.[111] Fractionated radiation *in vitro* can induce cisplatin resistance in surviving cells.[112]

Cisplatin can also enhance radiation effects on normal tissues. The MTD in the LAF mouse is 40 mg/m.^{2} At this dose, a DEF of 1.2 is seen in the lung and of 1.7 in the esophagus. With single doses at this level, no enhancement is seen in the kidney. Stewart et al. found a DEF of 1.1 when cisplatin was given 6 hours before but not after radiation.[113] Liliveld et al. demonstrated the highest degree of radiation enhancement of tumor cell kill when cisplatin was administered in a divided daily schedule before radiation.[114] That schedule also resulted in less enhancement of normal tissue toxicities, which is an important observation.

Synergism between cisplatin and 5-FU has been demonstrated in preclinical models *in vitro* and *in vivo*. Scanlon et al. have demonstrated[115] that cisplatin inhibits cellular uptake of methionine and stimulates endogenous synthesis of methionine from homocysteine, consequently increasing conversion of CH3-FH4 to FH4, a precursor of CH2-FH4. The resulting expanded reduced-folate pools enhance the inhibition of thymidylate synthase by FdUMP. Because both cisplatin and 5-FU have radiosensitizing properties, a rationale exists for using these agents in combination with radiotherapy.

Clinical Experience
Significant clinical experience with cisplatin as a radiation sensitizer exists. Trials in head and neck as well as cancer of the esophagus have shown improved outcome with com-

bined chemoradiation when cisplatin and 5-FU are given. The most compelling evidence for the effect of cisplatin alone as a chemosensitizer in locally advanced lung cancer comes from the EORTC,[17] which compared three groups treated with radiation alone, radiation plus weekly cisplatin (30 mg/m2), and radiation plus daily cisplatin (6 mg/m^2). Survival was significantly improved in the combined therapy arms, especially with the use of daily cisplatin (p = 0.0009). The fact that the most benefit was seen in the treatment arm with low-dose daily cisplatin (unlikely to have a direct cytotoxic effect) and that the benefit in survival was only caused by an improvement in local control, is very strong evidence for clinical benefits of radiation enhancement by cisplatin. Numerous studies have combined cisplatin with other drugs along with concomitant radiation, and a complete review is beyond the scope of this chapter. Lau et al. demonstrated excellent one- and two-year survival rates with combined cisplatin and etoposide and concurrent radiation for locally advanced NSCLC.[98] Of interest is that only one randomized trial of sequential chemoradiation versus concomitant chemoradiation has been published in locally advanced NSCLC. This trial demonstrated statistically improved two-year survival rates for the concomitant arm, suggesting a role for radiosensitization and improved survival by improving local control.[116]

Carboplatin

Preclinical Data with Radiation
The interaction between moderate-dose radiation and carboplatin was studied in cisplatin-sensitive (GLC4) and -resistant (GLC4-CDDP) human SCLC cell lines.[117] The radiosensitizing effect of the platinum drugs was expressed as an enhancement ratio calculated directly from survival levels of the initial slope of the curve. Carboplatin showed increased enhancement with prolonged incubation up to 1.21 in GLC4 and was equally effective as cisplatin in GLC4-CDDP. According to the isobologram analysis, prolonged incubation with both platinum drugs showed at least additivity with radiation for both cell lines at clinically achievable doses. The radiosensitizing capacity on both lung cancer cell lines did not depend on their platinum sensitivity. This study showed that the interaction of radiation with the clinically less toxic carboplatin can be improved by prolonged low-dose exposure before irradiation and is as potent as cisplatin in the resistant lung cancer cell line. Evidence for radiosensitization by carboplatin with an enhancement ratio of 1.8 is reported in Chinese hamster lung cells (V79) irradiated in culture under hypoxic conditions.[118] Potentiation of radiotherapy in mice bearing a transplanted mouse mammary tumor (MTG-B) is reported as a supraadditive tumor growth delay when 60 mg/kg carboplatin is administered either 30 minutes before or immediately after 20 Gy of irradiation. Carboplatin is believed to be more effective than cisplatin as a sensitizing agent because higher concentrations of the drug are achieved in free solution. Thus radiation enhancement, which is concentration dependent, might occur more rapidly with carboplatin than with cisplatin.

Clinical Experience
A phase II study of daily carboplatin (25 mg/m^2) given along with accelerated fractionated irradiation to 60 Gy over 4 weeks for locally advanced NSCLC demonstrated a response rate of 84% in 31 patients.[119] Similarly, a phase II study of split-dose radiation along with carboplatin given on day 1 of week 1 and week 6 has been performed with a response rate of 53%.[120] Responders had a significantly higher area under the curve (AUC) of carboplatin than nonresponders in this study. A phase III trial of accelerated radiation therapy with and without carboplatin (350 mg/m^2 day 1, every 28 days) in locally advanced NSCLC is ongoing.[121] Interim analysis showed increased hematologic and esophageal toxicities when carboplatin was added. Trials have also been conducted with the combination of carboplatin and etoposide given along with radiation.

Antimetabolites

Because methotrexate and other antimetabolites are cell-cycle specific, their administration alters the kinetics of surviving cells. Cells in the late S-phase of the cycle are known to be less sensitive to radiation therapy. Certain antimetabolites, however, are active against these cells.

Methotrexate

Mechanisms of Action
Methotrexate (MTX), a synthetic analog of folic acid, is a potent inhibitor of dihydrofolate reductase (DHFR), a key enzyme in folate metabolism. Inhibition of DHFR results in depletion of cellular-reduced folates and interferes with vital cellular enzymes that require reduced folate cofactors (including enzymes of the thymidylate and purine synthesis and amino acid metabolism). Intracellularly, methotrexate is metabolized to active polyglutamate metabolites, which inhibit DHFR and several other cellular enzymes, including enzymes that catalyze formyl transfer reactions in purine biosynthesis.

Preclinical Data with Radiation
Dose-response curves in an experimental mammary tumor indicate that MTX generally kills less than one log of cells using an *in vivo/in vitro* assay and exhibits a mild linear reduction with dose as evidenced by increasing growth delay. Experiments in a rat rhabdomyosarcoma cell line with MTX and radiation showed no evidence of a supraadditive effect.[122] An *in vivo* lung experimental system with MTX has shown a DEF of 1.6 (1.3 to 2).[123] In this experiment, MTX was given at high doses (2.1 gm/m^2) 2 hours before

irradiation. No significant effect was seen on esophageal or renal toxicities with these doses. Using a normal intestinal crypt system, MTX yielded a DEF of 1 to 1.8, depending on dose, with the higher value at the higher doses.

Clinical Experience

MTX has been shown to enhance late CNS damage when used in high doses and with whole-brain irradiation. Similar effects can be seen with intrathecal methotrexate when combined with radiation. MTX has also been shown to enhance skin and mucosal toxicity when given with radiation in head and neck cancer patients. The cyclophosphamede methotrexcite and 5–fleurouracil (CMF) regimen containing methotrexate when given with breast radiation in the adjuvant setting increases pulmonary toxicity. Trials of methotrexate with radiation in lung cancer are almost all in the setting of combination chemotherapy, and thus the sole effect of methotrexate cannot be determined. However, a trial reported in the early 1970s that combined methotrexate with radiation therapy for squamous cell carcinoma of the lung suggested no clinical tumor interaction.

Alkylating Agents

Because alkylating agents have been shown to be ineffective in patients with NSCLC,[15] their clinical use in this setting has largely been abandoned. Additionally, alkylating agents can cause pulmonary toxicity. They are used extensively in other malignancies, so their interactions with radiation are reviewed here.

Mechanisms of Action

Alkylating agents are polyfunctional compounds that have the ability to substitute alkyl groups for hydrogen ions. These compounds react with phosphate, amino, hydroxyl, sulfhydryl, carboxyl, and imidazole groups, which are part of the molecular makeup of the body. In neutral or alkaline solution, these drugs ionize and produce positively charged ions that attach to susceptible nuclear proteins, with the most likely site of alkylation being the N-7 position of guanine. This alkylation reaction can have multiple effects, including abnormal base pairing with cleavage of the imidazole ring of guanine; cross-linking of DNA with interference with DNA replication and transcription of RNA; and the disruption of nucleic acid function. Disruption of DNA adducts represents the predominant mechanism of cytotoxicity. The alkylating agents are not cell cycle–specific agents.

Cyclophosphamide

Preclinical Data with Radiation

Byfield concluded from *in vitro* experiments that cyclophosphamide had no effect on radiation survival curves and that effects were strictly additive.[124] Experiments with *in vivo* spheroids reveal that cyclophosphamide is more effective

against the superficial cells but is additive to radiation at all depths.[125] Experimentally in rat hepatoma, Looney et al. showed that alternating chemotherapy with cyclophosphamide and radiation induces a maximal amount of tumor response.[126] Several studies have evaluated cyclophosphamide with radiotherapy and have shown increased injury in the normal tissues, including CNS, lung, bladder, small intestine, esophagus, and skin. The maximum tolerance dose (MTD) in mice is 250 mg/m.[2] At this dose, cyclophosphamide exhibits a DEF of 2.1 for pulmonary lethality but shows little interaction in the normal esophagus. With delayed irradiation, residual cyclophosphamide effect on the DEF was seen at up to 6 months.[127]

Nitrosureas

Preclinical Data with Radiation

In vitro studies indicate increased cell killing, which in some cases is additive, and in others, supraadditive. Decreases in the initial slope and in the final slope of the survival curve are noted. Radiation induces O6 alkyl-transferase, which creates resistance to N,N^1–bio(2-chlomethyl–)N–nitrosourea (BCNU), greatest at 48 hours after irradiation. The production of radiation-induced single-strand breaks is enhanced in human glioma tumor cell lines.[128] The induction of sister chromatid exchanges by radiation and BCNU appears only to be additive. *In vivo* experimental tumors, including the 9L brain tumor, the KHT sarcoma, and the EMT6 tumor, have shown increased animal survival, decreased metastases, and improved locoregional response with BCNU plus irradiation. In the EMT6 tumor, the greatest effect was seen with drug after irradiation, and the effect was supraadditive. Others[129] suggest that nitrosureas fix radiotherapy-induced DNA damage and that BCNU should be given 6 to 16 hours before or after radiation so that DNA cross-linking products can interact. In the LAF1 mouse, the MTD of BCNU is 75 mg/m.[2] The dose does not appear to enhance radiation injury to the lung, but it does increase the esophageal reaction with a DEF of 1.4. It shows no significant effect in the kidney.

Antitumor Antibiotics

Anthracyclines

Mechanisms of Action

Interference with the action of DNA topoisomerase II in regions of transcriptionally active DNA is the most widely cited and generally accepted mechanism of action of the anthracyclines. This enzyme acts by binding to DNA and nicking one of its strands, thus allowing the supercoiled macromolecule to relax as the opposite strand passes through the break. The enzyme then reanneals the broken ends. Anthracyclines are thought to act by stabilizing the topoisomerase-DNA complex in the cleaved configuration.

This event not only maintains the DNA single-strand breaks but also helps to create further DNA double-strand breaks. The ability of these drugs to generate free radicals, which are cytotoxic, has attracted much attention. Anthracyclines are reactive with heavy metal ions. In the cell, adriamycin binds to ferric iron, which then generates highly reactive hydroxyl radical species. This complex binds to cell membranes and causes oxidative cell damage; most tissues possess adequate defenses against this type of event and are able to repair the damage. Cardiac tissue is notably deficient in this respect and is highly vulnerable to oxidative attack.

Preclinical Data with Radiation

In vitro experiments reveal that doxorubicin reduces the cellular capacity to accumulate and repair radiation damage throughout the cell cycle. Double-strand break repair is inhibited.[130] These findings are similar for resistant and sensitive cell lines.[131] Indeed, no evidence exists for an induction of adriamycin resistance by previous irradiation. Experiments in spheroids suggest that drug exposure before irradiation gives maximal enhancement.[132] In the LAFI mouse, the MTD is 24 mg/m.^{2} At this dose, the DEF is 1.3 in lung, 1.9 in kidney, and 1.2 for intestinal crypt cells but not significantly elevated in esophagus. Maximal cell kill occurs when doxorubicin is delivered 12 hours after irradiation. Doxorubicin decreases SLDR in intestinal crypt cells by 10%. The greatest degree of reaction occurs with simultaneous administration; however, prolonged residual effects have been noted, as tested by delayed radiation exposure.

Clinical Experience

Clinically, in both NSCLC and SCLC, adriamycin has been used in different combination chemotherapy regimens with and without radiation. No trial of adriamycin alone with radiation in lung cancer has been performed. Enhanced cardiac toxicity with mediastinal radiation and doxorubicin treatment is well established. Furthermore, the radiation recall phenomenon is well established for this agent.

Mitomycin C

Mechanisms of Action

Mitomycin C is a bioreductive alkylating agent requiring *in vivo* activation to the cytotoxic species.

Preclinical Data with Radiation

Mitomycin C has been shown experimentally to interact with radiation through killing of hypoxic cells. This activity is probably not major at doses achievable in the clinic. Various *in vitro* experiments have described additive or supraadditive effects with radiation.[133,134] *In vivo* studies reveal both additive and supraadditive effects. Mitomycin does not change the shape of the radiation survival curve. Acute radiation reactions of skin and soft tissues are enhanced by mitomycin.[135]

Clinical Experience

Mitomycin C has been shown to be an integral component of treatment of squamous cell carcinoma of the anus when given along with 5-FU and radiation. A randomized trial of 5-FU and radiation with or without mitomycin C showed inferior results and increased local relapse in the group not receiving mitomycin C, suggesting that this agent has clinically relevant effects when given with radiation. Furthermore, the only trial in which concomitant chemoradiation was shown to be superior to sequential chemotherapy followed by radiation in locally advanced NSCLC used the MVP regimen, which contains mitomycin C. Multiple other studies have been performed in which mitomycin was used as part of the combination chemotherapy regimen.

REFERENCES

1. Steel GG. Terminology of clinical combined radiotherapy-chemotherapy. *Radiother and Oncol* 1989;14:315.
2. Phillips TL. Chemoradiotherapy. In: John MJ, Flam MS, Legha SS, et al. *Chemoradiation, an integrated approach.* Lea & Febiger, 1993:12.
3. Steel GG, Peckham MJ. Exploitable mechanisms in combined radiotherapy-chemotherapy: the concept of additivity. *Int J Rad Oncol Biol Phys* 1979;5(1):85.
4. Davis TW, Myers M, Wilson-Van Patten C, et al. Transcriptional responses to damage created by ionizing radiation: molecular sensors. In: Nickoloff JA and Hoekstra MF eds. *DNA damage and repair,* vol. 2. *DNA repair in higher eukaryotes.* Humana Press, 1998:223.
5. Cox JD, Azarnia N, Byhardt RW, et al. A randomized phase I/II trial of hyperfractionated radiation therapy with total doses of 60.0Gy to 79.2Gy: possible survival benefit with greater than or equal to 69.9Gy in favorable patients with Radiation Therapy Oncology Group stage III non-small-cell lung carcinoma: report of the Radiation Therapy Oncology Group 83–11. *J Clin Oncol* 1990;8(9):1543.
6. Begg AC, Fu KK, Kane LJ, et al. Single agent chemotherapy of a solid murine tumour assayed by growth delay and cell survival. *Cancer Res* 1980;40(1):145.
7. Hill BT. Interactions between antitumour agents and radiation and the expression of resistance. *Cancer Treatment Revs* 1991;18:149.
8. DeVita VT, Jr. The relationship between tumour mass and resistance to chemotherapy. *Cancer* 1988;51(7):1209.
9. Patel NH, Rothenberg ML. Multidrug resistance in cancer chemotherapy. *Invest New Drugs* 1994;12(1):1.
10. Carney DN, Mitchell JB, Kinsella TJ. *In vitro* radiation and chemotherapy sensitivity of established cell lives of human small cell lung cancer and its large cell morphologic variants. *Cancer Res* 1983;43:2806.
11. Munro AJ. An overview of randomised controlled trials of adjuvant chemotherapy in head and neck cancer. *Br J Cancer* 1997;71(1):83.
12. Goldie JH, Coldman AJ, Gudauskas GA. Rationale for use of noncross-resistant chemotherapy. *Cancer Treat Rep* 1982;66(3):439.
13. Day R. Treatment sequencing, uncertainty and asymmetry: Protocol strategies for combination chemotherapy. *Cancer Res* 1986;46(8):3876.
14. Tubiana M, Arriagada R, Cosset JM. Sequencing of drugs and

radiation. The integrated alternating regimen. *Cancer* 1985; 55(9 Suppl) 2131.

15. Non-small Cell Lung Cancer Collaborative Group. Chemotherapy in non-small cell lung cancer: a meta-analysis using updated data on individual patients from 52 randomised clinical trials. *BMJ* 1995;311(7010):899.

16. Dillman RO, Seagren SL, Propert KJ, et al. A randomized trial of induction chemotherapy plus high-dose radiation versus radiation alone in stage III non-small cell lung cancer. *N Engl J Med* 1990;323:940.

17. Schakke-Koning C, van den Bogaert W, Dalesio O, et al. Effects of concomitant cisplatin and radiotherapy on inoperable non-small-cell lung cancer. *N Engl J Med* 1992;326:524.

18. Saunders MI. Is control of the primary tumour worthwhile in non-oat cell carcinoma of the bronchus? *Clin Oncol* (RCR) 1991;3(4):185.

19. Saunders M, Dische S, Barrett A, et al. Continuous hyperfractionated accelerated radiotherapy (CHART) versus conventional radiotherapy in non-small cell lung cancer: a randomised multi-centre trial. *Lancet* 1997;350:161.

20. Tejedor M, Valerdi JJ, Lopez R, et al. Mitomycin, cisplatin and vindesine followed by radiotherapy combined with cisplatin in stage III non-small cell lung cancer: long-term results. *Int J Rad Oncol Biol Phys* 1995;31(4):813.

21. Burkes RL, Ginsberg RJ, Shepherd FA, et al. Induction chemotherapy with mitomycin, vindesine, and cisplatin for stage III unresectable non-small cell lung cancer: results of the Toronto phase II trial. *J Clin Oncol* 1992;10(4):580.

22. von Pawel J, Wagner H, Niederle N, et al. Phase II study of paclitaxel and cisplatin in patients with non-small cell lung cancer. 1996, *Semin Oncol* 23(6 Suppl 16):47.

23. Blanke C, Ansari R, Mantravadi R, et al. Phase III trial of thoracic irradiation with or without cisplatin for locally advanced unresectable non-small-cell lung cancer: a Hoosier Oncology Group Protocol. *J Clin Oncol* 1995;13(6):1425.

24. Trovo MG, Minatel E, Giovanni F, et al. Radiotherapy versus radiotherapy enhanced by cisplatin in stage III non-small cell lung cancer. *Int J Rad Oncol Biol Phys* 1992;24(1):11.

25. Trovo MG, Gigante M, Minatel E, et al. Combined modality treatment of locally advanced lung cancer. *Tumori* 1998;84:259.

26. Vokes EE, Leopold KA, Herndon J, et al. Investigations of new drugs in combination with cisplatin in stage III non-small cell lung cancer. *Semin Oncol* 1997;24(3) Suppl 8:42.

27. Langer CJ, Movsas B, Hudes R, et al. Induction paclitaxel and carboplatin followed by concurrent chemoradiotherapy in patients with unresectable, locally advanced non-small cell lung carcinoma: report of Fox Chase Cancer Centre study 94-001. *Semin Oncol* 1997;24(4) Suppl 12:89.

28. Isokangas OP, Joensuu H, Halme M, et al. Paclitaxel (Taxol) and carboplatin followed by concomitant paclitaxel, cisplatin and radiotherapy for inoperable stage III NSCLC. *Lung Cancer* 1998;20(2):127.

29. Choy H, Akerley W, Safran, et al. Multiinstitutional phase II trial of paclitaxel, carboplatin, and concurrent radiation therapy for locally advanced non-small-cell lung cancer. *J Clin Oncol* 1998;16(10):3316.

30. Socinski MA, Clark JA, Halle J, et al. Induction therapy with carboplatin/paclitaxel followed by concurrent carboplatin/paclitaxel and dose-escalating conformal radiotherapy in the treatment of locally advanced, unresectable non-small cell lung cancer: preliminary report of a phase I trial. *Semin Oncol* 1997; 24(4) Suppl 12:117.

31. Jeremic B, Shibamoto Y, Acimovic L, et al. Hyperfractionated radiation therapy with or without concurrent low dose daily Carboplatin/Etoposide for stage III non-small-cell lung cancer: a randomized study. *J Clin Oncol* 1996;14(4):1065.

32. Kelly K, Hazuka M, Pan Z, et al. A phase I study of daily carboplatin and simultaneous accelerated, hyperfractionated chest irradiation in patients with regionally inoperable non-small cell lung cancer. *Int J Rad Oncol Biol Phys* 1998;40(3):559.

33. Mirimanoff RO, Moro D, Bolla M, et al. Alternating radiotherapy and chemotherapy for inoperable stage III non-small-cell lung cancer: long-term results of two Phase II GOTHA trials. Groupe d'Oncologie Thoracique Alpine. *Int J Rad Oncol Biol Phys* 1998;42(3):487.

34. Clamon G, Herndon J, Cooper R, et al. Radiosensitization with carboplatin for patients with unresectable stage III non-small-cell lung cancer: a phase III trial of the Cancer and Leukemia Group B and the Eastern Cooperative Oncology Group. *J Clin Oncol* 1999;17(1):4.

35. Vokes EE, Masters GA, Mauer AM, et al. Clinical Studies of Docetaxel (Taxotere) and Concomitant Chest Radiation Therapy. *Semin Oncol* 1997;24(4) Suppl 14:26.

36. Lamond JP, Kinsella TJ, Boothman DA. Concentration and timing dependence of lethality enhancement between topotecan, a topoisomerase I inhibitor, and ionizing radiation. *Int J Rad Oncol Biol Phys* 1996;36(2):361.

37. Pignon JP, Arriagada R, Ihde DC, et al. A meta-analysis of thoracic radiotherapy for small-cell lung cancer. *N Engl J Med* 1992;327:1618.

38. Murray N, Coy P, Pater J, et al. Importance of timing for thoracic irradiation in the combined modality treatment of limited-stage small-cell lung cancer. *J Clin Oncol* 1993;11(2):336.

39. Turrisi A III, Johnson DH, Comis RL. In: Small cell lung cancer. John MJ, Flam MS, Legha SS, et al. *Chemoradiation, an integrated approach.* Philadelphia: Lea & Febiger, 1993:347.

40. Johnson BE, Bridges JD, Sobczeck M, et al. Patients with limited-stage small-cell lung cancer treated with concurrent twice-daily chest radiotherapy and etoposide/cisplatin followed by cyclophosphamide, doxorubicin and vincristine. *J Clin Oncol* 1996;14(3):806.

41. Thomas CR Jr, Giroux DJ, Stelzer KJ, et al. Concurrent cisplatin, prolonged oral etoposide, and vincristine plus chest and brain irradiation for limited small cell lung cancer: a phase II study of the Southwest Oncology Group (SWOG-9229). *Int J Rad Oncol Biol Phys* 1998;40(5)1039.

42. Gregor A, Drings P, Burghouts J, et al. Randomized trial of alternating versus sequential radiotherapy/chemotherapy in limited-disease patients with small-cell lung cancer: a European Organization for Research and Treatment of Cancer Lung Cancer Cooperative Group Study. *J Clin Oncol* 1997;15(8):2840.

43. Beith JM, Clarke SJ, Woods RL, et al. Long-term follow-up of a randomised trial of combined chemoradiotherapy induction treatment, with and without maintenance chemotherapy in patients with small cell carcinoma of the lung. *Eur J Cancer* 1996; 32A(3):438.

44. Giaccone G, Dalesio O, McVie GJ, et al. Maintenance chemotherapy in small-cell lung cancer: long-term results of a randomized trial. European Organization for Research and Treatment of Cancer Lung Cancer Cooperative Group. *J Clin Oncol* 1993; 11(7):1230.

45. Arriagada R, Le Chevalier T, Borie F, et al. Prophylactic cranial irradiation for patients with small-cell lung cancer in complete remission. *J Natl Canc Inst* 1995;87(3):183.

46. Gregor A, Cull A, Stephens RJ, et al. Prophylactic cranial irradiation is indicated following complete response to induction therapy in small cell lung cancer; results of a multicentre randomised trial. *Eur J Cancer* 1997;33(11):1752.

47. Yarbro JW. Mechanism of action of hydroxyurea. *Semin Oncol* 1992;19(suppl 9):1.
48. Donehower RC. An overview of the clinical experience with hydroxyurea. *Semin Oncol* 1992;19(suppl 9):11.
49. Kuo ML, Kinsella TJ. Expression of ribonucleotide reductase following ionizing radiation in human cervical carcinoma cells. *Cancer Res* 1998;58:2245.
50. Fram RJ, Kufe DW. Inhibition of DNA excision repair and the repair of x-ray induced DNA damage by cytosine arabinoside and hydroxyurea. *Pharmacol Ther* 1985;31:165.
51. Kuo ML, Kunugi KA, Lindstrom MJ, et al. The interation of hydroxyurea and ionizing radiation in human cervical carcinoma cells. *Cancer J Sci Amer* 1997;3:163.
52. Moran RG, Danenberg PV, Heidelberger C. Therapeutic response of leukemic mice treated with fluorinated pyrimidines and inhibitors of deoxyuridylate synthesis. *Biochem Pharmacol* 1982;31:2929.
53. Kuo ML, Kunugi KA, Lindstrom MJ, et al. The interaction of hydroxyurea and iododeoxyuridine on the radiosensitivity of human bladder cancer cells. *Cancer Res* 1995;55:2800.
54. Lerner HJ. Concomitant hydroxyurea and irradiation. Clinical experience with 100 patients with advanced head and neck cancer at Pennsylvania hospital. *Am J Surg* 1977;134:505.
55. Levin VA, Silver P, Hannigan J, et al. Superiority of post-radiotherapy adjuvant chemotherapy with CCNU, procarbazine and vincristine over BCNU for anaplastic gliomas:NCOG 6G61 final report. *Int J Radiat Oncol Biol Phys* 1990;18:321.
56. Piver MS, Barlow JJ, Vongtama V, et al. Hydroxyurea as a radiation sensitizer in women with carcinoma of the uterine cervix. *Am J Obstet Gynecol* 1977;129:379.
57. Stehman FB, Bundy BN, Thomas G, et al. Hydroxyurea versus misonidazole with radiation in cervical carcinoma: long-term follow-up of a Gynecologic Oncology Group trial. *J Clin Oncol* 1993;11:1523.
58. Vokes EE. 5-FU/oral leucovorin/hydroxyurea with concomitant radiotherapy for stage III non-small cell lung cancer. *Cancer* 1990;66:437.
59. Vokes EE. 5-FU, leucovorin, hydroxyurea and escalating doses of continuous infusion cisplatin with concomitant radiotherapy: a clinical and pharmacologic study. *Cancer Chemother Pharmacol* 1992;29:178.
60. Huang P, Chubb S, Hertel LW, et al. Action of 2'-2'-difluorodeoxycytidine on DNA synthesis. *Cancer Res* 1991;51:6110.
61. Shewach DS, Hahn TM, Chang E, et al. Metabolism of 2',2'-difluoro-2'-deoxycytidine and radiation sensitization of human colon carcinoma cells. *Cancer Res* 1994;54:3218.
62. Lawrence TS, Chang EY, Hahn TM, et al. Radiosensitization of pancreatic cancer cells by 2',2'-difluoro-2'-deoxycytidine. *Int J Radiat Oncol Biol Phys* 1996;34:846.
63. Lawrence TS, Eisbruch A, Shewach DS. Gemcitabine-mediated radiosensitization. *Semin Oncol* 1997;24(suppl 7):24.
64. Kinsella TJ. An approach to the radiosensitization of human tumors. *Cancer J Sci Amer* 1996;2:184.
65. Eisbruch A, Shewach DS, Urba S, et al. Phase I trial of radiation concurrently with low-dose gemcitabine for head and neck cancer, high mucosal and pharyngeal toxicity. *Proc Am Soc Clin Oncol* 1997;16:A1377.
66. Gregor A. Gemcitabine plus radiotherapy for non-small cell lung cancer. *Semin Oncol* 1997;24(suppl 8):39.
67. Vokes EE, Leopold KA, Herndon JE, et al. A CALGB randomized phase II study of gemcitabine or paclitaxel or vinorelbine with cisplatin as induction chemotherapy and concomitant chemoradiotherapy in stage IIIB non-small cell lung cancer: Feasibility data. *Proc Am Soc Clin Oncol USA* 1997;16:A1636.
68. Rice TW, Adelstein DJ, Koka A, et al. Accelerated induction therapy and resection for poor prognosis stage III non-small cell lung cancer. *Ann Thorac Surg* 1995;60:586.
69. Plunkett W, Gandhi V, Huang P, et al. Fludarabine: pharmacokinetics, mechanisms of action, and rationales for combination therapies. *Semin Oncol* 1993;20(suppl 7):2.
70. Kim JH, Alfieri AA, Kim SH, et al. The potentiation of radiation response on murine tumor by fludarabine phosphate. *Cancer Lett* 1986;36:369.
71. Gregoire V, Hunter N, Milas L, et al. Potentiation of radiation-induced regrowth delay in murine tumors by fludarabine. *Cancer Res* 1994;54:468.
72. Gregoire V, Van NT, Stephens LC, et al. The role of fludarabine-induced apoptosis and cell cycle synchronization in enhanced murine tumor radiation response in vivo. *Cancer Res* 1994;54:6201.
73. Gregoire V, Hunter N, Brock WA, et al. Fludarabine improves the therapeutic ratio of radiotherapy in mouse tumors after single-dose irradiation. *Int J Radiat Oncol Biol Phys* 1994;30:363.
74. Van Rijn J, van den Berg J, Meijer OW. Proliferation and clonal survival of human lung cancer cells treated with fractionated irradiation in combination with paclitaxel. *Int J Radiat Oncol Biol Phys* 1995;33:635.
75. Rosenthal DI, Close LG, Lucci JA, et al. Phase I studies of continuous-infusion paclitaxel given with standard aggressive radiation therapy for locally advanced solid tumors. *Semin Oncol* 1995;22(suppl 9):13.
76. Zanelli GD, Quaia M, Robieux I, et al. Paclitaxel as a radiosensitiser: a proposed schedule of administration based on in vitro data and pharmacokinetic calculations. *Eur J Cancer* 1997;33: 486.
77. Vokes EE, Harf DJ, Stenson K, et al. The role of paclitaxel in the treatment of head and neck cancer. *Semin Oncol* 1995; 22(suppl 12):8.
78. Safran H, King T, Choy H, et al. p53 mutations do not predict response to paclitaxel/radiation for non-small cell lung carcinoma. *Cancer* 1996;78:1203.
79. Rosenthal DI, Okani O, Corak J, et al. Seven-week continuous-infusion paclitaxel plus concurrent radiation therapy for locally advanced non-small cell lung cancer: a phase I study. *Semin Oncol* 1997;24(suppl 12):96.
80. Herscher LL, Hahn SM, Kroog G, et al. Phase I study of paclitaxel as a radiation sensitizer in the treatment of mesothelioma and non-small cell lung cancer. *J Clin Oncol* 1998;16:635.
81. Lau DH, Ryu JK, Gandara DR, et al. Twice-weekly paclitaxel and radiation for stage III non-small cell lung cancer. *Semin Oncol* 1997;24:106.
82. Choy H, Yee L, Cole BF. Combined-modality therapy for advanced non-small cell lung cancer: paclitaxel and thoracic irradiation. *Semin Oncol* 1995;22(suppl 15):38.
83. Glantz MJ, Choy H, Akerley W, et al. Weekly paclitaxel with and without concurrent radiation therapy: toxicity, pharmacokinetics, and response. *Semin Oncol* 1996;23(suppl 16):128.
84. Belani CP, Aisner J, Bahri S, et al. Chemoradiotherapy in non-small cell lung cancer: paclitaxel/carboplatin/radiotherapy in regionally advanced disease. *Semin Oncol* 1996;23(suppl 16):113.
85. Choy H, Akerley W, Safran H, et al. Multiinstitutional phase II trial of paclitaxel, carboplatin, and concurrent radiation therapy for locally advanced non-small cell lung cancer. *J Clin Oncol* 1998;16:3316.
86. Choy H, Rodriguez F, Koester S, et al. Synergistic effects of Taxol/Taxotere on radiation sensitivity on human tumor cell. *Int J Radiant Oncol Biol Phys* 1992;24:A1059.
87. Hennequin C, Giocanti N, Favaudon V. Interactions between ionizing radiations and brief exposure to docetaxel or paclitaxel in HeLa cells. 9th International Congress on Anti-Cancer Chemotherapy (SOMPS), Paris. 1995;124:A0335.

88. Watanabe A, Nishiwaki K, Hasegawa Y, et al. Effects of docetaxel and of irinotecan (CPT-11) combined with radiation on lung cancer cell lines. *Proc Am Soc Clin Oncol USA* 1995;14: A1617.

89. Mason K, Hunter N, Abbruzzese J, et al. In vivo enhancement of tumor response by Taxotere. *Proc Am Soc Clin Oncol USA* 1997;16:A775.

90. Aamdal S, Wibe E, Hallen MN, et al. Phase I study of concomitant docetaxel and radiation in locally advanced non-small cell lung cancer. *Proc Am Soc Clin Oncol USA* 1997;16:A1654.

91. Koukourakis MI, Kourousis C, Androulakis S, et al. Accelerated radiotherapy and weekly docetaxel for non-small cell lung cancer. *Proc Am Soc Clin Oncol USA* 1997;16:A1700.

92. Edelstein MP, Wolfe LA, Duch DS. Potentiation of radiation therapy by vinorelbine in non-small cell lung cancer. *Semin Oncol* 1996;23 (suppl 5):41.

93. Masters GA, Haraf DJ, Hoffman PC, et al. Phase I study of vinorelbine, cisplatin, and concomitant thoracic radiation in the treatment of advanced chest malignancies. *J Clin Oncol* 1998; 16:2157.

94. Lallev A, Anachkova B, Russev G. effect of ionizing radiation and topoisomerase II inhibitors on DNA synthesis in mammalian cells. *Eur J Biochem* 1993;216:177.

95. Clarke AR, Purdie CA, Harrison DJ, et al. Thymocyte apoptosis induced by p53-dependent and independent pathways. *Nature* 1993;362:849.

96. Giocanti N, Hennequin C, Balosso J, et al. DNA repair and cell cycle interactions in radiation sensitization by the topoisomerase II poison etoposide. *Cancer Res* 1993;53:2105.

97. Grau C, Overgaard J. Effect of etoposide, carmustine, vincristine, 5-fluorouracil, or methotrexate on radiobiologically oxic and hypoxic cells in C3H mouse mammary carcinoma in situ. *Cancer Chemother Pharmacol* 1992;39:227.

98. Albain KS, Rush VN, Crowley JJ, et al. Concurrent cisplatin etoposide plus chest radiotherapy followed by surgery for stages IIIA and IIIB non small cell lung cancer. *J Clin Oncol* 1995; 13:1880.

99. Kirichenko AV, Rich TA, Newman RA, et al. Potentiation of murine MC1-4 carcinoma radioresponse by 9-amino-20(S)-camptothecin. *Cancer Res* 1997;57:1929.

100. Lamond JP, Wang M, Kinsella TJ, et al. Radiation lethality enhancement with 9-amino camptothecin: Comparison to other topoisomerase I inhibitors. *Int J Rad Oncol Biol Phys* 1996; 36:369.

101. Change AYV, Gu Z, Keng R, et al. Radiation (XRT) sensitizing effects of topoisomerase (Topo) I and II inhibitors. *Proc Am Assoc Can Res* 1991;32:A2313.

102. Kim JH, Kim SH, Kolozsvary A, et al. Potentiation of radiation response in human carcinoma cells in vitro and murine fibrosarcoma in vivo by topotecan, an inhibitor, and ionizing radiation. *Int J Rad Oncol Biol Phys* 1992;22:515.

103. Lamond JP, Wang M, Kinsella TJ, et al. Concentration and timing dependence of lethality enhancement between topotecan, a topoisomerase I inhibitor, and ionizing radiation. *Int J Rad Oncol Biol Phys* 1996;36:361.

104. Marchesina R, Colombo A, Caserini C, et al. Interaction of ionizing radiation with topotecan in two human tumor cell lines. *Int J Cancer* 1996;66:342.

105. Boscia RE, Korbut T, Olde AS, et al. Interaction of topoisomerase I inhibitors with radiation in cis-diaminedichloroplatinum(II)-sensitive and -resistant cells in vitro and in the FSAIIC fibirosarcoma in vivo. *Int J Cancer* 1993;53:118.

106. Graham MV, Jahanzeb M, Dressler CM, et al. Results of a trial with topotecan dose escalation and concurrent thoracic radiation therapy for locally advanced, inoperable nonsmall cell lung cancer. *Int J Rad Oncol Biol Phys* 1996;36:1215.

107. Tamura K, Takada M, Kawase I, et al. Enhancement of tumor radio-response by irinotecan in human lung tumor xenografts. *Jap Cancer Res* 1997;88:218.

108. Omura M, Torigoe S, Kubota N. SN-38, a metabolite of the camptothecin derivative CPT-11, potentiates the cytotoxic effect of radiation in human colon adenocarcinoma cells grown as spheroids. *Radioth Oncol* 1997;43:197.

109. Yokoyama A, Kurita Y, Saijo, N, et al. Dose-finding study of irinotecan and cisplatin plus concurrent radiotherapy for unresectable stage III non-small-cell lung cancer. *Br J Cancer* 1998; 78:257.

110. Wheeler RH, Spencer S. Cisplatin plus radiation therapy. *J Infusional Chermother* 1995;5:61.

111. Korbelik M, Skov KA. Inactivation of hypoxic cells by cisplatin and radiation at clinically relevant doses. *Radiat Res* 1989;119: 145.

112. Dempke WC, Shellard SA, Hosking LK, et al. Mechanisms associated with the expression of cisplatin resistance in a human ovarian tumor cell line following exposure to fractionated X-irradiation in vitro. *Carcinogenesis* 1992;13:1209.

113. Stewart FA, Bartelink H, van der Voet GB, et al. Renal damage in mice after sequential cisplatin and irradiation: the influence of prior irradiation on platinum elimination. *Radiother Oncol* 1991;21:277.

114. Liliveld P, Scoles MA, Brown JM, et al. The effect of treatment in fractionated schedules with the combination of irradiation and six cytotoxic drugs on the RIF-1 tumor and normal mouse skin. *Int J Radiat Oncol Biol Phys* 1985;11:111.

115. Scanlon KJ, Safirstein RN, Thies H, et al. Inhibition of amino acid transport by cis-diamminedichloroplatinum (II) derivatives in L1210 murine leukemia cells. *Cancer Res* 1983;43:4211.

116. Furuse K, Fukuoka M, Takada Y, et al. A randomized phase III study of concurrent versus sequential thoracic radiotherapy in combination with mitomycin, vindesine, and cisplatin in unresectable stage III non-small cell lung cancer. *Proc Am Soc Clin Oncol USA* 1997;16:A1649.

117. Groen HJ, Sleijfer S, Meijer, et al. Carboplatin- and cisplatin-induced potentiation of moderate-dose radiation cytotoxicity in human lung cancer cell lines. *Br J Cancer* 1995;72:1406.

118. Douple EB, Richmond RC, O'Hara JA, et al. Carboplatin as a potentiator of radiation therapy. *Cancer Treat Rev* 1985; 12(suppl A):111.

119. Kunitoh H, Watanabe K, Nagatomo A, et al. Concurrent daily carboplatin and accelerated hyperfractionated thoracic radiotherapy in locally advanced non-small cell lung cancer. *Int J Radiat Oncol Biol Phys* 1997;37:103.

120. Wolf M, Goerg C, Goerg K, et al. Carboplatin and simultaneous radiation in the treatment of stage IIIA/B non-small cell lung cancer. *Oncolog* 1992;49(suppl 1):71.

121. Ball D, Bishop J, Smith J, et al. A phase III study of accelerated radiotherapy with and without carboplatin in non-small cell lung cancer: an interim toxicity analysis of the first 100 patients. *Int J Radiat Oncol Biol Phys* 1995;31:267.

122. Kipp JB, Kal HB, van Gennip AH, et al. Treatment of the rate R-1 rhabdomyosarcoma with methotrexate and radiation: effects of the action of radiation (10 Gy 300-kV x-rays) and methotrexate. *J Cancer Res Clin Oncol* 1993;119:215.

123. Phillips TL, Margolis L. Radiation pathology and the clinical response of lung and esophagus. *Front Radiat Ther Oncol* 1972; 6:254.

124. Byfield JE, Lynch M, Kulhanian F. Exclusive of an interactive effect of combined x-irradiation and activated cyclophosphamide in tissue culture. *Int J Radiat Oncol Biol Phys* 1986;12: 1441.

125. Olive PL. Response to spheroids implanted in the peritoneal

cavity of mice exposed to cyclophosphamide and ionizing radiation. *Br J Cancer* 1987;56:321.

126. Looney WB, Longerbeam MG, Hopkins HA, et al. Solid tumor models for the assessment of different treatment modalities. XXI. Comparison of different radiation dose schedules alone or in combination with cyclophosphamide. *Cancer* 1983;51:1012.

127. Travis EL, Bucci L, Fang MZ. Residual damage in mouse lungs at long intervals after cyclophosphamide in intestinal crypt cells. *Cancer Res* 1990;50:2139.

128. Ali-Osman F, Srivenugopal K, Berger MS, et al. DNA interstrand crosslinking and strand break repair in human glioma cell lines of varying [1,3-bis(2-chloroethyl-1-nitrosourea] resistance. *Anticancer Res* 1990;10:677.

129. Tofilon PJ, Williams ME, Deen DF. The effects of x-rays on BCNU-induced DNA crosslinking. *Radiat Res* 1984;99:165.

130. Bonner JA, Lawrence TS. Doxorubicin decreases the repair of radiation-induced DNA damage. *Int J Radiat Biol Phys* 1990; 57:55.

131. Zhang Y, Sweet KM, Sognier MA, et al. Interaction between radiation and drug damage in mammalian cells. 13. Radiation and doxorubicin age-response function of doxorubicin-sensitive and -resistant Chinese hamster cells. *Radiat Res* 1992;32:105.

132. Durand RE, Vanderbyl SL. Sequencing radiation and Adriamycin exposures in spheroids to maximize therapeutic gain. *Int J Radiat Oncol Biol Phys* 1989;17:345.

133. Rockwell S. Cytotoxicities of mitomycin-C and x-rays to aerobic and hypoxic cells in vitro. *Int J Radiat Oncol Biol Phys* 1982; 8:1035.

134. Dobrowsky W, Dobrowsky E, Rauth AM. Mode of interaction of 5-fluorouracil, radiation, and mitomycin C: in vitro studies. *Int J Radiat Onocol Biol Phys* 1992;22:875.

135. Fu KK, Lam KN. Early and late effects of mitomycin C and continuous low-dose-rate irradiation on the mouse skin and soft tissues of the leg. *Int J Radiat Oncol Biol Phys* 1991;21:1523.

16

IMMUNOLOGY OF LUNG CANCER

ROBERT K. BRIGHT

Increasing genetic evidence indicates that cancers arise from a series of molecular changes that lead to transformation and unrestrained cellular growth, often resulting in lethal tumor burdens. These changes are frequently manifested as the "aberrant" expression of proteins (mutated, upregulated, or expression of those normally silent) by the tumor cells marking them as potentially foreign, dangerous, or at least "altered" in contrast to the "normal" tissue cells from which the tumor(s) arose. The immune system is endowed with the ability to sort out these changes and distinguish between healthy and diseased, hence "normal" and malignant cells. Thus the proteins encoded by the aberrantly expressed genes of a tumor cell represent targets for the cells of the immune system, serving as tumor rejection or regression antigens. In this light, much effort has turned to the study of the manipulation of the immune response to tumors in the clinical setting. Transfer of immune cells and therapeutic vaccination represent two areas of active research that utilize methods of eliciting lymphocytes with specificity for antigens aberrantly expressed by tumor cells.

It is evident after a review of the literature that hundreds if not thousands of studies have been published on some aspect of tumor immunology or immunotherapy, from animal tumor models to human malignancies. Any attempt to compile all that has been investigated in the field would be a herculean task and beyond the scope or intent of this chapter. Therefore the following text represents an overview of the specific endeavors in immunotherapy alluded to above, namely immune cell transfer and active vaccination. The absence or inclusion of any study or studies was done without prior intent or favoritism, and the author apologizes in advance to those whose excellent and valuable contributions to the field of tumor immunology have been inadvertently missed.

HISTORICAL EVIDENCE FOR THE IMMUNOLOGIC REJECTION OF TUMORS

Early studies that form the foundation on which tumor immunology stands were conducted prior to current understanding of the cellular and molecular mechanisms of immunity. Therefore, it seems appropriate first to review the history of tumor immunity, then to define the cellular players and their roles in the immunologic destruction of cancer.

A prevailing question that puzzled investigators such as Peyton Rous[1] in the early days of tumor immunology (prior to the 1950s) was whether or not the tumor rejection observed in experimental animals was due to rejection of the tissue transplant or the tumor itself (being aware of the fact that a tumor arose from once healthy tissue). In other words, do tumors elicit an immune response that recognizes the tumor as a tumor or simply as a tissue graft that is all too commonly rejected. Due in part to difficulties is distinguishing between tumor immunity and transplant immunity (truly inbred strains of mice were not yet available), the field leaned toward tissue graft rejection (immunogenic differences involving the major histocompatibility antigens) as an explanation, if not *the* mechanism, for tumor rejection, a paradigm that dominated until the early 1950s.

During the late nineteenth century, while tumor transplantation rejection was being studied in animals, a surgeon by the name of William Coley was testing a vaccine preparation known as "Coley's toxin" on lymphoma and sarcoma patients at New York's Memorial Hospital (known today as the Memorial Sloan Kettering Cancer Center). Coley had observed tumor regression and remission in patients who suffered a nosocomial bacterial infection following resection of their tumors. He subsequently isolated the bacterium (later the active component) and demonstrated that this "toxin," when administered to sarcoma and lymphoma patients, could mediate tumor regression in nearly 50% of his cases.[2] The mechanism of action of this toxin-based vaccine is now believed to be mediated by cytokines that are induced following its administration, an observation that likely influenced the current tumor-cell vaccine strategies involving the engineering of tumor cells to express cytokine transgenes. Regardless, Coley recorded perhaps the earliest example of cancer therapy based on the deliberate manipulation of the immune system. However, with the advent of radiation and chemotherapies, along with difficulties in reproducing Coley's results, *immunotherapy* was sidelined for nearly 50 years.

In 1953 the paradigm was challenged when E.J. Foley

published his landmark work on the antigenic properties of methylcholanthrene (MCA) induced tumors in mice.[3] Foley eloquently demonstrated that when MCA tumors were ligated to induce necrosis, protection from a subsequent challenge with the same tumor was observed, while tumors grew quite well in unmanipulated animals. Certainly this phenomenon could not be attributed to differences in multiple histocompatibility complex (MHC) molecules (i.e., graft rejection) because the experiments were conducted using syngeneic mice. Excitement grew over the observation that tumors could be rejected by (presumed) immune recognition of antigens *uniquely* expressed on tumor cells. Four years later Prehn and Main confirmed and extended Foley's results by demonstrating that skin grafts were tolerated when mice of the same inbred strain were used. Moreover, ligated and necrosing syngeneic tumors induced protection from subsequent tumor challenge.[4] The conclusive proof of tumor antigenicity came in 1960, when George Klein and co-workers published a series of truly brilliant experiments in which surgical removal of tumors (as opposed to ligation) followed by tumor challenge resulted in protection.[5] More striking was their demonstration that tumor protection was obtained by injection of irradiated (inactivated) tumor cells prior to challenge; this experiment remains today as the standard for assessing tumor cell immunogenicity *in vivo*. Collectively, these experiments established that immune-mediated tumor rejection in inbred strains of mice was not a consequence of histocompatibility differences, but rather a result of tumor antigen recognition.

Numerous studies expounding the complexities of the immunologic rejection of solid tumors were published during the decades of the 1960s and 1970s. The majority of these studies focused on experimental tumor models in mice. As progress was made toward the feasibility of employing the immune system against human cancer, theories concerning the biology and progression of cancer as it relates to incidence and *natural* control of occurrence were also being developed. At the forefront was the *immune surveillance theory*.[6] This theory holds that all tumor cells express antigenic markers capable of eliciting immune responses resulting in tumor destruction, and that this process occurs continuously, preventing the outgrowth of malignant cells in most healthy individuals. As a person ages, the immune system declines, allowing the growth of tumors, hence one explanation for the increased incidence of cancer in people over the age of 50. Conceptually this theory would be difficult to prove *in vivo,* and certainly other mechanisms may participate in controlling cellular transformation and tumor formation in the *healthy* individual (e.g., events at the molecular and genetic level within the nascent tumor cell). Nonetheless, the power of the immune system lies within its ability to discriminate between self and nonself or, more appropriately, a normal cell from a tumor cell, and thereby selectively and specifically eliminating tumor cells while leaving normal cells intact. The arm of the immune system that is primarily responsible for tumor-specific immunity is classically referred to as the *adaptive* immune response. Adaptive immunity employs a subset of cells of the lymphocyte lineage as the primary effectors responsible for the mechanisms of tumor-specific killing.

T-CELL–MEDIATED IMMUNE RESPONSES

The intent of this review is to focus on the topic of tumor immunology in the context of therapy. However, an overview of the process and components of cellular immunity is essential to the understanding of immune responses to tumor cells as well as the manipulation of tumor immunity through vaccination, for example. In the interest of space, this will be an overview, and some of these concepts are also covered in Chapter 17.

Immunologic rejection of tumors is believed to be executed primarily by lymphocytes, the common position being that T-lymphocyte (cell) mediated immunity is essential for the destruction of most solid tumors. T-cells are typically subdivided into two main groups: (a) those that provide a "helper" function (CD4 + T-cells) for immune responses following recognition of peptide antigens processed and presented, typically from exogenous proteins that have been endocytosed or phagocytosed, in the context of class II major histocompatibility antigens (MHC-II) on professional antigen presenting cells (APCs)—dendritic cells, macrophages and B-lymphocytes, for example; and (b) those that directly mediate tumor destruction (CD8 + cytotoxic T-cells) resulting from recognition of peptide antigens (usually derived from endogenously expressed proteins) in the context of MHC-I molecules expressed on the surface of the tumor cells. MHC-I molecules are normally expressed on all somatic cells in the body, including fibroblasts and epithelial cells, which give rise to sarcomas and carcinomas respectively.

Typically CD4 + T-cells are noncytolytic yet have been shown to play a role in tumor rejection by providing the necessary help for CD8 + cytotoxic T-lymphocyte (CTL) activation and lytic activity. For example, tumor immunity was attributed to the induction of CD4 + T-cells in a murine melanoma model where tumors were engineered to express the human p97 gene,[7] as well as a model for disseminated MHC-II negative lymphoma[8] Topalian and colleagues identified CD4 + T-cells with specificity for tyrosinase, a shared tumor antigen associated with human malignant melanoma.[9] Although there is evidence for the role of CD4 + MHC-II-restricted T-cells in tumor immunity, the vast majority of tumor-reactive T-cells defined for human systems and in animal models are CD8 + MHC-I-restricted CTLs.[10,11]

CTLs recognize peptide fragments (8 to 10) amino acids in length) of intracellular protein antigens in the context of MHC-I molecule heavy chains in association with beta-2 microglobulin. These trimolecular complexes are expressed on the tumor (target) cell surface, giving an extracellular presentation of endogenously expressed and enzymatically processed protein fragments for a CTL to engage using its antigen-specific receptor(s) (T-cell receptor [TCR]).[12] The role of CTLs in tumor destruction has been demonstrated in numerous murine tumor models by inducing tumor-antigen–specific immune responses following immunization with; antigen-coated beads,[13] recombinant viruses,[14] synthetic peptides,[15] or naked plasmid DNA.[16] The presence of tumor-antigen–specific CD8 + CTLs within a developing tumor was first demonstrated for humans by growing the tumor-infiltrating lymphocytes (TIL) from resected melanomas.[17] The *in vitro* growth and adoptive transfer of TILs has become a viable and available therapy for patients with malignant melanoma. These studies (and numerous others) have clearly demonstrated that CTLs can be recruited via immunization or *in vitro* manipulation and deployed against tumors, resulting in complete protection or treatment of tumors in murine models or objective clinical responses for cancer patients. In light of the potential of immunotherapy we are left with the question: Why aren't more tumors immunologically rejected? Unfortunately, much of the skepticism regarding tumor immunology is based on the contention that the immune system has been taught to fight infection (foreign) not cancer (self) and cannot be educated otherwise. Mounting data, however, indicate that the cellular arm of the immune system can be taught to kill cancer and that the tumors themselves are often actively involved in the tactics of immunologic escape and evasion.

MECHANISMS OF TUMOR ESCAPE FROM IMMUNOLOGIC REJECTION

Without question, tumors—both spontaneous and viral induced—express *unique* (foreign or aberrantly expressed) antigenic targets capable of inducing tumor-destructive immune responses. Thus it is reasonable to presume that some form of *immune surveillance* is contributing to the control of tumor formation *in vivo*. However, it is also painfully clear that the incidence of lethal forms of cancer remains high. Perhaps the clinical occurrence of cancer represents those not-so-usual circumstances when the immune system is ineffective. The process of tumor progression in the absence of an apparent immune response is classically referred to as *tumor escape*. Much speculation is given to the mechanism(s) by which tumors escape and evade immune destruction. Although there exists a number of studies describing many possible mechanisms of tumor escape (few however, without accompanying contradictory reports), we will focus on mechanisms most likely to impact the development of immunotherapies, such as vaccines and adoptive cell transfer.

Down-Regulation of MHC-I Expression

As alluded to above, the common belief is that CD8 + CTLs comprise the primary and perhaps the most important arm of immune-mediated defense against solid tumors. The removal or down-regulation of MHC-I molecules from the surface of a tumor cell renders it incapable of presenting MHC-I molecules complexed with antigenic peptides and removes the means by which a CTL recognizes the tumor cell and subsequently destroys it. Indeed, some clinical studies using tumor sections and immunocytochemistry have shown that primary tumors sometimes exhibit detectable decreases in MHC-I expression compared to adjacent normal tissue. Interestingly, metastatic tumors do not seem to be any different from their parent (primary) tumors with respect to the level of MHC-I expression, though they have escaped immune destruction, as evidenced by the metastatic event. Examination of multiple human and experimental tumors has demonstrated that MHC-I expression is often retained on tumors from patient to patient or between tumor histologies; thus it has proven difficult to correlate tumorigenicity, or lack thereof, with MHC-I expression or down-regulation. Nonetheless, animal studies have demonstrated that tumorigenic cells lines capable of forming tumors *in vivo* become less tumorigenic in immunocompetent hosts when MHC-I expression is increased, typically accomplished by cytokine induction or MHC-I gene transfection.[18] The corollary assumption, again supported by data, is that MHC-I expression leaves a tumor cell nontumorigenic (due to increased immunogenicity) in syngeneic, immunocompetent animals. This assumption may not be true in some experimental tumor models. Often tumor models in murine systems include a tumorigenic cell line that expresses MHC-I, as well as an immunogenic tumor antigen capable of eliciting tumor-destructive immunity.[19,20] Although conclusions conflict concerning MHC-I down-regulation and its role as a mechanism of tumor escape, caution directs that it be given careful consideration when developing immunologic therapies for cancer that rely on induction of MHC-I–restricted CTLs.

Absence of Costimulation

It has become clear in recent years that T-cells require *secondary* signals in addition to those obtained through TCR-MHC-peptide engagement (the primary signal or signal 1) in order to become active effector cells. The B7 family of gene products (which include B7.1 and B7.2) have been identified as key elements that provide the second signal known as *costimulation*. The B7 ligand is found primarily on professional APCs such as dendritic cells and B-cells, and has not been demonstrated on somatic cells such as those giving rise to most solid tumors. The receptor for B7 is the CD28 molecule, which is found on T-cells. When CD28 on a T-cell is engaged by B7, following TCR engage-

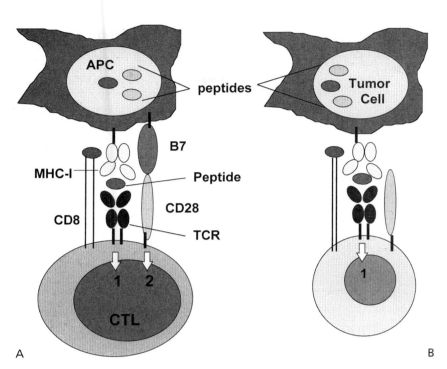

FIGURE 16.1. Schematic representation of T-cell recognition of an antigenic peptide in the context of an MHC-I molecule. **A:** Illustration of the events leading up to successful T-cell activation following effective delivery of signal 1 and signal 2 *costimulation* (see text for details). **B:** Illustration of the induction of T-cell anergy following delivery of signal 1 in the absence of signal 2 (see text for details). APC, antigen-presenting cell (e.g., dendritic cells); MHC-I, class I major histocompatibility antigen; CTL, CD8+ cytotoxic T-cell; TCR; T-cell antigen receptor.

ment of an MHC-peptide complex, the necessary 1,2 signals are delivered to the T-cell, resulting in its activation and proliferation (Figure 16.1). Experiments have demonstrated that the first (MHC-peptide) and second (B7-CD28) signals are most efficiently delivered when expressed on the same APC.[21] However, it is possible to deliver the appropriate costimulation *in vitro* by employing the B7 molecule on a third-party cell (author's unpublished observation). When resting or naive T-cells are engaged with a specific MHC-peptide complex through their TCR in the absence of B7 and CD28 engagement the result is *peripheral tolerance* or *anergy*.[22] Since tumors don't express B7 molecules (B-cell malignancies are an exception), tumor-cell antigen presentation to T-cells results in anergy, or functional unresponsiveness, hence the premise for absence of costimulation as a mechanism for tumor escape. Tumor cells that lack B7 expression and fail to stimulate T-cells can be engineered to express B7 and successfully stimulate tumor-specific T-cells.[23] Indeed, tumor cells expressing a B7 transgene are being explored as a "new generation" of whole-tumor-cell vaccines.

Tolerance

As described above, absence of costimulation represents a mechanism of immunologic tolerance to tumor cells. The primary mechanism of establishing peripheral tolerance is neonatal exposure to antigens during ontogeny. This process, involving thymic mechanisms of positive and negative selection,[24] provides the necessary environment for immu-

nologic tolerance of *self*-antigens and the prevention of autoimmune disease. Studies have demonstrated that tumor antigens encountered early enough in fetal development are tolerated by the adult animal and thus are no longer immunogenic. Viral-induced breast tumors in virus-bearing versus virus-free animals represent one instance.[25] Another example is SV40 large tumor antigen (Tag) transgenic mice that develop spontaneous tumors that remain Tag-positive and grow unchecked even though Tag is highly immunogenic in mice.[26] Tumor formation in the SV40 Tag transgenic system is difficult to define as *tolerance* to Tag, since Tag-positive tumors transplanted to syngeneic adult immunocompetent mice grow progressively, resulting in death unless an immune response to Tag is induced prior to transplantation.[19] In addition, when hemagglutinin (HA) of influenza virus was expressed in the pancreas of transgenic mice, driven by a tissue-specific promoter, the viral antigen was well tolerated and no autoimmune disease was evident even when the animals were immunized against HA. Interestingly, when these HA-transgenic mice were immunized with HA, followed by a lethal challenge with HA-expressing tumor cells, the tumors were rejected and HA-specific immunity was demonstrated, yet the pancreas was left healthy and functional.[27] Conversely, when lymphocytic choriomeningitis virus glycoprotein (LCMV), or LCMV-glycoprotein (GP) was expressed in the pancreas of transgenic mice to study the induction of autoimmunity against a defined antigen, tolerance was broken, resulting in autoimmune diabetes following immunization with dendritic cells that express LCMV-GP.[28] The implication here for cancer treatment is that therapeutic immunization against antigens that are not tumor-specific (most of the candidate tumor antigens for human cancer defined thus far are not tumor-specific) could result in autoimmune disease.

Though tolerance is clearly an obstacle in the path of many tumor immunotherapy approaches, complete understanding surrounding the involvement of tolerance in tumor immunity, as well as methods to overcome or manipulate it, require further investigation.

Tumor-Secreted Factors

Cultured tumor cells have been shown to secrete numerous cytokines and various growth factors. Some of these secreted factors are suppressive to the cells of the immune system. An example is transforming growth factor-beta (TGF-β). TGF-β is a family of molecules first identified as supporting transformation as defined by cell growth in soft agar. Many tumor cells secrete TGF-β, which sets up an immunosuppressive microenvironment around the tumor by inhibiting T-cell proliferation and CTL maturation. Tumors may secrete various cytokines as well. Cytokines have been shown to influence or drive T-helper cell function to support either cellular (CTL) or humoral (antibody) immunity.[29] Since CTLs are important for tumor cell killing, a cytokine profile (influenced by cytokines secreted by the tumor) that favors humoral versus cellular immunity could be detrimental to the successful immunologic rejection of the tumor. Therapies employed in such an environment may be aided by administration of anticytokine antibodies, recombinant cytokines (or tumor cells engineered to secrete cytokines), or cytokine analogues that block cytokine receptors on immune cells (e.g., T-cells) that drive a cellular immune response.

ACTIVE MANIPULATION OF THE IMMUNE RESPONSE TO ELIMINATE TUMORS

A realistic goal for the immunologic treatment of cancer is to administer immunotherapy as an adjuvant therapy to surgical resection of the primary tumor, the premise being first to minimize the tumor burden by "de-bulking" the patient's disease. It is clear from animal studies that there is a threshold for effective immunologic rejection of tumors with respect to tumor burden. The larger the existing tumor, the more difficult it is to treat or cure with immunotherapy. Current progress in improving early detection of cancer (with minimal burden and decreased likelihood of metastasis) will provide new opportunities to apply immunotherapy in a setting that should favor remarkable results.

Immunotherapy can be divided into two categories: active and passive strategies. Active approaches comprise both specific and nonspecific strategies, while passive methods involve the transfer of antigen-specific antibodies. Antibod-

ies have been useful clinically as diagnostic tools in the context of enzyme linked immunosorbent assays (ELISAs) or immunocytochemistry on tissue sections. The power of antibodies in this capacity comes by exploiting their ability to recognize surface proteins that are either unique on tumor tissues or overexpressed on tumor cells compared to normal cells. Antibodies have demonstrated potential as immunotherapeutic agents as well, by complexing the antibody with toxins (immunotoxins),[30] radioactive molecules,[31] or as free antibody presumably inducing mechanisms of antibody-dependent cell-mediated cytotoxicity (ADCC).[32] ADCC, for example, is a possible mechanism that is employed during therapy with tiastuzumab (Herceptin), a new passive immunotherapy for breast cancer that targets the HER-2/neu tumor antigen on breast cancer cells with an antigen-specific monoclonal antibody.

Active nonspecific immunotherapy of cancer involves the induction of immune cells that do not rely on tumor antigen recognition and MHC-I restriction. Generally the therapy involves administration of cytokines or immune stimulatory adjuvants such as bacille Calmette-Guérin (BCG) or *Cryptosporidium parvum*, resulting in the subsequent activation of nonspecific effectors such as natural killer (NK) cells or lymphokine-activated killer (LAK) cells. LAK cells have demonstrated limited efficacy as immunotherapeutic agents when activated *in vitro* and adoptively transferred back to the patient.

Countless studies have demonstrated that protective immune responses can be elicited by vaccination with candidate synthetic tumor antigens or peptide fragment(s) (epitopes) from the tumor antigen.[33] In this light, strategies for the development of new therapies for the treatment of human cancer based on the identification and characterization of a target tumor antigen(s) and the MHC-I–binding peptides from the tumor antigen(s) include: (a) *in vitro*–generated antitumor −CD8 + CTLs that may be useful for adoptive cellular transfer immunotherapy, and (b) active immunization with synthetic peptide epitope(s) as subunit therapeutic cancer vaccines.

Adoptive Transfer of Tumor-Specific T-Cells

Adoptive immunotherapy has been defined as the acquisition of immunity in a naive subject as the result of the administration of immunologically activated lymphoid cells.[34] The process of adoptive transfer of tumor-specific lymphocytes involves obtaining T-cells from the patient to be treated, culturing the T-cells *in vitro* to activate and expand them, and finally infusing them back into the patient. As alluded to above, T-cells that infiltrate solid tumor masses (e.g., melanomas and renal cell carcinomas) have proven to be a powerful source of tumor-reactive T-cells for adoptive cellular transfer. These T-cells, designated *tumor-infiltrating lymphocytes* (TILs), have been used successfully to treat patients with malignant melanoma. However, there are reasons why TIL transfer therapy has not seen wider application. For example, not all solid tumors are a source of TILs. In addition, administration of cytokines such as the T-cell growth factor IL-2 with the TILs is often necessary to maintain the T-cells *in vivo,* and it is often difficult to acquire enough autologous tumor cells to use as a source of tumor antigen for *in vitro* activation and expansion. One alternative is to collect lymph-node draining T-cells following immunization with autologous tumor and adjuvant, and to stimulate them *in vitro* with anti-CD3 (the signaling portion of the TCR) antibody.[35,36] This provides an effective method for generating sufficient numbers of tumor-reactive CTLs for adoptive transfer.

Active Specific Induction of Tumor Immunity

The identification of human tumor antigens and the availability of synthetic peptides representing selected immunogenic/immunodominant peptides from those antigens have made possible the generation of human tumor-specific CTLs. For example, repeated exposure of peripheral blood lymphocytes (PBLs) from melanoma patients to an immunodominant peptide from the shared melanoma antigen MART-1 (methods for antigen identification will be discussed below) resulted in the generation of CTLs that were from 50 to 100 times more potent in specific tumor killing than activated infiltrating lymphocytes harvested from the patients' tumors.[37] A separate study demonstrated the generation of CTL with specificity for the shared human melanoma antigen gp100 by *in vitro* stimulation of patient's PBLs with synthetic peptides representing CTL epitopes on gp100.[38] In addition, a number of studies demonstrated the feasibility of inducing tumor-reactive CTLs *in vitro* by coculturing PBLs from cancer patients with tumor cell lines expressing matched or autologous MHC-I antigens.[39,40–42] Most striking were the results from a recent clinical trial involving melanoma CTL-MHC-I peptides as a therapeutic vaccine administered to patients with advanced metastatic disease. Therapeutic-peptide vaccination resulted in a higher percentage of clinical responses (including complete responses) in patients than has previously been seen for any other therapy for melanoma.[43]

Indeed, this and other studies underway are clearly demonstrating the power and potential of therapeutic-peptide-based vaccines for the treatment of advanced cancer. In spite of the evidence for the existence of tumor-reactive CTLs in patients with cancer and in murine tumor models, as well as the potential of peptide-based therapeutic vaccines, most efforts to demonstrate an ongoing CTL response against tumor antigens in humans have failed. However, it is of the utmost importance to remember that in most murine tumor models (e.g., the Balb/c SV40 tumor model) the tumor of interest, though it expresses a highly immunogenic tumor-specific antigen (e.g., SV40 Tag) and MHC-I molecules, grows rapidly and aggressively *in vivo,* ultimately killing the immunocompetent host if an antigen-specific immune response is not present prior to or concurrent with tumor transplantation.[19]

IMMUNOTHERAPY OF LUNG CANCER

Of all the malignant diseases that plague humans lung cancer is the number one killer, second only to heart-related illness in overall mortality. Despite newfound optimism for high-dose chemotherapy for certain types of lung cancer (namely, small cell lung cancer),[44] overall treatment options are limited. This seemingly desperate situation demands investigation into new treatments and reevaluation of treatments such as immunotherapy with the application of new advances in technology. Typically, tumor immunotherapies can be divided into nonspecific and specific approaches. Nonspecific therapies primarily involve the administration of bacterium or components of bacterium with the expectation that an ensuing inflammatory immune response will result in accompanying immunity against the tumor. Specific immunotherapy involves either the passive transfer of tumor-reactive immune cells or antibodies that target and destroy the tumor, or active induction of tumor-destroying immunity following injection (vaccination) with inactivated tumor cells or molecular components of tumor cells (antigens).

Nonspecific Immunotherapy

The nonspecific immunotherapy of lung cancer dates back to the 1970s and 1980s, with trials showing little to no benefit.[45] Most efforts focused on the administration of BCG or *C. parvum* with limited success clinically. More recently, O'Brien and colleagues began trials to evaluate the efficacy of treating lung cancer patients with a different species of *Mycobacterium* (*M. vaccae*) devoid of toxicity, in combination with chemotherapy.[46]

Administration of cytokines represents another arm of nonspecific immunotherapy for cancer. Cytokine therapy for lung cancer had its origin with the T-cell growth factor interleukin-2 (IL-2) administered alone or in combination with LAK cells. Interferons (IFN) have also been explored as possible nonspecific immunotherapies against lung cancer. In recent years, recombinant IFN-α has been reevaluated clinically as a maintenance therapy following chemotherapy. Overall, the use of nonspecific approaches of immunotherapy has been disappointing and the hope in such treatments has waned. As the use of nonspecific immunotherapy declines, efforts to target tumors actively and specifically with cytolytic immune responses is on the rise.

Passive Specific Immunotherapy

As alluded to above, passive immunotherapy has traditionally involved either the infusion of tumor-specific antibodies or transfer of tumor-reactive immune cells. For passive antibody therapy, monoclonal antibodies (mAb) have seen the greatest utility. Antibodies have been administered alone—for example, L6 mAh, which recognizes a surface carbohydrate antigen on non–small cell lung cancer (NSCLC)[47]—or complexed to toxic molecules such as *Pseudomonas* exotoxin-A[48] or ricin for (SCLC).[49] Antibodies, for the most part, have not demonstrated much usefulness as therapies for lung cancer but remain valuable as diagnostic and prognostic tools.

The adoptive transfer of tumor-reactive immune cells into patients with advanced cancer was pioneered by Rosenberg and colleagues.[50] The earliest efforts involved the *ex vivo* expansion of lymphocytes in the presence of high-dose IL-2; the resulting effectors were designated lymphokine-activated killer cells or LAK cells. LAK cells behave somewhat like natural killer (NK) cells in that they are not MHC-restricted T-cells but do exhibit an increased propensity to kill tumor cells. In time, LAK cells were replaced by more potent, tumor-specific, MHC-I-restricted CTLs isolated from resected tumor following culture of the tumor in the presence of IL-2. Again pioneered by Rosenberg and colleagues, these CTLs, known as tumor-infiltrating lymphocytes (TILs), have demonstrated objective clinical responses when transfered into patients with malignant melanoma or renal cell carcinoma.[51] Gene therapy using cytokines is described in Chapter 17.

In the past, adoptive transfer trials for lung cancer involved LAK cells alone or with IL-2 or in combination with different chemotherapies. Though most these efforts were disappointing, it was reported by Kimura and colleagues, that LAK cells and IL-2 showed a significant survival benefit over radiotherapy, chemotherapy, or radiochemotherapy when administered to 105 randomized patients under going noncurative resection for lung cancer.[52] Adoptive transfer trials for melanoma have demonstrated that TILs are more potent that LAK cells; however, TILs have been difficult to isolate from malignancies other than melanoma (examples include breast, prostate, and lung cancer). A recent strategy to generate tumor-specific CTLs is to immunize patient with his or her own tumor cells in the presence of an immunostimulant such as the cytokine GM-CSF, then isolate and culture CTLs from the patient's draining lymph nodes or peripheral blood for expansion *in vitro* and subsequent transfer back to the patient.[53] Small-scale studies to evaluate this strategy for the therapy of lung cancer are just beginning; time will reveal their usefulness. Because most of the more common and deadly tumors do not easily (if at all) give rise to TILs, and the generation of CTLs *in vivo* as alluded to above is labor-intensive, taking weeks to accomplish, much effort has turned to active specific immunotherapy involving *tumor vaccines*.

Active Specific Immunotherapy

Early studies demonstrated that immunization of mice with inactivated tumor cells resulted in protection from a subsequent lethal tumor challenge, prompted trials to evaluate *whole-tumor-cell vaccines* in lung cancer patients. This early approach to tumor vaccination usually involved injection of irradiated autologous or allogeneic tumor cells alone or with an adjuvant such as BCG (more recently cytokines such as GM-CSF have been used). Unfortunately, like the nonspecific immunotherapy approaches to treating lung cancer, whole-tumor vaccines have not produced very promising results.[54] One explanation is that there are components of a whole-tumor cell that are at the very least detrimental if not suppressive to concomitant immunity. In this light, much effort has turned to the development of molecularly defined tumor vaccines. For example, Garbrilovitch and colleagues have recently begun evaluation of lung cancer vaccines comprised of either mutated *ras* oncogene products or mutated *p53* tumor suppressor gene products in an attempt to take advantage of the aberrant expression of these proteins in human lung cancers.[55] These and other studies are beginning to reveal the importance of identifying tumor-associated antigens (TAA) toward their development as defined therapeutic tumor vaccines. (See Chapter 17.)

TUMOR-ASSOCIATED ANTIGENS

A hallmark of active immunity that has formed the foundation of the field of *vaccinology* (pioneered for infectious disease such as polio and smallpox) is the ability of the immune system specifically to target and destroy invaders or diseased cells while leaving adjacent healthy cells intact. Specificity arises from immune cell recognition of defined targets, or *antigens,* on diseased cells (as described above, T-cell antigens are comprised of a peptide in the groove of an MHC molecule). As mentioned previously, the first evidence for antigens on tumor cells came from the pioneering work of Foley and Prehn and Main. For decades since, researchers have hunted for evidence of tumor-associated antigens (TAAs) on human tumors with the hope of employing the power and specificity of the immune system specifically to destroy tumor cells. The premise was that if TAAs could be identified that were exclusively expressed on tumor cells, then the immune response could be manipulated against these TAAs much as had been demonstrated for infectious agents, namely viruses. In this light, the hunt for tumor viruses began.

Viral Proteins

Certain cancers are believed to be caused by viral infection, although a direct causal relationship is difficult to define.

TABLE 16.1. VIRUS-ENCODED TUMOR-SPECIFIC ANTIGENS (TSA)

Virus	Candidate TSA	Tumor Association
EBV	EBNA 1–4, LMP	Burkitt's lymphoma Naso-pharyngeal carcinoma
HBV	HBsAg	Hepatocellular carcinoma
HHV-8*	(none yet)	Kaposi's sarcoma
HTLV-I	tax, gp46	T-cell lymphoma
HPV-16, 18	E6, E7	Cervical carcinoma
SV40†	Tag	Mesothelioma, Osteosarcoma, Ependymoma, Glioblastoma

* May not be involved in tumorigenesis.
† Involvement and association remains unclear.
EBV, Epstein-Barr virus; HBV, Hepatitis B virus; HHV, human herpes virus; HPV, human papilloma virus; SV40, simian virus 40; EBNA, Epstein-Barr nuclear antigen; LMP, late membrane protein; HBsAg, Hepatitis B virus surface antigen; Tag, large tumor antigen.

Some viruses considered to be associated with human malignancies include HBV with hepatocellular carcinoma, HTLV-I with T-cell lymphoma, EBV with Burkitt's lymphoma, and the human (HPV) with cervical papillomavirus carcinoma.[56] Viruses by nature possess the ability to alter host cell function and directly influence the multi-step process that leads to transformation. Viral-induced transformation may occur through the induction of genetic aberrations resulting from physical interaction of viral DNA with the host genome or through viral gene products expressed following infection. Since viral infection (in permissive as well as nonpermissive hosts) often results in the expression of viral-encoded protein antigens, cancers with true viral etiologies or associations represent prime candidates for the development of targeted, specific, immunologic therapies (Table 16.1).

The foremost example of targeting viral antigens for the immunotherapy of human cancer is that of HPV and cervical carcinoma. Clinical studies of malignant lesions indicate that greater than 90% of cervical carcinomas contain HPV genetic sequences.[57] The induction of tumor-killing CTLs by vaccination with MHC-1 peptides from E6 and/or E7 has been demonstrated most notably in murine models for HPV-16–induced cervical carcinoma.[58] Taken together, such information has led to clinical trials involving the vaccination of cervical carcinoma patients with peptides from the E6 or E7 oncoproteins of HPV. A second virus from the papovavirus family, simian virus 40, has recently been implicated in several different human malignancies.

Simian virus 40-like DNA sequences (in particular the SV40 large tumor antigen, *Tag,* gene) have been amplified from human tumors of the bone (osteosarcomas), brain (ependymomas and glioblastomas), and mesothelium, with over 60% percent of ependymomas exhibiting expression of

the SV40 Tag protein.[59] Further, reports have demonstrated that 60% of malignant pleural mesotheliomas (MPM) contain SV40 Tag genetic sequences and proteins.[60,61] The viral genes and gene products, though present in MPM tumors, could not be found in the normal mesothelium of the same patient. Studies involving other papovaviruses such as HPV as targets for immunotherapy of cervical carcinoma, along with data from murine models demonstrating the immunotherapeutic potential of SV40 Tag against Tag-positive tumors,[19] suggest that SV40 Tag represents a shared tumor-specific antigen that may be a target for the immunotherapy of MPM in humans. In spite of the enthusiasm surrounding the immunologic targeting of HPV and SV40 for the therapy of certain human cancers, it has become clear that viruses do not represent candidates for immunotherapy in the majority of human malignancies.

Oncogene and Tumor-Suppressor Gene Products

The tumor immunology specters of tolerance and autoimmunity have historically driven TAA hunting in the direction of antigens that are "non-self," such as viral antigens, or at least tumor-specific, such as mutated cellular proteins. With the dimming light of hope for finding tumor viruses to target in the more common human cancers (e.g., lung, breast, and prostate cancer), the next logical place to turn was to the proteins linked to the process of transformation and oncogenesis. Oncogene products provide the desired tumor-specific and also the potential for being a target that is shared among tumors of multiple histologies. The following are a few of the more common examples of TAAs from expressed oncogenes or tumor-suppressor genes.

The transmembrane tyrosine kinase *HER2/neu* has been demonstrated to be overexpressed in several clinically important human malignancies, including cancers of the breast, ovary, colon, and lung (see also Chapter 4). Although *HER2/neu* is expressed on some "normal" tissues and cells, it exhibits a significant increase in expression in some tumors compared to the corresponding normal tissue. This overexpression or upregulation has been demonstrated to be sufficient to elicit an immune response against *HER2/neu*. CTLs with specificity for *HER2/neu* epitopes have been identified in the peripheral blood of breast cancer patients,[62] and antibodies against an extracellular domain of *HER2/neu* have formed the basis for an antibody-based therapy, (Herceptin), recently approved by the FDA for certain breast cancers.

Oncogenes of the *ras* family are the most frequently expressed oncogenes in human cancers, including lung cancer (details on *ras* function and expression are covered in Chapter 4) *Ras* proteins that are involved in malignant transformation often differ from the normally expressed gene products by a single amino acid substitution. Studies have demonstrated that CTLs can be generated that recognize an epitope (containing a single amino acid substitution) on tumor cells that express mutated-activated *ras*, resulting in tumor protection *in vivo*.[63] Though single amino acid substitutions limit the number of possible peptide epitopes that may drive CTL-mediated killing of corresponding tumors (particularly with respect to the differences in peptide motif specificities demonstrated for the various human HLA molecules), the data suggest that activated *ras* may be a shared TAA target for the immunotherapy of multiple human cancers. Yet another tumor-specific antigen derived from a mutation in the normal protein resulting in a single amino acid substitution is that of β-catenin.[64] This candidate TAA, a cell adhesion protein, was cloned from melanoma cells using TILs generated *in vitro* from a surgically resected melanoma.

Similarly, mutations in the tumor suppressor *p53* have been identified in an increasing number of human cancers making it the leading shared TAA discovered for human malignancies to date.[65] (See also Chapter 6). The single amino acid substitutions that comprise the increased immunogenicity of "mutated" *p53* come with the same caution as that discussed above for mutated *ras* proteins, that is, they provide a limited number of potential targets for immunotherapy. However, a more recent study demonstrated that CTL immunity can be directed against nonmutated or "normal" epitopes in the *p53* protein, suggesting that tolerance can be broken against *p53*, making it a more viable shared candidate TAA.[66] Moreover, immunologic reactivity to normal *p53*, as well as other normal self TAAs to be discussed below, in the absence of apparent autoimmune-related pathology will expand the list of potential TAAs beyond that of foreign or tumor-specific/unique to include normal tissue differentiation antigens.

Antigens Cloned from Melanoma

The vast majority of TAAs discovered thus far for human cancers have been cloned from malignant melanoma. In general the melanoma antigens can be divided into two main categories. One group includes the MAGE, BAGE, and GAGE gene family of TAAs expressed on melanomas and a variety of other tumors, including lung cancers, but not on normal cells (the exception are the testes),[67] and the other group is comprised of normal melanocyte differentiation or lineage antigens (involved in skin pigmentation) which include tyrosinase, MART-1, gp100, and tyrosinase-related proteins-1 (TRP-1).[68] Several tumor antigens from each of the groups are currently being evaluated in clinical trials as therapeutic vaccines for melanoma (expanded on below).

Other Antigens

There are TAAs that have been identified and characterized that are distinct from viral proteins, mutated oncogenes, or

TABLE 16.2. TUMOR ANTIGENS ASSOCIATED WITH HUMAN LUNG CANCER

Tumor Antigen	Tumor Association
K-*ras*	NSCLC
p53	NSCLC, SCLC
HER2/neu	NSCLC
CEA	NSCLC, SCLC
MUC-1	NSCLC, SCLC

CEA, carcinoembryonic antigen; NSCLC, non–small cell lung cancer (may include histologies such as squamous cell adenocarcinoma); SCLC, small cell lung cancer.

the melanoma antigens discussed above (see Table 16.2.) The *mucin* family of genes and carcinoembryonic antigen (CEA) are examples of such TAAs. MUC-1 is a mucin found on malignant as well as normal ductal epithelial cells of the breast, ovary, pancreas, lung, and prostate.[69,70] Tumors will express a MUC-1 that is aberrantly glycosylated compared to MUC-1 on normal tissues. The altered glycosylation renders MUC-1 immunogenic, as has been demonstrated in animal tumor models.[71] CEA is normally silent in healthy adults but is expressed on many of the same tumors as MUC-1. This dual association[72] could lead to vaccine trials targeting CEA and MUC-1 in breast cancer patients.

In the past 5 to 7 years alone, great strides have been made toward the definition of relevant molecular targets on human tumor cells that may serve as TAAs for immunotherapy. Although the list of candidate TAAs has grown rapidly, it is nowhere near complete or inclusive of all malignancies. Yet, the growing list of TAAs on many human cancers has given investigators the necessary reagents to explore strategies of active immunotherapy against human cancer, namely therapeutic cancer vaccines.

CANCER VACCINES (TABLE 16.3)

The twofold premise for the development of therapeutic cancer vaccines is that there are differences in tumor and normal cells—differences that are manifested as abnormally expressed genes (TAAs)—and that there exist in patients the immune cells (CTLs) capable of discriminating between the normal and tumor cells though TAA recognition, resulting in CTL-mediated tumor killing. It is reasonable to speculate that these conditions exist for all human tumors and the patients who harbor the disease. With candidate TAAs in hand (for a limited number of cancers) and empirical evidence that antigen-specific tumor-killing CTLs exist in cancer patients, the challenge for investigators is to use the TAAs to elicit therapeutic immune responses in patients. However, in order to expand the study of cancer vaccines beyond tumors such as melanoma, investigators are faced

TABLE 16.3. TUMOR VACCINE STRATEGIES

Vaccine Source	Vaccine Design
Cell-based	Whole-tumor cells (modified with cytokine genes)
	DC-pulsed with peptide, protein, mRNA or transduced with recombinant retrovirus
Protein-based	HSPs
	recombinant protein in adjuvant
Peptide-based	T-cell epitopes in adjuvant
	B-cell epitopes in adjuvant
Plasmid DNA	naked plasmid DNA
	DNA-coated particles (ballistic*)
Viral vectors	recombinant vaccinia, other pox viruses
	recombinant adenovirus
	recombinant AAV

HSP, Heat Shock Proteins; DC, dendritic cells; AAV, adeno-associated virus (AAV is a less immunogenic vector).
* Gene gun.

with an additional challenge; to develop methods for identifying TAAs in the more common cancers to include cancers of the lung (Table 16.3).

Whole-Tumor Cells

As alluded to above for the immunotherapy of lung cancer, trials with inactivated whole-tumor cells administered as vaccines have been at best disappointing. It has been surmised that the reason for the ineffectiveness of whole-tumor cell vaccines in humans is the lack of costimulatory molecules on tumor cells and/or lack of secretion of the cytokines necessary for activating professional APCs (e.g., dendritic cells). To this end, tumor cells have been modified to express costimulatory molecules such as B7.1, cytokines such as GM-CSF, TNF-α, IFN-γ, or one of several interleukins.[73] Animal studies have demonstrated that immunization with GM-CSF–secreting inactivated tumor cells resulted in increased antitumor immunity *in vivo*.[74] Data such as these have led to the recent evaluation of GM-CSF-modified tumor cells as vaccines for several human cancers, including renal cell carcinoma.

Proteins or Peptides

Purified protein vaccines against cancer have primarily consisted of artificially engineered tumors with model antigens in murine tumor systems, for example, solid tumors expressing ovalbumin (OVA)[75] or the bacterial enzyme beta-galactosidase (β-gal).[76] Although these TAAs are completely artificial and the tumor models are irrelevant to real-life cancers, the information gained through these studies has and will continue to prove invaluable to the field of cancer vaccine development. Recombinant viral proteins (e.g., SV40 Tag and HPV) have also been tested as protein vaccines in ani-

mal tumor models.[77,78] Information gathered form these studies may be directly applied to human cancers with the corresponding viral association (see section on viral tumor antigens).

Synthetic peptide epitopes from cloned tumor antigens would be valuable for clinical trials for the following reasons: (a) peptides can be easily produced with minimal cost in large quantities that are stable and free of contaminating substances; (b) such peptides could be used to stimulate and expand CTLs from patients *ex vivo* for therapeutic transfer back to the same patient; (c) these anticancer CTL-inducing peptides could be developed as vaccines to be delivered parenterally for therapeutic treatment of cancer. A striking example is a recent clinical trial involving melanoma-derived TAA peptides as a therapeutic vaccine administered to patients with advanced metastatic disease. Peptide immunization resulted in a higher percentage of clinical responses (including complete responses) in patients than had previously been seen for any other therapy for melanoma.[43] Investigators are hopeful that peptide-vaccine studies currently underway will demonstrate the power and potential of therapeutic peptide-based vaccines for the treatment of cancer.

Nucleic Acids and Recombinant Viruses

Advances in recombinant DNA technology have ushered in some novel and exciting approaches for anti-cancer vaccine development, namely nucleic acid vaccination.[79] Injection of plasmid DNA-encoding TAAs has been successful in inducing tumor immunity in animal models when administered either ballistically as DNA-coated gold particles[80] or as "naked" DNA in saline.[16]

Viruses have long been known to be potent inducers of CTL-mediated immunity.[81] Efforts to deliver TAAs as vaccines with the greatest potential for CTL induction have employed recombinant viruses. Some examples include recombinant adenoviruses that express murine homologues to human melanoma antigens[82] and recombinant pox viruses including vaccinia, canary pox, or modified vaccinia viruses (MVA). Recombinant vaccinia viruses expressing model tumor antigens have not only been successful inducing protective immunity to tumor challenge, but also in treating established tumors in mice.[83,84]

Heat-Shock Proteins

A series of recent studies has revealed a new and potentially powerful source of TAAs as well as a novel strategy for vaccination against cancer. Srivastava and colleagues have demonstrated that heat-shock proteins (HSP) chaperone peptides from the cytosol of tumor cells to the endoplasmic reticulum, thereby playing an active role in the process of antigen presentation. More strikingly was their demonstration that purified heat-shock proteins (bearing peptides from intracellularly digested TAAs) effectively serve as vaccines against the tumor from which they were purified.[85] These studies have led to trials involving the extraction of HSPs from tumors resected from patients followed by therapeutic immunization with the purified HSPs.

Dendritic Cells

Dendritic cells (DCs) are arguably the most potent of antigen-presenting cells, expressing both MHC-I and MHC-II molecules, as well as a full complement of costimulatory molecules.[86] Therefore it is not surprising that DCs have been a recent focus of experimental cell-based cancer vaccines. Briefly, DC-based tumor vaccines include: DCs pulsed with recombinant protein TAAs, synthetic peptides[87] or mRNA-encoding TAAs,[88] DCs transduced with retroviruses expressing TAAs,[89] or DCs fused to tumor cells forming a DC-tumor hybrid cell vaccine.[90]

CONCLUSION

The overall rise in cancer incidence, coupled with a high mortality rate for many forms of cancer, necessitates the need for alternative therapies for treatment and prevention. Immunotherapeutic strategies for cancer treatment represent attractive alternatives to standard protocols for the following reasons: (a) The immune system has the ability to recognize changes as small as a single amino acid in a complex protein as well as distinguish "normal self" from "nonself" or "diseased self," thereby eliminating the overwhelming and sometimes fatally toxic side effects associated with most of the available conventional therapies. (b) The immune system is by nature systemic, that is, the cells and products of an immune response possess the ability to reach tissue sites harboring microscopic metastatic deposits of tumor cells not detectable or resectable using standard procedures. In this capacity immunotherapy holds great promise in the near future as a follow-up therapy for surgical resection of primary tumors. (c) Possibly the most powerful hallmark of the immune system is its unique ability to mount an amnestic response. This attribute has made possible, through vaccination, the eradication of deadly viral diseases such as polio and smallpox.

The widespread utilization of treatment modalities designed to induce an active immune response against human cancer has yet to be clinically realized. Progress to this end has been hampered, in part, by difficulties in identifying TAAs. With the exception of melanoma, very few candidate tumor antigens have been defined for human malignancies. Interestingly, the majority of melanoma antigens have been identified by screening cDNA libraries (generated from autologous or allogeneic melanoma cell lines) with CTLs from melanoma patients possessing melanoma-specific reactivities. The two key elements that made these antigen discovery efforts successful were melanoma cell lines and a source

of "primed" T-cells from patients (e.g., TILs). Unfortunately, tumor cell lines have been difficult to generate for the more common malignancies (e.g., breast, prostate, and lung cancer), and the generation of TILs has not been convincingly demonstrated for any cancers other than melanoma (an exception might be renal cell carcinoma). Thus new approaches (Table 16-4) are needed to identify candidate TAAs for the more common cancers such as breast, prostate, and lung cancer.

One approach is to screen libraries from tumor cells using tumor-specific antibodies from cancer patients.[91] Another is to use biochemistry and mass spectrometry to examine the peptide profile eluted from the MHC-I molecules expressed on tumor cells.[92] Finally, tumor-specific or upregulated TAAs could be identified by analysis of differentially expressed genes in tumor cells compared to normal cells of the same histology. This could be accomplished by (a) generating normal cell subtracted, tumor cell cDNA libraries (requires large amounts of mRNA, so normal and tumor cell lines are critical); (b) using serial analysis of gene expression (SAGE) techniques,[93] or (c) differential display, RT-PCR[94] (see also Chapter 1). Sequence information from cloned differentially expressed genes would allow investigators to test whether a series of candidate antigens are capable

---

TABLE 16.4. STRATEGIES FOR TUMOR ANTIGEN DISCOVERY

T-cell–based
- cDNA library from tumor cell lines screened for recognition with tumor-specific T-cells.
- Examples of cloned TAAs*. MAGE, BAGE, GAGE, MART-1, gp100, tyrosinase, *β*-catenin.

Antibody-based
- Phage expression library from tumor cells screened with patient antisera.
- Examples of cloned TAAs: NY-ESO-1, NY-CO-1 to 48, SSX2, MAGE, tyrosinase.

Biochemistry-based (mass spectrometry and HPLC)
- Elution of peptides from MHC-I on tumor cells followed by purification and sequencing.
- Examples of TAAs identified: tyrosinase, gp100.

Molecular Differential Analysis of Gene Expression†
- Differences in expressed genes (mRNA) from tumor cells compared to normal cells.
- Examples of methods to clone differential expressed TAAs:
  subtracted cDNA libraries
  DD-RT-PCR
  SAGE

---

* See antigens cloned from melanoma, above.
† Requires large amounts of mRNA from paired normal and tumor tissue or cell lines.
TAA, tumor-associated antigen; ESO, esophageal cancer; CO, colon cancer; HPLC, high-pressure liquid chromatography; MHC-I, type one major histocompatibility antigens; DD-RT-PCR, differential display reverse transcription polymerase chain reaction. (From Liang P, Pardee AB. Science 1992;257:967); SAGE, serial analysis of gene expression (Velculescu VE, Zhang L, Vogelstein, B, et al. *Science* 1995;270:484, with permission.)

of stimulating PBLs to generate CTLs (via *in vitro* peptide stimulation) that are capable of killing the tumor cells from which the TAAs were originally cloned.

It is evident that a single shared TAA that could be applied against cancer in general does not exist. It is also becoming clear that there may be multiple candidate TAAs for any one type of cancer (as with melanoma). Taken together, this information supports the possibility of multiple TAAs that may be clinically useful for specific tumor immunotherapy. However, it is likely that the number of candidate TAAs is finite and definable for a given type of cancer. Future clinical application may consist of early detection screening, at which time a tissue specimen could be examined for expression (molecular biology techniques, perhaps microchip arrays) of any one or more of the defined TAAs for that type of cancer (see also Chapter 1). The patient could then be treated with a vaccine (made up of TAAs expressed by the tumor) at a time point where tumor burden (minimal, perhaps following resection of primary lesion) and immune status of the patient would not undermine the efficacy of the therapy and subsequent response.

REFERENCES

1. Rous P. An experimental comparison of transplanted tumor and a transplanted normal tissue capable of growth. *J Exp Med* 1910; 12:344.
2. Coley WB. The treatment of malignant tumors by repeated inoculums of erysipelas. *Am J Med Sci* 1893;105:487.
3. Foley EJ. Antigenic properties of methylcholanthrene-induced tumors in mice of the strain of origin. *Cancer Res* 1953;13:835.
4. Prehn RT, Main JM. Immunity to methylcholanthrene-induced sarcomas. *J Natl Cancer Inst* 1957;18:769.
5. Klein G, Sjogren HO, Klein E, et al. Demonstration of resistance against methylcholanthrene-induced sarcomas in the primary autochthonous host. *Cancer Res* 1960;20:1561.
6. Burnet FM. Immunologic surveillance in neoplasia. *Transplant Rev* 1971;7:3.
7. Kahn M, Sugawara H, Mcgowan P, et al. CD4 + T cell clones specific for the human p97 melanoma-associated antigen can eradicate pulmonary metastases from a murine tumor expressing the p97 antigen. *J Immunol* 1991;146:3235.
8. Greenberg PD. Adoptive T cell therapy of tumors: mechanisms operative in the recognition and elimination of tumor cells. *Adv Immunol* 1990;49:281.
9. Topalian SL, Gonzales MI, Parkhurst M, et al. Melanoma-specific CD4 + T cells recognize nonmutated HLA-DR-restricted tyrosinase epitopes. *J Exp Med* 1996;183:1965.
10. Boon T, Cerottini J-C, Van den Eynde B, et al. Tumor antigens recognized by T lymphocytes. *Annu Rev Immunol* 1994;12:337.
11. Rosenberg SA. The development of new cancer therapies based on the molecular identification of cancer regression antigens. *The Cancer Journal, Sci Am* 1995;2:90.
12. Davis MM, Boniface JJ, Reich Z, et al. Ligand recognition by $\alpha\beta$ T cell receptors. *Annu Rev Immunol* 1998;16:523.
13. Kovacsovics-Bankowski M, Clark K, Benacerraf B, et al. Efficient major histocompatibility class I presentation of exogenous antigen upon phagocytosis by macrophages. *Proc Natl Acad Sci USA* 1993;90:4942.
14. Roa JB, Chamberlain RS, Bronte V, et al. IL-12 is an effective adjuvant to recombinant vaccinia virus-based tumor vaccines. *J Immunol* 1996;156:3357.
15. Feltkamp MCW, Smits HL, Vierboom MPM, et al. Vaccination with a cytotoxic T lymphocyte-containing peptide protects against a tumor induced by human papillomavirus type 16-transformed cells. *Eur J Immunol* 1993;23:2242.
16. Bright RK, Beames B, Shearer MH, et al. Protection against a lethal tumor challenge with SV40-transformed cells by the direct injection of DNA-encoding SV40 large tumor antigen. *Cancer Res* 1996;56:1126.
17. Rosenberg SA, Yannelli JR, Yang JC, et al. Treatment of patients with metastatic melanoma using autologous tumor-infiltrating lymphocytes and interleukin-2. *J Nat Cancer Inst* 1994;86:1159.
18. Wallich R, Bulbuc N, Hammerling GJ, et al. Abrogation of metastatic properties of tumor cells by *de novo* expression H-2^k antigens following H-2 gene transfection. *Nature* 1985;315:301.
19. Bright RK, Shearer MH, Pass HI, et al. Immunotherapy of SV40-induced tumors in mice: a model for vaccine development. *Dev Biol Stand* 1998;94:341.
20. Kast WM, Offringa R, Peters PJ, et al. Eradication of adenovirus E1-induced tumors by E1a-specific cytotoxic T lymphocytes. *Cell* 1989;59:603.
21. Schwartz RH. Costimulation of T lymphocytes: the role of CD28, CTLA-4, and B7/BB1 in interleukin-2 production and immunotherapy. *Cell* 1992;71:1065.
22. Schwartz RH. A cell culture model for T lymphocyte clonal anergy. *Science* 1990;248:1349.
23. Townsend SE, Allison JP. Tumor rejection after direct costimulation of CD8 + T cells by B7-transfected melanoma cells. *Science* 1993;259:368.
24. Kappler JW, Roehm N, Marrack P. T cell tolerance by clonal elimination in the thymus. *Cell* 1987;49:273.
25. Le Bon A, Desaymard C, and Papiemik M. Neonatal impaired response to viral superantigen encoded by MMTV(SW) and MTv-7. *Int Immunol* 1995;12:1897.
26. Husler MR, Kotopoulis KA, Sundberg JP, et al. Lactation-induced WAP-SV40 Tag transgene expression in C57BL/6J mice leads to mammary carcinoma. *Transgenic Res* 1998;7:253.
27. Morgan DJ, Kreuwel HTC, Fleck S, et al. Activation of low avidity CTL specific for a self epitope results in tumor rejection but not autoimmunity. *J Immunol* 1998;160:643.
28. Ludewig B, Odermatt B, Landmann S, et al. Dendritic cells induce autoimmune diabetes and maintain disease via *de novo* formation of local lymphoid tissue. *J Exp Med* 1998;188:1493.
29. Mossman TR, Coffman RL. Th1 and Th2 cells: different patterns of lymphokine secretion lead to different functional properties. *Annu Rev Immunol* 1989;7:145.
30. Krolick KA, Uhr JW, Slavin S, et al. *In vivo* therapy of a murine B cell tumor BCL1 using antibody-ricin A chain immunotoxins. *J Exp Med* 1982;155:1797.
31. Goldenberg DM. New developments in monoclonal antibodies for cancer detection and therapy. *CA Cancer J Clin* 1994;44:43.
32. Bright RK, Shearer MH, Kennedy RC. Immunization of BALB/c mice with recombinant SV40 large tumor antigen induces antibody-dependent cell-mediated cytotoxicity (ADCC) against SV40 transformed cells: an antibody based mechanism for tumor immunity. *J Immunol* 1994;153:2064.
33. Melief CJ, Offringa R, Toes RE, et al. Peptide-based cancer vaccines. *Curr Opin Immunol* 1996;8:651.
34. Shu SS, Plautz GE, Krauss JC, et al. Tumor immunology. *JAMA* 1997;278:1972.
35. Yoshizawa H, Chang AE, Shu S. Specific adoptive immunotherapy mediated by tumor-draining lymph node cells sequentially activated with anti-CD3 and IL-2. *J Immunol* 1991;147:729.
36. Chang AE, Aruga A, Cameron MJ, et al. Adoptive immunother-

apy with vaccine-primed lymph node cells secondarily activated with anti-CD3 and IL-2. *J Clin Oncol* 1997;15:796.

37. Parkhurst MR, Salgaller ML, Southwood S, et al. Improved induction of melanoma-reactive CTL with peptides from the melanoma antigen gp 100 modified at HLA-A*0201-binding residues. *J Immunol* 1996;157:2539.

38. Salgaller ML, Afshar A, et al. Recognition of multiple epitopes in the human melanoma antigen gp 100 by peripheral blood lymphocytes stimulated *in vitro* with synthetic peptides. *Cancer Res* 1995;55:4972.

39. Herin M, Lemoine C, Weynants P, et al. Production of stable cytolytic T-cell clones directed against autologous human melanoma. *Int J Cancer* 1987;39:390.

40. Slingluff CL, Darrow TL, Seigler HF. Melanoma-specific cytotoxic T cells generated from peripheral blood lymphocytes. *Ann Surg* 1989;210:194.

41. Crowley NJ, Slinghuff CL, Darrow TL, et al. Generation of human autologous melanoma-specific cytotoxic T-cells using HLA matched allogeneic melanomas. *Cancer Res* 1990;50:492.

42. Stevens EJ, Jacknin L, Robbins PF, et al. Generation of tumor-specific CTLs from melanoma patients by using peripheral blood stimulated with allogeneic melanoma tumor cell lines. *J Immunol* 1995;154:762.

43. Rosenberg SA, Yang JC, Schwartzentruber DJ, et al. Immunologic and therapeutic evaluation of a synthetic peptide vaccine for the treatment of patients with metastatic melanoma. *Nat Med* 1998;4:269.

44. Thatcher N, Sambrook RJ, Stephens RJ. First results of a randomized trial of dose intensification with G-CSF in small cell lung cancer. *Lung* 1997;18:7.

45. Al-Moundhri M, O'Brien M, Souberbielle BE. Immunotherapy of lung cancer. *Br J Cancer* 1998;78:282.

46. O'Brien MER, Bromelow K, Prendiville J, et al. A study of SRL 172 (Mycobacterium vaccae) as the first component of a tumour vaccine with immunological changes and clinical activity in patients with lung cancer. *Lung* 1997;18:163.

47. Goodman GE, Hellstrom I, Yelton D, et al. Phase I trial of chimeric monoclonal antibody L6 in patients with non small cell lung, colon, and breast cancer. *Cancer Immunol Immunother* 1993;36:267.

48. Pai L, Batra J, Fitzgerald D. Antitumor activities of immunotoxin made of mab B3 and various forms of pseudomonas exotoxin. *Proc Natl Acad Sci USA* 1991;88:3358.

49. Lynch TJ. Immunotoxin therapy of small cell lung cancer. N901 blocked ricin for relapsed small cell lung cancer. *Chest* 1993;103:436s.

50. Rosenberg SA, Lotze MT, Muul LM, et al. Observations on the systemic administration of autologous lymphokine-activated killer cells and recombinant interleukin-2 to patients with metastatic cancer. *N Engl J Med* 1985;313:1485.

51. Topalian SL, Muul LM, Solomon D, et al. Expansion of human tumor infiltrating lymphocytes for use in immunotherapy trials. *J Immunol Methods* 1987;102:127.

52. Kimura H, Yamaguchi Y. Adjuvant immunotherapy with interleukin-2 and lymphokine-activated killer cells after noncurative resection of primary lung cancer. *Lung Cancer* 1995;13:31.

53. Wakimoto H, Abe J, Tsunoda R, et al. Intensified antitumor immunity by a cancer vaccine that produces granulocyte-macrophage colony-stimulating factor plus interleukin-4. *Cancer Res* 1996;56:1828.

54. Hollinshead A, Stewart TH, Takita H, et al. Adjuvant specific active lung cancer immunotherapy trials. Tumor-associated antigens. *Cancer* 1987;60:1249.

55. Gabrilovich D, Kavanaugh D, Ishida T, et al. Induction of p53/ras specific cellular immunity in patients with common solid tumors. *Lung* 1997;18:90.

56. Rudden RW. Tumor immunology: immunologic approaches to the diagnosis and treatment of cancer. In: Rudden RW, ed. *Cancer biology.* 3rd ed. New York: Oxford University Press, 1995:442.

57. Resnick RM, Cornelissen MT, Wright DK, et al. Detection and typing of human papillomavirus in archival cervical cancer specimens by DNA amplification with consensus primers. *J Natl Cancer Inst* 1990;82:1477.

58. Melief CJM, Kast WM. T-cell immunotherapy of tumors by adoptive transfer of cytotoxic T lymphocytes and by vaccination with minimal essential epitopes. *Immunol Rev* 1995;146:167.

59. Bersagel DJ, Finegold MJ, et al. DNA sequences similar to those of simian virus 40 in ependymomas and choroid plexus tumors of childhood. *N Engl J Med* 1992;326:988.

60. Carbone M, Pass HI, et al. Simian virus 40 like DNA sequences in human pleural mesothelioma. *Oncogene* 1994;9:1781.

61. Pass HI, Kennedy RC, Carbone M. Evidence for and implications of SV40-like sequences in human mesotheliomas. In: DeVita V, Hellman, and Rosenberg SA, eds. *Important advances in oncology.* Philadelphia: Lippincott-Raven, 1996.

62. Linehan DC, Goedegebuure PS, Peoples GE, et al. Tumor-specific and HLA-A2-restricted cytolysis by tumor-associated lymphocytes in human metastatic breast cancer. *J Immunol* 1995;155:4486.

63. Fenton RG, Longo DL. Danger versus tolerance: paradigms for future studies of tumor-specific cytotoxic T lymphocytes. *J Natl Cancer Inst* 1997;89:272.

64. Robbins PF, El-Gamil, Li YF, et al. A mutated beta-catenin gene encodes a melanoma-specific antigen recognized by tumor infiltrating lymphocytes. *J Exp Med* 1996;183:1185.

65. Levine AJ, Momand J, Finlay CA. The p53 tumour suppressor gene. *Nature* 1991;351:453.

66. Vierboom MPM, Nijman HW, Offringa R, et al. Tumor eradication by wild-type p53-specific cytotoxic T lymphocytes. *J Exp Med* 1997;186:695.

67. Boon T, van der Bruggen P. Human tumor antigens recognized by T lymphocytes. *J Exp Med* 1996;183:725.

68. Rosenberg SA. Cancer vaccines based on the identification of genes encoding cancer regression antigens. *Immunol Today* 1997;18:175.

69. Zhang S, Zhang HS, Cordon-Cardo C, et al. Selection of tumor antigens as targets for immune attack using immunohistochemistry: protein antigens. *Clin Cancer Res* 1998;4:2669.

70. Wei WZ, Pauley R, Lichlyter D, et al. Neoplastic progression of breast epithelial cells—a molecular analysis. *Br J Cancer* 1998;78:198.

71. Henderson RA, Konitsky WM, Barratt-Boyes SM, et al. Retroviral expression of MUC-1 human tumor antigen with intact repeat structure and capacity to elicit immunity *in vivo. J Immunother* 1998;21:247.

72. Coveney EC, Geraghty JG, Sherry F, et al. The clinical value of CEA and CA15-3 in breast cancer management. *Int J Biol Markers* 1995;10:35.

73. Jaffee EM, Hurwitz, Pardoll DM. Gene modification of tumors. In: DeVita VT, Hellman S, Rosenberg SA, eds. *Biological therapy of cancer.* 2nd ed. Philadelphia: Lippincott, 1995:774.

74. Dranoff G, Jaffee E, Lazenby A, et al. Vaccination with irradiated tumor cells engineered to secrete murine granulocyte-macrophage colony-stimulating factor stimulates potent, specific, and long-lasting anti-tumor immunity. *Proc Natl Acad Sci USA* 1993;90:3539.

75. Young JW, Inaba K. Dendritic cells as adjuvants for class I major histocompatibility complex-restricted antitumor immunity. *J Exp Med* 1996;183:7.

76. Wang M, Bronte V, Chen PW et al. Active immunotherapy of cancer with a non-replicating recombinant fowlpox virus encod-

ing a model tumor-associated antigen. *J Immunol* 1995;154: 4685.

77. Shearer MH, Bright RK, Lanford RE, et al. Immunization of mice with baculovirus-derived recombinant SV40 large tumor antigen induces protective tumor immunity to a lethal challenge with SV40-transformed cells. *Clin Exp Immunol* 1993;91:266.

78. Ji H, Chang EY, Lin KY, et al. Antigen-specific immunotherapy for murine lung metastatic tumors expressing human papillomavirus type 16 E7 oncoprotein. *Int J Cancer* 1998;78:41.

79. Xiang ZQ, Pasquini S, He Z, et al. Genetic vaccines—a revolution in vaccinology? *Springer Semin Immunopathol* 1997;19:257.

80. Irvine KR, Rao JB, Rosenberg SA, et al. Cytokine enhancement of DNA immunization leads to effective treatment of established pulmonary metastases. *J Immunol* 1996;156:238.

81. Irvine KR, Restifo NP. The next wave of recombinant and synthetic anticancer vaccines. *Semin Cancer Biol* 1995;6:337.

82. Zhai Y, Zang JC, Kawakami Y, et al. Development and characterization of recombinant adenoviruses encoding MARTI or gp100 for cancer therapy. *J Immunol* 1996;156:700.

83. Bronte V, Tsung K, Rao JB, et al. IL-2 enhances the function of recombinant poxvirus-based vaccines in the treatment of established pulmonary metastases. *J Immunol* 1995;154:5282.

84. Xie YC, Hwang C, Overwijk W, et al. Induction of tumor antigen-specific immunity *in vivo* by a novel vaccinia vector encoding safety-modified simian virus 40 T antigen. *J Natl Cancer Inst* 1999;91:169.

85. Srivastava PK, Udono H. Heat-shock protein-peptide complexes in cancer immunotherapy. *Curr Opin Immunol* 1994;6:728.

86. Steinman RM. The dendritic cell system and its role in immunogenicity. *Annu Rev Immunol* 1991;9:271.

87. Porgador A, Gilboa E. Bone marrow-generated dendritic cells pulsed with a class I-restricted peptide are potent inducers of cytotoxic T lymphocytes. *J Exp Med* 1995;182:255.

88. Boczkowski D, Nair SK, Snyder D, et al. Dendritic cells pulsed with RNA are potent antigen-presenting cells *in vitro* and *in vivo*. *J Exp Med* 1996;184:465.

89. Specht JM, Wang G, Do MT, et al. Dendritic cells retrovirally transduced with a model antigen gene are therapeutically effective against established pulmonary metastases. *J Exp Med* 1997;186:1213.

90. Wang J, Saffold S, Cao X, et al. Eliciting T cell immunity against poorly immunogenic tumors by immunization with dendritic cell-tumor fusion vaccines. *J Immunol* 1998;161:5516.

91. Chen YT, Scanlan MJ, Sahin U, et al. A testicular antigen aberrantly expressed in human cancers detected by autologous antibody screening. *Proc Natl Acad Sci USA* 1997;94:1914.

92. Slingluff CL Jr, Hunt DE, Engelhard VH. Direct analysis of tumor-associated peptide antigens. *Curr Opin Immunol* 1994;6:733.

93. Velculescu VE, Zhang L, Vogelstein B, et al. Serial analysis of gene expression. *Science* 1995;270:484.

94. Liang P, Pardee AB. Differential display of eukaryotic mRNA by means of the polymerase chain reaction. *Science* 1992;257:967.

17

GENE THERAPY

CHOON-TAEK LEE
SAMIR KUBBA
KEITH COFFEE
DAVID P. CARBONE

Lung cancer continues to be a major cause of cancer death all over the world. Despite recent advances in chemotherapy, radiation therapy, surgery, and a host of combinations of these, only relatively small real advances have been achieved in improving the likelihood of surviving lung cancer. Major advances, however, are being made in the field of molecular biology and the understanding of the genetic basis of this disease, and the hope is that this information will ultimately lead to rationally designed treatments that improve the outcomes of lung cancer patients. Gene therapy is an early attempt at utilizing molecular biology in lung cancer therapeutics, and the status of the field and its specific application to this disease will be reviewed in this chapter.

Gene therapy is the treatment of cancer using genetic material as a therapeutic agent. The basic approaches of gene therapy can be broadly classified into one of two groups: (a) modification of the host response to the tumor, for example by inducing immunity or altering angiogenenic responses, or (b) production of a direct antitumor action in which the introduced genetic material directly affects the cancer cell to halt its growth or kill it. These two approaches will be discussed separately.

MODIFICATION OF HOST RESPONSES TO TUMORS

Improving Immunologic Recognition

During the process by which a normal cell becomes a neoplastic cell, a series of genetic lesions occur that result in the loss of normal growth regulation and the acquisition of the ability to avoid immune surveillance. Many of these genetic lesions directly or indirectly result in the expression of potential tumor antigens. Cytotoxic T-cell responses specific for several of these can be detected or artificially induced, but it is very clear that clinically evident tumors have managed to avoid induction of an effective immune response. Gene therapy techniques can be used to deliver biologically active genes intended to alter the tumor's local immunologic microenvironment, increasing the immunogenicity of cancer cells or the responsiveness of T-cells, improving antigen presentation, or providing missing paracrine factors.

MHC Molecules

The chromosomal region containing the MHC was originally identified because of the ability of genes in this region to mediate transplant rejection as well as to control the immune response of mice and guinea pigs to simple antigens (see also Chapter 16). The analogous genetic region in humans was subsequently shown to encode the genes called the human leukocyte antigens, or HLA molecules. The proximate function of the HLA molecules encoded within the MHC is the presentation of antigenic peptides to T-cells. HLA class I and class II molecules are cell surface glycoproteins, anchored to the membrane by hydrophobic transmembrane segments. HLA class I molecules bind to endogenously synthesized peptide fragments and present them on the cell surface for recognition by the T-cell receptor (TCR) on CD8+ T-cells. HLA class II molecules are primarily involved in presenting foreign antigens to CD4+ T-cells during the initiation and propagation of the immune response. HLA class I molecules are distributed widely among most somatic cells of the body, with the exception of red blood cells. Class II molecules have a much more restricted tissue distribution, generally limited to cells of the immune system such as B cells, macrophages, dendritic cells, and some subsets of T-cells. Class II interaction induces the production of cytokines necessary for the expansion of cytotoxic effectors.

Tumor cells have some level of expression of MHC class I molecules on their surface, but in many tumor cells expression of MHC may be low. Allogenic MHC class I genes have been introduced into tumor cells, and this results in the expected induction of allo-MHC-specific cytotoxic T-cells. Importantly, responses against endogenous tumor antigens are also induced. The allo-MHC-specific T-cells presumably assist in the generation of T-cells specific for previously silent tumor-specific antigens by producing cytokines in the tumor microenvironment. In a murine lung cancer system (3LL/3) from C57BL/6 mice (MHC type H-2[b]), transfection of the allogenic MHC molecule H-2L[d] caused a reduction in tumorigenicity and protection against unmodified 3LL/3.[1] Plautz and colleagues[2] showed that expression of a murine class I H-2K[s] gene in CT26 mouse colon adenocarcinoma (H-2K[d]) or MCA 106 fibrosarcoma (H-2K[b]) induced a cytotoxic T-cell response to H-2K[s] and, more importantly, to other antigens present on unmodified tumor cells which had not been recognized previously. Recently, allogenic MHC transfection has been applied to humans with HLA-B7 gene transfer. Nabel and colleagues[3] reported the reduction of tumor size in a melanoma patient after the direct gene transfer of an HLA-B7 gene in a liposome complex. Clinical protocols of HLA-B7 gene transfer by lipofection in advanced cancer including melanoma, renal cell cancer, and colon cancer have shown immune responses and tumor shrinkage.[4-10] Shrinkage of noninjected tumors was also reported in some of these studies.

Therapeutic transfection of syngeneic MHC class I and II molecules has been attempted in several different tumor model systems. Transfection of syngeneic MHC class II (A) in sarcoma cells induced an immune response against both transfected tumor cells and nontransfected tumor cells.[11] This finding suggests that transfected MHC class II molecules can induce T-helper cells specific to nontransfected tumor cells as well.

Low MHC class I molecule expression in some tumors may lead to decreased presentation of tumor-specific antigens on the cell surface, which could be one mechanism for their escape from immune surveillance. Transfection of syngeneic MHC class I molecules could induce or increase the presentation of endogenous peptide fragments derived from tumor-specific antigens, leading to generation of CD8 + CTLs specific for parental tumor antigens. Once induced, this response can cause recognition and lysis of nongene modified cells with lower levels of MHC expression. Increased MHC class I expression on tumor cells may thus result in enhanced immunogenicity and decreased tumorigenicity of tumor cells. Plaskin and co-workers[12] showed that high expression of a transfected H-2K[b] MHC gene in highly metastatic Lewis lung carcinoma cell (3LL) resulted in the conversion of a high metastatic phenotype to a nonmetastatic or low-metastatic phenotype and protection against the metastatic spread of 3LL.

Costimulatory Molecules (B7)

For the induction of T-cell–dependent cellular and humoral immune responses, there is a requirement for two different types of stimuli. The first is antigen-specific engagement of the T-cell receptor (TCR) with the antigen/MHC complex, and the second is the antigen-independent stimulation of another set of receptors called costimulatory molecules. This second signal is transmitted by the antigen-independent binding of costimulatory molecules on antigen-presenting cells (APC) with their corresponding receptors on T-cells. This signal is required to induce primary T-cell proliferation and other effector functions of the immune response.

The most extensively characterized costimulatory molecules are CD28 and CTLA-4 on T-cells and their ligands, CD80 (B7/BB1, B7-1) and CD86 (B70, B7-2), on professional APC. Ligation of CD28 on T-cells by its counter-receptors, CD80 (B7-1) and CD86 (B7-2), leads to the secretion of cytokines such as IL-2 and induces cytolytic T-cells. One of the reasons that professional antigen-presenting cells such as dendritic cells are such potent inducers of immunity is the high levels they express of both MHC and costimulatory molecules. Tumor cells may have tumor-specific antigens and MHC class I expression but only rarely express B7, and thus are extremely poor direct inducers of immune responses. The rationale of transfection of B7 into tumor cells is to provide or supplement the necessary costimulation for effective immune induction. Townsend and colleagues[13] demonstrated that B7-transfection into MHC class I and II positive melanoma induced the rejection of tumors *in vivo*. This rejection was mediated by CD8 + T-cells and did not require CD4 + T-cells.

Kato and co-workers[14] augmented the antitumor effect against existing tumors by the combination of B7 and interleukin 12 (IL-12) gene transfer, and found that these modified tumor cells could induce the rejection of metastatic tumors in syngeneic mice. They first transfected mouse lung carcinoma 3LL with mouse B7 using a plasmid vector and established transfectants expressing cell surface B7 (B7/3LL). Subsequently, interleukin-12 (IL-12) was transduced into these cells using retroviral vectors encoding two subunits of murine IL-12—p35 and p40 respectively—generating stable transfectants producing IL-12 (IL-12/3LL and IL-12/B7/3LL). Four weeks after 3LL inoculation, lung metastasis was significantly reduced, with a mean metastatic colony number of 55.2 with B7/3LL compared to 23.8 with IL-12/B7/3LL. These results indicate that potent therapeutic antitumor immunity can be induced by combination of costimulatory B7 and IL-12, and that this approach could potentially be useful for cancer gene therapy.

Carcinoembryonic antigen (CEA) is an oncofetal protein expressed by many adenocarcinomas, including those of lung origin. Recently, cotransduction of recombinant vaccinia virus expressing RVB7-1 and one expressing CEA (RV-CEA) resulted in CEA-specific T-cell responses and antitumor immunity against a murine carcinoma expressing human CEA. These findings suggest that B7 increased the immunogenicity of CEA.[15] B7 transduction into murine fibrosarcomas expressing a *p53* mutation resulted in the induction of mutant p53-specific CTL and loss of tumorigenicity as well as protective immunity against challenge by untransduced tumors.[16] Similar induction of immunity was found for the P1A epitope in the P815 (murine plasmacytoma) tumor model. Another study demonstrated that B7 and CD28 interaction provide costimulatory signals not only for T-cells but also for natural killer (NK) cells.[17] Tumor cell resistance to NK cells is associated with high expression of MHC class I molecules; B7:CD28 interaction induced by B7 transfection can overcome the MHC class I–mediated inactivation of NK cells, increasing their tumoricidal activity. All of these studies provide the experimental groundwork for attempts to utilize B7 in cancer gene therapeutic approaches.

Cytokines

Since the 1970s, immunotherapy against lung cancers using cytokine-gene–modified cancer cells has been studied as a novel approach for anticancer immunotherapy in many laboratories. Rosenberg was the first to report that systemic administration of IL-2 with or without *in vitro* expanded autologous lymphokine-activated killer cells (LAK) in advanced cancer patients was associated with significant antitumor responses.[18] However, the toxicities of systemic cytokine administration interfered with the popularization of this approach. To avoid systemic side effects and, more important, to approximate normal physiological conditions, gene therapy has been used to insert cytokine genes into tumor cells and induce local production of cytokines in the vicinity of tumors. These altered immunological microenvironments are then postulated to provide favorable conditions for host immune detection of tumor cells and previously unrecognized tumor-specific antigens. Effective recognition of these antigens and induction of a response can therefore allow detection and killing of nongene-modified tumor cells with the same tumor-specific antigen, even though they may be located far from the site of gene modification.

A number of cytokines have been tested for efficacy in animal models of cytokine gene therapy. IL-2, IL-4, IL-6, IL-7, IL-12, IFN-γ, TNF-α, G-CSF, and GM-CSF, among others, have been investigated. Basic experiments revealed that the subcutaneous injection of cancer cells modified by cytokine genes such as IL-2,[19–22] IL-4,[21,23,24] IL-6,[25] IL-7,[26] GM-CSF,[27] IFN-α, β, γ,[19,22,28] and TNF[29] induced tumor-specific immunity.

IL-2 in particular has been investigated extensively. Fearon and associates[30] demonstrated that IL-2 cDNA transfected into murine colon carcinoma (CT26) resulted in the loss of tumorigenicity and bypassed deficient T-helper function in the generation of an antitumor response. Ley and colleagues[31] showed that IL-2–transfected murine mastocytoma (P815) cells induced P815-specific CTL which led to regression of established tumors. Using a highly malignant and poorly immunogenic Lewis lung carcinoma, IL-

2 production by retrovirally transduced tumor cells induced antitumor CTL and eliminated the generation of lung metastasis.[32] In natural immune responses, IL-2 is produced by CD4 + T-cells activated by the binding of TCR and antigens presented by MHC class II molecules on APC. Secreted IL-2 will activate CD8 + T-cell precursors to cytotoxic T-cells. IL-2 secretion by gene-modified tumor cells may activate CD8 + T-cells directly, bypassing T-helper cells. IL-2 can overcome defects in signal transduction of T-cells of tumor-bearing patients caused by the decreased levels of p56[lck], and p59[fyn].[33] Early-phase clinical trials of IL-2 cytokine gene therapy have been performed, and immune responses as well as disease stabilization have been reported.[34–40]

IL-4 also shows antitumor effects in animal tumor models. IL-4 is produced by Th2 subset of helper T-cells and mast cells, and has many functions. It can induce LAK cells, stimulate B-cell proliferation and maturation, and activate endothelial cells to express vascular cell adhesion molecules.[41] Tepper and co-workers[42] demonstrated that IL-4 production from transfected tumor cells had antitumor effects in various tumor cell lines. This effect is blocked by anti–IL-4 antibody related to the level of the production, and is evident in nude mice. Infiltration of the transduced tumor site with macrophages and eosinophils suggested that inflammatory mechanisms were involved.

IL-6 is the pleiotropic cytokine that can stimulate the differentiated functions of B-cells and T-cells and induce the production of mature myeloid cells and megakaryocytes.[43] IL-6 has antitumor effects on murine models of lung cancer. The immunization of inactivated, IL-6–transfected Lewis lung carcinoma cells induced antitumor CTL and reduced the metastatic potential of these cells.[25]

IL-7 is a bone marrow stromal-cell–derived cytokine that stimulates pre–B-cell expansion. IL-7 also functions as a growth factor for thymocytes and CD4 + and CD8 + T-cells. IL-7 can enhance the antigen presentation indirectly by increasing expression of costimulatory cell adhesion molecules such as ICAM-1 and inhibit the production of immunosuppressive cytokines such as TGF-β.[44] The production of IL-7 by retroviral transduction in fibrosarcomas can decrease tumorigenicity and induce protective immunity against unmodified tumor challenge, and IL-7 transduction of immunogenic tumors can cause the regression of established lung metastasis.[26] A clinical trial of cytokine gene therapy with IL-7 is planned in lung cancer, but no preliminary results are available.

Interferon-γ produced by activated T-cells can modulate the immune response in a number of ways. IFN-γ can induce MHC class I and II molecules which will increase the presentation of antigen on the cell surface, and can induce the activation of macrophages.[45] Low expression of MHC molecules on tumor cells is one postulated mechanism by which tumors escape from host immune surveillance. Increased expression of MHC molecules by IFN-γ should increase the presentation of tumor-specific antigens and assist the induction of antigen-specific CTL. Transduction of a weakly immunogenic tumor (CMS-5) by retroviral IFN-γ induced the abrogation of tumorigenicity and persistent and specific antitumor immunity against the unmodified CMS-5 challenge.[46] The effect of IFN-γ has also been demonstrated in the 3LL mouse lung cancer model. Retroviral IFN-γ gene insertion into poorly immunogenic 3LL-D122 showed a significant decrease in tumorigenicity and metastatic potential, and induced tumor-specific CTL when modified tumor cells were injected after irradiation.[28]

Tumor necrosis factor has direct cytolytic effects on tumor cells and attracts and augments the tumoricidal activity of macrophages.[47] Systemic administration of TNF, however, was too toxic to achieve significant *in vivo* antitumor effects. Local production of TNF-α by retroviral transduction into the TNF-insensitive tumor cell line (J558L) drastically suppressed tumorigenicity in a syngeneic animal, even though it did not appreciably affect growth *in vitro*.[48] Administration of an anti–type-3 complement factor receptor to block the migration of inflammatory cells abolished the antitumor effects of TNF-α, which suggested the involvement of an inflammatory mechanism including the activation of macrophages.[48] The antitumor effect of TNF-α was also proven in human lung cancer cell lines, even though most human tumor cells are resistant to TNF-α. Insertion of human TNF-α cDNA into several human lung cancer cells resulted in decreased tumorigenicity in nude mice.[49] Furthermore, injection of a mixture of 50% gene-modified and 50% parental cells also showed decreased tumor formation. These data suggest that local production of TNF-α can induce antitumor effects on human lung cancer cell growth, and every tumor cell need not be gene-modified to produce local antitumor effects.

GM-CSF appears to be one of the most active cytokines in the induction of antitumor immunity. In a comparison of the efficacy of a number of cytokines using retroviral vectors, GM-CSF demonstrated the most potent, specific, and long-lasting antitumor immunity.[27] The antitumor immunity induction after gene therapy with GM-CSF was dependent on both CD4 + and CD8 + T-cells. This activity may be related to its ability to promote the differentiation of hematopoietic precursors to dendritic cells and other professional antigen-presenting cells.[50] Because culture and stable transduction of human tumors are problematic, "paracrine" GM-CSF release from gelatin-chondroitin microspheres mixed with irradiated tumor cells was tested and found to evoke antitumor immunity comparable to a GM-CSF–transduced tumor vaccine.[51] We have designed and produced an adenovirus-GM-CSF vector that also overcomes many of the limitations of *in vitro* culture of primary human tumors. Transduction of 3LL with this adenovirus-GM-CSF vector eliminated its tumorigenicity and induced tumor-specific CTL and the regression of established 3LL tumors.[52] Furthermore, we showed that this was associated with an increased number of dendritic cells in the tumor vaccine injection site. Simons and co-workers reported the result of a phase I trial of renal cell carcinoma vaccine transduced with GM-CSF. They showed the infiltration of dendritic cells and delayed type hypersensitivity reaction with one partial response.[53]

IL-12 is a new cytokine with dramatic antitumor effects and relatively modest systemic toxicity in animal models. IL-12 has the ability to promote the differentiation of uncommitted T-cells to Th1 cells, thought to be key to the production of effective antitumor immunity.[54] IL-12 also activates the CD8 + T-cells and NK cells and generates LAK cells.[55] Tahara and colleagues[56] demonstrated that IL-12-retroviral transduction of murine sarcomas showed suppression of tumorigenicity, induction of protective antitumor immunity, and suppression of preinjected nontransduced tumors. This group has also completed a phase I trial of IL-12–transduced autologous fibroblasts.[57] The efficacy of IL-12 was confirmed when delivered via recombinant vaccinia virus[58] and adenovirus.[59] In addition, IL-12 transduction of dendritic cells may improve their function in cancer patients.

To improve and facilitate the clinical application of cytokine gene therapy, several modifications of the published animal model tumor systems are being evaluated. Most animal studies and some human trials have used *in vitro* cultured autologous tumor cells as targets for gene transfer. In practice this approach has serious limitations in a clinical setting, in that generating an autologous tumor-cell line from each patient's tumor is difficult, expensive, and time-consuming, and not possible in many circumstances. However, the key to cytokine gene therapy appears to be the production of appropriate cytokines in the vicinity of tumors, and not necessarily from tumor cells themselves. Several types of cells have been used for gene transfer, including fibroblasts, tumor infiltrating lymphocytes (TILs), endothelial cells,[60] and dendritic cells. Transduction of fibroblasts has many advantages over transduction of autologous cancer cells, as they can be obtained from skin biopsies, grow easily in culture for many passages, and can be efficiently transduced with viral vectors *in vitro*. Fakhrai and colleagues[61] showed that immunization with a mixture of irradiated tumor cells and IL-2–transduced fibroblasts induced protective antitumor immunity and remission of established tumors. A similar result was reported for IL-12.[62]

Further improvements in immune effectors to increase cytotoxicity have been explored. Various protocols based on gene transfer into tumor-infiltrating lymphocytes (TILs), tumor cells, or fibroblasts to express cytokine genes have been initiated. TILs are lymphocytes within a tumor mass which have localized to the tumor. Rosenberg and co-workers[63,64] have utilized TNF-gene–transduced autologous TILs in advanced cancer patients and demonstrated enhanced antitumor effects with less toxicity than systemic administration. Transduction with chimeric T-cell receptor and antibody has the potential to improve targeting and killing by these effectors as well.[64]

To augment antitumor effect, a combination of two different immunogenes has been used to obtain a synergistic effect. Kato and co-workers[65] transfected mouse B7 and/or IL-12 into mouse lung carcinoma 3LL. CTL activity induced by the inoculation of IL-12/B7/3LL was increased about tenfold compared to parental 3LL inoculation. Four weeks after 3LL inoculation, lung metastasis was significantly reduced by IL-12/B7/3LL postinoculation, indicating that potent therapeutic antitumor immunity can be induced by combination with costimulators B7 and IL-12. Combination of syngeneic MHC class I transfection and IL-2 transduction in the mouse melanoma cells also showed synergistic effects on the eradication of established lung metastasis by the combined effects of efficient CTL induction and NK/LAK activity compared with single-gene–modified tumor cells.[66,67]

Genetic Immunization

For defined target antigens, induction of epitope-specific immunity has typically been accomplished using synthetic peptides.[68,69] A variety of strategies have been employed to enhance the efficacy of peptide-based vaccines because the use of peptides as immunogens is complicated by their weak inherent immunogenicity and variable chemical and physical properties.[70–73] The chemical and physical problems of protein-or peptide-based vaccines can be avoided by the use of "genetic vaccines," purified plasmid DNA expression vectors encoding the entire cloned open reading frame of proteins introduced into living animals. These DNA vaccine vectors may generate substantial humoral and cellular immunity with little or no toxicity.[74–78] We have shown the induction of T-cell epitope-specific (mutant p53) cellular immune responses and antitumor effects after introduction of a "genetic epitope" vaccine consisting of an expression cassette containing only an oligonucleotide coding for the desired epitope.[79] In this study we used a particle gun which traumatically delivers microscopic gold particles coated with the plasmid DNA into the shaved skin of living animals. A plasmid vector containing the adenovirus E3 leader sequence was constructed, which facilitates transport of the mutant p53 epitope into the endoplasmic reticulum, showing that it can be important for optimal CTL induction and tumor-protective immunity. The use of epitope-minigene genetic vaccines may thus have significant potential for the induction of responses against identified T-cell epitopes in tumors. Direct mechanical introduction of genes into the skin is also effective.[80]

When genes are introduced into the skin or tissues to induce immunity, it is very likely that the cell that is responsible for induction is the dendritic cell or its cutaneous counterpart, the Langerhans cell (see also Chapter 16). Dendritic cells (DCs) are the most effective antigen-presenting cells

(APCs) and another important target for gene therapy directed at induction of antitumor immunity. Defective antigen-presenting function of DCs in advanced cancer patients has been demonstrated, and vascular endothelial growth factor (VEGF) produced by tumor cells is one of the factors responsible for this defective DC function.[81] DCs also have the ability to produce several cytokines that are critically involved in tumor antigen presentation by APC. DCs can be generated from human peripheral blood cells cultured with GM-CSF and IL-4. Due to their pivotal role in the induction of immunity, DCs are an important target for cancer gene therapy. Unfortunately, transfection into DCs is not easy. Retrovirus, liposome, and calcium phosphate have been used with low transfection rate. Adenovirus has shown the better transduction rate into DCs.[82] Polylysine-modified adenovirus has also been shown to be effective.[83] A variety of antigens have been transduced into dendritic cells, and this results in highly efficient induction of immunity.[84] Transduction of tumor-specific antigen (MART-1) by adenovirus could induce melanoma-specific CTL.[85,86] Minigenes encoding mutant forms of *p53*[87] or wild-type *p53*-expressing adenovirus-transduced DCs[88] have been able to induce specific CTL. Transduction of cytokine genes such as IL-12 could also be a powerful method to induce tumor-specific CTL.[89]

To date, many protocols have been conducted or are underway worldwide designed to augment the immune response against cancers by gene therapy (i.e., by vaccine or direct cytokine or costimulatory molecule gene transduction). It remains to be seen whether the theory developed in animal models can be successfully applied to the therapy of human cancer. It is likely, however, that combinations of approaches along with vaccine therapy will be the most successful, especially those that are aimed at reversing cancer-associated immune defects.

Antiangiogenic Gene Therapy

Of the approximate 200 gene therapy trials currently underway, about half target the cancer cell. These strategies include the introduction of genes that (a) produce a toxic molecule when expressed in tumor cells, (b) attempt to correct or prevent a genetic mutation, (c) attempt to make tumor cells more sensitive to chemotherapeutic drugs, and (d) increase the immunogenecity of tumor cells. Another emerging branch of gene therapy focuses on tumor antiangiogenesis. While most gene therapy protocols directed against cancer must overcome (a) the limitations of access to tumor cells, (b) varying populations of tumor cells, (c) selection of resistant cells, and (d) dependence on cell cycling, antiangiogenic gene therapy is directed against the endothelial cells that are recruited to provide blood supply to the developing tumor. Antiangiogenic gene therapy is attractive because it has potentially less systemic toxicity, does not require that the gene enter the tumor cells, is independent of growth fraction or tumor cell heterogeneity, and does not induce drug resistance.[90]

Strategies for antiangiogenic gene therapy include local versus systemic therapy. In a review of this subject, Kong and Crystal[91] argue that this approach should be used exclusively in a local or regional setting. This argument rests on the possibility that (a) the bystander effect of antiangiogenic gene therapy may be greater than other forms of gene therapy directed only against the cancer cell, and (b) potential side effects of systemically administered antiangiogenic gene therapy may be avoided. Potential systemic side effects include delayed wound healing and effects on endometrial maturation and neonatal growth; however, some data suggest that these side effects are dependent on the specific gene used.[92–94]

Lin and colleagues report on studies investigating Tie2, an endothelium-specific receptor tyrosine kinase known to play a role in tumor angiogenesis.[95] An adenoviral vector was constructed to deliver a recombinant, soluble Tie2 receptor capable of blocking activation of the Tie2 receptor on endothelial cells. Plasma concentration of the soluble receptor was maintained for about eight days, and growth of two different primary tumors was significantly inhibited following a single injection of the Tie2 adenovirus. Mice that were coinjected with tumor cells and the Tie2 adenovirus developed few grossly apparent metastases compared to numerous large, well-vascularized lung metastases in mice that received a control virus.

Several studies have demonstrated that interference of VEGF-mediated angiogenesis with either anti-VEGF antibodies[96–98] or antisense[99] is sufficient to inhibit tumor growth and metastasis (see also Chapter 11). Goldman and associates also report on studies in which tumor cells were transfected with cDNA encoding the native soluble FLT-1–truncated VEGF receptor, which can function by sequestering VEGF and by forming inactive heterodimers with membrane-spanning VEGF receptors in a dominant negative fashion.[100] Transient transfection of the truncated FLT-1 receptor significantly inhibited the implantation and growth of human fibrosarcoma cells in nude mice. Survival was also significantly improved in mice injected intracranially with human glioblastoma cells stably transfected with the FLT-1 dominant negative receptor.

As with most forms of gene therapy, limitations exist to these approaches using antiangiogenesis vectors. The adenovirus typically yields only short-term expression that limits its use for antiangiogenic therapy. Newer vectors, including adeno-associated virus and lentivirus, under development should increase expression to weeks or months. If the concerns surrounding systemic therapy are satisfied through further studies, antiangiogenic gene therapy could become an important adjunct therapy, for example following surgery to prevent recurrence or metastases, in combination with conventional chemotherapy, vaccine therapy, immunotherapy, or other types of gene therapy.

Drug Resistance Genes

Various groups are attempting to enhance marrow protection during chemotherapy by transducing the multiple drug resistance gene (MDR1) into normal bone marrow or blood-derived stem cells. The MDR1 gene produces p-glycoprotein, which functions as a cellular efflux pump and may be responsible for the resistance of some tumor cells to various hydrophobic cytotoxic drugs. Insertion of the MDR1 gene into normal marrow stem cells produces a population of cells that can be selected for resistance to a systemically administered chemotherapeutic agent and thus permit higher doses of chemotherapy to be given with less toxicity and more efficacy. Retrovirus-mediated expression of the DNA repair protein O-methylguaonidine-DNA-methyltransferase protected mouse primary hematopoietic cells from nitrosourea-induced toxicity. Marrow from mice expressing methotrexate-resistant dihydrofolate reductase was protective against methotrexate toxicity in recipient syngeneic mice. Breast and ovarian cancer protocols using MDR1 alteration have been initiated using Pac (Taxol) as the chemotherapeutic agent. This approach does have the disadvantage of higher doses of medications, may not infer higher response, nonhematologic toxicities may be dose-limiting, and the therapy may be complicated by the prior contamination of the marrow with the tumor cells.

DIRECT-ACTING GENE THERAPY

Genetic abnormalities have been found in the cancer cell that functionally contribute to the process of carcinogenesis. Introducing genetic material can directly inhibit tumor growth by replacing a damaged tumor-suppressor gene, decreasing the expression of activated or overexpressed dominant oncogenes, or by introduction of an enzymatic activity that confers sensitivity to an otherwise nontoxic drug.

Tumor-Suppressor Gene Therapy

Recent advances in the cellular and molecular biology of lung cancer have identified many genetic alterations that represent potential new molecular targets for cancer therapy.[101] Cells are chronically faced with decisions to divide, differentiate, or undergo programmed cell death (apoptosis). Two major classes of genes are known to affect this process: dominant oncogenes and recessive oncogenes (tumor-suppressor genes). Protooncogenes (the normal homologues of dominant oncogenes) participate in critical cell functions, which include signal transduction and transcription. Only a single mutant oncogene allele is required to induce malignant transformation. Modifications of the dominant oncogenes that confer gain of transforming function include point mutation, amplification, translocation, and rearrangement. Tumor-suppressor genes that are frequently found to be mutated in lung cancer include *p53*, usually altered by a point mutation combined with loss of the associated wild-type allele, or *RB*, which is usually inactivated by deletions.

Tumor-suppressor gene products appear to play a role in governing proliferation by their regulation of transcription and cell-cycle control (see also Chapter 2). Replacement of inactivated tumor-suppressor genes by gene therapy has been extensively investigated, and several tumor suppressors are potential candidates for this approach. The inactivation of *p53* may be the most common genetic alteration in human tumors and is found in human lung cancer with high frequency.[102,103] The *p53* gene encodes a nuclear phosphoprotein which controls cell proliferation and suppresses neoplastic transformation. The wild-type (wt) p53 protein delays S-phase entry in the case of DNA damage, allowing for DNA repair and preventing the propagation of mutations and chromosomal rearrangements to the next cell generations.[104,105] Normal cells tolerate this cycle arrest, but cancer cells that are driven by activating mutations in dominant oncogenes undergo apoptosis and die. Thus in order for cancer cells to survive, they often mutate *p53* and are thus resistant to this sort of apoptotic cell death. One copy of the chromosomal region 17p13 which contains *p53* is frequently deleted in both small cell lung cancer (SCLC) and non–small cell lung cancer (NSCLC), and mutational inactivation of the remaining allele occurs in more than 90% of SCLC and 50% of NSCLC.[102–104,106] The complexities of the three-dimensional structure of the p53 tumor-suppressor gene product and the radical changes in this structure induced by a single point mutation makes it extremely difficult to restore its function with pharmaceuticals. Thus the basic concept of tumor-suppressor gene thereapy utilizing *p53* is to reintroduce a functionally active copy of the defective genes in the cancer cell by direct gene transfer to directly induce cell death by apoptosis. Reintroducing a wild-type *p53* gene into lung cancer cells, including bronchioloalveolar lung cancer (BAC), dramatically inhibits tumor cell growth and promotes tumor cell death despite the presence of mutations in multiple other genes.[106] Preclinical *in vitro* and *in vivo* murine studies in head and neck cancer and NSCLC demonstrated a significant antitumor effect of Ad-*p53*. Replacement of *p53* via retroviral vectors to human lung cancer cell lines with mutated *p53* resulted in stable expression of p53 protein and apoptosis *in vitro*.[107,108] In an orthotopic lung cancer model produced by intratracheal inoculation of human lung cancer cell lines into immunodeficient mice, direct intratracheal administration of retroviral-wt *p53* expression vectors inhibited tumor growth.[109] The difficulties associated with retroviruses have led most investigators to use a recombinant adenovirus. Initial experiments in which the H358 (a p53-null BAC cell line), H322 (p53 mutant), and H460 (p53- wild-type) human NSCLC cell lines were treated with Ad-p53 resulted in significant inhibition of cell growth in the H358 and

H322 lines.[110] Direct peritumoral injection of adenovirus-p53 also inhibits solid tumor growth in nude mice.[111] In these studies, the antitumor effect of *p53* introduction appears to be primarily cell-cycle arrest followed by the induction of apoptosis.

Several human clinical trials are under way using wild-type *p53*. A trial of retrovirus expressing wild-type p53 directly injected into NSCLC endobronchial or intrapulmonary nodules has recently been completed at MD Anderson.[112] The results from the first nine patients on the retroviral p53 protocol have been reported. All nine patients (median age 68 years: range 51 to 73 years) had a history of primary NSCLC carcinoma. Of these nine patients, four had recurrent endobronchial lesion (three squamous cell carcinomas and one adenocarcinoma) and were treated with bronchoscopic injections of the retroviral *p53* expression vector ITRp53A. Another four patients had chest wall lesions (two large cell carcinomas, one squamous cell carcinoma, and one adenocarcinoma) and were treated with percutaneous injection under CT or fluoroscopic guidance. The ninth patient had a left adrenal metastasis from a large cell carcinoma, which was treated with percutaneous injection of the vector under CT guidance. All patients in the study had failed existing treatments and had cancers that were growing progressively. Three of the seven patients evaluable for response showed evidence of tumor regression in the treated lesions. In the remaining four evaluable patients, tumor growth stabilized in three patients for periods ranging from eight to nine weeks. The fourth patient had a chest wall lesion that continued to progress after the first cycle of treatment. Each of these four patients had other sites of disease not treated by gene replacement that continued to progress during treatment with the vector.

Swisher and colleagues have recently completed a protocol in which an adenovirus vector was utilized (personal communication). Fifty-three patients were enrolled in this study and were treated by intratumoral injection at monthly intervals for six cycles. Patients were treated by direct assignment with or without CDDP 80 mg per m^2 intravenously over two hours and given three days before Ad-p53 injection. No significant vector-related toxicity was seen with up to six monthly injections. The severity of CDDP-associated toxicity (grade II or higher) was not increased with coadministration of Ad-p53. At the initial assessment at two months, four patients (8%) had a partial remission, while 33 patients (65%) had stable disease.

Major tumor regression in lung cancer has been documented independently by Nemunitis and associates (PRN Research, Dallas TX), who have entered patients in a current phase I trial. Of the first 35 patients on whom complete data is available, five of 14 (36%) receiving Ad-p53 alone had growth arrest of their tumor for more than four months. Six of 15 (40%) patients receiving Ad-p53 plus CDDP had growth arrest of their tumor for more than four months despite three of the six progressing on CDDP or carboplatin. Thus the above three human trials showed responses by p53 introduction with minimal vector-associated toxicity.

A study has recently being activated by Swisher and colleagues (personal communication) for stage III NSCLC in those patients who cannot tolerate surgery due to cardiac or pulmonary compromise, consisting of docetaxel (Taxotere) 20 mg per m^2 weekly for a total dose of 100 mg per m^2, along with 60 cGy radiation with concomitant Ad-p53 intratumoral instillation on weeks 1, 3, and 5. End points are local control at three months and will be compared to historical controls currently at only about 20%.

In all of these studies, it has been difficult to deliver recombinant virus into solid tumors so as to transduce a significant fraction of the tumor cells, and the effect is limited to the injected nodule, which may be of limited real clinical benefit. This is because adenovirus has a limited diffusion range in a solid tissue. Thus many investigators are focusing on clinical situations where improved transduction efficacy might be achieved with meaningful clinical results. Examples might include pleural effusions or peritoneal carcinomatosis, where small volume disease is limited to a closed body cavity, or BAC. BACs are chemoresistant and radioresistant.[113–115] In this disease, cancer cells grow initially as a thin monolayer along the pulmonary alveoli and bronchiolar surfaces without destruction of the underlying lung structure. This biology results in progressive shortness of breath and death by suffocation in the majority of these patients, but also makes this tumor uniquely appropriate for delivery of therapeutic agents directly to the tumor cells via the airways. The authors of this chapter have begun a pilot phase 1 trial of an adenovirus p53 gene delivered via bronchoalveolar lavage in patients with locally advanced BAC. Endobronchial delivery of recombinant wtp53 adenovirus via bronchoalveolar lavage may be a highly efficient means of gene transfer and a highly effective local therapeutic in this disease. Effective local palliation could well translate into significant clinical benefit. While BAC is only a subset of all NSCLC, the large numbers of NSCLC deaths each year and the complete lack of good therapeutic options for unresectable or recurrent BAC make the potential clinical impact of this therapy significant.

Systemic gene therapy with liposome-p53 complexes has been reported to cause a significant reduction of greater than 60% in primary tumor volume as compared to a control group.[116] Nude mice inoculated with breast carcinoma cells were injected every 10 to 12 days with liposome p53 via the tail vein. Analyses of the growth pattern revealed that the majority of the p53-treated animals had tumor regression. Induction of p21, marked histological changes, and increased apoptosis were present in the tumors of the p53-treated group. In addition, the p53-treated group had significantly fewer lung metastases. Introduction of p53 via liposomes was effective in the treatment of early endobronchial cancer in mice[117] and was shown to enhance radiation sensi-

tivity in head and neck cancers.[118] The endobronchial use of p53 liposomes may be less toxic than the use of adenovirus vectors in this situation and deserves further clinical exploration.

Other tumor-suppressor genes have also been used therapeutically. These include the retinoblastoma protein (*RB*), which is mutant in the majority of SCLCs and about 20% of NSCLCs.[119,120] *RB* introduction has definite antitumor effects which appear to depend on the extracellular environment of the tumor.[121] A p53-inducible inhibitor of cyclin-dependent kinases, WAF/CIP1, is another candidate gene for the replacement therapy.[122] A large part of the growth regulatory action of p53 appears to be mediated by this protein, which also known as p21. Overexpression of these two genes can arrest the cell cycle in G1 phase.[122] Adenovirus-p21 therapy of p53-deleted mouse prostate cancer cell lines induced growth arrest and resulted in a reduction of CDK2 kinase activity. Intratumoral injection with adenovirus-p21 but not with adenovirus-p53 prolonged the survival of tumor-bearing mice.[123,124] Inhibitory activity was also found in human NSCLC cell lines.[125]

p16 is another tumor-suppressor gene that can also be a candidate for tumor-suppressor gene therapy. Genetic abnormalities of *p16* have been found frequently in NSCLC but rarely in SCLC. Homologous deletion or point mutations have been found in 10% to 40% of NSCLC. Furthermore, hypermethylation in the 5′ CpG island of *p16* allele without genetic alteration will explain the high prevalence (30% to 70%) of absent p16 protein expression in lung cancer.[126] Introduction of a *p16* gene by a recombinant adenoviral vector induced growth arrest and G1 arrest. In lung cancer, adenovirus-mediated *p16* gene transfer could inhibit the proliferation of p16-negative lung cancer cell lines and induce dephospholylation of pRb.[127]

Combined tumor-suppressive gene therapy with adenovirus-p53 and adenovirus-p16 could cooperate to induce cancer cell apoptosis and suggests potentials for development of new cancer gene therapy strategy.[128]

p27 is another possible tumor-suppressor gene even though it is rarely mutated in human cancers, including lung cancer, but low levels of p27 are associated with poor prognosis in NSCLC.[129] Catzavelos and colleagues showed that alteration of p27 levels played an important role in lung tumor progression, and low levels of p27 not related with *ras* mutations may have independent poor prognostic significance in NSCLC.[130] Overexpression of p27 after transduction with an adenoviral vector induced growth arrest and apoptosis in breast cancer cell lines.[131] A comparison study of several adenoviral vectors with cyclin kinase inhibitors showed Ad-p27 induced potent suppressive effect on tumorigenicity.[132] From the above studies, p27 overexpression in NSCLC may be another replacement gene therapy modality.

The major conceptual problem with tumor-suppressor gene replacement therapy is that all clonogenic tumor cells would theoretically need to receive the therapeutic tumor-suppressor gene in order for there to be an observable clinical therapeutic impact. This is readily accomplished in tissue culture but it is obviously very difficult or impossible to achieve in patients, except perhaps in special clinical circumstances such as BAC, as outlined above, or after multiple applications of the gene. It is clear from chemotherapeutic studies that even single-log reduction of tumor bulk (90% cell kill) has only marginal clinical significance, so much work on delivery systems needs to be accomplished before this is more generally applied to clinical problems.

Ionizing Radiation and Gene Therapy

Tumor necrosis factor-α (TNF-α) is a cytokine that activates the cellular immune response and is directly cytotoxic to some tumor cells. Mechanism of direct cell killing by TNF-α involves both apoptosis and necrosis. When combined with radiation *in vivo*, TNF-α is reported to enhance tumor control through immune modulation. Hallahan and co-workers have reported that TNF-α enhances direct tumor cell killing *in vivo* and *in vitro* following exposure to ionizing radiation, and a clinical study that combined systemically (intravenously) administered TNF-α and therapeutic local/regional radiation demonstrated promising results in local tumor control. Systemic toxicity attributed to TNF-α limited the therapeutic efficacy of the treatment regimen. Hallahan and co-workers selected the CArG elements of the Egr-1 promoter (425 bp upstream from the transcription site) to regulate TNF-α because these elements are inducible by radiation in several types of human tumor cell lines.[133] They ligated a region containing the six CarG elements of the promoter enhancer region of the Egr-1 gene upstream to a TNF-α cDNA. A replication-defective adenovirus type 5 (Ad5) was used to deliver the Egr-TNFα genetic construct to tumors. It was observed that production of TNF-α in human tumor xenografts infected with the Ad.Egr-TNFα and treated with radiation enhanced tumor control as compared with radiation alone. A tenfold increase in TNF-α protein was observed after radiation.

Gene activation targeted by ionizing radiation is a new concept for cancer treatment whereby transcription of therapeutic genes is localized and regulated by ionizing radiation. The combination of proteins produced by targeted genes with the cytotoxic effect of ionizing radiation may enhance tumor cures without a significant increase in local or systemic toxicity. Temporally fractionated radiation provides a method for repeated gene induction resulting in prolonged, accentuated gene expression and thus may have wider applications in gene therapy and cancer treatment.

Drug-Sensitizing Gene Therapy

This approach has been used to induce selective transduction of tumor cells with a gene whose product can convert a relatively nontoxic prodrug administered systemically to a toxic metabolite in the cancer cell expressing the transduced gene product. Since Moolten originally suggested the potential utility of herpes simplex virus thymidine kinase (HSV-TK) gene for cancer treatment, drug sensitivity gene therapies have been widely adopted in animal and human therapeutic approaches.[134] Tumor cells that express the activating enzyme are killed, and cells without the transduced gene and enzyme are not affected. Several drug-resistant genes and drug combinations have been tested, including HSV-TK and ganciclovir, cytosine deaminase and 5-fluorouracil, and cytochrome P450 2B1 gene and cyclophosphamide.

The HSV-TK and ganciclovir combination has been the most widely investigated. Good responses have been observed in animal studies.[135] Thymidine kinase is the enzyme responsible for phosphorylation of thymidine and is involved in the salvage pathway for DNA synthesis. In contrast to cellular thymidine kinase, HSV-TK has an ability to phosphorylate not only thymidine but also several nucleoside analogues, including the guanosine analogue ganciclovir. Ganciclovir can be phosphorylated by HSV-TK to the triphosphorylated form. This triphosphorylated GCV enters the DNA synthesis pathway instead of the guanosine triphosphate, blocking DNA synthesis and inducing cell death. *In vitro* tumor cell line experiments have shown that ganciclovir sensitivity in HSV-TK gene–transduced tumors is at least 1,000 times greater than control, nontransduced tumor cell lines. Furthermore, HSV-TK–transduced tumors showed regression after ganciclovir treatment in animal tumor models. In a study done by Kumagai and colleagues, herpes simplex gene was ligated with four repeats of the Myc-Max response elements (a core nucleotide sequence CACGTG), rendering c-, L-, and N-*myc* overexpressing SCLC cell lines significantly suppressed by ganciclovir.[136]

It has been observed by this technique that a small fraction of tumor cells may be affected by HSV-TK, but the cytotoxic effect of transduced cells occurs on nontransduced cells too. This is termed the "bystander effect." Thus all tumor cells in a solid tumor need not be transduced in order to get 100% killing. The precise mechanism of this bystander effect has not been fully elucidated, but there are several mechanisms. The transfer of apoptotic vesicles by endocytosis from killed HSV-TK–positive cells to adjacent HSV-TK–negative tumor cells has been identified in some cases.[137] Recently metabolic cooperation between cells via gap junctions has been demonstrated, making the cell-to-cell passage of small molecules, including toxic metabolites of GCV, possible.[138] Another mechanism that may play a role in some circumstances is the induction of an immune response by the recruitment of macrophages and CD4 and CD8 T-cells to the tumor site.

There are more than 20 protocols using this strategy. More than 100 patients have been entered in these ongoing protocols.[139] Major tumor regression has been reported in eight of 62 patients in various kinds of tumors.

Cytosine deaminase (CD) and 5-fluorocytosine (5-FC) make up another well-studied drug sensitizing gene system. CD-expressing cells can deaminate the relatively nontoxic prodrug 5-FC to highly toxic drug, 5-fluorouracil, resulting in the killing of CD-expressing cells and adjacent cells by the bystander effect. The efficacy of CD and 5-FC has been proven in lung cancer model. Hoganson and associates compared three different toxin genes (HSV-TK, CD, and human deoxycytidine kinase) in human lung adenocarcinoma and reported that CD was the most promising.[140] They also reported that CD gene transfer followed by prolonged 5-FC could inhibit the growth of a lung adenocarcinoma in an animal model.[141]

The combination of drug-sensitizing therapy and cytokine gene therapy has been tried as well. The release of tumor-specific antigen by tumor cell death due to drug-sensitizing genes and the attraction of immune effector cells to tumor cells by cytokine may synergistically enhance the chance of generating tumor-specific CTL. Kwong and co-workers reported that combination of HSV-TK and IL-2 via adenoviral vectors could prevent the metastasis of murine lung cancer and improve animal survival.[142] Combination gene therapy of HSV-TK and GM-CSF plus bone-marrow–derived dendritic cells to improve the antigen presentation ability has been shown to lead to regression of established lung tumors in mice and confers protective immunity against rechallenge of parental tumors.[143]

Antisense cDNA and Oligonucleotide Approaches

Various efforts are under way to develop and apply oligonucleotides for therapy of a number of diseases. The phosphodiester backbone in the oligonucleotide is often modified to methyl-phosphonate or phosphorothioate to reduce degradation by nucleases. There are three principal types of *in vitro* and *in vivo* applications of this methodology: (a) Antisense oligodeoxynucleotide (ODN), which binds specifically to a target mRNA and prevent translation. Treatment with antisense nucleic acids attempts to block expression of the endogenous messenger RNA through the formation of translationally inactive RNA-specific duplexes. Plasmid or viral vectors have been used for transfering an open reading frame fragment of the desired gene oriented backwards (3' to 5') behind a powerful promoter, resulting in the production of an antisense RNA. Antisense RNA transcribed from these constructs forms an RNA duplex with sense mRNA, inhibiting translation.[144] (b) Triplex ODN, which bind specifically to double-stranded DNA and prevent transcription. These modified antisense oligonucleotides can enter tumor cells by endocytosis and form DNA-RNA duplexes with endogenous sense mRNA, inhib-

iting translation. (c) Antiprotein ODN, or "Aptamers," which bind to proteins and exert a biologic effect.

A variety of genes and cellular pathways have been targeted by this approach, including activated oncogenes such as K-*ras* and c-*myb*, and growth factors such as HER2/neu or insulinlike growth factors (IGF) and the IGF-1 receptor. The specific cell cycle regulatory proteins are also reasonable targets for cancer gene therapy. (See also Chapter 2) The tumor-suppressor genes *p53* and *RB*, discussed earlier, directly down-regulate progression through the cell cycle, but a number of cyclins and growth factors act to promote proliferation and thus are reasonable targets for gene-specific inhibition. Cyclin G1 (CYG1) is one member of the G1 cyclins that is overexpressed in human osteosarcoma. Antisense cyclin G1 (CYG1) delivered via a retroviral vector showed inhibition of growth of human osteogenic sarcoma cells.

Insulinlike growth factors are often essential for the maintenance of the malignant phenotype, and in lung cancer the IGF-1 receptor (IGF-1r) is often expressed at high levels.[145] Stable transfection of antisense plasmids expressing the first 300 bp of the IGF-1r reduces the tumorigenicity of a variety of tumor cell lines and has been reported to induce systemic antitumor effects on established, nongene-modified tumors in animal system models.[146] We have constructed an adenovirus-expressing antisense IGF-1r (Ad-IGF-1r/as), and a single transduction of this into human lung cancer cell line NCI H460 cells decreased the receptor number by about 50% and decreased soft agar clonogenic ability by almost ten fold. The intraperitoneal treatment of nude mice bearing established i.p. NCI H460 cells resulted in prolonged survival compared to that of nude mice treated with a reporter virus.[147] This suggests that Ad-IGF-1r/as has a therapeutic effect on established human lung cancer xenografts and may represent an effective and practical cancer gene therapy. Clearly there is potential for the antisense approach for therapy of lung cancer.

BCL2 is often overexpressed in small cell lung cancer, and antisense oligonucleotides spanning the length of the open reading frame were tested by Stahel and colleges for antitumor activity.[148,149] In these studies, an oligonucleotide from an internal portion of the protein was found to be the most effective and produced highly efficient killing and chemosensitization of a number of SCLC cell lines *in vitro*.

Epidermal growth factor (EGF) and its receptor (EGFR) have an important role in the pathogenesis of NSCLC. Blockade of EGFR by monoclonal antibody has been shown to suppress the growth of NSCLC overexpressing EGFR.[150] In human squamous cell carcinoma of head and neck, direct inoculation of EGFR antisense plasmid inhibited tumor growth and increased apoptosis by suppressing EGFR protein expression.[151]

Ribozymes

Ribozymes can be engineered to cleave selectively to a wide variety of RNA targets, thus modifying gene expression. The hairpin ribozyme is a 50 nt RNA enzyme under current development as a promising agent for sequence-specific RNA inactivation in gene therapy. Ribozymes are essentially antisense oligonucleotides that contain an RNAse active site. A ribozyme possessing this activity allows catalytic gene ablation by sequence-specific cleavage of the target transcript. This ability of ribozymes to confer gene "knock-out" at the mRNA level and inhibit normal gene expression by targeted cleavage of RNA renders them as valuable tools in fundamental studies of gene function both in cells *in vitro* and in transgenic models. Ribozymes have been used in cancer therapeutic approaches to inhibit activated oncogenes (*ras* and *bcr*-abl), oncogenic viruses, and the MDR1 gene as alluded to earlier.[152–155]

Dominant Inhibitory Growth Factor Receptors

For the uncontrolled proliferation of tumor cells, strong growth stimulation through the growth factor pathway is essential. Cancer cells acquire a growth advantage by active secretion of growth factors and overexpression of those receptors. Cancer cells are uniquely dependent on these autocrine or paracrine growth-signaling pathways and thus they can be targets for cancer therapy. Antisense intervention acts by inhibiting translation of the receptor protein, but this does not affect protein that is already present in the cell, even low levels of which may allow cancer cell survival. Mutant forms of these receptors can be introduced into cancer cells that can inactivate signaling through preexisting receptors, and these are called "dominant negative" receptors. An example of this is the design of defective IGF-IR or soluble mutant of IGF-IR that suppresses tumorigenicity and progression of tumors by a dominant negative mechanism.[156,157]

Intracellular Antibody

Overexpressed oncoproteins in cancer cells can be targeted in cancer cells by the delivery of a gene encoding for what is known as an "intracellular antibody."[158] The introduced gene encodes for a single chain Fv which, when expressed and translated intracellularly, recognizes and entraps the oncoprotein, inhibiting its function. This has been successfully applied to *erbB-2* in ovarian cancer.[159,160] Dramatic growth inhibition and prolonged survival of human tumors in xenografted animals was observed after delivery of the gene with a recombinant adenovirus. As this oncoprotein is also expressed in breast and lung cancers, it has therapeutic potential for these tumor sites as well.[161–163]

Oncolytic Virus

In gene therapy, viruses have been used for the delivery of therapeutic genes to tumor cells. Typical viral vectors in gene therapy have been designed to deliver a therapeutic gene and to be unable to replicate by themselves, even though wild-type forms of the virus can replicate and destroy the infected cells. Many investigators have begun to develop strains of virus that can specifically replicate in and destroy cancer cells directly and then propagate to adjacent cancer cells and kill them as well. Several viruses, such as herpes simplex type 1 virus and Newcastle virus, have been used for that purpose.

Adenovirus has been the best studied for this approach. For the replication of wild-type adenovirus in the host cells, it is essential to inactivate host p53 protein by the adenoviral E1B 55kD protein. Frank McCormick and colleague generated a mutant adenovirus lacking the E1B-55kD gene (ONYX-015), designed to replicate and lyse p53-deficient human tumor cells but not cells with functional p53.[164] More than a half of human tumors but no normal human cells have inactivated p53 function. The potential utility of this virus would be enormous. They also showed that ONYX-015 could cause tumor-specific lysis and also augment the efficacy of standard chemotherapeutic agents.[165] In the preliminary data of phase II trials in patients with head and neck cancer, intra- and peritumoral injection of ONYX-015 showed that p53-mutant tumors have undergone remarkable destruction (4% to 100% reduction), but no damage to adjacent normal tissue has been found.[166] The similarity of head and neck cancer and lung cancer in the pathogenesis and p53 mutation rate suggests the potential use of this strategy in lung cancer. Possible obstacles of this approach are the heterogenity of p53 status in human tumors and the generation of antiadenoviral humoral immunity that can prevent the replication of ONIX-015. Combination of ONYX-015 and other gene therapies, such as HSV-TK and/or CD, could be an another alternative.[167]

SUMMARY

Cancer arises when mutations occur in genes that control cell growth, DNA repair, and cell death. Novel treatments targeting these genetic lesions include gene therapy. Lung cancer, the leading cancer killer in the United States, is refractory to many types of therapy and is thus in need of such novel approaches. However, its poor immunogenicity and frequent metastases make the problem more difficult.

While gene therapy has received much attention, it has also been met with significant (and sometimes justified) skepticism for many of the reasons outlined above. Early trials of gene therapy have seen some promising results that we feel deserve more rigorous development. The practical contribution of gene therapy to clinical oncology is still minimal, but we believe that judicious application of gene therapy to specific clinical situations may ultimately improve lung cancer patient outcomes.

REFERENCES

1. Itaya T, Yamagiwa S, Okada F, et al. Xenogenization of a mouse lung carcinoma (3LL) by transfection with an allogenic class I major histocompatibility complex gene (H-2Ld). *Cancer Res* 1987;47:3136.
2. Plautz GE, Yang ZY, Wu BY, et al. Immunotherapy of malignancy by *in vivo* gene transfer into tumors. *Proc Natl Acad Sci U S A* 1993;90:4645.
3. Nabel GJ, Nabel EG, Yang ZY, et al. Direct gene transfer with DNA-liposome complexes in melanoma: expression, biological activity, and lack of toxicity in humans. *Proc Natl Acad Sci U S A* 1993;90:11307.
4. Bishop DK, DeBruyne LA, Chang AE, et al. Altered immune response following direct transfer of a foreign MHC gene in human melanoma [Meeting abstract]. Anti-Cancer Treatment, Sixth International Congress, 1996;92:6.
5. Gleich LL, Gluckman JL, Armstrong S, et al. Alloantigen gene therapy for squamous cell carcinoma of the head and neck: results of a phase-1 trial. *Arch Otolaryngol Head Neck Surg* 1998;124:1097.
6. Heo DS, Yoon SJ, Kim WS, et al. Locoregional response and increased natural killer activity after intratumoral injection of HLA-B7/beta2-microglobulin gene in patients with cancer. *Hum Gene Ther* 1998;9:2031.
7. Hersh E, Stopeck A, Harris D, et al. Long-term follow-up and retreatment studies on patients with metastatic malignant melanoma (MM) treated in a phase I/II study of direct intratumoral injection of the HLA-B7/beta2M gene (allovectin-7) in a cationic lipid vector [Meeting abstract]. *Proc Annu Meet Am Soc Clin Oncol* 1996;15:235.
8. Silver HK, Klasa RJ, Bally MB, et al. Phase I gene therapy study of HLA-B7 transduction by direct injection in malignant melanoma [Meeting abstract]. *Proc Annu Meet Am Assoc Cancer Res* 1996;37:342.
9. Stopeck AT, Hersh EM, Akporiaye ET, et al. Phase I study of direct gene transfer of an allogeneic histocompatibility antigen, HLA-B7, in patients with metastatic melanoma. *J Clin Oncol* 1997;15:341.
10. Vogelzang NJ, Sudakoff G, Hersh EM, et al. Clinical experience in phase I and phase II testing of direct intratumoral administration with allovectin-7: a gene-based immunotherapeutic agent [Meeting abstract]. *Proc Annu Meet Am Soc Clin Oncol.* 1996;15:235.
11. Ostrand-Rosenberg S, Thakur A, Clements V. Rejection of mouse sarcoma cells after transfection of MHC class II genes. *J Immunol* 1990;144:4068.
12. Plaskin D, Gelber C, Feldman M, et al. Reversal of the metastatic phenotype in Lewis lung carcinomas after transfection with syngeneic H-2Kb gene. *Proc Natl Acad Sci U S A* 1988;85:4463.
13. Townsend SE, Alison JP. Tumor rejection after direct costimulation of CD8 + T cells by B7-transfected melanoma cells. *Science* 1993;259:368.
14. Kato K, Okumura K, Yagita H. Immunoregulation by B7 and IL-12 gene transfer. *Leukemia* 1997;11[Suppl 3]:572.
15. Hodge JW, McLaughlin JP, Abrams SI, et al. Admixture of a recombinant vaccinia virus containing the gene for the costimulatory molecule B7 and a recombinant vaccinia virus containing a tumor-associated antigen gene results in enhanced specific T-cell responses and antitumor immunity. *Cancer Res* 1995;55:3598.
16. Lee CT, Ciernik IF, Wu S, et al. Increased immunogenicity of tumors bearing mutant p53 and P1A epitopes after transduction of B7-1 via recombinant adenovirus. *Cancer Gene Ther* 1996;3:238.
17. Geldhof AB, Raes G, Bakkus M, et al. Expression of B7-1 by a highly metastatic mouse T lymphoma induces optimal natural killer cell-mediated cytotoxicity. *Cancer Res* 1995;55:2730.
18. Rosenberg SA. Immunologic manipulation can mediate the regression of cancers in humans. *J Clin Oncol* 1988;6:403.
19. Belldegrun A, Tso CL, Sakata T, et al. Human renal carcinoma line transfected with interleukin-2 and/or interferon alpha gene(s): implications for live cancer vaccines. *J Natl Cancer Inst* 1993;85:207.
20. Gansbacher B, Zier K, Daniels B, et al. Interleukin 2 gene transfer into tumor cells abrogates tumorigenicity and induces protective immunity. *J Exp Med* 1990;172:1217.
21. Ohe Y, Podack ER, Olsen KJ, et al. Combination effect of vaccination with IL2 and IL4 cDNA transfected cells on the induction of a therapeutic immune response against Lewis lung carcinoma cells. *Int J Cancer* 1993;53:432.
22. Rosenthal FM, Cronin K, Bannerji R, et al. Augmentation of antitumor immunity by tumor cells transduced with a retroviral vector carrying the interleukin-2 and interferon-gamma cDNAs. *Blood* 1994;83:1289.
23. Ohira T, Ohe Y, Heike Y, et al. *In vitro* and *in vivo* growth of B16F10 melanoma cells transfected with interleukin-4 cDNA and gene therapy with the transfectant. *J Cancer Res Clin Oncol* 1994;120:631.
24. Golumbek PT, Lazenby AJ, Levitsky HI, et al. Treatment of established renal cancer by tumor cells engineered to secrete interleukin-4. *Science* 1991;254:713.
25. Porgador A, Tzehoval E, Katz A, et al. Interleukin 6 gene transfection into Lewis lung carcinoma tumor cells suppresses the malignant phenotype and confers immunotherapeutic competence against parental metastatic cells. *Cancer Res* 1992;52:3679.
26. McBride WH, Thacker JD, Comora S, et al. Genetic modification of a murine fibrosarcoma to produce interleukin 7 stimulates host cell infiltration and tumor immunity. *Cancer Res* 1992;52:393.
27. Dranoff G, Jaffee E, Lazenby A, et al. Vaccination with irradiated tumor cells engineered to secrete murine granulocyte-macrophage colony-stimulating factor stimulates potent, specific, and long-lasting anti-tumor immunity. *Proc Natl Acad Sci U S A* 1993;90:3539.
28. Porgador A, Bannerji R, Watanabe Y, et al. Antimetastatic vaccination of tumor-bearing mice with two types of IFN-gamma gene-inserted tumor cells. *J Immunol* 1993;150:1458.
29. Asher AL, Müle JJ, Kasid A, et al. Murine tumor cells transduced with the gene for tumor necrosis factor-alpha. Evidence for paracrine immune effects of tumor necrosis factor against tumors. *J Immunol* 1991;146:3227.
30. Fearon ER, Pardoll DM, Itaya T, et al. Interleukin-2 production by tumor cells bypasses T helper function in the generation of an antitumor response. *Cell* 1990;60:397.
31. Ley V, Langlade DP, Kourilsky P, et al. Interleukin 2-dependent activation of tumor-specific cytotoxic T lymphocytes *in vivo*. *Eur J Immunol* 1991;21:851.
32. Porgador A, Gansbacher B, Bannerji R, et al. Anti-metastatic vaccination of tumor-bearing mice with IL-2-gene-inserted tumor cells. *Int J Cancer* 1993;53:471.
33. Salvadori S, Gansbacher B, Pizzimenti AM, et al. Abnormal signal transduction by T cells of mice with parental tumors is not seen in mice bearing IL-2-secreting tumors. *J Immunol* 1994;153:5176.

34. Veelken H, Mackensen A, Lahn M, et al. A phase-I clinical study of autologous tumor cells plus interleukin-2-gene-transfected allogeneic fibroblasts as a vaccine in patients with cancer. *Int J Cancer* 1997;70:269.

35. Galanis E, Hersh EM, Stopeck, et al. Immunotherapy of advanced malignancy by direct gene transfer of an interleukin–2 DNA/DMRIE/DOPE lipid complex: phase I/II experience. *J Clin Oncol* 1999;17:3313.

36. Stingl G, Brocker EB, Mertelsmann R, et al. Phase I study to the immunotherapy of metastatic malignant melanoma by a cancer vaccine consisting of autologous cancer cells transfected with the human IL-2 gene. *J Mol Med* 1997;75:297.

37. Stingl G, Brocker EB, Mertelsmann R, et al. Phase I study to the immunotherapy of metastatic malignant melanoma by a cancer vaccine consisting of autologous cancer cells transfected with the human IL-2 gene. *Hum Gene Ther* 1996;7:551.

38. Sobol RE, Shawler DL, Carson C, et al. Interleukin 2 gene therapy of colorectal carcinoma with autologous irradiated tumor cells and genetically engineered fibroblasts: a Phase I study. *Clin Cancer Res* 1999;5:2359.

39. Das Gupta TK, Cohen EP, Richards JM. Phase I evaluation of interleukin-2-transfected irradiated allogeneic melanoma for the treatment of metastatic melanoma: appendix 1: protocol. *Hum Gene Ther* 1997;8:1701.

40. Belli F, Arienti F, Sule-Suso J, et al. Active immunization of metastatic melanoma patients with interleukin-2-transduced allogeneic melanoma cells: evaluation of efficacy and tolerability. *Cancer Immunol Immunother* 1997;44:197.

41. Paul WE. Interleukin 4/B cell stimulatory factor 1: one lymphokine, many functions. *FASEB J* 1987;1:456.

42. Tepper RI, Pattengale PK, Leder P. Murine interleukin-4 displays potent anti-tumor activity *in vivo. Cell* 1989;57:503.

43. Kishimoto T. The biology of interleukin 6. *Blood* 1989;74:1.

44. McBride WH, Dougherty GJ, Dubinett SM, et al. Interleukin-7 mediated cancer gene therapy. In: Sobol and Scanlon, eds. *The internet book of gene therapy.* Stamford, CT: Appleton and Lange, 1995, 105.

45. Collins T, Korman AJ, Wake CT, et al. Immune interferon activates multiple class-II major histocompatibility complex genes and the associated invariant chain gene in human endothelial cells and dermal fibroblasts. *Proc Natl Acad Sci U S A* 1984;81:4917.

46. Gansbacher B, Bannerji R, Daniels B, et al. Retroviral vector-mediated gamma-interferon gene transfer into tumor cells generates potent and long lasting antitumor immunity. *Cancer Res* 1990;50:7820.

47. Beutler B, Cerami A. The biology of cachectin/TNF: a primary mediator of host response. *Annu Rev Immunol* 1989;7:625.

48. Blankenstein T, Qin ZH, Uberla K, et al. Tumor suppression after tumor cell-targeted tumor necrosis factor alpha gene transfer. *J Exp Med* 1991;173:1047.

49. Han SK, Brody SL, Crystal RG. Suppression of *in vivo* tumorigenicity of human lung cancer cells by retrovirus-mediated transfer of the human tumor necrosis factor-alpha cDNA. *Am J Respir Cell Mol Biol* 1994;11:270.

50. Inaba K, Inaba M, Romani N, et al. Generation of large numbers of dendritic cells from mouse bone marrow cultures supplemented with granulocyte/macrophage colony-stimulating factor. *J Exp Med* 1992;176:1693.

51. Golumbek PT, Azhari R, Jaffee EM, et al. Controlled release, biodegradable cytokine depots: a new approach in cancer vaccine design. *Cancer Res* 1993;53:5841.

52. Lee C-T, Wu S, Ciernik IF, et al. Genetic immunotherapy of established tumors with adenovirus-murine granulocyte-macrophage colony-stimulating factor. *Hum Gene Ther* 1997;8:187.

53. Simons JW, Jaffee EM, Weber CE, et al. Bioactivity of autolo-gous irradiated renal cell carcinoma vaccines generated by *ex vivo* granulocyte-macrophage colony-stimulating factor gene transfer. *Cancer Res* 1997;57:1537.

54. Hsieh CS, Macatonia SE, Tripp CS, et al. Development of TH1 CD4 + T cells through IL-12 produced by Listeria-induced macrophages [see comments]. *Science* 1993;260:547.

55. Scott P. IL-12: initiation cytokine for cell-mediated immunity [Comment]. *Science* 1993;260:496.

56. Tahara H, Lotze MT. Antitumor effects of interleukin-12 (IL-12): applications for the immunotherapy and gene therapy of cancer. *Gene Ther* 1995;2:96.

57. Tahara H, Zitvogel L, Storkus, et al. Phase I clinical trial of interleukin-12 (IL-12) gene therapy using direct injection of tumors with genetically engineered autologous fibroblasts [Meeting abstract]. *Proc Annu Meet Am Soc Clin Oncol* 1996; 15:427.

58. Meko JB, Yim JH, Tsung K, et al. High cytokine production and effective antitumor activity of a recombinant vaccinia virus encoding murine interleukin 12. *Cancer Res* 1995;55:4765.

59. Fernandez NC, Levraud JP, Haddada H, et al. High frequency of specific CD8 + T cells in the tumor and blood is associated with efficient local IL-12 gene therapy of cancer. *J Immunol* 1999;162:609.

60. Schmidt-Wolf GD, Schmidt-Wolf IG. Cytokines and gene therapy. *Immunol Today* 1995;16:173.

61. Fakhrai H, Shawler DL, Gjerset R, et al. Cytokine gene therapy with interleukin-2-transduced fibroblasts: effects of IL-2 dose on anti-tumor immunity. *Hum Gene Ther* 1995;6:591.

62. Zitvogel L, Tahara H, Robbins PD, et al. Cancer immunotherapy of established tumors with IL-12. Effective delivery by genetically engineered fibroblasts. *J Immunol* 1995;155:1393.

63. Hwu P, Rosenberg SA. The use of gene-modified tumor-infiltrating lymphocytes for cancer therapy. *Annal NY Acad Sci* 1994;31:188.

64. Hwu P, Rosenberg SA. The genetic modification of T cells for cancer therapy: an overview of laboratory and clinical trials. *Cancer Detect Prev* 1994;18:43.

65. Kato K, Yamada K, Wakimoto H, et al. Combination gene therapy with B7 and IL-12 for lung metastasis of mouse lung carcinoma. *Cancer Gene Ther* 1995;2:316s.

66. Coughlin CM, Wysocka M, Kurzawa HL, et al. B7-1 and interleukin 12 synergistically induce effective antitumor immunity. *Cancer Res* 1995;55:4980.

67. Porgador A, Tzehoval E, Vadai E, et al. Combined vaccination with major histocompatibility class I and interleukin 2 gene-transduced melanoma cells synergizes the cure of postsurgical established lung metastases. *Cancer Res* 1995;55:4941.

68. Ishioka GY, Colon S, Miles C, et al. Induction of class I MHC-restricted, peptide-specific cytotoxic T cells by peptide priming *in vivo. J Immunol* 1989;143:1094.

69. Carbone F, Bevan M. Induction of ovalbumin-specific cytotoxic T cells by *in vivo* peptide immunization. *J Exp Med* 1989;169: 603.

70. Deres K, Schild H, Wiesmüller K-H, et al. *In vivo* priming of virus-specific cytotoxic T lymphocytes with synthetic lipopeptide vaccine. *Nature* 1989;342:561.

71. Gupta RK, Relyveld EH, Lindblad EB, et al. Adjuvants—a balance between toxicity and adjuvanticity. *Vaccine* 1993;11: 293.

72. Romero P, Cerottini J-C, Luescher I. Efficient *in vivo* induction of CTL by cell-associated covalent H-2Kd-peptide complexes. *J Immunol Methods* 1994;171:73.

73. Berzofsky JA. Epitope selection and design of synthetic vaccines: molecular approaches to enhancing immunogenecity and cross-reactivity of engineered vaccines. *Ann NY Acad Sci* 1993;690: 256.

74. Tang D, DeVit M, Johnston SA. Genetic immunization: A simple method for eliciting an immune response. *Nature* 1992; 356:152.

75. Ulmer JB, Donnelly JJ, Parker SE, et al. Heterologous protection against influenza by injection of DNA encoding a viral protein. *Science* 1993;259:1745.

76. Eisenbraun MD, Heydenburg Fuller D, Haynes JR. Examination of parameters affecting the eliction of humoral immune response by particle bombardment-mediated genetic immunization. *DNA Cell Biol* 1993;12:791.

77. Wang B, Ugen KE, Srikantan V, et al. Gene inoculation generates immune response against human immunodeficiency virus type 1. *Proc Natl Acad Sci USA* 1993;90:4156.

78. Fynan EF, Webster RG, Fuller DH, et al. DNA vaccines: Protective immunization by parental, mucosal and gene-gun inoculation. *Proc Natl Acad Sci USA* 1993;90:11478.

79. Ciernik IF, Berzofsky JA, Carbone DP. Induction of cytotoxic T lymphocytes and anti-tumor immunity with DNA vaccines expressing single T cell epitopes. *J Immunol* 1996;156:2369.

80. Ciernik IF, Krayenbuhl BH, Carbone DP. Puncture-mediated gene transfer to the skin. *Hum Gene Ther* 1996;7:893.

81. Gabrilovich DI, Chen HL, Girgis KR, et al. Production of vascular endothelial growth factor by human tumors inhibits the functional maturation of dendritic cells. *Nat Med* 1996;2: 1096.

82. Arthur JF, Butterfield LH, Roth MD, et al. A comparison of gene transfer methods in human dendritic cells. *Cancer Gene Ther* 1997;4:17.

83. Mulders P, Pang S, Dannull J, et al. Highly efficient and consistent gene transfer into dendritic cells utilizing a combination of ultraviolet-irradiated adenovirus and poly(L-lysine) conjugates. *Cancer Res* 1998;58:956.

84. Song W, Kong HL, Carpenter H, et al. Dendritic cells genetically modified with an adenovirus vector encoding the cDNA for a model antigen induce protective and therapeutic antitumor immunity. *J Exp Med* 1997;186:1247.

85. Butterfield LH, Jilani SM, Chakraborty NG, et al. Generation of melanoma-specific cytotoxic T lymphocytes by dendritic cells transduced with a MART-1 adenovirus. *J Immunol* 1998;161: 5607.

86. Ribas A, Butterfield LH, McBride WH, et al. Genetic immunization for the melanoma antigen MART-1/Melan-A using recombinant adenovirus-transduced murine dendritic cells. *Cancer Res* 1997;57:2865.

87. Ishida T, Gabrilovich DI, Chen H, et al. Mutant p53 minigene modified human dendritic cells stimulate tumor-specific cytotoxic T cells [Meeting abstract]. *Proc Annu Meet Am Assoc Cancer Res* 1997;38:632.

88. Ishida T, Stipanov M, Chada S, et al. Dendritic cells transduced with wild type p53 gene elicit potent antitumor immune responses. *Clin Exp Immunol* 1999;117:224.

89. Nishioka Y, Surin M, Robbins PD, et al. Effective tumor immunotherapy using bone-marrow derived dendritic cells genetically engineered to express interleukin-12. *J Immunother* 1997;20: 149.

90. Boehm T, Folkman J, Browder T, et al. Antiangiogenic therapy of experimental cancer does not induce acquired drug resistance [see comments]. *Nature* 1997;390:404.

91. Kong HL, Crystal RG. Gene therapy strategies for tumor antiangiogenesis [see comments]. *J Natl Cancer Inst* 1998;90:273.

92. O'Reilly MS, Boehm T, Shing Y, et al. Endostatin: an endogenous inhibitor of angiogenesis and tumor growth. *Cell* 1997; 88:277.

93. O'Reilly MS, Holmgren L, Shing Y, et al. Angiostatin: a novel angiogenesis inhibitor that mediates the suppression of metastases by a Lewis lung carcinoma [see comments]. *Cell* 1994;79: 315.

94. Klauber N, Rohan RM, Flynn E, et al. Critical components of the female reproductive pathway are suppressed by the angiogenesis inhibitor AGM-1470. *Nat Med* 1997;3:443.

95. Lin P, Buxton JA, Acheson A, et al. Antiangiogenic gene therapy targeting the endothelium-specific receptor tyrosine kinase Tie2. *Proc Natl Acad Sci U S A* 1998;95:8829.

96. Warren RS, Yuan H, Matli MR, et al. Regulation by vascular endothelial growth factor of human colon cancer tumorigenesis in a mouse model of experimental liver metastasis. *J Clin Invest* 1995;95:1789.

97. Melnyk O, Shuman MA, Kim KJ. Vascular endothelial growth factor promotes tumor dissemination by a mechanism distinct from its effect on primary tumor growth. *Cancer Res* 1996;56: 921.

98. Asano M, Yukita A, Matsumoto T, et al. Inhibition of tumor growth and metastasis by an immunoneutralizing monoclonal antibody to human vascular endothelial growth factor/vascular permeability factor 121. *Cancer Res* 1995;55:5296.

99. Claffey KP, Brown LF, del Aguila LF, et al. Expression of vascular permeability factor/vascular endothelial growth factor by melanoma cells increases tumor growth, angiogenesis, and experimental metastasis. *Cancer Res* 1996;56:172.

100. Goldman CK, Kendall RL, Cabrera G, et al. Paracrine expression of a native soluble vascular endothelial growth factor receptor inhibits tumor growth, metastasis, and mortality rate. *Proc Natl Acad Sci U S A* 1998;95:8795.

101. Carbone DP. The biology of lung cancer. *Semin Oncol* 1997; 24:388–401.

102. Chiba I, Takahashi T, Nau MM, et al. Mutations in the p53 gene are frequent in primary, resected non–small cell lung cancer. *Oncogene* 1990;5:1603.

103. D'Amico D, Carbone D, Mitsudomi T, et al. High frequency of somatically acquired p53 mutations in small cell lung cancer cell lines and tumors. *Oncogene* 1992;7:339.

104. Greenblatt MS, Bennett WP, Hollstein M, et al. Mutations in the p53 tumor supressor gene, clues to cancer etiology and molecular pathogenesis. *Cancer Res* 1994;54:4855.

105. Kastan MB, Onyekwere O, Sidransky D, et al. Participation of p53 protein in the cellular response to DNA damage. *Cancer Res* 1991;51:6304.

106. Takahashi T, Carbone D, Takahashi T, et al. Wild-type but not mutant p53 suppresses the growth of human lung cancer cells bearing multiple genetic lesions. *Cancer Res* 1992;52:2340.

107. Cai DW, Mukhopadhyay T, Liu Y, et al. Stable expression of the wild-type p53 gene in human lung cancer cells after retrovirus-mediated gene transfer. *Hum Gene Ther* 1993;4:617.

108. Fujiwara T, Grimm EA, Mukhopadhyay T, et al. A retroviral wild-type p53 expression vector penetrates human lung cancer spheroids and inhibits growth by inducing apoptosis. *Cancer Res* 1993;53:4129.

109. Fujiwara T, Cai DW, Georges RN, et al. Therapeutic effect of a retroviral wild-type p53 expression vector in an orthotopic lung cancer model. *J Natl Cancer Inst* 1994;86:1458.

110. Zhang WW, Fang X, Mazur W, et al. High-efficiency gene transfer and high-level expression of wild-type p53 in human lung cancer cells mediated by recombinant adenovirus. *Cancer Gene Ther* 1994;1:5.

111. Wills KN, Maneval DC, Menzel P, et al. Development and characterization of recombinant adenoviruses encoding human p53 for gene therapy of cancer. *Hum Gene Ther* 1994;5:1079.

112. Roth JA, Nguyen D, Lawrence DD, et al. Retrovirus-mediated wild-type p53 gene transfer to tumors of patients with lung cancer [see comments]. *Nat Med* 1996;2:985.

113. Barkley JE, Green MR. Bronchioloalveolar carcinoma. *J Clin Oncology* 1996;14:2377.
114. Delarue NC, Anderson W, Sanders D. Bronchiolar carcinoma, a reappraisal after 24 years. *Cancer* 1972;29:90.
115. Luddington LG, Verska JJ, Howard T. Bronchiolar carcinoma (alveolar cell) another great imitator, a review of 41 cases. *Chest* 1972;61:622.
116. Xu M, Kumar D, Srinivas S, et al. Parenteral gene therapy with p53 inhibits human breast tumors *in vivo* through a bystander mechanism without evidence of toxicity. *Hum Gene Ther* 1997; 8:177.
117. Zou Y, Zong G, Ling YH, et al. Effective treatment of early endobronchial cancer with regional administration of liposome-p53 complexes [see comments]. *J Natl Cancer Inst* 1998;90: 1130.
118. Xu L, Pirollo KF, Chang EH. Transferrin-liposome-mediated p53 sensitization of squamous cell carcinoma of the head and neck to radiation *in vitro*. *Hum Gene Ther* 1997;8:467.
119. Harbour JW, Lai S-L, Whang-Peng J, et al. Abnormalities in structure and expression of the human retinoblastoma gene in SCLC. *Science* 1988;241:353.
120. Horowitz J, Park S-H, Bogenmann E, et al. Frequent inactivation of the retinoblastoma anti-oncogene is restricted to a subset of human tumor cells. *Proc Natl Acad Sci U S A* 1990;87:2775.
121. Kratzke RA, Shimizu E, Geradts J, et al. RB-mediated tumor suppression of a lung cancer cell line is abrogated by an extract enriched in extracellular matrix. *Cell Growth Differ* 1993;4:629.
122. el-Deiry WS, Tokino T, Velculescu VE, et al. WAF1, a potential mediator of p53 tumor suppression. *Cell* 1993;75:817.
123. Eastham JA, Hall SJ, Sehgal I, et al. *In vivo* gene therapy with p53 or p21 adenovirus for prostate cancer. *Cancer Res* 1995; 55:5151.
124. Yang C, Cirielli C, Capogrossi MC, et al. Adenovirus-mediated wild-type p53 expression induces apoptosis and suppresses tumorigenesis of prostatic tumor cells. *Cancer Res* 1995;55:4210.
125. Inoue F, Hamada K, Kataoka M, et al. Growth inhibition of non–small cell lung cancer cells by a recombinant adenovirus-mediated transfer of the p21 gene. *Cancer Gene Ther* 1995;2: 339s.
126. Sekido Y, Fong KM, Minna JD. Progress in understanding the molecular pathogenesis of human lung cancer. *Biochim Biophys Acta* 1998;1:F21.
127. Lee JH, Lee CT, Yoo CG, et al. The inhibitory effect of adenovirus-mediated p16INK4a gene transfer on the proliferation of lung cancer cell line. *Anticancer Res* 1998;18:3257.
128. Sandig V, Brand K, Herwig S, et al. Adenovirally transferred p16INK4/CDKN2 and p53 genes cooperate to induce apoptotic tumor cell death. *Nat Med* 1997;3:313.
129. Esposito V, Baldi A, De Luca A, et al. Prognostic role of the cyclin-dependent kinase inhibitor p27 in non–small cell lung cancer. *Cancer Res* 1997;57:3381.
130. Catzavelos C, Tsao MS, DeBoer G, et al. Reduced expression of the cell cycle inhibitor p27Kip1 in non–small cell lung carcinoma: a prognostic factor independent of *ras*. *Cancer Res* 1999; 59:684.
131. Katayose Y, Kim M, Rakkar AN, et al. Promoting apoptosis: a novel activity associated with the cyclin-dependent kinase inhibitor p27. *Cancer Res* 1997;57:5441.
132. Schreiber M, Muller WJ, Singh G, et al. Comparison of adenovirus vectors expressing cyclin kinase inhibitors p16INK4A, p18INK4C, p19INK4D, p21WAF1/CIP1 and p27KIP1 in inducing cell cycle arrest, apoptosis and inhibition of tumorigenicity. *Oncogene* 1999;18:1663.
133. Hallahan DE, Dunphy E, Virudachalan S, et al. C-jun and Erg-1 participate in DNA synthesis and cell survival in response to ionizing radiation exposure. *J Biol Chem* 1995;270:30303.
134. Moolten FL. Tumor chemosensitivity conferred by inserted herpes thymidine kinase genes: paradigm for a prospective cancer control strategy. *Cancer Res* 1986;46:5276.
135. Moolten FL. Drug sensitivity ("suicide") genes for selective cancer chemotherapy. In: Sobol and Scanlon, eds. *The internet book of gene therapy: cancer therapeutics.* Stamford, CT: Appleton & Lange, 1995.
136. Kumagai T, Tanio Y, Osaki T, et al. Eradiation of Myc-overexpressing small cell lung cancer cells transfected with herpes simplex virus thyridine kinase gene containing Myc-Max response elements. Cancer Res 1996;56:354.
137. Freeman SM, Abboud CN, Whartenby KA, et al. The bystander effect: tumor regression when a fraction of the tumor mass is genetically modified. *Cancer Res* 1993;53:5274.
138. Bi WL, Parysek LM, Warnick R, et al. *In vitro* evidence that metabolic cooperation is responsible for the bystander effect observed with HSV tk retroviral gene therapy. *Hum Gene Ther* 1993;4:725.
139. Culver KW, Ram Z, Wallbridge S, et al. *In vivo* gene transfer with retroviral vector-producer cells for treatment of experimental brain tumors. *Science* 1992;256:1550.
140. Hoganson DK, Batra RK, Olsen JC, et al. Comparison of the effects of three different toxin genes and their levels of expression on cell growth and bystander effect in lung adenocarcinoma. *Cancer Res* 1996;56:1315.
141. Hoganson DK, Matsui H, Batra RK, et al. Toxin gene-mediated growth inhibition of lung adenocarcinoma in an animal model of pleural malignancy. *Hum Gene Ther* 1998;9:1143.
142. Kwong YL, Chen SH, Kosai K, et al. Combination therapy with suicide and cytokine genes for hepatic metastases of lung cancer. *Chest* 1997;112:1332.
143. Sharma S, Miller PW, Stolina M, et al. Multicomponent gene therapy vaccines for lung cancer: effective eradication of established murine tumors *in vivo* with interleukin-7/herpes simplex thymidine kinase-transduced autologous tumor and *ex vivo* activated dendritic cells. *Gene Ther* 1997;4:1361.
144. Mercola D, Cohen JS. Antisense approaches to cancer gene therapy. In: Sobol and Scanlon, eds. *The internet book of gene therapy: cancer therapeutics.* Stamford, CT: Appleton & Lange, 1995.
145. Baserga R. The insulin-like growth factor I receptor: a key to tumor growth? *Cancer Res* 1995;55:249.
146. Resnicoff M, Sell C, Rubini M, et al. Rat glioblastoma cells expressing an antisense RNA to the insulin-like growth factor-1 (IGF-1) receptor are nontumorigenic and induce regression of wild-type tumors. *Cancer Res* 1994;54:2218.
147. Lee C-T, Wu S, Gabrilovich D, et al. Antitumor effects of an adenovirus expressing antisense insulin-like growth factor 1 receptor on human lung cancer cell lines. *Cancer Res* 1996;56: 3038.
148. Ziegler A, Luedke GH, Fabbro D, et al. Induction of apoptosis in small-cell lung cancer cells by an antisense oligodeoxynucleotide targeting the *Bcl-2* coding sequence [see comments]. *J Natl Cancer Inst* 1997;89:1027.
149. Zangemeister-Wittke U, Schenker T, Luedke GH, et al. Synergistic cytotoxicity of *bcl*-2 antisense oligodeoxynucleotides and etoposide, doxorubicin and cisplatin on small-cell lung cancer cell lines. *Br J Cancer* 1998;78:1035.
150. Lee M, Draoui M, Zia F, et al. Epidermal growth factor receptor monoclonal antibodies inhibit the growth of lung cancer cell lines. *Monogr Natl Cancer Inst* 1992;13:117.
151. He Y, Zeng Q, Drenning SD, et al. Inhibition of human squamous cell carcinoma growth *in vivo* by epidermal growth factor receptor antisense RNA transcribed from the U6 promoter. *J Natl Cancer Inst* 1998;90:1080.
152. Kashani-Sabet M, Funato T, Florenes VA, et al. Suppression

of the neoplastic phenotype *in vivo* by an anti-*ras* ribozyme. *Cancer Res* 1994;54:900.

153. Feng M, Cabrera G, Deshane J, et al. Neoplastic reversion accomplished by high efficiency adenoviral-mediated delivery of an anti-*ras* ribozyme. *Cancer Res* 1995;55:2024.

154. Mitsudomi T, Steinberg SM, Oie HK, et al. *ras* gene mutations in non–small cell lung cancers are associated with shortened survival irrespective of treatment intent. *Cancer Res* 1991;51:4999.

155. Mitsudomi T, Viallet J, Mulshine JL, et al. Mutations of *ras* genes distinguish a subset of non-small-cell lung cancer cell lines from small-cell lung cancer cell lines. *Oncogene* 1991;6:1353.

156. Dunn SE, Ehrlich M, Sharp NJ, et al. A dominant negative mutant of the insulin-like growth factor-I receptor inhibits the adhesion, invasion, and metastasis of breast cancer. *Cancer Res* 1998;58:3353.

157. Hongo A, Yumet G, Resnicoff M, et al. Inhibition of tumorigenesis and induction of apoptosis in human tumor cells by the stable expression of a myristylated COOH terminus of the insulin-like growth factor I receptor. *Cancer Res* 1998;58:2477.

158. Deshane J, Loechel F, Conry RM, et al. Intracellular single-chain antibody directed against erbB2 down-regulates cell surface erbB2 and exhibits a selective anti-proliferative effect in *erb*B2 overexpressing cancer cell lines. *Gene Ther* 1994;1:332.

159. Deshane J, Cabrera G, Grim JE, et al. Targeted eradication of ovarian cancer mediated by intracellular expression of anti-*erb*B-2 single-chain antibody. *Gynecol Oncol* 1995;59:8.

160. Deshane J, Siegal GP, Alvarez RD, et al. Targeted tumor killing via an intracellular antibody against *erb*B-2. *J Clin Invest* 1995;96:2980.

161. Wodrich W, Volm M. Overexpression of oncoproteins in non–small cell lung carcinomas of smokers. *Carcinogenesis* 1993;14:1121.

162. Yu D, Wang SS, Dulski KM, et al. c-*erb*B-2/neu overexpression enhances metastatic potential of human lung cancer cells by induction of metastasis-associated properties. *Cancer Res* 1994;54:3260.

163. Tsai CM, Chang KT, Perng RP, et al. Correlation of intrinsic chemoresistance of non-small-cell lung cancer cell lines with HER-2/neu gene expression but not with ras gene mutations. *J Natl Cancer Inst* 1993;85:897.

164. McCormick F, Myers P. From genetics to chemistry: tumor suppressor genes and drug discovery. *Chem Biol* 1994;1:7.

165. Heise C, Sampson-Johannes A, Williams A, et al. ONYX-015, an E1B gene-attenuated adenovirus, causes tumor-specific cytolysis and antitumoral efficacy that can be augmented by standard chemotherapeutic agents [see comments]. *Nat Med* 1997;3:639.

166. Kirn D, Hermiston T, McCormick F. ONYX-015: clinical data are encouraging [Letter]. *Nat Med* 1998;4:1341.

167. Freytag SO, Rogulski KR, Paielli DL, et al. A novel three-pronged approach to kill cancer cells selectively: concomitant viral, double suicide gene, and radiotherapy. *Hum Gene Ther* 1998;9:1323.

EXPERIMENTAL MODELS OF LUNG CANCER

18

INITIATION OF CELL CULTURES FROM LUNG TUMOR BIOPSIES

HERBERT K. OIE
ADI F. GAZDAR

COLLECTION AND TRANSPORT OF TUMOR SPECIMENS

Lung cancer is the most common malignancy in the world and the cause of most cancer deaths in the United States.[1] The four major types of lung cancers described by the World Health Organization classification[2] are small cell lung cancer (25% of lung cancers), adenocarcinoma (30%), squamous cell carcinoma (25%), and large cell carcinoma (15%). All four major lung cancers are generally believed to have endodermal origins.

Squamous cell carcinoma, large cell carcinoma, and adenocarcinoma are usually grouped as non-small cell lung cancers (NSCLCs) based on differences in natural history, clinical behavior, and biologic properties but mainly because treatment centers follow different treatment policies for these malignancies.[3] Small cell lung cancer (SCLC) has attracted widespread interest because of its unique biologic and clinical properties. SCLC expresses many neuroendocrine features, most interestingly the secretion of many hormones and neuropeptides.[4,5] Some of the neuropeptides (e.g., gastrin-releasing peptide)[6,7] may function as autocrine growth factors. A detailed understanding of the mechanisms that mediate their mitogenic actions may provide alternate ways of treating these cancers.

Truly representative characterization of a tumor cell type would require large numbers of cell lines. Toward this end, we established and characterized more than 200 lung cancer cell lines (Table 18.1). Much of the available knowledge, especially of SCLC biology and molecular genetics, has come from studies utilizing these cell lines. It is hoped that more extensive studies on larger numbers of each lung cancer cell type will lead to more effective strategies for the treatment of lung malignancies.

In this chapter, we describe in detail the procedures and techniques that have evolved by modifying existing methods and devising new techniques (Table 18.2). Using these methods, we have succeeded in establishing many cell lines, mostly from SCLC and NSCLC specimens but also from a variety of other human cancers (Table 18.1).

Tumor specimens obtained for *in vitro* cultivation are basically solid tissues (i.e., cancer masses from the lung, lymph node, and extrapulmonary sites) or fluid samples (i.e., pleural and pericardial effusions, ascites, and bone marrow aspirates). The samples may be from primary or metastatic lesions. Generally, the resected specimen was taken to the pathology laboratory where the tissue was divided for distribution; the largest portion was fixed in formalin, and the remainder was apportioned to the various researchers. If the specimen for cultivation was small (i.e., obtained by needle biopsy), it was put between sterile, saline-moistened pieces of gauze to keep it from drying, placed in a sterile container, and transported to the cell culture laboratory.

Larger samples were put into sterile specimen jars containing cell culture medium (e.g., RPMI 1640, Eagle's MEM), with or without antibiotics. Occasionally, serum, albumin, or polyvinylpyrollidone were used to preserve cell viability.

Because of the extensive handling and occasional lapse in sterility, the interval between surgical removal of the tumor and the distribution of the samples for transport to the cell culture laboratory presents the best opportunity for the introduction of contaminants into the tissue samples. Probably the best scenario for obtaining viable tumor tissue for cultivation is as follows: with the mutual consent of surgeon and pathologist, the investigator desiring a specific tumor specimen for culture attends the operation, accepts the entire resection in a sterile covered tray, takes the specimen to pathology, and designates to the pathologist the area of the resection he or she thinks would most likely yield viable tumor cells for culture. A cross section or a wedge-shaped piece providing as much of the tumor edge as possible is most likely to yield aggressively growing tumor cells.

Before any specimen is obtained for culture, a detailed explanation of the intended usage of the sample should be presented to the patient and, if necessary, a consent form signed.

Any specimen that cannot be transported to the cell cul-

TABLE 18.1. CELL LINES ESTABLISHED FROM HUMAN TUMOR SPECIMENS (1976–1990)

Tumor Specimens	Number of Cell Lines
Lung cancers	224
SCLC	126
NSCLC	92
Mesothelioma	6
B-lymphocytes*	50
Colorectal cancers	18
Other cancers	7
Myeloma	2
Estesioneuroblastoma	1
Adrenocortical carcinoma	1
Gastric cancer	1
Breast cancer	2

NSCLC, non–small cell lung cancer; SCLC, small cell lung cancer.
* B-lymphocytes isolated from specimens cultured for tumor cell growth.

TABLE 18.2. PROCEDURES FOR THE ESTABLISHMENT OF HUMAN LUNG CANCER CELL LINES

Tumor Specimens
Solid tumors
Bone marrow aspirates
Pleural, pericardial, and ascitic effusions

Transport Methods
Solid tumors—in culture medium
Bone marrow aspirates—with heparin
Effusions—with heparin

Processing Methods
Solid tumors—mechanical spillout method
Bone marrow aspirates—Ficoll gradient separation
Effusions—Ficoll gradient separation

Culture Media
SCLC—HITES, H2, SCLC-2, R10, ACL4(5)
NSCLC—ACL4, ACL4(5), SCCRh, R10, H2
Mesothelioma—ACL4(5), SCCRh, R10, H2
B-lymphocytes—R10, ACL4(5), SCCRh, H2

Isolation Methods
Selective media (HITES, ACL4, SCCRh)
Differential trypsinization
Colony picking
Transfer of floating tumor aggregates
Removal of floating normal cells
Tumor cell overgrowth

Maintenance
Routine culture (split every 7–10 days)
Freeze isolated cells early and at several passages
Characterization

SCLC, small cell lung cancer; NSCLC, non–small cell lung cancer; FBS, fetal bovine serum; HITES, serum-free defined medium for SCLC; R10, RPMI 1640 + 10% FBS; H2, HITES + 2% FBS; SCLC-2, HITES plus cholera toxin, epidermal growth factor, bombesin, and bovine serum albumin; ACL4, serum-free defined medium for adenocarcinoma; ACL4(5), ACL4 plus 5% FBS; SCCRh, special medium for squamous cell carinoma.

ture laboratory within 1 hour is stored in a refrigerator. In collecting fluid specimens, special care should be taken to prevent clotting. Preservative-free heparin 5 μg/mL is added to pleural, pericardial, and ascitic effusions. Bone marrow aspirates are collected with a heparin-coated syringe and needle, deposited into tubes containing heparin, and transported to the cell culture laboratory.

Tumor specimens submitted to the cell culture laboratory from outside sources are collected as described previously, packed in wet ice, and delivered by overnight express service.

Many solid tumors contain necrotic tissue, which releases enzymes that are detrimental to cell viability. To reduce cell destruction from this source, specimens can be put into media containing polyvinylpyrollidone or methylcellulose and kept on ice from the time of collection and during transport, until the tissue is processed for culture.

Sodium bicarbonate-buffered tissue culture media require CO_2 to maintain a desired pH. Exposure to the air results in the medium becoming alkaline, a condition not favorable for cell viability. It is preferable to use a bicarbonate-free medium, such as L-15, initially supplemented with serum or a serum-substitute polyvinylpyrollidone to preserve cell viability.[8]

PROCESSING TUMOR SPECIMENS FOR CULTURE

Specimens should be processed for culture as soon as possible after arrival in the cell culture laboratory. If this is not possible, the samples should be refrigerated.

Solid Tumors

Solid tumors with adequate masses are disaggregated by mechanical procedures, proteolytic enzyme digestion, or a combination of the two methods. After placing the specimen in a Petri dish with a small amount of medium to keep the tissue wet, necrotic tissue, blood clots, fatty tissue, and connective tissue are trimmed from the specimen with scissors. The tissue is then cut into small, 1- to 3-mm squares, either with scissors or by cross-cutting with two scalpels. In many cases, this process of mincing the tissue released tumor aggregates into the medium. Several washes of these tissue pieces usually yield sufficient tumor cell aggregates for culture.

Several different enzyme mixtures have been used to disaggregate tumor tissues. Duchesne and colleagues[9] used a combination of pronase, DNase, and collagenase for lung cancer disaggregation. Rheinwald and Beckett[10] digested squamous cell carcinoma of the tongue, pharynx, and skin with 0.2% trypsin and 0.2% collagenase. Twentyman[3] combined mechanical and enzymatic methods to obtain cell suspensions for culture. Using either the cross-cutting scalpel method or scissors, the tumor tissue was chopped into fragments 1 mm square or smaller and then digested with bacterial neutral protease (1 mg/mL) at room temperature for 1 hour.

Although trypsin or a combination of trypsin and EDTA was widely used by early cell culturists, its harsh mode of action has resulted in its replacement with milder enzymes or enzyme combinations. During early years of attempting to culture SCLC from resected tissues, trypsin and EDTA digestion was found to be unsatisfactory because of poor recovery of viable cells. Additionally, resulting suspensions contained both tumor and normal cells in monodispersion, which produced a culture of tumor and normal cells uniformly distributed over the flask surface. Generally, the normal cells, usually fibroblasts, had the advantage of faster growth and overgrew the slower proliferating tumor cells.

Mechanical methods for disaggregating solid tumors have been used by several groups to establish cancer cell lines. Campling and colleagues[11] disaggregated lung cancer tissue by forcing small pieces through a wire mesh and separating the live cells from debris by Ficoll-Hypaque density gradient centrifugation. Kirkland and Bailey[12] obtained tumor cell clumps from colorectal adenocarcinoma tissue by "gentle teasing." The Dartmouth Medical School group led by Pettengill[13] initiated cultures of SCLC by seeding minced biopsy or autopsy specimens.

We have found that the simplest, fastest, and least traumatic method of processing not only SCLC but also NSCLC and other tumor specimens is by the mechanical spillout method.[8] Tumor tissue is chopped into small pieces using cross-cutting scalpels or scissors. The aggregates of tumor cells released by this mincing process are harvested by several series of choppings and washings. The washings are pooled and centrifuged. If necessary, erythrocytes and debris can be removed by Ficoll density gradient separation. The minced tissue suspension usually contains sufficient tumor cells for culturing without further processing.

The mechanical spillout method allows the harvesting of mostly tumor cell aggregates because normal cells are not easily dislodged from the tissue matrix by simply mincing. Because colonies of tumor cells develop from clumps instead of isolated single cells, the tumor cells are given a better start and are better able to compete with normal fibroblasts for growth.

Bone Marrow Aspirates

Because bone marrow specimens are usually quite bloody, the samples are subjected to Ficoll gradient separation to remove the erythrocytes as well as to concentrate live tumor cells. Usually 1 to 3 mL of aspirate is received. After diluting the specimen at least two to five times with serum-free medium in a 15-mL conical centrifuge tube, 2-mL Ficoll is carefully deposited at the bottom of the tube. The tube is then centrifuged in a refrigerated table-top Beckman GPR

centrifuge at 1,500 rpm for 15 minutes at 4°C. Cells at the interface are harvested with a pipet, pelleted by centrifugation, washed twice in 10 mL of medium at 1,000 rpm for 5 minutes, and cultured in 25-cm² flasks in 4 mL of media per flask containing penicillin 100 U/mL, streptomycin 100 μg/mL, gentamicin 5μg/mL, and fungizone 5 μg/mL.

Pleural, Pericardial, and Ascitic Effusions

Effusions may be received in volumes as little as a few milliliters or as large as 2 to 3 L. Cells from small volumes are centrifuged and, without further processing, placed into culture flasks. Large volumes are concentrated by centrifugation, and if large amounts of erythrocytes are present, the cell suspensions are subjected to Ficoll gradient separation. The interface layer of cells is harvested, washed twice with medium, and seeded into 25-cm² flasks.

The pellets from the gradients usually contain large aggregates, which break through the gradient and pellet with the erythrocytes. The pellets can be resuspended in medium and allowed to stand at room temperature so that the heavier cell aggregates sediment by gravitation. By removing the supernatant fluid, much of the erythrocytes are removed. Repeating this process results in a relatively erythrocyte-free tumor aggregate suspension suitable for cultivation.

CULTIVATION, ISOLATION, AND ESTABLISHMENT OF LUNG CANCER CELL LINES

Small Cell Lung Cancer

HITES is the acronym derived from the five growth factors (hydrocortisone, insulin, transferrin, estradiol, and selenium) added to the defined medium (RPMI 1640) to produce the selective medium for the growth of SCLC cells.[14] Other commercially available defined media such as Ham's F-12, Eagle's MEM, or DMEM can also be used. Duchesne and colleagues[9] used Ham's F-12 plus the HITES ingredients to grow lung cancer cells. Most other investigators used RPMI 1640, the defined medium used to develop the HITES medium.

Our experience has shown that in some cases, the specimen submitted for culture contains a mixture of lung cancer cell types. Hence, when sufficient tissue is available, the specimen is routinely seeded into 25-cm² flasks containing the following media: HITES, HITES plus 2.5% fetal bovine serum (FBS), squamous cell carcinoma Rheinwald (SCCRh),[15] RPMI 1640 plus 10% FBS (R10), and adenocarcinoma lung lines (ACL4)[16] plus 5% FBS. Cells from a very small percentage of SCLC specimens do poorly in all of the aforementioned media. These cells may require cholera toxin, bombesin, or epidermal growth factor for *in vitro* proliferation. Therefore, we include a flask containing the medium SCLC-2,[17] which contains all of these growth factors.

Most early epithelial cell cultures grew attached to the flask surface. Oboshi and colleagues[18] reported the first human SCLC line that grew as a floating culture. Most of the SCLC cell lines we have established in HITES and R10 grow as floating aggregates. In contrast, the cell lines developed in Waymouth's MB 752/1 medium supplemented with 20% FBS by the Dartmouth Medical School group were mainly adherent cultures.[13] Pettengill attributes the high calcium content in Waymouth's medium and the attachment factors present in FBS to the large number of adherent SCLC lines established by the Dartmouth group.[13]

SCLC tumors are rarely resected; therefore, most SCLC cell lines are derived from metastatic sources, including bone marrow aspirates, pleural effusions, and lymph nodes. Usually, SCLC clumps are microscopically observed as tightly packed, floating spheroids in the classic aggregate morphology. Individual cells in the aggregates are difficult to distinguish. Other aggregates are formed of loosely packed cells in the variant morphology. The lack of substrate attachment and strong cell-to-cell adhesion may be the result of the production of neural cell adhesion molecule (NCAM).[19,20]

Most SCLC cells grow as floating aggregates or as loosely attached colonies. In contrast, stromal cells require firm attachment to flask surfaces to proliferate. It is a simple matter to detach the loosely adhering SCLC colonies by gently rapping the flask, harvesting the detached aggregates, and transferring them to new flasks. A series of these transfers usually yields pure SCLC cultures. Although most SCLC cells grow as floating aggregates even in serum-containing medium, a few cell lines usually contain adherent cells. By repeatedly removing the floaters, adherent cell lines can be eventually isolated. Whether attached or floating, the properties characterizing SCLC cells are usually retained.

The development of a serum-free, growth factor-supplemented HITES medium has enhanced the ability to establish SCLC cell lines. The absence of serum significantly reduces the growth of stromal cells, and the additives promote the proliferation of most SCLC cells.

The more difficult cell contaminants to cope with in growing SCLC cells are the proliferating B lymphocytes (BL), which, similar to SCLC cells, grow as floating aggregates (Fig. 18.1). Proliferating BL cells are Epstein-Barr virus-transformed B-lymphoblastoid cells, which are present in some bone marrow aspirates, and lymph node biopsy specimens, the most common specimens obtained from SCLC patients.

BL aggregates are relatively easy to differentiate from SCLC cell clumps; the BL cells are loosely aggregated and have spikelike structures (uropods) projecting radially from the aggregates. These cells grow rapidly and cause acidification of the medium. Because BL cells require serum for proliferation, isolation of SCLC cells from a mixed culture is achieved by growing the cells in serum-free HITES me-

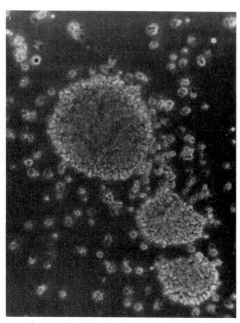

FIGURE 18.1. Proliferating B-lymphocytes, present as floating aggregates in culture, occasionally contaminate small cell lung cancer primary tissue cultures (100 × magnification).

dium. BL cells can be isolated by growing the mixed culture in the selective medium ACL4, in which BL cells grow well but SCLC cells do poorly (Fig. 18.2). Paired SCLC cell lines and "normal" BL cell lines from the same patients prove to be very useful in studies comparing the changes that occur in tumor cells, such as cytogenetic alterations.

The addition of serum diminishes the selective property of HITES medium. However, the growth of most SCLC cells is enhanced by the addition of small amounts of serum, suggesting that HITES medium, although supplying the minimum requirements for SCLC growth, lacks certain factors for optimum *in vitro* growth.

Non-Small Cell Lung Cancer

Early lung cancer cell lines can be established from NSCLC specimens because of the availability of large amounts of resected tissue. Most cell lines are grown and established in commercially available defined media (i.e., MEM, DMEM, McCoy's 5A, Ham's F-10, Ham's F-12) supplemented with 10% to 20% FBS, although several NSCLC lines have been developed in HITES medium plus 2.5% FBS.[3,11,21] Among the early NSCLC cell lines still in widespread use are A-549 and A-427[22] and Calu-1 and SK-MES-1.[23]

The NSCLC group includes three of the four major cell types of lung cancer—adenocarcinoma, squamous cell carcinoma, and large cell undifferentiated carcinoma; SCLC is the fourth major type. The diversity of these cell types presents a more complex problem in cultivation than the

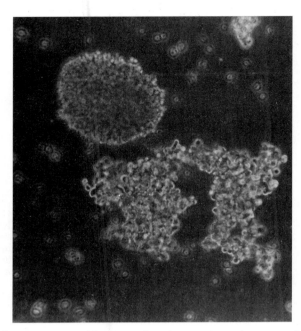

FIGURE 18.2. Proliferating B-lymphocytes (*round aggregate*) in a culture with variant small cell lung cancer (*irregularly shaped cellular aggregate*). These lymphocytes can serve as "normal cells" for molecular genetic studies if they can be isolated and grown free of the tumor cells (100 × magnification).

growing of SCLC cells. The development of the serum-free medium ACL4[16] for the selective growth of adenocarcinoma and of SCCRh,[15] a medium originally developed for the growth of skin keratinocytes that has proven useful in growing squamous cell carcinoma cells, helps to enhance the culturing of these two cell types. No special medium has been developed for large cell carcinoma.

To ensure that media for all cell types are provided, the NSCLC specimens should be grown in ACL4, ACL4 plus 5% FBS, SCCRh, R10, and HITES plus 2% FBS. The inclusion of serum in SCCRh medium allows normal cells to grow, but this medium is especially useful in initiating cultures from specimens containing a mixture of adenocarcinoma and squamous cell carcinoma. Addition of FBS to ACL4 reduces its selective capabilities, but many adenocarcinoma cells grow better in this medium with serum. Therefore, we have adopted the procedure of initially growing the specimens in serum-free media to suppress normal cell growth while the tumor cell colonies establish themselves. After the tumor colonies are fairly large, serum is added to help enhance tumor cell growth.

Because both NSCLC cells and normal cells grow as adherent colonies, isolation of tumor cells is a major problem. Various methods are used to obtain pure tumor cell cultures. One method utilizes the relative difference in attachment rates to separate tumor cells from normal cells. In some cases, small aggregates of tumor cells attach to the

flask surfaces within four to six hours, while the normal cells are still in suspension. By removing the medium, a reduction in the amount of contaminating stromal cells and erythrocytes is achieved. With pleural effusions, the normal cells (e.g., mesothelial cells, monocytes) usually attached faster, so by removing the floating aggregates of tumor cells and transferring them to new flasks, the number of normal cells is reduced. Erythrocytes can be eliminated by routine media changes. The use of several of these manipulations can result in the isolation of tumor cells.

Culturing of tumor cell aggregates obtained by the mechanical spillout method for processing solid tumor specimens produces adherent colonies of tumor and normal cells randomly distributed over the flask surface (Fig. 18.3). Tumor cells can be isolated in several ways under these circumstances. Well-isolated tumor colonies are dislodged by scraping the wall of the flask with the bent tip of a Pasteur pipet, aspirating the colonies into the pipet, and depositing them into the wells of a 24- or 96-well cell culture plate. Tumor cells can also be harvested by taking advantage of the differences in cell susceptibility to the action of trypsin and/or the chelating agent EDTA. By exposing a mixed culture of tumor and normal cell colonies to low concentrations of trypsin, EDTA, or both, cells are selectively detached from the flask surface. If normal cells are detached, the trypsinate is removed and discarded. The attached tumor cells are washed once with medium and refed with growth medium. Trypsinates containing mainly tumor cells are transferred to tubes and centrifuged. The pellets of cells are washed once with medium, centrifuged again, resuspended in growth medium, and seeded into new flasks. The old flask containing attached normal cells is then discarded.

Some adenocarcinoma colonies, when completely surrounded by fibroblasts, produce aggregates of cells loosely attached to the tumor cell colony in response to the impediment of lateral growth by fibroblasts (Fig. 18.4). Gentle rapping of the flask easily dislodges these aggregates, which are harvested and cultured in new flasks.

Some NSCLC cells, especially large cells and squamous cells, produce densely packed colonies. The peripheral cells continue to grow and migrate laterally, infiltrating the surrounding fibroblast monolayer and eventually, if bacterial or fungal contamination can be avoided, displacing the fibroblast cells. This displacement of fibroblasts after long periods of cultivation can be attributed to the ceasing of fibroblast growth as a result of contact inhibition, which eventually results in the deterioration of fibroblast cells by aging.

MAINTENANCE OF CELL LINES

We arbitrarily designate isolated tumor cell cultures as cell lines only after 25 passages and six months of continuous *in vitro* culture. The cells are maintained in 75-cm^2 tissue

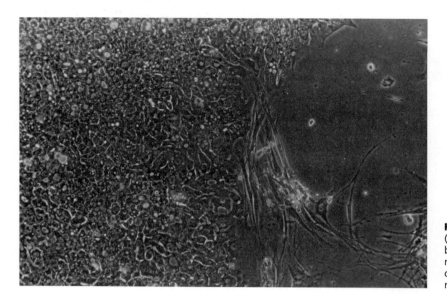

FIGURE 18.3. A culture of adenocarcinoma cells (**left**) contaminated with spindle-shaped fibroblasts. Adjusting serum concentrations and using mechanical methods of cloning can rid the culture of these contaminating normal cells (100 × magnification).

culture flasks, usually in the medium of isolation, and passaged every 7 to 10 days at low split ratios (1:2 or 1:3). For passaging, adherent cells are treated with a warm solution of 0.4% trypsin and 0.02% EDTA in Ca^{2+}- and Mg^{2+}-free phosphate-buffered saline (PBS) for one to two minutes at room temperature following a single wash with warm PBS to remove serum and divalent ions (Ca^{2+} and Mg^{2+}). The serum contains trypsin inhibitors, and divalent ions are used by cells for attachment. Fresh serum-containing medium is added to the detached cells to stop the action of trypsin, and the cells are triturated with a pipet to break up cell clumps and sedimented by centrifugation. The cell pellet

is resuspended in growth medium and distributed into new flasks.

Feeding adherent cultures is achieved by aspirating the spent medium with a suction apparatus fitted with heat-sterilizable platinum tubing. Platinum is ideal for this purpose because it heats and cools rapidly. Flasks of floating aggregate cultures are placed on a specially designed wooden block with a V-notch cut into it. The bottom corner of a flask is placed in this notch, and the cells are allowed to sediment to this corner by gravitation. Spent medium is aspirated by the suction apparatus and replaced with fresh medium. Alternatively, the cell aggregates are broken into

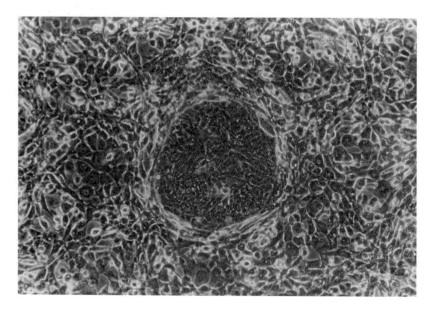

FIGURE 18.4. Colonies of adenocarcinoma (**center**) are surrounded by normal mesothelial cells (100 × magnification).

smaller clumps by trituration, transferred to new flasks at lower densities, and refed with fresh medium.

The cultures are fed once during the 7- to 10-day period, usually 3 to 4 days after passaging. Established cultures are fed with antibiotic-free medium so that periodic mycoplasma testing can be done using Gen-Probe.

It is important to freeze isolated cultures early and at several passages to prevent loss of these early cultures to laboratory accidents (e.g., bacterial, fungal, or mycoplasma contamination, wrongly prepared medium). Freezing medium consists of filter-sterilized 40% RPMI 1640, 10% dimethyl sulfoxide, and 50% FBS. Cells are stored at 135°C or lower in nitrogen or a compressor-driven ultra-low-temperature freezer, preferably in several freezers located at different sites to prevent loss of frozen cell stocks to freezer breakdown. A large stock of frozen cells is essential for cell lines that can only be used for limited passages.

CHARACTERISTICS FOR EARLY IDENTIFICATION

Identification of a tumor begins long before a sample of the tumor reaches the cell culture laboratory (Table 18.3). Information on the tumor type submitted with the specimen is invaluable in selecting the processing method and media. This is especially true in choosing a selective medium. If only a small sample is available, the wrong choice of selective medium usually results in loss of the specimen.

TABLE 18.3. CHARACTERISTICS FOR EARLY IDENTIFICATION OF HUMAN LUNG CANCER CELLS

Tumor Cells	Characteristics
SCLC	Phase microscopy: small cells forming tight spheroids or loose aggregates
	Cytospin preparation: small cells with scant cytoplasm and inconspicuous nucleoli
	Culture: serum-free defined medium HITES
	Biochemical markers: DDC, CK-BB, NSE, BLI
Large cell carcinoma	Phase microscopy: adherent cells; large, fairly uniform in size; no evidence of squamous cell or adenocarcinoma differentiation
Squamous cell carcinoma	Phase microscopy: adherent cells; forms whorls resembling keratin pearls; cornified envelopes in multilayered cultures
Adenocarcinoma	Phase microscopy: adherent cells or floating aggregates; large cells of varying size; floaters form glandular structures; mucin production appears in small vacuoles or goblet cells; dome formation in monolayer cultures
	Biochemical marker: DDC
	Culture: serum-free defined medium ACL4
B-lymphocytes	Phase microscopy: floating aggregates with spikelike protrusions (uropods) radiating from aggregates
	Cytospin preparation: nuclear EBV antigen
	Culture: requires serum for growth

BLI, bombesinlike immunoreactivity; CK-BB, creatine kinase brain-type isoenzyme; DDC, L-dopa decarboxylase; EBV, Epstein-Barr virus; NSE, neuron-specific enolase.

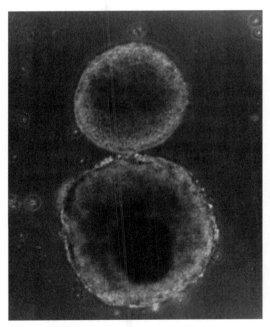

FIGURE 18.5. Classic cell aggregate morphology of small cell lung cancer in culture is characterized by floating, tightly packed spheroids (100 × magnification).

SCLCs grow in the serum-free, defined medium HITES as floating aggregates, which can be tightly packed spheroids in the classic morphology (Fig. 18.5) or more loosely structured aggregates in the variant morphology (Fig. 18.6). The cells are positive for L-dopa decarboxylase (DDC), creatine kinase brain-type isoenzyme, neuron-specific enolase, and bombesinlike immunoreactivity.[24-27] Variants usually have barely detectable or no DDC activity but retain the other biochemical markers. Cytospin preparations of SCLC cells show small round cells with scanty cytoplasm and a few inconspicuous nucleoli. Variant cells are slightly larger, with more cytoplasm and more prominent nucleoli.

Large cell carcinoma cells grow as attached epithelial cells that are generally uniform in size (Fig. 18.7). These cells show no evidence of squamous cell or adenocarcinoma differentiation.

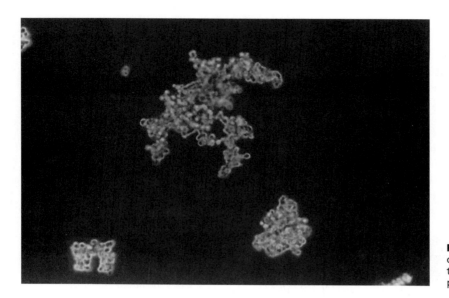

FIGURE 18.6. Cell aggregates of variant small cell lung cancer in culture have more loosely structured appearances compared with the classic morphology (100 × magnification).

Squamous cell carcinoma cells grow as adherent cultures, forming whorls that resemble keratin pearls (Fig. 18.8). Cornified envelope formation is the most distinguishing characteristic of squamous cells, which are only seen in multilayered cultures. Unfortunately, cornified envelope formation is a terminal event. Only cultures that can be maintained in a delicate balance of dividing undifferentiated cells and nonreplicating differentiated cells survive.

Adenocarcinoma cells grow in the selective medium ACL4 as adherent cultures. The cells are large and vary in size. Mucin production ranges from a few small vacuoles to goblet cell production. A few adherent cultures produce domes, which occur when fluid lifts the cells off the substrate (Fig. 18.9). Some adenocarcinomas grow as floating aggregates and produce glandular structures. Approximately 20% of adenocarcinomas show neuroendocrine phenotype,[3] and these cells usually are DDC-positive.

BLs grow as floating aggregates resembling variant SCLC clumps. They form loose aggregates and characteristically have spikelike protrusions (uropods) radiating outward from the aggregates. Giemsa-stained smears show cells with abundant cytoplasm and large nucleoli. BL cells express Ep-

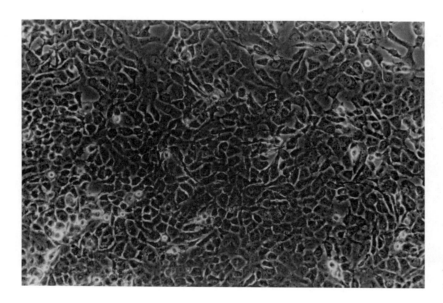

FIGURE 18.7. Large cell lung cancer in culture. These cell lines appear epithelial and uniform in size (100 × magnification).

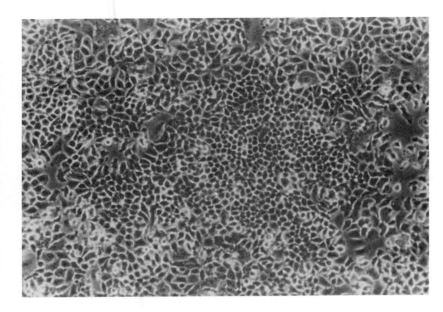

FIGURE 18.8. A monolayer culture of squamous cell lung cancer (100 × magnification).

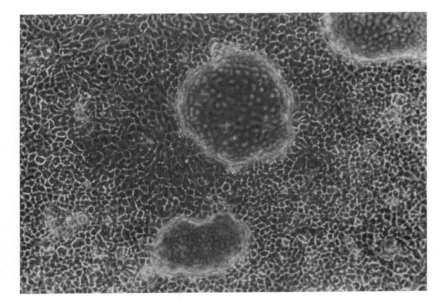

FIGURE 18.9. Adherent culture of adenocarcinoma of the lung. Dome formation is also seen (100 × magnification).

stein-Barr virus nuclear antigen. These cells require serum for growth, so they could be easily suppressed by growing them in serum-free HITES or ACL4 medium.

CONCLUSIONS

Earlier attempts to establish lung cancer cell lines were greatly impeded by the need to use serum-containing media, which favored fibroblast cell growth. Hence, fibroblasts outgrew and overgrew the slower growing carcinoma cells. The development of the serum-free, growth factor—supplemented media HITES for the selective growth of SCLC cells and ACL4 for the culturing of adenocarcinoma cells eliminates this problem. As a result, large panels of well-characterized SCLC and adenocarcinoma cell lines have been established. The easy availability of large numbers of well-characterized cell lines has generated an intense interest in lung cancers, resulting in a rapid accumulation of knowledge regarding the biology and molecular genetics of lung cancer.

The development of new technologies in cell culture and the determination of nutritional requirements for an ever-increasing number of tumor cell types will make cell lines from most human tumors available.

REFERENCES

1. Minna JD, Glatstein EJ, Pass HI, et al. Cancer of the lung. In: DeVita VT Jr, Hellman S, Rosenberg SA, eds. *Cancer: principles and practice of oncology.* Philadelphia: JB Lippincott, 1989:591.
2. The World Health Organization. Histological typing of lung tumors. *Am J Clin Pathol* 1982;77:123.
3. Twentyman PR. Lung cancer. In: Masters JRW, ed. *Human cancer in primary culture.* Netherlands: Kluwer Academic, 1991:199.
4. Sorenson GD, Pettengill OS, Brinck-Johnsen T, et al. Hormone production by cultures of small-cell carcinoma of the lung. *Cancer* 1981;47:1289.
5. Maurer LH. Ectopic hormone syndrome in small cell carcinoma of the lung. *Clin Oncol* 1985;4:1289.
6. Sausville E, Carney D, Battey J. The human vasopressin gene is linked to the oxytocin gene and is selectively expressed in a cultured lung cancer cell line. *J Biol Chem* 1985;260:10236.
7. Cuttitta F, Carney DN, Mulshine J, et al. Bombesin-like peptides can function as autocrine growth factors in human small-cell lung cancer. *Nature* 1985;316:823.
8. Leibovitz A. Development of tumor cell lines. *Cancer Genet Cytogenet* 1986;19:11.
9. Duchesne GM, Eady JJ, Peacock JH, et al. A panel of human lung carcinoma lines: establishment, properties and common characteristics. *Br J Cancer* 1987;56:287.
10. Rheinwald JG, Beckett MA. Tumorigenic keratinocyte lines requiring anchorage and fibroblast support cultured from human squamous cell carcinoma. *Cancer Res* 1981;41:1657.
11. Campling BG, Haworth AC, Baker HM, et al. Establishment and characterization of a panel of human lung cancer cell lines. *Cancer* 1992;69:2064.
12. Kirkland SC, Bailey IG. Establishment and characterization of six human colorectal adenocarcinoma cell lines. *Br J Cancer* 1986;53:779.
13. Pettengill OS, Carney DN, Sorenson GD, et al. Establishment and characterization of cell lines from human small cell carcinoma of the lung. In: Becker KL, Gazdar AF, eds. *The endocrine lung in health and disease.* Philadelphia: WB Saunders, 1984:460.
14. Simms E, Gazdar AF, Abrams PG, et al. Growth of human small cell (oat cell) carcinoma of the lung in serum-free growth factor supplemented medium. *Cancer Res* 1980;40:4356.
15. Erim TJ, Beckett MA, Miller D, et al. Clonal growth and serial passage of head and neck squamous cell carcinoma. *Proc Am Soc Clin Oncol USA* 1982:195.
16. Brower M, Carney DN, Oie HK, et al. Growth of cell lines and clinical specimens of human non-small cell lung cancer in a serum-free defined medium. *Cancer Res* 1986;46:798.
17. Oie HK, Brower M, Carney DN. Growth factor requirements for in vitro growth of small cell and other lung cancers in serum-free defined medium. In: Becker KL, Gazdar AF, eds. *The endocrine lung in health and disease.* Philadelphia: WB Saunders, 1984:469.
18. Oboshi S, Tsugawa S, Seido T, et al. A new floating cell line derived from human pulmonary carcinoma of oat cell type. *Gann Japanese Journal* 1971;64:505.
19. Doyle LA, Borges M, Hussain A, et al. An adherent subline of a unique small-cell lung cancer cell line down regulates antigens of the neural cell adhesion molecule. *J Clin Invest* 1990;86:1848.
20. Carbone DP, Koros AM, Linnoila RI, et al. Neural cell adhesion molecule expression and messenger RNA splicing patterns in lung cancer cell lines are correlated with neuroendocrine phenotype and growth morphology. *Cancer Res* 1991;51:6142.
21. Baillie-Johnson H, Twentyman PR, Twentyman PR, Fox NE, et al. Establishment and characterization of cell lines from patients with lung cancer (predominantly small cell carcinoma). *Br J Cancer* 1985;52:495.
22. Giard D, Aaronson SA, Todaro GJ, et al. In vitro cultivation of human tumors: establishment of cell lines from a series of solid tumors. *J Natl Cancer Inst* 1973;51:1417.
23. Fogh J, Trempe G. New human tumor cell lines. In: Fogh J, ed. *Human tumor cells in vitro.* New York: Plenum Press, 1975:115.
24. Gazdar AF, Carney DN, Russell EK, et al. Establishment of continuous, clonable cultures of small-cell carcinoma of the lung which have amine precursor uptake and decarboxylation cell properties. *Cancer Res* 1980;40:3502.
25. Gazdar AF, Zweig MH, Carney DN, et al. Levels of creatine kinase and its BB isoenzyme in lung cancer specimens and cultures. *Cancer Res* 1981;42:2773.
26. Marangos PJ, Gazdar AF, Carney DN. Neuron specific enolase in human small cell carcinoma cultures. *Cancer Lett* 1982;15:67.
27. Moody TW, Pert CB, Gazdar AF, et al. High levels of intracellular bombesin characterize human small-cell lung carcinoma. *Science* 1981;214:1246.

19

ANIMAL MODELS FOR STUDYING LUNG CANCER AND EVALUATING NOVEL INTERVENTION STRATEGIES

ALVIN M. MALKINSON
STEVEN A. BELINSKY

"Pulmonary carcinogenesis is studied in animals in order to determine the pathogenesis, prevention, early detection, and treatment of this disease on behalf of man."[1] Lung tumors in domestic animals were periodically observed by veterinarians, but it was not until Livingood's histologic description 100 years ago of a papillary tumor in a mouse[2] that the use of animals as experimental tools began. Genetically homozygous mice were established in the 1920s following generations of inbreeding, and inbred strains could be distinguished by their susceptibility or resistance to spontaneous or chemically induced lung tumor development. Procedures for testing putative carcinogens in rodent bioassays became more standardized, and are used today by regulatory agencies to assess carcinogenic risk. The most commonly used species in experimental respiratory carcinogenesis are mice, rats, hamsters, and dogs.[3] This chapter describes how animal models help in understanding lung cancer: by revealing the biology and molecular events during experimental pulmonary oncogenesis, by delineating genes that regulate tumor development, and by providing a convenient testing ground for innovative chemopreventative and chemotherapeutic strategies.

EXPERIMENTAL ADVANTAGES OF ANIMAL MODELS

Animal models allow discovery of genotoxic compounds which induce tumors and nongenotoxic agents that modulate carcinogenesis. Genes that regulate susceptibility to these agents and the timing of molecular events during tumor progression can be elucidated. Because different species develop different types of tumors, several animal models may prove valuable for delineating the biochemical changes that characterize a particular class of lung tumor.

Defined Exposure to Tobacco or Compounds with Related Mechanisms

People are continuously exposed to potentially harmful mixtures of chemicals and physical agents. The laboratory environment allows controlled administration of these environmental toxicants to animals (Table 19.1). Experimental variables typically include dosage, dosing frequency (e.g., lifetime exposure, a single injection of a rapidly metabolized substance), and host factors at the time of exposure (e.g., age, genetic background, and nutritional and proliferative status). Inbred strain A/J mice given a single intraperitoneal injection of 4-(methylnitrosamino)-1-(3-pyridyl)-1-butanone (NNK), a carcinogenically potent tobacco-derived nitrosamine, at any time after birth, develop dozens of benign lung adenomas within a few months.[4] When more time elapses following carcinogen administration, many of these induced tumors progress to adenocarcinomas that are histopathologically indistinguishable from human adenocarcinomas.[5]

In order for the full complex mixture of cigarette smoke to induce adenomas and adenocarcinomas in A/J mice, chronic exposure (e.g., six hours per day, five days per week for five to six months) followed by a recovery period in air for over four months is necessary.[5]

Modulations of Tumor Formation by Nongenotoxic Chemicals

The antioxidant, butylated hydroxytoluene (BHT), a widely used food additive, inhibits both tumor incidence and multiplicity in adult A/J mice receiving this agent prior to carcinogen administration.[6] Antioxidants inhibit lung tumor formation by interfering with the conversion of an inactive carcinogen to a more chemically reactive metabolite. Conversely, BHT, but not other antioxidants, can be converted through cytochrome P450 metabolism to an oxidative species that causes pneumotoxicity. Interestingly, if repeated

TABLE 19.1. CATEGORIES OF AGENTS THAT STIMULATE OR DISCOURAGE LUNG TUMOR DEVELOPMENT IN ANIMALS

Inducing and Promoting Agents	Protective or Regression-Inducing Agents
Cigarette components	Antioxidants (e.g., butylated hydroxytoluene)
Nitrosamines in smoke	Cruciferous vegetables (e.g., cabbage)
Polycyclic aromatic hydrocarbons in tar	
^{210}Po in tobacco	Retinoids
Carbonaceous particles	Anti-inflammatory drugs (e.g., sulindac)
Phenols	
Diesel exhaust	*cis*-platinum
Heavy metals (e.g., uranium)	Isothiocyanates
Fibers (e.g., asbestos)	Tea polyphenols
Radionuclides (e.g., radon particles)	Glucocorticoids
Carbamates (e.g., urethane)	Farnesyltransferase inhibitors
Butylated hydroxytoluene	Sulindac sulfone

doses of BHT are administered after carcinogen exposure, tumor multiplicity is enhanced.[7] One current explanation for this seemingly paradoxical behavior is that growth factors released at the injury site selectively stimulate the division of mutated cells. For example, in BALB/C mice exposed to 3-methylcholanthrene (MCA), a polycyclic aromatic hydrocarbon (PAH) found in cigarette smoke, tumors do not develop in the absence of BHT treatment.[8] This corresponds to a classic initiation/promotion protocol.

The experimental advantage is that the promotion stage is reversible, involving only altered gene expression, and does not include additional irreversible changes to DNA structure, such as those that cause oncogene activation or tumor-suppressor gene inactivation. The promotion stage is thus amenable to chemoprevention strategies. Among the changes BHT elicits that would encourage the growth of initiated cells are inflammation,[9] altered apoptosis,[10] and diminished cell to cell communication.[11] A role of inflammation in lung tumor development may account for the efficacy of anti-inflammatory drugs and tea polyphenols in inhibiting tumor formation (Table 19.1). Isothiocyanates inhibit lung tumorigenesis at the initiation stage by altering carcinogen metabolism. Cruciferous vegetables accelerate carcinogen clearance from the body. Farnesylation inhibitors prevent the *KRAS* oncogene product activated by an initiating mutation from binding to the plasma membrane to exert its activity.

Dissection of the Complex Ways That Cancer-Related Genes Respond to Environmental Agents

A/J mice develop tumors by the end of their lifetimes even in the absence of any applied carcinogen, but C57BL/6J mice do not. C57BL/6J mice are also resistant to lung carcinogens, even if they are given at a high dose or in multiple doses.[12] Similar or identical genes probably regulate susceptibility to both spontaneous and chemically induced lung

tumor development. Susceptibility to a complete carcinogen such as urethane and susceptibility to a promoting, nongenotoxic agent such as BHT are regulated by different genes, however. Tumor multiplicity is affected by BHT in only some of the strains of mice that respond to urethane.[9]

Evaluating the Temporal Sequence of Tumorigenesis

Because tumorigenesis is initiated by the experimenter, each stage of neoplasia (i.e., hyperplasia, benign tumor formation, and the benign-to-tumor transition) can be studied independently. Thus the researcher can distinguish between molecular changes that precede the onset of hyperplastic foci and those that characterize the evolution of malignancy from a benign stage, and thereby identify phenotypes that might be used for preclinical diagnosis.

PRIMARY LUNG TUMORS IN MICE

Mice are the most frequently studied animals in lung tumor research. Mice are less expensive to maintain, even for lifetime studies, than other species. Susceptible strains of mice develop lung tumors within a few months after carcinogen administration. The scientific advantages of mouse lung tumors as an experimental tool are their similarity to human adenocarcinomas[13,14] and the ability to apply genetic analytical techniques. A disadvantage is that mechanisms underlying small cell lung cancer (SCLC) and squamous cell carcinoma cannot be examined, because these classes of tumors do not occur in murine models.

Histogenesis

The only type of lung tumor that develops in the mouse is the peripheral adenoma, which often progresses to adeno-

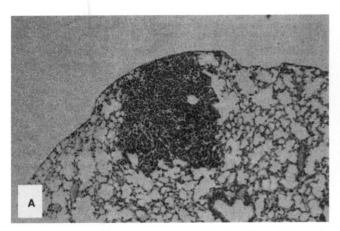
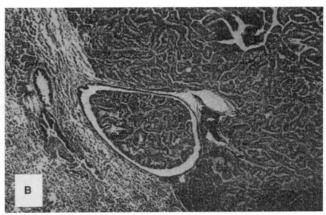

FIGURE 19.1. A: Solid or lepidic and **(B)** papillary tumors induced by urethane in A/J mouse lung. Hematoxylin and eosin stain; (50 × magnification). (From Thaete LG, Gunning WT, Stoner GD, et al. Cellular derivation of lung tumors in sensitive and resistant strains of mice: results at 28 and 56 weeks after urethane treatment. *J Natl Cancer Inst* 1987;78:743, with permission.)

carcinoma. Adenomas are benign, glandular structures with no evidence of invasion into the surrounding adjacent tissue. These adenomas can be of a solid lepidic pattern and grow along the alveolar septae without compression, or they can adopt a papillary, fingerlike growth pattern (Fig. 19.1). Most mice contain both adenoma types, but the relative proportion of these types within a single mouse depends on the length of time following carcinogen application, the genetic strain used, the age of the mouse at the time of administration, and the nature of the carcinogen. Among inbred strains, adenoma growth patterns vary from all papillary to all solid. In each strain, however, the percentage of papillary adenomas increases as a function of time following carcinogen administration.[15] Papillary adenomas tend to have a longer latency period than solid adenomas, and malignant tumors have been observed to arise within a papillary adenoma.[16] When adult A/J mice are treated with urethane, 80% to 85% of the adenomas present 14 weeks later are solid. Following transplacental carcinogenesis, however, all tumors formed are papillary.[17] Because the proportion of the two histologic tumor types is not related to the tumor multiplicity that is characteristic of a particular strain, a unique set of genes for pulmonary adenoma histologic type (*paht*),[18] has been hypothesized to regulate lung tumor phenotype.

These observations imply that the differentiation status of the lung at the time of carcinogen application determines adenoma histology. The cells within solid tumors have ultrastructural and biochemical features (i.e., round nuclei and lamellar bodies that synthesize surfactant) that typify alveolar Type II pneumocytes.[19] These are the stem cells of the alveoli; when the fragile Type I cells that compose more than 90% of the alveolar surface are injured and die, the Type II cells divide and differentiate to replace them. Type II cells are one of the few pulmonary cell types that prolifer-

ate in an unstimulated lung or following the release of growth factors during injury.

Three hypotheses have been advanced regarding the cellular origins of papillary tumors.[20] First, these tumors may arise by direct neoplastic conversion of nonciliated Clara cells, the putative stem cell of the bronchiole. The cells within these tumors have many features of Clara cells, including ultrastructure, enzyme and isozyme composition, and cytokeratin content. Clara cells metabolize carcinogens and undergo hyperplasia following carcinogen injection.[21] Other species, such as humans[22] and hamsters,[23] develop adenomas from Clara cells. The second hypothesis is that papillary tumors are the more aggressive structures to which some solid tumors progress and, therefore, like the solid adenomas, also arise from type II cells.[24] This hypothesis is based on the longer latency of the papillary tumors, the fact that type II cells can also metabolize carcinogens, a Clara cell-like morphology of some neoplastic type II cells, and the absence of CC10 (Clara cell-derived protein of 10,000 to 16,000 molecular weight, also called CC16); this is a secreted uteroglobin frequently used as a cellular biomarker for Clara cells. The third hypothesis is that developmental precursor cells, either multipotential stem cells that can differentiate into a Type II or Clara cell, or type II-specific precursors whose differentiative fate is altered by a carcinogen-induced activation of a protooncogene, are the papillary cells of origin. The main support for this hypothesis is the predominantly papillary tumor composition following transplacental carcinogenesis,[17] an ontogenetic stage in which a presumably high content of these precursor cells exist. The plasticity of type II and Clara cell structures (i.e., the wide range of structures that these cells can assume), the changes in cell composition that occur upon neoplastic transformation, and the many similarities between these two cell types make it difficult to distinguish among these possibilities.

The *paht* genes either determine which cell type is more susceptible to neoplastic growth or regulate the progression of a benign solid adenoma to an aggressive papillary adenoma that may become malignant. It is also important to clarify this phenotypic diversity because it has been postulated that a large portion of human adenocarcinomas arise from type II and Clara cells because many adenocarcinomas express genes characteristic of these cell types.[22,25–27] Over the past few decades, both the absolute incidence and relative incidence of adenocarcinoma among non–small cell lung cancer (NSCLC) patients have increased, whereas the relative frequency of squamous cell carcinoma has decreased. Adenocarcinoma is now the most frequent histologic type of human lung cancer in the United States and Japan. The incidence of lung cancer among nonsmokers has become the eighth most commonly diagnosed human cancer, and adenocarcinoma is the main tumor type in these people. The etiologic cause for this increased incidence of adenocarcinoma is unknown.

Molecular and Biochemical Changes during Mouse Lung Tumor Progression

Figure 19.2 illustrates the timing of some of the molecular and biochemical changes that occur in the course of mouse lung tumor progression; they are described in the following sections. Inbred strains vary at several points along this temporal pathway, and these variations can be used to understand the role of each change.

The biochemical changes detectable in neoplastic lung cells encourage cellular autonomy by increasing their resistance to normal host-mediated control mechanisms and to applied chemotherapeutic agents. The neoplastic mouse lung cell demonstrates the following factors:

1. *Enhanced ability to proliferate.* Mutant *KRAS* p21 allows continuous stimulation of downstream protein kinases, which leads to increased expression of proteins that stimulate cell proliferation. *MYC* expression enhances cell proliferation and is frequently overexpressed in lung tumor cells. *p53* mutation increases the half-life of *MYC*, and *p53* is a proliferative stimulus. *RB1* is a cell-cycle brake; its deletion and inactivation by mutation interfere with cell-cycle control.
2. *Resistance to negative growth factors.* The disturbances in cAMP signal transduction, as well as other pathways that allow cells to respond to environmental change (e.g., glucocorticoids, protein kinase C, gap junctions), may permit these cells to ignore or misperceive signals emanating from outside the cell that instruct the cells to stop dividing.
3. *Resistance to agents that might cause cell death.* These agents include the losses of constitutive and inducible P450 isozymes and NADPH-dependent quinone oxidoreductase (NQO1), all of which modulate the toxicity of foreign compounds.

DNA Structure and Behavior Are Modified Within 24 Hours After Carcinogen Application

The earliest alterations that have been detected are *DNA methylation,* covalent binding of an unmodified or metabolically altered form of the carcinogen to DNA, and diminished cell proliferation. The methylation of cytosines, par-

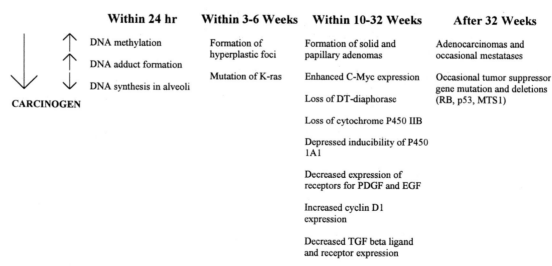

FIGURE 19.2. Time scale of mouse lung tumorigenesis. Sequential molecular changes following carcinogen application. Increased (↑) and decreased (↓) activity are indicated. *RB1, P53,* and *p16* are tumor-suppressor genes.

ticularly those associated with CpG islands within the promoter regions of genes, is emerging as a fundamental mechanism for transcriptional repression of tumor-suppressor and regulatory genes in cancer.[28] Changes in the balance of methylation within the cell have been linked in part to increased activity of DNA-methyltransferase (DNA-MTase), the enzyme that catalyzes DNA methylation at CpG sites.[29] Exposure to NNK results in increased DNA-MTase activity and genomic 5-methylcytosine levels, indicative of hypermethylation, in alveolar Type II cells isolated from A/J mice.[30] This change was detected seven days after carcinogen treatment, occurred in Type II cells but not Clara cells, and was specific to sensitive A/J mice; these changes were not seen in cells isolated from resistant C3H mice. In addition, DNA-MTase activity increased incrementally during lung cancer progression in A/J mice and coincided with increased expression of the DNA-MTase gene in hyperplasias, adenomas, and carcinomas. Thus increased DNA-MTase activity and concomitant hypermethylation are strongly associated with neoplastic development and may constitute a key step in carcinogenesis and a biomarker for premalignancy.

The persistence of DNA *adduct formation* has been correlated with lung tumor incidence. For example, NNK forms significantly more O^6-methylguanine adducts (O^6MG) in Clara and type II cells than in whole lung.[25] Additionally, the activating mutation in the *KRAS* protooncogene can be correlated with the particular DNA adduct formed by a carcinogen. NNK causes a G→A transition in the second base of codon 12 in *KRAS,* which could result from base mispairing caused by O^6MG.[31]

A rough estimate of the carcinogenicity of a compound is its effect on the proliferation of the target cell population.[32] Administration of many tissue-damaging agents to an animal causes a rapid but transient decrease in the ^{3}H-thymidine *labeling index* of the target cell population. This reduced level of ^{3}H-thymidine incorporation into DNA probably reflects the removal of cells that have been fatally damaged by the toxicant. Both lung-tumor–susceptible and –resistant strains exhibit a similar decrease in the labeling index of their Type II cell populations.[33] Strains vary, however, in their proliferative behavior after this initial reduction. Lung-tumor–susceptible strains such as A/J contain more dividing type II cells seven to 14 days after urethane treatment than prior to carcinogen administration.[33,34] Resistant strains, such as C57, merely recover their original proliferative level, and the timing of this recovery occurs later. Strains of mice with intermediate susceptibility (i.e., those that develop fewer tumors than A/J mice) show a smaller "overshoot" than A/J mice. These areas of intense proliferative activity are regionally localized and constitute the hyperplastic foci that will give rise to tumors. The relative basal proliferative rates (i.e., cell division in the absence of carcinogen treatment) of the alveolar type II and bronchiolar Clara cells in these strains correlate with tumor mul-

tiplicity.[35] It is easy to imagine how an increased proliferative rate could enhance the actions of carcinogenic inducers. For example, when a cell divides before a DNA adduct can be repaired, this increases the likelihood that the adduct will cause improper base pairing during DNA replication.

Biochemical Alterations Have Occurred by the Time the Benign Tumor Stage Is Reached

When DNA from benign tumors is transfected into NIH 3T3 cells, multilayered cell islands accumulate; growth above a monolayer is a neoplastic characteristic. The gene responsible for this neoplastic transformation is usually *KRAS.*[31] In fact, mutations in *KRAS* can be detected if hyperplastic foci are microdissected from tissue sections (see also Chapter 27), their DNA is extracted and amplified by the polymerase chain reaction (PCR), and the DNA is then sequenced.[25,36] It is probable, therefore, that mutation of *KRAS* is one of the events that initiates the tumorigenic process. The mutations in *KRAS* are in codon 12 or 61, the same sites where activating mutations typically occur in many human adenocarcinomas.[37] Moreover, the mutational spectrum seen in lung tumors from A/J mice relates directly to the specific mutagenic adducts formed as a result of carcinogen activation.[31] Spontaneous lung tumors have *KRAS* mutations at these same codon sites, but in contrast to chemical activation, mutational specificity is not observed. The resulting conformational change in the mutated *KRAS* p21 protein product interferes with GTP hydrolysis and renders the *KRAS* molecular switch in a permanently "on" position. This allows the transcription of genes associated with proliferation without growth factors.[38]

Although most chemically induced tumors in A/J mice contain *KRAS* mutations, activation of this gene is not always observed in lung tumors induced in other mouse strains. Half of the lung tumors induced in the CD-1 mouse by diethylnitrosamine (DEN) do not contain mutant *KRAS.*[39] The AXB and BXA recombinant inbred strains derived from A/J and C57 display a continuous pattern of lung tumor susceptibilities; some strains are as susceptible as A/J, some as resistant as C57, with the others in between. Tumors induced in those strains with the highest tumor multiplicities all had *KRAS* mutations, whereas the mutation incidence in strains with lower susceptibility was less.[40] The identity of the activated oncogene or oncogenes responsible for tumorigenesis when *KRAS* retains its wild-type structure is unknown. When ascertained, this will stimulate a search for a similar oncogene in those human adenocarcinomas that lack *KRAS* mutations and may lead to new prognostic strategies.

No mutation in any other oncogene has been identified, although enhanced expression of *MYC* is frequent. Mutations or deletions in the tumor-suppressor genes have been noted in mouse lung carcinomas. *P53* mutations were found in adenocarcinomas but rarely in adenomas, suggesting that this alteration might drive the benign-to-malignant transition.[36] Loss of heterozygosity involving the p16 gene on chromosome 4 is also frequent in malignant but not in benign mouse lung tumors.[41,42] In addition, cell lines derived from these mouse lung tumors often have homozygous deletion[42,43] of the p16 gene, implying that inactivation of this tumor-suppressor gene is a late event in murine lung carcinogenesis. This contrasts with recent studies in the rat and human where inactivation of p16 appears to be a critical early event.[44]

A characteristic of neoplasms is their *resistance to chemotherapeutic agents.* There are numerous mechanisms for this resistance, including enhanced transcription of the glycoprotein that pumps certain classes of xenobiotics out of cells. Another mechanism is a reduction in the content of enzymes that activate prodrugs. This is particularly relevant to mouse lung tumors, because Clara and type II cells are the main pulmonary sites of xenobiotic metabolism. The content of various cytochrome P450 isozymes, such as the phenobarbital-inducible IIB isozyme, is reduced in mouse lung adenomas.[21] The PAH-inducible IA1 isozyme is negligibly present in mammalian lungs but is highly inducible. The extent of IA1 induction in adenomas is lower than in control lung; by the carcinoma stage, IA1 induction is not detected.[21] There is thus a gradient of P450-mediated xenobiotic resistance of these tumors from the benign to the malignant stages. A functional consequence of a diminished ability of neoplastic tissue to respond to toxicants is exemplified by the decreased CYP2E1-dependent metabolism of 1,1-dichloroethylene (DCE), a chemical that injures Clara cells in mice. Formation of the glutathione-conjugated product of the DCE epoxide, which occurs at a high rate in Clara cells, was deficient in Clara cell hyperplasias, adenomas, and carcinomas.[45] NQO1 detoxifies quinones by catalyzing a two-electron reduction to form a hydroquinone, thereby preventing oxygen radical formation. For some chemotherapeutic drugs, such as mitomycin C, this could result in bioactivation. NQO1 localizes to type II cells, as determined by histochemical assay.[46] By the adenoma stage, no NQO1 activity is detectable,[46] and cell lines derived from these tumors also lack NQO1 activity. This loss in NQO1 activity is one of few characteristics of mouse lung tumors that are dissimilar from human adenocarcinomas. In fact, there is a marked increase in NQO1 activity and NQO1 mRNA content in many types of human NSCLC relative to normal lung or to SCLC.[47] This tumor-specific increase in NQO1 content has stimulated the design of quinones requiring bioactivation by NQO1 that potently inhibit the growth of NSCLC xenografts[48] and are now in clinical trials. It is noteworthy that practical consequences might ensue from the mouse lung tumor model even in this case, where a feature of the model differed from the human equivalent because the mouse studies led to the pursuit of these human investigations.

In addition to becoming relatively autonomous from en-

vironmental stimuli by decreasing the concentration of their xenobiotic-metabolizing enzymes, tumor cells also show derangements in their *signal transduction machinery.* As mouse lung tumors advance toward malignancy, several changes in cAMP-dependent protein kinase (PKA), which mediates the actions of cAMP in cells, have been observed. These changes include altered cAMP binding affinity, an enhanced degree of degradation of the regulatory (R) subunits of PKA by the Ca^{2+}-dependent protease calpain, and altered regulation of R-subunit autophosphorylation.[49] These changes make the tumor cells less responsive to hormone- or growth factor-induced elevations in cAMP content. cAMP derivatives inhibit the growth of the mouse lung epithelial cells.[50] Cell lines have been established from normal mouse lung explants.[51] They are immortalized but have features common to other nontumorigenic cell lines, such as anchorage dependence and contact inhibition. Spontaneous transformants of these nontumorigenic cells have been selected, and additional tumorigenic cell lines have been derived from mouse lung tumors.[52] These neoplastic cell lines grow as tumors when injected into syngeneic or immunocompromised mice, and are anchorage-independent; most of them have mutant *KRAS*.[53] Interestingly, these neoplastic lines with less PKA are less sensitive to cAMP-mediated growth inhibition than their nontumorigenic parental cell lines.[50] When the signal-transducing properties of neoplastic cell lines are compared to the nontumorigenic cells, defects in cAMP synthesis, caused by decreased β-adrenergic receptor function and decreased Gsα (the alpha subunit of the stimulatory GTP-binding trimeric complex that transduces hormonal occupation of a receptor to activate adenylate cyclase) function are observed.[54] Depressed R-subunit protein and mRNA content and altered regulation of R-subunit message stability complete this pattern of unresponsiveness.[55] Additional signaling pathways are compromised in these neoplastic cells, as seen by a decreased content of glucocorticoid hormone receptors,[56] epidermal growth factor receptors (EGFR),[57] platelet-derived growth factor receptors (PDGFR),[58] and protein kinase C.[59] Finally, these lung tumor cell lines have a reduced capacity for the intercellular communication that occurs via passage of small molecules from cell to cell through gap junctions.[60]

Genetic Basis of Susceptibility to Lung Tumor Growth

Inbred Strains

"The close genomic organization and functional relationship between the mouse and human genomes make the mouse an ideal mammal for the study of human disease and the disease process. Homologous genes are linked in both the mouse and human. Mutations in identical genes often produce identical or similar phenotypes in both species."[61] Inbred strains of mice provide populations with genetically identical members. Inbred strains are derived by mating brothers and sisters over several generations, and the strains differ from each other at many loci as the result of random loss or retention of allelic forms of each gene. Inbreeding has eliminated genetic variability as an experimental problem and generated differences among strains which can be used to understand the molecular basis of phenotypes. Identification of the genes underlying a particular pathology leads to their possible use in prevention, diagnosis, or therapy.

The genes responsible for determining whether untreated mice develop lung tumors may also regulate responsiveness to carcinogens, because the same strain distribution describes inheritance of spontaneous and chemically induced tumors.[12] Tumor susceptibility is organ-specific; a strain such as A/J is highly susceptible to lung tumor development but resistant to hepatocarcinogenesis.[62] Analysis of strain differences in lung tumor incidence and multiplicity by conventional Mendelian crosses indicates that this is a polygenic trait. Recombinant inbred (RI) strains are a useful tool for genetic analysis. When two different inbred strains are mated, their alleles are randomly shuffled among the F2 progeny, which are then inbred to establish strains with different allelic assortments. The continuous gradient of tumor multiplicities among the RI strains derived from susceptible A/J and resistant C57 strains confirmed the polygenic character of lung tumors.[63]

KRAS

Polymorphisms have been found among inbred strains in the structure of the *KRAS* protooncogene. DNA digestion with the EcoRI restriction endonuclease resulted in fragments of two different sizes, depending upon the strain. When the susceptibility to lung tumor development was compared to the distribution of this restriction fragment length polymorphism (RFLP) (see also Chapter 1) among inbred and RI strains, a good correlation was seen.[64] This indicates that *KRAS* is one of the genes determining susceptibility, referred to as the pulmonary adenoma susceptibility (*Pas*) genes. The basis of the RFLP is a 37 bp tandem repeat present in the second intron of *KRAS;* resistant strains have two repeats of this segment, whereas susceptible strains have a single copy.[65] Because the several dozen inbred and RI strains examined had either one or two copies of this sequence, but neither had zero nor more than two copies, and because this 37 bp sequence was unique to the *KRAS* intron, this is not a random transposition. Linkage analysis using F2 or backcross mice produced from crosses between sensitive A/J and a resistant strain also suggested that a major susceptibility site mapped near the *KRAS* gene on chromosome 6.[40,66-69] These quantitative trait locus (QTL) mapping studies indicated that the *KRAS* locus, or a gene linked very close to it, accounted for about two thirds of the variation in tumor multiplicity between sensitive and resistant strains.[69]

KRAS is a *pas* gene and is also the site of the probable initiating mutation. The number of copies of this 37 bp sequence often reflects the susceptibility to lung tumor induction. The polymorphism does not change the structure of the *KRAS* protein product because of its location within an intron. Rather, the presence or absence of a second 37 bp copy may regulate transcription.[65,66,70] If a mutant oncogene is not expressed, the mutation will be phenotypically silent.[71] The polymorphic difference within intron 2 has been used to determine which *KRAS* allele contains mutations in NNK-induced lung tumors from the C3A mouse (F1 hybrid cross between the C3H and A/J mice). The A/J allele was mutated and overexpressed in 90% of the lung tumors from carcinogen-treated C3A mice.[65] This predominance of mutations within the A/J allele from hybrid mice could stem from higher rates of transcription of the A/J allele compared with the C3H allele. However, this is not the sole mechanism for selective clonal expansion of the mutated allele from A/J mice. The effects on *KRAS* transcription of reporter gene constructs containing the K-*ras* promoter from either A/J or C3H mice ligated to the intron 2 polymorphic region from each strain were compared through transfection into tumor-derived cell lines from sensitive, intermediate, and resistant mouse strains. No significant differences were found in promoter activity.[72]

Other Gene Candidates for Susceptibility

Congenic strains of mice are selectively bred to be genetically identical except at a single site. Studies of mice congenic for the H-2 locus, which is the mouse equivalent of the human HLA major histocompatibility genes that regulate macrophage-lymphocyte interactions, indicate that H-2 affects lung tumor multiplicity. A/J mice whose H-2 alleles have been replaced by those of the resistant C57 strain get fewer tumors than normal A/J mice.[73] Lung tumors are mildly immunogenic, and this effect of H-2 suggests that some of the factors regulating lung tumor development involve interactions of nascent tumor cells with immune cells. Lymphocytic and macrophage infiltrations into lung tumors have been observed. Genetically or surgically immunocompromised mice acquire more lung tumors,[74] which is consistent with a role of immune factors. The H-2 region, however, also contains genes with functions not confined to the immune system. The structural gene for the glucocorticoid receptor also maps to the H-2 region, and the amount of circulating corticosterone influences tumor multiplicity to the same quantitative extent as does H-2 variation.[75] A urethane-treated, adrenalectomized A/J mouse develops about 30% more lung tumors than a sham-operated mouse, and mice implanted with a pellet that continuously releases excess corticosterone develop 30% fewer tumors.[76] Further, inhalation of budesonide, a synthetic glucocorticoid, nearly abolishes benzo(a)pyrene-induced lung tumor formation.[77] Also, the TNFα gene is located at H-2, and this cytokine regulates growth and differentiation of many cell types. Finally, linkage studies have indicated that susceptibility loci are contained within the H-2 region.[69]

Several chromosomal regions contain genes that confer sensitivity or resistance to lung tumorigenesis (Table 19.2). When the F1 generation resulting from an intercross between a sensitive and a resistant strain is injected with a lung carcinogen, the hybrid mice may contain the arithmetic mean of the tumor multiplicities of their parents.[78] In this case, the sensitive and resistant alleles are contributing

TABLE 19.2. CANDIDATE GENES FOR THE *PAS* AND *PAR* LOCI AND THEIR HOMOLOGOUS REGIONS ON THE HUMAN CHROMOSOME

Mouse Chromosome QTLs	Named Loci	Homologous Human Chromosomal Sites
1		1q31–q32
		1q25.2–q25.3
		1q22–q23
4		9p21
		9p22
		1p31–p32
6	Par4	7q31
6		2p12–p11.1
		2p13
6	Pas1	12p12.1
9		6p12
		15q24–q25
		3p11
10		6q25.1
		6q21
		6q21–q23.2
11	Par1	17q21.3–q23
		17q21.1
		17q21
12	Par3	14q11–q24
		3q11–q12
		14q24.3–q31
13		5q31–q35
		9q21.3–q22.1
		5p15.3–p15.2
17	Pas2	6p21–p21.2
		6p21.3
		6p21.3
18	Par2	5q31–q32
19	Pas3	11q13
		9q11–q22
19		10q34–q24
		10q24.3
		10q24–q26

From Fijneman RJA, Jansen RC, van der Valk, MA, et al. High frequency of interactions between lung cancer susceptibility genes in the mouse: mapping of *Sluc5* to *Sluc14*. *Cancer Res* 1998;58:4794, with permission.
Sites in boldface are frequently deleted or amplified in human adenocarcinoma.

equally to the susceptibility phenotype and are designated as *pas* (pulmonary adenoma susceptibility) alleles, or the resistant allele can display dominant inheritance, and the allele at that gene is described as *pas* (pulmonary adenoma resistance).[78] These chromosomal assignments were made using various mapping strategies that involve linkage analysis, which consists of breeding mice according to various schemes, phenotyping the progeny to see which mice carry the trait (i.e., lung tumor multiplicity), and genotyping them to find where within the genome they map based on their colocalization with previously assigned markers. A class of DNA polymorphisms known as microsatellites has recently been used in human and mouse genetic studies. These consist of simple, tandemly repeated, mononucleotide-to-tetranucleotide sequence motifs flanked by unique sequences, which serve as primers for PCR amplification. Inbred strains frequently vary in the number of repeat units in this motif at many chromosomal sites randomly distributed throughout the genome.[79] The resulting size differences allow visualization on agarose or acrylamide gels.

Hundreds of genes are contained within each of the chromosomal intervals, identified by linkage analysis, and identifying the single gene within each interval that regulates susceptibility is a daunting task. A further complication is that genes regulating susceptibility can interact with each other (epistasis) and either synergize or antagonize each other's contributions.[80] Many of the genes known to map within the *pas* and *par* loci have functions consistent with a role in susceptibility, such as encoding signaling molecules (i.e., receptors, protein kinases, G proteins, transcription factors, etc.), enzymes that catalyze metabolic activation and detoxification of carcinogens, and cytokines that modulate the immune response and inflammation.[81] Interestingly, many of these sites are deleted in human lung adenocarcinoma, supporting a role for them in neoplastic progression. The reason for expending such effort in identifying these tumor modifier genes is to learn what makes mice resistant to lung cancer, information that will yield new preventive and therapeutic drugs. This has been referred to by Dr. Richard Klausner, Director of the National Cancer Institute, as "the next great revolution in cancer research." The ultimate test of a candidate susceptibility gene, in addition to its polymorphic status between sensitive and resistant strains and its under- or overexpression in the tumors, is using it as a transgene to confer, say, resistant status to a normally sensitive strain.[81]

Transgenes and Targeted Genes with Induced Mutations

Lung tumors can be induced in transgenic mice with a mutated oncogene or tumor-suppressor genes as the transgene. Two relevant transgenic models involve the *HRAS* protooncogene[82] and the SV40 virus large T-antigen.[83] The *HRAS* transgene was attached to a variety of promoter-enhancer elements (e.g., albumin, mouse mammary tumor virus, immunoglobulin). SV40 T-antigen was ligated to promoters that should be preferentially expressed in type II (the surfactant apo-C promoter) or Clara (CC10) cells. The mice generated with either transgene were born with lung tumors or developed lung tumors soon after birth. Because the original genetic backgrounds of the host mice were resistant, these activated oncogenes overcame this inherited resistance. The tumors were adenomas at early stages of growth which later became carcinomas with structural and biochemical features resembling those lung tumors that arise in nontransgenic mice. These mice, genetically engineered to develop lung tumors, have been used to test putative lung carcinogens[84] and for exploring tumor histogenesis. Individual tumors in mice made transgenic with the SV40 T-antigen targeted with an apo-C promoter were heterogeneous with regard to expression of CC10 or SPC. Some cells contained both of these peripheral respiratory epithelial markers, some cells contained one but not the other marker, and some cells expressed neither.[83] This suggests that type II or Clara cells or precursor cells committed to these phenotypes underlie lung tumorigenesis. Other potential uses are to delineate key steps in the cellular dysregulations leading to multistep carcinogenesis, to examine interactions between known genes with oncogenic potential with each other, and to assess the functioning of these genes in different genetic backgrounds. Investigation into key steps in tumor development have used both transgenic and knock-out mice. Overexpression of prostacyclin synthase raises the levels of prostacyclin, which has anti-inflammatory effects in the lung, and diminishes lung tumor multiplicity in response to carcinogens, implying a role for inflammation in tumor development.[85] Inactivation of O^6-methylguanine-DNA methyltransferase (*Mgmt*), an enzyme that catalyzes adduct removal, gave rise to mice especially sensitive to lung tumorigenesis,[86] emphasizing the critical need for DNA repair in preventing lung cancer.

PRIMARY LUNG TUMORS IN RATS

In the early 1970s, the National Cancer Institute developed a protocol using rodents to evaluate the carcinogenic potential of chronic exposure to environmental agents. This protocol was adopted and refined by the National Toxicology Program and employed the F344 rat and the B6C3F1 hybrid mouse (C57BL/6J × C3H/HeJ). More than 400 chemicals have been tested for carcinogenicity, and these data constitute the primary database available today for the evaluation of mammalian carcinogenesis. The F344 rat appears to be a good model for evaluating the ability of environmental exposures to induce pulmonary neoplasia. In contrast to the A/J mouse, which exhibits a 95% frequency of spontaneous tumors by 20 months of age, the frequency of spontaneous lung tumors in this rodent is only around

2%.[87] In addition, both of the two major histologic forms of human NSCLC, adenocarcinoma and squamous cell carcinoma, can be induced in this animal model by chemical carcinogens.

Histogenesis

Spontaneous neoplasms of the lung in the rat are primarily alveolar-bronchiolar adenomas or carcinomas. The major histologic types induced by carcinogen exposure are alveolar-bronchiolar adenomas or carcinomas and squamous cell carcinomas. The predominant histological type identified from chemical exposure is the adenocarcinoma, whereas squamous cell carcinomas are more prevalent in animals exposed to high doses of radiation.[88] Cells within adenomas and carcinomas grow in a solid, papillary, or mixed solid and papillary pattern. As in mice, adenomas with a solid growth pattern tend to remain benign, whereas the papillary pattern has been associated with differentiation to the malignant state.[89]

Progenitor Cells

Lung neoplasms in the F344 rat originate in the lung periphery from a proliferation of epithelial cells along the alveolar septae. Examination of the ultrastructure of hyperplasias induced following exposure to either NNK[89] or plutonium[90] reveals morphologic features characteristic of type II pneumocytes. These cells typically contain numerous, prominent, cytoplasmic lamellar bodies and large round mitochondria. Ultrastructural examination of several adenomas and adenocarcinomas induced by these exposures also exhibit type II features. The malignant adenocarcinomas identified in the F344 rat lung appear to develop by the progression of alveolar hyperplasia to adenoma and ultimately carcinoma. Adenomas can be detected within hyperplasias, and carcinomas have been observed arising within adenomas.[89]

Determining the origin of the squamous cell carcinoma is complicated by the fact that no squamous epithelium is present in the normal tracheobronchial tree. The tumors exhibit all the ultrastructural characteristics of human squamous cells (i.e., tonofilament bundles, keratin, keratohyaline granules, desmosomes). Development of squamous cell carcinomas is not restricted to a single region of the pulmonary parenchyma; it occurs in both the bronchial and alveolar regions of the lung. However, the squamous cell tumors exhibit ultrastructural characteristics of the type II pneumocyte and do not demonstrate immunoreactivity with Clara cell antigen. These data suggest that the cuboidal epithelial cells that comprise some adenocarcinomas could transdifferentiate to a squamous cell phenotype.[90]

Identification of the type II pneumocyte as the major progenitor cell for lung neoplasia in the F344 rat may prove to be a good model for studying the development of environmentally induced human lung cancers. Adenocarcinoma of the lung is rapidly becoming the most prevalent histologic type of tumor in the world. The reduction of tar and nicotine concentrations in cigarettes has led to a significant increase in puff volume and hence a greater exposure of the alveolar epithelium to the chemical carcinogens present in tobacco. Approximately 50% of human adenocarcinomas are mucin-secreting and consist of tall columnar cells,[26] whereas the remaining tumors have little or no mucin. Electron microscopy of these non–mucin-secreting tumors shows cells with morphologic features consistent with those of either a Clara cell or a type II cell. The ability to isolate specific lung cell populations from the rat following exposure to environmental carcinogens[89] provides an opportunity to study and identify genetic and epigenetic changes associated with tumor initiation and development.

Environmental Exposures

The contribution of mixtures, rather than of a single component, to the induction of pulmonary neoplasia is an active area of research. The most important mixture contributing to human lung cancer is tobacco, which contains over 4,000 chemicals, gases, and volatiles. Developing an animal model for tobacco-induced cancer has generally relied on carcinogenicity studies of single components such as NNK (described below). However, in recent studies (Nikula et al., unpublished) where F344 rats were exposed to mainstream cigarette smoke equivalent to three to four packs per day, a significant increase in lung tumors was seen. Studying the mechanisms underlying lung tumor development in this cigarette-smoke model may be invaluable for dissecting the process of tobacco-induced cancer in people.

F344 rat lungs are also susceptible to pulmonary neoplasia following inhalation or systemic exposure to specific environmental and occupational chemicals; for example, intraperitoneal injection of rats with NNK-induced tumors at concentrations of NNK ranging from 1.5 to 750 mg.[89] The lowest amount of NNK mimics exposure to this nitrosamine by habitual cigarette smokers (two packs per day). Inhalation of tetranitromethane, a reagent used in industrial nitrosating processes, at concentrations similar to occupational limits induced lung tumors in F344 rats.[91] Thus, the F344 rat lung is a good model in which to study the molecular mechanisms underlying environmentally induced neoplasia.

Gene Dysfunctions

Examination of gene dysfunctions in lung tumors induced in the F344 rat has focused on both genetic and epigenetic mechanisms. Genetic studies have been restricted mostly to evaluating mutation frequency of the *KRAS* and *P53* genes. The prevalence and specificity for activation of *KRAS* vary markedly among environmental carcinogens. Activation of

this gene by a GGT-to-GAT transition was observed in 100% of the lung tumors induced by tetranitromethane.[91] *KRAS* was mutated in 40% of plutonium-induced lung tumors, with a GGT-to-AGT transition as the predominant base substitution.[92] In contrast, activation of this gene was observed in only 10% of the lung tumors induced by beryllium metal[93] and none of the lung tumors induced by NNK.[94] Although activated *RAS* genes were not detected in lung tumors induced by NNK, DNA from seven of ten tumors induced subcutaneous tumors in a nude mouse tumorigenicity assay. The presence of an active transforming gene that is not *KRAS* was inferred by the detection of rat repetitive sequences in DNA from these primary nude mouse tumors. Since mutation of *KRAS* occurs in only 30% of human adenocarcinomas,[37] the identification of non-*RAS* transforming genes in pulmonary tumors induced by NNK may aid in defining the process of neoplastic transformation in human lung tumors.

Alterations within the conserved region (exons 5 through 8) of the *P53* gene do not appear to be a common event in rodent pulmonary neoplasia. No adenocarcinomas induced by inhaled beryllium or injected NNK contained a mutation within this conserved region. In contrast, *P53* dysfunction has been detected at variables frequencies (5% to 40%) in squamous cell carcinomas induced by either NNK, x-rays, diesel exhaust, or carbon black.[95] These results are in sharp contrast to the high prevalence of *P53* mutations (50% to 65%) observed in human adenocarcinomas and squamous cell carcinomas.[96] Genes within the *P53* pathway (e.g., *MdmII* or *Waf1*) did not appear to be altered in rodent lung tumors.[95]

The promoters of approximately 60% of human genes are located within areas rich in the CG dinucleotide, referred to as CpG islands. Recent studies[28] have demonstrated an inactivation of critical regulatory genes in cancer cells as a result of promoter methylation. Studies conducted in animal models address several important mechanistic questions concerning whether environmental exposures target genes for methylation, the timing of the corresponding gene inactivations, and the concordance with human studies. Promoter methylation of the estrogen receptor varied in rat lung tumors, being most frequent (80%) in plutonium-exposed animals but inactivated in only 20% of lung tumors induced by NNK.[97] Similar results were observed in lung tumors induced in A/J mice by NNK and human NSCLC associated with tobacco. The mechanisms that inactivate the tumor suppressor gene in human tumors, homozygous deletion and aberrant promoter methylation, also occur in primary rat lung cancers and derived cell lines. Promoter methylation clearly originates in the primary tumor. Inactivation of p16 by aberrant methylation is an early event in rodent carcinogenesis, occurring at a high frequency in alveolar hyperplasias resulting from NNK.[98] Analogously, p16 methylation has been detected at early stages of human squamous cell carcinoma development.[44] Thus inactivating genes by methylation is recapitulated in rodent lung tumors. Future studies of genes such as p16 and estrogen receptor in rodent carcinogenesis models will be invaluable for understanding their roles in neoplastic progression and in defining the mechanisms associated with targeting genes for inactivation by this epigenetic process.

PRIMARY LUNG TUMORS IN HAMSTERS

Hamsters rarely develop spontaneous tumors and display little pulmonary inflammation, so that tumor yield is strictly a function of the experimental treatment. Mixtures of different carcinogens, such as PAHs and nitrosamines, gave an enhanced tumor yield, and combinations of chemicals similar to those found in cigarette smoke can potentially be instilled in these mixtures.

Problems associated with the use of hamsters in carcinogenesis studies include the following: their short tails preclude intravenous injections and make them difficult to handle, they may be aggressive and difficult to maintain, the hibernating status of the animals affects tumorigenesis, and concurrent infections can lead to variable tumor incidences.[99]

Histogenesis

Adenocarcinomas are the main tumor types induced in mice and rats by administration of individual or combinations of chemical carcinogens through any route. Although adenocarcinoma is currently the most common human lung cancer type, in the mid-twentieth century squamous carcinoma was most prevalent. Thus there was great excitement 30 years ago when bronchogenic carcinoma was produced in Syrian golden hamsters after intratracheal instillation of PAHs attached to ferric oxide particles.[100] The metaplastic and dysplastic changes that preceded the formation of frank malignancy resembled those associated with human carcinomas, although whether they are preneoplastic lesions *per se* or markers of chronic injury was not clear. These changes include replacing the goblet cells in the tracheobronchial epithelium with mucous cells, followed by the formation of multiple layers of cuboidal cells on top of a basal cell layer.[101] This change is referred to as "epidermoid metaplasia" because of the keratinization of the surface layer and the presence of a high concentration of desmosomes, as is found in skin. This response to injury is similar to that in humans.

Tumors in hamster trachea and stem bronchi correspond to human bronchial carcinomas, whereas hamster lobar bronchial and bronchiolar carcinomas resemble human peripheral adenocarcinomas.[102] Different tumors are induced by systemic versus topical application of chemicals. For example, subcutaneous or intraperitoneal injection of nitrosamines, such as DEN, induces peripheral tumors with Clara cell cytologic characteristics. These adenocarcinomas frequently contain mutated *KRAS,* but rarely exhibit mutated *p53.*[103] Intratracheal absorption of ^{210}Po, a radioactive soil contaminant present in cigarette smoke, also induces Clara cell adenocarcinomas.[23] DNA adducts can be found in Clara cells after carcinogenesis treatment.[104]

Neuroendocrine Tumors

Neuroendocrine tumors can be induced from a combination of nitrosamines plus continuous hypoxia or hyperoxia.[105] The theory is that the damage caused by aberrant arterial oxygen pressure will stimulate secretion of autocrine growth factors as part of the regenerative response.[106] This proliferation would augment the action of the carcinogen. The hypoxia would mimic the oxygen deficit caused by chronic obstructive pulmonary disease or smoking. Initial reports of hamsters treated in this manner described a 100% incidence of tumors with neuroendocrine features such as the secretion of bombesin, serotonin, calcitonin, and gastrin-releasing peptide. Subsequent studies by other investigators have not reproduced this observation, however, finding instead a marked but transient proliferation of peripheral neuroendocrine cells.[107] Whether this represents division of mature neuroendocrine cells, recruitment from a stem cell along a neuroendocrine route of differentiation, or transdifferentiation from a different cell type, such as Type II cells, is not clear.[108]

Inbred Strains

The number of tumors, the type of tumor induced, and their pulmonary location vary with the carcinogen used and the size of the carrier particles used to absorb the carcinogens in intratracheal instillation studies. Some improved techniques involve deposition of nitrosoureas onto a defined area of the trachea through a catheter to eliminate the need for particulate carriers,[109] and continuous carcinogen release from endobronchially implanted silastic carriers.[110] Perhaps most critical, however, is the fact that outbred hamsters are used in most research, and genetic variations are seen even when animals are purchased from the same vendor. Different outbred Syrian golden hamsters develop different distributions of spontaneous tumor types at various anatomic sites and vary in their susceptibilities to viral infections. An initial report of the use of inbred Syrian golden hamsters for respiratory carcinogenesis is very encouraging.[111] Tumors histologically analogous to those in humans were observed, and strains varied in their tumor susceptibility.

PRIMARY LUNG TUMORS IN THE BEAGLE

The advent of the nuclear age opened up a new era of research dedicated to assessing the biologic risks from radioactive fallout. Extensive studies using many internally deposited radionuclides were initially conducted in the rat and mouse. Based on data collected from these studies, external exposure limits and internal deposition limits for a large number of radionuclides were established. However, because these data were compiled using small animals with limited life spans, extrapolations to human risk were considered tenuous. The main criticism of the rodent studies was centered around an uncertainty of whether these animal models would exhibit the full array of late-developing effects that were characteristic of low-level radiation exposures in humans. In an attempt to circumvent these problems, lifespan studies were initiated in the beagle by the Atomic Energy Commission beginning in the early 1950s. These studies were designed to compare the long-term toxicity of a variety of radionuclides[112] administered in either single or repeated exposures.

Histogenesis

The overall incidence of spontaneous lung tumors in beagles is approximately 0.1% per dog-year up to the age of 12 years, and increases to 0.7% after 13 years of age.[113] Spontaneous canine neoplasms are mainly adenocarcinomas and, to a lesser extent, adenosquamous cell carcinomas. Several different histologic tumor types are induced by radiation. Papillary adenocarcinoma is the most common tumor induced by $^{239}PuO_2$. These tumors originate in the peripheral lung and are associated with plutonium deposits, fibrosis, and bronchioloalveolar metaplasia.[114] Bronchioloalveolar carcinoma, adenosquamous carcinoma, and epidermoid carcinomas are also induced by plutonium. A similar histologic spectrum of tumors has been observed in dogs chronically inhaling radon daughters and uranium ore dust.[115]

Progenitor Cells and Tumor Morphology

Radiation-induced lung tumors in beagles appear to originate primarily in the lung periphery. Although detailed morphologic analyses have not been conducted, the anatomic location of the neoplasms suggests that the tumors arise from Clara cells, Type II cells, or both. Squamous cell carcinomas may arise by squamous metaplasia of the subpleural lung. Preneoplastic lesions observed in the dog include atypical hyperplasia of the alveoli and bronchial metaplasia of the terminal airways. As in humans, adenomas are rarely detected in the beagle. Most adenocarcinomas exhibit a papillary growth pattern; solid growth patterns are only occasionally present.

Gene Dysfunctions

The analysis of gene dysfunctions in dogs has focused primarily on spontaneous and plutonium-induced tumors. The prevalence for activation of *KRAS* was examined in 21 spontaneous canine tumors.[116] The overall mutation frequency was 25%, and nucleotide substitutions were distributed randomly within codons 12 and 61. Mutation of this gene was not detected in plutonium-induced tumors in dogs.[117] These results contrast with the 40% frequency of *KRAS* mutation in lung tumors induced in the F344 rat by plutonium and in human adenocarcinomas associated with radon exposure.[118]

The expression of *EGFR*[119] and *TGFA*[120] has been examined in spontaneous and plutonium-induced lung tumors; *EGFR* is the receptor for *TGFA*. Overexpression of *EGFR* and *TGFA*[120] was observed in approximately 55% of tumors, irrespective of etiology. A positive association between increased expression of both the ligand and its receptor was not observed within the same tumor. However, 27% of radiation-induced proliferative foci expressed *TGFA*, and one third of these foci also expressed *EGFR*. Increased expression of a growth factor, its receptor, or both in these foci may indicate preneoplastic lesions with a heightened propensity for progressing to neoplasia. The possibility for selective growth advantage of pulmonary lesions via the EGF pathway has also been described in human NSCLC.[121]

Altered expression of *p53* protein has been determined by immunohistochemical analysis. Similar to the rat, the prevalence of *p53* dysfunction was low (less than 15%) in both spontaneous and plutonium-induced tumors and was restricted largely to adenosquamous and squamous histologic types.[117] In contrast, activation of the *p53* gene is detected in 40% to 55% of human lung tumors associated with radon exposure.[122] Species differences in *KRAS* and *p53* mutation frequencies suggest that multiple pathways exist for the development of cancers induced by high-LET (low energy transfer) radiation (plutonium, radon).

PERSPECTIVES FOR THE FUTURE

Chemoprevention and Intervention Using Animal Models

One major challenge in the study of lung cancer is the development of new intervention strategies to prevent and inhibit the spread of this disease in humans. Despite numerous radiation and chemotherapy protocols over the past 20 years, the median survival for nonresectable lung cancers is still only nine months.[123] When the pathways involved in the genesis of this disease are delineated, new therapies can be developed that focus not on cell killing but on modulating enzymes whose deregulation is responsible for cell transformation. New intervention strategies are usually evaluated *in vitro* using epithelial cell lines derived from a variety of human and rodent tumors or using cells injected into athymic nude mice.[124] *In vitro* systems lack endogenous factors (e.g., hormones, cytokines) that could influence therapeutic responsiveness and do not allow for the evaluation of pharmacokinetic variables such as delivery of the therapeutic agent to target cells, a factor that can profoundly influence drug efficacy.

The use of an animal model such as the A/J mouse to evaluate promising new intervention protocols affords an opportunity to study the responsiveness of pulmonary lesions at different stages of progression to chemotherapeutic intervention. The efficacy of this animal model has been evaluated using a classic chemotherapy agent with potential synergistic compounds.[125] Mice containing lung lesions (i.e., hyperplasia, adenoma, carcinoma) induced by NNK were treated for up to eight weeks with *cis*-platinum alone or in combination with indomethacin, metoclopramide, or both, and the effects on tumor growth were assessed. The most dramatic effects were observed in lungs from mice treated for eight weeks. *Cis*-platinum treatment reduced the size of carcinomas by 37%, whereas tumor mass was reduced by 50% to 60% with *cis*-platinum in combination with indomethacin, metoclopramide, or both. As is often observed with a majority of human lung tumors that respond to chemotherapy, tumor mass was reduced in the lungs of A/J mice, but few malignant tumors were completely eliminated. This *in vivo* model is suitable for studying and developing new chemointervention therapies.

13-cis-retinoic acid is used to prevent oral premalignancies and second primary head and neck tumors in humans,[126] and the scientific basis for this application was upper respiratory tract carcinogenesis in hamster models. Squamous metaplasia can largely be prevented in hamsters by simultaneous treatment with retinoids, carotenoids, and selenium along with the carcinogen.[127] Deletion of vitamin A from the hamster diet constitutes a model for squamous metaplasia that is reversed on readdition of this retinoid. Retinoids induce a pathway of mucociliary differentiation (i.e., the production of ciliated and goblet cells from mucous cell precursors), but a retinoid deficiency leads to squamous differentiation and cornification of the tracheobronchial epithelium.[128]

Several dozen compounds have been tested for their abilities to inhibit chemically induced lung tumors in A/J mice,[99,129] but few were potent enough to nearly abolish tumor formation. Budesonide, a synthetic glucocorticoid, reduced benzo(a)pyrene-induced tumor multiplicity by 90% when budesonide was administered through a nose-only nebulizer beginning one week following treatment with the inducer.[77] The convenience of this mode of administration of a chemopreventive agent suggests its practical use for humans at high risk of cancer development, and clinical trials are proceeding. Sulindac sulfone is a metabolite of the NSAID, sulindac, that, unlike its parent compound, fails to inhibit cyclooxygenase activity and the subsequent production of prostaglandins that inhibit neoplastic growth. Nonetheless, this derivative can prevent the formation of different tumor types in various animal models, possibly by stimulating apoptosis through its elevation of cGMP levels.[130] While the sulfone is equal to or less potent than

sulindac at inhibiting rat models of mammary and colon tumors, respectively, it was much more effective than sulindac at inhibiting lung tumor formation in mice.[131] Its relative lack of toxic side effects has resulted in the initiation of phase I clinical trials to test the efficacy of sulindac sulfone in humans at high risk.

The next century will see lung cancer incidence in the world reach epidemic proportions due to the escalation of smoking in Asia and the failure of smoking cessation programs for many addicted smokers. In the United States alone, 40% of the population are either current or former smokers; half of the lung cancer patients seen in the clinic are former smokers. Thus some of the major challenges over the next decade will be dissecting the pathways of lung cancer pathogenesis, identifying biomarkers that detect early lung cancer, developing novel prevention and intervention therapies for high-risk people, and improving the management of disseminated disease. Completion of the human genome and murine genome projects over the next five years will provide a database rich in sequences that await functional studies. Some of the most promising new technologies for gene discovery include serial analysis of gene expression (SAGE), which identifies and quantifies hundreds of thousand of gene transcripts from tumor cells[132] and methylated CpG island amplification for the cloning of differentially methylated genes.[133] In addition, the development of microarrays and silicon-based chips[134,135] will facilitate the analysis of tumors for hundreds of gene alterations. The animal models developed for studying the progression of lung cancer following defined environmental exposures are amenable to this new technology. Novel intervention and prevention approaches need to be developed to reduce the high mortality from lung cancer. Animal models have and will continue to be valuable tools for testing new interventions through oral, intravenous, and inhalation routes.

ACKNOWLEDGMENTS

This chapter was supported in part by USPHS grant CA 33497 and the Office of Biological and Environmental Research, U.S. Department of Energy, under Cooperative Agreement No. FC-0496AL76406.

REFERENCES

1. Crocker TT, Chase JE, Wells SA, et al. Preliminary report on experimental squamous carcinoma of the lung in hamsters and in a primate (Galago crassicaudatus). In: Nettesheim P, Hanna MG Jr, Detherage JW Jr, eds. *Morphology of experimental respiratory carcinogenesis.* Oak Ridge, TN: Atomic Energy Commission, 1970:317.
2. Livingood LE. Tumors in the mouse. *Johns Hopkins Bull* 1896; 66/67:177.
3. Reznik-Schuller HM. *Comparative respiratory tract carcinogenesis.* Boca Raton: CRC Press, 1993.

4. Hecht SS, Morse MA, Amin SG, et al. Rapid single dose model for lung tumor induction in A/J mice by 4-(methylnitrosamino)-1-(3-pyridyl)-1-butanone and the effect of diet. *Carcinogenesis* 1989;10:1901.

5. Witschi H. Tobacco smoke as a mouse lung carcinogen. *Exp Lung Res* 1998;24:385.

6. Wattenberg LW. Inhibition of chemical carcinogen-induced pulmonary neoplasia by butylated hydroxyanisole. *J Natl Cancer Inst* 1973;50:1541.

7. Witschi H, Williamson D, Lock S. Enhancement of urethan tumorigenesis in mouse lung by butylated hydroxytoluene. *J Natl Cancer Inst* 1977;58:301.

8. Malkinson AM, Koski KM, Evans WA, et al. Butylated hydroxytoluene exposure is necessary to induce lung tumors in BALB mice treated with 3-methylcholanthrene. *Cancer Res* 1997;57:2832.

9. Miller A, Dwyer CK, Auerbach LD, et al. Strain-related differences in the pneumotoxic effects of chronically administered butylated hydroxytoluene on protein kinase C and calpain. *Toxicology* 1994;90:141.

10. Dwyer-Nield LD, Thompson JA, Peljak G, et al. Selective induction of apoptosis in mouse and human lung epithelial cell lines by the *tert*-butyl hydroxylated metabolite of butylated hydroxytoluene: a proposed role in tumor promotion. *Toxicology* 1998;130:115.

11. Guan X, Hardenbrook J, Fernstrom MJ, et al. Downregulation by butylated hydroxytoluene of the number and function of gap junctions in epithelial cell lines derived from mouse lung and rat liver. *Carcinogenesis* 1995;16:2575.

12. Shimkin MB, Stoner GD. Lung tumors in mice: application to carcinogenesis bioassay. *Adv Cancer Res* 1975;21:1.

13. Malkinson AM. Primary lung tumors in mice: an experimentally manipulable model of human adenocarcinoma. *Cancer Res* 1992;53:2670s.

14. Malkinson AM. Molecular comparison of human and mouse pulmonary adenocarcinomas. *Exp Lung Res* 1998;24:541.

15. Thaete LG, Gunning WT, Stoner GD, et al. Cellular derivation of lung tumors in sensitive and resistant strains of mice: results at twenty-eight and fifty-six weeks after urethane treatment. *J Natl Cancer Inst* 1987;78:743.

16. Foley JF, Anderson MW, Stoner GD, et al. Proliferative lesions of the mouse lung: progression studies in strain-A mice. *Exp Lung Res* 1991;17:157.

17. Branstetter DG, Stoner GD, Budd C, et al. Effect of gestational development on lung tumor size and morphology in the mouse. *Cancer Res* 1988;48:379.

18. Thaete LG, Nesbitt MN, Malkinson AM. Lung tumor structure among inbred strains of mice: the pulmonary adenoma histologic type (pah) genes. *Cancer Lett* 1991;61:15.

19. Kauffman SL, Alexander L, Sass L. Histological and ultrastructural features of the Clara cell adenoma of mouse lung. *Lab Invest* 1979;40:708.

20. Malkinson AM. Genetic studies on lung tumor susceptibility and histogenesis in mice. *Environ Health Perspect* 1991;93:149.

21. Forkert PG, Parkinson A, Thaete LG, et al. Resistance of murine lung tumors to xenobiotic-induced cytotoxicity. *Cancer Res* 1992;52:6797.

22. Gazdar AF, Linnoila TR, Foley JF, et al. Peripheral airway cell differentiation in human lung cancer cell lines. *Cancer Res* 1990;50:5481.

23. Kennedy AR, McGandy RB, Little JB. Histochemical, light microscopic study of polonium-210 induced peripheral tumors in hamster lungs: evidence implicating the Clara cell as the cell of origin. *Eur J Cancer* 1977;13:1325.

24. Rehm S, Ward JM, Ten Have-Opbroek AAW, et al. Mouse papillary lung tumors transplacentally induced by N-nitrosoethylurea: evidence of alveolar type II cell origin by comparative light microscopic, ultrastructural, and immunohistochemical studies. *Cancer Res* 1988;48:148.

25. Belinsky SA, Devereux TR, Foley JF, et al. The role of the alveolar type II cell in the development and progression of pulmonary tumors in the A/J mouse. *Cancer Res* 1992;52:3164.

26. Gazdar AF, Linnoila RI. The pathology of lung cancer: changing concepts and newer diagnostic techniques. *Semin Oncol* 1988;15:215.

27. Dail DH, Hammar SP, Colby TV. *Pulmonary pathology—tumors.* New York: Springer-Verlag, 1995.

28. Baylin SB, Herman JG, Graff JR, et al. Alterations in DNA methylation: a fundamental aspect of neoplasia. *Adv Cancer Res* 1998;143:69.

29. Bestor T, Laudano A, Mattaliano R, et al. Cloning and sequencing of a cDNA encoding DNA methyltransferase of mouse cells. *J Mol Biol* 1988;971:203.

30. Belinsky SA, Nikula KJ, Baylin SB, et al. Increased cytosine DNA-methyltransferase activity is target-cell-specific and an early event in lung cancer. *Proc Natl Acad Sci U S A* 1996;4045:93.

31. You M, Candrian U, Maronpot RR, et al. Activation of the Ki-*ras* protooncogene in spontaneously occurring and chemically induced lung tumors of the strain A mouse. *Proc Natl Acad Sci U S A* 1989;86:3070.

32. Wheeler GP, Alexander JA. Rate of DNA synthesis as an indication of drug toxicity and as a guide for scheduling cancer therapy. *Cancer Treat Rep* 1978;62:755.

33. Shimkin MB, Sasaki T, McDonough M, et al. Relation of thymidine index to pulmonary tumors in mice receiving urethane and other carcinogens. *Cancer Res* 1969;29:994.

34. Thaete LG, Beer DG, Malkinson AM. Genetic variation in the proliferation of murine pulmonary type II cells: basal rates and alterations following urethane treatment. *Cancer Res* 1986;46:5335.

35. Thaete LG, Ahnen DJ, Malkinson AM. Proliferating cell nuclear antigen (PCNA/cyclin) immunocytochemistry as a labelling index in mouse lung tissues. *Cell Tissue Res* 1989;256:167.

36. Horio Y, Schrump DS, Chen A, et al. KRAS and P53 mutations are early and late events, respectively, in urethane-induced pulmonary carcinogenesis in A/J mice. *Mol Carcinog* 1996;17:217.

37. Rodenhuis S, Slebos RJC, Boot AJM, et al. Incidence and possible clinical significance of K-ras oncogene activation in adenocarcinoma of the human lung. *Cancer Res* 1988;48:5738.

38. Medema RH, Bos JL. The role of p21ras in receptor tyrosine kinase signalling. *Crit Rev Oncog* 1993;4:615.

39. Manam S, Storer RD, Prahalada S, et al. Activation of the Ki-ras gene in spontaneous and chemically induced lung tumors in CD-1 mice. *Mol Carcinog* 1992;6:68.

40. Lin L, Festing MFW, Devereux TR, et al. Additional evidence that the KRAS protooncogene is a candidate for the major mouse pulmonary adenoma susceptibility (Pas-1) gene. *Exp Lung Res* 1998;24:481.

41. Herzog CR, Wiseman RW, You M. Deletion mapping of a putative tumor suppressor gene on chromosome 4 in mouse lung tumors. *Cancer Res* 1994;4007:54.

42. Herzog CR, Soloff EV, McDoniels AL, et al. Homozygous codeletion and differential decreased expression of $p15^{INK4b}$, $p16^{INK4a}$-α and $p16^{INK4a}$-β in mouse lung tumor cells. *Oncogene* 1996;1885:13.

43. Belinsky SA, Swafford DS, Middleton SK, et al. Deletion and differential expression of $p16^{INK4a}$ in mouse lung tumors. *Carcinogenesis* 1997;115:18.

44. Belinsky SA, Nikula KJ, Palmisano WA, et al. Aberrant methylation of $p16^{INK4a}$ is an early event in lung cancer and a potential

biomarker for early diagnosis. *Proc Natl Acad Sci U S A* 1998; 95:11891.

45. Forkert P-G, Malkinson AM, Rice P, et al. Diminished CYP2E1 expression and formation of 2-S-glutathionyl acetate, a glutathione conjugate derived from 1,1-dichloroethylene epoxide, in murine lung tumors. *Drug Metab Dispos* 1999;27:68.

46. Thaete LG, Siegel D, Malkinson AM, et al. Quinone oxidoreductase (DT-diaphorase) activities in normal and neoplastic mouse lung epithelia. *Int J Cancer* 1991;49:145.

47. Malkinson AM, Siegel D, Forrest GL, et al. Elevated DT-diaphorase activity and mRNA content in human non−small cell lung carcinoma: relationship to the response of lung tumor xenografts to mitomycin C. *Cancer Res* 1992;52:4752.

48. Winski SL, Hargreaves RHJ, Butler J, et al. A new screening system for NAD(P)H: quinone oxidoreductase (NQO1)-directed antitumor quinones: identification of a new aziridinylbenzoquinone, RH1, and a NQO1-directed antitumor agent. *Clin Cancer Res* 1998;4:3083.

49. Butley MS, Stoner GD, Beer DS, et al. Protein kinases during the progression of urethane-induced mouse lung tumors. *Cancer Res* 1985;45:3677.

50. Banoub RW, Fernstrom M, Malkinson AM, et al. Enhancement of gap junctional intercellular communication by dibutyrl cyclic AMP in mouse lung epithelial cells. *Anticancer Res* 1996;16: 3715.

51. Bentel JM, Lykke AWJ, Smith GJ. Cloned murine non-malignant spontaneously transformed and chemical tumor-derived cell lines related to the type 2 pneumocyte. *Cell Biol Rep* 1989; 13:729.

52. Malkinson AM, Dwyer-Nield LD, Rice PL, et al. Mouse lung epithelial cell lines—tools for the study of differentiation and the neoplastic phenotype. *Toxicology* 1997;123:53.

53. Hanson LA, Nuzum EO, Jones BC, et al. Expression of the glucocorticoid receptor and K-ras genes in urethane-induced mouse lung tumors and cell lines. *Exp Lung Res* 1991;17:371.

54. Lange-Carter CA, Droms KA, Vuillequez JJ, et al. Differential responsiveness to agents which stimulate cAMP production in normal versus neoplastic mouse lung epithelial cells. *Cancer Lett* 1992;67:139.

55. Lange-Carter CA, Malkinson AM. Differential regulation of the stability of cAMP-dependent protein kinase mRNA in normal vs. neoplastic mouse lung epithelial cells. *Cancer Res* 1991;51: 6699.

56. Droms KA, Hanson LA, Malkinson AM, et al. Altered dexamethasone responsiveness and loss of growth control in tumorigenic mouse lung cell lines. *Int J Cancer* 1993;53:1017.

57. Smith GJ, Morris C, Leigh D, et al. EGF-receptor and extracellular matrix changes in mouse pulmonary carcinogenesis. *Exp Lung Res* 1991;17:327.

58. Rice PL, Porter SE, Koski KM, et al. Reduced receptor expression for platelet-derived growth factor and epidermal growth factor in dividing mouse lung epithelial cells. *Mol Carcinog* 1999; in press.

59. Nicks KM, Droms KA, Fossli T, et al. Altered functions of protein kinase C and cyclic AMP-dependent protein kinase in a cell line derived from a mouse lung tumor. *Cancer Res* 1989; 49:5191.

60. Ruch RJ, Cesen-Cummings K, Malkinson AM. Role of gap junctions in lung neoplasia. *Exp Lung Res* 1998;24:523.

61. Sharp JJ, Davisson MT. The Jackson Laboratory induced mutant resource. *Lab Anim* 1994;23:32.

62. De Munter HK, Den Engelse L, Emmelot P. Studies on lung tumors IV. Correlation between [^{3}H]thymidine labeling of lung and liver cells and tumor formation in GRS/A and C3Hf/A male mice following administration of dimethylnitrosamine. *Chem Biol Interact* 1979;24:299.

63. Malkinson AM, Nesbitt MN, Skamene E. Susceptibility to urethane-induced pulmonary adenomas between A/J and C57BL/6J mice: use of AXB and BXA recombinant inbred lines indicating a three-locus genetic model. *J Natl Cancer Inst* 1985; 7:971.

64. Ryan J, Barker PE, Nesbitt MN, et al. K-ras2 as a genetic marker for lung tumor susceptibility in inbred mice. *J Natl Cancer Inst* 1987;79:1351.

65. You M, Wang Y, Stoner GD, et al. Parental bias of Ki-ras oncogenes detected in lung tumors from mouse hybrids. *Proc Natl Acad Sci U S A* 1992;89:5805.

66. Malkinson AM, You M. Working hypothesis: the intronic structure of cancer-related genes regulates susceptibility to cancer. *Mol Carcinog* 1994;10:61.

67. Gariboldi M, Manenti G, Canzian F, et al. A major susceptibility locus to murine lung carcinogenesis maps on chromosome 6. *Nat Genet* 1993;3:132.

68. Devereux TR, Wiseman RW, Kaplan N, et al. Assignment of a locus for mouse lung tumor susceptibility to proximal chromosome 19. *Mamm Genome* 1994;5:749.

69. Festing MFW, Yang AL, Malkinson AM. At least four genes are associated with susceptibility to urethane-induced pulmonary adenomas in mice. *Genet Res* 1994;64:99.

70. Chen B, Johanson L, Wiest JS, et al. The second intron of the K-ras gene contains regulatory elements associated with mouse lung tumor susceptibility. *Proc Natl Acad Sci U S A* 1994;91: 1589.

71. Finney RE, Bishop JM. Predisposition of neoplastic transformation caused by gene replacement of H-ras1. *Science* 1993;260: 1524.

72. Jones-Bolin SE, Johansson E, Palmisano WA, et al. Effect of promoter and intron 2 polymorphisms on murine lung K-ras gene expression. *Carcinogenesis* 1998;1503:19.

73. Oomen LCJM, Demant P, Hart AAM, et al. Multiple genes in the H-2 complex affect differently the number and growth rate of transplacentally induced lung tumors in mice. *Int J Cancer* 1983;31:447.

74. Malkinson AM. The genetic basis of susceptibility to lung tumors in mice. *Toxicology* 1989;54:241.

75. Oomen LCJM, Van der Valk MA, Hart AAM, et al. Glucocorticoid hormone effect on transplacental carcinogenesis and lung differentiation: influence of histocompatibility-2 complex. *J Natl Cancer Inst* 1989;81:512.

76. Droms KA, Fernandez CA, Thaete LG, et al. Effects of adrenalectomy and corticosterone administration on mouse lung tumor susceptibility and histogenesis. *J Natl Cancer Inst* 1988;80:365.

77. Wattenberg LW, Widemann TS, Estensen RD, et al. Chemoprevention of pulmonary carcinogenesis by aerosolized budesonide in female A/J mice. *Cancer Res* 1997;57:5489.

78. Malkinson AM, Beer DS. A single gene in BALB/cBy mice with a major effect on susceptibility to urethane-induced pulmonary adenoma. *J Natl Cancer Inst* 1983;70:981.

79. Paterson AB. *Molecular dissection of complex traits*. Boca Raton: CRC Press, 1998.

80. Fijneman RJA, Jansen RC, van der Valk, MA, et al. High frequency of interactions between lung cancer susceptibility genes in the mouse: Mapping of Sluc5 to Sluc14. *Cancer Res* 1998; 58:4794.

81. Malkinson AM. Inheritance of pulmonary adenoma susceptibility in mice. *Prog Exp Tumor Res* 1999;35:78.

82. Maronpot RR, Palmiter RD, Brinster RC, et al. Pulmonary carcinogenesis in transgenic mice. *Exp Lung Res* 1991;17:305.

83. Wikenheiser KA, Clark JC, Linnoila RI, et al. Simian virus 40 large T antigen directed by transcriptional elements of the human surfactant protein C gene produced pulmonary adenocarcinomas in transgenic mice. *Cancer Res* 1992;52:5342.

84. Tennant RW. Evaluation and validation issues in the development of transgenic mouse carcinogenicity bioassays. *Environ Health Perspect* 1998;106:S473.

85. Keith RL, Miller YE, Malkinson AM, et al. Selective pulmonary prostacyclin synthase overexpression in transgenic mice is chemoprotective against lung tumorigenesis. *Am J Resp Crit Care Med* 1999;159:A206.

86. Sakumi K, Shiraishi A, Shimizu S, et al. Methylnitrosourea-induced tumorigenesis in MGMT gene knockout mice. *Cancer Res* 1997;57:2415.

87. Haseman JK, Huff J, Boorman GA. Use of historical control data in carcinogenicity studies in rodents. *Toxicol Pathol* 1984; 12:126.

88. Hahn FF, Lundgren DL. Pulmonary neoplasms in rats that inhaled cerium-144 dioxide. *Toxicol Pathol* 1992;20:169.

89. Belinsky SA, Foley JF, White CM et al. Dose response relationship between O^6-methylguanine formation in Clara cells and induction of pulmonary neoplasia in the rat by 4-(methylnitrosamino)-1-(3-pyridyl)-1-butanone. *Cancer Res* 1990;50: 3772.

90. Herbert RA, Hahn FF, Gillett NA, et al. Immunohistochemical and ultrastructural features of plutonium-induced proliferative lesions and pulmonary epithelial neoplasms in the rat. Evidence for their origin from type II pneumocytes. *Vet Pathol* 1994;31: 366.

91. Stowers SJ, Glover PL, Reynolds SH, et al. Activation of the K-ras protooncogene in lung tumors from rats and mice chronically exposed to tetranitromethane. *Cancer Res* 1987;47:3212.

92. Stegelmeier BL, Gillett NA, Rebar AH, et al. The molecular progression of plutonium-239-induced rat lung carcinogenesis: Ki-ras expression and activation. *Mol Carcinog* 1991;4:43.

93. Nickell-Brady C, Hahn FF, Finch GL, et al. Analysis of K-ras, P53 and c-raf-1 mutations in beryllium-induced rat lung tumors. *Carcinogenesis* 1994;15:257.

94. Belinsky SA, Devereux TR, White CM, et al. Role of Clara cells and type II cells in the development of pulmonary tumors in rats and mice following exposure to a tobacco-specific nitrosamine. *Exp Lung Res* 1991;17:263.

95. Belinsky SA, Swafford DS, Finch GL, et al. Alterations in the K-ras and p53 genes in rat lung tumors. *Environ Health Perspect* 1997;901:105.

96. Hollstein M, Sidransky D, Vogelstein B, et al. P53 mutations in human cancers. *Science* 1991;253:49.

97. Issa J-P J, Baylin SB, Belinsky SA. Methylation of the estrogen receptor CpG island in lung tumors is related to the specific type of carcinogen exposure. *Cancer Res* 1996;3655:56.

98. Swafford DS, Middleton SK, Palmisano WA, et al. Frequent aberrant methylation of p16^{INK4a} in primary rat lung tumors. *Mol Cell Biol* 1997;1306:17.

99. Benfield, JR, Schuller HM, Malkinson AM, et al. Preclinical models of lung cancer. In: Kane, MA, Bunn, PA, Jr, eds. *Biology of lung cancer.* New York: Marcel Dekker, Inc., 1998;9:247.

100. Saffiotti V, Celis F, Kolb LH. A model for the experimental induction of bronchogenic carcinoma. *Cancer Res* 1968;161: 607.

101. Becci PJ, McDowell EM, Trump BF. The respiratory epithelium. VI. Histogenesis of lung tumors induced by benzo(a)pyrene-ferric oxide in the hamster. *J Natl Cancer Inst* 1979;48:473.

102. Reznik-Schuller HM. Cancer induced in the respiratory tract of rodents by N-nitroso compounds. In: Reznik-Schuller HM, ed. *Comparative respiratory tract carcinogenesis.* Boca Raton: CRC Press, 1983;109.

103. Oreffo VIC, Lin HW, Gumerlock PH, et al. Mutational analysis of a dominant oncogene (c-Hi-ras-2) and a tumor suppressor gene (P53) in hamster lung tumorigenesis. *Mol Carcinog* 1993; 6:199.

104. Fong AT, Rasmussen RE. Formation and accumulation of O^6-ethylguanine in DNA of enriched populations of Clara cells, alveolar type II cells, and macrophages of hamsters exposed to diethylnitrosamine. 1987;43:289.

105. Schuller HM, Becker KL, Witschi HP. Animal model for neuroendocrine lung cancer. *Carcinogenesis* 1988;9:293.

106. Schuller HM. Mechanisms of neuroendocrine lung carcinogenesis. In: Thomassen DG, Nettesheim P, eds. *Biology, toxicology, and carcinogenesis of respiratory epithelium.* New York: Hemisphere Publishing Corporation, 1990:195.

107. Sunday ME, Willett CG. Induction and spontaneous regression of internal pulmonary neuroendocrine cell differentiation in a model of preneoplastic lung injury. *Cancer Res* 1992;82:26775.

108. Nylen ES, Becker KL, Joshi PA, et al. Pulmonary bombesin and calcitonin in hamsters during exposure to hyperoxia and diethylnitrosamine. *Am J Respir Cell Mol Biol* 1990;2:25.

109. Grubbs CJ, Moon RC, Norikane K. 1-methyl-1-nitrosurea induction of cancer in a localized area of the Syrian golden hamster trachea. *Prog Exp Tumor Res* 1979;24:345.

110. Hammond WG, Benfield JR. Hamster bronchial carcinogenesis induced by carcinogen-containing sustained release implants placed endobronchially: a clinically relevant model. *J Cell Biochem* 1993;17F[Suppl]:104.

111. Hammond WG, Gabriel A, Paladugu RR, et al. Differential susceptibility to bronchial carcinogenesis in syngeneic hamsters. *Cancer Res* 1987;47:5202.

112. Thompson RC. *Life-span effects of ionizing radiation in the beagle dog.* Washington, DC: U.S. Department of Energy, 1989.

113. Taylor GN, Shabestari L, Angus W, et al. Primary pulmonary tumors in beagles. *Am J Vet Res* 1979;40:1316.

114. Park JF, Sanders CL, Weller RE, et al. Comparative toxicology of inhaled $^{239}PuO_2$ in dogs and rats. *Health Phys* 1989;57:31.

115. Cross FT, Palmer RF, Filipy RE, et al. Carcinogenic effects of radon daughters, uranium ore dust and cigarette smoke in beagle dogs. *Health Phys* 1982;42:33.

116. Kraegel SA, Gumerlock PH, Dungworth DL, et al. K-ras activation in non–small cell lung cancer in the dog. *Cancer Res* 1992; 52:4724.

117. Tierney LA, Hahn FF, Lechner JF. P53, erbB-2 and K-ras gene alterations are rare in spontaneous and plutonium-239-induced canine lung neoplasia. *Radiat Res* 1996;181:145.

118. McDonald JW, Taylor JA, Watson MA, et al. p53 and K-ras in radon-associated lung adenocarcinoma. *Cancer Epidemiol Biomed Prev* 1995;791:4.

119. Gillett NA, Stegelmeier BL, Kelly G, et al. Expression of epidermal growth factor receptor in plutonium-239-induced lung neoplasms in dogs. *Vet Pathol* 1992;29:46.

120. Gillett NA, Stegelmeier BL, Chang IY, et al. Expression of transforming growth factor α in plutonium-239-induced lung neoplasms in dogs: investigations of autocrine mechanisms of growth. *Radiat Res* 1991;126:289.

121. Cerny T, Barnes DM, Hasleton P, et al. Expression of epidermal growth factor receptor (EGF-R) in human lung tumors. *Br J Cancer* 1986;54:265.

122. Vahakangas KH, Samet JM, Metcalf RA, et al. Mutations of P53 and ras genes in radon-associated lung cancers from uranium miners. *Lancet* 1992;339:576.

123. Dillman RO, Seagren SL, Proppert KJ, et al. A randomized trial of induction chemotherapy plus high dose radiation versus radiation alone in stage III non-small-cell lung cancer. *N Engl J Med* 1990;323:940.

124. Sklar MD. Increased resistance to cis-diaminedichlororplatinum (II) in NIH 3T3 cells transformed by ras oncogenes. *Cancer Res* 1988;48:793.

125. Belinsky SA, Stefanski SA, Anderson MW. The A/J mouse lung

as a model for developing new chemointervention strategies. *Cancer Res* 1993;53:410.

126. Lippman SM, Hong WK. 13-cis-retinoic acid and cancer chemoprevention. Biology and novel therapeutic approaches for epithelial cancer of the aerodigestive tract. *J Natl Cancer Inst Monograph* 1992:111.

127. Harris CC, Sporn MB, Kaufman DG. Histogenesis of squamous metaplasia in the hamster tracheal epithelium caused by vitamin A deficiency or benzo(a)pyrene ferric oxide. *J Natl Cancer Inst* 1979;48:473.

128. Jetten AM, Nervi C, Vollberg TM. Control of squamous differentiation in tracheobronchial epidermal and epithelial cells: role of retinoids. Biology and novel therapeutic approaches for epithelial cancer of the aerodigestive tract. *J Natl Cancer Inst Monograph* 1992:13:93.

129. Herzog CR, Lubet RA, You M. Genetic alterations in mouse lung tumors: implications for cancer chemoprevention. *J Cell Biochem* 1997;Suppl28/29:49.

130. Thompson WJ, Pamukou TR, Liu L, et al. Exisulind (Prevatac™) induced apoptosis in cultured colonic tumor cells involves inhibition of cyclic GMP (cG) phosphodiesterase (PDE). *Proc Am Assoc Cancer Res* 1999;40:4.

131. Malkinson AM, Koski KM, Dwyer-Nield LD, et al. Inhibition of 4-(methylnitrosamino)-1-(3-pyridyl)-1-butanone (NNK)-induced mouse lung tumor formation by FGN-1 (sulindac sulfone). *Carcinogenesis* 1998;19:1353.

132. Zhang L, Zou W, Velculescu VE, et al. Gene expression profiles in normal and cancer cells. *Science* 1997;1268:276.

133. Toyota M, Ho C, Ahuja N, et al. Identification of differentially methylated sequences in colorectal cancer by methylated CpG island amplification. *Cancer Res* 1999;2307:59.

134. Brown PO, Botstein D. Exploring the new world of the genome with DNA microarrays. *Nat Genet* 1999;33:21.

135. Lipshutz RJ, Fodor SPA, Gingeras TR, et al. High density synthetic oligonucleotide arrays. *Nat Genet* 1999;20:21.

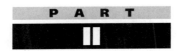

PART

II

ETIOLOGY/EPIDEMIOLOGY/ SCREENING/EARLY DETECTION/PREVENTION

20

ETIOLOGY AND EPIDEMIOLOGY OF LUNG CANCER

DAVID SCHOTTENFELD

Lung cancer is the leading cause of cancer mortality in men and women in the United States, accounting for 28 percent of all cancer deaths each year. Whereas lung cancer accounted for only 3 percent of all female cancer deaths in 1950, by 1995 it accounted for an estimated 24 percent of all female cancer deaths. In 1994, the age-adjusted mortality rate per 100,000 was 70.9 for men, and 33.8 for women. In reviewing lung cancer mortality trends between 1990 and 1994, the age-adjusted rate in men decreased by about 1.4 percent per year and in women increased by about 1.7 percent per year. The age-adjusted lung cancer death rates in the United States surpassed those of breast cancer in white women in 1986 and in black women in 1990. Lung cancer is the most common cause of cancer mortality among men in Western industrialized nations.

The incidence patterns, because of persistently poor survival rates, parallel closely the mortality rates; currently, 15 percent of incidence cancers in men and 13 percent in women are attributed to lung cancer. During 1990 to 1994, the average annual age-adjusted lung cancer incidence per 100,000 in United States white men was 76.0, which was exceeded only by prostate cancer (134.7); the average annual lung cancer incidence rate in white women was 41.5, which was second to that of breast cancer (111.8). The United States Surveillance, Epidemiology and End Results (SEER) lung cancer incidence trends from 1973 to 1994 demonstrated, for ages 65 and over, a percentage increase for women (220.5%) that was substantially greater than that for men (18.2%). The age-specific lung cancer incidence rates in men under 65 years of age have declined 16.1 percent since 1973, whereas in women, the rates have increased 58.2 percent.[1]

Lung cancer incidence and mortality patterns follow, after a latency interval of 20 or more years, the temporal patterns of cigarette smoking. In older men in the United States, lung cancer has displaced coronary heart disease as the leading cause of excess mortality among smokers.[2] The risk of dying from lung cancer is associated with age of initiation and duration of cigarette smoking, and with the number and tar concentration of cigarettes smoked each day or as a regular pattern.

Smoking is currently estimated to be the cause of 85 percent of lung cancer deaths.[3] Exposures to other environmental and occupational respiratory carcinogens may be interactive with cigarette smoking, and may also influence trends of lung cancer incidence and mortality.

DESCRIPTIVE EPIDEMIOLOGY

Age and Gender

Throughout the world, the age-adjusted incidence rates of lung cancer among men exceed, by twofold or more, that among women. In the United States, the age-adjusted incidence rates in men began to plateau and then declined in the 1980s. The pattern in women differed significantly from that in men. Age-adjusted incidence in women increased on average by 4.1 percent per year between 1973 and 1994, but during 1990 to 1994, the average annual increase was only 0.2 percent. This pattern is attributable to lower prevalences of smoking in cohorts of men born prior to 1910 and of women born prior to 1920. Age-specific rates increase exponentially until the rates plateau and then decline after the age of 80 in men and the age of 70 in women (Figure 20.1). Only 5% to 10% of lung cancer cases are diagnosed under 50 years of age. Epidemiologic studies of lung cancer in young adults emphasize the predominance of adenocarcinomas and the importance of a positive family history. The current smoking pattern and magnitude of relative risk due to smoking in women in the United States are converging on the smoking pattern and risk evident in similarly aged males.[4,5]

Compared with women, men generally began smoking cigarettes at an earlier age, smoked more cigarettes per day and for a longer duration, inhaled more deeply, and consumed cigarettes with higher tar content. With increasing tobacco smoking in women after World War II, lung cancer mortality increased substantially in North America and

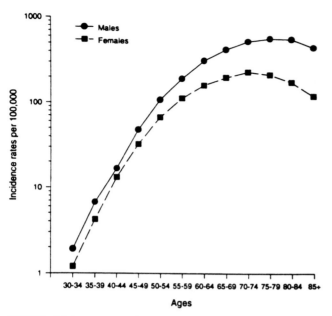

FIGURE 20.1. Age-specific lung cancer incidence rates per 100,000 males and females, United States, 1994.

TABLE 20.1. AGE-ADJUSTED (1970 U.S. STANDARD) LUNG CANCER INCIDENCE PER 100,000, 1975, 1980, 1985, 1990, 1994 IN SEER REGISTRY AREAS, BY RACE AND SEX

Year of Diagnosis	White		Black	
	Men	Women	Men	Women
1975	75.9	21.8	101.2	20.6
1980	82.2	28.2	131.0	33.8
1985	82.1	35.9	131.3	40.2
1990	80.7	42.5	118.7	47.0
1994	72.6	43.3	110.6	48.0

of death, ranking below coronary heart disease. The excess mortality from lung cancer among black men, compared with white men, was greatest for the age interval 35 to 64 years. Cohorts of white men born before 1900 had higher (50%) age-specific rates than black men; but this pattern reversed after 1915.

During 1975 to 1990, the age-adjusted lung cancer incidence in United States black women was 10% to 20% higher than that in white women (Table 20.1). The increase since 1975 was 120% in black and 89% in white women. Since 1985, the incidence rates have continued to increase at an average annual rate of 2.4% for black and 2.2% for white women.

The SEER program of the National Cancer Institute enables a comparison of risks for the period 1988 to 1992 among various racial and ethnic groups in the United States (Table 20.2). The lowest age-adjusted lung cancer incidence rates in men and women were registered for the Native Americans, Hispanics, and Japanese; the highest rates were reported in blacks, native Hawaiians, and non-Hispanic whites. The ratio of male to female incidence rates reflected elevated risks in men that were 2.5 to 3.5 times the rates in women from the various racial and ethnic groups. Al-

Western Europe. Several recent case-control studies have even suggested that female smokers have a higher relative risk of lung cancer than male smokers, after adjusting for age and average daily intensity of smoking exposure.[6,7,8] In a prospective study conducted in Copenhagen, Denmark, although rate ratios for all histologic types of lung cancer increased with number of pack-years of exposure for both men and women, the relative risks did not differ between men and women after adjusting for age and duration and intensity of smoking.[9] The case-control design and the method of estimation of odds ratios in women may have been susceptible to recall bias, underreporting of amount smoked by the cases, and differences in baseline risks of lung cancer between male and female nonsmoking controls (i.e., occupational risk factors, nutritional risk factors, unmeasured exposure to environmental tobacco smoke, etc.). However, the question of gender differences in susceptibility to tobacco smoking merits further investigation. Prospective studies are required to derive unconfounded incidence measures of absolute or attributable risk that may be compared in smoking and nonsmoking men and women.

Race and Ethnicity

The risk of lung cancer in United States black men has been about 50 percent higher than that in white men in the past 10 to 15 years, but the annual rate of decline since 1985 in black men (−3.1%) has been greater than that in white men (−1.2%) (Table 20.1). Among United States black men, lung cancer mortality was the second leading cause

TABLE 20.2. TOTAL AND LUNG CANCER INCIDENCE RATES (PER 100,000) BY GENDER, RACE, AND ETHNICITY, UNITED STATES SEER, 1988–1992*

Race/Ethnicity	Males		Females	
	Total	Lung	Total	Lung
African American	560	117.0	326	44.2
Hawaiian	340	89.0	321	43.1
Non-Hispanic White	469	76.0	346	41.5
Chinese	282	52.1	213	25.3
Japanese	322	43.0	241	15.2
Hispanic	319	41.8	243	19.5
Native American (New Mexico)	196	14.4	180	**

* Incidence rate age-adjusted to the 1970 United States standard population.
** Fewer than 25 cases.

though the ratio of age-adjusted lung cancer incidence rates varied substantially by ethnicity (1.3 to 8.1), the percentage of all cancer deaths attributed to lung cancer in men and women combined was as high in Native Americans (27.7%) as in African Americans (26.1%).

It is generally assumed that the differences in rates of lung cancer can be partially explained by different lifetime patterns of cigarette smoking. Compared with white males, a higher percentage of blacks were current smokers, smoked cigarettes with greater yield of tar and nicotine, and preferred to smoke mentholated cigarettes, which may promote deeper inhalation of cigarette smoke. However, among current smokers, black males smoked fewer cigarettes per day and tended to start smoking at a slightly later age. Reports, which were not confounded by differences in smoking habits, of higher serum cotinine levels, or of 4-aminobiphenyl-hemoglobin adduct levels, in black smokers when compared with white smokers suggested that there may also be differences in susceptibility between blacks and whites as expressed in the metabolism of tobacco smoke.[10]

The age-adjusted lung cancer incidence was 32% lower in Hispanic than in non-Hispanic white men. The percent of current smokers was comparable for Hispanic and non-Hispanic white men, but Hispanic men smoked about half as many cigarettes per day. In a case-control study in New Mexico, where most of the Hispanics were American-born, the estimates of relative risk of smoking and lung cancer were similar for Hispanic and non-Hispanic white males. However, the cigarette smoking patterns in the Hispanic controls indicated that there were substantial ethnic differences in average daily exposure levels.[6,11,12]

Socioeconomic Status

Various studies have reported an inverse association between lung cancer mortality and socioeconomic status. A twofold gradient in mortality was observed between low and high social class, as measured by occupation, income, or education. Smoking patterns accounted for part of the differential risk by social class, with smoking prevalence rates increased among "blue-collar" workers and among those with lower levels of education.[13,14] Socioeconomic status may also serve as a surrogate measure for other risk factors such as occupation, diet, and ambient air pollutants, or may influence the quality, access, and utilization of health care services.

International Patterns

Global lung cancer incidence is increasing at a rate of 0.5% per year, and as a consequence, lung cancer is the leading cause of cancer incidence and mortality in European countries, accounting for about 21% of all cancer cases in men.[15,16] In most parts of the world, rates were higher in urban than in rural areas, and two to six times higher in men than in women. The varying levels of age-adjusted

TABLE 20.3. AGE-ADJUSTED LUNG CANCER MORTALITY RATES* PER 100,000 POPULATION FOR SELECTED COUNTRIES, IN MALES AND FEMALES, 1992–1995

Country	Males	Country	Females
Hungary	84.0	United States	26.3
Poland	71.4	Denmark	24.9
Netherlands	64.8	Canada	22.9
Italy	56.2	United Kingdom	20.9
United States	55.3	Hungary	17.9
Canada	52.5	Ireland	17.6
United Kingdom	51.8	New Zealand	17.6
Denmark	50.4	China	15.8
Greece	49.8	Australia	13.2
Spain	47.9	Netherlands	12.6
Germany	47.3	Norway	10.9
France	47.0	Sweden	10.8
Ireland	45.4	Czech Republic	10.3
Finland	44.2	Austria	9.7
Bulgaria	42.9	Switzerland	9.3
Austria	42.8	Israel	8.4
Switzerland	41.9	Japan	8.3
China	37.3	Italy	7.9
Norway	31.6	Finland	6.9
Japan	31.0	Greece	6.9
Israel	27.0	Bulgaria	6.6
Sweden	22.9	Mexico	5.8
Mexico	16.1	Spain	3.6

* Rates are age-adjusted to the World Health Organization standard population.

(world standard) lung cancer mortality rates summarized in Table 20.3 were, in general, correlated with cigarette smoking practices that were prevalent at least ten years prior to diagnosis. Worldwide, it has been estimated that 47% to 52% of men and 10% to 12% of women smoke tobacco. In developed countries, 51% of men and 21% of women smoke. The prevalence of smoking men and women, the types of cigarettes and amounts smoked, ages at initiation and duration of smoking exposure, and proportions of heavy smokers in the population, were important determinants of geocultural variations in lung cancer incidence. Recent trends in lung cancer mortality in men exhibited declining rates in all European countries except in France, Greece, Portugal, and Spain. Cigarette smoking in China has followed a pattern similar to that among adults in the United States, although the significant pattern of increase, particularly among men, occurred 40 years later. Of the Chinese deaths attributed to tobacco, 15% are due to lung cancer and 45% to chronic obstructive lung disease. The relatively elevated rates of adenocarcinoma of the lung among Chinese women in China and Singapore have been attributed to exposures to smoking tobacco and to environmental pollutants other than smoking tobacco (e.g., fossil fuel combustion products and cooking oils in the home).[17,18]

TABLE 20.4. LUNG CANCER INCIDENCE RATES (PER 100,000) BY HISTOLOGICAL TYPE, RACE, AND SEX IN FIVE UNITED STATES SEER AREAS*

Race/Sex	Squamous Cell			Adenocarcinoma		
	1969–1971	1984–1986	% Increase	1969–1971	1984–1986	% Increase
Whites						
Males (M)	21.7	27.2	25.3	9.3	19.6	110.8
Females (F)	2.7	6.9	155.6	3.5	11.2	220.0
M/F Ratio	8.0	3.9		2.7	1.8	
Blacks						
Males (M)	33.8	50.6	49.7	11.5	28.9	151.3
Females (F)	3.4	10.5	208.8	3.8	12.2	221.1
M/F Ratio	9.9	4.8		3.0	2.4	

* From Devesa SS, Blot WJ, Stone BJ, et al. Age-adjusted to the 1970 standard population. Areas included Atlanta, Detroit, San Francisco/Oakland, and states of Iowa and Connecticut.

Histopathology

The distribution of cell types of lung carcinoma based on the SEER program in 1990 were, for male cases: squamous cell (epidermoid) (31.2%), adenocarcinoma (22.7%), small cell (16.6%), large cell (9.3%), bronchioloalveolar (2.5%), and other including adenosquamous and mixed small and large cell (17.7%) (see also Chapter 26). Cumulative exposure to cigarette smoking increases the risks for squamous cell carcinoma, adenocarcinoma, small cell carcinoma and large cell carcinoma, although prior to 1965, the risk tended to increase less steeply in men in relation to intensity and duration of cigarette smoking for adenocarcinoma, when compared with squamous cell and small cell carcinoma. In the early 1970s, data from the SEER program indicated that there were among white males more than twice as many squamous cell carcinomas as adenocarcinomas, whereas among white females, the incidence of adenocarcinoma exceeded that of squamous cell carcinoma by 30% (Table 20.4). By the mid-1980s, because of substantial increases in the incidence of adenocarcinoma in white males, the excess of squamous cell carcinoma decreased to 39%; among white females, the incidence of adenocarcinoma from 1984 to 1986 was 62% higher than that of squamous cell carcinoma. Small cell and non–small cell carcinoma incidence in United States white and African American men peaked around 1984 and then began to decline. Lung cancer incidence in white females, however, increased beyond 1990 for all histologic subtypes. The annual incidence of bronchioloalveolar carcinoma was approximately 1.5 per 100,000, and the epidemiologic features were more characteristic of adenocarcinoma than of squamous cell carcinoma. The increasing age-adjusted incidence rates for lung cancer that were evident during the previous two decades have included increases for the most common histologic types, but were proportionately greater for adenocarcinomas. Similar patterns have been described in Switzerland, Holland, Hong Kong, Korea, Israel, and Japan. The percentage of lung cancer cases classified as adenocarcinoma was higher in Asia than in North American or Europe. Adenocarcinoma is currently the most prominent form of lung cancer in younger persons, women of all ages, lifetime nonsmokers and long-term former smokers.

There is no single satisfactory explanation for the changing histologic patterns over the past two decades. The proportionate and absolute increases in incidence trends for adenocarcinoma have occurred in conjunction with declining incidence of the classification "other and unspecified histology." Increasing use of mucin stains and immunocytochemical staining for antibodies to carcinoembryonic antigen has contributed to enhanced recognition of adenocarcinomas. The alterations in histologic patterns have also been interpreted as signaling the effects of changing composition and filtration of cigarette tobacco, with increasing production of volatile nitrosamines and their deposition upon deeper inhalation in terminal bronchioles and alveoli. The tobacco-specific nitrosamine 4-(methylnitrosamino)-1-(3-pyridyl)-1-butanone is bloodborne and activated or metabolized in the liver. The deposition of cigarette particulates containing polycyclic aromatic hydrocarbons in proximal lung bronchi is associated with the development of squamous cell carcinoma.[19–22]

LIFESTYLE AND ENVIRONMENTAL RISK FACTORS

Tobacco

The causal relationship between tobacco smoking and lung cancer was established by epidemiologic studies conducted in the 1950s and 1960s.[23,24] The complexity of tobacco smoke, with over 3,000 different chemicals, has made it difficult to identify the contribution of the more than 40 putative carcinogenic agents. The carcinogens in tobacco smoke include the polynuclear aromatic hydrocarbons

(PAHs), N-nitrosamines, aromatic amines, other organic (e.g., benzene, acrylonitrile) and inorganic (e.g., arsenic, acetaldehyde) compounds, and polonium 210. The composition of the smoke depends on the ambient conditions of smoking, the blend of tobacco leaf, filtration, additives, paper wrapping, and so on. Tobacco smoke produced by the tobaccos in pipes and cigars is both harsher and more alkaline than that produced by cigarettes. The majority of the compounds in tobacco are produced in an oxygen-deficient, hydrogen-rich environment, arising from pyrolysis and distillation, in the region immediately behind the burning tip of the cigarette.[25]

As mainstream cigarette smoke emerges from the cigarette, it has approximately 10^9 to 10^{10} particles per ml. The aerodynamic diameters of the particles, ranging in size from 0.1 to 1.0 micrometer, determine the sites of deposition in the airways and alveolar regions of the lung. The fraction of smoke retained varies markedly with the pattern of inhalation. The chemical analysis of tobacco smoke is separated into particulate, or "tar," and gaseous phases. Filter tips of cellulose acetate remove volatile nitrosamines and phenols selectively. The neutral fraction of the particulate phase contains potentially important tumor initiators such as the PAHs.

In 1964, the first Surgeon General's report on smoking summarized existing evidence and declared cigarette smoking to be the major cause of lung cancer among American men.[26] In the ensuing 30 years, epidemiologic studies have established that there were increasing risks in women and underscored the relationships with onset, duration, intensity, and cessation of smoking. Three major prospective studies demonstrated a rising trend in lung cancer death rates with increasing average amounts smoked per day in current smokers (Table 20.5).[27–29] The initial emphasis of epidemiologic studies of lung cancer and smoking was on men who, in almost all countries, began smoking earlier, consumed greater quantities of tobacco, and exhibited higher relative risks than women.

In the past 20 years, the prevalence of cigarette smoking in many countries, including the United States, has increased significantly among women; concomitantly, changes in smoking practices have been accompanied by increasing relative and attributable risks for lung cancer.[30,31] In a follow-up study of approximately 600,000 women conducted in the 1980s by the American Cancer Society, the relative risk of dying of lung cancer in current smokers was 12.7; for those who smoked 30 or more cigarettes per day, the relative risk was increased 22.3 times compared with the never smoker.[32] In 1985, cigarette smoking accounted for an estimated 82 percent of lung cancer deaths, or 31,600 deaths. The International Agency for Research on Cancer estimated that the smoking-attributable fraction of lung cancer deaths occurring in the United States and in England and Wales was 92% in men and 78% in women.[25] In 1995, an estimated 47 million U.S. adults and 4.5 million U.S. adolescents were cigarette smokers.

Lower tar content and the use of filters are factors that may result in reduced lung cancer risks in those who smoke. In the earlier American Cancer Society (ACS) Twenty-Five State Study, males who smoked "low-tar" (i.e., less than 22 mg) cigarettes experienced 20% lower risk of dying of lung cancer when compared with males who continued to smoke high-tar cigarettes. The excess lung cancer risk for current smokers was directly proportional to the estimated milligrams of tar consumed daily: standardized mortality ratio (SMR) = 100 + 1.731 × milligrams of tar per day.[33] In the more recent ACS Fifty State Study, Garfinkel and Stellman[34] concluded that doubling the cigarette tar yield would result in a 40% increase in the relative risk of dying of lung cancer, independently of the amount smoked or depth of inhalation. The Federal Trade Commission estimated that the current average sales-weighted tar content of cigarettes manufactured in the United States was about 12 to 13 mg of tar per cigarette, compared with nearly 40 mg in the early 1950s. Lifelong filter cigarette smokers have experienced 20% to 40% lower risk of lung cancer than lifelong nonfilter smokers, after adjusting for differences in the amount smoked.[35,36]

While these studies suggested that switching to filtered or low-tar cigarettes may modestly reduce the risk of lung

TABLE 20.5. RELATIVE RISKS OF DEATH FROM LUNG CANCER AMONG MALE SMOKERS ACCORDING TO NUMBER OF CIGARETTES SMOKED

Number of Cigarettes Smoked per Day	American Cancer Society (ACS) Volunteers	United States Veterans	British Physicians
Nonsmokers	1.0	1.0	1.0
Current cigarette smokers*	9.2	12.1	14.0
1–9	4.6	5.5	7.8
10–19	8.6	9.9	17.4
20–39	14.7	17.4	25.1
40+	18.8	23.9	

* Classification of current smokers refers to ACS study. The categories for United States Veterans were 1–9, 10–20, 21–39, and 40+, and for the British Physicians were 1–14, 15–24, and 25+ per day.

TABLE 20.6. RELATIVE RISKS OF LUNG CANCER AMONG MALES ACCORDING TO YEARS AFTER QUITTING SMOKING

Cohort	Years after Smoking Cessation					
	0	1–4	5–9	10–14	15–19	20+
British Physicians	15.8	16.0	5.9	5.3	------2.0------	
U.S. Veterans	11.3	18.8	7.5	5.0	5.0	2.1
American Cancer Society*	13.7	12.0	7.2		------1.1------	

All risks relative to lifelong nonsmokers.
* Excludes those who smoked less than one pack of cigarettes per day.

cancer, the more significant reduction in risk would be derived from cessation of smoking. Whereas 25% of smoking adults in the United States continue to smoke, an additional 40% to 50% have become former smokers. As shown in Table 20.6, the relative risk of lung cancer among ex-smokers decreased significantly after five years of smoking cessation. In the initial one to four years after quitting smoking, however, the relative risk of lung cancer among ex-smokers may have been higher than among current smokers, presumably because a proportion of individuals may have stopped smoking because of illness or premonitory symptoms of lung cancer.

It has been suggested that the risk of lung cancer in former smokers will approximate but never equal that of lifelong nonsmokers. The baseline risk of lung cancer in lifelong nonsmokers increases in relation to age raised to the fourth or fifth power. In the British Physicians Study, Doll showed that the incidence of lung cancer in cigarette smokers increased approximately in proportion to the fourth power of duration of smoking, and was multiplicative with the previously described exponential increase with age among never-smokers.[37] The percentage reduction in risk after quitting depended on the prior duration and average amount smoked each day, being more readily demonstrable among lighter smokers and smokers of lesser duration or those who quit at a younger age.[38] Lung cancer results from a multi-step process in which persistent genetic lesions accumulate at specific chromosomal loci. The vast majority of current or former smokers, in contrast to never-smokers, exhibit loss of heterozygosity at multiple chromosomal sites (e.g., 3p14, 9p21, p16, p53) in both normal and metaplastic or dysplastic bronchial epithelium[39] (see also Chapter 18).

Pipe and cigar smoking were linked to lung cancer, but the estimated relative risks, compared with people who never smoked, were considerably lower than the risks reported among cigarette smokers; the risks among exclusively pipe or cigar smokers in the United States or England varied from no increased risk in some studies, to twofold or higher risks in other studies. In countries such as Sweden, Switzerland, and Holland, where pipe or cigar smoking was nearly as common as cigarette smoking, the relative risks of lung cancer were equally high for all forms of smoked tobacco.[40,41] Differences in the manner in which pipes and cigars were smoked in different countries, i.e., depth of inhalation or amount smoked, may provide an explanation for differences in the estimated risks. Risks of lung cancer also varied with the type of tobacco used. Dark tobaccos were associated with greater risk of lung cancer than light tobaccos, and with formation of higher levels of 4-aminobiphenyl-hemoglobin adducts.[42]

Environmental Tobacco Smoke

Environmental tobacco smoke (ETS) is comprised of sidestream smoke (about 80%) released from burning tobacco in between puffs and from the exhaled smoke (about 20%) of the smoker. The smoke that the smoker inhales is known as mainstream smoke. Other minor contributors to ETS include the smoke that escapes during puffing from the burning cone, and gaseous components that diffuse through the cigarette paper. These components are diluted by the ambient air and when inhaled, in particular by nonsmokers, are referred to as "passive" or "involuntary" smoking. ETS contains various toxic agents, including mutagens and carcinogens, which, for some chemicals (e.g., nitrosamines, 4-aminobiphenyl, benzo(a)pyrene), have been measured at higher concentrations than in mainstream smoke. Estimates of ETS exposure, based on serum or urinary measurements of cotinine, the metabolite of nicotine, suggest that involuntary smokers absorb about 0.5% to 1% of the nicotine that active smokers absorb, or smoke the equivalent of about one half a cigarette a day. Studies of 4-aminobiphenyl-hemoglobin adduct levels indicate that passive smokers have approximately 14% of the concentration of active smokers.[43]

Table 20.7 lists the relative risks of lung cancer among nonsmoking women based on a review of epidemiologic studies in various countries which have evaluated dose-response trends.[44–61] The risks increased with amounts smoked by husbands, with about 30% to 150% increases in relative risk experienced in general among those women most heavily exposed. A weighted analysis of 37 published epidemiological studies resulted in the conclusion that there was an elevated risk of 24% (95% confidence interval, 13%

TABLE 20.7. RELATIVE RISK OF LUNG CANCER AMONG NONSMOKING WOMEN ACCORDING TO LEVEL OF HUSBAND'S SMOKING

Author	No. of Lung Cancers	Husband's Smoking Status	
		Light	Heavy*
Hirayama, 1981[44]	201	1.4	1.9
Trichopolous et al., 1983,[45] 1984[46]	77	1.9	2.5
Garfinkel, 1981[47]	153	1.3	1.1
Correa et al., 1983[48]	22	1.2	3.5
Koo et al., 1984[49]	88	1.9	1.2
Wu et al., 1985[50]	28	1.2	2.0
Garfinkel et al., 1985[51]	134	1.1	2.0
Akiba et al., 1986[52]	94	1.4	2.1
Pershagen et al., 1987[53]	67	1.0	3.2
Lam et al., 1987[54]	199	1.9	2.1
Gao et al., 1987[55]	406	1.2	1.7
Janerich et al., 1990[56]	191	0.8	1.1
Fontham et al., 1991[57]	420	1.1	1.3
Brownson et al., 1992[58]	432	0.9	1.3
Stockwell et al., 1992[59]	210	1.5	2.4
Fontham et al., 1994[60]	651	1.1	1.8
Boffetta et al., 1998[61]	509	0.6	1.3

* Definitions of heavy smokers varied by study, but typically included those who smoked 20 or more cigarettes per day.

to 36%) among nonsmoking wives of *smoking* husbands, when compared with nonsmoking wives of *nonsmoking* husbands.[62] Workplace exposures to ETS are measured with less precision than spousal exposures; however, some studies have suggested that there is a dose-response relationship when combining workplace and spousal sources of ETS. It has been suggested that when using biological markers of nicotine exposure in studies of ETS and lung cancer, about 5% of female respondents who were in fact smokers may have reported that they were nonsmokers. Correcting for this bias, however, would result in an adjusted relative risk in nonsmoking women who were living with smokers of about 1.15 to 1.20. The report of the National Research Council concluded that about 20% of lung cancers occurring in nonsmoking women and men, or 3,000 cases per year, may be attributable to exposure to ETS; in the context of lung cancer cases diagnosed each year in smokers and nonsmokers, 2% to 3% may be attributable to ETS.[63]

Air Pollution

Pollutants in the urban air other than from tobacco have been investigated as potential causal agents in the epidemic rise of lung cancer in industrialized nations. The products of fossil fuel combustion, principally polycyclic hydrocarbons, have been of particular concern. Other sources of ambient air pollution have been motor vehicle and diesel engine exhausts, power plants, and industrial and residential emissions. The ratio of urban to rural age-adjusted lung cancer mortality rates in many industrialized nations has varied

between 1.1 and 2.0. It has been suggested that the net attributable risk effect of protracted exposure to urban air pollutants in men with average smoking habits would be ten cases of lung cancer per 100,000 per year. In most countries, however, a major fraction (i.e., 80% or greater) would be attributable to cigarette smoking, and the independent association with urban residence, or the "urban factor," could not be assessed without controlling for the confounding effect of differences in smoking practices between urban and rural residents. In addition, the "urban factor" has yet to be defined, but is undoubtedly a complex mixture of interacting chemical compounds and elements that vary by geographic area and over time.[64,65] Exposure to combustion-source ambient air pollution has been associated with declining pulmonary function, increased rates of hospitalization for respiratory illnesses, and increased rates of cardiopulmonary diseases mortality.[66]

Evidence in support of the potential association of air pollution with lung cancer may be provided by occupational studies of workers exposed to combustion products from fossil fuels. Workers exposed to emissions from retort coal gas plants manifested smoking-adjusted relative risk of lung cancer that was approximately twice that in unexposed workers.[67] Roofers exposed to coal tar fumes while working outdoors had an approximately 50% increase in lung cancer risk after 20 years of exposure and 150% increase after 40 years.[68]

Benzo(a)pyrene has been used as a surrogate index of ambient urban air exposure produced by fossil fuel combustion and correlated with lung cancer mortality rates. However, putative carcinogenic agents present in ambient urban air may include inorganic particles or fibers (e.g., arsenic, asbestos, chromium, nickel, uranium); radionuclides (e.g., ^{210}Pb, ^{212}Pb, ^{222}Ra); and organic gaseous and particulate combustion products (e.g., dimethylnitrosamine, benzene, benzo(a)pyrene, 1,2-benzanthracene). In the longitudinal study of the American Cancer Society, age-, occupational-, and smoking-standardized rates for lung cancer were computed according to residence. Minimal differences in mortality were observed between urban and rural residential areas, or among cities categorized by indices of pollution.[69] The World Health Organization International Agency for Research on Cancer has declared diesel engine exhaust a *probable carcinogen*.[70] In studies of railroad workers exposed to diesel exhaust, Garshick and colleagues[71] described a 40% increase in the smoking-adjusted relative risk of lung cancer.

In a rural area in Yunan Province in China, an excess risk of lung cancer among men and women was attributed to indoor pollution because of burning soft, smoky coal in poorly ventilated homes.[72] In Shanghai, the elevated risk of lung cancer was hypothesized to be due to prolonged exposure to oil vapors, particularly from rapeseed oil that was used in high-temperature wok cooking.[73] In urban Shenyang in northeastern China, indoor pollution from coal-burning heating devices gave rise to an age-, education-, and tobacco-smoking-adjusted relative risk of 2.3 for lung cancer in the highest exposure group.[74,75]

Indoor Radon

Radon (^{222}Ra), with a half-life of 3.8 days, is an inert, radioactive, colorless, and odorless gas at usual environmental temperatures that can percolate through the earth's crust and accumulate in residential dwellings. At sufficiently high concentrations, radon and its α-particle–emitting decay products, polonium-214 and polonium-218, have been shown to cause lung cancer in cigarette smoking and nonsmoking uranium, tin, and iron-ore miners. These observations have been replicated by conducting experimental studies in rats.[76] Indoor radon exposure accounts for about 50% to 80% of the total radiation received on average in the United States. It has been estimated, based on extrapolations from high-risk miner studies, that indoor radon may cause between 6,000 to 36,000 lung cancer deaths per year in the United States.[77] Joint exposures to tobacco smoke and radon gas have been interpreted to yield risks of lung cancer that were greater than linear and additive and approximated multiplicative or log linear effects.

There have been at least eight epidemiologic case-control studies conducted in five countries of lung cancer risk from exposure to residential radon.[78] Axelson and colleagues[79] noted an increased risk of lung cancer among persons living in stone compared to wood houses in Sweden. In a later study by Pershagen and co-workers,[80] it was concluded that the smoking-adjusted risk of lung cancer increased in rela-

tion to the cumulative and time-weighted exposure to radon. The relative risk was 1.3 (95% confidence interval, 1.1–1.6) for average radon concentrations over a period of about 30 years of 3.8 to 10.8 pico Curies (pCi) per liter; for exposure in excess of 10.8 pCi per liter, the relative risk was 1.8 (95% confidence interval, 1.1–2.9). Moreover, there was evidence that the joint effect of radon exposure and tobacco smoking was multiplicative rather than additive. In a study conducted in New Jersey, the risk of lung cancer was increased more than two-fold among women living in homes with radon levels exceeding 4 pCi per liter.[81] However, in a case-control study of women who were recently diagnosed with lung cancer in China, no association was demonstrated between increasing residential radon exposure and lung cancer; 20% of the year-long radon measurements exceeded 4 pCi per liter, the level above which remedial action is recommended in the United States.[82] Conclusions to those from the study in China were recently presented based on a study by Létourneau and colleagues in Canada.[83] Thus, although radon and its α-particle–emitting decay products are classified as a human lung carcinogen, there is uncertainty about whether residential radon exposure levels contribute to the lung cancer burden to the extent predicted based on extrapolations from studies of underground miners. Epidemiologic studies of indoor radon in the United States must be interpreted with caution because of limitations in estimating lifetime exposures based on current exposure measurements and because average residential exposure levels are generally low, with extrapolated relative risk estimates of less than 1.2, thus potentially confounded by effects of active and environmental tobacco smoke inhalation or of other residential environmental pollutants. Notwithstanding these caveats, recent publications are supportive of risks of lung cancer associated with residential radon exposure that are consistent with extrapolations of risk using underground mining-based models.[78,84]

Occupational Respiratory Carcinogens

Although smoking is the major cause of lung cancer, other respiratory tract carcinogens have been identified, or are suspect, and may enhance the carcinogenic effects of tobacco smoke. Notable among these independent determinants of lung cancer are chemical and physical agents that have been identified in the workplace (Table 20.8). An example of an occupational lung cancer was described in central Europe in the latter part of the nineteenth century in underground metal miners. The likely cause of what was described historically as "mountain disease" has been attributed to the miner's inhalation of radon and α-emitting radon daughters. At that time, lung cancer was a rare disease, and the prevalence of cigarette smoking was low. Other occupational agents classified as Group 1 carcinogens by the International Agency for Research on Cancer include arsenic, asbestos, bis (chloromethyl) ether, chromium (hexavalent), nickel and nickel compounds, polycyclic aromatic compounds (PAHs), and vinyl chloride. Currently, occupational exposures have been estimated to account for 5% to 20% of lung cancers occurring among men and women of different cultures and nations.[85]

Asbestos

The association between asbestos exposure and lung cancer has been established by epidemiological and animal experimental studies. It has been estimated that since the beginning of World War II, up to 8 million persons in the United States have been exposed to asbestos in the workplace. In the United States, more than 90% of the production and consumption of asbestos is represented by the serpentine or curly form of fiber known as chrysotile ("white asbestos"). The bronchopulmonary neoplasms of various cell types induced by asbestos tend to originate peripherally and in the lower lobes, accompanied frequently by the fibrosis of asbestosis.

Asbestos is a general term used to describe a variety of naturally occurring hydrated silicates that produce mineral fibers upon mechanical processing. In addition to the serpentine group described previously, there are the amphiboles, a larger family of straight, needlelike fibers that includes anthophyllite, tremolite and amosite ("brown asbestos"), and crocidolite ("blue asbestos"). The vast majority of mesotheliomas are associated with exposure to crocidolite asbestos. Because of unique physical and chemical properties, such as noncombustibility, withstanding temperatures of over 500°C, resistance to acids, high tensile strength, and use in thermal and acoustic insulation, asbestos has had wide applications in commercial products. Such products include textiles, cement, paper, wicks, ropes, floor and roofing tiles, water pipes, wallboard, fireproof clothing, gaskets, and brake linings.

A variety of morphologic, biochemical, and molecular techniques have been utilized to document events that might be associated with asbestos toxicity at the cellular level. Prolonged exposure to asbestos results in the accumulation of macrophages and inflammatory cells in the alveoli, which is accompanied by the release of oxygen free radicals, the peroxidation of cell membranes, and damage to DNA and other macromolecules. Asbestos fibers that cross the alveolar epithelium may be translocated to the pleura by macrophages. The shape, length, and persistence of fibers may be important in eliciting cellular responses intrinsic to carcinogenesis. Longer, rodlike fibers (i.e., more than 5 to 10 micrometers in length and less than 0.25 microns in diameter) appear to be more cytotoxic than shorter, coarse fibers. Electrostatic charge on the fiber surface may enhance deposition in lung tissue, and the surface biochemistry may also impact the inflammatory response. Experimentally, in tracheobronchial epithelial culture systems, asbestos exhibits the characteristics of a tumor promoter; chronic exposure to

asbestos, subsequent to the introduction of subcarcinogenic amounts of dimethyl benzanthracene (DMBA), has resulted in increased DNA synthesis, basal cell hyperplasia, squamous metaplasia, and a low incidence (about 5%) of squamous cell carcinoma. In the induction of mesotheliomas and pleural sarcomas, asbestos is a complete carcinogen.[86,87]

The risk of lung carcinoma in cigarette smokers has been examined in a number of asbestos-exposed populations. In 1968, Selikoff and colleagues[88] reported on the effects of combined exposures to cigarette smoking and asbestos in insulation workers; the relative risk for lung cancer significantly exceeded the level of risk expected if each exposure were to have acted only independently (noninteractively). The synergy resulting from combined exposures to tobacco and asbestos has been demonstrated in asbestos factory workers, Quebec miners and millers, amosite asbestos factory workers, and Finnish anthophyllite miners and millers.[89] Although most studies have concluded that the resulting relative risks were close to multiplicative, as in exposures, to smoking and radon combined, a study among Canadian chrysotile miners and millers concluded that the effect of each agent was independent and additive.[90] Various sources have concluded that asbestos exposure, in the absence of tobacco smoking, increases the risk of both squamous cell carcinoma and adenocarcinoma of the lung. It is assumed that the dose-response relationship is linear and without an apparent threshold.

Mesothelioma has a protracted latency period averaging 35 to 40 years. Unlike carcinoma of the lung, smoking does not contribute to the development of mesothelioma in asbestos workers. Statistics on the incidence and mortality of mesothelioma are not reported routinely, because of problems in histopathologic classification of mesothelial cell hyperplasia and malignant neoplasia and the distinction from metastatic sarcomas or adenocarcinomas. A combination of histochemistry, immunocytochemistry, and electron microscopy may be necessary to achieve a precise and valid diagnosis. In the SEER program, consisting of population-based cancer registries that cover about 10% of the total United States population, the average annual age-adjusted incidence of mesothelioma (per 100,000 population) from 1985 to 1989 was 1.6 among white males and 0.4 among white females. In developed countries, approximately one mesothelioma case occurs concurrently with 100 lung carcinoma cases. The rates in nonwhites were too low to yield reliable estimates during this period of time. As reported in other countries, pleural exceeded peritoneal mesotheliomas by a ratio of 9 : 1 in males and 3 : 1 in females.[91] The tumors arise rarely in the pericardium. In the SEER areas over the period from 1973 to 1984, the age-adjusted annual incidence of mesothelioma increased by nearly 12% per year in males and by 1% in females. The incidence rates appeared to have peaked among those born around 1910, and have declined among cohorts born subsequently. Projections for

TABLE 20.8. CHEMICALS AND INDUSTRIAL PROCESSES ASSOCIATED WITH HUMAN LUNG CANCER*

Agent	Human Target Organs	Epidemiology	Toxicology
Arsenic	Lung Skin Urinary tract	Over 95% of arsenic produced in the United States is by-product of copper, lead, zinc and tin ore smelting. Excess lung cancer reported in association with use and production of inorganic trivalent arsenic-containing pesticides. Dose-response trends have been validated by measuring concentrations in air and urine. In review of published studies, combined relative risk reported as 3.69 (95% CI, 3.06–4.46). Joint action with tobacco smoking appears to be more than additive and less than multiplicative. Latency of 10–35 years.	No satisfactory animal model. In tissue culture systems: chromosomal aberrations inhibition of DNA repair increased sister chromatid exchanges. The current OSHA standard for airborne inorganic arsenic is 10 micrograms/m³.
Asbestos	Lung Mesothelium or serosa of pleura, pericardium, and peritoneum ?GI tract ?Larynx	Various workers in asbestos industries at increased risk—miners, millers, textile, insulation, shipyard, cement. Average latency period of 25 to 30 years for carcinoma of lung. Length in interval varies with type of fiber, exposure intensity and duration, host factors. Dose-response relationship which is approximately linear in form across mid to upper levels of exposure. Relative risk of lung cancer appears to decrease following cessation of exposure. Synergistic relationship with cigarette smoking, which is more than additive and close to multiplicative. Asbestos exposure in the United States accounts for approximately 5% of lung cancer deaths in men.	Asbestos minerals are divided into: (a) the amphiboles, including amosite, crocidolite, anthophyllite, and tremolite; (b) serpentine class which is represented by chrysotile. All types of commercial asbestos fibers are carcinogenetic in mice, rats, hamsters, and rabbits; after inhalation, or intrapleural and intraperitoneal administration, cancers of the lung and bronchus, and/or mesotheliomas have been induced. The current OSHA standard is 0.1 fibers per ml for fibers greater than 5 microns in length.
Bis (chloromethyl) ether, and chloromethyl methyl ether	Lung	Used in manufacture of ion exchange resins, polymers, plastics; tumor cell type was primarily (85%) small-cell (oat-cell) carcinoma. Changes in industrial process from open-kettle to closed hermetically isolated systems in 1971 have markedly reduced exposure and were accompanied by declining risk of lung cancer. Increasing risk with increasing intensity and duration of exposure.	Highly carcinogenic in rodents by inhalation, skin application, or subcutaneous injection. BCME is a more potent carcinogen than CMME.
Chromium and compounds	Lung Nasal and paranasal sinuses	Used in metal alloys, electroplating, lithography magnetic tapes, paint pigments, cement, rubber, photoengraving, composition floor covering, and as oxidant in synthesis of organic chemicals. Excess risk, threefold and higher, was demonstrated for all cell types of lung cancer in the chromate-producing industry, producers of chromate paints, and chromate plating workers, particularly during 1930–1945. Risks in other occupational settings, with lower intensity exposures, have not been consistently or substantially increased.	Epidemiologic and experimental data implicate hexavalent and not trivalent chromium compounds. The OSHA standard for chromic acid and hexavalent chromates is 0.1 mg/m³.

Agent	Target organ(s)		
Nickel and compounds	Lung Nasal and paranasal sinuses Larynx	Used in electroplating, manufacturing of stainless steel and other alloys, ceramics, storage batteries, electric circuits, petroleum refining, and oil hydrogenation. Risk associated with earliest stage of refining, involving heavy exposure to dust from relatively crude ore. In some nickel refineries, high levels of PAHs, arsenic, or other agents may have contributed to increased risks. In mining for nickel, workers may be exposed to asbestos.	Animal studies indicate that nickel compounds can produce local sarcomas by injection, and pulmonary tumors by inhalation and intratracheal instillation. Several forms of nickel may be carcinogenic, and include oxides, sulfites and soluble nickel. The OHSA standard is 0.1 mg/m^3 for soluble compounds, and 1 mg/m^3 for nickel metal and insoluble nickel compounds.
Polycyclic aromatic hydrocarbons (PAHs)	Lung Skin and scrotum Urinary bladder	These chemicals may result from ferrochromium production and smelting of nickel-containing ores; aluminum production, iron and steel founding, coke production, and coal gasification; coal tars, coal tar pitches, untreated mineral oils; soots from cumbustion and diesel engine exhausts. In relation to coke oven emissions, risk of lung cancer highest in workers on the topside of coke ovens. Among the most heavily exposed, lifetime risk could reach 40%. Combined relative risk, based on six studies, of 1.31 (95% CI, 1.13–1.44) for diesel-exposed workers.	PAHs result from pyrolysis or incomplete combustion of organic compounds. Benzo(a)pyrene-DNA adducts, a marker of PAH exposure, have been detected in the blood samples of coke oven workers. Diesel exhaust, the particulate phase, has been demonstrated to be a lung carcinogen in animals.
Radon	Lung	Increased risks of lung cancer have been observed among underground miners in North America, Europe, and Asia, and quantitatively related to the inhalation of radon daughter products. Although small-cell cancers predominate, all cell types are affected. Radiation and cigarette smoking are interactive with relative risks somewhat less than multiplicative. Exposure levels in miners associated with elevated risks generally exceeded 100 Working Level Months (about 0.5 Gy). Linear nonthreshold dose-response. For the same cumulative dose, prolonged exposures at low dose rates appear more hazardous than shorter exposures at higher dose rates.	Dose of high LET alpha particles to individual cells will vary with respiratory dynamics, thickness of the epithelial cell and overlapping mucous layers, and the clearance rate of absorbed radioactive particles. Cellular DNA damage depends on the type of radiation, amount of energy deposited per volume of tissue, the rate at which the energy is deposited, and the time over which a given dose is accumulated.
Vinyl chloride	Liver (angiosarcoma) Lung Brain Lymphoreticular (?)	Principal use is in production of plastics, packaging materials, and vinyl asbestos floor tiles. A review of 12 cohort studies of men employed at synthetic plastics or polyvinyl chloride polymerization plants reported SMRs for lung cancer indicating an overall observed-to-expected lung cancer ratio of 1.12 (95% confidence interval from 1.0 to 1.2).	Inhalation of vinyl chloride monomer and polyvinyl chloride in experimental animals causes pulmonary fibrosis and adenomas, skin appendage tumors, and osteochondromas.

* Agents are those classified as known carcinogens (Group 1) by the International Agency for Research on Cancer.

the United States are approximately 2,000 new cases per year in the 1990s.[92]

There are well-documented areas of elevated incidence of mesothelioma, such as the coastal area of Virginia, England and Wales, and Japan, where there were shipbuilding centers; among women in areas where during World War II gas masks with asbestos filters were manufactured; or in South Africa, where excess mesothelioma incidence was concentrated in mining districts. Mesotheliomas may result from neighborhood or environmental (nonoccupational) exposures to asbestos industries and from household contact with asbestos dust, primarily through the laundering of work clothing.[93–97]

All types of asbestos have the potential for causing mesothelioma, although the risks in humans are two to four times more significant for amphibole fibers, such as crocidolite and amosite, than for the serpentine fibers of chrysotile. The mechanisms of induction appear related to the physical properties of fiber size and dimension. The amphibole straight rodlike fibers can more readily be transported or penetrate to peripheral segments of the lung. The pathogenesis in mesothelial cells is accompanied by induced protooncogene expression and the formation of oxygen radical species.[98,99]

The association between the physical structure of asbestos fibers and carcinogenicity has raised concerns regarding possible hazards of other fibers, whether natural or synthetic. Inorganic synthetic vitreous substances derived from glass, rock, slag, or clay are used primarily in the manufacture of thermal and acoustic insulation materials. Intrapleural injection of such fibers is associated with mesothelioma or sarcoma of the pleura of laboratory animals. In 1987, the World Health Organization declared that glass wool, rock wool, slag wool, and ceramic fibers were to be classified as 2B agents, namely agents possibly carcinogenic to humans.[100] This category is generally used for agents for which there is limited evidence in humans and where there is the absence of sufficient evidence in experimental animals. Epidemiologic studies of the association of occupational exposures to synthetic vitreous fibers and the risk of lung cancer have not shown a consistent pattern of risk in relation to duration of employment, average intensity and cumulative exposure dose levels, or latency interval. Further, many of the studies have not controlled adequately for confounding by cigarette smoking habits or exposure to other workplace respiratory carcinogens.[101,102]

Nutrition: Antioxidants and Fat

Epidemiologic studies have provided evidence about the nature of dietary deficiencies and excesses that have influenced the risk of lung cancer. The most consistent association, gathered from case-control and cohort studies, was that increased consumption of fresh vegetables, fruits, and carotenoids lowered the risk in men and women, in current or former smokers, and for all histologic types. The higher levels of consumption, as specified by tertile, quartile, or quintile categories, when compared with the lower levels, tended to be associated with 40% to 50% reduction in the smoking-age-gender–adjusted relative risk of lung cancer of various cell types. Various antioxidants were considered as putative chemopreventive nutrients, but a major focus has been on the carotenoids, particularly β-carotene.[103–115] Some investigators have reported that β-carotene was most protective in current or heavy smokers, whereas others have found that β-carotene or carotenoids were most protective in former smokers or in nonsmokers. In a population-based case-control study of lung cancer in nonsmokers conducted in New York State, Mayne and co-workers[116] concluded that the increased consumption of raw (not cooked) fruits and vegetables was associated with a significantly reduced risk for lung cancer. Dietary β-carotene (odds ratio = 0.70; 95% CI = 0.50 to 0.99), but not dietary retinol (vitamin A), was significantly associated with risk reduction for lung cancer in nonsmoking men and women.

By the mid-1980s, large-scale randomized clinical trials of β-carotene, β-carotene plus retinol, or β-carotene and/or vitamin E were initiated in subjects at increased risk of lung cancer. The α-tocopherol/β-carotene trial (ATBC) in Finland was a primary prevention trial among over 29,000 male smokers of 50 to 69 years of age.[117] The 2×2 factorial design evaluated 20 mg β-carotene and/or 50 International Units of α-tocopherol (vitamin E) daily for 6.5 years. These doses represented a fivefold excess over the median intake of α-tocopherol and a tenfold excess over the median intake of β-carotene in the general population. When compared with placebo groups, supplementation with vitamin E did not alter lung cancer incidence; however, participants receiving β-carotene alone or in combination with α-tocopherol had significantly higher lung cancer incidence (relative risk = 1.18; 95% CI, 1.03 to 1.36). The excess lung cancer incidence was demonstrable after the initial 18 months, and the randomized design and analysis controlled for cigarette smoking history.

The β-carotene and retinol efficacy trial (CARET) was a multicenter randomized trial to test whether oral administration of the combination of β-carotene (30 mg per day) and retinyl palmitate (25,000 IU per day) would decrease lung cancer incidence in high-risk populations of women smokers and men smokers and/or exposed asbestos workers. In the treatment group, when compared with the placebo group, the relative risk, after an average follow-up of four years, of death from lung cancer was 1.46 (95% CI, 1.07 to 2.00). The point estimates exceeded 1.1 for the current smokers, asbestos-exposed men, and current women smokers.[118,119]

The Physicians' Health Study was a long-term trial organized to test the effect of aspirin on cardiovascular disease incidence. β-carotene (50 mg) was added in a 2×2 design. In this healthy male population with 11% current cigarette smokers, and after an average follow-up of 12.5 years, the investigators concluded that the intervention did not reduce or increase the incidence of lung cancer (relative risk = 0.93).[120,121]

It is disturbing and challenging to reflect about the lack of demonstrable benefit or even an adverse outcome of increased risk of lung cancer in smoking men and women participating in various chemoprevention clinical trials. The results of these clinical trials would appear to contradict the epidemiologic observational studies. β-carotene is only one of many carotenoids ingested in vegetables and fruits and, under conditions of increased oxidative stress as in exposure to cigarette smoke or asbestos, β-carotene can be oxidized to an epoxide or reactive electrophilic derivative that would be mitogenic rather than inhibitory of cell proliferation.[122] Handelman and associates exposed human plasma to the gas phase of cigarette smoke and observed oxidative disruption of carotenoids and α-tocopherol.[123] In addition to carotenoids, fresh fruits and vegetables contain other micronutrients including vitamin C, folic acid, flavones, isoflavonoids (e.g., soy products), protease inhibitors, thiocyanates, and indoles (e.g., indole-3-carbinol in *Brassica* vegetables).[124] Folic acid, methionine, and choline are interrelated in methyl group metabolism. Selective growth and transformation of cells can result from imbalances in DNA hypomethylation and overexpression of protooncogenes, or hypermethylation of promoter regions that may attenuate the expression of tumor suppressor genes.

Various chemopreventive mechanisms of action by micronutrients and nonnutritive phytochemicals in fruits and vegetables have been suggested by *in vitro* and animal feeding experimental studies. The complex interrelated mechanisms by which substances in vegetables and fruits may inhibit carcinogenesis include regulation of cell differentiation; "quenching" or "trapping" of oxygen or hydroxyl free radicals; preventing the formation of electrophilic metabolites from precursor compounds by inhibiting the enzymatic activation pathway (e.g., cytochrome P450) or by inducing the detoxification pathway (e.g., glutathione S-transferase); enhancing DNA methylation; inhibiting the expression of oncogenes; and stimulating immune function[125] (see also Chapters 21, 25).

Lung cancer mortality is significantly positively correlated in various countries with per capita fat availability and consumption. An excess of lung cancer has been reported in case-control studies among persons with high dietary intake of foods rich in fat and cholesterol, including whole milk and eggs. However, the positive association of dietary cholesterol and lung cancer risk has not been reflected in studies of serum cholesterol levels. Shekelle and colleagues[126] have hypothesized that a low, not elevated, serum cholesterol is predictive of increased risk of lung cancer, particularly in the subgroup of the population with low intake of β-carotene. Studies of the effects of dietary cholesterol and total and saturated fat have attempted to control

for the confounding effects of gender, smoking status, and intake of energy, fruits, vegetables, and carotenoids.[127] Despite the positive association with dietary fat, lung cancer risk is not associated with increasing body mass; indeed, several studies have described elevated risks in subgroups in the lowest categories of body mass index. Dietary lipids have been postulated to affect carcinogenesis by promoting mechanisms that affect cell proliferation and gap junction intercellular communication.

Previous Nonneoplastic Lung Disease

Lung cancer risk has been reported to be increased among persons with a history of tuberculosis, pulmonary fibrosis as in silicosis, or chronic bronchitis and emphysema. An increased risk of lung cancer following the diagnosis of tuberculosis has been reported in cohort and case-control studies. For example, in a population-based case-control study of lung cancer that was conducted in Shanghai, Zheng and associates[128] reported that the age-sex-smoking–adjusted odds ratio or relative risk of lung cancer was increased by 50% (95% CI, 1.2 to 1.8) among all survivors of tuberculosis, and by 100% among those diagnosed with tuberculosis within the previous 20 years. Among males, prior infection was reported by 26% of the cases and by 20% of the controls. The relative risk of lung cancer was higher for adenocarcinoma than for squamous or oat-cell carcinoma, and the locations of the granulomatous fibrotic lesions were highly correlated with that of the lung cancers. Based on the estimation of relative risk and the proportion of the population in Shanghai exposed to pulmonary tuberculosis, 9% of lung cancer cases were attributed to prior infection. In a case-control study by Hinds and colleagues,[129] the relative risk of lung cancer in never-smoking women in Hawaii with prior tuberculosis was increased significantly (odds ratio 8.2, 95% CI, 1.3 to 54.4).

The International Agency for Research on Cancer (IARC) has classified silica as a "probable" lung carcinogen (2A). Inhalation of silica causes both lung fibrosis and cancer in rats, but fibrosis in the absence of cancer has been observed in mice. For workers exposed to crystalline silica with clinical indication of pneumoconiosis, as reported in 15 cohort (12) and case-control (3) studies, the combined relative risk of lung cancer was 1.33 (95% CI, 1.12 to 1.45).[130] In a metaanalysis of lung cancer mortality among patients with silicosis, Smith and co-workers[131] reported a pooled estimated relative risk of 2.2 (95% CI, 2.1 to 2.4). Relative risks have been elevated in workers with increased exposure to silica dust that is incurred in mining and quarrying, and in the granite, ceramics and glass, and foundry industries. In underground mining, exposure to silicon dioxide or crystalline silica may be confounded by exposure to radon and its α-particle progeny, diesel fumes, asbestos, and other occupational carcinogens, and/or to tobacco smoke. Increased risk appears to vary with the severity of pulmonary fibrosis, or with clinical signs of obstructive lung diseases that accompany chronic silicosis.[132] The excess risk of lung cancer reported in previous studies has persisted after adjusting for smoking or has not been associated with excess risks for other smoking-related cancers, as in the upper digestive or urinary tract organs.

Cigarette smoking may result in chronic bronchitis and/or emphysema (COPD) and/or lung cancer. In the early 1960s, Passey[133] hypothesized that it was the irritating properties of tobacco smoke, resulting in chronic bronchitis and inflammatory destruction of lung tissue, that was of pathogenic significance in the causal pathway of lung cancer, rather than any direct action by volatile and particulate carcinogens in tobacco smoke. The experiments of Kuschner,[134] however, suggested an alternative explanation; namely, that bronchial and bronchiolar inflammation, accompanied by reactive proliferation, squamous metaplasia, and dysplasia in basal epithelial cells, provided a cocarcinogenic mechanism for neoplastic cell transformation upon exposure to polycyclic aromatic hydrocarbons.

Although cigarette smoking is the predominant cause of COPD, with an estimated attributable risk fraction exceeding 80% in smoking individuals, perhaps only 10% to 15% of current smokers will eventually develop clinically significant sequellae of productive cough, exertional dyspnea, and cardiovascular disease.[135] There are at least ten cohort studies that have reported that chronic obstructive airway disease is an independent predictor of lung cancer risk (Table 20.9).[136–145]

Chronic cigarette smoking retards mucociliary clearance of foreign particulates and respiratory tract secretions, evokes an inflammatory response accompanied by fibrosis and thickening in the membranous and respiratory bronchioles, and causes mucus gland hypertrophy, hyperplasia, and dysplasia in the proximal airways.[146] The manifestations of COPD signal the extent of bronchopulmonary structural and functional damage arising from the interaction of sustained exposure to toxic products of tobacco combustion and host susceptibility. In this context, COPD is a biomarker of both exposure dose level and tissue susceptibility. A more controversial issue would be that of how COPD impacts the development of lung cancer. A conceptual model is proposed that incorporates the potential cocarcinogenic effects of chronic obstructive pulmonary disease in the causal pathway of cigarette smoke and lung cancer (Figure 20.2). The molecular events in the natural history of lung cancer comprise multiple genetic mutations that are determinants of neoplastic transformation and tumor progression, and the elaboration of autocrine growth factors that influence the clonal behavior and morphologic features of neoplastic cells. Chronic inflammation in the proximal and distal bronchial airways is an important cause of obstructive symptoms and provides the dynamic setting for oxidative stress and the formation of free radicals that accompany the reparative proliferative response. Increased proliferation kinetics and the interaction of hydroxyl radicals with DNA augment the likelihood of DNA structural and transcriptional errors.

GENETIC PREDISPOSITION

In a study of familial aggregation of lung cancer, Tokuhata and Lilienfeld[147] reported a significantly increased risk of

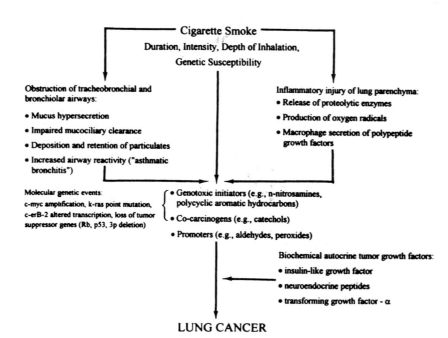

FIGURE 20.2. Enhancement of the causal pathway of cigarette smoke and lung cancer by the association with chronic obstructive pulmonary disease. (From Islam SS, Schottenfeld D. Declining FEV1 and chronic productive cough in cigarette smokers: a 25-year prospective study of lung cancer incidence in Tecumseh, Michigan. *Cancer Epidemiol Biomarkers Prev* 1994;3:289, with permission.)

TABLE 20.9. REVIEW OF COHORT STUDIES OF CHRONIC OBSTRUCTIVE PULMONARY DISEASE AND LUNG CANCER

	Sources of Exposed and Nonexposed	Person-Years and Interval (Years) of Follow-Up	Index of Risk	Age, Smoking-Adjusted Relative Risk (95% C.I.)	Commentary
Peto et al.,[136]	2,718 British men identified in random surveys conducted between 1954–1961, 25–64 years of age.	20–25 years of follow-up		When index of air-way obstruction exceeded 2 S.D. below average (108 men) risk of lung cancer mortality increased, 1.3.	Mucus hypersecretion was not predictive of COPD mortality, but was correlated with lung cancer mortality.
			maximal value for: $FEV_1 \div$ standing height[3] chronic phlegm production by questionnaire.	Mucus hypersecretion was predictive of 40% increased risk of lung cancer, after adjustment for FEV_1/Ht^3.	
Skillrud et al., 1986[137]	93 men, 20 women, 45–59 years of age from rural area of S.E. Minnesota; 123 controls treated for fractures, dental extractions. Matched on age, sex, occupation, smoking history.	1973–74 until 1984	% predicted $FEV_1 \leq 70\%$ compared with $FEV_1 \geq 85\%$	10-year cumulative probability in men: $$\frac{0.108}{0.025} = 4.32$$ $(0.93, 19.99)$	No lung cancer cases in women.
Tockman et al., 1987[138]	Screening and early detection for lung cancer clinical trial at Johns Hopkins—3,728 white males, 45 yrs and older, who smoked at least 1 pack of cigarettes per day. Intermittent positive pressure breathing trial, 667 white males, 30–74 years of age, with COPD.	Lung cancer screening: 4,436 p-yrs or less than 2 yrs IPPB trial: 2,001 p-yrs or 3 yrs followed.	FEV_1 greater than 60% of predicted value compared with less than or equal to 60%. $FEV_1/FVC \leq 60\%$. chronic cough or shortness of breath.	lung cancer screening trial: 2.72 (0.98, 7.55) IPPB trial: 4.85	Presence of symptoms of chronic cough or shortness of breath did not contribute significantly to lung cancer risk after adjustment for FEV_1 % predicted.
Tenkanen et al., 1987[139]	3 urban and 3 rural areas in Finland; 4,452 men, selected by sampling birth cohorts, 1898–1902, 1903–1907, 1908–1917, from electoral lists.	Follow-up period, 1964–1980	Phlegm, all day for at least three months each year. Shortness of breath when walking. Wheezing	Phlegm = 1.9 (P < .001) Shortness of breath = 1.6 (0.05 < P < 0.10) (controlling for other symptoms, smoking, age). Severe wheezing alone was not associated with significant increase in risk of lung cancer.	Significant lung cancer risk was associated with severe level of phlegm production, even after controlling for smoking, shortness of breath, and wheezing.

(continued)

TABLE 20.9. *Continued.*

	Sources of Exposed and Nonexposed	Person-Years and Interval (Years) of Follow-Up	Index of Risk	Age, Smoking-Adjusted Relative Risk (95% C.I.)	Commentary
Kuller et al., 1990[140]	Cigarette smoking males (n = 8,194) participating in the Multiple Risk Factor Intervention Trial. Of the above, 6,075 (75%) had satisfactory pulmonary function measurements. Aged 35–57 years at entry.	Average follow-up, 10.5 years (1973–1984). However, the FEV_1 measurements were obtained at year three, thus allowing for 0.5 years of follow-up.	FEV_1 levels distributed into quintiles. For example, lowest quintile included ≤2,670 ml, highest quintile ≥3,749ml.	FEV_1 (lowest) ÷ FEV_1 (highest) = 3.57(.94, 12.5). Proportional hazards model was compatible with 40% reduction in risk with increase in FEV_1 of 1,000 ml.	Production of phlegm for greater than 3 months in a year was a significant predictor of lung cancer, after adjusting for age, smoking and FEV_1. There was no relation between baseline shortness of breath and subsequent lung cancer mortality.
Lange et al., 1990[141]	Population-based sample of 7,573 women and 6,373 men who were participants in the Copenhagen City Heart Study.	Average follow-up period of about 10 years.	% predicted FEV_1, FEV_1/FVC %, chronic phlegm (3 months each year for more than one year).	Cox regression model controlling for age, sex, cigarette smoking. % predicted FEV_1: 40–79 = 2.1 (1.3, 3.4) <40 = 3.9(2.2, 7.2) FEV_1 ÷ FVC <0.6 = 2.6	Regression coefficients did not differ between women and men. Among subjects who reported chronic phlegm at enrollment only 54% reported it on reexamination 5 years later.
Vestbo et al., 1991[142]	Random sample (6.6%) of all men, 46–69 years of age, living in city in Denmark, 1973. n = 876.	1974–1985, 12,134 p-yrs Cancer incidence was based on the Danish Cancer Registry.	Chronic phlegm (lasting at least three months), cough or shortness of breath. FEV_1 per liter, under the expected FEV_1 given the height. Chronic bronchitis (defined as cough and phlegm lasting three months or more for at least two years).	Cox regression model using age as the underlying time scale: FEV_1 = 2.1 (1.3, 3.4) cough = 2.5 (1.3, 5.0) dyspnea = 2.2 (1.0, 4.9) phlegm = 1.2 (0.5, 3.0) chronic bronchitis = 0.8 (0.3, 2.7).	Dyspnea was significant predictor of COPD and overall mortality.

Reference	Population	Methods	Analysis	Results
Nomura et al., 1991[143]	6,317 Japanese-American men residing on Hawaiian island of Oahu, who were 45–68 years of age at entry.	19-year follow-up survey subsequent to examination in 1965–1968.	% predicted FEV$_1$ quartile distribution. Highest quartile category (>103.5%) was baseline in estimating relative risk.	Lowest quartile % predicted FEV$_1$ = 2.1 (1.3, 3.5) (<84.5%). Only 2 percent of the cohort had % predicted FEV$_1$ of less than 60%. The data suggested that subjects with % predicted FEV$_1$ below 94.5%, after controlling for age and smoking, were at increased risk of lung cancer (95% C.I., 1.3–4.1).
Islam & Schottenfeld, 1994[144]	2,099 women and 1,857 men, 25 years of age or older when first examined from 1962 to 1965 in Tecumseh, Michigan.	25-year prospective relation to baseline ventilatory lung function and cigarette smoking status; average annual decline in FEV$_1$ (ml/years); Cox proportional hazards regression model with % predicted FEV$_1$.	Among smoking men and women, those in lowest quartile % FEV$_1$ were at 2.7 times the risk of lung cancer compared with highest quartile. With each 10% decrease in % FEV$_1$, the risk of lung cancer increased 1.17 times, after controlling for age, sex, and cigarette smoking intensity.	Rapidly declining ventilatory function in conjunction with persistent symptoms of chronic bronchitis in current smokers is predictive of increased risk of lung cancer.
Hole et al., 1996[145]	7,058 men and 8,353 women, aged 45–64 years at baseline screening 1972 to 1976, as part of a general population study in Renfrew and Paisly, Scotland.	Minimum of 15 years of follow-up.	FEV$_1$ relative to the predicted value, in relation to cause-specific mortality, adjusted for age, sex, social class, cigarette smoking. Cox proportional hazards regression model, with hazard ratios relative to highest quintile of FEV$_1$.	Hazard ratios for lung cancer in subjects in the lowest quintile of FEV$_1$ distribution: men: 2.53 (1.69, 3.79) women: 4.37 (1.84, 10.42). Significant trends were observed among life time never smokers with impaired FEV$_1$ for ischemic heart disease, stroke and lung cancer. The gradients of risk of dying for a nonsmoker with a low % FEV$_1$ were similar to the relative risks for heavy smokers but with high quintile levels of pulmonary expiratory function.

lung cancer mortality among nonsmoking relatives of lung cancer cases when compared with nonsmoking relatives of age-race-and-sex—matched controls. Other investigators have reported two-to fourfold increased risks of lung cancer among close relatives of lung cancer patients. In a segregation analysis involving 337 high-risk families with lung cancer, Sellers and colleagues[148] described a pattern of autosomal codominant inheritance, and hypothesized that segregation at this gene locus would account for 69% of the lung cancer cases diagnosed in persons up to age 50 years. Samet and associates[149] concluded that the personal risk of lung cancer was increased more than fivefold if at least one parent had had lung cancer. In a study of families of women with lung cancer, an odds ratio gradient was noted: never-smoker with a positive family history (5.7); smoker with a negative family history (15.1); and smoker with a positive family history (30.0).[150] Familial aggregation of lung cancer may be attributed to shared mainstream and sidestream tobacco smoking or other environmental and/or heritable determinants. On the assumption that a lung cancer susceptibility gene with a frequency of 0.3 to 0.5 would increase the risk of lung cancer in carriers, then an autosomal recessive model of inheritance would predict that siblings of cases would manifest a two-to fourfold increased relative risk of lung cancer.[151]

Multiple inherited and acquired mechanisms of susceptibility to lung cancer have been proposed (a detailed discussion of these mechanisms is reviewed in Chapter 21). Individual susceptibility to tobacco-induced lung cancer may be dependent on competitive gene-enzyme interactions that affect activation or detoxification of procarcinogens and levels of DNA adduct formation, or on the integrity of endogenous mechanisms for repairing lesions in DNA.[152] Nicotine is converted to cotinine in a two-step enzymatic process for which the rate-limiting step is the drug-metabolizing enzyme cytochrome P-450, a genetically polymorphic enzyme. Glucuronyl transferase enzymes conjugate and inactivate carcinogenic compounds, including NNK, a potent procarcinogen in tobacco smoke. In a case-control study by Nakachi and colleagues[153] in which they assessed DNA polymorphisms in the cytochrome P4501A1 gene in relationship to squamous cell lung carcinoma, persons with the susceptible genotype had a relative risk of 7.31 after adjusting for cigarette smoking history. DNA polymorphisms in the cytochrome P450 gene (CYP1A1), or aromatic hydrocarbon hydroxylase, which is responsible for the metabolic activation of benzo(a) pyrene and other polyaromatic hydrocarbons, may represent a locus of a susceptibility gene for lung cancer. Increased activity of CYP1A1 has been demonstrated in lung cancer cells when compared with normal tissue in the same patient, suggesting that dysregulation of the gene may occur in carcinogenesis. However, no association between lung cancer and CYP1A1 polymorphisms was reported in studies in Finland conducted by Hirvonen and co-workers.[154,155]

The genetically controlled ability to metabolize the antihypertensive agent debrisoquine has been linked to the risk of lung cancer. The P450 gene (CYP2D6) that regulates debrisoquine metabolism appears to influence the metabolism of nicotine to cotinine and metabolic activation of 4(methylnitrosamino)-1-(3-pyridyl)-1-butanone (NNK), a tobacco-specific nitrosamine, which is a potent carcinogen in experimental animals. Those who are extensive metabolizers in the hydroxylation of a 10 mg test dose of debrisoquine, a dominant trait affecting up to 90% of the United States white population, have been characterized as being at increased risk of lung cancer. Caporaso and associates[156] had initially estimated the smoking-adjusted relative risk to be increased sixfold, but more recently, studies have suggested more modest increases that are twofold or have failed to demonstrate an association using either the debrisoquine metabolic phenotype or PCR assays for detecting the genotype.[157,158]

Other biomarkers of susceptibility may include glutathione-S-transferase (GST) gene polymorphisms. Isoenzymes of glutathione-S-transferase have been identified, and the presence of the GST-μ isoenzyme is dominantly inherited.[159] Several case-control studies have suggested that subjects with deficiency of the GST-μ isoenzyme or the GSTM1 null genotype, may have a 10% to 60% increase in lung cancer risk. Some studies have also evaluated potential interactions between CYP1A1 and GSTM1 genotypes.[160] Studies in Japan have reported that subjects with the combined GSTM1 null genotype and CYP1A1 polymorphisms were at increased risk.[161]

It is now clear that human tumors result from a complex sequence of mutational events. The bronchial epithelium of sustained smokers progresses from squamous metaplasia, to dysplasia, to invasive carcinoma, which is accompanied by progressive genomic instability. Many of the genetic defects that have been described in somatic cells of lung neoplasms are acquired during adult life, and are related to exposures to environmental carcinogens. Some genetic events, however, are inherited in a Mendelian fashion. Individuals with combinations of alleles that control enzyme systems regulating activation or detoxification pathways may be at increased risk of lung cancer when exposed to even low dose levels of tobacco smoke or other mutagens. However, the importance of these phenotypic biochemical manifestations in predicting human lung cancer risk is questionable. In a cohort study of monozygotic and dizygotic twin pairs followed in the National Academy of Sciences/National Research Council Twin Registry, it was concluded that inherited predisposition was not demonstrable in relationship to smoking-induced lung cancer diagnosed in men older than 50 years.[162] If one were to assume that 50% of lung cancer deaths before age 50 years were due to genetic predisposition, this would represent only 5% of lung cancer deaths.

REFERENCES

1. Ries LAG, Kosary CL, Hankey BF, et al. *SEER cancer statistics review: 1973–1994.* Bethesda, MD: National Cancer Institute. NIH Pub. No. 97–2789, 1997.
2. Shopland DR, Eyre HJ, Pechacek TF. Smoking-attributable cancer mortality in 1991. Is lung cancer now the leading cause of death among smokers in the United States? *J Natl Cancer Inst* 1991;83:1142.
3. U.S. Department of Health and Human Services. *A report of the surgeon general: the health benefits of smoking cessation.* U.S. Department of Health and Human Services, Public Health Service, Centers for Disease Control, Center for Chronic Disease Prevention and Health Promotion, Office on Smoking and Health. DHSS Pub. No. (CDC) 90–8416, 1990.
4. Kreuzer M, Kreienbrock L, Gerken M, et al. Risk factors for lung cancer in young adults. *Am J Epidemiol* 1998;147:1028.
5. Schwartz AG, Yang P, Swanson GM. Familial risk of lung cancer among nonsmokers and their relatives. *Am J Epidemiol* 1996; 144:554.
6. Brownson RC, Chang JC, Davis JR. Gender and histologic type variations in smoking-related risk of lung cancer. *Epidemiology* 1992;3:61.
7. Risch HA, Howe GR, Jain M, et al. Are female smokers at higher risk for lung cancer than male smokers? A case-control analysis by histologic type. *Am J Epidemiol* 1993;138:281.
8. Zang EA, Wynder EL. Differences in lung cancer risk between men and women: examination of the evidence. *J Natl Cancer Inst* 1996;88:183.
9. Prescott E, Osler M, Hein HO, et al. Gender and smoking-related risk of lung cancer. *Epidemiology* 1998;9:79.
10. Wagenknecht LE, Cutter GR, Haley NH, et al. Racial differences in serum cotinine levels among smokers in the coronary artery risk development in young adults study. *Am J Public Health,* 1990;80:1053.
11. Markides KS, Coreil J, Ray LA. Smoking among Mexican Americans: a three generation study. *Am J Public Health* 1987; 77:708.
12. Marin G, Perez-Stable EJ, Marin BV. Cigarette smoking among San Francisco Hispanics: the role of acculturation and gender. *Am J Public Health* 1989;79:196.
13. Novotny TE, Warner KE, Kendrick JS, et al. Smoking by blacks and whites: socioeconomic and demographic differences. *Am J Public Health* 1989;78:1187.
14. Pierce JP, Fiore MC, Novotny TE, et al. Trends in cigarette smoking in the United States: educational differences are increasing. *JAMA* 1989;261:56.
15. Kurihara M, Aoki K, Hisamichi S. *Cancer mortality statistics in the world, 1950–1985.* Nagoya: Nagoya University Press, 1989.
16. Magrath I, Litvak J. Cancer in developing countries: opportunity and challenge. *J Natl Cancer Inst* 1993;85:862.
17. Law CH, Day NE, Chanmugaratnam K. Incidence rates of specific histological types of lung cancer in Singapore Chinese dialect groups, and their etiological significance. *Int J Cancer* 1976;17:304.
18. MacLennan R, DaCosta J, Day NE, et al. Risk factor for lung cancer in Singapore Chinese, a population with high female incidence rates. *Int J Cancer* 1977;20:854.
19. Shraufnagel D, Peloquin A, Pare J, et al. Differentiating bronchioloalveolar carcinoma from adenocarcinoma. *Am Rev Respir Dis* 1982;125:74.
20. Lubin JH, Blot WJ. Assessment of lung cancer risk factors by histologic category. *J Natl Cancer Inst* 1984;73:383.
21. Devesa SS, Shaw GL, Blot WJ. Changing patterns of lung cancer incidence by histologic type. *Cancer Epidemiol Biomarkers Prev* 1991;1:29.

22. Charloux A, Quoix E, Wolkove N, et al. The increasing incidence of lung adenocarcinoma: reality or artifact? A review of the epidemiology of lung adenocarcinoma. *Int J Epidemiol* 1997; 26:14.
23. Doll R, Hill AB. A study of the etiology of carcinoma of the lung. *Br Med J* 1952;2:1271.
24. Levin ML, Goldstein H, Gerhardt PR. Cancer and tobacco smoking: a preliminary report. *JAMA* 1950;143:336.
25. International Agency for Research on Cancer (IARC). *Tobacco smoking.* IARC Monographs on the Evaluation of Carcinogenic Risk of Chemicals to Humans. Vol. 38, Lyon: IARC, 1986.
26. Advisory Committee to the Surgeon General of the U.S. Public Health Service. *Smoking and health.* Washington, DC: Public Health Service Publication No. 1103, U.S. Government Printing Office, 1964.
27. Hammond EC. Smoking in relation to the death rates of one million men and women. *Natl Cancer Inst Monogr* 1966;19: 127.
28. Doll R, Peto R. Mortality in relation to smoking: 20 years' observations on male British doctors. *Br Med J* 1976;2:1525.
29. Rogot E, Murray JL. Smoking and causes of death among US veterans: 16 years of observation. *Public Health Rep* 1980;15: 213.
30. Harris JE. Cigarette smoking among successive birth cohorts of men and women in the United States during 1900–1980. *J Natl Cancer Inst* 1983;71:473.
31. Fiore MC, Novotny TE, Pierce JP, et al. Trends in cigarette smoking in the United States: the changing influence of gender and race. *JAMA* 1989;261:49.
32. Garfinkel L, Stellman SD. Smoking and lung cancer in women: findings in a prospective study. *Cancer Res* 1988;48:6951.
33. Stellman SD, Garfinkel L. Lung cancer risk is proportional to cigarette tar yield: evidence from a prospective study. *Prev Med* 1989;18:518.
34. Stellman SD, Garfinkel L. Smoking habits and tar levels in a new American Cancer Society prospective study of 1.2 million men and women. *J Natl Cancer Inst* 1986;76:1057.
35. Lubin JH, Blot WJ, Berrino F, et al. Patterns of lung cancer risk according to type of cigarette smoked. *Int J Cancer* 1984; 33:569.
36. Wilcox H, Schoenberg J, Mason T, et al. Smoking and lung cancer: risk as a function of cigarette tar content. *Prev Med* 1988;17:263.
37. Doll R, Peto R. Cigarette smoking and bronchial carcinoma: dose and time relationships among regular smokers and lifelong nonsmokers. *J Epidemiol Community Health* 1978;32:303.
38. Halpern MT, Gillespie BW, Warner KE. Patterns of absolute risk of lung cancer mortality in former smokers. *J Natl Cancer Inst* 1993;85:457.
39. Mao L, Lee JS, Kurie JM, et al. Cloned genetic alterations in the lungs of current and former smokers. *J Natl Cancer Inst* 1997;89:857.
40. Abelin T, Gsell OR. Relative risk of pulmonary cancer in cigar and pipe smokers. *Cancer* 1967;20:1288.
41. Damber LA, Larsson LG. Smoking and lung cancer with special regard to type of smoking and type of cancer. A case-control study in north Sweden. *Br J Cancer* 1986;53:673.
42. Bryant MS, Vineis P, Skipper P, et al. Hemoglobin adducts of aromatic amines: associations with smoking status and type of tobacco. *Proc Natl Acad Sci* 1988;85:9788.
43. U.S. Surgeon General. *The health consequences of involuntary smoking.* Washington, DC: United States Department of Health and Human Services, Centers for Disease Control, Pub No. 87–8398, 1986.
44. Hirayama T. Non-smoking wives of heavy smokers have a

higher risk of lung cancer: a study from Japan. *Br Med J* 1981; 282:183.

45. Trichopoulos D, Kalandidi A, Sparros L. Lung cancer and passive smoking: conclusion of the Greek study. *Lancet* 1983;2: 677.

46. Trichopoulos D, Kalandidi A, Sparros L. Passive smoking and lung cancer. *Lancet* 1984;1:684.

47. Garfinkel L. Time trends in lung cancer mortality among nonsmokers and a note on passive smoking. *J Natl Cancer Inst* 1981; 66:1061.

48. Correa P, Pickle LW, Fontham E, et al. Passive smoking and lung cancer. *Lancet* 1983;2:595.

49. Koo LC, Ho JH, Saw D. Is passive smoking an added risk factor for lung cancer in Chinese women? *J Exp Clin Cancer Res* 1984; 3:277.

50. Wu AH, Henderson BE, Pike MC, et al. Smoking and other risk factors for lung cancer in women. *J Natl Cancer Inst* 1985; 74:747.

51. Garfinkel L, Auerbach O, Joubert L. Involuntary smoking and lung cancer: a case-control study. *J Natl Cancer Inst* 1985;79: 463.

52. Akiba S, Kato H, Blot WJ. Passive smoking and lung cancer among Japanese women. *Cancer Res* 1986;46:4806.

53. Pershagen G, Hrubec Z, Svensson C. Passive smoking and lung cancer in Swedish women. *Am J Epidemiol* 1987;125:17.

54. Lam TH, Kung IT, Wong EM, et al. Smoking, passive smoking and histological types of lung cancer in Hong Kong Chinese women. *Br J Cancer* 1987;56:673.

55. Gao YT, Blot WJ, Zheng W, et al. Lung cancer among Chinese women. *Int J Cancer* 1987;40:604.

56. Janerich DT, Thompson WD, Varela LR, et al. Lung cancer and exposure to tobacco smoke in the household. *N Engl J Med* 1990;323:632.

57. Fontham ET, Correa P, Wu-Williams A, et al. Lung cancer in nonsmoking women: a multicenter case-control study. *Cancer Epidemiol Biomarkers Prev* 1991;1:35.

58. Brownson RC, Alavanja MC, Hook ET, et al. Passive smoking and lung cancer in nonsmoking women. *Am J Pub Health* 1992; 82:1525.

59. Stockwell HG, Goldman AL, Lyman GH, et al. Environmental tobacco smoke and lung cancer risk in nonsmoking women. *J Natl Cancer Inst* 1992;84:1417.

60. Fontham ETH, Correa P, Reynolds P, et al. Environmental tobacco smoke and lung cancer in nonsmoking women. A multicenter study. *JAMA* 1994;271:1752.

61. Boffetta P, Agudo A, Ahrens W, et al. Multicenter case-control study of exposure to environmental tobacco smoke and lung cancer in Europe. *J Natl Cancer Inst* 1998;90:1440.

62. Hackshaw AK, Law MR, Wald NJ. The accumulated evidence on lung cancer and environmental tobacco smoke. *Br Med J* 1997;315:980.

63. National Research Council. *Environmental tobacco smoke,* Washington, DC: National Academy Press, 1986.

64. Doll R. Atmospheric pollution and lung cancer. *Environ Health Perspect* 1978;22:23.

65. Friberg L, Cederlof R. Late effects of air pollution with special reference to lung cancer. *Environ Health Perspect* 1978;22:45.

66. Pope CA III, Dockery DW, Schwartz J. Review of epidemiological evidence of health effects of particulate air pollution. *Inhal Toxicol* 1995;7:1.

67. Doll R, Vessey MB, Beasley RWR, et al. Mortality of gas workers—final report of a prospective study. *Br J Ind Med* 1972; 29:394.

68. Hammond EC, Selikoff IJ, Lawther PL, et al. Inhalation of benzpyrene and cancer in man. *Ann NY Acad Sci* 1976;271: 116.

69. Hammond EC, Garfinkel L. General air pollution and cancer in the United States. *Prev Med* 1980;9:169.

70. IARC. Diesel and gasoline exhausts and some nitroarenes. In: *Evaluation of carcinogenic risk of chemicals to man.* Vol. 46, Lyon: International Agency for Research on Cancer, 1989.

71. Garshick E, Schenker MB, Munoz A, et al. A retrospective cohort study of lung cancer and diesel exhaust exposure in railroad workers. *Am Rev Respir Dis* 1988;137:820.

72. Mumford JL, He XZ, Chapman RS, et al. Lung cancer and indoor air pollution in Xuan Wei, China. *Science* 1987;235: 217.

73. Gao YT, Blot WJ, Zheng W, et al. Lung cancer and smoking in Shanghai. *Int J Epidemiol* 1988;17:277.

74. Xu ZY, Blot WJ, Xiao HP, et al. Smoking, air pollution, and the high rates of lung cancer in Shenyang, China. *J Natl Cancer Inst* 1989;81:1800.

75. Wu-Williams AH, Dai XD, Blot WJ, et al. Lung cancer among women in northeast China. *Br J Cancer* 1990;62:982.

76. Cross FT. Residential radon risks from the perspective of experimental animal studies. *Am J Epidemiol* 1994;140:333.

77. Lubin JH, Boice JD Jr, Edling C, et al. Lung cancer in radon-exposed miners and estimation of risk from indoor exposure. *J Natl Cancer Inst* 1995;87:817.

78. Lubin JH, Boice JD Jr. Lung cancer risk from residential radon: meta-analysis of eight epidemiologic studies. *J Natl Cancer Inst* 1997;89:49.

79. Axelson O, Anderson K, Desai G, et al. Indoor radon exposure and active and passive smoking in relation to the occurrence of lung cancer. *Scand J Work Environ Health* 1988;14:286.

80. Pershagen G, Akerblom G, Axelson O, et al. Residential radon exposure and lung cancer in Sweden. *N Engl J Med* 1994;330: 159.

81. Schoenberg JB, Klotz JB, Wilcox HB, et al. Case-control study of residential radon and lung cancer among New Jersey women. *Cancer Res* 1990;50:6520.

82. Blot WJ, Zu ZY, Boice JD, et al. Indoor radon and lung cancer in China. *J Natl Cancer Inst* 1990;82:1025.

83. Létourneau EG, Krewski D, Choi NW, et al. Case-control study of residential radon and lung cancer in Winnipeg, Manitoba, Canada. *Am J Epidemiol* 1994;140:310.

84. Darby S, Whitley E, Silcocks P, et al. Risk of lung cancer associated with residential radon exposure in south-west England: a case-control study. *Br J Cancer* 1998;78:394.

85. Samet JM, Lerchen ML. Proportion of lung cancer caused by occupation: a critical review. In: Gee JBL, Morgan WKC, Brooks SM, eds. *Occupational lung disease.* New York: Raven Press, 1984:55.

86. Hughes JM, Weill H. Asbestos and man-made fibers. In: Samet JM, ed. *Epidemiology of lung cancer.* New York: Marcel Dekker, Inc., 1994:185.

87. Mossman BT. Carcinogenic potential of asbestos and nonasbestos fibers. *J Environ Sci Health* 1988;6:151.

88. Selikoff IJ, Hammond EC, Churg J. Asbestos exposure, smoking and neoplasia. *JAMA* 1968;204:104.

89. Saracci R. The interactions of tobacco smoking and other agents in cancer etiology. *Epidemiol Rev* 1987;9:175.

90. McDonald JC, Liddell FDK, Gibbs GW, et al. Dust exposure and mortality in chrysotile mining, 1910–75. *Br J Indust Med* 1980;37:11.

91. Zwi AB, Reid G, Landau SP, et al. Mesothelioma in South Africa, 1976–84: incidence and case characteristics. *Int J Epidemiol* 1989;18:320.

92. Lilienfeld DE, Mandel JS, Coin P, et al. Projection of asbestos-related diseases in the United States, 1985–2009. *Br J Med* 1988;45:283.

93. Tagnon I, Blot WJ, Stroube RB, et al. Mesothelioma associated

with the shipbuilding industry in coastal Virginia. *Cancer Res* 1980;40:3875.

94. Mossman BT, Gee JBL. Asbestos-related diseases. *N Engl J Med* 1989;320:1721.

95. Churg A. Lung asbestos content in long-term residents of a chrysotile mining town. *Am Rev Respir Dis* 1986;134:125.

96. Council of Scientific Affairs, American Medical Association. Asbestos removal, health hazards, and the EPA. *JAMA* 1991; 255:696.

97. Acheson ED, Gardner MJ, Pippard EC, et al. Mortality of two groups of women who manufactured gas-masks from chrysotile and crocidolite asbestos: A 40-year follow-up. *Br J Indust Med* 1982;39:344.

98. Beru KA, Quinlan TR, Moulton G, et al. Comparative proliferative and histopathologic changes in rat lungs after inhalation of chrysotile or crocidolite asbestos. *Toxicol Appl Pharmacol* 1996;137:67.

99. Brody AR. Asbestos-induced lung disease. *Environ Health Perspect* 1993;100:21.

100. International Agency for Research on Cancer (IARC). *Man-made mineral fibers and radon.* Vol. 43. Lyon, France: IARC, 1988:39.

101. Marsh GM, Enterline PE, Stone RA, et al. Mortality among a cohort of U.S. man-made mineral fiber workers: 1985 follow-up. *J Occup Med* 1990;32:594.

102. Lee I-M, Hennekens CH, Trichopoulos D, et al. Man-made vitreous fibers and risk of respiratory system cancer: a review of the epidemiologic evidence. *J Occup Environ Med* 1995;37: 725.

103. Bjelke E. Dietary vitamin A and human lung cancer. *Int J Cancer* 1975;15:561.

104. Mettlin C, Graham S, Swanson M. Vitamin A and lung cancer. *J Natl Cancer Inst* 1979;62:1435.

105. Hirayama T. Diet and cancer. *Nutr Cancer* 1979;1:67.

106. Kvale G, Bjelke E, Gart JJ. Dietary habits and lung cancer risk. *Int J Cancer* 1983;31:397.

107. Samet JM, Skipper BJ, Humble CG, et al. Lung cancer risk and vitamin A consumption in New Mexico. *Am Rev Respir Dis* 1985;131:198.

108. Pisani P, Berrino F, Macaluso M, et al. Carrots, green vegetables and lung cancer: A case-control study. *Int J Epidemiol* 1986; 15:4.

109. Ziegler RG, Mason TJ, Stemhagen A, et al. Carotenoid intake, vegetables, and the risk of lung cancer among white men in New Jersey. *Am J Epidemiol* 1986;123:1080.

110. Byers T, Graham S, Haughney BP, et al. Diet and lung cancer risk: Findings from the Western New York Diet Study. *Am J Epidemiol* 1987;125:351.

111. Paganini-Hill A, Chao A, Ross RK, et al. Vitamin A, β-carotene and the risk of cancer: a prospective study. *J Natl Cancer Inst* 1987;79:3.

112. Le Marchand L, Yoshizawa CN, Kolonel LN, et al. Vegetable consumption and lung cancer risk: a population-based case-control study in Hawaii. *J Natl Cancer Inst* 1989;81:1158.

113. Fraser GE, Beeson WL, Phillips RL. Diet and lung cancer in California Seventh-Day Adventists. *Am J Epidemiol* 1991;133: 683.

114. Le Marchand L, Hankin JH, Kolonel LN, et al. Intake of specific carotenoids and lung cancer risk. *Cancer Epidemiol Biomarkers Prev* 1993;2:183.

115. Steinmetz KA, Potter JD, Folsom AR. Vegetables, fruit and lung cancer in the Iowa Women's Health Study. *Cancer Res* 1993;53:536.

116. Mayne ST, Janerich DT, Greenwald P, et al. Dietary beta carotene and lung cancer risk in U.S. nonsmokers. *J Natl Cancer Inst* 1994;86:33.

117. The Alpha-Tocopherol, Beta Carotene Cancer Prevention Study Group. The effect of vitamin E and beta carotene on the incidence of lung cancer and other cancers in male smokers. *N Engl J Med* 1994;330:1029.

118. Omenn GS, Goodman GE, Thornquist MD, et al. Risk factors for lung cancer and for intervention effects in CARET, the Beta-Carotene and Retinol Efficacy Trial. *J Natl Cancer Inst* 1996;88:1550.

119. Omenn GS. Chemoprevention of lung cancer: the rise and demise of beta-carotene. *Annu Rev Public Health* 1998;19:73.

120. Steering Committee of the Physicians' Health Study Research Group. Final report on the aspirin component of the ongoing Physicians' Health Study. *N Engl J Med* 1989;321:129.

121. Hennekens CH, Buring JE, Manson JE, et al. Lack of effect of long-term supplementation with beta-carotene on the incidence of malignant neoplasms and cardiovascular disease. *N Engl J Med* 1996;334:1145.

122. Mayne ST, Graham S, Zheng TZ. Dietary retinol: prevention or promotion of carcinogenesis in humans? *Cancer Causes Control* 1991;2:443.

123. Handelman GJ, Packer L, Cross CE, et al. Destruction of tocopherols, carotenoids and retinol in human plasma by cigarette smoke. *Am J Clin Nutr* 1996;63:559.

124. Ziegler RG, Mayne ST, Swanson CA. Nutrition and lung cancer. *Cancer Causes Control* 1996;7:157.

125. Khuri FR, Lippman SM, Spitz MR et al. Molecular epidemiology and retinoid chemoprevention of head and neck cancer. *J Natl Cancer Inst* 1997;89:199.

126. Shekelle RB, Tangney CC, Rossof AH, et al. Serum cholesterol, beta-carotene, and risk of lung cancer. *Epidemiology* 1992;3: 282.

127. Alavanja MCR, Brown CC, Swanson C, et al. Saturated fat intake and lung cancer risk among nonsmoking women in Missouri. *J Natl Cancer Inst* 1993;85:1906.

128. Zheng W, Blot WJ, Liao ML, et al. Lung cancer and prior tuberculosis infection in Shanghai. *Br J Cancer* 1987;56:501.

129. Hinds MW, Cohen HI, Kolonel LN. Tuberculosis and lung cancer risk in nonsmoking women. *Am Rev Respir Dis* 1982; 125:776.

130. Steenland K, Loomis D, Shy C, Simonsen N. Review of occupational lung carcinogens. *Am J Indust Med* 1996;29:474.

131. Smith AH, Lopipero PA, Barroga VR. Meta-analysis of studies of lung cancer among silicotics. *Epidemiology* 1995;6:617.

132. Pairon JC, Brochard P, Jaurand MC, et al. Silica and lung cancer: a controversial issue. *Eur Respir J* 1991;4:730.

133. Passey RD. Some problems of lung cancer. *Lancet* 1962;2:107.

134. Kuschner M. The J Burns Amberson Lecture: the causes of lung cancer. *Am Rev Respir Dis* 1968;98:573.

135. U.S. Department of Health and Human Services. *The health consequences of smoking: chronic obstructive lung disease.* A report of the Surgeon General. U.S. Department of Health and Human Services, Office on Smoking and Health. DHHS Pub. No. 84–50205, 1984.

136. Peto R, Speizer FE, Cochrane AL, et al. The relevance in adults of air-flow obstruction, but not of mucus hypersecretion, to mortality from chronic lung disease. Results from 20 years of prospective observation. *Am Rev Respir Dis* 1983;128:491.

137. Skillrud DM, Offord KP, Miller D. Higher risk of lung cancer in chronic obstructive pulmonary disease. *Ann Intern Med* 1986; 105:503.

138. Tockman MS, Anthonisen NR, Wright EC, et al. Airways obstruction and the risk for lung cancer. *Ann Intern Med* 1987; 106:512.

139. Tenkanen L, Hakulinen T, Teppo L. The joint effect of smoking and respiratory symptoms on risk of lung cancer. *Int J Epidemiol* 1987;16:509.

140. Kuller LH, Ockene J, Meilhan E, et al. Relation of forced expiratory volume in one second (FEV$_1$) to lung cancer mortality in the multiple risk factor intervention trial (MRFIT). *Am J Epidemiol* 1990;132:265.

141. Lange P, Nyboe J, Appleyard M, et al. Ventilatory function and chronic mucus hypersecretion as predictors of death from lung cancer. *Am Rev Respir Dis* 1990;141:613.

142. Vestbo J, Knudsen KM, Rasmussen FV. Are respiratory symptoms and chronic airflow limitation really associated with an increased risk of respiratory cancer? *Int J Epidemiol* 1991;20:375.

143. Nomura A, Stemmermann GN, Chyou P-H, et al. Prospective study of pulmonary function and lung cancer. *Am Rev Respir Dis* 1991;144:307.

144. Islam SS, Schottenfeld D. Declining FEV1 and chronic productive cough in cigarette smokers: a 25-year prospective study of lung cancer incidence in Tecumseh, Michigan. *Cancer Epidemiol Biomarkers Prev* 1994;3:289.

145. Hole DJ, Watt GCM, Davey-Smith G, et al. Impaired lung function and mortality risk in men and women: findings from the Renfrew and Paisley prospective population study. *Br Med J* 1996;313:711.

146. Wanner A, Salathe M, Oriordan TG. Mucociliary clearance in the airways. *Am J Resp Crit Care Med* 1996;154:1868.

147. Tokuhata GK, Lilienfeld AM. Familial aggregation of lung cancer among hospital patients. *Pub Health Rep* 1963;78:277.

148. Sellers TA, Bailey-Wilson JE, Elston RC, et al. Evidence for Mendelian inheritance in the pathogenesis of lung cancer. *J Natl Cancer Inst* 1990;82:1272.

149. Samet J, Humble C, Pathak D. Personal and family history of respiratory disease and lung cancer risk. *Am Rev Respir Dis* 1986;134:466.

150. Horwitz RI, Smaldone LF, Viscoli CM. An ecogenetic hypothesis for lung cancer in women. *Arch Intern Med* 1988;148:2609.

151. Peto J. Genetic predisposition to cancer. In: Cairns J, Lyon J, Skolnick M, eds. *Cancer incidence in defined populations.* Cold Spring Harbor, NY: Cold Spring Harbor Laboratory, 1980:203.

152. Wei Q, Cheng L, Hong WK, et al. Reduced DNA capacity in lung cancer patients. *Cancer Res* 1996;56:4103.

153. Nakachi N, Imai K, Hayashi S, et al. Genetic susceptibility to squamous cell carcinoma of the lung in relation to cigarette smoking dose. *Cancer Res* 1991;51:5177.

154. Hirvonen K, Husgafvel-Pursianen K, Karjalainen A, et al. Point mutational Msp1 and 11e-Val polymorphisms closely linked in the CYP1A1 gene: lack of association with susceptibility to lung cancer in a Finnish study population. *Cancer Epidemiol Biomarkers Prev* 1992;1:485.

155. Hirvonen A, Husgafvel-Pursianen K, Antilla S, et al. PCR based CYP2D6 genotyping for Finnish lung cancer patients. *Pharmacogenetics* 1993;3:19.

156. Caporaso NE, Tucker MA, Hoover RN, et al. Lung cancer and the debrisoquine metabolic phenotype. *J Natl Cancer Inst* 1990;82:1264.

157. Shaw GL, Falk RT, Deslauriers J, et al. Debrisoquine metabolism and lung cancer risk. *Cancer Epidemiol Biomarkers Prev* 1995;4:41.

158. Shaw GL, Falk RT, Frame JN, et al. Genetic polymorphism of CYP2D6 and lung cancer risk. *Cancer Epidemiol Biomarkers Prev* 1998;7:215.

159. Nazar-Stewart V, Motulsky AG, Eaton DL, et al. The glutathione S-transferase μ polymorphism as a marker for susceptibility to lung carcinoma. *Cancer Res* 1993;53:2313.

160. Garcia-Closas M, Kelsey KT, Wiencke JK, et al. A case-control study of cytochrome P4501A1, glutathione S-transferase M1, cigarette smoking and lung cancer susceptibility. *Cancer Causes Control* 1997;8:544.

161. Hayashi S, Watanabe J, Kawajiri K. High susceptibility to lung cancer analyzed in terms of combined genotypes of P4501A1 and Mu-class glutathione S-transferase genes. *Jpn J Cancer Res* 1992;83:866.

162. Braun MM, Caporaso NE, Page WF, et al. Genetic component of lung cancer: cohort study of twins. *Lancet* 1994;344:440.

21

GENETIC SUSCEPTIBILITY TO LUNG CANCER

ANN G. SCHWARTZ

Lung cancer has long been considered a disease determined solely by environmental exposures. It is estimated that 80% to 90% of lung cancer incidence can be attributed to cigarette smoking.[1] However, only 10% to 15% of all smokers develop lung cancer[2] and 10% to 15% of all lung cancers occur among nonsmokers. Clearly, individual differences exist in susceptibility to lung carcinogens. This chapter explores whether individual differences in susceptibility to lung cancer are inherited.

EVIDENCE SUPPORTING AN INHERITED COMPONENT TO RISK

The search for evidence supporting an inherited component for disease begins by adressing the following three questions:[3] (a) Does the disease aggregate or cluster in families? (b) Is familial aggregation related to shared environmental exposures, biologically inherited susceptibility, or cultural inheritance of risk factors? (c) What is the pattern of inheritance of genetic susceptibility? If evidence supports an inherited component of disease, then the next set of questions focuses on the localization of disease genes and mechanisms of carcinogenesis.

Familial Aggregation

Familial aggregation or clustering of a disease provides the first piece of evidence supporting the possibility of an inherited component to that disease. More than 30 years ago, Tokuhata and Lilienfeld[4] observed that the number of deaths caused by lung cancer was higher among relatives of lung cancer cases than among relatives of controls. Several other studies since then have demonstrated a familial component to lung cancer risk[5-11] (Table 21.1) (see also Chapter 20) with odds ratios (OR) associated with family history ranging from 1.3 to 7.2. These studies have used traditional case-control designs, in which familial risk is indicated by cases being more likely than controls to report a family history of lung cancer. The consistent demonstration of

lung cancer aggregation in families can have several interpretations, including: (a) an inherited component to lung cancer risk; (b) environmental risk factors such as cigarette smoking shared among family members; or (c) family structure (i.e., family size and ages) differs between cases and controls affecting the risk profile of the family. To understand the reasons behind familial aggregation of lung cancer, exposure to cigarette smoke and other risk factors among relatives and the age structure of the family must be known.

The Causes of Familial Aggregation

Only three studies of familial aggregation of lung cancer have been done using a detailed family study approach,[12] collecting risk factor data for family members. These studies are summarized in Table 21.2. In a study of families of 270 lung cancer cases and a similar number of controls, Tokuhata and Lilienfeld[4] observed that the number of deaths caused by lung cancer was four times that expected among non-cigarette-smoking relatives of lung cancer cases and two times that expected among cigarette-smoking relatives. The effect of smoking on lung cancer risk was greater than the familial effects in males, whereas the reverse was true in females. The effect of family history was stronger among nonsmokers than among smokers. Cigarette smoking and family history interacted, resulting in very high risk of lung cancer among persons with both characteristics.

The second study was conducted among residents of 10 parishes in Louisiana, with families of 336 persons dying from lung cancer in a four-year period.[5] After adjusting for age, sex, smoking history, and occupational exposures for each relative, a 2.4-fold excess of lung cancer was reported among relatives of lung cancer cases as compared to relatives of spouse controls. Parents of cases had a four-fold increased risk of developing lung cancer. Relatives were also at excess risk for cancers of the nasal cavity, mid-ear, and larynx (Relative Risk [RR] = 4.6); trachea, lung, and bronchus

TABLE 21.1. CASE-CONTROL STUDIES OF FAMILY HISTORY OF LUNG CANCER

Author	Study Population	Familial Risk OR (95% CI)	Family History of Lung Cancer Definition
Ooi et al., 1986[5]	336 population-based lung cancer deaths 307 spouse controls	3.1 (1.9–5.5)	At least one first-degree relative
Samet et al., 1986[6]	518 population-based incident lung cancer cases 769 population-based controls	5.3 (2.2–12.8)	Parental history
Wu et al., 1988[7]	336 population-based, female, incident lung cancer cases with adenocarcinoma 336 neighborhood controls	3.9 (2.0–7.6)	Parental or sibling history
Shaw et al., 1991[8]	937 population-based incident lung cancer cases 955 population-based controls	1.8 (1.3–2.5) 2.8 (1.2–6.6)	At least one first-degree relative Two or more first-degree relatives
Osann et al., 1991[9]	217 female lung cancer cases selected from participants in an HMO's multiphasic checkup 213 female controls participating in the checkup	1.9 (0.7–5.6)	At least one first-degree relative
Schwartz et al., 1996[10]	257 population-based, nonsmoking, incident lung cancer cases 277 population-based, nonsmoking controls	1.4 (0.8–2.5) 7.2 (1.3–39)	At least one first-degree relative At least one first-degree relative of subjects age 40–59
Wu et al., 1996[11]	646 population-based, nonsmoking, female incident lung cancer cases 1,252 population-based controls	1.3 (0.9–1.9) 2.8 (0.9–8.3)	Parental or sibling history History in mother

TABLE 21.2. FAMILY STUDIES OF FAMILIAL RISK OF LUNG CANCER

Author	Study Population	Familial Risk
Tokuhata and Lilienfeld, 1963	2,110 first-degree relatives of 270 hospital-based cases 1,995 first-degree relatives of 270 neighborhood controls	35 observed lung cancer deaths in case relatives/13.3 expected (Obs/Exp = 2.6, p = 0.0006) Obs/Exp for nonsmokers = 3.8 (p = 0.004) Obs/Exp for smokers = 2.3 (p = 0.01)
Ooi et al., 1986[5]	2,720 first-degree relatives of 336 population-based deaths 2,230 first-degree relatives of 307 spouse controls	RR* = 2.4 (p < 0.05) all relatives RR* = 4.4 (p < 0.05) parents
Schwartz et al., 1996[10]	2,252 first-degree relatives of 257 nonsmoking, population-based, incident cases 2,408 first-degree relatives of 277 nonsmoking, population-based controls	RR* = 1.3 (0.7–2.2) all relatives RR* = 6.1 (1.1–33) relatives of cases age 40–59
Schwartz (preliminary data)	1,502 first-degree relatives of 236 population-based, incident lung cancer cases under age 45 2,172 first-degree relatives of 354 population-based controls under age 45	RR* = 2.1 (1.2–3.7) all relatives

* RR, Relative risks of lung cancer in relatives of cases as compared to relatives of controls, adjusting for each relative's lung cancer risk factors.

(RR = 3.0); skin (RR = 2.8); and uterus, placenta, ovary, and other female organs (RR = 2.1.)[13]

The third study, the author's Family Health Study in Detroit, was designed to focus on individuals likely to have risk most strongly associated with genetic factors (early-onset cases under age 45) and individuals who demonstrate increased susceptibility to low levels of exposure (nonsmoking and early-onset cases). Population-based, incident lung cancer cases were identified through the Metropolitan Detroit Cancer Surveillance System (MDCSS) of the Karmanos Cancer Institute, a participant in the National Cancer Institute's (NCI's) Surveillance, Epidemiology, and End Results (SEER) program, and population-based controls were selected through random digit dialing.[10]

Excess risk of lung cancer, after adjustment for each relative's age, sex, race, smoking status, occupation, industry, and history of other lung diseases, was limited to first-degree relatives of nonsmoking lung cancer cases 40 to 59 years of age (RR = 6.1; 95% Cl 1.1–33.4)[10] and relatives of early-onset cases (RR = 2.1; 95% Cl 1.2–3.7) (unpublished preliminary findings). Although not statistically significant, offspring of the nonsmoking cases had seven times the risk of lung cancer,[10] siblings of early-onset cases were at sixfold increased risk, and relatives of younger, female nonsmoking cases with adenocarcinoma of the lung were at the highest risk with a RR of 22.3.[14]

In characterizing lung cancer families in Detroit, other cancers were observed among first-degree relatives. Relatives of nonsmoking cases were 20% more likely to develop any cancer than relatives of controls (RR = 1.19; 95% Cl 0.94–1.50).[15] A similar excess risk of cancer was seen for all sites excluding lung cancer (RR = 1.19, 95% Cl 0.94–1.51). Risk among first-degree relatives of cases was approximately 1.4-fold or higher than that of relatives of controls for cancers of the digestive system (RR = 1.52; 95% Cl 1.02–2.27), breast (RR = 1.72; 95% Cl 0.90–2.22), and tobacco-related sites, including respiratory

system, oral cavity and pharynx, esophagus, bladder, and kidney (RR = 1.42; 95% Cl 0.93–3.18). A positive family history of lung cancer at a very early age (less than 40 years) also increased the risk of any cancer 80% (95% Cl 1.2–2.7) and breast cancer 5.1-fold (95% Cl 1.7–15.1)[16] after adjusting for age, race, sex, and smoking status of each relative and sex and age of the proband.

The role for inherited susceptibility of lung cancer is suggested by these findings of familial aggregation, exceeding that associated with familial clustering of smoking habits and considering family size and structure. The findings of stronger aggregation when onset of disease is early are indicative of an inherited component to risk. These studies also provide evidence that susceptibility to cancer among relatives of lung cancer cases may not be limited to cancers of the lung. The most prevalent cancers in lung cancer families include tobacco-related cancers and cancers of the digestive tract and breast.

Patterns of Inheritance

These case-control family-based studies add to the evidence supporting an inherited susceptibility to lung cancer but do not explicitly address genetic models, which may underlie familial aggregation. The third question to be addressed, given familial aggregation of lung cancer, is what is the pattern of inheritance of genetic susceptibility? The Louisiana study and the nonsmoking portion of the Detroit study, both described previously, are the only two studies that have addressed this question (Table 21.3). Segregation analysis was used to determine if the pattern of disease occurrence in relatives is consistent with Mandelian dominant, codominant, or recessive inheritance of a major gene, transmission of environmental factors, or is sporadic, after considering the age, sex, and environmental exposures among family members.

In the Louisiana study, the pattern of lung cancer occur-

TABLE 21.3. SEGREGATION STUDIES OF MODE OF INHERITANCE OF LUNG CANCER IN FAMILIES

Author	Study Population	Mode of Inheritance	Risk Allele Frequency
Louisiana			
Sellers et al., 1990[17]	337 population-based families	Mendelian codominant	q(a) = 0.052
Sellers et al., 1992[18]	106 population-based families of cases < age 60	Mendelian codominant	q(a) = 0.062
	231 population-based families of cases ≥ age 60	Mendelian inheritance, mode of transmission not distinguished	
Metropolitan Detroit			
Yang et al., 1997[20]	257 population-based families of nonsmoking cases	Environmental model	
Yang et al., 1999[21]	47 population-based families of nonsmoking cases age 40–59	Mendelian codominant	q(a) = 0.004
	210 population-based families of nonsmoking cases age 60–84	Environmental model	

rence in families of persons dying from lung cancer was consistent with Mendelian codominant inheritance of a rare autosomal gene with variable age at onset.[17] This putative gene is estimated to be responsible for 69% of the lung cancer at age 50, 47% at age 60, and 22% at age 70. Heterogeneity in inheritance patterns based on age at death of the lung cancer proband was also noted.[18] In the subset of families of probands dying before age 60, the model predicts that virtually all lung cancer occurs among cigarette-smoking gene carriers. Aggregation of smoking-associated cancers (i.e., lung, oral cavity, esophagus, nasopharynx, larynx, cervix, bladder, kidney, and pancreas) in case families was also consistent with Mendelian inheritance.[19]

In the Detroit study of families of nonsmoking lung cancer cases, complex segregation analysis performed for the entire sample of 257 nonsmoking cases and their 2,219 family members, found an environmental model with homogeneous risk across generations best explained the observed data.[20] Both the hypothesis that lung cancer occurrence was sporadic and the hypothesis that a genetic predisposition accounts for the familial aggregation were rejected.

To further investigate heterogeneity by age of the proband, the segregation analysis was repeated, stratified by age of the proband.[21] A Mendelian codominant model, with significant modifying effects of smoking and chronic bronchitis, best explained the observed data in the families of 47 nonsmoking probands 40 to 59 years of age. The estimated risk allele frequency was 0.004. Homozygous individuals with the risk allele are rare in the study population (1.6/100,000), making the attributable risk very low, even considering very high penetrance of early-onset lung cancer (85% in males and 74% in females by age 60). Heterozygous individuals constitute 1% of the study population and have a relatively low risk of lung cancer unless they are smokers with chronic bronchitis. Those homozygous for the low-risk allele were estimated to be at 6% and 2% risk of lung cancer in males and females, respectively, by age 80 if they smoked and had a history of chronic bronchitis. These findings point to a high-risk gene contributing to early-onset lung cancer. The attributable risk associated with the high-risk allele declines with age because the role of tobacco smoking and chronic bronchitis become more important. No evidence suggested a major gene segregating in families of nonsmoking cases age 60 to 84 years.

GENES FOR LUNG CANCER

Consistent evidence suggests that lung cancer aggregates in families, that aggregation is not completely accounted for by clustering of environmental risk factors or family structure, and that the pattern of cancer occurrence in some families is consistent with Mendellan inheritance of a rare major gene, particularly when onset is early. The studies of

familial risk described (a) support the existence of a single gene for lung cancer acting in a subset of families, with penetrance modified by environmental exposures, and (b) are consistent with common susceptibility genes acting to moderately increase cancer risk. Single genes and susceptibility genes are distinguished from one another based on several characteristics.[22] Single genes are necessary and sufficient to cause disease, are rare in the population, and are associated with strong familial aggregation and large relative risks, with onset of disease at an early age. Examples of single gene/cancer associations include *RB* and retinoblastoma[23] and *BRCA1* and breast cancer.[24] Susceptibility genes are neither necessary nor sufficient for disease occurrence, are often common (gene frequencies greater than 1%), and are associated with moderate familial aggregation. Common susceptibility genes, at frequencies of greater than 0.20, occur so often in the population that distinct familial aggregation may not be observed.[25]

Single Genes for Lung Cancer

A single gene for lung cancer has not yet been identified. Lung cancer has been shown to occur, on occasion, in Li-Fraumeni families, associated with inherited p53 mutations.[26] Although some lung cancer families may carry a mutated p53 gene, and breast cancer has been seen in conjunction with lung cancer, an excess of childhood cancers has not been noted, suggesting that inherited p53 mutations do not account for all the observed aggregation.

A genome-wide search for a lung cancer gene can proceed along two paths: linkage studies and relative-pair based studies.[27] Genetic linkage studies aim to localize a disease gene to a chromosomal region by identifying cosegregation of a marker gene and a putative disease gene in families more often than expected. Linkage studies require the accrual of large, multigeneration pedigrees with multiple affected family members and knowledge of the mode of disease transmission. This strategy is powerful when genetic loci are highly penetrant, but power decreases when susceptibility alleles become more common and less penetrant.[28] Relative-pair based methods are also used to detect linkage by demonstrating that affected relatives inherit an identical chromosomal region more often than expected by chance. This approach does not require specification of a mode of inheritance or the collection of large pedigrees, but it may be less powerful than a correctly specified linkage model. The difficulties in pursuing either of these approaches with lung cancer are that lung cancer families are rare, with cases having two or more first-degree relatives affected occurring in only 1% of the population, onset is usually in the mid to late 60s, and because of the high case fatality for lung cancer, affected relatives are typically deceased, requiring the used of fixed tissue for genotyping. Because of the large environmental component to risk, smoking data must be collected on all family members, many of whom may also be deceased.

The Genetic Epidemiology of Lung Cancer Consortium (GELCC) was formed in 1996 and recently funded by the NCI to conduct the first multicenter linkage study to identify a gene for lung cancer. Participating centers include the University of Cincinnati College of Medicine, Karmanos Cancer Institute/Wayne State University School of Medicine, Johns Hopkins University, MD Anderson Cancer Center, University of Texas Southwestern Medical Center, Medical College of Ohio, University of Colorado Health Sciences Center, and the National Human Genetics Research Institute. The GELCC plans to identify high-risk lung cancer families, to genotype informative family members using 400 markers evenly spaced throughout the genome, and to map a gene for lung cancer using genetic linkage analysis.

Susceptibility Genes for Lung Cancer

The existence of common susceptibility genes for lung cancer is also supported by findings of moderate familial aggregation. Candidate susceptibility genes include those associated with carcinogen metabolism, DNA repair, and alpha-1-antitrypsin.

Metabolic Enzyme Polymorphisms

Several genetically determined polymorphisms in the microsomal mixed-function oxidases (cytochrome P450s/phase I) and phase II enzymes have been studied. Phase I enzymes metabolically activate procarcinogens to genotoxic electrophilic intermediates that can bind DNA (Figure 21.1). DNA adducts, if not repaired or removed, can lead to mutations within oncogenes or tumor-suppressor genes initiating the carcinogenic process. Phase II enzymes detoxify genotoxic intermediates by conjugation, forming water-soluble compounds that are excreted by the cell (Figure 21.1). Individual differences in susceptibility to carcinogens are thought to result from the balance between the formation of genotoxic intermediates and detoxification. Individuals who rapidly move through phase I metabolism and are defi-cient in phase II metabolism, resulting in the accumulation of genotoxic intermediates, are presumed to be at increased risk of lung cancer.

The most widely studied polymorphic loci coding for enzymes involved in the activation and conjugation of tobacco smoke constituents are the cytochrome P450, phase I enzymes CYP1A1, CYP2E1, and the phase II glutathione S-transferases (GSTM1, GSTT1, GSTP1), and N-acetyltransferases (NAT2). Although only limited evidence indicates that CYP2D6 is involved in the metabolism of carcinogens in tobacco smoke, polymorphisms at this locus have also been studies in relation to lung cancer.[29] Several reviews of the associations among these genetic polymorphisms and lung cancer risk have been published, and only a brief overview will be given.[29-32]

Evidence for an association between *CYP1A1* polymorphisms and risk of lung cancer has come primarily from studies in Japanese populations with risks increased more than two-fold[33] and more recently in a population in Hawaii, which included Caucasians, Japanese, and Hawaiians.[34] Risk associated with *CYP1A1* genotype has not been detected in studies of populations in Brazil,[35] Norway,[36] Finland,[37] or the United States.[38] Frequencies of variant alleles differ markedly by ethnicity, with higher frequencies in the Japanese population. Studies in populations with lower frequencies of variant alleles may be underpowered to detect risk differences.

A recent metaanalysis of studies of *CYP2D6* polymorphisms and lung cancer concludes that individuals characterized as poor metabolizers, either by phenotype or genotype, are at reduced risk of lung cancer (odds ratio (OR) = 0.69; 95% Cl 0.52–0.90).[39] Expressed in terms of risk associated with extensive metabolism, extensive metabolizers are at 1.4-fold increased risk of developing lung cancer. Two other reviews have estimated that lung cancer risk associated with extensive metabolism is increased 2.3-fold (95% Cl 1.6–3.4)[40] or not increased at all (OR = 1.05; 95% Cl 0.75–1.47).[41] Bouchardy et al.[42] demonstrated that increased lung cancer risk was only associated with *CYP2D6* phenotype in heavy smokers. Variations by smoking status may explain some of the conflicting findings.

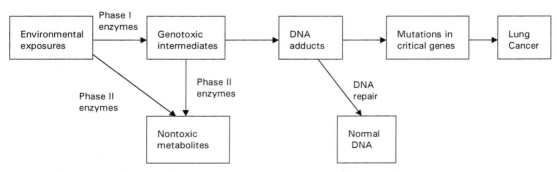

FIGURE 21.1. The role of phase I and phase II enzymes and DNA repair in lung carcinogenesis.

Variants of *CYP2E1* have not been associated with increased risk of lung cancer in Japan,[43] Brazil,[35] or Finland.[37] A recent study in Hawaii reported a 10-fold decrease in risk of lung cancer in individuals homozygous for the variant alleles.[34]

Glutathione S-transferases, examples of phase II enzymes, occur in several classes. *GSTM1* occurs in the null form in approximately 50% of the population. The most recent metaanalysis estimates an overall OR of 1.13 (95% Cl 1.04–1.25), suggesting modest increased risk associated with the *GSTM1* null genotype.[44] An earlier review provides a slightly larger OR of 1.41 (95% Cl 1.23–1.61), concluding that *GSTM1* deficiency accounts for approximately 17% of all lung cancer cases.[45] Polymorphisms in *GSTT1*[46] and *GSTP1* have not been as well studied. Individuals carrying the null *GSTT1* genotype have not been shown to be at increased risk of lung cancer unless also carrying the *GSTM1* null genotype.[47,48] In two studies, the *GSTP1* low-activity allele has been associated with an approximately twofold increased risk.[49,50]

Only a few studies have been conducted of *NAT2* genotype and lung cancer risk; two studies have had negative findings.[51,52] Cascorbi et al.[53] found a 2.4-fold (95% Cl 1.05–5.32) excess risk when *NAT2*4/*4*, was overexpressed yielding fast acetylation. One study found increased risk for slow acetylators among never smokers but an increased risk for rapid acetylators among smokers.[54] The dual role of *NAT2* in both activation and deactivation of arylamines complicate these studies.

The results from several of these studies suggest that the effects of a metabolic enzyme phenotype or genotype may be more evident at low levels of exposure to carcinogens.[35,55,56] At high exposure levels, saturation of enzyme activity may occur among both rapid and slow metabolizers.[57] This activity may not occur among those individuals with lower exposures, so the effects of genotype are more likely to be evident.

The identification of nonsmoking and early-onset lung cancer cases may serve to characterize families with altered metabolism of carcinogens and increased susceptibility. In the author's Detroit study, preliminary analyses of the polymorphisms in *CYP1A1, CYP2E1,* and *CYP1B1* have been conducted. Among nonsmokers, individuals carrying at least one copy of the exon 7 Val allele in *CYP1A1* were at twofold increased risk of developing lung cancer (95% Cl 0.6–6.6) after adjusting for age, race, sex, and environmental tobacco smoke exposure.[58] When the analysis was limited to nonsmokers with passive smoke exposure, the OR was somewhat higher, 2.3 (95% Cl 0.7–8.1). Excess risk associated with the *CYP1A1* variant allele was highest among nonsmokers under age 60 (OR = 3.6; 95% Cl 0.7–19.7). Although these findings are not statistically significant, they suggest that the *CYP1A1* exon 7 polymorphism may contribute to risk of early-onset lung cancer among nonsmokers. No increased risk of lung cancer was

associated with the *CYP2E1* Rsal polymorphism in nonsmokers (OR = 0.69; 95% Cl 0.08–6.29). These analyses are continuing, and the larger sample sizes, with the associated increase in power, will allow for a more complete evaluation and exploration of gene-environment and gene-gene interactions.

Cytochrome P4501B1 is a newly identified enzyme that activates polycyclic aromatic hydrocarbons (PAHs) (see also Chapter 3), several aryl amines, and heterocyclic amines to genotoxic metabolites[59,60] and is present in the lung. A polymorphism in the gene coding for this enzyme, a C-to-G transversion in exon 3, results in an amino acid change from Leu-432 to Val.[61,62] In preliminary analysis, nonsmokers in the Detroit study carrying the Val/Val genotype have been shown to be at five times higher risk of lung cancer than nonsmokers carrying either the Leu/Leu or Leu/Val genotype (95% Cl 2.4–14.9)(63). Sixty-four percent of these cases reported exposure to environmental tobacco smoke. A statistically insignificant twofold increased risk of early-onset lung cancer was associated with the Val/Val genotype. Eighty percent of the early-onset cases were smokers. This is the only study to date to investigate the relationship between *CYP1B1* and lung cancer risk. These data suggest that when exposure is low, the contribution of low-penetrant susceptibility genes may be revealed.

In general, studies of metabolic enzyme polymorphisms have yielded conflicting results. Conclusions from these studies have been limited by the low frequency of some polymorphisms in the population, variability in allele frequencies by ethnicity, the potential for heterogeneity by histologic type of lung cancer, and variation in risk associated with level of exposure to tobacco smoke. One genotype is unlikely to have a strong effect on risk and interactions between *CYP1A1* and *GSTM1*,[64,65] and *GSTM1* and *GSTT1*[47,48] have been reported. To fully evaluate the role of these polymorphisms in lung cancer risk, alterations at several loci, gene-gene interactions, and gene-environment interactions must be considered, necessitating extremely large, well-designed studies.

Mutagen Sensitivity and DNA Repair Capacity

Individual variability in DNA repair capacity may contribute to inherited susceptibility to lung cancer, with individuals who are unable to repair DNA damage, or do so at a slower rate, accumulating mutations that may modulate risk (Figure 21.1). The mutagen sensitivity assay measures chromatid breaks in cultured lymphocytes after exposure to bleomycin[66] or BPDE (Benzo[a]pyrene Diol Epoxide)[67] as an indirect measure of DNA excision repair effectiveness. The extent of genetic damage in lymphocytes is thought to reflect damage in target tissues.[68] Increased numbers of bleomycin or BPDE-induced breaks have been associated with a 4.3- and 7.3-fold increased risk of lung cancer, respectively.[69] As has been shown for some metabolic enzyme polymorphisms, risk of lung cancer associated with mutagen sensitivity in nonsmokers and light smokers was higher than that seen for smokers and higher in younger as compared to older individuals. These findings suggest that those who are mutagen sensitive may be susceptible at earlier ages and at lower exposures than individuals with fewer mutagen-induced breaks.

Mutagen sensitivity has been shown to correlate with DNA repair capacity.[70] In a pilot study of 51 lung cancer patients and 56 controls, DNA repair capacity was measured using the host-cell reactivation assay.[71] Cases were more likely to have reduced DNA repair capacity (OR = 5.7; 95% Cl 2.1–15.7) after adjustment for age, sex, ethnicity, and smoking status. Amino acid substitution variants have been identified in several DNA repair genes (i.e., ERCC1, XPD, XPF, XRCC3, and XRCCl), and studies of these polymorphisms and risk of lung cancer are warranted.[72]

α-1-Antitrypsin

α-1-Antitrypsin is an inhibitor of serine proteinases, protecting the lower respiratory system from damage by neutrophil elastase. A deficiency in this enzyme, associated with the *Pi* S or Z alleles, increases risk of emphysema.[73] Chronic obstructive pulmonary disease (COPD) and lung cancer share risk factors, can both be familial, and the presence of a history of COPD increases risk of lung cancer (See also Chapters 20, 22),[74–76] suggesting that α-1-antitrypsin might also be important in the development of lung cancer, especially in those individuals with low levels of exposure to tobacco smoke. In a recent study, the frequency of α-1-antitrypsin deficiency (α1AD) in a hospital-based series of lung cancer patients was compared to published α1AD frequencies of 7%.[77] Overall, lung cancer patients had a higher α1AD frequency (12.3%). The 34 nonsmoking lung cancer cases in the study had an α1AD rate of 20.6%. This study was unable to adjust for ethnicity, tobacco exposure, or other potential confounders, such as COPD, because it lacked a control group.

In preliminary analyses of the Detroit data for nonsmokers, individuals carrying either the *Pi* S or Z alleles were at 2.6-fold increased risk of lung cancer (95% Cl 0.7–9.1).[78] The carrier frequency was 15.6% in the nonsmoking cases and 5.8% in nonsmoking controls. In nonsmokers under age 60 years, the OR was 13.8 (95% Cl 1.4–137), whereas in nonsmokers 60 years of age or older the OR was 1.7 (95% Cl 0.3–8.3) after adjustment for age, sex, race, and environmental tobacco smoke exposure. These analyses need to be completed for the entire data set, but the findings suggest that α1AD may be associated with earlier onset lung cancer among nonsmokers.

Results from case-control studies of polymorphic loci and cancer risk must be interpreted with caution. If disease incidence and allele frequencies vary by ethnicity, spurious results might arise.[79] Proper selection of control populations

and stratification by ethnicity in the analysis are essential. It should be emphasized that there is likely to be tremendous heterogeneity in lung cancer cause, and the role of lung cancer susceptibility genes should not be underestimated. These genes may be of high frequency and associated with a substantial attributable risk in the population, even when the relative risk of lung cancer is increased only moderately. Large numbers of nonsmoking and early-onset lung cancer patients have not been studied at these candidate loci, and these subgroups may provide the most insight. African Americans and females have also been under-represented, even though, in younger age groups, the incidence of lung cancer among African Americans is higher than in whites, and women have rates comparable to men. The inclusion of multiple polymorphic loci studied within the same population will allow for the study of gene-gene interactions.

SUMMARY

Substantial evidence supports an inherited component to lung cancer. Familial aggregation has been demonstrated, and contributions by a major gene for lung cancer have been suggested. Although a single gene for lung cancer has not yet been identified, several susceptibility genes have been associated with moderately increased risk. Future studies need to consider a wide range of design strategies, including (a) family-based studies with the collection of family history beyond first-degree relatives to further evaluated modes of inheritance and heterogeneity by age at diagnosis; (b) large population-based studies of candidate susceptibility genes and gene-gene and gene-environment interactions; and (c) linkage studies with genome-wide searches for single genes to more fully understand the role of inherited susceptibility in lung cancer. Lung cancer is one of the major cancers, for which only minimal progress has been made in early detection and treatment. Because it is the leading cause of death from cancer, it is exceedingly important to identify high-risk populations. Once high-risk individuals with a genetic predisposition can be identified, they can be targeted for early education, access to developing screening methods, and close medical follow-up.

REFERENCES

1. Hammond EC, Seidman H. Smoking and cancer in the United States. *Prev Med* 1980;9:169.
2. Mattson ME, Pollack ES, Cullen JW. What are the odds that smoking will kill you? *Am J Public Health* 1987;77:425.
3. King, MC, Lee GM, Spinner NB, et al. Genetic epidemiology. *Am Rev Public Health* 1984;5:1.
4. Tokuhata GK, Lilienfeld AM. Familial aggregation of lung cancer in humans. *J Natl Cancer Instit* 1963;30:289.
5. Ooi WL, Elston RC, Chen VW, et al. Increased familial risk for lung cancer. *J Natl Cancer Instit* 1986;76:217.
6. Samet J, Humble C, Pathak D. Personal and family history of respiratory disease and lung cancer risk. *Am Rev Respir Dis* 1986; 134:466.

7. Wu AH, Yu MC, Thomas DC, et al. Personal and family history of lung disease as risk factors for adenocarcinoma of the lung. *Cancer Res* 1988;48:279.

8. Shaw GL, Falk RT, Pickle LW, et al. Lung cancer risk associated with cancer in relatives. *J Clin Epidemiol* 1991;44(4/5):429.

9. Osann KE. Lung cancer in women: the importance of smoking, family history of cancer, and medical history of respiratory diseases. *Cancer Res* 1991;51:4893.

10. Schwartz AG, Yang P, Swanson GM. Familial risk of lung cancer among nonsmokers and their relatives. *Am J Epidemiol* 1996; 144:554.

11. Wu AH, Fontham ETH, Reynolds P, et al. Family history of cancer and risk of lung cancer among lifetime nonsmoking women in the United States. *Am J Epidemiol* 1996;143:535.

12. Khoury MJ, Beaty TH, Cohen BH. *Fundamentals of genetic epidemiology.* New York: Oxford University Press, 1993.

13. Sellers TA, Ooi WL, Elston RC, et al. Increased familial risk for non-lung cancer among relatives of lung cancer patients. *Am J Epidemiol* 1987;126(2):237.

14. Lesnick TG, Yang P, Schwartz AG. Familial aggregation of adenocarcinoma of the lung in female nonsmoking probands. *Am J Hum Genet* 1997;61:A204.

15. Schwartz AG, Rothrock M, Yang P, et al. Increased cancer risk among relatives of nonsmoking lung cancer cases. *Genet Epidemiol* 1999;17:1.

16. Schwartz AG, Seigfried JM, Weiss L. Familial aggregation of breast cancer with early onset lung cancer. *Gene Epidemiol.* 17; 274.

17. Sellers TA, Bailey-Wilson JE, Elston RC, et al. Evidence for Mendelian inheritance in the pathogenesis of lung cancer. *J Natl Cancer Inst* 1990;82:1272.

18. Sellers TA, Bailey-Wilson JE, Potter JD, et al. Effect of cohort differences in smoking prevalence on models of lung cancer susceptibility. *Genet Epidemiol* 1992;9:261.

19. Sellers TA, Chen P-L, Potter JD, et al. Segregation analysis of smoking-associated malignancies: evidence for Mendelian inheritance. *Am J Med Gene* 1994;52:308.

20. Yang P, Schwartz AG, McAllister AE, et al. Genetic analysis of families with nonsmoking lung cancer probands. *Gene Epidemiol* 1997;14:181.

21. Yang P, Schwartz AG, McAllister AE, et al. Lung cancer risk in families of nonsmoking probands: heterogeneity by age at diagnosis. *Gene Epidemiol.* 17;253.

22. Caporaso N, Goldstein A. Cancer genes: single and susceptibility: exposing the difference. *Pharmacogenet* 1995;5:59.

23. Cavenee WK, Koufos A, Hansen MF. Recessive mutant genes predisposing to human cancer. *Mutat Res* 1986;168:3.

24. Miki Y, Swensen J, Shattuck-Eidens D, et al. Isolation of BRCA1, the 17q-linked breast and ovarian cancer susceptibility gene. *Science* 1994;266:66.

25. Easton D, Peto J. The contribution of inherited predisposition to cancer incidence. *Cancer Surveys* 1990;3:396.

26. Malkin D, Li FP, Strong LC, et al. Germ line p53 mutations in a familial syndrome of breast cancer sarcomas and other neoplasms. *Science* 1990;250:1233.

27. Lander ES, Shork NJ. Genetic dissection of complex traits. *Science* 1994;265:2037.

28. Risch N, Merikanges K. The future of genetic studies of complex human diseases. *Science* 1996;273:1516.

29. Hecht SS. Tobacco smoke carcinogens and lung cancer. *J Natl Cancer Inst* 1999;91:1194.

30. Nebert DW, McKinnon RA, Puga A. Human drug-metabolizing enzyme polymorphisms: effects on risk of toxicity and cancer. *DNA Cell Biol* 1996;15:273.

31. Hengstler JG, Arand M, Herrero ME, et al. Polymorphisms of N-acetyltransferases, glutathione S-transferases, microsomal epoxide hydrolase and sulfotransferases: influence on cancer susceptibility. *Recent Results Cancer Res* 1998;154:47.

32. Hirvonen A. Polymorphisms of xenobiotic-metabolizing enzymes and susceptibility of cancer. *Environ Health Perspect* 1999; 107(Suppl 1):37.

33. Kawajiri K, Nakachi K, Imai K, et al. Identification of genetically high risk individuals to lung cancer by DNA polymorphisms of the cytochrome P450IA1 gene. *FEBS* 1990;263:131.

34. LeMarchand L, Sivaraman L, Pierce L, et al. Associations of CYP1A1, GSTM1, and CYP2E1 polymorphisms with lung cancer suggest cell type specificities to tobacco carcinogens. *Cancer Res* 1998;58:4858.

35. Sugimura H, Hamada GS, Suzuki I, et al. CYP1A1 and CYP2E1 polymorphisms and lung cancer, a case-control study in Rio de Janeiro, Brazil. *Pharmacogenet* 1995;5:S145.

36. Tefre T, Ryberg D, Haugen A, et al. Human CYP1A1 (cytochrome P_1450) gene: lack of association between the MspI RFLP and incidence of lung cancer in a Norwegian population. *Pharmacogenet* 1991;1:20.

37. Hirvonen A, Husgafvel-Pursianinen K, Antilla S, et al. Metabolic cytochrome P450 genotypes and assessment of individual susceptibility to lung cancer. *Pharmacogenet* 1992;2:259.

38. Shields PG, Caporaso NE, Falk RT, et al. Lung cancer, risk, and a CYP1A1 genetic polymorphism. *Cancer Epidemiol Biomarkers Prev* 1993;2:481.

39. Rostami-Hodjegan A, Lennard MS, Woods HF, et al. Meta-analysis of studies of the CYP2D6 polymorphism in relation to lung cancer and Parkinson's disease. *Pharmacogenet* 1998;8:227.

40. Amos CI, Caporaso NE, Weston A. Host factors in lung cancer risk: a review of interdisciplinary studies. *Cancer Epidemiol Biomarkers Prev* 1992;1:505.

41. Christensen PM, Gotzsche PC, Brosen K. The sparteine/debrisoquine (CYP2D6) oxidation polymorphism and the risk of lung cancer: a meta-analysis. *Eur J Clin Pharmacol* 1997;51:389.

42. Bouchardy C, Benhamou S, Dayer P. The effects of tobacco on lung cancer risk depends on CYP2D6 activity. *Cancer Res* 1996; 56:251.

43. Watanabe J, Yang JP, Eguchi H, et al. An RsaI polymorphism in the CYP2E1 gene does not affect lung cancer risk in a Japanese population. *Jpn J Cancer Res* 1995;86:245.

44. Houlston RS. Glutathione S-transferase M1 status and lung cancer risk: a meta-analysis. *Cancer Epidemiol Biomarkers Prev* 1999; 8:675.

45. McWilliams JE, Sanderson BJS, Harris EL, et al. Glutathione S-transferase MI (GSTM1) deficiency and lung cancer risk. *Cancer Epidemiol Biomarkers Prev* 1995;4:589.

46. Rebbeck TR. Molecular epidemiology of the human glutathione S-transferase genotype GSTM1 and GSTT1 in cancer susceptibility. *Cancer Epidemiol Biomarkers Prev* 1997;6:733.

47. Kelsey KT, Spitz MR, Zuo Z-F, et al. Polymorphisms in the glutathione S-transferase class mu and theta genes interact and increase susceptibility to lung cancer in minority populations. *Cancer Causes Control* 1997;8:554.

48. Jourenkova N, Reinikanen M, Bouchardy C, et al. Effects of glutathione S-transferase GSTM1 and GSTT1 genotypes on lung cancer risk in smokers. *Pharmacogenet* 1997;7:515.

49. Ryberg D, Skaug V, Hewer A, et al. Genotypes of glutathione transferase M1 and P1 and their significance for lung DNA adduct levels and cancer risk. *Carcinogenesis* 1997;18:1285.

50. Harries LW, Stubbins MJ, Forman D, et al. Identification of genetic polymorphism at the glutathione S-transferase Pi locus and association with susceptibility to bladder, testicular and prostate cancer. *Carcinogenesis* 1997;18:641.

51. Roots I, Brockmoller J, Drakoulis N, et al. Mutant genes of cytochrome P-450IID6, glutathione S-transferase class mu, and

arylamine N-acetyltransferase in lung cancer patients. *Clin Investig* 1992;70:307.

52. Martinez C, Agundez JAG, Olivera M, et al. Lung cancer and mutations at the polymorphic NAT2 gene locus. *Pharmacogene* 1995;5:207.

53. Cascorbi I, Brockmoller J, Mrozikiewicz PM, et al. Homozygous rapid arylamine N-acetyltransferase (NAT2) genotype as a susceptibility factor for lung cancer. *Cancer Res* 1996;56:3961.

54. Nyberg F, Hou SM, Hemminki K, et al. Glutathione S-transferase 1 and N-acetyltransferase 2 genetic polymorphisms and exposure to tobacco smoke in nonsmoking and smoking lung cancer patients and population controls. *Cancer Epidemiol Biomarkers Prev* 1998;7:875.

55. Nakachi K, Imai K, Hayashi S, et al. Genetic susceptibility to squamous cell carcinoma of the lung in relation to cigarette smoking dose. *Cancer Res* 1991;51:5177.

56. Vineis P, Martone T. Genetic-environmental interactions and low-level exposure to carcinogens. *Epidemiol* 1995;6:455.

57. Vineis P, Bartsch H, Caporaso N, et al. Genetically based N-acetyltransferase metabolic polymorphism and low level environmental exposure to carcinogens. *Nature* 1994;369:154.

58. Schwartz AG, Lassige D, Gillen-Caralli D, et al. CYP1A1 and CYP2E1 polymorphisms and lung susceptibility among nonsmokers. *Am J Epidemiol* 1998;147:S21.

59. Shimad T, Hayes CL, Yamazaki H, et al. Activation of chemically diverse procarcinogens by human cytochrome P450 1B1. *Cancer Res* 1996;56:2979.

60. Spink DC, Spink BC, Cao JQ, et al. Differential expression of CYP1A1 and CYP1B1 in human breast epithelial cells and breast tumor cells. *Carcinogenesis* 1998;19:291.

61. Stoilov I, Akarsu AN, Sarfarazi M. Identification of three different truncating mutations in cytochrome P4501B1 (CYP1B1) as the principle cause of primary congenital glaucoma (Buphthalmos) in families linked to the GLC3A locus on chromosome 2p21. *Human Molec Genet* 1997;6:641.

62. Tang YM, Green B, Chen GF, et al. Genetic polymorphisms of human CYP1B1 gene. *Proc Am Assoc Cancer Res USA* 1998;39:626.

63. Schwartz AG, Lassige D, Gillen-Caralli D, et al. CYP1B1 and risk of early Onset and non-cigarette smoking associated lung cancer. *Proc Am Assoc Cancer Res USA* 1999;40:90.

64. Hayashi S, Watanabe J, Kawajiri K. High susceptibility to lung cancer analyzed in terms of combined genotypes of P4501A1 and Mu-class glutathione S-transferase genes. *Jpn J Cancer Res* 1992;83:866.

65. Alexandrie A-K, Sundberg MI, Seidegard J, et al. Genetic susceptibility to lung cancer with special emphasis on CYP1A1 and GSTM1: a study on host factors in relation to age at onset, gender and histological cancer types. *Carcinogenesis* 1994;15:1785.

66. Hsu TC, Johnson DA, Cherry LM, et al. Sensitivity of geneotoxic effects of bleomycin in humans: possible relationship to environmental carcinogenesis. *Int J Cancer* 1989;43:403.

67. Wei Q, Gu J, Cheng L, et al. Benzo(a)pyrene diol epoxide-induced chromosomal aberrations and risk of lung cancer. *Cancer Res* 1996;56:3975.

68. Hagmar I, Brogger A, Hansteen IL, et al. Cancer risk in humans predicted by increased levels of chromosomal aberrations in lymphocytes: nordic study group on the health risk of chromosome damage. *Cancer Res* 1994;54:2919.

69. Amos CI, Xu W, Spitz MR. Is there a genetic basis for lung cancer susceptibility? *Recent Results Cancer Res* 1999;151:3.

70. Wei Q, Spitz MR, Gu J, et al. DNA repair capacity correlates with mutagen sensivity in lymphoblastoid cell lines. *Cancer Epidemiol Biomarkers Prev* 1996;5:199.

71. Wei Q, Cheng L, Hong WK, et al. Reduced DNA repair capacity in lung cancer patients. *Cancer Res* 1996;56:4103.

72. Shen MR, Jones IM, Mohrenweiser H. Nonconservative amino acid substitution variants exist at polymorphic frequency in DNA repair genes in healthy humans. *Cancer Res* 1998;58:604.

73. Crystal RG, Brantly ML, Hubbard RC, et al. The alpha-antitrypsin gene and its mutations: Clinical consequences and strategies for therapy. *Chest* 1989;95:196.

74. Wu AH, Fontham ET, Reynolds P, et al. Previous lung diseases and risk of lung cancer among lifetime nonsmoking women in the United States. *Am J Epidemiol* 1995;141:1023.

75. Cohen BH, Graves CG, Levy DA, et al. A common familial component in lung cancer and chronic obstructive pulmonary disease. *Lancet* 1977;September:523.

76. Alavanja MCR, Brownson RC, Boice JD, et al. Preexisting lung disease and lung cancer among nonsmoking women. *Am J Epidemiol* 1992;136:623.

77. Yang P, Wentzlaff KA, Katzman JA, et al. Alpha-antitrypsin deficiency allele carriers among lung cancer patients. *Cancer Epidemiol Biomarkers Prev* 1999;8:461.

78. Schwartz AG, Lassige D, Gillen-Caralli D, et al. Alpha-1-antitrypsin carrier status and lung cancer risk among nonsmokers. *Am J Epidemiol* 1998;147:S21.

79. Khoury MJ, Flanders WD. Nontraditional epidemiologic approaches in the analysis of gene-environment interaction: case-control studies with no controls! *Am J Epidemiol* 1996;144:207.

22

EARLY DIAGNOSIS AND INTERVENTION IN LUNG CANCER: CLINICAL STUDIES

THOMAS L. PETTY
YORK E. MILLER

Lung cancer is the most common fatal malignancy in both men and women in the United States. In 1999, an estimated 171,600 patients will be diagnosed. Because the diagnosis is most commonly made in later stages, including presentations that manifest as distant metastasis, approximately 158,900 deaths will occur in 1999, if the current survival statistics continue. Today, lung cancer is the third most common cause of death in the world. Worldwide, lung cancer was responsible for more than 900,000 deaths in 1990.[1]

Studies examining the efficacy of screening for lung cancer carried out in the 1970s and 1980s have led to a nihilistic attitude regarding the early diagnosis of lung cancer. Easily obtained clinical indices that can be used to identify individuals at high risk for the development of lung cancer were not appreciated at the time of design of the large screening trials. Unfortunately, these trials were carried out in populations that are not at greatly increased risk for lung cancer and may have yielded falsely discouraging results. The purpose of this chapter is to present an approach to early identification and intervention that could dramatically alter the course and outcome of lung cancer today.

HISTORICAL PERSPECTIVE

The association between chronic lung disease and lung cancer was recognized more than 40 years ago (see also Chapter 20). Advanced emphysema, chronic bronchitis, and chronic tuberculosis antedated the diagnosis of lung cancer in 45 of 86 patients over a 10-year period. More than 90% of these 86 patients had a chronic cough prior to the diagnosis of lung cancer. Ironically, in that era, chest x-rays and sputum cytology screening for lung cancer were advised.[2,3] Later, it was again emphasized that lung cancer commonly accompanied chronic lung diseases such as chronic bronchitis.[4]

On December 4, 1951, the Philadelphia Neoplasm Research Project was initiated to study the natural history of bronchogenic carcinoma in a population of older men by semiannual chest mini photofluorograms and a symptom questionnaire. By December 1965, the project was completed. In all, 6,137 male smokers were enrolled. One hundred fifty-six histologically confirmed lung cancers had been identified; 66 on enrollment and 90 after enrollment.[5] Upon completion of this study, The Philadelphia Neoplasm Research Project concluded that early diagnosis of lung cancer was impractical and did not result in reduced mortality.

In the mid-1970s, the National Cancer Institute (NCI) funded three studies, which were conducted at the Johns Hopkins Medical School,[6] the Memorial Sloan-Kettering Cancer Center,[7] and the Mayo Clinic.[8] These studies enrolled men in a screening program using serial chest x-rays and sputum cytologic studies. At the end of these studies, it was again concluded that screening for lung cancer does not reduce mortality from lung cancer. A study of men at high risk in Czechoslovakia also concluded a lack of benefit from semiannual screening.[9]

With the benefit of hindsight, it is now clear that serious deficiencies existed in the design of these studies. All sought to study high-risk smokers, but the association of airflow obstruction with susceptibility to lung cancer was not widely appreciated at the time of design of these studies and was therefore not exploited to define a high-risk group. The entrance criteria for tobacco use were not high enough to guarantee a high risk for lung cancer (only one pack-year of smoking was required before entry in some cases). Women, who are now believed to be of higher susceptibility than men to lung cancer, were not included.

An important shortcoming was that it was believed to be unethical to have an unscreened control population, so none of the studies carried out in the United States had an unscreened control group. The Memorial Sloan-Kettering and Johns Hopkins studies compared yearly with more intensive screening regimens, and the Mayo study compared screening every three months with a recommendation to have yearly screening. It was hoped that the control group (recommended to have yearly screening), would contain a sizable subgroup that did not comply with this recommendation, but this subgroup was not as large as hoped. It is important to appreciate that at the time these studies were conducted, the yearly chest radiograph was a standard component of health care. In summary, the current practice of not performing any studies on high-risk smokers or ex-smokers with airflow obstruction, sputum production, or additional exposures to carcinogens such as asbestos or radon daughters has not been shown to be equally efficacious as screening; the question has not been studied.

The results of the Mayo Clinic study have now been revisited.[8] Strauss has concluded that, in fact, early identification did result in improved survival in patients found with early stages of disease. Perhaps the Johns Hopkins study is even more revealing because it showed that many cases of lung cancer that were missed might have been diagnosed using more modern techniques applied to libraried sputum cytology specimens.[11]

The NCI studies resulted in a shift of diagnosis to more early stages of disease, and meaningful improvements were made in resectability, survival, and fatality of lung cancer. Although overall mortality was not improved by screening, these studies did demonstrate higher 5-year survival rates than expected. Nonetheless, the current dogma is that screening for lung cancer is not worthwhile, and it is not recommended for even large populations of high-risk smokers.[12]

THE ASSOCIATION BETWEEN CHRONIC AIRFLOW OBSTRUCTION AND LUNG CANCER

The strong association between the presence of airflow obstruction and lung cancer has been known for more than two decades.[13,14] More recent studies have strengthened this association.[15,16] An interesting observation of the Lung Health Study sheds additional light on this relationship. In a sample of middle-aged men and women, over the age of 35, but not yet 60, with only mild degrees of airflow obstruction and with the requirement of smoking at least a pack a day for 10 years (i.e., 10 pack-years), 5,887 patients were followed for 5 years.[17] The main objective of this study was to learn the impact of intervention via smoking cessation and the use of a bronchodilating anticholinergic aerosol on the rate of decline of ventilatory function. In brief, those patients (approximately 22%) who were sustained quitters throughout the 5-year follow-up had a slight improvement in lung function, followed by only a minor decline (Figure 22.1). At the end of 5 years, ventilatory function as judged by FEV was only slightly below the mean FEV, levels at enrollment. By contrast, those patients who continued to smoke had much more rapid rates of decline. One of the most interesting features of this study was the cause of death, presented in Table 22.1. Fifty-seven, or 1%, had died of lung cancer by the end of 5 years. At this writing, another group of patients have emerged with lung cancer in a late

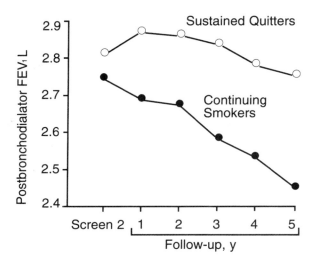

FIGURE 22.1. Mean postbronchodilator forced expiratory volume at 1 second (FEV1) for participants in the smoking intervention and placebo group who were sustained quitters (○) and continuing smokers (●). The two curves diverge sharply after baseline. (From Anthonisen NR, Connett JE, Kiley JP, et al. Effects of smoking intervention and the use of an inhaled anticholinergic bronchodilator on the rate of decline in FEV$_1$. The Lung Health Study. *JAMA* 1994;272:1,497, with permission.)

follow-up. Now, more than 100 (i.e., approximately 2%), have either died or developed lung cancer. One would have expected that heart attack or stroke might be the most common cause of mortality, but this was not the case, (n = 37). Thus 20 more lung cancer deaths than heart attack and stroke deaths were reported during the follow-up. Unfortunately, no chest x-rays were done during the Lung Health Study to learn whether or not lung cancer was present at the time of enrollment. One can conclude from all of these studies linking airflow obstruction to lung cancer that the increased risk is approximately four- to six-fold, compared to when no airflow obstruction is present, with all other factors including smoking history, occupational exposures, age, sex, and family history taken into consideration.

The new wave of enthusiasm for lung volume reduction surgery has also demonstrated the strong association be-

TABLE 22.1. THE LUNG HEALTH STUDY: DEATHS WITHIN FIVE YEARS*

Cause	Special Intervention	Usual Care	Total
Lung cancer	38	19	57
Cardiovascular disease	25	12	37
Other	35	20	55
Total	98	51	149

* Randomization 2:1 special intervention to usual care.

tween advanced emphysema and lung cancer.[18] In resected tissues, 6.4% had cancer, of which several were identified only by pathologic examination. Survival at short-term follow-up was excellent.[18]

RISK FACTORS

By far, the most powerful risk factor in lung cancer is smoking. Approximately 1 in 10 smokers develop bronchogenic carcinoma over a lifetime.[19] Although no safe level of smoking exists, historical tradition has offered the notion that smoking a pack a day for 20 years (i.e., 20 pack-years) or more indicates the populations at highest risk. In general, the year that one starts to smoke and the intensity of smoking over a lifetime magnifies the smoking-related risk.[20] Passive smoking is also an established risk factor for lung cancer.[21]

Certain occupations, such as asbestos mining, those involving asbestos dust exposure, and uranium mining, along with exposure to arsenic, nickel, acrylonitrile, chromium, beryllium, cadmium, chloromethyl ether solvents, and possibly silica, are known occupational risks.[22] Diesel exhaust is considered a risk factor and may explain the increase risk of lung cancer among different types of professional drivers in Denmark.[23] Family history is a definite risk factor, as it is for many organ-associated carcinomas.[24] Consumption of a diet low in fruits and vegetables (possibly because of antioxidant content), may magnify risk.[25] HIV infection may result in lung cancer occurring at a young age, often occurring after a less intense exposure to tobacco than in patients who are not HIV-infected.[26]

IDENTIFICATION OF ROENTGENOGRAPHICALLY OCCULT LUNG CANCER

Chest X-rays

Although the chest x-ray is the time-tested method of identifying lung cancer, a reassessment of the outcome of the screening studies has offered renewed hope that case finding with x-rays or screening in high-risk populations may be beneficial. The course and prognosis of cancer so identified has led to only a modest improvement in overall cancer mortality.[27] This sad reality has called for new approaches to the identification of early lung cancer.[27]

Sputum Cytology

Many years ago, Saccomanno perfected and championed the use of Papanicolaou staining of exfoliated bronchial epithelial cells to identify roentgenographically occult lung cancer. Saccomanno and others studied the evolution and development of progressive stages of dysplasia (mild,

moderate, and severe) as a prelude to carcinoma *in situ* and invasive carcinoma.[28–30] Squamous carcinomas tend to be central and exfoliate early. By contrast, adenocarcinomas, which are peripheral, do not exfoliate quite as readily. Peripheral adenocarcinomas may be more readily identified by newer imaging techniques (see following section). Sputum cytology has been considered the first step in the diagnosis of suspicious pulmonary shadows and nodules, and is less expensive in identifying the presence of malignancy, by far, than fiberoptic bronchoscopy, which is the gold standard for diagnosis today. Bronchoscopic procedures, of course, are appropriate for further confirmation of the histologic type of malignancy and staging. Newer fluorescence-intensified bronchoscopy increases the diagnostic yield in tiny tumors that are difficult to visualize by standard white light bronchoscopy. Sputum cytology is a logical first step in identifying malignancy, which could be further evaluated by invasive techniques.

RESULTS OF SCREENING FOR EARLY LUNG CANCER

Although early-stage lung cancers clearly have a better prognosis than more advanced stage tumors, this outcome may be partly a reflection of innate tumor biology. In other words, the more indolent tumors may spend more time in early-stage disease than do more aggressive tumors. Intensive screening efforts would then be expected to discover biologically more aggressive tumors at an apparently early stage, and stage-specific survival would then decrease. Several reports of outcomes from relatively small series in which an effort to diagnose early-stage lung cancer was made demonstrate excellent survival, which would not be the case if screening were ineffective for this reason.

United States

Pulmonologists working in a modest-sized rural community hospital in western Colorado (St. Mary's in Grand Junction) sought to identify cancer based on clinical clues or other risk factors. In this community, 51 consecutive patients with roentgenographically occult lung cancer were identified.[31] Forty-three men and eight women were identified between the ages of 46 and 81 (mean age 64.2); all but two were smokers. Whether or not environmental tobacco smoke could have played a role in the two nonsmokers is not known. Thirty-nine of these patients were smokers with symptoms of cough, increasing dyspnea, family history, or an x-ray lesion that appeared to be a healed scar. Patients with hemoptysis were not included in this series because hemoptysis is a known sentinel sign and symptom for lung cancer. Twelve cancer patients were screened based on occupational risks, with eleven having had significant uranium mining experience at a time when uranium was mined on the Colorado plateau. One was an asbestos worker.

In this study, sputum cytology revealed either carcinoma *in situ* or invasive carcinoma in some of the patients. Establishing the source of these abnormal cytologic findings by fiberoptic bronchoscopy was the next step. Thirty-one cancers (61%) were found on the first biopsy. Additional biopsies were required for confirmation of cancer, with two bronchoscopies required in eight cases (17%), three in another eight cases (17%), and more than three in three patients. Thus the knowledge of lung cancer, as demonstrated by sputum cytology, urged the physicians in their bronchoscopic approaches to confirmation, preparatory to surgery or other therapies. In this series, 86% were squamous carcinomas, 6% were adenocarcinomas, 4% were large cell carcinoma, and 4% were undifferentiated carcinoma. This histologic destruction reflected the fact that squamous carcinomas are central and tend to exfoliate early. As revealed in the study, sputum cytology does not identify all patients with adenocarcinoma. The cancer stage was *in situ* in 7 (14%), stage I in 38 (74%), and stage II or stage II-A in 2 (4%). Thus only four (8%) patients were at a stage precluding a surgical cure. Twenty-seven of the patients received curative surgical therapy. Their outcome is presented in Figure 22.2. Only three patients had died of cancer at 5 years. Total mortality was only nine patients. Nineteen additional patients were candidates for ablative radiation therapy. Taken together, both surgical and radiation treatments resulted in a much better lung cancer survival rate, with only 9 deaths at 5 years, and total mortality of 21

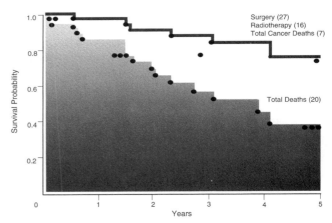

FIGURE 22.3. Actual survival in all 46 patients who received treatment with expectation of cure (27 surgery and 19 by radiation; Kaplan-Meier life table method). Both cancer deaths and deaths from all causes are included. Circles indicate time of death. Vertical lines indicate survival observation at the time of original report. (From Bechtel JJ, Kelley WR, Petty TL, et al. Outcome of 51 patients with roentgenographically occult lung cancer detected by sputum cytologic testing: a community hospital program. *Arch Intern Med* 1994;154:975, with permission.)

deaths in 5 years (Figure 22.3). This result is far better than in cancers identified either accidentally or on the basis of symptoms, where the overall cancer mortality rate is approximately 85% at 5 years.

Japan

The results of surgical treatment for roentgenographically occult bronchogenic squamous cell carcinomas has also been reported to be excellent.[32] Ninety-four such patients received surgical resection. The survival over 5 years is presented in Figures 22.4 and 22.5. A total of seven patients

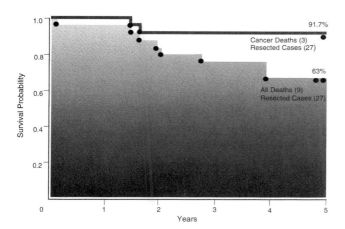

FIGURE 22.2. Survival predictions based on actuarial experience of the 27 patients who received resectional surgery for cure (Kaplan-Meier life table method). Both cancer deaths and deaths from all causes are listed. Circles indicate time of death. Vertical lines indicate survival at the time of original report. (From Bechtel JJ, Kelley WR, Petty TL, et al. Outcome of 51 patients with roentgenographically occult lung cancer detected by sputum cytologic testing: a community hospital program. *Arch Intern Med* 1994; 154:975, with permission.)

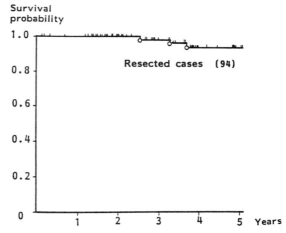

FIGURE 22.4. Survival probability of patients with resected roentgenographically occult bronchogenic SCC (time of death from lung cancer).

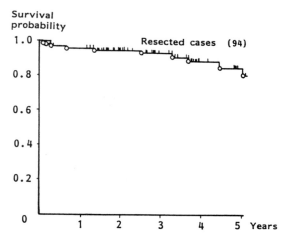

FIGURE 22.5. Survival probability of patients with resected roentgenographically occult bronchogenic SCC (time of death from all causes).

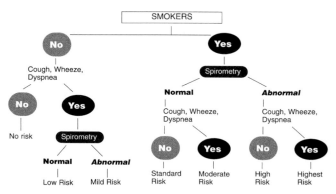

FIGURE 22.6. Algorithm to assist in the determination of level of risk of lung cancer of smokers versus non-smokers. Assumes no additional risk; for example, asbestos exposure, uranium mining, chloro methyl ethyl ether exposure, or family history of lung cancer.

with a subsequent primary cancer had surgical resection with no recurrence after the second operation. Two deaths from lung cancer occurred. These favorable results included an 80.4% survival rate at 5 years, including deaths from all causes, and a 93.5% survival rate considering only lung cancer deaths. Although subsequent primary cancers remained a challenge, the reliability of sputum cytology to identify the presence of roentgenographically occult lung cancer was exceedingly good.[32]

Scandinavia

The long-term survival of patients with lung cancer from a defined geographic area in Sweden, before and after radiologic screening, showed a much better survival with carcinoma identified with semiannual screening, compared to when it was identified following symptoms.[33] Combined survival at 4 years was 41.7%, compared to 10.3% for those discovered by symptoms (P < 0.001). Thus it seems certain that the early identification of lung cancer, either roentgenographically or by sputum cytology, will identify patients with early-stage carcinoma who are suitable for curative therapy, either by surgery or by radiation therapy.

A PRAGMATIC APPROACH TO SCREENING IN HIGH-RISK POPULATIONS

Because heavy smokers (i.e., those with airflow obstruction) and symptomatic patients are most apt to develop lung cancer, a systematic approach to stratified screening has been proposed.[34] This approach has resulted in the development of two simple algorithms, by which it was proposed that a high yield of lung cancer could be obtained in a targeted

population (Figures 22.6 and 22.7). That this approach can result in a relatively high yield of occult lung cancer was shown in a study of 613 patients, where sputum cytology was obtained at home, with mall-in specimen containers.[35] Five carcinomas *in situ* and six invasive carcinomas, both squamous and adenocarcinoma, were identified (Table 22.2). Three patients with severe atypia can also be considered to have pre- or early-stage carcinoma. Thus the yield in smokers of 30 pack-years or more with airflow obstruction is well above the yield of other screening tests for lethal malignancies such as breast cancer, where the overall yield is approximately 0.23% in women age 50 to 54 to 0.48% in women 75 to 79 years.[36] Interestingly, four more carcinomas have already been identified in the group with only moderate atypia. At this writing, the entire cohort is being followed to identify the final yield that will occur in the targeted population of heavy smokers with associated airflow obstruction.

Peripheral lung cancers, which are most often adenocarcinomas, can be readily identified by spiral CT scans, which

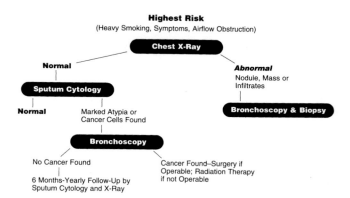

FIGURE 22.7. Practical diagnostic approach to lung cancer.

TABLE 22.2. RESULTS OF SPUTUM CYTOLOGY IN HIGH-RISK PATIENTS

Dysplasia Grade	Number	Percentage
None	72	12.0%
Regular metaplasia	63	11.0%
Mild atypia	309	50.0%
Moderate atypia	155	25.0%
Severe atypia	3	.2%
Carcinoma *in situ*	5	1.8%
Invasive carcinoma	6	
Total:	**613**	

From Kennedy TC, Proudfoot SP, Franklin WA, et al. Cytopathological analysis of sputum in patients with airflow obstruction and significant smoking histories. *Cancer Res* 1996;56:4, 673, with permission.

can be completed in 15 seconds with a single breath hold. The dose of irradiation is similar to that associated with mammography. Screening trials for lung cancer utilizing low-dose spiral CT scans are currently underway.[37,38] Recently, a new mobile CT scanner unit has been used in a population-based study that involved mass screening for lung cancer in Japan.[38] Five thousand, four hundred eighty-three people between 40 and 74 years old volunteered. This program was promoted by public announcements by local governments and by leaflets. For comparison, two control groups, from the annual general health survey (n = 10,966), were matched by sex and age within 2 years, and included the smoking habits for smokers of at least 30 pack-years. Of the 5,483 participants, 3,967 underwent CT scans and photofluorography. This group included 64% men and 36% women. Nineteen patients were diagnosed as having lung cancer (0.48%), which is significantly higher than previous standard mass assessments done in the same area. CT missed one case that was found solely on the basis of sputum cytology. Several clinically significant benign lesions were also identified in the study.

Among the 19 patients in whom the workup showed lung cancer, 18 had surgery and one refused surgery but later developed metastasis. The most frequent cell type was adenocarcinoma. Of the 19 patients, 16 were stage I and three were stage IV. It is a fact that the mini-photofluorography had shown no evidence of cancer in 18 of the 19 patients. It should be pointed out that this trial was done in rural Japan where the rate of lung cancer is reported to be low (i.e., only 30 to 50 cases expected per 100,000 in population). The authors found the CT identified almost 10 times as many cancers as were identified by standard mass screening previously done. This study strongly suggests that CT scanning may replace chest x-rays in early case finding or in screening of high-risk populations.

Most recently, the results of the Anti-Lung Cancer Association screening program were presented. From 1975 to 1993, 26,338 examinations with chest x-rays and sputum cytology were performed, with a detection rate of lung cancer at 0.16%. When low-dose spiral CT examinations were added from 1993 to 1998, 35 lung cancer cases were found in 9,452 (0.37%) examinations. Moreover, this translated to a 3-year survival of 83% from 1993 to 1998 compared to 56% in the former period.[39]

The results of the Early Lung Cancer Action Project (ELCAP) have been reported[40] and are complementary at the Japanese data. ELCAP was designed to evaluate baseline and annual repeat screening by low-radiation-dose computed tomography (low-dose CT) in people at high risk of lung cancer. One thousand symptom-free volunteers, 60 years or older, with at least 10 pack-years of cigarette smoking and no previous cancer, who were medically fit to undergo thoracic surgery were enrolled. Chest radiographs and low-dose CT were done for each participant, and noncalcified pulmonary nodules were investigated using short-term high-resolution CT follow-up for the smallest noncalcified nodules. Noncalcified nodules were detected in 23% of the participants by low-dose CT at baseline, compared to 7% by chest radiography. Malignant disease was detected in 2.7% by CT and 0.7% by chest radiography. Of the 27 CT-detected cancers, 26 were resectable. Biopsies were done on 28 of the 233 participants with noncalcified nodules; 27 had malignant noncalcified nodules and one had a benign nodule. No participant had thoracotomy for a benign nodule. These data point to the utility of low-dose CT in detecting small noncalcified nodules, which could prove to be lung cancer at an earlier and potentially more curable stage. Plans are under way for a multicenter national trial to verify these results.

DEVELOPMENT OF MOLECULAR APPROACHES TO EARLY LUNG CANCER DETECTION

Development of new approaches to identify lung cancer in sputum is being pursued. Sputum, bronchial washings, and bronchoalveolar lavage fluid are complex specimens containing a wide variety of soluble and cellular components, only a portion of which are epithelial derived. Novel techniques to derive epithelial cell–enriched specimens from sputum are being developed.[41] Computerized image analysis of Feulgen-stained exfoliated cells has shown significant promise in improving diagnostic capabilities.[41] Encouraging reports of increased sensitivity of monoclonal antibodies for detecting malignant cells in sputum have not been duplicated by additional groups, but further development of this assay is underway.[41,43] Several additional novel markers are under evaluation (see also Chapter 23), including mutation detection targeted at p53 and *ras* genes. In addition, DNA methylation is often aberrant in lung tumors,[43] and a polymerase chain reaction–based method of methylation detection has recently been applied to sputum. Although considerable excitement, has been generated regarding the application of molecular markers to the early detection of lung cancer, none of the tests developed to date are currently ready for large-scale application. Prior to applying any molecular marker to early detection of lung cancer, test characteristics, such as reproducibility (both within a laboratory and between laboratories) sensitivity, and specificity when tested in appropriate disease and control groups, need to be determined.

In addition to early detection, molecular markers have a high potential to achieve clinical application to identify high-risk individuals in whom other screening techniques might be applied for surveillance.[45] Several genetic aberrations have been described in the respiratory epithelial cells of lung cancer patients and current or ex-smokers without lung cancer,[46,47] p53 mutations affecting nonmalignant respiratory epithelial cells have only rarely been described in individuals without lung cancer and might define a group of smokers at extremely high risk for the development of cancer.[48] (see also Chapter 6) Loss of heterozygosity of chromosomes 3p and 9p can be found in most smokers studied to date and might therefore be a less attractive risk marker (see also Chapters 23, 28).[46,47] Either specific combinations or the total number of mutations detectable in respiratory epithelium may be prognostic.

A panel of biomarkers instead of a single marker will likely be required to identify occult lung cancer. The cancer gene marker may be present in exfoliated cells, which appear morphologically normal. This marker is an important new area of outcomes research, which could lead to algorithms that may increase the efficiency and reduce the cost of case finding or screening.[49,50]

ADVANCED IMAGING TECHNIQUES

Recently, F-fluorodeoxyglucose PET scanning has revealed a high degree of sensitivity and specificity in lung cancer identification,[51–54] with positive predictive values greater than 90% and negative predictive values approaching 100%. The finding of a metabolically active nodule is highly indicative of malignancy.[51] Whole-body PET scanning can be used in the staging of non–small cell cancer[54] (see also Chapter 30).

ENHANCED BRONCHOSCOPY TECHNIQUES

The best outcome in lung cancer management is treatment when the lesion is discovered in preinvasive stages. However, the intraepithelial neoplastic lesions are somewhat difficult to localize by conventional white light bronchoscopy, particularly if the bronchoscopist is not highly experienced in searching for subtle changes that may indicate lung cancer, as was the case in the Grand Junction Study.[31]

Autofluorescence bronchoscopy was introduced to detect high degrees of dysplasia or in carcinoma *in situ*[55,56] (see also Chapters 23, 24). Conventional white light bronchoscopy uses illuminated light that is reflected backscattered absorbed, but it does not induce tissue fluorescence, a process known as *reflectance imaging*. The tissue autofluorescence is not visible to the unaided eye because the intensity is low and obscured by the backscattered light. With suitable instruments, however, the autofluorescence reflected to create an image, which indicates a high likelihood of malignancy.[56] In a recent study, autofluorescence bronchoscopy, when used as an adjunct to standard white light bronchoscopy, enhanced the bronchoscopist's ability to localize small, subtle lesions, which were often malignancies, that were confined to the epithelium (i.e., *in situ* or preinvasive).[57] It is virtually certain that a cure of these lesions with surgery, radiation, and/or laser therapy will be likely. In addition, a novel new therapeutic approach, photodynamic therapy, may also achieve a cure for *in situ* and stage I carcinoma.[58,59] Fluorescent bronchoscopy can be used in surveillance of subsequent carcinomas and sputum markers, either molecular or cytomorphologically, which suggest a second or recurrent lung cancer. Surveillance employing malignancy-associated changes (MACs) is also under study as a method of detecting small peripheral adenocarcinomas and as an indication of lung cancer recurrence.[60,61]

A NEW, EXCITING APPROACH TO THE EARLY IDENTIFICATION OF LUNG CANCER

Individual cases of lung cancer must be diagnosed on the basis of clinical suspicion, bolstered by the necessary technology to prove presence and location and to determine the histologic type of malignancy. Suspicion must be based on smoking histories, family histories, occupational exposures, and symptoms. When a high-risk individual is identified (i.e., heavy smoking with any of the following: airflow obstruction, positive family history, additional carcinogenic exposures, or symptoms), systematic studies to identify the presence or absence of lung cancer seem reasonable, given the lack of currently available scientific information that attempts at early identification are not useful in this patient group. The algorithms shown in Figures 22.6 and 22.7, although overly simplistic, may be useful in this regard. Either sputum markers of malignancy using cytomorphology or standard chest x-rays or CT scans will identify the presence of a premalignant or malignant lesion (sputum), or an airway or peripheral abnormality (CT imaging). The next step is to identify the site through white light bronchoscopy or if that modality is unrevealing, with fluorescent endoscopy. When the tumor is located, a biopsy should be performed, and staging should proceed thereafter.

The phenomena of MACs may add still another surveillance tool (see also Chapter 23).[60,61] MACs are subtle alterations in the size, shape, or texture of the cell nucleus of nonmalignant exfoliated calls that appear to be a result of growth factors produced by nearby lung cancer cells. Their presence may be used in early identification or for surveillance of recurrent lung cancer.[60,61]

Today, the main diagnostic focus should be on early lesions that are amenable to cure. It is distinctly possible that early intraepithelial lesions can be dealt with by photodynamic therapy,[58,59] or other methods such as electrocautery, cryotherapy, or thermoablation, with a YAG laser or brachytherapy. Indeed, the identification of premalignant lesions would expand the possibility of controlled clinical trials in chemoprevention, using the premalignant lesions as endpoints[62,63] (see also Chapter 25).

Thus far, the growing problem of lung cancer, caused primarily by smoking, has eluded prevention, in part because of persistence of transformed epithelial cells lining the airways of aging former smokers. Recent studies have reported that similar numbers of new lung cancer cases arise from former smokers compared to current smokers.[64]

The continued seduction of 3,000 teenagers daily into the bondage of tobacco addiction with advertising financed by a tobacco industry bent on sustaining its economic success unfortunately ensures that lung cancer will remain a major clinical problem for many years, even if all recruitment of new smokers were to stop immediately. The growing tobacco epidemic has created the most vexing and recalcitrant cancer of our time. With tobacco smoking out of control in large countries such as China, we face a true global disaster. These frightening realities pose an immense challenge to clinicians and scientists who aim to reduce the socioeconomic impact of lung cancer as we approach the new millennium.

REFERENCES

1. Parkin DM, Pisani P, and Farlay J. Global cancer statistics. California, 1999;49:33.
2. Finke W. Chronic pulmonary disease in patients with lung cancer. *NY State J Med* 1958;58:3,783.
3. Lemon AH. Program for early diagnosis of cancer. *Rev Mod Med* 1959;265.
4. Rimington J. Smoking, chronic bronchitis, and lung cancer. *Br Med J* 1971;2:373.
5. Weiss W, Boucot KR, Cooper DA. Growth rate in the detection and prognosis of bronchogenic carcinoma. *JAMA* 1966;198: 1,246.
6. Frost JK, Ball WC Jr., Levin ML, et al. Early lung cancer detection: results of the initial (prevalence) radiologic and cytologic screening in the Johns Hopkins study. *Am Rev Respir Dis* 1984; 130:549.
7. Flehinger BJ, Melamed MR, Zaman MB, et al. Early lung cancer detection: results of the initial (prevalence) radiologic and cytologic screening in the Memorial Sloan-Kettering study. *Am Rev Respir Dis* 1984;130:555.
8. Fontana RS, Sanderson DR, Taylor WF, et al. Early lung cancer detection: results of the initial (prevalence) radiologic and cyto-

9. logic screening in the Mayo Clinic study. *Am Rev Respir Dis* 1984;130:561.
9. Kubik A, Parkin DM, Khlat M, et al. Lack of benefit from semi-annual screening for lung cancer of the lung: follow-up report of a randomized controlled trial on a population of high-risk males in Czechoslovakia. *Int J Cancer* 1990;45:26.
10. Strauss GM, Gleason RE, Sugarbaker DJ. Screening for lung cancer. Another look; a different view. *Chest* 1997;111:754.
11. Tockman MS, Gupta PK, Myers JD, et al. Sensitive and specific monoclonal antibody recognition of human lung cancer antigen on preserved sputum cells: a new approach to early lung cancer detection. *J Clin Oncol* 1988;6:1,685.
12. Eddy DM. Screening for lung cancer. *Ann Intern Med* 1989;111: 232.
13. Cohen BH, Diamond EL, Graves CG, et al. A common familial component in lung cancer and chronic obstructive pulmonary disease. *Lancet* 1977;2:523.
14. Cohen BH. Is pulmonary dysfunction the common denominator for the multiple effects of cigarette smoking? *Lancet* 1978;2: 1,024.
15. Skillrud DM, Offord DP, Miller RD. Higher risk of lung cancer in chronic obstructive pulmonary disease: A prospective, matched, controlled study. *Ann Intern Med* 1986;105:503.
16. Tockman MS, Anthonisen NR, Wright EC, et al. Airways obstruction and the risk for lung cancer. *Ann Intern Med* 1987; 106:512.
17. Anthonisen NR, Connett JE, Kiley JP, et al. Effects of smoking intervention and the use of an inhaled anticholinergic bronchodilator on the rate of decline in FEV_1. The Lung Health Study. *JAMA* 1994;272:1,497.
18. Hazelrigg SR, Boley TM, Weber D, et al. Incidence of lung nodules found in patients undergoing lung volume reduction. *Ann Thorac Surg* 1997;64:303.
19. Spivack SD, Fasco MJ, Walker VE, et al. The molecular epidemiology of lung cancer. *Crit Rev Toxicol* 1997;27:319.
20. Boucot KR, Weiss W, Seidman H, et al. The Philadelphia Pulmonary Neoplasm Research Project: basic risk factors of lung cancer in older men. *Am J Epidemiol* 1972;95:4.
21. Reynolds P, Fontham ET. Passive smoking and lung cancer. *Ann Med* 1995;27:633.
22. Steenland K, Loomis D, Shy C, et al. Review of occupational lung carcinogens. *Am J Ind Med* 1996;29:474.
23. Hansen J, Raaschou-Nielsen O, Olsen JH. Increased risk of lung cancer among different types of professional drivers in Denmark. *Occupat Environ Med* 1998;55:115.
24. Schwartz AG, Yang P, Swanson GM. Familial risk of lung cancer among nonsmokers and their relatives. *Am J Epidemiol* 1996; 144:554.
25. Colditz GA, Stampfer MJ, Willett WC. Diet and lung cancer. A review of the epidemiologic evidence in humans. *Arch Intern Med* 1987;147:157.
26. Wistuba II, Behrens C, Milchgrub S, et al. Comparison of molecular changes in lung cancers in HIV-positive and HIV-indeterminate subjects. *JAMA* 1998;279:1,554.
27. Roth JA. New approaches to treating early lung cancer. *Cancer Res* 1992;52:2,652S.
28. Saccomanno G, Sanders RP, Ellis H, et al. Concentration of carcinoma or atypical cells in sputum. *Acta Cytol* 1963;7:305.
29. Saccomanno G, Sanders RP, Archer VE, et al. Cancer of the lung: the cytology of sputum prior to the development of carcinoma. *Acta Cytol* 1965;9:413.
30. Greenberg SD. Diagnosis of sputum atypias by cell image analysis: a review. *Surg Synth Path Res* 1983;229.
31. Bechtel JJ, Kelley WR, Petty TL, et al. Outcome of 51 patients with roentgenographically occult lung cancer detected by sputum

cytologic testing: a community hospital program. *Arch Intern Med* 1994;154:975.

32. Saito Y, Nagamoto N, Ota S, et al. Results of surgical treatment for roentgenographically occult bronchogenic squamous cell carcinoma. *J Thorac Cardiovasc Surg* 1992;104:401.

33. Hillerdal G. Long-term survival of patients with lung cancer from a defined geographical area before and after radiological screening. *Lung Cancer* 1996;15:21.

34. Petty TL. Lung cancer screening. *Compr Ther* 1995;21:432.

35. Kennedy TC, Proudfoot SP, Franklin WA, et al. Cytopathological analysis of sputum in patients with airflow obstruction and significant smoking histories. *Cancer Res* 1996;56:4,673.

36. Salzmann P, Kerlikowske K, Phillips K. Cost-effectiveness of extending screening mammography guidelines to include women 40 to 49 year of age. *Ann Intern Med* 1997;127:955.

37. Kaneko M, Egucki K, Ohmatsu H, et al. Peripheral lung cancer: screening and detection with low-dose spiral CT versus radiography. *Radiology* 1996;201:798.

38. Sone S, Takashima S, Li F, et al. Mass screening for lung cancer with a mobile spiral computer tomography scanner. *Lancet* 1998; 351:1,242.

39. Kaneko M. CT screening for lung cancer in Japan. In: Proceedings of International Conferences on Prevention and Early Diagnosis of Lung Cancer. Dominioni L, Strauss G., eds. Italy, 1998, p. 144.

40. Henschke CI, McCauley DI, Yankelevitz DF, et al. Early Lung Cancer Action Project: overall design and findings from baseline screening. *Lancet* 1999;354:99.

41. Tockman MS, Qiao Y, Li L, et al. Safe separation of sputum cells from mucoid glycoprotein. *Acta Cytol* 1995;39:1,128.

42. Ikeda N, MacAulay C, Lam S, et al. Malignancy associated changes in bronchial epithelial cells and clinical application as a biomarker. *Lung Cancer* 1998;19:161.

43. Qiao YL, Tockman MS, Li L, et al. A case-cohort study of an early biomarker of lung cancer in a screening cohort of Yunnan tin miners in China. *Cancer Epidemiol Biomarkers Prev* 1997;6: 893.

44. Belinsky SA, Nikula KJ, Baylin SB, et al. Increased cytosine DNA-methyltransferase activity is target-cell-specific and an early event in lung cancer. *Proc Natl Acad Sci USA* 1996;93:4,045.

45. Miller YE, Franklin WA. Molecular events in lung carcinogenesis. *Hematol Oncol Clin North Am* 1997;11:215.

46. Mao L, Lee JS, Kurie JM, et al. Clonal genetic alterations in the lungs of current and former smokers. *J Natl Cancer Inst* 1997; 89:857.

47. Wistuba II, Lam S, Behrens C, et al. Molecular damage in the bronchial epithelium of current and former smokers. *J Natl Cancer Inst* 1997;89:1,366.

48. Franklin WA, Gazdar AF, Haney J, et al. Widely dispersed p53 mutation in respiratory epithelium. A novel mechanism for field carcinogenesis. *J Clin Invest* 1997;100:2,133.

49. Mulshine JL, Scott FM, Zhou J, et al. Development of molecular approaches to early lung cancer detection. *Sem Rad Oncol* 1996; 6:72.

50. Zhou J, Mulshine JL, Unsworth EJ, et al. Purification and characterization of a protein that permits early detection of lung cancer. Identification of heterogeneous nuclear ribonucleoprotein-A2/B1 as the antigen for monoclonal antibody 703D4. *J Biol Chem* 1996;271:10,760.

51. Hughes JM. 18F-fluorodeoxyglucose PET scans in lung cancer. *Thorax* 1996;51:16S.

52. Sazon DA, Santiago SM, Soo Hoo GW, et al. Fluorodeoxyglucose-positron emission tomography in the detection and staging of lung cancer. *Am J Respir Crit Care Med* 1996;153:417.

53. Chin R Jr., Ward R, Keyes JW, et al. Mediastinal staging of non-small-cell lung cancer with positron emission tomography. *Am J Respir Crit Care Med* 1995;152:2,090.

54. Bury A, Dowlati A, Paulus P, et al. Whole body 18FDG positron emission tomography in the staging of non-small cell lung cancer. *Eur Respir J* 1997;10:2,529.

55. Lam S, MacAulay C, Hung J, et al. Detection of dysplasia and carcinoma in situ using a lung imaging fluoroscopic endoscopy (LIFE) device. *J Thorac Cardiovasc Surg* 1993;105:1,035.

56. Lam S, MacAulay C, LeRiche JE, et al. Early localization of bronchogenic carcinoma. *Diag Thor Endosc* 1994;1:75.

57. Lam S, Kennedy T, Unger M, et al. Localization of bronchial intraepithelial neoplastic lesions by fluorescence bronchoscopy. *Chest* 1998;113:696.

58. Kato H, Okunaku T, Shimatani H. Photodynamic therapy for early stage bronchogenic carcinoma. *J Clin Laser Med Surg* 1996; 14:235.

59. Cortese DA. Bronchoscopic photodynamic therapy of radiologically occult lung cancer: the American experience. In: Herzel MR, ed. *Minimally invasive techniques in thoracic medicine and surgery.* London: Chapman & Hall, 1995:173.

60. MacAulay C, Lam S, Payne PW, et al. Malignancy-associated changes in bronchial epithelial cells in biopsy specimens. *Anal Quant Cytol Histol* 1995;17:55.

61. Palcic B, Payne PW, MacAulay CM, et al. Malignancy associated changes (MACs) as diagnostic and prognostic indicators—recent results from the lung and cervix. *Acta Cytol* 1995;39:341S.

62. Greenwald P, Kelloff G, Burch-Whitman C, et al. Chemoprevention. *CA Cancer J Clin* 1995;45:31.

63. Hennekens CH, Buring JE, Manson JE, et al. Lack of effect of long-term supplementation with beta carotene on the incidence of malignant neoplasms in cardiovascular disease. *N Engl J Med* 1996;334:1,145.

64. Strauss G, DeCamp M, Dibiccaro E, et al. Lung cancer diagnosis is being made with increasing frequency in former cigarette smokers. *Proceedings of ASCO* 1995;14:362.

23

MOLECULAR AND CYTOLOGIC TECHNIQUES OF EARLY DETECTION

ADI F. GAZDAR
STEPHEN LAM
IGNACIO I. WISTUBA

Lung cancer is the most frequent cause of cancer deaths in both men and women in the United States,[1] and tobacco smoking is accepted as the number one cause of this devastating disease.[2] Lung cancer is classified into two major clinic-pathological groups, namely small cell lung carcinoma (SCLC) and non–small cell lung carcinoma (NSCLC).[3] Squamous cell carcinoma, adenocarcinoma, and large cell carcinoma are the major histologic types of NSCLC.[3] Large cell carcinoma probably represents poorly differentiated variants of the other NSCLC types.[3]

As with other epithelial malignancies, lung cancers are believed to arise after a series of progressive pathological changes (preneoplastic lesions).[4] Many of these preneoplastic changes are frequently detected accompanying lung cancers[5] and in the respiratory mucosa of smokers.[6] Although many molecular abnormalities have been described in clinically evident lung cancers,[7] relatively little is known about the molecular events preceding the development of lung carcinomas and the underlying genetic basis of tobacco-related lung carcinogenesis. The risk population for targeting early detection and chemoprevention efforts to has been defined as current and heavy smokers, and patients who have survived one cancer of the upper aerodigestive tract. However, conventional morphologic methods for the identification of premalignant cell populations in the airways have limitations. This has led to a search for other biological properties of respiratory mucosa that may provide new methods for assessing the risk of developing invasive lung cancer in smokers, for early detection, and for monitoring their response to chemopreventive regimens. These markers (also referred as "intermediate markers") include genetic abnormalities in bronchial epithelial cells.

Less than 15% of patients with lung cancer today will survive their disease.[8] Survival of patients with advanced disease has not improved significantly over the last three decades.[9] Essentially, the only patients who achieve long-term survival are those with stage 0 or stage I disease. The five-year survival for patients with stage 0 disease is more than 90%.[9] Unfortunately, patients with stage 0 disease constitute only a minority of the lung cancer population;[10] less than 0.6% of patients with lung cancer are currently diagnosed at this stage because these small cancers do not usually produce any symptoms.

Examination of the age-standardized mortality rate for all cancers shows an interesting difference between men and women.[11] While the overall cancer mortality rate, has remained relatively unchanged among men in the last two decades, there has been a gradual decline in the mortality rate among women. This is thought to be due to improvements in the detection of preinvasive lesions by means of the Papanicolaou (Pap) smear for cervical cancer[12] and screening mammography for breast cancer,[13] followed by the subsequent removal of these lesions. The success of screening in these tumor sites offers hope that a similar strategy may also lead to a reduction in lung cancer mortality.

Sputum cytology examination is currently the only non-invasive method that can detect early lung cancer and premalignant lesions. Preinvasive and microinvasive cancers that are found by sputum cytology examination are very amenable to curative treatment such as surgery,[14,15] laser hyperthermia with the Nd:YAG laser,[16] cryotherapy,[17] electrocautery,[18] or photodynamic therapy with porfimer sodium (Photofrin).[19] Unfortunately, enthusiasm for the use of sputum cytology as a technique for early detection of lung cancer has been dampened by the negative screening studies in the 1970s, which failed to show a survival benefit.[20–24] However, the reasons why sputum cytology as practiced two decades ago fails to be the equivalent of the Pap cervical smear need to be examined critically in order to understand how modern methods can improve the usefulness of exfoliated sputum cells as an early detection tool.

SPUTUM CYTOLOGY EXAMINATION

Since the 1930s, sputum cytology examination has been used for the diagnosis of advanced and early lung cancer.[20–27] The range of sensitivity varies from 20% to nearly 100%. In screening studies, the sensitivities are usually in the 20% to 30% range, while the higher numbers are from studies in patients with invasive lung cancer. The average sensitivity and specificity from a review of the literature was 64.5% and 97.9% respectively.[28] There is no obvious trend of improvement in the sensitivity of sputum cytology between 1940 to 1990, as one might expect with better experience and training. One possible obstacle to improving the sensitivity of sputum is the present classification system. The present system is based upon years of careful observation of patients who developed lung cancer and is derived partially from similar observations in uterine cervix. Individuals are trained to recognize abnormal cells and place them into discrete categories. These categories are often based upon subjects who developed lung cancer and are divided into seven categories: (a) normal, (b) squamous cell metaplasia, (c) squamous cell metaplasia with mild atypia, (d) squamous cell metaplasia with moderate atypia, (e) squamous cell metaplasia with marked atypia, (f) carcinoma *in situ*, and (g) invasive carcinoma.[4] Although based upon extensive observation and with reasonable correlation to histology, there is considerable interobserver variation in the diagnosis. The agreement is good for the normal and invasive carcinoma categories but poor for the intervening categories.[4,29] Among the reasons for the interobserver variability in classifying specimens is that observers place emphasis on different cellular features. This may also account for the difference in the reported spontaneous regression rate of preinvasive lesions, which vary from 20% to 80% for marked atypia.[30,31]

Another reason for the low sensitivity of sputum cytology in previous screening studies may lie in the selection of loose enrollment criteria. For example, in the NCI Early Lung Cancer Cooperative Group study, the inclusion criteria were 45 years of age and smoking at least one package of cigarettes daily at the time of enrollment or within the previous year.[20] Using a stricter smoking history (greater than or equal to 40 pack-years) and the addition of airflow obstruction (FEV_1 per FVC less than 70%) as another enrollment criteria, Kennedy and coworkers recently reported that 0.9% of their patients with chronic obstructive pulmonary disease were found to have carcinoma *in situ;* invasive cancer was found in another 0.9%.[32] This detection rate is much higher than the 0.2% to 0.3% in the NCI prevalence screening study.

Other factors were found to influence the sensitivity of sputum cytology examination. The yield is highest in those with squamous cell carcinoma and lowest in adenocarcinoma.[31] The location of the tumor and the size of the lesion are also important. The yield is higher for tumors that are located centrally or in a lower lobe and with lesions that are greater than 2 cm in diameter.[33,34] The yield is lower for peripheral tumors and for lesions in the upper lobe or those that are smaller than 2 cm. For example, in a screening setting in subjects with predominantly small peripheral cancers detected by spiral CT, only 11% of the lung cancers were detected by sputum cytology examination alone, with another 15% detected by both methods.[35]

NEWER DETECTION METHODS USING SPUTUM CELLS

To improve the sensitivity of sputum test as a population screening tool for the detection of early lung cancer, three approaches are currently under development: immunostaining of transformed epithelial cells, polymerase chain reaction (PCR)-based assays to detect oncogene mutations, and computer-assisted image analysis of exfoliated sputum cells.

A nuclear ribonucleoprotein—hnRNP A2/B1—was found to be overexpressed in most lung cancer cell types as well as transformed epithelial cells.[36,37] In a retrospective study using sputum specimens that were collected during the Johns Hopkins Lung Project, 64% of the subjects whose sputum samples showed moderate atypia and positive immunostaining for hnRNP A2/B1 developed lung cancer on follow-up while 88% of those with negative immunostaining did not.[38] The sensitivity increased to 91% with no change in the specificity if the sputum specimens were limited to those that preceded the clinical appearance of lung cancer by less than two years.

Two prospective studies were carried out to evaluate hnRNP A2/B1 overexpression for the detection of preclinical lung cancer: one in patients with completely resected stage I lung cancer and the second among tin miners in China.[37,39] At the end of the first year of follow-up, the positive predictive value of hnRNP overexpression in sputum cells was 67%. The sensitivity and specificity for predicting the development of second primary lung cancer were 77% and 82% respectively. For the development of primary lung cancer, the corresponding figures were 82% and 65% respectively among the tin miners.

PCR-based assays can detect one mutant-containing cell among an excess of 100,000 normal cells.[40–42] A retrospective study in ten patients with adenocarcinoma—eight with K-*ras* mutation and two with *p53* mutation, eight showed an identical mutation in the sputum cells one to 13 months prior to clinical diagnosis.[40] These mutations were absent in samples from control subjects without lung cancer and those that were collected more than 24 months prior to diagnosis. Another study using enriched PCR identified K-*ras* mutation in 47% of the sputum samples from patients with non–small cell lung cancer.[43–45] However, 12.5% of the control subjects without lung cancer also carried this mutation. Because a given mutation is found in only a proportion of the patients with lung cancer and because these genomic alterations may also be present in a significant number of smokers without lung cancer,[46,47] the use of PCR-based assays to detect genetic mutations needs to be evaluated in a prospective manner in a large population of smokers with and without lung cancer. There are as yet no long-term follow-up studies to determine the risk of lung cancer when one or more of these mutations are found. Furthermore, for some mutations such as K-*ras,* a very limited number of mutations occur in human cancers.[48] Such mutations can be readily detected by a wide variety of methods, including some highly sensitive ones.[49] In contrast, many different mutations have been described in the *p53* gene, and methods to detect the wide range of mutations need to be utilized.[50]

Immunostaining and PCR-based methods require the presence of premalignant or malignant cells (or DNA shed from these cells) for diagnosis. Preinvasive cancers, especially peripheral adenocarcinomas, typically do not exfoliate many cells into the bronchial lumen. The number of epithelial cells from the lower respiratory tract in an expectorated specimen is also influenced by the subject's performance and collection method. For example, a study by the Lung Cancer Early Detection Working Group showed that with sputum induction using hypertonic saline, 19.6% of the specimens from current smokers and 28.9% of the specimens from former smokers were unsatisfactory.[51]

The use of nongenetic changes in normal cells that are induced by the presence of malignant cells in the vicinity, such as malignancy associated changes (MACs),[52] may overcome the problems discussed above. MACs refer to subvisual or nonobvious changes in the distribution of DNA in the nuclei of normal cells due to the presence of preinvasive or invasive cancer in the vicinity. These changes can be quantitated by computer-assisted image analysis.[53] In a study using bronchial biopsies taken from the opposite lung or from a lobe different from the primary tumor, MACs were found to be present in 86% of the normal-appearing specimen.[54] A retrospective analysis of sputum cytology slides that were collected during the Mayo Lung Project[55] revealed that MACs alone correctly identified 74% of the subjects who later developed lung cancer. Furthermore, the presence of MACs was found to precede clinical diagnosis by 12 months or more. The advantage of this approach is that the method is not dependent on the presence of malignant cells in the sputum, although the presence of atypical or malignant cells can improve the sensitivity of detection to over 90%.[55]

DETECTION OF PERIPHERAL LUNG CANCER

On a spiral chest CT, lesions as small as 1 mm can be seen. Despite this sensitivity, preinvasive lung cancers in the central airways are usually not detectable because these early lesions are only a few cell layers thick.[56,57] Chest CT however, may be better for the detection of tumors in the *peripheral* airways. Although spiral CT is several times more sensitive than standard chest x-ray,[58] lesions smaller than 10 mm that are discovered by this means present a diagnostic challenge. In one of the largest studies using CT detection of early lesions,[35,59] 7% of patients found to have abnormal CTs required further investigations such as thin-section CT, and 13% required biannual follow-up examinations. Lung biopsy procedures such as bronchoscopy, CT-guided fine-needle aspiration biopsy, or video-assisted thoracoscopy was performed in only 3% of the subjects for tissue diagnosis. Of those that had a lung biopsy procedure, approximately 10% turned out to have a nonmalignant lesion. The use of molecular markers or MAC in exfoliated sputum cells to improve the diagnostic accuracy of chest CT needs to be investigated further. Newer studies incorporating helical CT are discussed in Chapter 22.

FLUORESCENCE BRONCHOSCOPY FOR LOCALIZATION OF EARLY LUNG CANCER

Only 30% to 40% of carcinoma *in situ* are visible to an experienced endoscopist on conventional white-light bronchoscopy.[57] A new development in bronchoscopic localization of intraepithelial neoplastic lesion is fluorescence bronchoscopy.[60] When the bronchial surface is illuminated by light, the light can be reflected, back-scattered, absorbed, or induce tissue fluorescence. Conventional white-light bronchoscopy makes use of the first three optical phenomena. The tissue autofluorescence is not visible because the intensity is very low and overwhelmed by the background illuminating light. However, with suitable instrumentation, the tissue autofluorescence can be made visible to enhance our ability to localize areas of intraepithelial neoplasia in the tracheal bronchial tree.

When the bronchial surface is illuminated by violet or blue light (400 to 440 nm) normal tissues have significantly higher fluorescence intensity compare to dysplastic lesions or carcinoma *in situ,* especially in the green region of the emission spectrum.[61] There are several reasons for the decrease in autofluorescence in precancerous and cancerous tissues.[62,63] The major portion of the fluorescence signal comes from the submucosa. A decrease in the extracellular matrix in the submucosa, such as from the secretion of cancerous tissues[64] will result in a decrease in the amount of fluorophores or the quantum yield of these molecules. Recently it was observed that the microvascular density is increased in dysplastic lesions and *in situ* carcinoma.[65] Due to the increased absorption of the blue light and the fluorescent light by blood, the fluorescence intensity of these lesions is decreased. A third reason for the decrease in autofluorescence in dysplastic tissues and carcinoma *in situ* is the increase in thickness of the epithelial layer.[63] This thickening impedes transmission of the blue light to the submucosa and the fluorescent light from the submucosa to the bronchial surface. These effects are particularly pertinent to the green region of the autofluorescence spectra because the absorption characteristics of bronchial tissue and blood favor the absorption of green light. These differences in the autofluorescence property of normal, preneoplastic, and neoplastic tissues were used in the development of the lung imaging fluorescence endoscopy (LIFE) device for the detection and localization of intraepithelial neoplasia.[66,67] The procedure is part of a standard fiber-optic bronchoscopy, except that the illuminating light is white, not blue, and a special camera is used. The fluorescence examination adds an average of ten minutes to the diagnostic bronchoscopic procedure under a local anesthetic.

Worldwide experience, including a recently completed multicenter trial in the United States and Canada, showed that the addition of the LIFE-Lung examination to conventional white-light bronchoscopy improved the sensitivity of detecting intraepithelial neoplastic lesions by several-fold.[68–72] (LIFE bronchoscopy is discussed further in Chapter 24).

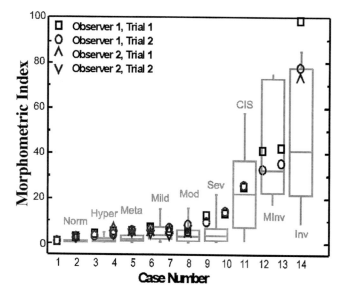

FIGURE 23.1. Morphometric index reproducibility: correlation of morphometric index with pathology grade and index reproducibility. The boxes indicate the central 50th percentile and the error bars show the central 95th percentile for each category.

NUCLEAR MORPHOMETRY OF BRONCHIAL BIOPSIES

A problem that is common to all early detection and chemo-prevention programs is how to diagnose intraepithelial (pre-invasive) neoplasia accurately and reproducibly. For example, a review of over 700 bronchial biopsies obtained in a multicenter early-detection clinical trial[72] by two experienced reference pathologists showed little disagreement in the interpretation of normal biopsies and invasive cancer but considerable disagreement about the preinvasive lesions. The classification by pathologists from different institutions agreed with those by the reference pathologists in only 34.8% of the biopsies.[73]

The morphological criteria for the histopathology of intraepithelial neoplasia of the bronchus developed several decades ago[4,74,75] have not been critically examined, particularly in terms of reproducibility of the diagnosis and, more important, as a grading system that would reflect the biological behavior of these lesions. Recently, the Armed Forces Institute of Pathology in the United States pioneered an effort to define preinvasive lesions to be included in the new World Health Organization (WHO) classification.[76] However, the current histopathology classification does not lend itself to quantitative analysis readily.

In an attempt to overcome the problems of intra- and interobserver variation in the grading of intraepithelial neoplastic lesions, computer-assisted image analysis has been used to quantitate the morphometric changes in tissue sections.[77] Quantitative nuclear morphometry is performed in normal and invasive cancer biopsies in order to generate a

morphometric index which separates these two groups. This index was tested on 377 bronchial biopsies (Figure 23.1). This test set confirms the wide variation in the diagnosis of preinvasive lesions using conventional histopathology criteria. However, using quantitative nuclear morphometry, a morphometric index of 7.5 was found to separate the dysplasia groups from the carcinoma *in situ* and the invasive cancer group. An index of 2.66 was found to separate the biopsies that were graded as normal, hyperplasia, or metaplasia from the dysplasia biopsies. This method is highly reproducible (Figure 23.1). A change in the absolute morphometric index of three or more represents a significant change. These results suggest that quantitative morphometric measurements may provide a better method to grade intraepithelial neoplastic lesions objectively.

OVERVIEW OF MOLECULAR ABNORMALITIES IN LUNG CANCER

Several cytogenetic, allelotyping, and comparative genomic hybridization (CGH) studies have revealed that multiple genetic changes (estimated to be between 10 and 20) are found in clinically evident lung cancers and involve known and putative recessive oncogenes as well as several dominant oncogenes.[7]

Dominant Oncogenes

Examples of abnormal dominant oncogenes in lung cancer are the *ras* family members (K-*ras*, H-*ras* and N-*ras*) (see also Chapter 4), the *myc* family members (C-*myc*, N-*myc*, and L-*myc*) (see also Chapter 5), and the *HER-2/neu* gene. *ras* mutations occur in approximately 20% of NSCLC, mainly in adenocarcinomas (90% involving K-*ras* gene at codon 12), while *ras* mutations have not been detected in any SCLC tumor or cell line.[7,78] Another example of a dominant oncogene in lung cancer would be overexpression of the *myc* family of genes, which occurs in nearly all SCLCs and in many NSCLCs.[79–81] Recent CGH studies have shown that lung cancer cell lines and tumor tissues demonstrate increased copy numbers consistent with amplification of underlying dominant oncogenes at several chromosomal regions, including 1p, 1q, 2p, 3q, 5q, 11q, 16p, 17q, 19q, and Xq.[82–86] Some of these regions, like 1p32 (L-*myc*), 2p25 (N-*myc*), and 8q24 (C-*myc*), contain known dominant oncogenes, while in others, the genes need to be identified.

Recessive Oncogenes

The list of recessive oncogenes that are involved in lung cancer is likely to include as many as ten to 15 known and putative genes.[7] These include changes in *TP53* (17p13), *RB* (13q14), *CDKN2* (9p21), and new candidate recessive oncogenes in the short arms of chromosome 3 (3p) at 3p12 (*DUTT1* gene),[87] 3p14.2 (*FHIT* gene),[88,89] 3p21 (*BAP-1* gene), and 3p25 regions.[7] Recessive oncogenes are believed to be inactivated via a two-step process involving both alleles. Knudson has proposed that the first "hit" is frequently a point mutation, while the second allele is subsequently inactivated via a chromosomal deletion, translocation, or other event such as methylation.[90] Two key examples in lung cancer are the *TP53* and the *RB* genes. Mutations of *TP53* gene are very common in lung cancer, occurring in over 90% of SCLCs and approximately 50% of NSCLCs.[7] There is evidence that *TP53* gene mutations occur in association with specific carcinogen exposure and that specific carcinogens predispose to specific mutations. Of interest, a coincidental mutational hotspot at the *TP53* gene has been found between invasive lung carcinomas and adduct hotspots caused by benzo(α)pyrene metabolites derived from cigarette smoke.[91] Another well-documented genetic change that occurs frequently in lung cancer is that of the *RB* gene. In more than 80% of SCLCs and some 20% to 30% of NSCLCs the protein has been mutated, so it cannot fulfill its normal cell cycle regulatory function.[92–94]

Many recessive oncogenes remain to be identified, although in most instances their chromosomal locations are known from cytogenetic and molecular analysis. Loss of heterozygosity analysis (LOH) using polymorphic microsatellite markers is frequently used to identify allelic losses at specific chromosomal regions, suggesting the involvement of other tumor-suppressor genes in lung cancer pathogenesis (see also Chapter 28).[95] The chromosomal regions include 1q, 2q, 5q, 6p, 6q, 8p, 8q, 9q, 10q, 11p, 11q, 14q, 17q,

18q, and 22q.[95–103] Although several of these chromosomal arms contain known or candidate tumor-suppressor genes (such as MCC and APC at 5q21, TSCI at 9q34, WT1 at 11q13, DCC at 18q221, and NF2 at 22q12), these genes are not known to be mutated in lung cancer. Recently, two new candidate tumor-suppressor genes called PTEN/MMAC1[104] and PPP2R1B,[105] located at 10q23 and 11q22–24 respectively, have demonstrated frequent somatic alterations in lung cancer.[105,106]

Tumor-Type-Specific Genetic Changes Are Found in Lung Cancers

Studies of large numbers of lung cancers have demonstrated different patterns of involvement between the two major groups of lung carcinomas (SCLC and NSCLC)[95] and between the three major histologic types of lung carcinomas (SCLC, squamous cell carcinomas, and adenocarcinomas) (Wistuba et al., unpublished data).[98,107] Thus genetic abnormalities in lung cancer can be classified into two groups; those that are common to all lung cancers and those that are associated with a specific histologic type of lung cancer. *RB* mutations are usually limited to SCLCs, *CDKN2* mutations to NSCLCs, and *RAS* mutations to adenocarcinomas. Our published[95,107] and unpublished results of allelotyping lung cancer cell lines and microdissected invasive primary tumors indicate that SCLCs demonstrate more frequent losses at 4p, 4q, 5q21 (APC-MCC region), 10q, and 13q14 (*RB*), while losses at 9p21 and 8p21–23 are more frequent in NSCLCs. Of interest, is that we have found different patterns of allelic loss involving the two major types of NSCLC (squamous cell and adenocarcinoma), with higher incidences of deletions at 17p13 (*TP53*), 13q14 (*RB*), 9p21 (*CDKN2*), 8p21–23, and several 3p regions in squamous cell carcinomas. These results suggest that more genetic changes accumulate during tumorigenesis in squamous cell carcinomas than in adenocarcinomas. These differences may be related to differences in tumorigenic mechanisms, such as etiologic factors (for instance, type and extent of smoking exposure), operating via separate pathways. In fact, different patterns of allelic losses[98] and *TP53* gene mutations have been reported in lung carcinomas arising in nonsmokers versus smokers.[108]

PRENEOPLASIA AND THE DEVELOPMENT OF LUNG CANCER

Lung cancers are believed to arise after a series of progressive pathological changes (preneoplastic or precursor lesions) in the respiratory mucosa.[4] While the sequential preneoplastic changes have been defined for centrally arising squamous carcinomas,[4] they have been poorly documented for large cell carcinomas, adenocarcinomas, and SCLCs.[3]

Mucosal changes in the large airways that may precede

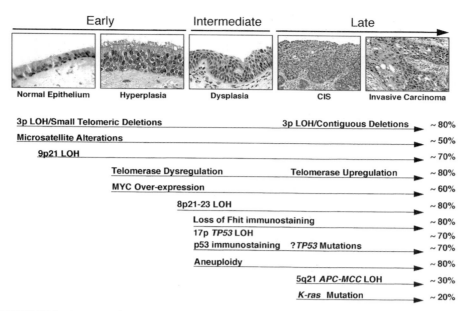

FIGURE 23.2. Sequential histologic and molecular changes during the multistage pathogenesis of lung cancer. Molecular changes occurring during lung cancer pathogenesis may commence early (normal or slightly abnormal epithelium), at an intermediate (dysplasia) stage, or relatively late (carcinoma *in situ*, CIS, or invasive carcinoma).

or accompany invasive squamous cell carcinoma include hyperplasia (basal cell hyperplasia and goblet cell hyperplasia), squamous metaplasia, squamous dysplasia, and carcinoma *in situ* (Figure 23.2).[4] Because all forms of lung cancers are strongly smoking-associated, the sequential preneoplastic changes associated with squamous carcinomas may also be present in adenocarcinomas and SCLCs. Hyperplasia of the bronchial epithelium and squamous metaplasia are extremely common reactive findings and occur in response to cigarette smoking[6,109] as well with a variety of other stimuli, such as chronic infection, asthma, and so on. These changes are reversible and are not, in the strict sense, truly premalignant. Squamous dysplasia and carcinoma *in situ* are the changes most frequently associated with the development of squamous cell lung carcinomas.[5] Because dysplasia and carcinoma *in situ* are seldom visible to the naked eye, their reported frequencies may be underestimated.

Adenocarcinomas may be accompanied by changes, including atypical adenomatous hyperplasia (AAH),[110] in peripheral airway cells, although the malignant potential of these lesions has not been demonstrated. However, lesions with AAH features are frequently detected accompanying adenocarcinomas, especially when a bronchioloalveolar carcinomatous pattern is seen at the edge of less differentiated adenocarcinomas.[110,111] The concept of the adenoma-carcinoma sequence as it applies to AAH and adenocarcinoma of the lung suggests there is a continuum from AAH to peripherally arising adenocarcinomas.

Bronchiolar neuroendocrine cell hyperplasia represents a proliferation of neuroendocrine cells in and around small airways.[112] Because of their association with peripheral carcinoid tumors, it has been suggested that they are precursors to the carcinoid tumors.[112] While no specific preneoplastic changes have been described for SCLC, smoking-related changes, including squamous dysplasia and carcinoma *in situ*, may be found in association with these tumors.[113]

Currently available information suggests that lung preneoplastic lesions are frequently extensive and multifocal throughout the lung, indicating a field effect ("field cancerization") by which much of the respiratory epithelium has been mutagenized, presumably from exposure to carcinogens.[114] Thus lung carcinomas may occur anywhere in the vast and anatomically complicated respiratory tree, including the peripheral lung, and second tumors are relatively frequent after one upper aerodigestive tract carcinoma.[115]

GENETIC ABNORMALITIES DURING THE MULTISTAGE DEVELOPMENT OF LUNG CANCER

Although our knowledge of the molecular events in invasive lung cancer is relatively extensive, until recently we knew little about the sequence of events in preneoplastic lesions. A few studies have provided suggestions that molecular lesions can be identified at early stages of the pathogenesis of lung cancer.[40,116–122] *MYC* and *RAS* upregulation, cyclin D1 expression, *p53* immunostaining, and DNA aneuploidy have been detected in dysplastic epithelium adjacent to invasive lung carcinomas.[121,123–129] *KRAS* mutations have been also detected in atypical adenomatous hyperplasia,[130] which may be a potential precursor lesion of adenocarcinoma. *TP53* gene abnormalities (including mutations, deletions and overexpression) have been demonstrated in nonmalignant epithelium of lung specimens resected for lung cancer.[120,121] They also occur in the histologically normal and abnormal epithelium of smokers.[46,47] Recently, Franklin and colleagues described an identical *p53* gene mutation widely dispersed in normal and preneoplastic epithelium of a smoker without lung cancer.[131]

To further understand the sequential molecular changes involved in lung cancer pathogenesis, we have developed a scheme to search systematically for mutations in preneoplastic lesions and normal epithelium using archival paraffin-embedded materials (Figure 23.3).[132] Microsections from lung cancer resections and bronchoscopic biopsies containing preneoplastic lesions and normal respiratory epithelium are examined for the presence of genetic changes. Using a precise microdissection technique (micromanipulator or laser capture microdissection)[116,133] (see also Chapter 27) under direct microscopic observation, a variable number of cells from these areas are precisely isolated along with invasive primary tumor and stromal lymphocytes (as a source of normal constitutional DNA). Using PCR-based techniques, these different specimens are examined for point mutations and allelic losses at chromosomal regions frequently mutated or deleted in clinically evident lung carcinomas.

MUTATIONS FOLLOW A SEQUENCE

Our data have demonstrated that in lung cancer the developmental sequence of molecular changes is not random (Figure 23.2), with LOH at one or more 3p regions (especially telomeric regions 3p21, 3p22–24, and 3p25) and 9p21, and to a lesser extent at 8p21–23, 13q14 (*RB*), and 17p13 (*TP53*), being detected frequently very early in pathogenesis in histologically normal epithelium (Figure 23.4).[134] In contrast, LOH at 5q21 (APC-MCC region) and K-*ras* mutations were detected only at the carcinoma

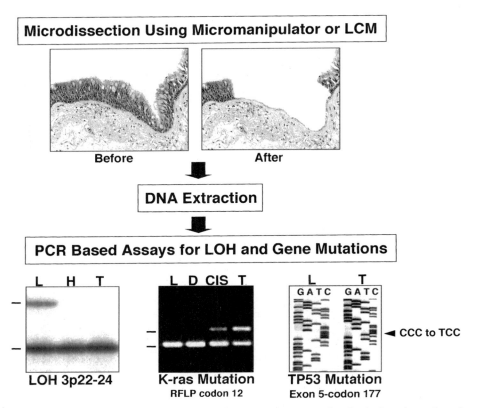

FIGURE 23.3. Schema outlining procedures for investigating molecular lesions in preinvasive lesions and invasive cancers of the respiratory tract. **Top:** representative example of microdissection of hyperplastic lesion. **Bottom:** molecular analyses of microdissected invasive carcinoma (T) and preneoplastic lesion (H). Normal lymphocytes (L) are used as source of constitutional DNA. Representatives examples of loss of heterozygosity (LOH) (**left**); designed restriction fragment length polymorphism for K-*ras* mutation analysis at codon 12 (**center**); and sequencing of *TP53* gene showing mutation at exon 5, codon 177 (**right**).

Lung Cancer Patient   Smoker

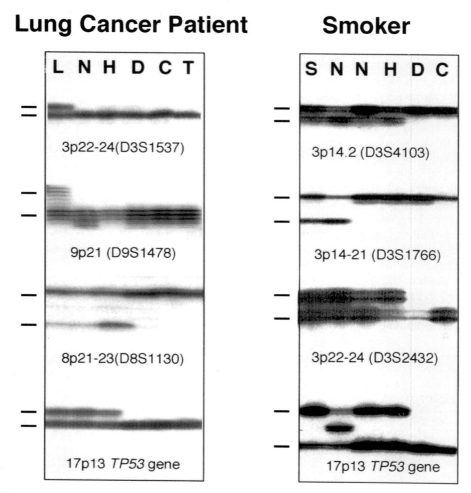

FIGURE 23.4. Representative autoradiographs of microsatellite analyses for loss of heterozygosity (LOH) and microsatellite alterations (MAs) at four chromosomal regions of a lung squamous cell carcinoma case and its corresponding bronchial histologically normal epithelium and preneoplastic lesions (**left**), and biopsy specimens representing a constellation of normal and premalignant areas from four smoker subjects. *L* and *S*, lymphocytes (as source of constitutional DNA); *N*, histologically normal epithelium; *H*, hyperplasia; *D*, dysplasia; *C*, carcinoma *in situ*; and *T*, invasive carcinoma.

in situ stage, and *TP53* mutations appear at variable times. Detailed examination of all our material suggests that the order of events (allelic losses) is usually either 3p→9p→8p or 3p→8p→9p deletions followed by *TP53* deletions. In early lesions (normal epithelium to metaplasia), the 3p losses are small and multifocal, commencing at the distal half of the chromosomal arm.[134] In later lesions (carcinoma *in situ* and invasive cancers), all or almost the entire chromosome is lost.

Recent attention has focused on the *FHIT* gene at 3p14.2, a candidate tumor-suppressor gene for lung and other cancers, which spans FRA3B, the most common of the aphidocolin-inducible fragile sites (see also Chapter 8).[89,135,136] We speculated that breaks at FRA3B destabil-

ize the entire short arm of chromosome 3, leading to multiple deletions and loss of the entire arm. However, our data indicated that allelic losses at other more telomeric 3p regions (3p21, 3p22–24, and 3p25) appeared at earlier morphological stages than losses within and around the *FHIT* gene.[134] This is in agreement with the recently published findings of loss of the Fhit protein expression (as demonstrated by immunostaining) from the dysplasia stage.[137]

Our data also indicate that different patterns of sequential deletions are detected in the pathogenesis of the major histologic types of lung cancers. Overall, more cumulative and earlier allelic loss at 9p21, 17p (*TP53*), 13q14 (*RB*), and at different 3p regions are found in centrally arising

SCLCs and squamous cell carcinomas than in peripheral adenocarcinomas (Wistuba et al., in preparation).

ACCUMULATION OF GENETIC CHANGES IN THE DEVELOPMENT OF LUNG CANCER

The development of epithelial cancers requires multiple mutations,[138] the stepwise accumulation of which may represent a mutator phenotype.[139,140] Thus it is possible that those preneoplastic lesions that have accumulated multiple mutations are at higher risk for progression to invasive cancer. Of interest is that using a panel of microsatellite markers targeting chromosomal regions frequently deleted in invasive lung carcinomas, we have detected similar incidences of LOH between histologically normal epithelium and slightly abnormal epithelial changes (hyperplasia and squamous metaplasia) accompanying lung carcinomas,[134] indicating that the latter foci may represent reactive foci and are not at higher risk for progression to invasive carcinomas. However, high-grade dysplasias and carcinoma *in situ* accompanying invasive squamous cell lung carcinomas demonstrated a significant increase of total number of allelic losses,[134] suggesting that the accumulation of mutations correlates with the morphologic changes and may lead to development of invasive carcinomas (sequential theory of lung cancer development). In particular, the allelic loss patterns of carcinoma *in situ* lesions were identical or nearly identical to those present in the corresponding invasive carcinomas.[134] As some specimens of histologically normal or mildly abnormal epithelia, especially accompanying SCLCs, have demonstrated a very high incidence of allelic loss, equal or greater than that present in some high-grade dysplasia and carcinoma *in situ* samples, we suggest that, in some cases, especially SCLC, carcinoma *in situ* and invasive carcinoma may arise directly from histologically normal or from mildly abnormal epithelium without passing through the entire histologic sequence (parallel theory of cancer development).

Of great interest is that our detailed allelotyping analyses of chromosome arms 3p[134] and 8p[141] during the multistage development of squamous cell carcinomas have demonstrated that the extent of the deletions increases with progressive histologic changes (Figure 23.5). Thus in all squamous cell invasive carcinomas and carcinoma *in situ* lesions, most of the 3p and 8p arms were deleted, and in all patients the extent of the losses in carcinoma *in situ* and invasive carcinomas was greater that the 3p and 8p allelic losses found in the corresponding normal and preneoplastic foci.

Analysis of our data indicated that four patterns of allelic loss could be identified (negative; early; intermediate; advanced) in histologically normal epithelium and precursor lesions accompanying squamous cell lung carcinomas (Figure 23.6).[134] Histologically normal or mildly abnormal foci had a negative pattern (no allelic loss) or early pattern of

loss, while all foci of carcinoma *in situ* and invasive tumor had an advanced pattern. However, dysplasias demonstrated the entire spectrum of allelic loss patterns and were the only histologic category having the intermediate pattern. These findings suggest that dysplasias represent a heterogeneous group of lesions at a molecular level. As only a fraction (10% of moderate dysplasia, 40% to 80% of severe dysplasias) are believed to progress to cancer,[30,142,143] molecular studies may aid in the identification of the subgroups of smokers with dysplasia who are at the greater risk of progression to lung cancer.

Our findings demonstrate that despite similar smoking exposures, different pathways and genotypic changes are involved in the pathogenesis of the three major histologic types of lung carcinoma, namely SCLC, squamous cell carcinoma and adenocarcinoma. It appears that more allelic deletions accumulate during the tumorigenesis in centrally arising SCLCs and squamous cell carcinomas than in peripherally located adenocarcinomas. The findings of different patterns of LOH in the three major types of lung cancers are consistent with their different clinical characteristics.

LUNG CANCER PRECURSOR LESIONS REPRESENT OUTGROWTH OF MULTIPLE CLONES

Molecular analyses suggested that precursor lesions represented outgrowths of multiple clones, a finding compatible with the field effect theory.[144] Our recent analysis of 58 normal and noninvasive foci accompanying 12 invasive squamous cell carcinomas having one or more molecular abnormalities, indicated that 30 (52%) probably arose as independent clonal events, while 28 (48%) were potentially of the same clonal origin as the corresponding tumor. If the potentially clonal lesions are truly clonal in origin, subclonal drift[145] must have occurred as an early and widespread event, as only four foci (6%) (from two subjects) of 62 lesions had identical patterns of mutations. However, we cannot exclude the possibility that some other earlier molecular event (for which we did not examine) occurred in a single cell whose progeny were dispersed widely throughout the bronchial epithelium and subsequently gave rise to all of the foci we examined. If this event occurred, then subclonal drift[145] must have occurred as an early and widespread event. In addition, our recent genetic analysis of the histologically normal or mildly abnormal (hyperplasia and squamous metaplasia) bronchial epithelium adjacent to invasive lung cancers indicated that multiple small clones of cells (up to 400) having identical pattern of LOH are frequently detected (Park et al., in preparation). These findings suggest that histologically normal bronchial epithelium and lung cancer precursor lesions having smoking-related genetic damage represent outgrowths of multiple small clones of

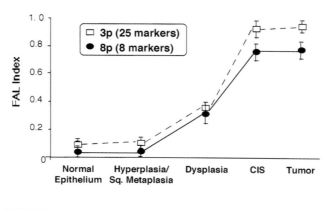

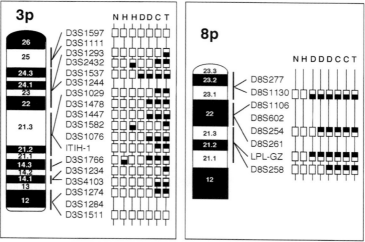

FIGURE 23.5. **Top:** loss of heterozygosity (LOH) expressed in terms of the means of Fractional Allelic Loss (FAL) Index (i.e., fraction of microsatellite loci showing LOH in each epithelial sample) of chromosome 3p and 8p21–23 regions. **Bottom:** examples of allelotyping analysis at the chromosome 3p and 8p21–23 regions of normal epithelium and precursor lesions accompanying resected squamous cell carcinomas using eighteen 3p (**left**) and eight 8p (**right**) microsatellite markers. □, No LOH; ◧, lower allele lost; ◧ upper allele lost. They demonstrate progression in the size of the chromosome 3p and 8p deletions in the invasive carcinomas and their accompanying normal epithelium and precursor lesions. Notice that the same allele is lost in preneoplastic, noninvasive, and invasive lesions. **N**, histologically normal epithelium; **H**, hyperplasia; **D**, dysplasia; **CIS**, carcinoma *in situ;* and **T**, invasive carcinoma.

genetically abnormal cells, a finding compatible with the field effect theory.

SIMILAR GENETIC CHANGES ARE DETECTED IN INVASIVE LUNG CANCERS AND THEIR PRECURSOR LESIONS

We and others have noted that the specific parental allelics lost in chromosomal deletions present in preneoplastic lesions and their accompanying cancers are similar (Figures 23.4 and 23.5).[116,117,121,134] We have referred to this phenomenon as allele-specific mutations (ASM). Others have noted ASM in advanced bronchial (severe dysplasias) lesions,[121] which are believed to be the immediate precursors

of invasive cancers and which were located adjacent to centrally arising squamous cell carcinomas. We have detected ASMs in preneoplastic lesions located in all regions of the respiratory epithelium (bronchi, bronchioles, and alveoli) involving several differentiated cell types (mucous cells, metaplastic squamous cells, Clara cells, and type II alveolar pneumocytes).[116,117,134] In addition, we have detected this phenomenon in a wide spectrum of preneoplastic lesions, including hyperplasia, squamous metaplasia, dysplasia, and carcinoma *in situ*.[116,117,134] Of great interest is that we have detected ASMs in smoking-related damaged epithelium, even in biopsy samples obtained from different lungs.[47]

What is the mechanism by which ASMs arise? We have proposed two possibilities. First, the lesions could be clonal in origin: a single cell or small clone of cells develops loss

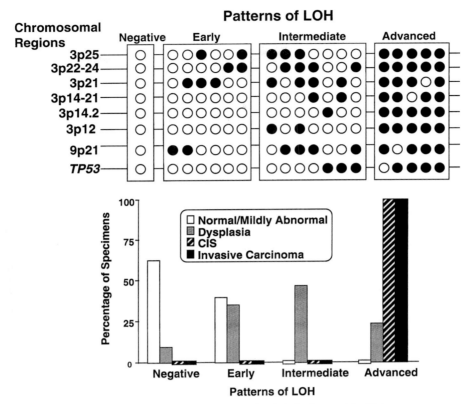

FIGURE 23.6. **Top:** patterns of loss of heterozygosity (LOH) observed in 12 lung squamous cell carcinomas and their corresponding histologically normal epithelium, preneoplasias, and carcinoma *in situ* lesions. ○, No LOH; ●, LOH. **Bottom:** relationship between histologic categories and patterns of LOH. Only dysplasias demonstrated the entire spectrum of patterns and were the only histologic category having the intermediate patterns.

or point mutations at a specific allele at one or more loci, migrates widely throughout the respiratory epithelium of both lungs, and eventually gives rise to a tumor. For the reasons stated above, this is highly unlikely. This possibility would require an unexpected fluidity of the bronchial epithelial cells or at least of those cells in which initial genetic changes arise. The second possibility is that in individuals, one of any pair of alleles has a greater tendency to be lost, perhaps as a result of some form of genomic imprinting or the presence of fragile sites, resulting in an inherited propensity to lose one of the two alleles.

However, some studies support alternative theories by which ASMs may arise. Multicentric development of lesions is supported by a study by Sozzi and associates of five patients with multiple lesions in their bronchial tree. The authors detected losses of different alleles of chromosome 3p regions and different mutations in the *TP53* and K-*ras* genes between invasive lung tumors and accompanying preneoplastic lesions.[119] In addition, as previously mentioned, Franklin and colleagues studied the entire bronchial tree of a smoker dying without lung carcinoma.[131] A single, identical point mutation, G-to-T transversion in codon 245, was

identified in the bronchial epithelium from seven of ten widely dispersed bilateral epithelial tissues. The morphology of the involved sites varied from normal to squamous metaplasia to moderate dysplasia. These findings support the alternative theory that a single clone of cells can become widely dispersed throughout the respiratory epithelium. Our recent findings of the ASM phenomenon in lung cancer precursor lesions that appeared to be of independent clonal origin suggests that ASM occurs via an alternative mechanism.[134] Whatever its mechanism, ASM is likely to be a phenomenon of major biological significance.

GENOMIC INSTABILITY IN THE PATHOGENESIS OF LUNG CANCER

In addition to the specific genetic changes discussed above, other evidence indicates that genomic instability occurs in lung cancer and its preneoplastic lesions. This evidence includes our finding of widespread aneuploidy throughout the respiratory epithelium of lung cancer patients.[126] Another molecular change frequently present in a wide variety of cancer types is microsatellite alterations (MAs) (also known as genomic alterations).

In hereditary nonpoplyposis colon cancer (HNPCC), inherited defects in DNA mismatch repair enzymes result in large-scale genetic instability, with the formation of a ladderlike pattern replacing the normal allele pattern.[146] Another form of microsatellite change, where only a single band of altered size is found, has been described in many forms of sporadic cancers, including lung cancer at frequencies of 0% to 45%).[147–150] We and others refer to these changes as microsatellite alterations.[134,147,151–153] While the relationship of MAs to defects in the DNA repair mechanism has not been established, MAs probably represent evidence of some form of genomic instability.[154] Because they arise in noncoding regions of the genome, they are not in the direct pathway of tumorigenesis. MAs represent changes in the size of polymorphic microsatellite markers compared to the normal germ line in individual persons. Nevertheless, MAs are attractive candidates for the early molecular detection of lung and other cancers.[147,152,155] Our data demonstrated the presence of MAs in a subset (50%) of lung carcinomas,[134,153] as well as in their accompanying preneoplastic lesions and normal appearing epithelium.[134] Unlike allelic losses, the frequency of MAs did not increase with more advanced histologic changes. Of interest is that MAs, when present in nonmalignant foci, were always of a different size from those present in the corresponding invasive tumors. These findings indicate either that the preneoplastic lesions are not clonally related to the corresponding tumors or that the MAs arose during subclonal evolution. The finding of MAs in exfoliated cells present in sputum[152] from cancer patients suggest that they may be markers for lung cancer or for subjects at increased risk of developing lung cancer.

TELOMERASE DYSREGULATION IN THE PATHOGENESIS OF LUNG CANCER

Telomerase is currently recognized as a nearly ubiquitous tumor marker. Telomerase is a specialized ribonucleoprotein polymerase that adds TTAGGG repeats at the ends of vertebrate chromosomal DNA called telomeres.[156] Human telomeres undergo progressive shortening with cell division through replication-dependent sequence loss at DNA termini.[157] Telomerase is thought to compensate for the loss of telomeric repeats and is associated with the acquisition of the immortal phenotype. A variety of immortal cell lines, malignant tumors, and testicular cells have been found specifically to express telomerase activity,[158–161] whereas most normal somatic cells do not express this activity.[162,163] Most NSCLC and SCLC tumors are telomerase-positive (see also Chapter 9).[159]

Telomerase has been detected in preinvasive lesions in a number of tumor systems, including lung.[164] In the lung, low levels of telomerase activity have been detected in hyperplasia, dysplasia, and carcinoma *in situ*, compared to invasive cancer. While weak telomerase RNA expression is detected in basal layers of normal and hyperplastic epithelium from lung cancer patients, dysregulation of telomerase expression increases with tumor progression, with moderate to strong expression throughout the multilayered epithelium in metaplasia, dysplasia, and carcinoma *in situ*.[164] Of interest, foci of intense telomerase upregulation are seen in carcinoma *in situ* lesions in the vicinity of the invasive component of lung cancers. In addition, similar patterns of dysregulation of telomerase expression with increasing histologic grade have also been noted in bronchoscopic biopsies of smoking-damaged epithelium of current and former smokers, suggesting that telomerase could be also used as a potential marker for risk assessment (Rahti et al, in preparation).

MOLECULAR MARKERS FOR EARLY DETECTION OF LUNG CANCER

Mutant K-*ras* and *TP53* genes have been detected in the sputum some months prior to diagnosis of cancer,[40] and K-*ras* mutations have been detected in bronchoalveolar lavage fluids from patients with adenocarcinoma (56%) but not in patients with squamous cell carcinoma or with other diagnosis.[44] Recently, Ahrendt and co-workers[165] have reported that molecular assays could identify cancer cells in bronchoalveolar lavage fluid from patients with early-stage lung cancers. Using PCR-based assays for K-*ras* and *TP53* gene mutations, CpG-island methylation of the *CDKN2* gene, and microsatellite instability, they were able to detect identical molecular abnormalities in the bronchoalveolar fluid and corresponding tumors in 23 of 43 (53%) of the cases. These findings suggest that molecular strategies may detect the presence of neoplastic cells in the central and peripheral airways in patients with early-stage lung carcinomas.

SMOKING-DAMAGED BRONCHIAL EPITHELIUM

It has been established that advanced lung preneoplastic changes occur far more frequently in smokers than in nonsmokers and increase in frequency with amount of smoking, adjusted by age.[5,6] Although morphologic recovery occurs after smoking cessation,[5,166] elevated lung cancer risk persists.[167] Changes in bronchial epithelium, including metaplasia and dysplasia, have been utilized as surrogate end points for chemoprevention studies.[168,169] Risk factors that identify normal and premalignant bronchial tissue at risk for malignant progression need to be better defined. However, most of the molecular studies of lung preneoplastic lesions have been performed in material from small numbers of subjects with concurrent lung cancer, and only scant information is available about molecular changes in the respiratory epithelium of smokers without cancer.[46,47,121,122]

Two independent studies describing genetic changes in bronchial biopsy specimens from current and former smokers have been reported.[46,47] Mao and colleagues[46] described their analyses of the LOH and histologic abnormalities present in biopsies from 54 current and former smokers and nine nonsmokers. In each of the current and former smokers, bronchoscopy biopsies from six preselected sites demonstrated histologic changes, including squamous metaplasia and dysplasia. In addition, LOH using three microsatellite markers at chromosomal region 3p14, 9p21, and 17p13 (*TP53*) were used as surrogate markers of tumor-suppressor gene inactivation in the tissues. Although some differences were seen when the specimens of current smokers were compared with those of former smokers, allelic losses were surprisingly common in the nonmalignant lung epithelial tissue of both groups. Of the 76% of smokers who demonstrated allelic loss at one or more of the three chromosomal regions analyzed, deletions were detected in 75%, 57%, and 18% of the subjects at 3p14, 9p21, and 17p13 (*TP53*), respectively.

Our results,[47] which are in agreement with the above-described findings, also indicate that genetic changes similar to those found in lung cancers can be detected in nonmalignant bronchial epithelium from current and former smokers

and may persist for many years after smoking cessation. In our study, multiple biopsy specimens were obtained from 18 current smokers, 24 former smokers, and 21 nonsmokers. PCR-based assays for fifteen polymorphic microsatellite DNA markers were used to examine eight chromosomal regions (3p14.2 at the *FHIT* gene, 3p14–21, 3p21, 3p22–24, 5q21 at the APC-MCC region, 9p21, 13q14 at *RB,* and 17p13 at *TP53*) for genetic changes (LOH and MAs). High frequencies of LOH and MAs were observed in biopsies from current and former smokers and no significant differences were observed between the two groups. Of great interest is that no molecular changes were detected in nonsmoking subjects. Among individuals who smoked, 86% demonstrated LOH in one or more biopsies and 24% showed LOH in all biopsies. Somewhat surprisingly, about half of the histologically normal epithelium showed LOH; however, the frequency of LOH and the severity of histologic changes did not correspond until the carcinoma *in situ* stage (Figure 23.7). A subset of the biopsies from smokers with either normal or preneoplastic histology showed LOH at multiple chromosomal sites, a phenomenon frequently observed in carcinoma *in situ* and invasive cancer. Our findings suggest that carcinoma *in situ* and other histologically normal and abnormal foci having multiple regions of allelic loss are at increased risk for progressing to invasive cancer. As has been observed in epithelial foci accompanying

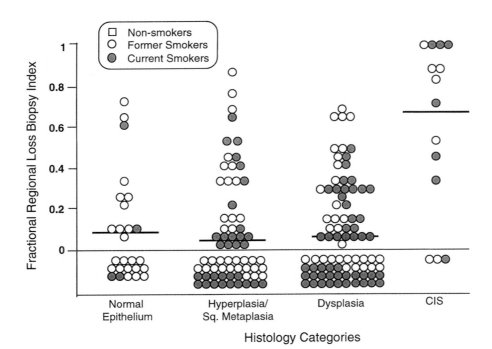

FIGURE 23.7. Loss of heterozygosity (LOH) in individual biopsy specimens obtained from current and former smokers according to smoking status and histologic categories. LOH is expressed in terms of the fractional regional loss index by biopsy specimen (i.e., the fraction of chromosome regions showing LOH in each biopsy specimen, range 0 to 1). Horizontal bars indicate the mean for each histologic category.

invasive lung carcinoma,[134] allelic losses on chromosome 3p and 9p were more frequent than deletions in chromosomes 5q21, 17p13 (*TP53* gene), and 13q14 (*RB* gene).

All these findings suggest the hypothesis that identifying biopsies with extensive or certain patterns of allelic loss may provide new methods for assessing the risk in smokers of developing invasive lung cancer and for monitoring response to chemoprevention. As with all diagnostic tests, this concept will need to be validated in clinical trials.

ACKNOWLEDGMENT

Supported by contract N01-CN-45580-01 from the Early Detection Research Network, and Specialized Program of Research Excellence grant 1-P50-CA70907-01 from the National Cancer Institute, Bethesda, MD.

REFERENCES

1. Parker SL, Tong T, Bolden S, et al. Cancer statistics, 1997. *CA Cancer J Clin* 1997;47:5.
2. Parkin DM, Pisani P, Lopez AD, et al. At least one in seven cases of cancer is caused by smoking. Global estimates for 1985. *Int J Cancer* 1994;59:494.
3. Colby TV, Koss MN, Travis WD. Tumors of the lower respiratory tract, 3rd. series, Fascicle 13. In: Rosai J, Sobin LH, eds. *Atlas of tumor pathology.* Washington, DC: Armed Forces Institute of Pathology, 1995:1.
4. Saccomanno G, Archer VE, Auerbach O, et al. Development of carcinoma of the lung as reflected in exfoliated cells. *Cancer* 1974;33:256.
5. Auerbach O, Stout AP, Hammond EC, et al. Changes in bronchial epithelium in relation to smoking and cancer of the lung. *N Engl J Med* 1961;265:253.
6. Auerbach O, Hammond EC, Garfinkel L. Changes in bronchial epithelium in relation to cigarette smoking, 1955–1960 vs. 1970–1977. *N Engl J Med* 1979;300:381.
7. Sekido Y, Fong KM, Minna JD. Progress in understanding the molecular pathogenesis of human lung cancer. *Biochim Biophys Acta* 1998;1378:F21.
8. Landis SH, Murray T, Bolden S, et al. Cancer statistics, 1998. *CA Cancer J Clin* 1998;48:6.
9. Minna JD. Neoplasms of the lung. In: Braunwald E, Isselbacher K, Petersdorf R, et al., eds. *Harrison's principles of internal medicine.* New York: McGraw-Hill, 1997:1221.
10. Fry WA, Menck HR, Winchester DP. The National Cancer Data Base report on lung cancer. *Cancer* 1996;77:1947.
11. Anon. *Canadian cancer statistics.* Toronto, Canada: National Cancer Institute, 1996.
12. Anderson GH, Boyes DA, Benedet JL, et al. Organization and results of the cervical cytology screening programme in British Columbia, 1955–85. *Br Med J (Clin Res Ed)* 1988;296:975.
13. Kerlikowske K, Grady D, Rubin SM, et al. Efficacy of screening mammography. A meta-analysis. *JAMA* 1995;273:149.
14. Cortese DA, Pairolero PC, Bergstralh EJ, et al. Roentgenographically occult lung cancer. A ten-year experience. *J Thorac Cardiovasc Surg* 1983;86:373.
15. Bechtel JJ, Kelley WR, Petty TL, et al. Outcome of 51 patients with roentgenographically occult lung cancer detected by sputum cytologic testing: a community hospital program. *Arch Intern Med* 1994;154:975.
16. Cavaliere S, Foccoli P, Farina PL. Nd:YAG laser bronchoscopy. A five-year experience with 1,396 applications in 1,000 patients. *Chest* 1988;94:15.
17. Ozenne G, Vergnon JM, Roulier A, et al. Cryotherapy of in-situ or microinvasive bronchial carcinoma. *Chest* 1990;98:105S.
18. van Boxem TJ, Venmans BJ, Schramel FM, et al. Radiographically occult lung cancer treated with fibreoptic bronchoscopic electrocautery: a pilot study of a simple and inexpensive technique. *Eur Respir J* 1998;11:169.
19. Furuse K, Fukuoka M, Kato H, et al. A prospective phase II study on photodynamic therapy with photofrin II for centrally located early-stage lung cancer. The Japan Lung Cancer Photodynamic Therapy Study Group. *J Clin Oncol* 1993;11:1852.
20. Frost JK, Ball WJ, Levin ML, et al. Early lung cancer detection: results of the initial (prevalence) radiologic and cytologic screening in the Johns Hopkins study. *Am Rev Respir Dis* 1984;130:549.
21. Flehinger BJ, Melamed MR, Zaman MB, et al. Early lung cancer detection: results of the initial (prevalence) radiologic and cytologic screening in the Memorial Sloan-Kettering study. *Am Rev Respir Dis* 1984;130:555.
22. Fontana RS, Sanderson DR, Woolner LB, et al. Screening for lung cancer. A critique of the Mayo Lung Project. *Cancer* 1991;67:1155.
23. Kubik A, Parkin DM, Khlat M, et al. Lack of benefit from semi-annual screening for cancer of the lung: follow-up report of a randomized controlled trial on a population of high-risk males in Czechoslovakia. *Int J Cancer* 1990;45:26.
24. Edell ES, Cortese DA, McDougall JC. Ancillary therapies in the management of lung cancer: photodynamic therapy, laser therapy, and endobronchial prosthetic devices. *Mayo Clin Proc* 1993;68:685.
25. Dudgeon LS, Wrigley CH. On the demonstration of particles of malignant growth in the sputum by means of the wet-film method. *J Laryngol Otol* 1935;50:752.
26. Farber SM, McGrath AK, Benioff MA, et al. Evaluation of cytologic diagnosis of lung cancer. *JAMA* 1950;144:1.
27. Pilotti S, Rilke F, Gribaudi G, et al. Sputum cytology for the diagnosis of carcinoma of the lung. *Acta Cytol* 1982;26:649.
28. Bocking A, Biesterfeld S, Chatelain R, et al. Diagnosis of bronchial carcinoma on sections of paraffin-embedded sputum. Sensitivity and specificity of an alternative to routine cytology. *Acta Cytol* 1992;36:37.
29. Holiday DB, McLarty JW, Farley ML, et al. Sputum cytology within and across laboratories. A reliability study. *Acta Cytol* 1995;39:195.
30. Band PR, Feldstein M, Saccomanno G. Reversibility of bronchial marked atypia: implication for chemoprevention. *Cancer Detect Prevent* 1986;9:157.
31. Risse EK, van't Hof MA, Laurini RN, et al. Sputum cytology by the Saccomanno method in diagnosing lung malignancy. *Diagn Cytopathol* 1985;1:286.
32. Kennedy TC, Proudfoot SP, Franklin WA, et al. Cytopathological analysis of sputum in patients with airflow obstruction and significant smoking histories. *Cancer Res* 1996;56:4673.
33. Ng AB, Horak GC. Factors significant in the diagnostic accuracy of lung cytology in bronchial washing and sputum samples. *Acta Cytol* 1983;27:397.
34. Umiker WO, DeWeese MS, Lawrence GH. Diagnosis of lung cancer by bronchoscopic biopsy, scalene lymph node biopsy, and cytology smears: a report of 42 histologically proven cases. *Surgery* 1957;41:705.

35. Kaneko M, Eguchi K, Ohmatsu H, et al. Peripheral lung cancer: screening and detection with low-dose spiral CT versus radiography. *Radiology* 1996;201:798.

36. Zhou J, Mulshine JL, Ro JY, et al. Expression of heterogeneous nuclear ribonucleoprotein A2/B1 in bronchial epithelium of chronic smokers. *Clin Cancer Res* 1998;4:1631.

37. Tockman MS, Zhukiv T, Erozan YS, et al. Monoclonal antibody detection of premalignant lesions of the lung. In: Martinet Y, Hirsch FR, Martinet N, et al., eds. *Biological basis of lung cancer prevention.* Basel, Switzerland,: Birkhauser Verlag AG, 1997.

38. Tockman MS, Gupta PK, Myers JD, et al. Sensitive and specific monclonal antibody recognition of human lung cancer antigen on preserved sputum cells. *J Clin Oncol* 1988;6:1685.

39. Tockman MS, Mulshine JL. Sputum screening by quantitative microscopy: a new dawn for detection of lung cancer? *Mayo Clin Proc* 1997;72:788.

40. Mao L, Hruban RH, Boyle JO, et al. Detection of oncogene mutations in sputum precedes diagnosis of lung cancer. *Cancer Res* 1994;54:1634.

41. Sidransky D, Von Eschenbach A, Tsai YC, et al. Identification of *p53* gene mutations in bladder cancers and urine samples. *Science* 1991;252:706.

42. Sidransky D, Tokino T, Hamilton SR, et al. Identification of *ras* oncogene mutations in the stool of patients with curable colorectal tumors. *Science* 1992;256:102.

43. Mills NE, Fishman CL, Rom WN, et al. Ras oncogene detection in bronchioloalveolar lavage fluid from patients with lung cancer. *Lung Cancer* 1994[Suppl 1]:11.

44. Mills NE, Fishman CL, Scholes J, et al. Detection of K-ras oncogene mutations in bronchoalveolar lavage fluid for lung cancer diagnosis. *J Natl Cancer Inst* 1995;87:1056.

45. Yakubovskaya MS, Spiegelman V, Luo FC, et al. High frequency of K-*ras* mutations in normal appearing lung tissues and sputum of patients with lung cancer. *Int J Cancer* 1995;63:810.

46. Mao L, Lee JS, Kurie JM, et al. Clonal genetic alterations in the lungs of current and former smokers. *J Natl Cancer Inst* 1997;89:857.

47. Wistuba II, Lam S, Behrens C, et al. Molecular damage in the bronchial epithelium of current and former smokers. *J Natl Cancer Inst* 1997;89:1366.

48. Bos JL. *ras* oncogenes in human cancer: a review. *Cancer Res* 1989;49:4682.

49. Gazdar AF, Virmani A. Sensitive methods for the detection of *ras* mutations in lung cancer: some answers, more questions. *Clin Chem* 1998;44:1376.

50. Chiba I, Takahashi T, Nau MM, et al. Mutations in the *p53* gene are frequent in primary, resected non–small cell lung cancer. *Oncogene* 1990;5:1603.

51. Tockman MS, Erozan YS, Gupta P, et al. The early detection of second primary lung cancers by sputum immunostaining. LCEWDG Investigators. Lung Cancer Early Detection Group. *Chest* 1994;106:385S.

52. Nieburgs HE, Goldberg AF, Bertini B, et al. Malignancy associated changes (MAC) in blood and bone marrow cells of patients with malignant tumors. *Acta Cytol* 1967;11:415.

53. Palcic B, Macaulay C. Malignancy associated changes: can they be employed clinically? In: Weid GL, Bartels PH, Rosenthal DL, et al., eds. *Compendium on the computerized cytology and histology laboratory.* Chicago: Tutorials of Cytology, 1994:157.

54. MacAulay C, Lam S, Payne PW, et al. Malignancy-associated changes in bronchial epithelial cells in biopsy specimens. *Anal Quant Cytol Histol* 1995;17:55.

55. Payne PW, Sebo TJ, Doudkine A, et al. Sputum screening by quantitative microscopy: a reexamination of a portion of the National Cancer Institute Cooperative Early Lung Cancer Study. *Mayo Clin Proc* 1997;72:697.

56. Nagamoto N, Saito Y, Imai T, et al. Roentgenographically occult bronchogenic squamous cell carcinoma: location in the bronchi, depth of invasion and length of axial involvement of the bronchus. *Tohoku J Exp Med* 1986;148:241.

57. Woolner LB. Pathology of cancer detected cytologically. In: Group NCICELC, ed. *Atlas of early lung cancer.* Tokyo: Igaku-Shoin, 1983:107.

58. Sone S, Takashima S, Li F, et al. Mass screening for lung cancer with mobile spiral computed tomography scanner. *Lancet* 1998; 351:1242.

59. Kanazawa K, Kawata Y, Niki N, et al. Computer-aided diagnosis for pulmonary nodules based on helical CT images. *Comput Med Imaging Graph* 1998;22:157.

60. Lam S, D. BH. Future diagnostic procedures. *Chest Surg Clin N Am* 1996;6:363.

61. Hung J, Lam S, LeRiche JC, et al. Autofluorescence of normal and malignant bronchial tissue. *Lasers Surg Med* 1991;11:99.

62. Qu J, MacAulay C, Lam S, et al. Optical properties of normal and carcinoma bronchial tissue. *Appl Optics* 1994;33:7397.

63. Qu J, MacAulay CE, Lam S, et al. Laser induced fluorescence spectroscopy at endoscopy: tissue optics; Monte Carlo modelling and *in vivo* measurements. *Optical Engineering* 1995;34: 3334.

64. Bolon I, Gouyer V, Devouassoux M, et al. Expression of c-ets-1, collagenase 1, and urokinase-type plasminogen activator genes in lung carcinomas. *Am J Pathol* 1995;147:1298.

65. Fontanini G, Vignati S, Bigini D, et al. Neoangiogenesis: a putative marker of malignancy in non-small-cell lung cancer (NSCLC) development. *Int J Cancer* 1996;67:615.

66. Palcic B, Lam S, Hung J, et al. Detection and localization of early lung cancer by imaging techniques. *Chest* 1991;99:742.

67. Lam S, MacAulay C, Hung J, et al. Detection of dysplasia and carcinoma in situ with a lung imaging fluorescence endoscope device. *J Thorac Cardiovasc Surg* 1993;105:1035.

68. Lam S, MacAulay C, LeRiche JC, et al. Early localization of bronchogenic carcinoma. *Diagn Therapeut Endos* 1994;1:75.

69. Khanavkar B, Gnudi F, Muti A, et al. [Basic principles of LIFE—autofluorescence bronchoscopy. Results of 194 examinations in comparison with standard procedures for early detection of bronchial carcinoma—overview]. *Pneumologie* 1998;52: 71.

70. Yokomise H, Yanagihara K, Fukuse T, et al. Clinical experience of lung imaging fluorescence endoscope (LIFE) on lung cancer patients. *J Bronchol* 1997;4:205.

71. Ikeda N, Kim K, Okunaka, et al. Early localization of bronchogenic cancerous/precancerous lesions with lung imaging fluorescence endoscope. *Diagn Therapeut Endos* 1997;3:197.

72. Lam S, Kennedy T, Unger M, et al. Localization of bronchial intraepithelial neoplastic lesions by fluorescence bronchoscopy. *Chest* 1998;113:696.

73. Vermylen P, Roufosse C, Pierard P. Detection of preneoplastic lesions with fluorescence bronchoscopy (FB). *Eur Respir J* 1997; 10:425S.

74. Auerbach O. Cancerous and precancerous lung changes: a slide review. *CA Cancer J Clin* 1969;19:138.

75. Auerbach O, Saccomanno G, Kuschner M, et al. Histologic findings in the tracheobronchial tree of uranium miners and non-miners with lung cancer. *Cancer* 1978;42:483.

76. Travis WD, Colby TV, Corrin B, et al. *World Health Organiza-*

tion classification of lung and pleural tumors. International Histological Classification of tumors. Berlin: Springer-Verlag, 1999.

77. Lam S, MacAulay CE. Endoscopic localization of preneoplastic lung lesions. In: Martinet Y, Hirsch FR, Martinet N, et al., eds. *Clinical and biological basis of lung cancer prevention.* Basel: Birkhauser Verlag, 1998:231.

78. Mitsudomi T, Viallet J, Mulshine JL, et al. Mutations of *ras* genes distinguish a subset of non-small-cell lung cancer cell lines from small-cell lung cancer cell lines. *Oncogene* 1991;6:1353.

79. Nau MM, Carney DN, Battey J, et al. Amplification, expression and rearrangement of c-*myc* and N-*myc* oncogenes in human lung cancer. *Curr Top Microbiol Immunol* 1984;113:172.

80. Nau MM, Brooks BJ, Carney DN, et al. Human small cell lung cancers show amplification and expression of the N-*myc* gene. *Proc Natl Acad Sci U S A* 1986;83:1092.

81. Little CD, Nau MM, Carney DN, et al. Amplification and expression of the c-*myc* oncogene in human lung cancer cell lines. *Nature* 1983;306:194.

82. Levin NA, Brzoska P, Gupta N, et al. Identification of frequent novel genetic alterations in small cell lung carcinoma. *Cancer Res* 1994;54:5086.

83. Levin NA, Brzoska PM, Warnock ML, et al. Identification of novel regions of altered DNA copy number in small cell lung tumors. *Genes Chromosomes Cancer* 1995;13:175.

84. Petersen I, Bujard M, Petersen S, et al. Patterns of chromosomal imbalances in adenocarcinoma and squamous cell carcinoma of the lung. *Cancer Res* 1997;57:2331.

85. Petersen I, Langreck H, Wolf G, et al. Small-cell lung cancer is characterized by a high incidence of deletions on chromosomes 3p, 4q, 5q, 10q, 13q and 17p. *Br J Cancer* 1997;75:79.

86. Schwendel A, Langreck H, Reichel M, et al. Primary small-cell lung carcinomas and their metastases are characterized by a recurrent pattern of genetic alterations. *Int J Cancer* 1997;74:86.

87. Sundaresan V, Chung G, Heppell-Parton A, et al. Homozygous deletions at 3p12 in breast and lung cancer. *Oncogene* 1998;17:1723.

88. Ohta M, Inoue H, Cotticelli MG, et al. The *FHIT* gene, spanning the chromosome 3p14.2 fragile site and renal carcinoma-associated t(3;8) breakpoint, is abnormal in digestive tract cancers. *Cell* 1996;84:587.

89. Sozzi G, Veronese ML, Negrini M, et al. The *FHIT* gene at 3p14.2 is abnormal in lung cancer. *Cell* 1996;85:17.

90. Knudson AG. Hereditary cancers: clues to mechanisms of carcinogenesis. *Br J Cancer* 1989;59:661.

91. Denissenko MF, Pao A, Tang M-S, et al. Preferential formation of benz[a]pyrene adducts in lung cancer mutational hotspots in *p53. Science* 1996;274:430.

92. Horowitz JM, Yandell DW, Park SH, et al. Point mutational inactivation of the retinoblastoma antioncogene. *Science* 1989;243:937.

93. Harbour JW, Sali SL, Whang-Peng J, et al. Abnormalities in structure and expression of the human retinoblastoma gene in SCLC. *Science* 1988;241:353.

94. Hensel CH, Hsieh CL, Gazdar AF, et al. Altered structure and expression of the human retinoblastoma susceptibility gene in small cell lung cancer. *Cancer Res* 1990;50:3067.

95. Virmani AK, Fong KM, Kodagoda D, et al. Allelotyping demonstrates common and distinct patterns of chromosomal loss in human lung cancer types. *Genes Chromosomes Cancer* 1998;21:308.

96. D'Amico D, Carbone DP, Johnson BE, et al. Polymorphic sites within the MCC and APC loci reveal very frequent loss of

heterozygosity in human small cell lung cancer. *Cancer Res* 1992;52:1996.

97. Ohata H, Emi M, Fujiwara Y, et al. Deletion mapping of the short arm of chromosome 8 in non–small cell lung carcinoma. *Genes Chromosomes Cancer* 1993;7:85.

98. Sato S, Nakamura Y, Tsuchiya E. Difference of allelotype between squamous cell carcinoma and adenocarcinoma of the lung. *Cancer Res* 1994;54:5652.

99. Shiseki M, Kohno T, Nishikawa R, et al. Frequent allelic losses on chromosomes 2q, 18q, and 22q in advanced non–small cell lung carcinoma. *Cancer Res* 1994;54:5643.

100. Bepler G, Garcia-Blanco MA. Three tumor-suppressor regions on chromosome 11p identified by high-resolution deletion mapping in human non-small-cell lung cancer. *Proc Natl Acad Sci U S A* 1994;91:5513.

101. Iizuka M, Sugiyama Y, Shiraishi M, et al. Allelic losses in human chromosome 11 in lung cancers. *Genes Chromosomes Cancer* 1995;13:40.

102. O'Briant KC, Bepler G. Delineation of the centromeric and telomeric chromosome segment 11p15.5 lung cancer suppressor regions LOH11A and LOH11B. *Genes Chromosomes Cancer* 1997;18:111.

103. Suzuki K, Ogura T, Yokose T, et al. Loss of heterozygosity in the tuberous sclerosis gene associated regions in adenocarcinoma of the lung accompanied by multiple atypical adenomatous hyperplasia. *Int J Cancer* 1998;79:384.

104. Li J, Yen C, Liaw D, et al. PTEN, a putative protein tyrosine phosphatase gene mutated in human brain, breast and prostate cancer. *Science* 1997;275:1943.

105. Wang SS, Esplin ED, Li JL, et al. Alterations of the PPP2R1B gene in human lung and colon cancer. *Science* 1998;282:284.

106. Forgacs E, Biesterveld EJ, Sekido Y, et al. Mutation analysis of the PTEN/MMAC1 gene in lung cancer. *Oncogene* 1998;17:1557.

107. Shivapurkar N, Virmani AK, Wistuba II, et al. Deletions of chromosome 4 at multiple sites are frequent in malignant mesothelioma and small cell lung carcinoma. *Clinical Cancer Res* 1999;5:17.

108. Takeshima Y, Seyama T, Bennett WP, et al. p53 mutations in lung cancers from non-smoking atomic-bomb survivors. *Lancet* 1993;342:1520.

109. Peters EJ, Morice R, Benner SE, et al. Squamous metaplasia of the bronchial mucosa and its relationship to smoking. *Chest* 1993;103:1429.

110. Shimosato Y, Noguchi M, Matsumo Y. Adenocarcinoma of the lung: its development and malignant progression. *Lung Cancer* 1993;9:99.

111. Mori M, Chiba R, Takahashi T. Atypical adenomatous hyperplasia of the lung and its differentiation from adenocarcinoma. Characterization of atypical cells by morphometry and multivariate cluster analysis. *Cancer* 1993;72:2331.

112. Miller RR, Muller NL. Neuroendocrine cell hyperplasia and obliterative bronchiolitis in patients with peripheral carcinoid tumors. *Am J Surg Pathol* 1995;19:653.

113. Gazdar AF, Cohen MH, Ihde DC, et al. Bronchial epithelial changes in association with small cell carcinoma of the lung. In: Muggia F, Rozencweig M, eds. *Proceedings of the Second National Cancer Institute Conference on Lung Cancer Treatment.* Vol. 10. New York: Raven Press, 1979:167.

114. Slaughter DP, Southwick HW, Smejkal W. "Field cancerization" in oral stratified squamous epithelium: clinical implications of multicentric origin. *Cancer* 1953;6:963.

115. Johnson BE. Second lung cancers in patients after treatment for an initial lung cancer. *J Natl Cancer Inst* 1998;90:1335.

116. Hung J, Kishimoto Y, Sugio K, et al. Allele-specific chromosome 3p deletions occur at an early stage in the pathogenesis of lung carcinoma. *JAMA* 1995;273:558.

117. Kishimoto Y, Sugio K, Mitsudomi T, et al. Allele specific loss of chromosome 9p in preneoplastic lesions accompanying non–small cell lung cancers. *J Natl Cancer Inst* 1995;87:1224.

118. Sozzi G, Miozzo M, Tagliabue E, et al. Cytogenetic abnormalities and overexpression of receptors for growth factors in normal bronchial epithelium and tumor samples of lung cancer patients. *Cancer Res* 1991;51:400.

119. Sozzi G, Miozzo M, Pastorino U, et al. Genetic evidence for an independent origin of multiple preneoplastic and neoplastic lung lesions. *Cancer Res* 1995;55:135.

120. Sozzi G, Miozzo M, Donghi R, et al. Deletions of 17p and p53 mutations in preneoplastic lesions of the lung. *Cancer Res* 1992; 52:6079.

121. Sundaresan V, Ganly P, Hasleton P, et al. p53 and chromosome 3 abnormalities, characteristic of malignant lung tumours, are detectable in preinvasive lesions of the bronchus. *Oncogene* 1992;7:1989.

122. Thiberville L, Payne P, Vielkinds J, et al. Evidence of cumulative gene losses with progression of premalignant epithelial lesions to carcinoma of the bronchus. *Cancer Res* 1995;55:5133.

123. Nuorva K, Soini Y, Kamel D, et al. Concurrent *p53* expression in bronchial dysplasias and squamous cell lung carcinomas. *Am J Pathol* 1993;142:725.

124. Bennett WP, Colby TV, Travis WD, et al. p53 protein accumulates frequently in early bronchial neoplasia. *Cancer Res* 1993; 53:4817.

125. Hirano T, Franzen B, Kato H, et al. Genesis of squamous cell lung carcinoma. Sequential changes of proliferation, DNA ploidy, and *p53* expression. *Am J Pathol* 1994;144:296.

126. Smith AL, Hung J, Walker L, et al. Extensive areas of aneuploidy are present in the respiratory epithelium of lung cancer patients. *Br J Cancer* 1996;73:203.

127. Li ZH, Zheng J, Weiss LM, et al. c-k-*ras* and *p53* mutations occur very early in adenocarcinoma of the lung. *Am J Pathol* 1994;144:303.

128. Satoh Y, Ishikawa Y, Nakagawa K, et al. A follow-up study of progression from dysplasia to squamous cell carcinoma with immunohistochemical examination of p53 protein overexpression in the bronchi of ex-chromate workers. *Br J Cancer* 1997; 75:678.

129. Betticher DC, Heighway J, Thatcher N, et al. Abnormal expression of CCND1 and RB1 in resection margin epithelia of lung cancer patients. *Br J Cancer* 1997;75:1761.

130. Westra WH, Baas IO, Hruban RH, et al. K-*ras* oncogene activation in atypical alveolar hyperplasias of the human lung. *Cancer Res* 1996;56:2224.

131. Franklin WA, Gazdar AF, Haney J, et al. Widely dispersed *p53* mutation in respiratory epithelium. *J Clin Invest* 1997;100: 2133.

132. Gazdar AF, Carbone DP. *The biology and molecular genetics of lung cancer.* Austin: RG Landes Co., 1994:1.

133. Simone NL, Bonner RF, Gillespie JW, et al. Laser-capture microdissection: opening the microscopic frontier to molecular analysis. *Trends Genet* 1998;14:272.

134. Wistuba II, Behrens C, Milchgrub S, et al. Sequential molecular abnormalities are involved in the multistage development of squamous cell lung carcinoma. *Oncogene* 1999;18:643.

135. Fong KM, Biesterveld EJ, Virmani A, et al. *FHIT* and FRA3B 3p14.2 allele loss are common in lung cancer and preneoplastic bronchial lesions and are associated with cancer-related FHIT cDNA splicing aberrations. *Cancer Res* 1997;57:2256.

136. Ohta M, Inoue H, Cotticelli MG, et al. The *FHIT* gene, spanning the chromosome 3p14.2 fragile site and renal carcinoma-associated t(3;8) breakpoint, is abnormal in digestive tract cancers. *Cell* 1996;84:587.

137. Sozzi G, Pastorino U, Moiraghi L, et al. Loss of *FHIT* function in lung cancer and preinvasive bronchial lesions. *Cancer Res* 1998;58:5032.

138. Fisher JC. Multiple mutation theory of carcinogenesis. *Nature* 1958;181:651.

139. Loeb LA. Mutator phenotype may be required for multistage carcinogenesis. *Cancer Res* 1991;51:3075.

140. Loeb LA. Cancer cells exhibit a mutator phenotype. *Adv Cancer Res* 1998;72:25.

141. Wistuba II, Behrens C, Virmani AK, et al. Allelic losses at chromosome 8p21–23 are early and frequent events in the pathogenesis of lung cancer. *Cancer Res* 1999;59:1973.

142. Frost JK, Ball WJ, Levin ML, et al. Sputum cytopathology: use and potential in monitoring the workplace environment by screening for biological effects of exposure. *J Occup Med* 1986; 28:692.

143. Risse EK, Vooijs GP, van't Hof MA. Diagnostic significance of "severe dysplasia" in sputum cytology. *Acta Cytol* 1988;32: 629.

144. Strong MS, Incze J, Vaughan CW. Field cancerization in the aerodigestive tract—its etiology, manifestation, and significance. *J Otolaryngol* 1984;13:1.

145. Nowell PC. The clonal evolution of tumor cell populations. *Science* 1976;194:23.

146. Liu B, Parsons R, Papadopoulos N, et al. Analysis of mismatch repair genes in hereditary non-polyposis colorectal cancer patients. *Nat Med* 1996;2:169.

147. Mao L, Lee DJ, Tockman MS, et al. Microsatellite alterations as clonal markers for the detection of human cancer. *Proc Natl Acad Sci U S A* 1994;91:9871.

148. Fong KM, Zimmerman PV, Smith PJ. Microsatellite instability and other molecular abnormalities in non–small cell lung cancer. *Cancer Res* 1995;55:28.

149. Adachi J-I, Shiseki M, Okazaki T, et al. Microsatellite instability in primary and metastatic lung carcinomas. *Genes Chromosomes Cancer* 1995;14:301.

150. Merlo A, Mabry M, Gabrielson E, et al. Frequent microsatellite instability in primary small cell lung cancer. *Cancer Res* 1994; 54:2098.

151. Orlow I, Lianes P, Lacombe L, et al. Chromosome 9 allelic losses and microsatellite alterations in human bladder tumors. *Cancer Res* 1994;54:2848.

152. Miozzo M, Sozzi G, Musso K, et al. Microsatellite alterations in bronchial and sputum specimens of lung cancer patients. *Cancer Res* 1996;56:2285.

153. Wistuba II, Behrens C, Milchgrub S, et al. Comparison of molecular changes in lung cancers arising in HIV positive and HIV indeterminate subjects. *JAMA* 1998;279:1554.

154. Loeb LA. Microsatellite instability: marker of a mutator phenotype in cancer. *Cancer Res* 1994;54:5059.

155. Mao L, Schoenberg MP, Scicchitano M, et al. Molecular detection of primary bladder cancer by microsatellite analysis. *Science* 1996;271:659.

156. Morin GB. The human telomere terminal transferase enzyme is a ribonucleoprotein that synthesizes TTAGGG repeats. *Cell* 1989;59:521.

157. Hastie ND, Dempster M, Dunlop MG, et al. Telomere reduction in human colorectal carcinoma and with ageing. *Nature* 1990;346:866.

158. Chadeneau C, Hay K, Hirte HW, et al. Telomerase activity associated with acquisition of malignancy in human colorectal cancer. *Cancer Res* 1995;55:2533.

159. Hiyama K, Hiyama E, Ishioka S, et al. Telomerase activity in small-cell and non-small-cell lung cancers. *J Natl Cancer Inst* 1995;87:895.

160. Hiyama E, Yokoyama T, Tatsumoto N, et al. Telomerase activity in gastric cancer. *Cancer Res* 1995;55:3258.

161. Hiyama E, Gollahon L, Kataoka T, et al. Telomerase activity in human breast tumors. *J Natl Cancer Inst* 1996;88:116.

162. Counter CM. The roles of telomeres and telomerase in cell life span [review]. *Mut Res Rev Genet Toxicol* 1996;366:45.

163. Yashima K, Maitra A, Timmons CF, et al. Expression of the RNA component of telomerase during human development and differentiation. *Cell Growth Differ* 1998;9:805.

164. Yashima K, Litzky LA, Kaiser L, et al. Telomerase expression in respiratory epithelium during the multistage pathogenesis of lung carcinomas. *Cancer Res* 1997;57:2373.

165. Ahrendt SA, Chow JT, Xu L-H, et al. Molecular detection of tumor cells in bronchoalveolar lavage fluid from patients with early-stage lung cancer. *J Natl Cancer Inst* 1999;17:332.

166. Bertram JF, Rogers AW. Recovery of bronchial epithelium on stopping smoking. *Br Med J* 1981;283:1567.

167. US Centers for Disease Control, Office of Smoking and Health. *Morbidity and mortality weekly report* 1994;43.

168. Schantz SP. Chemoprevention strategies: the relevance of premalignant and malignant lesions of the upper aerodigestive tract. *J Cell Biochem Suppl* 1993;17F:18.

169. Boone CW, Kelloff GJ. Intraepithelial neoplasia, surrogate endpoint biomarkers, and cancer chemoprevention. *J Cell Biochem Suppl* 1993;17F:37.

24

THE USE OF LIGHT FOR THE EARLY DETECTION AND TREATMENT OF LUNG CANCER

HARVEY I. PASS
DENIS A. CORTESE
ERIC S. EDELL
STEPHEN LAM
HARUBUMI KATO

Light has been the subject of medical treatments since the ancient Greeks.[1] Raab first described the phenomenon in 1900 by documenting the death of paramecia with acridine and light,[2] and Tappeiner coined the term "photodynamic therapy" (PDT).[3] Skin cancer was treated with eosin and light in 1903,[3] Hausman found in 1910 that *porphyrins*, naturally occurring iron-or magnesium-free respiratory pigments present in the protoplasm of plant and animal cells, promoted photochemically induced cell death.[4] In the late 1950s, hematoporphyrin derivative (HpD) was prepared by Lipson and Baldes[5] based on a personal recommendation by Dr. Samuel Schwartz that the tumor-localizing properties of crude hematoporphyrin may be improved by using the supernatant that results from the preparation of hematoporphyrin. HpD concentrated in squamous cell carcinomas and adenocarcinomas,[6] and Lipson was the first to report that endoscopic fluorescence could be observed in patients with endobronchial tumors using HPD as the sensitizer.[7] In 1966, Lipson and colleagues were also the first to report a therapeutic response in a patient with recurrent breast cancer using multiple sessions of PDT with HpD.[8] The tumor was not eradicated, but objective evidence indicated a cytotoxic effect. Ensuing studies by Dougherty and others explored the use of PDT in the treatment of various animal and human malignancies,[9–15] and in 1982, Hayata was the first to use HpD to treat endobronchial tumors using a fiberoptic bronchoscope.[16]

PHOTODYNAMIC THERAPY: BASIC PRINCIPLES

PDT is based on the photochemical reaction that occurs when a sensitizing drug is exposed to light in the presence of oxygen. Absorbed light energy converts the sensitizer to an excited state, which in turn interacts with molecular oxygen to form singlet oxygen or oxygen-free radicals. Singlet oxygen is a powerful oxidizing agent that damages plasma membranes and other subcellular organelle (Figure 24.1). PDT is of no value unless all three components of a photochemical reaction—light, oxygen, and sensitizer—are simultaneously present when treating disease.

Components of Photodynamic Therapy

Light

Light is high-velocity energy transmitted in electromagnetic waves, which displays particulate characteristics by delivering energy in discrete measurable units called photons. The absorption of photons by a photosensitizer is the first reaction of a photodynamic system, and photochemical reactions can occur only if light is absorbed.[17] The *action spectrum* of a sensitizer defines the rate of a photochemical reaction when the sensitizer is stimulated by a given wavelength of light and usually corresponds to the absorption spectrum of the sensitizer. The *absorption spectrum* of a sensitizer determines the wavelength of light, measured in nanometers (nm), which is used to achieve the maximum photodynamic effect, and generally falls within the visible light spectrum between ultraviolet (UV) and infrared (IR) light. *Porphyrin sensitizers* have an intense absorption band at the UV end of the spectrum called the Soret band,[17] which maximally excites a sensitizer. The energy of light is *inversely related to its wavelength,* with lower wavelengths delivering more energy. However, shorter wavelengths are attenuated by hemoglobin as they pass through tissue, and the depth of tissue penetration by light is also inversely proportional to wavelength (Figure 24.2). Therefore, light at the *infrared* end of the spectrum penetrates much deeper

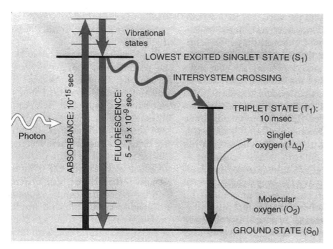

FIGURE 24.1. Energy states and interaction of photosensitizing agents. Before exposure to light, a molecule of sensitizer is in the ground state. When a photon of the appropriate wavelength is absorbed, an electron is raised to a higher energy level. The molecule then rearranges to a stable excited state. At this point, there are two possibilities. The excited molecule can fluoresce, emitting a photon and dropping back to the ground state, or an intersystem crossing can change the spin of an electron. During the lifetime of the resulting triplet state, absorbed energy can be passed along to molecular oxygen in tissue, activating the oxygen molecule to the singlet state. Singlet oxygen can oxidize any oxidizable biologic molecule with which it is in contact. (From Kessel D. Photodynamic therapy. *Sci Med* 1998;5:46, with permission.) (See Color Figure 24.1.)

into a tumor than *UV* light. Although stimulation of a porphyrin sensitizer with blue-violet light may result in more energy production, the tissue penetration of less than 1 mm is inadequate to treat malignancy. Therefore, PDT with porphyrin-based sensitizers is usually performed with 630 nm red light or higher wavelengths, which give tissue penetration of at least 10 mm.

The *total energy delivered* depends on the *duration* of light delivery and the *dose-rate* of light. The dose-rate, or power density, of light is usually expressed in mW/cm.^{2} *In vitro*, higher dose-rate delivery to tumor cells at a given total energy results in greater PDT cytotoxicity.[18] The relative inefficiency of PDT at lower dose-rates may result from the ability of tumor cells to repair sublethal damage or buffer toxic oxidative stresses.

Light Delivery

The appropriate method of light delivery for PDT depends on the experimental or clinical situation. An x-ray view box covered with a ruby red acetate filter can be used for *in vitro* PDT experiments,[18] whereas an argon-pumped dye laser exciting either Kiton Red or rhodamine B producing up to 15 watts of red light or a less expensive diode laser or LED array will be used as a typical light source for PDT in the clinical environment. The light source is coupled to one or more fiberoptic cables used to convey light with minimal energy loss to the treatment field. The end of the

cable is fitted with a tip designed to disperse light in a pattern appropriate for the clinical application. A cleaved tip projects light forward for treating flat surfaces, and a bulbous tip projects light in an isotropic spherical distribution for illuminating large cavities. A tip specially coated with cylindrical scattering material disperses light perpendicular to the axis of the fiber. This type of tip can be used for intraluminal applications, such as endobronchial PDT.

Oxygen

Although a few photodynamic systems are oxygen-independent, molecular oxygen is required to achieve cytotoxicity with porphyrin-based PDT.[19,20] PDT kills cells by selective destruction of essential molecules through photooxidative reactions via the production of singlet oxygen (see following sections). Several studies corroborate the importance of oxygen to photochemical systems. Using sodium dithionate to remove oxygen from the system, Lee showed that tumor cytotoxicity correlates directly with oxygen concentration.[20]

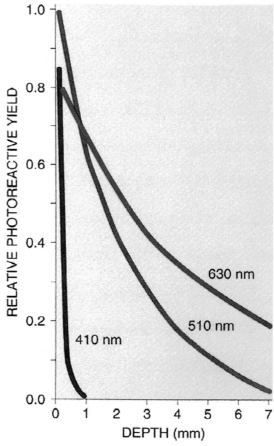

FIGURE 24.2. The relative phototoxic effect of a sensitizer is a function of irradiation wavelength. Longer wavelengths penetrate tissue to a greater depth. (From Kessel D. Photodynamic therapy. *Sci Med* 1998;5:46, with permission.) (See Color Figure 24.2.)

Mitchell used a customized glass Petri system to demonstrate that cells treated in hypoxic conditions are extremely resistant to PDT.[19] Similar studies have been performed *in vivo*. Gomer found that restricting the blood flow to the hind limb of albino mice inhibited the photosensitizing effects of porphyrin PDT.[21] Although attempts to directly quantitate singlet oxygen *in vivo* have been unsuccessful,[22,23] investigators have used transcutaneous oxygen-detecting electrodes to measure microcirculatory damage after PDT.[24,25] This technology may one day be used to determine the clinical effectiveness of photochemical systems.

Photosensitizers

Maximal quantum yield of a photochemical system occurs with light wavelengths that correspond to the sensitizer's Soret band, which for porphyrin sensitizers such as Photofrin II (PII) is in the 400 nm region. The absorption spectra for PII is characterized by this absorption peak at 405 nm that stimulates *fluorescence,* enabling the chemical to act as a tumor marker. To balance maximal quantum yield with deepest tissue penetration, PDT is performed at higher wavelengths (more than 590 nm) corresponding to minor peaks further along the absorption spectrum of the sensitizer. Under these conditions, PDT sensitizers generate singlet oxygen with quantum yield of 0.2 to 0.6 with tissue penetration up to 10 mm.

Uptake and retention of the porphyrin compounds has been studied in murine models. Levels are highest in the liver, adrenal glands, and urinary bladder, with lower levels declining in the following order: pancreas, kidney, spleen, stomach, bone, lung, heart, muscle, and brain.[26,27,28] In these animal models, intravenous injections result in higher tumor concentration than is obtained by intraperitoneal injections. In addition, these chemicals are heavily concentrated in phagocytic cells, lymphoid tissue, and regenerating tissues such as biopsy sites. Importantly, PII accumulates and is retained by vascular endothelium through the mechanism of endocytosis.[29] In addition, PII appears to be associated predominantly with low-density lipoproteins, but some components are also bound to albumin.[30,31] Structural proteins, such as collagen, also may have an effect on the distribution of PII. Ultimately, the intracellular accumulation of these photosensitizers is the result of a complex relation of all of these factors, which include both vascular and cellular components. The serum half-life in humans is 20 to 30 hours, but the photosensitizing component is retained in the skin, at low levels, for up to 6 weeks. Other photosensitizing agents under investigation include chlorins, phthalocyanines, tetraphenylporphine sulfate, the texaphyrins, benzoporphyrins, and cationic sensitizers, such as Rhodamine-123. Some of these second-generation sensitizers have an increased quantum yield at longer wavelengths and have much shorter periods for skin photosensitivity.[32]

Biophysical Basis for Photodynamic Therapy

Selective Retention of Photosensitizers

Selective retention of photosensitizer by malignant tissue is the central and most intriguing component of PDT. In 1948, Figge and colleagues[33] showed that crude hematoporphyrin was retained in tumors. In the 1960s, Lipson and colleagues[5,8,34,35] showed that HpD was retained by tumor tissue to a greater extent than crude hematoporphyrin. The measurements were based on fluorescence yield when tumor-containing HpD was irradiated with light of the appropriate wavelength. Since then, several investigators have demonstrated that both HpD and PII have a greater retention in tumor than in normal tissues by measuring fluorescence as a function of time after injection of the photosensitizer. However, the ratios of fluorescence within solid tumors versus various normal tissues varies widely. Overall, it appears that the tumor/normal tissue ratio is greater than 1 for PII 24 to 48 hours after intravenous injection in humans. However, some of the earliest work by Lipson and colleagues[34] showed that malignant tissue fluoresced within three hours of intravenous injection, well before normal tissue began to fluoresce. In fact, the three-hour time interval has been used for the detection and localization of lung cancer.[36,37] For purposes of cancer therapy, a time interval of between 24 and 72 hours is commonly used.

The reasons that tumor tissues selectively retain PII are unknown. There are several theories, but the explanation is still a subject of ongoing research. *In vitro* cell culture studies show that both normal and cancerous cells concentrate the photosensitizers and are killed by PDT. Transformed and nontransformed cells have identical PDT survival curves.[38] Perry and colleagues[39] found no differences in survival for thoracic cancer cells compared to normal lung fibroblasts during *in vitro* PDT experiments. This information would indicate that cancer and transformed cells do not selectively increase or retain photosensitizers in the *in vitro* situation. However, differences in *in vivo* retention of sensitizer between tumor and normal tissues have been demonstrated on numerous occasions. Selective retention within tumor tissue and cells may be related *in vivo* to a low pH found in tumors. Sensitizers are more soluble at low pH and, therefore, may be selectively retained. Neoplastic angiogenesis results in blood vessels with incomplete endothelium, which may have an increased permeability to porphyrin macromolecules. Increased concentrations of porphyrin have been noted along the vascular stroma of solid tumor tissue. The lack of normal lymphatic drainage could increase sensitizer concentration within tumor interstitial spaces. Proliferating cancer cells have higher levels of low-density lipoprotein receptors, which may facilitate the endocytosis of low-density lipoprotein-bound sensitizer components relative to normal tissues. Finally, macrophages and tumor-associated monocytes reconcentrate and retain photosensitizers within tumors. Intravenous injection of these photosensitizers leads to a higher uptake than that obtainable by intraperitoneal injection when tumors are located outside the abdominal cavity. On the other hand, Tochner and colleagues[40] found that intraperitoneal injection of HpD in an ovarian cancer ascites model resulted in higher therapeutic effect because there was no dependence on vascular delivery. Some components of photosensitizers, such as monomers, bind to albumin and globulin and are found to localize in the stroma of tumor tissue, whereas other components bind to lipoproteins. Albumin and high-density lipoprotein-bound components are not transported into the cell directly but are deposited on the cell membrane. Low-density lipoprotein-bound sensitizers appear to be transported into the cytoplasm quickly and accumulate in the lysosomal compartments.

Effects of Photodynamic Therapy in Vitro

Cytotoxicity

A wide variety of cell lines show sensitivity to PDT.[2,39,41–49] Comparison of different lung cancer histologies reveals few real differences in the characteristics that influence PDT cytotoxicity,[39] and the survival curves for a variety of thoracic malignancies, including adenocarcinoma, squamous cell carcinoma, large cell carcinoma, small cell carcinoma, and mesothelioma, are quite similar.[39]

The most impressive effect seen *in vitro* soon after cells are treated with PDT is damage to the plasma membrane.[49,59] Membranes are the primary targets of PDT, partly because of the water-lipid partition coefficient of PII. Porphyrins bind initially to the plasma membrane, followed by migration to intracellular regions. In only a few hours after PDT, normal cellular movement stops and large membrane blebs form on the cell surface.[51] These large balloonlike structures, often as large as the cell itself, indicate severe membrane damage and are the first visible sign of photooxidation in the cell.[52,53] This disruption of the integrity of the plasma membrane results in leakage of intracellular contents out of the cell.[54,55] After membrane blebbing occurs, cell division comes to a halt and cell lysis begins. As alluded to earlier, PDT damages other membranes in addition to the plasma membrane. Because of these effects on cell membranes, PDT may injure the nucleus, lysosomes, Golgi apparatus, endoplasmic reticulum, and mitochondria. Mitochondrial damage after PDT may involve inhibition of oxidative phosphorylation and electron transport with subsequent reduction in ATP production.[56,57] One cellular target that appears to escape serious damage by PDT is nuclear DNA. Although PDT can induce DNA strand breaks, this reaction does not lead to cell death. PDT does not appear to be mutagenic.[58]

Resistance of cells to PDT may one day determine the clinical efficacy of PDT in cancer treatment. Several investigators have begun to examine the role of the multidrug resistance (MDR) phenotype in PDT resistance. In MDR associated with chemotherapy, a membrane pump actively transports drug out of the cell. Conceivably, this mechanism could transport photosensitizer out of the cell, thereby reducing the photodynamic effect at treatment. This process could become a particular problem when treating patients with combined chemotherapy-photodynamic therapy regimens. Similarly, patients who have previously failed chemotherapy might likewise develop cross-resistance to PDT. Studies comparing the sensitivities of cells that express MDR versus wild-type cells from the same cell line revealed no cross-resistance to PDT.[59] Using cells made resistant to PDT by repeated exposure to PDT, investigators have shown that this resistance is not caused by decreased intracellular levels of sensitizer, the mechanism of action of classic MDR.[60,61] MDR may be associated with cross-resistance to PDT depending on the sensitizer used.[62] A more plausible explanation for PDT resistance involves the mechanism of action of PDT. Buffering of toxic oxygen radicals by free-radical scavengers could explain the induced resistance of cells to PDT. Studies by Ryter have shown that PDT can enhance transcription and translation of oxidative stress genes.[83] Many studies involving chemotherapy resistance have shown that free-radical buffering enzymes such as glutathione can protect cells against drugs that produce free radicals. Although no one knows how cells become resistant to PDT, mechanisms other than MDR are probably involved.

In Vivo Cytotoxicity

Flank tumors in mice regress completely by 2 days after treatment with PDT. Soon after PDT, blood flow stasis occurs in both arterioles and venules.[64,65] A vascular effect is one of the main components of tumor destruction with many of the presently investigated sensitizers. Vasoconstriction of arterioles, thrombosis of venules, and edema of perivascular tissues accompany the reduction in blood flow. Ben Hur suggests that PDT induces the endothelium to release vasoconstrictors and clotting factors, which cause local coagulation and stasis.[29] This reaction begins a cascade in which local blood flow stasis and endothelial damage retain red blood cells in the treatment field longer, thereby exposing them to higher doses of PDT. Subsequent damage results in red cell agglutination, which further exacerbates the low-flow state. Neutrophils and platelets bind to damaged endothelium with release of prostaglandins and arichidonates, which also act on the microvasculature. Other factors such as von Willebrands factor, platelet-activating factor, and nitric oxide may also be involved. The photodynamic process itself may lead to alterations in tumor blood flow.[66] A positive feedback cycle of oxygen depletion by the photooxidative system, acidosis, increased intratumoral swelling with decreased blood flow, and worsening hypoxia could account for static blood flow followed by tumor necrosis. Nuclear magnetic resonance studies examining tumor energy substrate levels during and after PDT indicate that ATP levels are virtually undetectable by 2 to 4 hours[67–69] and appear to decline in a dose-dependent fashion.[70]

The antitumor effect of PDT may be partly caused by modulation of the immune system. Various studies have documented the release of vasoactive agents such as prostaglandins, thromboxane, and histamine from murine peritoneal macrophages and mast cells.[71–73] These mediators could contribute to the vascular and metabolic effects of PDT in mediating tumor necrosis. PDT also induces macrophages to release tumor necrosis factor (TNF) in a dose-dependent fashion[74] and conversely, PDT may exert a net inhibitory effect on the immune system. Contact hypersensitivity remains suppressed 2 weeks after PDT,[75] and this effect is adoptively transferred by macrophages.[76] PDT also inhibits the mitogen-stimulated division of human peripheral blood lymphocytes.[77] Therefore, although PDT can induce nonspecific immune cells to produce substances such as TNF, prostaglandins, thromboxanes, and histamines that could either directly or indirectly mediate tumor necrosis, the overall effect of PDT on the immune system is unknown.

Increased specificity and sensitivity of photodynamic therapy resulting in an improved tumor/normal treatment index may result by treating tumors with antibody-sensitizer conjugates. A photosensitizing agent could be combined with a monoclonal antibody with idiotypic specificity for a known tumor. Theoretically, this treatment would increase the specificity of the sensitizer for the tumor, resulting in increased tumor cytoxicity with reduced side effects in normal tissues. Mew demonstrated this concept by showing that monoclonal antibody-photosensitizer conjugates effectively mediated tumor regression *in vivo* and kills a variety of cell lines *in vitro*.[78,79] PDT using monoclonal antibody-sensitizer conjugates appears to result in greater tumor specificity, longer remission, and less normal tissue toxicity in murine subcutaneous tumors.[80] Similar constructs have demonstrated selective killing of human ovarian carcinoma and melanoma cells[81,82] but work in this area remains highly investigational.

CLINICAL APPLICATIONS OF PDT IN THORACIC CANCER

Detection of *In Situ* Lung Cancer

Localization of lung cancer at the *in situ* or microinvasive stage can generally be accomplished by direct visual examination of the tracheobronchial tree using the flexible fiberoptic bronchoscope. The procedure is usually done with only topical anesthesia. Occasionally a cancer is difficult to see at its earliest stage, and, therefore, a more detailed and careful endoscopic examination using general anesthesia is necessary. General anesthesia permits the endoscopist time

to inspect the mucosal surfaces for signs of early cancer, such as thickening, irregularity, erythema, and pallor.

Rarely, these routine bronchoscopy procedures fail to confirm the localization of an early-stage squamous cell carcinoma, either *in situ* or early microinvasive, because they are difficult to see. To facilitate the localization of these tumors, various bronchoscopic instruments have been devised during the past 15 years. The earliest instruments used laser-induced fluorescence from PII or HpD-containing tumor. Historically, low-dose PII techniques were described, and most recently, a new technique relying on tissue autofluorescence without the use of a sensitizer has revolutionized this discipline.

In the early 1980s, special instrumentation systems were developed to be used with the photosensitizers PII and HpD. These systems were necessary to overcome technical problems of fluorescence detection and now serve as an historical footnote. Nevertheless, the principles guiding their development remain intact. It was known that chemical fluorescence from small superficial tumors could not be seen with the conventional flexible fiber bronchoscope because of the combination of a low concentration of chemical in the tumor, a low fluorescence yield, and high optical losses in the fiberoptic bundles. Each of the detection systems developed relied on amplification of a fluorescence signal, which was then displayed as either an audio signal or visual image. With the use of an image-intensifying, wavelength-detecting device, wavelengths of approximately 405 nM (blue-violet) were used to selectively produce characteristic reddish fluorescence from tissue containing significant amounts of the sensitizer. Either the endoscopist could image the areas of red fluorescence as distinct from the green autofluoresence, or a ratio for different areas of red to green fluorescence were calculated with the areas of highest ratios indicating the likely sites of tumor. The overall experience using these detection systems demonstrated that HpD and PII may be helpful in localizing tumors that are both roentgenographically and bronchoscopically occult. The detection of fluorescence, however, was not specific for carcinoma. Areas of cellular atypia ranging from moderate to marked were also sites of low-level fluorescence. Therefore, the bronchoscopist must biopsy all suspicious areas of fluorescence in order to confirm the localization of a cancer to a specific site.

The original Tokyo Medical College system, the University of California system, and the Mayo system were each successful in detecting the fluorescence from cancer foci; however, distinguishing between tumor fluorescence and nonspecific autofluorescence of the normal bronchial mucosa was difficult. A Japanese system actually displayed the wave pattern of light detected and distinguished the fluorescence between HpD and that of autofluorescence. The endoscopist alternated between white light for visual confirmation and a Krypton or excimer dye laser system to excite the sensitizer. Other systems described by Lam, Profio, and

Balchum were variations on the theme of a "ratioing fluorometer probe." The probe consisted of two fiberoptics of a two-channel bronchoscope: one for conducting the exciting violet light to the tip of the scope and the other to transmit the emitted light. The emitted light was split by a beam splitter through a red filter and a green filter. An analog divider ratioed the red fluorescence to the green autofluorescent intensity. An audio signal pitch in this system was proportional to the red/green ratio. By using this probe, there was decreased dependence on distance or angle from the end of the scope to the lesion. Bronchi with increased red/green ratios were presumed to be involved with tumor. After taking readings throughout the bronchial tree, all surfaces were next inspected under white light and fluorescence bronchoscopy to correlate positive localized fluorescence with increased ratios. This system was similar to another system developed by Laser Therapeutics, which allowed video images of the red and green fluorescence.

The most striking disadvantage of this technique was the requirement that patients receiving the sensitizer avoid sunlight for 4 to 6 weeks to avoid severe skin burn. Lam subsequently reported the use of low-dose (0.25 mg/kg) PII instead of the usual 2 to 3 mg/kg dose in conjunction with a ratioing fluorometer probe. The red/green ratios of known normal areas was .9 to 1.8, whereas the red/green ratios in biopsy-proven tumor areas was 4.8 (3.0 to 9.5). Increasing the dose of PII by 700% (to 2 mg/kgm) increased the ratio in the tumor area by only 64% (to 7.9). Moreover, skin photosensitivity testing after the .25 mg/km PII but prior to the additional 1.75 mg/gm revealed no skin reaction to as high a dose as 30 J/cm^2, a light dose commonly used to eradicate recurrent skin malignancies (after giving the patient the usual 2 mg/kg dose of sensitizer). Lam's involvement with autofluorescence (see following sections) relegated these observations to historical interest.

The original system used by the Mayo Clinic used violet excitation alternating with white light to illuminate the areas in question. The resulting fluorescence of the tissue caused by excitation of the previously given sensitizer was detected by a fiberoptic guide linked to a photomultiplier. The fluorescence signal was amplified as an audio signal whose intensity was proportional to the amount of fluorescence detected. The system allowed the endoscopist to view the field using the white light and to guide brushings and biopsies by the intensity of the "fluorescence pitch."

Success in detecting these occult neoplasms was reported from all centers involved in their development. Nevertheless, the systems lacked specificity because areas of cellular atypia or moderate or marked degrees would also concentrate sensitizer and have low levels of fluorescence. Moreover, the improvement in the signal-to-noise ratio in small, thin preinvasive lesion was only 1.5 to 2-fold at best,[83] and false positives in areas of inflammation or metaplasia were on the order of 27% to 50%.

At the same time that Lam and colleagues were working on low-dose fluorescence detection with the sensitive-ratio fluorometric measurements, they extended their observations to the possibility of using *in vivo* spectroscopy. The guiding principle was to explore the use of autofluorescence spectra of normal tissue and carcinoma *in situ* to facilitate localizing cancer in the bronchial tree. A difference exists between the *in vivo* autofluorescence spectra of normal bronchial mucosa and carcinoma *in situ* induced by a helium-cadmium laser at 442 nm (Figure 24.3). Fluorescence spectroscopy for normal tissue characteristically has a high intensity at 500 nm, which gradually decreases at longer wavelengths. On the other hand, *in situ* carcinoma demonstrates a relatively low intensity of fluorescence at 500 nm and remains low throughout the longer wavelengths. The investigators developed a device called the lung imaging fluorescence endoscope (LIFE). LIFE consists of a helium cadmium laser as a light source (442nm), two image-intensified CCD cameras with green (520 nm) and red (more than 630 nm) filters, respectively, a computer with an imaging board, and a color video monitor. Two images at different wavelengths are simultaneously captured in precise registration by the imaging board. The images are then combined and processed by an imaging board using a specially designed algorithm that allows normal tissue to be clearly distinguished from malignant tissue when displayed as a pseudocolor image on the video monitor. The computed image is displayed in real time. The detection of lung tumors is based on the observation that tumors *in vivo* have considerably lower autofluorescence in the green range than normal tissue, whereas emission in the red range is similar. The computed image is independent of the distance between the bronchoscope tip and the bronchial wall. The processed image can be displayed as desired (e.g., normal tissue as green and tumor as brown or brownish red) allowing guided biopsy under direct vision for pathologic confirmation.

This technique was first described by Profio and colleagues[84] in 1984 for use with sensitizer-induced fluorescence and is now used to differentiate cancer from normal tissue based on tissue autofluorescence. The system was tested *in vivo* by using it to detect squamous cell cancers and precancerous lesion in a hamster cheek pouch mode,[85] and spectral differences between precancerous, cancerous, and normal bronchial mucosa in 32 patients were documented using the LIFE system.[86] These observations were validated[87] in 82 volunteers recruited from occupational groups at risk for development of lung cancer. The premise was that one could determine differences in tissue autofluorescence between normal and malignant bronchial tissues in order to improve the sensitivity of standard fiberoptic bronchoscopy in detecting dysplasic and carcinoma *in situ* (CIS). This study consisted of 25 nonsmokers, 40 ex-smokers, and 17 current smokers with mean ages of 52, 55, and 49 years, respectively. One or more sites of moderate or severe dysplasia were found in 12% of the ex-smokers and current smokers but in none of the nonsmoker volunteers.

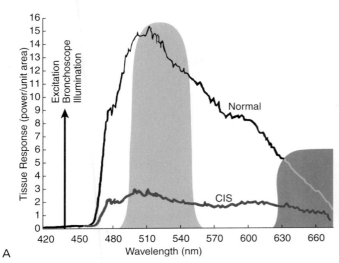

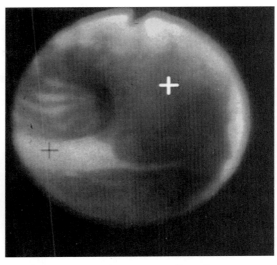

FIGURE 24.3. A: Autofluorescence spectra of normal bronchial mucosa and squamous cell carcinoma *in situ.* **B:** Reddish brown fluorescence of carcinoma *in situ* distinguished from the green fluorescence of normal bronchial mucosa. (Courtesy of XILLIX Technologies Corporation, British Columbia, Canada.) (See Color Figure 24.3B.)

CIS was found in two of the ex-smokers. The sensitivity of fluorescence bronchoscopy (86%) was found to be 50% better than that of conventional white light bronchoscopy (52%) in detecting dysplasia and CIS.

Most recently, a multicenter trial was performed to determine if autofluorescence bronchoscopy, when used as an adjunct to white light bronchoscopy, could improve the bronchoscopist's ability to locate and remove biopsy specimens from areas suspicious of intraepithelial neoplasia.[88] White light bronchoscopy was followed by fluorescence examination with the lung imaging device in 173 subjects known or suspected to have lung cancer. Biopsy specimens were taken from all areas suspicious of moderate dysplasia or worse on white light bronchoscopy or LIFE examination. In addition, random biopsy specimens were also taken from other parts of the bronchial tree. The relative sensitivity for the combination of white light and LIFE bronchoscopy compared to white light examination alone was 6.3 for intraepithelial neoplastic lesions and 2.71 when invasive carcinomas were also included. This translated to a 171% increase in sensitivity for the combination of white light and LIFE bronchoscopy over white light examination alone. The positive predictive value was 0.33 and 0.39 and the negative predictive value was 0.89 and 0.83, respectively, for the combination versus white light bronchoscopy alone. These studies led to FDA approval of this device for the detection of preneoplastic lesions of the airway.

This technology is an important addition to the armamentarium for early detection and prevention of lung cancer; however, its limitations must be noted. These include: (a) limitation to the detection of high-grade preinvasive lesions such as moderate/severe dysplasia and carcinoma *in*

situ. Autofluorescence is not useful in the detection of metaplasia or mild dysplasia; (b) pathologic interpretation must be consistent with classification of airway lesions; (c) a learning curve probably exists with the instrument so that subjective interpretation of fluorescence images becomes uniformly objective; and (d) the population studied influences the results of the examination for former smokers and has a lower prevalence of mild dysplasia and metaplasia compared to current smokers, whereas high-grade lesions persist after smoking stops. Moreover, women have a lower prevalence of high-grade lesions than men (13% versus 31%).[89]

The early detection of lung cancer with PDT will probably be reserved for those difficult clinical situations such as high-risk asymptomatic patients with positive sputum cytologies but negative radiologic evaluations and negative bronchoscopy. Other potential beneficiaries of these techniques might be patients with positive margins for carcinoma *in situ* after resection for bronchial carcinoma. These techniques are limited, however, in specificity because cellular atypia and metaplasia retain sensitizer and fluoresce on stimulation. Sensitivity is also restricted in that current systems require bronchoscopes too large to examine small diameter airways. Continued investigation into digital imaging combined with fluorescence detection and miniaturization of equipment may one day obviate these current weaknesses.

Photodynamic Therapy as a Treatment for Lung Cancer

Bronchoscopic PDT has been an investigational treatment for lung cancer since 1980. The technique is relatively sim-

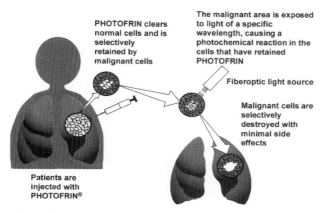

FIGURE 24.4. Schema of photodynamic therapy for bronchial lesions. See text for details. (Courtesy of Dr. Jeffrey Wiemann, Louisville, Kentucky.) (See Color Figure 24.4.)

ple and can be performed under local or general anesthesia using a standard flexible bronchoscope (Figure 24.4). The treatment does not result in the loss of lung tissue and can be used safely in patients with complicating medical illnesses such as heart disease and chronic obstructive lung disease. Empirical observations have shown that light doses as high as 600 J/cm and intravenous Photofrin doses of 2 mg/kg were not associated with any serious complications. *In vivo* animal experiments investigating the effect of PDT on a normal trachea have shown no apparent damage to the cartilage and suggest that PDT is unlikely to cause perforation or collapse of normal major airways.[90] Bronchoscopic PDT is presently approved for use in the the palliation of symptoms caused by endobronchial disease in higher stage lung cancer, as well as for primary treatment of microinvasive lung cancer in nonsurgical candidates.

Photodynamic Treatment of Early-Stage Lung Cancer

Several findings from the large-scale U.S. lung cancer screening projects indicate that a treatment modality such as PDT might be perfect for the treatment of early, superficial squamous cell cancers.[91] In patients with positive sputum cytologies and negative chest films, most lesions are confined to the bronchial wall with no extrabronchial involvement. The depth of these lesions, approximately 5 mm, corresponds to the tissue penetration of red light. These lesions detected by screening techniques tend to be centrally located squamous cell cancers. Because of their central location, major operations such as sleeve resection or even pneumonectomy are often required to manage early, noninvasive lesions. Photodynamic therapy possesses the ability to selectively treat large surface areas at risk without the problems associated with major resections that may not be curative. After an initial curative attempt, many patients, approxi-

mately 4% per year, will recur with second primary lesions, indicating the failure of localized surgery to cure a more generalized disease. If large-scale screening efforts are targeted to this high-risk population (i.e., patients who have had a previous curative stage I resection) localization of the endobronchial source of the abnormal sputums could be followed by PDT.

Other candidates for endobronchial PDT besides those found to have radiographically occult lung cancer would be those patients who refuse operative therapy or who are unable to have surgical resection because of high surgical risk limited pulmonary function, or multicentricity of lesions.

Several phase II clinical trials have examined the role of PDT in the treatment of early-stage lung bronchial cancer. Since 1980 at the Tokyo Medical College, 251 patients have had 297 lung cancers treated with photocynamic therapy. These data led to the approval of PDT for early-stage lung cancer in Japan in 1994, and have been updated since a previous report of the experience.[92] Ninety-five patients with 116 early cancers have been treated with endobronchial PDT. An argon laser coupled to a dye laser employing Rhodamine-B dye or an Excimer dye laser was used to generate 630-nm laser light. Endoscopic PDT was performed with topical anesthesia and intravenous sedation approximately 48 hours after an intravenous injection of 2 mg/kg of Photofrin II. A laser beam was transmitted through a fiber inserted through the instrument channel of a fiberoptic bronchoscope. The fiber tip was maintained 1 to 2 cm from the lesion, yielding a circular area of illumination estimated to be between 4 and 8 mm. Power output at the fiber tip was adjusted to range from 80 to 400mW when using the argon dye laser. When the Excimer laser was used, the frequency was set at 30 Hz with the energy adjusted to 4 mJ/pulse. Illumination time ranged from 10 to 40 minutes, giving energy densities of 100 to 800 J/cm². Tumor response to PDT was evaluated endoscopically, roentgenographically, cytologically, and histologically at periodic intervals after treatment. In resected specimens or at autopsy, the treated areas were examined macroscopically and histologically. After PDT complete remission, no evidence of tumor by any of the previously mentioned criteria was obtained in 77 patients (81%). Patients who ultimately had a complete remission often required an additional course of PDT to accomplish this outcome. The recurrence rate has been recorded as 16%. Complete remission was not obtained in the lesions that were anatomically difficult to photoradiate, in those lesions in which it was not possible to obtain an angle of irradiation of 90 degrees to the surface, or in lesions invading beyond the cartilage. Furuse reported similar results in 54 patients with 64 centrally located early-stage lung cancers. An 85% complete response rate was reported after a single session of PDT, and length of the longitudinal tumor was the only independent prognostic factor for a complete response.[93] In summarizing his experience with endobronchial PDT, McCaughan reported 16 patients with clinical stage I disease treated with PDT because they were ineligible for surgery. A remarkable estimated five-year survival of 93% was reported, but median time of follow-up was only 39 months for the 11 patients reported as still alive with no evidence of disease.[94]

The Mayo experience with PDT in patients with lung cancer has been slightly different than the Tokyo experience. However, the clinical observations are similar and complementary in nature. PDT at Mayo Clinic uses HpD rather than Photofrin. The laser technology is an argon pump dye laser using Rhodamine-B dye. The fiberoptics are the same. Photoradiation is usually delivered between 3 and 5 days (usually 3 days) after intravenous injection of 2.5 to 5 mg/kg of HpD. Laser power and total joules are similar to those described by the Tokyo group. Since 1980, more than 120 patients have been treated with this therapy at the Mayo Clinic. This experience includes a subset of 58 nonsurgical patients with an 84% complete response and fulfills the following criteria: (a) are roentgenographically occult, (b) are squamous cell carcinoma, (c) appear to be superficial mucosal tumors by bronchoscopic examination, and (d) are less than estimated 3 cm² in surface area. Nineteen patients (39%) have recurred after a single treatment, with a median time to tumor recurrence of 4.1 years. Eleven patients (22%) have recurred after a second treatment, and the median survival is 3.5 years (Edell, personal communication, 1999).

A comparison of the long-term results of surgery or PDT in patients who could have a potentially curative surgical resection has not been subjected to a randomized trial. In a preliminary study, however, 13 patients, with a total of 14 cancers, were considered surgical candidates and underwent PDT as an alternative to surgery.[95] The patients were treated with the understanding that if residual cancer was present after no more than two sessions of PDT, performed at three-month intervals, they would receive standard surgical therapy. In the group of 13 patients, 12 (92%) demonstrated a complete response, meaning that the carcinoma had disappeared bronchoscopically, by biopsy of the treated region, by brushings, and by washing cytology. Ten of the fourteen cancers (70%) demonstrated a complete response after the first photodynamic treatment. Three other cancers demonstrated a complete response after the second treatment. In total, 13 of the 14 cancers (93%) demonstrated a complete response after the two treatments. All 13 cancers were superficial and appeared to be spreading over the mucosa based on bronchoscopic examination. One cancer of the 14 (7%) failed to show a complete response. This cancer was a bulky, exfoliative lesion by bronchoscopic examination.

Of the 13 cancers that demonstrated a complete response, 3 (23%) recurred during the first 2 years of follow-up. Two of the cancers were then surgically resected. The third cancer, which initially demonstrated complete response after only one session of PDT, underwent a second

PDT treatment and has not recurred since. Ten of the thirteen cancers that showed a complete response have not recurred for up to 5 years of follow-up. In total, 10 of the 13 patients (77%) were spared an operation. The three patients with persistent cancer underwent surgical resection, and in each case, the postsurgical stage for each cancer was T1, N0, M0.

These data from the Mayo Clinic have now been extended to 21 patients, of which 15 (71%) had a complete response after one PDT treatment. With a follow-up of 24 to 116 months (median, 72 months), 4 patients (19%) have recurred after their first PDT session.[109]

In September 1997, the Oncologic Drug Advisory Committee recommended approval of PDT for *microinvasive lung cancer* for nonsurgical candidates in the United States. This approval was based on the data from three open label studies involving a total of 102 patients receiving PDT for early-stage lung cancer. On review of the data, 24 of the 102 patients, by external review, were thought to be neither radiation nor surgical candidates. Analysis of the data with regard to histologic complete tumor response, time to recurrence, overall survival and disease-specific survival revealed striking similarities between the whole group and the subset, as well as when the data were compared to the previously mentioned Japanese and Mayo data. Complete response rate after one PDT course was 92% and 75%, recurrences were 46% and 44% at median times to recurrence of 2.7 and 2.8 years, and median survivals were 3.4 and 2.5 years, for the subset versus all patients, respectively (Quadralogics Technologies, personal communication, 1999).

The most common complication after PDT treatment of early lung cancer remains photosensitivity reactions (23%). Other mild adverse events include transient obstructive symptoms caused by exudate and edema formation related to the PDT inflammatory response. Dyspnea can be life-threatening in a minority (4%) of cases and is usually related to bilateral PDT treatments simultaneously. Frequent clean-up bronchoscopies with attention to debridement may be necessary.

Palliation of Endobronchial Obstruction

The most common use of PDT in the treatment of patients with lung cancer has been in the palliation of symptoms caused by endobronchial tumor[39] (Figure 24.5). Multiple phase II studies documenting the safety and efficacy of PDT for relieving endobronchial obstruction have been performed.[96–104]

In attempting to summarize the overall experience in treating patients with obstructing carcinoma of the tracheobronchial tree, PDT appears to be most effective in the treatment of polypoid tumors. A poor response occurs with submucosal and peribronchial disease.[105,106] The median duration of complete response appears to be approximately 22 weeks if more than one-half of the airway obstruction

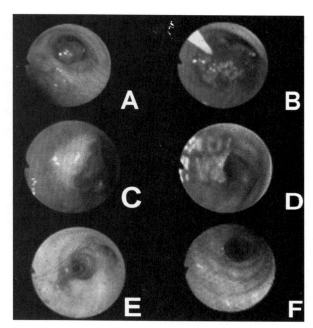

FIGURE 24.5. Photodynamic therapy for a patient with partial obstruction of the right mainstem bronchus. **A:** 90% obstructive non–small cell lung cancer 0.5 cm from the main carina. **B:** Laser fiber is positioned for interstitial treatment 48 hours after the patient received Photofrin II. **C:** Appearance of the lesion 48 hours after treatment before any debridement of the avascular base. **D:** Appearance of the lesion base after bronchoscopic debridement revealing the right upper lobe orifice to the right and the bronchus intermedius straight ahead. **E:** Appearance of the airway 2 months later. Only a superficial ulcer is present at the site of the original lesion **F:** Appearance of the airway 3 months after treatment. A histological complete response was documented. (See Color Figure 24.5.)

is caused by a mucosal process. However, the median duration is only 7 weeks if the tumor is predominantly submucosal or peribronchial. In addition, lack of perfusion or reduced perfusion out of proportion to the reduction in ventilation is associated with peribronchial involvement and poor outcome. Extraluminal tumor compression on CT scan also indicates a poor response.[107,108] One of the largest and most representative series of patients who had PDT for obstructing airway cancers has been reported by McCaughan.[94] Patients were treated with Photofrin, 2 mg/kg administered intravenously 48 hours before surface irradiation, as well as implantation techniques using power densities chiefly at 400 mW/cm of fiber. Light doses were modified depending on the airway treated: 400 J/cm of fiber for trachea and main bronchi, 300 J/cm for lobar bronchi, and 200 J/cm for segmental bronchi. A total of 492 bronchoscopic sessions delivering the therapy to 673 airway sites with 1,128 treatments, were performed in 175 patients over a 14-year period. Aggressive clean-up bronchoscopies were performed on the first and third days after treatment, and repeat endoscopic evaluation was performed 1 month after the treatment. The indications for PDT use in this population include endobronchial obstruction, hemoptysis of a

chronic and not massive nature, and treatment of bronchial stump recurrences. Although no intraoperative deaths occurred in McCaughan's series, eight patients died within the first 30 days, four from pulmonary hemorrhage. In fact, fatal massive hemoptysis (FMH) has been described in this treatment setting by several different investigators, and the rate of FMH is comparable to that seen with endobronchial brachytherapy and YAG laser therapy. It is generally agreed that in experienced hands, the FMH seen with PDT is probably caused by progression of disease.

FDA approval of endobronchial phototherapy for malignant disease came in 1999 after reviewing the results of a phase III trial comparing Photofrin PDT to YAG laser for the palliation of endobronchial lung cancer for 211 patients, of whom 75% had stage III–IV disease (Wiemann J, personal communication, 1999). Patients were randomized to receive either PDT or YAG. At month 1 or later after treatment, the objective tumor response rate was significantly higher with PDT (60%, 60/102) compared to Nd:YAG (41%, 45/109). Marked improvement ($\geq$2 grades) in dyspnea was observed in 23% (14/60) of PDT-treated patients with moderate to severe symptoms at baseline compared to 13% (9/68) of Nd:YAG-treated patients. Cough improved in 24% (15/63) of PDT-treated patients versus 8% (5/65) of patients who received Nd:YAG. Hemoptysis improved in 79% (19/24) of PDT-treated patients compared to 35% (11/31) of Nd:YAG-treated patients. Adverse events reported in patients receiving PDT (n = 99) were dyspnea (32%), hemoptysis (18%), bronchitis (11%), and photosensitivity reactions (20%). Patients receiving Nd:YAG (n = 99) reported dyspnea (17%), hemoptysis (12%), and bronchitis (3%). Life-threatening adverse effects including FMH and respiratory insufficiency were comparable in both populations. Early deaths and overall survival were similar. Based on these results, PDT with porfimer sodium was considered to be as effective as YAG for palliation of symptoms from obstructing endobronchial non–small cell lung cancer and in reduction of luminal obstruction. The PDT safety profile in this patient population was acceptable, and clinically important benefit was seen in approximately one-third of patients with moderate to severe symptoms at baseline.

CONCLUSIONS

The early detection of lung cancer using photodynamic techniques is evolving, and the LIFE scope has had FDA approval since the first edition of this book. The complementary nature of the LIFE scope and similar systems with PDT now add a powerful tool not only in the detection of lung cancer but also in defining airway carcinogenesis. More accurate means of biopsying and immortalizing bronchial cells reflective of airway events will eventually help in the definition of lung cancer biomarkers.

Photodynamic therapy for the treatment of lung cancer

in various settings has been approved in France, the Netherlands, Japan, the United States, and the United Kingdom. The therapy is still in its infancy with regard to appropriate sensitizers and light delivery systems, and it is predicted that all components of the therapy will be more efficient and, in fact, less morbid in the future. The morbidity at the present time is limited to transient inflammatory events in the airway as well as photosensitivity of the skin. Fatal massive hemoptysis, although a rare associated event, must be carefully explained to the patient as a possibility. One can foresee a future in which new sensitizers will have better tumor-associated retention and localizing properties and will have skin photosensitivity measured in hours. Future sensitizers will be able to be activated at greater depths within tissue. Moreover, total outpatient treatment, with sensitizer and light delivery performed only hours apart, will probably be the norm within the next 5 years.

REFERENCES

1. Daniell MD, Hill JS. A history of photodynamic therapy. *Aust N Z J Surg* 1991;61:340.
2. Raab O. Uber die Wirkung Fluoreszierenden Stoffen. *Infusoria Z Biol* 1900;39:524.
3. Jesionek A, Tappeiner VH. Zur Behandlung der hautcarcinomit mit fluorescierenden stoffen. *Muench Med Wochenshr* 1903;47:2042.
4. Hausman W. Die sensibilisierende Wirkung des hematoporphyrins. *Biochem Z* 1911;30:276.
5. Lipson RL, Baldes EJ. The photodynamic properties of a particular hematoporphyrin derivative. *Arch Dermatol* 1960;82:508.
6. Gregorie HG, Horger EO, Ward JL, et al. Hematoporphyrin derivative for detection and management of cancer. *Ann Surg* 1968;167:82.
7. Lipson RL, Baldes EJ. Hematoporphyrin derivative: a new aid for endoscopic detection of malignant disease. *J Thorac Cardiovasc Surg* 1961;42:623.
8. Lipson RL, Gray MJ, Baldes EJ. Hematoporphyrin derivative for detection and management of cancer. *Proc 9th Int Cancer Cong Tokyo, Japan* 1966;393.
9. Dougherty RJ. Activated dyes vs anti-tumor agents. *J Natl Cancer Inst* 1974;51:1333.
10. Dougherty TJ, Crindley GE, Fiel R, et al. Photoradiation therapy II. Cure of animal tumors with hematoporphyrin and light. *J Natl Cancer Inst* 1975;55:115.
11. Dougherty TJ, Kaufman JE, Goldfarb A, et al. Photoradiation therapy for the treatment of malignant tumors. *Cancer Res* 1978;38:2628.
12. Dougherty TJ. Photoradiation therapy. *Urol Suppl* 1984;23:61.
13. Mang TS, Dougherty TJ, Potter WR, et al. Photobleaching of porphyrins used in photodynamic therapy and implications for therapy. *Photochem Photobiol* 1987;45:501.
14. Dougherty TJ. Photosensitizers: therapy and detection of malignant tumors. *Photochem Photobiol* 1987;45:874.
15. Kelly JF, Snell NE, Berenbaum MC. Photodynamic destruction of human bladder carcinoma. *J Urol* 1976;115:150.
16. Hayata Y, Kato H, Konaka C, et al. Hematoporphyrin derivative and laser photoradiation in the treatment of lung cancer. *Chest* 1982;81:269.
17. Spikes JD. Photobiology of porphyrins. In: Doiron DR, Gomer CJ, eds *Porphyrin localization and treatment of tumors.* New York: Alan R. Liss, 1984.
18. Matthews W, Cook J, Pass HI. *In vitro* photodynamic therapy of human lung cancer: investigation of dose-rate effects. *Cancer Res* 1989;49:1718.
19. Mitchell JB, McPherson S, DeGraff W, et al. Oxygen dependence of hematoporphyrin derivative-induced photoinactivation of Chinese hamster cells. *Cancer Res* 1985;45:2008.
20. Lee See K, Forbes IJ, Betts WH. Oxygen dependency of phototoxicity with haematoporphyrin derivative. *Photochem Photobiol* 1984;39:631.
21. Gomer CJ, Razum NJ. Acute skin response in albino mice following porphyrin photosensitization under oxic and anoxic conditions. *Photochem Photobiol* 1984;40:435.
22. Gomer CJ. Preclinical examination of first and second generation photosensitizers used in photodynamic therapy. *Photochem Photobiol* 1991;54:1093.
23. Patterson MS, Madsen SJ, Wilson BC. Experimental tests of the feasibility of singlet oxygen luminescence and monitoring *in vivo* during photodynamic therapy. *J Photochem Photobiol* 1990;5:69.
24. Tromberg BJ, Orenstein A, Kimel S, et al. *In vivo* tumor oxygen tension measurements for the evaluation of the efficiency of photodynamic therapy delivery. *Photochem Photobiol* 1990;52:375.
25. Reed MW, Mullens AP, Anderson GL, et al. The effect of photodynamic therapy on tumor oxygenation. *Surgery* 1989;106:94.
26. Bugelski PJ, Porter CW, Dougherty TJ. Autoradiographic distribution of hematoporphyrin derivative in normal and tumor tissue of the mouse. *Cancer Res* 1981;41:4606.
27. Little FM, Gomer CJ, Hyman S, et al. Observations in studies of quantitative kinetics of tritium labelled hematoporphyrin derivatives (HpD_I and HpD_{II}) in the normal and neoplastic rat brain model. *J Neurooncol* 1984;2:361.
28. Gomer CJ, Ferrario A. Tissue distribution and photosensitizing properties in mono-aspartyl chlorin e6 in a mouse tumor model. *Cancer Res* 1990;50:3985.
29. Ben Hur E, Orenstein A. The endothelium and red blood cells as potential targets in PDT-induced vascular stases. *Int J Radiat Biol* 1991;60:293.
30. Barel A, Jori G, Perin A, et al. Role of high-, low-, and very low-density lipoproteins in the transport and tumor-delivery of hematoporphyrin, *in vivo. Cancer Lett* 1986;32:145.
31. Mazière JC, Morlière P, Santus R. The role of the low density lipoprotein receptor pathway in the delivery of lipophilic photosensitizers in the photodynamic therapy of tumors. *J Photochem Photobiol B* 1991;8:351.
32. Kreimer-Birnbaum M. Modified porphyrins, chlorins, pthalocyanines, and purpurins: second-generation photosensitizers for photodynamic therapy. *Sem Hematol* 1989;26:157.
33. Figge FHJ, Weiland GS, Manganiello LOJ. Cancer detection and therapy. Affinity of neoplastic embryonic and traumatized tissue for porphyrins and metalloporphyrins. *Proc Soc Exp Biol Med* 1948;68:640.
34. Lipson RL, Baldes EJ. The use of a derivative of hematoporphyrin in tumor detection. *J Natl Cancer Inst* 1961;26:1.
35. Grey M, Lipson RL, Mack JVS, et al. Use of hematoporphyrin derivative in detection and management of cervical cancer. *Am J Obstet Gynecol* 1967;9:766.
36. Edell ES, Cortese DA. Detection and phototherapy of lung cancer. In: Morstyn G, Kaye A, eds. *Phototherapy of cancer.* London: Harwood Academic 1990:185.
37. Benson RC, Jr., Farrow GM, Kinwey JH, et al. Detection and localization of in situ carcinoma of the bladder with hematoporphyrin derivative. *Mayo Clin Proc* 1982;57:548.
38. Pass HI, Evans S, Matthews WA, et al. Photodynamic therapy

of oncogene-transformed cells. *J Thorac Cardiovasc Surg* 1991; 101:795.

39. Perry RR, Matthews W, Pass HI, et al. Sensitivity of different human lung cancer histologies to photodynamic therapy. *Cancer Res* 1990;50:4272.

40. Tochner Z, Mitchell JB, Smith P, et al. Photodynamic therapy of ascites tumours within the peritoneal cavity. *Br J Cancer* 1986;53:733.

41. Keller SM, Taylor PD, Weese JL. *In vitro* killing of human malignant mesothelioma by photodynamic therapy. *J Surg Res* 1990;48:337.

42. Roberts WG, Berns MW. *In vitro* photosensitization I. Cellular uptake and subcellular localization of MONO-L-aspartyl chlorin e6, chloro-aluminum sulfonated phthalocyanine, and Photofrin II. *Lasers Surg Med* 1989;9:90.

43. Matthews EK, Cui Z. Photodynamic action of sulfonated aluminum phthalocyanines (SALPCS) on AR4-2J cells, a carcinoma cell line of rat exocrine pancreas. *Br J Cancer* 1990;61: 695.

44. Sery TW, Shield JA, Augsburger JJ, et al. Photodynamic therapy of human ocular cancer. *Ophthalmic Surg* 1987;18:413.

45. Pope AJ, Masters W, MacRobert AJ. The photodynamic effect of a pulsed dye laser on human bladder carcinoma cells *in vitro*. *Urol Res* 1990;18:267.

46. Jamieson CH, McDonald WN, Levy JG. Preferential uptake of benzoporphyrin derivative by leukemia versus normal cells. *Leuk Res* 1990;14:209.

47. Rogers DW, Lanzafame RJ, Hinshaw JR. Effect of argon laser and Photofrin II on murine neuroblastoma cells. *J Surg Res* 1991;50:255.

48. West CML. Size-dependent resistance of human tumor spheroids to photodynamic treatment. *Br J Cancer* 1989;59:510.

49. Kessel D. Sites of photosensitization by derivatives of hematoporphyrin. *Photochem Photobiol* 1986;44:489.

50. Volden G, Christensen T, Moan J. Photodynamic membrane damage of hematoporphyrin derivative-treated NHIK 3025 cells in vitro. *Photochem Photobiophys* 1981;3:105.

51. Jewell SA, Bellomo G, Thor H, et al. Bleb formation in hepatocytes during drug metabolism is caused by disturbances in thiol and calcium ion homeostasis. *Science* 1982;217:1257.

52. Borrelli MJ, Wong RSL, Dewey WC. A direct correlation between hyperthermia-induced blebbing and survival in synchronous G₁ CHO cells. *J Cell Physiol* 1986;126:181.

53. Dubbelman TMAR, Smeets M, Boegheim JP. J. Cell models. In: Moreno G, Potter RH, Truscott TG, eds. *Photosensitization: molecular and medical aspects.* NATO AST, 1992.

54. Sonoda M, Murali-Krishna C, Riesz P. The role of singlet oxygen in the photochemolysis of red blood cells sensitized by phthalocyanine sulfonates. *Photochem Photobiol* 1987;46:635.

55. Hilf R, Murant RS, Narayanan U, et al. Hematoporphyrin derivative-induced photosensitivity of mitochondrial succinate dehydrogenase and selected cytosolic enzymes of R3230AC mammary adenocarcinomas of rats. *Cancer Res* 1984;44:1483.

56. Hilf R, Murant RS, Narayanan U, et al. Relationship of mitochondrial function and cellular adenosine triphosphate levels to hematoporphyrin derivative-induced photosensitization in R3230AC mammary tumors. *Cancer Res* 1986;46:211.

57. Gomer CJ. DNA damage and repair in CHO cells following hematoporphyrin photoradiation. *Cancer Lett* 1980;11:161.

58. Ben-Hur E, Fujihara T, Suzuki F, et al. Genetic toxicology of the photosensitization of Chinese hamster cells by phthalocyanines. *Photochem Photobiol* 1987;45:227.

59. Kessel D, Erickson C. Porphyrin photosensitization of multidrug resistant cell types. *Photochem Photobiol* 1992;55:397.

60. Singh G, Wilson BC, Sharkey SM, et al. Resistance to photodynamic therapy in radiation induced fibrosarcoma. *Photochem Photobiol* 1991;54:307.

61. Luna MC, Gomer CJ. Isolation and initial characterization of mouse tumor cells resistant to porphyrin-mediated photodynamic therapy. *Cancer Res* 1991;15:4243.

62. Diddens H. Role of multidrug resistance in photodynamic therapy. Proceeding of optical methods for tumor treatment detection. Mechanisms and techniques in photodynamic therapy. *SPIE* 1992;45:115.

63. Ryter SW, Gomer CS, Ferrario A, et al. Cellular stress responses following photodynamic therapy. In: Henderson BW, Dougherty TJ, eds. *Photodynamic therapy: basic principles and clinical applications.* New York: Marcel Dekker, 1992:55.

64. Stern SJ, Flock S, Small S, et al. Chloraluminum sulphonated phthalocyanine versus dihematoporphyrin ether: early vascular events in the rat window chamber. *Laryngoscope* 1991;101:1219.

65. Wieman TJ, Mang TS, Fingar VS, et al. Effect of photodynamic therapy on blood flow in normal and tumor vessels. *Surgery* 1988;104:512.

66. Bellnier DA, Henderson BW. Determinants for photodynamic tissue destruction. In: Henderson BW, Dougherty TJ, eds. *Photodynamic therapy.* New York: Marcel Dekker, 1992:117.

67. Dodd NJF, Moore JV, Poppitt G, et al. *In vivo* magnetic resonance imaging of the effects of photodynamic therapy. *Br J Cancer* 1989;60:164.

68. Moore JV, Dodd NJF, Wood B. Proton nuclear magnetic resonance imaging as a predictor of the outcome of photodynamic therapy of tumors. *Br J Radiol* 1989;62:869.

69. Mattiello J, Evelhoch JL, Brown E, et al. Effect of photodynamic therapy on RIF-1 tumor metabolism and blood flow examined by 31P and 2H NMR spectoscopy. *NMR Biomed* 1990;3:64.

70. Chopp M, Hetzel FW, Jiang Q. Dose dependent metabolic response of mammary carcinoma to photodynamic therapy. *Radiat Res* 1990;121:288.

71. Henderson BW, Donovan JM. Cellular prostaglandin E release after photodynamic therapy. *Lasers Med Sci* 1988;3:103.

72. Fingar VH, Wieman TJ, Doak KW. Role of thromboxane and prostacycline release on photodynamic therapy-induced tumor destruction. *Cancer Res* 1990;50:2599.

73. Ortner MJ, Abhold RH, Chignell CF. The effect of protoporphyrin on histamine secretion by rat peritoneal mast cells: a dual phototoxic reaction. *Photochem Photobiol* 1981;33:355.

74. Evans S, Matthews W, Perry R, et al. Effect of photodynamic therapy on tumor necrosis factor production by murine macrophages. *J Natl Cancer Inst* 1990;82:34.

75. Elmets CA, Bowen KD. Immunological suppression in mice treated with hematoporphyrin derivative photoradiation. *Cancer Res* 1986;46:1608.

76. Lynch DH, Haddad S, King VJ, et al. Systemic immunosuppression induced by photodynamic therapy (PDT) is adoptively transferred by macrophages. *Photochem Photobiol* 1989;49:453.

77. Kol R, Ben Hur E, Marko R, et al. Inhibition of human lymphocyte stimulation by visible light and phthalocyanine sensitization: nitrogen and wavelength dependency. *Int J Radiat Biol* 1989;55:1015.

78. Mew D, Wat CK, Levy JG. Photoimmunotherapy: treatment of animal tumors with tumor-specific monoclonal antibody—hematoporphyrin conjugates. *J Immunol* 1983;130: 1473.

79. Mew D, Lum CK, Wat GH, et al. Ability of specific monoclonal antibodies and conventional antisera conjugated to hematoporphyrin to label and kill selective cell lines subsequent to light activation. *Cancer Res* 1985;45:4380.

80. Pogrebniak HW, Matthews W, Black C, et al. Targeted phototherapy with sensitizer-monoclonal antibody conjugate and light. *Surg Oncol* 1993;2:31.

81. White EA, Schambelan M, Rost CR, et al. Use of computed tomography in diagnosing the cause of primary aldosteronism. *N Engl J Med* 1980;303:1503.

82. Thibonnier M, Sassano P, Joseph A, et al. Diagnostic value of a single dose of captopril in renin-and aldosterone-dependent, surgically curable hypertension. *Cardiovasc Rev Rep* 1982;3:1659.

83. Lam S. Bronchoscopic, photodynamic, and laser diagnosis and therapy of lung neoplasms. *Curr Opin Pulm Med* 1999;2:271.

84. Profio AE, Doiron DR, Samaik J. Fluorometer for endoscopic diagnosis of tumors. *Med Phys* 1984;11:516.

85. Kluftinger AM, Davis NL, Quenville NF. Detection of squamous cell cancer and precancerous lesions by imaging of tissue autofluorescence in the hamster cheek pouch model. *Surg Oncol* 1992;1:183.

86. Hung J, Lam S, LeRiche JC, et al. Autofluorescence of normal and malignant bronchial tissue. *Lasers Surg Med* 1991;11:99.

87. Lam S, Hung JY, Kennedy SM, et al. Detection of dysplasia and carcinoma in situ by ratio fluorometry. *Am Rev Respir Dis* 1992;146:1458.

88. Lam S, Kennedy T, Unger M, et al. Localization of bronchial intraepithelial neoplastic lesions by fluorescence bronchoscopy. *Chest* 1998;113:696.

89. Lam S, Palcic B. Re: Autofluorescence bronchoscopy in the detection of squamous metaplasia and dysplasia in current and former smokers. *J Natl Canc Inst* 1999;91:561.

90. Smith SGT, Bedwell J, MacRobert AJ, et al. Experimental studies to assess the potential of photodynamic therapy for the treatment of bronchial carcinomas. *Thorax* 1993;48:474.

91. Woolner LB, Fontana RS, Cortese DA, et al. Roentgenographically occult lung cancer: pathologic findings and frequency of multicentricity during a ten year period. *Mayo Clin Proc* 1984;59:453.

92. Kato H, Okunaka T, Shimatani H. Photodynamic therapy for early stage bronchogenic carcinoma. *J Clin Laser Med Surg* 1996;14:235.

93. Furuse K, Fukuaka M, Kato H, et al. A prospective phase II study on photodynamic therapy with photofrin II for centrally located early-stage lung cancer. *J Clin Oncol* 1993;11:1852.

94. McCaughan J, Williams T. Photodynamic therapy for endobronchial malignant disease: a prospective fourteen year study. *J Thorac Cardio Surg* 1997;114:940.

95. Edell ES, Cortese DA. Photodynamic therapy in the management of early superficial squamous cell carcinoma as an alternative to surgical resection. *Chest* 1992;102:1319.

96. Pass HI, Delaney T, Smith PD, et al. Bronchoscopic phototherapy at comparable dose rates: early results. *Ann Thorac Surg* 1989;47:693.

97. Kato H. Lung cancer. In: Hayata Y, Dougherty TJ, eds. *Lasers and hematoporphyrin derivative in cancer.* Tokyo: Kgaka-Shion, 1983:39.

98. Doiron DR, Balchum OJ. Hematoporphyrin derivative photoradiation therapy of endobronchial lung cancer. In: Andreoni A, Bucedda R, eds. *Porphyrin in tumor phototherapy.* New York: Plenum Press, 1984:195.

99. Balchum OJ, Doiron DR, Huth GC. Photodynamic therapy of obstructing lung cancer. In: Doiron DR, Gomer CJ, eds. *Porphyrin localization and treatment of tumors.* New York: Alan R. Liss, 1984:721.

100. Balchum OJ. Photodynamic therapy of endobronchial lung tumors. Clayton Foundation Conference, 1987.

101. Vincent RG, Dougherty TJ, Rao U. Photoradiation therapy in the treatment of advanced carcinoma of the trachea and bronchus. In: Doiron DR, Gomer CJ, eds. *Porphyrin localization and treatment of tumors.* New York: Alan R. Liss, 1984:759.

102. Forbes IJ, Ward AD, Jackal FJ, et al. Multidisciplinary approach to phototherapy in tumors. In: Doiron DR, Gomer CJ, eds. *Porphyrin localization and treatment of tumors.* New York: Alan R. Liss, 1984:693.

103. Lam S, Kostashuk EC, Coy P, et al. A randomized comparative study of the safety and efficacy of photodynamic therapy using Photofrin II combined with palliative radiotherapy alone in patients with inoperable non-small cell bronchogenic carcinoma: a preliminary redport. *Photochem Photobiol* 1987;5:893.

104. Hugh-Jones P, Gardner WN. Laser photodynamic therapy for inoperable bronchogenic carcinoma. *J Med* 1987;243:565.

105. LoCicero J, Metzdorff M, Almgren C. Photodynamic therapy in the palliation of late stage obstructing non-small cell lung cancer. *Chest* 1990;98:97.

106. Sutedja T, Baas P, Stewart F. A pilot study of photodynamic therapy in patients with inoperable non-small cell lung cancer. *Eur J Cancer* 1992;28A:1370.

107. Lam S, Muller NL, Miller RR, et al. Predicting the response of obstructive endobronchial tumors to photodynamic therapy. *Cancer* 1986;58:2298.

108. Zwirewich CV, Muller NL, Lam S. Photodynamic laser therapy to alleviate complete bronchial obstruction: comparison of CT and bronchoscopy to predict outcome. *AJR* 1988;151:897.

109. Cortese DA, Edell ES, Kinsey JH. Photodynamic therapy for early stage squamous cell carcinoma. *Mayo Clin Proc* 1997;72:595.

25

CHEMOPREVENTION: SCIENTIFIC RATIONALE AND CLINICAL STUDIES

ROY S. HERBST

FADLO R. KHURI

WAUN KI HONG

Lung cancer is among the most common malignancies in the world and the leading cause of cancer-related mortality.[1] Although the five-year survival rate for patients with lung cancer has improved significantly since the early 1970s, this disease has retained a high mortality rate, making all aspects of lung cancer research a priority for clinicians, researchers, and the public. Despite advances in standard therapies—surgery, radiotherapy, and chemotherapy—the five-year survival rate of patients with lung cancer remains approximately 14%. For many years the number one cancer killer in men, lung cancer has just recently (within the last five years) become the preeminent cause of cancer-related death in women. This is due to an increased incidence of smoking in women during the late sixties and early seventies. As detailed in Chapter 20, there is usually a 20-year lag between increases in smoking patterns and subsequent increases in lung cancer incidence. Most patients present with metastatic or locally advanced disease for which therapy has demonstrated limited benefit. Ongoing clinical trials continue to be the method by which new compounds and new combinations of chemotherapy and radiation treatments are evaluated; however, given the slow progress, there has been an increased focus on lung cancer prevention strategies.

Since 90% of lung cancers are tobacco-related, primary prevention of lung cancer by smoking cessation remains an important objective. However, given the rising trend in worldwide tobacco consumption and the fact that former smokers still have higher lung cancer risk than nonsmokers (more than 50% of lung cancer occurs in former smokers),[2] lung cancer will remain a formidable problem well into the next century. We now know from molecular studies that, even after the cessation of tobacco use, genetic scars and alterations persist.[3] Chemoprevention is defined by Michael A. Sporn as the use of specific natural or synthetic compounds to reverse, suppress, or prevent carcinogenic progression to invasive cancer.[4]

Chemoprevention using 13-cis-retinoic acid (13cRA) has been demonstrated to be effective in preventing second primary tumors of the head and neck,[5] and this pivotal study, albeit small, set the stage for numerous clinical trials to evaluate similar agents for their chemopreventive ability in a variety of solid tumors, including those of the breast, colon, rectum, cervix, prostate, bladder, head and neck, and, of course, lung. In this chapter, we will review chemopreventive strategies exclusively as they relate to the prevention of lung cancer and second primary tumors in lung cancer patients.

THE RELATIONSHIP OF LUNG CANCER AND SMOKING: PRIMARY PREVENTION

The relationship between lung cancer and smoking has been established in an increasingly compelling fashion over the last five decades, and few would question this association. The association between cigarette smoke and lung cancer was first observed and cited by Ochsner and DeBakey in their landmark treatise in 1942.[6] In the 1950s, two large, well-designed epidemiologic studies further established a strong link between smoking and lung cancer.[7–9] The importance, however, of the histologic changes that were observed in smokers with lung cancer was reported by Auerbach and colleagues.[10] This group sectioned the entire tracheobronchial trees of deceased smokers and of individuals in whom lung cancer had developed, reporting three major types of epithelial changes: an increase in hyperplasia, a primary loss of cilia, and the presence of atypical cells. Perhaps most striking was the finding of carcinoma *in situ;* lesions composed entirely of atypical cells without cilia, whose average thickness was five or more cell rows, were observed in 15% of the tissue sections from patients who died of lung cancer. Of note is that carcinoma *in situ* lesions were never found by Auerbach and his collaborators in the pathologic specimens of nonsmokers, and few were found in the bronchial trees of light smokers.[10] In addition, a dose-response effect was demonstrated, because the changes were observed in 4.3% of bronchial sections from patients who had smoked one to two packs of cigarettes per day and in 11.4% of the sections from those who smoked two or more packs of cigarettes per day. Others have subsequently established such findings in the bronchial tissue of passive smokers.[11]

Recent studies attribute approximately 87% of lung cancers to tobacco exposure. The relative risk for developing lung carcinoma in current smokers is 24-fold greater than that for people who have never smoked.[12] However, the relative lung carcinoma risk in all cohorts of former smokers, although lower than for current smokers, remains greater than for those who have never smoked.[12] This close correlation between smoking status and lung cancer resulted in the National Cancer Institute's Division of Cancer Prevention and Control's emphasis on instituting cancer prevention as the major strategy in the control of lung cancer. The result of these campaigns to educate the public about the hazards of cigarette smoking has been a substantial reduction in the percentages of adults who actively smoke in the United States.[13] A survey of data from 1965 through 1991 reveals that these and other campaigns have had a substantial impact. In fact, the most recent data available from 1998 reveal that 29.9% of adult men and 19% of adult women were estimated to be former smokers, representing a 77.2% decrease from 1965 in the percentage of Americans who actively smoke.[13] This change has been attributed both to smoking cessation (the rate of which has doubled over the last three to four decades) and a decrease in the number of people who actually commence smoking.

LUNG CANCER AND FORMER SMOKERS

With the decrease in smoking, it becomes even more imperative to develop strategies for at-risk former smokers. In the most recent estimate conducted in 1991, 43.5 million adults in the United States were estimated to be former smokers, of whom 15.3 million are 45 to 64 years old. Of this group, 10.9 million are above the age of 65.[13] Astonishingly, although smoking cessation has helped reduce the absolute number of smokers, as many as 48.5% of people who have ever smoked are now considered former smokers. While it is clear that the risk of developing lung cancer decreases in individuals who stop smoking, the magnitude of the problem in former smokers is great. Two surveys of patients with lung cancer performed recently at the University of Texas M. D. Anderson Cancer Center and the Brigham and Women's Hospital respectively[2,14] demonstrate that more than 50% of lung cancer cases seen at these centers occurred in former smokers. This clearly shows a population presenting a significant public health problem for the United States, where there appears to be an increasing number of former smokers who will remain at substantial lifetime risk of cancer development.

SCREENING FOR LUNG CANCER

Screening is another approach to decreasing lung cancer mortality. Because patients with early-stage disease have higher cure rates, there has been the theory that effective screening programs could potentially have a significant impact on overall survival. However, screening strategies with chest radiographs and standard sputum cytology have to date all failed to alter overall survival rates in this disease.[14]

While intense controversy regarding screening for breast, colorectal, and prostate cancer still exists, a consensus does exist regarding lung cancer screening. All major organizations involved in public health recommend against any efforts to detect early lung cancer because each of the four randomized controlled clinical trials has failed to demonstrate a significant reduction in lung cancer mortality as a result of screening. Trials for lung cancer screening conducted at Memorial Sloan-Kettering Cancer Center, John Hopkins Hospital, and the Mayo Clinic were negative.[15–17] Many physicians feel that with new screening techniques and other diagnostic techniques, such as spiral low-dose CT scans, sputum cytology, and bronchial brushing, it may be possible to establish lung cancer diagnoses earlier enough to make an impact on overall survival rates in the context of this dreaded disease (for further details of lung cancer screening, see also Chapter 22).

FIELD CANCERIZATION

Chemoprevention represents an effort to arrest carcinogenesis and prevent the development of a malignancy by the administration of specific compounds. The rationale for chemoprevention of lung cancer is based on two principles of tumor biology common to most epithelial cancers: field cancerization and multi-step carcinogenesis, which are demonstrated in Figure 25.1 and Figure 25.2, respectively. Field cancerization (Figure 25.1) was first described by Slaughter and colleagues, who identified epithelial hyperplasia, hyperkeratinization, and atypia in grossly normal appearing epithelium adjacent to cancers of the oral cavity. Notably, multiple tissue sections were also found to contain carcinoma *in situ*. Such histologic changes throughout the oral epithelium suggest that steps in the development of malignancy occurred elsewhere in the aerodigestive tract (Figure 25.1). This concept is important in the chemoprevention of lung cancer, for it suggests that the development of an aerodigestive tract malignancy is not a random event but rather the result of diffuse changes that are present throughout the epithelium.

The existence of diffuse premalignant changes in the aerodigestive tract suggests the important clinical finding

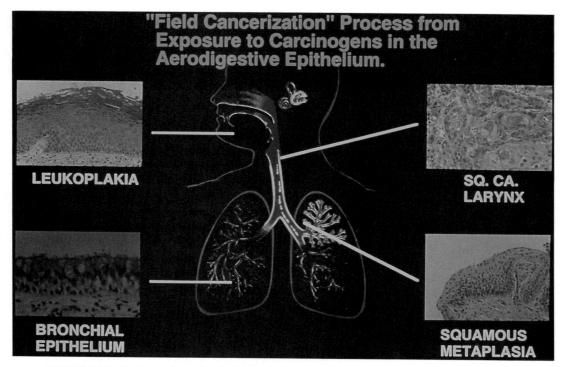

FIGURE 25.1. A schematic and pathologic representation of the Concept of Field Cancerization: Epithelium throughout the respiratory tract is affected by similar toxins, hence the concern about second primary cancer prevention. (See Color Figure 25.1.)

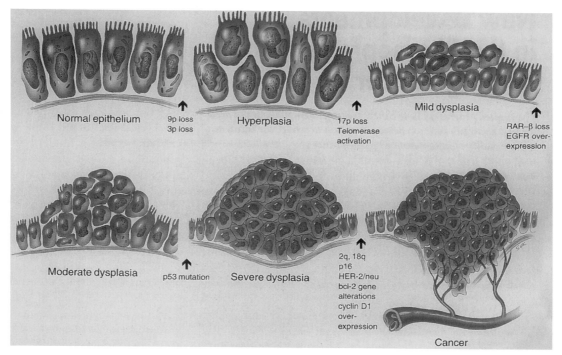

FIGURE 25.2. Multi-step process of lung carcinogenesis: A schema of molecular changes that have been reported to occur during the multi-step lung carcinogenic process. While representing potential points for intervention (i.e., chemoprevention), these events could potentially (once available) serve as biomarkers of cancer risk and intermediate end points for clinical studies. (From Papadimitrakopoulou VA. New developments in the chemoprevention of lung cancer. *Prim Care Cancer* 1998;18[Suppl. 1]:52, with permission.) (See Color Figure 25.2.)

that patients who survive an initial diagnosis of cancer in one region are subsequently susceptible to the development of second primary tumors. More specifically, it is now known that specific genetic alterations are most likely involved in this process. For example, Hung and colleagues[18] have demonstrated that highly specific deletions in the short arm of chromosome 3 occur during hyperplasia, the earliest stage in the pathogenesis of lung cancer, and that they can be found throughout the respiratory tract. Furthermore, Kishimoto and associates[19] noted similar evidence for allele-specific losses on the short arm of chromosome 9 in the earliest stages of lung cancer pathogenesis. This work was consistent with earlier work by Sozzi and co-workers,[20] who detected deletions of the short arm of chromosome 17 and of the *p53* gene in premalignant lung lesions. Further work by Sozzi and her colleagues has followed up on Hung's previous work and has demonstrated that one of the genes on chromosome 3p that is most likely lost in lung carcinogenesis is the fragile histidine triad (*FHIT*) gene[21,22] (See also Chapter 8).

Compelling evidence supporting the field carcinogenesis theory comes from studies of genetic alterations throughout the respiratory tract in paraffin-embedded tissue sections using a chromosome *in situ* hybridization technique[23,24] and in DNA content analyses after Feulgen staining.[25] Using biotinylated chromosome 7–17 specific centromeric DNA probes, investigators at the University of Texas M. D. Anderson Cancer Center demonstrated that chromosomal polysomies were found not only in tumor cells but also in histologically defined premalignant lesions such as oral leukoplakia[24] and in nonmalignant epithelial lesions adjacent to tumors.

MULTI-STEP CARCINOGENESIS

Although the series of genetic events leading to the development of lung cancer are not as well defined as in some systems (that is colorectal cancer),[26] lung cancer seems to result from multiple genetic events. Multiple studies have reported that invasive squamous cell carcinomas of the lung arise in association with areas of carcinoma *in situ*.[9,10,27,28] These progressive changes from metaplasia to carcinoma have been accepted as the hallmark of an orderly carcinogenic progress that ultimately leads to the development of squamous cell carcinoma (one such model is shown in Figure 25.2). Some initial findings in this regard were documented by Saccomanno and colleagues,[29] who examined serial sputum samples of uranium miners. Their subsequent cytologic examination of exfoliated bronchial cells in the sputum of these miners led the researchers to conclude that human lung cancers develop through a series of readily identifiable stages. Saccomanno and his colleagues further divided these stages into squamous cell metaplasia, squamous cell metaplasia with atypia (mild, moderate, or marked),

carcinoma *in situ,* and invasive squamous cell carcinoma. Quantitative cytochemical studies in human and animal models have further supported these findings with the demonstration of increasing amounts of DNA in exfoliated cells from abnormal epithelia.[30,31] Thus mildly atypical cells were found to exhibit a diploid-tetraploid range of DNA content, thereby most likely representing normal proliferative activity, whereas moderately and severely dysplastic cells had DNA content that was far greater than that encountered in the diploid population.

The data supporting this rely on the facts that complex cytogenetic abnormalities are consistently found in tumor cells[32,33] and that similar genetic abnormalities are found in normal and nonmalignant lung tissue samples from patients with lung cancer.[34] Along these lines, work by Mao and associates[35] demonstrated that *ras* mutations could be detected in the sputum of smokers prior to the actual diagnosis of lung cancer, thereby postulating a potential role for molecular screening where radiographic screening had previously failed to be effective. This genetic evidence was further strengthened by the fact that the number of chromosomal or genetic alterations in lung cancers seems to involve both the activation of dominant cellular oncogenes and the inactivation or chromosomal deletion of tumor-suppressor genes.[36] Since the inactivation of tumor-suppressor genes requires at least two genetic changes to inactivate both alleles, lung cancer cells must undergo several distinct genetic events to progress from the premalignant stage to active lung cancer. Conservative estimates based on both the cytogenetic and molecular genetic changes place the total number of genetic events required for lung carcinogenesis at between ten and 20 events[34] (Figure 2). Data from Mao and associates[35] have demonstrated loss of heterozygosity (LOH) on chromosomes 3p, 9p, and also (but less frequently) 17p not only in the bronchial biopsy tissue of patients who have cancer but also in the bronchial tissue of current and former smokers in whom there is no clinical evidence of disease or even, in some cases, of histologic abnormalities. This data establishes that tobacco use produces long-term irreversible (and reversible) effects and illustrates the persistent genetic damage found in the airways of former smokers. Mao's data indicate that 67% of former smokers demonstrate evidence of persistent genetic abnormalities in bronchial epithelium. These data lead one to believe that there are stable genetic alterations that can persist in the airway long after smoking cessation. Most critically, the fact that LOH at 9p and 17p persists even in patients who quit smoking suggests that these may be markers of stable genetic damage caused by cigarette smoke, unlike LOH at 3p, which appears to be largely reversible following smoking cessation. It is this persistent genetic injury that may, in fact, be the fingerprint of subsequent carcinogenic progression.

Mao and associates used microsatellite DNA studies at three specific loci—chromosomes 3p14, 9p21, and

17p13—to evaluate individual smokers (40 current smokers and 14 former smokers).[35] Genetic alterations at chromosomal sites containing putative tumor-suppressor genes (3p14 and the *FHIT* gene, 9p21 and the *p16* gene, and 17p13 and the *p53* gene) were frequently found even in the histologically normal or minimally altered bronchial epithelium of chronic or former smokers. Wistuba and colleagues[37] have verified that these and other similar genetic alterations, while present in the airways of current and former smokers, are never seen in the normal bronchial epithelium of nonsmokers (see also Chapter 23).

While squamous metaplasia was initially identified as a potentially reversible premalignant lesion and was studied in multiple chemopreventive trials,[30,31] the data of Mao and associates[35] and Wistuba and associates[37] demonstrated that persistent genetic abnormalities can be found even in the absence of squamous metaplasia. Therefore the reliability of squamous metaplasia as a putative premalignancy model for lung cancer has become questionable. The development of a comprehensive model of premalignancy will likely require integration of recent molecular observations of persistent genetic abnormalities such as those demonstrated by Mao and associates[3] with a reexamination of putative histologic subtypes of premalignancy, including bronchial metaplasia.

CHEMOPREVENTION

The rationale for a chemopreventive intervention in former smokers is clear from the evidence of persistent genetic damage in the airway as well as the etiologic role that tobacco plays in causing smoking-related genetic changes. With an increasing ability to detect and evaluate histologic abnormalities in bronchial tissue, the overall goal remains to develop agents that can be effective as chemopreventive compounds.[4]

The concept of using chemopreventive agents to reduce cancer risk stems both from epidemiologic and laboratory evidence. Epidemiological studies have demonstrated that vitamin A deficiency as well as decreased amounts of vitamin E and β-carotene are associated with an increased incidence of lung cancer in humans.[38] Vitamin A deficiency was long ago reported to induce squamous metaplasia in the mucosa of the upper aerodigestive tract[39] that is similar to the premalignant changes in this mucosa found in heavy smokers.[9] Dietary vitamin supplementation reversed squamous metaplasia in the trachea of vitamin A–deficient animals *in vivo,*[40] and various retinoids exhibited a similar activity *in vitro.*[41] Among other functions, these compounds are felt to exert anticarcinogenic activity by causing antioxidant effects and scavenging free radicals that are the by-products of many normal metabolic functions, thereby preventing cancer-causing damage to DNA. However, no clear-cut evidence of the specific effectiveness of vitamins A and E or

β-carotene has been demonstrated, and epidemiologic data cannot discount the possibility that other constituents of vegetables and fruits may provide the anticarcinogenic effects of these foods. While suggestive of effect, epidemiologic evidence taken alone cannot substitute for a randomized, double-blind, clinical study.

A number of problems and pitfalls with lung cancer chemoprevention studies involve (or revolve around) using the end point of cancer incidence in patients at increased but still marginal risk of cancer. These studies generally require a large number of patients and take years to decades to complete. The intermediate end points, such as those discussed in this paper, are helpful; however, these biomarkers have yet to be fully validated. It will take the efforts of a large group of subjects and investigators to expedite the validation of intermediate end point biomarkers and tailor clinical chemopreventive trials along these lines.

Retinoids

Vitamin A derivatives, or retinoids, are a family of compounds that have complex biologic effects, including the modulation of differentiation, proliferation, and apoptosis within both normal and neoplastic tissues.[42,43] The complexity of their function depends not only on the diversity of the retinoid ligands but also on the diversity of the nuclear retinoid receptors that mediate their activity. Retinoids bind to DNA and activate retinoid receptors, which function then as cellular transcription factors. These receptors are expressed at varying levels in different cell types, and their differential expression affects downstream gene expression. There exist two classes of nuclear retinoid receptors: the retinoic acid receptors (RARs), and the retinoid X receptors (RXRs). Within these two classes, there are three subclasses—α, β, and γ—which are subsequently divided further into a large number of isoforms produced through differential promoter usage and alternative splicing of receptor transcripts.[42,43] Specific isoforms of RARs and RXRs appear to have different functions, activating alternate downstream target genes. RXRs form homodimers and heterodimers with RARs or a host of other receptors, such as those for vitamin D and thyroid hormones, and with a variety of orphan receptors.[42] Because RXR is a ligand-binding partner in combination with orphan receptors, RXR ligands appear to be more versatile than RAR ligands in the activation of retinoic acid and other pathways.

The natural and synthetic retinoids, including all-trans, 13-cis, and 9-cis retinoic acid, all exist as stereoisomers, spontaneously interconverting in the intracellular space. For that reason, treatment with these retinoids nonselectively activates both RARs and RXRs. In contrast, several of newer synthetic retinoids are being developed that are capable of binding specifically to individual nuclear retinoids, thus allowing a degree of selectivity in the enhancement of the desired effects of certain retinoids with reduced side effects.

For example, a retinoid specific only for RAR-β may avoid inducing dermatologic side effects that have been caused by activation of RAR-γ. The overall goal is to enhance the potential therapeutic effects of specific retinoids while limiting the toxic effects caused by the widely used natural retinoids.[44]

Retinoid receptors affect gene transcription either directly or indirectly. This phenomenon is illustrated by the receptor interaction with activator protein-1 (AP-1), which is an important regulator of cellular proliferation and inflammation.[45–47] The mechanism of this interaction was explored by Kamei and co-workers[48] who demonstrated that retinoid-mediated inhibition of AP-1 activity appears to be the result of competition between nuclear retinoid receptors and AP-1 for binding to a transcriptional coactivator. This coactivator is found in limited quantities in the cell and thus is the rate-limiting step for both the retinoid receptors and AP-1.[48] Synthetic retinoids have been developed that selectively inhibit AP-1 without activating nuclear receptors.[49] These AP-1 (transcriptional activator protein-1) selective synthetic retinoids have been found to be potent antiproliferative agents in a number of tumor-derived cell lines[45,49] and are capable of reversing the squamous differentiation of bronchial epithelial cells.[50] Their toxicity profile may be favorable compared with their less-specific precursors, as retinoid toxicity has been linked to retinoid receptor activation.

Recent evidence suggests that the loss of specific of RARs might be involved in the promotion of lung carcinogenesis. Xu and colleagues examined transcripts of nuclear retinoid receptors using digoxigenin-labeled riboprobes specific for RAR-α, RAR-β, and RAR-γ in formalin-fixed, paraffin-embedded specimens from 79 patients with non–small cell lung cancer (NSCLC) and as a control in specimens from 17 patients without lung cancer.[51] Northern blotting and *in situ* hybridization techniques were used. All receptors were expressed in at least 89% of control normal bronchial tissue. RAR-α, RXR-α, and RXR-γ were expressed in more than 95% of the NSCLC specimens. In contrast, RAR-β, RAR-γ, and RXR-β expression was detected in only 42%, 72%, and 76% of NSCLC samples, respectively. These data suggest that the expression of RAR-β and possibly also of RAR-γ and RXR-β is suppressed in a large percentage of patients with lung cancer.

Further work in the area of retinoid biology and pharmacology has focused on the study of retinoid resistance. Clinical *de novo* retinoid resistance occurs in 40% of oral premalignant lesions and appears to develop over time in many lesions that had previously responded to retinoid treatment.[44] The mechanisms that underlie retinoid resistance are not yet well defined. However, the frequency with which clinical resistance is encountered has resulted in the evaluation of novel retinoids such as 4-N-(hydroxyphenyl) retinamide (4-HPR), which does not appear to bind any of the retinoid receptors but is a potent *in vitro* inducer of apoptosis.[44,52] Retinoids also appear to have potent effects when combined with other cytotoxic or cytostatic agents. Shalinsky and colleagues.[53] demonstrated that 9-cRA combined with cisplatin in human oral squamous carcinoma xenografts in nude mice shows enhanced antitumor efficacy bordering on synergism. Thus retinoids alone or in combination with other cytotoxic[53] or biologic[54,55] agents have the intriguing potential to reverse preneoplastic lesions. The preclinical demonstration of efficacy as well as the extensive epidemiologic data previously cited has led to the integration of retinoids into clinical chemoprevention trials in upper aerodigestive tract cancers as well as lung cancer.

Carotenoids

β-carotene is of interest because it is a natural agent with few toxic effects and is the prototype of a class of compounds known as carotenoids. Epidemiologically, several retrospective and prospective trials have demonstrated an inverse correlation between dietary carotenoid intake (largely in vegetables and fruits) and the incidence of lung cancer, most specifically squamous cell carcinoma.[56–58] The main known side effect of β-carotene was thought to be yellowing of the skin.

Other Agents

N-acetylcysteine, a substance that decreases glutathione levels, is also being evaluated in some lung cancer trials.[59] Another often-studied agent is α-tocopherol (vitamin E), which is a natural agent with strong antioxidant properties. Epidemiologic evidence suggests that α-tocopherol intake has an inverse correlation with the incidence of lung cancer. A recent clinical trial with this agent showed its efficacy in patients with oral leukoplakia.[60] The toxicity of α-tocopherol (vitamin E) is minimal, and there is some evidence to suggest α-tocopherol may abrogate the toxicity of retinoids, making this type of combination of α-tocopherol with a retinoid extremely promising for future clinical development.[61]

The success of chemopreventive clinical trials in patients with head and neck cancers spawned interest in chemopreventive strategies for lung cancer. Both cancers occur in the aerodigestive tract, and tobacco use is a likely cause in both diseases (Field Cancerization, Figure 25.1). Exposure of the entire aerodigestive tract to repeated carcinogenic insult (that is, smoke) results in field cancerization or changes throughout the field. These changes yield multiple independent foci of premalignant lesions that progress at different rates to form multiple primary cancers. The 4% to 7% annual incidence of second primary tumors in patients with lung and head and neck cancer supports this theory.

STUDY END POINTS IN CHEMOPREVENTION TRIALS

Using cancer development as an end point (still a rare event) results in large, costly randomized studies. One approach to reducing the number of subjects required to demonstrate activity in chemoprevention trials is to use intermediate biologic end points to define the activity of an agent before its evaluation in large clinical studies with cancer as a primary end point. This is often referred to as reversal of premalignancy. Potential intermediate markers could include general changes in the epithelium, such as metaplasia, or more specific markers, such as cytogenetic or molecular changes.

Reversal of Premalignancy

One of the major problems in studies attempting to reverse premalignancy has been the difficulty in defining consistent premalignant changes in the bronchial epithelium. Investigators have used both cytologic changes in sputum and histologic changes in bronchial biopsy samples from metaplasia to dysplasia as markers of risk. Reversal of these premalignant changes to normal tissue has been regarded as a potential intermediate end point for the chemoprevention of lung cancer. Saccomanno and colleagues were among the first to evaluate changes in sputum cytology induced by retinoids.[62] Patients with at least moderately atypical metaplasia were treated with 13cRA, 1 to 2.5 mg per kg per day. Sputum atypia did not improve with retinoid treatment, but alterations were noted in cellular morphology.

In general, studies focusing on sputum analysis from chronic smokers have shown a wide spontaneous variation in the degree of atypia over time and no consistent effect from retinoids[30,31,60–64] (Table 25.1).

In an effort to develop a more dependable, semiquantitative assay, Mathe and co-workers described the metaplasia index (MI) to quantitate the degree of squamous metaplasia in bronchial biopsies from six specific anatomic sites.[63] The MI was defined as the number of samples with metaplasia divided by the total number of samples analyzed, multiplied by 100. MIs were documented pre- and posttreatment in a single-arm trial of smokers receiving etretinate (25 mg per day for six months).[63] This trial demonstrated a decrease in the MI following etretinate therapy from 34.57% to 26.96% after six months of treatment. Of note was that MI decreased to 0% in four patients who ceased smoking, though these patients were excluded from the overall analysis. While the difference was significant, there was unfortunately no control group to assess the natural history of bronchial metaplasia in untreated patients. Arnold and associates, in a study that evaluates the efficacy of etretinate, used atypia in sputum cytology specimens as an end point.[65] Patients with moderate or severe sputum atypia were randomized to receive either etretinate (25 mg per day) or a placebo. At the completion of six months of treatment, an improvement in sputum atypia was noted in subjects in both the etretinate and placebo groups (32.3% and 29.8% of the patients, respectively), and no real benefit was seen.

These findings, however, were confirmed by those of Lee and colleagues.[31] In this trial, 93 smokers with metaplasia or dysplasia quantitated at baseline using the MI were randomized to 13-cis retinoic acid (13cRA, 1 mg per kg per day) or placebo for six months.[31] Subjects completed the trial and underwent repeat bronchoscopy. Posttreatment biopsy samples demonstrated a similar rate of decrease in the MI in both trial arms that was most strongly associated with smoking cessation. Clearly, future trials of this sort will need to be placebo-controlled to correct for multiple variables such as smoking cessation, sampling differences, and spontaneous regression that can influence the final outcome.

TABLE 25.1.   COMPLETED RANDOMIZED CHEMOPREVENTION TRIALS IN LUNG CANCER

First Author or Study Group (Year)	Study Endpoint	Study Design (Phase)	Number of Patients	Therapy	Outcome
Heimburger (1988)[30]	Metaplasia or sputum atypia	II	73	Vitamin B12 plus folic acid	Positive
Arnold (1992)[65]	Metaplasia (bronchial tissue)	III	150	Etretinate	No benefit
van Poppel (1992)	Micronuclei (sputum)	III	114	Beta-carotene	Positive
Lee (1994)[31]	Metaplasia (bronchial tissue)	III	87	Isotretinoin	No benefit
McLarty (1995)[64]	Metaplasia or sputum atypia	III	755	Beta-carotene plus retinol	No benefit
Alpha-tocopherol, Beta-carotene Cancer Prevention Study Group (1994)	Lung cancer and other cancers	III	29,133 (smokers)	Alpha-tocopherol, beta-carotene	Harmful[a][b]
Hennekens (1996)[69] Physicians Health Study	Malignant neoplasms and cardiovascular disease	III	22,071 (smokers)	Beta-carotene	No benefit[c]
Omenn (1996) CARET trial	Lung cancer and cardiovascular disease	III	18,314 (healthy males)	Beta-carotene and retinol	Harmful[a][b]

[a] Increased incidence of lung cancer detected in smokers receiving beta-carotene.
[b] Duration of intervention was six years.
[c] Duration of intervention was 12 years.

PRIMARY PREVENTION IN HIGH-RISK POPULATIONS

Based on epidemiologic data, which indicated an inverse correlation between cancer risk and dietary β-carotene, β-carotene has been the major agent studied in primary prevention of lung cancer.[58,66-69] Three large primary prevention trials using β-carotene with or without α-tocopherol or retinol have been completed. Interestingly, two of the three trials have documented an increased incidence of lung cancer in the treatment arms with β-carotene (Table 25.1), certainly an unexpected result.

The Finnish ATBC trial, the largest of its kind, randomized 29,133 male smokers in southwest Finland aged 50 to 69 years to one of four regimens, using a 2×2 factorial design. The regimens were α-tocopherol (50 mg per day) alone, β-carotene (20 mg per day) alone, both agents, or placebo.[66] The participants in the ATBC trial continued the interventions for five to eight years; compliance was excellent as more than 80% of subjects took at least 95% of their assigned medications. The median length of follow-up on the study was 6.1 years. Over the course of the study, 876 new cases of lung cancer were diagnosed. Patients receiving β-carotene had an 18% increased incidence of lung cancer (p = 0.01) and an 8% increased mortality rate. α-tocopherol administration failed significantly to alter either lung cancer incidence or overall mortality rate. The primary cause of increased mortality in the β-carotene group included lung cancer, ischemic heart disease, and hemorrhagic strokes. Subsequent analysis of these data demonstrated a trend to increased risk after β-carotene treatment in heavy smokers (more than or equal to one pack per day) and in those who had high ethanol intake (more than 11 g per day).[67] The surprising results from this study were not only the failure of β-carotene to demonstrate a protective effect but also the suggestion that supplemental pharmacologic doses of β-carotene might be harmful to smokers. Therefore, this study demonstrates that caution must be used when relying completely on epidemiologic data to design large randomized clinical trials.

Accrual to another primary prevention trial performed in the United States was stopped early due to similar findings. This study, conducted by the University of Washington at Seattle, was designated the Carotene and Retinol Efficacy Trial (CARET) study and randomized a total of 18,314 smokers, former smokers, and people with a history of asbestos exposure to a combination of β-carotene (30 mg per day) and retinol (25,000 IU per day), in the form of retinyl palmitate (vitamin A), or placebo in a double-blind fashion.[68,70] Toxic effects were not a significant problem and consisted mostly of mild skin yellowing in subjects who received β-carotene. After a mean follow-up period of four years, accrual was suspended due to an increased relative risk of lung cancer and death due to lung cancer in the treatment arm (hazard ratio 1.28 versus 1.46, respectively).

As in the ATBC trial, excess lung cancer incidence was most associated with current smoking and the highest quartile of ethanol intake.[70]

The mechanism of enhancement of lung carcinogenesis by supplemental β-carotene (alone or in combination with retinol) in smokers has not yet been defined. The most plausible theory at this time suggests a pro-oxidant effect of β-carotene in the damaged lungs of individuals who continue to smoke heavily,[71] but this has yet to be firmly established. In light of the data from the CARET and ATBC trials, current smokers should not use β-carotene supplements.

A third trial, of male physicians in the United States, of whom only 11% were current smokers, randomized 20,071 participants to β-carotene (50 mg four times per day) or placebo.[69] Neither benefit nor harm was demonstrated from the intervention in terms of the incidence of malignant neoplasms, cardiovascular disease, or death from all causes.

Several pilot studies are currently looking at patients previously exposed to asbestos fibers or tin dust. A pilot study of 816 patients was recently completed evaluating daily doses of retinyl palmitate (25,000 IU) and β-carotene (30 mg).[72] Tin miners in southern China have an annual incidence of lung cancer exceeding 1%. In a pilot study in this population, 358 people were randomized to receive vitamin A (25,000 IU), β-carotene (50 mg), vitamin E (800 IU), selenium (400 μg), or placebo in a trial with a 2×4 factorial design. Compliance has exceeded 90%, and toxicity has not been a problem.[72] Results from this study are pending.

PREVENTION OF SECOND PRIMARY TUMORS

As previously discussed, patients with a prior history of aerodigestive tract malignancies are at an increased risk of developing a second primary tumor (SPT), particularly lung cancer, making this population perhaps at the highest risk for developing lung cancers. Three randomized trials designed to reduce the incidence of second primary tumors in patients with an index cancer lesion of the head and neck or lung have now been completed. Two of these three trials have demonstrated an impact on tobacco-related cancer with retinoid treatment (Table 25.2).

In a study by Hong and colleagues[5] in 1991, 103 patients with the prior diagnosis of squamous cell cancer of the head and neck treated with surgery, radiotherapy, or both were randomized to receive either high-dose 13cRA (50 to 100 mg per m^2 per day) or a placebo for one year. Although originally conceived as an adjuvant trial, this study did not demonstrate any impact of treatment on locoregional recurrence or metastatic disease. However, with a median follow-up period of 32 months, second primary tumors developed in only two (4%) of the treated patients as opposed to 12 (24%) of patients receiving placebo. Of particular note,

TABLE 25.2. RANDOMIZED TRIALS OF RETINOIDS IN HUMAN CANCER CHEMOPREVENTION OF SECOND PRIMARY CANCERS

Reference	Population	Intervention	No. Patients	End Point	Result	P Value
Hong (1990, 1994)[5,38]	US—prior HNSCC	13 cRA (50–100 mg/m²/day) Placebo	49 51	Second primary tumor	4% (32 mo); 14% (55 mo) 24% (32 mo); 31% (55 mo)	.005 (32 mo) .042 (55 mo)
Pastorino (1993)[76]	Italy—prior NSCLC	Retinyl Palmitate (300,000/IU/day) No treatment control	150 157	Second primary lung tumors	Longer time to second primary tumor development	.045
Bolla (1994)[75]	France—prior HNSCC	Etretinate (50/25 mg/day) Placebo	156	Second primary tumor	18% 18% (41 mo)	NS

HNSCC, head and neck squamous cell carcinoma; NSCLC, non–small cell lung cancer; RP, retinyl palmitate; 13 cRA, 13-cis-retinoic acid.

93% (13 of 14) of the second primary tumors observed were in the carcinogen-exposed field of the upper aerodigestive tract, lungs, and esophagus. Recent reanalysis of this trial at a median follow-up period of 4.5 years demonstrated 16 second primary tumors in the placebo group and only seven in the 13cRA group.[73] Three lung cancers were found in the retinoid group versus nine in the placebo group. Therefore the effect of 13cRA persisted for approximately two years after the cessation of 13cRA in the retinoid arm. These promising results are offset somewhat by the significant toxic effects on mucocutaneous tissues associated with 13cRA that necessitated a marked dose reduction among one third of the patients during one year of therapy (from 100 to 50 mg per m² per day). Despite the decreased dose, toxicity in this study remained significant. Unfortunately, 13cRA at the dose used is difficult to tolerate for extended periods of time, and many patients are unwilling to continue taking the medication, especially populations at lower risk of developing cancer. Recent trials of 13cRA in the treatment of patients with oral leukoplakia have demonstrated a possible way to decrease toxicity using lower doses for more prolonged periods.[74] Hence newer studies in lung cancer chemoprevention, including a large randomized phase III study, now use a lower dose.

A second trial, by Bolla and colleagues,[75] randomized 316 patients with prior squamous cell cancer of the oral cavity or oropharynx to etretinate (50 mg per day for one month, followed by 25 mg per day for two years) or a placebo. After a median follow-up time of 41 months, treatment was not observed to affect incidence of either SPT or recurrent disease. The results of this trial were notable for the high rate of SPT (23% of patients), 79% of which were clearly tobacco-related.

In the only completed chemoprevention study of patients with an index diagnosis of lung cancer, Pastorino et al.[76] randomized 307 patients who had been surgically cured of stage I NSCLC to receive either high-dose retinyl palmitate (300,000 IU per day for one year) or a placebo. The retinyl palmitate (vitamin A) was well tolerated in this study; only

five patients required cessation of drug because of toxic effects. Fewer primary disease recurrences were noted in the group that received retinyl palmitate, but the difference was not statistically significant. The retinyl palmitate treatment was associated with an overall reduction in SPT: there were 18 in that group (12%) versus 29 (18%) in the retinyl palmitate and placebo arms, respectively. Considering only tobacco-related tumors, the data are more striking, with 13 SPT in the retinoid arm versus 25 in the placebo arm, and this difference achieved statistical significance. In contrast to 13cRA, the retinyl palmitate was well tolerated by patients, and compliance over one year of treatment exceeded 80%.

Building on the results of these two positive trials, two large trials are underway to determine definitively the role of retinoids in preventing second primary tumors (Table 25.3). These current trials include a National Cancer Institute (U.S.) sponsored phase III trial of low-dose 13cRA (30 mg per day for three years) versus placebo in patients who have undergone curative resection for stage I NSCLC. Patients will receive follow-up care for four years after treatment ends to assess reduction in SPT incidence. Accrual of patients to this study was completed in April of 1997, with approximately 1,485 patients registered.[77] Similarly, the Euroscan study is evaluating the efficacy of retinyl palmitate (300,000 IU per day) and the antioxidant N-acetylcysteine (600 mg per day) in the prevention of SPT following the definitive therapy of early-stage squamous cell carcinoma of the head and neck or fully resected stage I, II, or IIIA (T3N0 only) NSCLC (based on the prior study already described).[78] This study has a 2 × 2 factorial design; study participants received either retinyl palmitate alone or N-acetylcysteine alone, both drugs, or placebo for two years and then four years' follow-up care.[78] As of the most recent report of the data on 2,440 participants (1,449 head and neck cases, 991 lung cases), there have been 204 recurrences (27% in the patients with lung cancer). There were a total 133 SPTs (5.5%) with 83 in the head and neck group (5.7%) and 50 in lung group (5.0%).[78]

TABLE 25.3. SELECTED ONGOING CHEMOPREVENTION TRIALS IN LUNG CANCER AND HEAD AND NECK CANCER

Trial	Patients	No. Patients Accrued/Goal	Agents	Goals
Euroscan	Fully resected stage I–IIIA NSCLC	2600	NAC Retinyl palmitate (30,000 IU/day) versus placebo	Prevention of SPT
Intergroup Study	Fully resected stage I NSCLC	1453/1453	13-cis-retinoic acid (30 mg/day) versus placebo	Prevention of SPT
M. D. Anderson Cancer Center	Former smokers (quit for > 12 mos) with or without early stage aerodigestive cancers	110/225	13-cis-retinoic acid (1 mg/kg/day) + α-tocopherol (1,200 IU/day) versus 9-cis-retinoic acid (50 mg/day) vs placebo	Reversal of bronchia or dysplasia and g markers

FUTURE DIRECTIONS

Future directions include improved epidemiological models of lung cancer risk to identify high-risk patients for studies. Following this, we will need better to define those patients most likely to benefit from these interventions and target them for chemoprevention studies.

The ongoing phase III trials offer a combination of caution and promise. Given the dismal five-year survival rates of patients with an established diagnosis of lung cancer and the failure of early detection methods to affect overall survival rates, careful construction of a molecular model of lung carcinogenesis is vital to the development and testing of effective chemopreventive compounds. Although epidemiologic data have provided clues to compounds that may functionally retard the carcinogenic processing lung tissue, the β-carotene trials warn against the direct application of epidemiologic data into the clinical setting.

Most promising is the study of intermediate end point markers that could substantially reduce the cost, effort, and time required to complete large randomized chemoprevention trials. Trials that use cancer incidence as their primary end point usually require thousands of patients and cost several million dollars to complete. No less significant is the time required, with a minimum of five to ten years needed to ascertain whether the intervention was successful, equivocal, or harmful. The discovery of potentially valuable intermediate end point markers such as RAR-β is of pivotal importance. Other important genetic markers, including LOH at chromosomes 3p, 9p, and 17p and the potential role of the *p53* tumor-suppressor gene (as well as other tumor-suppressor genes such as the retinoblastoma gene) need to be carefully and prospectively studied to further clarify the biology and molecular genetics of lung carcinogenesis. With knowledge of lung cancer biology, the physician can select useful intermediate end point markers with which to study promising chemopreventive compounds. Once these compounds are shown to be effective in the reversal of preneoplastic disease, they can be taken to larger primary prevention trials. This careful marriage between

molecular biology and clinical investigation is likely to provide the framework for development of chemopreventive regimens for individuals at high risk for lung cancer.

The magnitude of the lung cancer problem (in most cases due to tobacco use) has inspired research into lung cancer causation and the active development of specific agents capable of reversing the carcinogenic process. The fact that former smokers remain at increased risk for lung cancer development[2,11,79,80] epidemiologically and the now proven fact that known genetic mechanisms for this process exist[20,37,80] have led to an increased focus on chemopreventive trials in former smokers. Given the increased lung cancer incidence in active smokers who received β-carotene[66,67,69,70] current chemopreventive interventions are increasingly targeting former smokers, and chemopreventive strategies at this time have no role in standard practice outside the context of a clinical trial.

Two large randomized lung cancer prevention trials are underway. Currently investigators at the M. D. Anderson Cancer Center have launched a randomized, placebo-controlled, double-blind trial of 13cRA plus α-tocopherol (to attenuate toxicity)[81] versus a novel retinoid, 9-cis-retinoic acid, which binds both RAR-RXR heterodimers and RXR-RXR homodimers, versus placebo in former smokers with or without cancer. Because former smokers can have persistent genetic deletions even in the absence of visible histologic abnormalities, all former smokers who have smoked at least 20 pack-years are eligible for participation in this study. The study population will comprise 225 former smokers, and accrual is expected to be complete in the year 2000.[81] Among the parameters being evaluated are the reversal of metaplasia, dysplasia, or both, the presence of persistent genetic lesions at the sites of specific tumor suppressor genes, and the loss of and possible upregulation of RAR-β.

Data from Oridate and associates[82] indicate that 4-HPR, a novel synthetic retinoid that does not appear to bind nuclear retinoid receptors, can induce apoptosis in cervical carcinoma cells by inducing reactive oxygen species. This work has been applied to lung cancer cell lines, and it appears that 4-HPR may be more effective than all-*trans* retinoic acid in inducing apoptosis in head and neck squamous carcinoma cell lines.[51] This has led to increased enthusiasm for the incorporation of such novel and nontoxic retinoids into chemoprevention trials.

Furthermore, recent data[49] have identified several synthetic retinoids that can specifically activate retinoid response networks, thereby selectively inducing specific biologic responses. These molecules appear preferentially to cause the induction of apoptosis in human lung cancer cells *in vivo* in animal models, thereby providing a potential role for selective retinoids in lung cancer therapy as well as chemoprevention.

Finally, other small molecules and routes of delivery may be equivalent and possibly even superior to oral retinoids. Recent compelling data from Wiedmann and colleagues on the use of budesonide, an aerosolized glucocorticoid, in the reversal of lung adenomas in mice, suggest that aerosolized delivery of chemopreventive compounds may be a provocative and ultimately more successful approach to lung chemoprevention.[83] The addition of other biologic agents, such as interferon or other antiangiogenic agents, is also being explored.

Hence the challenge of the next few years is to employ selective and highly specific chemopreventive compounds against new molecular targets.[84] The careful design and implementation of clinical chemoprevention trials, along with continued advances in the understanding of the principles of lung carcinogenesis and the development of novel, increasingly effective compounds with improved drug delivery techniques, should lead to significant advances in lung cancer chemoprevention.

REFERENCES

1. Ginsberg RJ, Kris MG, Armstrong JG. Cancer of the lung. In: DeVita VT, Hellman S, Rosenberg SA, eds. *Cancer: Principles and Practice of Oncology*, 4th ed. Philadelphia, PA: Lippincott, 1994:673.
2. Khuri JM, Spitz MR, Hong WK. Lung cancer chemoprevention: targeting former rather than current smokers. *Cancer Prev Int* 1995;2:55.
3. Mao L, Lee JS, Khuri JM, et al. Clonal genetic alterations in the lungs of current and former smokers. *J Nat Cancer Inst* 1997;89:857.
4. Sporn MB, Dunlop NM, Newton DL, et al. Prevention of chemical carcinogenesis by vitamin A and its synthetic analogs (retinoids). *Fed Proc* 1976;35:1332.
5. Hong WK, Lippman SM, Itri LM, et al. Prevention of second primary tumors with isotretinoin in squamous cell carcinoma of the head and neck. *N Engl J Med* 1990;323:795.
6. Ochsner A, DeBakey M. Carcinoma of the lung. *Arch Surg* 1941;42:209.
7. Doll R, Hill AB. Smoking and carcinoma of the lung [Preliminary report]. *Br Med J* 1950;2:739.
8. Wynder EL, Graham EA. Tobacco smoking as a possible etiologic factor in bronchogenic carcinoma: a study of six hundred and eighty four proved cases. *JAMA* 1950;143:329.
9. Auerbach O, Gere JB, Forman JB, et al. Changes in bronchial epithelium in relation to smoking and cancer of the lungs: a report of progress. *N Engl J Med* 1957;256:97.
10. Auerbach O, Stout AP, Hammond EC, et al. Changes in bronchial epithelium in relation to cigarette smoking and in relation to lung cancer. *N Engl J Med* 1961;256:253.
11. Trichopoulus D, Mollo F, Tomatis L, et al. Active and passive smoking and pathological indicators of lung cancer risk in an autopsy series. *JAMA* 1992;268:1697.
12. Shopland DR, Eyre HJ, Pechacek TF. Smoking atributable cancer mortality in 1991: is lung cancer now the leading cause of death among smokers in the United States. *J Nat Cancer Inst* 1991;83:1142.
13. Office of Smoking and Health, US Centers for Disease Control. *MMWR* 1994:43.
14. Strauss GM. Measuring effectiveness of lung cancer screening: from consensus to controversy and back. *Chest* 1997;112;4S[Suppl]:216S.
15. Martini N. Results of the Memorial-Sloan Kettering Study in screening for early lung cancer. *Chest* 1986;89:325S.
16. Tockman MS. Survival and mortality from lung cancer in a screened population: the John Hopkins Study. *Chest* 1986;89:324S.
17. Sanderson DR. Lung cancer screening: the Mayo study. *Chest* 1986;89:324.
18. Hung J, Kishimoto Y, Sugio K, et al. Allele-specific chromosome 3p deletions occur at an early stage in the pathogenesis of lung cancer. *JAMA* 1995;273:558.
19. Kishimoto Y, Sugio K, Hung JY, et al. Allele-specific loss in chromosome 9p loci in preneoplastic lesions accompanying non–small cell cancer. *J Natl Cancer Inst* 1995;87:1224.
20. Sozzi G, Miozzo M, Donghi R, et al. Deletions of 17p and p53 mutations in preneoplastic lesions of the lung. *Cancer Res* 1991;51:400.
21. Sozzi G, Rornielli S, Tagliabue E, et al. Absence of FHIT protein in primary lung tumors and cell lines with FHIT gene abnormalities. *Cancer Res* 1997;57:5207.
22. Muller CY, O'Boyle JD, Fong KM, et al. Abnormalities of fragile histidine triad genomic and complementary DNAs in cervical cancer: association with human papillomavirus subtype. *J Natl Cancer Inst* 1998;90:433.
23. Kim SY, Lee JS, Ro JY, et al. Interphase cytogenetics in parafin sections of lung tumors by non-isotopic in-situ hybridization: mapping genotype/phenotype heterogenicity. *Am J Pathol* 1993;142:307.
24. Voravud N, Shin DM, Ro JY, et al. Increased polysomies of chromosome 7 and 17 during head and neck multistage tumorigenesis. *Cancer Res* 1993;52:2874.
25. Gazdar AF, Hung J, Walker L, et al. Extensive areas of dysplasia and aneuploidy of the entire bronchial mucosal tract accompanies non–small cell lung cancers (NSCLC) and provides evidence for the field cancerization theory. *Proc Am Soc Clin Oncol* 1993;12:334.
26. Vogelstein B, Fearon ER, Hamilton SR, et al. Genetic alterations during colorectal tumor development. *N Engl J Med* 1988;319(9):525.
27. Auerbach O, Hammond CE, Garfinkel L. Changes in bronchial epithelium in relation to cigarette smoking, 1955–1960 vs. 1970–1977. *N Engl J Med* 1979;300:381.
28. Black H, Ackerman LV. Importance of epidermoid carcinoma *in situ* in histogenesis of carcinoma of the lung. *Am Surg* 1952;136:44.
29. Saccomanno G, Archer VE, Auerbach O, et al. Development of carcinoma of the lung as reflected in exfoliated cells. *Cancer* 1974;33:256.
30. Heimburger DC, Alexander CB, Burch R, et al. Improvement

in bronchial squamous metaplasia in smoking treated with folate and vitamin B12. Report of a preliminary randomized, double-blind intervention trial. *JAMA* 1988;259:1525.

31. Lee JS, Lippman SM, Benner SE, et al. Randomized placebo controlled trial of isotretinoin in chemoprevention of bronchial squamous metaplasia. *J Clin Oncol* 1994;12:937.

32. Hittelman WN, Wang ZQ, Cheong N, et al. Premature chromosome condensation and cytogenics of human solid tumors. *Cancer Bull* 1989;41:298.

33. Sozzi G, Miozzo M, Tagliabue E, et al. Cytogenetic abnormalities and overexpression of receptors for growth factors in normal bronchial epithelium and tumor samples of lung canr patients. *Cancer Res* 1991;51:400.

34. Ihde DC, Minna JD. Non–small cell lung cancer. Part I. Biology, diagnosis and staging. *Curr Probl Cancer* 1991;15:61.

35. Mao L, Hruban RH, Boyle JO, et al. Detection of oncogene mutations in sputum precedes diagnosis of lung cancer. *Cancer Res* 1994;54:1634.

36. Inman DS, Harris CC. Oncogenes and tumor suppressor genes in human lung carcinogenesis. *Crit Rev Oncog* 1991;2:161.

37. Wistuba II, Lam S, Behrens C, et al. Molecular damage in the bronchial epithelium of current and former smokers. *J Nat Cancer Inst* 1997;89:1366.

38. Hong WK, Itri LM. Retinoids and human cancers, In: Sporn MB, Roberts AB, Goodman DS, eds. *The retinoids.* New York: Raven Press, 1994:597.

39. Wolbach SB, Howe PR. Tissue changes following deprivation of fat-soluable A vitamin. *J Exp Med* 1925;62:753.

40. Wolbach SB. Effects of vitamin A deficiency and hypervitaminosis in animals. In: Sebrell, WH; Harris, RS, eds. *The vitamins.* Vol. 1. New York: Academic Press, 1956:106.

41. Sporn MB, Newton DL. Chemoprevention of cancers with retinoids. *Fed Proc* 1979;38:2528.

42. Mangelsdorf DJ, Umesono K, Evans RM. The retinoid receptors. In: Sporn MB, Roberts AB, Goodman DS, eds. *The retinoids.* New York: Raven Press, 1994:319.

43. Chambon P. The retinoid signaling pathway: molecular and genetic analyses. *Semin Cell Biol* 1994;5:115.

44. Mayne ST, Lippman SM. Retinoids and carotenoids. In: DeVita VT, Hellman S, Rosenberg SA, eds. *Cancer: principles and practice of oncology,* 5th ed. Philadelphia, PA: Lippincott, 1997.

45. Fanjul A, Dawson MI, Hobbs PD, et al. A new class of retinoids with selective inhibition of AP-1 inhibits proliferation. *Nature* 1994;372:107.

46. Li JJ, Dong Z, Dawson MI, et al. Inhibition of tumor promoter–induced transformation by retinoids that transrepress AP-1 without transactivating retinoic acid response element. *Cancer Res* 1996;56:483.

47. Angel P, Karin M. The role of Jun, Fos and the AP-1 complex in cell-proliferation and transformation. *Biochim Biophys Acta* 1991;1072.

48. Kamei Y, Xu I, Heinzel T, et al. A CBP integrator complex mediates transcriptional activation and AP-1 inhibition by nuclear receptors. *Cell* 1996;85:403.

49. Lu XP, Fanjul A, Pricard N, et al. Novel retinoid-related molecules as apoptosis inducers and effective inhibitors of human lung cancer cells *in vivo. Nat Med* 1997;3:686.

50. Lee HY, Dawson MI, Walsh GL, et al. Retinoic acid receptor- and retinoid x receptor-selective retinoids activate signaling pathways that converge on AP-1 and inhibit squamous differentiation in human bronchial epithelial cells. *Cell Growth Differ* 1996;7:997.

51. Xu XC, Sozzi G, Lee JS, et al. Suppression of retinoic acid receptor β in non-small-cell lung cancer *in vivo*: implications for lung cancer development. *J Natl Cancer Inst* 1997;89:624.

52. Oridate N, Lotan D, Xu XC, et al. Differential induction of

apoptosis by all-trans-retinoic acid and N-(4hydroxyphenyl) retinamide in human head and neck squamous cell carcinoma cell lines. *Clin Cancer Res* 1996;2:855.

53. Shalinsky DR, Bishoff EE, Gregory MD, et al. Enhanced antitumor efficacy of cisplatin in combination with ALRT 1057 (9-*cis* retinoic acid) in human oral squamous carcinoma xenografts in nude mice. *Clin Cancer Res* 1996;2:511.

54. Lippman SM, Kavanagh JJ, Parades-Espinoza M, et al. 13-*cis*-retinoic acid plus interferon alpha-2a: Highly active systemic therapy for squamous cell carcinoma of the cervix. *J Natl Cancer Inst* 1992;84:241.

55. Lippman SM, Parkinson DR, Itri LM, et al. 13-*cis*-retinoic acid and interferon alpha-2a: effective combination therapy for advanced squamous cell carcinoma of the skin. *J Natl Cancer Inst* 1992;84:235.

56. Peto R, Doll R, Buckley JD, et al. Can dietary beta-carotene materially reduce human cancer rates? *Nature* 1987;290:201.

57. Willett WM, McMahon B. Diet and cancer: an overview. *N Engl J Med* 1984;310:633.

58. Ziegler RG, Subar AF, Craft NE, et al. Does β-carotene explain why reduced cancer risk is associated with vegetable and fruit intake? *Cancer Res* 1992;52:2060S.

59. Greenwald P, Cullen JW, Kelloff G, et al. Chemoprevention of lung cancer. *Chest* 1989;96:14S.

60. Benner SE, Winn RJ, Lippman SM, et al. Regression of oral leukoplakia with alpha-tocopherol: a community clinical oncology program chemoprevention study. *J Nat Cancer Inst* 1993;85:44.

61. Dimery IW, Hong WK, Lee JJ, et al. Phase I trial of alpha-tocopherol effects on 13-cis-retinoic acid toxicity. *Ann Oncol* 1997;8:85.

62. Saccomanno G, Moran PG, Schmidt RD, et al. Effect of 13-*cis* retinoids on premalignant and malignant cells of lung origin. *Acta Cytol* 1982;26:78.

63. Mathe G, Gouveia J, Hercend TM, et al. Correlation between precancerous bronchial metaplasia and cigarette consumption, and preliminary results of retinoid treatment. *Cancer Detect Prev* 1982;5:461.

64. McLarty JW, Holiday DB, Girard WM, et al. β-Carotene, vitamin A, and lung cancer chemoprevention: results of an intermediate endpoint study. *Am J Clin Nutr* 1995;62:1431S.

65. Arnold AM, Browman GP, Levin MN, et al. The effect of synthetic retinoid etretinate on sputum cytology: results from a randomized trial. *Br J Cancer* 1992;65:737.

66. The Alpha-Tocopherol BCCPSG. The effect of vitamin E and beta carotene on the incidence of lung cancer and other cancers in male smokers. *N Engl J Med* 1994;330:1030.

67. Albanes D, Heinonem OP, Taylor PR, et al. Alpha-tocopherol, beta carotene cancer prevention study: effects of baseline characteristics and study compliance. *J Natl Cancer Inst* 1996;88:1560.

68. Omenn GS, Goodman GE, Thornquist MD, et al. The carotene and retinol efficacy trial (CARET) to prevent lung cancer in high risk populations: pilot study with asbestos-exposed workers. *Cancer Epidemiol Biomarkers Prev* 1993;2:381.

69. Hennekens CH, Buring JE, Manson JE, et al. Lack of long-term supplementation with beta-carotene on the incidence of malignant neoplasms and cardiovascular disease. *N Engl J Med* 1996;334:1145.

70. Omenn GS, Goodman GE, Thornquist MD, et al. Risk factors for lung cancer and for intervention effects in CARET, the Beta-Carotene and Retinol Efficacy Trial. *J Natl Cancer Inst* 1996;88:1500.

71. Mayne ST, Handleman GJ, Beecher G. β-carotene and lung cancer promotion in heavy smokers: a plausible relationship. *J Natl Cancer Inst* 1996;88:1513.

72. Xuan XZ, Schatakin A, Mao BL, et al. Feasibility of conducting a lung cancer chemoprevention trial among tin miners in Yunnan, PR China. *Cancer Coverage Central* 1991;2:175.

73. Benner TF, Sr., Lippman SM, et al. Prevention of second primary tumors with isotretinoin in patients with squamous cell carcinoma of the head and neck: long-term follow-up. *J Natl Cancer Inst* 1994;86:140.

74. Lippman SM, Batsakis JG, Toth BB, et al. Comparison of low-dose isotretinoin with beta carotene to prevent oral carcinogenesis. *N Engl J Med* 1993;328:15.

75. Bolla M, Lefur R, Ton Van J, et al. Preventation of second primary tumors with etretinate in squamous cell carcinoma of the oral cavity and oropharynx. Results of a multicentric double-blind randomized study. *Eur J Cancer* 1994;30:767.

76. Pastorino U. Nutrition and chemoprevention controversies. *Ann Oncol* 1993;4:117.

77. Winn RJ, CCOP Central Office. Personal communication. November, 1997.

78. Van Zanderÿk N, Pastorino V, De Vries N, et al. Randomized trial of chemoprevention with vitamin A and N-acetylcysteine in patients with cancer of the upper and lower airways: The Euroscan study [Abstract]. *Proc ASCO* 99; p464a, 1788.

79. Thun MJ, Lally CA, Flannery JT, et al. Cigarette smoking and changes in the histopathology of lung cancer. *J Natl Cancer Inst* 1997;89:1580.

80. Denissenko MF, Pao A, Tung M, et al. Preferential formation of benzo[a]pyrene adducts at lung cancer mutational hotspots in p53. *Science* 1996;274:430.

81. Hong WK. Personal communication. February, 1998.

82. Oridate N, Suzuki S, Higuchi M, et al. Involvement of reactive oxygen species in N-(4-hydroxyphenyl) retinamide-induced apoptosis in cervical carcinoma cells. *J Natl Cancer Inst* 1997; 89:1191.

83. Wiedmann TS, Estensen RE, Zimmerman CL, et al. Chemoprevention of pulmonary carcinogenesis by aerosolized budesonide in female A/J mice. *Cancer Res* 1997;57:5489.

84. Hong WK, Sporn MB. Recent advances in chemoprevention of cancer. *Science* 1997;278:1073.

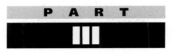

PART

III

PATHOLOGY

26

CLASSIFICATION, HISTOLOGY, CYTOLOGY, AND ELECTRON MICROSCOPY

WILLIAM D. TRAVIS
JAMES LINDER
BRUCE MACKAY

CLASSIFICATION

Lung cancer is currently the most common worldwide cause of major cancer incidence and mortality.[1] It is estimated that lung cancer will account for more than 187,000 new cases in the United States during 1999 and more than 164,000 cancer deaths.[2] Although lung cancer incidence in the United States began to decline in males in the early 1980s,[3] it continues to increase in women.[4]

Accurate pathologic classification of lung cancer is essential for patients to receive the appropriate therapy. Although classification of the vast majority of lung cancers is straightforward, areas of controversy and diagnostic challenges remain. Lung cancer diagnosis is based primarily on light microscopy, but useful information can be obtained from special techniques such as immunohistochemistry and electron microscopy. This chapter focuses primarily on histologic and cytologic approaches to the diagnosis and classification of the major subtypes of lung cancer, with special attention on neuroendocrine lung tumors. Electron microscopy is also discussed in detail in this chapter. Immunohistochemistry, flow cytometry, and molecular biology are mentioned only briefly because they are addressed in other chapters.

The most widely accepted histologic classification for lung tumors is that proposed by the World Health Organization (WHO) which was revised in 1999 (Table 26.1). The major histologic types of lung cancer are squamous cell carcinoma, adenocarcinoma, small cell lung carcinoma (SCLC), and large cell carcinoma. These four tumors can be subclassified into more specific subtypes such as the bronchioloalveolar carcinoma (BAC) variant of adenocarcinoma.[6] In addition, there are other less common lung tumors, such as carcinoid tumors (Table 26.1). A more extensive discussion of the pathology of lung tumors with greater detail on uncommon lung tumors than is possible here can be found in several textbooks.[6–10]

SHIFTS IN HISTOLOGIC TYPE BY SEX, RACE, AND AGE

The sex and race distribution for the various histologic subtypes of lung cancer has shifted over the past several decades (Figure 26.1).[11] Population-based data gathered by the National Cancer Institute's (NCI) Surveillance, Epidemiology, and End Results (SEER) Program demonstrated that the age-adjusted rate (AAR) for lung cancer for all race-sex groups combined has risen sharply since 1950.[11,12] From 1969 to 1991, the overall AAR of lung cancer incidence rose from 37.8 to 68.2 per 100,000.[3] However, the percentage increase has diminished in recent years.[2–4] Lung cancer rates for both black and white men peaked and began to decrease around 1984. Although rates continue to increase for women of both races, this decrease has diminished in recent years.[3,4,11]

In white and black males, the rates of squamous cell carcinoma, SCLC, and large cell carcinoma declined after peaks in 1981 and 1982, 1986 and 1987, and 1986 and 1988, respectively.[3] In addition, the rates for adenocarcinoma in black males peaked in 1987, whereas the rates in white males appeared to have plateaued between 1989 and 1991.[3] Lung carcinoma AAR among white and black females continued to increase for all histologic types, except for large cell carcinoma among whites and BAC among whites and blacks. Most of these changes reflect past cigarette smoking patterns. Demonstration of declines and tapering increases among several population subgroups suggests that reductions will occur soon in the overall incidence and mortality rate for this highly fatal cancer.

These shifts in the AAR have resulted in adenocarcinoma surpassing squamous cell carcinoma as the most common histologic type of lung cancer for all sex-race groups (Table 26.2, Figure 26.2).[13–15] The change is caused by not only an increase in adenocarcinoma but also a decrease in squamous cell carcinoma in men. Carcinoid tumors represent the most common lung malignancy in patients under 30 years of age.[11]

TABLE 26.1. WHO/IASLC HISTOLOGIC CLASSIFICATION, 3rd ED., 1999*

Preinvasive Lesions
  Squamous dysplasia/carcinoma *in situ*
  Atypical adenomatous hyperplasia
  Diffuse idiopathic pulmonary neuroendocrine cell
    hyperplasia
Squamous cell carcinoma
  Variants
    Papillary
    Clear cell
    Small cell
    Basaloid
Small cell carcinoma
  Combined small cell carcinoma
Adenocarcinoma
  Acinar
  Papillary
  Bronchioloalveolar carcinoma
    Nonmucinous
    Mucinous
    Mixed mucinous and nonmucinous or indeterminate
  Solid adenocarcinoma with mucin
  Adenocarcinoma with mixed subtypes
    Variants
      Well-differentiated fetal adenocarcinoma
      Mucinous ("colloid") adenocarcinoma
      Mucinous cystadenocarcinoma
      Signet ring adenocarcinoma
      Clear cell adenocarcinoma
Large cell carcinoma
  Variants
    Large cell neuroendocrine carcinoma
      Combined large cell neuroendocrine carcinoma
    Basaloid carcinoma
    Lymphoepithelioma-like carcinoma
    Clear cell carcinoma
    Large cell carcinoma with rhabdoid phenotype
Adenosquamous carcinoma
Carcinomas with pleomorphic, sarcomatoid, or sarcomatous
  elements
  Carcinomas with spindle and/or giant cells
    Pleomorphic carcinoma
    Spindle cell carcinoma
    Giant cell carcinoma
  Carcinosarcoma
  Pulmonary blastoma
  Other
Carcinoid tumor
  Typical carcinoid
  Atypical carcinoid
Carcinomas of salivary gland type
  Mucoepidermoid carcinoma
  Adenoid cystic carcinoma
  Others
Unclassified carcinoma

WHO = World Health Organization; IASLC = International Association for the Study of Lung Cancer
* From Travis WD, Colby TV, Corrin B, et al. in collaboration with pathologists from 14 countries. *Histological typing of lung and pleural tumors.* 3rd ed. Berlin: Springer Verlag, 1999, with permission.

TABLE 26.2. FREQUENCY AND AGE-ADJUSTED RATE (AAR) PER 100,000 POPULATION FOR ALL RACES, BOTH SEXES: 1983–87*

	No. Cases (%)	AAR
Adenocarcinoma	19,087 (31.5)	16.7
Adenocarcinoma (NOS) and other specific ADC	15,545 (25.7)	13.7
Bronchioloalveolar carcinoma	1,561 (2.6)	1.4
Papillary adenocarcinoma	400 (0.7)	0.3
Adenosquamous carcinoma	870 (1.4)	0.8
Other	659 (1.1)	0.6
Bronchial gland carcinoma	52 (0.1)	0
Adenoid cystic carcinoma	16 (<0.1)	0
Mucoepidermoid carcinoma	36 (0.1)	0
Squamous Cell Carcinoma	17,789 (29.4)	15.3
Other Specific Carcinoma	11,586 (19.1)	10.1
Giant cell and spindle cell carcinoma	179 (0.3)	0.2
Small cell carcinoma	10,786 (17.8)	9.4
Carcinoid	616 (1.0)	0.5
Other	5 (<0.1)	0
Unspecified Carcinoma	10,798 (17.8)	9.4
Large cell carcinoma	5,577 (9.2)	4.9
Undifferentiated carcinoma	1,052 (1.7)	0.9
Other unspecified carcinoma	4,169 (6.9)	3.6
Sarcoma and Other Soft Tissue Tumors	84 (0.1)	0.1
Other Specified Types	47 (0.1)	0
Carcinosarcoma	39 (0.1)	0
Other	8 (<0.1)	0
Unspecified	1,123 (1.9)	0.9

* From Travis WD, Travis LB, Devesa SS. Lung Cancer. *Cancer* 1995; 75:191, with permission.

One study by El-Torky et al. suggested a substantial increase in the frequency of SCLC in women.[16] Although data from the SEER program indicated that the AAR for SCLC increased between 1973–1987, only a slight increase occurred in its relative frequency in both men and women.[11]

Several studies have suggested that the frequency of BAC is increasing.[17,18] However, this theory was not confirmed by data from the SEER program, which showed a slight decrease in the percentage of lung cancers diagnosed as BAC and no significant change in the AAR.[11]

The peak age-specific rates for the 1983–1987 year period in the SEER data occurred at approximately 70 to 74 years of age for each major histologic type of lung cancer.[11] Squamous cell carcinoma was the most common histologic type among persons 65 years and older, whereas adenocarcinoma predominated among younger individuals.

These shifts in histologic types and sex/race distribution may result from differences in smoking habits or other dietary, host, environmental, and/or occupational factors.

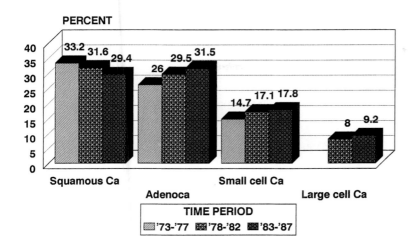

FIGURE 26.1. Age-adjusted rates per 100,000 person years for all races and both sexes for each five-year time period (1973–1977, 1978–1982, and 1983–1987) for all lung carcinomas as well as for the four major histologic subtypes of lung carcinoma. (From Travis WD, Travis LB, Devessa LS. Lung Cancer. *Cancer* 1995;75:191, with permission.)

PATHOLOGY

General Pathologic Features

The pathologic diagnosis of lung cancer can be established by examination of cytologic or surgical pathology specimens.[6] The certainty of the diagnosis may depend on the amount of tumor in the specimen and how well the tumor cells are preserved. In general, surgical pathology specimens are more likely to provide diagnostic material than cytologic specimens; however, in some cases cytology may provide more diagnostic information than the histology of biopsies. Histologic specimens may be from bronchoscopic or needle biopsies and open biopsy procedures such as thoracoscopy, excisional wedge biopsy, lobectomy, or pneumonectomy.

The location of the tumor and the condition of the patient may influence the type of specimen that can be obtained. Central tumors are often best sampled with bronchoscopic biopsies or sputum cytology, whereas specimens from peripheral tumors may be more readily procured sampled by transbronchial biopsies or fine-needle biopsies.

Pathologic Staging

Pathologic characteristics important for staging of lung cancer can be considered according to the various T categories (Table 26.3) (see also Chapter 32). TX tumors are diagnosed by cytology alone in patients without a radiographically detectable or bronchoscopically visible tumor. Tumor size is important in separating T1 from T2 lesions because T1 tumors are 3 cm or less in greatest dimension. Visceral pleural invasion is absent in T1 tumors, but its presence in a tumor of any size makes the tumor at least a T2 lesion. If a tumor involves the main bronchus, 2 cm or more distal to the carina, it is regarded as a T2 lesion. The presence of atelectasis or obstructive pneumonitis that extends to the hilar region but involves less than an entire lung also makes a tumor of any size at least a T2 lesion. A tumor of any size is regarded as a T3 lesion if it extends into the chest wall (including superior sulcus tumors), the diaphragm, the mediastinal pleura or parietal pericardium without involving the heart, great vessels, trachea, esophagus, or vertebral body. If it causes atelectasis or obstructive pneumonitis of

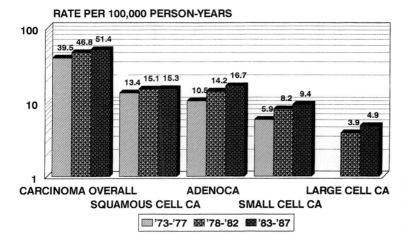

FIGURE 26.2. Percent histology distribution of the four major subtypes of lung cancer for all races and both sexes over the three time intervals 1973–1977, 1978–1982, and 1983–1987. (From Travis WD, Travis LB. Devessa LS. Lung Cancer. *Cancer* 1995;75:191, with permission.)

TABLE 26.3. ANATOMIC CHARACTERISTICS OF THE PRIMARY TUMOR IMPORTANT FOR STAGING

T-Primary Tumor

TX Primary tumor cannot be assessed, or tumor proven by the presence of malignant cells in sputum or bronchial washings but not visualized by imaging or bronchoscopy

T0 No evidence of primary tumor

Tis Carcinoma *in situ*

T1 Tumor 3 cm or less in greatest dimension, surrounded by lung or visceral pleura, without bronchoscopic evidence of invasion more proximal than the lobar bronchus (i.e., not in)

T2 Tumor with *any* of the following features of size or extent:
—More than 3 cm in greatest dimension
—Involves main bronchus, 2 cm or more distal to the carina
—Invades visceral pleura
—Associated with atelectasis or obstructive pneumonitis that extends to the hilar region but does not involve the entire lung

T3 Tumor of any size that directly invades any of the following: chest wall (including superior sulcus tumors), diaphragm, mediastinal pleura, parietal pericardium; or tumor in the main bronchus less than 2 cm distal to the carina,[19] but without involvement of the carina; or associated atelectasis or obstructive pneumonitis of the entire lung.

T4 Tumor of any size that invades any of the following: mediastinum, heart, great vessels, trachea, esophagus, vertebral body, carina; separate tumor nodule(s) in the same lobe; tumor with malignant pleural effusion[19]

Notes

1. The uncommon superficial spreading tumor of any size with its invasive component limited to the bronchial wall, which may extend proximal to the main bronchus, is also classified as T1.
2. Most pleural effusions with lung cancer are caused by tumor. In a few patients, however, multiple cytopathologic examinations of pleural fluid are negative for turnout, and the fluid is nonbloody and is not an exudate. Where these elements and clinical judgment dictate that the effusion is not related to the tumor, the effusion should be excluded as a staging element, and the patient should be classified as T1, T2, or T3.

N-Regional Lymph Nodes

NX Regional lymph nodes cannot be assessed

N0 No regional lymph node metastasis

N1 Metastasis in ipsilateral peribronchial and/or ipsilateral hilar lymph nodes and intrapulmonary nodes, including involvement by direct extension

N2 Metastasis in ipsilateral mediastinal and/or subcarinal lymph node(s)

N3 Metastasis in contralateral mediastinal, contralateral hilar, ipsilateral or contralateral scalene, or supraclavicular lymph node(s)

M-Distant Metastasis

MX Distant metastasis cannot be assessed

M0 No distant metastasis

M1 Distant metastasis, includes separate tumor nodule(s) in a different lobe (ipsilateral or contralateral)

PTNM Pathological Classification

The pT, pN, and pM categories correspond to the T, N, and M categories.

pN0 Histologic examination of hilar and mediastinal lymphadenectomy specimen(s) ordinarily include six or more lymph nodes.

G-Histopathologic Grading

GX Grade of differentiation cannot be assessed

G1 Well differentiated

G2 Moderately differentiated

G3 Poorly differentiated

G4 Undifferentiated

Stage Grouping

Occult carcinoma	TX	N0	M0
Stage O	TIS	N0	M0
Stage IA	T1	N0	M0
Stage IB	T2	N0	M0
Stage IIA	T1	N1	M0
Stage IIB	T2	N1	M0
	T3	N0	M0
Stage IIIA	T1	N2	M0
	T2	N2	M0
	T3	N1, N2	M0
Stage IIIB	Any T	N3	M0
	T4	Any N	M0
Stage IV	Any T	Any N	M1

the entire lung, it is also regarded as a T3 lesion. A tumor of any size is a T4 lesion if it invades the mediastinum, heart, great vessels, trachea, esophagus, vertebral body, or the carina. Lung cancers are also regarded as T4 lesions if they cause separate tumor nodule(s) in the same lobe or a malignant pleural effusion.[19]

Assessment of lymph node involvement is also important. NX is applicable if regional lymph nodes cannot be assessed. N0 signifies no lymph node metastases. N1 indicates metastases to ipsilateral peribronchial and/or ipsilateral hilar lymph nodes and intrapulmonary nodes, including involvement by direct extension. N2 applies to cases with metastases to ipsilateral mediastinal lymph nodes or subcarinal lymph nodes. N3 corresponds to metastases to contralateral hilar or mediastinal, ipsilateral or contralateral scalene or supraclavicular lymph nodes. All lymph nodes submitted with a surgical resection specimen should be examined histologically. Grading of tumors is based on the area of worst differentiation. GX is used when the grade of differentiation cannot be assessed. G1, G2, and G3 represent well, moderately, and poorly differentiated, respectively. G4 represents an undifferentiated tumor.[6]

Synchronous Primary Lung Cancers and Intrapulmonary Satellite Lesions

Synchronous primary lung cancers occur in approximately 0.5% of lung cancer patients.[20-24] By definition, synchronous primary lung cancers consist of concurrent, separate, malignant lung epithelial neoplasms with different histology or tumors of similar histology arising in different locations (segments, lobes, or lung).[20] Some definitions also require that tumors of the same histology not only be in a different segment of a lobe or the lung, but that the following criteria also be met: (a) origin from carcinoma *in situ* (b) no carcinoma in lymphatics common to both, and (c) no extrapulmonary metastases at the time of diagnosis.[25] A recent study found synchronous non–small cell lung carcinoma (NSCLC) in 0.8% of 3,034 lung cancer patients and suggested that the prognosis for patients with synchronous NSCLC may not be dismal if both tumors are resectable and stage I or II.[26]

Satellite nodules can be encountered in 8% to 10% of resected lung cancer specimens.[27,28] They are defined as well-circumscribed foci of carcinoma adjacent to but clearly separated from the main tumor by normal lung parenchyma.[27] The satellite nodule should have the same histology as the main tumor, but it should not represent an intrapulmonary lymph node metastases.[27] The presence of satellite nodules has a significantly adverse effect on prognosis, especially for patients with stage I disease.[27]

General Histologic Features

The major histologic subtypes of lung cancer include squamous cell carcinoma, adenocarcinoma, SCLC, and large cell

carcinoma (Table 26.1),[6] but because major differences exist in the therapeutic approach to patients with SCLC versus NSCLC, the major question often asked of pathologists is whether a lung cancer is an SCLC or an NSCLC. This differential diagnosis is discussed in a following section under the topic of SCLC.

The majority of lung cancers are histologically heterogeneous, which impacts on diagnosis of lung cancer because it is a potential source of variation in interobserver interpretation.[6] It is seldom recognized in bronchoscopic biopsy specimens because of the small sample of tissue. Histologic heterogeneity was thoroughly documented in a study of 100 surgically resected (n = 65) or autopsy (n = 35) lung cancer specimens reviewed by five lung pathologists.[28] Only 34% of the cases were homogeneous according to the majority of the panelists. Major heterogeneity (adenocarcinoma versus squamous cell carcinoma) was identified in 45% of the cases. Minor (subtype) heterogeneity (e.g., mixtures of acinar and papillary patterns in adenocarcinoma) was found in 21% of the cases.[29] Histologic heterogeneity also contributes to the "discrepancy" between the bronchoscopic biopsy interpretation compared to the pathologic diagnosis in subsequent resection specimens, which can occur in up to 38% of cases.[30] Therefore, in small bronchoscopic biopsy specimens, if unequivocal squamous cell or adenocarcinomatous differentiation is not seen and the tumor is an NSCLC, the best diagnosis is often "*non–small cell carcinoma.*"

Heterogeneity also exists at the ultrastructural level.[31-35] Several ultrastructural studies have shown that electron microscopy is more sensitive in detecting features of squamous or glandular differentiation than light microscopy.[31-35] Thus by electron microscopy, lung cancers appear even more heterogeneous than by light microscopy. Also, by electron microscopy a high percentage of large cell carcinomas show features of squamous cell or adenocarcinoma.[32,35] Thus the percentage of lung carcinomas classified as adenosquamous carcinomas by electron microscopy is much greater than by light microscopy.[31]

PREINVASIVE LESIONS

In the 1999 WHO International Association for the Study of Lung Cancer (ASLC) histologic classification of lung tumors, preinvasive lesions include squamous dysplasia/carcinoma *in situ* atypical adenomatous hyperplasia (AAH), and diffuse idiopathic pulmonary neuroendocrine cell hyperplasia (DIPNECH).[6] AAH and DIPNECH are two new lesions that were added since the 1981 classification was proposed. They are thought to be precursor lesions for adenocarcinomas and carcinoids, respectively.

In Situ Squamous Cell Carcinoma

In situ carcinoma of the bronchial epithelium is recognized for squamous cell carcinoma but not for the other histologic subtypes of lung carcinoma. It is the cytologically malignant end of the spectrum of squamous dysplasia and carcinoma *in situ*. By gross examination, *in situ* squamous cell carcinoma is characterized by loss of the normal longitudinal ridges of the bronchial mucosa, often with mucosal thickening and erythema.[36] In a resected specimen, careful mapping of the bronchial lesions and serial blocking of the bronchi may be helpful to document the extent of the process. Invasive carcinoma is often found in association with *in situ* carcinoma. If the invasion is early, it may appear grossly as a nodular mucosal thickening or ulceration.

Histologically, *in situ* carcinoma is characterized by full-thickness cytologic atypia of squamous epithelium. The cells show an increased nuclear to cytoplasmic ratio and nuclear hyperchromasia. Mitoses may be seen extending up to the surface of the squamous epithelium. Rarely, one may encounter a thin layer of maturation at the surface of the epithelium over the *in situ* carcinoma. Although the adjacent mucosa may show signs of dysplasia, in most cases an abrupt transition occurs from normal epithelium to *in situ* carcinoma.[36] *In situ* carcinoma can involve submucosal glands without penetrating the subepithelial basement membrane. Squamous dysplasia and *in situ* carcinoma does not necessarily progress to invasive carcinoma; evidence suggests that they may regress to normal mucosa.[37-40]

The concept of roentgenographically occult carcinoma is applied to those lung cancers that are not visible on chest x-ray but shed tumor cells into the sputum.[41-43] Virtually all of these tumors are squamous cell carcinomas and many have some degree of *in situ* cancer.[41-43] In a study of 68 surgically resected specimens from such patients, Woolner et al. classified these cases into the following categories: carcinoma *in situ* (34%), intramucosal invasion: less than 0.1 cm (18%), invasion to bronchial cartilage: 0.11–0.30 cm (16%), deep invasion to full thickness of the bronchial wall: 0.31–0.5 cm (14%), and extrabronchial invasion: more than 0.5 cm (18%).[44] Nagamoto et al. divided occult squamous cell carcinoma into a creeping and a penetrating type.[45] Most cases are the creeping type, which shows extensive superficial growth. The penetrating type shows a marked downward growth and tends to become advanced more rapidly.[45] Metastases are not seen in tumors that do not invade beyond the subepithelial basement membrane.[44,46,47] According to Nagamoto, lymph node metastases are seen only in radiographically occult lung cancers with a length of longitudinal extension greater than 20 mm.[42] These patients are at increased risk for multicentric synchronous or metachronous lung carcinomas.[44,48]

Atypical Adenomatous Hyperplasia

AAH is a bronchioloalveolar proliferation that is worrisome but does not meet criteria for bronchioloalveolar carcinoma.[48,49,50] It is considered a precursor to adenocarcinoma (Figure 26.3A and B).[51] They are most often discovered incidentally as millimeter-sized histologic findings in lung cancer resection specimens.

Other published terminology for these lesions includes alveolar cell hyperplasia,[52] atypical alveolar hyperplasia,[53] atypical bronchioloalveolar cell hyperplasia,[54] alveolar epithelial hyperplasia,[55] and bronchioloalveolar adenoma.[56,50]

AAH may be found in 5.7% to 21.4% of lung cancer resection specimens. The variable percentage probably results from differences in effort made to look for the lesions as well as variation in diagnostic criteria.[50,54,55,57]

Because of their small size, AAH are usually incidental histologic findings, but they may be detected grossly, especially if they are 0.5 cm or larger. Processing the specimen in Bouin's fixative accentuates the gross visibility of AAH.[50] The lesions appear as ill-defined nodules usually less than 5 mm in diameter. Rarely, AAH may exceed 0.5 cm in diameter, and cases have been reported up to 1.0 cm.[50,54] Weng et al. found multiple lesions in 6.7% of lung cancer resection specimens and 2% of lung specimens resected for metastases.[54]

Histologically, AAH is a discrete, but ill-defined bronchioloalveolar proliferation (Figure 26.3A) in which the alveoli and respiratory bronchioles are lined by monotonous, slightly atypical cuboidal to low-columnar epithelial cells (Figure 26.3B). Focally, the alveolar walls may be altered to show a papillary growth pattern. Gaps usually exist between the cells. Nucleoli are inconspicuous or absent, but nuclear cytoplasmic inclusions may be seen. The alveolar septa may be slightly thickened with interstitial fibrosis, a mild lymphocytic infiltrate, and occasional lymphoid aggregates.

Although AAH has a distinct place in the classification of preinvasive lesions, in many cases it is very difficult to separate from nonmucinous BAC because of the great deal of morphologic overlap.[58] AAH must be distinguished primarily from the nonmucinous subtype of BAC and type II pneumocyte hyperplasia with interstitial inflammation and/or fibrosis.[59-62] Separation of AAH from small nonmucinous BAC may be very difficult.[6,49,63] The diagnosis of adenocarcinoma is favored if there is marked crowding of cells and/or overlapping of nuclei, nuclear atypia, and prominent papillary or invasive growth. Size is useful in that lesions 0.5 cm or greater in diameter with cytologic atypia are more likely to represent BAC, but in the absence of atypia, the diagnosis of AAH is still possible.[50]

It has not been shown that AAH alters the prognosis of patients with lung cancer.[64] Moreover, little data proves that AAH presenting in patients without lung carcinoma will subsequently develop a lung carcinoma. For this reason, a conservative approach is recommended in patients who

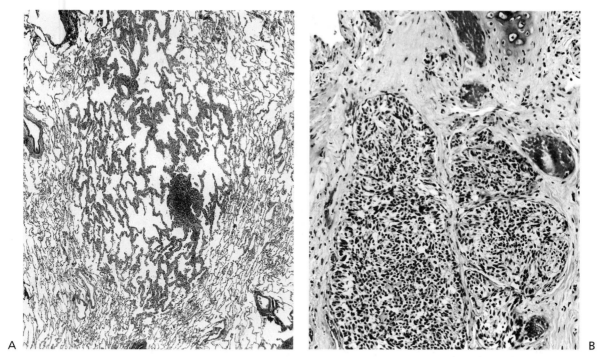

FIGURE 26.3. Atypical adenomatous hyperplasia. **A:** This millimeter-sized bronchioloalveolar proliferation is ill defined with mild thickening of the alveolar walls. A lymphoid aggregate is present (hematoxylin and eosin, 30 × magnification). **B:** The alveolar walls show mild fibrous thickening, the hyperplastic pneumocytes show minimal atypia, and gaps are present between the cells (hematoxylin and eosin, 300 × magnification). (From Travis WD. Pathology of pulmonary incipient neoplasia. In: Albores-Saavedra J, Henson DE, eds. *Pathology of incipient neoplasia.* Philadelphia: WB Saunders, 2000 (*in press*), with permission. Case contributed by Dr. M. Noguchi, University of Tsukuba, Japan.)

are incidentally found to have AAH in the absence of an associated lung carcinoma.

Diffuse Idiopathic Pulmonary Neuroendocrine Cell Hyperplasia

DIPNECH is a rare condition in which neuroendocrine cells proliferate throughout the peripheral airways in the form of neuroendocrine cell hyperplasia, tumorlets, and sometimes carcinoid tumors.[6,65–67] Clinically, it is associated with obstructive airways disease because of the bronchiolar fibrosis. This condition is regarded as a precursor to carcinoid tumors because a subset of these patients has one or more carcinoid tumors.[6]

In DIPNECH, the neuroendocrine cell hyperplasia and tumorlets are thought to be a primary proliferation in contrast to the much more common situation where these lesions are seen as a reactive secondary lesion in the setting of airway inflammation and/or fibrosis.[68–71] Carcinoid tumors are arbitrarily separated from tumorlets if the neuroendocrine proliferation is 0.5 cm or larger.[6,10]

In DIPNECH, the histologic findings consist of increased numbers of scattered single cells, small nodules (neuroendocrine bodies), or linear proliferations of neuroendocrine cells within the bronchiolar epithelium (Figure 26.4A and B). Confluent micronodular proliferations of neuroendocrine cells represent tumorlets, and if they are 0.5 cm in size or greater, they are called carcinoid tumors. Airway narrowing is often caused by fibrosis or the neuroendocrine proliferations and tumorlets (Figure 26.4B).

Squamous Cell Carcinoma

Squamous cell carcinoma accounts for approximately 30% of all lung cancers (Table 26.2).[1] Two-thirds of squamous cell carcinomas present as central lung tumors, whereas many among the remaining one-third are peripheral.[10,72] Most cavitating lung cancers are squamous cell carcinomas, and virtually all cases show intravascular tumor cells adjacent to the tumor.[73] Intercellular bridging, squamous pearl formation, and individual cell keratinization characterize squamous differentiation in squamous cell carcinomas. (Fig-

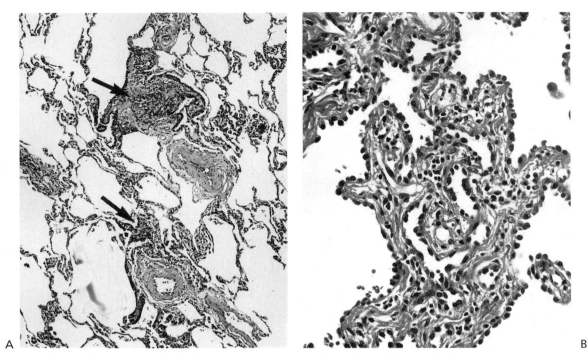

FIGURE 26.4. Diffuse idiopathic neuroendocrine cell hyperplasia. **A:** Nodules of hyperplastic neuroendocrine cells are present around the bronchioles *(arrows)*. **B:** This tumorlet is associated with a bronchus (cartilage—*top right*) and consists of a nodule of neuroendocrine cells. (Case contributed by Dr. Anthony A. Gal, Emory University, Atlanta, GA.)

ure 26.5) In well-differentiated tumors, these features are readily apparent; however, in poorly differentiated tumors, they are difficult to find (Figure 26.6).[74] Squamous cell carcinomas are commonly believed to arise from a progression of squamous metaplasia or basal cell hyperplasia with

atypia, through dysplasia, carcinoma *in situ,* and microinvasive carcinoma.[75] However, it is also possible that squamous cell carcinoma can develop *de novo* in normal bronchial mucosa.[46] Squamous cell carcinoma arises most often in

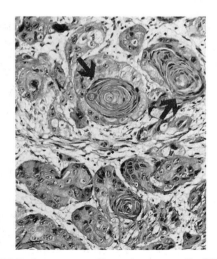

FIGURE 26.5. Squamous cell carcinoma, well differentiated. These tumor cells have abundant eosinophilic keratinized cytoplasm and form nests and keratin pearls *(arrows)* characteristic of squamous differentiation (hematoxylin and eosin, 200 × magnification).

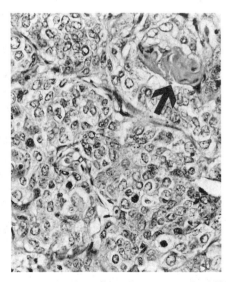

FIGURE 26.6. Squamous cell carcinoma, poorly differentiated. This tumor is growing in sheets and shows focal keratinization *(arrow)* (hematoxylin and eosin, 400 × magnification).

segmental bronchi, and involvement of lobar and mainstem bronchi occurs by extension.[46] The histologic subtypes of squamous cell carcinoma include papillary, clear cell, small cell,[76] and basaloid variants.[6] Papillary squamous cell carcinomas often show a pattern of exophytic endobronchial growth.[77,78] Rarely, squamous cell carcinoma of the lung arises in nonirradiated patients with laryngotracheobronchial papillomatosis, and these tumors have been shown to contain human papillomavirus DNA.[79,80] A minute squamous cell carcinoma has been reported, arising in the wall of a congenital lung cyst.[81]

Adenocarcinoma

Adenocarcinomas account for a little more than 30% of all lung cancers (Table 26.2).[11] According to the 1999 World Health Organization (WHO) classification, adenocarcinomas can be subclassified into five major subtypes: acinar (gland forming), papillary, bronchioloalveolar, solid with mucous formation, and mixed adenocarcinoma.[5] In addition, several unusual variants of adenocarcinoma include well-differentiated fetal adenocarcinoma,[82] mucinous ("colloid") adenocarcinoma,[83] mucinous cystadenocarcinoma,[84–87] signet ring carcinoma,[88] and clear cell adenocarcinoma.[6] The WDFA was previously regarded as the epithelial pattern of pulmonary blastoma as defined in the 1981 WHO classification.[188] However, subsequent studies have shown that it represents a variant of adenocarcinoma.[8,90] The term *pulmonary blastoma* is reserved for the biphasic tumors that have a component of WDFA and a primitive sarcomatous component.[6] Two unusual gross patterns of adenocarcinoma include the endobronchial polypoid adenocarcinoma[91] and pseudomesotheliomatous adenocarcinoma.[92–94] A single case of adenocarcinoma involving the bronchial epithelium in a pattern similar to that of Paget's disease has been reported.[95] Adenocarcinomas have also been reported arising in cystic lung lesions.[96,97]

Most adenocarcinomas are histologically heterogeneous, consisting of two or more of the histologic subtypes; therefore, most adenocarcinomas fall into the mixed subtype. Adenocarcinomas form acinar (glandular) (Figure 26.7) or papillary structures. When they grow in a purely lepidic fashion, they are regarded as BAC (see following). Solid adenocarcinomas with mucin closely resemble large cell carcinoma, except for the production of intracytoplasmic mucin that should be present in at least five cells in at least two high-power fields. Adenocarcinomas are often associated with scarring fibrosis. At the periphery, many adenocarcinomas show a focal BAC-like pattern. Psammoma bodies may be seen in up to 10% of tumors with a papillary component.[98]

The concept of scar carcinoma was proposed for those lung cancers associated with dense fibrotic scars.[99–101] The classic description of a scar carcinoma is a peripheral tumor

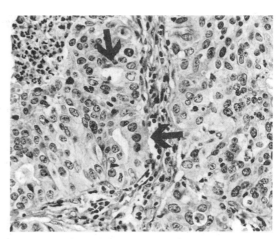

FIGURE 26.7. Adenocarcinoma, poorly differentiated. Focal gland formation *(arrows)* is present in this tumor, which otherwise consists of sheets of undifferentiated large cells (hematoxylin and eosin, 400 × magnification).

causing thickening and often puckering of the overlying pleura, with common anthracotic pigment and cholesterol clefts within the scar, and necrosis.[102] Although scars can be found in association with any histologic type of lung cancer, we have chosen to discuss this concept here because most of these tumors are adenocarcinomas.[99,100,103] Scar carcinomas reportedly have distinctive clinical features such as a higher distribution of adenocarcinoma, frequent presentation with nonpulmonary symptoms related to metastases, and presentation as radiographically occult lung cancer.[104] It has been proposed that patients with scar carcinomas have a worse prognosis than tumors without scarring,[104] although other studies suggest that no difference in prognosis exists compared to similar histologic cell types devoid of scarring.[105,106]

Shimosato and colleagues have shown that the scars in most of these tumors are most likely caused by the tumors,[100] and the concept that the lung cancer developed as a result of a pulmonary scar is incorrect. Multiple subsequent studies have supported this impression,[101,103,107] although it is likely that lung carcinomas may arise in the setting of certain pulmonary fibrotic conditions.[108–112]

Bronchioloalveolar Carcinoma

BAC is defined as an adenocarcinoma of the lung, which grows in a lepidic fashion along the alveolar septae without invasive growth (Figure 26.8). In the new 1999 WHO/IASLC classification, the lack of invasive growth was added as an essential criterion[6] because data suggests that such patients may be curable by surgical resection.[113] Although a BAC-like pattern of spread is common at the edge of conventional adenocarcinomas, histologically pure BAC

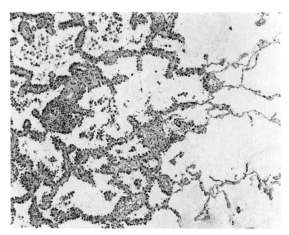

FIGURE 26.8. Adenocarcinoma, bronchioloalveolar type, non–mucin-producing. This tumor consists of uniform cuboidal cells proliferating along the alveolar septae. The alveolar architecture is preserved. The tumor contrasts with the normal alveolar walls *(right)* (hematoxylin and eosin, 100 × magnification).

is uncommon, accounting for only 3% of all invasive lung malignancies (Table 26.2).[11] Controversy exists whether histologic, histogenetic, or clinical dissimilarity is present between classic adenocarcinomas and bronchioloalveolar carcinoma.[114–117] However, much of the literature on the subject of BAC needs to be reevaluated based on the new definition of BAC. One of the problems resulting from the previous WHO classifications is that the percentage of lepidic growth pattern required to make the diagnosis of BAC was not specified.[89,118] As a result, some authors regarded tumors with only a minor component of lepidic growth to represent BAC.[118] Another problem with BAC is that metastatic adenocarcinomas can mimic the histologic appearance of BAC, especially the mucinous variant.[120]

More than 50% of BACs may be associated with focal scars, and the tumor often grows around the edge of the scar.[121] However, if the tumor shows irregular tumor cell nests and a desmoplastic stromal reaction, it is regarded as having a component of acinar or solid adenocarcinoma and is no longer a pure BAC.[10,121]

There are two major histologic types of BAC: nonmucinous and mucinous.[8] Rarely, BAC may consist of a mixture of mucinous and nonmucinous subtypes, or it may be difficult to make a precise distinction between the two subtypes.[6] Approximately 41% to 60% are mucin-producing, 21% to 45% are non–mucin-producing, 12 to 14% are a mixture, and in up to 7% of cases, it may be difficult to classify the tumor.[121,122] The mucin-producing tumors show gross and microscopic mucin production and tend to be multicentric.[122] They may also cause lobar consolidation resembling pneumonia on gross examination. Histologically, these tumors consist of tall columnar cells with abun-

dant apical cytoplasmic mucin and small basally oriented nuclei. The tumor cells grow along thin alveolar septae. The surrounding airspaces are often filled with mucin, sometimes creating a colloidlike appearance.

The nonmucinous BAC are more likely to be solitary.[122] Histologically, these tumors are composed of cuboidal cells proliferating along alveolar septae. A hobnail or saw-toothed appearance is often seen. Nuclear inclusions may be found in up to 56% of cases and are usually seen in nonmucinous tumor cells. These inclusions show the following properties: (a) they are PAS-positive; (b) they stain with immunohistochemistry for surfactant apoprotein; and (c) by ultrastructure they appear to consist of a network of 40-nm branching microtubules thought to arise from the inner nuclear membrane.[120,123] Nonmucinous BAC may consist of either Clara cells or type II pneumocytes; however, this distinction is not important for histologic classification.

Several pathologic variations of BAC may be encountered. A sclerosing variant is recognized, in which the alveolar septae are thickened by fibrosis without loss of the alveolar architecture.[124] The fibrosis in such cases may be rich in elastic fibers.[113] However, the presence of focal scarring within a BAC should raise concern for possible invasive growth. BAC may be cystic, and it rarely presents as multiple, diffuse, bilateral, cystic, cavitary lesions.[125] Tumors characterized by extensive mucin production have been described as mucinous or so-called colloid carcinomas.[83] Dekmezian et al. reported a single case of a BAC with myoepithelial cells.[126]

It can be difficult to separate BAC from a variety of other lesions, including reactive epithelial hyperplasias in fibrotic lung conditions, atypical adenomatous hyperplasia,[49,50, 55,57] and metastatic carcinomas. Because of the new WHO/IASLC definition, a final diagnosis of BAC can be achieved only in a surgical resection specimen. For this reason, bronchoscopic or needle biopsies showing an adenocarcinoma with a lepidic growth pattern may suggest only the possibility of BAC and are insufficient to exclude the presence of invasive growth.

Various pathologic features have been described as prognostic factors for BAC. Many of these need to be reevaluated given the new definition of BAC. Formerly described prognostic factors included cell type, with nonmucinous tumors having a much better survival than mucinous tumors.[121,122] The presence of multiple tumors,[121] alveolar spread,[120,124] size greater than 3 cm,[124] the sclerosing variant of BAC,[124] high histologic grade,[127] pleural invasion,[124] and lymph node metastases[124] also were shown to correlate with a poor prognosis. Daly et al. found that the presence of dense collagen within the tumor was associated with a better prognosis.[121] Linnoila et al. found that peripheral airway immunohistochemic markers such as surfactant-associated protein and 10kD Clara cell protein were independent prognostic factors for survival in patients with NSCLCs including

BAC.[128] Although patients with solitary nonmucinous tumors less than 3 cm in diameter have an excellent prognosis, patients with advanced-stage BAC have a poor prognosis comparable to other lung adenocarcinomas.[129,130]

Small Cell Carcinoma

Pathologic Features

SCLC accounts for 20% of all lung cancers (Table 26.2), and approximately 30,000 new cases occur in the United States each year.[11] Approximately two-thirds of SCLCs present as a perihilar mass. SCLCs are typically situated in a peribronchial location with infiltration of the bronchial submucosa and peribronchial tissue. Bronchial obstruction is usually caused by circumferential compression, although rarely endobronchial lesions can occur. Because the diagnosis is usually established on transbronchial biopsy and/or cytology, it is unusual to encounter SCLC as a surgical specimen. Extensive lymph node metastases are common. The tumor is white-tan, soft, friable, and often shows extensive necrosis. With advanced disease, the bronchial lumen may be obstructed by extrinsic compression. In up to 5% of cases, SCLC presents as a peripheral coin lesion.[131,132]

Subclassification of SCLC has evolved considerably over the past two decades. In 1981 the WHO proposed that SCLC be subclassified into three subtypes: (a) oat cell carcinoma, (b) intermediate cell type, and (c) combined oat cell carcinoma.[5] However, expert lung cancer pathologists could not reproduce this subclassification, and significant differences in survival could not be shown. For these reasons, in 1988 the IASLC proposed that the intermediate cell type category be dropped and added the category of mixed small cell/large cell carcinoma because it appeared that these patients might have a worse prognosis than other SCLC patients.[133] They continued to use the category of combined SCLC for tumors mixed with adenocarcinoma or squamous cell carcinoma and proposed that all tumors lacking a non–small cell component be called SCLC.[133] Because subsequent data suggested that the prognosis for mixed small cell/large cell carcinoma might actually be better, and because there are problems in reproducibility for this subtype,[134] in the new WHO/IASLC classification, combined SCLC is the only subtype of SCLC (Table 26.1).[6]

By light microscopy, SCLC consists of tumor cells characterized by small size, a round to fusiform shape, scant cytoplasm, finely granular nuclear chromatin, and absent or inconspicuous nucleoli (Figure 26.9A).[6] Nuclear molding and smearing of nuclear chromatin caused by crush artifact may be conspicuous. Mitotic figures are common, sometimes exceeding 100 mitoses per 10 high-power fields. The tumor often grows in sheets without a specific pattern, but rosettes, peripheral palisading, organoid nesting, streams, ribbons, and rarely, tubules or ductules may be present.[135] Necrosis is usually extensive. Mitotic rates are high. Hematoxyphilic encrustation of vessel walls (Azzopardi effect) is a common finding (Figure 26.9B).[135]

Although no absolute upper limit exists for cell size in the diagnosis of SCLC, it has been suggested that the cells should measure approximately the diameter of two to three small resting lymphocytes.[136] Within the entity of SCLC, cell size range includes cases that have larger cells approaching the size of large cell carcinoma. This problem was addressed by the 1981 WHO/IASLC classification for lung tumors that proposed the category of intermediate cell type of SCLC.[133] Vollmer et al. used morphometry to demonstrate a gradual transition in cell size from the smallest SCLC to large cell carcinoma.[137] Thus cases that fall in the middle of the spectrum cannot be distinguished according to cell size alone. This finding may account, in part, for the difficulty in interobserver reproducibility of the intermediate subtype category of SCLC as proposed by the 1981 WHO classification.[137]

According to the morphometric study by Vollmer et al., the size of SCLC cells also appears greater in larger biopsy specimens.[137] Thus the tumor cells of SCLC appear larger in well-fixed open biopsies than in transbronchial biopsy specimens.

Subsequent to chemotherapy, biopsy specimens from 15% to 45% of patients with SCLC can show an admixture of components of large cell, squamous, giant cell, or adenocarcinoma.[138–140]

Combined SCLC

Less than 10% of SCLCs show a mixture with another histologic component type of NSCLC. A combination of SCLC and large cell carcinoma (Figure 26.10) is found in approximately 4% to 6% of cases.[133] Approximately 1% to 3% of SCLCs may be combined with adenocarcinoma or squamous cell carcinoma.[133,134,139,141] Mixtures of SCLC can also occur with spindle cell carcinoma,[142,143] giant cell carcinoma,[143] and carcinosarcoma.[144] It remains to be proven whether these patients have significant differences in clinical features, prognosis, and response to therapy.[141] Some evidence suggests a survival benefit for patients who undergo resection.[141]

Clinical Features and Prognosis

SCLC has a very aggressive clinical course with frequent widespread metastases. It is considered a distinct clinicopathologic entity because of the many characteristic clinical manifestations, the unique pathologic features, and the sensitivity to chemotherapy.

Untreated patients with limited-stage and extensive-stage SCLC have a median survival of 3 and 1.5 months, respec-

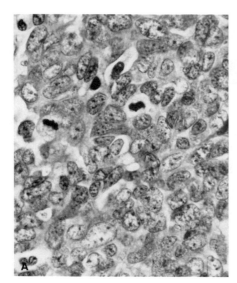
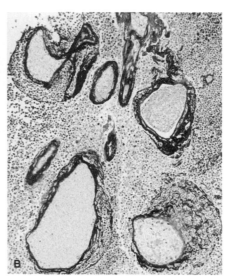

FIGURE 26.9. Small cell carcinoma. **A:** This tumor consists of densely packed small tumor cells with scant cytoplasm, finely granular nuclear chromatin, inconspicuous or absent nucleoli, and multiple mitoses (hematoxylin and eosin, 100 × magnification). **B:** This small cell carcinoma is extensively necrotic and shows the Azzopardi effect or hematoxyphillic staining of the vascular walls caused by DNA encrustation (hematoxylin and eosin, 100 × magnification).

tively. With combination chemotherapy and chest radiotherapy, the median survival is improved to 10–16 months for patients with limited-stage disease, and 6–11 months for patients with high-stage disease.

Differential Diagnosis

Because major differences exist in therapeutic approach to patients with SCLC versus NSCLC, the major question

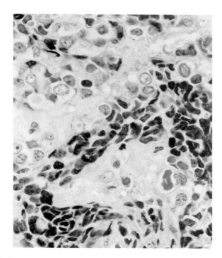

FIGURE 26.10. Combined small cell and large cell carcinoma. This tumor consists of large cells with abundant cytoplasm and vesicular nuclei with prominent nucleoli admixed, with small cells having scant cytoplasm and finely granular chromatin (hematoxylin and eosin, 630 × magnification).

asked of pathologists is whether the tumor is an SCLC or an NSCLC. The distinction of SCLC from large cell carcinoma or large cell neuroendocrine carcinoma (LCNEC) should not rest on a single criteria such as cell size or nucleoli; multiple additional features should be assessed, including nuclear to cytoplasmic ratio, nuclear chromatin, nucleoli, nuclear molding, cell shape (fusiform versus polygonal), and hematoxylin vascular staining (Table 26.4).[137,145]

Morphologic separation of SCLC from NSCLC can be difficult. In the study by Reglue et al. agreement for the diagnosis of SCLCs for all five observers was 93% and for at least four or five observers it was 98%.[29] Disagreement among expert lung cancer pathologists over the distinction between SCLC and NSCLC may occur in up to 5% to 7% of cases.[28,145]

The poor agreement (only 72%) for the subtyping of SCLCs (e.g., oat cell versus intermediate) is one of the reasons for the recent revised classification of SCLC, which was proposed to replace the histologic subtyping in the second edition. WHO classification (Table 26.1).[133]

In small, crushed biopsy specimens, SCLC can be difficult to distinguish from carcinoid tumors, lymphocytic infiltrates, or poorly differentiated NSCLC. In some cases, comparison with cytology specimens taken at the time of bronchoscopy enables a definitive diagnosis. Lymphoid infiltrates, whether caused by small lymphocytic lymphoma or chronic inflammation, can be distinguished from SCLC by their discohesive pattern of growth, contrasting with the epithelial clustering and nuclear molding of SCLC. In addition, immunohistochemistry for keratin (epithelial marker)

TABLE 26.4. LIGHT MICROSCOPIC FEATURES FOR DISTINGUISHING SMALL CELL CARCINOMA AND LARGE CELL NEUROENDOCRINE CARCINOMA

Histologic Feature	Small Cell Carcinoma	Large Cell Neuroendocrine Carcinoma
Cell size	Smaller (less than diameter of 3 lymphocytes)	Larger
Nuclear/cytoplasmic ratio	Higher	Lower
Nuclear chromatin	Finely granular, uniform	Coarsely granular or vesicular Less uniform
Nucleoli	Absent or faint	Often (not always) present May be prominent or faint
Nuclear molding	Characteristic	Less prominent
Fusiform shape	Common	Uncommon
Polygonal shape with ample pink cytoplasm	Uncharacteristic	Characteristic
Nuclear smear	Frequent	Uncommon
Basophilic staining of vessels and stroma	Occasional	Rare

and common leukocyte antigen (lymphoid marker) can be very useful. If the biologic behavior of a tumor raises doubts about the diagnosis of SCLC, additional biopsies may be helpful to establish the diagnosis.[147]

Large Cell Carcinoma

Large cell carcinoma is a poorly differentiated carcinoma that does not have features of squamous cell carcinoma, adenocarcinoma, or SCLC. Thus it is a diagnosis of exclusion, and a spectrum of morphology is encompassed by this histologic subtype. Most tumors consist of large cells with abundant cytoplasm and large nuclei with prominent nucleoli and/or vesicular nuclei (Figure 26.11).[10,148–151] Several variants of large cell carcinoma are recognized in the

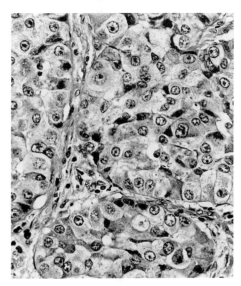

FIGURE 26.11. Large cell carcinoma. This tumor consists of sheets and nests of large cells with abundant cytoplasm and vesicular nuclei with prominent nucleoli (hematoxylin and eosin, 400 × magnification).

new WHO/IASLC histologic classification of lung cancer, including LCNEC[6,145,152] basaloid carcinoma,[153] lympho-epithelial-like carcinoma,[154–156] clear cell carcinoma,[157] and large cell carcinoma with rhabdoid phenotype.[158]

Many poorly differentiated adenocarcinomas or squamous cell carcinomas may show a component of large cell carcinoma. Because such tumors are classified according to their best differentiated component, no combined adenocarcinoma or squamous cell carcinoma/large cell carcinoma exists. Therefore, a small bronchial biopsy may reveal large cell carcinoma, whereas the subsequent resected specimen may enable more specific classification as a squamous cell carcinoma or an adenocarcinoma.[30,31,159] For this reason, if clear-cut morphologic criteria cannot be satisfied for subclassification as squamous cell or adenocarcinoma, the general diagnosis of "lung cancer, non–small cell type" should be made. Positive staining of intracytoplasmic mucin with the mucicarmine or periodic-acid-Schiff with diastase digestion (DPAS) stains separate the solid variant of adenocarcinoma with mucin production from large cell carcinoma. If large cell carcinoma is mixed with SCLC, it is regarded primarily as a variant of SCLC: mixed small cell/large cell carcinoma.[133]

Several variants of large cell carcinoma include clear cell carcinoma,[160] lymphoepithelioma-like carcinoma,[15,161,162] and LCNEC.[145] This discussion focuses primarily on LCNEC and its relationship to SCLC. Spindle and giant cell carcinomas and the concept of pleomorphic carcinoma are also mentioned.

Large cell carcinoma accounts for 9% of all lung carcinomas.[11] These tumors may be central or peripheral, and by gross examination they often appear as large necrotic tumors. Histologically, the tumors usually consist of sheets and nests of large polygonal cells with vesicular nuclei and prominent nucleoli.[5] They may have a somewhat squamous or adenocarcinoma appearance, but they fall short of criteria for those tumors. By electron microscopy, a high percentage of large cell carcinomas show features of squamous cell or adenocarcinoma.[32,35,163]

Large Cell Neuroendocrine Carcinoma

Pathologic Features

Approximately two-thirds of LCNECs are peripheral, with the remainder being centrally located. The average size is 4.0 cm with a range from 0.7 cm up to 9 cm. They are usually circumscribed, nodular masses with a necrotic, tan, red cut surface.

LCNECs are defined by the following histologic criteria: (a) light microscopic features commonly associated with neuroendocrine tumors such as organoid, palisading, trabecular, or rosettelike growth patterns (Figure 26.12A); (b)

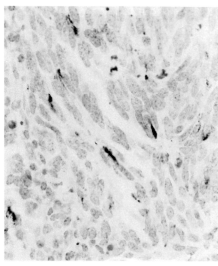

FIGURE 26.13. Large cell neuroendocrine carcinoma. Focally, the tumor cells stain positively for chromogranin (chromogranin, 630 × magnification).

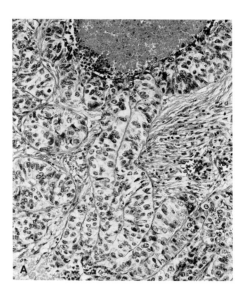

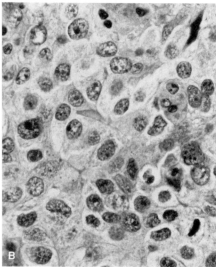

FIGURE 26.12. Large cell neuroendocrine carcinoma. **A:** Organoid nests and trabecular growth patterns give this tumor a neuroendocrine morphologic appearance. Necrosis is also conspicuous *(top, bottom)* (hematoxylin and eosin, 400 × magnification). **B:** The tumor cells have abundant cytoplasm and some show vesicular nuclei and/or prominent nucleoli. A mitotic figure is present (hematoxylin and eosin, 800 × magnification).

tumor cells of large size, polygonal shape, low nuclear to cytoplasmic ratio, coarse or vesicular nuclear chromatin, and frequent nucleoli (Figure 26.12B); (c) high mitotic rate (>10/10 HPF) with a mean of 60 mitoses per 10 HPF and some exceeding 100 per 10 HPF; (d) frequent necrosis; and (e) neuroendocrine features by immunohistochemistry (Figure 26.13) or electron microscopy.[145] The term *large cell carcinoma, with neuroendocrine morphology* can be used for tumors resembling LCNEC by light microscopy but lacking proof of neuroendocrine differentiation by electron microscopy or immunohistochemistry.

The term *combined LCNEC* is used for those tumors associated with other histologic types of NSCLC (Table 26.1). Most often this represents a component of adenocarcinoma. If a component of SCLC exists, then the tumor becomes a combined SCLC.

Clinical Features

The median age for patients with LCNEC is 62 years (range 33 to 87 years). Virtually all patients are cigarette smokers and most have over a 40 pack-year history of smoking.[145] Ectopic hormone production is uncommon in cases of LCNEC and has not been observed in any reported cases.[145]

LCNEC is an aggressive malignancy with a prognosis approaching the dismal outlook for SCLC. Fifty percent of patients are dead at 1.2 years, and the 5- and 10-year survival is 23% and 11%, respectively. Therefore, patients with LCNEC also have a worse outlook than for adenocarcinoma. Some patients with LCNEC, particularly those with stage I or II tumors, may do well. The optimal therapy remains to be defined because these tumors are rare and few institutions have accumulated enough patients to make definite therapeutic recommendations. Until more information is known about the clinical behavior of LCNEC and its response to chemotherapy, resectable tumors should be removed surgically. Some patients with advanced-stage disease have responded to chemotherapy so that adjunctive chemotherapy may be beneficial following surgery.

Differential Diagnosis

LCNEC must be distinguished from adenocarcinoma, SCLC, large cell carcinoma, and large cell carcinoma with neuroendocrine differentiation (LCC-ND). Mitotic counts are one of the most useful criteria for distinguishing adenocarcinoma from LCNEC.[145] According to the new WHO/IASLC criteria for adenocarcinoma, the upper limit of mitoses should be 10 mitoses per 2 mm^2 (10 high-power fields on some microscopes).[6,164] This limit contrasts with the mitotic rate of LCNEC, which should have a mitotic count greater than 11 per 2 mm^2 (10 high-power fields, but typically ranges between 50 to 100 mitoses per 10 high-power fields.[145] The extent of necrosis in LCNEC is generally more extensive than in adenocarcinoma, where it usually consists of punctate foci within organoid nests of tumor cells. Nuclei of adenocarcinoma usually show a finely granular chromatin, whereas most LCNEC have a vesicular or coarse chromatin. Thus adenocarcinoma is histologically intermediate grade, whereas LCNEC is histologically high grade. Separation of LCNEC from SCLC requires consideration of multiple histologic features rather than a single criterion (Table 26.4).

Large cell carcinomas can be separated into those that have neuroendocrine features by light microscopy as well as immunohistochemistry and/or electron microscopy (LCNEC), those with a neuroendocrine morphology (NEM) but lacking neuroendocrine differentiation by electron microscopy or immunohistochemistry (LCC-NEM), those with no neuroendocrine pattern by light microscopy or special studies (classic LCC), and those with neuroendocrine differentiation (NED) by special studies (LCC-NED).[6,145] LCC-NEDs differ from LCNECs histologically in that they lack neuroendocrine morphologic characteristics by light microscopy, such as prominent organoid nesting, trabecular, palisading, or rosette-like patterns.

Further data regarding the spectrum of clinical and pathologic features of LCNEC are awaiting larger series of cases. We hope this research will further define the differences in survival and response to therapy for LCNEC compared to adenocarcinoma, large cell carcinoma, LCC with NEM, LCC-NED, and SCLC.

Data is conflicting regarding the issue of whether NSCLC-NED may be responsive to SCLC chemotherapy regimens[165-167] or whether expression of neuroendocrine markers may be an unfavorable prognostic factor.[168-175] The significance of separation of LCNEC, LCC-NEM, and LCC-NED remains to be determined.

Adenosquamous Carcinoma

Adenosquamous carcinoma accounts for 0.6% to 2.3% of all lung cancers.[176-180] According to the new WHO/IASLC criteria, the tumor should consist of a mixture of at least 10% adenocarcinoma and squamous carcinoma.[8] Ishida described three subtypes of adenosquamous carcinoma, including a predominantly glandular type, a predominantly squamous type, and a mixed type.[177] Although some studies have suggested a worse survival for adenosquamous carcinoma,[178,180] others indicate no difference from other NSCLCs.[177,179]

Carcinomas with Pleomorphic, Sarcomatoid, or Sarcomatous Elements

Carcinomas with pleomorphic, sarcomatoid, and sarcomatous elements represent a continuum of differentiation in poorly differentiated carcinomas. In the 1981 WHO classification, spindle cell carcinoma was classified as a variant of squamous cell carcinoma, and giant cell carcinoma was regarded as a variant of large cell carcinoma.[5] However, the concept of pleomorphic carcinoma was reported by Fishback et al. and emphasized that most carcinomas with spindle cell and/or giant cell differentiation were associated with patterns of other major subtypes of lung carcinoma, such as squamous cell carcinoma, adenocarcinoma, or large cell carcinoma.[143] Pleomorphic carcinomas tend to be large, peripheral tumors that often invade the chest wall. Because of the prominent histologic heterogeneity of this tumor, adequate sampling is important and should consist of at least one section per centimeter of the tumor diameter. In the new WHO/IASLC classification, at least a 10% component of the spindle cell and/or giant cell component must be present for a diagnosis of pleomorphic carcinoma.[6]

Giant and spindle cell carcinomas account for 0.3% of all invasive lung malignancies.[11] If the tumor has a pure giant cell pattern, the term *giant cell carcinoma* can be used. Giant cell carcinoma consists of huge, bizarre pleomorphic and multinucleated tumor giant cells (Figure 26.14).[181-183] The tumor cells of giant cell carcinoma are very large, measuring approximately two to three times the size of those in ordinary NSCLCs.[182] The nuclei may be single or multiple; sometimes they are bizarre with atypical mitotic figures. The cells are often discohesive and infiltrated by inflammatory cells. Neutrophil emperipolesis characterized by cytoplasmic infiltration by neutrophils is a distinctive feature (Figure 26.14). Fishback et al. recognized that 98% of giant cell carcinomas are associated with one or more other histologic subtypes such as spindle cell carcinoma (65%), adenocarcinoma (44%), large cell carcinoma (29%), squamous cell carcinoma (6%), and SCLC (2%). Therefore, pure giant cell carcinoma is rare, accounting for only 2% of cases of pleomorphic spindle and/or giant cell carcinomas.[143]

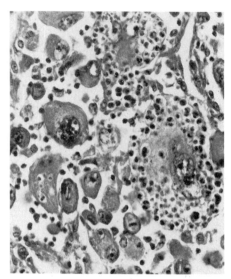

FIGURE 26.14. Giant cell carcinoma. These giant tumor cells are discohesive and infiltrated by numerous neutrophils, which show emperipolesis. Although none of these cells is multinucleated, they are huge with abundant eosinophilic cytoplasm and atypical large nuclei (hematoxylin and eosin, 400 × magnification).

If the carcinoma consists of a pure spindle cell pattern, it can be regarded as spindle cell carcinoma (Figure 26.15).[184–186] however, Fishback et al. showed that only 9% of spindle cell carcinomas are associated with squamous cell carcinoma. Many cases were associated with a mixture of other histologic subtypes, with 52% showing a component of giant cell carcinoma, 47% adenocarcinoma, 24% large cell carcinoma, and 2% SCLC.[143] Only 10% of cases showed a pure spindle cell pattern.[143] Although immuno-

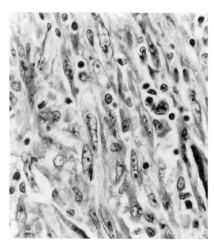

FIGURE 26.15. Spindle cell carcinoma. These spindle-shaped tumor cells have hyperchromatic atypical nuclei and were positive with immunohistochemic staining for keratin (hematoxylin and eosin, 630 × magnification).

histochemistry for epithelial markers such as keratin can be helpful in confirming epithelial differentiation, the new WHO/IASLC requires only light microscopic criteria.[6] Nevertheless, immunohistochemistry and less often electron microscopy can be helpful.[184–186] In some cases, multiple epithelial markers may be necessary to demonstrate epithelial differentiation because these tumors are poorly differentiated. However, immunohistochemistry can be problematic because some sarcomas may express keratin. It is important to sample spindle cell carcinomas extensively to exclude the presence of recognizable carcinomatous foci that would allow for classification as pleomorphic carcinoma. If such foci cannot be found by light microscopy, one should perform immunohistochemistry for epithelial markers such as keratin, EMA, or CEA.

The study by Fishback et al. of pleomorphic carcinomas showed that spindle cell and giant cell carcinoma coexist in 40% of cases.[143] These tumors were often associated with other histologic subtypes (more than 90% for spindle cell carcinoma and more than 97% for giant cell carcinoma). They typically presented as large peripheral lung masses in elderly male smokers and had a poor prognosis with a 10% five-year survival.[143]

Carcinosarcoma and Pulmonary Blastoma

Although carcinosarcoma and pulmonary blastoma were placed under the category of miscellaneous tumors in the 1981 WHO classification,[5] in the new WHO/IASLC classification they are regarded as types of carcinoma of the lung.[6] The new WHO/IASLC classification defines carcinosarcoma as a tumor consisting of a mixture of carcinoma and sarcoma that should show heterologous elements such as malignant cartilage, bone, or skeletal muscle. Pulmonary blastomas consist of a glandular component that resembles well-differentiated fetal adenocarcinoma and a primitive sarcomatous component.[6]

OTHER NEUROENDOCRINE TUMORS

Although SCLC represents one of the four major histologic subtypes of lung cancer, it is also generally regarded as a part of the spectrum of pulmonary neuroendocrine neoplasia. Other neuroendocrine lung tumors include typical and atypical carcinoid and LCNEC (Table 26.5). The clinical aspects of carcinoids and LCNEC are addressed briefly in this chapter because they are not specifically addressed elsewhere in this textbook.

The classification of pulmonary neuroendocrine tumors of the lung is perplexing. Although a spectrum of clinical and histologic features of malignancy exist among these tumors, this complexity is compounded by a bewildering variety of terms and criteria in the literature.[6,10,145]

TABLE 26.5. TERMINOLOGY FOR PULMONARY NEUROENDOCRINE LESIONS*

Common Neoplasms with a Neuroendocrine Light Microscopic Appearance
  A. Typical Carcinoid
  B. Atypical Carcinoid
  C. Large Cell Neuroendocrine Carcinoma (LCNEC)†
      LCNEC (if confirmed by immunohistochemistry or electron microscopy)
      Combined LCNEC
  D. Small Cell Carcinoma
      Combined small cell carcinoma

Non-small Cell Lung Carcinoma with Neuroendocrine Differentiation (NSCLC-NED)
    (Adenocarcinoma, squamous cell carcinoma, or large cell carcinoma with neuroendocrine features not seen by light microscopy but detected by immunohistochemistry or ultrastructure)

† Large cell neuroendocrine carcinoma with neuroendocrine morphology (if special studies negative or not available)
* From Travis WD, Colby TV, Corrin B, et al. *Histological typing of lung and pleural tumors.* 3rd ed. Berlin: Springer Verlag, 1999, with permission.

Lung tumors with neuroendocrine morphology include the low-grade typical carcinoid (TC), intermediate-grade atypical carcinoid (AC), and the high-grade LCNEC and SCLC. This classification has substantial reproducibility, with the greatest difficulty in separating TC from AC and LCNEC from SCLC.

Neuroendocrine differentiation may be detected by immunohistochemical or ultrastructural studies in 10% to 20% of histologically ordinary NSCLCs such as squamous cell carcinomas, adenocarcinomas, or large cell carcinomas (Table 26.5). The term *NSCLC-NE* is sometimes used for these cases.[145]

Typical and Atypical Carcinoid

Pathologic Features

Carcinoid tumors are often divided into central and peripheral tumors. The percentage of peripheral tumors varies from 16% to 40%,[187,188] with the remaining tumors being centrally located. Central carcinoids often have a large endobronchial component, with a fleshy, smooth, polypoid mass protruding into the bronchial lumen. Necrosis or extensive hemorrhage are characteristic of AC. Peripheral carcinoids are situated in the subpleural parenchyma, and they often do not bear an anatomic relationship to a bronchus.

Central carcinoids tend to be larger than peripheral tumors, with a mean diameter of 3.1 cm (range 0.5 to 10 cm) versus 2.4 cm (range 0.5 to 6 cm).[188] ACs are larger than TCs with a mean diameter of 3.6 cm for ACs compared to 2.3 cm for TCs.[188]

Both TCs and ACs are characterized histologically by an organoid growth pattern and uniform cytologic features, consisting of moderate eosinophilic, finely granular cytoplasm with nuclei possessing a finely granular chromatin pattern (Figure 26.16) (Table 26.6). Nucleoli are inconspicuous in most TCs but they may be more prominent in ACs. A variety of histologic patterns may occur in both AC and TC, including spindle cell (Figure 26.17), trabecular, palisading, rosettelike, papillary, sclerosing papillary, glandular, and follicular patterns.[145] The tumor cells of pulmonary carcinoid tumors may have oncocytic, acinic cell-like, signet-ring, mucin-producing, or melanocytic features.[145]

The original criteria for AC, as defined by Arrigoni et al.[164] were recently modified to a carcinoid tumor with mitoses between 2 and 10 per 2 mm^2 area of viable tumor (10 high-power fields in certain microscopes) or the presence of necrosis (Figure 26.18).[152] The presence of features such as pleomorphism, vascular invasion, and increased cellularity are not as helpful in separating TC from AC. In contrast, TC may have focal cytologic pleomorphism, but necrosis is absent and mitotic figures are rare (Table 26.6).[145,164] The necrosis in AC usually consists of small foci centrally located within organoid nests of tumor cells; uncommonly, the necrosis may form larger confluent zones. Criteria for separation of TC from AC are summarized in Table 26.6.

Clinical Features

Carcinoid tumors are low-grade malignant neoplasms of neuroendocrine cells, which constitute 1% to 2% of all lung tumors.[136] They are divided into typical and atypical types, with the latter possessing more malignant histologic and clinical features.[164]

The indolent nature of carcinoid tumors is reflected by

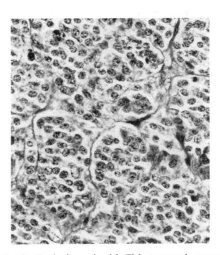

FIGURE 26.16. Typical carcinoid. This tumor is growing in organoid nests and consists of uniform medium-sized cells with a moderate amount of eosinophilic cytoplasm (hematoxylin and eosin, 500 × magnification).

TABLE 26.6. TYPICAL AND ATYPICAL CARCINOID: DISTINGUISHING FEATURES

Histologic or Clinical Feature	Typical Carcinoid	Atypical Carcinoid
Histologic patterns: organoid, trabecular, palisading, and spindle cell	Characteristic	Characteristic
Mitoses	Absent or <2 per 2 mm² area of viable tumor (10 high-power fields on some microscopes)	2–10 per 2 mm² of area of viable tumor (10 high-power fields on some microscopes)
Necrosis	Absent	Characteristic, usually focal or punctate
Nuclear pleomorphism, hyperchromatism	Usually absent, not sufficient by itself for diagnosis of AC	Often present
Regional lymph node metastases at presentation	5–15%	40–48%
Distant metastases at presentation	Rare	20%
Survival at 5 years	90–95%	58%
Disease-free survival at 10 years	90–95%	35%

the finding that 51% of patients are asymptomatic at presentation.[188] The most common pulmonary manifestations include hemoptysis in 18%, postobstructive pneumonitis in 17%, and dyspnea in 2% of patients.[188] Various paraneoplastic syndromes can occur with carcinoid tumors including the carcinoid syndrome,[188,189] Cushing's syndrome,[190] and acromegaly.[191] Bronchial carcinoids occur with equal frequency in men and women.[188,192] The mean age is 55 years with a range up to 82 years.[188] Bronchial carcinoids are the most common lung tumor in childhood.[183]

Surgery is the primary approach to management of bronchial carcinoids.[187,183] Patients with TC have an excellent prognosis and rarely die of tumor.[188,194] The finding of metastases should not be used as a criteria for distinguishing TC from AC because 5% to 20% of TCs have regional lymph node involvement.

Compared to TCs, ACs have a larger tumor size, a higher rate of metastases, and the survival is significantly reduced. The mortality reported in most series is approximately 30%, ranging from 27 to 47%.[164,188,195,196]

Prognosis in carcinoid tumors has been correlated with various clinical and pathologic features, including lack of surgical therapy, advanced stage, large tumor size (greater than 3 cm), lymph node metastases, vascular invasion, atypical versus typical histology, intraluminal versus extrabron-

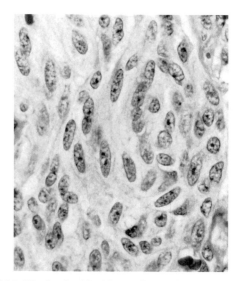

FIGURE 26.17. Carcinoid with spindle cell features. These tumor cells are prominently spindle-shaped and show the finely granular nuclear chromatin and moderate amount of eosinophilic cytoplasm characteristic of carcinoid tumors (hematoxylin and eosin, 1,000 × magnification).

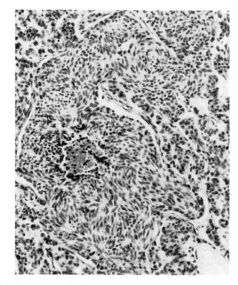

FIGURE 26.18. Atypical carcinoid. A punctate focus of necrosis is present in one of the organoid nests of spindle-shaped tumor cells. This feature is characteristic of atypical carcinoids (hematoxylin and eosin, 200 × magnification).

chial spread, aneuploidy, S-phase, and integrated optical density measurement of nuclear DNA content.[188,192,195–198]

Differential Diagnosis

It can be difficult to distinguish TC from AC (and occasionally SCLC) in small, crushed biopsy specimens; therefore, one should be careful when interpreting transbronchial biopsies if the tumor cells are not well preserved. Although a spindle cell pattern is more common in AC and SCLC, it should not be used as a criterion for malignancy because it also occurs in TC. Spindle cell carcinoids differ from other non-neuroendocrine tumors composed of spindle-shaped cells, such as smooth muscle tumors (leiomyoma, leiomyosarcoma), chemodectoma, and spindle cell carcinoma. Separation of these tumors from carcinoid can be made by recognition in the latter of an organoid pattern, finely granular nuclear chromatin, and positive immunohistochemical staining for neuroendocrine markers or dense core granules by electron microscopy.

IMMUNOHISTOCHEMISTRY, AND FLOW CYTOMETRY

Immunohistochemistry plays an important role in the evaluation of neuroendocrine neoplasms of the lung. Many antibodies, including neuroendocrine, hormonal, epithelial, and other markers, can be used to immunohistochemically stain neuroendocrine lung tumors.

Small Cell Lung Carcinoma

Recent studies have shown that the most useful neuroendocrine markers for SCLC in formalin-fixed, paraffin-embedded tissue sections are chromogranin A, synaptophysin, Leu-7, and certain neural cell adhesion molecules (NCAMs).[145,199,200] Guinee et al. found staining for chromogranin in 60% versus 47%, NSE in 60% versus 33%, Leu-7 in 40% versus 24%, and synaptophysin in 5% versus 19% of open lung versus transbronchial biopsy specimens of SCLC.[199] The NCAM antibody 123C3 has shown promise in paraffin-embedded tissue sections.[201,202] Although NSE has been advocated as a useful marker for neuroendocrine differentiation, it is relatively nonspecific because it stains up to 60% of NSCLCs.[145] Bombesin or gastrin-related peptide (GRP) can be demonstrated immunohistochemically in a high percentage of SCLCs.[145,199]

Keratin (AE1/AE3) and membrane antigen (EMA) stain virtually all SCLCs in both open lung biopsy and transbronchial biopsy specimens.[145,199] Therefore, if keratin staining is negative in a suspected SCLC, one should be careful to exclude other possibilities, such as chronic inflammation,

lymphoma, primitive neuroectodermal tumor, or small round cell sarcoma. Nevertheless, some SCLCs may be negative for keratin, and varied staining results may be caused by the antibody and/or methods used and the preservation of the material. Occasionally, a punctate perinuclear "do like" pattern of keratin staining may be encountered in SCLC, but this pattern is not specific and is found in the minority of keratin-positive cases.

Despite extensive efforts to identify monoclonal antibodies that will reliably distinguish SCLC from NSCLC, so far no antibodies have been proven to be effective in routinely processed, formalin-fixed, paraffin-embedded sections.[203,204] Up to 10% to 20% of NSCLCs exhibit neuroendocrine differentiation detectable by immunohistochemistry or electron microscopy. It is important, however, to remember that the WHO criteria for classification of lung cancer are based on conventional light microscopy, and data obtained by electron microscopy may not be comparable to data obtained by light microscopy alone.

DNA analysis of SCLC reveals a high percentage of aneuploidy, ranging up to 85% of cases,[145,197,205] but aneuploidy does not appear to correlate well with prognosis.[197,205] A high nuclear/cytoplasmic ratio in lung neuroendocrine tumors, which selects for SCLC, correlates strongly with prognosis.[206] High nucleolar organizer region values in lung neuroendocrine tumors also correlate with poor prognosis.[207]

Large Cell Neuroendocrine Carcinoma

LCNECs stain immunohistochemically with neuron specific enolase (NSE) (100%), chromogranin (80%), Leu-7 (40%), synaptophysin (40%), bombesin (40%), CEA (100%), and keratin (100%).[145] The immunohistochemic staining is often focal. Aneuploidy can be found in 75% of LCNECs.[145] Several molecular studies have shown that a high frequency of chromosomal abnormalities (p53, 3p, 9p, 5q and 11q) exist in the high-grade LCNECs and SCLCs with low and intermediate percentages of molecular changes in TC and AC, respectively.[208–212]

Carcinoid Tumors

Of the various types of pulmonary neuroendocrine tumors, the highest percentage, distribution, and intensity of immunohistochemic staining for neuroendocrine and hormonal markers can be found in TC. Chromogranin is the most useful immunohistochemic marker of neuroendocrine differentiation, followed by synaptophysin and Leu 7.[145]

Aneuploidy can occur in both TC and AC. It has been found in 5%–32% of TC and 16%–79% of AC.[145,192,197,213,214] Aneuploidy is significantly more frequent in AC than TC.[192,213,214] and it correlates with poor prognosis.[213] However, all aneuploid carcinoid tumors do not behave aggressively; in one study, 58% of patients with aneuploid carcinoid tumors survived five years.[213]

ELECTRON MICROSCOPY

Most lung carcinomas are diagnosed without the aid of ultrastructural study, but the electron microscope provides more information on the structure of the tumor cells than can be obtained from hematoxylin/eosin sections, and it is often helpful when the light microscopy alone is not adequate. A fine-needle aspiration biopsy can provide sufficient material, but the specimen must be handled properly to yield good results.[215] The electron microscope can also be useful in research studies on lung tumors. The detailed morphology of cell lines can be documented, and it is possible to perform precise immunocytochemistry, *in situ* hybridization, and image analysis using electron microscopic preparations. A brief account of the ultrastructure of the major types of primary lung tumors is included in this chapter to complement the descriptions of the light microscopy and cytology.

Squamous Carcinoma

Squamous cell carcinomas from different parts of the body look basically similar by light and electron microscopy. Variations in their appearance are mainly caused by the degree of keratinization and the level of differentiation. No specific differences separate a primary squamous cell carcinoma of the lung from one that has metastasized to the lung from a cutaneous or mucosal site. A considerable range of appearances can nonetheless be seen with the electron microscope among squamous cell lung carcinomas. This ability is partly because the fine structure of the tumor cells undergoes marked changes with loss of differentiation. It also reflects the fact that many NSCLCs of the lung are heterogeneous in their composition and show both squamous and glandular differentiation. A mixture of the two lines of maturation is sometimes evident by electron microscopy, so examination of only a few cells does not always reveal whether the tumor is predominantly a squamous cell or adenocarcinoma. The small sample studied by electron microscopy is nevertheless usually sufficiently representative to provide an accurate diagnosis.[34]

In a differentiated squamous carcinoma, the cells are more or less round, although they look polygonal when packed together. The cells are often separated from their neighbors by a slender gap (Figure 26.19). Nuclei have slightly irregular profiles, and the chromatin is coarsely clumped. The cells possess considerable amounts of cytoplasm, which contains the usual organelles—mitochondria, cisternae of endoplasmic reticulum—in moderate quantities. The better differentiated squamous tumors arising in the lung show evidence of keratinization, and the cells then contain thin bundles of cytokeratin filaments, which course through the cytoplasm and attach to the cell junctions. The latter are mature desmosomes, and when the cells are not intimately apposed, they are connected through short protrusions of the surface cytoplasm with desmosomes at their

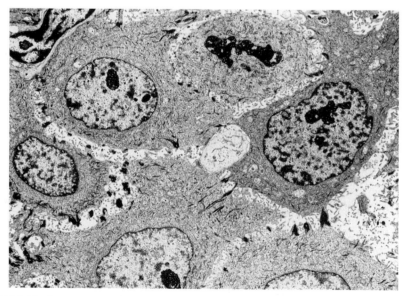

FIGURE 26.19. Squamous carcinoma, moderately differentiated, ultrastructure. The cells of this tumor contain many thin bundles of tonofilaments. Within the clefts between the cells, desmosomes are conspicuous by their dense appearance (4,000 × magnification).

tips, creating the so-called intercellular bridges that are helpful to the light microscopist. Bridges will not be visible if the cell surfaces are closely apposed, so they are not always seen in well-differentiated tumors. Fragments of basal lamina may surround groups of tumor cells.[216]

The distinctive features of the differentiated squamous tumors are progressively lost as the tumors dedifferentiate, and variations in the level of differentiation can often be seen within a small group of cells. Uniform spacing of the cells, abundant tonofilaments, and numerous mature desmosomes can, within the space of a few cells, be replaced by irregular gaps, wispy strands of keratin, and scattered, poorly constructed attachment sites. The number of cell junctions in lung carcinomas appears to relate to clinical stage and survival time.[217] The end stage of the process of dedifferentiation is cells with no cytokeratin and few or no junctions: attachment sites that are present are mere paired tiny densities of the cell membranes. Along with these alterations, the amount of cytoplasm and number of organelles diminish. The ultrastructure of truly dedifferentiated squamous cells thus does not betray their squamous lineage.

Adenocarcinoma

Much more variety in histology and ultrastructure is seen in the cells of bronchogenic adenocarcinomas compared to the squamous tumors. Cells in the better differentiated adenocarcinomas may contain some cytokeratin filaments, but they are rarely plentiful. The surfaces of adjacent cells are connected by desmosomes, which are fewer and smaller than in squamous carcinomas. Adenocarcinomas commonly have a glandular architecture that is manifested ultrastructurally by lumens bordered by cells with microvilli on their apical surfaces (Figure 26.20). The cell membranes, particularly when the cells are columnar, fuse where they reach the lumen, forming a tight junction that seals off the intercellular space from the lumen. The tight junctions are beltlike in that they encircle the cell, in contrast to desmosomes, which are small disks, like tiny spot welds between the cell surfaces.

The number, length, and appearance of the microvilli in bronchogenic adenocarcinomas is variable. They are often irregular in distribution and size, whereas in a typical epithelial mesothelioma, the long, slender, often curving and branching microvilli are distinctive.[218] In a few of the peripheral lung adenocarcinomas that show bronchioloalveolar differentiation, the microvilli are more numerous and straight, and they contain slender cores of actin filaments that extend downward into the apical cytoplasm (Figure 26.20). These microvilli are identical in appearance to the ones on gastrointestinal cells, therefore, using this feature to identify a metastatic gastric or intestinal adenocarcinoma within the lung is not reliable.[219]

Part of the variety in appearance among adenocarcinoma cells is produced by the presence of secretory products within their cytoplasm. There may be accumulations of glycogen or mucin, and the latter occupy diffuse electronlucent zones or form discrete droplets that accumulate in the apical cytoplasm (Figure 26.20).

Bronchioloalveolar adenocarcinomas differentiate in the direction of cells found in the distal respiratory passages, and they consequently show a various appearances by electron microscopy. The most common form of differentiation in this type of adenocarcinoma is toward the nonciliated bronchiolar or Clara cell, which in the normal lung forms a protein secretion that contributes to the pulmonary surfactant. The dense-core granules in these cells are of exocrine

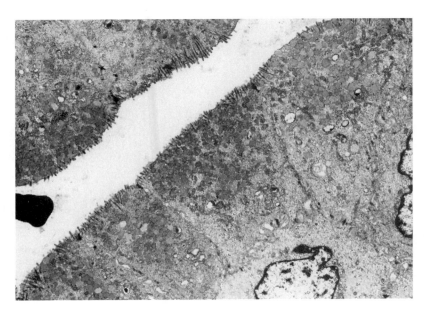

FIGURE 26.20. Bronchioloalveolar adenocarcinoma, ultrastructure. These tumor cells border on a slender lumen. The indistinct bodies in the cytoplasm are mucin droplets. Microvilli are highlighted by cores of microfilaments that extend into the subjacent cytoplasm (6,000 × magnification).

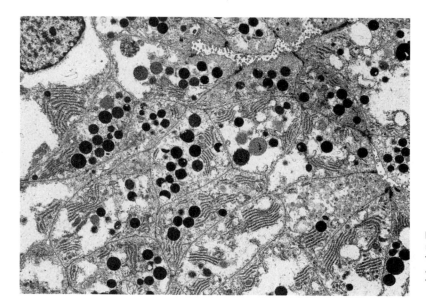

FIGURE 26.21. Bronchioloalveolar adenocarcinoma, ultrastructure. The plane of section passes through the apices of the tumor cells, and small slits of lumen are visible. This tumor is showing Clara cell differentiation, manifested by the large secretory granules (5,500 × magnification).

caliber, and they gather in the apical cytoplasm (Figure 26.21). Mucin can also be present in small quantities in the apical cytoplasm in tumor cells with Clara-cell differentiation, but in some bronchioloalveolar adenocarcinoma, the cells are filled with mucin. Ciliated cells are unusual in a lung adenocarcinoma,[220] although they are rarely seen in a bronchioloalveolar adenocarcinoma. Another distal respiratory passage cell that is infrequently found in these tumors is the type II pneumocyte. Its distinctive lamellar bodies, which provide the lipid component of the surfactant, are

found in the apical cytoplasm (Figure 26.22). It can be difficult to distinguish reactive type II pneumocytes from neoplastic cells because the former may be entrapped within the tumor, or they can be from the rim of reactive cells, which are commonly present around the mass of tumor cells. The nuclear inclusions that are seen in a small proportion of bronchioloalveolar adenocarcinomas are produced by an elaborate replication of the inner of the paired membranes that form the nuclear envelope.[7] Although myoepithelial cells occur in the ducts and acini of normal bronchial

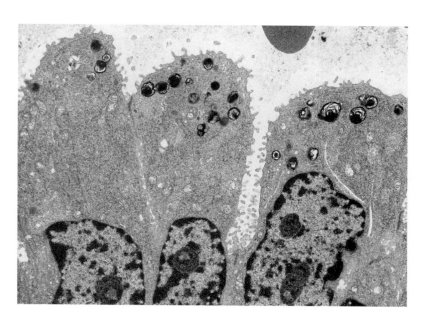

FIGURE 26.22. Bronchioloalveolar adenocarcinoma, ultrastructure. The presence of lamellar bodies in the upper cytoplasm of the cells of this tumor indicates type II pneumocyte differentiation. Note also how the cells protrude into the lumen (9,300 × magnification).

glands, they are only rarely a component of a bronchogenic adenocarcinoma.[126]

Small Cell Carcinoma

Ultrastructural studies have helped to define the light microscopic features of this tumor, and they have clarified its position in the classification of lung tumors and the validity of the subtypes that have been created by light microscopists. Information on the fine structure of SCLCs has also come from the study of cell lines, although it is not always possible to extrapolate *in vitro* findings to *in vivo* observations.

The typical SCLC cell is smaller than those of most NSCLCs, but morphometric studies performed on low-magnification electron micrographs have shown that overlap occurs in cell and nuclear size between the two groups, and the best discriminator is the nuclear/cytoplasmic ratio.[221] The amount of cytoplasm is SCLCs is generally scanty (Figure 26.23). The cells are ovoid rather than round, and they can become elongated. The shape of the nucleus parallels that of the cell, and the chromatin is generally finely aggregated and uniformly dispersed; its homogeneous distribution can often be appreciated in paraffin sections. The cell surface is smooth and devoid of microvilli, although in some cases the cytoplasm forms short, tubular extensions. Cells tend to be closely apposed, and some cell junctions can almost always be located. They range in maturity from small desmosomes to mere apposed densities on the cell membranes.

Generally only a few organelles are present in the cytoplasm of SCLC cells, in contrast to the moderate numbers that are seen in better differentiated NSCLCs. A few mitochondria and some slender cisternae can usually be found. Dense-core granules are plentiful in only a few tumors, and it is often necessary to examine several cells before granules are found. In approximately one-third of SCLCs granules cannot be detected, although they may subsequently become evident in cell lines. The granules are of neuroendocrine caliber and appearance, which means they are consistently small, of the order of 100 to 120 nm, with a distinct limiting membrane. If the granules in a tumor are larger than this limit, carcinoid should be suspected. Unlike the situation in many extrapulmonary SCLCs, granules do not commonly congregate in dendritic processes. Increasing numbers of SCLCs, with and without neuroendocrine features, are being described in extrapulmonary sites, and they must be considered in the differential diagnosis when SCLC is suspected in material procured from an apparent metastasis.

Most pathologists utilize the terminology for SCLC subtypes that has accumulated over the years from light microscopic observations. Electron microscopy has not shown any consistent features that will serve to subclassify SCLC, offering support for the view that the terms *oat-cell, lymphocyte-like,* and *intermediate cell* should be discarded.[133] The cells of SCLC can transform following therapy, showing more variability in cell and nuclear size and shape and even simulating a large cell carcinoma, so subtyping is of dubious value in material from a treated patient. It has been suggested that two variants of SCLC should continue to be recognized.[133] One, the combined form of SCLC, contains areas of differ-

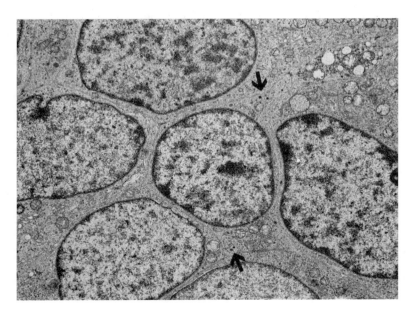

FIGURE 26.23. Small cell lung carcinoma, ultrastructure. The cells are closely apposed, and they have scanty cytoplasm and sparse organelles with only occasional small dense-core granules. The finely clumped but uniformly dispersed chromatin is characteristic (9,200 × magnification).

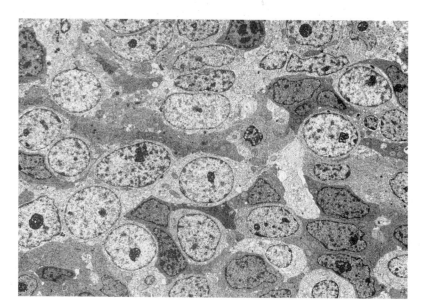

FIGURE 26.24. Large cell carcinoma, ultrastructure. An intimate admixture of small dense cells is present in this large cell carcinoma, but their nuclear features are not typical of a small cell lung carcinoma and they did not contain neuroendocrine granules (3,000 × magnification).

entiated NSCLC. The other has been designated as mixed small cell/large cell carcinoma, but it may be questioned whether such a tumor truly exists in untreated patients because the appearance can be simulated by a large cell carcinoma with a content of smaller cells (Figure 26.24).

Large Cell Carcinoma

With loss of differentiation, the specific features that characterize squamous and glandular lung carcinomas are progressively lost, and the cells tend to become smaller with less cytoplasm and fewer organelles than more differentiated tumors. When this process of dedifferentiation is complete, no features will then serve to identify the tumor as either squamous or adenocarcinoma, and it is a true undifferentiated large cell carcinoma. The cells generally have sparse organelles, and cell junctions are hard to find. Some evidence of differentiation in the form of small collections of microvilli within tiny lumens (Figure 26.25) or sandwiched between cells, or collections of cytokeratin filaments, are often seen with the electron microscope in tumors that were called large cell carcinoma by light microscopy. This minimal level of differentiation probably does not have any significance as far as the behavior or response to therapy of the tumors are concerned, and no compelling reason suggests reclassifying the tumors based on the ultrastructural findings.

Electron microscopy can be helpful in the study of pleomorphic tumors in the lung.[222] The multilobated nuclei are seen to good advantage in electron micrographs (Figure 26.26). A few poorly constructed cell junctions are often found, where the pleomorphic cells come into contact, and some microvilli may be detected. The extensive cytoplasm often contains many organelles including lysosomes. These findings are not specific, and it may be impossible to distinguish between a primary lung tumor and a metastatic pleomorphic carcinoma or sarcoma by electron microscopy alone.

Sarcomatoid Carcinomas

A small percentage of NSCLCs undergo sarcomatoid change. This is a form of dedifferentiation, and the cytologic characteristics of the initial differentiated tumor are progressively lost in the transformation process. The cells become spindle-shaped and may form crude fascicles; the tumor must then be distinguished from a sarcoma or a spindle cell mesothelioma. This differential diagnosis can be difficult because a complex spectrum of fine structure is seen in sarcomas, and mesotheliomas show much variation in cell structure. Immunostaining is the best approach, but electron microscopy may reveal small wisps of cytokeratin filaments or scattered desmosomes and absence of the luxuriant microvilli of an epithelial mesothelioma, and therefore offer some support for a light microscopic diagnosis of carcinoma.[184,223]

Large Cell Neuroendocrine Carcinoma

Ultrastructurally, LCNECs have a few dense-core granules that are often focal or patchy in distribution[145] and show glandular differentiation or squamous features.[145] The distinction of LCNEC from NSCLC with neuroendocrine fea-

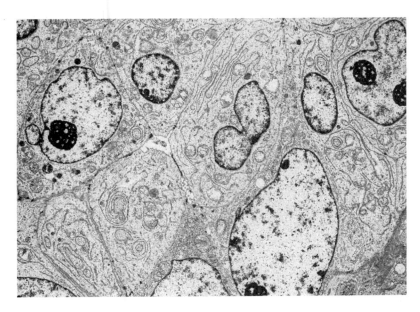

FIGURE 26.25. Large cell carcinoma, ultrastructure. In a large cell carcinoma, no evidence of differentiation exists at the light microscope level, but electron microscopy may reveal tiny lumens containing a few microvilli (5,000 × magnification).

tures is based on light microscopic morphology rather than electron microscopy.

Non–Small Cell Carcinoma With Neuroendocrine Features

This poorly understood variant of NSCLC has usually been identified by immunostaining for neuroendocrine markers, notably neuron-specific enolase and the more reliable chromogranin. The tumor cells are at least twice the size of those seen in SCLCs.[224] Electron microscopy has shown granules of endocrine caliber, although they are less numerous than in a typical carcinoid. The tumor is probably underdiagnosed because only a small minority of lung tumors are examined ultrastructurally, but as many as 10% of NSCLCs may possess some neuroendocrine features.[145,200,225] Insight into these tumors is also being obtained from studies of cell lines.[226] It can be anticipated that the current classification of neuroendocrine lung neoplasms will be modified as more information about the tumors is obtained.[227]

Carcinoid Tumors

A variety of patterns is seen among typical carcinoid tumors in light microscopic sections, but at the ultrastructural level,

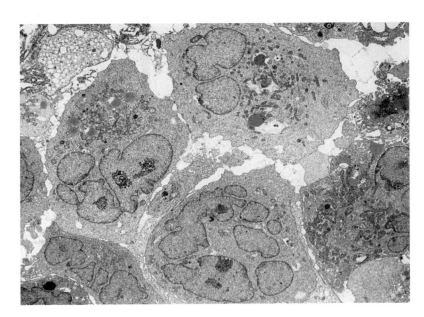

FIGURE 26.26. Large cell (pleomorphic) carcinoma, ultrastructure. The multilobated nuclei of a pleomorphic large cell carcinoma are seen to good advantage with the electron microscope (3,900 × magnification).

considerable uniformity in the appearance of the cells is present. In a particular tumor, they are predominantly either round or fusiform and compactly grouped. The smooth cell surfaces are apposed, but filopodia are sometimes seen, and a few tumors contain aggregates of microvilli on some cell surfaces, which may project into a small lumen.

Neighboring cells are fairly similar in appearance. The round or ovoid nuclei are centrally placed and surrounded by more cytoplasm than is seen in most SCLCs, and the cytoplasm is richer in organelles: mitochondria and slender cisternae can be abundant. The nuclear chromatin tends to form coarser clumps than in a typical SCLC cell. In atypical and more aggressive carcinoid tumors, variations in nuclear and cell size and shape are generally evident at the ultrastructural level, although they are seen to better advantage by light microscopy, where more cells can be examined and the pattern of the tumor is more readily assessed. Cell junctions in the typical carcinoids are mostly small desmosomes, which are present in moderate numbers. Cell junctions are fewer and more primitive in the atypical tumors, and they may only be minute thickenings of the cell membranes.

Carcinoid tumors form hormonal polypeptides and certain other products, and dense-core granules are a prominent feature of the cytoplasm (Figure 26.27). The granules are numerous in most of the cells of a tumor, but they can vary in number from cell to cell, and they are often sparse in the atypical carcinoids. Many mitochondria pack the cytoplasm in the so-called oncocytic variant.[228] A few carcinoids contain discrete aggregates of intermediate filaments within the cytoplasm of their cells, and granules are then fewer in number and more difficult to find. Cells of the uncommon chemodectoma of the lung also contain many filaments, but granules are not present.[229]

The size and appearance of the granules in carcinoid tumors is of some importance in differential diagnosis. The granules in lung carcinoid cells are generally round, but they are angular in approximately 5% of the tumors. Secretory granules in lung tumor cells range from large exocrine-type granules similar to those seen in Clara cells to the small uniform granules of some SCLCs and most endocrine cell granules are intermediate in caliber between these two extremes. Some overlap does occur, however. In a morphometric examination of granules in bronchial carcinoids, the range of diameters was found to be from 98 to 391 nm with a mean of 175 nm.[221] The smallest granules in carcinoids thus overlap in size those seen in SCLC, and consequently they alone do not serve to discriminate between the two tumors. It should still be possible to effect this distinction by electron microscopy from the other features of the cells, although it becomes more difficult with the loss of differentiation that takes place in the more aggressive carcinoid tumors.

CYTOLOGY

Historical Background

The diagnosis of lung cancer by cytologic methods is of historical interest because it was an early demonstration that malignancy could be diagnosed through the examination of exfoliated cells. As reviewed by Johnston, Donne and Walsh separately noted in 1845 that exfoliated respiratory cells occurred in sputum.[230] The first major series of patients

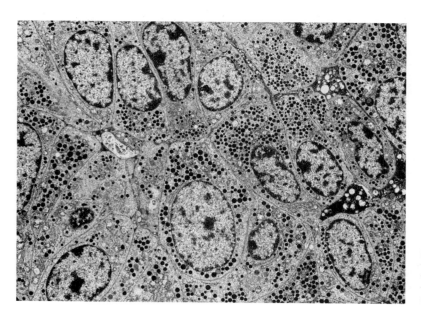

FIGURE 26.27. Typical carcinoid tumor, ultrastructure. Granules fill the cytoplasm in a typical carcinoid tumor. The granules are close to the upper limit of the size range seen in endocrine tumor cells (4,000 × magnification).

where the examination of sputum led to a diagnosis of lung cancer was by Hamplen in 1919. In this study, 13 of 25 cases were successfully diagnosed. After several years of quiescence, pulmonary cytology enjoyed a period of rapid development in the 1950s. Particularly important was the demonstration that lung cancer diagnosis was possible by percutaneous biopsy of the chest wall. In the 1960s, Dahlgren and Nordenstrom published a monograph reporting an 87% success rate in the diagnosis of lung tumors by transthoracic biopsy.[231] These important studies were part of a growing awareness that indicated fine-needle aspiration biopsy as a standard diagnostic tool. Further studies in the 1970s and 1980s validated needle aspiration as an alternative to open lung biopsy or transbronchial biopsy for the diagnosis of pulmonary malignancy, as well as other infectious and inflammatory lung diseases.[232,233] During this time, technical advances in radiologic technique permitted the imaging of small lesions and guided aspiration biopsy.[234–236] The design of bronchoscopes—improved smaller diameter, flexible bronchoscopes—opened an entirely new avenue for the investigation of lung disease.[237,238]

Diagnostic Techniques

Five major techniques are used to obtain cellular material for the diagnosis of carcinoma of the lung.[239,240] The oldest and most fundamental technique is sputum collection, which depends on the spontaneous exfoliation of cells. Three bronchoscopic techniques include bronchial washing, bronchial brushing, and bronchoalveolar lavage. Finally, needle aspiration techniques can be performed through the chest wall under radiographic guidance or transbronchoscopically. Cytology can also be performed on bronchial biopsy rinse fluid to improve the diagnostic yield.[241]

No single technique is necessarily superior to the others. The choice of cell collection technique is affected by many factors. The personal preference of the physician, which usually reflects where she or he received postgraduate training, is key. Thus some physicians are quick to opt for bronchoscopy or fine-needle aspiration, whereas others choose a more measured approach of collecting sputum on an outpatient basis. Understandably, the approach to the diagnosis of pulmonary disease may change with the economic effects of health-care reform.

The type of disorder that is clinically suspected may favor one sampling method over another. A diffuse abnormality in the lung that is presumed to be inflammatory may be better evaluated by the examination of sputum or bronchial washing or bronchoalveolar lavage than would a focal abnormality.[242,243] The location of a suspect lesion within the pulmonary or thoracic cavity affects the diagnosis method chosen. Different methods have potentially important differences in the diagnostic sensitivity, based on tumor location.[237,244] Finally, the clinical condition of the patient may also dictate the method chosen. Critically ill patients may

require rapid diagnosis afforded by invasive procedures. Others, however, may be so debilitated that bronchoscopic procedures are hazardous, and the simple collection of sputum desired.

Although substantial similarity exists among the morphology of cells obtained by these different techniques, important differences relate to cell preservation. A discussion of the attributes of different specimen collection techniques and their effects on cellular morphology follows.

Sputum

The strongest appeal for sputum examination is the ease of specimen collection. Sputum examination also has relatively high diagnostic sensitivity, particularly when multiple specimens have been collected.[245,246] Sputum may be spontaneously expectorated or induced by artificial means. Spontaneous specimens are produced by a deep cough initiated by the patient without extrinsic stimuli, whereas induced sputa rely on irritation of the respiratory tract, usually through inhalation of vaporized saline and propylene glycol. With few exceptions, induced sputa provide a more representative sample of lower respiratory tract cells.[247] In a study of patients with proven cancer, Khajota et al. found that induced sputum was diagnostic in 84%, whereas only 52% of noninduced sputum specimens contained malignant cells.[248] This does not mean that spontaneous sputa are unacceptable, but a greater proportion of specimens is unsatisfactory for diagnostic purposes.[249] The number of carbon-containing macrophages in the material determines the adequacy of a sputum specimen.[250] Specimens lacking pulmonary macrophages are unsatisfactory for evaluation. The absence of cancer cells in a patient with a lung lesion may simply be caused by a sampling error, reflecting that the specimen is saliva rather than sputum.

Different options are available for the subsequent processing of the sputum specimen. If the specimen is brought to the laboratory soon after collection, fresh material can be processed without fixation. Fresh specimens should be examined for particulate material or blood-strained tissue fragments. These elements of the specimen, because they often harbor cancer cells, are selected with forceps and used to prepare a smear between two glass slides. These slides are immediately fixed in 95% ethanol for approximately 30 minutes. Air-drying of the slide should be vigorously avoided because this technique causes the loss of detailed nuclear morphology. After fixation, slides are stained by a Papanicolaou technique. This staining method, which uses a combination of orange-G, eosin, and hematoxylin, is favored by most cytopathologists. The Papanicolaou stain offers excellent rendition of nuclear morphology, which is essential for determining whether a cell is benign or malignant. It also differentially stains the cytoplasm of epithelial cells, permitting the classification of cells as squamous or nonsquamous in differentiation.

Alternatives for the fixation of specimens can be used if the sputum cannot be processed when fresh. The simplest alternative is providing the patient with a container of 70% solution of ethanol. Although this provides some cell preservation, the material unfortunately tends to congeal, which limits the exposure of cells to the ethanol. The variation in fixation causes artifacts in the nuclear morphology that can create difficulty in interpreting the cells. Also, the rubbery quality of alcohol-fixed sputum complicates the specimen processing because smears cannot be made.

Saccomanno proposed an alternative method for cell fixation in 1963.[251] This approach, which uses a mixture of 50% ethanol and 2% carbowax for the prefixation of cells, is particularly suited for the collection of sputa in an outpatient situation. The patient can expectorate consecutive deep morning cough specimens into the same container over several days. When this specimen is returned to the laboratory, it can be processed in aggregate. Blending of Saccomanno-preserved materials is required to homogenize the specimen. The resulting material can be used for the preparation of smears, membrane filters, or cytocentrifuge slides.

The sensitivity of detecting lung cancer differs between freshly smeared and fixed, blended sputum. Much of this difference is attributable to artifacts caused by the mechanical blending of the specimen. Studies differ on the issue of which technique has superior sensitivity.[252] Some suggest a similar sensitivity for detecting squamous carcinoma between fresh, unfixed sputum and material for the Saccomanno technique but lower sensitivity with small cell undifferentiated carcinoma and adenocarcinoma. The mechanical blending disrupts cell fragments and shears mucin-containing vacuoles from cells, thus complicating the diagnosis of adenocarcinoma. Blending also disperses the cells of small cell undifferentiated carcinoma, so that finding cells among a background of inflammatory cells is difficult. In a report by Rizzo et al., the blended technique had a greater sensitivity than the manual smearing method for the detection of lung cancer.[253] The addition of dithiothreitol to the sample may also aid processing and improve sensitivity.[254]

Another option for specimen processing that we mention for completeness more than for advocacy is the histologic sectioning of paraffin-embedded sputum. Bocking and colleagues recently described this approach to the screening of 1,889 patients, 219 of whom had bronchial carcinoma. A sensitivity of 84.5% was reported, when at least three specimens were collected. These authors suggest that this method might be suitable for mass screening programs.[255]

The decision of which processing method to use is dictated less by choice and more by whether or not the laboratory receives fresh or fixed specimens. A drawback to blending methods is the generation of aerosols that pose a risk to laboratory personnel, particularly if *Mycobacterium tuber-*

culosis or other infectious agents are present. For this reason, all respiratory specimens should be processed following universal precautions, including biohazard containment hoods, if available.

The sensitivity of detecting lung cancer by sputum examination increases with the number of specimens obtained.[230,250] Different studies suggest that the sensitivity of single sputum specimens for detection of lung cancer is approximately 50%, whereas the examination of three or more specimens raises sensitivity to nearly 90%. The type of tumor and anatomic location further affects sensitivity of lung cancer diagnosis in sputum specimens. The highest sensitivity can be expected with centrally located squamous carcinoma. These tumors often involve the bronchial mucosa, and when poorly differentiated, the poor cohesion between tumor cells results in the exfoliation of many tumor cells. By comparison, the sensitivity of sputum examination in the diagnosis of SCLC is low.[239,246] The bulk of the tumor is often in the bronchial submucosa, so that cells are not shed into respiratory secretions. Also, because individual cells of this tumor can resemble small lymphocytes, more cells may be required for their identification to be made with confidence.

The situation where sputum examination appears to be the preferred method for the diagnosis of lung carcinoma is when an immediate diagnosis is not mandatory, so that multiple specimens can be collected on an outpatient basis. A diagnosis is possible, without the cost of hospitalization or bronchoscopic lung examination. If one is successfully able to diagnose lung cancer by the examination of sputum, the cost of diagnosis may be dramatically reduced. Raab and Hornberger reported that sputum cytology, as a first test for central lesions, was cost effective and lowered mortality without affecting long-term survival.[257] Cytologic diagnosis requires an experienced pathologist who is capable of rendering a definitive diagnosis of malignancy on sputum materials. Appropriate use of lung cytology presumes that surgeons, oncologists, or others responsible for the patient's management will pursue definitive therapy based on the cytologic diagnosis. If the pathologist is only willing to interpret such specimens as "suspicious," or the clinical staff requires tissue biopsy before therapy, the examination of sputum only duplicates other diagnostic efforts and adds to cost. The validity of using lung cytology as a definitive technique for the planning of therapy has been recently discussed by Caya et al.[258] Even when bronchoscopy is planned, the collection of prebronchoscopic sputa can increase the diagnostic yield. Miura et al. described 17 of 114 patients where the diagnosis of adenocarcinoma could be made in the prebronchoscopy sputum, but the bronchoscopic examination was normal.[259]

Sputum collection can also aid the diagnostic evaluation of elderly or debilitated patients in whom bronchoscopy might be considered hazardous, or where such facilities are not available.[247]

Bronchial Washing and Brushing

Bronchoscopy has been the most popular method to diagnose lung cancer in recent years. Increased numbers of internal medicine physicians have received training in pulmonology. Bronchoscopes have been improved, allowing the direct visualization of endobronchial abnormalities deeper into the lung. In addition modern bronchoscopic technique allows the bronchoscopist to collect multiple specimens during a single procedure, so that a transbronchial or endobronchial tissue biopsy can be taken in conjunction with any cytologic examination.

Bronchoscopes may be rigid or flexible and are available in various diameters.[260] Although flexible bronchoscopes are much more popular among pulmonologists, rigid bronchoscopy may be necessary to sample certain anatomic locations within the lung. Bronchial washing or brushing refers to the sampling of lesions arising in the first- second- and third-order bronchi that are directly visualized and sampled.[261,262] Washing of the bronchi is achieved by the instillation of 3 to 10 mL of sterile saline, which is immediately reaspirated and taken for cytologic analysis. The resulting specimen is processed by the standard cytologic method for body fluids, which includes the preparation of cytocentrifuge slides, smears of large-tube centrifugation, or membrane filter preparations.

Bronchial brushing is suitable to sample any lesion that can be directly visualized by the bronchoscopist.[263,264] Thus endobronchial tumors are relatively easily diagnosed by this method. Either a disposable or reusable brush may be used, both offering similar diagnostic yield.[265] The brush used to sample the lesion can be smeared onto a glass slide, which is rapidly fixed in ethanol and/or rinsed into normal saline.[266] In some laboratories, the material obtained by brushing is rinsed into Saccomanno's preservative. These specimens are then processed in the laboratory by the Papanicolaou technique. It is preferable to perform the washing before the brushing because brushing may lead to bleeding which obscures cellular material. Bronchial washing and brushing is often performed in conjunction with endobronchial biopsy of exophytic lesions within the lung. This method maximizes the quantity of material available for evaluation. In large studies, the sensitivity of single bronchial washing and brushing for detecting lung cancer is approximately 65%. This sensitivity is similar to endobronchial or transbronchial biopsy of the lung. Recent studies have shown that combining sputum examination with bronchial brushing achieves sensitivity greater than either method alone.[267]

Bronchoalveolar Lavage

Many similarities exist between bronchoalveolar lavage and bronchial washing. Both depend on bronchoscopic methods and use fluid to collect cells from the lung. The most substantive difference is that a narrow diameter bronchoscope used in the lavage procedure can be passed into fifth- or sixth-order bronchi. When the bronchoscope is placed into a wedged position, so that the lumen of the bronchus is obstructed, saline can be instilled through the bronchoscope. Saline mixes with the epithelial lining fluid of the bronchi and alveoli, effectively washing out normal and neoplastic cells, infectious organisms, and chemical constitutes from the lung.

The fluid obtained by lavage can be subjected to multiple types of chemical, microbiologic, immunologic, or cytologic analysis.[268,269] The latter is achieved by the preparation of either membrane filters or cytocentrifuge slides for Papanicolaou staining and the preparation of cytocentrifuge slides for a Romanowsky stain, such as Diff-Quik or Wright-Giemsa.

Bronchoalveolar lavage is an important tool for the diagnosis of alveolar-based lung diseases. Interest in bronchoalveolar lavage grew out of the experimental studies of immunologic lung diseases, such as idiopathic pulmonary fibrosis in the 1960s and the 1970s. The historical development of lavage has been summarized by several authors.[268–270] In the 1980s, the popularity of bronchoalveolar lavage grew because it offered a rapid and highly sensitive method to diagnose opportunistic infection in immunosuppressed individuals. The number of these patients grew exponentially during this time, reflecting the emergence of the acquired immune deficiency syndrome (AIDS) and large numbers of iatrogenically immunosuppressed individuals caused by cancer chemotherapy or organ transplantation. Not until the late 1980's was there substantial recognition that bronchoalveolar lavage was well suited for the diagnosis of lung cancer.[271–273] Bronchoalveolar lavage for the diagnosis of lung cancer has been studied in several hundred patients.[271,274–277] Different investigators have reported the sensitivity of lavage to range from 30% to 65% for the detection of pulmonary malignancy. The differences in these studies likely reflect methodologic variation because relatively little standardization of the lavage method or the manner that the specimen is processed after collection currently exists. Bronchoalveolar lavage can reasonably be expected to yield a diagnosis of lung cancer in approximately 60% of patients who have a tumor. In this sense, lavage has a similar sensitivity to other cytologic or bronchial biopsy methods. The sensitivity of cancer detection in an individual patient is related to the type of lung cancer. Lavage has a higher diagnostic yield for the diagnosis of peripheral lung lesions that cannot be reached by traditional bronchial washing or brushing.[275,276] Lavage is particularly suited for the diagnosis of bronchoalveolar adenocarcinoma, where tumor cells within the alveoli are readily washed out by the procedure.[271,277]

Fine-Needle Aspiration Biopsy

No technique has affected the utilization of diagnostic cytopathology more than fine-needle aspiration biopsy. Although fine-needle aspiration biopsy is best recognized for its suitability in the diagnosis of superficial tumors that arise in the breast and thyroid, transthoracic needle aspiration biopsy under fluoroscopic or computed topographic (CT) guidance is widely performed for the diagnosis of pulmonary masses[278–281] and can be coupled with CT examination for staging.[282] In the fine-needle aspiration procedure, a 22- to 28-gauge needle is passed into a mass, negative pressure is applied with a syringe, and a cutting motion is used to dislodge tumor cells from the mass. Cells and small tissue fragments are drawn into the hub of the needle or into the syringe. This material is expelled onto the glass slide, and then smeared between two slides. Optimally, both fixed and air-dried smears should be prepared. Rapid immersion of the slide in 95% ethanol is suitable for fixation of material that can be subsequently stained by the Papanicolaou technique. The air-dried slide can be stained by a Romanowsky method. Rapid assessment of the suitability of an aspirated specimen can also be performed in the radiology suite.[283,284]

Often, visible tissue fragments are obtained by the aspiration, particularly if larger bore cutting needles are used in the aspiration procedure.[285,286] These fragments contain valuable information, and they should always be embedded into a cell block for tissue sectioning and hematoxylin and eosin staining. The dual examination of the cytologic aspirate and the tissue section improves the sensitivity of the aspiration by several percentage points and can result in more accurate classification of the histologic type of malignancy.[287]

Another means to increase the sensitivity is by washing the bore of the needle used in the procedure.[288] Diagnostic material that coats the internal lumen can be rinsed out with saline, and then used to prepare membrane filters or liquid-based cytologic preparations (e.g., ThinPrep, Cytyc Corporation, Boxborough, MA; Autocyte Prep, Autocyte, Elon College, NC).[289] The importance of fine-needle aspiration biopsy as a diagnostic tool is its ability to sample localized lung lesions anywhere in the thoracic cavity. Peripheral lung lesions that are inaccessible by bronchoscopic methods can be sampled by fine-needle aspiration biopsy under radiographic guidance. Also, aspiration techniques can safely assess centrally located lesions that are next to vital organs. When small-diameter needles are used in the aspiration procedure, vital structures such as the aorta can usually be punctured without adverse consequence. Also, the technique is highly accurate. The sensitivity of fine-

needle aspiration biopsy in the detection of lung cancer exceeds 85%.[278,290]

Although most fine-needle aspiration biopsy procedures are done through the chest wall, a modification of the technique can sample mediastinal and peribronchial masses through transbronchial aspiration. This technique, pioneered by Wang, requires placement of the tip of the bronchoscope against the bronchial wall, then passage of the fine needle through the channel of the bronchoscope.[291] Wang needle biopsy has a diagnostic yield of 25% to 40%.[292,293] This method is particularly helpful in the staging of patients with lung cancer and to assess mediastinal or peribronchial lymph nodes. In collecting such specimens, care must be taken not to contaminate the transbronchial specimen with intraluminal carcinoma, which results in false staging.[294]

Another use of fine-needle aspiration is in the intraoperative evaluation of tumors. The major advantage of this technique is its ability to sample a lesion that may be inaccessible to incisional biopsy or be located next to a blood vessel or vital structure.[295] In a recent study by Guarda, a large series of consecutive intraoperative cytology was compared with the synchronous frozen section. Agreement of diagnosis occurred in approximately 99% of cases.[296] Another report described only two cases where the cytologic and frozen section results were discrepant.[297] The better morphologic detail of cytologic smears can aid the interpretation of frozen sections.

The contraindications of fine-needle aspiration biopsy are few. Aspiration should be avoided in patients with a hemorrhagic diathesis, with uncontrollable cough, or those who may harbor a pulmonary ecchinococcal cyst. A final word of caution is that the pathologist must maintain an open mind for all differential diagnostic possibilities because virtually any malignant or benign neoplasm or inflammatory process can be sampled by fine-needle aspiration biopsy.[298]

Normal and Reactive Cells

The cytomorphologic diagnosis of lung cancer requires an understanding of the normal and non-neoplastic reactive cells in respiratory cytology specimens. The broad categories of "normal" cells are bronchial epithelial cells, pneumocytes that line alveoli and terminal bronchi, macrophages, and inflammatory cells.

The bronchial epithelial cells, which provide a protective covering for the upper portions of the airways, are distinguished by their columnar shape, having a longer axis than width and a basally oriented nucleus. Bronchial epithelial cells may be either ciliated or nonciliated. The cilia that project from the apex of the columnar epithelial cell are an important morphologic feature of benign cells. Cilia are anchored to the cell by virtue of a terminal bar, which appears as a linear, eosinophilic thickening at the cell apex. Columnar epithelial cells can have extreme morphologic atypia in response to irritants, such as chemotherapy or inflammation. In cytologic material, columnar epithelial cells occur singly or in cohesive clusters. The latter pose a threat to be misinterpreted as carcinoma. However, the presence of cilia or a terminal bar in a cell constitutes an absolute cytomorphologic marker that the cell is benign no matter how atypical it may appear. If a single ciliated cell is observed within a cluster, it is best to interpret all cells in that cluster as benign. Reparative epithelial atypia is a significant consideration in lung cancer diagnosis, which is discussed subsequently.

Goblet cells are pear-shaped, nonciliated bronchial epithelial cells with a large mucin-containing cytoplasmic vacuole. This mucin causes cell fragility and accounts for their shearing during cytopreparation. Distorted goblet cells can potentially be mistaken for the mucin-containing cells of adenocarcinoma. This diagnosis is particularly problematic when increased numbers of goblet cells are present, such as occurs with bronchial irritation, chronic bronchitis, and asthma.

The cytomorphology of alveolar pneumocytes and macrophages is similar. Both are single cells, ranging from 10 to 15 microns in diameter, with a single centrally located nucleus. The rounded nucleus has pale, uniformly dispersed chromatin, which is often hypochromatic. Multinucleated macrophages are common, particularly in irritated airways caused by cigarette smoking. Often, a single small rounded nucleolus is present. The distinguishing feature of the pulmonary macrophage reflects its function. Intracytoplasmic debris, consisting of phagocytized carbon, dusts, red cells, iron, and other material indicate that the cell is a macrophage. Otherwise, it is difficult to discriminate macrophages from the type I or type II pneumocytes that line alveoli.[298] As discussed elsewhere in this text, pulmonary pneumocytes have the potential to assume bizarre morphologic appearance in response to lung injury, and reparative terminal bronchiolar cells can mimic the bronchioloalveolar type of adenocarcinoma.

Inflammatory cells are the final group of normal cells in respiratory material to discuss. Neutrophils, eosinophils, basophils, and lymphocytes are present in different proportions within the lung. Increased numbers of one or another type of inflammatory cells serves as a marker of pulmonary infection, immunologic lung disease, or nonspecific tissue injury.[299] It has been suggested that lymphocytic inflammation is a marker of cancer within the lung.[300] Inflammation may be a consequence of bronchial obstruction, reflect a yet undefined immunologic response against the carcinoma, or be incidental. In the routine practice of cytopathology, however, the identification of inflammatory cells provides little clue about the presence of pulmonary neoplasia. One possible exception may be the high percentage of lymphocytes seen in the differential cell count of the bronchoalveolar lavage of patients with primary or metastatic Hodg-

kin's disease, or in the slide background of fine-needle aspiration in Hodgkin's disease.[301,302]

One important aspect of lymphocytic inflammation is the potential of lymphocytes to be misinterpreted as SCLC, which is discussed in more detail in the following section.

Pulmonary Malignancy

Carcinomas of the lung, pulmonary sarcomas, extranodal lymphomas, and metastatic tumors constitute the gamut of malignancy within the lung. The morphology of lung tumors has been well described in books and monographs.[269,303,304] Our discussion focuses on lung carcinoma, except for the mention of differential diagnostic considerations.

Squamous Cell Carcinoma In Situ

As discussed elsewhere in this chapter, squamous cell carcinoma appears to arise from a multistage carcinogenesis model where reserve cell hyperplasia, squamous metaplasia, and atypical squamous metaplasia precede the development of *in situ* squamous carcinoma, which in turn precedes invasive carcinoma.[46] This sequence bears similarity to the process that occurs in the uterine cervix, although our understanding of the pulmonary counterpart is less complete. The classic cytologic studies of the development of squamous cell carcinoma *in situ* are those of Saccomanno, who documented progressive changes in the epithelial cells of uranium workers who smoked cigarettes.[251] Many others have described the occurrence of *in situ* carcinoma of the bronchi.[305,306] Morphologically, the tumor sheds small, rounded single cells, with nuclear features of malignancy—high nuclear to cytoplasmic ratio, hyperchromasia, and irregular thickening and thinning of the nuclear envelope. A thick band of chromatin is often present along the periphery of the nucleus. Bizarre cells, and a necrotic slide background that typifies invasive carcinoma, are not features of *in situ* squamous cell carcinoma.

There has been substantial interest in the use of cytologic screening to identify persons at risk for invasive squamous carcinoma, with the hope that the dramatic reduction in mortality that was observed with cervical cancer could be duplicated in the lung.[246,307–809] Several major lung cancer screening projects have been undertaken. Most notable are the Mayo Clinic Lung Project, and those at Johns Hopkin's University and Memorial Sloan-Kettering. These studies indicate that *in situ* or early invasive carcinoma can be detected by cytologic screening. While a tendency existed to identify patients with a lower stage of disease with a greater survivorship in those screened, no significant difference in lung cancer mortality rate existed between screened and control groups. The conclusion of these studies is that results do not justify recommending large-scale radiologic or cytologic screening for early lung cancer.[308] Recent reanalysis of these

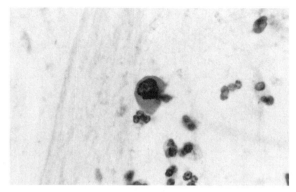

FIGURE 26.28. Squamous cell carcinoma, cytology. Although this cell is not particularly large, it has atypical nuclear morphology. Squamous cell carcinoma is characterized by variably sized keratinized cells. The chromatin in this cell is heavily condensed, and the nucleus is irregularly shaped.

studies, however, has questioned this conclusion and advocated additional trials assessing the utility of screening (see also Chapter 22).

Squamous Cell Carcinoma

The cytologic diagnosis of this tumor rests on two separate observations: (a) the recognition of abnormal nuclear morphology to affirm that a population of malignant cells is present, and (b) the identification of squamous differentiation within the cytoplasm. In respiratory cytologic material, the nuclear morphology of squamous cell carcinoma is diverse. Nuclei may be large or small, round or irregularly shaped, and have chromatin that is dispersed throughout the nucleus, coarse, or condensed so that the nucleus is totally opacified (Figure 26.28). Cells with these sharply angulated and opacified nuclei most typify squamous cell carcinoma (Figure 26.28). Although macronucleoli are most characteristic for pulmonary adenocarcinomas, nucleoli are often present in cells with squamous differentiation.

Cells of squamous cell carcinoma assume various shapes, from the classic polygonal cell to bizarre triangular or tadpole-shaped cells. The tadpole-shaped cells may contain a unique cytoplasmic manifestation—the Herxheimer spiral, which represents condensed keratin proteins. Cells may be single, or more commonly, in a sheet.

The defining quality of squamous cell carcinoma is cytoplasmic keratinization of tumor cells (Figure 26.28) that is morphologically manifested by cytoplasmic orangophilia or deep cytoplasmic cyanophilia with the Papanicolaou stain. The keratin imparts a refractile quality to the cytoplasm, which is best appreciated by lowering the condenser of the microscope. A hallmark feature of squamous cells is so-called endo-ectoplasmic ringing—a deep cyanophilic or eosinophilic band of keratin material that is deposited along

the periphery of the cell. Ultrastructurally, this band corresponds to the tonofibrillar bundles that are involved in anchoring the cells through desmosomal attachments. The keratin fibrils are responsible for the well-defined, sharp cytoplasmic border of squamous cells. Although orangophilia is a feature of keratinization, it is incorrect to presume that all orangophilic cells are from a squamous cell carcinoma. Metaplastic cells, macrophages, or pneumocytes are deeply orangophilic when they are air-dried.

Squamous cell carcinoma undergoes cavitation more often than other primary lung tumors, which results in the exfoliation of many cells into respiratory specimens.[73,310] Tumor-rich specimens, combined with the tendency of squamous cell carcinoma to arise in the central portion of the lung, make the cytologic diagnosis of this tumor relatively straightforward.

The manner in which the cytologic specimen is collected affects tumor cell morphology. With squamous cell carcinoma, the major effect is degeneration of cells expectorated in the sputum. These cells are smaller, have opacified chromatin, and are more likely to be orangophilic than cells obtained by the direct sampling of a tumor by fine-needle aspiration or bronchoscopic techniques.

The differential diagnosis of invasive squamous cell carcinoma includes squamous cell carcinoma *in situ,* other types of lung cancer, atypical squamous metaplasia, and reparative cellular reactions. Each type is discussed elsewhere in this chapter.

Adenocarcinoma

Three cytologic types of pulmonary adenocarcinoma are recognized: acinar, bronchioloalveolar, and papillary. The common acinar cell type typifies the general concept of adenocarcinoma as a gland-forming tumor. In cytologic material, glands are three-dimensional cell clusters (Figure 26.29). By changing the plane of focus of the microscope,

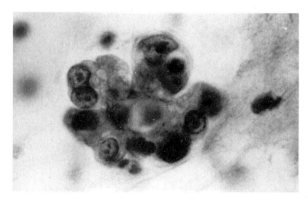

FIGURE 26.29. Adenocarcinoma, cytology. This cluster of tumor cells has a broad depth of focus. Mucin within the cytoplasm imparts a soap-bubble quality. Tumor cells have centrally placed macronucleoli.

the lumen of the glandular acinus can be demonstrated. Adenocarcinoma cells have a rounded to polygonal shape with a large nucleus. In comparison to squamous cell carcinoma, the chromatin of pulmonary adenocarcinoma is less condensed and may assume a bland, water-clear quality. This appearance often complicates the diagnosis of pulmonary adenocarcinoma because reactive bronchial epithelial cells and stimulated macrophages can have similar nuclear chromatin. A single rounded eosinophilic macronucleolus in the center of the nucleus is a feature of adenocarcinoma (Figure 26.29). Although nucleoli occur in other types of lung cancer, they are often multiple, smaller, or irregularly distributed throughout the cell.

The cytoplasm of adenocarcinoma cells is cyanophilic, with cells having an indistinct border. Mucin within the cytoplasm can impart a foamy quality to the cytoplasm or coalesce into one or more large vacuoles (Figure 26.29). Complex internal structure to these vacuoles is an aid in distinguishing mucin-containing vacuoles from imbibition vacuoles that occur in the cytoplasm of macrophages as they drink in fluid. An assessment of the relationship between the large cytoplasmic vacuoles and the nucleus can aid the diagnosis of malignancy. The ease with which malignant nuclei are deformed allows the nucleus to mold around the vacuole, which imparts a sharp edge to the nucleus.

The bronchioloalveolar cell type of adenocarcinoma arises in the distal portions of the respiratory tract. This type of adenocarcinoma has several morphologic features that distinguish it from the acinar cell type. Although cell clusters with extreme depth of focus may be present, these do not contain three-dimensional acini. These cell clusters may assume a papillary configuration, although a central fibrovascular stalk is not present. Aside from numerous single cells, small flower petal or floret clusters of cells are typical of bronchioloalveolar cell carcinoma. If one word were chosen to describe the nuclear morphology of this tumor, it would be "bland." The nuclei are rounded or bean-shaped with gentle folds and contain finely granular chromatin and small nucleoli. The blandness of the tumor cells often proves challenging in separating macrophages and reactive cells that have originated in the terminal portions of the bronchus.

Reactive terminal bronchiolar cells are an enormous potential diagnostic pitfall, as discussed following. Psammoma bodies accompany some cases of bronchioloalveolar carcinoma. Although they are important to stimulate the search for tumor, they may occur with reactive bronchial epithelium or other pulmonary tumors.

The papillary type of adenocarcinoma is among the most uncommon primary pulmonary neoplasms, accounting for 9% of adenocarcinoma in a WHO series.[117] The defining feature of this tumor is the three-dimensional architectural structure of tumor cells supported on a fibrovascular stalk.[311] Only scattered reports of the cytology of this tumor exist, one of which described psammoma bodies within the

tumor.[312] Similar to bronchioloalveolar cell carcinoma, the nuclear morphology of the cells is relatively bland. These two tumors can be difficult to distinguish because papillary structures occur in both.

As discussed elsewhere in this chapter, adenocarcinoma of the lung has been diagnosed with increasing frequency in recent years. Because the predominant location of pulmonary adenocarcinoma is in the periphery of the lung, techniques that are best suited toward this diagnosis include percutaneous needle aspiration and bronchoalveolar lavage.

Small Cell Carcinoma

At the opposite end of the size spectrum is SCLC. The WHO in 1981 described three subtypes, including the oat cell type, intermediate cell type, and combined type.[5] This classification was modified by the IASLC in 1988, who proposed three categories: (a) SCLC (b) mixed small cell/large cell carcinoma, and (c) combined SCLC.[133] The small cells are rounded or carrot-shaped (Figure 26.30). The diameter of cells from SCLC is approximately one-and-a-half to two times that of a small lymphocyte. At low magnification, tumor cells appear to lack cytoplasm, but at high magnification, a thin rim of cytoplasm can be discerned in well-preserved cells. Cells of SCLC can occur singly, in a linear arrangement within respiratory mucus, or in loosely cohesive clusters (Figure 26.30). The most characteristic features of SCLC are found in these clusters. One feature is the molding of tumor cells around each other, the result of the rapid growth rate of the tumor within the confined space of the submucosa (Figure 26.30). Another diagnostic feature is the necrosis of individual tumor cells within cell clusters. These pyknotic tumor cells are surrounded by neutrophils. Cells within the cluster may have nuclear crush artifact, similar to the crush artifact well known to pathologists in bronchial biopsy material.[313]

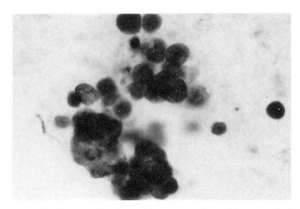

FIGURE 26.30. Small cell carcinoma, cytology. Tumor cells from small cell carcinoma have negligible cytoplasm. Cells are closely apposed to each other, creating the nuclear molding that typifies this tumor.

SCLC includes cases that have a larger cell size, with a diameter approximately three times the diameter of a lymphocyte. These cases correspond to those cases regarded as the intermediate subtype of SCLC as defined by the WHO in 1981.[5] Distinguishing this tumor from poorly differentiated NSCLCs can be difficult. A particular challenge is the so-called large cell type of neuroendocrine carcinoma that has close similarity to large cell carcinoma.

The combined type of SCLC poses another diagnostic problem. This tumor harbors both SCLC and NSCLC in significant proportions. The latter component may be squamous cell carcinoma, adenocarcinoma, or large cell carcinoma, individually or in combination. This entity is relatively common because a NSCLC component occurs in 5% to 10% of cases of SCLC.[133] This percentage may be higher when more comprehensive evaluation is computed of the tumor by multiple sections. Patients with combined tumor may have a prognosis poor than those with SCLC.[314]

The major differential diagnostic considerations with SCLC are reserve cell hyperplasia, inspissated mucus, lymphocytes, and other small cell tumors. By far the most common problem is reserve cell hyperplasia. Reserve cells normally lie along the basement membrane of the epithelium, where they serve as progenitors for bronchial epithelial cells. Irritation of the airways stimulates reserve cell proliferation. Several features correctly identify reserve cells. They are approximately the size of a small lymphocyte, with dense chromatin that lacks the granularity or micronucleoli that can be found in SCLC. Reserve cells are almost always tightly clustered, and cells within the cluster usually retain cell boundaries, without the extreme nuclear molding that characterizes SCLC.

Although crushed lymphocytes are more often a differential diagnostic problem in bronchial biopsy specimens, they can be problematic in cytologic material. Of particular note are the changes of bronchial-associated lymphoid tissue that follow infection or bronchial irritation. The expansion of germinal centers with immune stimulation sheds lymphoid cells that are similar in size to SCLC. However, lymphoid cells are usually well-rounded and have a characteristic chromatin pattern.

Large Cell Carcinoma

The cytologic diagnosis of large cell carcinoma is one of exclusion. This tumor is defined by the *absence* of cytologic features that are characteristic of either squamous cell carcinoma or adenocarcinoma. Thus the cells from this tumor lack evidence of cell keratinization, endoplasmic ringing, or cytoplasmic mucin. Large cell carcinomas usually display ample malignant characteristics within the nucleus. There are marked aberrations in the chromatin pattern, coarse chromatin, irregular nuclear contours, and large irregular nucleoli. The nuclear to cytoplasmic ratio is high, with tumor cells having a scant cytoplasm with an ill-defined

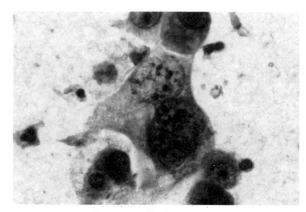

FIGURE 26.31. Large cell carcinoma, cytology. Cells of large cell carcinoma are markedly pleomorphic with multiple nucleoli. No features of squamous or glandular differentiation are present.

cytoplasmic border (Figure 26.31). The tumor often exfoliates many highly malignant cells. However, poorly differentiated adenocarcinomas and squamous cell carcinomas can also exfoliate many single cells, so that further sampling of the tumor may reveal inconsistencies between the cytologic diagnosis of large cell carcinoma and the subsequent histologic diagnosis. A variation of large cell carcinoma is giant cell carcinoma, which consists of multinucleated tumor cells that are many-fold the diameter of surrounding cells.

Neuroendocrine Tumors

Pulmonary carcinoid tumors are well known to diagnostic pathologists. However, in a study by Anderson et al., approximately one-quarter of typical carcinoids were misdiagnosed as either non-Hodgkin's lymphoma or as normal lung cells in aspirated material.[315] Appreciating the cytologic features of this tumor, the stripped cytoplasm, course chromatin, and plexiform vascularity is important for correct diagnosis.[316,317] The spindle cell variant of carcinoid tumor poses a different problem in needle aspiration material because it may be mistaken for sarcoma, spindle cell variants of carcinoma, and benign mesenchymal cells.[318]

Accuracy of Lung Cancer Diagnosis by Cytologic Methods

Several aspects recur in any discussion of the diagnostic accuracy of lung cytology. The first is the issue of sensitivity—how often any one cytologic method accurately identifies lung cancer in a patient when tumor is actually present. This issue has been thoroughly reviewed by Johnston and Bossen, leading these authors to conclude that an unequivocal cytologic diagnosis could generally be made in approximately 50% of cases where sputum or bronchial material was obtained.[256] The diagnosis was facilitated by the examination of multiple lower respiratory tract specimens with optimum sensitivity, requiring examination of up to five specimens. These authors also noted that examination of multiple specimen types, a combination of both sputum and bronchial material, were essential for maximum diagnostic accuracy, and that sputum examination was equal to if not superior to bronchoscopic exam. Fine-needle aspiration, as mentioned previously, has a higher sensitivity of approximately 90%. The most comprehensive analysis of pulmonary fine-needle aspiration was reported as part of the College of American Pathologists Q-probe Quality Assurance Program. In this study of 13,094 lung fine-needle aspirates at 436 institutions, the sensitivity of the fine-needle aspiration procedure was 89%, with 96% specificity, 99% positive predictive value, and 70% negative predictive value. The false-positive rate was 0.8%, and the false-negative rate was 8%.[319] The issue of false-negative cytology is vexing for pathologists because the absence of abnormal cells may be caused by either sampling error (no abnormal cells were collected) or interpretive errors (abnormal cells on the slide were not correctly identified).[320] In a recent study of negative predictive value of lung needle aspiration cytology by Zakowski et al. the recommendation of repeat aspiration was made when no specific benign diagnosis was made.[321]

The sensitivity of lung cancer detection may be aided by the simultaneous measurement of carcinoembryonic antigen in respiratory specimens.[322,323] Immunohistochemic staining for CEA, or other markers, can be performed directly on slides that have been previously stained by the Papanicolaou technique.[324]

Comparative studies have assessed the relative sensitivity of bronchial washing/brushing with bronchial biopsy. Naryshkin et al. described 224 cases where 75% correlated completely. In the remainder, biopsy and cytology were diagnostic in relatively equal proportions, leading the authors to conclude that a specific diagnosis was obtained more often from the combination of cytology and biopsy than from either alone.[325] Others, in comparing diagnostic techniques, have reached a similar conclusion.[237]

The issue of specificity has two elements (a) how often, when a diagnosis of malignancy is rendered, is this interpretation correct, and (b) how successful is cytology in predicting the classic histologic types of malignancy. Avoiding poor specificity, where many false-positive malignant diagnoses are made, requires a careful attention to the nuclear morphologic features that classically predict malignancy. Nevertheless, even expert cytopathologists may render a false-positive diagnosis. In large series, the reported false-positive rate because of atypical forms of metaplasia and reactive and reparative changes ranges from of 0% to 2%.

The other aspect of specificity relates to the correlation between different types of respiratory tract specimens. Comparisons may be made among sputum, bronchial cytologic specimens, fine-needle aspiration, and histologic materials. In a large study by Johnston, the prediction of histologic type of primary lung cancer from sputum and bronchial material was compared with histologic diagnosis. The rate of concordance was 85% with squamous cell carcinoma, 79% with adenocarcinoma, 30% with large cell carcinoma, 93% with SCLC, and 30% with adenosquamous carcinoma.[326] Recent studies have confirmed this observation.[327] As mentioned previously, the variable sampling of different areas within a tumor accounts for most of the poor correlation between cytologic and histologic diagnoses. Fortunately, a relatively high correlation rate exists between the histologic and cytologic diagnosis of SCLC. As discussed elsewhere in this book, the distinction between SCLC versus NSCLC is important for selection of therapy.

Previously, we mentioned the disadvantage of overusing the "suspicious" diagnosis. The definitive diagnosis and classification of cancer by cytology permits prompt planning of therapy. However, "suspicious" or "suspect" is useful as a diagnostic category because some respiratory specimens contain abnormal cells that lack definitive diagnostic features of malignancy.[328] At least 50% of these patients will have carcinoma on subsequent evaluation.

Differential Diagnostic Problems in Pulmonary Cytology

The preceding discussion has mentioned several problems that complicate the diagnosis of lung cancer. These issues have recently been reviewed in a monograph addressing errors and pitfalls in diagnostic cytology.[329] A common and treacherous problem is that of reactive airway epithelial cells from altered lining epithelium.[330] A wide variety of external stimuli of infectious agents and other relatively nonspecific factors can cause abnormal cell morphology. Previously, we discussed the problems posed by squamous metaplastic or by hyperplastic reserve cells, mimicking squamous carcinoma and SCLC, respectively. A greater problem is atypia of bronchial epithelial cells, where individual cells or cells in clusters simulate NSCLC. Reactive bronchial epithelial cells may have a nuclear diameter five to ten times that of a resting columnar epithelial cell. The cytoplasm does not proportionately increase in quantity, so that gross changes in nuclear to cytoplasmic ratio are common. As discussed previously, the presence of cilia or a terminal bar on these cells is key to correctly interpreting their reactive nature.

Unfortunately, a definitive marker such as cilia does not exist for atypical terminal bronchiolar cells. When irritated, cells that line alveoli and terminal bronchioles assume a morphology that is similar to bronchioloalveolar adenocarcinoma.[231] Reactive cells of terminal bronchiolar origin occur with pulmonary infection, pulmonary infarction, and virtually any cause of diffuse alveolar damage.[332]

The differential diagnosis of lung cancer must also include consideration of metastatic carcinoma, sarcomas, and hematolymphoid malignancies. Each of these diseases can shed cells that resemble lung carcinoma into the respiratory tract.[333]

REFERENCES

1. Parkin DM, Pisani P, Ferlay J. Global cancer statistics. *CA-A Cancer J Clin* 1999;49(1):33.
2. Landis SH, Murray T, Bolden S, et al. Cancer statistics, 1999. *CA-A Cancer J Clin* 1999;49(1):8.
3. Travis WD, Lubin J, Ries L, et al. United States lung carcinoma incidence trends: declining for most histologic types among males, increasing among females. *Cancer* 1996;77:2464.
4. Wingo PA, Ries LA, Giovino GA, et al. Annual report to the nation on the status of cancer, 1973–1996, with a special section on lung cancer and tobacco smoking. *J Natl Cancer Inst* 1999; 91(8):675.
5. World Health Organization. *Histological typing of lung tumors*, 2nd ed. Geneva: World Health Organization, 1981.
6. Travis WD, Colby TV, Corrin B, et al. in collaboration with pathologists from 14 countries. Histological typing of lung and pleural tumors, 3rd ed. Berlin: Springer Verlag, 1999.
7. Mackay B, Lukeman JM, Ordónez NG. *Tumors of the lung*, 1st ed. Philadelphia: WB Saunders, 1991.
8. Dail DH, Hammar SP. *Pulmonary pathology*, 2nd ed. New York: Springer-Verlag, 1994.
9. Saldana MJ. *Pathology of pulmonary disease*, 1st ed. Philadelphia: JB Lippincott, 1994.
10. Colby TV, Koss MN, Travis WD. *Tumors of the lower respiratory tract; Armed Forces Institute of Pathology fascicle,* third series. Washington, D.C.: Armed Forces Institute of Pathology, 1995.
11. Travis WD, Travis LB, Devesa SS. Lung cancer [published erratum appears in *Cancer* 1995;75(12):2979]. *Cancer* 1995;75: 191.
12. Devesa SS, Blot WJ, Fraumeni JF, Jr. Declining lung cancer rates among young men and women in the United States: a cohort analysis. *J Natl Cancer Inst* 1989;81:1568.
13. Vincent RG, Pickren JW, Lane WW, et al. The changing histopathology of lung cancer: a review of 1682 cases. *Cancer* 1977; 39:1647.
14. Valaitis J, Warren S, Gamble D. Increasing incidence of adenocarcinoma of the lung. *Cancer* 1981;47:1042.
15. Cox JD, Yesner RA. Adenocarcinoma of the lung: recent results from the Veterans Administration Lung Group. *Am Rev Respir Dis* 1979;120:1025.
16. el-Torky M, el-Zeky F, Hall JC. Significant changes in the distribution of histologic types of lung cancer. A review of 4928 cases. *Cancer* 1990;65:2361.
17. Auerbach O, Garfinkel L. The changing pattern of lung carcinoma. *Cancer* 1991;68:1973.
18. Barsky SH, Grossman DA, Ho J, et al. The multifocality of bronchioloalveolar lung carcinoma: evidence and implications of a multiclonal origin. *Mod Pathol* 1994;7:633.
19. *TNM classification of malignant tumours,* 5th ed. New York: Wiley, 1997.
20. Ferguson MK. Synchronous primary lung cancers. *Chest* 1993; 103:398S.
21. Carey FA, Donnelly SC, Walker WS, et al. Synchronous primary lung cancers: prevalence in surgical material and clinical implications. *Thorax* 1993;48:344.
22. Deschamps C, Pairolero PC, Trastek VF, et al. Multiple primary lung cancers. Results of surgical treatment. *J Thorac Cardiovasc Surg* 1990;99:769; discussion 777–8.
23. Mathisen DJ, Jensik RJ, Faber LP, et al. Survival following resection for second and third primary lung cancers. *J Thorac Cardiovasc Surg* 1984;88:502.
24. Wu SC, Lin ZQ, Xu CW, et al. Multiple primary lung cancers. *Chest* 1987;92:892.
25. Martini N, Melamed MR. Multiple primary lung cancers. *J Thorac Cardiovasc Surg* 1975;70:606.
26. Pommier RF, Vetto JT, Lee JT, et al. Synchronous non-small cell lung cancers. *Am J Surg* 1996;171:521.
27. Deslauriers J, Brisson J, Cartier R, et al. Carcinoma of the lung. Evaluation of satellite nodules as a factor influencing prognosis after resection. *J Thorac Cardiovasc Surg* 1989;97:504.
28. Kunitoh H, Eguchi K, Yamada K, et al. Intrapulmonary sublesions detected before surgery in patients with lung cancer. *Cancer* 1992;70:1876.
29. Roggli VL, Vollmer RT, Greenberg SD, et al. Lung cancer heterogeneity: a blinded and randomized study of 100 consecutive cases. *Hum Pathol* 1985;16:569.
30. Chuang MT, Marchevsky A, Teirstein AS, et al. Diagnosis of lung cancer by fibreoptic bronchoscopy: problems in the histological classification of non-small cell carcinomas. *Thorax* 1984; 39:175.
31. Auerbach O, Frasca JM, Parks VR, et al. A comparison of World Health Organization (WHO) classification of lung tumors by light and electron microscopy. *Cancer* 1982;50:2079.
32. Churg A. The fine structure of large cell undifferentiated carcinoma of the lung. Evidence for its relation to squamous cell carcinomas and adenocarcinomas. *Hum Pathol* 1978;9:143.
33. McDowell EM, Trump BF. Pulmonary small cell carcinoma showing tripartite differentiation in individual cells. *Hum Pathol* 1981;12:286.
34. Mooi WJ, Dingemans KP, Wagenaar SS, et al. Ultrastructural heterogeneity of lung carcinomas: representativity of samples for electron microscopy in tumor classification. *Hum Pathol* 1990;21:1227.
35. Horie A, Ohta M. Ultrastructural features of large cell carcinoma of the lung with reference to the prognosis of patients. *Hum Pathol* 1981;12:423.
36. Carter D. Pathology of early squamous cell carcinoma of the lung. *Pathol Annual* 1978;13 Pt 1:131.
37. Topping DC, Griesemer RA, Nettesheim P. Development and fate of focal epithelial lesions in tracheal mucosa following exposure to 7,12-dimethylbenz(a)anthracene. *Cancer Res* 1979;39: 4829.
38. Topping DC, Griesemer RA, Nettesheim P. Quantitative assessment of generalized epithelial changes in tracheal mucosa following exposure to 7,12-dimethylbenz(a)anthracene. *Cancer Res* 1979;39:4823.
39. Ono J, Auer G, Caspersson T, et al. Reversibility of 20-methylcholanthrene-induced bronchial cell atypia in dogs. *Cancer* 1984;54:1030.
40. Auer G, Ono J, Nasiell M, et al. Reversibility of bronchial cell atypia. *Cancer Res* 1982;42:4241.
41. Early lung cancer detection: summary and conclusions. *Am Rev Respir Dis* 1984;130:565.
42. Nagamoto N, Saito Y, Ohta S, et al. Relationship of lymph node metastasis to primary tumor size and microscopic appearance of roentgenographically occult lung cancer. *Am J Surg Pathol* 1989; 13:1009.
43. Cortese DA, Pairolero PC, Bergstralh EJ, et al. Roentgenographically occult lung cancer. A ten-year experience. *J Thorac Cardiovasc Surg* 1983;86:373.
44. Woolner LB, Fontana RS, Cortese DA, et al. Roentgenographically occult lung cancer: pathologic findings and frequency of multicentricity during a 10-year period. *Mayo Clin Proc* 1984; 59:453.
45. Nagamoto N, Saito Y, Suda H, et al. Relationship between length of longitudinal extension and maximal depth of transmural invasion in roentgenographically occult squamous cell carci-

noma of the bronchus (nonpolypoid type). *Am J Surg Pathol* 1989;13:11.

46. Melamed MR, Zaman MB, Flehinger BJ, et al. Radiologically occult in situ and incipient invasive epidermoid lung cancer: detection by sputum cytology in a survey of asymptomatic cigarette smokers. *Am J Surg Pathol* 1977;1:5.

47. Carter D, Marsh BR, Baker R, et al. Relationships of morphology to clinical presentation in ten cases of early squamous cell carcinoma of the lung. *Cancer* 1976;37:1389.

48. Morales FM, Matthews JI. Diagnosis of parenchymal Hodgkin's disease using bronchoalveolar lavage. *Chest* 1987;91:785.

49. Kitamura H, Kameda Y, Ito T, et al. Atypical adenomatous hyperplasia of the lung. Implications for the pathogenesis of peripheral lung adenocarcinoma [In Process Citation]. *Am J Clin Pathol* 1999;111(5):610.

50. Miller RR. Bronchioloalveolar cell adenomas. *Am J Surg Pathol* 1990;14:904.

51. Noguchi M, Shimosato Y. The development and progression of adenocarcinoma of the lung. *Cancer Treat Res* 1995;72:131.

52. Rao SK, Fraire AE. Alveolar cell hyperplasia in association with adenocarcinoma of lung. *Mod Pathol* 1995;8:165.

53. Kerr KM, Carey FA, King G, et al. Atypical alveolar hyperplasia: relationship with pulmonary adenocarcinoma, p53, and c-erbB-2 expression. *J Pathol* 1994;174:249.

54. Weng SY, Tsuchiya E, Kasuga T, et al. Incidence of atypical bronchioloalveolar cell hyperplasia of the lung: relation to histological subtypes of lung cancer. *Virchows Arch A Pathol Anat Histopathol* 1992;420:463.

55. Nakanishi K. Alveolar epithelial hyperplasia and adenocarcinoma of the lung. *Arch Pathol Lab Med* 1990;114:363.

56. Kushihashi T, Munechika H, Ri K, et al. Bronchioloalveolar adenoma of the lung: CT-pathologic correlation. *Radiology* 1994;193:789.

57. Carey FA, Wallace WA, Fergusson RJ, et al. Alveolar atypical hyperplasia in association with primary pulmonary adenocarcinoma: a clinicopathological study of 10 cases. *Thorax* 1992;47:1041.

58. Mori M, Chiba R, Takahashi T. Atypical adenomatous hyperplasia of the lung and its differentiation from adenocarcinoma. Characterization of atypical cells by morphometry and multivariate cluster analysis. *Cancer* 1993;72:2331.

59. Meyer EC, Liebow AA. Relationship of interstitial pneumonia, honeycombing, and atypical epithelial proliferation to cancer of the lung. *Cancer* 1965;18:322.

60. Raeburn C, Spencer H. A study of the origin and development of lung cancer. *Thorax* 1953;8:1.

61. Spencer H, Raeburn C. Pulmonary (bronchiolar) adenomatosis. *J Pathol Bacteriol* 1956;71:145.

62. Fraire AE, Greenberg SD. Carcinoma and diffuse interstitial fibrosis of lung. *Cancer* 1973;31:1078.

63. Ritter JH. Pulmonary atypical adenomatous hyperplasia. A histologic lesion in search of usable criteria and clinical significance. *Am J Clin Pathol* 1999;11:587.

64. Suzuki K, Nagai K, Yoshida J, et al. The prognosis of resected lung carcinoma associated with atypical adenomatous hyperplasia: a comparison of the prognosis of well-differentiated adenocarcinoma associated with atypical adenomatous hyperplasia and intrapulmonary metastasis. *Cancer* 1997;79(8):1521.

65. Brown MJ, English J, Muller NL. Bronchiolitis obliterans due to neuroendocrine hyperplasia: high-resolution CT—pathologic correlation. *Am J Roentgenol* 1997;168(6):1561.

66. Sheerin N, Harrison NK, Sheppard MN, Hansell DM, Yacoub M, Clark TJ. Obliterative bronchiolitis caused by multiple tumourlets and microcarcinoids successfully treated by single lung transplantation. *Thorax* 1995;50:207.

67. Aguayo SM, Miller YE, Waldron JA, Jr. et al. Brief report: idiopathic diffuse hyperplasia of pulmonary neuroendocrine cells and airways disease. *N Engl J Med* 1992;327:1285.

68. Pelosi G, Zancanaro C, Sbabo L, et al. Development of innumerable neuroendocrine tumorlets in pulmonary lobe scarred by intralobar sequestration. Immunohistochemical and ultrastructural study of an unusual case. *Arch Pathol Lab Med* 1992;116:1167.

69. Ranchod M. The histogenesis and development of pulmonary tumorlets. *Cancer* 1977;39:1135.

70. Whitwell F. Tumourlets of the lung. *J Pathol Bacteriol* 1955;70:529.

71. Canessa PA, Santini D, Zanelli M, et al. Pulmonary tumourlets and microcarcinoids in bronchiectasis. *Monaldi Arch Chest Dis* 1997;52(2):138.

72. Tomashefski JF, Jr, Connors AF, Jr, Rosenthal ES, et al. Peripheral vs central squamous cell carcinoma of the lung. A comparison of clinical features, histopathology, and survival. *Arch Pathol Lab Med* 1990;114:468.

73. Chaudhuri MR. Primary pulmonary cavitating carcinomas. *Thorax* 1973;28:354.

74. Carlile A, Edwards C. Poorly differentiated squamous carcinoma of the bronchus: a light and electron microscopic study. *J Clin Pathol* 1986;39:284.

75. Carter D. Squamous cell carcinoma of the lung: an update. *Semin Diagn Pathol* 1985;2:226.

76. Churg A, Johnston WH, Stulbarg M. Small cell squamous and mixed small cell squamous—small cell anaplastic carcinomas of the lung. *Am J Surg Pathol* 1980;4:255.

77. Dulmet-Brender E, Jaubert F, Huchon G. Exophytic endobronchial epidermoid carcinoma. *Cancer* 1986;57:1358.

78. Sherwin RP, Laforet EG, Strieder JW. Exophytic endobronchial carcinoma. *J Thorac Cardiovasc Surg* 1962;43:716.

79. Byrne JC, Tsao MS, Fraser RS, et al. Human papillomavirus-11 DNA in a patient with chronic laryngotracheobronchial papillomatosis and metastatic squamous-cell carcinoma of the lung. *N Engl J Med* 1987;317:873.

80. Helmuth RA, Strate RW. Squamous carcinoma of the lung in a nonirradiated, nonsmoking patient with juvenile laryngotracheal papillomatosis. *Am J Surg Pathol* 1987;11:643.

81. Usui Y, Takabe K, Takayama S, et al. Minute squamous cell carcinoma arising in the wall of a congenital lung cyst. *Chest* 1991;99:235.

82. Kodama T, Shimosato Y, Watanabe S, et al. Six cases of well-differentiated adenocarcinoma simulating fetal lung tubules in pseudoglandular stage. Comparison with pulmonary blastoma. *Am J Surg Pathol* 1984;8:735.

83. Moran CA, Hochholzer L, Fishback N, et al. Mucinous (So-called colloid) carcinomas of lung. *Mod Pathol* 1992;5:634.

84. Dixon AY, Moran JF, Wesselius LJ, et al. Pulmonary mucinous cystic tumor. Case report with review of the literature. *Am J Surg Pathol* 1993;17:722.

85. Higashiyama M, Doi O, Kodama K, et al. Cystic mucinous adenocarcinoma of the lung. Two cases of cystic variant of mucus-producing lung adenocarcinoma. *Chest* 1992;101:763.

86. Kragel PJ, Devaney KO, Meth BM, et al. Mucinous cystadenoma of the lung. A report of two cases with immunohistochemical and ultrastructural analysis. *Arch Pathol Lab Med* 1990;114:1053.

87. Kragel PJ, Devaney KO, Travis WD. Mucinous cystadenoma of the lung. *Arch Pathol Lab Med* 1991;115:740.

88. Kish JK, Ro JY, Ayala AG, et al. Primary mucinous adenocarcinoma of the lung with signet-ring cells: a histochemical comparison with signet-ring cell carcinomas of other sites. *Hum Pathol* 1989;20:1097.

89. Histological typing of lung tumours. *Tumori* 1981;67:253.

90. Koss MN. Pulmonary blastomas. *Cancer Treat Res* 1995;72: 349.

91. Kodama T, Shimosato Y, Koide T, et al. Endobronchial polypoid adenocarcinoma of the lung. Histological and ultrastructural studies of five cases. *Am J Surg Pathol* 1984;8:845.

92. Lin JI, Tseng CH, Tsung SH. Pseudomesotheliomatous carcinoma of the lung. *South Med J* 1980;73:655.

93. Harwood TR, Gracey DR, Yokoo H. Pseudomesotheliomatous carcinoma of the lung. A variant of peripheral lung cancer. *Am J Clin Pathol* 1976;65:159.

94. Koss MN, Travis WD, Moran C, et al. Pseudomesotheliomatous adenocarcinoma: a reappraisal. *Semin Diagn Pathol* 1992;9:117.

95. Higashiyama M, Doi O, Kodama K, et al. Extramammary Paget's disease of the bronchial epithelium. *Arch Pathol Lab Med* 1991;115:185.

96. Benjamin DR, Cahill JL. Bronchioloalveolar carcinoma of the lung and congenital cystic adenomatoid malformation. *Am J Clin Pathol* 1991;95:889.

97. Prichard MG, Brown PJ, Sterrett GF. Bronchioloalveolar carcinoma arising in longstanding lung cysts. *Thorax* 1984;39:545.

98. Matthews MJ, Mackay B, Lukeman J. The pathology of non-small cell carcinoma of the lung. *Semin Oncol* 1983;10:34.

99. Auerbach O, Garfinkel L, Parks VR. Scar cancer of the lung: increase over a 21 year period. *Cancer* 1979;43:636.

100. Shimosato Y, Suzuki A, Hashimoto T, et al. Prognostic implications of fibrotic focus (scar) in small peripheral lung cancers. *Am J Surg Pathol* 1980;4:365.

101. Cagle PT, Cohle SD, Greenberg SD. Natural history of pulmonary scar cancers. Clinical and pathologic implications. *Cancer* 1985;56:2031.

102. Friedrich G. Periphere Lungenkerbse auf dem Boden pleuranaher Narben. *Virchows Arch [Pathol Anat]* 1939;304:230.

103. Kung IT, Lui IO, Loke SL, et al. Pulmonary scar cancer. A pathologic reappraisal. *Am J Surg Pathol* 1985;9:391.

104. Bakris GL, Mulopulos GP, Korchik R, et al. Pulmonary scar carcinoma. A clinicopathologic analysis. *Cancer* 1983;52:493.

105. Freant LJ, Joseph WL, Adkins PC. Scar carcinoma of the lung. Fact or fantasy? *Ann Thorac Surg* 1974;17:531.

106. Ochs RH, Katz AS, Edmunds LH, Jr et al. Prognosis of pulmonary scar carcinoma. *J Thorac Cardiovasc Surg* 1982;84:359.

107. el-Torky M, Giltman LI, Dabbous M. Collagens in scar carcinoma of the lung. *Am J Pathol* 1985;121:322.

108. Nagai A, Chiyotani A, Nakadate T, et al. Lung cancer in patients with idiopathic pulmonary fibrosis. *Tohoku J Exp Med* 1992; 167:231.

109. Turner-Warwick M, Lebowitz M, Burrows B, et al. Cryptogenic fibrosing alveolitis and lung cancer. *Thorax* 1980;35:496.

110. Case BW, Dufresne A. Asbestos, asbestosis, and lung cancer: observations in Quebec chrysotile workers. *Environ Health Perspect* 1997;105 Suppl 5:1113.

111. Hillerdal G, Henderson DW. Asbestos, asbestosis, pleural plaques and lung cancer. *Scand J Work Environ Health* 1997; 23(2):93.

112. Yoneda K. Scar carcinomas of the lung in a histoplasmosis endemic area. *Cancer* 1990;65:164.

113. Noguchi M, Morikawa A, Kawasaki M, et al. Small adenocarcinoma of the lung. Histologic characteristics and prognosis. *Cancer* 1995;75:2844.

114. Bennett DE, Sasser WF. Bronchiolar carcinoma: a valid clinicopathologic entity? A study of 30 cases. *Cancer* 1969;24:876.

115. Kimula Y. A histochemical and ultrastructural study of adenocarcinoma of the lung. *Am J Surg Pathol* 1978;2:253.

116. Schraufnagel D, Peloquin A, Paré JA, et al. Differentiating bronchioloalveolar carcinoma from adenocarcinoma. *Am Rev Respir Dis* 1982;125:74.

117. Sorensen JB, Hirsch FR, Olsen J. The prognostic implication of histopathologic subtyping of pulmonary adenocarcinoma according to the classification of the World Health Organization. An analysis of 259 consecutive patients with advanced disease. *Cancer* 1988;62:361.

118. World Health Organization. *Histological typing of lung tumours,* 1st ed. Geneva: World Health Organization, 1967.

119. Barsky SH, Cameron R, Osann KE, et al. Rising incidence of bronchioloalveolar lung carcinoma and its unique clinicopathologic features. *Cancer* 1994;73:1163.

120. Clayton F. Bronchioloalveolar carcinomas. Cell types, patterns of growth, and prognostic correlates. *Cancer* 1986;57:1555.

121. Daly RC, Trastek VF, Pairolero PC, et al. Bronchoalveolar carcinoma: factors affecting survival. *Ann Thorac Surg* 1991;51: 368; discuss.

122. Manning JT, Jr, Spjut HJ, Tschen JA. Bronchioloalveolar carcinoma: the significance of two histopathologic types. *Cancer* 1984;54:525.

123. Singh G, Scheithauer BW, Katyal SL. The pathobiologic features of carcinomas of type II pneumocytes. An immunocytologic study. *Cancer* 1986;57:994.

124. Clayton F. The spectrum and significance of bronchioloalveolar carcinomas. *Pathol Annu* 1988;23 Pt 2:361.

125. Ohba S, Takashima T, Hamada S, et al. Multiple cystic cavitary alveolar-cell carcinoma. *Radiology* 1972;104:65.

126. Dekmezian R, Ordóñez NG, Mackay B. Bronchioloalveolar adenocarcinoma with myoepithelial cells. *Cancer* 1991;67:2356.

127. Tao LC, Delarue NC, Sanders D, et al. Bronchiolo-alveolar carcinoma: a correlative clinical and cytologic study. *Cancer* 1978;42:2759.

128. Linnoila RI, Jensen SM, Steinberg SM, et al. Peripheral airway cell marker expression in non-small cell lung carcinoma. Association with distinct clinicopathologic features. *Am J Clin Pathol* 1992;97:233.

129. Feldman ER, Eagan RT, Schaid DJ. Metastatic bronchioloalveolar carcinoma and metastatic adenocarcinoma of the lung: comparison of clinical manifestations, chemotherapeutic responses, and prognosis. *Mayo Clin Proc* 1992;67:27.

130. Harpole DH, Bigelow C, Young WG, Jr et al. Alveolar cell carcinoma of the lung: a retrospective analysis of 205 patients. *Ann Thorac Surg* 1988;46:502.

131. Kreisman H, Wolkove N, Quoix E. Small cell lung cancer presenting as a solitary pulmonary nodule. *Chest* 1992;101:225.

132. Gephardt GN, Grady KJ, Ahmad M, et al. Peripheral small cell undifferentiated carcinoma of the lung. Clinicopathologic features of 17 cases. *Cancer* 1988;61:1002.

133. Hirsch FR, Matthews MJ, Aisner S, et al. Histopathologic classification of small cell lung cancer. Changing concepts and terminology. *Cancer* 1988;62:973.

134. Fraire AE, Johnson EH, Yesner R, et al. Prognostic significance of histopathologic subtype and stage in small cell lung cancer. *Hum Pathol* 1992;23:520.

135. Azzopardi JG. Oat-cell carcinoma of the bronchus. *J Pathol Bacteriol* 1959;78:513.

136. Carter D, Eggleston JC. *Tumors of the lower respiratory tract. Atlas of Tumor Pathology,* second series, fascicle 17. Washington, D.C.: Armed Forces Institute of Pathology, 1980.

137. Vollmer RT. The effect of cell size on the pathologic diagnosis of small and large cell carcinomas of the lung. *Cancer* 1982;50: 1380.

138. Bégin P, Sahai S, Wang NS. Giant cell formation in small cell carcinoma of the lung. *Cancer* 1983;52:1875.

139. Sehested M, Hirsch FR, Osterlind K, et al. Morphologic variations of small cell lung cancer. A histopathologic study of pretreatment and posttreatment specimens in 104 patients. *Cancer* 1986;57:804.

140. Bepler G, Neumann K, Holle R, et al. Clinical relevance of histologic subtyping in small cell lung cancer. *Cancer* 1989;64: 74.

141. Mangum MD, Greco FA, Hainsworth JD, et al. Combined small-cell and non-small-cell lung cancer. *J Clin Oncol* 1989;7: 607.

142. Tsubota YT, Kawaguchi T, Hoso T, et al. A combined small cell and spindle cell carcinoma of the lung. Report of a unique case with immunohistochemical and ultrastructural studies. *Am J Surg Pathol* 1992;16:1108.

143. Fishback NF, Travis WD, Moran CA, et al. Pleomorphic (spindle/giant cell) carcinoma of the lung. A clinicopathologic correlation of 78 cases. *Cancer* 1994;73:2936.

144. Sümmermann E, Huwer H, Seitz G. Carcinosarcoma of the lung, a tumour which has a poor prognosis and is extremely rarely diagnosed preoperatively. *J Thorac Cardiovasc Surg* 1990; 38:247.

145. Travis WD, Linnoila RI, Tsokos MG, et al. Neuroendocrine tumors of the lung with proposed criteria for large-cell neuroendocrine carcinoma. An ultrastructural, immunohistochemical, and flow cytometric study of 35 cases. *Am J Surg Pathol* 1991; 15:529.

146. Vollmer RT, Ogden L, Crissman JD. Separation of small-cell from non-small-cell lung cancer. The Southeastern Cancer Study Group pathologists' experience. *Arch Pathol Lab Med* 1984;108:792.

147. Marchevsky AM, Chuang MT, Teirstein AS, et al. Problems in the diagnosis of small cell carcinoma of the lungs by fiberoptic bronchoscopy. *Cancer Detect Prev* 1984;7:253.

148. Delmonte VC, Alberti O, Saldiva PH. Large cell carcinoma of the lung. Ultrastructural and immunohistochemical features. *Chest* 1986;90:524.

149. Yesner R. Large cell carcinoma of the lung. *Semin Diagn Pathol* 1985;2:255.

150. Downey RS, Sewell CW, Mansour KA. Large cell carcinoma of the lung: a highly aggressive tumor with dismal prognosis. *Ann Thorac Surg* 1989;47:806.

151. Ishida T, Kaneko S, Tateishi M, et al. Large cell carcinoma of the lung. Prognostic implications of histopathologic and immunohistochemical subtyping. *Am J Clin Pathol* 1990;93:176.

152. Travis WD, Rush W, Flieder DB, et al. Survival analysis of 200 pulmonary neuroendocrine tumors with clarification of criteria for atypical carcinoid and its separation from typical carcinoid. *Am J Surg Pathol* 1998;22(8):934.

153. Brambilla E, Moro D, Veale D, et al. Basal cell (basaloid) carcinoma of the lung: a new morphologic and phenotypic entity with separate prognostic significance. *Hum Pathol* 1992;23:993.

154. Butler AE, Colby TV, Weiss L, et al. Lymphoepithelioma-like carcinoma of the lung. *Am J Surg Pathol* 1989;13:632.

155. Chan JK, Hui PK, Tsang WY, et al. Primary lymphoepithelioma-like carcinoma of the lung. A clinicopathologic study of 11 cases. *Cancer* 1995;76(3):413.

156. Pittaluga S, Wong MP, Chung LP, et al. Clonal Epstein-Barr virus in lymphoepithelioma-like carcinoma of the lung. *Am J Surg Pathol* 1993;17:678.

157. Katzenstein AL, Prioleau PG, Askin FB. The histologic spectrum and significance of clear-cell change in lung carcinoma. *Cancer* 1980;45:943.

158. Cavazza A, Colby TV, Tsokos M, et al. Lung tumors with a rhabdoid phenotype. *Am J Clin Pathol* 1996;105:182.

159. Haratake J, Horie A, Tokudome S, et al. Inter- and intra-pathologist variability in histologic diagnoses of lung cancer. *Acta Pathol Jpn* 1987;37:1053.

160. Edwards C, Carlile A. Clear cell carcinoma of the lung. *J Clin Pathol* 1985;38:880.

161. Bëgin LR, Eskandari J, Joncas J, et al. Epstein-Barr virus related lymphoepithelioma-like carcinoma of lung. *J Surg Oncol* 1987; 36:280.

162. Weiss LM, Movahed LA, Butler AE, et al. Analysis of lymphoepithelioma and lymphoepithelioma-like carcinomas for Epstein-Barr viral genomes by in situ hybridization. *Am J Surg Pathol* 1989;13:625.

163. Kodama T, Shimosato Y, Koide T, et al. Large cell carcinoma of the lung—ultrastructural and immunohistochemical studies. *Jpn J Clin Oncol* 1985;15:431.

164. Arrigoni MG, Woolner LB, Bernatz PE. Atypical carcinoid tumors of the lung. *J Thorac Cardiovasc Surg* 1972;64:413.

165. Linnoila RI, Jensen SM, Steinberg SM, et al. Neuroendocrine (NE) differentiation in non-small cell lung cancer (NSCLC) correlates with favorable response to chemotherapy. *Proc Am Soc Clin Oncol* 1989;3:248.

166. Graziano SL, Mazid R, Newman N, et al. The use of neuroendocrine immunoperoxidase markers to predict chemotherapy response in patients with non-small-cell lung cancer. *J Clin Oncol* 1989;7:1398.

167. Gazdar AF, Kadoyama C, Venzon D, et al. Association between histological type and neuroendocrine differentiation on drug sensitivity of lung cancer cell lines. *Monogr Natl Cancer Inst* 1992;191.

168. Berendsen HH, de Leij L, Poppema S, et al. Clinical characterization of non-small-cell lung cancer tumors showing neuroendocrine differentiation features. *J Clin Oncol* 1989;7:1614.

169. Kibbelaar RE, Moolenaar KE, Michalides RJ, et al. Neural cell adhesion molecule expression, neuroendocrine differentiation and prognosis in lung carcinoma. *Eur J Cancer* 1991;27:431.

170. Schleusener JT, Tazelaar HD, Jung SH, et al. Neuroendocrine differentiation is an independent prognostic factor in chemotherapy-treated nonsmall cell lung carcinoma. *Cancer* 1996;77: 1284.

171. Addis BJ. Neuroendocrine differentiation in lung carcinoma [editorial]. *Thorax* 1995;50:113.

172. Kiriakogiani-Psaropoulou P, Malamou-Mitsi V, Martinopoulou U, et al. The value of neuroendocrine markers in non-small cell lung cancer: a comparative immunohistopathologic study. *Lung Cancer* 1994;11:353.

173. Linnoila RI, Piantadosi S, Ruckdeschel JC. Impact of neuroendocrine differentiation in non-small cell lung cancer. The LCSG experience. *Chest* 1994;106:367S.

174. Carles J, Rosell R, Ariza A, et al. Neuroendocrine differentiation as a prognostic factor in non-small cell lung cancer. *Lung Cancer* 1993;10:209.

175. Skov BG, Sorensen JB, Hirsch FR, et al. Prognostic impact of histologic demonstration of chromogranin A and neuron specific enolase in pulmonary adenocarcinoma. *Ann Oncol* 1991; 2:355.

176. Fitzgibbons PL, Kern WH. Adenosquamous carcinoma of the lung: a clinical and pathologic study of seven cases. *Hum Pathol* 1985;16:463.

177. Ishida T, Kaneko S, Yokoyama H, et al. Adenosquamous carcinoma of the lung. Clinicopathologic and immunohistochemical features. *Am J Clin Pathol* 1992;97:678.

178. Naunheim KS, Taylor JR, Skosey C, et al. Adenosquamous lung carcinoma: clinical characteristics, treatment, and prognosis. *Ann Thorac Surg* 1987;44:462.

179. Sridhar KS, Raub WA, Jr. Duncan RC, et al. The increasing recognition of adenosquamous lung carcinoma (1977–1986). *Am J Clin Oncol* 1992;15:356.

180. Takamori S, Noguchi M, Morinaga S, et al. Clinicopathologic characteristics of adenosquamous carcinoma of the lung. *Cancer* 1991;67:649.

181. Addis BJ, Dewar A, Thurlow NP. Giant cell carcinoma of the

lung—immunohistochemical and ultrastructural evidence of dedifferentiation. *J Pathol* 1988;155:231.

182. Ginsberg SS, Buzaid AC, Stern H, et al. Giant cell carcinoma of the lung. *Cancer* 1992;70:606.

183. Chejfec G, Candel A, Jansson DS, et al. Immunohistochemical features of giant cell carcinoma of the lung: patterns of expression of cytokeratins, vimentin, and the mucinous glycoprotein recognized by monoclonal antibody A-80. *Ultrastruct Pathol* 1991;15:131.

184. Matsui K, Kitagawa M. Spindle cell carcinoma of the lung. A clinicopathologic study of three cases. *Cancer* 1991;67:2361.

185. Nappi O, Wick MR. Sarcomatoid neoplasms of the respiratory tract. *Semin Diagn Pathol* 1993;10:137.

186. Ro JY, Chen JL, Lee JS, et al. Sarcomatoid carcinoma of the lung. Immunohistochemical and ultrastructural studies of 14 cases. *Cancer* 1992;69:376.

187. Stamatis G, Freitag L, Greschuchna D. Limited and radical resection for tracheal and bronchopulmonary carcinoid tumour. Report on 227 cases. *Eur J Cardiothorac Surg* 1990;4:527.

188. McCaughan BC, Martini N, Bains MS. Bronchial carcinoids. Review of 124 cases. *J Thorac Cardiovasc Surg* 1985;89:8.

189. Ricci C, Patrassi N, Massa R, et al. Carcinoid syndrome in bronchial adenoma. *Am J Surg* 1973;126:671.

190. Pass HI, Doppman JL, Nieman L, et al. Management of the ectopic ACTH syndrome due to thoracic carcinoids. *Ann Thorac Surg* 1990;50:52.

191. Scheithauer BW, Carpenter PC, Bloch B, et al. Ectopic secretion of a growth hormone-releasing factor. Report of a case of acromegaly with bronchial carcinoid tumor. *Am J Med* 1984;76:605.

192. el-Naggar AK, Ballance W, Karim FW, et al. Typical and atypical bronchopulmonary carcinoids. A clinicopathologic and flow cytometric study. *Am J Clin Pathol* 1991;95:828.

193. Lack EE, Harris GB, Eraklis AJ, et al. Primary bronchial tumors in childhood. A clinicopathologic study of six cases. *Cancer* 1983;51:492.

194. Warren WH, Gould VE. Long-term follow-up of classical bronchial carcinoid tumors. Clinicopathologic observations. *Scand J Thorac Cardiovasc Surg* 1990;24:125.

195. Paladugu RR, Benfield JR, Pak HY, et al. Bronchopulmonary Kulchitzky cell carcinomas. A new classification scheme for typical and atypical carcinoids. *Cancer* 1985;55:1303.

196. Bonato M, Cerati M, Pagani A, et al. Differential diagnostic patterns of lung neuroendocrine tumours. A clinico-pathological and immunohistochemical study of 122 cases. *Virchows Arch A Pathol Anat Histopathol* 1992;420:201.

197. Jackson-York GL, Davis BH, Warren WH, et al. Flow cytometric DNA content analysis in neuroendocrine carcinoma of the lung. Correlation with survival and histologic subtype. *Cancer* 1991;68:374.

198. Smolle-Jüttner FM, Popper H, Klemen H, et al. Clinical features and therapy of "typical" and "atypical" bronchial carcinoid tumors (grade 1 and grade 2 neuroendocrine carcinoma). *Eur J Cardiothorac Surg* 1993;7:121; discussion 125.

199. Moskaluk CA, Pogrebniak HW, Pass HI, et al. Surgical pathology of the lung in chronic granulomatous disease. *Am J Clin Pathol* 1994;102:684.

200. Linnoila RI, Mulshine JL, Steinberg SM, et al. Neuroendocrine differentiation in endocrine and nonendocrine lung carcinomas. *Am J Clin Pathol* 1988;90:641.

201. Lantuejoul S, Moro D, Michalides RJ, et al. Neural cell adhesion molecules (NCAM) and NCAM-PSA expression in neuroendocrine lung tumors. *Am J Surg Pathol* 1998;22(10):1267.

202. Kaufmann O, Georgi T, Dietel M. Utility of 123C3 monoclonal antibody against CD56 (NCAM) for the diagnosis of small cell carcinomas on paraffin sections. *Hum Pathol* 1997;28(12):1373.

203. Souhami RL, Beverley PC, Bobrow LG. Antigens of small-cell lung cancer. First International Workshop. *Lancet* 1987;2:325.

204. Tome Y, Hirohashi S, Noguchi M, et al. Preservation of cluster 1 small cell lung cancer antigen in zinc-formalin fixative and its application to immunohistological diagnosis. *Histopathology* 1990;16:469.

205. Oud PS, Pahlplatz MM, Beck JL, et al. Image and flow DNA cytometry of small cell carcinoma of the lung. Cancer 1989;64:1304.

206. Battlehner CN, Saldiva PH, Carvalho CR, et al. Nuclear/cytoplasmic ratio correlates strongly with survival in non-disseminated neuroendocrine carcinoma of the lung. *Histopathology* 1993;22:31.

207. Böhm J, Kacic V, Gais P, et al. Prognostic value of nucleolar organizer regions in neuroendocrine tumours of the lung. *Histochemistry* 1993;99:85.

208. Roncalli M, Doglioni C, Springall DR, et al. Abnormal p53 expression in lung neuroendocrine tumors. Diagnostic and prognostic implications. *Diagn Mol Pathol* 1992;1:129.

209. Onuki N, Wistuba II, Travis WD, et al. Genetic changes in the spectrum of neuroendocrine lung tumors. *Cancer* 1999;85(3):600.

210. Pryzygodzki R, Finkelstein S, Zeren H, et al. p53 analysis of neuroendocrine (NE) tumors: discriminating factors in atypical carcinoid within the NE spectrum. *Mod Pathol* 1994;7:153A.

211. Brambilla E, Negoescu A, Gazzeri S, et al. Apoptosis-related factors p53, Bcl2, and Bax in neuroendocrine lung tumors. *Am J Pathol* 1996;149(6):1941.

212. Rusch VW, Klimstra DS, Venkatraman ES. Molecular markers help characterize neuroendocrine lung tumors. *Ann Thorac Surg* 1996;62:798.

213. Jones DJ, Hasleton PS, Moore M. DNA ploidy in bronchopulmonary carcinoid tumours. *Thorax* 1988;43:195.

214. Caulet S, Capron F, Ghorra C, et al. Flow cytometric DNA analysis of 20 bronchopulmonary neuroendocrine tumours. *Eur Respir J* 1993;6:83.

215. Mackay B, Fanning T, Bruner JM, et al. Diagnostic electron microscopy using fine needle aspiration biopsies. *Ultrastruct Pathol* 1987;11:659.

216. Havenith MG, Dingemans KP, Cleutjens JP, et al. Basement membranes in bronchogenic squamous cell carcinoma: an immunohistochemical and ultrastructural study. *Ultrastruct Pathol* 1990;14:51.

217. McDonagh D, Vollmer RT, Shelburne JD. Intercellular junctions and tumor behavior in lung cancer. *Mod Pathol* 1991;4:436.

218. Bedrossian CW, Bonsib S, Moran C. Differential diagnosis between mesothelioma and adenocarcinoma: a multimodal approach based on ultrastructure and immunocytochemistry. *Semin Diagn Pathol* 1992;9:124.

219. Burgart LJ, Heller MJ, Reznicek MJ, et al. Cytomegalovirus detection in bone marrow transplant patients with idiopathic pneumonitis. A clinicopathologic study of the clinical utility of the polymerase chain reaction on open lung biopsy specimen tissue. *Am J Clin Pathol* 1991;96:572.

220. Nakamura S, Koshikawa T, Sato T, et al. Extremely well differentiated papillary adenocarcinoma of the lung with prominent cilia formation. *Acta Pathol Jpn* 1992;42:745.

221. Mackay B, Ordóñez NG, Bennington JL, et al. Ultrastructural and morphometric features of poorly differentiated and undifferentiated lung tumors. *Ultrastruct Pathol* 1989;13:561.

222. Damjanov I, Tuma B, Dominis M. Electron microscopy of large cell undifferentiated and giant cell tumors. *Pathol Res Pract* 1989;184:137.

223. Matsui K, Kitagawa M, Miwa A. Lung carcinoma with spindle cell components: sixteen cases examined by immunohistochemistry. *Hum Pathol* 1992;23:1289.

224. Wick MR, Berg LC, Hertz MI. Large cell carcinoma of the lung with neuroendocrine differentiation. A comparison with large cell "undifferentiated" pulmonary tumors. *Am J Clin Pathol* 1992;97:796.

225. Piehl MR, Gould VE, Warren WH, et al. Immunohistochemical identification of exocrine and neuroendocrine subsets of large cell lung carcinomas. *Pathol Res Pract* 1988;183:675.

226. Kasai K, Kameya T, Kadoya K, et al. A pulmonary large cell carcinoma cell line expressing neuroendocrine cell markers and human chorionic gonadotropin alpha-subunit. *Jpn J Cancer Res* 1991;82:12.

227. Hammar SP, Bockus D, Remington F, et al. The unusual spectrum of neuroendocrine lung neoplasms. *Ultrastruct Pathol* 1989;13:515.

228. Matsumoto S, Muranaka T, Hanada K, et al. Oncocytic carcinoid of the lung. *Radiat Med* 1993;11:63.

229. Torikata C, Mukai M. So-called minute chemodectoma of the lung. An electron microscopic and immunohistochemical study. *Virchows Arch A Pathol Anat Histopathol* 1990;417:113.

230. Johnston WW, Frable WJ. The cytopathology of the respiratory tract. A review. *Am J Pathol* 1976;84:372.

231. Dahlgren S. Aspiration biopsy cytology. I. Cytology of supradiaphragmatic organs. Lungs. *Monogr Clin Cytol* 1974;4:195.

232. Donat EE, Wood J, Tao LC. The application of fine needle aspiration cytology in the diagnosis of multiple primary malignant tumors. *Acta Cytol* 1989;33:800.

233. Johnston WW. Fine needle aspiration biopsy versus sputum and bronchial material in the diagnosis of lung cancer. A comparative study of 168 patients. *Acta Cytol* 1988;32:641.

234. Flehinger BJ, Melamed MR, Zaman MB, et al. Early lung cancer detection: results of the initial (prevalence) radiologic and cytologic screening in the Memorial Sloan-Kettering study. *Am Rev Respir Dis* 1984;130:555.

235. Johnson RD, Gobien RP, Valicenti JF, Jr. Current status of radiologically directed pulmonary thin needle aspiration biopsy. An analysis of 200 consecutive biopsies and review of the literature. *Ann Clin Lab Sci* 1983;13:225.

236. Nordenström BE. Technical aspects of obtaining cellular material from lesions deep in the lung. A radiologist's view and description of the screw-needle sampling technique. *Acta Cytol* 1984;28:233.

237. Popp W, Merkle M, Schreiber B, et al. How much brushing is enough for the diagnosis of lung tumors? *Cancer* 1992;70:2278.

238. Zavala DC. Diagnostic fiberoptic bronchoscopy: techniques and results of biopsy in 600 patients. *Chest* 1975;68:12.

239. Jay SJ, Wehr K, Nicholson DP, et al. Diagnostic sensitivity and specificity of pulmonary cytology: comparison of techniques used in conjunction with flexible fiber optic bronchoscopy. *Acta Cytol* 1980;24:304.

240. Healy TM, Borrie J. Lung cancer diagnosis: evaluation of diagnostic techniques. *N Z Med J* 1975;81:423.

241. Rosell A, Monso E, Lores L, et al. Cytology of bronchial biopsy rinse fluid to improve the diagnostic yield for lung cancer. *Eur Respir J* 1998;12(6):1415.

242. Buccheri G, Barberis P, Delfino MS. Diagnostic, morphologic, and histopathologic correlates in bronchogenic carcinoma. A review of 1,045 bronchoscopic examinations. *Chest* 1991;99:809.

243. Popovich J, Jr. Kvale PA, Eichenhorn MS, et al. Diagnostic accuracy of multiple biopsies from flexible fiberoptic bronchoscopy. A comparison of central versus peripheral carcinoma. *Am Rev Respir Dis* 1982;125:521.

244. Edell ES, Cortese DA. Bronchoscopic localization and treatment of occult lung cancer. *Chest* 1989;96:919.

245. Mehta AC, Marty JJ, Lee FY. Sputum cytology. *Clin Chest Med* 1993;14:69.

246. Shepherd FA. Screening, diagnosis, and staging of lung cancer. *Curr Opin Oncol* 1993;5:310.

247. Jack CI, Sheard JD, Lippitt B, et al. Lung cancer in elderly patients: the role of induced sputum production to obtain a cytological diagnosis. *Age Ageing* 1993;22:227.

248. Khajotia RR, Mohn A, Pokieser L, et al. Induced sputum and cytological diagnosis of lung cancer. *Lancet* 1991;338:976.

249. Pedersen B, Brons M, Holm K, et al. The value of provoked expectoration in obtaining sputum samples for cytologic investigation. A prospective, consecutive and controlled investigation of 134 patients. *Acta Cytol* 1985;29:750.

250. Risse EK, Vooijs GP, van't Hof MA. Relationship between the cellular composition of sputum and the cytologic diagnosis of lung cancer. *Acta Cytol* 1987;31:170.

251. Saccomanno G, Saunders R, Ellis H, et al. Concentration of carcinoma or atypical cells in sputum. *Acta Cytol* 1963;7:305.

252. Risse EK, van't Hof MA, Laurini RN, et al. Sputum cytology by the Saccomanno method in diagnosing lung malignancy. *Diagn Cytopathol* 1985;1:286.

253. Rizzo T, Schumann GB, Riding JM. Comparison of the pick-and-smear and Saccomanno methods for sputum cytologic analysis. *Acta Cytol* 1990;34:875.

254. Tang CS, Tang CM, Lau YY, et al. Sensitivity of sputum cytology after homogenization with dithiothreitol in lung cancer detection. Two years of experience. *Acta Cytol* 1995;39(6):1137.

255. Böcking A, Biesterfeld S, Chatelain R, et al. Diagnosis of bronchial carcinoma on sections of paraffin- embedded sputum. Sensitivity and specificity of an alternative to routine cytology. *Acta Cytol* 1992;36:37.

256. Johnston WW, Bossen EH. Ten years of respiratory cytopathology at Duke University Medical Center. I. The cytopathologic diagnosis of lung cancer during the years 1970 to 1974, noting the significance of specimen number and type. *Acta Cytol* 1981;25:103.

257. Raab SS, Hornberger J, Raffin T. The importance of sputum cytology in the diagnosis of lung cancer: a cost-effectiveness analysis. *Chest* 1997;112(4):937.

258. Caya JG, Gilles L, Tieu TM, et al. Lung cancer treated on the basis of cytologic findings: an analysis of 112 patients. *Diagn Cytopathol* 1990;6:313.

259. Miura H, Konaka C, Kawate N, et al. Sputum cytology-positive, bronchoscopically negative adenocarcinoma of the lung. *Chest* 1992;102:1328.

260. Paolini A, Tosato F, Casella MC, et al. The role of fiberoptic bronchoscopy in the diagnosis of pulmonary cancer. *Minerva Chir* 1979;34:947.

261. Ng AB, Horak GC. Factors significant in the diagnostic accuracy of lung cytology in bronchial washing and sputum samples. II. Sputum samples. *Acta Cytol* 1983;27:397.

262. Mak VH, Johnston ID, Hetzel MR, et al. Value of washings and brushings at fibreoptic bronchoscopy in the diagnosis of lung cancer. *Thorax* 1990;45:373.

263. Fennessy JJ. Bronchial brushing and transbronchial forceps biopsy in the diagnosis of pulmonary lesions. *Dis Chest* 1968;53:377.

264. Bibbo M, Fennessy JJ, Lu CT, et al. Bronchial brushing technique for the cytologic diagnosis of peripheral lung lesions. A review of 693 cases. *Acta Cytol* 1973;17:245.

265. Kinnear WJ, Wilkinson MJ, James PD, et al. Comparison of the diagnostic yields of disposable and reusable cytology brushes in fibreoptic bronchoscopy. *Thorax* 1991;46:667.

266. Augusseau S, Mouriquand J, Brambilla C, et al. Cytological

survey of bronchial brushings and aspirations performed during fiberoptic bronchoscopy. *Arch Geschwulstforsch* 1978;48:245.

267. Sing A, Freudenberg N, Kortsik C, et al. Comparison of the sensitivity of sputum and brush cytology in the diagnosis of lung carcinomas. *Acta Cytol* 1997;41(2):399.

268. Reynolds HY. Bronchoalveolar lavage. *Am Rev Respir Dis* 1987; 135:250.

269. Linder J, Rennard S. *Bronchoalveolar lavage,* 1st ed. Chicago: American Society of Clinical Pathologists, 1988.

270. Rossi GA. Bronchoalveolar lavage in the investigation of disorders of the lower respiratory tract. *Eur J Respir Dis* 1986;69: 293.

271. Greco RJ, Steiner RM, Goldman S, et al. Bronchoalveolar cell carcinoma of the lung. *Ann Thorac Surg* 1986;41:652.

272. Linder J, Radio SJ, Robbins RA, et al. Bronchoalveolar lavage in the cytologic diagnosis of carcinoma of the lung. *Acta Cytol* 1987;31:796.

273. Rennard SI. Bronchoalveolar lavage in the assessment of primary and metastatic lung cancer. *Respiration* 1992;59 Suppl 1:41.

274. Wongsurakiat P, Wongbunnate S, Dejsomritrutai W, et al. Diagnostic value of bronchoalveolar lavage and postbronchoscopic sputum cytology in peripheral lung cancer. *Respirology* 1998; 3(2):131.

275. de Gracia J, Bravo C, Miravitlles M, et al. Diagnostic value of bronchoalveolar lavage in peripheral lung cancer. *Am Rev Respir Dis* 1993;147:649.

276. Pirozynski M. Bronchoalveolar lavage in the diagnosis of peripheral, primary lung cancer. *Chest* 1992;102:372.

277. Springmeyer SC, Hackman R, Carlson JJ, et al. Bronchiolo-alveolar cell carcinoma diagnosed by bronchoalveolar lavage. *Chest* 1983;83:278.

278. Bonfiglio TA. Fine needle aspiration biopsy of the lung. *Pathol Annu* 1981;16 Pt 1:159.

279. Johnston WW. Percutaneous fine needle aspiration biopsy of the lung. A study of 1,015 patients. *Acta Cytol* 1984;28:218.

280. Kato H, Konaka C, Kawate N, et al. Percutaneous fine-needle cytology for lung cancer diagnosis. *Diagn Cytopathol* 1986;2: 277.

281. Denley H, Singh N, Clelland CA. Transthoracic fine needle aspiration cytology of lung for suspected malignancy: an audit of cytological findings with histopathological correlation. *Cytopathology* 1997;8(4):223.

282. Akamatsu H, Terashima M, Koike T, et al. Staging of primary lung cancer by computed tomography-guided percutaneous needle cytology of mediastinal lymph nodes. *Ann Thorac Surg* 1996;62(2):352.

283. Pak HY, Yokota S, Teplitz RL, et al. Rapid staining techniques employed in fine needle aspirations of the lung. *Acta Cytol* 1981; 25:178.

284. Stewart CJ, Stewart IS. Immediate assessment of fine needle aspiration cytology of lung. *J Clin Pathol* 1996;49(10):839.

285. Greene R, Szyfelbein WM, Isler RJ, et al. Supplementary tissue-core histology from fine-needle transthoracic aspiration biopsy. *Am J Roentgenol* 1985;144:787.

286. Weisbrod GL, Herman SJ, Tao LC. Preliminary experience with a dual cutting edge needle in thoracic percutaneous fine-needle aspiration biopsy. *Radiology* 1987;163:75.

287. Yang PC, Lee YC, Yu CJ, et al. Ultrasonographically guided biopsy of thoracic tumors. A comparison of large-bore cutting biopsy with fine-needle aspiration. *Cancer* 1992;69:2553.

288. Henry-Stanley MJ, Stanley MW. Processing of needle rinse material from fine-needle aspirations rarely detects malignancy not identified in smears. *Diagn Cytopathol* 1992;8:538.

289. Burt AD, Smillie D, Cowan MD, et al. Fine needle aspiration cytology: experience with a cell block technique [letter]. *J Clin Pathol* 1986;39:114.

290. Barbazza R, Toniolo L, Pinarello A, et al. Accuracy of bronchial aspiration cytology in typing operable (stage I-II) pulmonary carcinomas. *Diagn Cytopathol* 1992;8:3.

291. Wang KP, Marsh BR, Summer WR, et al. Transbronchial needle aspiration for diagnosis of lung cancer. *Chest* 1981;80: 48.

292. Schenk DA, Bryan CL, Bower JH, et al. Transbronchial needle aspiration in the diagnosis of bronchogenic carcinoma. *Chest* 1987;92:83.

293. Wagner ED, Ramzy I, Greenberg SD, et al. Transbronchial fine-needle aspiration. Reliability and limitations. *Am J Clin Pathol* 1989;92:36.

294. Cropp AJ, DiMarco AF, Lankerani M. False-positive transbronchial needle aspiration in bronchogenic carcinoma. *Chest* 1984; 85:696.

295. DeCaro LF, Pak HY, Yokota S, et al. Intraoperative cytodiagnosis of lung tumors by needle aspiration. *J Thorac Cardiovasc Surg* 1983;85:404.

296. Guarda LA. Intraoperative cytologic diagnosis: evaluation of 370 consecutive intraoperative cytologies. *Diagn Cytopathol* 1990;6:235.

297. Kontozoglou TE, Cramer HM. The advantages of intraoperative cytology. Analysis of 215 smears and review of the literature. *Acta Cytol* 1991;35:154.

298. Machicao CN, Sorensen K, Abdul-Karim FW, et al. Transthoracic needle aspiration biopsy in inflammatory pseudotumors of the lung. *Diagn Cytopathol* 1989;5:400.

299. Hunninghake GW, Gadek JE, Kawanami O, et al. Inflammatory and immune processes in the human lung in health and disease: evaluation by bronchoalveolar lavage. *Am J Pathol* 1979; 97:149.

300. Fedullo AJ, Ettensohn DB. Bronchoalveolar lavage in lymphangitic spread of adenocarcinoma to the lung. *Chest* 1985;87:129.

301. Flint A, Kumar NB, Naylor B. Pulmonary Hodgkin's disease. Diagnosis by fine needle aspiration. *Acta Cytol* 1988;32:221.

302. Wisecarver J, Ness MJ, Rennard SI, et al. Bronchoalveolar lavage in the assessment of pulmonary Hodgkin's disease. *Acta Cytol* 1989;33:527.

303. Bonfiglio T. Transthoracic thin needle aspiration biopsy. *Diagnostic cytopathology* Vol. 4, 1st ed. Bucher O, ed., Paris: Masson, 1983.

304. Johnston WW, Frable WJ. Diagnostic respiratory cytopathology. 1993.

305. Saito Y, Imai T, Nagamoto N, et al. A quantitative cytologic study of sputum in early squamous cell bronchogenic carcinoma. *Anal Quant Cytol Histol* 1988;10:365.

306. Tao LC, Chamberlain DW, Delarue NC, et al. Cytologic diagnosis of radiographically occult squamous call carcinoma of the lung. *Cancer* 1982;50:1580.

307. Eddy DM. Screening for lung cancer. *Ann Intern Med* 1989; 111:232.

308. Fontana RS, Sanderson DR, Woolner LB, et al. Screening for lung cancer. A critique of the Mayo Lung Project. *Cancer* 1991; 67:1155.

309. Shields TW. Screening, diagnosis, and staging of non-small cell lung cancer and consideration of unusual primary tumors of the lungs. *Curr Opin Oncol* 1992;4:299.

310. Chiu FT. Cavitation in lung cancers. *Aust N Z J Med* 1975;5: 523.

311. Zusman-Harach SB, Harach HR, Gibbs AR. Cytological features of non-small cell carcinomas of the lung in fine needle aspirates. *J Clin Pathol* 1991;44:997.

312. Chen KT. Psammoma bodies in fine-needle aspiration cytology of papillary adenocarcinoma of the lung. *Diagn Cytopathol* 1990;6:271.

313. Davenport RD. Diagnostic value of crush artifact in cytologic

specimens. Occurrence in small cell carcinoma of the lung. *Acta Cytol* 1990;34:502.

314. Fushimi H, Kikui M, Morino H, et al. Detection of large cell component in small cell lung carcinoma by combined cytologic and histologic examinations and its clinical implication. *Cancer* 1992;70:599.

315. Anderson C, Ludwig ME, O'Donnell M. Fine needle aspiration cytology of pulmonary carcinoid tumors. *Acta Cytol* 1990;34:505.

316. Mitchell ML, Parker FP. Capillaries. A cytologic feature of pulmonary carcinoid tumors. *Acta Cytol* 1991;35:183.

317. Gephardt GN, Belovich DM. Cytology of pulmonary carcinoid tumors. *Acta Cytol* 1982;26:434.

318. Fekete PS, Cohen C, DeRose PB. Pulmonary spindle cell carcinoid. Needle aspiration biopsy, histologic and immunohistochemical findings. *Acta Cytol* 1990;34:50.

319. Zarbo RJ, Fenoglio-Preiser CM. Interinstitutional database for comparison of performance in lung fine-needle aspiration cytology. A College of American Pathologists Q-Probe Study of 5264 cases with histologic correlation. *Arch Pathol Lab Med* 1992;116:463.

320. Caya JG, Clowry LJ, Wollenberg NJ, et al. Transthoracic fine-needle aspiration cytology. Analysis of 82 patients with detailed verification criteria and evaluation of false-negative cases. *Am J Clin Pathol* 1984;82:100.

321. Zakowski MF, Gatscha RM, Zaman MB. Negative predictive value of pulmonary fine needle aspiration cytology. *Acta Cytol* 1992;36:283.

322. Goldstein N, Lippmann ML, Goldberg SK, et al. Usefulness of tumor markers in serum and bronchoalveolar lavage of patients undergoing fiberoptic bronchoscopy. *Am Rev Respir Dis* 1985;132:60.

323. Pinto MM, Ha DJ. Carcinoembryonic antigen content in fine needle aspirates of the lung. A diagnostic adjunct to cytology. *Acta Cytol* 1992;36:277.

324. Travis WD, Wold LE. Immunoperoxidase staining of fine needle aspiration specimens previously stained by the Papanicolaou technique. *Acta Cytol* 1987;31:517.

325. Naryshkin S, Daniels J, Young NA. Diagnostic correlation of fiberoptic bronchoscopic biopsy and bronchoscopic cytology performed simultaneously. *Diagn Cytopathol* 1992;8:119.

326. Johnston WW, Bossen EH. Ten years of respiratory cytopathology at Duke University Medical Center. II. The cytopathologic diagnosis of lung cancer during the years 1970 to 1974, with a comparison between cytopathology and histopathology in the typing of lung cancer. *Acta Cytol* 1981;25:499.

327. DiBonito L, Colautti I, Patriarca S, et al. Cytological typing of primary lung cancer: study of 100 cases with autopsy confirmation. *Diagn Cytopathol* 1991;7:7.

328. Caya JG, Wollenberg NJ, Clowry LJ. Respiratory cytology: significance of "suspect" results in a series of 435 patients. *South Med J* 1985;78:701.

329. Linder J. Errors and pitfalls in lung and pleural cytology. *Monogr Pathol* 1997;(39):40.

330. Naryshkin S, Young NA. Respiratory cytology: a review of non-neoplastic mimics of malignancy. *Diagn Cytopathol* 1993;9:89.

331. Johnston WW. Type II pneumocytes in cytologic specimens. A diagnostic dilemma. *Am J Clin Pathol* 1992;97:608.

332. Stanley MW, Henry-Stanley MJ, Gajl-Peczalska KJ, et al. Hyperplasia of type II pneumocytes in acute lung injury. Cytologic findings of sequential bronchoalveolar lavage. *Am J Clin Pathol* 1992;97:669.

333. Bardales RH, Powers CN, Frierson HF, Jr et al. Exfoliative respiratory cytology in the diagnosis of leukemias and lymphomas in the lung. *Diagn Cytopathol* 1996;14(2):108.

334. Travis WD. Pathology of pulmonary incipient neoplasia. In: Albores-Saavedra J, Henson DE, ed. *Pathology of incipient neoplasia*. Philadelphia: WB Saunders, 2000 (*in press*).

27

TECHNIQUES AND APPLICATIONS OF TISSUE MICRODISSECTION

JOHN W. GILLESPIE
NICOLE L. SIMONE
ROBERT F. BONNER
LANCE A. LIOTTA
MICHAEL R. EMMERT-BUCK

Human tissues consist of multiple interacting cell populations in a complex three-dimensional arrangement, with each cellular phenotype determined by a unique profile of mRNA and protein expression. Molecular analysis of specimens geared toward an understanding of individual cell types requires methods and approaches that permit histopathologically defined cell types to be selectively studied. This approach is particularly important for pathologic processes where the diseased cells constitute only a small percentage of the total cells present in a sample, or, as in the case of tumor progression, the disease evolves through stages represented by discrete microscopic foci. To date, this goal has been accomplished primarily through immunohistochemical and *in situ* hybridization studies. Although these techniques have been useful tools to examine tissue specimens, they are limited to single gene analysis and in general do not allow qualitative studies (mutation, deletion analysis) of DNA, mRNA, or proteins to be performed. Thus microdissection has become an increasingly useful method to study defined cell types from tissue samples.[1] In concert with newly developing molecular analytical techniques, this approach allows for a highly sensitive and specific means to study disease processes as they exist *in vivo*. Many techniques of microdissection have been developed and are briefly described in following sections. The present chapter focuses primarily on laser capture microdissection, a new technology invented at the National Institutes of Health, which has been developed into an automated and high-throughput system, with examples of its use in lung neoplasms.

DEVELOPMENT OF TISSUE MICRODISSECTION TECHNIQUES

The concept of tissue microdissection is simple; that is, procuring a specific population of cells from a heterogeneous tissue sample under direct microscopic visualization. However, in practice the approach is technically challenging. Early efforts entailed grossly removing tissue from a frozen section slide or utilizing a scalpel blade to scrape sections and procure cells of interest.[2,3] Subsequently, the use of a manual or micromanipulator-guided needle with an adhesive tip was developed, which improved the accuracy and reliability of microdissection.[4,5] A technical advance known as selective ultraviolet radiation fractionation (SURF) was developed using ink to protect against ultraviolet irradiation and obliterating the genetic material of the unwanted surrounding tissue.[6] A similar method was developed for isolating single cells, which utilizes a high-energy ultraviolet laser microbeam to obliterate the unwanted cells. The desired cells are then retrieved by a needle.[7] Another laser-based method called non-contact laser microdissection of membrane-mounted native tissue was developed, which involves placing a tissue section onto a membrane on a glass slide and using a high-intensity ultraviolet beam to cut out an area of tissue/membrane that can subsequently be recovered.[8,9]

LASER CAPTURE MICRODISSECTION

Laser capture microdissection (LCM) is a positive selection method that was developed at the National Institutes of Health (NIH) and designed to permit simple, fast, and reliable microdissection of tissue.[10,11] The system utilizes an infrared laser integrated into a standard microscope with alignment into the optics subsystem. The technique relies on the use of a thermoplastic transparent film, which lies on the surface of a routinely prepared tissue section on a glass slide. The investigator examines the tissue section microscopically and activates the laser when the desired cells underlie the target. This laser activates the film with subsequent binding and procurement of the cells of interest (Fig-

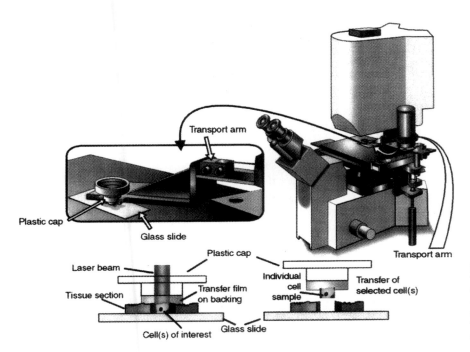

FIGURE 27.1. Laser capture microdissection (LCM) system showing the process of microdissection of cells from tissue. The laser beam activates the thermoplastic film embedding the underlying cells, which can then be separated from the tissue. (See Color Figure 27.1.)

ure 27.1). The laser pulse is brief (approximately 5 msec) and the membrane is activated at 90°C, thus the tissue experiences only a brief thermal transient as the heat generated from the membrane is rapidly dissipated. LCM allows for visualization and image capturing of tissue as it is microdissected including images of the tissue before and after microdissection. This ability is critical in maintaining an accurate record of each dissection and correlating histopathology with subsequent molecular results. In the following sections, the principles of tissue handling, staining, and dissection using LCM are discussed. Current and regularly updated protocols can be found on the websites listed in the Web Resources section at the end of the chapter. Examples of research studies utilizing LCM are also presented at the end of the chapter in the References section.

TISSUE PROCESSING FOR LCM

The importance of specimen handling for tissues to be used for molecular analysis cannot be overstated. Factors such as the time interval between surgical removal and sample processing, type of fixative and embedding medium, and length of fixation time have a significant impact on the recovery of nucleic acids and proteins. If the investigator is unaware of the time interval between surgery and sample processing, the quality of macromolecules in each specimen needs to be determined empirically. As a practical approach in this situation, we start with a scrape of a tissue section to assess the quality of DNA, RNA, or proteins of the specimen before utilization of the tissue in a study. Thus cases that

are sufficient for a given analysis can be identified prior to the time and effort involved in microdissection.

After tissue is removed from a patient, it can be either frozen or placed in fixative and embedded. Both approaches have advantages and disadvantages. The major advantage of tissue freezing is the excellent preservation of DNA, RNA, and proteins, including active enzymes. The disadvantages include the relatively poor histologic detail on examination and the logistic problems associated with storing blocks and recut slides in freezers. The advantages of studying fixed and embedded tissue include ease of use, optimal histology, and generally abundant amount of archival patient material available for study. The major disadvantage is the generally lower quality macromolecules that can be recovered from fixed and embedded samples.

Frozen Tissue

Immediately after removal from the patient, the tissue should be subdivided into thin pieces and immediately snap frozen in embedding compound and stored at −80°C. Cutting sections is performed using a standard cryostat at −20°C and standard noncoated glass slides. The recut sections can be temporarily stored in the cryostat while being cut; however, the slides must not be left at room temperature for any length of time because the tissue will stick irreversibly to the slide and interfere with subsequent LCM.

Embedded Tissue

The critical element of tissue fixation and embedding is to maintain excellent histologic detail while preserving the biomacromolecules and allow for practical handling of the embedded blocks. The standard protocol of formalin-fixation and paraffin-embedding of tissue seriously limits studies of mRNA and protein. However, the tissue can still be used for DNA analysis. If cases have been properly fixed and processed, then excellent polymerase chain reaction (PCR) amplification occurs in close to 100% of cases. We and other groups are currently examining the effects of various fixatives and embedding compounds on recovery of biomacromolecules. Strategies using non–cross-linking fixatives and low-temperature embedding compounds appear promising.[12–14]

Staining

Slide staining should be conducted immediately before microdissection is performed. Hematoxylin and eosin staining as performed in a histopathology laboratory is the standard for LCM; however, elimination of hematoxylin improves

subsequent DNA amplification by PCR. Recently, an adjunct protocol using immunohistochemical staining to improve cell targeting has been developed[15] Staining reagents are changed on a daily basis to avoid cross contamination between cases.

LCM

Once the tissue has been properly processed, sectioned, and stained, it is ready for microdissection. The tissue is visualized under the microscope and an initial roadmap image as well as predissection, postdissection, and cap images are taken to document the histology, the steps of microdissection, and the microdissected cells, respectively. The laser beam size may be adjusted from 7.5 μm to 30 μm to allow microdissection of either groups of cells or single cells depending on the investigator's needs. For example, Figure 27.2 shows microdissection of normal bronchiolar epithelium, and Figure 27.3 shows microdissection of a single

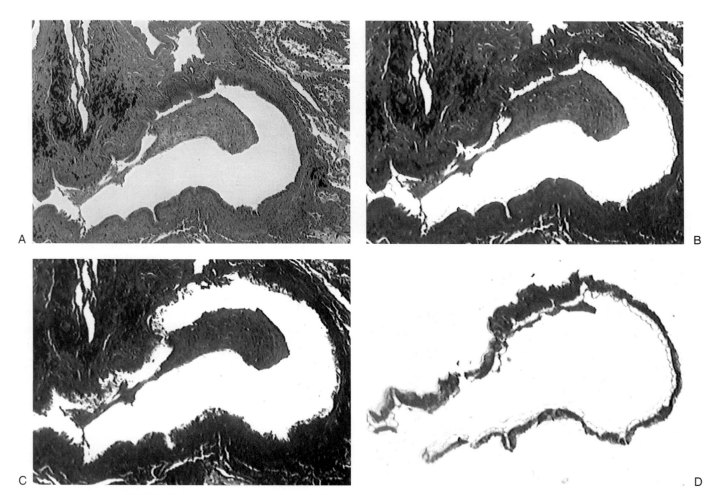

FIGURE 27.2. Microdissection of normal bronchiolar epithelium. **A:** roadmap, **(B)** before microdissection, **(C)** after microdissection, and **(D)** cap with dissected tissue (200 X magnification). (See Color Figure 27.2.)

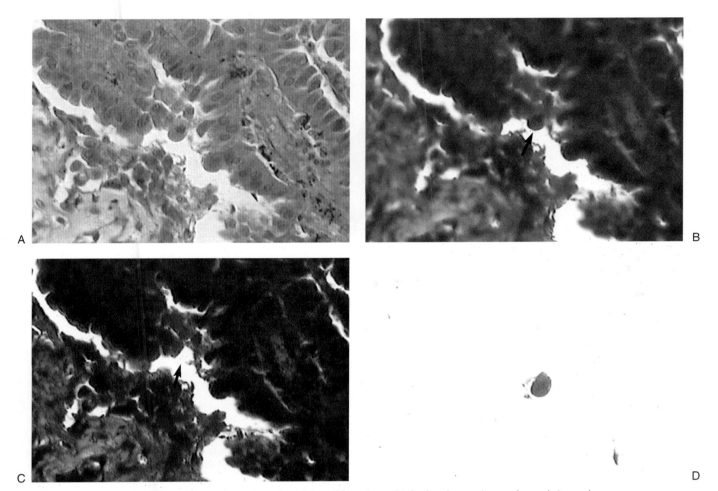

FIGURE 27.3. Microdissection of a single cell from bronchioloalveolar carcinoma *(arrow)*. **A:** roadmap, **(B)** before microdissection, **(C)** after microdissection, and **(D)** cap demonstrating microdissected cell (1000 X magnification). (See Color Figure 27.3.)

bronchioloalveolar carcinoma cell. The total number of cells procured depends on the molecular analytical technique being employed. After the microdissection is complete, the cap with microdissected cells is placed onto an Eppendorf tube containing the appropriate buffer for molecular analysis. The tube is then inverted to allow the lysis of the cells, and the sample is ready for molecular analysis.

EXAMPLES OF TISSUE MICRODISSECTION

The combination of tissue microdissection and emerging molecular analysis technologies significantly expands the opportunities for study of pathologic processes such as cancer. For example, as illustrated in Figure 27.4 many techniques can be applied to LCM-derived cell samples to examine the DNA mutational events that occur during tumorigenesis as well as the patterns of gene expression at each stage of disease progression. Examples of two applica-

tions of tissue microdissection in cancer research performed in the Pathogenetics Unit of the Laboratory of Pathology, National Cancer Institute (NCI) are presented as follows.

Multiple Endocrine Neoplasia Type I

Multiple endocrine neoplasia type I (MENI) is an inherited syndrome characterized by development of multiple neuroendocrine (NE) tumors in affected individuals. To precisely localize the genomic location of the gene on chromosome 11q13, we performed loss of heterozygosity (LOH) analysis in 188 tumors from 81 patients using tissue microdissection.[16] Six tumors (three MENI, three sporadic) were identified, which provided important gene location boundaries and indicated that the gene was located between markers PYGM and D11S4936, a region of approximately 300 kb. Subsequent DNA sequencing from the identified minimal interval on chromosome 11q13 identified the *MENI* gene,

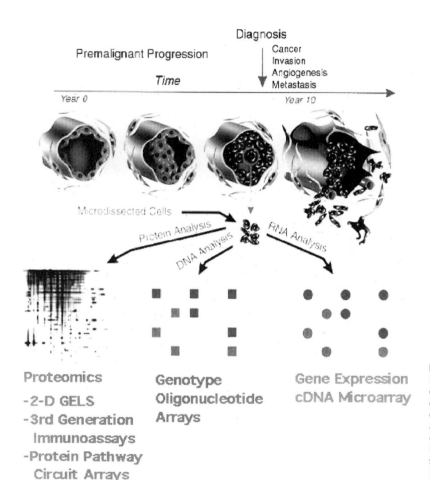

FIGURE 27.4. Application of LCM to study the molecular events associated with cancer progression. The expression pattern of proteins (two-dimensional gel electrophoresis or immunoassays), RNA (differential display, microarray hybridization, or cDNA libraries), and DNA genotype (mutational analysis, loss of heterozygosity, comparative genomic hybridization) can be compared within the same patient. In the tissue section, normal precursor epithelium, premalignant lesions, and invasive cancer foci can be microdissected and compared. (See Color Figure 27.4.)

which contains 10 exons and encodes a ubiquitously expressed 2.8 kb transcript.[17]

To investigate the role of the *MEN1* gene in lung neuroendocrine cancers NE tumors, we studied a series of sporadic lung tumors (11 carcinoids, 13 large cell [LCNECs], 9 primary small cell lung cancer [SCLC], 35 SCLC cell lines) to determine if *MEN1* gene inactivation was involved in the pathogenesis of these lesions.[18,19] Each tumor was analyzed for allelic deletions and mutations of the *MEN1* gene using tissue microdisection combined with dideoxy fingerprinting (ddF) for mutational screening, and LOH analysis at the locus of the gene on chromosome 11q13. In 4 of 11 (36%) carcinoids both copies of the *MEN1* gene were inactivated. All four tumors showed the presence of a mutation in one allele of the gene and LOH of the second allele. Observed mutations included a 1 bp insertion, a 1 bp deletion, a 13 bp deletion, and a single nucleotide substitution affecting a donor splice site. Each mutation predicts truncation of menin. The remaining seven carcinoids showed neither the presence of an *MEN1* gene mutation nor 11q13 LOH. All SCLCs and cell lines were negative for *MEN1* gene mutations. LOH at 11q13 was detected in

20% of SCLCs and cell lines, most likely a consequence of genomic instability not specifically related to *MEN1* gene inactivation. None of the 13 LCNECs showed 11q13 LOH. Interestingly, one LCNEC case showed a 1 bp frameshift deletion of the *MEN1* gene predicting protein truncation. This finding is the first demonstrated mutation in a tumor outside the usual MEN1-associated realm, and the first mutation to be observed in a tumor that does not demonstrate loss of the second allele. In summary, the data implicate the *MEN1* gene in the pathogenesis of sporadic lung carcinoids, representing the first defined genetic alteration in these tumors. *MEN1* gene inactivation was found to occur infrequently in LCNEC, and was not observed in SCLC.

NCI Cancer Genome Anatomy Project

An understanding of the *in vivo* gene expression profiles that occur in normal and tumor cells has multiple uses in the fight against human cancer, from promoting new insights and hypotheses regarding fundamental tumor development to identifying new diagnostic and therapeutic markers.[20] To promote efforts to understand cancer development and progression at a molecular level, the NCI recently began the Cancer Genome Anatomy Project (CGAP). The primary goals of the project are: (a) discovery of novel human genes toward a complete human unigene set; and (b) assessment of the technical challenges associated with creating molecular fingerprints of cancer progression, and development of appropriate technologic and informatics tools to facilitate this process.

cDNA libraries were prepared from lung, colon, prostate, breast, and ovarian tumors using tissue microdissection and subjected to 3′ end sequencing.[21,22] All data from the project are immediately made available to the public and can be viewed on the CGAP website (http://www.ncbi.nlm.nih.gov//ncicgap/) along with analysis tools to analyze patterns of gene expression.

REFERENCES

1. Emmert-Buck MR, Lubensky IA, Chuaqui RF, et al. Applications of tissue microdissection in molecular pathology. In: Hanausek M, Walaszek Z eds. *Methods in molecular medicine, Vol. 14: Tumor marker protocols,* Totowa, NJ: Humana Press, 1997: 269.
2. Fearon E, Hamilton SR, Vogelstein B. Clonal analysis of human colorectal tumors. *Science* 1987;238:193.
3. Radford D, Fair K, Thompson AM, et al. Allelic loss on chromosome 17 in ductal carcinoma in situ of the breast. *Cancer Res* 1993;53:2947.
4. Going J, Lamb RF. Practical histological microdissection for PCR analysis *J Pathol* 1996;179:121.
5. Emmert-Buck MR, Roth MJ, Zhuang Z, et al. Increased gelatinase A (MMP-2) and cathepsin B activity in invasive tumor regions of human colon cancer samples. *Am J Pathol* 1994; 145(6):1285.
6. Shibata D, Hawes D, Li Z, et al. Specific genetic analysis of microscopic tissue after selective ultraviolet radiation fractionation and the polymerase chain reaction. *Am J Pathol* 1992;141(3): 539.
7. Becker I, Becker K, Rohrl MH, et al. Laser-assisted preparation of single cells from stained histological slides for gene analysis. *Histochem Cell Biol* 1997;108:447.
8. Bohm M, Wieland I, Schutze K, et al. Non-contact laser microdissection of membrane-mounted native tissue. *Am J Pathol* 1997;151(1):63.
9. Schutze K, Labr G. Identification of expressed genes by laser-mediated manipulation of single cells. *Nat Biotech* 1998;16:737.
10. Emmert-Buck M, Bonner RF, Smith PD, et al. Laser capture microdissection. *Science* 1996;274:998.
11. Bonner RF, Emmert-Buck MR, Cole K, et al. Laser capture microdissection: molecular analysis of tissue. *Science* 1997; 278(21):1481.
12. Goldsworthy SM, Stockton PS, Trempus CS, et al. Effects of fixation on RNA extraction and amplification from laser capture microdissected tissue. *Molecular Carcinogenesis* 1999;25:86.
13. Cole KA, Krizman DB, Emmert-Buck MR. The genetics of cancer—a 3D model. *Nat Genet* 1999;21(1):38.
14. Pretlow TP, O'Riordan MA, Spancake KM, et al. Two types of putative preneoplastic lesions identified by hexosaminidase activity in whole-mounts of colons from F344 rats treated with carcinogen. *Am J Pathol* 1993;142(6):1695.
15. Fend F, Emmert-Buck MR, Chuaqui R, et al. Immuno LCM: laser capture microdissection of immunostained frozen sections for mRNA analysis. *Am J Pathol* 1999;154(1):61.
16. Emmert-Buck MR, Lubensky IA, Dong Q, et al. Localization of the multiple endocrine neoplasia type I (MENI) gene based on tumor deletion mapping. *Cancer Res* 1997;15:1855.
17. Chandrasekharappa SC, Guru SC, Manickam P, et al. Positional cloning of the gene for multiple endocrine neoplasia-type 1. *Science* 1997;276:404.
18. Debelenko LV, Brambilla E, Agarwal SK, et al. Identification of *MENI* gene mutations in sporadic carcinoid tumors of the lung. *Hum Mol Genet* 1997;6(13):2285.
19. Debelenko LV, Swalwell JI, Kelley MJ, et al. *MENI* gene mutation analysis of high grade neuroendocrine lung carcinoma *submitted*).
20. Strausberg RL, Dahl CA, Klausner RD. New opportunities for uncovering the molecular basis of cancer. *Nat Genet* 1997;15: 415.
21. Krizman DB, Chuaqui RF, Meltzer PS, et al. Construction of a representative cDNA library from prostatic intraepithelial neoplasia. *Cancer Res* 1996;56:5380.
22. Peterson LA, Brown MR, Carlisle AJ, et al. An improved method of directionally cloned cDNA libraries from microdissected cells. *Cancer Res* 1998;58:5326.

28

GENOMIC IMBALANCES IN LUNG CANCER

ALESSANDRA TOSOLINI
JOSEPH R. TESTA

Clonal, somatic chromosome alterations are well documented in many human cancers and may be indicative of molecular events critical in tumorigenesis. Some of these chromosome abnormalities, mainly balanced reciprocal translocations, are associated specifically with certain types of leukemias, lymphomas, and sarcomas.[1–3] Specific reciprocal translocations have been found that alter the expression of dominantly acting oncogenes or other cell-growth-related genes located at or very near the site of chromosomal exchange. For example, in Burkitt's lymphoma, the translocation-mediated juxtaposition of the *MYC* protooncogene, located in chromosome 8, and one of the immunoglobulin loci, located in chromosomes 2, 14, and 22, leads to the deregulated expression of *MYC*. Other reciprocal translocations produce fusion genes, such as the *ABL-BCR* rearrangement, caused by a specific translocation between chromosomes 9 and 22, which is observed in some types of leukemia. As a result of this rearrangement, a hybrid mRNA transcript and a novel protein with tyrosine kinase activity are produced. In many of these malignancies, a balanced rearrangement is the only cytogenetic abnormality present. In contrast, in lung carcinomas and other common types of epithelial tumors, the karyotypes often exhibit multiple genetic alterations. Tumor-suppressor genes (TSGs) are important in these neoplasms, but oncogenes (e.g., members of the *RAS* and *MYC* families) can also be involved in these tumors. A paradigm for such malignancies is colorectal cancer, in which tumorigenesis proceeds through a stepwise series of genetic changes involving TSGs such as *APC* and *TP53* and oncogenes such as KRAS.[4]

Lung carcinomas are now the leading cause of cancer mortality among both men and women in the United States, projected to account for more than 171,000 deaths in 1998.[5] Cytogenetic and molecular cytogenetic analyses of lung tumors can reveal specific genomic imbalances that can have clinical significance with regard to prognosis and therapy. Despite the high incidence of lung cancer, the cytogenetic data available are rather limited in this neoplasm compared to that available for the hematologic malignancies.[3] Primary lung tumor specimens often have a low mitotic index, which makes obtaining an adequate number of metaphase cells suitable for detailed karyotypic analysis difficult. Moreover, the karyotypes can be extremely complex with many additional chromosomes, complicating efforts to identify consistent changes. Reports describing detailed karyotypes of primary small cell lung cancer (SCLC) specimens have been limited to only a few cases.[6–8] Whang-Peng and colleagues were the first to describe a consistent clonal abnormality, deletion of the short arm of chromosome 3 (3p), in tumor cells from SCLC patients.[9] Other recurrent deletions have also been reported in SCLC.[8,10] In addition, extrachromosomal double minutes (dmins) and intrachromosomal homogeneously staining regions (hsrs), two cytogenetic manifestations of gene amplification, have been observed in SCLC, particularly in cell lines derived from these tumors.[8,11,12] Prior to 1994, detailed reports of karyotypes of primary non–small cell lung cancers (NSCLCs) were limited to several small series, usually of fewer than 10 patients,[13–17] or several selected cases or case reports.[18–23] Other early descriptions of cytogenetic changes in NSCLC have been made,[24–33] but these either did not provide complete karyotypes or reported on metastatic tumors, effusions, or established cell lines that had been cultured for many passages. Since 1994, several large series have described karyotypes from short-term cultures of primary NSCLCs.[24–27] Even though karyotypes in NSCLC are generally very complex, recurrent cytogenetic changes have been identified. For example, Lukeis and colleagues described a nonrandom chromosomal abnormality, deletion of the short arm of 9, in 9 of 10 NSCLCs,;s[5] and frequent numerical loss of chromosome 9 has also been reported.[34,35] Recently, several other recurrent chromosome alterations have been identified in NSCLCs.

This chapter summarizes cytogenetic studies of lung carcinomas performed by the authors and by other investigators worldwide. In addition, the importance of recent advances in molecular cytogenetics, especially comparative genomic hybridization (CGH) analysis,[39] and their applications to the study of lung carcinomas are discussed. The karyotypic and molecular cytogenetic findings indicate that both SCLC and NSCLC are characterized by the accumulation of multiple genomic imbalances. The molecular implications of recurrent chromosomal changes found in lung tumors are discussed.

METHODOLOGY

Cell Culture Aspects

To ensure that any karyotypic alterations are representative of the *in vivo* situation, direct preparations of tumor specimens and short-term cultures are preferable to long-term cultures. In our experience, however, mitoses are generally very sparse in direct preparations, and most of our successful analyses are from tumor cells cultured for 1 day to several weeks. Because metastases are presumably representative of a more progressive form of the neoplasm, and because lengthy *in vitro* culture can lead to additional chromosomal abnormalities,[1] it is important to document aberrations in primary tumor specimens harvested after a short *in vitro* culture period.[40]

Solid lung tumor tissue obtained from resections can be disaggregated by mechanical means.[41] The specimen is placed in culture medium containing 10% fetal bovine serum (FBS) and minced using scalpels. Hard tissue that is refractory to mincing is incubated with gentle shaking for 3 to 5 hours in complete medium to which collagenase A (0.5 mg/ml) has been added. Cells are then washed in a balanced salt solution, and single cells and cell aggregates are plated directly into plastic tissue culture flasks containing medium plus 10% FBS. Individual cultures are harvested for karyotypic analysis after 1, 2, and 3 days *in vitro* by overnight exposure to 10 ng/ml colcemid. The growth of several additional cultures of NSCLC cells is monitored daily with an inverted microscope; harvesting of metaphases is performed when adequate numbers of dividing cells are present, as indicated by a rounded morphology.

Methods for establishing SCLC cell lines are described in detail elsewhere.[42–44] For solid tumor specimens, single-cell suspensions are prepared from tumor tissues by mincing the specimen, passing it through a stainless-steel mesh, and gently pipeting the cells in the presence of culture medium. Bone marrow specimens are diluted to 10 mL with medium, and tumor cells are obtained by layering the specimen over Ficoll-Hypaque, followed by centrifugation at 500 xg for 20 minutes. Cells are cultured at a density of approximately 1×10^6 cells/ml in culture medium consisting of serum-free medium (HITES),[42] HITES plus 5% FBS, or McCoy's modified 5A, 10% FBS, and 20% heat-inactivated human effusion fluid.[44] Once the cell lines are well established (i.e., in 3 to 6 months), they may be maintained in RPMI 1640 supplemented with 10% FBS. SCLC specimens and cell lines are harvested for cytogenetics as described previously.

Chromosome Banding and Karyotypic Analysis

Monolayers of NSCLC cells are removed from the culture surface by trypsinization prior to treatment with a hypo-tonic solution consisting of 0.075M KCl or a 4 : 1 mixture of 0.075M KCl and 1% sodium citrate for 20 minutes at 37°C. The cells are then fixed in three changes of a 3 : 1 mixture of methanol-glacial acetic acid chilled to −20°C. Metaphase spreads are prepared by dropping two to three drops of the fixed cell suspension onto clean, wet slides. The slide preparations are dried briefly (~1 minute) over a steam bath and then placed in a dry oven at 55°C for 5 to 7 days. Chromosomes are treated with trypsin-EDTA (0.006%) and Wright stain to produce G-bands. For each specimen, we attempt to obtain chromosome counts on at least 20 metaphase spreads, five to ten of which are photographed and used to prepare karyotypes.

Chromosome identification and karyotypic designations are based on the consensus reached at several international meetings and as published in two authoritative documents.[45,46] A tumor is considered to be karyotypically abnormal if a clone of aberrant cells is found. The observation of a minimum of two or more cells with the same extra chromosome or structural rearrangement or of three or more cells with the same missing chromosome is considered evidence for an abnormal clone.

Fluorescence *In Situ* Hybridization

Fluorescence *in situ* hybridization (FISH) permits investigators to rapidly map the chromosomal location of genes and is helpful in interpreting the centromeric origin and breakpoints of complicated structural abnormalities and in determining the identity of chromosomal material whose origin is uncertain by routine cytogenetic banding techniques. Interphase cytogenetics involves the use of nonisotopic DNA probes to examine interphase nuclei for chromosomal alterations. For example, FISH with satellite DNA probes to the centromere of specific chromosomes can be used to detect numeric abnormalities within interphase nuclei of human solid tumors. Using such a fluorescence-based detection system, hybridization of an alpha-satellite probe to a specific interphase chromosome appears as a brightly fluorescent spot. The number of spots corresponds to the centromeric copy number of a specific chromosome in a given cell nucleus.

For studies of interphase nuclei, we use cell suspensions of tumor specimens that have been disaggregated mechanically. The cell suspensions are processed directly, without culture, treated with 0.075 M KCl hypotonic solution for 20 minutes at 37°C, and then fixed in a 3 : 1 mixture of methanol:acetic acid. Chromosome-specific probes such as α-satellite centromere probes may be labeled with biotin or digoxigenin by nick translation. Hybridization of biotinylated probes may be detected with fluorescein isothiocyanate (FITC)-avidin.[47] Hybridization of digoxigenin-labeled probes may be detected with anti-digoxigenin-rhodamine. The probes can be hybridized individually to interphase nuclei, or they may be co-hybridized to the same slide preparation. For each specimen, several hundred nuclei are counted, and the number of bright fluorescent spots per nucleus is scored. For each probe, hybridization and counting are also carried out on a normal diploid control (e.g., normal lymphocytes or fibroblasts) to ensure the reliability of the probe and hybridization conditions.

Comparative Genomic Hybridization

Comparative genomic hybridization (CGH) analysis represents a valuable approach for overcoming the considerable technical difficulties encountered by cytogeneticists studying chromosome changes in lung cancers. This technique is a valuable molecular cytogenetic tool for identifying losses, gains, and amplification of chromosomal segments in solid tumors.[39,48]

In a CGH analysis, DNA from a tumor and from a normal reference tissue are labeled separately with different haptens, (e.g., biotin and digoxigenin). Identical amounts of both tumor DNA and reference DNA are hybridized simultaneously to normal metaphase chromosome spreads together with an excess of unlabeled Cot-1 blocking DNA to prevent the ubiquitous hybridization of interspersed repetitive sequences contained in the tumor and reference DNA probes. Hybridization of the labeled DNA is detected by two different fluorophores (e.g., green-fluorescing FITC for the tumor DNA and red-fluorescing rhodamine for the reference DNA). The relative amounts of tumor and reference DNA bound to a given chromosomal region depend on the relative abundance of those sequences in the respective DNA samples; these amounts can be quantified by measuring the ratio of green to red fluorescence, using a digital image analysis system. Under- or overrepresentation of chromosomal sequences in the tumor genome is reflected by differences in the fluorescence intensity values of the respective fluorochromes.

We perform CGH analyses basically according to the method described by Kallioniemi and colleagues.[39] Genomic DNA from a normal male donor is labeled with digoxigenin-11-dUTP by nick translation or by random priming; tumor DNA is labeled accordingly with biotin-11-dUTP. After preannealing the specimens to an excess of Cot-1 DNA, biotinylated total tumor DNA and digoxigenin-labeled normal genomic reference DNA are hybridized simultaneously to normal male metaphase spreads for 3 to 4 days at 37°C. The Cot-1 DNA inhibits binding of labeled DNA to the centromeric and heterochromatic regions; therefore these regions are excluded from the analysis.[39] After posthybridization washing of the slides, biotinylated sequences are detected with FITC-avidin, and digoxigenin-labeled sequences are detected with anti-digoxigenin-rhodamine. Alternatively, tumor and normal DNAs can be directly labeled, using SpectrumGreen™-dUTP and TexasRed™-dUTP (Vysis). Chromosomes are counterstained with DAPI for chromosome identification. The FITC and rho-

damine fluorescence specific for the tumor genome and reference genome, respectively, are quantified as gray level images by a cooled charge-coupled device camera interfaced to a computer workstation for image acquisition. A software program integrates the green and red fluorescence signals orthogonally to the chromosomal axis, subtracts local background fluorescence, and calculates the intensity profiles for each color and the ratio of the two colors along individual chromosomes to indicate gains or losses in tumor DNA. A software package is used to compute FITC-rhodamine ratio profiles along chromosomes, such that monosomy of a chromosome in a tumor would theoretically result in a ratio value of 0.5 and trisomy in a value of 1.5. The means of the individual ratio profiles from at least five metaphase spreads per tumor are calculated, and the average values are plotted as profiles alongside individual chromosome ideograms. The three vertical lines beside individual chromosome ideograms indicate different threshold values between tumor DNA and normal reference DNA. The line on the left corresponds to a threshold value of 0.75, which would exist if 50% of the cells from a near diploid tumor had monosomy of a given chromosome. The center line indicates a balanced state. The line on the right represents a threshold value of 1.25, which would occur if 50% of the cell population exhibited trisomy for that chromosome. Overrepresentation defined by a sharp peak is considered indicative of DNA amplification.

Loss of Heterozygosity Analysis

Frequent loss of heterozygosity (LOH) involving a specific chromosomal region, in a given malignancy, is often used as an indicator of the presence of a TSG, whose loss/inactivation can contribute to tumorigenesis. Such analyses of allelic loss are performed using highly polymorphic microsatellite DNA markers. DNA from tumor and blood pairs are amplified using the polymerase chain reaction (PCR) technique with appropriate primer sets. We customarily body label the PCR product with $[^{32}P]$-dCTP. The radiolabeled DNA is then size-fractionated by electrophoresis through a 6% denaturing polyacrylamide gel and subjected to autoradiography. Detailed examination of a series of lung tumors for LOH at various polymorphic loci distributed along a chromosome can reveal a common minimal region of deletion where a putative TSG potentially important in lung tumorigenesis may reside.

KARYOTYPIC CHANGES IN SMALL CELL LUNG CANCER

In SCLCs, karyotypic changes are usually quite extensive, even in newly diagnosed primary tumors. Our laboratory has performed karyotypic analyses of fresh specimens and early passage cell lines from 18 SCLC patients.[8,49] Many

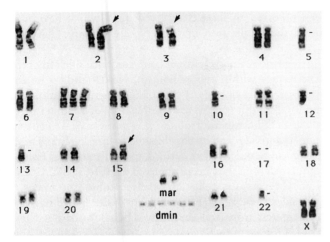

FIGURE 28.1. Karyotype of a Giemsa (G)-banded metaphase spread from a small cell lung cancer (SCLC) cell line that displays multiple cytogenetic alterations, including each of the abnormalities commonly found in SCLC (i.e., losses of 3p, 5q, 13q, 17p) and the presence of double minutes (dmin). An unbalanced translocation exists between 3p and 17q, monosomy 5 and monosomy 13 (numerical losses), and 17q and 15p. Both copies of 17p appear to be lost as a result of the two unbalanced translocations involving the two chromosome 17 homologues. This karyotype also has several other clonal changes, including a structurally altered chromosome 2 (2q+), trisomy 7, and monosomies of chromosomes 10, 12, and 22. Unidentified marker chromosomes (mar) and dmin are shown at the bottom. Arrows indicate structurally rearranged chromosomes 2, 3, and 15. (From Testa JR, Graziano SL. Molecular implications of recurrent cytogenetic alterations in human small cell lung cancer. *Cancer Detection Prevention* 1993;17:267, with permission.)

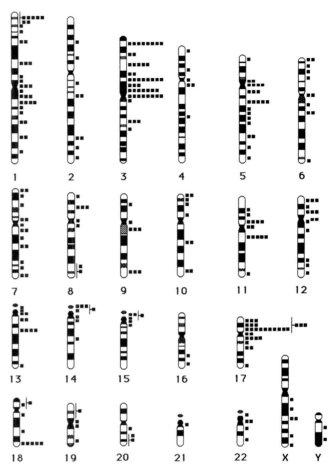

FIGURE 28.2. Ideogram depicting breakpoints (■) of clonal chromosome rearrangements seen in 38 reported small cell lung cancers (SCLCs) (see text). Whenever a single case contained two or more rearrangements with breaks at identical bands, only one of these breakpoints is shown. (From Testa JR, Liu Z, Feder M. Advances in the analysis of chromosome alterations in human lung carcinoma. *Cancer Genet Cytogenet* 1997;95:20, with permission.)

SCLCs have modal chromosome numbers in the triploid range (13 of 18 cases in our series). In many of these cases, most or all of the recurrent chromosome abnormalities described in the following sections occurred in combination (Figure 28.1). The total number of these changes ranged from 11 to more than 60 per tumor.

Figure 28.2 depicts the breakpoint sites of clonal chromosome rearrangements seen in a total of 38 fresh SCLC specimens and early passage SCLC cell lines for which complete karyotypic details have been reported.[6–8,10,49] As shown in Figure 28.2, some chromosomes often participate in structural rearrangements in SCLC; prominent among these are chromosomes 1, 3, 5, and 17. Among the 18 SCLC specimens that we have examined, breakpoints clustered at 3p, 5q, 1p, and 17p. Recurrent losses from each of these arms have been observed.

Chromosome Losses

Loss of 3p

In 1982, Whang-Peng and colleagues reported a nonrandom chromosomal alteration, del(3p), in tumor cells from patients with SCLC.[9] They observed this abnormality in

20 of 20 SCLC cell lines and fresh tumor specimens derived from bone marrow. An interstitial deletion of 3p in SCLC was consistently identified in several other studies as well.[6,8, 11,43,44,50–52] However, in other reports only a minority of SCLC cell lines exhibited a 3p deletion.[10,12,24] DeFusco and colleagues examined fresh SCLC tumors grown in short-term culture and found alterations of 3p in only 5 of 11 cases.[7] However, LOH analysis of 3p markers confirms an almost universal loss of genetic material in this region.[53–55]

Of the 18 SCLC tumors and cell lines that we analyzed, cytogenetic evidence for loss of 3p was found in 16 cases.[8,49] Among cases with structural changes affecting 3p, three had terminal or interstitial deletions, seven had one or more unbalanced derivative chromosomes involving partial loss of 3p [i.e., der(3)], three had an i(3q)(q10), two had both a deletion and either a der(3) or an i(3q), and one near-tetraploid tumor had an i(3q), a der(3), and a numerical loss of 3. Another specimen had an unbalanced translocation derivative in which breakage occurred in the long arm of chromosome 3, resulting in loss of 3pter->q21. The deletions were large in 15 of these 16 cases, with the shortest region of overlap (SRO) of losses being 3p21->25; the remaining case had a derivative with loss of 3p25->pter. Two tumors did not have a visible alteration affecting 3p; LOH analysis performed on one of these cases revealed that allelic losses had occurred at both DNA markers tested, one located at 3p21 and the other at 3p25. Only one of the 18 SCLC specimens did not have a visible structural alteration of chromosome 3. LOH analysis of this case revealed allelic losses at both the DNF15S2 (chromosome band 3p21) and *RAF1* protooncogene (3p25) loci.[8] Taken collectively, the cytogenetic and LOH findings indicate that all 18 of these SCLC cases had losses involving 3p.

At least some of the discrepancies among laboratories may be explained by differences in the interpretation of karyotypes.[44] Thus whereas interstitial or terminal deletions of 3p are not uniformly seen in SCLC, losses of 3p by other mechanisms such as unbalanced translocations or isochromosome formation have a comparable net result.[56] In our series, only five cases had intrachromosomal deletions of 3p (accompanied by another altered chromosome 3 in two cases), and eleven others showed losses of 3p caused by other types of unbalanced rearrangements. The remaining case had allelic losses of 3p that were not evident from the karyotype. The SRO of 3p losses among these cases was found to be at 3p21-p25. In other reports, the SRO has been placed at 3p14-p23,[9] 3p21-p22,[55] or 3p23-p24.[57] Some of these interlaboratory differences can be attributed to difficulties in precisely assigning breakpoints in some cases, particularly when the quality of the chromosome preparation is suboptimal. In contrast to these reports, our interpretation of the minimal 3p deletion extends more distally to 3p25 and agrees with molecular analyses demonstrating consistent LOH at the *RAF1* locus at band 3p25 in SCLC.[44,58,59] In addition, other reports of LOH have demonstrated that almost all SCLC tumors exhibit allelic losses from the chromosomal region 3p14-p21, as well.[53-55] Virmani and colleagues identified three hot spots at 3p12, 3p14.2, and 1p13 in SCLC.[60] In many of their cases, most of the 3p arm was lost. Therefore, the deleted segment in SCLC usually is very large. This consistent allelic loss at 3p strongly supports the hypothesis that one or more TSGs important in the pathogenesis of SCLC reside within this chromosomal region. Several groups have searched for rare homozygous 3p deletions in lung cancers as an approach to locate such a gene(s). At least three distinct regions at homozygous losses have been identified. Rabbits and colleagues identified a homozygous deletion of 3p in the DNA of the SCLC cell line U2020; the deletion removed a chromosomal segment of approximately eight megabases within 3p12-p13.[61-67] Overlapping homozygous deletions have been observed in three SCLC cell lines, which have narrowed the localization of one of these putative TSGs to <350 kb within 3p21.3.[64-67] The semaphorin A(V) gene, which encodes a nerve growth cone guidance signaling protein, resides within this region and was found to be expressed in only one of 23 SCLC cell lines.[65] In addition, mutations of this gene were identified in 3 of 40 lung cancer cell lines. The function of the semaphorin A(V) gene in nonneural tissues and its possible role in lung carcinogenesis remains to be determined. A third, more distal site of homozygous deletions has been observed in several SCLC and NSCLC cell lines as well as in two direct tumor specimens.[64]

Besides these sites of homozygous losses, there has also been interest in several candidate TSGs located elsewhere in 3p. One prominent example is the *FHIT* gene, which encompasses the fragile site *FRA3B,* located at 3p14.2. Sozzi and colleagues reported abnormalities in RNA transcripts of *FHIT* in 80% of SCLCs and 40% of NSCLCs[68] (see also Chapter 8). In addition, 76% of their lung tumors exhibited loss of *FHIT* alleles, and Southern blot analysis revealed rearranged *Bam*HI fragments in several cases. Deletion within intron 5 of the *FHIT* gene was found in 100% of the SCLC cases analyzed by Virani and colleagues.[60] The role of *FHIT* in lung carcinogenesis is currently the subject of intense investigation.

Loss of 5q

We previously reported that alterations of 5q are often involved in SCLC.[8] In addition, our review of karyotypic data presented in two earlier reports revealed losses of 5q in approximately one-half of all SCLC specimens examined.[7,10] Among the 18 SCLC cases that we have analyzed, 16 showed either a numerical loss of chromosome 5, an i(5p) resulting in loss of the entire long arm of chromosome 5, a der(5) resulting in loss of part of 5q, or an interstitial deletion of 5q. In 15 cases, the SRO of deleted segments was 5q13->21; the remaining case had a breakpoint in 5q13, with loss of 5pter->q13. Thus losses involving 5q13 were found in 12 cases overall.

This recurrent loss of 5q13-q21 suggests that this region may contain a TSG contributing to the pathogenesis of SCLC. Several cell-regulatory genes are located at band 5q13, including the gene-encoding phosphatidylinositol-3 kinase-associated protein, p85α, which has been shown to modulate interactions between certain activated receptors and the phosphatidylinositol-3 kinase,[69,70] and the *RASA* locus, which encodes the GTPase-activating protein involved in signal transduction. In addition, the putative TSGs *MCC* and *APC*, which have been shown to be somatically altered in some colorectal tumors, are located at 5q21.[71] Allelic losses of *MCC* and *APC* occur in approximately 80% of SCLCs; however, no mutations or homozygous deletions of these genes have been documented in SCLC.[72]

Loss of 13q

Loss of chromosome 13 has been described in some studies of SCLC.[8,10] Numerical losses of chromosome 13 in the absence of structural change have been observed in 11 of the 18 SCLC cases we examined. Another three cases had structural alterations with breakpoints at 13q14, which is the site of the retinoblastoma susceptibility gene, *RB1*. Thus 14 of our 18 (78%) SCLC cases had changes that affect 13q14. Interestingly, a similar proportion (nearly 80%) of SCLC tumors exhibit absent or very low levels of expression of *RB1*,[73] suggesting that in many SCLC cases, cytogenetic changes could unveil an inactivated *RB1* gene on the remaining, karyotypically normal chromosome 13 homolog.

Loss of 17p

Morstyn and colleagues reported abnormalities of chromosome 17 in eight of ten SCLC cell lines they examined,[10] but the specific types of alterations and breakpoints were not described. In another report, rearrangements of chromosome 17 were described in four of eleven SCLC specimens, including three cases with breakpoints at 17p11-p13 resulting in losses of part of 17p.[7] Loss of part or all of 17p was observed in 14 of 18 specimens from my series. In four of these cases, the only alteration of chromosome 17 was a numerical loss. Another 10 specimens had structural alterations that were interpreted as unbalanced rearrangements that would result in loss of part or all of band 17p13; nine of these specimens had partial deletions or various derivative chromosomes with breakpoints in 17p or proximal 17q, and one tumor had both a dicentric (15p;17p) and a der(17).

Yokota and colleagues reported LOH from 17p in five of five SCLC specimens they examined.[74] *TP53* is located at band 17p13.1 and has been shown to be a common target for molecular alteration in lung cancer.[75,76] The finding of common cytogenetic losses of 17p appears to be consistent with this molecular evidence because a mutated *TP53* allele may exist on the remaining copy of 17p. Virani and colleagues noted allelic losses at the *TP53* locus in all 11 informative SCLC cell lines they examined.[60] Loss of the intron 1 and the telomeric region of the *TP53* gene was documented in 86% of these cases.

Gene Amplification

Dmin and hsr have been reported in some SCLCs, particularly cell lines derived from these tumors. Such novel cytogenetic alterations were reported in 3 of 16 (19%) SCLC cell lines studied by Whang-Peng and colleagues[11] and in 5 of 18 (28%) cases examined by our research group.[8,49] The incidence of dmins may be much higher in SCLC specimens obtained late in the disease course. For example, Wurster-Hill et al. observed dmins or hsrs in 11 of 15 SCLC specimens from heavily pretreated patients with extensive distant metastases; 7 of the 15 samples were obtained at autopsy.[12]

It is now well documented that dmin and hsr are associated with amplification of oncogenes and genes involved in drug resistance.[77,78] Southern blot analysis revealed amplification of specific oncogenes in each of our four cell lines displaying dmin. Two of these cases exhibited a 5- to 10-fold level of amplification of either *MYC* or *MYCN* oncogenes. In each of the latter two cell lines, dmin were observed in a minority of the cells examined cytogenetically. The level of amplification of *MYC* or *MYCN* was approximately 60-fold in the other two cell lines. In each of the latter cases, all of the metaphase spreads examined contained a large hsr or multiple dmin, including a few mitoses with more than 100 of these tiny bodies. FISH of a nonisotopically labeled *MYCN* probe to metaphase cells of the SCLC tumor having −60-fold amplification of this gene demonstrated that the amplified sequences reside within the dmin and hsr.

In SCLC cell lines, amplification of various members of the *MYC* family of oncogenes is relatively common.[79–81] However, such amplification appears to be less common in primary tumors. In a study of primary SCLCs, amplification of *MYC* or *MYCN* was reported in only 5 of 45 (11%) SCLC specimens.[82] In studies carried out in our laboratory, cytogenetic evidence for gene amplification was found in four of our eight established cell lines, but in only one of twelve fresh specimens. Among the four patients whose tumor cells contained dmin and hsr, three received prior cytotoxic therapy. Overall, such cytogenetic alterations were identified in four of six specimens from previously treated patients versus only one of twelve (8%) from untreated patients. Similarly, Brennan and colleagues detected amplification of one of the *MYC* family genes in 28% of tumor specimens from previously treated SCLC patients, compared to only 8% of specimens from untreated patients.[83] This finding and the relatively low incidence of *MYC* family gene amplification in primary tumors[82] implies that such amplification is unlikely to represent an initial, transformation-related event in SCLC.

KARYOTYPIC CHANGES IN NON–SMALL CELL LUNG CANCER

In NSCLC, cytogenetic changes are often extensive, with many numerical and structural changes. We have carried out detailed cytogenetic analyses of primary tumors from 70 NSCLC patients.[34] Only three of these tumors had fewer than 10 clonal chromosomal changes, and some tumors showed as many as 60 to 70 different structural and numerical changes. The number of cytogenetic changes per tumor was similar among different histologic subgroups. Other large series have also demonstrated numerous chromosomal alterations in most primary NSCLC cases.[15,16,31,35–37]

In some karyotypic studies of NSCLC, only clones displaying a single numerical change (i.e., gain of chromosomes 7 or 12) were observed.[13,18,22] The significance of these findings is uncertain because cell populations carrying an extra chromosome 7 as the only karyotypic change have been described in cultures from several malignant disorders of the bladder, brain, colon, and kidney as well as in cultured cells from nonneoplastic tissue obtained from the lung, brain, kidney, and placenta and in patients with Dupuytren contracture or Peyronie disease.[84,85] In some series, approximately 10% of cultured cells from all nonneoplastic kidney samples examined displayed trisomy 7,[84,85] and trisomy 7 and trisomy 10 have been shown to characterize subpopulations of tumor-infiltrating lymphocytes in kidney tumors and in the surrounding kidney tissue.[86] In ovarian cancer, trisomy 12 has been found to represent a recurrent chromosome aberration in benign ovarian tumors, particularly in fibromas, rather than in tumors of epithelial origin.[87] Thus in NSCLC it is presently unclear whether clones exhibiting simple karyotypes with gains of either chromosome 7 or chromosome 12 actually reflect changes in the malignant cell population. Johansson and colleagues reported pseudodiploid karyotypes with one or a few clonal structural rearrangements in two adenosquamous carcinomas, leading them to conclude that this relatively rare histologic subtype differs from other lung cancers by having simple pseudodiploid or near-diploid instead of massively aneuploid tumor cells.[22]

Among our 70 NSCLC cases, the modal chromosome number was near-diploid in 18 cases (26%), near-triploid in 40 cases (57%), and near-tetraploid to near-hexaploid in 12 cases (17%). Near-triploidy was the most common ploidy in each of the histologic categories (45% of adenocarcinomas, 63% of squamous cell carcinomas, and 83% of other NSCLCs).

Overall, the available data indicate that karyotypes in NSCLC generally are very complicated, even in newly diagnosed primary tumors. We have focused investigations on samples obtained prior to initiating cytotoxic therapy. Thus the complicated cytogenetic pattern seen in these cases appears to be part of the natural course of NSCLC. Moreover, it is unlikely that this genomic complexity can be attributed to *in vitro* karyotypic evolution because most of our analyses were from relatively short-term cultures of tumor cells.

Numerical Changes

In NSCLC, all chromosomes contribute to numerical changes. In our series of 70 cases, losses of chromosomes 9 (47 cases, 67%) and 13 (45 cases, 64%) were the two most common numerical changes. Loss of the Y chromosome was observed in 29 of 49 (59%) tumors from male patients. Gain of chromosome 7 was also a common numerical change (28 of 70 cases, 40%). Other chromosomes commonly involved in numerical gains were numbers 5 and 12, each of which was identified in approximately 20% of the

cases examined. Polysomy for all or part of chromosome 7 in NSCLC has been reported at varying frequencies by several investigators.[13–15,19,25,33,35–37] Lee and colleagues proposed that trisomy 7 is a very early change in NSCLC that can be found in premalignant lung tissue in a subset of patients.[13] Lukeis and colleagues reported loss of material from the short arm of chromosome 9 in nine of ten NSCLCs suggesting that this change is a potentially important event in lung carcinogenesis.[15] In other reports, common numerical losses of chromosome 9 have been described.[14,38] Losses of chromosomes 13 and Y have also been observed in other studies of primary NSCLC.[14,15]

Structural Abnormalities

Balanced translocations are rarely reported in NSCLCs, whereas losses resulting from missing chromosomes or unbalanced rearrangements (i.e., deletions and derivative chromosomes) are often observed. Figure 28.3 depicts 1,826 breakpoint sites of clonal chromosome rearrangements seen in short-term cultures from 185 primary NSCLC specimens for which complete karyotypic details are available. Included in this summary are data from 70 specimens examined in our laboratory and 115 cases reported by other investigators.[13–15,17–23,35–37] The most common sites of chromosomal breakage were at or near the heterochromatic centromere regions of chromosomes 1, 3, 5, 6, 7, 8, 9, 11, 13, 14, 15, and 17. Other regions of chromosomes 1, 3, 6, 7, 9p, 11, and 19 were also prone to rearrangement.

The chromosome arm most often contributing to losses was 9p (59 of 70 tumors, 84%). Other chromosome arms lost in at least 60% of cases included 3p, 6q, 8p, 9q, 13q, 17p, 18q, 19p, 21q, 22q, and the short arms of each of the acrocentric chromosomes. The chromosome arms most often involved in gains were 7p and 7q. Among the entire 70 tumors, gains of part or all of 7p and 7q were observed in 61% and 60% of cases, respectively. Extra copies of chromosome arms 1p, 1q, 3q, 5p, 11q, and 12q were also common.

We evaluated the relationship between clonal chromosome alterations and various clinical parameters in 70 NSCLC patients for whom detailed karyotypic assessment was possible.[88] Clinical features investigated were diagnosis, tumor stage and grade, gender, smoking history measured in pack-years, and survival. Certain chromosome abnormalities were significantly associated with histologic subtype, tumor grade, stage, and prognosis. Rearrangements involving chromosome arms 2p and 3q were more common in squamous cell carcinoma than in adenocarcinoma. Loss of 3p was observed more often in squamous cell carcinomas. Gain of 7p was more common in adenocarcinomas. Rearrangement of 17p was associated with a lower tumor grade. Rearrangement of Xp and loss of chromosome 12 or 22 were each associated with higher tumor stage. Rearrangement of

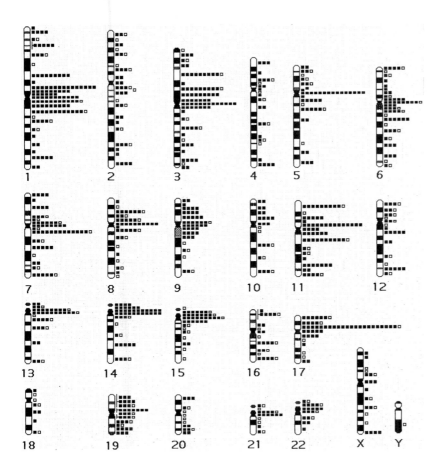

FIGURE 28.3. Ideogram showing breakpoints of clonal chromosome rearrangements seen in short-term cultures of primary tumor specimens from 185 non–small cell lung cancers (NSCLCs). Each closed box (■) represents breakpoints in two different cases; each open box (□) indicates a breakpoint from a single case. Whenever a single case had two or more rearrangements with breaks at the same band, only one of these breakpoints is depicted. (From Testa JR, Liu Z, Feder M. Advances in the analysis of chromosome alterations in human lung carcinoma. *Cancer Genet Cytogenet* 1997;95:20, with permission.)

3p or 6q was correlated with a better survival outlook. In contrast, loss of chromosomes 4 or 22 portended a poor prognosis. An increased number of marker chromosomes was observed in patients having a higher number of pack-years. Overall, our data indicate that chromosome abnormalities can have clinical and pathologic significance in NSCLC.

Chromosome Losses

Loss of 3p

Loss of all or part of the short arm of 3 was identified in approximately 75% of the NSCLC cases that we examined. LOH from 3p has been reported in 25% to 100% of NSCLC cases in different reports.[54,55,74,89–91] The SRO of chromosome losses appears to be at 3p21.[34] Allelic loss at 3p21 has been reported in all major types of lung cancer.[54,55] However, LOH from 3p can occur at a significantly higher frequency in squamous cell carcinomas than in adenocarcinomas.[92] Although deletion of 3p14-p23 was initially reported as a specific chromosome aberration in SCLC,[8] subsequent studies have revealed frequent deletions

of 3p in several other malignancies, including renal cell carcinoma, mesothelioma, ovarian cancer, and breast cancer.[3] Thus loss of 3p may represent an important generalized tumorigenic event common to various solid tumors, including NSCLC.

Loss of 9p

As noted earlier, 9p was the most common lost chromosome segment in our NSCLC series, and deletion of 9p has been proposed as a critical change in this neoplasm.[15] Only a minority of our cases had either an interstitial deletion or terminal deletion of 9p, but many other tumors had either an apparently unbalanced rearrangement (i.e., various derivatives) affecting 9p or had less than the expected number of copies of chromosome 9 (e.g., only two copies of chromosome 9 in a triploid tumor). Homozygous losses of DNA sequences from 9p21-p22 have been reported in some NSCLCs, suggesting that loss or inactivation of a TSG(s) located within this region may contribute to the pathogenesis of some of these tumors.[93] The TSG *p16/CDKN2A* is located at 9p21, and homozygous deletions or mutations of this gene occur in many NSCLC cell lines and in 20% to 30% of tumor specimens from NSCLC patients.[94,95]

Loss of 17p

Rearrangement of 17p is a very common finding in NSCLC. In fact, 17p11 represents the most common chromosomal breakpoint site in karyotypic studies of NSCLC (Figure 28.3). The structural changes of 17p include partial deletions and various derivative chromosomes. DNA analyses have demonstrated that loss of alleles from 17p is a common occurrence in NSCLC.[89] Our data suggest that visible cytogenetic changes may be the cause of the allelic loss detected by molecular methods, at least in some cases. As in SCLC, the cytogenetic and molecular evidence suggests that loss of 17p containing a normal *TP53* allele could unmask a remaining, mutant allele on the other remaining, cytogenetically normal homolog.

Other Abnormalities

Isochromosomes

Although no nonrandom balanced reciprocal translocations have been reported in NSCLC, several recurrent isochromosomes have been found. In our studies, the most common isochromosome was an i(5p), which was observed in nine tumors, eight of which had adenomatous features. An i(8q) was identified in six of our NSCLC cases, including five adenocarcinomas and one large cell lung carcinoma. Several other groups have also reported isochromosomes of 5p and 8q in NSCLC.[14,15,19,27,28,30,31] Other isochromosomes seen in our series of NSCLCs include i(1q), i(3q), i(6p), i(7p), i(13q), and i(14q), each seen in several cases.

An association between i(8q) and adenocarcinoma of the lung has been reported by several investigators.[19,96] Even though i(8q) and i(5p) appear to be recurrent changes in adenocarcinoma of the lung, they are not specific for this tumor. An i(8q) has been reported in various types of leukemia and in several different solid tumors; likewise, i(5p) has been observed in several different solid malignancies and appears to be particularly common in tumors of the uterus and bladder.[3] Among the SCLC cases studied by our laboratory, one case had an i(5p) and another had an i(8q).[8] It has been suggested that i(8q) could represent a primary change in NSCLC.[19] However, in a NSCLC cell line that we studied, the only abnormality of chromosome 8 found at passage 9 was trisomy 8, whereas at a later passage, a minority of cells contained two normal homologs and an i(8q).[16] In addition, i(8q) was found in only a single cell or in a minority of karyotyped cells in another two cases. Taken collectively, these findings suggest that i(8q) may be a secondary event in NSCLC.

Gene Amplification

Variable numbers of dmins were seen in 7 of our 70 (10%) specimens. Two cases had an hsr, including one of the seven cases that had dmins. Tumor material was available for Southern blot analysis in five of our eight NSCLC cases that exhibited dmins, hsrs, or both. The DNA studies revealed amplification of *MYC* in two cases and *EGFR* in one case. Eight different oncogene probes were tested in the other two cases, but an amplified sequence was not identified. In two other series of NSCLC specimens examined by Southern blot analysis, amplification of the *MYC* oncogene was documented in 3 of 36 (8%) and 4 of 25 (16%) cases.[97,98] Amplification of *KRAS2* has also been reported in a case of NSCLC having dmins.[99]

Metastatic Tumors

Two series focused on karyotypic changes in metastatic tumors from NSCLC patients.[31,33] In one study of NSCLC cell lines mostly derived from metastatic lesions, statistical analysis revealed that structural alterations were nonrandomly distributed among the chromosomes.[31] A statistically significant number of clonal breakpoints were observed at chromosome regions 1q1, 1q3, 3p1, 3p2, 3q1, 3q2, 7q1, 13p1, 14p1, 15p1, and 17q1. Most of these regions undergo frequent rearrangement in primary tumors as well, although breakage at 1q3 does not appear to be a prominent change in primary tumors (Figure 28.3). Furthermore, breakage at 5cen, 6p1->6q1, 8cen->8p1, 9p2, 11p1->11q1, 17p1, and 19p1 appeared to be much less common in these metastatic tumors than in primary tumors. Whether these discrepancies are caused by karyotypic evolution during tumor progression, evolution occurring during prolonged growth *in vitro,* or difference in cytogenetic interpretation is uncertain at this time.

In the second report, pleural effusions containing metastatic or invasive tumor cells were examined.[33] Recurrent breakpoint regions included 1p1, 3p10-p21, 3q11-q25, 6p11-p25, 6q13-q23, 7q11-q36, 9q32-q34, 11p1, 11q13-q24, 13p, 14p, 15p, 17p, and 19p. Most of these regions are also often involved in primary tumors, although breakage at 3q11-q25 and 6p11-p25 has not been reported to be nonrandomly involved in primary tumors. A lower frequency of 9p loss was observed in pleural effusions than in primary tumors, whereas breakpoints at 9q32-q34 were found almost exclusively in effusions and, therefore, could represent a change associated with tumor progression.[33] Four other metastatic tumors from NSCLC patients have been reported to have a breakpoint at this region.[30,31] Lukeis and colleagues also observed that loss of chromosome 8 or 8p, loss of Y, and rearrangement of 5q are less common in effusions than in primary tumors, whereas extra or rearranged chromosome 7, extra chromosome 20, loss of chromosome 22, and dmin occur at a higher frequency in effusions than in primary tumors.[15,33]

MOLECULAR CYTOGENETICS

Fluorescence *In Situ* Hybridization Analysis

Although technical advances in cell culture and cytogenetics have improved the overall success rate and quality of chromosome studies in lung cancer, it has not been possible to examine karyotypes of the malignant cells in every specimen. In many cases, the mitotic rate of the tumor cells is very low, and analyzable abnormal metaphase spreads are not found. Karyotypic analysis is time consuming, and it is not feasible to routinely cut out karyotypes of large numbers of metaphase spreads. Furthermore, *in vitro* culturing of tumor cells may result in selective growth of cells that may not represent the whole tumor cell population. FISH can overcome many of these problems. This procedure permits investigators to directly examine interphase cells from

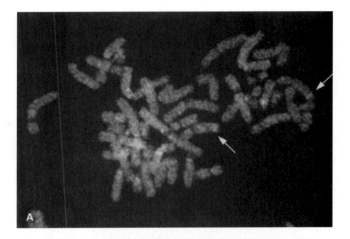

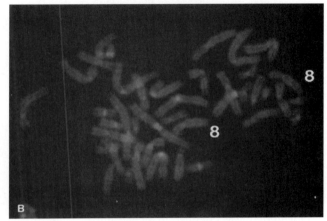

FIGURE 28.5. **A:** Computer-generated fluorescence ratio image of a normal human metaphase spread after comparative genome hybridization with biotin-labeled DNA, detected by fluorescein isothiocyanate (FITC), from a lung cancer cell line, and digoxigenin-labeled DNA, detected by rhodamine, from normal placenta. Yellow-green indicates balance between the FITC and rhodamine values. Bright green indicates overrepresentation of DNA in the tumor, and red represents underrepresentation of tumor DNA. Intense green fluorescence on chromosome 8q24 (*arrows*) suggests that the MYC protooncogene located in this band may be amplified in the lung cancer cells. **B:** The same metaphase spread, stained with diamidino-2-phenylindole, which permits the identification of each chromosome. The two copies of chromosome 8 are indicated by numbers. (See Color Figure 28.5.)

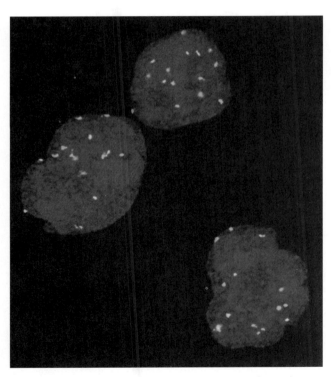

FIGURE 28.4. Fluorescence *in situ* hybridization of two chromosome-specific centromere repeat probes to interphase cell nuclei, counterstained blue with diamidino-2-phenylindole, from a human non-small cell lung cancer specimen. DNA probes labeled with biotin or digoxigenin hybridizing to complementary centromere sequences within the nuclei were detected by immunofluorescence using fluorophores emitting green (fluorescein isothiocyanate) or red (rhodamine). The nuclei exhibit abnormally high numbers of chromosome 7 (red spots) and chromosome 18 (green) fluorescent signals, indicative of gains of these chromosomes. (See Color Figure 28.4.)

tissue sections or cell suspensions of tumor specimens. Because of the relative ease of analyzing FISH preparations, it is possible to rapidly count the number of target sites in a large number of tumor cells. In addition to enhancing karyologic investigations of tumor specimens, such interphase cytogenetics techniques may represent a useful approach to assess "noninvolved" bronchial tissues and premalignant lesions for the presence of cells with early (primary) chromosome changes. Example of FISH analyses are seen in Figures 28.4, 28.5, and 28.6.

To determine the feasibility of FISH for the analysis of genetic changes in lung cancer, we used a panel of centro-

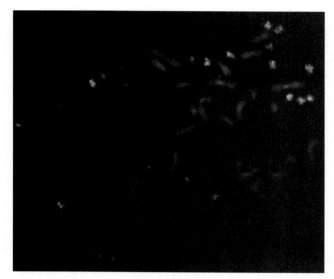

FIGURE 28.6. Fluorescence *in situ* hybridization of a MYCN probe to a partial metaphase spread from the small cell lung cancer cell line. Multiple fluorescent signals are observed on each of the double minutes, indicating that the amplified *MYCN* oncogene resides within these small chromatin bodies. (See Color Figure 28.6.)

meric DNA probes specific for the autosomes 6, 7, 8, 9, 12, 17, and 18 to analyze 17 primary NSCLCs.[100] Evidence for aneuploidy was obtained in all specimens. Gain of part or all of chromosome 7 was especially prominent, occurring in a large population of cells in each of 14 tumors (82%). Extra centromeric copies of chromosomes 6, 12, and 17 were also common, being observed in nine to eleven cases each. Gain of chromosome 9 was infrequent three tumors). In two cases, most of the nuclei had only a single chromosome 9 fluorescent signal. Karyotypic findings were available for six cases and were generally consistent with the FISH data. Both methods revealed considerable heterogeneity within individual tumors. NSCLC specimens from 26 males were assayed with a Y-specific centromeric sequence; loss of the Y was observed in 13 cases (50%). These investigations demonstrate the feasibility of interphase FISH for the successful analysis of numerical chromosome changes in NSCLCs.

Comparative Genomic Hybridization Analysis

Reid and colleagues performed a CGH analysis of 13 primary SCLC specimens.[101] They demonstrated frequent chromosome losses expected in this tumor type (i.e., 3p-, 13q-, and 17p-), as well as several recurrent abnormalities that had not been recognized in previous karyotypic studies of SCLC: 4q-, 10q-, and amplification of 19q13. In another

CGH analysis of 18 SCLC cell lines, Levin and colleagues observed recurrent decreases in the copy number of 3p, 13q, and 17p.[102] These investigators also identified overrepresentation of the chromosomal sites 1p22->32, 2p24->25, and 8q24, sites of the genes *MYCL, MYCN,* and *MYC,* respectively, which are often amplified in SCLC cell lines. Novel copy number increases were detected at 5p, 1q24, and Xq26, and decreases involved 22q12.1->13.1, 10q26, and 16p11.2. Some of the DNA copy number changes, including gains of 1p22->32, 2p24->25, and 3q22->25 and loss of 18p, were found to occur preferentially in "variant" SCLC lines, suggesting that genes may reside at these sites whose overexpression or inactivation contributes to the radiation-resistant phenotype or aggressive growth properties characteristic of this SCLC subtype. An example of amplification of 2p24-p25 in an SCLC cell line with 60-fold amplification of *MYCN* is shown in Figure 28.7. Levin and colleagues also used CGH to identify DNA copy number changes in seven primary tumors and three metastases from

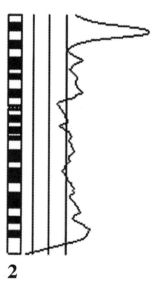

2

FIGURE 28.7. Comparative genomic hybridization (CGH) analysis of chromosome 2 from a small cell lung cancer (SCLC) cell line displaying amplification of 2p23.3-p24, encompassing the site of the *MYCN* locus at 2p24. Most of the remainder of chromosome 2 is overrepresented, whereas the distal portion of the long arm of 2q is underrepresented. Southern blot analysis demonstrated that *MYCN* is amplified approximately 60-fold in this cell line (not shown). CGH ratio profile represents the average fluorescence ratios calculated for chromosome 2 from a total of five metaphase spreads. Note that the three vertical lines beside individual chromosome ideograms indicate different threshold values between tumor DNA and normal reference DNA. The line on the left represents the threshold value corresponding to a chromosomal loss. The center line indicates a balanced state. The line on the right represents the threshold value corresponding to a chromosomal gain. Overrepresentation defined by a sharp peak is considered indicative of DNA amplification. (From Testa JR, Liu Z, Feder M. Advances in the analysis of chromosome alterations in human lung carcinoma. *Cancer Genet Cytogenet* 1997;95:20, with permission.)

eight SCLC patients.[103] Frequent overrepresentation of chromosome arms 5p, 8q, 3q, and Xq, and underrepresentation of chromosome arms 3p, 17p, 5q, 8p, 10q, 13q, and 4p were identified, confirming the existence of many of the chromosome changes previously identified by conventional karyotypic analysis of SCLC lines. Each of the reports of CGH analyses of SCLCs has identified a recurrent region of chromosomal loss at 10q24->26, suggesting that a putative TSG important in the pathogenesis of SCLC may reside at this location.

Recently, a putative TSG *PTEN/MMAC1* was identified at 10q23.3 and found to be deleted or mutated in a wide variety of human malignancies such as glioma, melanoma meningioma, glioblastoma, and carcinomas of the prostate, breast, and kidney. Yokomizo and colleagues found alterations in *PTEN/MMCA1,* gene in 18% of SCLC cell lines and in 10% of primary SCLC samples.[104] These abnormalities included point mutations, small fragment deletions, and large homozygous deletions. None of the 23 NSCLC specimens and cell lines tested displayed alterations of *PTEN/MMCA1,* suggesting that the inactivation of this

gene contributes to the pathogenesis of SCLC but not NSCLC.

We performed CGH analysis on 20 NSCLC biopsies and cell lines to identify recurrent chromosomal imbalances in this malignancy.[105] The chromosome arms most often overrepresented were 3q (85%), 5p (70%), 7p (65%), and 8q (65%), which were observed at high copy numbers in many cases. Other common overrepresented sites were 1q, 2p, and 20p. DNA sequence amplification was often observed, with the most common site being 3q26 (six cases). Other recurrent sites of amplification included 8q24, 3q13, 3q28-qter, 7q11.2, 8p11-12, 12p12, and 19q13.1-13.2. The most common underrepresented segment was 3p21 (50%); other recurrent sites of autosomal loss included 8p21-pter, 15q11.2-13, 5q11.2-15, 9p, 13q12-14, 17p, and 18q21-qter (Figure 28.8). These regions of copy number decreases are also common sites of allelic loss, further implicating these sites as locations of TSGs. Although some of the overrepresented segments harbor known or suspected oncogenes/growth-regulatory genes, we have identified 3q and 5p as new sites that are often overrepresented in

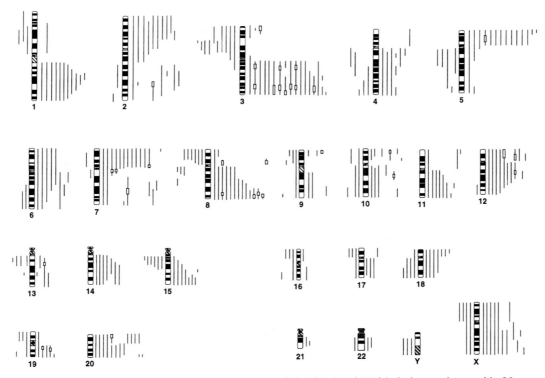

FIGURE 28.8. Summary of comparative genomic hybridization (CGH) imbalances detected in 20 non–small cell lung cancer (NSCLC) tumor specimens and early passage cell lines. Vertical lines on the left of each chromosome ideogram represent loss of genetic material in a given tumor, whereas those on the right correspond to gains. For each chromosome, smaller copy number aberrations (CNAs) are placed farthest from the ideogram for ease of identification of minimal regions of overlap (e.g., overrepresentation at 1q25–31, 2p16–21, 3q26–qter, 8q24, and 12p11.2–12). (From Balsara B, Sonoda G, du Manoir S, et al. Comparative genomic analysis detects frequent, often high-level overrepresentation of DNA sequences at 3q, 5p, 7p, and 8q in human non-small cell lung carcinoma. *Cancer Res* 1997;57:2116, with permission.)

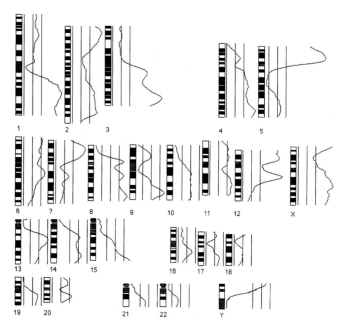

FIGURE 28.9. CGH fluorescence ratio profile of a non–small cell lung cancer (NSCLC) cell line showing the recurrent alterations observed in NSCLC. Overrepresentation of part or all of chromosome arms 1q, 2p, 2q, 3q, 4q, 5p, 7p, 8q, 12p, and amplification of 3q13, 3q26–27, 8p11.2, 8q24, 9q33, 12q14–15, and underrepresentation of part or all of 8p, 9p. The profile represents the average fluorescence ratios calculated for each chromosome from a total of 10 metaphase spreads.

NSCLC. Many of the common genomic imbalances occurred in combination in a given tumor (Figure 28.9).

Petersen and colleagues carried out CGH analyses on 50 NSCLCs (25 adenocarcinomas and 25 squamous cell carcinomas).[106] The chromosome arms most often underrepresented were 1p, 3p, 4q, 5q, 6q, 8p, 9p, 13q, 18q, and 21q. The chromosomal sites most often overrepresented were 5p, 8q, 11q13, 16p, 17q, and 19q. Adenocarcinomas showed more common gains of chromosome 1q and losses of chromosomes 3q, 9q, 10p, and 19, whereas squamous cell carcinomas were characterized by an increased incidence of gains of chromosome arms 3q and 12p as well as losses of chromosome arm 2q. These investigators also reported a correlation between 20q13 gain and invasiveness in adenocarcinomas.

Gains of 1q, 3q, 5p, and 8q and loss of 3p were each observed in at least 50% of cases in each of these two CGH studies. Overrepresentation of 3q26 was the most prominent change observed, which appears to be particularly common in squamous cell carcinomas. Amplification of 3q26 was identified in three of nine squamous cell carcinomas of the lung analyzed by reverse chromosome painting.[107] Moreover, increased copy number at 3q26-27 has also been reported as a recurrent change in various other tumors including SCLCs,[101] ovarian cancers,[108] and advanced cervi-

cal carcinomas.[109] A candidate gene located at 3q26.3, whose product may contribute to the control of cell proliferation and malignant transformation, is *PIK3CA*. *PIK3CA* encodes the catalytic subunit of phosphatidylinositol-3 kinase, a critical component of several cell signaling pathways including those of epidermal growth factor and platelet-derived growth factor. *SKP2,* a potentially relevant gene located in 5p, encodes a protein associated with the CDK2–cyclin A complex. This protein has been found to be essential for S-phase entry.

CONCLUSIONS

Classic and molecular cytogenetic analysis has demonstrated that numerous somatic genetic events are involved in the pathogenesis of lung carcinomas. The karyotypes of these neoplasms often have extensive changes, even in newly diagnosed primary tumors, but the pattern and biologic implications of recurrent chromosome alterations are beginning to emerge. Chromosomal losses are often observed, and some of these changes (e.g., deletions of 3p, 5q, 10q, and 17p in SCLC; deletions of 3p, 9p, and 17p in NSCLC) occur at the location of known or suspected TSGs, whose loss and/or inactivation may play a fundamental role in lung tumorigenesis. Other alterations (e.g., dmins, hsrs) represent cytogenetic manifestations of oncogene amplification, and the net effect of such changes may be an increase in a gene product that provides an added proliferative advantage. Other chromosomal imbalances, (e.g., gains of 1q, 3q, 5p, 7, and 8q in NSCLC) could have a similar effect. The complex pattern of cytogenetic changes often seen in newly diagnosed lung carcinomas emphasizes the need for future investigations of "normal" bronchus or premalignant lesions in order to identify primary genetic changes important for early detection and intervention in this aggressive neoplasm.

In future cytogenetic investigations, it will be important to determine whether such genomic imbalances are correlated with clinical parameters such as metastatic behavior and prognosis. Furthermore, as the understanding of chromosome alterations in lung cancer increases, it should be possible to establish a useful panel of nonisotopic DNA probes to facilitate the rapid diagnostic assessment of lung tumor specimens. Germane to this achievement, considerable recent excitement has been generated regarding emerging microarray technologies.[110–112] It will now be possible to develop gridded arrays of relevant genomic fragments to quickly assess individual tumors for mutations or DNA copy at precise chromosomal locations. Similarly, arrays of cDNAs will facilitate comparisons of gene expression profiles of malignant versus normal lung tissues.

ACKNOWLEDGEMENTS

This work was supported by NIH grants CA-58184 and CA-06927, by an appropriation from the Commonwealth of Pennsylvania, and by a gift from the Ann Ricci Memorial Fund.

REFERENCES

1. Heim S, Mitelman F. *Cancer cytogenetics,* 2nd ed. New York: Alan R. Liss, 1995.
2. Sandberg AA. *The chromosomes in human cancer and leukemia,* 2nd ed. New York: Elsevier North Holland, 1990.
3. Mitelman F. *Catalog of chromosome aberrations in cancer,* 5th ed. New York: Alan R. Liss, 1994.
4. Fearon ER, Vogelsten B. A genetic model for colorectal tumorigenesis. *Cell* 1990;61:759.
5. Landis SH, Murray T, Bolden S, et al. Cancer statistic, 1998. *CA—Cancer J Clinicians* 1998;48:6.
6. Sozzi G, Bertoglio MG, Borrello MG, et al. Chromosomal abnormalities in a primary small cell lung cancer. *Cancer Genet Cytogenet* 1987;27:45.
7. DeFusco PA, Frytak S, Dahl RJ, et al. Cytogenetic studies in 11 patients with small cell carcinoma of the lung. *Mayo Clin Proc* 1989;64:168.
8. Miura I, Graziano SL, Cheng JQ, et al. Chromosome alterations in small cell lung cancer: frequent involvement of 5q. *Cancer Res* 1992;52:1322.
9. Whang-Peng J, Kao-Shan CS, Lee EC, et al. Specific chromosome defect associated with human small-cell lung cancer: deletion of 3p(14-23). *Science* 1982;215:181.
10. Morstyn G, Brown J, Novak U, et al. Heterogeneous cytogenetic abnormalities in small cell lung cancer cell lines. *Cancer Res* 1987;47:3322.
11. Whang-Peng J, Bunn PA Jr, Kao-Shan CS, et al. A nonrandom chromosomal abnormality, del 3p(14-23), in human small cell lung cancer (SCLC). *Cancer Genet Cytogenet* 1982;6:119.
12. Wurster-Hill DH, Cannizzaro LA, Pettengill OS, et al. Cytogenetics of small cell carcinoma of the lung. *Cancer Genet Cytogenet* 1984;13:303.
13. Lee JS, Pathak S, Hopwood V, et al. Involvement of chromosome 7 in primary lung tumor and nonmalignant normal lung tissue. *Cancer Res* 1987;47:6349.
14. Viegas-Pequignot E, Flury-Herard A, De Cremoux H, et al. Recurrent chromosome aberrations in human lung squamous cell carcinomas. *Cancer Genet Cytogenet* 1990;49:37.
15. Lukeis R, Irving L, Garson M, et al. Cytogenetics of non-small cell lung cancer: analysis of consistent non-random abnormalities. *Genes Chrom Cancer* 1990;2:116.
16. Miura I, Siegfried JM, Resau J, et al. Chromosome alterations in 21 non-small cell lung carcinomas. *Genes Chrom Cancer* 1990;2:328.
17. Flury-Herard A, Viegas-Pequignot E, De Cremoux H, et al. Cytogenetic study of five cases of lung adenosquamous carcinomas. *Cancer Genet Cytogenet* 1992;59:1.
18. Liang JC, Kurzrock R, Gutterman JU, et al. Trisomy 12 correlates with elevated expression of p21^{ras} in a human adenosquamous carcinoma of the lung. *Cancer Genet Cytogenet* 1986;23:183.
19. Jin Y, Mandahl N, Heim S, et al. Isochromosomes i(8q) or i(9q) in three adenocarcinomas of the lung. *Cancer Genet Cytogenet* 1988;33:11.
20. Ronne M, Elberg JJ, Shibasaki Y, et al. A case of squamous cell lung carcinoma with tetrasomy 7 and chromosome 1 C-band polymorphism. *Anticancer Res* 1989;9:1101.
21. Pejovic T, Heim S, Orndal C, et al. Simple numerical chromosome aberrations in well-differentiated malignant epithelial tumors. *Cancer Genet Cytogenet* 1990;49:95.
22. Johansson M, Jin Y, Heim S, et al. Pseudodiploid karyotypes in adenosquamous carcinomas of the lung. *Cancer Genet Cytogenet* 1992;63:95.
23. Drouin V, Viguie F, Debesse B. Near-haploid karyotype in a squamous cell lung carcinoma. *Genes Chrom Cancer* 1993;7:209.
24. Zech L, Bergh J, Nilsson K. Karyotypic characterization of established cell lines and short-term cultures of human lung cancers. *Cancer Genet Cytogenet* 1985;15:335.
25. Fan Y-S, Li P. Cytogenetic studies of four human lung adenocarcinoma cell lines. *Cancer Genet Cytogenet* 1987;26:317.
26. Rey JA, Bello MJ, de Campos JM, et al. Deletion 3p in two lung adenocarcinomas metastatic to the brain. *Cancer Genet Cytogenet* 1987;25:355.
27. Bello MJ, Moreno S, Rey JA. Involvement of chromosomes 1, 3, and i(8q) in lung adenocarcinoma. *Cancer Genet Cytogenet* 1989;38:133.
28. Cagle PT, Taylor LD, Schwartz MR, et al. Cytogenetic abnormalities common to adenocarcinoma metastatic to the pleura. *Cancer Genet Cytogenet* 1989;39:219.
29. Kadowaki MH, Ferguson MK. The role of chromosome 3 deletions in lung cancer. *Lung Cancer* 1990;6:165.
30. Erdel M, Peter W, Spiess E, et al. Karyotypic characterization of established cell lines derived from a squamous cell carcinoma and an adenocarcinoma of human lung cancers. *Cancer Genet Cytogenet* 1990;49:185.
31. Whang-Peng J, Knutsen T, Gazdar A, et al. Non-random structural and numerical chromosome changes in non-small-cell lung cancer. *Genes Chrom Cancer* 1991;3:168.
32. Law E, Gilvarry U, Lynch V, et al. Cytogenetic comparison of two poorly differentiated human lung squamous cell carcinoma lines. *Cancer Genet Cytogenet* 1992;59:111.
33. Lukeis R, Ball D, Irving L, et al. Chromosome abnormalities in non-small cell lung cancer pleural effusions: cytogenetic indicators of disease subgroups. *Genes Chrom Cancer* 1993;8:262.
34. Testa JR, Siegfried JM, Liu Z, et al. Cytogenetic analysis of 63 non-small cell lung carcinomas: recurrent chromosome alterations amid frequent and widespread genomic upheaval. *Genes Chrom Cancer* 1994;11:178.
35. Johansson M, Dietrich C, Mandahl N, et al. Karyotypic characterization of bronchial large cell carcinomas. *Int J Cancer* 1994;57:463.
36. Johansson M, Karauzum SB, Dietrich C, et al. Karyotypic abnormalities in adenocarcinomas of the lung. *Inter J Oncol* 1994;5:17.
37. Johansson M, Jin Y, Mandahl N, et al. Cytogenetic analysis of short-term cultured squamous cell carcinomas of the lung. *Cancer Genet Cytogenet* 1995;81:46.
38. Testa JR, Siegfried JM. Chromosome abnormalities in non-small cell lung cancer. *Cancer Res* 1992;52:2702.
39. Kallioniemi A, Kallioniemi OP, Sudar D, et al. Comparative genomic hybridization for molecular cytogenetic analysis of solid tumors. *Science* 1992;258:818.
40. Siegfried JM, Hunt JD, Zhou J-Y, et al. Cytogenetic abnormalities in non-small cell lung carcinoma: similarity of findings in conventional and feeder cell layer cultures. *Genes Chrom Cancer* 1993;6:30.
41. Siegfried JM, Ellison DJ, Resau JH, et al. Correlation of modal chromosome number of cultured non-small cell lung carcinomas with DNA index of solid tumor tissue. *Cancer Res* 1991;51:3267.
42. Carney DN, Gazdar AF, Bepler G, et al. Establishment and identification of small cell lung cancer cell lines having classic and variant features. *Cancer Res* 1985;45:2913.
43. Graziano SL, Cowan BY, Carney DN, et al. Small cell lung

cancer cell line derived from a primary tumor with a characteristic deletion of 3p. *Cancer Res* 1987;47:2148.

44. Graziano SL, Pfeifer AM, Testa JR, et al. The involvement of the RAF1 locus, at band 3p25, in the 3p deletion of small-cell lung cancer. *Genes Chrom Cancer* 1991;3:283.

45. ISCN (1991). *Guidelines for cancer cytogenetics, supplement to an international system for human cytogenetic nomenclature.* Mitelman F, ed. Basel: S Karger, 1991.

46. ISCN (1995). *An international system for human cytogenetic nomenclature.* Mitelman F, ed. Basel: S Karger, 1995.

47. Pinkel D, Straume T, Gray JW. Cytogenetic analysis using quantitative, high-sensitivity, fluorescence hybridization. *Proc Natl Acad Sci USA* 1986;83:2934.

48. du Manoir S, Speicher MR, Joos S, et al. Detection of complete and partial chromosome gains and losses by comparative genomic *in situ* hybridization. *Hum Genet* 1993;90:590.

49. Testa JR, Graziano SL. Molecular implications of recurrent cytogenetic alterations in human small cell lung cancer. *Cancer Detect Prev* 1993;17:267.

50. de Leij L, Postmus PE, Buys CHCM, et al. Characterization of three new variant type cell lines derived from small cell carcinoma of the lung. *Cancer Res* 1985;45:6024.

51. Falor WH, Ward-Skinner R, Wegryn S. A 3p deletion in small cell lung carcinoma. *Cancer Genet Cytogenet* 1985;16:175.

52. Bepler G, Jaques G, Koehler A, et al. Markers and characteristics of human SCLC cell lines. *J Cancer Res Clin Oncol* 1985;113:253.

53. Naylor SL, Johnson BE, Minna JD, et al. Loss of heterozygosity of chromosome 3p markers in small-cell lung cancer. *Nature* 1987;329:451.

54. Brauch H, Johnson B, Hovis J, et al. Molecular analysis of the short arm of chromosome 3 in small-cell and non-small-cell carcinoma of the lung. *N Engl J Med* 1987;317:1109.

55. Kok K, Osinga J, Carritt B, et al. Deletion of a DNA sequence at the chromosomal region 3p21 in all types of lung cancer. *Nature* 1987;330:578.

56. Cavenee WK, Dryja TP, Phillips RA, et al. Expression of recessive alleles by chromosomal mechanisms in retinoblastoma. *Nature* 1983;305:779.

57. Ibson JM, Water JJ, Twentyman NM, et al. Oncogene amplification and chromosomal abnormalities in small cell lung cancer. *J Cell Biochem* 1987;33:267.

58. Sithanandam G, Dean M, Beck T, et al. Loss of heterozygosity at the c-*raf* locus in small cell lung carcinoma. *Oncogene* 1989;4:451.

59. Brauch H, Tory K, Kotler F, et al. Molecular mapping of chromosome 3p deletion sites in human lung cancer. *Genes Chrom Cancer* 1990;1:240.

60. Virani AK, Fong KM, Kodagoda D, et al. Allelotyping demonstrates common and distinct patterns of chromosomal loss in human lung cancer types. *Genes Chrom Cancer* 1998;21:308.

61. Rabbitts P, Bergh J, Douglas J, et al. A submicroscopic homozygous deletion at the D3S3 locus in a cell line isolated from a small cell lung carcinoma. *Genes Chrom Cancer* 1990;2:231.

62. Latif F, Tory K, Modi WS, et al. Molecular characterization of a large homozygous deletion in the small cell lung cancer cell line U2020: a strategy for cloning the putative tumor suppressor gene. *Genes Chrom Cancer* 1992;5:119.

63. Todd S, Roche J, Hahner L, et al. YAC contigs covering an 8-megabase region of 3p deleted in the small-cell lung cancer cell line U2020. *Genomics* 1995;25:19.

64. Roche J, Boldog F, Robinson M, et al. Distinct 3p21.3 deletions in lung cancer and identification of a new human semaphorin. *Oncogene* 1996;12:1289.

65. Sekido Y, Bader S, Latif F, et al. Human semaphorins A(V) and IV reside in the 3p21.3 small cell lung cancer deletion region and demonstrate distinct expression patterns. *Proc Natl Acad Sci USA* 1996;93:4120.

66. Wei MH, Latif F, Bader S, et al. Construction of a 600-kilobase cosmid clone contig and generation of a transcriptional map surrounding the lung cancer tumor suppressor gene (TSG) locus on human chromosome 3p21.3: progress toward the isolation of a lung cancer TSG. *Cancer Res* 1996;56:1487.

67. Yamakawa K, Takahashi T, Horio Y, et al. Frequent homozygous deletions in lung cancer cell lines detected by a DNA marker located at 3p21.3-p22. *Oncogene* 1993;8:327.

68. Sozzi G, Veronese ML, Negrini M, et al. The *FHIT* gene 3p14.2 is abnormal in lung cancer. *Cell* 1996;85:17.

69. Cannizzaro LA, Skolnik EY, Margolis B, et al. The human gene encoding phosphatidylinositol-3 kinase associated p85a is at chromosome region 5q12-13. *Cancer Res* 1991;51:3818.

70. Escobedo JA, Navankasattusas S, Kavanaugh WM, et al. cDNA cloning of a novel 85 kD protein that has SH2 domains, and regulates binding of PI3 kinase to the PDGF b-receptor. *Cell* 1991;65:75.

71. Nishisho I, Nakamura Y, Miyoshi Y, et al. Mutations of chromosome 5q21 genes in FAP and colorectal cancer patients. *Science* 1991;253:665.

72. D'Amico D, Carbone DP, Johnson BE, et al. Polymorphic sites within the *MCC* and *APC* loci reveal very frequent loss of heterozygosity in human small cell lung cancer. *Cancer Res* 1992;52:1996.

73. Harbour JW, Lai S-L, Whang-Peng J, et al. Abnormalities in structure and expression of the human retinoblastoma gene in SCLC. *Science* 1988;241:353.

74. Yokota J, Wada M, Shimosato Y, et al. Loss of heterozygosity on chromosomes 3, 13, and 17 in small-cell carcinoma and on chromosome 3 in adenocarcinoma of the lung. *Proc Natl Acad Sci USA* 1987;84:9252.

75. Takahashi T, Nau MM, Chiba I, et al. p53: A frequent target for genetic abnormalities in lung cancer. *Science* 1989;246:491.

76. Nigro JM, Baker SJ, Preisinger AC, et al. Mutations in the p53 gene occur in diverse human tumour types. *Nature* 1989;342:705.

77. Kaufman RJ, Brown PC, Schimke RT. Amplified dihydrofolate reductase genes in unstably methotrexate-resistant cells are associated with double minute chromosomes. *Proc Natl Acad Sci USA* 1979;76:5669.

78. Lin CC, Alitalo K, Schwab M, et al. Evolution of karyotypic abnormalities and c-*myc* oncogene amplification in human colonic carcinoma cell lines. *Chromosoma* 1985;92:11.

79. Little CD, Nau MM, Carney DN, et al. Amplification and expression of the c-*myc* oncogene in human lung cancer cell lines. *Nature* 1983;306:194.

80. Nau MM, Brooks BJ, Battey J, et al. L-*myc*, a new *myc*-related gene amplified and expressed in human small cell lung cancer. *Nature* 1985;318:69.

81. Nau MM, Brooks BJ, Carney DN, et al. Human small-cell lung cancers show amplification and expression of the N-*myc* gene. *Proc Natl Acad Sci USA* 1986;83:1092.

82. Wong AJ, Ruppert JM, Eggleston J, et al. Gene amplification of c-*myc* and N-*myc* in small cell carcinoma of the lung. *Science* 1986;233:461.

83. Brennan J, O'Connor T, Makuch RW, et al. *Myc* family DNA amplification in 107 tumors and tumor cell lines from patients with small cell lung cancer treated with different combination chemotherapy regimens. *Cancer Res* 1991;51:1708.

84. Elfving P, Lundgren R, Cigudosa JCC, et al. Trisomy 7 in nonneoplastic kidney tissue cultured with and without epidermal growth factor. *Cancer Genet Cytogenet* 1992;64:99.

85. Elfving P, Cigudosa JC, Lundgren R, et al. Trisomy 7, trisomy

10, and loss of the Y chromosome in short-term cultures of normal kidney tissue. *Cytogenet Cell Genet* 1990;53:123.

86. Dal Cin P, Aly MS, Delabie J, et al. Trisomy 7 and trisomy 10 characterize subpopulations of tumor-infiltrating lymphocytes in kidney tumors and in the surrounding kidney tissue. *Proc Natl Acad Sci USA* 1992;89:9744.

87. Pejovic T, Heim S, Mandahl N, et al. Trisomy 12 is a consistent chromosomal aberration in benign ovarian tumors. *Genes Chrom Cancer* 1990;2:48.

88. Feder M, Siegfried MJ, Blashem A, et al. Clinical relevance of chromosome abnormalities in non-small cell lung cancer. *Cancer Genet Cytogenet* 1998;102:25.

89. Weston A, Willey JC, Modali R, et al. Differential DNA sequence deletions from chromosomes 3, 11, 13, and 17 in squamous-cell carcinoma, large-cell carcinoma, and adenocarcinoma of the human lung. *Proc Natl Acad Sci USA* 1989;86:5099.

90. Rabbitts P, Douglas J, Daly M, et al. Frequency and extent of allelic loss in the short arm of chromosome 3 in nonsmall-cell lung cancer. *Genes Chrom Cancer* 1989;1:95.

91. Viallet J, Minna JD. Dominant oncogenes and tumor suppressor genes in the pathogenesis of lung cancer. *Am J Respir Cell Mol Biol* 1990;2:225.

92. Tsuchiya E, Nakamura Y, Weng SY, et al. Allelotype of non-small cell lung cancer: comparison between loss of heterozygosity in squamous cell carcinoma and adenocarcinoma. *Cancer Res* 1992;52:2478.

93. Olopade OI, Buchhagen DL, Malik K, et al. Homozygous loss of the interferon genes defines the critical region on 9p that is deleted in lung cancers. *Cancer Res* 1993;53:2410.

94. de Vos S, Miller CW, Takeuchi S, et al. Alterations of *CDKN2 (p16)* in non-small cell lung cancer. *Genes Chrom Cancer* 1995;14:164.

95. Washimi O, Nagatake M, Osada H, et al. In vivo occurrence of *p16 (MTS1)* and *p15 (MTS2)* alterations preferentially in non-small cell lung cancers. *Cancer Res* 1995;5:514.

96. Miura I, Resau J, Tomiyasu T, et al. Isochromosome (8q) in four patients with adenocarcinoma of the lung. *Cancer Genet Cytogenet* 1990;48:203.

97. Yokota J, Wada M, Yoshida T, et al. Heterogeneity of lung cancer cells with respect to the amplification and rearrangement of *myc* family oncogenes. *Oncogene* 1988;2:607.

98. Gemma A, Nakajima T, Shiraishi M, et al. *Myc* family gene abnormality in lung cancers and its relation to xenotransplantability. *Cancer Res* 1988;48:6025.

99. Miyaki M, Sato C, Matsui T, et al. Amplification and enhanced expression of cellular oncogene c-Ki-*ras*-2 in a human epidermoid carcinoma of the lung. *Jpn J Cancer Res (Gann)* 1985;76:260.

100. Taguchi T, Zhou J-Y, Feder M, et al. Detection of aneuploidy in interphase nuclei from non-small cell lung carcinomas by fluorescence in situ hybridization using chromosome-specific repetitive DNA probes. *Cancer Genet Cytogenet* 1996;89:120.

101. Ried T, Petersen I, Holtgreve-Grez H, et al. Mapping of multiple DNA gains and losses in primary small cell lung carcinomas by comparative genomic hybridization. *Cancer Res* 1994;54:1801.

102. Levin NA, Brzoska P, Gupta N, et al. Identification of frequent novel genetic alterations in small cell lung carcinoma. *Cancer Res* 1994;54:5086.

103. Levin NA, Brzoska PM, Warnock ML, et al. Identification of novel regions of altered DNA copy number in small cell lung tumors. *Genes Chrom Cancer* 1995;13:175.

104. Yokomizo A, Tindall DJ, Drabkin H, et al. PTEN/MMAC1 mutations identified in small cell, but not in non-small cell lung cancers. *Oncogene* 1998;17:475.

105. Balsara B, Sonoda G, du Manoir S, et al. Comparative genomic analysis detects frequent, often high-level overrepresentation of DNA sequences at 3q, 5p, 7p, and 8q in human non-small cell lung carcinoma. *Cancer Res* 1997;57:2116.

106. Petersen I, Bujard M, Petersen S, et al. Patterns of chromosomal imbalances in adenocarcinoma and squamous cell carcinoma of the lung. *Cancer Res* 1997;57:2331.

107. Brass N, Ukena I, Remberger K, et al. DNA amplification on chromosome 3q26.1-q26.3 in squamous cell carcinoma of the lung detected by reverse chromosome painting. *Eur J Cancer* 1996;32A:1205.

108. Sonoda G, Palazzo J, du Manoir S, et al. Comparative genomic hybridization detects frequent overrepresentation of chromosomal material from 3q26, 8q24, and 20q13 in human ovarian carcinomas. *Genes Chrom Cancer* 1997;20:320.

109. Heselmeyer K, Schrock E, du Manoir S, et al. Gain of chromosome 3q defines the transition from severe dysplasia to invasive carcinoma of the uterine cervix. *Proc Natl Acad Sci USA* 1996;93:479.

110. DeRisi J, Penland L, Brown PO, et al. Use of a cDNA microarray to analyse gene expression patterns in human cancer. *Nature Genet* 1996;14:457.

111. Hacia JG, Brody LC, Chee MS, et al. Detection of heterozygous mutations in BRCA1 using high density oligonucleotide arrays and two-colour fluorescence analysis. *Nature Genet* 1996;14:441.

112. Pinkel D, Segraves R, Sudar D, et al. High resolution analysis of DNA copy number variation using comparative genomic hybridization to microarrays. *Nature Genet* 1998;20:207.

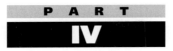

CLINICAL PRESENTATION, DIAGNOSIS, STAGING, AND PROGNOSIS

29

CLINICAL PRESENTATION

MICHAEL KRAUT
ANTOINETTE WOZNIAK

Lung cancer is a common disease, both in the United States and in those countries throughout the world in which cigarette smoking is prevalent. Although the incidence of the disease is about equal to that of breast cancer and prostate cancer, the lethality of lung cancer distinguishes it. Lung cancer is by far the most common cause of cancer death in the United States, representing the leading cause of cancer death in both men and women. In the United States approximately 171,000 new cases of lung cancer will be diagnosed in 1999, and nearly 160,000 will die of the disease.[1] An estimated more than one million people developed lung cancer in 1990, the most recent year for which worldwide statistics are available.[2] Given the trends in tobacco use, more than one million people will certainly die of lung cancer throughout the world during 1999.

Although lung cancer remains predominantly a disease of men in Europe, in the United States the number of women contracting lung cancer has risen dramatically over the past two decades. At present, the ratio of men to women with the disease is approximately three to two.

Because lung cancer is a common disease, all clinicians need to be familiar with its manifestations. Moreover, because so many patients are stricken with the disease, clinicians must be aware that a significant minority will present with unusual manifestations. The presentation of the lung cancer patient ranges from the asymptomatic and mundane to the difficult diagnostic dilemma.

MANIFESTATIONS OF LOCAL DISEASE

Asymptomatic

In its early stages, lung cancer is asymptomatic. The lung parenchyma is not generously supplied with pain fibers, and primary lung cancers can reach considerable size without causing any symptoms. This lack of symptoms is particularly true for more peripheral lesions. Less than 5% of lung cancers are discovered in patients who have no symptoms of the disease.[3] These lesions are often discovered during the investigation of an unrelated complaint, or on a chest radiograph done as part of a preoperative evaluation or as part of an extended physical examination.[4,5]

Methods to identify a greater proportion of lung cancer patients while still asymptomatic have been the focus of much effort. Screening of the entire adult population is not practical, and previous efforts were unable to demonstrate an increase in survival.[6] Attempts had been made to use high-resolution fast CT for screening[7] as well as autofluorescence endoscopy (see also Chapters 22, 24).

Cough

Cough is the most common symptom reported at presentation by patients with lung cancer. Cough is present at diagnosis in 50% or more of patients, and eventually develops in nearly all patients who are not successfully cured by surgery.[8] Because the majority of lung cancer patients are smokers, the cough may initially be no more than an insidious change from baseline. In most cases, however, worsening of cough leads patients to seek medical attention for presumed bronchitis or pneumonia. The typical patient receives one, two, or occasionally more courses of outpatient oral antibiotics before a chest x-ray is performed, revealing the true nature of the underlying pathology. Unfortunately, even after the clear demonstration of a mass lesion, some patients continue to receive antibiotic therapy, perhaps as an exercise in wishful thinking.

The development of a new or worsening cough in a patient with a significant (i.e., greater than 40 pack-years) smoking history should prompt the performance of a chest radiograph to assess for underlying lung cancer. This evaluation is particularly true if the cough is not associated with fever and coryza or other signs of upper respiratory infection (URI), or if the symptoms continue beyond the 5 to 7 days that a viral URI would be likely to persist. The patient who exhibits high fever, chills, and pleuritic chest pain in addition to cough warrants a chest x-ray for the evaluation of pneumonia, independent of other factors.

Hemoptysis

Hemoptysis varies greatly in severity, ranging from a few streaks to massive exsanguination. The typical presentation

TABLE 29.1. PRINCIPAL SYMPTOMS OF LOCAL DISEASE[3,4,5,6]

Symptom	Approx % Present at Diagnosis
Cough	45–75
Weight Loss	20–70
Dyspnea	40–60
Chest Pain	30–45
Hemoptysis	25–35
None	2–5

is that of blood-streaked or blood-tinged sputum. Because this symptom is far more likely to be caused by bronchitis than by cancer, patients with this symptom are typically managed with oral antibiotics initially. The index of suspicion is raised when the patient has a significant smoking history or when the problem persists or recurs despite conservative therapy. If a chest radiograph does not reveal an obvious cause, these patients with persistent hemoptysis should undergo fiberoptic bronchoscopy.[9]

The management of hemoptysis caused by lung cancer depends on the severity. Blood-streaked sputum is common and requires no specific therapy beyond reassurance. More serious hemoptysis, manifest as frank blood, often produced in the range of 5 to 10 mL per hour, requires more aggressive intervention. Cough suppression with narcotics is essential; acetaminophen with codeine (e.g., Tylenol #4) is a good choice because this drug is often easier for the patient to obtain than codeine alone. The patient should be instructed to keep the good (unaffected) side of the lung up when lying down. Fiberoptic bronchoscopy is sometimes necessary to localize the source of the bleeding. In patients with unresectable or metastatic disease, radiotherapy is the preferred treatment for moderately severe hemoptysis. This treatment is effective and generally well tolerated.[10]

The patient who develops hemoptysis after previous radiotherapy presents a greater challenge. In certain instances, an emergent thoracotomy with resection of the affected area may be the best therapy. More commonly, however, the technical difficulty of this intervention or the general condition of the patient dictates a different approach. In a clinical setting where skilled interventional radiologists are available, selective embolization of bronchial arteries feeding the area of hemorrhage can be very effective.[11,12]

Massive hemoptysis, such as occurs with tumor erosion into the main pulmonary arteries, is usually immediately fatal. If the patient survives the initial episode, intubation is required to protect the central airways and to allow effective suctioning because hypoxia caused by filling of alveoli with blood leads to rapid respiratory failure. The choices for management of the hemorrhage are as noted previously.

Management of hemoptysis requires experience and sound clinical judgement. Many patients with this problem have a limited life expectancy, and the interventions chosen must be consistent with realistic goals for the patient.

Chest Pain

Chest pain is a common symptom in early-stage lung cancer, and it is often present without frank evidence of invasion of the pleura, chest wall, or mediastinum. Because the lung parenchyma is not well supplied with pain fibers, the origin of this type of pain is not clear. This pain is not a poor prognostic sign and it typically responds well to management of the underlying tumor. Analgesics should be employed pending more definitive therapy; similar to management of any pain, the simplest treatment that is effective should be employed, but this should not preclude the use of narcotics if they are necessary to control the pain in an individual case.

It is not unusual for a patient with this type of pain to undergo an evaluation for angina, including coronary catheterization. Given the prevalence of coronary artery disease, especially among smokers, it is not surprising that such patients have been discovered to have lung cancer from chest radiographs performed pre- or postoperatively for coronary artery bypass grafting. Often, however, catheterization is negative or shows only minimal disease, prompting further investigation, which eventually uncovers the underlying lung malignancy.

Dyspnea

Dyspnea in lung cancer can result from a variety of causes and is often multifactorial. Many patients with lung cancer have some degree of underlying chronic lung disease, and the development of cancer may cause worsening of baseline dyspnea because of further loss of effective lung parenchyma. Obstructive airway disease is an independent risk factor for the development of lung cancer and is the most common concomitant lung disease in pulmonary malignancy.[13] The development of significant atelectasis, especially of an entire lobe, may result in dyspnea; this problem is also worse in patients with underlying lung disease. The differential diagnosis of dyspnea is wide and includes cardiac and pericardial disease in addition to pulmonary complications. Several complications of locally advanced disease can result in dyspnea (see Table 29.2).

Management of dyspnea involves identification and treatment of any underlying bronchospasm and elimination, if possible, of the causative lesion. Specific intervention depends on the cause. Hypoxia can be treated with oxygen. In patients with dyspnea caused by uncorrectable underlying problems, such as pulmonary entrapment by diffuse pleural disease, or progressive parenchymal involvement by advancing tumor, small doses of morphine are most effective, with the dose titrated to the desired effect. In the patient who is near death, sedatives may be useful as well.

TABLE 29.2. CAUSES OF DYSPNEA

Loss of Alveolar Space due to Extensive Tumor
Atelectasis/Obstruction
Lymphangitic Tumor Spread
Pleural Effusion
Pericardial Effusion or Constriction
Hemoptysis with Aspiration
Pneumonia (including Postobstructive)
Bronchospasm
Emphysema
Cardiac Failure
Pulmonary Embolism
Other

Dyspnea is a symptom that is extremely distressing to patient and family alike; it is incumbent upon the physician to eliminate this unpleasant situation to the maximum extent possible. Unfortunately, many patients are inadequately treated for this problem.

Wheezing

Localized wheezing may be the presenting symptom in patients with disease in the major airways, particularly in the mainstem bronchi. This symptom should be distinguished from the generalized wheezing of bronchospasm; this type of wheezing is often localized, and the patient is often able to tell from which side it is emanating. This type of lesion is almost always associated with a debilitating cough.

Lesions that are primarily endobronchial but that are too proximal for resection often require special management techniques. The armamentarium of the radiation oncologist, thoracic surgeon, and pulmonologist has been expanded in recent years by the addition of new or improved treatments. High dose-rate brachytherapy can be extremely effective in palliating central endobronchial lesions, either alone or in combination with external beam radiation (see also Chapter 49). Photodynamic therapy techniques have improved recently with the development of better photosensitizing agents and can be effectively employed in this setting (see also Chapter 24).[14] In skilled hands, laser therapy can also be useful for this problem, particularly when previous therapies have failed.[15]

Weight Loss

Weight loss is a common symptom of lung cancer at presentation, but it is not necessarily a sign of advanced disease. Among those with squamous cell carcinoma, approximately one-third of early-stage patients report weight loss of 10 pounds or more. Cachexia may develop in patients at all stages of disease when the tumor is actively synthesizing hormonally active compounds, such as tumor necrosis factor (see following section, Paraneoplastic Syndromes).

MANIFESTATIONS OF LOCALLY ADVANCED DISEASE

Hoarseness

Hoarseness in association with lung cancer is almost always caused by involvement of the left recurrent laryngeal nerve. Because of a quirk of embryogenesis, the left recurrent laryngeal nerve passes under the arch of the aorta; in this location, it is susceptible to damage from advanced primary tumors and from lymphadenopathy in the aorto-pulmonary window. New-onset hoarseness caused by left vocal cord paralysis is always indicative of surgically unresectable disease.

Some patients with left vocal cord paralysis develop significant problems of aspiration. This symptom can become a vexing clinical problem; occasionally, patients require a feeding tube to prevent recurrent bouts of pneumonitis. Teflon injection of the affected cord may be beneficial in some patients.[16]

Hoarseness occasionally improves with treatment of the causative malignancy, but more often it persists because of either inadequate control of the tumor or irreversible damage to the nerve. In the patient fortunate enough to survive locally advanced disease, Teflon injection of the paralyzed cord can improve voice quality.

Phrenic Nerve Paralysis

The phrenic nerve courses along the pericardium bilaterally and is subject to injury caused by invasion by primary tumor or bulky adenopathy. The left phrenic nerve is more commonly affected than the right, probably because of the relatively greater proximity of the left phrenic nerve to lymph nodes of the aorto-pulmonary window. Damage to the left phrenic nerve results in paralysis of the left hemidiaphragm, with consequent volume loss in the left hemithorax. Because the left hemidiaphragm is normally lower than the right, this condition has a rather characteristic x-ray appearance. The proximity of the left recurrent laryngeal nerve to the phrenic nerve in the aorto-pulmonary window occasionally results in coexisting hoarseness and left diaphragmatic paralysis. Phrenic nerve paralysis is always indicative of locally advanced disease. This condition is normally not reversible.

Dysphagia

Dysphagia can result from esophageal obstruction by bulky mediastinal adenopathy. Although bulky adenopathy is a relatively common occurrence, this symptom is surprisingly uncommon. Another potential cause of dysphagia is recurrent laryngeal nerve injury. In addition to hoarseness, recurrent laryngeal nerve damage can lead to dysfunction of the pharyngeal swallowing mechanism; this problem may be associated with aspiration as well (see previous section Hoarseness).

Treatment of the mediastinal adenopathy with radiotherapy (with or without concurrent chemotherapy) may improve dysphagia caused by this mechanism. Selected patients may require nutritional support until effective swallowing is reestablished.

Stridor

Stridor results from compromise of the lumen of the trachea. It can be caused by invasion of the trachea by tumor, or less commonly, bilateral vocal cord paralysis. An aggressive approach to management of stridor is necessary because this problem is life-threatening and extremely distressing. Prompt initiation of treatment, including radiotherapy or brachytherapy, with or without chemotherapy, is essential. For lesions located high in the trachea, or stridor caused by vocal cord paralysis, a tracheostomy may permit placement of a rigid canula beyond the obstruction. Because flow is related to diameter in an exponential fashion, a small increase in diameter can result in a dramatic improvement in symptoms; this increase can sometimes be accomplished via laser fulguration.[17,18]

Symptoms can be eased by the use of a helium-oxygen mixture (70:30) in place of room air or oxygen alone; helium has a much lower viscosity than nitrogen, thus reducing obstruction to flow.[19] Patients whose disease progresses despite therapy may require significant doses of morphine for control of symptoms.

Superior Vena Cava Syndrome

Superior vena cava (SVC) syndrome is a relatively common complication of lung cancer. It is generally a consequence of obstruction of the superior vena cava by right paratracheal adenopathy or central extension of a primary tumor in the right upper lobe. The syndrome is characterized by facial swelling, flushing, cough, and neck and chest wall vein distention. The extent and severity of symptoms greatly depends on how rapidly the obstruction progresses and on the speed and extent of the development of collateral circulation. Rapidly developing obstruction is most dangerous because it can result in central nervous system symptoms, including coma and death. Much more commonly, however, the onset is insidious, with swelling of the face, upper extremities, and breasts, causing the patient to seek medical attention.

In the undiagnosed patient, the principal differential diagnosis is between lung cancer and lymphoma. Approximately 80% of patients with SVC syndrome in the United States have an underlying diagnosis of lung cancer, divided approximately equally between small cell and non–small cell histologies.[20] In countries where tuberculosis is more prevalent, this disease is also a significant cause of SVC syndrome. Once considered an emergency, current practice is to obtain a tissue diagnosis expeditiously prior to the initiation of appropriate therapy.[21] Bronchoscopy, medias-

tinoscopy, or mediastinotomy usually yields a diagnosis with little risk to the patient. Radiotherapy remains the preferred treatment for non–small cell lung cancer (NSCLC); in selected situations, concurrent chemotherapy may be appropriate. Small cell lung cancer (SCLC) is best approached with chemotherapy (with or without concurrent radiotherapy),[22] (see also Chapters 53, 54).

Pleural Effusion

Approximately 15% to 20% of lung cancer patients present with pleural effusion. Although most of these effusions are ultimately determined to be malignant, about one-half are initially cytologically negative. Diagnostic thoracentesis should be performed to determine the origin of the effusion, with an adequate amount of fluid sent for cytology. The differential diagnosis for causes of effusion can include atelectasis, pneumonia, tuberculosis, and congestive heart failure, among others. It is important to identify malignant effusion if possible. Proper classification of an effusion can both prevent the application of ineffective local measures (i.e., surgery or radiotherapy) as well as ensure that resectable patients are not denied the benefits of surgery.

The management of malignant pleural effusion varies greatly depending on the clinical situation. Patients with good performance status and reasonable life expectancy can benefit from aggressive interventions such as video-assisted thoracoscopy and talc insufflation. Traditional thoracostomy tube placement can also be beneficial to patients who are in good physical condition.[23,24,25] Patients with more advanced stages of disease are better served by placement of a flexible small-bore catheter, which does not require hospitalization.

Pleural effusions may resolve with effective chemotherapy, especially in patients with SCLC. In selected patients with NSCLC, chemotherapy may be tried as initial management of effusion, but most patients in this category require more aggressive local measures at some point (see also Chapter 59).

Pericardial Effusion

Pericardial effusion develops in 5% to 10% of patients with lung cancer. Its dramatic clinical symptoms can be readily alleviated by relatively simple interventions, so recognizing this complication is important. Pericardial effusion typically occurs in the setting of progressive locally advanced disease. The onset is usually insidious, with shortness of breath and orthopnea as the initial symptoms. The symptoms and signs progress to severe dyspnea, anxiety, tachycardia, substernal chest tightness or pain, jugular venous distention, pulsus paradoxus, hepatomegaly, and azotemia, and ultimately hypotension and death.

It is important to recognize that pericardial tamponade can be difficult to diagnose, and that the diagnosis is missed antemortem in as many as one-third of patients. Patients can be relatively asymptomatic except for dyspnea and anxiety until very late in the course of the disease. The symptoms are relatively nonspecific and are often attributed to progression of parenchymal lung disease. The finding of dyspnea without concurrent hypoxia in an anxious, dyspneic patient with locally advanced lung cancer should always prompt an investigation for pericardial disease.

Two-dimensional echocardigraphy is the best diagnostic test in the evaluation of the patient with suspected pericardial tamponade. The test is universally available and gives rapid results. When a significant effusion is identified, the choice of therapy depends on whether right-sided collapse typical of tamponade is seen. The patient with tamponade requires immediate intervention; unless the patient's life expectancy is very limited, the preferred treatment is pericardiotomy (pericardial window) via a subxiphoid approach.[26] Patients with a very short expected survival, or in whom thoracic surgical intervention is not immediately available, can be approached with pericardiocentesis. In institutions where skilled radiologic interventional teams are available, the placement of a small-bore pericardial catheter can be effective. This catheter can be used to instill a pericardial sclerosing agent, with many patients achieving good control of the effusion[27] (see also Chapter 60).

Pericardial effusion is a late complication of radiation therapy and combined chemoradiotherapy to the mediastinum, particularly when significant portions of the pericardium are included in the field.[28] This complication can occur in patients who are cured of their malignancy; pericardial window is life-saving in this circumstance. As greater numbers of patients receive aggressive chemoradiotherapy regimens for stage III NSCLC, we can expect to see increasing numbers of patients with late benign pericardial effusion requiring intervention.

Pancoast Syndrome

Pancoast syndrome is the occurrence of shoulder and upper chest wall pain caused by the presence of a tumor in the apex of the lung with invasion of adjacent structures. It can be accompanied by Horner's syndrome, brachial plexopathy, and reflex sympathetic dystrophy. The typical patient has symptoms for one year or more before a diagnosis of malignancy is made. The patient is often evaluated by an orthopedic surgeon or a rheumatologist for persistent shoulder pain, and many patients receive steroid injections of the shoulder joint before a chest x-ray reveals the underlying cause of the problem.

The pain is usually caused by direct invasion of the chest wall and the first and second ribs, and in some cases by invasion of the transverse processes and bodies of the upper thoracic vertebrae. Spinal cord compression can occur by direct invasion of the spinal canal at this level, requiring aggressive intervention. Invasion of the lower roots of the brachial plexus results in pain in the arm, radiating down to the fourth and fifth digits. Destruction of the superior cervical ganglion causes Horner's syndrome, which is the triad of ipsilateral ptosis, meiosis, and anhydrosis that results from loss of sympathetic innervation of the affected side of the face. When the upper sympathetic chain is also destroyed, autonomic innervation to the affected limb is lost, leading to reflex sympathetic dystrophy, a condition characterized by pain and swelling resulting from loss of vascular tone regulation.

Patients with Pancoast tumors have often experienced long periods of poorly controlled pain by the time the diagnosis is made. Pain control can be problematic, and these patients often require large doses of long-acting narcotics to achieve comfort.

Treatment of Pancoast tumors depends on the stage at presentation. Patients without involvement of mediastinal lymph nodes can achieve long-term survival after preoperative radiotherapy or chemoradiotherapy followed by aggressive surgical resection.[29] When mediastinal lymph nodes are present, treatment is palliative, and the primary focus shifts to the significant problem of controlling symptoms, especially pain. Radiotherapy is the mainstay of treatment, with or without chemotherapy, in this setting (see also Chapter 39). Pain control is usually transient, however, and most patients require further intervention. Achieving adequate control of pain is challenging in this situation, and many patients require high doses of systemic narcotics. Some patients achieve significant relief by placement of an epidural or intradural catheter.

Lymphangitic Spread

Lymphangitic spread of the tumor through the parenchyma of the lung is an ominous development, usually portending the imminent demise of the patient. This problem is characterized by the development of progressive dyspnea, cough, and hypoxia associated with an expanding infiltrate. Fever is often a component as well. High-dose corticosteroids are often transiently effective in relieving dyspnea caused by this complication.

Lymphangitic spread often presents a diagnostic dilemma. The nonspecific nature of the infiltrate often results in uncertainty regarding the diagnosis, and the differential diagnosis typically includes infection and radiation pneumonitis. In some cases, high-resolution computed tomography (CT) scanning may reveal characteristic changes associated with lymphangitic spread.[30] Bronchoscopy with bronchoalveolar lavage can also be useful in establishing a diagnosis. Although open lung biopsy is usually definitive, its use must be weighed against the morbidity of the procedure. Empiric use of antibiotics and high-dose steroids may be preferable in many patients.

MANIFESTATIONS OF EXTRATHORACIC SPREAD

Brain Metastases

Lung cancer is the most common cause of brain metastases. Approximately one-half of SCLC patients develop brain metastases during the course of their disease. Lesser numbers of NSCLC patients develop this complication, but the incidence is increased in certain clinical settings, particularly after resection of locally advanced disease.

The manifestations of brain metastases are variable and depend on the location of the lesion and the amount of associated edema or hemorrhage. Patients may present with focal weakness, generalized or focal seizures, confusion or dementia, dysphasia, visual disturbances, or ataxia. Leptomeningeal disease may present as cranial nerve palsies or *cauda equina* syndrome.

CT scanning is useful in identifying the presence of metastases, especially in symptomatic patients. Magnetic resonance imaging (MRI) is clearly the gold standard for identifying central nervous system (CNS) disease, however, and is more sensitive than CT. MRI with gadolinium contrast is particularly important for identifying other, smaller lesions when resection is being contemplated; it is also useful for spotting potential leptomeningeal involvement.

Initial management of symptomatic brain metastases consists of corticosteroids (usually dexamethasone), given intravenously at first in very symptomatic patients, otherwise orally. Patients with seizures should receive diphenylhydantoin, but this drug is not recommended prophylactically because of a high potential for side effects.[33] Subsequent management depends on the size, number, and location of the lesions and general condition of the patient. Of particular importance in deciding on an aggressive intervention is the status of the lung cancer in the rest of the body; widespread uncontrolled disease contraindicates the use of resection or other aggressive measures.[31,32]

Resection of one to three metastatic lesions is reasonable in patients who are in good general condition. Resection followed by whole-brain irradiation results in better long-term control than radiotherapy alone. Patients with posterior fossa lesions are particularly likely to benefit from resection. Stereotactic radiosurgery (gamma knife) may have a similar role; studies to investigate this treatment are ongoing (see also Chapter 58).

Leptomeningeal carcinomatosis represents a particularly difficult challenge in patients with lung cancer. It is poorly responsive to treatment, and most patients deteriorate rapidly, even with aggressive interventions such as Ommaya reservoir placement and intrathecal chemotherapy. Except in carefully selected patients, leptomeningeal disease should be approached conservatively, with an emphasis on comfort.[34]

Bone Metastases

Bone is a common site of metastatic involvement in lung cancer. Management of metastases depends on the condition of the patient and the location of the disease. Metastases to weight-bearing areas should be considered for radiotherapy, whereas non–weight-bearing sites can be treated with systemic chemotherapy, with radiotherapy reserved for progression. In contrast to breast cancer, lung cancer patients do not typically survive long enough to benefit from aggressive interventions such as hip joint replacement for metastatic disease; such approaches should be limited to carefully selected cases.

Bone pain caused by metastases may require significant doses of narcotics for control; these patients may benefit from the addition of a nonsteroidal antiinflammatory drug (NSAID), which can be quite effective and which may result in a reduction of the narcotic dose.

Liver and Adrenal Metastases

Lung cancer commonly spreads to the liver and adrenal glands in addition to the brain and skeletal system. Except for some reports regarding resection of solitary adrenal metastases, results of surgical resection are uniformly disappointing.[35] The sensitivity of the liver and surrounding organs to radiotherapy limits the use of this modality as well, although patients with rapidly expanding livers can sometimes obtain palliation of pain. Systemic therapy may be effective, but benefits tend to be short lived.

Other Metastatic Sites

Because lung cancer is so common, metastases are occasionally seen at a variety of other sites, some very unusual, including skin, soft tissue, bowel, thyroid, ovary, and pancreas, among others. Management of other metastatic sites is typically symptomatic.

PARANEOPLASTIC SYNDROMES

Carcinomas of the lung most often present with symptoms related to the locoregional effects of the primary tumor or to the manifestation of extrathoracic spread. However, remote effects of the primary cancer, termed paraneoplastic syndromes, result in organ dysfunction.[36] Several different paraneoplastic syndromes are clinically apparent in 10% to 20% of patients with bronchogenic carcinoma. The more common syndromes associated with lung cancer are listed in Table 29.3.

Cachexia

Cancer cachexia syndrome is characterized by anorexia, weight loss and weakness resulting in impaired immune

TABLE 29.3. PARANEOPLASTIC SYNDROMES ASSOCIATED WITH LUNG CANCER

Endocrinologic	Hematologic/Vascular
Hypercalcemia (PTH-RP)	Anemia
Hyponatremia (SIADH)	Autoimmune Hemolytic
Cushing's Syndrome	Anemia
(ACTH)	Leukocytosis
Gynecomastia (βhCG)	Eosinophilia
Galactorrhea (prolactin)	Monocytosis
Hypoglycemia (insulinlike	Thrombocytosis
substance)	Idiopathic Thromboctopenic
Acromegaly (growth	Purpura
hormone)*	Trousseau's Syndrome
Calcitonin**	Nonbacterial Thrombotic
Thyroid Stimulating	Endocarditis
Hormone**	Vasculitis
Neurologic	**Miscellaneous**
Lambert-Eaton	Cachexia
Myasthenic Syndrome	Hyperuricemia/Hyporuricemia
Peripheral Neuropathy	Fever
Cerebellar Degeneration	Hypertension (renin)
Limbic Encephalitis	Membranous Nephropathy
Encephalomyelitis	
Stiff-Man Syndrome	
Opsoclonus/Myoclonus	
Retinopathy	
Muskuloskeletal	
Clubbing	
Hypertrophic Pulmonary	
Osteoarthropathy	
Dermatomyositis	
Polymyostitis	
Myopathy	
Mucocutaneous	
See Table 29.2	

* Associated with carcinoid tumors.
** No significant clinical syndrome.

status, tissue wasting, and decline in performance status.[37] This syndrome occurs commonly in lung cancer patients but usually in the case of advanced disease. The origin of cancer cachexia is not totally understood but is probably multifactorial. Several cytokines, tumor factors, and hormones have been implicated, including tumor necrosis factor alpha, interleukins, proteoglycan, insulin, corticotropin, epinephrine, human growth factor and insulinlike growth factor.[38,39] The cancer patient may also have a maladaptive metabolism resulting in a poor utilization of nutrients, in addition to decreased caloric intake.[40] Anorexia can be potentiated by pain, gastrointestinal involvement by tumor, development of food aversions, and the systemic effect of cancer treatment.[41]

The cachexia syndrome is not easily managed. Simply increasing nutritional support even by enteral or parenteral means is not clinically efficacious.[42] Several pharamacologic agents have been utilized to improve anorexia in cancer patients. The most commonly used agent is megestrol ace-

tate. In a trial by Loprinzi, a positive dose-response effect on appetite resulted with increasing doses of megestrol acetate (no benefit beyond 800 mg/day), and a trend toward non–fluid weight gain was apparent.[43] Steroids have limited benefit; tetrahydrocannabinol derivatives may be useful in improving appetite and symptoms of nausea. A better understanding of the mechanism of cancer-related anorexia/cachexia will clearly be needed before more advances can be made.

ENDOCRINOLOGIC SYNDROMES

Hypercalcemia

Hypercalcemia is a fairly common metabolic problem associated with malignancies. Several pathologic mechanisms have been proposed, including osteolytic bone metastases or humoral and cytokine factors such as parathyroid hormone-related protein, transforming growth factor α, interleukin-1, tumor necrosis factor, prostaglandins, and lymphotoxin.[44] Some of the more common cancers associated with hypercalcemia include breast, lung, kidney, head, and neck, and hematologic malignancies such as multiple myeloma and lymphomas.[45] Bender and Hansen reviewed 200 consecutive cases of bronchogenic lung cancer and found a 12.5% incidence of hypercalcemia.[46] Hypercalcemia associated with carcinoma of the lung can occur with bone metastases but often occurs in the absence of osseous involvement. Squamous cell carcinoma is the most common histology associated with this paraneoplastic presentation, generally in advanced-stage disease.[47] Hypercalcemia rarely occurs in small cell carcinoma even though other paraneoplastic syndromes are common in this malignancy.[48] Benign conditions may be responsible for hypercalcemia in cancer patients. An example of this relationship would be coexistence of primary hyperparathyroidism with the malignancy.[49]

Calcium is controlled by the interaction of parathyroid hormone (PTH), 1,25-dihydroxyvitamin D, and calcitonin in the bone, kidney, and gastrointestinal tract. PTH stimulates bone resorption, renal calcium reabsorption in the distal renal tubules, and production of vitamin D by the kidney. Patients with cancer-related hypercalcemia can have increased PTH activity in their blood.[50] Immunoreactive PTH levels are usually low or normal, however a PTH-related protein (PTH-RP) can be detected in the serum. This protein product is homologous with PTH at the amino-terminus, which is the portion that binds to the PTH receptor.[51] The gene responsible for PTH-RP expression is located on the short arm of chromosome 12. PTH-RP acts as a hormone that stimulates bone resorption and renal phosphate wasting, resulting in hypercalcemia and hypophosphatemia.

Clinical symptoms associated with hypercalcemia can be variable depending on the level of serum calcium and rapidity with which the level was achieved. Early manifestations can include nausea and vomiting, fatigue, lethargy, anorexia, muscle weakness, constipation, pruritis, polyuria, and polydypsia. The symptoms may not be recognized because they can be related to the existing malignancy, treatment toxicities (i.e., chemotherapy, narcotics), and other comorbid conditions. If untreated, patients can become severely dehydrated, subsequently developing renal insufficiency. Glomerular filtration is decreased, and a reversible defect in the kidney can result in loss of urine-concentrating ability.[52] Neurologic manifestations can also be significantly worsened, resulting in confusion, obtundation, psychosis, seizures, and coma. Further effects on the gastrointestinal tract can lead to obstipation and ileus. Electrocardiographic changes can occur with a prolonged PR interval, shortened QT interval, and a wide T-wave. These changes can result in bradycardia and atrial or ventricular arrhythmias. Poor performance status, advanced age, and preexisting renal and hepatic dysfunction can add to the effects of hypercalcemia.

Patients who have serum calcium levels higher than 13 mg/dl or who exhibit symptoms related to hypercalcemia usually require treatment. Goals of treatment should include hydration, inhibition of bone resorption and/or promotion of calcium excretion, and treatment of the underlying malignancy.[53]

Because hypercalcemic patients are often dehydrated, rehydration has become a mainstay of treatment. Vigorous hydration with isotonic saline (200 to 400 mL/hr) can be used for several hours to restore intravascular volume and glomerular filtration and to promote calcium excretion.[54] Care must be taken in the patient with cardiovascular compromise or renal insufficiency to avoid volume overload. Slower hydration may be more appropriate in this population. In cases of renal failure, dialysis may have to be employed. Diuretics should be used judiciously once rehydration is achieved. Thiazide diuretics should be avoided because they can increase calcium resorption in the distal tubule. Furosemide is the diuretic of choice and can promote calcium excretion by interfering with calcium reabsorption in the ascending limb of Henle's loop. Diuretics should be used primarily to balance fluid intake and output. The use of saline hydration and forced diuresis for treatment of hypercalcemia is no longer recommended. Along with hydration, a pharmaceutical agent that helps decrease bone resorption should be employed.

The biphosphonates are the most common drugs used for the treatment of hypercalcemia. These compounds are structural analogues of pyrophosphate and by binding to hydroxyapatite are potent inhibitors of bone crystal dissolution and osteoclast resorption.[54] Pamidroniate is the most widely used biphosphonate. It is generally administered at a dose of 60 or 90 mg as a 2- to 4-hour infusion. Onset of action is 24 to 48 hours and side effects are minimal (i.e., venous irritation, flu like symptoms). Pamidronate has been shown to be more effective than a first-generation biphos-

phonate etidronate.[55] Other more potent biphosphonates are currently undergoing clinical trials.

Gallium nitrate is a potent inhibitor of bone resorption via inhibition of an ATPase-dependent pump in the osteoclast.[56] It may also play a role in bone formation.[57] Gallium nitrate is usually administered at a dose of 100 to 200 mg/m^2/day by continuous infusion for up to five days. Onset of action is usually within 24 to 48 hours. Clinical trials indicate gallium's superiority over etidronate and calcitonin.[58,59] Urine output has to be maintained during administration, and nephrotoxic drugs should be avoided because of a potential for renal toxicity.

Calcitonin exerts its hypocalcemic effect by inhibiting bone resorption and promoting calcium excretion.[45] Its main advantage is that it has a rapid onset of action (2 to 4 hours) and can be used in critically ill patients even if they have renal insufficiency. A very rare incidence of hypersensitivity has been associated with administration. The main disadvantage of the drug is that the hypocalcemic effect is weak and rapidly wears off. It usually needs to be combined with another hypocalcemic agent for prolonged effect. The maximum dose of calcitonin is 8 IU/kg intramuscularly or subcutaneously every six hours.[60]

Plicamycin (mithramycin) is an antineoplastic agent that is toxic to osteoclasts.[61] The usual dose is 25 μg/kg given as a brief infusion. Dose adjustment have to be made in patients with renal and/or hepatic insufficiency. Because of potential side effects of nausea and vomiting, bone marrow suppression, nephrotoxicity, and hepatotoxicity, it is no longer commonly used unless the patient has hypercalcemia resistant to other agents.

Corticosteroids are useful agents in patients whose diseases are often treated with these drugs (i.e., hematologic malignancies, breast cancer). Steroids are not particularly effective in lung cancer–related hypercalcemia.

Ultimately successful treatment of the malignancy controls the hypercalcemia. This goal is particularly difficult in the case of advanced lung cancer. No effective oral agents, are available for maintenance of a desired serum calcium level. Patients who have continued problems with symptomatic hypercalcemia may require intermittent treatment with one of the hypocalcemic agents. Pamidronate can easily be given as an outpatient infusion for this purpose.

Syndrome of Inappropriate Antidiuretic Hormone

The syndrome of inappropriate antidiuretic hormone (SIADH) is most commonly associated with SCLC. Other cancers including NSCLC, prostate, adrenal cortex, esophageal, pancreas, colon, head and neck, thymoma, mesothelioma, bladder, carcinoid tumors, and hematologic malignancies have been associated with SIADH.[62] Nonmalignant conditions, such as an intracranial process (i.e., trauma, cerebral vascular accident, infection), pulmonary infection, or drug-related toxicity, can also be associated with SIADH. Chemotherapeutic agents (vincristine, cisplatin, cyclophosphamide), narcotics, chlorpropramide, thiazides, chlofibrate, and carbomazepines have all been implicated.[63] Other causes for hyponatremia in the lung cancer patient include cardiac, liver and renal disease, adrenal insufficiency, hypothyroidism, and gastrointestinal and renal losses that are not SIADH related.

The patient with SIADH usually presents with hyponatremia. The diagnosis requires several clinical criteria to be present, including euvolemia, serum hyposmolality with inappropriate urine hyperosmolality and urinary sodium, and normal renal, adrenal, and thyroid function. Other causes of hyponatremia need to be ruled out, particularly drug-related causes. A serum measurement of ADH is not necessary to make the diagnosis of SIADH.

Patients are generally asymptomatic, but the degree of symptoms is related to the rate of fall of the serum sodium. Patients often present with nonspecific complaints of nausea, generalized weakness, anorexia, headache, and lethargy. When the serum sodium falls below 115 mEq/L, altered mental status, psychosis, seizures, focal neurologic signs, and coma can result.

Mild hyponatremia with little or no symptoms can be managed by fluid restriction of 500 to 1,000 mL per day.[62] Because it is often difficult to accomplish fluid restriction on an outpatient basis, demeclocycline may be used. Demeclocycline at 600 mg/day partially inhibits the action of vasopressin by producing a reversible diabetes insipidus.[64] The drug can take up to two weeks to be effective. Patients may experience gastrointestinal upset, and renal function should be monitored while the patient is on treatment.

In patients with severe symptoms related to hyponatremia, such as mental status changes, treatment with hypertonic 3% saline and furosemide may be required. The goal is not to correct the serum sodium too rapidly. The recommended correction rate is 1 mEq/L/hour to avoid the potential complication of central pontine demyelinosis.[65,66] Patients must be monitored carefully in this situation, preferably in an intensive care unit setting.

Because the majority of cancer patients who present with SIADH have SCLC, treatment with systemic chemotherapy should be instituted. More than 80% of the patients will normalize their serum sodium within six weeks of treatment.[67] The presence of SIADH is not a prognostic factor with regard to tumor response or patient outcome.[68] Some patients actually develop SIADH postchemotherapy.[67] In the treated patient, the redevelopment of a low serum sodium may herald the recurrence of disease.

Ectopic Adrenocorticotropin Hormone Syndrome

Most normal tumor tissues produce a precursor adrenocorticotropin hormone (ACTH) molecule, whereas carcinomas produce this same precursor in much larger quantities. Some neoplasms convert the precursor ACTH to biologically active ACTH, resulting in clinically apparent Cushing's syndrome.[69] The most common malignancy associated with ectopic Cushing's syndrome is SCLC. Other lung cancer histologies tend to produce precursor ACTH that does not result in Cushing's.[70] Other neoplasms associated with ectopic ACTH production include carcinoid tumors, thymic cancer, islet cell tumors, pheochromocytoma, neuroblastoma, medullary carcinoma of the thyroid, and various malignancies.[71]

The clinical features associated with Cushing's disease and Cushing's syndrome from ectopic ACTH production are not entirely identical. Both may have truncal obesity, moon facies, weakness, hypertension, hirsutism, and metabolic disturbances. Purple striae and a buffalo hump are not usually seen in patients with malignancies because they do not live long enough to develop these physical findings. Hyperpigmentation occurs in ectopic ACTH related to Cushing's syndrome. Metabolic alkalosis, glucose intolerance, and hypokalemia are the biochemical abnormalities. The hypokalemia can be very severe. In cancer-related Cushing's, the hypokalemia is caused by the mineralocorticoid (aldosterone) receptor binding of cortisol.[72]

The goal of diagnosis is to distinguish between pituitary adenoma, ectopic ACTH production, and adrenal disorders. Radioassays of the ACTH plasma level are elevated in pituitary-related Cushing's and ectopic ACTH production. The elevated ACTH rules out primary adrenal disease. A dexamethasone suppression test is usually the next step.

The low-dose dexamethasone suppression test (0.5 mg every 6 hours for 8 doses) does not suppress either ectopic ACTH secretion or patients with Cushing's disease. The high-dose dexamethasone suppression test (2 mg every 6 hours for 8 doses) suppresses cortical production in patients with pituitary-related Cushing's disease and usually does not suppress production related to ectopic ACTH production. Because these tests do not ensure the origin of the ACTH production, metyrapone and corticotropins releasing hormone suppression tests have been used.[73,74] Inferior petrosal venous sampling, although invasive, can show a gradient as compared to peripheral samples in Cushing's disease.[75]

In patients with SCLC, approximately 5% develop Cushing's syndrome.[76] In these cases, treatment should initially include systemic chemotherapy. Patients with SCLC and Cushing's syndrome appear to have inferior response to treatment and shortened survival.[77] It is postulated that this observation may relate to increased complications, such as infections related to exposure to high-dose corticosteroids. For control of symptoms related to Cushing's syndrome, medications can be used along with antineoplastic treatment. Ketoconazole is probably the medical treatment of choice because of its effectiveness and low incidence of side effects. The drug exerts its effect by blocking corticosteroid production via inhibition of 17-hydroxylase and 11-

hydroxylase.[78] The dose is 400 to 1,200 mg/day. Hypoadrenalism has been reported with prolonged treatment. Other agents such as mitotane, metyrapone, and aminoglutethemide have been used, but they either are not as effective as ketoconazole or they have less favorable toxicity profiles. The somatostatin analogue octreotide has been used in the suppression of ACTH release associated with carcinoid tumors.[79]

Other Endocrinologic Paraneoplastic Syndromes

Lung cancers, particularly SCLCs, can produce other hormonal substances, but this process does not always result in a clinically significant paraneoplastic syndrome. SCLCs and carcinoids can produce calcitonin, but hypocalcemia is rarely seen.[80] Gonadotropin secretion can occur from bronchogenic carcinomas.[80] Production of the β-subunit of human chronic gonadotropin can result in a male patient presenting with gynecomastia. Other causes of βhCG elevation, such as germ cell tumors, should be ruled out in this situation. Galactorrhea as a result of increased prolactin level has been reported.[81] Thyroid-stimulating hormone can be produced by tumors but rarely results in clinical hyperthyroidism. Acromegaly has been attributed to the release of a growth hormone–releasing factor by a bronchial carcinoid.[82] Hypoglycemia is rarely associated with non–islet cell malignancies. Mesothelioma is the most common neoplasm associated with hypoglycemia. The suspected cause is the tumor secretion of a nonsuppressable insulin-like substance.[83]

Neurologic Syndromes

Neurologic paraneoplastic syndromes are relatively rare and can involve any portion of the nervous system. Effects can be relatively focal or widespread. These syndromes may often develop before the actual diagnosis of the cancer. SCLC is the most common histologic type associated with neurologic paraneoplastic syndromes.

The origin of most neurologic paraneoplastic syndromes is thought to be related to an autoimmune process. The tumor produces substances that are similar to those normally expressed by the nervous system. It is hypothesized that autoantibodies are produced by the immune system in reaction to the foreign substances produced by the tumor, and these autoantibodies cross-react with neuronal antigens, thus causing damage to normal tissue.

Several autoantibodies have been characterized in patients with neurologic paraneoplastic syndromes. Anti-Hu antibodies are expressed in patients with SCLC.[84] The antibody is a 35 to 40 kD protein that has activity against the neuronal nucleus. Low titers are often present with no clinically evident paraneoplastic syndrome. Their presence may be indicative of better response to chemotherapy and

improved survival.[85] Anti-Hu is associated with the clinical syndromes of encephalomyelitis, sensory neuropathy, cerebellar degeneration, autonomic neuropathy, limbic encephalitis, and opsoclonus/myoclonus.[84] Other antibodies that have been identified in SCLC include anti-Yo (cerebellar degeneration), anti-Ri (opsoclonus/myoclonus, cerebellar degeneration), anti-VGCC (Lambert-Eaton myasthenic syndrome), antiretinal (cancer-associated retinopathy), and antiamphiphisin (stiff-man syndrome).[86]

Lambert-Eaton Myasthenic Syndrome (LEMS) can occur in up to 3% of SCLC patients.[87] Most patients usually present with weakness of the proximal muscles associated with aches and stiffness. Patients may also complain of autonomic dysfunction (i.e., dry mouth, constipation, impotence)[88] and paresthesias. Cranial nerve findings can occur but are usually mild. The findings of a diminished compound muscle action potential at rest, and an incrementing response with rapid, repetitive nerve stimulation or maximum voluntary muscle contraction is pathonomonic of the syndrome.[89] Treatment of LEMS has included plasmapheresis, IVIG, 3–4 diaminopyridine, pryridostigmin, and immunosuppressive therapy. Successful treatment of the malignancy usually improves the symptoms.

Several types of peripheral neuropathy can occur as paraneoplastic syndromes: motor, sensory, sensorimotor, and autonomic.[90] The motor neuropathies have more often been seen in Hodgkin's and non-Hodgkin's lymphoma. The sensory neuropathies are more commonly associated with SCLC. The sensory loss usually begins distally and extends proximally. The symptoms can become quite severe, resulting in significant disability. No specific treatment is available, and antineoplastic therapy may or may not be beneficial. The syndrome of pseudo-obstruction of the bowel is the best-characterized autonomic neuropathy usually associated with SCLC.[91] Additional symptoms of autonomic neuropathy include gastroparesis, esophageal dismotility, orthostatic hypotension, urinary retention, impotence, and dry mouth.

Paraneoplastic cerebellar degeneration usually presents with abrupt onset of cerebellar symptoms, such as ataxia and dysarthria. Mild to moderate dementia can also develop. As previously described, several antibodies have been associated with this disorder. Pathologic changes are associated with loss of Purkinje cells.[92] This disorder is rare and usually predates the development of the malignancy. Cerebellar degeneration may be part of a more generalized encephalomyelitis in SCLC that is associated with anti-Hu antibody.[84] Limbic encephalitis is another rare paraneoplastic syndrome that may be isolated or associated with encephalomyelitis.[93] Symptoms can include memory loss, personality changes, confusion, hallucinations, and seizures.

Myotonia and stiff-man syndrome, consisting of severe muscle stiffness and cramping, have been reported with SCLC.[94] Treatment of the cancer and steroids may help the symptoms. Opsoclonus/myoclonus, which is a syndrome more common in children with neuroblastoma, has been seen in adults with lung cancer.[95] Finally, cancer-associated retinopathy is a rare paraneoplastic syndrome reported with SCLC. It is characterized by loss of the rods, cones, and ganglion cells of the retina.[96] Symptoms include photosensitivity, scotomatous visual loss, impaired color vision, and nightblindness. Steroids may help stabilize symptoms.

Musculoskeletal Paraneoplastic Syndromes

Hypertrophic pulmonary osteoarthopathy (HPO) has long been associated with carcinoma of the lung. It is characterized by both digital clubbing and periostosis of the tubular bones.[97] Digital clubbing involves paronychial soft tissue expansion with loss of the angle between the base of the nail bed and cuticle and can involve both fingers and toes. Clubbing can present as an isolated finding but must be associated with periostosis to diagnose HPO. Nonmalignant conditions can be associated with HPO, but the most common neoplastic cause is bronchogenic carcinoma. Adenocarcinoma and large cell are the most common histologies, with SCLC accounting for a small number of cases.[98] The origin of HPO is not really known. It has been suggested that a humoral mechanism, specifically growth hormone, may be involved.[99]

Diagnosis is made with radiographs of the long bones, which show periosteal elevation. A radioisotope bone scan can be very sensitive in detecting HPO before it is evident on radiographs. Patients often present with arthralgias, which can be very debilitating. Treatment of the malignancy does not usually alleviate symptoms because patients often have advanced NSCLC. NSAIDs can be useful in treating the pain.

Dermatoyositis and polymyositis are inflammatory conditions characterized by muscle weakness and tenderness, and skin changes, in the case of dermatomyositis. Breast and lung cancers are the most common associated malignancies. Most cases are idiopathic in nature and unrelated to cancer. Some controversy exists about whether an actual increase in cancer risk is related in patients who have either condition.[101,102] The course of these conditions may not parallel the course of the malignancy. Immunosuppressives, particularly steroids, have been used for treatment.

Mucocutaneous Manifestations

Many cutaneous syndromes are associated with cancer. Many of these skin lesions are uncommon, and the association with malignancy is stronger. Some of the cutaneous findings are common and may be associated with benign conditions. It is beyond the scope of this review to describe

TABLE 29.4. MUCOCUTANEOUS SYNDROMES ASSOCIATED WITH LUNG CANCER

Pigmented/Keratoses
  Acanthosis Nigricans
  Tripe palms
  Generalized melanosis (ACTH production)
  Bazex's disease
  Acquired Tylosis
Erythema
  Erythema annulare centrifugum
  Erythema gyratum repens
Miscellaneous
  Dermatomyositis
  Pachydermoperiostosis
  Hypertrichosis languignosa
  Pruritis
  Scleroderma

all of these mucocutaneous manifestations. Table 29.4 shows a compilation of the syndromes associated with lung cancer.[63–102]

Hematologic Syndromes and Vascular Manifestations

Anemia is a common problem in cancer patients, with many possible causes such as bleeding, nutritional deficiencies, and bone marrow involvement by the malignancy. Anemias with no apparent cause can be termed *paraneoplastic*. Red blood cells are usually normochromic or slightly hypochromic, ferritin levels and iron stores are normal or increased, and erythropoetin levels and reticulocyte counts are inappropriately low. The anemia may be related to several cytokines that blunt erythropoetin response.[103] Rarely, autoimmune hemolytic anemia, red cell aplasia, and microangiopathic hemolytic anemia have been associated with lung cancers.[104,105]

Leukocytosis is observed in some patients and may be related to the effects of IL-1 or granulocyte-stimulating factor.[106] Leukopenia is rare. Both eosinophilia and monocytosis can occur infrequently. Thrombocytosis is a fairly common occurrence and may be related to cytokine release of IL-6 or thrombopoetin.[107,108] An idiopathic thrombocytopenia purpuralike syndrome can rarely be seen in lung cancer.[109]

Trousseau's syndrome is one of the earliest paraneoplastic syndromes described. It represents an association between thrombosis and malignancy. It is seen in several malignancies, including gastrointestinal, lung, breast, ovarian, and prostate cancers.[110] Deep vein thrombosis of the lower extremities and pulmonary embolism are the most common presentations, although unusual location of thromboses can occur. The origin is probably multifactorial and can include release of procoagulant materials (particularly from mucin), release of cytokines that have procoagulant activity, platelet hyperactivity, and the release of tissue factors via abnormal tumor vasculature.[111] Therapy with heparin and/or coumadin may not provide satisfactory treatment.

Nonbacterial thrombotic endocarditis is associated with sterile verrucous fibrin platelet lesions in the left-sided heart valves. It is most commonly associated with adenocarcinoma of the lung.[112] This syndrome can cause tumor embolisms to the brain and other organs. Anticoagulants are usually not useful.

REFERENCES

1. Landis S, Murray T, Bolden S, et al. Cancer Statistics: 1999. *CA Cancer J Clin* 1999;49(1):8.
2. Parkin DM, Pisani P, Ferlay J. Global cancer statistics. *CA Cancer J Clin* 1999;49(1):33.
3. Chute CG, Greenberg ER, Baron J, et al. Presenting conditions of 1539 population-based lung cancer patients by cell type and stage in New Hampshire and Vermont. *Cancer* 1985;56:2107.
4. Hyde L, Hyde CI. Clinical manifestations of lung cancer. *Chest* 1974;65:299.
5. Grippi MA. Clinical aspects of lung cancer. *Semin Roentgenol* 1990;25(1):12.
6. Frost JK, Ball WC Jr, Levin MI et al. Early lung cancer detections: results of the initial (prevalence) radiologic and cytologic screening in the Johns Hopkins study. *Am Rev Respir Dis* 1984;130(4):549.
7. Henschke CI, McCauley DI, Yankelevitz DF, et al. Early Lung Cancer Action Project: overall design and findings from baseline screening. *Lancet* 1999;354(9173):99.
8. Patel AM, Peters SG. Clinical manifestations of lung cancer. *Mayo Clin Proc* 1993;68:273.
9. Poe RH, Israel RH, Marin MA et al. Utility of fiberoptic bronchoscopy in patients with hemoptysis and a nonlocalizing chest roentgenogram. *Chest* 1988;93(1):70.
10. Hoegter D. Radiotherapy for palliation of symptoms in incurable cancer. *Curr Probl Cancer* 1997;21(3):129.
11. Cremaschi P, Naseimbene C, Vitulo P, et al. Therapeutic embolization of bronchial artery: a successful treatment in 209 cases of relapse hemoptysis. *Angiology* 1993;44(4):295.
12. Hayakawa K, Tanaka F, Torizuka T, et al. Bronchial artery embolization for hemoptysis: immediate and long term results. *Cardiovasc Intervent Radiol* 1992;15(3):154.
13. Tockman MS, Anthonisen NR, Wright EC, et al. Airways obstruction and the risk for lung cancer. *Ann Intern Med* 1987;106(4):512.
14. Moghissi K, Dixon K, Stringer M, et al. The place of bronchoscopic photodynamic therapy in advanced unresectable lung cancer: experience of 100 cases. *Eur J Cardiothorac Surg* 1999;15(1):1.
15. Lui JS, Amemiya R, Chung FM, et al. The present status of bronchoscopic Nd: YAG laser. *J Clin Laser Med Surg* 1991;9(1):63.
16. Kraus DH, Ali MK, Ginsberg RJ, et al. Vocal cord medialization for unilateral paralysis associated with intrathoracic malignancies. *J Thorac Cardiovasc Surg* 1996;111(2):334.
17. Torre M, Amari D, Barbieri B, et al. Emergency laser vaporization and helium oxygen administered for acute malignant tracheobronchial obstruction. *Am J Emerg Med* 1989;7(3):294.
18. Chen K, Baron J, Wenker OC. Malignant airway obstruction: recognition and management. *J Emerg Med* 1998;16(1):83.
19. Curtis JL, Mahlmeister M, Fink JB, et al. Helium-oxygen gas therapy. Use and availability for the emergency treatment of inoperable airway obstruction. *Chest* 1986;90(3):455.
20. Rodrigues N, Straus MJ. Superior vena caval syndrome. In Straus MJ, ed. *Lung cancer: clinical diagnosis and treatment.* Philadelphia: Grune & Stratton 1983;323.
21. Schraufnagel D, Hill R, Leech J, et al. Superior vena caval obstruction. Is it a medical emergency? *Am J Med* 1981;70:1169.
22. Sculier JP, Evans WK, Feld R, et al. Superior vena caval obstruction syndrome in small cell lung cancer. *Cancer* 1986;57:847.
23. Light RW. Malignant pleural effusion. In: *Pleural effusion.* Philadelphia: Williams & Wilkens, 1990;94.
24. Lynch TJ Jr. Management of malignant pleural effusions. *Chest* 1993;103(4 Suppl):385S.
25. Ronson RS, Mittar JT Jr. Video-assisted thoracoscopy for pleural disease. *Chest Surg Clin N Am.* 1998;8(4):919.
26. Park JS, Rentsehler R, Wilbur D. Surgical management of pericardial effusion in patients with malignancies. Comparison of subxiphoid window versus pericardiectomy. *Cancer* 1991;67(1):76.
27. Bellon RJ, Wright WH, Unger EC. CT-guided pericardial drainage catheter placement with subsequent pericardial sclerosis. *J Comput Assist Tomogr* 1995;19(4):672.
28. Caret RW, Sawicka JM, Choi NC. Cytologically negative pericardial effusion complicating combined modality therapy for localized small-cell carcinoma of the lung. *J Clin Oncol* 1987;5(5):818.
29. Paulson D. Carcinomas in the superior pulmonary sulcus. *J Thorac Cardiovasc Surg* 1975;70:109.
30. Munk PL, Muller NL, Miller RR, et al. Pulmonary lymphangitic carcinomatosis: CT and pathologic findings. *Radiology* 1988;166:705.
31. Davey P. Brain metastases. *Curr Prob Cancer* 1999;23(2):59.
32. Kelly K, Bunn PA Jr. Is it time to reevaluate our approach to the treatment of brain metastasis in patients with non-small cell lung cancer. *Lung Cancer* 1998;20(2):85.
33. Cohen N, Strauss G, Lew R, et al. Should prophylactic anticonvulsants be administered to patients with newly diagnosed cerebral metastases? A retrospective analysis. *J Clin Oncol* 1988;6(10):1621.
34. Grossman SA, Krabak MJ. Leptomeningeal carcinomatosis. *Cancer Treat Rev* 1999;25(2):103.
35. Lo CY, van Heerden JA, Soreide JA, et al. Adrenalectomy for metastatic disease to the adrenal glands. *Br J Surg* 1996;83(4):528.
36. Hall TC, ed. Paraneoplastic syndromes. *NY Acad Sci Ann* 1974;230:1.
37. Nathanson L, Puccio M. The cancer cachexia syndrome. *Semin Oncol* 1997;24:277.
38. Socher SH, Martinez D, Craig JB, et al. Tumor necrosis factor not detectable in patients with clinical cancer cachexia. *J Natl Cancer Inst* 1988;80:595.
39. Todorov P, Cariuk P, McDevitt T, et al. Characterization of a cancer cachetic factor. *Nature* 1996;379:739.
40. Heber D, Tchekmedyian NS. Mechanisms of cancer cachexia. *Contem Oncol* 1995;6.
41. Nelson KA, Walsh D, Sheehan FA. The cancer anorexia-cachexia syndrome. *J Clin Oncol* 1994;12:213.
42. Klein S. Clinical efficacy of nutritional support in patients with cancer. *Oncology* 1993;7(suppl 11):87.
43. Loprinzi CL, Michalak JC, Schaid DJ, et al. Phase III evaluation of four doses of megestrol acetate as therapy for patients with cancer, anorexia and/or cachexia. *J Clin Oncol* 1993;11:762.
44. Mundy GR. Hypercalcemic factors other than parathyroid hormone-related protein. *Endocrinol Metab Clin North Am* 1989;18:795.

45. Mundy GR, Martin TJ. The hypercalcemia of malignancy: pathogenesis and management. *Metabolism* 1982;31:1247.
46. Bender RA, Hansen H. Hypercalcemia in bronchogenic carcinoma. *Ann Intern Med* 1974;80:325.
47. Coggeshall J, Merrill W, Hande K, et al. Implications of hypercalcemia with respect to diagnosis and treatment of lung cancer. *Am J Med* 1986;80:325.
48. Hayward ML, Howell DA, O'Donnell JF, et al. Hypercalcemia complicating small-cell carcinoma. *Cancer* 1981;48:1643.
49. Farr HW, Fahey TJ Jr, Nash AG, et al. Primary hyperthyroidism and cancer. *Am J Surg* 1973;126:539.
50. Goltzman D, Stewart AF, Broadus AE. Malignancy associated hypercalcemia: evaluation with a cytochemical bioassay for parathyroid hormone. *J Clin Endocrinol Metab* 1981;53:899.
51. Suva LJ, Winslow GA, Wettenhall RE, et al. A parathyroid hormone-related protein implicated in malignant hypercalcemia: cloning and expression. *Science* 1987;237:893.
52. Bajournas DR. Clinical manifestations of cancer-related hypercalcemia. *Semin Oncol* 1990;17:16.
53. Bilezebian JP. Management of acute hypercalcemia. *N Engl J Med* 1992;326:1196.
54. Ritch PS. Treatment of cancer-related hypercalcemia. *Semin Oncol* 1990;17:26.
55. Gucalp R, Ritch P, Wiernik PH, et al. Comparative study of pamidronate disoduim and etidronate disoduim in the treatment of cancer-related hypercalcemia. *J Clin Oncol* 1991;9:1467.
56. Blair HC, Teitelbaum SL, Tan H-L, et al. Reversible inhibition of osteoclastic activity by bone-bound gallium (III). *J Cell Biochem* 1992;48:401.
57. Bockman RS, Bosley A, Blumenthal NC, et al. Gallium increases bone calcium and crystallite perfection of hydroxyapatite. *Calif Tissue Int* 1986;39:376.
58. Warrell RP Jr, Israel R, Frisone M, et al. A randomized double-blind study of gallium nitrate versus calcitonin for acute treatment of cancer-related hypercalcemia. *Ann Intern Med* 1988;108:669.
59. Warrell RP Jr, Heller G, Murphy WP, et al. A randomized double-blind study of gallium nitrate compared to etidronate for acute control of cancer-related hypercalcemia. *J Clin Oncol* 1991;9:1467.
60. Warrell RP Jr. Oncologic emergencies: metabolic emergencies. In: DeVita VT Jr, Hellman S, Rosenberg SA, eds. *Cancer: principles and practice of oncology.* 5th ed. Philadelphia: JB Lippincott, 1997;2486.
61. Kiang DT, Loken MK, Kennedy BJ. Mechanism of the hypocalcemic effect of mithramycin. *J Clin Endocrinol Metab* 1979;48:341.
62. Glover DJ, Glick JH. Metabolic oncologic emergencies. *CA* 1987;37:302.
63. John WJ, Foon KA, Patchell RA. Parancoplastic syndromes. In: DeVita VT Jr, Hellman S, Rosenberg SA, eds. *Cancer: principles and practice of oncology.* 5th ed. Philadelphia: JB Lippincott, 1997;2397.
64. Cherrill DA, Stote RM, Birge JR, et al. Demeclocycline treatment in the syndrome of inappropriate antidiuretic hormone secretion. *Ann Intern Med* 1975;83:654.
65. Wright DG, Laureno R, Victor M. Pontine and extrapontine myelinosis. *Brain* 1979;102:361.
66. Ayres JC, Krothapalli RK, Arieff A. Treatment of symptomatic hyponatremia and its relation to brain damage. *N Engl J Med* 1987;317:1190.
67. List AF, Hainsworth JD, Davis BW, et al. The syndrome of inappropriate secretion of antidiuretic hormone in small cell lung cancer. *J Clin Oncol* 1986;4:1191.
68. Bondy PK, Gilby ED. Endocrine function in small cell undifferentiated carcinoma of the lung. *Cancer* 1982;50:2147.
69. Odell WD. Endocrine/metabolic syndromes of cancer. *Semin Oncol* 1997;24:299.
70. Yalow RS, Eastridge CE, Higgins G Jr et al. Plasma and tumor ACTH in carcinoma of the lung. *Cancer* 1979;44:1789.
71. Liddle GW, Island DP, Ney RL, et al. Non-pituitary neoplasms and Cushing's syndrome. *Arch Intern Med* 1963;11:471.
72. Howlett TA, Drurg PL, Perry L, et al. Diagnosis and management of ACTH-dependent Cushing's syndrome: comparison of the features in ectopic and pituitary ACTH production. *Clin Endocrinol* 1986;24:699.
73. Avgerinos PC, Wanovski JA, Oldfield EH, et al. The metyrapone and dexamethasone suppression tests for the differential diagnosis of the adrenocorticotropin-dependent Cushing's syndrome: a comparison. *Ann Intern Med* 1994;121:318.
74. Nieman LK, Chrousos GP, Oldfield EH, et al. The ovine corticotropin-releasing hormone stimulation test and the dexamethasone suppression test in the differential diagnosis of Cushing's syndrome. *Ann Intern Med* 986;105:862.
75. Midgette AS, Aron DC. High dose dexamethasone suppression testing versus inferior petrosal sign and sampling and the differential diagnosis of adrenocorticotropin-dependent Cushing's syndrome: a decision analysis. *Am J Med Sci* 1995;309:162.
76. Hansen M, Pederson AG. Tumor markers in patients with lung cancer: incidence of SIADH and ectopic ACTH. *Chest* 1986;89:2195.
77. Shepherd FA, Laskey J, Evans WK, et al. Cushing's syndrome associated with ectopic corticotropin production and small cell lung cancer. *J Clin Oncol* 1992;10:21.
78. Sonio N. The use of Ketoconazole as an inhibitor of steroid production. *N Engl J Med* 1987;317:812.
79. Bertagna X, Favrod-Coune C, Escouralle H, et al. Suppression of ectopic adrenocorticotropin secretion by the long-acting somatostatin analog octreotide. *J Clin Endocrinol Metab* 1989;68:988.
80. Silva OL, Broder, LE, Doppman JL, et al. Calcitonin as a marker for bronchogenic cancer: a prospective study. *Cancer* 1979;44:680.
81. Faiman C, Colwell JA, Ryan RJ, et al. Gonadotropin secretion from a bronchogenic carcinoma. *N Engl J Med* 1967;277:1395.
82. Blackman MR, Rosen SW, Weintraub BD. Ectopic hormones. *Adv Intern Med* 1978;23:85.
83. Scheithauer BW, Block B, Carpenter PC, et al. Ectopic secretion of a growth hormone-releasing factor: Report of a case of acromegaly with bronchial carcinoid tumor. *Am J Med* 1984;76:605.
84. Gordon P, Hendricks GM, Kahn CR, et al. Hypoglycemia associated with non-islet cell tumor and insulin-like growth factors. *N Engl J Med* 1981;305:1452.
85. Dalman J, Graus F, Rosenblum MK, et al. Anti-Hu-associated paraneoplastic encephalomyelitis/sensory neuronopathy. A clinical study of 71 patients. *Medicine* 1992;71:59.
86. Posner JB, Malats N, René R, et al. Anti-Hu antibodies as a prognostic marker for SCLC response to therapy. *J Invest Med* 1996;44:234A.
87. Dalman JO, Posner JB. Paraneoplastic syndromes affecting the nervous system. *Semin Oncol* 1997;24:318.
88. Van Oosterhout AGM, Van de Pal M, Ten Velde GPM, et al. Neurologic disorders in 203 consecutive patients with small cell lung cancer. *Cancer* 1996;77:1434.
89. O'Neill JH, Murray NM, Newsom-Davis J. The Lambert-Eaton Myasthenic syndrome. A review of 50 cases. *Brain* 1988;111:577.
90. Sanders DB. Lambert-Eaton Myasthenic syndrome: clinical di-

agnosis, immune-mediated mechanisms, and update on therapies. *Ann Neurol* 1995;37:635.

91. Sillevis-Smitt P, Posner JB. Paraneoplastic peripheral neuropathy. *Báilliere's Clin Neurol* 1995;4:443.

92. Colemont LJ, Camilleri M. Chronic intestinal pseudo-obstruction: diagnosis and treatment. *Mayo Clin Proc* 1989;64:60.

93. Posner JB. Paraneoplastic syndromes. In: Posner JB, ed. *Neurologic complications of cancer.* Philadelphia: FA Davis, 1995:353.

94. Brennan LV, Craddock PR: Limbic encephalopathy as a nonmetastic complication of oat cell lung cancer. Its reversal after treatment of the primary lung lesion. *Am J Med* 1983;75:518.

95. Humphrey JG, Hill ME, Gordon AS, et al. Myotonia associated with small cell carcinoma of the lung. *Arch Neurol* 1976;33: 375.

96. Digre KB. Opsoclonus in adults. Report of three cases and review of the literature. *Arch Neurol* 1996;43:1165.

97. Jacobson DM, Thirkill CE, Tipping SJ. A clinical trial to diagnose paraneoplastic retinopathy. *Ann Neurol* 1990;28:162.

98. Martinez-Lavin M, Matucci-Cerinic M, Jajic J, et al. Hypertrophic osteoarthropathy: consensus on its definition, classification, assessment and diagnostic criteria. *J Rheumatol* 1993;20:1386.

99. Stenseth JH, Clagett OT, Woolner LB. Hypertrophic pulmonary osteoarthropathy. *Dis Chest* 1967;52:62.

100. Ennis CG, Cameron DP, Burger HG. On the etiology of hypertrophic pulmonary osteoarthropathy in bronchogenic carcinoma: lack of relationship to elevated growth hormone levels. *Aust NZ J Med* 1973;3:157.

101. Sigurgeirsson B, Lindelof B, Edhag O, et al. Risk of cancer in patients with dermatomyositis or polymyositis: a population-based study. *N Engl J Med* 1992;326:363.

102. Lakhampal S, Bunch TW, Ilstrup DM, et al. Polymyositis-dermatomyositis and malignant lesions: does an association exist? *Mayo Clin Proc* 1986;61:645.

103. Cohen PR, Kurzrock R. Mucocutaneous paraneoplastic syndromes. *Semin Oncol* 1997;24:334.

104. Spivak JL. Cancer-related anemia: its causes and characteristics. *Semin Oncol* 1994;21:3.

105. Spira MA, Lynch EC. Autoimmune hemolytic anemia and carcinoma: an unusual association. *Am J Med* 1979;67:753.

106. Antman KH, Skarin AT, Mayer RJ, et al. Microangiopathic hemolytic anemia and cancer: a review. *Medicine* 1979;58:377.

107. Shimasaki AK, Hirata T, Kawamura T, et al. The level of serum granulocyte colony-stimulating factor in cancer patients with leukocytosis. *Internal Med* 1992;31:861.

108. Gastl G, Plante M, Finstead CI, et al. High IL-6 levels in ascitic fluid correlate with reactive thrombocytosis with epithelial ovarian cancer. *Br J Hematol* 1993;83:433.

109. Estrov Z, Talpaz M, Maligit G, et al. Elevated plasma thrombopoietin activity in patients with cancer related thrombocytosis. *Am J Med* 1995;98:551.

110. Doan C, Bouroncie BA, Wiseman BK. Idiopathic and secondary thrombocytopenic purpura: clinical study and evaluation of 381 cases over a period of 28 years. *Ann Intern Med* 1960;53: 861.

111. Sack GH, Levin J, Bell WR. Trousseau's syndrome and other manifestations of chronic disseminate coagulopathy in patients with neoplasms. *Medicine* 1977;56:1.

112. Green KB, Silverstein RL. Hypercoagulability in cancer. *Hematol Oncol Clin North Am* 1996;10:506.

30

IMAGING

LESLIE E. QUINT
ISAAC R. FRANCIS
RICHARD L. WAHL
BARRY H. GROSS

Bronchogenic carcinoma is generally first imaged (and often first detected) by chest radiography. Chest radiography is the preferred initial imaging modality because of its availability, low cost, low radiation dose, and sensitivity.[1] Computed tomography (CT) and occasionally magnetic resonance (MR) imaging of the chest and abdomen are used to stage a known or suspected lung cancer. Various nuclear medicine procedures may be employed to aid in the staging process and to assess the patient's medical status for operability, including cardiac and pulmonary function. These techniques are all described in further detail in the following sections.

MORPHOLOGIC APPEARANCES OF LUNG CANCER

For the purpose of this discussion, solitary pulmonary nodule (SPN) is defined as a lesion up to four cm in diameter; larger lesions are designated as masses. Lung cancer morphology depends, to a certain extent, on cell type. Although prediction of cell type from morphology is far from 100% accurate, the following generalizations are often correct:[2]

1. Adenocarcinoma usually presents as an SPN, and most malignant SPNs are adenocarcinomas. Squamous cell is also a common SPN, while SPN is the typical manifestation of alveolar cell carcinoma.
2. Large central masses frequently represent squamous cell carcinoma or small cell carcinoma; small cell especially involves mediastinal and hilar lymph nodes, sometimes without a recognizable parenchymal lesion, while squamous cell is generally centered at or adjacent to the hilum.
3. A large peripheral mass most commonly represents large cell carcinoma or squamous cell carcinoma; adenocarcinoma occasionally manifests this way. Large cell is usually a large a peripheral mass, but a large central mass is its next most common manifestation.

4. Multiple nodules generally occur with alveolar cell carcinoma; adenocarcinoma has also manifested this way.[3] With alveolar cell carcinoma, multiple nodules are a late manifestation, usually reflecting aerogenous (or less commonly hematogenous) dissemination.
5. Airspace disease is another late manifestation of alveolar cell carcinoma. It may be focal, lobar, or more diffuse (Figure 30.1).

LUNG CANCER SCREENING

Given the success of mammographic screening for breast cancer, it seems intuitively obvious that there should be a similar benefit to chest radiographic screening for lung cancer. However, precise figures for sensitivity and specificity of chest radiography are nearly impossible to come by. In fact, sensitivity is particularly dependent on the size of the lesion, its position in the lung, and its morphology. Individual centers participating in large-scale screening of high-risk men for lung cancer have reported detection of more early stage lesions compared to newly diagnosed cancers in the typical nonscreened population.[1,4] For example, the Mayo Clinic screened men 45 years of age or older who smoked more than one pack of cigarettes per day, using chest radiography and sputum cytology every four months. In 4,593 screened patients, 92 lung cancers were detected, and more than half were American Joint Committee stage I lesions.[4] Screening at Memorial-Sloan Kettering Cancer Center produced similar results, with 40% of detected cancers still in stage I; in the two years following cessation of the screening program, this dropped to 20%.[1]

However, the real benefit of screening must be improved survival. Two analyses of the Mayo Lung Project have shown no such improvement;[5,6] the lung cancer death rate was calculated at 3.1 per 1000 person-years in the screened population, as opposed to 3.0 per 1000 person-years in a control group.[5] Furthermore, screening results in cost beyond the expense of radiography and the delivered radiation

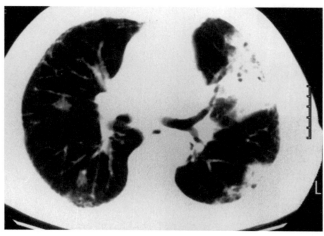

FIGURE 30.1. Multifocal, bilateral airspace disease in alveolar cell carcinoma.

dose; there are false-positive results in 5% of screening chest radiographs and in 0.5% of screening sputum cytologies.[5] A separate lung cancer screening study[7] of 305,934 participants noted a low detectability rate of stage I adenocarcinoma and late recognition of rapidly growing small cell and squamous cell carcinomas. Thus these three studies[5–7] all concluded that "a policy of periodic screening cannot yet be endorsed." In fact, the best description of lung cancer screening may be as an unproven but not a discredited practice.[8] Chapters 22 and 24 discuss new methods in lung cancer screening.

Recent studies have suggested that low-dose CT scanning might be an alternative way to screen for various pulmonary parenchymal abnormalities.[9–11] Based on initial small studies that demonstrated minimal (if any) decrement in detection of lung nodules with this technique compared to conventional-dose CT,[12–14] a recent report[15] specifically addressed the issue of low-dose CT detection of lung nodules in comparison to conventional CT images. Simulated nodules were displayed in 144 of 200 image panels, each reviewed by six radiologists independently. Nodules were detected with similar sensitivity (60% versus 63%) and specificity (88% versus 91%) by low-dose CT. Helical CT is a further technical refinement that may make low-dose CT screening a practical alternative[16–20] (see also Chapter 22).

MISSED LUNG CANCER

Experience teaches that larger lesions are more easily diagnosed than smaller lesions, and peripheral lesions are more readily detected than central lesions. Radiologic diagnosis is facilitated by the presence of typical radiographic features;

uncommon manifestations of lung cancer (such as spontaneous regression) may prove misleading.[21,22] In one study of 27 missed lung cancers, the single most frequently identified cause of missed diagnoses was failure of the radiologist to compare the current chest radiographs with previous chest radiographs.[23] Other important factors were upper lobe location of the lesion (81%) and female gender of the patient (67%).

In the Mayo Clinic lung cancer screening article cited above,[4] each radiographic study was reviewed by two (and often three) trained and interested observers (chest radiologists or chest physicians) specifically to answer the question: "Is there lung cancer?" Amazingly, 45 of 50 peripheral carcinomas that they diagnosed were visible in retrospect, with 18 visible for more than one year and four for more than two years; one was visible in retrospect for 53 months! Furthermore, 12 of 16 perihilar carcinomas and 13 of 20 carcinomas presenting as hilar or paratracheal lymph node enlargement were visible in retrospect, although not generally for as long as the peripheral carcinomas. The authors concluded that ". . . failure to detect a small pulmonary nodule on a single examination should not constitute negligence or be the basis for malpractice litigation."

SOLITARY PULMONARY NODULE (SPN)

In the setting of a previous extrapulmonary primary cancer, the relative likelihood that a new SPN is a solitary metastasis versus a new lung cancer depends on the histology of the previous primary tumor. In some instances the odds favor a new lung primary, such as for head and neck carcinoma (15.8:1), bladder carcinoma (8.3:1), and cervical carcinoma (6:1).[11] In fact, with some primaries, all malignant SPNs in one series were lung cancers (prostate, 26 patients; stomach, 7 patients; esophagus, 4 patients; pancreas, three patients). In other cases, a solitary metastasis is favored, such as in patients with soft tissue sarcoma (17.5:1), osteosarcoma (6.7:1), melanoma (4.1:1), and testicular carcinoma (2:1). With most primaries the answer is in between, but slightly favoring lung cancer; examples include breast carcinoma (1.7:1), colon carcinoma (1.4:1), renal cell carcinoma (1.2:1), and endometrial carcinoma (1.1:1).[24]

The SPN is a common presentation of lung cancer. However, most SPNs are benign. Summarizing five large series[25–29] of resected SPNs, Siegelman[30] noted that 53.9% were granulomas, 28.3% were bronchogenic carcinomas or other primary malignancies, 6.6% were hamartomas, and 3.5% were metastases. An even higher percentage of all SPNs are presumably benign, because nodules that are clearly calcified on chest radiographs are rarely resected.

The challenge in evaluating SPNs is to avoid invasive procedures in patients who have benign nodules without allowing potentially curable bronchogenic carcinomas the time to progress to more advanced or even unresectable disease. This is an area of active, ongoing research.[31–36] The many approaches that have been tried attest to the lack of complete success for any one modality to date. A proper SPN evaluation acknowledges the following key points:

1. Imaging at a single point in time relies heavily on morphologic characteristics in distinguishing benign from malignant SPNs.
2. Calcification is the single best morphologic indicator of benignancy.
3. Behavior (that is, lack of growth) is *far* better than any morphologic criterion at predicting benignancy.
4. Any predictor of benignancy must err on the side of intervention—it is better to resect a benign SPN unnecessarily than erroneously to call a malignant SPN benign.

With the above in mind, and realizing the significant expense (and in some cases radiation dose) of radiologic tests, it is always best to start the evaluation of the SPN by seeking old radiographs for comparison. This saves money, radiation, and often time, and provides the possibility for proving that a lesion is benign, no matter what its morphology is. A lesion that is stable for two years or more *is* benign—end of discussion. The flip side is that almost no matter what the morphology is, a growing lesion has declared itself to be one that should be resected. The lack of vigor with which old films are pursued is generally disappointing; if the patient were a close relative, we would all try a lot harder to spare him/her unnecessary tests that involve (potentially fatal) injection of intravenous contrast. And consider this—how many adults 40 years of age or older have never had a prior chest radiograph? In the United States the number must be vanishingly small.

When a lesion is stable, but for less than two years, the situation is less clear-cut. Follow-up radiography to two years may suffice, especially when the period of stability is already close to that standard. If only short-term (that is, less than three months) stability is established, it may be best to proceed as though no prior studies had been available.

When comparison studies are not available, demonstration of calcification is the best way to attempt to establish a benign etiology. However, not all calcifications are benign; for example, eccentric calcification of a nodule at chest radiography is unrevealing as to the nature of the nodule. The demonstration of calcification on chest radiographs has been made more difficult by current widely used techniques that employ high kVp. For that reason, chest fluoroscopy with low kVp spot films would be a good next step in looking for calcification. Unfortunately, few centers still perform chest fluoroscopy. Computed chest radiography with selective windowing may be an alternative possibility.[37]

At the current time, most patients with an SPN at chest radiography and no previous comparison films go to CT. Thin-section CT densitometry with or without a reference phantom (a cylinder filled with a calcium-containing substance that serves as a standard of comparison to assess density of a patient's nodule) facilitates the detection of calcification that could be missed on chest radiographs. In a large cooperative study, 65 of 118 (55%) benign nodules were shown by CT to contain previously unsuspected calcification.[38] In 28 of these 65 patients, the calcification was directly visible on thin-section CT images; in 37, it was detected by comparison to the reference phantom. Many centers, however, have found the phantom to be significantly less helpful, and in current practice it is rarely used.

Thin-section CT without the reference phantom has significant potential to prevent unnecessary thoracotomies. At Johns Hopkins, more than 40% of SPNs without plain film evidence of calcification proved to be benign, and more than 50% of these were correctly assessed by CT by the detection of diffuse calcification; for lesions under 2 cm in size, the likelihood both of benignancy and of correct assessment by CT increased.[39] In the absence of nodule calcification, thin-section CT can still occasionally establish a benign diagnosis. Fat in a pulmonary nodule makes hamartoma the almost certain diagnosis.[40]

In some centers, nodules that are indeterminate at CT densitometry may be percutaneously aspirated; high accuracies have been reported, with a positive predictive value of 99%. The real challenge, of course, is to make a negative cytologic aspiration accurate and furthermore to establish a specific benign diagnosis. Using systematic staining and culture schemes, high negative predictive values have been reported for patients in whom a specific benign diagnosis could be made.[41] However, the negative predictive value is generally lower in patients with a biopsy showing nonspecific inflammation. Recent published studies have reported overall negative predictive values ranging from 52% to 84%.[42,43]

Given these results, surgeons at many institutions believe that a negative fine-needle aspiration biopsy of an SPN is not sufficiently reliable due to sampling error, and they will resect the nodule regardless of the biopsy results. Therefore, preoperative biopsy is generally not indicated at such institutions. An exception would occur in the patient with a history of previous extrathoracic primary neoplasm. At other institutions, it is advocated that a nonspecific negative fine-needle aspiration biopsy of an SPN be followed by a repeat biopsy. If the repeat biopsy is also negative for neoplasm, then close follow-up is advised. Some investigators have suggested the use of core biopsies to increase the yield of specific benign diagnoses.[44,45]

Before the SPN comes to thoracotomy there is still the possibility of following the lesion radiographically at close intervals. This is where the radiologic discussion ends; follow-up radiography versus histologic sampling is a clinical, not a radiologic decision. If follow-up radiography is elected, it might start at two to three month intervals, which might later increase to six-month intervals if the SPN remains stable. The ultimate goal is to demonstrate two years of stability, proving benignancy.

An overview of the recent literature reveals many interesting and innovative approaches to proving that an SPN is benign. Preliminary studies with follow-up of noncalcified SPNs have reported that all or nearly all malignant SPNs enhance by at least 20 Hounsfield units (HU) within two to four minutes after contrast injection; few benign SPNs enhance to that degree.[46–48] Based on these promising preliminary results, a multicenter study recently evaluated 356 SPNs that were greater than or equal to 5 mm, solid, relatively spherical, homogeneous, and without calcification or fat on noncontrast images. Contrast-enhanced images were obtained at one, two, three, and four minutes after onset of injection (3 mm collimation, 420 mgl per kg, 300 mgl per ml administered at 2 ml per sec).[49] Although final results have not yet been published, an abstract of this study reports 98% sensitivity, 58% specificity, and 77% accuracy in diagnosing malignancy, using a threshold of 15 HU. Prevalence of malignancy in this patient group was 48% (171 of 356 nodules). Given the high sensitivity found by these studies, it is somewhat surprising that this has not become a standard tool in the workup of SPNs. A recent study demonstrated overlap in enhancement of malignant lesions and benign, active inflammatory lesions,[50] which may explain the low specificity and the current minor role of this technique.

Spiral (helical) CT is a new modality with greater ability to depict three-dimensional anatomy than conventional CT. Spiral CT surface evaluation of vascular involvement by SPNs was carried out in 29 patients with noncalcified SPNs of less than 3 cm in size.[36] Eighteen SPNs were malignant (nine bronchogenic carcinoma, nine metastatic) and eleven were benign (six granulomas, two hamartomas, one mixed granuloma, one arteriovenous malformation, one inflammatory infiltrate). Venous involvement was present in all 18 malignant SPNs, but also in four of 11 benign SPNs. Arterial involvement was seen in all nine bronchogenic carcinomas, in five of nine metastatic lesions, and in two of 11 benign SPNs. Thus vascular involvement does not distinguish between benign and malignant SPNs.

Magnetic resonance imaging findings in two patients with tuberculomas were potentially helpful in one study.[33] Imaging after injection of gadolinium-DTPA revealed thin rim enhancement with a low-intensity center. There was no similar appearance in a retrospective review of 20 bronchogenic carcinomas. Interestingly, the MR appearance of tuberculomas is strikingly similar to the CT appearance of tuberculous mediastinal lymph nodes after injection of intravenous contrast material.[51] Another study of 28 patients with SPNs has suggested that signal intensity measurements of nodules on dynamic contrast-enhanced MR studies may provide information about the nature of the nodules.[52]

There have been several interesting nuclear medicine approaches to the SPN using SPECT and positron emission tomography (PET). PET has shown significant promise in

several studies due to its reliance on the metabolic behavior of the nodule rather than its morphology; these studies are described in the nuclear medicine section later in this chapter.

STAGING OF LUNG CANCER

Preoperative tumor staging in patients with non–small cell lung cancer (NSCLC) is important in order to identify those patients with localized disease who are likely to benefit from surgical resection. The TNM staging system, revised in 1997, is the most widely accepted and used classification system for pre- and postoperative staging.[53,54] In the TNM staging classification, T1 tumors are 3 cm or less in diameter, are surrounded by lung or visceral pleura, and are without bronchoscopic evidence of invasion more proximal than the lobar bronchus. T2 tumors show one or more of the following features: larger than 3 cm; involvement of a mainstem bronchus of 2 cm or more distal to the carina; invasion of visceral pleura; atelectasis extending to the hilum, without involvement of the entire lung. T3 tumors show invasion of the chest wall, diaphragm, pericardium, mediastinal pleura, or mainstem bronchus (less than 2 cm distal to the carina), or have atelectasis of an entire lung. T4 cancers invade the mediastinum, heart, great vessels, trachea, esophagus, or vertebral body, have an associated malignant pleural effusion, have satellite nodule(s) within the ipsilateral primary-tumor lobe of the lung. Metastatic spread to lymph nodes is classified as N1 for peribronchial or ipsilateral hilar nodes and for intrapulmonary nodes involved by direct extension of the primary tumor. Metastatic disease to ipsilateral mediastinal or subcarinal nodes falls into the N2 category, and into the N3 category for involvement of contralateral mediastinal or hilar nodes, and ipsilateral or contralateral scalene or supraclavicular lymph nodes.

Stage I tumors have no lymph node metastases. Stage II tumors either have no lymph node metastases or spread is confined to hilar lymph nodes. Stage IIIA includes tumors with spread to ipsilateral mediastinal or subcarinal nodes, whereas stage IIIB includes tumors with involvement of contralateral mediastinal or hilar nodes, and ipsilateral or contralateral scalene or supraclavicular lymph nodes. Tumors with distant metastases are classified as stage IV.

COMPUTED TOMOGRAPHY (CT)

Evaluation of the Primary Tumor

Pleural Invasion

A pleural effusion in a patient with lung cancer may be malignant, caused by pleural metastases, or it may be benign, particularly in a patient with postobstructive pneumo-

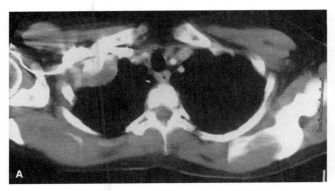
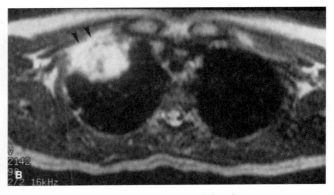

FIGURE 30.2. **A:** CT shows right upper lobe mass encasing and destroying a rib. **B:** T2-weighted MR image reveals high-signal-intensity material within the anterior chest wall (*arrowheads*) indicative of tumor invasion.

nia. The hallmark for a malignant effusion is soft-tissue nodularity along the pleural surfaces, accompanying the effusion, although this finding is not always present. It has been reported that pleural nodularity and/or fissural thickening are indicative of pleural metastases, even in the absence of pleural effusion.[55] Pleural tumor dissemination is classified as T4 disease and is generally considered unresectable.

Chest Wall Invasion

CT has shown somewhat disparate results in assessing for chest wall invasion by tumor, with sensitivity ranging from 38% to 87% and specificity from 40% to 90%.[56–62] Signs of invasion may include bone destruction with mass extending into the chest wall, pleural thickening, loss of the extrapleural fat plane, obtuse angle between mass and chest wall, and greater than 3 cm of contact between mass and chest wall (Figures 30.2, 30.3, 30.4). In a series of 112 patients

with cancers adjacent to the pleural surface, Ratto and colleagues[59] found that CT was 83% sensitive and 80% specific for chest wall invasion using a cutoff of 0.9 for the ratio between the length of tumor-pleura contact and tumor diameter. They also found that obliteration of the extrapleural fat plane was 85% sensitive and 87% specific for invasion. However, they noted that the extrapleural fat plane was not always visible, particularly when the tumor contacted the ribs; on the other hand, this plane was usually visible when the tumor contacted the pleural surface in between the ribs. Length of tumor-pleura contact, angle between the tumor and the pleura, presence of soft tissue mass involving the chest wall, and rib destruction were less accurate indicators of chest wall invasion in this series. Pennes and associates[58] noted that in their series of 33 patients with peripheral pulmonary malignancies, five patients showed encroachment on or increased density of the extrapleural fat; however, only three of these five had chest wall or pleural invasion

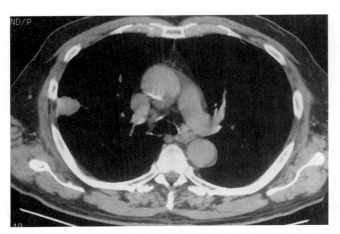

FIGURE 30.3. Peripheral right lung mass is indeterminate for chest wall invasion at CT. Surgical specimen showed no pleural invasion.

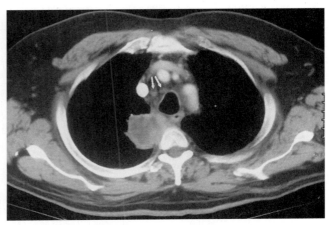

FIGURE 30.4. False-negative CT for spine invasion and mediastinal lymph node metastases (*arrows* point to normal-sized mediastinal nodes).

at surgery. In the other two patients, lymphoid aggregates were present in the extrapleural fat, suggesting that nonspecific inflammatory processes involving the pleura may extend into the adjacent extrapleural soft tissues. Pleural thickening was a very sensitive (100%) indicator of chest wall invasion in this study, although very poor specificity (44%) led to poor accuracy (58%). In the 20 patients with peripheral lung malignancies studied by Pearlberg and co-workers[62], definite bone destruction at CT showed 100% positive predictive value (11 of 11). Tumor extension around ribs into fat or muscle of the chest wall had a positive predictive value of 33% (three of nine). In each of these six false-positive cases, fibrous, inflammatory, and/or hemorrhagic changes were shown in the adjacent pleural or extrapleural tissues, but no tumor extension was seen.

Some investigators have employed artificial (that is, induced) pneumothorax in order to increase the accuracy of CT in diagnosing chest wall and mediastinal pleural invasion (Figure 30.5). For example, Watanabe and colleagues[63]

found 100% sensitivity, 80% specificity and 88% accuracy for CT using this technique in 12 patients. In one patient with no separation between the tumor and the mediastinal pleura, only adhesions were found at surgery, with no mediastinal tumor invasion. In a different study of 43 patients with equivocal chest wall invasion on routine CT, artificial pneumothorax yielded 100% accuracy for diagnosing chest wall invasion and 76% accuracy for mediastinal invasion.[64] These authors noted difficulty when the tumor was near the root of the pulmonary arteries and veins, because it was occasionally hard to introduce air into this region of the pleural space.

Other techniques for diagnosing chest wall invasion rely on the absence of relative movement between the chest wall and the adjacent tumor during respiration. Investigators have used inspiratory/expiratory CT, ultrasonography, and cine-MR during deep breathing to evaluate this feature, with moderately successful results.[65–67]

In summary, these studies suggest that the best and the

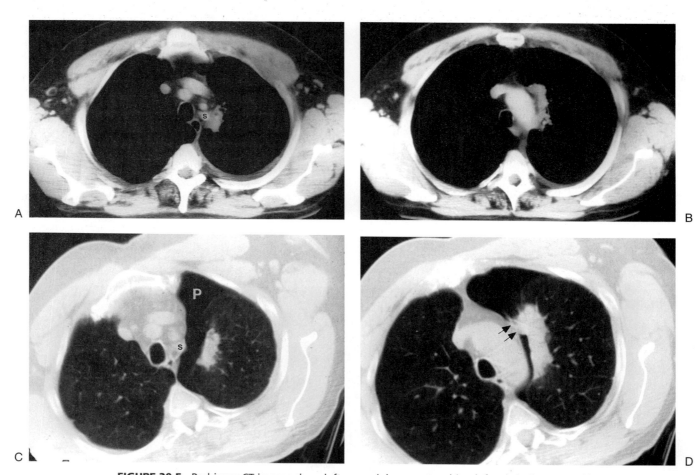

FIGURE 30.5. Prebiopsy CT images show left upper lobe mass touching left subclavian artery (s) (**A**) and mediastinal pleura (**B**), suggestive of invasion of these structures. Postbiopsy CT images reveal a left pneumothorax (*P*) with separation of the mass from the left subclavian artery (s) (**C**), proving lack of invasion of the artery. However, the mass remains adherent to the mediastinal pleura (*arrows*) (**D**). At surgery there was no mediastinal invasion. (From Quint L, Francis I. Radiologic staging of lung cancer. *J Thorac Imaging* 1999:14;235, with permission.)

only reliable criterion for diagnosing chest wall invasion with routine CT is definite bone destruction, with or without tumor mass extending into the chest wall. Thin sections (3 to 5 mm) and bone window photography are often helpful in making this assessment. It should be noted that chest wall invasion does not preclude surgical resection, because the surgeon can perform en bloc resection and chest wall reconstruction. However, this procedure is associated with increased operative morbidity and mortality. In addition, patients with known mediastinal nodal metastases and chest wall invasion are felt to have a very poor prognosis (7% reported five-year survival following surgical resection), and surgery is usually not advocated in these patients.[68,69] Superior sulcus tumors invading extrapleurally are usually treated with radiation therapy followed by surgical resection.

Mediastinal Invasion

Although invasion of the mediastinum falls into the T4 category in the TNM staging classification, minimal invasion of fat only (without invasion of vascular or other structures) is generally considered resectable by many surgeons. Therefore it is not usually necessary preoperatively to diagnose mediastinal fat invasion. On the other hand, a reliable diagnosis of invasion of mediastinal vessels, trachea, esophagus, and/or vertebral body would preclude surgical resection. Several studies have investigated the usefulness of CT in detecting mediastinal invasion and in predicting resectability of the primary tumor.[56,60,70–77] Accuracy for distinguishing between T0–2 and T3–4 tumors has been reported to be 56% to 89%.[74–77] However, this information is not particularly helpful, because the clinically important distinction is between resectable (T3) and unresectable (T4) cancers.

In one retrospective study of 80 patients with an indeterminate CT for mediastinal invasion (that is, mass contig-

uous with the mediastinum but without definite infiltration into the mediastinal fat or extension around the central vessels or mainstem bronchi), the authors were able to identify a large group of masses that were likely to be technically resectable using one or more of the following criteria: contact of 3 cm or less with mediastinum, less than 90 degrees of contact with aorta, and mediastinal fat between the mass and mediastinal structure.[70] Thirty-six of 37 masses in this category were resectable; 28 of 36 masses had no mediastinal invasion, and eight of 36 had focal limited invasion. However, more than 3 cm contact with mediastinum, more than 90 degrees of contact with aorta, obliteration of the fat plane between the mass and mediastinal structures, presence of mass effect on adjacent mediastinal structures, and pleural or pericardial thickening were not reliable signs of either invasion or unresectability. Kameda and colleagues[72] studied 52 patients with lung cancer, including 21 with central tumors. CT was 100% sensitive although not specific (60% to 67%) in evaluating for superior vena cava or right pulmonary artery invasion. For the left pulmonary artery and the left atrium or pulmonary vein, CT had high specificity (94% to 100%) but poor sensitivity (56% to 62%). In a CT study of 108 patients, Izbicki and associates reported one false-positive case for aortic invasion and multiple false-negative cases for invasion of an atrium, pulmonary artery, superior vena cava, or mediastinal bronchus.[73] Choe and colleagues found that obliteration of the superior pulmonary vein at CT was consistent with intrapericardial extension of tumor through the pulmonary vein in ten of ten patients.[78] On the other hand, only four of nine patients with obliteration of the inferior pulmonary vein at CT showed intrapericardial tumor extension at surgery.

In summary, CT diagnosis of mediastinal fat or mediastinal structure invasion is generally unreliable, and a patient should not be denied surgery based on unproven CT findings (Figures 30.6, 30.7, 30.8, 30.9). Gross medi-

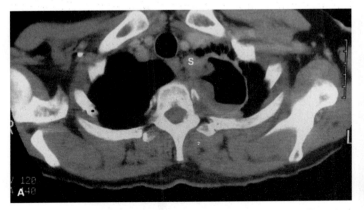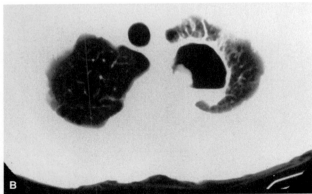

FIGURE 30.6. A,B: Cavitary squamous cell carcinoma obliterates margins of left subclavian artery (s), suggesting invasion. No invasion present at surgery.

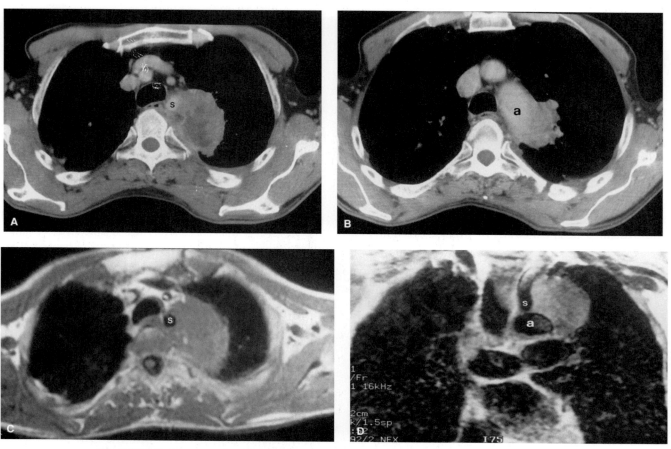

FIGURE 30.7. Lung mass invades mediastinal fat and touches left subclavian artery (s) and aortic arch (a) on axial CT (**A,B**), axial MR (**C**), and coronal MR (**D**) images. Surgery revealed left subclavian artery invasion, although the aortic arch was intact.

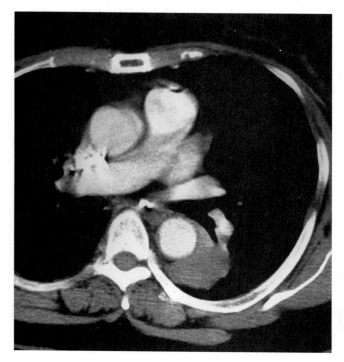

FIGURE 30.8. Left lower lobe mass contacts the aorta over a large portion of its circumference, suggesting aortic invasion. At surgery the aorta was not invaded. (From Quint L, Francis I. Radiologic staging of lung cancer. *J Thorac Imaging* 1999:14;235, with permission.)

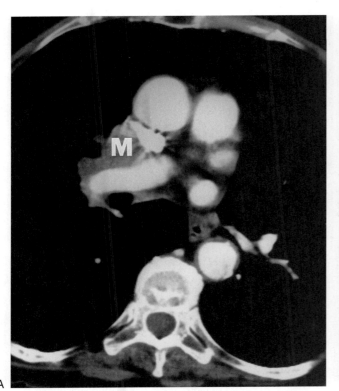
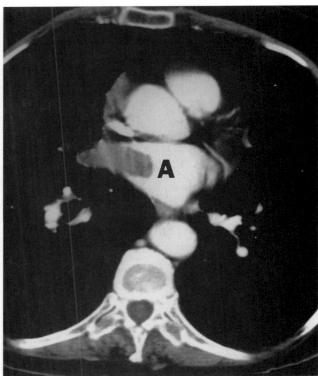

A   B

FIGURE 30.9. **A,B:** Right hilar mass (*M*) invades into the left atrium (*A*) via the right superior pulmonary vein.

astinal fat invasion may be proved via mediastinoscopy or transbronchial Wang needle biopsy. Findings suggestive of central tracheobronchial invasion at CT are usually further evaluated using bronchoscopy. CT and bronchoscopy are complementary procedures: bronchoscopy is superior to CT in evaluating the mucosal surface of the airway, whereas CT is superior in visualizing tumor spread extraluminally and occasionally within the wall of the bronchus.

Prediction of Need for Lobectomy versus Pneumonectomy

Tumor invasion of central pulmonary arteries and veins, as well as tumor extension across the major fissure (anywhere on the left; above the minor fissure on the right), are findings that would generally require pneumonectomy for resection rather than lobectomy. In many cases, tumor involvement of a mainstem bronchus also necessitates pneumonectomy (Figure 30.10), although some of these tumors may be resected with lobectomy using a sleeve resection and bronchoplasty (Figure 30.11, 30.12). The assessment of the need for lobectomy versus pneumonectomy is important in the patient with poor pulmonary function who

cannot tolerate a pneumonectomy. Quint and colleagues[79] found CT to be inaccurate in making this assessment (Figure 30.13), although thin sections (1.5 to 3.0 mm) helped in evaluating for tumor spread across a fissure (Figure 30.14). Preliminary work done by this group suggested that three-dimensional CT reconstructions in this setting may improve accuracy in evaluating central pulmonary vascular invasion.[80] Thin sections (less than or equal to 3 mm) are probably necessary to evaluate the central bronchi optimally. Newer CT scanners using helical or spiral scanning modes will enable acquisition of large numbers of thin sections during a single breath hold. These capabilities may facilitate analysis of tumor invasion into adjacent structures, particularly using sagittal, coronal, and off-axis planar reconstructed images.

Differentiation between Tumor and Adjacent Atelectasis/Pneumonia

Another use for CT in evaluating local extension of the primary tumor is in distinguishing central tumor from adjacent collapsed lung. After an intravenous bolus of urographic contrast material, the atelectatic lung may enhance much more than the adjacent tumor, thus giving a more

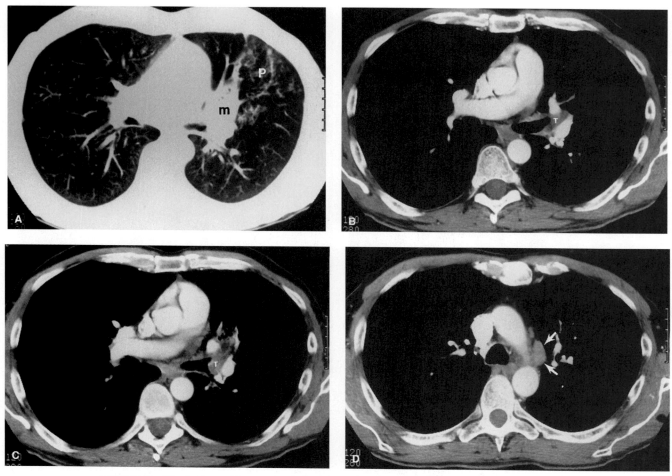

FIGURE 30.10. **A:** Central lung mass (m) with postobstructive pneumonitis (P). **B,C:** Tumor (*T*) involves upper and lower lobe bronchi. Invasion of left main stem bronchus seen at bronchoscopy; pneumonectomy performed. **D:** Enlarged aortopulmonary window lymph nodes (*arrows*) were benign at histological analysis.

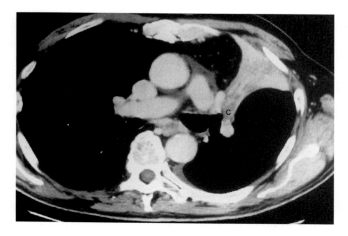

FIGURE 30.11. Left upper lobe carcinoma (*C*) with postobstructive atelectasis. Invasion of left mainstem bronchus necessitated resection via sleeve lobectomy.

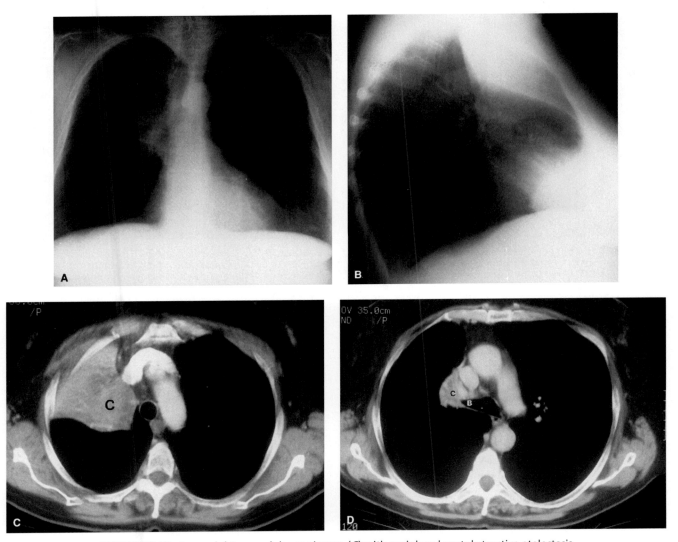

FIGURE 30.12. Large right upper lobe carcinoma (*C*) with peripheral postobstructive atelectasis. Chest radiographs (**A,B**) demonstrate right upper lobe collapse. CT (**C,D**) shows occlusion of right upper lobe bronchus and narrowing of right mainstem bronchus (*B*). Right upper lobectomy performed using sleeve resection.

accurate assessment of tumor size[81] (Figures 30.15, 30.16). However, in many cases it remains difficult to distinguish tumor from adjacent postobstructive atelectasis or pneumonia (Figures 30.17, 30.18).

CT Evaluation of Hilar and Mediastinal Lymph Nodes

Significance

Metastatic disease to hilar lymph nodes (N1 disease) adversely affects patient prognosis, although it does not generally affect resectability. Usually, involved hilar nodes can be easily removed from the hilar vessels at surgery. Thus, while preoperative detection of tumor spread to hilar nodes is useful, it is generally not crucial in directing surgical treat-

ment planning. Moreover, the presence or absence of hilar node metastases is an unreliable indicator of mediastinal node metastases.[82,83]

In the past, the presence of mediastinal node metastases has been considered a contraindication to thoracotomy, and preoperative detection of mediastinal spread of disease has generally precluded surgical resection. However, some investigators have found reasonable three- and five-year survival rates for patients with positive ipsilateral mediastinal nodes, and many surgeons now feel that certain groups of patients with limited N2 disease may be surgical candidates.[84–86] Naruke and colleagues[87] found significantly increased five-year survival in patients with N2 disease (14%) as compared to patients with N3 disease (0%) following pulmonary resection in 1,479 patients with no distant metastatic disease. It has been suggested that resection may be

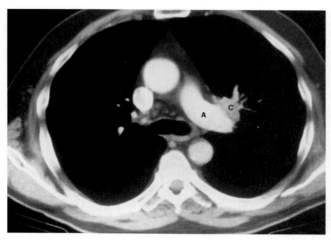

FIGURE 30.13. Left upper lobe cancer (*C*) abutting left main pulmonary artery (*A*). Arterial invasion present at surgery. (From Quint L, Glazer G, Orringer M. Central lung masses: prediction with CT of need for pneumonectomy versus lobectomy. *Radiology* 1987;165:735, with permission.)

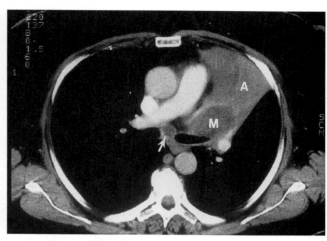

FIGURE 30.15. Contrast enhanced CT reveals low-density, central left upper lobe mass (*M*) with higher-density postobstructive atelectasis (*A*). Enlarged subcarinal lymph node (*arrow*).

worthwhile in patients with ipsilateral mediastinal nodal disease as long as the nodes are not in the high paratracheal region, are not numerous or bulky, and can be completely resected.[88,89] Some groups have advocated surgical resection in conjunction with postoperative radiation therapy in patients with mediastinal metastases.[82,90,91] Other investigators have suggested that patients with N2 or N3 disease may benefit from chemotherapy or combined chemotherapy and radiation, either alone or prior to surgical resection.[92–97]

CT Criteria for Detection of Lymph Node Metastases

Given the importance of preoperative nodal staging for treatment planning, a noninvasive imaging modality such as CT is of great potential value for assessment of mediastinal nodes, both ipsilateral and contralateral to the primary lung tumor. Mediastinal lymph nodes are generally identified on axial CT images as nonenhancing, oval, soft tissue densities surrounded by mediastinal fat. Nodal size can be estimated by measuring the short and long-axis diameters of a node as seen on the axial images. Glazer and colleagues[98] stated

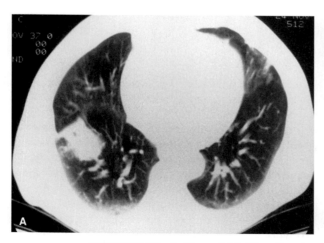

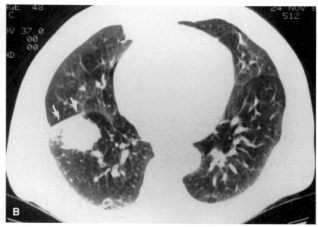

FIGURE 30.14. A: 10 mm thick CT section shows right lower lobe mass in region of major fissure. **B:** 3 mm thick CT section shows tumor confined to the lower lobe, without transfissural tumor spread (*arrows* define fissure). Findings surgically confirmed. (From Quint L, Gross B, Glazer G. Primary and metastatic malignancy. *Lung biology, health and disease.* 46 vol. Marcel Dekker, 1990: 1999, with permission.)

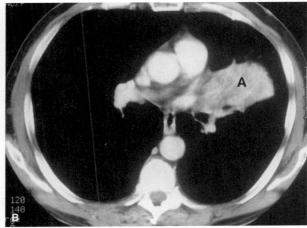

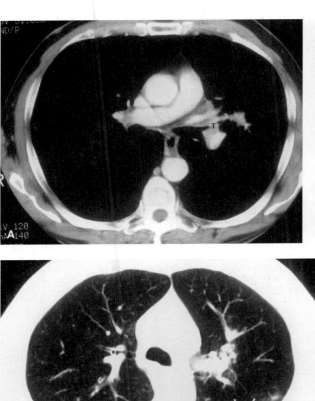

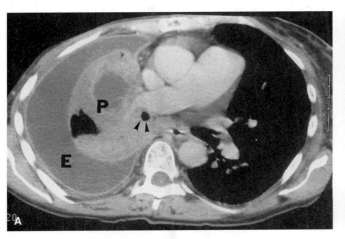

FIGURE 30.16. Patient with two separate lung cancers. **A:** Left upper lobe endobronchial tumor (*T*). **B:** Note high-density, branching vessels in postobstructive atelectasis (*A*). **C:** Additional cancer in the superior segment of the left lower lobe (*arrows*).

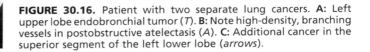

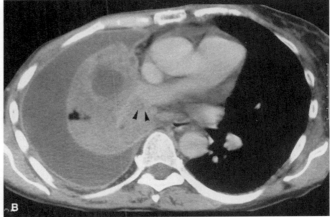

FIGURE 30.17. Small tumor in bronchus intermedius with necrotic, postobstructive pneumonia (*P*) simulating large lung tumor (*E, benign pleural effusion*). **A:** Superior portion of bronchus intermedius is patent (*arrowheads*). **B:** More inferiorly, the bronchus is occluded by tumor (*arrowheads*).

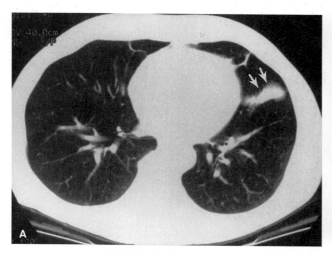
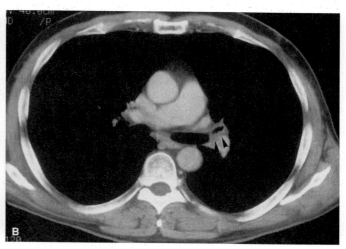

FIGURE 30.18. Postobstructive atelectasis simulating a peripheral cancer. **A:** Lingular opacity (*arrows*) originally interpreted as an enlarging lung nodule on serial chest radiographs and CT scans. **B:** The true cancer is a small endobronchial lesion (*arrowheads*) obstructing the lingular bronchus.

that the short-axis diameter is a more accurate predictor of nodal size than the long-axis diameter, because long-axis measurements are more dependent on the spatial orientation of the node. The long-axis diameter is accurate on transverse CT images only when the longest axis of the ovoid, three-dimensional lymph node is oriented in the plane of section that is, the transverse plane. If the lymph node is vertically oriented, the long-axis diameter on CT has no relation to the true long-axis measurement of the lymph node. Short-axis diameters are also affected by nodal orientation, although to a lesser extent. In a CT/autopsy correlation study, Quint and co-workers[99] found that the short-axis diameter of the nodes at CT was the best predictor of actual nodal volume.

CT criteria for lymph node malignancy theoretically in-clude morphological features such as nodal density and margination, as well as nodal size. In practice, however, most of these features are not helpful, and increased nodal size is the only useful criterion for malignancy (Figure 30.19). One exception to this rule is the occasional finding of central nodal low density, suggesting necrosis (Figure 30.20); this is a good indicator for malignant nodal disease. Rarely the central low density will show the attenuation of fat, and this finding is reliable for benignancy (Figure 30.21). In addition, a recent study has suggested that rounding of the contour of a hilar lymph node, where it meets the lung margin, is indicative of metastatic disease.[100]

Several groups have investigated the normal size limits for mediastinal lymph nodes, studying normal patients and those with lung cancer. Genereux and Howie[101] studied CT scans of normal patients and compared their findings with dissection of 12 cadaver mediastina. The largest medi-

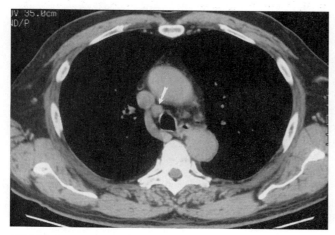

FIGURE 30.19. Mildly enlarged right paratracheal lymph node (*arrow*) containing proven metastasis.

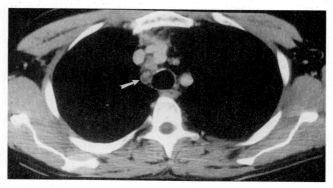

FIGURE 30.20. Mildly enlarged tumor containing right paratracheal lymph nodes, one showing central necrosis (*arrow*).

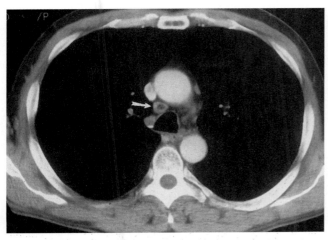

FIGURE 30.21. Central fat density within an enlarged mediastinal lymph node (*arrow*) is reliable for benignancy.

astinal nodes at CT were in the precarinal/subcarinal and aortopulmonary regions, and at autopsy, the largest nodes were in the pretracheal and precarinal/subcarinal regions. These authors measured long-axis lymph node diameters at CT and found that 95% were less than 11 mm. In another CT study by Schnyder and Gamsu,[102] the mean diameter of normal lymph nodes in the pretracheal, retrocaval space was 5.5 mm plus or minus 2.8 SD (short versus long axis not specified), with 91% (116 of 127) being less than or equal to 1 cm. A CT/autopsy study in five cadavers by Quint and colleagues[99] showed excellent correlation for the number of nodes in right-sided mediastinal regions, with poorer correlation in left-sided regions. Mean short-axis nodal diameters at CT ranged from 3.2 to 7.3 mm, depending on exact nodal location. Kiyono and colleagues[103] dissected 40 cadaver mediastina from patients without chest malignancy or infection, and recorded the number, size (short and long axes in the transverse plane), and ATS location of each lymph node identified. Based on their findings, these authors proposed standards for maximum short axis diameters as follows: 12 mm for ATS region 7 (subcarinal), 10 mm for ATS regions 4 (right lower paratracheal) and 10R (right tracheobronchial angle), and 8 mm for other regions. They found that maximum long-axis diameters showed a wider variation.

Glazer et al.[98] examined normal mediastinal lymph nodes on CT scans from 56 normal patients and tabulated the number and size of lymph nodes in each anatomical region as specified by the American Thoracic Society (ATS) lymph node mapping scheme. In this study, 1 cm was the optimal upper limit of normal for the short axis of a mediastinal node at CT, with slight variations according to specific location (range 7 to 11 mm). The largest nodes were in the subcarinal and right tracheobronchial regions, whereas the smallest nodes were in the upper paratracheal and left peri-

bronchial regions. A prior CT study by the same group involving patients with NSCLC similarly found 1 cm as the optimal size threshold for diagnosing metastatic disease in mediastinal nodes.[104] Platt and colleagues[105] confirmed 11 mm as the upper limit of normal size at CT for subcarinal lymph nodes in 46 patients with NSCLC.

In order to address the issue of lymph node size versus presence/absence of metastases, Gallardo and colleagues conducted a pathological study of lymph nodes resected from 67 patients with NSCLC.[106] The authors correlated lymph node size (as measured on the fresh, resected nodes in the pathology department) with presence or absence of tumor at histological examination. Using a size threshold of 10 mm (short versus long axis not specified), 73 of 167 (44%) patients had enlarged mediastinal nodes and 58 of 167 (35%) had enlarged hilar nodes. Eighteen of 73 (25%) and 12 of 58 (21%) patients had neoplastic involvement of mediastinal and hilar nodes at pathological examination, respectively (25% mediastinal nodal PPV). The PPV for enlarged mediastinal lymph nodes in squamous cell carcinoma was 23% and in adenocarcinoma was 18%. These low values were reflective of the large number of false-positive cases due to enlarged, benign lymph nodes.

These results highlight one pitfall in using a nodal size threshold to distinguish benign from malignant lymph nodes at CT. Benign nodes may be enlarged due to reactive hyperplasia, anthracosis, inflammation, or infection (Figure 30.22). Conversely, malignant nodes may be normal in size if they contain only microscopic metastases (Figure 30.4). Daly and associates[107] reported that enlarged, benign nodes were a particular problem for central tumors with postobstructive pneumonia. Gross and co-workers[108] addressed the issue of microscopic metastases to normal-sized nodes in a study of 39 patients with bronchogenic carcinoma. Five of 39 (13%) patients had metastases limited to normal-sized nodes as measured at surgery and pathology; however, two of these five patients showed enlarged nodes at CT owing to inaccurate CT depiction of nodal size in the subcarinal region. In one patient, multiple normal-sized subcarinal nodes containing metastatic tumor were visualized only as a single large mass at CT. In the second patient, a 10 × 9 mm subcarinal node containing metastatic tumor measured 12 × 11 mm at CT, and was therefore identified as abnormal. Thus metastatic disease to normal-sized mediastinal lymph nodes was missed at CT in only three of 39 (8%) patients, and the authors concluded that metastatic disease to normal-sized mediastinal lymph nodes is not a major problem in CT staging of lung cancer. Similarly, Daly and associates[107] reported that of 146 patients studied, only two of eight CT false-negative cases were attributable to microscopic metastases. On the other hand, ten of 25 (40%) patients with mediastinal metastases in one study[88] and seven of 11 (64%) patients in another study[109] had no enlarged nodes. There is no obvious explanation for these discrepant results.

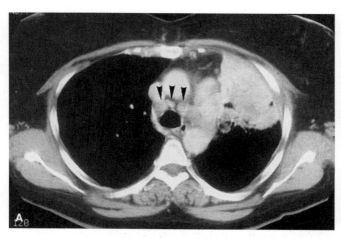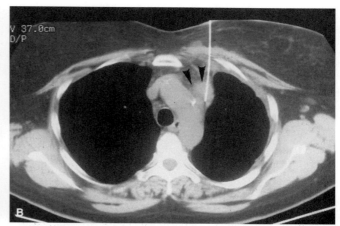

FIGURE 30.22. **A,B:** Left upper lobe cancer, postobstructive pneumonia, and bilaterally enlarged mediastinal lymph nodes (*arrowheads*). Right paratracheal lymph nodes (sampled via mediastinoscopy) and aortopulmonary window lymph nodes (sampled via CT guided aspiration biopsy) were benign. A single left lower paratracheal lymph node contained metastatic disease at thoracotomy.

Regardless of the actual frequency of microscopic lymph node metastases, it has been suggested that microscopic disease may have a better prognosis than metastases to enlarged nodes, and thus it may not be as crucial to detect microscopic spread of tumor preoperatively.[85,110] For instance, Pearson and colleagues[89] reported that the survival rate in patients whose N2 status was established at mediastinoscopy was significantly worse than in those with a negative mediastinoscopy, in whom the N2 status was established at subsequent thoracotomy. Similarly, Cybulsky and co-workers found that patients with false-negative CT studies for mediastinal nodal metastases did better than those with true-positive CT studies (five-year survival following resection was 13.5% versus 6.6%, respectively).[111] These differences may relate to the distinction between normal-sized nodes with microscopic metastases versus enlarged metastatic lymph nodes, because enlarged nodes are more likely to be detected by mediastinoscopy and called abnormal at CT. Moreover, in a study of 115 patients who had undergone resection for NSCLC, Ishida and colleagues found increased survival for patients with microscopic nodal metastases compared to those with moderate or gross nodal metastases.[112] These findings are supported by one small CT series which suggested that metastases to enlarged mediastinal nodes were more likely to have extracapsular spread of tumor than microscopic metastases to normal-sized nodes.[108] Because extracapsular spread is thought to be a poor prognostic indicator,[113,114] microscopic metastases to normal-sized nodes may have a less dire prognosis than enlarged malignant nodes.

In summary, although different size threshold values for normal mediastinal lymph nodes have been suggested, the current consensus is that this figure should generally be approximately 1 cm in short-axis diameter.[98,99,101,102,104,110,115–119] Some authors have preferred to use nodal size criteria that vary with the precise mediastinal nodal location, based on the studies described above.[120,121]

Evaluation of Hilar Lymph Node Metastases (N1 Disease)

Conventional radiography and tomography have been used extensively in the past to evaluate patients with bronchogenic carcinoma. In one study of 47 lung cancer patients, the reported sensitivity of conventional radiography for hilar disease was 53%, with specificity of 84% and accuracy of 71%.[118] In a subsequent study of 84 patients with suspected intrathoracic neoplasm, sensitivity and accuracy were 64% and specificity was 65%.[122] Conventional tomography has been only slightly better. Reported sensitivities have ranged from 47% to 85%, specificities from 60% to 80%, and accuracies from 74% to 80% in three studies.[118,122,123] Accuracy was not reported and could not be calculated in one additional series,[124] but must have fallen between 47% and 72%.

The accuracy of CT in detecting hilar lymph node metastases is unclear. Three lung cancer studies reported low sensitivity (45% to 63%) and positive predictive value (38% to 68%) and moderately high negative predictive value (79% to 85%).[73,125,126] Two of these studies showed high specificity (92% to 93%), whereas the other reported only 58% specificity. Accuracies ranged from 59% to 82%. One older report was more sanguine, with 90% accuracy, 88% positive predictive value, and 100% negative predictive value.[8]

Evaluation of Mediastinal Lymph Node Metastases (N2/N3 Disease)

The accuracy of conventional radiography and tomography in diagnosing mediastinal lymph node metastases has generally been quite low due to poor sensitivity (6% to 81% sensitivity for conventional radiographs and 20% to 73% for tomography).[75,107,110,117,118,124,127-131] Disparate results have been reported regarding the accuracy of CT in this setting (Table 30.1). Many studies have found fairly high sensitivity for CT (>85%)[8,61,76,104,116,118,120,124,131-134] and high negative predictive value (>85%)[8,120,121,126,132,133,135-137] (Table 30.1). Others have found high specificty (>85%).[73,107,119-121,128,132,133,136-141] On the other hand, other recent studies have shown low accuracy, resulting from both poor sensitivity and poor specificity.[56,74,125] Low sensitivity in some studies was attributed to the high frequency of microscopic metastases within normal-sized nodes.[73] Low specificity arose from the frequent occurrence of enlarged, hyperplastic nodes, particularly in patients with postobstructive pneumonitis.[125] Dales and colleagues[142] performed a metaanalysis of CT accuracy in staging mediastinal lymph nodes in NSCLC using data from studies published between 1980 and 1988. Pooled data revealed accuracy, sensitivity, and specificity figures that were approximately 80% each. They found no significant differences between the results from studies performed using fourth-generation versus third/second-generation CT scanners. Moreover, there is no data to suggest that the new helical/spiral scanners will improve CT accuracy in this setting.

Results within some of the individual studies quoted above varied according to the size and morphologic criteria used for diagnosing metastatic disease to mediastinal lymph nodes. For example, Seely and associates[136] found that sensitivity increased and specificity decreased if long-axis diameter measurements were used instead of short-axis measurements or if adjacent nodal stations were considered together instead of considering each nodal station alone. Buy and co-workers[120] found maximal sensitivity when individual size thresholds were used for each individual nodal station, rather than using a uniform 10 mm size cutoff. In contrast, the data of Ikezoe and colleagues showed slightly better sensitivity, albeit significantly worse specificity and accuracy, using a uniform 10 mm threshold rather than two separate criteria (13 mm for nodes in the subcarinal, precarinal, and tracheobronchial regions and 10 mm for nodes in other regions).[121] Specificity in the study of Buy and co-workers[120] was maximized when the criterion for nodal abnormality was defined as follows: the short axis of the largest mediastinal node in the lymphatic drainage territory of the cancer was greater than or equal to 10 mm and the difference between this node and the largest node in the other territories was greater than 5 mm. According to the investi-

gation of Ratto and colleagues,[133] specificity increased dramatically if nodes 10 to 15 mm in short-axis diameter were considered indeterminate and excluded from analysis. However, 36% (44 of 123) of patients fell into this category, limiting the usefulness of this criterion. These authors also found increased specificity if the criterion for abnormal nodes was modified to include nodes 10 to 20 mm in short axis diameter with central necrosis and/or a discontinuous capsule.

In some studies, CT accuracy also appeared to depend on the precise anatomic location within the mediastinum being analyzed. In the study of McLoud and colleagues,[125] sensitivity of CT using a single size criterion (10 mm short-axis diameter) varied for individual nodal stations, ranging from 17% to 83%. Highest sensitivity was found in ATS regions 4R and 5, and lowest in 7, 4L, 10R, 10L. Specificity ranged from 72% to 94%, being highest in 10L and lowest in 10R. Platt and associates compared staging of right and left lung tumors.[115] Although prior reports have shown that CT is more accurate in evaluating right-sided mediastinal lymph nodes,[99,143] Platt and colleagues found no statistically significant difference in staging accuracy between left and right lung cancers.[115] This is probably due to involvement of subcarinal and contralateral mediastinal lymph nodes, which are present more often in left lung cancers as compared to right-sided lesions.[144]

There were also some reported differences when the data were broken down according to cell type of the tumor. Ikezoe and colleagues[121] found that sensitivity for cases of adenocarcinoma (61%) was lower than that for squamous cell carcinoma (86%), but specificity for these two groups was almost the same (93% to 94%). There was an increased number of false-negative cases for adenocarcinomas, as compared to squamous cell carcinomas in both this study and two others;[73,111] the authors postulated that this probably indicated a higher frequency of microscopic metastases in adenocarcinomas. On the other hand, Ratto and colleagues[133] reported no difference in staging accuracy between squamous cell carcinoma and adenocarcinoma.

When calculated on a nodal station-by-station basis, results in some studies varied according to whether or not adjacent nodal stations were included in the analysis. For instance, inclusion of adjacent nodal stations led to an increase in sensitivity and a decrease in specificity in one investigation.[136] However, it is important to note that the clinical usefulness of a staging modality does not depend upon accurate detection of disease in any individual node or nodal group, but rather upon accurate detection of mediastinal nodal malignancy in the individual patient, either ipsilateral or contralateral to the neoplasm. Moreover, several authors have reported increased sensitivity in mediastinal lymph node evaluation when calculated on a patient-by-patient basis rather than on a nodal station-by-station basis.[108,125,136]

There are many possible reasons for the different re-

TABLE 30.1. CT STAGING OF MEDIASTINAL LYMPH NODE METASTASES IN PATIENTS WITH KNOWN OR SUSPECTED LUNG CANCER

Authors	No. of Patients	Patient Selection Criteria	Upper Limit Normal Lymph Node Size at CT (mm)	Basis	Prevalence (%)	Sensitivity (%)	Specificity (%)	Accuracy (%)	PPV (%)	NPV (%)
Lewis et al. (1990)[126]	418	Known lung cancer	10	Per patient	29	84	84	84	69	93
Ikezoe et al. (1990)[121]	208	Known lung cancer; only adeno-carcinoma and squamous cell carcinoma included	13 SAD for subcarinal, precarinal and tracheobronchial regions; 10 SAD other regions	Per patient	31	69	94	86	83	91
Ratto et al. (1990)[133]	123	Known non–small cell lung cancer; patients with proven N3 disease excluded	<10 SAD	Per patient	32.5	90	54	66	48	92
			<10 SAD*	Per patient	32.5	86‡	88‡	87‡	80‡	92‡
			<20 SAD†	Per patient	32.5	75	90	85	79	88
Webb et al. (1991)[74]	155	Known or suspected non–small cell lung cancer	NS	Per patient	21	52	69	65	31	84
Cybulsky et al. (1992)[111]	124	Proven N2 disease	<10 LAD	Per patient	NS	51	NS	NS	NS	NS
Izbicki et al. (1992)[73]	108	Known lung cancer	10 SAD	Per station	19#	24#	93#	80#	44#	84#
				Per patient	26#	NS	NS	58#	NS	NS
McLoud et al. (1992)[125]	143	Known or suspected lung cancer	10 SAD	Per station	15	44	85	79	34	89
				Per patient	31	64	62	63	44	79
Daly et al. (1993)[128]	681	Known lung cancer	<10–15¶	Per patient	NS	NS	NS	NS	NS	93
Seely et al. (1993)[136]	104	Known lung cancer; only T1 lesions	10 LAD	Per station	8	55	86	83	25	96
			10 SAD	Per station	8	41	93	89	35	95
			10 LAD	Per station including adjacent stations	8	77	73	71	14	98
			10 SAD	Per station including adjacent stations	8	59	91	88	36	96
			10 LAD	Per patient	21	77	73	74	44	92
			10 SAD	Per patient	21	59	91	85	65	89
Gdeedo et al. (1997)[36]	74	Known non–small cell lung cancer; negative mediastinoscopy	10 SAD	Per patient	9.5	43	57	55	9	90

SAD, short-axis diameter
LAD, long-axis diameter
PPV, positive predictive value
NPV, negative predictive value
NS, not specified
* nodes 10 to 15 mm SAD indeterminate and excluded from analysis; nodes ·15 mm considered abnormal.
† nodes 10 to 20 mm SAD also considered abnormal if central necrosis present or capsule is discontinuous.
‡ 44/123 (36%) patients excluded from analysis.
# excludes ATS region 10
¶ <10 mm 1987–1991; <15 mm (1979–1986).

ported CT accuracies among studies in detecting mediastinal metastases. Differences in patient populations and prevalence of mediastinal nodal disease would affect CT accuracy. Some investigations included all patients with known or suspected lung cancer, and some included only those with biopsy proven cancer. Others focused on clinical T1N0M0 cancers, that is, small lesions surrounded by lung parenchyma, with no conventional radiographic signs

of mediastinal disease. Seely and colleagues[136] found higher specificity in their study of T1 cancers as compared to historical controls for all cancers. They postulated that this was partly due to lack of obstructive pneumonitis with resultant enlarged, hyperplastic nodes.

In addition, there were substantial variations in scanning techniques. Some studies used older CT scanners (second-generation) with long scan times (18 to 20 seconds), resulting in image blur from biologic motion; studies done on third- and fourth-generation scanners did not have this problem. CT examinations were performed using different section thicknesses, section spacing, and methods of administration of intravenous urographic contrast material. Gaps between slices [139,140,145] and motion artifact from long scan times[117,138–140] probably contributed to insensitive detection of enlarged lymph nodes. There were no uniform criteria for interpreting the scans, and definitions of nodal enlargement ranged from "any visible node" to 2 cm diameter, with or without morphological nodal changes. Some investigators interpreted their results on a patient-by-patient basis, some on a nodal station-by-station basis, and some on a nodal station-by-station basis including adjacent nodal stations. It can be quite difficult at CT and surgery to precisely determine the boundaries between one nodal station and an adjacent one, and some studies, including the recent, large study of McLoud and associates[125] made no allowances for this pitfall. Many studies appeared to lack precise radiologic/surgical/pathologic correlation, and different methods of proof were employed. This is important because certain mediastinal node groups are accessible only at thoracotomy and would be missed at mediastinoscopy. Moreover, it is plausible that those studies employing thorough mediastinal lymph node dissection rather than nodal palpation and biopsy would show decreased CT sensitivity, due to the inability to detect microscopic metastases within normal sized lymph nodes. However, Daly and co-workers[107] were unable to substantiate this premise. They divided their patients into two surgical groups: in group I (51 cases) mediastinal nodes were removed only if palpably abnormal, if CT showed enlarged nodes, or if hilar nodes were grossly tumorous. In group II (97 cases) the mediastinum was explored in every patient and all nodes were resected. There was no statistically significant difference in CT sensitivity between these two groups (88% and 75%, respectively).

CT Evaluation of Distant Metastases

Several autopsy series have demonstrated an overall prevalence of distant metastases in patients with end-stage lung cancer as high as 93%. Key sites involved include liver (33% to 40%), adrenal (18% to 38%), brain (15% to 43%), bone (19% to 33%), kidney (16% to 23%), and abdominal lymph nodes (29%).[146–148] Autopsy studies performed in the immediate postoperative period as well as one report of abdominal exploratory surgery prior to thoracotomy for bronchogenic carcinoma have shown lower prevalences of metastatic spread to individual organs (liver 7% to 14%, adrenal 1% to 9%, brain 4%, bone 1% to 5%, kidney 0% to 4%, abdominal lymph nodes 5% to 8%). Nonetheless, the overall prevalence of occult metastatic disease was fairly high (18% to 36%) in these pre-CT-era studies[149–152]. One of these studies found that extrathoracic metastases were more common among men with adenocarcinoma than among those with squamous cell carcinoma.[149] A more recent autopsy report also found a

moderately high frequency (19% of 103, = 18%) of distant metastases in patients dying in the perioperative period after lung cancer resection.[150]

Out of 95 patients with newly diagnosed NSCLC and N0 disease at CT, one report demonstrated CT evidence of extrathoracic tumor spread in 24 of 95 (25%) patients. These included metastases to brain (ten), bone (eight), liver (six), adrenal (six), and soft tissue (two) (some patients had involvement at more than one site).[153] An additional, prospective study of 146 patients with potentially resectable NSCLC (clinical T3 or less and N2 or less)[154] revealed distant metastatic disease in 30 of 146 (30%) patients. These metastases were detected by chest or abdominal CT, brain CT, abdominal ultrasonography, and/or bone scan, and presumably each finding was proved. The lesions were distributed as follows: 13% bone, 13% brain, 12.3% liver, 7.5% adrenal, 1.4% kidney, and 1.4% subdiaphragmatic nodules (in 17 patients the metastases were "multiorganic"). The authors indicated that patients with nonsquamous cell carcinomas (adenocarcinoma or large cell carcinoma) were at significantly greater risk for metastases outside the thorax than those with squamous cell cancer (p = less than 0.5). No relationship was detected between the TN stage and the existence of metastases in adenocarcinoma and large cell adenocarcinoma. There was, however, an association between advanced N stage (IIIa) and presence of extrathoracic metastases for squamous cell cancers. None of the stage I intrathoracic squamous cell cancers had metastases. Many patients with metastases to brain, bone, liver, and adrenal were asymptomatic. Thus these authors advocated the routine performance of preoperative upper abdominal CT and/or ultrasonography in all patients except those with asymptomatic stage I squamous cell cancers. Brain CTs were suggested for all patients with adenocarcinoma and large cell carcinoma, as well as for those with squamous cell cancer and neurologic symptoms. Bone scanning was suggested only in those patients with clinical and laboratory indications of possible bone involvement by metastatic disease.

A recent study by Quint and colleagues found 21% overall prevalence of distant metastases in 348 patients with newly diagnosed NSCLC.[155] In 56% of patients with distant metastases, the lesions were detected using chest or abdominal CT. Brain, bone, liver, and adrenal glands were the most common sites of disease, in decreasing order. Brain metastases often occurred as an isolated finding. On the other hand, isolated liver metastases were uncommon, and therefore the incremental yield of abdominal CT over chest CT was quite small. Thus these authors concluded that abdominal CT does not appear to be an effective method of screening for metastases if chest CT has been performed.

Despite the high prevalence of adrenal metastases from bronchogenic carcinoma, approximately two thirds of adrenal masses in patients with NSCLC actually represent adenomas, rather than metastases.[156] Adrenal adenomas are found in about 3% to 9% of autopsies on adults,[157,158] and approximately 1% of patients undergoing abdominal CT have benign incidental adrenal masses larger than 1 cm.[159] In a recent study of 546 patients with lung cancer, 22 of 546 (4%) patients had one or more adrenal masses on preoperative CT.[160] Seventeen of 22 had proof of adrenal status via either biopsy or follow-up. Five of these 17 were malignant (29%) and 12 of 17 were benign (71%). These authors reported that adenomas were well defined and low in attenuation and showed a smooth, high attenuation rim and involvement of only part of gland. Features of metastases included a low attenuation, large (over 5 cm) mass without a rim and irregular, mixed attenuation.[160] Unfortunately, there is significant overlap in the appearance of adrenal metastases and benign adenomas on routine, contrast-enhanced CT. Therefore detection of an adrenal mass on such a study requires further workup. Considerable work has recently been done using noncontrast CT delayed enhanced CT, and MR in evaluating adrenal masses[161–165] (Figures 30.23, 30.24). Using these techniques, it is often possible definitively to diagnose benign adrenal cortical adenomas without biopsy. If these imaging studies suggest the presence of a metastasis, biopsy proof is generally required before altering therapy.

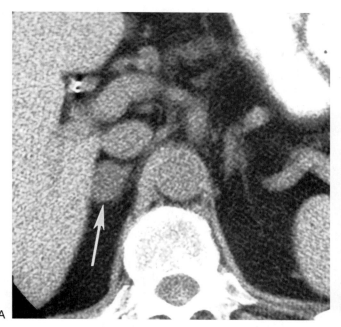

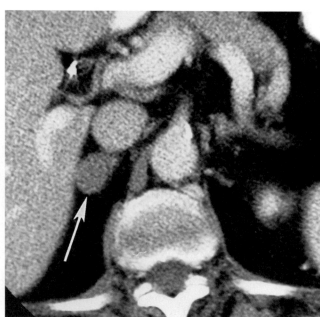

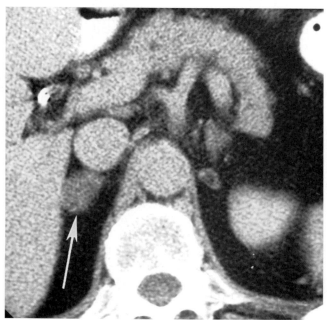

FIGURE 30.23. A: Benign adrenal cortical adenoma (arrow) showing typical density and enhancement characteristics at CT. Right adrenal nodule shows low density (14 HU) on a precontrast image. **B:** The nodule enhances significantly (65 HU) during administration of intravenous contrast. **C:** There is substantial washout on a 15-minute delayed image (29 HU).

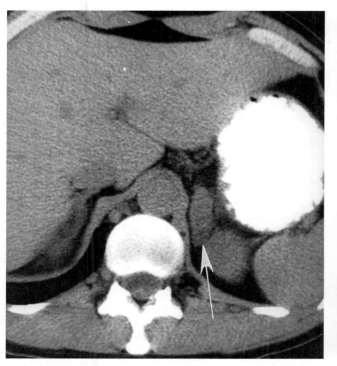

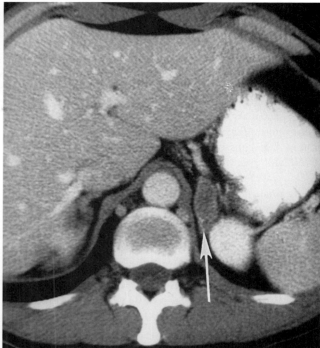

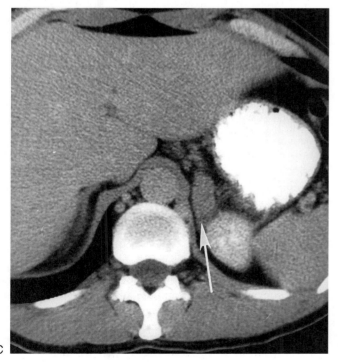

FIGURE 30.24. A: Adrenal metastasis (*arrow*) showing typical density and enhancement characteristics at CT. Right adrenal nodule shows soft tissue density (25 HU) on a precontrast image. **B:** The nodule enhances significantly (54 HU) during administration of intravenous contrast. **C:** There is little washout on a 15-minute delayed image (53 HU).

Usefulness of CT in Clinical T1N0M0 Patients

There is substantial controversy over the usefulness of CT in the preoperative evaluation of patients with radiographic T1N0M0 cancers. Reports in the surgical and radiologic literature give varying figures for the prevalence of proven mediastinal lymph node or distant metastases in this set of patients, ranging from 3% to 33%.[104,127,166–172] The lower prevalences may be underestimations, reflecting incomplete mediastinal nodal sampling and/or lack of good-quality preoperative abdominal CT scanning. Because distant metastases remain a contraindication to thoracotomy, and known mediastinal metastases will alter treatment at many institutions, CT is potentially useful by detecting such occult disease. In the series of Parker and associates[167] CT evidence for unresectable spread of disease was obtained in 12 of 36 patients with radiographic T1N0M0 disease, including metastases to the liver (four patients), the adrenal (one patient), an axillary lymph node (one patient), and mediastinal lymph nodes (eight patients). Conces and colleagues[172] reported CT signs of inoperability in 7 of 26 radiographic T1N0M0 cases with surgical correlation (27%). Metastatic disease was confirmed in four of these seven cases, including mediastinal metastases in three (3 of 26, 12% prevalence) and one contralateral lung malignancy. Of 31 radiographic T1N0M0 patients reported by Heavey and co-workers,[171] eight (26%) had proven spread of disease, including six patients with malignant mediastinal lymph nodes (19% prevalence), one with an adrenal metastasis, and one patient with a metastasis to the contralateral lung. CT detected five of these eight cases, thus preventing thoracotomy in five of 31 (16%) patients. As noted by Heavey and co-workers,[171] preventing thoracotomy in only 16% of patients resulted in significant overall cost savings, even when the cost of CT scans and prethoracotomy biopsies is taken into account. Thus these studies suggest that CT is highly useful in the preoperative workup of such patients.

On the other hand, another study of radiographic T1N0M0 tumors by Pearlberg and colleagues[170] found only two of 23 (8.7%) patients with proven mediastinal metastases; however, these patients did not undergo total mediastinal nodal sampling, and thus the true prevalence may have been somewhat higher. CT findings averted thoracotomy in only one patient, due to mediastinal adenopathy subsequently proven at mediastinotomy to contain metastatic disease. Becker et al.[168] in a prospective investigation of thirty-eight patients with presumed lung cancer (radiographic T1N0M0), found proven mediastinal nodal metastases in only one patient. Eleven of thirty-eight lesions turned out to be benign. Thus, preliminary data indicate that CT may be helpful and cost-effective in the preoperative assessment of patients with radiographic T1N0M0 lesions when the diagnosis of lung cancer has been proven.

Predicting Resectability with CT

Prediction of resectability depends upon accurate detection of T4, N3, and/or M1 tumors. One prospective study of 96 patients with lung cancer and preoperative CT found a 12% prevalence of unresectability.[173] CT criteria for unresectability included encasement of the proximal pulmonary arteries or carina, or gross mediastinal involvement by tumor, or widespread lymphadenopathy or distant metastases. Using these criteria, CT was 96% accurate and showed 97% positive predictive value and 50% negative predictive

value for resectability. Therefore CT was useful in the preoperative setting in this patient group.[173]

Current Usefulness of CT

In 1986, Epstein and associates surveyed 533 thoracic surgeons to see how CT has affected the preoperative evaluation of bronchogenic carcinoma in their practices.[174] Thirty-six percent of surgeons routinely requested CT and 62% requested CT selectively, depending on tumor size, location, and presence/absence of mediastinal abnormality on chest radiographs. Seventy-eight percent of surgeons used the CT information to direct nodal sampling at mediastinoscopy or mediastinotomy. However, nearly all (99%) would not accept enlarged mediastinal lymph nodes at CT as proof of unresectability. CT was used mainly to assess lymph node size, and secondarily to assess technical feasibility of tumor resection. Fifty-seven percent said a normal CT should eliminate prethoracotomy mediastinoscopy/mediastinotomy. Most surgeons still adhere to these premises, although it is now extremely rare for a patient to have lung cancer surgery without a preoperative CT.

It is important for the radiologist to know what treatment options are available at his or her particular institution and what features of the tumor or its spread would affect treatment decisions. At many institutions, proven T4, N3, or M1 disease is considered unresectable. Patients with N2 disease may be treated with preoperative chemotherapy and radiation therapy. CT findings are used to help define the extent of the primary mass, look for calcifications that might indicate benignancy, determine its relationships with nearby structures, assess for resectability, and suggest the type of surgery required for resection. If enlarged mediastinal lymph nodes are detected, CT may be used to direct preoperative lymph node sampling via transbronchoscopic Wang needle biopsy, mediastinoscopy, or mediastinotomy. Nodes accessible to transbronchoscopic Wang needle biopsy include the paratracheal, tracheobronchial, and subcarinal groups. Transbronchial Wang needle biopsy may be facilitated by ultrasound guidance. Nodes accessible to mediastinoscopy include pretracheal, anterior subcarinal, and anterior tracheobronchial groups. Lymph nodes in the aortopulmonary window are not accessible using these techniques, and tissue sampling requires other approaches such as thoracoscopy or anterior thoracotomy. As an alternative to surgical staging procedures, some groups advocate the use of CT-guided hilar and mediastinal lymph node biopsies,[174–177] although this is not common practice unless the nodal masses are large (Figure 30.22).

In summary, at many institutions, preoperative chest CT (including the adrenal glands) is routinely performed on all patients suspected of having NSCLC. Abdominal CT is not generally necessary, given the low frequency of isolated liver metastases. Intravenous contrast material is administered in order to help distinguish vessels from lymph nodes and to aid in evaluation of primary tumor extent.

Many CT studies have reported high negative predictive values in detecting metastatic disease to mediastinal lymph nodes. In addition, Daly and co-workers reported that overall projected two-year and five-year survival rates for 37 CT false-negative patients in their series were 40% and 28%, respectively.[135] Given this information, many investigators believe that a negative CT obviates the need for mediastinoscopy, and these patients should go directly to thoracotomy.[110,126,135] An exception may be made for patients with T3 tumors or central adenocarcinomas, due to the high incidence of positive mediastinal lymph nodes and low negative predictive value of CT in this setting.[135] In addition, patients with suspected chest wall invasion, including Pancoast tumors, should probably have mediastinoscopy regardless of CT findings, because mediastinal nodal metastases and chest wall invasion portend a poor prognosis, and these patients are not usually felt to be surgical candidates.[68,69] In a dissenting opinion, Pearson and colleagues recommended mediastinoscopy for all T2 and T3 tumors and for T1 adenocarcinomas and large cell carcinomas, even in the setting of a negative CT.[179] On the other hand, all patients with abnormal mediastinal lymph nodes at CT need lymph node biopsy; therapy should not be planned based upon unproven, positive CT findings.

MAGNETIC RESONANCE IMAGING

Magnetic resonance imaging (MRI) has been used by several investigators in the assessment of patients with lung cancer, although mainly as a problem-solving tool. Advantages of MRI over CT include superior contrast resolution, the ability directly to image in any desired plane, and the ability directly to image vascular structures without the use of intravascular contrast material. However, MRI has poorer spatial resolution, and calcifications are difficult to image. MRI quality suffers due to motion artifacts (mainly from cardiac and respiratory motion), as well as vascular pulsation and bulk patient motion. (Many of these artifacts, however, have been overcome by the recently introduced breath-hold techniques.) In addition, the relatively low signal from the air-containing lung parenchyma (on spin-echo MR images) hinders the evaluation of parenchymal abnormalities. Thus the role of MRI in the detection and staging of bronchogenic carcinoma has been limited. However, MRI maybe useful in certain circumstances for the staging of bronchogenic carcinoma.[180–186]

Primary Tumor

Differentiation between Tumor and Adjacent Atelectasis or Pneumonia

In central tumors associated with peripheral atelectasis or pneumonia due to endobronchial extension of tumor, MRI may be useful to differentiate between tumor and the associated parenchymal changes (Figure 30.25). Postobstructive pneumonitis appears as areas of high signal intensity on T2-weighted images due to the high water content, in contrast to the lower signal intensity of central tumors. This differentiation is possible in about 40% of cases.[81,187,188] However, if the patient develops organizing fibrous pneumonitis, the separation between tumor and atelectasis is not as readily performed, as areas of organizing pneumonitis may also have low signal intensity and thus resemble the central tu-

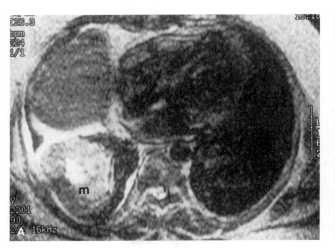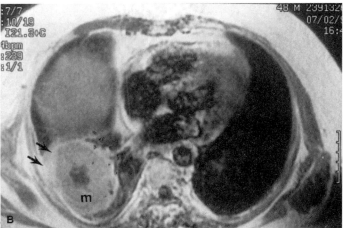

FIGURE 30.25. Right lower lobe tumor (*m*) with central necrosis and peripheral atelectasis. **A:** T2-weighted spin-echo image demonstrates difficulty in separating atelectasis from tumor. **B:** Atelectasis is of higher signal intensity (*arrows*) than tumor (*m*) on Gd-DTPA-enhanced T1-weighted image.

mors.[189,190] Kono and colleagues used gadolinium-enhanced imaging to distinguish between central tumors and postobstructive atelectasis: accuracy improved from 77% on the spin-echo T2-weighted images to between 85% and 89% on the Gd-DTPA enhanced images. In 67% of these cases, the signal intensity of the central tumors was lower than that of the atelectasis, and in 18% it was higher. The tumors tended to show gradual enhancement, whereas the atelectatic areas demonstrated rapid enhancement, reaching a peak after three minutes.[191]

Superior Sulcus Tumors

Superior sulcus tumors can result in chest wall extension and are considered clinically as a special category of lung carcinomas. They commonly involve the brachial plexus, and subclavian vessels as well as the vertebral bodies. Accurate assessment of tumor extension is critical for planning therapeutic options. CT has limitations in assessing the vertical extent of tumor due to the axial orientation of the images, the presence of beam-hardening artifacts from the adjacent bony structures, as well as poor contrast resolution. Sagittal and coronal MRIs often display the anatomic relationships in the apex more clearly than axial images, and thus are better suited to depicting apical tumor extent[192–196] (Figure 30.26). If MRI shows disruption or infiltration of the thin rim of extrapleural fat at the lung apex, tumor extension is to be suspected. These findings may be better depicted with the use of surface coils. Two published studies have reported on the relative merits of MRI as compared to CT in the evaluation of superior sulcus tumors. In a study of ten patients, seven of whom had surgical proof, MRI was accurate in depicting chest wall invasion in three, brachial plexus invasion in one, and subclavian artery encasement in one. In a study of superior sulcus tumors, Hee-

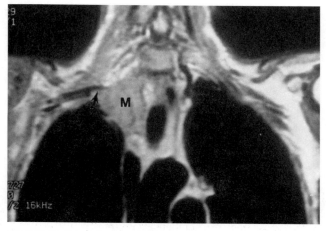

FIGURE 30.26. Relationships between apical tumor (*m*) and adjacent vascular structures (*arrow*) are clearly depicted on coronal T1-weighted spin-echo MR image.

lan and his colleagues demonstrated an accuracy rate of 94% with MRI as compared to 63% with CT for detecting tumor invasion beyond the lung apex.[197,198]

Chest Wall Invasion

Computed tomography is limited in its ability to predict chest wall invasion. Due to its superior contrast resolution, MRI is potentially capable of demonstrating subtle chest wall invasion and may be superior to CT in this regard. Chest wall invasion is best depicted as disruption of the normal extrapleural fat by moderate-intensity soft tissue on spin-echo T1-weighted images or as high-signal-intensity tissue on T2-weighted images (Figure 30.27). The use of surface coils can provide high resolution images depicting these changes. However, inflammatory change and tumor extension into the chest wall may have similar appearances on MRI, making it difficult to distinguish between the two entities. It remains to be seen if the administration of intravascular contrast agents can help make this differentiation easier.[181,183,185,186]

In a study of 13 patients with surgical and pathological proof, Haggar and colleagues demonstrated that spin-echo MRI had a negative predictive value of 100% for chest wall invasion (nine of nine patients). More importantly, in nine cases in which CT was equivocal, MRI accurately resolved the issue.[199] However, in the report of the Radiology Diagnostic Oncology Group trial (RDOG) involving twenty-three patients with surgical and pathological proof, CT and spin-echo MRI were equivalent. Areas under the receiver operating curve (ROC) were 0.857 (SE 0.036) for MRI as compared to 0.868 (SE 0.033) for CT.[74]

Padovani and colleagues reported their experience on the accuracy of MRI in detecting chest wall invasion in 34 patients with pathologic proof or CT evidence of bone destruction in areas contiguous with the tumor. Using spin-echo T1- and T2-weighted images, as well as gadolinium-enhanced T1-weighted spin-echo images, MRI had a sensitivity of 90% and a specificity of 86%. Contrast-enhanced and unenhanced spin-echo images showed equal sensitivity.[200]

Mediastinal Invasion

Both CT and MRI depict gross mediastinal invasion by lung carcinoma, although both techniques have the same limitations in distinguishing tumor contiguity from tumor extension into specific mediastinal structures.[70] Involvement of the cardiac chambers (although rare) and the pericardium can be easily evaluated with MRI. If the normal 2 to 3 mm curvilinear low-signal-intensity rim representing the pericardium is disrupted, then tumor extension into the pericardium is suspected, although this alone is not a contraindication to resection.[201,202]

In a surgical study that compared the accuracies of CT and MRI in detecting mediastinal invasion, the two modali-

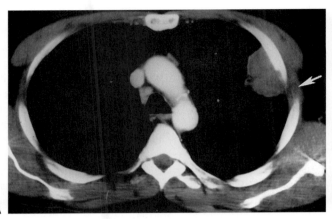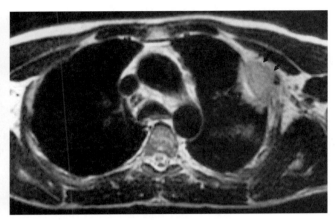

FIGURE 30.27. Left upper lobe carcinoma. **A:** CT demonstrates asymmetric soft tissue in an intercostal space of the left lateral chest wall (*arrow*), suggestive of chest wall invasion. **B:** Axial cardiac-gated T1-weighted MR image shows tumor extension (*arrows*) into the chest wall musculature. Chest wall invasion was confirmed via surgery and pathology.

ties showed similarly poor sensitivities (55% for CT, 64% for MRI).[75] In a more recent study from the Radiology Diagnostic Oncology Group (RDOG) trials, MRI showed slightly better accuracy than CT in diagnosing mediastinal invasion in a small group of patients (n = 11): areas under the ROC curves were 0.924 (SE 0.034) for MRI and 0.832 (SE 0.034) for CT.[74]

Evaluation of Mediastinal Lymph Nodes

In several studies that compared CT and MRI for the detection of mediastinal nodal metastases, the two modalities have had similar results (Figure 30.28). Because both studies depend on nodal size, they show low sensitivity and low specificity.[8,74,75,187,202–204] However there are some differences between CT and MRI that need to be addressed. Because of the poorer spatial resolution with MRI, small adjacent nodes that are discrete on CT can appear as one large, indistinct mass at MRI, leading to an erroneous diagnosis of nodal enlargement.[187] In addition, MRI is poor for detecting calcification, and thus enlarged benign nodes containing calcification may be misclassified as being malignant. On the other hand, MRI has potential advantages in evaluating the aortopulmonary window and subcarinal region owing to its ability to image in the coronal plane: coronal imaging helps to eliminate the partial-volume-averaging problems that occur with axial CT images.

CT is limited in its ability to detect normal-sized nodes containing metastases as well as in distinguishing between enlarged hyperplastic and enlarged malignant nodes. Early

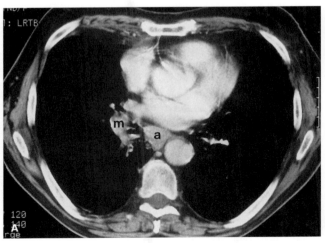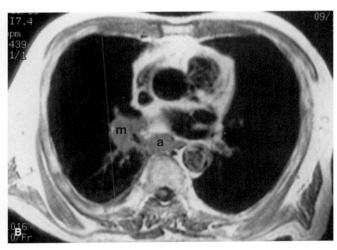

FIGURE 30.28. Right lower lobe mass (*m*) and enlarged mediastinal lymph nodes (*a*) are equally well seen at CT (**A**) and MRI (**B**).

on, it was hoped that MRI could distinguish between normal or hyperplastic nodes and tumor-containing nodes based on differences on signal-intensity characteristics. However it later became clear that signal-intensity characteristics did not correlate with tissue type.[205,206] More recently, MRI has been performed using intravenous infusion of contrast agents that are taken up by the reticuloendothelial system, in order to evaluate for malignancy in lymph nodes. A study by Anzai and colleagues of patients with head and neck cancer found 95% sensitivity and 84% specificity for detecting malignancy in lymph nodes using MRI with dextran-coated ultrasmall superparamagnetic iron oxide particles.[207,208]

Evaluation for Distant Metastases

Conventional contrast-enhanced CT has limitations in distinguishing between adrenal adenomas and metastases. Early reports using low- and mid-field MRI scanners noted that most adenomas were hypointense or isointense with the liver on T2-weighted sequences, whereas metastases were hyperintense.[209,210] On high-field-strength imagers, it was noted that some adenomas were of high signal intensity and thus simulated metastases.[211,212] Thus distinction between adenomas and metastases was not possible in some cases using spin-echo MR imaging.

Krestin and colleagues have used Gd-DTPA-enhanced breath-held gradient-recalled fast imaging to attempt to separate adenomas from malignant tumors. In this study, most adenomas showed early mild enhancement with quick washout, in contrast to malignant tumors, which showed early, strong, and persistent enhancement. However, there was misclassification in nearly 10% of patients in this study.[213]

Leroy-Willig and colleagues demonstrated that adenomas contain more lipid in comparison to malignant tumors, and thus differentiation between these two groups was possible on MR spectroscopic imaging.[214] Mitchell and colleagues were one of the first groups to use chemical-shift MRI to distinguish between adenomas and metastases. They were able accurately to classify adenomas and metastases in 96% of patients. On lipid-sensitive out-of-phase images, lipid-rich adenomas showed signal loss and appeared dark in comparison to a reference organ such as the spleen.[215] Most metastases, however, do not show this change on the out-of-phase images. This early work has now been corroborated by several other investigators and has an accuracy rate of more than 90% in the diagnosis of a lipid-rich adenoma[216–218] (Figure 30.29). More recently, unenhanced CT densitometry has been used to distinguish between lipid-rich adenomas and nonadenomatous masses. Using a threshold of 10 HU, an accuracy of over 90% can be achieved for the diagnosis of a lipid-rich adenoma.[162,219] In cases where unenhanced CT shows an adrenal mass with a density measurement of more than 10 HU or MRI shows a mass which does not lose signal intensity on opposed-phase images, the mass is classified as non-lipid rich and needs a biopsy or resection for further evaluation.

NUCLEAR MEDICINE

Introduction

As is discussed elsewhere in this chapter and text, after a pulmonary nodule is identified, it must be determined whether it is of malignant or benign etiology. If malignant, a careful assessment of the extent of the tumor is generally performed to determine if it is likely to be fully resectable.

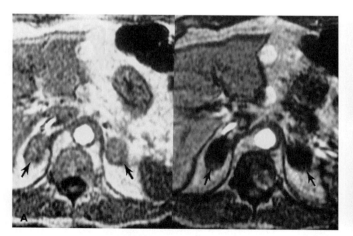
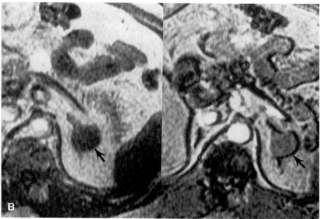

FIGURE 30.29. MR phase imaging of adrenal masses (left images, in phase; right images, out of phase). **A:** Bilateral adrenal cortical adenomas (*arrows*) lose signal and become dark on out-of-phase MR images, confirming that they contain lipid. **B:** In a different patient, the left adrenal metastasis (*arrows*) does not lose signal on the out-of-phase image.

This is done because only about 15% of patients with lung cancer will survive five years following surgery. Patients who die do so because the disease was not fully removed at the time of surgery. If the disease appears to be resectable, it is also necessary to determine whether the patient's cardiac and pulmonary function are sufficiently good to allow for survival of the requisite surgical procedure. After surgery, or if nonsurgical approaches to management are undertaken, assessments for recurrent disease and/or treatment response are generally undertaken. Nuclear medicine procedures can contribute to the aforementioned assessments. Many of the applications of nuclear medicine in lung cancer imaging are described in the following section. The discussion is divided by type of scan and its current and potential methods of clinical application. This is a relatively rapidly emerging area with several new techniques recently entering clinical practice. With US Medicare reimbursement for FDG PET imaging for the evaluation of both the solitary pulmonary nodule and for lung cancer staging, there has been rapidly growing use of the PET imaging method.

Ventilation/Perfusion Scintigraphy

Assessments of pulmonary perfusion/ventilation are an important part of the algorithm for determining if a patient with lung cancer will have adequate pulmonary function following thoracotomy. Since many patients who have lung cancer also have moderate to severe obstructive airways disease, loss of an entire lung at surgery may be sufficient to compromise already borderline pulmonary function to such an extent that they would become pulmonary cripples or not survive the operation due to the loss of lung function. While assessments of pulmonary function by spirometry are quite useful, these assessments provide an index of whole-lung function, not lateralizing information regarding pulmonary function.

While not fully studied in a prospective manner, a variety of studies have indicated that a minimum pulmonary function level compatible with life is about 0.8 to 1.0 liters exhaled in 1 second (FEV1).[220] Thus, after curative resection of lung cancer, this level of pulmonary function should be present to allow for satisfactory oxygenation. The general approach taken in attempts to predict pulmonary function postoperatively is to perform a ventilation/perfusion (or just perfusion) lung scan preoperatively to ascertain what fraction of total pulmonary ventilation or perfusion is from the lung which is to be removed. In brief, the quantitative fraction of perfusion or ventilation in the proposed residual lung is multiplied times the pre-operative FEV1 to result in the predicted post-operative FEV1.[221] If this number is more than 0.8 liters, the patient's predicted pulmonary function is considered adequate. Whether perfusion, as determined by Tc99m macroaggregated albumin distribution, or ventilation is chosen does not appear to make a large difference in outcome, as ventilation and perfusion are generally comparably impaired. In practice, fractional perfusion is most commonly used as a predictor in most centers, as this parameter is quite easily measured. While aerosols are being more commonly used in ventilation studies, data on the predictive value of aerosol ventilation studies are not yet available. Thus, in many centers, predictions are based on the fractional perfusion.[222] An example of a quantitative lung perfusion study is shown in Figure 30.30.

Bone Scanning

The use of the bone scan in the preoperative assessment of patients with newly diagnosed NSCLC cell lung cancer is somewhat variable based on practice locale. In general, it is agreed that surgical resection of the primary tumor in a patient with bone metastases is likely to be a fruitless undertaking. Gravenstein and colleagues reported death within six months in forty of forty-six patients with bone metastases.[223] Therefore, known bone metastases generally suggest an approach to therapy aimed at palliation, not cure. Thoracotomy entails the risk of death from surgery, pain, associated morbidity, and substantial costs of up to $40,000. Thus preventing an unnecessary thoracotomy can lead to large cost savings as well as improved medical care. Because a bone scan costs only about $400, to detect one patient with bone metastases, many studies can be performed potentially and still be cost-effective.

The literature surrounding this test is somewhat controversial, but two recent studies have suggested an incidence of bone metastases at presentation in patients with new NSCLC of about 15%.[222] With this level of prevalence, it is quite reasonable to believe that bone scanning would be a rational procedure in each patient prior to thoracotomy. Another study has suggested an approximately 9% prevalence of metastases in such patients.[225] Algorithms have emerged to suggest that, instead of performing a bone scan on all patients with newly diagnosed lung cancer, the numbers of scans could be reduced by 50% through selection of patients at "high risk" for metastases based on clinical and laboratory findings. These findings included bone pain, chest pain, pain or tenderness on motion, an elevated serum alkaline phosphatase, or an elevated serum calcium level. At least one of these findings was present in any patient identified with bone metastases in a series of 110 patients with NSCLC.[225] Others argue that a bone scan should be performed if the primary tumor is physically large or in any lung cancer with small cell histology.

Thus it can be recommended that an algorithm be adapted in which bone scans are performed in a higher prevalence subset of patients, who number about half of the total referred with lung cancer. Cost-benefit analysis appears to support this approach, though practice patterns may differ by institution. It should also be realized that additional costs beyond the bone scan will be incurred with a pattern of care including the use of bone scans. For exam-

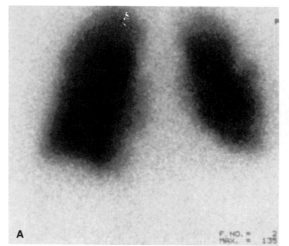

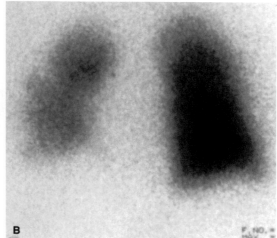

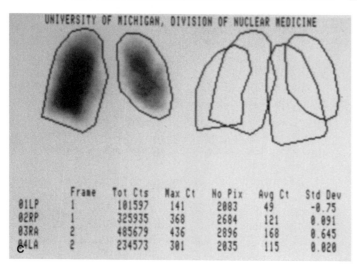

FIGURE 30.30. Preoperative anterior (**A**) and posterior (**B**) pulmonary perfusion study (Tc99m MAA, lung scan) in a patient with left lung cancer scheduled for pneumonectomy. Twenty-eight percent of perfusion goes to the left lung as determined by region of interest analysis (**C**). With a preoperative FEV1 of 2.0 liters, this scan predicts a postoperative FEV1 of 1.44 liters, well above the 0.8 liters considered sufficient for survival postoperatively.

ple, additional radiographs may be necessary in some instances to be certain that the abnormality seen on bone scan is a metastasis as opposed to a benign skeletal abnormality. A bone scan illustrating direct tumor involvement in the thoracic spine is shown in Figure 30.31.

The bone scan is also important in follow-up and is capable of demonstrating metastases to bone in symptomatic and asymptomatic patients. The degree of vigor chosen in pursuing skeletal metastases postoperatively is generally less than in the preoperative patient. As in most neoplasms, identification of large metastases in weight-bearing bones which are at increased risk of fracture and the detection of destructive vertebral lesions are of greatest importance. These lesions can be irradiated before damage such as spinal cord encroachment or pathological fracture occurs. Recently it has been suggested that PET imaging with FDG could supplant the bone scan for staging, but in most institutions

PET is not available, so the bone scan remains very commonly performed as a staging procedure.

Gallium, Thallium, and MIBI Imaging

67 gallium and 201 thallium have been used in lung cancer imaging for a number of years with variable clinical results. While there was substantial popularity of 67 Ga in the pre-CT era, its use has declined significantly with the availability of CT. The 67 Ga scan can, however, detect many primary and metastatic mediastinal foci of lung cancer.[226] In addition, SPECT imaging equipment is improving, and the use of multi-head SPECT systems should result in increased sensitivity for smaller lesions. At present, however, the relatively low uptake of 67 gallium in lung cancers makes reliable detection of tumor foci less than 2cm in diameter difficult. In addition to relatively poor sensitivity in small lesions, 67 gallium uptake occurs into some inflammatory

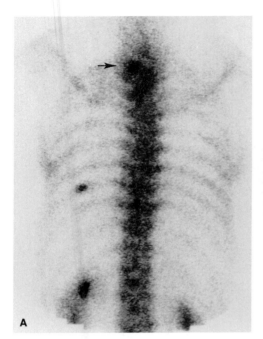
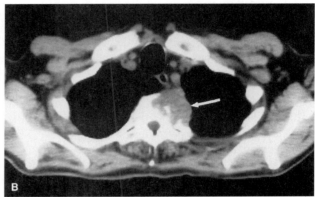

FIGURE 30.31. Posterior view from bone scan performed three hours after intravenous injection of Tc99m methylene diphosphonate (MDP) **A:** Focal increased uptake noted in left upper thoracic spine (*arrow*) and left seventh rib. CT showed tumor invasion into spine **B:** Patient judged unresectable and treated with radiation therapy.

lymph nodes, decreasing the specificity of the method. One prospective study showed 67 Ga to have a sensitivity of less than 25% and accuracy of about 60% in detecting mediastinal nodal metastases.[227] Thus, in most centers, 67 Ga is no longer used in the assessment of primary or metastatic lung cancer.

TI-201, a potassium analog, accumulates in viable cancer cells and can, especially with SPECT, image many larger primary lung cancers. The current literature suggests that the accuracy of lung cancer imaging with 201 TI appears to be somewhat superior to 67 Ga, but this tracer has not been as extensively explored in lung cancer imaging.[227] Preliminary data from two series of 9 and 37 patients, respectively, suggest that lesions in lymph nodes and primary tumors greater than 1.5 to 2 cm in diameter can be detected by tomographic techniques.[228,229] The detection sensitivity in smaller lesions is not as good, however.[228–230] In a larger series mainly using planar imaging, the sensitivity of TI-201 for primary lung cancers was 86%, but only a small fraction of mediastinal lymph node metastases was detected.[231] These observations led Sehwell and colleagues to conclude that TI-201, at least with planar imaging, was probably of limited value in lung cancer staging.[231] TI-201 has also been preliminarily evaluated in monitoring therapy for lung cancer patients.[232]

Suga and associates have examined the ability of TI-201 scintigraphy to separate benign from malignant solitary pulmonary nodules.[233] Images obtained fifteen minutes after

TI-201 injection showed no differential uptake between malignant and benign lesions, but imaging at three hours postinjection showed an 81% accuracy in separating the lesions of differing histologies. This difference was due to more avid retention of TI-201 in malignant than benign lesions. Additional studies in larger patient populations will be needed to determine the role of TI-201 in lung cancer imaging and staging. At present, in most clinical practices it remains an investigative tool.

SPECT using technetium-99m methoxyisobutylisonitrile (MIBI) has been used in the assessment of SPNs, with limited success. For example, Kao and colleagues used SPECT to evaluate fifty-four patients with SPNs and ten controls.[35] Of the SPNs, 46 were bronchogenic carcinomas and eight were benign. SPECT detected only thirty of the forty-six carcinomas, and also detected six of eight benign lesions. Thus this technique did not appear to be particularly helpful.

Myocardial Perfusion Imaging

While a major concern in the management of patients with newly diagnosed lung cancer is whether the disease is surgically resectable, it must also be determined whether the patient has an acceptable risk of surgery. A determination of operative risk as regards loss of pulmonary function using ventilation/perfusion scanning was discussed earlier in this chapter. However, an additional consideration is the potential of death during surgery or in the perioperative period due to a cardiac event such as myocardial infarction. Many patients with lung cancer are smokers. Smoking is a risk factor for lung cancer and coronary artery disease. Thus some patients will have both coronary artery disease and lung cancer. Patients with severe coronary artery disease are at an increased risk of death during major surgeries. While most of the literature regarding risk stratification for surgery has emerged in the setting of preoperative vascular surgery, it is clear that many physicians now apply preoperative myocardial perfusion imaging in an attempt to define patients at high and low risk of cardiac death following thoracotomy.[234] Brown has recently reviewed this general area, and concludes that patients considered for major surgery who have significant cardiac risk factors should be considered for myocardial perfusion scintigraphy preoperatively.[234] Patients with reversible myocardial perfusion defects on TI-201 stress scintigraphy are considered to be at a high risk of infarction/death, versus the group with normal or fixed defects on scan. Eagle and colleagues reported that, in 116 patients undergoing major abdominal vascular surgery, in an intermediate risk group those without redistribution on TI-201 scans showed a 3.2% risk of a cardiac event, while those with TI-201 redistribution had a much higher 29.6% risk of a cardiac event.[235] It is generally believed that correcting the cardiac perfusion defect will reduce the risk of perioperative morbidity/mortality, though this is not as well studied as the risk stratification power of TI-201. While detailed prospective study of the predictive value of myocardial perfusion scintigraphy in lung cancer patients is lacking, myocardial perfusion imaging is a powerful predictor of outcomes in patients who undergo other major surgical procedures. This technique is being applied to assessing patients

who are considered for surgery who may have coexistent coronary artery disease.

Adrenal and Hepatic Imaging

CT has revolutionized the anatomic evaluation of the upper abdomen, but despite its power, it is not a perfect test. Two areas of difficulty include adrenal masses and liver lesions. It has been possible to distinguish between malignant and benign adrenal lesions in many instances by evaluating the adrenal uptake of 131 I NP-59, an iodocholesterol analog. Metastases to the adrenal are not uncommon in patients with newly diagnosed lung cancer, presenting as an enlarged adrenal; however, benign nodules in the adrenal are common as well. Francis and associates studied this issue in twenty-eight patients with known cancer who had adrenal masses identified during their staging CT exam.[236] In this study, 131 NP-59 was administered intravenously, and several days later gamma images of the adrenals were obtained. Biopsy confirmation of diagnosis was obtained. Of the fourteen cases with increased ^{131}I NP-59 tracer uptake in the enlarged adrenal, all were adenomas. If there was decreased or symmetric uptake of tracer, metastatic tumor could not be excluded and was present on biopsy in ten cases. Adrenal cysts could also have diminished uptake. In some very large adrenal lesions, larger than 5 cm, increased tracer uptake can be seen due to adrenal cancer, though this is a rare occurrence. In brief, if there is increased uptake of NP-59 into a moderately enlarged adrenal gland, there is a very low probability that the lesion represents a lung cancer metastasis (Figure 30.32). If the adrenal is "cold" on NP-59, a biopsy would be necessary to determine the etiology of the lesion (Figure 30.33). Recent studies of the cost-benefit

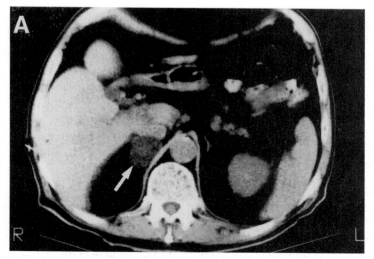
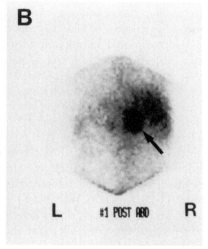

FIGURE 30.32. **A:** CT shows right adrenal mass in a patient with normal adrenal function. **B:** Posterior images four days postinjection of 131 I NP-59, an iodocholesterol analog, demonstrate intense tracer uptake in right adrenal mass ("concordant" pattern). Thus the mass represents functional adrenal tissue consistent with benign adrenal cortical adenoma, not a metastasis.

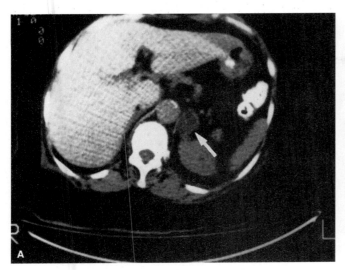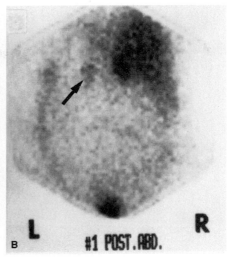

FIGURE 30.33. **A:** CT demonstrates left adrenal mass in a patient with lung cancer. **B:** NP-59 scan shows diminished tracer uptake on left and normal uptake on right ("discordant" pattern). This suggests that the left adrenal mass represents a metastasis. (From Gross M, Shapiro B, Bouffard J, et al. Distinguishing benign from malignant adrenal masses. *Ann Intern Med* 1988;109:613, with permission.)

of adrenal imaging with NP-59 have shown the method to be cost-effective. At present, this scan is available at only a few institutions, and many institutions without this agent perform CT-guided adrenal needle biopsies to resolve this problem. PET, however, is showing considerable promise as a radionuclide method to evaluate the adrenals and is already more widely available than the NP-59 method.

A second area of application of nuclear medicine studies is in the liver. Hepatic hemangiomas are commonly found in patients with cancer as incidental findings. While the CT findings are characteristic in most cases, 30% of these lesions are atypical in appearance. Ziessman and associates have shown, using triple-head SPECT, that imaging of red blood cells labeled with Tc99m allowed visualization of 20/20 hemangiomas greater than or equal to 1.4 cm in diameter.[237] This is in contrast to planar or single-head SPECT, where small lesions are commonly undetected. For example, with single-head SPECT, the sensitivity for hemangioma detection was only 38% for lesions between 1 and 2 cm in diameter, while for planar imaging, lesions under 3 cm in diameter were not uncommonly missed.[238] The hemangioma scan is highly specific for hemangioma in the liver, with only rare false positive cases including very large hepatomas, one carcinoid, and one hepatoblastoma reported to date. These are very uncommon, however, and in a series of 45 hepatomas studied in Japan, none of the patients had evidence of increased uptake of Tc-labeled red blood cells. This area has recently been reviewed by Rubin and colleagues.[239] Scan utilization patterns differ by institution, but the nuclear scan is much less expensive than an MRI

scan and is the procedure of choice for lesions of over 1.5 cm in diameter (Figure 30.34).

Antibody Scanning

The concept of imaging tumors with monoclonal antibodies reactive with specific tumor antigens is an attractive one which has been under study for the past 15 years.[240] The approach has clinical utility in imaging colorectal cancers and has been applied to lung cancer in several trials. At present, there is no FDA-approved radiolabeled monoclonal antibody for lung cancer imaging, though several clinical trials have demonstrated that there is potential for this methodology. These studies have involved anti-CEA (anti–carcinoembryonic antigen) antibodies and antibodies reactive with high-molecular-weight mucins. In NSCLC, several studies have shown that primary tumors can be imaged with 75% to 100% sensitivity, although some accumulation also occurred in nonmalignant tissues with specificities in the 25% to 75% range[241,242] and there was a problem in detecting tumors less than 2 cm in size in many instances. Thus, while feasible, this technique did not appear particularly helpful for the assessment of primary lung nodules.

A large prospective trial of the NRLU-10 murine antibody, which recognizes a 40 kD cell surface glycoprotein expressed by many epithelial cancers, was performed in the United States. With a Tc99m label, the Fab fragment of this antibody demonstrated a sensitivity for detection of the primary lesion of over 90%, detection of several more nodal metastases than seen by CT.[243,244] In a presurgical series,

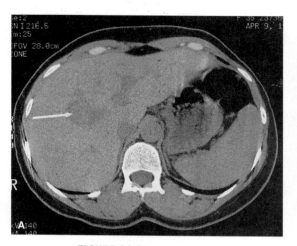
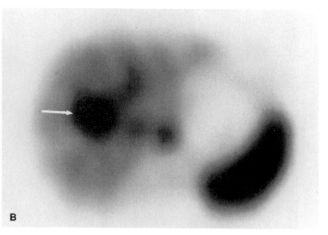

FIGURE 30.34. A: CT scan shows 3.5 cm right hepatic lesion (arrow) which is of indeterminate etiology in this lung cancer patient. **B:** Tc99m-labeled red blood cell triple-head SPECT scan obtained one hour after the injection shows intense tracer uptake in the liver, diagnostic for hemangioma. Intense activity also noted in spleen, portal vessels, descending aorta, and inferior vena cava.

Rusch and colleagues had five false-positive antibody scans of the mediastinum/hilum in a series of 21 patients.[245] Separation of blood pool activity from normal nodes has been problematic, but the results are at least as good as CT in staging the mediastinum (Figure 30.35).

An attractive aspect of nuclear medicine studies with tumor-avid agents is the potential for screening the entire body with a scan. This is becoming possible in NSCLC, with detection rates of known metastases in the area of the 90% range with the NRLU-10 mab, except in bone metastases, where the detection rate is substantially lower, with the antibody scan an inadequate substitute for the bone scan.[246]

Small cell lung cancer (SCLC) also expresses antigens on the surface which may be satisfactory targets for monoclonal antibody imaging. The staging procedure in SCLC is generally simpler than in NSCLC as SCLC is generally not a surgical condition. Rather, a decision has to be made if the disease is limited (to receive radiation therapy and chemotherapy) or extensive (to receive chemotherapy only). This

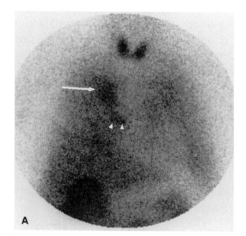
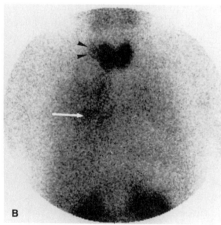

FIGURE 30.35. A: Anterior view from Tc99m NRLU-10 Fab (monoclonal antibody fragment) scan 17 hours post tracer injection shows uptake into right lung NSCLC (*arrow*) and mediastinal metastases (*arrowheads*) (proven at surgery). Uptake in thyroid and clearance of radiotracer through the gut/billary tree are normal findings. **B:** Scan with the same reagent in a different patient with small cell lung cancer. Uptake demonstrated in right thoracic primary lesion (*arrow*) and in tumor adjacent to the right lobe of the thyroid (*arrowheads*). (Images, courtesy of Dr. H. Breitz, Virginia Mason Medical Center, Seattle, WA.)

decision is often made by bone marrow biopsy. An imaging study of 96 patients from 21 sites was performed with the Tc99m NRLU-10 mab. In this study, the antibody scan was the single most accurate test when compared to CT, bone scan, or bone marrow aspirate. False-positives in this study were rare, with a positive predictive value of the test of more than 95% with about a 10% understaging rate.[246,247] Thus it is possible that in SCLC, the antibody scan might replace standard imaging methods for staging.

With antibodies, a concern exists that a foreign protein is being administered and the patient receiving the antibody may develop an immune response to the antibody. Indeed, up to 25% of patients with NSCLC developed an antimouse response to the antibody infusion.[245] This may limit follow-up studies. The antibody infusion was safe, however. To date, however, the utilization of this monoclonal antibody scan in staging lung cancer has been quite modest, and this method has not found general acceptance, despite being FDA-approved.

Small peptides reactive with receptors on the surface of SCLC have recently been used in clinical imaging studies and have demonstrated feasibility of concept. One of the peptides, reactive with the somatostatin receptor, is already an approved agent in Europe. The exact role of this agent in SCLC imaging requires further study, as not all of the tumors are receptor-positive.[248] This type of approach is attractive in that the peptides generally do not cause an immune response due to their small size, and can be given repeatedly. Recently, a Tc99m-labeled peptide (P-829) reactive with somatostatin receptors has been shown to be promising in assessing both NSCLC and SCLC.[249] It is possible that this agent may be clinically available for lung cancer imaging in late 1999, although the exact method for using this agent will be in evolution as clinical experience has been relatively modest. Preliminary data suggest the agent to be most useful in characterizing pulmonary lesions as malignant or benign, and the data suggest the agent will be useful in the more common non–small cell phenotype of lung cancer. The precise role of this agent in staging lung cancer is not yet developed.

Antibody, and potentially peptide, imaging may assume a growing role in the detection of lung cancer, with data very promising in SCLC and encouraging in NSCLC, especially for the Tc99m-labeled P-829 peptide. Clinical experience in lung cancer with both the peptides and antibodies remains limited, however. Nonetheless, this area of imaging has substantial potential.

Positron Emission Tomography (PET)

The most rapidly emerging application of nuclear medicine techniques for the assessment of solitary pulmonary nodules and possible metastases of lung cancer is positron emission tomography (PET). This method differs from standard nuclear medicine imaging in that short-lived isotopes are used

which emit positrons. The positrons then interact with normal tissue electrons to produce pairs of 511 KeV photons which then can be detected by the very sensitive positron emission tomographic camera.

Lung cancer has been successfully imaged in several trials using PET with both 11C methionine and FDG. Kubota and co-workers first reported successful imaging of lung cancer in eight of eight patients with primary lung cancers, with substantially more 11C methionine uptake in tumor than in normal lung tissue.[250] In a follow-up series of 16 patients, the investigative team from Tohoku University showed increased 11C methionine uptake in each case of primary lung cancer, with somewhat more 11C methionine uptake in the large cell than in the squamous cell carcinomas.[251]

Nolop and co-workers showed that FDG accumulated in 12 of 12 lung carcinomas studied with FDG, with all histologies imaging in the study. Mean tumor to nontumor ratios of over 6:1 were seen, and no obvious correlation was observed between tumor grade and FDG uptake in this small series.[252] Investigators from Tohoku University in Sendai, Japan, showed that about 85% to 90% of solitary pulmonary nodules are detected by PET with either FDG or methionine. They observed an elevated SUV (standardized uptake value) of tracer uptake with FDG and methionine in patients with lung cancer, while in benign lesions the SUV was significantly lower.[31] Similar results were recently reported by Gupta and colleagues, who showed that FDG uptake into primary lung cancers was significantly greater than that seen into benign pulmonary lesions, with SUV of 5.63 plus or minus 2.38 (SD) in malignant and 0.56 plus or minus 0.27 (SD) in benign lesions (p = less than 0.001).[32] Patz and colleagues demonstrated that FDG PET is very effective at separating primary lung cancers from inflammatory processes in the lung, based on the lesion SUV. In a series of 51 patients with focal pulmonary abnormalities (of which 38 were solitary pulmonary nodules), it was noted that the 33 malignant lesions had an SUV of 6.5 plus or minus 2.9 (SD), while benign lesions had an SUV of 1.7 plus or minus 1.2 (SD). Thus an excellent separation between benign and malignant lesions by SUV was possible.[253]

Kubota and colleagues also compared the accuracy of FDG and methionine PET in assessing pulmonary nodules. Both methionine and FDG were comparable in their imaging accuracies, with a 93% sensitivity, 60% specificity, and 79% accuracy for methionine, and an 83% sensitivity, 90% specificity, and 86% accuracy for FDG. Tumors less than 1 cm in diameter were noted to be particularly difficult to evaluate because of their small size relative to the resolution of the PET scanner.[31]

The ability of PET to separate malignant from benign lesions is high but not totally perfect. Thus high tracer uptake can sometimes be seen in an inflammatory or infectious process, such as aspergillosis or TB. Preliminary reports suggest that the smallest of pulmonary nodules may not be as well characterized by PET as larger nodules, possibly due to their motion in the PET scanner field of view and the incomplete signal recovery from small lesions. This results in underestimation of their SUV, unless a correction for scanner resolution is applied. The whole-body PET technique has also been applied to the detection of intrathoracic masses, and in the eight patients with bronchogenic carcinoma, there was clear visualization of the tumors by PET as areas of increased focal tracer accumulation.[255] Several metastatic lung nodules could also be detected by this approach, though it must be realized that quantification is not possible with this method. This method allows evaluation of the entire body.

A prospective multicenter trial of FDG PET was performed in eighty-nine patients in the assessment of solitary pulmonary nodules by Lowe and colleagues.[256] This study showed that, using SUV data, PET had an overall sensitivity and specificity for detection of malignant nodules of 92% and 90%, respectively. Some differences in sensitivity were seen with smaller lesions, so that for the smaller lesions (less than 1.5 cm) visual analysis, as opposed to quantitative analysis, was of greater sensitivity. A trial from Germany in

fifty-four pulmonary lesions-3 cm or less in diameter showed PET to be 90% sensitive and 83% specific in lesion characterization (as malignant or benign).[257] False-negatives included two bronchial carcinomas and one metastasis. With a prevalence of 4% to 10% false-negatives, there are risks of missing tumors if PET is the only test performed. Most would recommend follow-up imaging tests of solitary pulmonary nodules following a negative PET to exclude tumor growth, as a small percentage of patients with negative PET scans of SPN will have malignant tumors present. This seems to occur with greater frequency in bronchioloalveolar cell carcinomas, for example, which have considerably lower uptake of FDG than other lung cancers.[258] It is suggested that CT always be examined along with the PET study to be certain that bronchioloalveolar cell carcinomas are not missed on PET due to their lower tracer uptake. Nonetheless, PET is a very accurate, but not perfect, method for evaluating solitary pulmonary nodules noninvasively.

Another issue in lung cancer management is whether the tumor has spread to the mediastinal lymph nodes. This question is of substantial importance in NSCLC, where cure is generally possible only with complete excision of viable tumor from the thorax. In contrast, SCLC is more com-

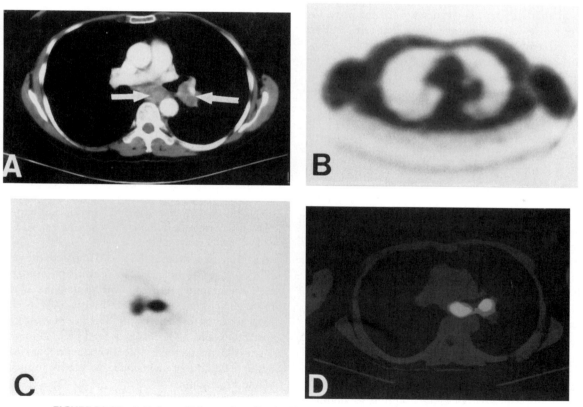

FIGURE 30.36. A: Enlarged hilar and mediastinal lymph nodes (*arrows*) on CT. **B:** Transmission PET image at the same level as in **(D)**. This patient had proven metastastic NSCLC in the mediastinum. **C:** Intense uptake of FDG on emission PET. **D:** Fusion image showing increased activity in the enlarged nodes.

monly treated nonsurgically by chemotherapy or irradiation. With NSCLC, it has been recognized that if there is tumor involvement of the mediastinum at the time of initial diagnosis, the patient's probability of survival for five years is reduced to just 5% to 10%. By contrast, if there is no mediastinal lymph node involvement, five-year survival is increased to a 40% to 50% probability. Knowing if there is mediastinal tumor involvement can alter the approach to management as in high-risk patients for surgery, thoracotomy may be inappropriately risky if there is a very high likelihood of mediastinal tumor involvement. There are only limited data published to date on this topic. A report on 25 patients studied with 11C methionine PET showed that there was higher 11C uptake in the tumor-involved lymph nodes than in the tumor-negative nodes (3.89 versus 2.38 mean SUV) (p = less than 0.001) and that with threshold setting post hoc, a nearly 90% accuracy in detecting mediastinal metastases could be defined.[259]

Data recently reported from the University of Michigan showed FDG PET to be significantly more accurate than CT in staging presumed NSCLC. In a prospective study of 23 patients, PET was about 82% accurate, while CT was 52% accurate (p = less than 0.05).[260] PET had the capability to detect tumor in some normal-sized lymph nodes and to exclude tumor involvement in enlarged lymph nodes in multiple instances. A preliminary report from Heidelberg, Germany, has shown even better accuracy for FDG PET but was performed with a PET scanner that had a limited field of view and thus was not able to evaluate the entire mediastinum at risk for metastases.[261] Application of quantification to the PET data may be of utility in additionally refining the accuracy of PET. It should be noted that accurately determining tracer uptake in mediastinal lymph nodes is difficult with PET, because count recovery is somewhat limited when the lymph nodes are small. Many studies on using PET for mediastinal staging have been reported in the past several years showing PET to be more accurate than CT for mediastinal staging. As an example, Vansteenkiste et al. showed the accuracy of CT and PET for mediastinal staging to be 68% and 94%, respectively.[262] A recent meta-analysis of the PET and CT literature by Dwamena, et al. has shown a sensitivity and specificity of 79% and 91%, respectively for PET, which is considerably higher than that for CT at 60% and 77%, respectively.[263] Examples of PET scan evaluating the mediastinum are shown in Figures 30.36, 30.37 and 30.38.

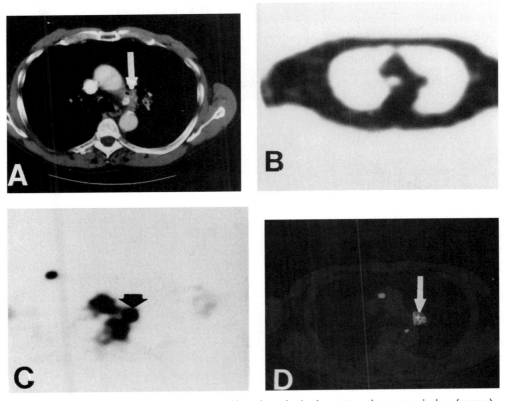

FIGURE 30.37. **A:** Normal-sized mediastinal lymph nodes in the aortopulmonary window (*arrow*) on CT. **B:** Transmission PET image at the same level as in (**D**). Tumor-involved, normal-sized nodes were proven at surgery in this patient with NSCLC. **C:** Increased FDG uptake in the left side of the mediastinum on emission PET. **D:** Fusion image showing increased activity in these normal sized lymph nodes (*arrow* and +).

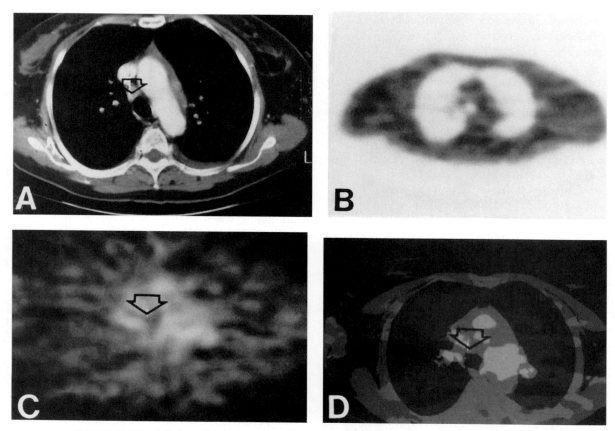

FIGURE 30.38. A: Enlarged lymph node in the right paratracheal region (*arrow*) on CT. **B:** Transmission PET image at the same level as in (**D**). This patient was found to have no tumor involvement of mediastinal lymph nodes. **C:** Enlarged lymph node in the right paratracheal region with no increased uptake over blood pool on emission PET. **D:** Fusion image confirms absence of increased FDG uptake within the enlarged node. (From Wahl R, Quint L, Greenough R, et al. Staging of mediastinal non–small cell lung cancer with FDG-PET, CT, and fusion images: preliminary prospective evaluation. *Radiology* 1994;191:371, with permission.)

Most recently, the prognostic importance of FDG PET in lung cancer has been investigated. In 125 potentially operable non-small cell lung cancer patients, the standardized uptake value (SUV), a semi-quantitative measurement of FDG uptake on PET scan, was analyzed. An SUV of greater than 7 was correlated with each survival. Moreover, the SUV of greater than 7 had the best discriminative value for prognoses, both in all patients and those detected. An SUV of less than 7 in stage Ia patients had a 2-year survival of 86%, but 2-year survival fell to 60% if the SUV was above 7. Nearly all detected tumors greater than 3 cm has SUVs of more than 7, with an expected 2-year survival of 43%.[264]

The published data regarding the ability of PET to detect visceral metastases from lung cancer are very encouraging. PET and bone scanning had, respectively, an accuracy of 96% and 66% in the evaluation of osseous involvement in 110 consecutive patients with NSCLC. The superior accuracy of PET was due to a much lower false-positive rate

than bone scan.[264] The specificity of bone scans can, of course, be enhanced by comparison with skeletal radiographs. Recently, an approximately 14% rate of finding additional metastases during lung cancer staging was reported by Weder and colleagues suggesting that PET should have a growing role in staging NSCLC patients before major surgery is undertaken.[265] Specific evaluation of adrenal metastases by PET has been undertaken. As an example, in evaluating possible adrenal metastases in patients with bronchogenic carcinoma, PET has shown a sensitivity of 100% with a specificity of 80% in a study of 33 patients.[266] PET, while a very useful method for staging the entire body, can fail to detect brain metastases (for example, as their uptake can be very similar to that of normal brain, meaning lesions can be hard to detect in some instances).[267] Thus anatomic imaging is recommended for such suspected lesions. Cost analysis studies have shown that using PET to stage lung cancer is cost-effective.[268]

While FDG has been used in treatment monitoring, it

should be noted that other tracers such as methionine have been employed. For example, in lung cancer treatment monitoring, declines in methionine uptake into tumors were commonly seen with effective therapy.[270] In some instances, the decline in methionine uptake was more predictive of the long-term survival of the patient than the change in tumor size. PET is rapidly emerging as a useful method in lung cancer management. Data are emerging to suggest PET plays a unique role in treatment management, both for chemotherapy and radiation therapy, but larger studies are needed to determine the precise role of PET in treatment response assessment.[271]

For all of the discussions of PET regarding lung cancer included in this chapter, the published literature has been based on dedicated PET scanning devices. In the last several years, lower-cost modified gamma camera devices capable of doing routine nuclear medicine studies (such as bone scans) and PET imaging have been developed and marketed. At present, the performance of these devices is not well characterized, but early data indicate they are considerably less accurate than dedicated PET for detecting small lesions in the chest and are particularly limited in the abdomen. As this technology emerges, performance will likely improve, but at present the limited literature available shows these devices to be inferior to dedicated PET in their accuracy. Thus, their place in clinical patient management will hinge on the accuracy determined for each device in prospective trials.

Summary

The role of nuclear medicine in the evaluation of the patient with a solitary pulmonary nodule suspected to represent lung cancer is rapidly evolving. PET and, to a somewhat lesser extent, SPECT techniques have demonstrated good accuracies in separating malignant from benign pulmonary nodules. At present, however, the accuracies are less than 100%, so they are not perfect substitutes for histological examination. At many centers, PET with a dedicated PET scanner is being applied in the more clinically difficult cases, such as the difficult-to-biopsy lesions or in patients who are a greater-than-usual risk of surgical assessment/biopsy. Data with SPECT and Tc99m-labeled peptides are emerging but are very limited as regards SPN characterization. Once the diagnosis of cancer is made, the bone scan is very important for assessing patients who have any signs or laboratory findings suggesting the presence of metastatic disease to bone. Detection of bone metastases would generally preclude operation. Recent data suggest PET to be more accurate than the bone scan in lung cancer staging. Staging the mediastinum and rest of the body with FDG PET alone is an increasingly attractive alternative to standard imaging methods. Staging of the entire patient with a single scan also appears to be possible with monoclonal antibodies reactive with SCLC—although this method is only infrequently applied at most centers. PET is expected to assume a greater role in lung cancer regional nodal staging, with recent data from many series indicating PET to be clearly more accurate than CT. It is not anticipated that PET will replace CT in the thorax, however, as anatomic information regarding the primary tumor stage will remain necessary to plan surgical procedures. Also, CT will help locate and characterize bronchioloalveolar cancers. PET can also survey the entire body with FDG, and it is possible that FDG whole-body imaging may become the only nuclear medicine staging test necessary for NSCLC (Figures 30.39, 30.40). 131 NP-59 scan-

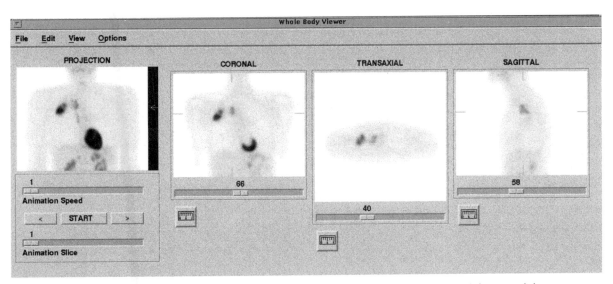

FIGURE 30.39. Projection, coronal, transverse, and sagittal PET images showing right upper lobe lung cancer and lymph node metastases in the right side of the mediastinum.

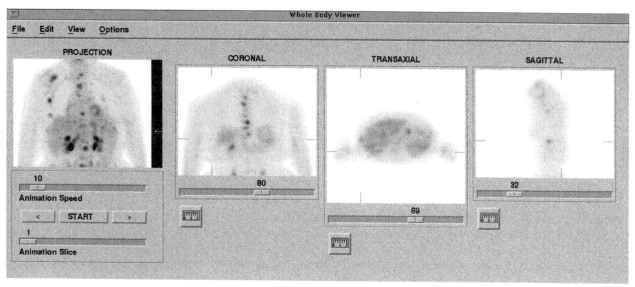

FIGURE 30.40. Projection, coronal, transverse, and sagittal PET images showing increased FDG uptake in multiple metastases in the liver, bone, and soft tissues.

ning has been shown to be effective in separating metastases to the adrenals from functioning adrenal tissue, saving patients from adrenal biopsies. But because of its limited availability, it is quite likely to be replaced by PET or other methods. Ventilation perfusion lung scanning can help determine whether the patient can be expected to have satisfactory pulmonary function postoperatively for respiratory survival, while myocardial perfusion studies can help identify patients at high risk for perioperative cardiac events, including death. In follow-up, bone scanning represents the most widely used nuclear medicine procedure, but the applications of PET are expected to grow rapidly as this technology becomes more widely available. Early data indicate a growing role for PET in assessing the postoperative or postradiation/chemotherapy-treated lung. Thus, nuclear medicine procedures are assuming increasing importance in the imaging management of patients with known or suspected lung cancer.

REFERENCES

1. Heelan R. Lung cancer imaging: primary diagnosis, staging, and local recurrence. *Semin Oncol* 1991;18:87–98.
2. McCarthy M, Ros P, Sobin L. Scientific exhibit—carcinoma of the lung: updated imaging—pathologic correlations. *RSNA* 1985:17.
3. Zwirewich C, Miller R, Muller N. Multicentric adenocarcinoma of the lung: CT-pathologic correlation. *Radiology* 1990; 176:185.
4. Muhm J, Miller W, Fontana R. Lung cancer detected during a screening program using four-month chest radiographs. *Radiology* 1983;148:609.
5. Eddy D. Screening for lung cancer. *Ann Int Med* 1989;111: 232.
6. Fontana R, Sanderson D, Woolner L. Screening for lung cancer: a critique of the Mayo lung project. *Cancer* 1991;67:1155.
7. Soda H, Tomita H, Kohno S, et al. Limitation of annual screening chest radiography for the diagnosis of lung cancer: a retrospective study. *Cancer* 1993;72:2341.
8. Heelan R, Martini N, Westcott J. Carcinomatous involvement of the hilum and mediastinum: computed tomographic and magnetic resonance evaluation. *Radiology* 1985;156:111.
9. Munden R, Pugatch R, Liptay M, et al. Small pulmonary lesions detected at CT: clinical importance. *Radiology* 1997;202:105.
10. Milla N, Ito K, Ikeda M, et al. Fundamental and clinical evaluation of chest computed tomography imaging in detectability of pulmonary nodule. *Nagoya J Med Sci* 1994;1994:127.
11. Hazelrigg S, Boley T, Weber D, et al. Incidence of lung nodules found in patients undergoing lung volume reduction. *Ann Thorac Surg* 1997;64:303.
12. Lee K, Primack S, Staples C, et al. Chronic infiltrative lung disease: comparison of diagnostic accuracies of radiography and low- and conventional-dose thin-section CT. *Radiology* 1994; 191:669.
13. Naidich D, Marshall C, Gribbin C, et al. Low-dose CT of the lungs: preliminary observations. *Radiology* 1990;175:729.
14. Diederich S, Lenzen H, Puskas Z, et al. Low dose computerized tomography of the thorax: experimental and clinical studies. *Radiology* 1996;36:475.
15. Rusinek H, Naidich D, McGuinness G, et al. Pulmonary nodule detection: low-dose versus conventional CT. *Radiology* 1998; 209:243.
16. Kaneko M, Eguchi K, Ohmatsu H, et al. Peripheral lung cancer: screening and detection with low-dose spiral CT versus radiography. *Radiology* 1996;201:798.
17. Mori K, Tominaga K, Hirose T, et al. Utility of low-dose helical CT as a second step after plain chest radiography for mass screening for lung cancer. *J Thoracic Imaging* 1997;12:173.
18. Itoh S, Ikeda M, Isomura T, et al. Screening helical CT for mass screening of lung cancer: application of low-dose and single-breath-hold scanning. *Radiat Med* 1998;16:75.
19. Sone S, Takashima S, Li F, et al. Mass screening for lung cancer

with mobile spiral computed tomography scanner. *Lancet* 1998; 351:1242.

20. Gartenschlager M, Schweden F, Gast K, et al. Pulmonary nodules: detection with low-dose vs. conventional-dose spiral CT. *Eur Radiol* 1998;8:609.

21. Felson B, Wiot J. Some less familiar roentgen manifestations of carcinoma of the lung. *Semin Roentgenol* 1977;12:187.

22. Woodring J. Unusual radiographic manifestations of lung cancer. *Radiol Clin North Am* 1990;28:599.

23. Austin J, Romney B, Goldsmith L. Missed bronchogenic carcinoma: radiographic findings in 27 patients with a potentially resectable lesion evident in retrospect. *Radiology* 1992;182:115.

24. Cahan W, Shah H, Castro E. Benign solitary lung lesions in patients with cancer. *Ann Surg* 1978;187:241.

25. Good C, Hood R, McDonald J. Significance of a solitary mass in the lung. *AJR* 1953;70:543.

26. Davis E, Peabody JJ, Katz S. The solitary pulmonary nodule. A ten-year study based on 215 cases. *J Thorac Surg* 1956;32: 728.

27. Walske B. The solitary pulmonary nodule. *Dis Chest* 1956;49: 302.

28. Taylor R, Rivkin L, Salyer J. The solitary pulmonary nodule. A review of 236 consecutive cases, 1944 to 1956. *Ann Surg* 1958;147:197.

29. Steele J. The solitary pulmonary nodule. *J Thorac Cardiovasc Surg* 1963;46:21.

30. Siegelman S, Zerhouni E, Leo F. CT of the solitary pulmonary nodule. *AJR* 1980;135:1.

31. Kubota K, Matsuzawa T, Fujiwara T, et al. Differential diagnosis of lung tumor with positron emission tomography: a prospective study. *J Nucl Med* 1990;31.

32. Gupta N, Frank A, Dewan N. Solitary pulmonary nodules: detection of malignancy with PET with 2-(F-18)-fluoro-2-deoxy-D-glucose. *Radiology* 1992;184:441.

33. Sakai F, Sone S, Maruyama A. Thin-rim enhancement in Gd-DTPA-enhanced magnetic resonance images of tuberculoma: a new finding of potential differential diagnostic importance. *J Thorac Imaging* 1992;7:64.

34. Swensen S, Morin R, Schueler B. Solitary pulmonary nodule: CT evaluation of enhancement with iodinated contrast material—a preliminary report. *Radiology* 1992;182:343.

35. Kao C, Wang S, Lin W. Differentiation of single solid lesions in the lungs by means of single-photon emission tomography with technetium-99m methoxyisobutylisonitrile. *Eur J Nuc Med* 1993;20:249.

36. Strunk V, Schweden F, Schild H, et al. Spiral CT with 3D surface reconstruction in assessing solitary pulmonary foci. *Rofo Fortschr Geb Rontgenstr Neuen Bildgeb Verfahr* 1993;158:26.

37. Sherrier R, Chiles C, Johnson G, et al. Differentiation of benign from malignant pulmonary nodules with digitized chest radiographs. *Radiology* 1987;162:645.

38. Zerhouni E, Stitik F, Siegelman S. CT of the pulmonary nodule: a cooperative study. *Radiology* 1986;160:319.

39. Siegelman S, Khouri N, Leo F. Solitary pulmonary nodules: CT assessment. *Radiology* 1986;160:307.

40. Siegelman S, Khouri N, Jr WS. Pulmonary hamartoma: CT findings. *Radiology* 1986;160:313.

41. Gobien R, Valicenti J, Paris B, et al. Thin-needle aspiration biopsy: methods of increasing the accuracy of a negative prediction. *Radiology* 1982;145:603.

42. Mitruka S, Landreneau R, Mack M, et al. Diagnosing the indeterminate pulmonary nodule: percutaneous biopsy versus thoracoscopy. *Surgery* 1995;118:676.

43. Rio F, Lobato S, Pino J, et al. Value of CT-guided fine needle aspiration in solitary pulmonary nodules with negative fiberoptic bronchoscopy. *Acta Radiol* 1994;35:478.

44. Klein J, Salomon G, Stewart E. Transthoracic needle biopsy with a coaxially placed 20-gauge automated cutting needle: results in 122 patients. *Radiology* 1996;198:715.

45. Hayashi N, Sakai T, Kitagawa M, et al. CT-guided biopsy of pulmonary nodules less than 3 cm: usefulness of the spring-operated core biopsy needle and frozen-section pathologic diagnosis. *AJR* 1998;170:329.

46. Swensen S, Brown L, Colby T, et al. Pulmonary nodules: CT evaluation of enhancement with iodinated contrast material. *Radiology* 1995;194:393.

47. Yamashita K, Matsunobe S, Tsuda T, et al. Solitary pulmonary nodules: preliminary study of evaluation with incremental dynamic CT. *Radiology* 1995;194:399.

48. Swensen S, Brown L, Colby T, et al. Lung nodule enhancement at CT: prospective findings. *Radiology* 1996;201:447.

49. Swensen S, Viggiano R, Midthun D, et al. Lung nodule enhancement at CT: multicenter study. *Radiology* 1998;209(P): 221.

50. Zhang M, Kono M. Solitary pulmonary nodules: evaluation of blood flow patterns with dynamic CT. *Radiology* 1997;205:471.

51. Im J, Song K, Kang H. Mediastinal tuberculous lympohadenitis: CT manifestations. *Radiology* 1987;164:115.

52. Guckel C, Schnabel K, Deimling M, et al. Solitary pulmonary nodules: MR evaluation of enhancement patterns with contrast-enhanced dynamic snapshot gradient-echo imaging. *Radiology* 1996;200:681.

53. Mountain C. Revisions in the International System for Staging Lung Cancer. *Chest* 1997;111:1710.

54. Mountain C, Dresler C. Regional lymph node classification for lung cancer staging. *Chest* 1997;111:1718.

55. Murayama S, Murakami J, Yoshimitsu K, et al. CT diagnosis of pleural dissemination without pleural effusion in primary lung cancer. *Radiat Med* 1996;14:117.

56. Gdeedo A, VanSchil P, Corthouts B, et al. Comparison of imaging TNM [(i)TNM] and pathological TNM [(p)TNM] in staging of bronchogenic carcinoma. *Eur J Cardiothorac Surg* 1997; 12:224.

57. Glazer H, Duncan MJ, Aronberg D. Pleural and chest wall invasion in bronchogenic carcinoma: CT evaluation. *Radiology* 1985;157:191.

58. Pennes D, Glazer G, Wimbish K, et al. Chest wall invasion by lung cancer: limitations of CT evaluation. *AJR* 1985;144:507.

59. Ratto G, Piacenza G, Frola C. Chest wall involvement by lung cancer: computed tomographic detection and results of operation. *Ann Thorac Surg* 1991;51:182.

60. Venuta F, Rendina E, Ciriaco P. Computed tomography for preoperative assessment of T3 and T4 bronchogenic carcinoma. *Eur J Cardiothorac Surg* 1992;6:238.

61. Rendina E, Bognolo D, Mineo T. Computed tomography for the evaluation of intrathoracic invasion by lung cancer. *J Thorac Cardiovasc Surg* 1987;94:57.

62. Pearlberg JL, Sandler MA, Beute GH, et al. Limitations of CT in evaluation of neoplasms involving chest wall. *J Comput Assist Tomogr* 1987;11:290.

63. Watanabe A, Shimokata K, Saka H, et al. Chest CT combined with artificial pneumothorax: value in determining origin and extent of tumor. *AJR* 1991;156:707.

64. Yokoi K, Mori K, Miyazawa N, et al. Tumor invasion of the chest wall and mediastinum in lung cancer: evaluation with pneumothorax CT. *Radiology* 1991;181:147.

65. Yokozaki M, Nawano S, Nagai K, et al. Cine magnetic resonance imaging, computed tomography and ultrasonography in the evaluation of chest wall invasion of lung cancer. *Hiroshima Med Sci* 1997;46:61.

66. Murata K, Takahashi M, Mori M, et al. Chest wall and medias-

tinal invasion by lung cancer: evaluation with multisection expiratory dynamic CT. *Radiology* 1994;191:251.

67. Suzuki N, Saito T, Kitamura S. Tumor invasion of chest wall in lung cancer: diagnosis with US. *Radiology* 1993;187:39.

68. Piehler J, Pairolero P, Weiland L, et al. Bronchogenic carcinoma with chest wall invasion: factors affecting survival following en bloc resection. *Ann Thorac Surg* 1982;34:684.

69. Paone J, Spees E, Newton C, et al. An appraisal of en bloc resection of peripheral bronchogenic carcinoma involving the thoracic wall. *Chest* 1982;81:203.

70. Glazer H, Kaiser L, Anderson D. Indeterminate mediastinal invasion in brochogenic carcinoma: CT evaluation. *Radiology* 1989;173:37.

71. Wursten H, Vock P. Mediastinal infiltration of lung carcinoma (T4NO-1): the positive predictive value of computed tomography. *Thorac Cardiovasc Surg* 1987;35:355.

72. Kameda K, Adachi S, Kono M. Detection of T-factor in lung cancer using magnetic resonance imaging and computed tomography. *J Thorac Imaging* 1988;3:73.

73. Izbicki J, Thetter O, Karg O. Accuracy of computed tomographic scan and surgical assessment for staging of bronchial carcinoma. *J Thorac Cardiovasc Surg* 1992;104:413.

74. Webb W, Gatsonis C, Zerhouni E, et al. CT and MR imaging in staging non-small cell bronchogenic carcinoma: report of the radiologic diagnostic oncology group. *Radiology* 1991;178:705.

75. Martini N, Heelan R, Westcott J. Comparative merits of conventional, computed tomographic, and magnetic resonance imaging in assessing mediastinal involvement in surgically confirmed lung carcinoma. *J Thorac Cardiovasc Surg* 1985;90:639–648.

76. Musset D, Grenier P, Carette M. Primary lung cancer staging: prospective comparative study of MR imaging with CT. *Radiology* 1986;160:607.

77. Laurent F, Drouillard J, Dorcier F. Bronchogenic carcinoma staging: CT versus MR imaging. Assessment with surgery. *Eur J Cardiothorac Surg* 1988;2:31.

78. Choe DH, Lee JH, Lee BH, et al. Obliteration of the pulmonary vein in lung cancer: significance in assessing local extent with CT. *J Comput Assist Tomogr* 1998;22:587.

79. Quint L, Glazer G, Orringer M. Central lung masses: prediction with CT of need for pneumonectomy versus lobectomy. *Radiology* 1987;165:735.

80. Quint L, McShan D, Glazer G, et al. Three dimensional CT of central lung tumors. *Clin Imaging* 1990;14:323.

81. Tobler J, Levitt R, Glazer H. Differentiation of proximal bronchogenic carcinoma from post-obstructive lobar collapse by magnetic resonance imaging: comparison with computed tomography. *Invest Radiol* 1987;22:538.

82. Kirsh M, Kahn D, Gago O. Treatment of bronchogenic carcinoma with mediastinal metastases. *Ann Thorac Surg* 1971;12:11.

83. Martini N, Flehinger B, Zaman M. Results of resection in non–oat cell carcinoma of the lung with mediastinal lymph node metastases. *Ann Surg* 1983;198:386.

84. Naruke T, Suemasu K, Ishikawa S. Lymph node mapping and curability at various levels of metastasis in resected lung cancer. *J Thorac Cardiovasc Surg* 1978;76:832.

85. Watanabe Y, Shimizu J, Oda M. Aggressive surgical intervention in N2 non–small cell cancer of the lung. *Ann Thoracic Surg* 1991;41:253.

86. Mountain C. Expanded possibilities for surgical treatment of lung cancer. *Chest* 1990;97:1045.

87. Naruke T, Goya T, Tsuchiya R. Prognosis and survival in resected lung carcinoma based on the new international staging system. *J Thorac Cardiovasc Surg* 1988;96:440.

88. McKenna R, Libshitz H, Mountain C. Roentgenographic evalu-

89. Pearson F, DeLarue N, Ilves R, et al. Significance of positive superior mediastinal nodes identified at mediastinoscopy in patients with resectable cancer of the lung. *J Thorac Cardiovasc Surg* 1982;83:1.

90. Martini N, Flehinger B. The role of surgery in N2 lung cancer. *Surg Clin North Am* 1987;67:1037.

91. Patterson G, Piazza D, Pearson F. Significance of metastatic disease in subaortic lymph nodes. *Ann Thorac Surg* 1987;43:155.

92. Taylor SI, Trybula M, Bonomi P. Simultaneous cisplatin fluorouracil infusion and radiation followed by surgical resection in regionally localized stage III, non–small cell lung cancer. *Ann Thorac Surg* 1987;43:87.

93. Faber L, Kittle C, Warren W. Preoperative chemotherapy and irradiation for stage III non–small cell lung cancer. *Ann Thorac Surg* 1989;47:669.

94. Skarin A, Jochelson M, Sheldon T. Neoadjuvant chemotherapy in marginally resectable stage III MO non–small cell lung cancer: long-term follow-up in 41 patients. *J Surg Oncon* 1989;40:266.

95. Sugarbaker D, Hemdon J, Kohman L, et al. Results of Cancer and Leukemia Group B protocol 8935: a multi-institutional phase II trimodality trial of stage HIA (N2) non–small cell lung cancer. *J Thorac Cardiovasc Surg* 1995;109:473.

96. Roth J. A randomized trial comparing perioperative chemotherapy and surgery with surgery done in resectable stage IIIA non–small cell lung cancer. *J Natl Cancer Inst* 1994;86:673.

97. Rosell R, Gomez-Codina J, Camps C, et al. A randomized trial comparing chemotherapy plus surgery with surgery alone in patients with non–small cell lung cancer. *N Engl J Med* 1994;330:153.

98. Glazer G, Gross B, Quint L, et al. Normal mediastinal lymph nodes: number and size according to American thoracic society mapping. *AJR* 1985;144:261.

99. Quint L, Glazer G, Orringer M, et al. Mediastinal lymph node detection and sizing at CT and autopsy. *AJR* 1986;147:469.

100. Shimoyama K, Murata K, Takahashi M, et al. Pulmonary hilar lymph node metastases from lung cancer: evaluation based on morphology at thin-section, incremental dynamic CT. *Radiology* 1997;203:187.

101. Genereux G, Howie J. Normal mediastinal lymph node size and number: CT and anatomic study. *AJR* 1984;142:1095.

102. Schnyder P, Gamsu G. CT of the pretracheal retrocaval space. *AJR* 1981;136:303.

103. Kiyono K, Sone S, Sakai F. The number and size of normal mediastinal lymph nodes: a postmortem study. *AJR* 1988;150:771.

104. Glazer G, Orringer M, Gross B, et al. The mediastinum in non–small cell lung cancer: CT-surgical correlation. *AJR* 1984;142:1101.

105. Platt J, Glazer G, Orringer M. Radiologic evaluation of the subcarinal lymph nodes: a comparative study. *AJR* 1988;151:279.

106. Gallardo J, Naranjo F, Cansino M, et al. Validity of enlarged mediastinal nodes as markers of involvement by non-small cell lung cancer. *Am Rev Respir Dis* 1992;146:1210.

107. Daly BJ, Faling L, Pugatch R. Computed tomography. An effective technique for mediastinal staging in lung cancer. *J Thorac Cardiovasc Surg* 1984;88:486.

108. Gross B, Glazer G, Orringer MB, et al. Bronchogenic carcinoma metastatic to normal-sized lymph nodes: frequency and significance. *Radiology* 1988;166:71.

109. Arita T, Matsumoto T, Kuramitsu T, et al. Is it possible to differentiate malignant mediastinal nodes from benign nodes

by size? Reevaluation by CT, transesophageal echocardiography, and nodal specimen. *Chest* 1996;110:1004.

110. Faling L, Pugatch R, Jung-Legg Y. Computed tomographic scanning of the mediastinum in the staging of bronchogenic carcinoma. *Am Rev Respir Dis* 1981;124:690.

111. Cybulsky I, Lanza L, Ryan M, et al. Prognostic significance of computed tomography in resected N2 lung cancer. *Ann Thorac Surg* 1992;54:533.

112. Ishida T, Tateishi M, Kaneko S, et al. Surgical treatment of patients with nonsmall-cell lung cancer and mediastinal lymph node involvement. *J Surg Oncol* 1990;43:161.

113. Bergh N, Schersten T. Bronchogenic carcinoma: a follow-up study of a surgically treated series with special reference to the prognostic significance of lymph node metastases. *Acta Chir Scand* 1965;347[Suppl]:1.

114. Fisher E, Gregorio R, Redmond C, et al. Pathologic findings from the National Surgical Adjuvant Breast Project (protocol no. 4). III. The significance of extranodal extension of axillary metastases. *Am J Clin Pathol* 1976;65:439–444.

115. Platt J, Glazer G, Gross B, et al. CT evaluation of mediastinal lymph nodes in lung cancer: influence of the lobar site of the primary neoplasm. *AJR* 1987;149:683.

116. Baron R, Levitt R, Sagel S, et al. Computed tomography in the preoperative evaluation of bronchogenic carcinoma. *Radiology* 1982;145:727.

117. Moak G, Cockerill E, Farber M, et al. Computed tomography vs standard radiology in the evaluation of mediastinal adenopathy. *Chest* 1982;82:69.

118. Osborne D, Korobkin M, Ravin C. Comparison of plain radiography, conventional tomography, and computed tomography in detecting intrathoracic lymph node metastases from lung carcinoma. *Radiology* 1982;142:157.

119. Rea H, Shevland J, House A. Accuracy of computed tomographic scanning in assessment of the mediastinum in bronchial carcinoma. *J Thorac Cardiovasc Surg* 1981;81:825.

120. Buy J, Ghossain M, Poirson F. Computed tomography of mediastinal lymph nodes in nonsmall cell lung cancer. *J Comput Assist Tomogr* 1988;12:545.

121. Ikezoe J, Kadowaki K, Morimoto S. Mediastinal lymph node metastases from nonsmall cell bronchogenic carcinoma: reevaluation with CT. *J Comput Assist Tomogr* 1990;14:340.

122. Glazer G, Francis I, Shirazi K. Evaluation of the pulmonary hilum: comparison of conventional radiography, 55 degree posterior oblique tomography, and dynamic computed tomography. *J Comput Assist Tomogr* 1983;7:983.

123. Glazer G, Gross B, Aisen A, et al. Imaging of the pulmonary hilum: a prospective comparative study in patients with lung cancer. *AJR* 1985;145:245.

124. Lewis JJ, Madrazo B, Gross S. The value of radiographic and computed tomography in the staging of lung carcinoma. *Ann Thorac Surg* 1982;34:553.

125. McLoud T, Bourgouin P, Greenberg R, et al. Bronchogenic carcinoma: analysis of staging in the mediastinum with CT by correlative lymph node mapping and sampling. *Radiology* 1992; 182:319.

126. Lewis J, Pearlberg J, Beute G. Can computed tomography of the chest stage lung cancer? Yes and no. *Ann Thorac Surg* 1990; 49:591.

127. Whitcomb M, Barham E, Goldman A, et al. Indications for mediastinoscopy in bronchogenic carcinoma. *Am Rev Respir Dis* 1976;113:189.

128. Patterson G, Ginsberg R, Poon P. A prospective evaluation of magnetic resonance imaging, computed tomography, and mediastinoscopy in the preoperative assessment of mediastinal node status in bronchogenic carcinoma. *J Thorac Cardiovasc Surg* 1987;94:679.

129. Muller N, Webb W, Gamsu G. Paratracheal lymphadenopathy: radiologic findings and correlation with CT. *Radiology* 1985; 156:761.

130. Thermann M, Poser H, Muller-Hermelink K. Evaluation of tomography and mediastinoscopy for the detection of mediastinal lymph node metastases. *Ann Thorac Surg* 1984;37:443.

131. Hirleman M, Yiu-Chiu V, Chiu L, et al. The resectability of primary lung carcinoma: a diagnostic staging review. *J Comput Tomogr* 1980;4:146.

132. Lahde S, Hyrynkangas K, Merikanto J, et al. Computed tomography and mediastinoscopy in the assessment of resectability of lung cancer. *Acta Radiol* 1989;30:169.

133. Ratto G, Frola C, Cantoni S, et al. Improving clinical efficacy of computed tomographic scan in the preoperative assessment of patients with non–small cell lung cancer. *J Thorac Cardiovasc Surg* 1990;99:416.

134. Richey H, Matthews J, Helsel R, et al. Thoracic CT scanning in the staging of bronchogenic carcinoma. *Chest* 1984;85:218.

135. Daly B, Mueller J, Faling L. N2 lung cancer: outcome in patients with false-negative computed tomographic scans of the chest. *J Thorac Cardiovasc Surg* 1993;105:904.

136. Seely J, Mayo J, Miller R, et al. T1 lung cancer: prevalence of mediastinal nodal metastases and diagnostic accuracy of CT. *Radiology* 1993;186:129.

137. Daly BJ, Faling L, Bite G. Mediastinal lymph node evaluation by computed tomography in lung cancer. *J Thorac Cardiovasc Surg* 1987;94:664.

138. Underwood GJ, Hooper R, Alelbaum S, et al. Computed tomographic scanning of the thorax in the staging of bronchogenic carcinoma. *N Engl J Med* 1979;300:777.

139. Modini C, Passariello R, Iascone C. TNM staging in lung cancer: role of computed tomography. *J Thorac Cardiovasc Surg* 1982;84:569.

140. Goldstraw P, Kurzer M, Edwards D. Preoperative staging of lung cancer: role of computed tomography. *J Thorac Cardiovasc Surg* 1983;38:10.

141. Khan A, Gersten K, Garvey J, et al. Oblique hilar tomography, computed tomography, and mediastinoscopy for prethoracotomy staging of bronchogenic carcinoma. *Radiology* 1985;156: 295.

142. Dales R, Stark R, Raman S. Computed tomography to stage lung cancer. *Am Rev Respir Dis* 1990;144:1096.

143. Ferguson M, MacMahon H, Little A, et al. Regional accuracy of computed tomography of the mediastinum in staging of lung cancer. *J Thorac Cardiovasc Surg* 1986;91:498.

144. Nohl H. An investigation into the lymphatic and vascular spread of carcinoma of the bronchus. *Thorax* 1956;11:172.

145. Nakata H, Ishimaru H, Nakayama C, et al. Computed tomography for preoperative evaluations of lung cancer. *J Comp Assist Tomogr* 1986;10:147.

146. Abrams HL, Spiro R, Goldstein N. Metastases in carcinoma. Analysis of 1000 autopsied cases. *Cancer* 1950;3:74.

147. Anderson EE. Nonfunctioning tumors of the adrenal gland. *Urol Clin North Am* 1977;4:263.

148. Matthews MJ. Problems in morphology and behavior of bronchopulmonary malignant disease. In: Israel L, Chahinian P, eds. *Lung cancer: natural history, prognosis and therapy.* New York: Academic Press, 1976:23.

149. Weiss W, Gillick JS. The metastatic spread of bronchogenic carcinoma in relation to the interval between resection and death. *Chest* 1977;71:725.

150. Smith RA. Evaluation of long-term results of surgery for bronchial carcinoma. *J Thorac Cardiovasc Surg* 1981;82:325.

151. Bell J. Abdominal exploration in one-hundred lung carcinoma suspects prior to thoracotomy. *Ann Surg* 1968;167:199.

152. Matthews MJ, Kanhouwa S, Pickren J, et al. Frequency of resid-

ual and metastatic tumor in patients undergoing curative surgical resection for lung cancer. *Cancer Chemother Rep* 1973;4(5): 63.

153. Salvatierra A, Baamonde C, Llamas JM et al. Extra thoracic staging of bronchogenic carcinoma *Chest* 1990;97:1052.

154. Sider L, Horejs D. Frequency of extrathoracic metastases from bronchogenic carcinoma in patients with normal-sized hilar and mediastinal lymph nodes on CT. *AJR* 1988;151:893.

155. Quint L, Tummala S, Brisson L, et al. Distribution of distant metastases from newly diagnosed non–small cell lung cancer. *Ann Thorac Surg* 1996;62:246.

156. Oliver TW, Bernardino ME, Miller JI, et al. Isolated adrenal masses in nonsmall-cell bronchogenic carcinoma. *Radiology* 1984;153:217.

157. Commons RR, Callaway CP. Adenomas of the adrenal cortex. *Arch Intern Med* 1948;81:37.

158. Hedeland H, Ostberg G, Hokfelt B. On the prevalence of adrenocortical adenomas in an autopsy material in relation to hypertension and diabetes. *Acta Medica-Scandinavica* 1968;184:211.

159. Glazer HS, Weyman PJ, Sagel SS, et al. Nonfunctioning adrenal masses: incidental discovery on computed tomography. *AJR* 1982;139:81.

160. Gillams A, Roberts CM, Shaw P, et al. The value of CT scanning and percutaneous fine needle aspiration of adrenal masses in biopsy-proven lung cancer. *Clin Radiol* 1992;46:18.

161. Korobkin M, Lombardi T, Aisen A, et al. Characterization of adrenal masses with chemical shift and gadolinium enhanced MR imaging. *Radiology* 1995;197:411.

162. Korobkin M, Brodeur F, Yutzy G, et al. Differentiation of adrenal adenomas from nonadenomas using CT attenuation values. *AJR* 1996;166:531.

163. Korobkin M, Brodeur F, Francis I, et al. Delayed enhanced CT for differentiation of benign from malignant adrenal masses. *Radiology* 1996;200:737.

164. Korobkin M, Giordano T, Brodeur F, et al. The relationship between histologic lipid and CT/MR findings in adrenal adenomas. *Radiology* 1996;200:743.

165. Korobkin M, Brodeur F, Francis I, et al. CT time-attenuation washout curves of adrenal adenomas and nonadenomas. *AJR* 1998;170:747.

166. Duncan KA, Gomersall LN, Weir J. Computed tomography of the chest in T1N0M0 non–small cell bronchial carcinoma. *Br J Radiol* 1993;66:20.

167. Parker LA, Mauro MA, Delany DJ, et al. Evaluation of T1N0M0 lung cancer with CT. *J Comput Assist Tomogr* 1991; 15:943.

168. Becker GL, Whitlock WL, Schaefer PS, et al. The impact of thoracic computed tomography in clinically staged T1, N0, M0 chest lesions. *Arch Intern Med* 1990;150:557.

169. Baker ME, Spritzer C, Blinder R, et al. Benign adrenal lesions mimicking malignancy on MR imaging: report of two cases. *Radiology* 1987;163:669.

170. Pearlberg J, Sandler M, Beute G, et al. T1N0M0 bronchgenic carcinoma: assessment by CT. *Radiology* 1985;157:187.

171. Heavey LR, Glazer GM, Gross BH, et al. The role of CT in staging radiographic T1N0M0 lung cancer. *AJR* 1986;146:285.

172. Conces DJ, Jr, Klink JF, Tarver RD, et al. T1N0M0 lung cancer: evaluation with CT. *Radiology* 1989;170:643.

173. Lahde S, Paivansalo M, Rainio P. CT for predicting the resectability of lung cancer. A prospective study. *Acta Radiol* 1991; 32:449.

174. Epstein D, Stephenson L, Gefter W. Value of CT in the preoperative assessment of lung cancer: a survey of thoracic surgeons. *Radiology* 1986;161:423.

175. Akamatsu H, Terashima M, Koike T, et al. Staging of primary lung cancer by computed tomography-guided percutaneous

176. Westcott J. Percutaneous needle aspiration of hilar and mediastinal masses. *Radiology* 1981;141:323.

177. Williams R, Haaga J, Karagiannis E. CT guided paravertebral biopsy of the mediastinum. *J Comput Tomogr* 1984'8:575.

178. Salazar A, Westcott J. The role of transthoracic needle biopsy for the diagnosing and staging of lung cancer. *Clin Ches Med* 1993;14:99.

179. Pearson F. Staging of the mediastinum. *Chest* 1993;103:346S.

180. Templeton P, Caskey C, Zerhouni E. Current uses of CT and MR imaging in the staging of lung cancer. *Radiol Clin North Am* 1990;28:631.

181. Gefter W. Magnetic resonance imaging in the evaluation of lung cancer. *Semin Roentgenol* 1990;25:73.

182. Webb W, Golden J. Imaging strategies in the staging of lung cancer. *Clin Chest Med* 1991;12:133.

183. Webb W, Sostman H. MR imaging of thoracic disease: clinical uses. *Radiology* 1992;182:621.

184. Kono M, Kusumoto M, Adachi S. Thoracic magnetic resonance imaging. *Curr Clin Chest Med* 1992;4:62.

185. White C, Templeton P, Belani C. Imaging in lung cancer. *Semin Oncol* 1993;20:142.

186. White C, Templeton P. Radiologic manifestations of bronchogenic cancer. *Clin Chest Med* 1993;14:55.

187. Webb W, Jensen B, Sollitto R. Bronchogenic carcinoma: staging with MR compared with staging with CT and surgery. *Radiology* 1985;156:117.

188. Levitt R, Glazer H, Roper C. Magnetic resonance imaging of mediastinal and hilar masses: comparison with CT. *AJR* 1985; 145:9.

189. Shioya S, Haida M, Ono Y. Lung cancer: differentiation of tumor, necrosis, and atelectasis by means of T1 and T2 values measured *in vitro*. *Radiology* 1988;167:105.

190. Bourgouin P, McLoud T, Fitzgibbon J. Differentiation of bronchogenic carcinoma from postobstructive pneumonitis by magnetic resonance imaging: histopathologic correlation. *J Thorac Imaging* 1991;6:22.

191. Kono M, Adachi S, Kusumoto M, et al. Clinical utility of Gd-DTPA-enhanced magnetic resonance imaging in lung cancer. *J Thorac Imaging* 1993;8:18.

192. Castagno A, Shuman W. MR imaging in clinically suspected brachial plexus tumor. *AJR* 1987;149:1219.

193. Takasugi J, Rapoport S, Shaw C. Superior sulcus tumors: the role of imaging. *J Thorac Imaging* 1989;4:41.

194. Rapoport S, Blair D, McCarthy S, et al. Brachial plexus: correlation of MR imaging with CT and pathologic findings. *Radiology* 1988;167:161.

195. Blair D, Rapoport S, Sostman H. Normal brachial plexus: MR imaging. *Radiology* 1987;165:763.

196. Freundlich I, Chasen M, Datla G. Magnetic resonance imaging of pulmonary apical tumors. *J Thorac Imaging* 1996;11:210.

197. Heelan R, Demas B, Caravelli J. Superior sulcus tumors: CT and MR imaging. *Radiology* 1989;170:637.

198. McLoud T, Filion R, Edelman R. MR imaging of superior sulcus carcinoma. *J Comput Tomogr* 1989;1989:233.

199. Haggar A, Pearlberg J, Froelich J. Chest-wall invasion by carcinoma of the lung: detection by MR imaging. *AJR* 1987;148: 1075.

200. Padovani B, Mouroux J, Seksik L, et al. Chest wall invasion by bronchogenic carcinoma: evaluation with MR imaging. *Radiology* 1993;187:33.

201. Barakos J, Brown J, Higgins C. MR imaging of secondary cardiac and paracardiac lesions. *AJR* 1989;153:47.

202. Amparo E, Higgins C, Farmer D. Gated MRI of cardiac and paracardiac masses: initial experience. *AJR* 1984;143:1151.

203. Grenier P, Dubray B, Carette M, et al. Preoperative thoracic staging of lung cancer. CT and MR evaluation. *Diagn Interv Radiol* 1989;1:23.

204. Bonomo L, Ciccotosto C, Guidotti A, et al. Lung cancer staging: the role of computed tomography and magnetic resonance imaging. *Eur J Radiol* 1996;23:35.

205. Dooms G, Hricak H, Moseley M. Characterization of lymphadenopathy by magnetic resonance relaxation times: preliminary results. *Radiology* 1985;155:691.

206. Glazer G, Orringer M, Chenevert T. Mediastinal lymph nodes: relaxation time/pathologic correlation and implications in staging of lung cancer with MR imaging. *Radiology* 1988;168:429.

207. Harisinghani M, Saini S, Hahn P, et al. MR imaging of lymph nodes in patients with primary abdominal and pelvic malignancies using ultra small superparamagnetic iron oxide (Combidex). *Acad Radiol* 1998;5[Suppl 1]:S167.

208. Anzai Y, Blackwell K, Hirschowitz S, et al. Initial clinical experience with dextran-coated superparamagnetic iron oxide for detection of lymph node metastases in patients with head and neck cancer. *Radiology* 1994;192:709.

209. Glazer G, Woolsey E, Borrello J. Adrenal tissue characterization using MR imaging. *Radiology* 1986;158:73.

210. Reinig J, Doppman J, Dwyer A. Adrenal masses differentiated by MR. *Radiology* 1986;158:81.

211. Kier R, McCarthy S. MR characterization of adrenal masses: field strengths and pulse sequence considerations. *Radiology* 1989;171:671.

212. Baker M, Blinder R, Spitzer C. MR evaluation of adrenal masses of 1.5T. *AJR* 1989;153:307.

213. Krestin G, Steinbrich W, Friedmann G. Adrenal masses: evaluation with fast gradient-echo MR imaging and gadolinium-DTPA enhanced dynamic studies. *Radiology* 1989;171:675.

214. Leroy-Willig A, Roucayrol J, Luton J. *In vitro* adrenal cortex lesions characterization by NMR spectroscopy. *Magn Reson Imaging* 1987;5:339.

215. Mitchell D, Crovello M, Matteucci T, et al. Benign adrenocortical masses: diagnosis with chemical shift MR imaging. *Radiology* 1992;185:345.

216. McNicholas M, Lee M, Mayo-Smith W, et al. An algorithm for the differential diagnosis of adrenal adenomas and metastases. *AJR* 1995;165:1453.

217. Mayo-Smith W, Lee M, McNicholas M, et al. Characterization of adrenal masses (<5 cm) by use of chemical shift MR imaging: observer performance versus quantitative measures. *AJR* 1995;165:91.

218. Outwater E, Siegelman E, Radecki P, et al. Distinction between benign and malignant adrenal masses: value of T1-weighted chemical-shift MR imaging. *AJR* 1995;65:579.

219. Lee M, Hahn P, Papanicolaou N, et al. Benign and malignant adrenal massess: CT distinction with attenuation coefficients, size and observer analysis. *Radiology* 1991;179:415.

220. Olsen G, Block A, Swenson E. Pulmonary function evaluation of the lung resection candidate: A prospective study. *Am Rev Resp Dis* 1975;111:379.

221. Ali M, Mountain C, Ewer M. Predicting loss of pulmonary function after pulmonary resection for bronchogenic carcinomas. *Chest* 1980;77:337.

222. Ryo U. Prediction of postoperative loss of lung function in patients with malignant lung mass. Quantitative regional ventilation-perfusion scanning. *Radiol Clin North Am* 1990;28:657.

223. Gravenstein S, Peltz M, Pories W. How ominous is an abnormal scan in bronchogenic carcinoma? *JAMA* 1979;241:2523.

224. Quinn DL, Ostrow LB, Porter DK, et al. Staging of non–small cell bronchogenic carcinoma. Relationship of the clinical evaluation to organ scans. *Chest* 1986;89:270.

225. Michel F, Soler M, Imhof E. Initial staging of non–small cell lung cancer: value of routine radioisotope bone scanning. *Thorax* 1991;46:469.

226. Bekerman C, Caride V, Hoffer P, et al. Noninvasive staging of lung cancer. Indications and limitations of gallium-67 citrate imaging. *Radiol Clin North Am* 1990;28:497.

227. McKenna R, Haynie T, Libshitz H, et al. Critical evaluation of the GA 67 scan for surgical patients with lung cancer. *Chest* 1985;1985:428.

228. Matsuno S, Tanabe M, Kawasaki Y. Effectiveness of planar image and single photon emission tomography of thallium-201 compared with gallium-67 in patients with primary lung cancer. *Eur J Nucl Med* 1992;19:86.

229. Tonami N, Hisada K, Watanabe Y. [201T1 single photon emission computed tomography in the diagnosis of lung cancer]. *Rinsho Hoshasen* 1990;35:825.

230. Ishibashi M, Honda N, Yoshioka F. Validation of single-photon emission computed tomography (SPECT) using thallium-201 in patients with lung cancer. *Kurume Med J* 1991;38:87.

231. Sehweil A, McKillop J, Milroy R. 201T1 scintigraphy in the staging of lung cancer, breast cancer and lymphoma. *Nucl Med Commun* 1990;11:263.

232. Duman Y, Burak Z, Erdem S. The value and limitations of 201T1 scintigraphy in the evaluation of lung lesions and post-therapy follow up of primary lung carcinoma. *Nucl Med Commun* 1993;14:446.

233. Suga K, Kume N, Orihashi N. Difference in 201T1 accumulation on single photon emission computed tomography in benign and malignant thoracic lesions. *Nucl Med Commun* 1993;14:107.

234. Brown K. Prognostic value of TI-201 myocardial perfusion imaging: a diagnostic tool comes of age. *Circulation* 1991;83:363.

235. Eagle K, Coley C, Newell J. Combining clinical and thallium data optimizes preoperative assessment of cardiac risk before major vascular surger. *Ann Int Med* 1989;110:859.

236. Francis I, Smid A, Gross M, et al. Adrenal masses in oncologic patients: functional and morphologic evaluation. *Radiology* 1988;166:353.

237. Ziessman H, Silverman P, Patterson J. Improved detection of small cavernous hemangiomas of the liver with high-resolution three-headed SPECT. *J Nucl Med* 1991;32:2086.

238. Tumeh S, Benson C, Nagel J, et al. Cavemous hemangioma of the liver: detection with single-photon emission computed tomography. *Radiology* 1987;164:353.

239. Rubin R, Lichtenstein G. Scintigraphic evaluation of liver masses: cavermous hepatic hemangioma [clinical reference]. *J Nucl Med* 1993;34:849.

240. Goldenberg D, DeLand F, Kim E. Use of radiolabeled antibodies to carcinoembryonic antigens for the detection and localization of disease by external photoscanning. *N Engl J Med* 1978;298:1384.

241. Krishnamurthy S, Morris J, Antonovic R. Evaluation of primary lung cancer with Indium 111 anti-carcino-embryonic antigen (ZCE-025) monoclonal antibody scintigraphy. *Cancer* 1990;65:458.

242. Biggi A, Gianfranco B, Ferrigno D. Detection of suspected primary lung cancer by scintigraphy with indium-111 anti-carcinoembryonic antigen monoclonal antibodies (type FO23C5). *J Nuc Med* 1991;32:2064.

243. Friedman S, Sullivan K, Salk D. Staging non–small carcinoma of the lung using technetium 99 m labeled monoclonal antibodies. *Hematol Oncol Clin North Am* 1990;4:1069.

244. Vansant J, Johnson D, O'Donnell D. Staging lung carcinoma with a Tc99m labeled monoclonal antibody. *Clin Nuc Med* 1992;17:431.

245. Rusch V, Macapinlac H, Heelan R. NR-LU-10 monoclonal antibody scanning. A helpful new adjunct to computed tomog-

raphy in evaluating non-small-cell lung cancer. *J Thorac Cardiovasc Surg* 1993;106:200.

246. Breitz H, Sullivan K, Nelp W. Imaging lung cancer with radiolabeled antibodies. *Semin Nucl Med* 1993;23:127.

247. AbdelNabi H, Abrams P, Ackerhalt R. Tc99m labeled monoclonal antibody imaging of small cell carcinoma of the lung. *J Nuc Med* 1989;309:818.

248. Balaban E, Walter B, Cox J. Radionuclide imaging of bone marrow metastases with a Tc99m labeled monoclonal antibody to small cell lung carcinoma. *Clin Nuc Med* 1991;16:732.

249. Kwekkeboom D, Krenning E, Bakker W. Radioiodinated somatostatin analog scintigraphy in small-cell lung cancer. *J Nucl Med* 1991;26:37.

250. Blum J, Handmaker H, Rinne N. The utility of a somatostatin-type receptor binding peptide radiopharmaceutical (P829) in the evaluation of solitary pulmonary nodules. *Chest* 1999;115:224.

251. Kubota K, Matsuzawa T, Ito M. Lung tumor imaging by positron emission tomography using C-11 L-methionine. *J Nucl Med* 1985;26:37.

252. Fujiwara T, Matsuzawa T, Kubota K. Relationship between histologic type of primary lung cancer and carbon-11-L-methionine uptake with positron emission tomography. *J Nucl Med* 1989;30:33.

253. Nolop K, Rhodes C, Brudin L. Glucose utilization *in vivo* by human pulmonary neoplasms. *Cancer* 1987;60:2682.

254. Patz EJ, Lowe V, Hoffman J. Focal pulmonary abnormalities: evaluation with F-18 fluorodeoxyglucose PET scanning. *Radiology* 1987;188:487.

255. Rege S, Hoh C, Glaspy J. Imaging of pulmonary mass lesions with whole-body positron emission tomography and fluorodeoxyglucose. *Cancer* 1993;72:82.

256. Lowe V, Fletcher J, Gobar L, et al. Prospective investigation of positron emission tomography in lung nodules. *J Clin Oncol* 1998;16:1075.

257. Prauer H, Weber W, Romer W, et al. Controlled prospective study of positron emission tomography using the glucose analogue [18f]fluorodeoxyglucose in the evaluation of pulmonary nodules. *Br J Surg* 1998;85.

258. Kim B, Kim Y, Lee K, et al. Localized form of bronchioloalveolar carcinoma: FDG PET findings. *AJR* 1998;170:935.

259. Miyazawa H, Arai T, Inagaki K, et al. Detection of mediastinal lymph node metastasis from lung cancer with positron emission tomography (PET) using 11C-methionine. *Nippon Kyobu Geka Gakkai Zasshi* 1992;40:2125.

260. Wahl R, Quint L, Greenough R, et al. Staging of mediastinal non-small cell lung cancer with FDG-PET, CT, and fusion images: preliminary prospective evaluation. *Radiology* 1994;191:371.

261. Knopp M, Bischoff H, Oberdorfer F, et al. Forshungs-schwerpunkt radiologishe diagnostik und therapie, deutsches krebsforschungszentrum, heidelberg. [Positron emission tomography of the thorax. The current clinical status] Positronenemissionstomographie des thorax. Derzeitiger klinischer stellenwert. *Radiologe* 1992;32:290.

262. Vansteenkiste J, Stroobants S, DeLeyn P, et al. Lymph node staging in non-small-cell lung cancer with FDG-PET scan: a prospective study on 690 lymph node stations from 68 patients. *J Clin Oncol* 1998;16:2142.

263. Dwamena B, Sonnad S, Angobaldo J, et al. Mediastinal staging of non-small cell lung cancer (NSCLC) in the nineteen nineties: a meta-analytic comparison of positron emission tomography and x-ray computed tomography. *Radiology* 1999;213:530.

264. Vansteenkiste J, Stroobants S, Dupont P, et al. Prognostic importance of FDG on PET-Scan in non small cell lung cancer. *Proc ASCO* 1999; p. 464a, abstract 1791.

265. Bury T, Barreto A, Daenen F, et al. Fluorine-18 deoxyglucose positron emission tomography for the detection of bone metastases in patients with non-small cell lung cancer. *Eur J Nucl Med* 1998;25:1244.

266. Weder W, Schmid R, Bruchhaus H, et al. Detection of extrathoracic metastases by positron emission tomography in lung cancer. *Ann Thoracic Surg* 1998;66:886.

267. Erasmus J, Jr., Patsy E, McAdams H, et al. Evaluation of adrenal masses in patients with bronchogenic carcinoma using 18F-fluorodeoxyglucose positron emission tomography. *AJR* 1997;168:1357.

268. Griffeth L, Rich K, Dehdashti F, et al. Brain metastases from non-central nervous system tumors: evaluation with PET. *Radiology* 1993;186:37.

269. Scott W, Shepherd J, Gambhir S. Cost-effectiveness of FDG-PET for staging non-small cell lung cancer: a decision analysis. *Ann Thor Surg* 1998;66:1876.

270. Kubota K, Yamada S, Ishiwata K. Evaluation of the treatment response of lung cancer with positron emission tomography and L-[methyl-11C]methionine: a preliminary study. *Eur J Nucl Med* 1993;20:495.

271. Hebert M, Lowe V, Hoffman J, et al. Positron emission tomography in the pretreatment evaluation and follow-up of non-small cell lung cancer patients treated with radiotherapy: preliminary findings. *Am J Clin Oncol* 1996;19:416.

31

TISSUE PROCUREMENT: BRONCHOSCOPIC TECHNIQUES

DEBORAH SHURE
JOHN F. CONFORTI

Bronchoscopy has long had a role in the diagnosis of bronchogenic carcinoma, beginning with the use of rigid bronchoscopy and the increased incidence of lung cancer in the 1950s.[1,2] With the advent of flexible fiberoptic bronchoscopy, the role of bronchoscopy expanded beyond the recognition of endobronchial disease possible with rigid bronchoscopy to sampling of peripheral masses not visible in the central airways but evident fluoroscopically. More recently, the reincarnation of bronchoscopic aspirating needles (first used through rigid bronchoscopes) in a flexible form has opened the area of mediastinal staging and enhanced more standard sampling applications of bronchoscopy.

The roles of bronchoscopy in patients with bronchogenic carcinoma can be grouped into the areas of diagnosis, staging, evaluation of therapeutic outcome, and endoscopic therapeutic intervention. Varying techniques are applicable to each group, so that an overall organized strategy is important. Some exciting, as yet experimental, techniques may well alter these approaches in the next decade.

DIAGNOSIS

Endobronchial Masses

Bronchogenic carcinoma often presents as an endobronchial exophytic mass (Figure 31.1) in the central airways (mainstem to subsegmental bronchi).[1,3] This presentation is typical of squamous cell and small cell carcinoma but can occur with any cell type.[4] This form of bronchogenic carcinoma is easy to recognize endoscopically and usually easy to biopsy with standard biopsy forceps. The yield with a minimum of three biopsies should be close to 100%.[5,6] Washing and brushing do not substantially increase the yield but are inexpensive and are usually performed in addition to the biopsies for the occasional added case.

Bronchoscopic needle aspiration can also be used to sample endobronchial masses, but the technique does not seem to offer an improved yield over traditional forceps biopsy. In one study of 60 patients with endobronchial lesions,

forceps biopsy had an 85% diagnostic yield, whereas needle aspiration had a 65% yield.[1] Another study of 60 patients had opposite results: 80% yield with needle aspiration and 60% with forceps biopsy. Because most studies find very high yields with biopsy alone, bronchoscopic needle aspiration is unlikely to substitute for forceps biopsy in these lesions. Nonetheless, it would seem to have some limited applications in endobronchial masses. It has been suggested that bronchoscopic needle aspiration may be useful in lesions that are very friable and may bleed excessively with forceps biopsy.[8] Occasionally, endobronchial biopsies may be nondiagnostic because extensive necrosis results in sampling error. Bronchoscopic needle aspiration may improve yield by sampling deeper tissue. It may also be useful in sampling lesions located in areas in which forceps tend to slip off the bronchial wall. Finally, rapid on-site cytopathology may provide an immediate diagnosis when deemed necessary.

Submucosal and Peribronchial Tumor

A less common presentation of bronchogenic carcinoma is submucosal spread or peribronchial involvement, which causes extrinsic compression or concentric narrowing of the bronchus.[1] In the case of submucosal spread, normal mucosal markings are often effaced and the surface may be covered with a fine network of engorged bronchial collateral vessels (Figure 31.2). This sort of tissue involvement is usually much firmer than the soft exophytic mass discussed previously and is consequently more difficult to biopsy. The diagnostic yield is considerably lower than with forceps biopsy of exophytic masses, probably because of the difficulty in sampling deeper tissue layers and because of a less dense carcinomatous process with a consequently greater sampling error.

Diagnosis of bronchogenic carcinoma in these lesions has been aided by the use of bronchoscopic needle aspiration. In one study, forceps biopsy detected 55% of such tumors, whereas bronchoscopic needle aspiration alone detected

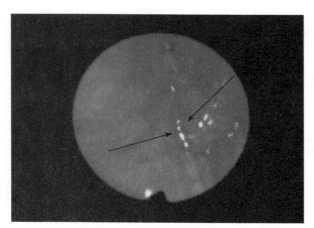

FIGURE 31.1. Endobronchial mass occluding a segmental bronchus. (See Color Figure 31.1)

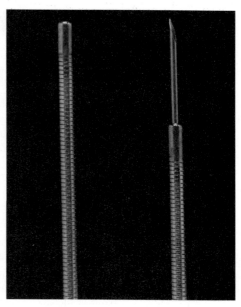

FIGURE 31.3. Bronchoscopic aspirating needle in retracted and advanced positions. (Olympus Corp. Lake Success, New York.)

71%.[9] The combination of forceps biopsy and needle aspiration detected 90%, and adding either a wash or a brush brought the yield to 97%. Interestingly, diagnostic yields are often incrementally increased by different sampling methods when the sampling error is higher.

The technique for sampling submucosal or peribronchial tissue is straightforward. The needle device is advanced through the bronchoscope channel in the retracted position. Once the tip of the device is 2 cm above the area to be sampled, the needle can be advanced from its sheath (Figure 31.3). At this point, it is usually helpful to withdraw the needle's sheath into the bronchoscope channel so that only the needle remains exposed. This maneuver allows the sheath to be supported by the bronchoscope channel and gives the operator greater control over the exact placement and advancement of the needle. The needle is then inserted

at an oblique angle into the submucosal layers or perpendicular to the wall in the case of suspected peribronchial disease. Once the needle is embedded in the tissue, it is moved vigorously back and forth (remaining in the site) while suction is applied to the proximal end of the device. It is, of course, important to remember to withdraw the needle into its sheath prior to removing the needle from the bronchoscope.

The optimal number of aspirations has not been studied, but the percentage of adequate aspirations can be increased by on-site processing of the aspirate by a cytopathologist. In one study, the percentage of specimens with malignant cells increased from 31% to 56%.[10] This increase occurred regardless of the location of the lesion (i.e., endobronchial, submucosal, or peripheral). In the absence of rapid evaluation of the aspirate, it appears useful to do at least three aspirations in the involved area.[11] Handling of the specimen can be done in various ways that appear to be equivalent, so it is best to coordinate handling with the cytopathologist to fit individual institutional needs.

Bronchoscopic needle aspiration is also useful in nonmalignant disease, which may be relevant in the evaluation of suspected malignancy. One study found an 87% yield in patients with HIV infection and intrathoracic adenopathy secondary to mycobacterial disease.[12] In 32%, needle aspiration was the exclusive means of diagnosis. This method has also been studied extensively in the diagnosis of sarcoidosis. Optimal diagnostic yields occurred when transbronchial lung biopsy was combined with bronchoscopic needle aspiration.[13]

Despite the demonstrated utility of bronchoscopic

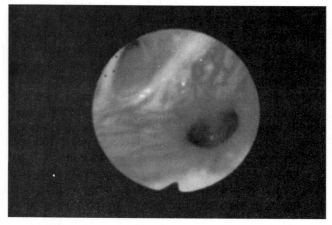

FIGURE 31.2. Submucosal infiltration of bronchogenic carcinoma. Normal bronchial markings are lost and engorged bronchial collateral vessels are prominent. (See Color Figure 31.2)

needle aspiration, it remains an underutilized technique. A computerized survey performed at the 1995 American College of Chest Physicians Fellows' Conference found that only 10% reported routinely performing bronchoscopic needle aspiration.[14] Reported limitations at their institutions included suboptimal technique (30%), technician support (1%), cytopathology support (14%), and a combination of all of these factors (25%). Thirty percent felt that this technique was not useful. A learning curve is also necessary when performing bronchoscopic needle aspiration. One study recorded their results during a 3-year period with serial multifaceted educational interventions. Their yields increased significantly from 21.4% to 47.6%, and fewer cytologically unsatisfactory specimens were obtained.[15] Thus improved experience in training programs and ongoing education is necessary for this technique to achieve its maximum utility.

Peripheral Masses

Peripheral lung masses (including solitary pulmonary nodules) have always presented more of a diagnostic problem than lesions in central airways, and reported diagnostic yields have generally been lower, in the range of 30% to 50%.[16-19] Transbronchial biopsy has been the mainstay of specimen sampling of peripheral masses. Its yield is partly affected by the number of biopsies performed. Optimal yields require at least four adequate samples[5,20] with small or large biopsy forceps. Optimal yields in discrete mass lesions (as opposed to diffuse interstitial disease) require the use of fluoroscopy in more than one plane to ensure accurate placement of the biopsy instrument. Biplane fluoroscopy, rotation of the C-arm of a fluoroscope, or rotating the patient in a fixed fluoroscope all provide adequate assessment of placement.

The yield of transbronchial biopsy is affected most by lesion size. In general, poor yields (<35%) are obtained in sampling lesions smaller than 2 cm in diameter,[16,17,20-22] probably because only one bronchus tends to supply lesions this size, whereas two or more bronchi are involved in lesions 2 cm and larger, increasing the likelihood of the forceps reaching the mass.[23] Computed tomographic evidence of a bronchus leading to the lesion, "bronchus sign," predicts a higher diagnostic yield with biopsy techniques.[24] An exception to increasing yield with increasing lesion size is the case of lesions larger than 6 cm in diameter. Very large lesions tend to have significant components of inflammation and necrosis, which increase the sampling error and decrease the yield despite the generous size of the mass.[16]

Although the statement is often made that lesions in the outer third of the lung are too far out to reach with the transbronchial biopsy technique, this impression is actually mistaken. In fact, forceps can often be passed close to the pleural surface, creating one mechanism of pneumothorax with bronchoscopy. Lesions in the inner third of the lung

may actually be more difficult to sample because of the tighter branching pattern of bronchi leading to the mass.

One remaining factor influencing diagnostic yield is the nature of the mass: primary versus metastatic. Primary bronchogenic carcinomas are bronchocentric in origin and, therefore, are more easily sampled by forceps passed through the airway. Metastatic nodules are usually hematogenous in origin and perivascular in location,[25] and the yield on transbronchial biopsy appears to be lower than for primary carcinomas.[19,26,27]

Two problems seem basic to the difficulty in sampling peripheral lesions: (a) the lack of direct peripheral visualization of the tumor and (b) the lack of adequate directional steering of the forceps in the periphery. Ultrathin bronchoscopes have been developed to achieve better peripheral visualization and appear to offer hope of increased range,[28] but they are unlikely to reach the level of most radiographically visible masses and have little prospect of offering any sampling capability. An older instrument, the single or double-hinged curette, actually provided some directional capability in the periphery but is somewhat fragile and has not met with widespread use, perhaps because of the cumbersomeness of the procedure.[29] Those using this device first use bronchography to map the bronchial tree leading to the mass. Because bronchography can effect cytologic results, the patients are not bronchoscoped for 2 weeks after the bronchogram. Fluoroscopy and the bronchogram are then used to manipulate the curette into the lesion. The ability to flex the hinges of the curette offers more directional control than traditional biopsy forceps. The process is, however, a long one and not clearly worth the time and expense considering other techniques.

More recently, two techniques have provided some improvement in sampling peripheral lesions without providing increased visualization or directional control. They are transbronchial needle aspiration and bronchoalveolar lavage (BAL). The technique of transbronchial needle aspiration of peripheral masses is similar to that of transbronchial biopsy. The device is passed under fluoroscopic guidance into the mass, and the needle is extended and moved back and forth in the lesion while aspirating at the proximal end. The needle is then removed from the mass, withdrawn into its sheath, and removed from the bronchoscope channel. It does not appear to be necessary to inject saline into the mass prior to aspiration.

Transbronchial needle aspiration significantly increases the yield of bronchoscopy in the diagnosis of peripheral masses 2 cm or larger in diameter.[20,23] In one study,[20] the yield for lesions less than 2 cm in diameter was the same with transbronchial biopsy and transbronchial needle aspiration (35%), but for larger lesions, transbronchial needle aspiration increased the yield over that of transbronchial biopsy from 52% to 76%. The technique was particularly useful for lesions that could not be penetrated by standard forceps so that transbronchial biopsies could not be performed.

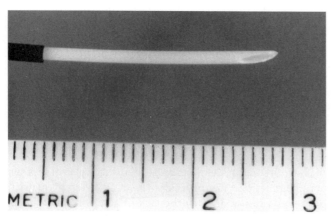

FIGURE 31.4. Plastic bronchoscopic aspirating needle. The needle is 18 g with no rigid section. (SoftCor, Microvasive Corp. Watertown, Massachusetts.)

Such cases are probably caused by a tumor extrinsically compressing the bronchus leading to it or by the tumor being situated outside a bronchial branching point. In this subset, the yield of transbronchial needle aspiration was 80%. In other studies, the technique enhances the yield of bronchoscopy in the diagnosis of metastatic nodules,[30] again illustrating the ability of the needle to pass through areas difficult to access with traditional biopsy forceps.

Two aspirating needles may particularly enhance the yield of bronchoscopy for peripheral lesions, although neither has been extensively studied. A plastic needle (Figure 31.4) with no rigid section at the distal end (e.g., SoftCor, Microvasive Corp, Watertown, Massachusetts) has been helpful in the authors' experience in accessing lesions in difficult locations such as the superior segment of the lower lobes or the medial aspect of the upper lobes. Maneuverability is improved by the absence of the 1- to 2-cm rigid distal section characteristic of most needles and forceps. It is also an 18-gauge device that offers the potential of a histologic specimen in addition to cytology. In most situations, the combination of histology and cytology produces a better yield than either alone. Using this needle, the author has achieved yields of 85% for lesions 2 cm or larger. The second needle is an 18-gauge metal needle that has been used primarily for mediastinal staging (see also Chapters 32, 35), again because of the potential for an improved yield with the added histology specimen.

BAL has yet to be fully explored as an adjunct to transbronchial biopsy or transbronchial needle aspiration in the assessment of peripheral masses, but recent reports suggest that it at least enhances the yield over that of transbronchial biopsy, brushing, and washing.[31–36] BAL is theoretically appealing because it is known to be able to obtain material from the alveolar level in diffuse lung diseases such as *Pneumocystis pneumonia* and sarcoidosis.[35] So far, yields in bronchogenic carcinoma have varied significantly from 33%[31]

to 65%,[33] and few studies have systematically compared yields from the common sampling procedures in the same patients. One study found a yield of 75% using a combination of transbronchial biopsy, BAL, and brushings.[37] In most studies, BAL provided the only bronchoscopic evidence of carcinoma in a meaningful number of cases (6% to 11%).[37] More studies will undoubtedly be published in the next few years, which we hope will sort out the best combination of sampling techniques. In the authors' experience (unpublished), the combination of transbronchial needle aspiration and BAL appears to provide a better yield than transbronchial biopsy with brushing and BAL.

Lymphangitic Carcinoma

Lymphangitic carcinoma represents a special case of diffuse lung disease and, as with other forms of diffuse disease, it is readily sampled by transbronchial biopsy. Transbronchial needle aspiration has not been tested in lymphangitic carcinoma, but it would appear unlikely to be useful in this setting because the technique is generally more suited to dense lesions than to diffuse parenchymal lesions.[38] BAL has been shown to add to the diagnostic yield in lymphangitic carcinoma,[32] although it has not been systematically compared to other sampling techniques.

Special Issues

Occasional disputes arise over the necessity for a preoperative diagnosis of lung cancer in cases of solitary pulmonary nodules, which are distinguished from a lung mass by the absence of radiographic findings other than a well-circumscribed round mass completely surrounded by lung. This particular presentation poses a dilemma because it can be caused by either benign or malignant processes, and surgery for benign disease should be avoided, if possible. Evidence of very long lesion doubling time (>2 years) from previous chest radiographs, radiographic evidence of a benign pattern of calcification, supports the diagnosis of a benign lesion. Many lesions (including benign ones) do not, however, meet these criteria.

In the absence of computed tomographic evidence of mediastinal adenopathy, some physicians have argued that bronchoscopy (or transthoracic needle aspiration) does not alter outcome.[39] Unfortunately, the issue is not clear-cut. In some populations, such as the Southwest United States, a significant number (up to 50%) of solitary nodules in patients over 50 years old may be caused by benign processes such as coccidioidomycosis, which can be detected by bronchoscopy,[40] so that the patient population must be considered. Second, the potential for mediastinal staging has not been accounted for in the algorithms. In addition, bronchogenic carcinoma is multicentric.[41] The reported incidence of simultaneous tumors has varied from 1.2%[42] to 10% to 22% in occult carcinoma.[43,44] Although a small study of solitary pulmonary nodules found no second (endobronchial lesions),[45] the actual incidence in the subset of patients with solitary nodules has not been reported. The ability to detect second lesions, which might influence the approach to therapy, would clearly affect the approach to preoperative diagnosis. One study using decision analysis to determine the effect of diagnostic strategy on survival found that immediate surgery had a very slight survival advantage if the likelihood of malignancy was very high; preoperative biopsy had a very slight advantage if the probability of cancer was intermediate; and observation had a very slight advantage if the probability of cancer was very low.[46]

A second special issue is the role of bronchoscopy in hemoptysis with a normal or nonlocalizing chest radiograph. A surprising number of studies have addressed this issue in the past ten years, with remarkably similar conclusions despite some small variations.[18,47–56] All studies have found that bronchoscopy is indicated in patients at risk for lung cancer: age over forty years, a significant smoking history, and male sex (although this factor has probably changed with the greatly increased incidence of bronchogenic carcinoma in women).

No consensus exists on the significance of the volume of hemoptysis. One study found a significant incidence of carcinoma only when the volume of hemoptysis was greater than 30 mL,[53] another when the volume was greater than 60 mL,[51] and a third found no relation to volume.[57] Bronchoscopy appears to be indicated in the presence of hemoptysis and a normal chest radiograph when any risk of cancer exists or symptoms of cancer are present, regardless of the volume of the bleeding.

A third issue is that of occult bronchogenic carcinoma; that is, positive sputum cytology with a normal chest radiograph. Bronchoscopy is the diagnostic procedure of choice in such situations. The majority of lesions are found on the first bronchoscopy.[44] If not, then most can be found on repeated bronchoscopies every three months.[44] If repeat bronchoscopy is needed, computed tomography may be useful to indicate suspicious areas,[58,59] although computed tomography is not sensitive to submucosal disease.[56] In unusual circumstances, bronchography may also be helpful.[60] In any case, most occult tumors not found on the initial bronchoscopy are carcinomas *in situ,* or minimally invasive tumors that have a good prognosis even when diagnosed up to 5 years after the initial positive sputum cytology.[44] Some experimental techniques involving fluorescence bronchoscopy may, however, provide more rapid accurate localization in the future (see also Chapters 22, 24).

A final special issue is the role of bronchoscopy in patients with pneumonia. Bronchoscopy is commonly believed to be indicated in nonresolving segmental or lobar pneumonia to detect an endobronchial obstruction. One study of patients with community-acquired pneumonia found an incidence of bronchogenic carcinoma of 14% in patients over age fifty on early bronchoscopy.[61] Again, the optimal timing of bronchoscopy has not been examined.

STAGING

Proximal Extent

It has long been known that the proximal extent of bronchogenic carcinoma influences resectability,[2,62] yet this aspect of staging is often neglected in routine diagnostic bronchoscopies and determined instead at the time of surgery. In some cases, surgery may not be indicated if the tumor has spread too centrally. Carinal biopsy has been shown to be useful in the presence of endobronchial tumor, even when the carina itself appears visually normal.[62] Approximately 5% of so-called blind carinal biopsies are positive in the presence of a central endobronchial tumor.[63,64] Although the incidence of positive blind biopsies is not particularly high, the biopsy procedure is brief with very little risk, and the implications of a positive biopsy are important.

A second important aspect of determining proximal spread is the assessment of submucosal involvement in the more distal airways. Biopsy of the next proximal bronchus to the bronchus containing an endobronchial mass has been found to be useful in determining resectability and was often done through rigid bronchoscopes,[1,65] but the procedure has not been popular with fiberoptic bronchoscopy for unclear reasons. More recently, transbronchial needle aspiration has been found to be useful and to compare favorably with surgical findings in assessing proximal submucosal spread of endobronchial tumors.[51]

Second Lesions

A careful search for second lesions should be part of a diagnostic bronchoscopy for lung cancer. Although the incidence of second lesions in the presence of solitary pulmonary nodules may not be high (see previous section, DIAGNOSIS, Special Issues), second lesions seem to occur with some frequency in patients presenting with occult carcinoma[43,44] and endobronchial primaries. Such a search is particularly important because chest radiographs are unlikely to detect endobronchial tumors until secondary signs of obstruction occur. In fact, even complete endobronchial obstruction may not be associated with radiographic signs of obstruction in up to 44% of patients.[66]

Mediastinal Staging

Transbronchial needle aspiration has enlarged the scope of bronchoscopy to include assessment of mediastinal adenopathy. Paratracheal, subcarinal, hilar, and aorticopulmonary window nodes can all be accessed through the flexible bronchoscope. The technique is similar regardless of the location. Similar to submucosal aspirates, the needle should be advanced proximal to the site to be aspirated, and the sheath should be pulled back to support the body of the device in the channel of the bronchoscope. The needle should then be moved to the area of interest determined either by the physical appearance of the area or by the suspicion of adenopathy based on chest radiographs or computed tomography. The needle should be firmly placed against the tissue to be aspirated to anchor it before advancing it with a jabbing motion into the deeper layers.[67] Aspiration is then performed while moving the needle back and forth within the tissue.

The most common problem with the transbronchial needle technique seems to be inadequate insertion of the needle in the tissue of interest. Because the insertion maneuver tends to push the distal tip of the bronchoscope back from the needle device, the operator can be too far from the needle to accurately determine its position. As a result, it is helpful to slide the bronchoscope over the needle to remain close enough to determine the depth of penetration. If the needle has not adequately penetrated, one simple maneuver is extremely helpful. With the needle embedded shallowly in the tissue, having the patient gently cough usually pushes the needle fully into the involved tissue.[68]

Aspiration of paratracheal lesions can also be problematic. It has been suggested that the needle should be passed perpendicular to the tracheal wall,[69] but this maneuver is often difficult to achieve. In practice, if the aspirating needle is long enough (approximately 1.3 cm), it can adequately penetrate the tracheal wall to sample surrounding nodes, even at an oblique angle. The needle must, however, be anchored between tracheal rings, rather than abutted against cartilage, before attempting to advance it. One technique that may be helpful in improving the angle of entry to the wall is to partially impale the needle at an oblique angle. Slowly advance the bronchoscope distally as the angle of the needle turns toward the wall, then advance the remainder of the needle and perform the aspiration as previously described. The coughing maneuver is almost essential to penetration of the tracheal wall. Again, it is important to confirm that the needle is adequately advanced in the site before performing the aspiration.

Various needle devices are available and suitable for transbronchial, transtracheal, or transcarinal aspiration. The length of the needle is important. Needles 1 cm in length tend to be inadequate, whereas 1.3 cm appears optimal. The needle gauge may also be important. Although good results have been reported with a 20-gauge (or 21-gauge thin-walled) needle,[70] larger gauge needles (18- or 19-gauge) offer the advantage of histologic specimens in addition to cytologic specimens and may increase the diagnostic yield of the procedure.[71–75] At least one study[75] has compared a 22-gauge needle to a 19-gauge needle in the same patients and found the 19-gauge needle superior in diagnostic yield (86% versus 53%).

The overall yield of bronchoscopic needle aspiration probably depends on the patient population and the screening procedures employed in determining the need for the aspiration. Studies in which all patients with suspected bronchogenic carcinoma undergo transcarinal needle aspira-

tion have found an overall yield of 15%.[70,76] Using selective criteria can increase the yield. Limiting transcarinal aspirations to patients with either endobronchial lesions or a widened carina increased the specificity of the aspirate to 25% to 40%, respectively.[70] Computed tomographic evidence of mediastinal adenopathy appears to provide the greatest specificity. Using computed tomography to determine the need for mediastinal aspirates, most studies are able to detect approximately two-thirds of the true positive nodes in patients with bronchogenic carcinoma.[30,68,71,75,77–79] These yields have been similar in routine use of the procedure (outside of protocol studies) in community-based hospitals[80] and teaching hospitals.[81] These yields are sufficiently high to be able to spare a significant number of patients with unresectable disease the risk and expense of more invasive staging procedures.[70] Newer techniques for guiding bronchoscopic needle aspiration are now available with limited data supporting their use. Endoscopic ultrasound and virtual bronchoscopy may be particularly useful for this purpose.

Although false-positive results have rarely been reported with mediastinal bronchoscopic aspirations,[82–84] care must be taken to avoid them because they could adversely influence therapeutic decisions. Simple measures include avoidance of the primary tumor prior to sampling the mediastinal nodes to prevent contamination of the bronchoscope channel by tumor cells. If the patient has a positive sputum cytology, it may be safest not to perform mediastinal aspiration because its interpretation could be difficult if it were positive. Similarly, if secretions well up from the lower airways, covering the area to be aspirated, the chances of contamination are too great to perform the aspirate. In all cases, adequacy of cellularity should be assessed by the cytopathologist. A specimen with a few free-floating malignant cells may not be reasonably distinguishable from contamination. Whenever significant doubt about the adequacy of the aspirate exists, conventional staging should be used rather than make a possibly inappropriate therapeutic decision.

One additional role of mediastinal aspiration is the primary diagnosis of small cell carcinoma. Mediastinal aspiration is often the only diagnostic sample in bronchoscopic examination of patients presenting with bulky central disease in small cell carcinoma without evident endobronchial lesions.[30]

EVALUATION OF THERAPY

A less common application of the diagnostic capabilities of fiberoptic bronchoscopy in bronchogenic carcinoma is in the evaluation of treatment efficacy. This application has been studied in patients with small cell carcinoma in comparing bronchoscopic findings during and after treatment to chest radiographic findings in patients whose presenting disease was endobronchial.[36,85–87] All studies have found that a significant percentage (25% to 35%) of patients have radiographic clearing but still have endoscopically evident disease. These findings are, perhaps, not surprising considering the high percentage of patients who can have major endobronchial obstruction without radiographic signs of obstruction.[66] More subtle changes would be even less likely to be detectable by chest radiography.

The role of computed tomography in relation to bronchoscopy in this patient population has not been reported, but it is likely to have some limitations as well because it tends to be less sensitive than bronchoscopy to the detection of submucosal disease[56] or small endobronchial lesions. The utility of bronchoscopy in evaluating treatment of patients with non–small cell carcinoma also remains to be studied. Again, it seems probable that it would be similarly useful.

ENDOSCOPIC THERAPEUTIC INTERVENTION

Through recent technologic advancements and renewed interest in older techniques, several therapeutic procedures may be performed to palliate central airway obstruction, including laser photoresection, stent placement, cryotherapy, brachytherapy, balloon dilation, and photodynamic therapy. Because many of these topics are discussed elsewhere in this textbook, we focus on stents and cryotherapy.

Stents

The deployment of stents to maintain luminal patency is a concept borrowed from vascular and biliary interventional experiences. Early attempts to maintain airway caliber in patients with subglottic stenosis involved modifications of endotracheal tubes and the development of the Montgomery T-Tube.[88] This T-shaped silicone tube requires a permanent tracheotomy and a dual-operator rigid deployment technique. Surgical implantation of a silicone-based Neville stent was also performed in segments of stenosis and malacia.[89] It was sutured in place during thoracotomy.

With improved vascular stenting techniques and the development of metallic alloys, airway stenting gained popularity. Stents were deployed using fluoroscopic guidance and a balloon dilated to the appropriate luminal size. Self-expandable stents such as the Gianturco (Cook Inc., Bloomington, Indiana) became the standard metal stent used in the airway. These stents, however, were permanent and associated with complications, including airway perforation, hemorrhage, fistula formation, and plugging with tumor growth and secretion.[90] Interest in the development of a stent that would maintain airway caliber, be easily deployed, and minimize complications has lead to the numerous present-day stents, which can be grouped into three major classes: silicone, metallic alloys, and hybrid stents.

Silicone stents were developed initially as modifications of the Montgomery T-Tube. The addition of a carinal branch,[91] modifications in size, shape, and flexibility,[92] and newer deployment techniques increased usage in patients with central airway obstruction. Deployment techniques involved fitting the stent over a smaller endotracheal tube or rigid bronchoscope, pushing the stent through the vocal cords, and then fitting it into place with a larger caliber tube. The pitfalls of this technique included laryngeal and vocal chord damage, submaximal dilation, and smaller stent placement.

Dumon designed a patented silicone stent (Axion, Aubagne, France, distribution Bryan Corp., Woburn, Massachusetts) to palliate both malignant and benign airway obstruction.[93] Regularly placed surface studs allow for anchoring in the tracheobronchial tree and limit the surface contact to minimize mucosal ischemia. The development of a patented tube-pusher delivery system (i.e., EFER, La Ciotat, France) addressed many of the pitfalls of early silicone stent deployment. The technique involves loading the folded stent into an introducer, placing the introducer through the barrel of a rigid bronchoscope, and expelling the stent with a tube pusher while slowly withdrawing the rigid bronchoscope.

The Dumon group placed more than 502 stents between 1987 and 1992.[94] Indications for stent placement were predominantly malignant airway disease and stenosis. Central airways (trachea, right and left mainstem bronchi) were the main sites stented. The mean stent duration was 14.18 months for benign disease and 3.35 months for malignant disease. Complications included migration (8.8%), granuloma (8.5%), and obstruction by secretions (4.8%). The advantages of the Dumon stent are that it provides extensive airway support and is easily removed. The disadvantages are that it is a thick tube, which limits the luminal diameter, has the potential to migrate, and requires rigid bronchoscopic deployment.

The two most popular metallic mesh stents are the Wallstent and the Ultraflex (Microvasive, Boston Scientific). The Wallstent is made of a cobalt super alloy woven into a cylindrical wire mesh. The deployment apparatus consists of a compressed elongated stent covered by an outer sheath attached to a valve body. The area to be stented is fluoroscopically labeled with surface markers. After a guidewire is bronchoscopically placed through the desired segment, the bronchoscope is removed, leaving the guidewire in place. The stent is loaded over the guidewire until the markers on the stent correlate with the surface markers. Because the Wallstent is compressed and elongated, shortening needs to be considered as the stent is deployed. The deployment technique consists of pulling back the valve body while observing fluoroscopically. Some bronchoscopists reinsert the bronchoscope and visualize the stent deployment. After half of the stent is deployed, positioning should be reevaluated prior to completing the deployment.

The Wallstent has sharp, pointy edges that may result in granulation tissue formation. Because the compressed stent is longer than the deployed stent, malposition is a potential complication. The Wallstent is also permanent and does not allow for repositioning once deployed. Tumor growth through the walls and limitation of mucociliary clearance may result in potential obstruction.

The Ultraflex stent is composed of a nitinol single strand with looped edges. Although plagued by many of the same complications as the Wallstent, it has some theoretical advantages. The smooth edges may cause less granulation tissue formation. The memory properties of the nitinol allow for the compressed stent to be the same length as the expanded stent, which may lead to more accurate placement. By grasping the string edge, the stent may be repositioned even after deployment. Once epithelialization occurs, however, the stent is not movable.

Hybrid stents represent a combination of silastic and metallic stents. Wallstents and Ultraflex stents are available coated, in an attempt to decrease tumor growth through the wire-mesh structure. This feature may expand the potential use of these stents to support the airway when small fistula exist. Another hybrid stent called the Dynamic-Y-Stent has theoretical advantages favoring its use. It has both a tracheal and bronchial component that can be trimmed according to the individual airway characteristics. The posterior tracheal component is thin and collapsible, allowing for changes in airway caliber with respiration and cough, which may facilitate mucous clearance and decrease the risk of secretion accumulation. The anterior tracheal component is supported with metal rings, simulating cartilage. Potential uses for this stent include complex airway lesions, lesions involving the carina, diffuse malacia, and airway fistula.

Unfortunately, no controlled, randomized, comparative studies for stent placement have been conducted. The data for metallic stents are limited to small patient groups, poorly controlled with the lack of long term follow-up; therefore, no consensus exists regarding stent selection for a specific airway lesion. Until large, prospective, randomized studies are performed, we are left with expert opinion as our only guide to many therapeutic airway interventions.

Cryotherapy

Cryotherapy is the therapeutic application of extreme cold for local destruction of living tissue. Historically, its use in the treatment of malignancy dates back to 1848, when James Arnott used cold application to palliate uterine carcinoma. Endoscopic cryotherapy is relatively new, made possible by recent improvements in bronchoscopic equipment and the development of cryotherapy probes for direct application. Cryotherapy utilizes the reverse principles of cryogenics, which preserves cellular function. It induces selective cell necrosis by rapidly cooling tissue, typically at a rate less than $-30°$ Celsius per minute, and by slowly thawing the tissue after a prolonged freeze time. Necrosis results from crystallization, cellular dehydration, and structural disruption followed by microthrombi formation.

Cryoprobes are utilized to directly administer cold to a specific location. The probe may be rigid, semirigid, or flexible. The rigid and semirigid probes can only be used through a rigid bronchoscope, whereas the flexible probes fit down the working channel of a flexible bronchoscope. The cryogen (cooling agent) used is typically nitrous oxide, although carbon dioxide and hydrocarbons are also effective. Capillary tubes inside the cryoprobe transfer the cryogen to the tip of the probe, where it expands from high pressure to atmospheric pressure. The gas expansion lowers the temperature of the fluid (the Joule effect) and produces droplets. This effect allows for direct, low-temperature application at the tip of the probe, producing temperatures of $-30°$ Celsius or lower.

Patient selection for cryotherapy requires an endoscopically visible lesion that is accessible to the bronchoscopist. The cryoprobe is inserted through the working channel and is advanced approximately 4 mm distal to the tip of the bronchoscope. The probe is applied to the lesion as the foot pedal is depressed, beginning the freeze cycle. Within fifteen seconds, an ice ball forms at the probe tip. One to three freeze-thaw cycles are applied to the tumor area, with each freeze lasting for one minute. At the end of each freeze cycle, the ice ball is observed until thawing is complete before the probe is removed. Gentle tugging of the probe safely facilitates removal.

The thrombotic and coagulation effects of cryotherapy are delayed, requiring approximately twenty-four to forty-eight hours. Thus debulking at the time of initial application is avoided because the tumor's vascular supply is intact and massive hemorrhage may result. Because cryotherapy may cause tissue swelling and edema, it is recommended that cryotherapy not be initially used for critical airway lesions that could obstruct completely.

Endoscopic cryotherapy is an excellent modality for the symptomatic improvement of malignant tracheobronchial lesions. More than 600 patients were treated with cryotherapy for malignant tracheobronchial lesions at the Harefield Hospital in Northern London. Overall, 78% noted subjective improvement. For those patients presenting with dyspnea, cough, hemoptysis, and stridor, approximately two-thirds noted improvement in their symptoms.[95]

EXPERIMENTAL TECHNIQUES AND FUTURE APPLICATIONS
Routine Bronchoscopy

Interestingly, new nonbronchoscopic technology may expand the role of standard fiberoptic bronchoscopy with forceps biopsy. Studies are beginning to emerge, demonstrating the adequacy of standard forceps biopsy sample for various genetic analyses, such as detection of p53[96] and the analysis of DNA content.[97] Others have explored the utility of BAL in the detection of several possibly significant markers for the diagnosis of lung cancer.[98–100]

Fluorescence Bronchoscopy

Fluorescence bronchoscopy emerged from the need to detect more subtle presentations of bronchogenic carcinoma, such as minimally invasive disease or carcinoma *in situ,* or to detect proximal submucosal spread of endobronchial disease for adequate staging. The bulk of the work has been done using a fluorescence-enhancing agent, a hematoporphyrin derivative (HpD), to concentrate a fluorescing agent in neoplastic tissue. HpD is injected intravenously and picked up by actively dividing tissue, including inflammatory tissue. After 3 days, it tends to concentrate in neoplastic or severely dysplastic cells. When exposed to an appropriate wavelength, usually delivered by a laser, the tissue concentrating the HpD produces a characteristic fluorescence.[101,102] This technique has also been used to treat carcinoma *in situ* and to debulk main airway obstruction. Oxidation reactions occur on treated surfaces, causing tissue destruction and tumor slough (see also Chapter 24). This technique is clearly capable of detecting lesions not visible by standard white light bronchoscopy,[103,104] but it has not become commonly applied. Possible reasons include the expense of the equipment and potential complications of HpD, mainly severe, prolonged photosensitivity.[106]

A newer technique, autofluorescence bronchoscopy, utilizes the well-known autofluorescence properties of neoplastic tissue[106–109] to achieve the same end. Neoplastic tissue fluorescs without a fluorescence-enhancing agent when exposed to the proper wavelengths. Detecting the fluorescence requires sophisticated image analysis and amplification. Using this technique, investigators have determined that autofluorescence bronchoscopy is 50% more sensitive than white light bronchoscopy in detecting severe dysplasia and carcinoma *in situ.*[110–112] A recent multicenter clinical trial was conducted in seven institutions in the United States and Canada, comparing white light bronchoscopy and fluorescence examination in 173 subjects with known or suspected lung cancer. Biopsy specimens taken from suspicious areas revealed that the relative sensitivity of white light bronchoscopy plus fluorescence endoscopy versus white light bronchoscopy alone was 6.3 for intraepithelial malignancy.[113]

Fluorescence endoscopy has great potential for detecting occult carcinoma and determining the true proximal spread of endobronchial disease. Further applications may include airway surveillance in high-risk patients, such as those in chemoprevention protocols or who have been previously treated for bronchogenic carcinoma (see also Chapter 24).

Ultrasound Bronchoscopy

Endoscopic applications of ultrasonography have been developed for intravascular use and are now beginning to be evaluated in the airways. The technique appears capable of detecting peripheral carcinomas, endobronchial tumors, mediastinal lymph nodes down to 3 mm in size, and hilar lesions.[114–116] It also has utility in determining the depth of tumor involvement in patients with carcinoma *in situ.*[117] Its greatest utility may be in improving diagnostic yields from bronchoscopic needle aspiration and decreasing the number of aspirates required. One study using on-site cytopathologic diagnosis found that bronchoscopic needle aspirations required fewer passes to diagnose carcinomas in paratracheal nodes. It will be interesting to see if the technique enhances diagnostic yields by providing better localization, particularly in peripheral carcinoma. Limitations to performing endoscopic ultrasound include equipment expense, appropriate training, technical difficulties in obtaining an adequate acoustic window, and the presence of anthracosilicosis.[115]

Virtual Bronchoscopy

Virtual bronchoscopy has emerged with the advent of improved techniques in thoracic imaging. Volumetric data acquisition offered by helical computed tomography has permitted the creation of computer-generated, three-dimensional surface renderings of the tracheobronchial tree. The ability to perform computer-simulated endoscopy has great potential in all facets of bronchoscopy. In preliminary studies, computer-simulated endoscopy accurately reflects major endobronchial anatomy when compared to standard bronchoscopy.[118] It is particularly useful in the diagnosis of high-grade stenosis, extraluminal compression,[119] and polypoid endobronchial lesions greater than 5 mm in diameter.[120] The technology is still, however, in developmental stages and awaits careful scientific scrutiny. Potential applications include guidance for bronchoscopic needle aspiration, improved diagnostic yields for peripheral carcinoma, precise airway measurements to plan stent placement and balloon dilation, and vascular localization to plan laser photoresection, cryotherapy, and electrocautery.

A DIAGNOSTIC APPROACH

Bronchoscopic diagnosis and staging of lung cancer can be approached systematically and tailored to the individual presentation. Patients presenting with endobronchial lesions should undergo biopsy of the primary lesion, a search for second lesions, and evaluation of the proximal spread of disease by submucosal aspirate of the proximal bronchus and biopsy of the carina. If computed tomography indicates the presence of significant adenopathy, bronchoscopic needle aspiration of the involved nodes (if accessible) can be performed during the initial diagnostic procedure.

Peripheral mass lesions can be sampled under fluoroscopic guidance by transbronchial biopsy, brushing, and transbronchial needle aspiration. BAL also appears to be very useful. Again, computed tomography can be used to guide aspiration of significant mediastinal adenopathy, and second lesions should be looked for routinely as part of the initial examination.

Similar to all procedures, their use should be conditioned by the individual case as well as the local skills and results of the operator. The patient's input is also important. Some patients would strongly prefer not to undergo more than one procedure, so that surgery, particularly for a solitary pulmonary nodule, may be appropriate without a preoperative diagnosis. Others may not consider surgery until a diagnosis of malignancy is clearly established. Here is where the art of medicine must merge with the statistics of procedure results to determine the best approach. Similarly, with the relatively new field of endoscopic palliative therapy, we must plan our therapeutic approaches with the individual clinical situation and anatomy in mind. We hope clearer guidelines will evolve with increasing clinical experience with these techniques.

REFERENCES

1. Cotton RE The bronchial spread of lung cancer. *Br J Dis Chest* 1959;53:142.
2. Rabin CB, Selikoff IR, Kramer R. Paracarinal biopsy in evaluation of operability of carcinoma of the lung. *Arch Surg* 1952; 65:822.
3. Rabinovitch J, Hochberg LA, Lederer M. Primary (bronchogenic) carcinoma of the lung. *J Thoracic Surg* 1940;9:332.
4. Caputi M, Filippo ADI, Ferraro G, et al. Endobronchial aspects of pulmonary neoplasia. *Pan Med* 1986;28:195.
5. Popovich J, Jr., Kvale PA, Eichenhorn MS, et al. Diagnostic accuracy of multiple biopsies from flexible fiberoptic bronchoscopy. *Am Rev Respir Dis* 1982;125:521.
6. Shure D, Astarita RW. Bronchogenic carcinoma presenting as an endobronchial mass. Optimal number of biopsy specimens for diagnosis. *Chest* 1983;83:865.
7. Lundgren R, Bergman F, Angstrom T. Comparison of transbronchial fine needle aspiration biopsy, aspiration of bronchial secretion, bronchial washing, brush biopsy and forceps biopsy in the diagnosis of lung cancer. *Eur J Respir Dis* 1983;64:378.
8. Givens CD, Marini JJ. Transbronchial needle aspiration of a bronchial carcinoid tumor. *Chest* 1985;88:152.
9. Shure D, Fedullo PF. Transbronchial needle aspiration in the diagnosis of peribronchial and submucosal bronchogenic carcinoma. *Chest* 1985;88:49.
10. Schmidt JA, Mizel SB, Cohen D, et al. Interleukin 1, a potential regulator of fibroblast proliferation. *J Immunol* 1982;128:2177.
11. Shure D. Fiberoptic bronchoscopy—diagnostic applications. *Clin Chest Med* 1987;8:1.
12. Harkin TJ, Ciotoli C, Addrizzo-Harris DJ, et al. Transbronchial needle aspiration (TBNA) in patients infected with HIV. *Am J Respir Crit Care Med* 1998;157:1913.
13. Leonard C, Tormey VJ, O'Keane C, et al. Bronchoscopic diagnosis of sarcoidosis [see comments]. *Eur Respir J* 1997;10:2722.
14. Haponik EF, Shure D. Underutilization of transbronchial needle aspiration—Experiences of current pulmonary Fellows. *Chest* 1997;112:251.
15. Haponik EF, Cappellari JO, Chin R, et al. Education and experience improve transbronchial needle aspiration performance. *Am J Respir Crit Care Med* 1995;151:1998.
16. Cortese DA, McDougall JC. Biopsy and brushing of peripheral lung cancer with fluoroscopic guidance. *Chest* 1979;75:141.
17. Ellis JH, Jr. Transbronchial lung biopsy via the fiberoptic bronchoscope. Experience with 107 consecutive cases and comparison with bronchial brushing. *Chest* 1975;68:524.
18. Hanson RR, Zavala DC, Rhodes ML, et al. Transbronchial biopsy via flexible fiberoptic bronchoscope: result in 164 patients. *Am Rev Respir Dis* 1976;114:67.
19. Fletcher EC, Levin DC. Flexible fiberoptic bronchoscopy and fluoroscopically guided transbronchial biopsy in the management of solitary pulmonary nodules. *West J Med* 1982;136:477.
20. Shure D, Fedullo PF. Transbronchial needle aspiration of peripheral masses. *Am Rev Respir Dis* 1983;128:1090.
21. Stringfield JT, Markowitz DJ, Bentz RR, et al. The effect of tumor size and location on diagnosis by fiberoptic bronchoscopy. *Chest* 1977;72:474.
22. Radke JR, Conway WA, Eyler WR, et al. Diagnostic accuracy in peripheral lung lesions. *Chest* 1979;76:176.
23. Wang KP, Haponik EF, Britt EJ, et al. Transbronchial needle aspiration of peripheral pulmonary nodules. *Chest* 1984;86:819.
24. Bilaçeroglu S, Kumcuoglu Z, Alper H, et al. CT bronchus sign-guided bronchoscopic multiple diagnostic: procedures in carcinomatous solitary pulmonary nodules and masses. *Respiration* 1998;65:49.
25. Wood DA, Miller M. The role of the dual pulmonary circulation in various pathologic conditions of the lung. *J Thoracic Surg* 1938;7:649.
26. Cortese DA, McDougall JC. Bronchoscopic biopsy and brushing with fluoroscopic guidance in nodular metastatic lung cancer. *Chest* 1981;79:610.
27. Mohsenifar Z, Chopra SK, Simmons DH. Diagnostic value of fiberoptic bronchoscopy in metastatic pulmonary tumors. *Chest* 1978;74:369.
28. Tanaka M, Kawanami O, Satoh M, et al. Endoscopic observation of peripheral airway lesions. *Chest* 1988;93:228.
29. Ono R, Loke J, Ikeda S. Bronchofiberscopy with curette biopsy and bronchography in the evaluation of peripheral lung lesions. *Chest* 1981;79:162.
30. Gay PC, Brutinel WM. Transbronchial needle aspiration in the practice of bronchoscopy. *Mayo Clin Proc* 1989;64:158.
31. de Gracia J, Curull V, Vidal R, et al. Diagnostic value of bronchoalveolar lavage in suspected pulmonary tuberculosis. *Chest* 1988;93:329.
32. Levy H, Horak DA, Lewis MI. The value of bronchial washings and bronchoalveolar lavage in the diagnosis of lymphangitic carcinomatosis. *Chest* 1988;94:1028.
33. Pirozynski M. Bronchoalveolar lavage in the diagnosis of peripheral, primary lung cancer [see comments]. *Chest* 1992;102:372.
34. Rennard SI, Spurzem JR. Bronchoalveolar lavage in the diagnosis of lung cancer [editorial; comment]. *Chest* 1992;102:331.
35. Stover DE, Zaman MB, Hajdi SI, et al. Bronchoalveolar lavage in the diagnosis of diffuse pulmonary infiltrates in the immunosuppressed host. *Ann Intern Med* 1984;107:1.
36. Tondini M, Rizzi A. Small-cell lung cancer: importance of fiberoptic bronchoscopy in the evaluation of complete remission. *Tumori* 1989;75:266.
37. Shiner RJ, Rosenman J, Katz I, et al. Bronchoscopic evaluation of peripheral lung tumours. *Thorax* 1988;43:887.
38. Shure D, Moser KM, Konopka R. Transbronchial needle aspiration in the diagnosis of pneumonia in a canine model. *Am Rev Respir Dis* 1985;131:290.
39. Torrington KG, Kern JD. The utility of fiberoptic bronchoscopy in the evaluation of the solitary pulmonary nodule. *Chest* 1993;104:1021.

40. Wallace JM, Catanzaro A, Moser KM, et al. Flexible fiberoptic bronchoscopy for diagnosing pulmonary coccidioidomycosis. *Am Rev Respir Dis* 1981;123:286.
41. Klinke F, Hohenberger E, Clarins P, et al. The multiple primary lung carcinoma. *Pan Med* 1986;28:321.
42. Kono M, Fujii M, Adachi S, et al. Multiple primary lung cancers: radiographic and bronchoscopic diagnosis. *J Thorac Imaging* 1993;8:63.
43. Saito Y, Nagamoto N, Ota S, et al. Results of surgical treatment for roentgenographically occult bronchogenic squamous cell carcinoma. *J Thorac Cardiovasc Surg* 1992;104:401.
44. Woolner LB, Fontana RS, Cortese DA, et al. Roentgenographically occult lung cancer: pathologic findings and frequency of multicentricity during a 10-year period. *Mayo Clin Proc* 1984; 59:453.
45. Goldberg SK, Walkenstein MD, Steinbach A, et al. The role of staging bronchoscopy in the preoperative assessment of a solitary pulmonary nodule. *Chest* 1993;104:94.
46. Cummings SR, Lillington GA, Richard RJ. Managing solitary pulmonary nodules. The choice of strategy is a "close call." *Am Rev Respir Dis* 1986;134:453.
47. Adelman M, Haponik EF, Bleecker ER, et al. Cryptogenic hemoptysis. Clinical features, bronchoscopic findings, and natural history in 67 patients. *Ann Intern Med* 1985;102:829.
48. Heaton RW. Should patients with haemoptysis and a normal chest X-ray be bronchoscoped? *Postgrad Med J* 1987;63:947.
49. Jackson CV, Savage PJ, Quinn DL. Role of fiberoptic bronchoscopy in patients with hemoptysis and a normal chest roentgenogram. *Chest* 1985;87:142.
50. Lederie FA, Nichol KL, Parenti CM. Bronchoscopy to evaluate hemoptysis in older men with nonsuspicious chest roentgenograms. *Chest* 1989;95:1043.
51. York EL, Jones RL, King EG, et al. The value of submucous needle aspiration in the prediction of surgical resection line of bronchogenic carcinoma. *Chest* 1991;100:1028.
52. O'Neil KM, Lazarus AA. Hemoptysis. Indications for bronchoscopy. *Arch Intern Med* 1991;151:171.
53. Poe RH, Israel RH, Marin MG, et al. Utility of fiberoptic bronchoscopy in patients with hemoptysis and a nonlocalizing chest roentgenogram. *Chest* 1988;93:70.
54. Santiago SM, Lehrman S, Williams AJ. Bronchoscopy in patients with haemoptysis and normal chest roentgenograms. *Br J Dis Chest* 1987;81:186.
55. Weaver LJ, Solliday N, Cugell DW. Selection of patients with hemoptysis for fiberoptic bronchoscopy. *Chest* 1979;76:7.
56. Set PA, Flower CD, Smith IE, et al. Hemoptysis: comparative study of the role of CT and fiberoptic bronchoscopy. *Radiology* 1993;189:677.
57. Johnston H, Reisz G. Changing spectrum of hemoptysis. Underlying causes in 148 patients undergoing diagnostic flexible fiberoptic bronchoscopy. *Arch Intern Med* 1989;149:1666.
58. Foster WL, Jr., Roberts L, Jr., McLendon RE, et al. Localized peribronchial thickening: a CT sign of occult bronchogenic carcinoma. *Am J Roentgenol* 1985;144:906.
59. Naidich DP, Lee JJ, Garay SM, et al. Comparison of CT and fiberoptic bronchoscopy in the evaluation of bronchial disease. *Am J Roentgenol* 1987;148:1.
60. Brown SD, Foster WL. Localization of occult bronchogenic carcinoma by bronchography. *Chest* 1991;100:1160.
61. Gibson SP, Weir DC, Burge PS. A prospective audit of the value of fibre optic bronchoscopy in adults admitted with community acquired pneumonia. *Respir Med* 1993;87:105.
62. Waltner JG. Inoperability of carcinoma of the lung established by carinal biopsy. *Ann Otol Rhinol Laryngol* 1961;70:1165.
63. Suratt PM, Smiddy JF, Gruber B. Deaths and complications associated with fiberoptic bronchoscopy. *Chest* 1976;69:747.
64. Shure D, Fedullo PF, Plummer M. Carinal forceps biopsy via the fiberoptic bronchoscope in the routine staging of lung cancer. *West J Med* 1985;142:511.
65. Griess DF, McDonald JR, Clagett OT. The proximal extension of carcinoma of the lung in the bronchial wall. *J Thoracic Surg* 1945;14:362.
66. Shure D. Radiographically occult endobronchial obstruction in bronchogenic carcinoma. *Am J Med* 1991;91:19.
67. Shure D. Transbronchial biopsy and needle aspiration. *Chest* 1989;95:1130.
68. Schenk DA, Bower JH, Bryan CL, et al. Transbronchial needle aspiration staging of bronchogenic carcinoma. *Am Rev Respir Dis* 1986;134:146.
69. Wang KP, Gupta PK, Haponik EF, et al. Flexible transbronchial needle aspiration. Technical considerations. *Ann Otol Rhinol Laryngol* 1984;93:233.
70. Shure D, Fedullo PF. The role of transcarinal needle aspiration in the staging of bronchogenic carcinoma. *Chest* 1984;86:693.
71. Wang KP. Flexible transbronchial needle aspiration biopsy for histologic specimens. *Chest* 1985;88:860.
72. Wang KP, Fuenning C, Johns CJ, et al. Flexible transbronchial needle aspiration for the diagnosis of sarcoidosis. *Ann Otol Rhinol Laryngol* 1989;98:298.
73. Wang KP. Transbronchial needle biopsy for histology specimens [editorial]. *Chest* 1989;96:226.
74. Schenk DA, Strollo PJ, Pickard JS, et al. Utility of the Wang 18-gauge transbronchial histology needle in the staging of bronchogenic carcinoma. *Chest* 1989;96:272.
75. Schenk DA, Chambers SL, Derdak S, et al. Comparison of the Wang 19-gauge and 22-gauge needles in the mediastinal staging of lung cancer. *Am Rev Respir Dis* 1993;147:1251.
76. Versteegh RM, Swierenga J. Bronchoscopic evaluation of the operability of pulmonary carcinoma. *Acta Otolaryng* 1962;56:603.
77. Schenk DA, Bryan CL, Bower JH, et al. Transbronchial needle aspiration in the diagnosis of bronchogenic carcinoma. *Chest* 1987;92:83.
78. Wang KP, Terry PB, Marsh BR. Bronchoscopic needle aspiration biopsy of paratracheal tumors. *Am Rev Respir Dis* 1978; 118:17.
79. Wang KP, Terry PB. Transbronchial needle aspiration in the diagnosis and staging of bronchogenic carcinoma. *Am Rev Respir Dis* 1983;127:344.
80. Harrow EM, Oldenburg FA, Jr., Lingenfelter MS, et al. Transbronchial needle aspiration in clinical practice. A five-year experience. *Chest* 1989;96:1268.
81. Salathé M, Solër M, Bolliger CT, et al. Transbronchial needle aspiration in routine fiberoptic bronchoscopy. *Respiration* 1992; 59:5.
82. Schenk DA, Chasen MH, McCarty MJ, et al. Potential false positive mediastinal transbronchial needle aspiration in bronchogenic carcinoma. *Chest* 1984;86:649.
83. Cropp AJ, DiMarco AF, Lankerani M. False-positive transbronchial needle aspiration in bronchogenic carcinoma. *Chest* 1984; 85:696.
84. Lodi M, Susa A, Cavallini G. False positive diagnosis of bronchogenic carcinoma based on bronchoscopic brushing and sputum cytology. A surgical point of view. *Ital J Surg Sci* 1988;18:385.
85. Ihde DC, Cohen MH, Bernath AM, et al. Serial fiberoptic bronchoscopy during chemotherapy for small cell carcinoma of the lung. *Chest* 1978;74:531.
86. Bye PTP, Harvey HPB, Woolcock AJ, et al. Fibre-optic bronchoscopy in small cell lung cancer: finding pre and post chemotherapy. *Aust NZ J Med* 1980;10:397.
87. Wang JS, Lia SL, Perng RP. Importance of fiberoptic bronchos-

copy before and during chemotherapy for small cell carcinoma of the lung in the evaluation of complete remission. *Chung Hua I Hsueh Tsa Chih* (Taipei). 1991;48:41.

88. Montgomery WW. T-tube tracheal stent. *Arch Otolaryngol* 1965;82:320.
89. Neville WE, Hamouda F, Andersen J, et al. Replacement of the intrathoracic trachea and both stem bronchi with a molded Silastic prosthesis. *J Thorac Cardiovasc Surg* 1972;63:569.
90. Nashef SA, Dromer C, Velly JF, et al. Expanding wire stents in benign tracheobronchial disease: indications and complications. *Ann Thorac Surg* 1992;54:937.
91. Westaby S, Jackson JW, Pearson FG. A bifurcated silicone rubber stent for relief of tracheobronchial obstruction. *J Thorac Cardiovasc Surg* 1982;83:414.
92. Duvall AJ, Bauer W. An endoscopically introducible T-tube for tracheal stenosis. *Laryngoscope* 1977;87:2031.
93. Dumon JF. A dedicated tracheobronchial stent. *Chest* 1990;97:328.
94. Dumon JF, Kovitz K, Dumon MC. Tracheobronchial Stents. In: Feinsilver SH, Fein AM, eds. *Textbook of bronchoscopy.* Baltimore: Williams and Wilkins, 1995:400.
95. Maiwand MO, Homasson JP. Cryotherapy for tracheobronchial disorders. *Clin Chest Med* 1995;16:427.
96. Mitsudomi T, Lam S, Shirakusa T, et al. Detection and sequencing of p53 gene mutations in bronchial biopsy samples in patients with lung cancer [see comments]. *Chest* 1993;104:362.
97. Haneda H, Miyamoto H, Isobe H, et al. Accuracy of the bronchoscopic DNA content analysis of non-small-cell lung carcinoma. *J Surg Oncol* 1992;49:182.
98. Yoss EB, Berd D, Cohn JR, et al. Flow cytometric evaluation of bronchoscopic washings and lavage fluid for DNA aneuploidy as an adjunct in the diagnosis of lung cancer and tumors metastatic to the lung. *Chest* 1989;96:54.
99. Slebos JC, Kibbelaar RE, Dalesio O, et al. K-ras oncogene activation as a prognostic marker in adenocarcinoma of the lung. *N Engl J Med* 1990;323:561.
100. LeFever A, Funahashi A. Elevated prostaglandin E2 levels in bronchoalveolar lavage fluid of patients with bronchogenic carcinoma. *Chest* 1990;98:1397.
101. Doiron DR, Profio AE, Vincent RG, et al. Fluorescence bronchoscopy for detection of lung cancer. *Chest* 1979;76:27.
102. Profio AE, Doiron DR. Laser fluorescence bronchoscope for localization of occult lung tumors. *Med Phys* 1979;6:523.
103. Profio AE, Doiron DR. A feasibility study of the use of fluorescence bronchoscopy for localization of small lung tumours. *Phys Med Biol* 1977;22:949.
104. Kinsey JH, Cortese DA, Sanderson DR. Detection of hematoporphyrin fluorescence during fiberoptic bronchoscopy to localize early bronchogenic carcinoma. *Mayo Clin Proc* 1978;53:594.
105. Deal CW, Louis E, Kerth WJ, et al. A method for measuring precapillary bronchopulmonary artery blood flow. *Ann Thorac Surg* 1967;3:365.
106. König K, Dietel W, Schubert H. In vivo autofluorescence investigations on animal tumors. *Neoplasma* 1989;36:135.
107. Harris DM, Werkhaven J. Endogenous porphyrin fluorescence in tumors. *Lasers Surg Med* 1987;7:467.
108. Yang YL, Ye YM, Li FM, et al. Characteristic autofluorescence for cancer diagnosis and its origin. *Lasers Surg Med* 1987;7:528.
109. Kluftinger AM, Davis NL, Quenville NF, et al. Detection of squamous cell cancer and pre-cancerous lesions by imaging of tissue autofluorescence in the hamster cheek pouch model. *Surg Oncol* 1992;1:183.
110. Palcic B, Lam S, Hung J, et al. Detection and localization of early lung cancer by imaging techniques. *Chest* 1991;99:742.
111. Lam S, MacAulay C, Hung J, et al. Detection of dysplasia and carcinoma in situ with a lung imaging fluorescence endoscope device. *J Thorac Cardiovasc Surg* 1993;105:1035.
112. Lam S, MacAulay C, Palcic B. Detection and localization of early lung cancer by imaging techniques. *Chest* 1993;103:12S.
113. Lam S, Kennedy T, Unger M, et al. Localization of bronchial intraepithelial neoplastic lesions by fluorescence bronchoscopy. *Chest* 1998;113:696.
114. Ono R, Suemasu K, Matsunaka T. Bronchoscopic ultrasonography in the diagnosis of lung cancer. *Jpn J Clin Oncol* 1993;23:34.
115. Schüder G, Isringhaus H, Kubale B, et al. Endoscopic ultrasonography of the mediastinum in the diagnosis of bronchial carcinoma. *Thorac Cardiovasc Surg* 1991;39:299.
116. Hürter T, Hanrath P. Endobronchial sonography: feasibility and preliminary results. *Thorax* 1992;47:565.
117. Becker HD. Endobronchial ultrasound—a new perspective in bronchology. *Ultraschall Med* 1996;17:106.
118. Salvolini L, Gasparini S, Baldelli S, et al. [Virtual bronchoscopy: the correlation between endoscopic simulation and bronchoscopic findings]. *Radiol Med* (Torino.) 1997;94:454.
119. Rapp-Bernhardt U, Welte T, Budinger M, et al. Comparison of three-dimensional virtual endoscopy with bronchoscopy in patients with oesophageal carcinoma infiltrating the tracheobronchial tree. *Br J Radiol* 1998;71:1271.
120. Summers RM, Selbie WS, Malley JD, et al. Polypoid lesions of airways: early experience with computer-assisted detection by using virtual bronchoscopy and surface curvature. *Radiology* 1998;208:331.

32

INTERNATIONAL STAGING SYSTEM FOR LUNG CANCER

CLIFTON F. MOUNTAIN

CONSIDERATIONS IN STAGING

History, Purpose, and General Principles

Physicians have been concerned with the problem of the clinical classification of malignant tumors for half a century.[1] The relationship between prognosis and the extent of disease at diagnosis derived initially from observations that crude survival, or apparent recovery, rates were higher for patients in whom the disease was localized than for those in whom the disease had extended beyond the organ of origin. This observation gave rise to designating groups of patients as "early" and "late" cases, implying, erroneously, some fixed progression with time. In 1944, Denoix[2] first emphasized the need for a flexible, reliable cancer classification system based on a generally acceptable description of the facts of a case. He proposed that "the initial descriptions must be definitive, common to all, and based on findings which anyone can confirm with as little margin for personal interpretation among surgeons as possible." From concentration on this common minimum, Denoix and colleagues developed the TNM system for describing characteristics of the primary tumor (the "T" component), the status of regional lymph nodes (the "N" component), and the presence or absence of distant metastasis (the "M" component).[3] Stage grouping of the TNM anatomic subsets came later, and a uniform clinical classification for all cancer sites was subsequently developed by Union Internationale Contre le Cancer (UICC) study groups[4] and special site task forces of the American Joint Committee on Cancer (AJCC).[5] A twofold purpose of clinical stage classification was defined as follows: First, to facilitate the accurate, concise description of the apparent extent of disease in a way that can be readily communicated to others or reproduced by them (the TNM classification), and second, to facilitate comparison of differing therapeutic approaches by combining patients with certain common attributes (TNM anatomic subsets) into groups (stages) with generally similar prognoses and treatment options.[6] These principles served

the clinical and research communities well over the years. Manuals published by the UICC[7-8] and the American Joint Committee AJCC,[9-10] and the works of others,[11-13] provided guidelines for clinical staging of lung cancer, recommendations for histopathologic staging, and data confirming the usefulness of the TNM and stage classifications.

THE INTERNATIONAL SYSTEM FOR STAGING LUNG CANCER

Staging and histologic classifications remain today as major indicators of the curative potential and limitations of available therapy for lung cancer. The value of these tools for predicting prognosis still depends on identifying consistent, reproducible patient groups that may be related to the end results of treatment. The International System for Staging Lung Cancer[14] was developed in response to a need for classification that would unify variations in staging definitions and that would have consistent meaning and interpretation among physicians and scientists throughout the world. The system proved effective for this purpose and has been used widely since 1986, when it was adopted by the UICC[15] and the AJCC.[16] In the subsequent decade, after ten years of applying the International System for Staging Lung Cancer, a requirement for more specific staging was recognized that (a) would meet clinical and sophisticated research needs, and (b) maintain the integrity of the present classification without major change, until diagnostic, treatment, and research advances could have a proven significant effect on prognosis. Two major problems emerged: First, heterogeneity existed with respect to the end results for the TNM subsets in stage I, stage II, and stage IIIA disease, and second, inconsistency resulted from the use of multiple systems for classifying regional lymph nodes. These problems were addressed with the least possible disruption of the International Staging System by revising the stage grouping rules for the TNM anatomic subsets and recommending a new schema for classifying regional lymph nodes.[17-18] The revisions in the staging system and recommendations for regional lymph node mapping were adopted by the UICC and the AJCC in May 1996, and have been published in the manuals of both organizations.[19–21]

THE REVISED INTERNATIONAL SYSTEM FOR STAGING LUNG CANCER

The revised staging system (Tables 32.1–32.5) consists of a change in the rules for stage grouping of the TNM anatomic subsets and an addition to the T4 and M1 descriptors to aid in classifying metastatic nodules (not lymph node metastasis) in the ipsilateral lung. Data that reconfirms the relationship of prognosis to specific disease extent categories[17] supports the revisions in stage grouping. (The data sources and stastistical methods are documented in Table 32.6 at the end of this chapter.)

Relationship To Clinical and Research Objectives

New prognostic factors for lung cancer are under intensive investigation in many centers throughout the world. Studies of molecular genetic markers, of growth factors and receptors, and of pathologic factors, such as angiogenesis and cell proliferation, provide a body of literature that documents good or bad outcomes according to the presence or absence of tumor and host factors.[22–23] In this milieu of evolving knowledge of the molecular biology of lung cancer—its initiation, growth, and metastasis—the stage of disease remains as a benchmark for evaluating the effect on survival durations of new factors derived from the research.[24–26] Within the next decade, new markers of prognosis and reproducible, cost-effective methodologies undoubtedly will be identified and confirmed; new approaches to treatment could render the staging concept obsolete (see also Chapter 33). At this time, however, biologic prognostic markers are not yet a reliable and proven clinical reality.[27] Anatomic staging continues to serve as the most valid indicator of prognosis, as a guide for treatment planning, and as a means for communicating the results of treatment for specific groups of patients.

Clinical, Surgical-Pathologic, and Retreatment Classifications

The clinical stage (cTNM-cStage), based on all information obtained before treatment is instituted or a decision for no treatment is made, is assigned to each patient, and is not changed throughout the course of the disease. Identical staging descriptors are useful and applicable at specific points in the life history of the cancer. For those patients assigned to undergo surgical treatment, surgical-pathologic staging (pTNM-pStage), based on information obtained from pathologic examination of resected specimens, is useful be-

cause of the more precise description of the extent of the primary tumor and regional lymph node metastasis. Except for identifying possible intrapulmonary metastasis, p-staging provides no additional information regarding the cM category. In multimodality therapy programs, retreatment staging (rTNM-rStage), evaluation of disease extent following initial or induction therapies, may be useful for assigning subsequent treatment steps, as well as for evaluating the end results. It is essential that identical definitions are used for each type of classification and that the type (i.e., clinical, c; surgical-pathologic, p; or retreatment, r) is specified in end results reports according to staging criteria.

Staging and Cell Type

The International System for Staging Lung Cancer is relevant for classifying the four major cell types of lung cancer; squamous cell carcinoma, adenocarcinoma (including bronchioalveolar carcinoma), large cell carcinoma, and small cell carcinoma. It also may be applied to "undifferentiated carcinomas" with no specific subtype identified. Although small cell carcinoma is commonly designated as "limited" or "extensive" disease, staging of this tumor according to the more specific TNM categories is useful and may be required for selecting patients for multimodality programs involving adjuvant surgery.[28] The proportion of patients achieving a complete response, the duration of the response, and recurrence after a complete response is directly related to the extent of the disease at diagnosis. New treatment plans are designed from the results achieved for specific groups of patients that are identified in terms of TNM and stage classifications.

TNM Descriptors and Stage Grouping

The numeric descriptors for each TNM component reflect increasing primary tumor size and invasiveness (T1-2-3-4), the absence or presence and extent of metastasis in regional lymph nodes (N0-1-2-3), and the absence or presence of tumor spread to distant lymph node or organ sites (M0-1). Definitions for the TNM descriptors, shown in Table 32.1, remain the same as defined in the International System for Staging Lung Cancer,[14] except for two minor additions to aid in classifying multiple lung nodules: T4 designates satellite tumor nodules in the ipsilateral primary tumor lobe of the lung; all other separate nodules in the nonprimary tumor lobes are classified M1.[17] Table 32.2 shows the 17 anatomic TNM subsets, according to stage group, that describe progressive levels of disease extent, from small, circumscribed "coin" lesions with no evidence of metastasis to the most extensive tumors with distant metastasis present.

Stage IA and Stage IB

The revised stage grouping rules (Table 32.2) designate small tumors, less than or equal to 3 cm in greatest dimen-

TABLE 32.1. TNM DESCRIPTORS

Primary Tumor (T)

TX Primary tumor cannot be assessed, or tumor proven by the presence of malignant cells in sputum or bronchial washings but not visualized by imaging or bronchoscopy

T0 No evidence of primary tumor

Tis Carcinoma *in situ*

T1 Tumor 3 cm or less in greatest dimension, surrounded by lung or visceral pleura, without bronchoscopic evidence of invasion more proximal than the lobar bronchus,* (i.e., not in the main bronchus)

T2 Tumor with any of the following features of size or extent:
More than 3 cm in greatest dimension
Involves main bronchus, 2 cm or more distal to the carina
Invades the visceral pleura
Associated with atelectasis or obstructive pneumonitis that extends to the hilar region but does not involve the entire lung

T3 Tumor of any size that directly invades any of the following: chest wall (including superior sulcus tumors), diaphragm, mediastinal pleura, parietal pericardium; or tumor in the main bronchus less than 2 cm distal to the carina, but without involvement of the carina; or associated atelectasis or obstructive pneumonitis of the entire lung

T4 Tumor of any size that invades any of the following: mediastinum, heart, great vessels, trachea, esophagus, vertebral body, carina; or tumor with a malignant pleural or pericardial effusion,** or with satellite tumor nodule(s) within the ipsilateral primary tumor lobe of the lung

Regional Lymph Nodes (N)

NX Regional lymph nodes cannot be assessed

N0 No regional lymph node metastasis

N1 Metastasis to ipsilateral peribronchial and/or ipsilateral hilar lymph nodes, and intrapulmonary nodes involved by direct extension of the primary tumor

N2 Metastasis to ipsilateral mediastinal and/or subcarinal lymph node(s)

N3 Metastasis to contralateral mediastinal, contralateral hilar, ipsilateral or contralateral scalene, or supraclavicular lymph node(s)

Distant Metastasis (M)

MX Presence of distant metastasis cannot be assessed

M0 No distant metastasis

M1 Distant metastasis present[†]

*Note: The uncommon superficial tumor of any size with its invasive component limited to the bronchial wall, which may extend proximal to the main bronchus, is also classified T1.
**Note: Most pleural effusions associated with lung cancer are caused by tumor. However, a few patients have multiple cytopathologic examinations of pleural fluid that are negative for tumor. In these cases, the fluid is nonbloody and is not an exudate. When these elements and clinical judgment dictate that the effusion is not related to the tumor, the effusion should be excluded as a staging element, and the patient should be staged T1, T2, or T3. Pericardial effusion is classified according to the same rules.
[†]Note: Separate metastatic tumor nodule(s) in the ipsilateral nonprimary tumor lobe(s) of the lung are also classified M1.
From Mountain CF. Revisions in the international staging system for lung cancer. *Chest* 1997;111:1710, with permission

TABLE 32.2. STAGE GROUPING—TNM SUBSETS

Stage	TNM Subset		
Stage 0	Carcinoma *in situ*		
Stage IA	T1 N0 M0		
Stage IB	T2 N0 M0		
Stage IIA	T1 N1 M0		
Stage IIB	T2 N1 M0		
	T3 N0 M0		
Stage IIIA	T3 N1 M0		
	T1 N2 M0	T2 N2 M0	T3 N2 M0
Stage IIIB	T4 N0 M0	T4 N1 M0	T4 N2 M0
	T1 N3 M0	T2 N3 M0	T3 N3 M0
	T4 N3 M0		
Stage IV	ANY T ANY N M1		

From Mountain CF. Revisions in the international system for staging lung cancer. *Chest* 1997;111:1710, with permission.

sion with no evidence of metastasis, T1 N0 M0 disease, as stage IA (Figure 32.1). An individual stage designation for this anatomic subset is warranted because the prognosis for patients with T1 N0 M0 tumors is significantly better than the outcome achieved for any other group of patients—an observation confirmed by end results studies according to both clinical and surgical-pathologic staging criteria. Table 32.3 shows that 61% of patients with cStage IA non–small

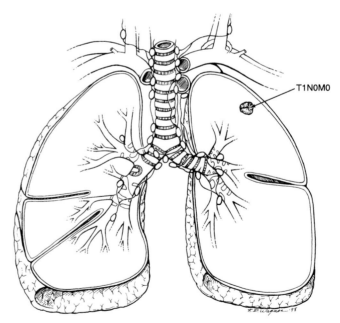

FIGURE 32.1. Stage IA (*T1N0M0*) lung cancer identifies tumors 3 cm or less in greatest dimension, surrounded by lung parenchyma, with no evidence of invasion proximal to a lobar bronchus and no evidence of metastasis. (From Mountain CF, Libshitz HI, Hermes KE. Lung cancer—handbook for staging, imaging, and lymph node classification. Houston: Clifton F. Mountain Foundation, 1999, with permission.)

TABLE 32.3. NON–SMALL CELL LUNG CANCER. CUMULATIVE PERCENT OF PATIENTS SURVIVING ACCORDING TO CLINICAL STAGING CRITERIA

Stage/TNM	Number	Cumulative % Surviving		
		1 Year	3 Years	5 Years
I A - T1N0M0	675	90	71	61
I B - T2N0M0	1,130	72	46	38
II A - T1N1M0	26	84	42	37
II B	329	60	33	24
T2N1M0	227	63	35	26
T3N0M0	102	54	30	21
III A	445	52	19	13
T3N1M0	38	58	12	9
T1-2-3N2M0	407	51	20	13
III B	836	33	7	5
T4 N0-1-2M0	396	34	8	7
Any T N3M0	440	32	6	3
IV	1,166	17	2	<1
Any T Any N M1				

Overall comparison: $p < 0.01$; pairwise comparison, all stages $p < 0.05$ except for cIB versus cIIA; see Table 32.6 for data source and statistical methods.

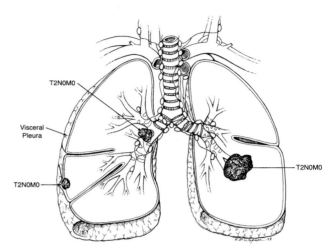

FIGURE 32.2. Stage IB (*T2N0M0*) lung cancer includes larger tumors or those of any size that invade the visceral pleura or main bronchus, greater than 2 cm from the carina, or that have atelectasis/pneumonitis extending to the hilar region. No evidence of metastasis is present. (From Mountain CF, Libshitz HI, Hermes KE. Lung cancer—handbook for staging, imaging, and lymph node classification. Houston: Clifton F. Mountain Foundation, 1999, with permission.)

cell lung cancer (NSCLC) and 67% of those with pStage IA non–small cell (NSC) lung tumors are expected to survive five years or more. Higher rates may be reported for selected patients entered into special studies.[28]

Patients with larger tumors or those of any size that invade the visceral pleura or main bronchus (>2 cm distal to the carina), with no evidence of metastasis, the T2 N0 M0 anatomic subset, are designated stage IB (Figure 32.2). A significant difference between the survival rates for patients with stage IA and those with stage IB NSCLC is documented ($p < 0.05$) according to both clinical and surgical-pathologic staging criteria; however, as shown in Tables 32.3–32.4, the disparity is greater in the clinical category. Thirty-eight percent of patients with larger, more invasive tumors, the cStage IB NSC group, are expected to survive 5 years or more after treatment. In the surgical-treatment group of patients, pStage IB NSCLC, a 57% cumulative survival rate is documented (Table 32.4). The difference in outcome for the cStage IB and pStage IB groups may be related to stage migration, based on the surgical-pathologic evaluation of regional lymph nodes.

Stage IIA and Stage IIB

Stage IIA includes patients with T1 tumors with metastasis present in peribronchial and/or hilar lymph nodes, the T1 N1 M0 anatomic subset (Figure 32.3). A clinical presentation of stage IIA lung cancer is seldom seen radiographically (n = 26 NSC tumors in this series) and, based on surgical findings, stage migration is a common observation. A larger proportion of patients classified pStage IIA was observed in

the surgical treatment group than was observed at clinical presentation. Stage IIB includes two anatomic subsets: First, T2 tumors with metastasis in peribronchial or hilar lymph nodes, T2 N1 M0, and second, T3 tumors with limited, circumscribed extrapulmonary extension, such as peripheral tumors invading the chest wall or mediastinum and with no evidence of metastasis, T3 N0 M0 (Figure 32.4) A significantly better prognosis ($p < 0.03$) is shown for patients

TABLE 32.4. NON–SMALL CELL LUNG CANCER. CUMULATIVE PERCENT OF PATIENTS SURVIVING ACCORDING TO SURGICAL-PATHOLOGIC STAGE OF DISEASE AND TNM SUBSET

pStage/TNM	Number	Cumulative % Surviving-Years After Treatment		
		1 Year	3 Years	5 Years
I A - T1N0M0	511	91	71	67
I B - T2N0M0	549	94	67	57
II A - T1N1M0	76	88	65	55
II B	375	77	47	39
T2N1M0	288	78	47	39
T3N0M0	87	76	47	38
III A	399	64	32	23
T3N1M0	55	65	30	25
T1-2-3N2M0	344	64	32	23

Overall comparison: $p < 0.01$; pairwise comparison, all stage groups $p < 0.05$ except for p1B versus pIIA; see Table 32.6 for data source and statistical methods. (From Mountain CF. Revisions in the international system for staging lung cancer. *Chest* 1997;111:1710, with permission.)

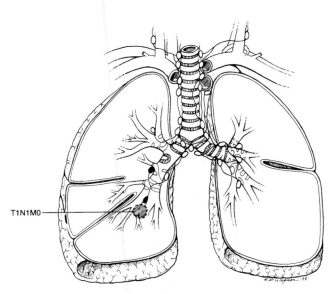

FIGURE 32.3. Stage IIA (*T1N1MO*) lung cancer identifies T1 tumors involving peribronchial or hilar lymph nodes by direct extension or metastasis. No evidence of further lymph node or distant metastasis is present. (From Mountain CF, Libshitz HI, Hermes KE. Lung cancer—handbook for staging, imaging, and lymph node classification. Houston: Clifton F. Mountain Foundation, 1999, with permission.)

with cStage IIA NSCLC compared to those classified as cStage IIB—37% and 24% of patients with NSCLC, respectively, expected to survive five years (Table 32.3). The difference in survival rates for patients with pStage IIA and pStage IIB tumors also is significant—55% and 39%, respectively, expected to survive five years after treatment, p < 0.05 (Table 32.4). The rationale for revised stage grouping rules that specifically identify T1 N1 M0 tumors as stage IIA is supported by the end results studies and because a specific category is needed to collect data for studying the outcome of a larger number of patients with a T1 N1 M0 clinical presentation.

The revised stage grouping that places T3 N0 M0 tumors in stage IIB rather than in stage IIIA is based on the following observations of prognosis. The relationship to survival rates is similar for both the clinically staged and surgical-pathologically staged anatomic subsets of NSC lung tumors: cT2 N1 M0 and cT3 N0 M0, 26% and 21%, respectively, expected to survive five years; pT2 N1 M0 and pT3 N0 M0, 39% and 38%, respectively, expected to survive five years after treatment (Tables 32.3–32.4). The rationale for the revision is also supported by a significant difference in the survival rates between the revised stage IIB and stage IIIA groups of patients.[17]

Stage IIIA

The stage IIIA category classifies tumors with limited, circumscribed extension of the primary tumor and involvement of intrapulmonary or hilar lymph nodes, T3 N1 M0 disease, and the presence of ipsilateral mediastinal lymph node metastasis, N2, in patients with T1, T2, or T3 primary tumors. Four subsets are involved: T3 N1 M0, T1 N2 M0, T2 N2 M0, and T3 N2 M0 (Figure 32.5). The deleterious effect on prognosis of clinically detectable lymph node metastasis is demonstrated in the cumulative survival rates for patients with NSCLC in the cT3 N1 M0 and cT1-2-3 N2 M0 anatomic subsets—9% and 13%, respectively, expected to survive five years (Table 32.3). In patients with N2 disease, the best outcome was shown for a small group with T1 primary tumors, whereas the poorest prognosis was observed for those with T3 tumors. The end results for the surgical-pathologically staged patients show the improved outcome that is achieved for selected patients with stage IIIA NSCLC whose disease is amenable to complete resection (Table 32.4). Similar cumulative survival rates were documented for patients with NSCLC in the pT3 N1 M0 and pT1-2-3 N2 M0 subsets, a cumulative 25% and 23%, respectively, surviving five years. The rationale for modifying the TNM subsets designated as stage IIIA is supported by the end results studies.

Stage IIIB

Stage IIIB includes lung cancer with extensive extrapulmonary extension, such as tumor invading mediastinal struc-

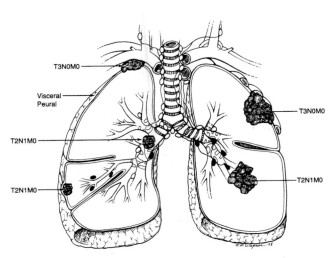

FIGURE 32.4. Stage IIB (*T2N1MO* and *T3NOMO*) lung cancer includes (1) tumors larger than 3 cm., or with other T2 characteristics, that involve peribronchial and/or hilar lymph nodes by direct extension or metastasis. No further lymph node or distant metastasis is present, and (2) tumors with limited, circumscribed, extrapulmonary extension, T3, such as peripheral tumors invading the chest wall or central tumors involving the pericardium, with no evidence of metastasis. (From Mountain CF, Libshitz HI, Hermes KE. Lung cancer—handbook for staging, imaging, and lymph node classification. Houston: Clifton F. Mountain Foundation, 1999, with permission.)

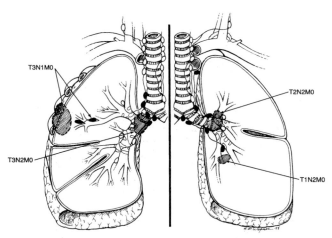

FIGURE 32.5. Stage IIIA (*T3N1MO* and *T1-2-3N2MO*) lung cancer identifies (1) tumors with localized, circumscribed extrapulmonary extension, T3, with metastasis involving peripbronchial and or hilar lymph nodes, and (2) T1-2-3 tumors with metastasis involving the ipsilateral mediastinal and subcarinal lymph nodes. No evidence of further lymph node or distant metastasis is present. Tumors involving the pericardium, with no evidence of metastasis. (From Mountain CF, Libshitz HI, Hermes KE. Lung cancer—handbook for staging, imaging, and lymph node classification. Houston: Clifton F. Mountain Foundation, 1999, with permission.)

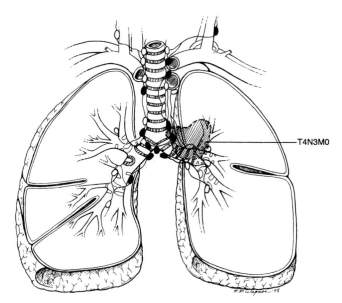

FIGURE 32.6. Stage IIIB (*T4AnyNMO* and *Any TN3MO*) classifies extensive extrapulmonary tumor invasion of mediastinal structures such as the trachea, esophagus, heart and major vessels, and metastasis involving the contralateral mediastinal and hilar lymph nodes, and the ipsilateral and contralateral supraclavicular/scalene lymph nodes. No distant metastasis is present. (From Mountain CF, Libshitz HI, Hermes KE. Lung cancer—handbook for staging, imaging, and lymph node classification. Houston: Clifton F. Mountain Foundation, 1999, with permission.)

tures—the esophagus, trachea, carina, heart, major vessels—or the vertebral body, or with malignant pleural effusion, all of which indicate T4 disease. Metastasis to contralateral hilar and ipsilateral and contralateral supraclavicular/scalene lymph nodes may be present, N3 disease; however, no evidence of distant metastasis is present. No revision in the stage grouping of the TNM subsets in stage IIIB was made, except for the modification of the T4 definition described earlier. The subsets include T4 N0 M0, T4 N1 M0, T4 N2 M0, and T1 N3 M0, T2 N3 M0, T3 N3 M0, and T4 N3 M0 (Figure 32.6). Only one-third of patients with cStage IIIB NSCLC are expected to survive 1 year and 5% for 5 years after treatment (Table 32.3). This outcome varies slightly according to the TNM category—a 7% cumulative survival rate was shown for the group with cT4 N0-1-2 M0 tumors and 3% for the cAnyT N3 M0 group. Although it may not be clinically relevant, the difference in survival rates between the cStage IIIB subsets and cStage IV is statistically significant, p < 0.01 (Table 32.3).

Stage IV

Stage IV is reserved for patients with distant metastasis, M1 disease. The M1 descriptor was modified by the addition of ipsilateral (non–lymph node) metastasis in nonprimary tumor lobe(s) as evidence for M1 disease. Clinical signs and symptoms of metastasis to distant organ sites usually are confirmed by imaging techniques; however, routine brain

and bone scans have not proved cost-effective for patients with NSC tumors. The significance of adrenal nodules imaged on abdominal computed tomography (CT) should be determined by biopsy. Positron emission tomography (PET) holds promise for making clinical estimates of metastatic disease more reliable; however, specific indications for its use and application of the findings remain under study.[30] The disastrous effect of metastasis to distant organ sites, such as liver, bone, brain, contralateral lung, or distant lymph nodes, is reflected in the survival rates for patients with NSCLC with this manifestation—only 17% expected to survive one year after treatment and less than 1% for five years. (The present data does not include patients with intrapulmonary metastasis classified as M1.)

RECOMMENDATIONS FOR STAGING WHEN THE RULES DON'T FIT

The outcome in patients with lung cancer may be influenced by many factors, and it would be impossible to design a workable staging system that accounted for all of them. In practice, we can use only a classification system that discriminates most patients within a definable subgroup. Thus limitations are imposed on the definitions and, unless such limitations are accepted, a hopelessly complex and unmanageable number of subcategories could result.

In the absence of a body of data that describes the prognostic implications of tumors with no applicable specific staging rule, the TNM and stage classifications must be assigned according to logic or convention. Some common questions and problems in staging lung cancer are as follows:

Discontinuous Tumor Foci in Visceral or Parietal Pleura

Tumor foci in the parietal or visceral pleura that are discontinuous from direct pleural invasion by the primary tumor should be staged T4. Discontinuous tumor lesions *outside* the parietal pleura in the chest wall or in the diaphragm are classified M1.

Invasion of the Phrenic Nerve

Invasion of the phrenic nerve is apparent clinically and usually represents limited direct extension of the primary tumor. As such, it indicates T3 disease and does not preclude surgical treatment, if no criteria for T4 pertain.

Invasion of the Vagus Nerve

Measures of disease extent that cannot be identified and applied to clinical staging should not be considered as staging elements. One does not generally perceive involvement of the vagus nerve clinically unless its recurrent branch (i.e., the recurrent laryngeal nerve) is affected, in which case the involvement is readily detectable. Recurrent laryngeal nerve symptoms are often caused by mediastinal lymph node metastasis, although they can be caused by primary tumor invasion. It is important to note, however, that (a) recurrent laryngeal nerve involvement usually indicates inoperability, and (b) the survival for such patients is similar to that for the IIIB-T4 stage group. Accordingly, we recommend a T4 classification for tumors with evidence of recurrent laryngeal nerve involvement.

Great Vessels

Tumor involvement of the great vessels is classified T4. The following are defined as "great vessels": (a) aorta; (b) superior caval vein; (c) inferior caval vein; (d) main pulmonary artery; (e) *intrapericardial portions* of the trunk of the right or left pulmonary arteries, and (f) *intrapericardial portions* of the superior or inferior right or left pulmonary veins. Involvement of more distal branches of the main arterial and venous trunks would be classified T3.

By virtue of the prognosis and treatment options associated with vena caval syndrome and esophageal and tracheal compression, these manifestations indicate stage IIIB not IIIA disease. It would be contradictory to the T4 definition

to routinely assign an N2 classification to these manifestations of disease extent. In the rare instance of a peripheral primary tumor that clearly is not in direct continuity with great vessels, evidence of compression of these structures may be caused by nodal disease. The T and N categories are then classified according to the established rules for these descriptors.

Involvement of the Vertebral Body

In most patients with superior sulcus or Pancoast's tumors with clinical evidence of vertebral body invasion, this extension of the disease indicates unresectability and a poor prognosis. Successful resection for tumors with localized invasion of a specific area of the vertebral body has been reported with a better prognosis than that anticipated for patients with unresectable disease. Investigational surgical programs, usually multidisciplinary efforts undertaken by thoracic and neurosurgeons, have addressed removal of part or all of the vertebra. Although a few patients may be found at operation to have resectable tumor invading the vertebral body, clinical evidence of this extent of disease is generally associated with nonsurgical treatment options and a prognosis consistent with the T4 category.

A tumor arising in the superior sulcus of the lung with evidence for a true Pancoast's syndrome (i.e., a Horner's syndrome and brachial plexus involvement) should be classified T4, whether or not vertebral body invasion is present.

Synchronous Multiple Primary Lung Cancers

Synchronous multiple primary lung cancers should be staged independently. The tumor with the highest stage of disease or more serious prognostic implications should be used for tumor registry entry of a single patient, and a specific field should be assigned for the identification of multiple primary lung cancers. Coding may then be expanded to include particular characteristics for each tumor, such as histology, treatment, and survival data. If synchronous multiple lung cancers have similar prognoses and staging characteristics, the tumor receiving first treatment should be selected for tumor registry data entry.

REGIONAL LYMPH NODE CLASSIFICATION FOR LUNG CANCER STAGING

A classification for regional lymph nodes that is compatible with the International System for Staging Lung Cancer, and that incorporates features of multiple systems previously in use, is shown in Figure 32.7 and Table 32.5. This lymph node mapping schema, developed by Mountain and Dresler,[18] provides a single system that incorporates features of the most commonly used lymph node maps—the schema

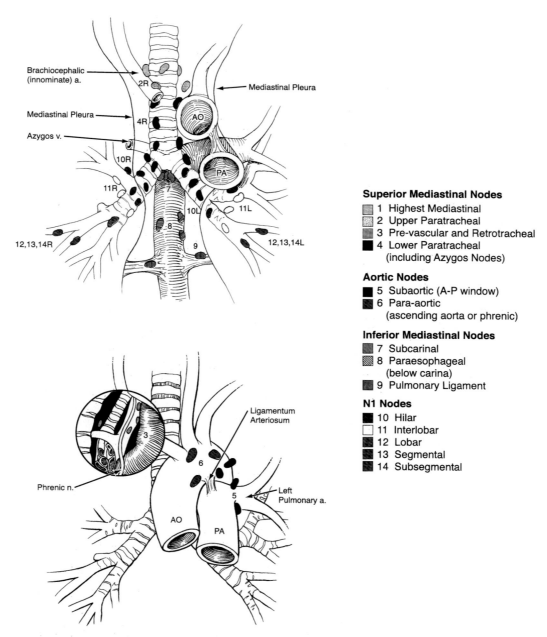

Superior Mediastinal Nodes

- 1 Highest Mediastinal
- 2 Upper Paratracheal
- 3 Pre-vascular and Retrotracheal
- 4 Lower Paratracheal
  (including Azygos Nodes)

Aortic Nodes

- 5 Subaortic (A-P window)
- 6 Para-aortic
  (ascending aorta or phrenic)

Inferior Mediastinal Nodes

- 7 Subcarinal
- 8 Paraesophageal
  (below carina)
- 9 Pulmonary Ligament

N1 Nodes

- 10 Hilar
- 11 Interlobar
- 12 Lobar
- 13 Segmental
- 14 Subsegmental

FIGURE 32.7. Regional Lymph Node Stations for Lung Cancer Staging. (From Mountain CF and Dresler CM, from Naruke,[31] and The American Thoracic Society/North American Lung Cancer Study Group,[32] (copyright 1996, Mountain and Dresler; may be reproduced for educational purposes without permission).[18]

developed by Naruke and which was based on data,[31] and the map proposed by the North American Lung Cancer Study Group, based on recommendations of the American Thoracic Society.[32] The schema has been adopted and recommended by the UICC[20] and the AJCC.[21] For clinical research study of the relationships among specific lymph node metastasis and primary tumor growth, cell type, patterns of recurrence or further metastasis, and biologic fac-

tors, a consistent, reproducible method for collecting and reporting data is required.

Lymph Node Mapping Schema

The definitions for staging the status of regional lymph nodes (the "N" component) in patients with lung cancer are shown in Table 32.1. Anatomic landmarks for 14 hilar,

TABLE 32.5. LYMPH NODE MAP DEFINITIONS[18]

Nodal Station: Anatomic Landmarks

N2 NODES—All N2 nodes lie within the mediastinal pleural envelope.

1 Highest Mediastinal Nodes: Nodes lying above a horizontal line at the upper rim of the bracheocephalic (left innominate) vein where it ascends to the left, crossing in front of the trachea at its midline

2 Upper Paratracheal Nodes: Nodes lying above a horizontal line drawn tangential to the upper margin of the aortic arch and below the inferior boundary of #1 nodes.

3 Prevascular and Retrotracheal Nodes: Pre- and retrotracheal nodes may be designated 3A and 3P. Midline nodes are considered to be ipsilateral.

4 Lower Paratracheal Nodes: The lower paratracheal nodes on the right lie to the right of the midline of the trachea between a horizontal line drawn tangential to the upper margin of the aortic arch and a line extending across the right main bronchus at the upper margin of the upper lobe bronchus, and contained within the mediastinal pleural envelope.

The lower paratracheal nodes on the left lie to the left of the midline of the trachea between a horizontal line drawn tangential to the upper margin of the aortic arch and a line extending across the left main bronchus at the level of the upper margin of the left upper lobe bronchus, medial to the ligamentum arteriosum and contained within the mediastinal pleural envelope.

Researchers may wish to designate the lower paratracheal nodes as #4s (superior) and #4i (inferior) subsets for study purposes. The #4s nodes may be defined by a horizontal line extending across the trachea and drawn tangential to the cephalic border of the azygos vein. The #4i nodes may be defined by the lower boundary of #4s and the lower boundary of #4, as described previously.

5 Subaortic (A–P window): Subaortic nodes are lateral to the ligamentum arteriosum or the aorta or left pulmonary artery and proximal to the first branch of the left pulmonary artery and lie within the mediastinal pleural envelope.

6 Para-aortic Nodes (ascending aorta or phrenic): Nodes lying anterior and lateral to the ascending aorta and the aortic arch or the innominate artery, beneath a line tangential to the upper margin of the aortic arch.

7 Subcarinal Nodes: Nodes lying caudal to the carina of the trachea but not associated with the lower lobe bronchi or arteries within the lung.

8 Paraesophageal Nodes (below carina): Nodes lying adjacent to the wall of the esophagus and to the right or left of the midline, excluding subcarinal nodes.

9 Pulmonary Ligament Nodes: Nodes lying within the pulmonary ligament, including those in the posterior wall and lower part of the inferior pulmonary vein.

N1 NODES—ALL N1 nodes lie distal to the mediastinal pleural reflection and within the visceral pleura.

10 Hilar Nodes: The proximal lobar nodes, distal to the mediastinal pleural reflection, and the nodes adjacent to the bronchus intermedius on the right. Radiographically, the hilar shadow may be created by enlargement of both hilar and interlobar nodes.

11 Interlobar Nodes: Nodes lying between the lobar bronchi.

12 Lobar Nodes: Nodes adjacent to the distal lobar bronchi.

13 Segmental Nodes: Nodes adjacent to the segmental bronchi.

14 Subsegmental Nodes: Nodes around the subsegmental bronchi.

From Mountain CF, Dresler CM. Regional lymph node classification for lung cancer staging. *Chest* 1997;111:1718, with permission.

intrapulmonary, and mediastinal lymph node stations and their accompanying definitions illustrate that all N2 nodes are contained within the mediastinal pleural envelope and that all N1 nodes lie distal to the mediastinal pleural reflection (Figure 32.7). It is difficult to show the anatomic relationships of the three-dimensional structures in the chest in an artistic rendition; therefore, it is important to relate the anatomic landmarks for each station shown on the map to the definitions in Table 32.5. The N2 nodes are numbered 1 through 9 and include the superior mediastinal nodes (numbers 1–4), the aortic nodes (numbers 5–6), and the inferior mediastinal nodes (numbers 7–8). The N1 nodes are numbered 10–14. Numbers 10L and 10R are the most proximal nodes in the N1 category and are designated hilar nodes; numbers 11R/L–14R/L are designated intrapulmonary nodes, with specific designations related to the location on or between the bronchi (Table 32.5). Depending on the location of the primary tumor, the ipsilateral nodes are designated right or left; midline prevascular and retrotracheal lymph nodes are considered ipsilateral. As noted in Table 32.5, researchers may wish to divide the lower paratracheal nodes into superior (4s) and inferior (4i) groups, as an aid to the study of metastasis to specific lymph node levels.

To confirm the extent of N1 and N2 disease, extended or total resection of all lymph node groups accessible to the

TABLE 32.6. APPENDIX—COLLECTED DATABASE FOR CLASSIFICATION RESEARCH[17]

Institution	Number of Cases
The University of Texas M. D. Anderson Cancer Center, 1975–1988*	4,351
Reference Center for Anatomic and Pathologic Classification of Lung Cancer, 1977–1982†	968
Total	5,319

* Consecutive patients treated for primary lung cancer, 1975–1980; surgical patients only, 1981–1982; consecutive patients (receiving no previous treatment) treated for non–small cell lung cancer, 1983–1988.
† Patients treated for primary lung cancer by the National Cancer Institute cooperative Lung Cancer Study Group—representative slide material and case documentation submitted to the Reference Center for Anatomic and Pathologic Classification of Lung Cancer at the University of Texas M. D. Anderson Cancer Center for confirmation of staging and histology. From Mountain CF. Revisions in the international staging system for lung cancer. *Chest* 1997;111:1718, with permission.
The Wilcoxon (Gehan) statistic was used for comparing the survival experience of patient groups.[34] Analysis was carried out using a software package (Statistical Program for the Social Sciences; SPSS, Inc., Chicago). The terminal event was death from cancer or unknown cause; deaths within 30 days of operation were excluded. The end results according to clinical stage are calculated from the date of first treatment or the decision for no treatment, and those according to surgical-pathologic stage are calculated from the date of first treatment.

surgeon is essential (see also Chapter 35). Pathologic assessment of pulmonary resection and lymphadenectomy specimens represents the highest order of reliability. Although most patients with lung cancer are not candidates for surgical treatment, the lymph node mapping schema is useful for clinical staging and correlative studies of diagnostic and evaluative procedures.

The prognostic implications of lymph node metastasis are well known; however, within the spectrum of the N1 and N2 categories, the relationship of the presence and extent of metastasis to the primary tumor status, the status of the lymph nodes (i.e., intranodal or extranodal disease), the number of levels of metastasis, and various histologic and biologic features are not fully understood. A unified lymph node mapping schema provides a means for collecting data to study these important facets of metastatic disease and to apply the information to clinical practice. Table 32.6 lists the database for the staging system used by the authors.

SUMMARY

The recommendations for staging lung cancer and for classifying regional lymph nodes provide a consistent, reproducible method for communicating information and comparing the results of differing treatments for lung cancer. The total tumor burden for a given patient cannot be precisely quantitated, and the balance between host defenses and tumor agressiveness cannot be precisely measured. However, our data support the tenet that patients can be grouped according to certain measurable common features of their disease so that within each stage, treatment options and survival expectations are generally similar. Survival patterns according to staging criteria are a measure of the efficacy of currently available therapy; therefore, the staging information serves as a valuable guide for treatment planning.

ACKNOWLEDGEMENTS

The author wishes to acknowledge the contribution of Kay E. Hermes, Biomedical Analyst, to the research and writing of this report. The work is supported by the Clifton F. Mountain Foundation.

REFERENCES

1. World Health Organization Technical Report Series, No. 53, July 1952, p. 47.
2. Denoix PF. Enquete permanent dans les centres anticancereux. *Bull Inst Nat Hgy* (France) 1944;1:1.
3. Union Internationale Contre le Cancer (UICC). The birth of TNM. *UICC Cancer Magazine* 1988;9.
4. Union Internationale Contre le Cancer (UICC). *TNM classification of malignant tumors* (Livre de Poche). Geneva: UICC, 1968.
5. Copeland M. American Joint Committee on Cancer staging and end results reporting. Objectives and progress. *Cancer* 1965;18:1637.
6. Union Internationale Contra le Cancer (UICC) (Committee on clinical stage classification and applied statistics). *The TNM system General rules*. Geneva: UICC, 1966.
7. Union Internationale Contre le Cancer (UICC). *TNM classification of malignant tumors*. Geneva: UICC, 1974.
8. Union Internationale Contre le Cancer (UICC). Harmer MH, ed. *TNM classification of malignant tumors*, 3rd ed. Geneva: UICC, 1978; enlarged and revised, Geneva: UICC 1982.
9. American Joint Committee for Cancer Staging and End Results Reporting, Task Force on the Lung. *Clinical staging of cancer of the lung*. Chicago: American College of Surgeons, 1973.
10. American Joint Committee on Cancer (AJCC) *Manual for staging cancer*, 1st ed. 1977, revised and reprinted 1978, 1980; 2nd ed., 1983, Chicago: American Joint Committee, 1983.
11. Mountain CF, Anderson WAD, Carr DT. A system for the clinical staging of lung cancer. *Am J Roentgenol and Radium Ther Nucl Med* 1974;120:130.
12. Mountain CF. Assessment of surgery for control of lung cancer. *Ann Thorac Surg* 1977;24:365.
13. Ishikawa S. Staging system on TNM classification for lung cancer. *Jpn J Clin Oncol* 1973;6:19.
14. Mountain CF. A new international staging system for lung cancer. *Chest* 1986;89:225s.
15. Union Internationale Contre le Cancer (UICC). Lung tumors. In: Hermanek P, Sobin LH, eds. *TNM classification of malignant tumors*, ed 4. Berlin: Springer-Verlag, 1987.
16. American Joint Committee on Cancer (AJCC). Lung. In: Beahrs OH, Hensen E, Hutter RVP, et al. eds. *Manual for staging cancer*. ed 4. Philadelphia: JB Lippincott, 1992.
17. Mountain CF. Revisions in the international system for staging lung cancer. *Chest* 1997;111:1710.
18. Mountain CF, Dresler CM. Regional lymph node classification for lung cancer staging. *Chest* 1997;111:1718.
19. International Union Against Cancer (UICC) Lung. In: Sobin LH, Wittekind CB, eds. *TNM classification of malignant tumors* 5th ed. New York: Wiley-Liss, 1997.
20. International Union Against Cancer (UICC): Lung and pleural tumors. In: Hermanek P, Hutter RVP, Sobin L, eds. *TNM atlas*. 4th ed. (Illustrated guide to the TNM/ptNM classification) New York: Wiley-Liss, 1997.
21. American Joint Committee on Cancer (AJCC). Lung. In: Fleming ID, Cooper JS, Hensen DE, et al., eds. *Manual for staging cancer*. Philadelphia: JB Lippincott, 1997.
22. Van Zandwijk N, Van't Veer LJ. The role of prognostic factors and oncogenes in the detection and management of non-small cell lung cancer. *Oncology* 1998;12:(1 Suppl 2):55.
23. Huang CL, Taki T, Adachi M, et al. Mutations of p53 and K-ras genes as prognostic factors for non-small cell lung cancer. *Int J Oncol* 1998;12:553.
24. Kwiatowski DJ, Harpole DH, Jr., Godleski JU. Molecular pathologic substaging in 244 stage I non-small cell lung cancer patients: clinical implications. *J Clin Oncol* 1998;16:2468.
25. Fontanni G, DeLaurentis M, Vignati S, et al. Evaluation of epidermal growth factor-related growth factors and receptors and of neoangiogenesis in completely resected stage I-IIIA non-small cell lung cancer: amphiregulin and microvessel count are independent prognostic indicators of survival. *Clin Cancer Res* 1998; 4:241.
26. Kawaguchi T, Yamamoto S, Kudoh S, et al. Tumor angiogenesis as a major prognostic factor in stage I lung adenocarcinoma. *Anticancer Res* 1997;17(5B):3743.
27. Mountain CF. New prognostic factors in lung cancer. Biologic prophets of cancer cell agression. *Chest* 1995;108:246.
28. Darling GE. Staging of the patient with small cell lung cancer. *Chest Surg Clin N Am* 1997;7:81.
29. Flehinger BJ, Kimmel M, Melamed MR. The effect of surgical

treatment on survival from early lung cancer; implications for screening. *Chest* 1992;101:1013.

30. Weber W, Schmid RA, Bruchhaus H, et al. Detection of extrathoracic metastases by positron emission tomography in lung cancer. *Ann Thorac Surg* 1998;66:886.

31. Naruke T, Suemasu K, Ishikawa S. Lymph node mapping and curability of various levels of metastases in resected lung cancer. *J Thorac Cardiovasc Surg* 1978;76:832.

32. American Thoracic Society. Clinical staging of primary lung cancer. *Am Rev Respir Dis* 1983;127:1.

33. Mountain CF, Libshitz HI, Hermes KE. Lung cancer—handbook for staging, imaging, and lymph node classification. Houston: Clifton F. Mountain Foundation, 1999.

34. Gehan EA. Statistical methods for survival time studies. In: Staquet MJ, ed. *Cancer therapy, prognostic factors and criteria of response.* New York: Raven Press, 1975;7.

33

CLINICAL AND MOLECULAR PROGNOSTIC FACTORS AND MODELS FOR NON–SMALL CELL LUNG CANCER

CHRISTINE L. LAU
THOMAS A. D'AMICO
DAVID H. HARPOLE, JR

The most important predictor of survival in non–small cell lung cancer (NSCLC) is the TNM stage at diagnosis, with the best chance for cure remaining complete surgical resection. Patients with clinical stage I (pathologic stage I, II, and microscopic IIIA) NSCLC who have undergone resection with a curative intent have an estimated 50% recurrence and cancer death rate at five years.[1,2] An understanding of tumor virulence on a molecular level may identify subsets of early-stage patients with poorer prognosis. If a definitive set of tumor markers that document early recurrence could be identified, earlier intervention (radiation therapy or re-resection for a local recurrence, chemotherapy or a novel therapy for a distant recurrence) may increase the overall survival. Additionally, markers capable of identifying patients with advanced or metastatic disease would prevent unnecessary surgical procedures in this group. This section focuses on identification of clinicopathologic and molecular factors that may be used in combination with the TNM staging system to provide a more accurate substaging system, therefore allowing stratification within a stage of patients at high risk for recurrence and death.

CLINICAL FACTORS

The current staging system does not consider clinical symptoms, histology, or biologic aggressiveness of tumors. The presence of symptoms even when corrected for stage, particularly weight loss and poor performance status at the time of diagnosis of lung cancer, have been found to have a significantly negative impact on survival in patients with NSCLC.[2] Harpole et al.[2] reported that the presence of symptoms in stage I NSCLC was a significant factor in predicting overall survival. In their analysis of 289 patients, 189 without symptoms had a five-year survival rate of 74% versus a 41% survival rate in the 100 patients with symptoms (p < 0.001). The presence of hemoptysis, cough, and chest pain were all found to be predictive of decreased survival.

Male sex has been found to be an adverse prognostic indicator in some studies;[2,4–6] however, much of this difference may be the result of tumor size at presentation because women tend to present with smaller tumors (as well as less smoking history and increased percentage with adenocarcinoma).[2] Others series have not shown male sex to be an adverse prognostic factor.[2]

Although clinical factors are beneficial in terms of predicting prognosis, their use is limited because of their low prevalence in early-stage lung cancer. Patients with early-stage disease often remain asymptomatic despite having biologically aggressive tumors. Furthermore, symptoms are descriptive in nature and thus subject to patient and physician bias.

HISTOPATHOLOGIC FACTORS

T Status/Tumor Size

In stage I NSCLC, the size of the primary tumor has been shown to significantly impact survival.[2,8,9] Five-year survivals of 67% to 83% for stage 1A (T1N0) and 50% to 65% for stage IB (T2N0) are reported.[2,5,9] More precise sizing of stage I tumors has also been shown to be prognostically significant with tumors 0 to 2 cm, 2 to 4 cm, and more than 4 cm having five-year survivals of 74%, 60%, and 45%, respectively, as shown in Fig. 33.1 (Harpole, unpublished data). Padilla et al.[7] further substaged T1 stage I disease into tumors 0.1 to 1.0 cm 1.1 to 2.0 cm, and 2.1 to 3.0 cm in size with reported survivals of 90%, 86.1%, and 65.4% (p = 0.0092). Tumor size in stage II lung cancer has also been shown to impact survival with T1N1 tumors having five-year survivals of 55% compared to T2N1 with five-year survivals of 39% (p < 0.05).[9] Martini et al.;[10] however, did not report a statistically significant survival

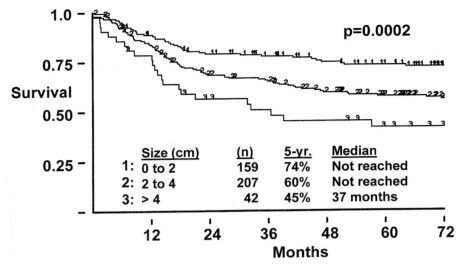

FIGURE 33.1. Survival by tumor size (cm).

difference between T1 and T2 stage II lung cancer, but they did report improved survival in stage II NSCLC with primary tumors ≤3 cm compared to those whose primary was ≥5 centimeters (p = 0.02). Based on the statistically significant survival advantage seen with T1 tumors, the revised international lung cancer staging system divides stage 1 into stage IA and IB and stage II into stage IIA (T1N1) and IIB (T2N1) (see also Chapter 32).

In early-stage lung cancer, the location of the tumor has been shown to be a prognostic factor. Visceral pleural involvement has been shown to correlate with poorer overall survival.[2,8,11] Because of this prognostic significance, tumors with visceral pleural involvement are considered T2 even when they are ≤3 centimeters in size.[9]

Lymph Node Status

For patients with stage II NSCLC, the number of N1 nodes with cancer and the location of these nodes is more important than the size of the primary tumor. Martini and colleagues[10] reported that single N1 node involvement in stage II NSCLC was a favorable prognostic factor compared to patients with multiple N1 node involvement (45% versus 31%; p = 0.016). Yano and colleagues[12] assessed 78 patients with stage II lung cancer and found a significant five-year survival advantage in patients with positive lobar N1 nodes (64.5%) compared to hilar N1 nodes (39.7%; p = 0.014). Additionally, in this study the patterns of metastatic spread were different based on location of involved N1 nodes; the brain was the most common site in patients with lobar N1 disease, whereas the lungs were the common site of spread in hilar N1 positive patients. Survival in stage IIIA (N2) NSCLC has also been shown to correlate with the

number of lymph nodes involved. Five-year survivals of 43% following primary tumor resection and mediastinal lymph node dissection in patients found to have microscopic metastatic disease in only one mediastinal lymph node has been reported as compared to the 23% to 25% five-year survival for surgically resected stage IIIA disease as a whole.[9,13,14]

Histologic Subtypes

Whether histologic subtyping of NSCLC according to the World Health Organization[15] into squamous cell carcinoma, adenocarcinoma, or large cell carcinoma has prognostic significance regarding overall survival is controversial. Harpole and colleagues[2] and others[7] reported no significant survival advantage for any histologic tumor type in patients with stage I NSCLC. Other groups have shown a significant five-year survival advantage to patients with squamous cell cancers compared to adenocarcinomas.[5,8] The Lung Cancer Study Group reported an increase in recurrence rates in patients with nonsquamous NSCLC.[16] Kwiatkowski and colleagues[6] found no survival differences among stage I lung cancer patients with different histologic types; however, when they subtyped adenocarcinomas, patients with the solid tumor with mucin type had a significantly decreased survival (p = 0.019) compared to patients with the other subtypes of adenocarcinoma.

Martini and colleagues[10] found no survival difference between squamous cell carcinoma and other histologies in 214 stage II NSCLC patients. This group did report a difference in patterns of recurrence based on histology, with squamous cell carcinomas recurring locally and adenocarcinomas distantly. In contrast to Martini et al.[10] Ichinose and colleagues[11] reported on 63 patients with stage II NSCLC and found that patients with squamous cell carcinomas had a significant survival advantage over patients with nonsquamous tumors. Looking at patients with N2 (stage IIIA), Martini and Flehinger[13] found no survival difference between patients with adenocarcinoma and patients with squamous cell carcinomas.

Tumor Differentiation

Tumors can be differentiated based on histologic and light microscopic findings into well, moderate, poor, or undifferentiated. Poorer differentiation is associated with decreased survival in NSCLC.[2,5,17,18] Ichinose and colleagues[11] reported that patients with well-differentiated stage I tumors had five-year survivals of 87% versus 71% five-year survival in patients with stage I tumors that were moderately or poorly differentiated (p = 0.0029). However, tumor differentiation was not found to be prognostically significant in patients with stage II or IIIA tumors in this study.

Lymphatic and Blood Vessel Invasion

The presence or absence of lymphatic or blood vessel invasion has been considered an indication of biologic aggressiveness in NSCLC. Kessler and colleagues[19] used light microscopy to assess blood vessel invasion, specifically the main venous or arterial parabronchial vessels. The presence of blood vessel invasion correlated with a significantly decreased survival in this series in agreement with others.[11,19,20] Ichinose and colleagues[11] reported that fifteen of seventeen patients with recurrence whose primary tumor had venous blood vessel invasion were distant, suggesting the veins as a source for metastatic spread. Harpole and colleagues[2] reported the presence of vascular invasion to be a highly significant factor in prognosis. More recently, Kwiatkowski and colleagues[6] found lymphatic invasion to be a significant negative predictor of survival, with five-year survival in stage I NSCLC patients of 74% if lymphatic invasion was absent, compared to a five-year survival of 54% if present (p = 0.0004).

Routine histologic and light microscopic techniques are used to evaluate tumor size, N-status, histology, differentiation, and vascular/lymphatic invasion, but these methods are limited by sensitivity and the experience of the pathologist. For example, histologically negative lymph nodes may contain micrometastatic disease in 15% of cases.[21]

MOLECULAR MARKERS

The change from normal bronchial epithelium to carcinoma is the end result of a series of acquired genetic mutations and alterations in normal cellular proteins. The critical regulatory genes mutated in NSCLC include various protooncogenes and tumor-suppressor genes. Carcinogenesis can occur with either activation or deletion of these important regulatory genes. Protooncogenes when altered may acquire transforming potential, leading to dysregulation of normal cell growth. Only one of the two alleles needs to be altered for the transforming effect and, therefore, protooncogenes are known as dominant genes. Tumor-suppressor genes have been implicated in lung cancer, with cellular transformation occurring by either elimination of both alleles or by mutation or functional abnormality of their protein products. The reader is referred to Chapters 1–11 for greater detail.

Carcinogenesis

Growth-regulating Proteins

Several genes normally control cell growth and development. Alterations in these genes can change the phenotype of a cell, allow the expression of abnormal signal transduction proteins, and activate multiple enzyme cascades in the cell. Growth-regulating genes whose protein products have been implicated in NSCLC include *ras* oncogenes, epidermal growth factor receptor gene, and *erb*B-2/*Her2-neu* oncogenes.

Ras Oncogenes

Ras oncogenes are a family of genes that code for a protein located on the inner surface of the cell membrane (see also Chapter 4). The protein known as p21 is involved in signal transduction and has guanosine triphosphatase activity. Mutations of *ras* genes result in blockage of guanosine triphosphatase activity, allowing a continued signal for proliferation. There are three main members of the *ras* oncogene family (K-*ras*, H-*ras*, and N-*ras*), and the vast majority of mutations involved in NSCLC occur in K-*ras* at codon 12 (other codons 13, 61). Mutations in K-*ras* have been found most commonly in adenocarcinomas and are linked with smoking and asbestos exposure.[22] Slebos and colleagues initially reported activation of K-*ras* oncogene as a strong negative prognostic factor in patients with resected adenocarcinomas.[23] Fukuyama and colleagues[24] reported that NSCLC patients with K-*ras* mutations at codon 12 had a relative risk of death of 5.6 compared to patients without the mutation. In addition to the prognostic significance of K-*ras* gene mutations, the overexpression of p21 has similarly been found to correlate with a negative survival. Harada and colleagues[25] found that NSCLC patients with p21-negative tumors (stained immunohistochemically using anti-*ras* p21 monoclonal antibody rp-35) had significantly longer survival times compared to patients whose tumors were p21 positive. More recently, however, Nemunaitis and colleagues[26] did not attribute significant negative prognostic value to elevated p21 in adenocarcinoma patients with normal *ras*-oncogenes. The majority of evidence, albeit in retrospective studies, indicates that K-*ras* mutations correlate with decreased survival, and therefore little controversy exists that it has value as a molecular marker.

Protooncogenes c-*erbB*-1 and c-*erbB*-2 (HER-2/*neu*)

The protooncogene c-*erbB*-1 encodes for epidermal growth factor receptor (EGFr), a tyrosine kinase-type membrane receptor (see also Chapter 4). Ligand binding to EGFr results in receptor dimerization, autophosphorylation, activation of cytoplasmic proteins, and eventually DNA synthesis.[27] Mutations in c-*erbB*-1 can result in constitutive activation of EGFr despite the absence of ligand, with the result being uncontrolled tumor growth. In NSCLC, elevated levels of EGFr have been shown to be present compared to normal lung tissue. Additionally, elevated levels of EGFr are found in later stage lung cancers and in lung cancers with mediastinal involvement,[28] but these levels have not been found to correlate with prognosis.[22,27,29] However, subset analysis (TINO) in one study evaluating a panel of immunohistochemical markers in resected stage I NSCLC did find a decreased survival rate in EGFr overexpressing tumors.[30,31] Based on the available data, although EGFr may play a role in initial tumorgenesis and may be a marker for advanced disease, increased expression of EGFr cannot currently be considered as a significant prognostic molecular marker in NSCLC.

C-*erbB*-2/*HER*-2/*neu* shares extensive homology (80%) with c-*erbB*-1 and encodes for a transmembrane tyrosine kinase (p185neu), which also functions as a growth factor receptor. Kern and colleagues[32] found that ten of twenty-nine patients with adenocarcinoma overexpressed p185*neu*, and this overexpression was associated with decreased survival. Following this initial report, several additional studies have confirmed these results with adenocarcinomas and NSCLC as a group.[4,31,33,34] Overexpression of p185*neu* is currently felt to be an independent negative prognostic factor in NSCLC.

Cell-cycle Specific Proteins

Normal bronchial epithelium is arrested in the G0 phase of the cell cycle, with a designated cell life. When it reaches the end of its life, an apoptotic cascade begins, allowing the senescent cell to die. Deletion or mutations in the genes involved in regulating the cell's lifespan can cause them to become resistant to apoptosis or "immortal." Apoptotic factors (p53, bcl-2) and cell cycle–regulating factors (Rb, Ki-67, and cyclins) are implicated in NSCLC (see also Chapters 2, 4, 6, 7).

P53 Tumor-Suppressor Gene

The tumor-suppressor gene *P53* encodes for a nuclear phosphoprotein involved in cell growth through regulation of transcriptional events. Mutations in *P53* are the most common mutations associated with human cancers,[3] and in NSCLC *P53* is found to be mutated or overexpressed in more than 50% of cases. Similar to abnormalities in K-ras, mutations in *P53* are associated with smoking.[22] Significant controversy remains over its use as a molecular prognostic indicator in NSCLC because in some studies mutation or protein expression of *P53* is associated with decreased survival,[4,6,31,34–39] some with no association to survival;[29,40] and some with increased survival.[41,42] Reasons for this controversy are unclear but may at least partially relate to whether gene mutation or protein expression is measured.[3,43] Overexpression does not necessarily mean that the *P53* gene is mutated, but it is an abnormal finding. Additionally, the group of NSCLC patients assessed may provide some explanation for the controversy. Dalquen and colleagues found *P53* expression to be a negative prognostic factor in node-negative but not node-positive NSCLC patients.[44] Along these lines, a study consisting of 408 stage I NSCLC patients confirmed the negative prognostic value of overexpression of *P53* with a 70% five-year survival for NSCLC patients with *P53* minus tumors compared to 52% survival for *P53*+ tumors (p = 0.001).[31]

BCL2 Protooncogene (Apoptotic Gene)

The protooncogene BCL2 encodes a protein that inhibits apoptosis (programmed cell death) and thus regulates cell viability. Overexpression of BCL2, surprisingly, has been associated with improved survival in NSCLC[45,46] or a trend toward improved survival.[6,31]

Retinoblastoma (RB) and p16^INK4a Tumor-Suppressor Genes

The *RB* gene encodes a nuclear protein that interacts with the protein product of *P53* in the nucleus and is involved with transcriptional events and cell cycle regulation (keeping the cell quiescent) (see also Chapter 7). This tumor-suppressor gene is located on a chromosomal region often found deleted in the childhood ocular cancer retinoblastoma. Loss of RB protein expression occurs commonly in NSCLC, most often seen in later stage tumors. Loss of RB protein expression has been associated with either a decrease in survival[31,47] or no correlation with survival.[6,48] Additionally, patients with both loss of RB protein expression and p53 protein overexpression (TP53 mutation) have an even worse prognosis.[31,47] D'Amico and colleagues[31] reported five-year survivals in 404 stage I NSCLC patients of 72%, 62%, and 48% for RB+/p53−; RB+/p53+; and RB−p53+ (protein expression) tumors, respectively. Therefore, the loss of RB is felt to be a negative prognostic factor.

A cyclin-dependent kinase inhibitor p16^INK4a is involved in keeping a cell in the quiescent state (G0). The mechanism by which the gene product of p16^INK4a inhibits entry into the cell cycle is through its inhibition of the cyclin-dependent kinase 4 mediated phosphorylation of the RB gene product. Inactivation of p16^INK4a results in unregulated cell growth and transformation. Worse survival has been seen in NSCLC patients whose tumors do not express $p16^{INK4a}$. Additionally, an inverse correlation has been appreciated between levels of RB and $p16^{INK4a}$.

Tumor Invasion

Two processes are necessary for a tumor colony to grow and become invasive: angiogenesis and basement membrane degradation. When a tumor colony expands, it outgrows its blood supply and central necrosis develops. The resultant ischemia stimulates angiogenesis within the cancer, resulting in ingrowth of capillaries and tumor growth. In order for an *in situ* tumor to invade surrounding tissues, the glycoprotein matrix that surrounds normal bronchial epithelium must be degraded by enzymes (matrix metalloproteinases, cathepsin B). These two processes allow cancer cells to enter the lymphatic or vascular spaces, thus setting the stage for the next phase: distant metastases.

Angiogenesis

Tumor-induced neovascularization (angiogenesis) is necessary for both tumor growth and metastatic spread, and a large research effort is currently being directed into studying its role in cancer development (see also Chapter 11). The number of microvessels in an NSCLC can be used to assess angiogenesis. Antibody to factor viii can be used to identify the number of microvessels in an NSCLC,[50] and the degree of angiogenesis as measured by viii staining has been shown to have significant negative prognostic implications. Harpole et al.[34] examined angiogenesis in 275 consecutive patients with stage I NSCLC and found that angiogenesis was the most significant prognostic factor in stage I NSCLC compared to *erb*B-2 (*HER-2/neu*), p53, and KI-67. Attempts to increase sensitivity and specificity using immunostaining for CD31(platelet/endothelial cell adhesion molecule) instead of factor viii did not prove successful, and its use did not correlate with prognosis.[51] Recently, an anti-CD34 monoclonal antibody specific for endothelial cells has been found useful in immunostaining of microvessels.[52,53] In contrast to anti-CD31, anti-CD34 antibody has been found to be more specific and reproducible than staining for factor viii. Fontanini et al.[52] prospectively analyzed a cohort of 407 patients with NSCLC, using anti-CD34 antibody to detect microvessels, and found that patients with more vascularized tumors experienced significantly decreased survivals ($p < 0.00001$). Patients with stage I lung cancers and highly vascularized tumors had 50% two-year survivals compared to 95% survival in this group of patients with the lowest microvessel counts. Besides using endothelial cell antigen antibodies to assess microvessel counts, Imoto et al.[54] reported on the prognostic significance of vascular endothelial growth factor expression in NSCLC

and found it to be a significant prognostic indicator, especially with squamous cell cancer.

Invasion/Extracellular Matrix Degradation

Matrix metalloproteinases have been implicated in the breakdown of vascular barriers, allowing tumor cells to infiltrate blood vessels. The matrix metalloproteinase, stromelysin-3, has received the greatest attention in NSCLC and has been found to be more abundant in NSCLC than in normal lung tissue.[55]

Plasminogen activators are members of the serine protease family and convert plasminogen to plasmin. Plasmin can degrade various proteins in the extracellular matrix. Plasminogen activators are regulated by plasminogen activator inhibitors. Yoshino and colleagues have found that decreased levels of plasminogen activator inhibitor 2 correlate with decreased survival and increased lymph node metastases in NSCLC patients.[56]

Cathepsin B is a cellular protein located in the lysosome (cysteine proteinase), and it is involved in protein degradation within the cell. It has been implicated in tumor cells in the digestion of the extracellular matrix. Because it can digest the extracellular matrix, it is involved in tumor invasion and metastases. Higher grade expression of cathepsin B has been prognostically correlated with decreased survival in NSCLC.[3,57] Sukoh and colleagues[57] reported that patients with stage I NSCLC whose tumors strongly expressed cathepsin B had decreased survival compared to patients whose tumors did not express cathepsin B. In contrast, Mori and colleagues[58] did not find high expression of cathepsin B in stage I NSCLC patients to correlate with survival.

Formation of Metastases

A carcinoma can invade surrounding structures, including blood vessels and lymphatic channels, allowing tumor cells to circulate throughout the body. The formation of metastatic lesions, however, requires that circulating tumor cells adhere to the endothelium of a distant capillary or lymph vessel and transgress the endothelial membrane of the target organ. Paget in 1889 identified that tumors require both the "correct seed and soil" for metastatic spread.[59] Therefore, only tumor cells that express the correct adhesion molecules (CD-44, siayl-Tn, blood group A) are able to successfully attach and invade a new location in the body.

Adhesion Molecules

Cluster designation 44 (CD-44), an integral membrane glycoprotein, is a receptor for hyaluronan (component of the extracellular matrix). CD-44 is involved in cell-to-cell and cell-to-extracellular matrix interactions and is correlated with metastatic spread. Expression of CD44 has been shown to be a negative prognostic factor in NSCLC.[31] Hirata and colleagues[60] reported that expression of a variant isoform of CD-44 negatively correlated with survival in stage I NSCLC patients. D'Amico and colleagues reported a five-year survival of 54% in patients with CD44 expression compared to a 67% survival in patients without CD44 expression (p = 0.05).[31]

Blood Group Antigens and Precursor Antigens

The loss of expression of blood group A allows immature blood group antigens to be exposed; these antigens have been implicated in cell motility and, therefore, have been speculated to be involved with metastatic spread. Lee and colleagues[61] assessed the presence of blood group antigens immunohistochemically in 164 patients with completely resected NSCLC. In this study, survival of the twenty-eight patients with blood group A or AB whose lung cancers lacked the blood group A antigen was significantly worse than survivals of patients with the blood group A antigen on their tumors or patients with blood group B or O. Miyake and colleagues[62] stained for the precursors of blood group A and B antigens (H/Le^y/Le^b) using the monoclonal MIA-15-5 (migration-inhibitory antibody; named for its ability to inhibit motility and metastatic ability of cancer cells) and reported that MIA-positive tumors had a significantly worse prognosis than MIA-negative tumors. The MIA-positive tumor patients had a five-year survival of 20.9% versus 58.6% for patients with MIA-negative tumors (p < 0.001). Additionally, Matsumoto and colleagues[63] found that loss of blood group antigens on lung cancer correlated with increased metastatic potential and worse prognosis. More recently, however, reports have not shown this prognostic correlation in early-stage lung cancer,[6,64] and one report even found that MIA-15-5–positive tumors had an increased survival.[29] Thus blood group antigens and their precursors are currently not felt to be important in the biologic aggressiveness of NSCLC.

Detection of Micrometastases by Molecular Biologic Markers

Occult micrometastatic disease in the lymph nodes and bone marrow not appreciable by routine histologic staining can be detected with the use of immunohistochemic techniques and reverse transcriptase–polmerase chain reaction techniques (rt-PCR) (see also Chapter 1). These techniques are able to detect the presence of one tumor cell in 10^5 to 10^8 normal cells.[65] Rt-PCR may be more sensitive than immunohistochemic staining for detection of micrometastases.[65] The markers used to detect micrometastases include cytokeratins, mucins (cell surface glycoprotein), and various molecular markers such as epidermal growth factor receptor and P53 expression. The use of epithelial elements is particularly appealing because they are directed toward the identification of epithelial elements that are not present in normal

lymph nodes and bone marrow. Detection of occult micrometastatic lymph node or bone marrow disease using rt-PCR or immunohistochemistry potentially may allow selection of a subset of patients who would benefit substantially from induction therapies.

Occult micrometastatic disease found using immunohistochemic staining has been shown to correlate with early relapse and worse prognosis.[66–69] Maruyama and colleagues[69] reported on the detection of micrometastases in lymph nodes using an anti-cytokeratin monoclonal antibody and the value of this detection in predicting early relapse in patients with stage I NSCLC. They identified cytokeratin-positive cells in lymph nodes of thirty-one out of forty-four (70.5%) stage I patients, restaging nineteen of these as N1 and 12 as N2 disease, respectively. In these patients with micrometastatic disease in the mediastinal lymph nodes, the disease-free survival rate was significantly shorter than in those with node-negative disease (p = 0.004). Immunohistochemic staining for the presence of EGFr or p53 has also been used in the detection of micrometastatic disease. The presence of these biologic markers in lymph nodes is correlated with decreased survival.[70]

Salerno and colleagues[65] used rt-PCR to detect the presence of messenger RNA transcripts for MUC1 in lymph nodes. Using this technique, they found occult metastases in 33 of 88 lymph nodes negative for metastatic disease based on light microscopy.

Several groups have been able to identify micrometastases of lung cancer in bone marrow. Using immunohistochemic techniques, Pantel and colleagues identified cytokeratin-positive cells in the bone marrow of patients with operable lung cancer and found that their presence correlated with cancer relapse (66.7% versus 36.6%, p < 0.05). This same group later[68] found that 60% with apparently localized disease had micrometastases in their bone marrow. Cote and colleagues, using immunohistochemic techniques to identify bone marrow metastases in 43 NSCLC patients, reported a significantly shorter time to tumor relapse with the presence of micrometastases in the bone marrow (7.3 versus 35.1 months, p = 0.0009).[71] Additionally, for patients with early-stage lung disease, the detection of occult bone marrow metastases was associated with a higher rate of recurrence. Most recently, in 139 patients with NSCLC of various stages, cytokeratin 18–positive cells were demonstrated in the bone marrow in 60%. In the sixty-six patients without lymph node metastases, occurence of two or more tumor cells in the bone marrow was an independent predictor of survival (B. Passlick, *personal communication*).

Markers of Tumor Proliferation

These markers estimate the proportion of tumor cells nearing mitosis and consist of assessment by light microscopy (mitotic index), flow cytometry (ploidy, S-phase), or immunohistochemic techniques (Ki-67, proliferating cell nuclear antigen.

Mitotic Index/Ploidy

Harpole and colleagues reported that tumors with ≥15 mitosis per high-power field had a significantly worse survival rate than tumors with a lower number of mitotic figures present.[2] Recently, however, Kwiatkowski[6] found no survival differences in stage I NSCLC patients whose tumors had mitotic index of 0 to 10, 10 to 20, 21 to 30, or more than 30, with five-year survival rates of 68%, 67%, 72%, and 60%, respectively. Investigation into DNA content by flow cytometry initially suggested that more biologically aggressive tumors were aneuploid, whereas those associated with a better prognosis appeared to be diploid.[18,72] Subsequent studies, however, have not confirmed this survival advantage with diploid tumors.[22,73] The prognostic significance of the number of cells in the S-phase (S-phase fraction) of the cell cycle has not been extensively studied in NSCLC. High S-phase fraction has been associated either with a decrease in survival[72] or with no correlation to survival.[3,74] Volm and colleagues[72] reported on 187 predominantly advanced-stage NSCLC patients and found that patients whose tumors had ≤8% of their cells in the S-phase had significantly improved survival compared to patients whose tumors had >8% of their cells in S-phase (p = 0.041). In comparison, Schmidt and colleagues[74] found no prognostic significance to S-phase percentage in T1N0 tumors.

Ki-67 Proliferation Marker

The tumor proliferation marker Ki-67, a nonhistone nuclear protein, is expressed by cells near mitosis and can be used to identify rapidly dividing tumors. Several series have noted a decrease in survival in association with higher levels of expression of Ki-67.[4,34,73] Pence and colleagues[73] evaluated Ki-67 proliferation indices in 61 predominantly early-stage lung cancer patients (stage I: 39 patients; stage II: 12 patients; stage III/IV: 10 patients) and found that patients with Ki-67 proliferation indexes of less than 3.5 had two-year survivals of 54% compared to 8% for patients with Ki-67 proliferation indexes of more than 3.5 (p = 0.01). In patients with stage I NSCLC, Harpole and colleagues[4] reported a 52% five-year survival in patients with a Ki-67 index greater than 10%, compared to a 68% five-year survival in patients with a ki-67 index of 0% to 5% (p < 0.02). Additionally, Ki-67 proliferation had a highly significant correlation with p53 overexpression. In a larger group of patients, D'Amico and colleagues[31] reported a trend that did not reach significance toward decreased survival in high- versus low-level Ki-67 expression (p = 0.071). In conclusion, higher Ki-67 proliferation indexes appear to inversely correlate with prognosis.

Proliferating Cell Nuclear Antigen

Proliferating cell nuclear antigen (PCNA) is a nuclear protein that binds to DNA polymerase. Because of its involvement with DNA replication, its presence is highest in rapidly growing cells, whereas its level is undetectable in quiescent cells. Ishida and colleagues found that positive staining for PCNA correlated with decreased survival in NSCLC patients.[3,75]

Serum Markers for Early Detection

Various serum markers may eventually be used to identify patients with NSCLC, to identify those with more advanced disease, and to predict prognostic information. Potential serum markers showing promise in NSCLC[76] are carcinoembryonic antigen (CEA),[77,78] CA-125,[79] Cyra21-1,[80] and sialyl Lewis X-I antigen.[81]

MULTIVARIATE MODELS

Because the NSCLCs are a diverse group of tumors, one molecular marker invariably can not predict increased biologic virulence 100% of the time. Adenocarcinomas, large cell carcinomas, and squamous cell carcinomas preferentially express various markers. For these reasons, molecular model systems consisting of a panel of molecular markers have the ability to optimize the sensitivity of biologic markers across the spectrum of NSCLC.

Kwiatowski and colleagues[6] evaluated 244 patients with stage I NSCLC and identified six independent variables that predicted tumor recurrence: (a) adenocarcinoma solid tumor with mucin subtype, (b) tumor diameter ≥4 cm, (c) lymphatic invasion, (d) p53 expression, (e) K-*ras* mutation, and (f) absence of H-*ras* expression. This group proposed a molecular pathologic substaging system in stage I NSCLC based on these variables. If patients had ≤ two factors, then they were assigned as grade 1a; if they had three factors, then they were assigned grade 1b; and if they had ≥4 factors, then they were assigned grade 1c. The basis of this substaging was based on the detected five-year cancer-free survival rates of 87%, 58%, and 21% for each proposed substage, respectively. Additionally, they showed that wedge resections were associated with a decrease in cancer-free survival and recommended that lobectomy be performed for stage I NSCLC, unless medically contraindicated.

Recently, D'Amico and colleagues[31] proposed a molecular model system consisting of five biologic markers affecting various points in the metastatic sequence (growth regulation, cell cycle regulation, apoptosis, angiogenesis, and metastatic adhesion factor) to further risk-stratify patients with NSCLC. The five biologic factors found to be significant predictors of survival in multivariable analysis were *erb*B-2, RB, p53, factor viii staining for angiogenesis, and CD-44.

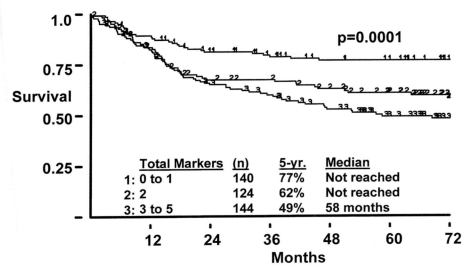

FIGURE 33.2. Survival by Multivariate Model.

Combining these factors, patients are stratified into substage 1, zero to one markers; substage 2, two markers, or substage 3, three to five markers, with five-year survivals of 77%, 62%, and 49%, respectively (p = 0.0001) (Figure 33.2).

CONCLUSIONS

The TNM stage of NSCLC at diagnosis remains the most important determinant of survival. Clinical factors, including symptoms, performance status, and weight loss, have definitive prognostic value and may be used to supplement the current staging system. Certain pathologic characteristics (tumor size, nodal involvement) of the tumor can be used to stratify patients into risk categories, whereas the role of other factors (histology, differentiation) is currently less defined. Particularly in early-stage lung cancer, the size of the primary tumor correlates with survival. Identifying T2N0 as high-risk stage I disease, the Cancer and Leukemia group B (CALGB) is currently sponsoring an intergroup trial (CALGB 9633) to address the role of adjuvant chemotherapy (taxol and carboplatin) in addition to surgery in this group of NSCLC patients.

Significant research is ongoing, investigating the biology of NSCLC, and the roles of protooncogenes, tumor-suppressor genes, angiogenic factors, extracellular matrix proteases, and adhesion molecules are being elucidated. Although evidence is accumulating that K-*ras*, c-*erb*B-2, p53, *bcl*-2, RB, neovascularization, and extracellular matrix proteases are involved in NSCLC tumor virulence, the current studies are fraught with small sample sizes, heterogeneous populations, and variations in techniques. Other biologic markers, such as EGFr, blood group antigens, and blood group precursor antigens, were initially felt to have prognos-

tic implications in NSCLC, but recent studies have not been able to confirm their value. Studies addressing the use of tumor proliferation markers as prognostic indicators have not conclusively proven their value. Prospective, large studies with homogenous groups designed to evaluate the role of these various markers should clarify their potential involvement in NSCLC.

REFERENCES

1. Strauss GM, Kwiatowski DJ, Harpole DH, et al. Molecular and pathologic markers in stage I non-small cell carcinoma of the lung. *J Clin Oncol* 1995;13:1265.
2. Harpole DH, Herndon JE, Young WG, et al. Stage I Nonsmall cell lung cancer: a multivariate analysis of treatment methods and patterns of recurrence. *Cancer* 1995;76:787.
3. Strauss GM. Prognostic markers in resectable non-small cell lung cancer. *Hematol/Oncol Clin N Am* 1997;1:409.
4. Harpole DH, Herndon JE, Wolfe WG, et al. A prognostic model of recurrence and death in stage I non-small cell lung cancer utilizing presentation, histopathology, and oncoprotein expression. *Cancer Res* 1995;55:51.
5. Nesbitt JC, Putnam JB, Walsh GL, et al. Survival in early-stage non-small cell lung cancer. *Ann Thorac Surg* 1995;60:466.
6. Kwiatowski DJ, Jr DHH, Godleski J, et al. Molecular pathologic substaging in 244 stage I non-small-cell lung cancer patients: clinical implications. *J Clin Oncol* 1998;16:2468.
7. Padilla J, Calvo V, Peñalver JC, et al. Surgical results and prognostic factors in early non-small cell lung cancer. *Ann Thorac Surg* 1997;63:324.
8. Gail MH, Eagan RT, Feid R, et al. Prognostic factors in patients with resected stage I non-small cell lung cancer: a report from the Lung Cancer Study Group. *Cancer* 1984;54:1802.
9. Mountain CF. Revisions in the international system for staging lung cancer. *Chest* 1997;111:1710.
10. Martini N, Burt ME, Bains MS, et al. Survival after resection of stage II non-small cell lung cancer. *Ann Thorac Surg* 1992;54:460.

11. Ichinose Y, Yano T, Asoh H, et al. Prognostic factors obtained by a pathologic examination in completely resected non-small cell lung cancer. *J Thorac Cardiovasc Surg* 1995;110:601.

12. Yano T, Yokoyama H, Inoue T, et al. Surgical results and prognostic factors of pathologic N1 disease in non-small-cell carcinoma of the lung. *J Thorac Cardiovasc Surg* 1994;107:1398.

13. Martini N, Flehinger BJ. The role of surgery of N2 lung cancer. *Surg Clin N Am* 1987;67:1037.

14. Martini N. Mediastinal lymph node dissection for lung cancer: The Memorial experience. *Chest Surg Clin N Am* 1995;5:189.

15. World Health Organization. Histological typing of lung tumors. In: World Health Organization, ed. *International histological classification of tumors,* No. 1. Geneva: World Health Organization, 1981.

16. Group TLCS, Thomas PA, Piantadosi S. Postoperative T1 N0 non-small cell lung cancer. *J Thorac Cardiovasc Surg* 1987;94:349.

17. Kadri MA, Dussek JE. Survival and prognosis following resection of primary non small cell bronchogenic carcinoma. *Eur J Cardiothoracic Surg* 1991;5:132.

18. Ichinose Y, Hara N, Ohta M, et al. Is T factor of the TNM staging system a predominant prognostic factor in pathologic stage I non-small cell lung cancer? a multivariate prognostic factor analysis of 151 patients. *J Thorac Cardiovasc Surg* 1993;106:90.

19. Kessler R, Gasser B, Massard G, et al. Blood vessel invasion is a major prognostic factor in resected non-small cell lung cancer. *Ann Thorac Surg* 1996;62:1489.

20. Macchiarini P, Fontanini G, Hardin MJ, et al. Blood vessel invasion by tumor cells predicts recurrence in completely resected T1 N0 M0 non-small-cell lung cancer. *J Thorac Cardiovasc Surg* 1993;106:80.

21. Chen Z-l, Perez S, Holmes EC, et al. Frequency and distribution of occult micrometastases in lymph nodes of patients with non-small cell lung carcinoma. *J Natl Canc Inst* 1993;85:493.

22. Rusch VW, Dmitrovsky E. Molecular biologic features of non-small cell lung cancer: clinical implications. *Chest Surg Clin N Am* 1995;5:39.

23. Slebos RJC, Kibbelaar R, Dalesio O, et al. K-ras oncogene activation as a prognostic marker in adenocarcinoma of the lung. *N Engl J Med* 1990;323:561.

24. Fukuyama Y, Mitsudomi T, Sugio K, et al. K-ras and p53 mutations are an independent unfavourable prognostic indicator in patients with non-small-cell lung cancer. *Br J Cancer* 1997;75:1125.

25. Harada M, Dosaka-Akita H, Miyamoto H, et al. Prognostic significance of the expression of ras oncogene product in non-small cell lung cancer. *Cancer* 1992;69:72.

26. Nemunaitis J, Klemow S, Tong A, et al. Prognostic value of K-ras mutations, ras oncoprotein, and c-erb B-2 oncoprotein expression in adenocarcinoma of the lung. *Am J Clin Oncol (CCT)* 1998;21:155.

27. Pfeiffer P, Nexo E, Bentzen SM. Enzyme-linked immunosorbent assay of epidermal growth factor receptor in lung cancer: comparisons with immunohistochemistry, clinicopahtological features, and prognosis. *Br J Cancer* 1998;78:96.

28. Fujino S, Enokibori T, Tezuka N, et al. A comparison of epidermal growth factor receptor levels and other prognostic parameters in non-small cell lung cancer. *Eur J Cancer* 1996;32A:2070.

29. Greatens TM, Niehans GA, Rubins JB, et al. Do molecular markers predict survival in non-small-cell lung cancer. *Am J Respir Crit Care Med* 1998;157:1093.

30. Pastorino U, Andreola S, Tagliabue E, et al. Immunohistochemical markers in stage I lung cancer: relevance to prognosis. *J Clin Oncol* 1997;15:2858.

31. D'Amico TA, Massey M, Herndon JE, et al. A biologic risk model for stage I lung cancer: immunohistochemical analysis of 408 patients using 10 molecular markers. *J Thorac Cardiovasc Surg* 1999;117:736.

32. Kern JA, Schwartz DA, Nordberg JE, et al. P185neu expression in human lung adenocarcinoma predicts shortened survival. *Cancer Res* 1990;50:5184.

33. Tateishi M, Ishida T, Mitsudomi T, et al. Prognostic value of c-erbB-2 protein expression in human lung adenocarcinoma and squamous cell carcinoma. *Eur J Cancer* 1991;27:1372.

34. Harpole DH, Richards WG, Herndon JE, et al. Angiogenesis and molecular biologic substaging in patients with stage I non-small cell lung cancer. *Ann Thorac Surg* 1996;61:1470.

35. Quinlan DC, Davidson AG, Summers CL, et al. Accumulation of p53 protein correlates with a poor prognosis in human lung cancer. *Cancer Res* 1992;52:4828.

36. Fujino M, Dosaka-Akita H, Harada M, et al. Prognostic significance of p53 and ras p21 expression in nonsmall cell lung cancer. *Cancer* 1995;76:2457.

37. David H, Harpole J, Marks JR, et al. Localized adenocarcinoma of the lung: oncogene expressiona of erbB-2 and p53 in 150 patients. *Clin Canc Res* 1995;1:659.

38. Horio Y, Takahashi T, Kuroishi T, et al. Prognostic significance of p53 mutations and 3p deletions in primary resected non-small cell lung cancer. *Cancer Res* 1993;53:1.

39. Mitsudomi T, Oyama T, Kusano T, et al. Mutations of the p53 gene as a predictor of poor prognosis in patients with non-small-cell lung cancer. *J Natl Canc Inst* 1993;85:2018.

40. McLaren R, Kuzu I, Dunnill M, et al. The relationship of p53 immunostaining to survival in carcinoma of the lung. *Br J Cancer* 1992;66:735.

41. Lee JS, Yoon A, Kalapurakal SK, et al. Expression of p53 oncoprotein in non-small cell lung cancer: a favorable prognostic factor. *J Clin Oncol* 1995;13:1893.

42. Passlick B, Izbicki JR, Haussinger K, et al. Immunohistochemical detection of p53 is not associated with a poor prognosis in non-small cell lung cancer. *J Thorac Cardiovasc Surg* 1995;109:1205.

43. Carbone DP, Minna JD. Molecular foundation of oncology. In: Broder S, ed. Baltimore: Williams and Wilkins, 1991: p. 79.

44. Dalquen P, Sauter G, Torhorst J, et al. Nuclear p53 overexpression is an independent prognostic parameter in node-negative non small cell lung carcinoma. *J Pathol* 1996;178:53.

45. Pezzella F, Turley H, Kuzu I, et al. bcl-2 protein in non-small cell lung carcinoma. *N Engl J Med* 1993;329:690.

46. Fontanini G, Vignati S, Bigini D, et al. Bcl-2 protein: a prognostic factor inversely correlated to p53 in non-small-cell lung cancer. *Br J Cancer* 1995;71:1003.

47. Xu H-J, Quinlan DC, Davidson AG, et al. Altered retinoblastoma protein expression and prognosis in early-stage non-small-cell lung carcinoma. *J Natl Canc Inst* 1994;86:695.

48. Reissman PT, Koga H, Takahashi R, et al. Inactivation of the retinoblastoma susceptibility gene in non-small cell lung cancer. *Oncogene* 1993;8:1913.

49. Kratzke RA, Greatens TM, Rubins JB, et al. Rb and p16INK4a expression in resected non-small cell lung tumors. *Cancer Res* 1996;56:3415.

50. Macchiarini P, Fontanini G, Hardin MJ, et al. Relation of neovascularisation to metastasis of non-small-cell lung cancer. *Lancet* 1992;340:145.

51. Duarte I, Buflin BL, Pennington MF, et al. Angiogenesis as a predictor of survival after surgical resection for stage I non-small-cell lung cancer. *J Thorac Cardiovasc Surg* 1998;115:652.

52. Fontanini G, Lucchi M, Vignati S, et al. Angiogenesis as a prognostic indicator of survival in non-small cell lung cancer. *J Natl Canc Inst* 1997;89:881.

53. Matsuyama K, Chiba Y, Sasaki M, et al. Tumor angiogenesis as a prognostic marker in operable non-small cell lung carcinoma. *Ann Thorac Surg* 1998;65:1405.

54. Imoto H, Osaki T, Taga S, et al. Vascular endothelial growth factor expression in non-small-cell lung cancer: prognostic significance in squamous cell carcinoma. *J Thorac Cardiovasc Surg* 1998; 115:1007.
55. Anderson IC, Sugarbaker DJ, Ganju RK, et al. Stromelysin-3 is overexpressed by stromal elements in primary non-small cell lung cancers and regulated by retinoic acid in pulmonary fibroblasts. *Cancer Res* 1995;55:4120.
56. Yoshino H, Endo Y, Watanabe Y, et al. Significance of plasminogen activator inhibitor 2 as a prognostic marker in primary lung cancer: association of decreased plasminogen activator inhibitor 2 with lymph node metastasis. *Br J Cancer* 1998;78:833.
57. Sukoh N, Abe S, Ogura S, et al. Immunohistochemical study of cathepsin B. prognostic significance in human lung cancer. *Cancer* 1994;74:46.
58. Mori M, Kohli A, Baker SP, et al. Laminin and cathepsin B as a prognostic factor in stage I non-small cell lung cancer: are they useful? *Modern Pathol* 1997;10:572.
59. Paget S. The distribution of secondary growths in cancer of the breast. *Lancet* 1889;1.
60. Hirata T, Fukuse T, Naiki H, et al. Expression of CD44 variant exon 6 in stage 1 non-small cell lung carcinoma as a prognostic factor. *Cancer Res* 1998;58:1108.
61. Lee JS, Ro JY, Sahin AA, et al. Expression of blood-group antigen A - a favorable prognostic factor in non-small cell lung cancer. *N Engl J Med* 1991;324:1084.
62. Miyake M, Taki T, Hitomi S, et al. Correlation of expression of H/Le/Le antigens with survival in patients with carcinoma of the lung. *N Engl J Med* 1992;327:14.
63. Matsumoto H, Muramatsu H, Shimotakahara T, et al. Correlation of expression of ABH blood group carbohydrate antigens with metastatic potential in human lung carcinomas. *Cancer* 1993;72:75.
64. Dresler CM, Ritter JH, Wick MR, et al. Immunostains for blood group antigens lack prognostic significance in T1 lung carcinoma. *Ann Thorac Surg* 1995;59:1069.
65. Salerno C, Frizelle S, Niehans G, et al. Detection of occult micrometastases in non-small cell lung carcinoma by reverse transcriptase-polymerase chain reaction. *Chest* 1998;113:1526.
66. Pantel K, Izbicki JR, Angstwurm M, et al. Immunocytological detection of bone marrow micrometastases in operable non-small-cell lung cancer. *Cancer Res* 1993;53:1027.
67. Passlick B, Izbicki JR, Kubuschok B, et al. Immunohistochemical assessment of individual tumor cells in lymph nodes of patients with non-small-cell lung cancer. *J Clin Oncol* 1994;12:1827.
68. Pantel K, Izbicki J, Passlick B, et al. Frequency and prognostic significance of isolated tumour cells in bone marrow of patients with non-small-cell lung cancer without overt metastases. *Lancet* 1996;347:649.
69. Maruyama R, Sugio K, Mitsudomi T, et al. Relationship between early recurrence and micrometastases in the lymph nodes of patients with stage I non-small-cell lung cancer. *J Thorac Cardiovasc Surg* 1997;114:535.
70. Dobashi K, Sugio K, Osaki T, et al. Micrometastatic p53-positive cells in the lymph nodes of non-small-cell lung cancer: prognostic significance. *J Thorac Cardiovasc Surg* 1997;114:339.
71. Cote RJ, Beattie EJ, Chaiwun B, et al. Detection of occult bone marrow micrometastases in patients with operable lung carcinoma. *Ann Surg* 1995;222:415.
72. Volm M, Hahn EW, Mattern J, et al. Five year follow-up study of independent clinical and flow cytometric prognostic factors for the survival of patients with non-small cell lung carcinoma. *Cancer Res* 1988;48:2923.
73. Pence JC, Kerns BM, Dodge RK, et al. Prognostic significance of the proliferation index in surgically-resected non-small cell lung cancer. *Arch Surg* 1993;128:1382.
74. Schmidt RA, Rusch VW, Piantadosi S. A flow cytometry study of non-small cell lung cancer classified as T1N0. *Cancer* 1992; 69:78.
75. Ishida T, Kaneko S, Akazawa K, et al. Proliferating cellnuclear antigen expression and argyrophilic nucleolar organizer regions as factors influencing prognosis of surgically treated lung cancer patients. *Cancer Res* 1993;53:5000.
76. Vinolas N, Molina R, Galan MC, et al. Tumor markers in response monitoring and prognosis of non-small cell lung cancer: preliminary report. *Anticancer Res* 1998;8:631.
77. Rubins JB, Dunitz J, Rubins HB, et al. Serum carcinoembryonic antigen as an adjunct to preoperative staging of lung cancer. *J Thorac Cardiovasc Surg* 1998;116:412.
78. Icard P, Regnard J-J, Essomba A, et al. Preoperative carcinoembryonic antigen level as a prognostic indicator in resected primary lung cancer. *Ann Thorac Surg* 1994;58:811.
79. Diez M, Torres A, Pollan M, et al. Prognostic significance of serum CA 125 antigen assay in patients with non-small cell lung cancer. *Cancer* 1993;73:1368.
80. Wieskopf B, Demangeat C, Purohit A, et al. Cyfra 21-1 as a biologic marker of non-small cell lung cancer: evaluation of sensitivity, specificity and prognostic role. *Chest* 1995;108:163.
81. Satoh H, Ishikawa H, Yamashita YT, et al. Predictive value of preoperative serum sialyl lewis X-i antigen levels in non-small cell lung cancer. *Anticancer Res* 1998;18:2865.

34

STAGING AND PROGNOSTIC FACTORS FOR SMALL CELL LUNG CANCER

RONALD FELD
URI SAGMAN
MICHAEL LeBLANC

The emergence of strategies employing combination chemotherapy and radiotherapy have contributed significantly to the management of patients with small cell lung cancer (SCLC) during the last two decades. Most patients respond to initial treatment. Unfortunately, most also subsequently relapse, and cure for most patients with SCLC remains elusive. As with most patients with human malignancies, patients with SCLC undergo staging investigations. An attempt to define disease outcome determinants has also been a goal of management of patients with SCLC. This chapter highlights the traditional approaches to staging and the assessment of prognostic factors in SCLC. Emphasis is given to the limitations of the current staging system and the use of available prognostic factors. Finally, efforts to achieve a consensus for a staging classification for SCLC and novel statistical methodologies are outlined.

STAGING

Even though systemic chemotherapy is the mainstay of treatment for patients with all stages of SCLC, accurate clinical staging is important to determine whether it is necessary to add other treatment modalities, such as radiotherapy, and less frequently to identify the small subpopulation of patients who may be eligible for surgical resection or bone marrow transplantation protocols. Another reason for staging is to determine prognosis. This ability is particularly important for patients who are participating in clinical trials because accurate staging ensures comparability of the patients in each treatment arm and identifies subgroups of varying prognoses that should be stratified to provide balance in the arms. The first revised TNM staging system,[1] when applied to patients with non–small cell lung cancer (NSCLC) resulted in well-defined subgroups of patients whose prognosis depends on tumor size (T), extent of hilar or mediastinal node involvement (N), and presence or absence of distant metastases (M). Because the TNM staging

system requires accurate surgical lymph node sampling, it has not been routinely applied to SCLC. Patients with this disease are seldom considered surgical candidates and commonly have radiologic evidence of hilar or mediastinal node involvement. At presentation, more than 90% of patients have stage III (locally advanced) or stage IV (systemic metastases) disease. For these reasons, patients are usually staged according to a simple two-stage system developed by the Veteran's Administration Lung Cancer Study Group.[2] This system classifies patients as having *limited disease* (LD) when the tumor is confined to one hemithorax and its regional lymph nodes, including the ipsilateral mediastinal, ipsilateral supraclavicular, and contralateral hilar nodes. In essence, LD may be defined simply as a localized tumor that may easily be encompassed within an acceptable radiotherapy portal. Tumors that present with ipsilateral pleura effusions, left laryngeal nerve involvement, or superior vena cava obstruction are still considered limited. Pericardial involvement and bilateral pulmonary parenchymal involvement are considered *extensive disease* (ED) because the radiotherapy portal required to encompass this bulk of disease would be too large and would be associated with a significant risk of unacceptable toxicity. Any evidence of disease outside the thorax is classified as ED. In 1982, an expert panel of the International Association for the Study of Lung Cancer (IASLC) reviewed the staging of SCLC and recommended no change in this two-stage system because no stage-specific treatment of lung cancer was required.[3]

Although this simple staging system has gained general acceptance, areas of controversy remain. With respect to nodal involvement, certain investigators believe that patients who have involvement of the contralateral mediastinal lymph nodes should be staged as ED, whereas others prefer to adopt a more liberal approach and recommend broadening the LD category to include not only contralateral mediastinal nodes but also contralateral supraclavicular nodes.[4] The staging of patients with ipsilateral pleural effusions also remains controversial. There is agreement that all patients with contralateral pleural effusions should be included in the ED category. Some investigators recommend inclusion of ipsilateral pleural effusions in the ED subgroup as well, whereas others suggest that such patients should be included only if the effusion demonstrates malignant cells on cytologic examination. A Southwest Oncology Group[5] analysis of outcome of patients with SCLC demonstrated that the survival of patients with isolated pleural effusions and no other evidence of systemic metastases was nearly identical to patients with LD. Further, the same group[6] had reported previously that the prognosis was not altered significantly even when the pleural effusion contained malignant cells.

In 1989, the IASLC published a consensus report that arose out of a workshop on staging for SCLC.[7] They recommended that LD should include patients with hilar, ipsilateral, and contralateral mediastinal and ipsilateral and contralateral supraclavicular lymph nodes as well as patients with ipsilateral pleural effusions both cytologically positive and negative. They based these conclusions on the observation that the prognosis of patients with contralateral adenopathy and ipsilateral pleural effusions is superior to patients with distant metastatic disease and more closely parallels that of patients with LD.

A new TNM staging system for lung cancer has recently been introduced based on data from a recent publication by Mountain.[8] (See also Chapter, 32) Both the old and the more up-to-date TNM staging system have not generally been applied to patients with SCLC, which is not likely to change in the near future. Although this is true, several groups have shown that TNM stage is prognostically important for the small subgroup of patients with SCLC who are able to undergo surgical resection.[9,10] In two large surgical series, Shepherd and colleagues[9] and Karrer and associates[10] reported five-year survivals of 68% and 62%, respectively, for patients with pathologically confirmed stage I tumors (T1-2, N0) treated by surgery and chemotherapy. In both these series, the survival of SCLC patients was similar to that of the same TNM subgroups of NSCLC patients. In an attempt to assess the impact of T and N staging on prognosis, the Toronto Group[11] undertook a retrospective study of 180 LD patients and identified a subgroup called *very limited disease* who had a more favorable prognosis. For these patients, who had no evidence of mediastinal or supraclavicular node involvement, obstructing tumors, or pleural effusions, the projected five-year survival was 25%. This unusually good prognostic group may be particularly important in the interpretation of clinical trials of new therapy.

In most series, about one-half to two-thirds of patients are found to have ED. This wide range is the result of variability in both the number of staging procedures undertaken and the sensitivity of the imaging modalities employed. With the introduction of more sensitive diagnostic techniques, more patients will be found to have ED. The removal of these "previously occult" ED patients from the LD group will result in an improvement in survival for both groups of patients (LD and ED), although the overall survival of the two groups will not change. This phenomenon of stage migration, or the Will Rogers phenomenon, in which increased sensitivity of staging techniques makes all stages of cancer patients appear to live longer, was first reported by Feinstein and colleagues.[12] Dearing and associates[13] analyzed the effect of changes in staging procedures on prognostic factors over a 14-year period. They reported that brain involvement was associated with significantly shorter survival in patients treated before 1979 but not in patients treated thereafter. Brain metastases were diagnosed by radionuclide scanning before 1979 and by computed tomography (CT) after 1979. In contrast, the introduction of CT scanning of the abdomen led to a reduction in the proportion of patients who underwent routine liver biopsy. The scan was less sensitive than blind biopsies, and this led to a poorer prognosis for patients with liver metastases identified by scan than for those identified by histologic examination of biopsy material.

Staging Procedures

The subject of staging of SCLC has recently been reviewed[13] and the author's recommendations go along with our approach to this subject. Table 34.1 lists the staging procedures that are most appropriate for patients who are undergoing standard therapy and for those who are on clinical trials. All patients should have a complete history and physical examination, a chest radiograph, simple blood tests, including hematology with white blood cell differential and platelet counts, and biochemistry, including electrolytes, liver function tests, and alkaline phosphatase and lactate dehydrogenase (LDH) levels. For patients who are not in a clinical trial, some level of further investigation is required to determine whether they have LD or ED because patients with localized tumors are potential candidates for combined modality treatment programs that incorporate thoracic irradiation. Because the determination of all sites of metastatic involvement does not influence the choice of therapy, it may not be necessary to undertake all scans for all patients. The most common sites of extrathoracic involvement are the bone, liver, bone marrow, and central nervous system. If abnormalities are detected on the baseline history, physical examination, or laboratory screening tests, the initial staging tests should be directed by those abnormalities. Once a staging test is positive and ED has been confirmed, it is not necessary to proceed with the rest of the staging investigations unless required for a clinical trial.[14,15]

As diagnostic procedures have become more sophisticated, the costs incurred to investigate patients with SCLC have also increased. In the absence of a specific therapeutic intervention that contributes significantly to long-term survival, these costly diagnostic procedures potentially only add to the cost of therapy without offering a significant benefit

TABLE 34.1. RECOMMENDED STAGING PROCEDURES FOR PATIENTS WITH SMALL CELL LUNG CANCER

Procedure	Standard	Recommended for Patients on Clinical Trials
Complete physical examination	Yes	Yes
Hematology with differential, WBC, and platelet count	Yes	Yes
Biochemistry with electrolytes, liver function tests, lactate dehydrogenase	Yes	Yes
Chest radiograph	Yes	Yes
Scan of thorax	Only for limited disease patients to facilitate radiotherapy planning	Yes
Ultrasound or CT scan of abdomen	Yes	Yes
Radionuclide bone scan	Yes	Yes
Skeletal radiographs	If bone scan is indeterminate	If bone scan is indeterminate
CT or MRI of brain	Yes	Yes
MRI of spine	Only if clinically indicated	Only if clinically indicated
Bone marrow aspiration and biopsies	Only if hematology is abnormal	Only for patients on limited disease trials
Bronchoscopy	Only if needed for diagnosis	Baseline only necessary for limited disease patients if posttreatment bronchoscopy is required to confirm complete response
Mediastinoscopy	Only if needed for diagnosis	Only if needed for diagnosis
Lumbar puncture	Only if clinically indicated	Only if clinically indicated
Liver biopsy	No	Only necessary if indeterminate results are obtained from CT or ultrasound of abdomen
Monoclonal antibody scans	No	No, unless the trial is specifically evaluating monoclonal antibodies
Biomarkers	No	No, unless the trial is specifically evaluating the role of biomarkers
Pulmonary function tests	Only if there is concern about the ability to deliver thoracic irradiation	Only if there is concern about the ability to deliver thoracic irradiation

* If one of these studies is positive, further tests are not necessary because extensive disease will have been confirmed. The decision as to which scan should be done first should be guided by any abnormalities detected on the baseline history, physical examination, and blood work.

in terms of outcome. In this era of increased competition for healthcare funds, greater fiscal responsibility on the part of the physician is essential, and it becomes increasingly necessary to limit diagnostic and therapeutic procedures to those that have significant impact on treatment decisions or treatment outcome. Richardson and colleagues[15] from the Navy Medical Oncology Branch of the National Cancer Institute developed an algorithm for staging SCLC patients. They recommend that patients should be staged using a sequence of procedures, rather than a standard battery of staging tests for all patients. They reported that approximately 20% of their patients were found to have ED on their initial history, physical examination, and routine biochemical screen. Those patients did not undergo any further scans. The patients who had no evidence of ED on their initial diagnostic evaluation underwent investigation of the bony skeleton first, followed by abdominal and then cranial CT. At each step, further testing was discontinued once a positive result was obtained. This series of staging procedures resulted in an overall cost saving of $1,418.00 per patient. The major factor in reducing costs was the concept of stopping subsequent staging procedures once a single site of distant metastatic disease had been identified.

Intrathoracic Staging

The plain posteroanterior and lateral chest radiograph is one of the most important diagnostic tests for patients with SCLC.[16] Its sensitivity, ease of performance, and low cost make this option the investigation of choice for repeated assessment of response during therapy. It is well recognized, though, that plain chest radiographs may underestimate the degree of chest wall invasion or involvement in the mediastinum either by direct extension of the tumor or by mediastinal lymph node metastases.

Computed Tomography

With the introduction of CT in the late 1970s, a giant step was taken in the ability to diagnose and stage lung cancer employing noninvasive imaging techniques. CT imaging confirms abnormalities seen on plain chest radiograph and can often detect lesions that cannot be resolved on chest radiograph. It also has played an important role in staging lung cancer, especially spread to areas of the mediastinum undetected on plain films, although perhaps it is more important for patients with NSCLC. There is a general agreement that normal mediastinal lymph nodes are less than 1 cm in transverse diameter. Any lymph node larger than this suggests lymphadenopathy and should be investigated further by more invasive techniques.[17,18]

CT also can suggest possible areas of local invasion of the primary tumor to chest wall, vertebrae, or mediastinal structures. Small pleural effusions or pleural nodules, often undetected on plain films and evident on CT, are of uncertain significance.[19,20]

An added advantage of CT scanning is the ability to detect abnormalities below the diaphragm, especially metastases to the liver and adrenal glands. CT for the investigation of lung cancer should include upper abdominal scanning to the level of the kidneys to include imaging of the liver and adrenal glands. With respect to determining metastatic spread to mediastinal lymph nodes, a large prospective study comparing the results of CT with pathologic staging of the mediastinum showed a sensitivity on a per-patient basis of 64% and a specificity of 62%. Although the likelihood of metastatic involvement increases with increasing size of lymph nodes, 15% of nodes less than 10 mm in size may contain tumor, and conversely, as many as one-third of lymph nodes measuring 2 to 4 cm in diameter may not contain tumor.[21–23] Although CT scans provide superior visualization of the soft tissues of the hila and mediastinum, confirmation of hilar or mediastinal lymph node involvement is not likely to alter treatment for most patients with SCLC. For that reason, CT scanning does not always play a critical role in the management of patients with this tumor, and the major uses of this diagnostic technique should be to plan radiotherapy for those patients found to have LD and to exclude patients with disease that cannot be encompassed in a tolerable radiotherapy port. In view of this, Richardson and colleagues[15] recommend delaying CT scanning until all other investigations have ruled out extrathoracic metastatic spread. This procedure could potentially reduce the number of CT scans needed by more than 60%. Unfortunately, however, many patients have already had a thoracic CT scan by the time they are referred to a medical oncologist. There is general agreement that magnetic resonance imaging (MRI) does not add significantly to plain chest radiograph or CT scanning for patients with SCLC.[24,25]

Although positron emission tomography (PET) is being explored extensively in NSCLC for staging purposes, very little information is presently available on its value in staging SCLC. Because of both the lack of data and the lack of PET scanners worldwide, its use for the staging of this malignancy must presently be considered experimental. Invasive staging procedures to define the extent of intrathoracic

tumor are seldom necessary for patients with SCLC. Fiberoptic bronchoscopy need not be undertaken, unless it is necessary to make a diagnosis. However, if bronchoscopic confirmation of complete response is required for patients participating in a research protocol, a pretreatment bronchoscopy is essential to compare results.[26] Similarly, mediastinoscopy is almost never required for patients with SCLC with the possible exception of the very small subgroup of patients with T1-2, N0 tumor who may be considered for surgical resection.[11]

Central Nervous System Metastases

Brain metastases are present at the time of initial diagnosis in approximately 10% of patients with SCLC[14,15] but may be present at autopsy in up to 65% of patients. Although MRI is probably superior to CT in the detection of brain and spinal cord metastases, CT scanning remains the most common staging investigation for the central nervous system. Because CT scanning is more sensitive than radionuclide scanning of the brain, it can identify considerably smaller tumor deposits. This method has the potential to significantly alter the prognostic implications of detecting metastatic disease in the brain. As shown by Dearing and colleagues[13] in their review of 411 patients with SCLC, brain involvement diagnosed by radionuclide scanning before December 1979 was associated with shorter survival, but this was not the case for patients treated thereafter who had their brain metastases documented by CT scanning. For the 19 patients in this series who presented with brain involvement as the only site of ED, survival was only slightly less than that of the LD patients. Other investigators have also reported that patients who have asymptomatic brain metastases diagnosed incidentally through staging procedures have a survival similar to that of LD patients.[27]

Leptomeningeal involvement and carcinomatous meningitis are infrequent at the time of initial diagnosis of SCLC. Therefore, lumbar puncture and cytologic analysis of the cerebral spinal fluid should not be considered a routine staging procedure and should be undertaken only if indicated by clinical symptoms. Several lumbar punctures may be required to confirm the meningeal involvement. MRI may contribute significantly to the diagnosis of carcinomatous meningitis and may be more helpful than myelography, which will not demonstrate the tumor unless nodular lesions are present along the nerve root sleeves or the spinal cord.

Abdominal Staging

The liver and adrenal glands are common sites of metastatic involvement in SCLC.[14,15,28] Radionuclide scanning of the liver has virtually been abandoned in favor of ultrasound and CT scanning, which have the potential to detect not only liver metastases but also adrenal and other abdominal metastases. Hirsch and colleagues[28,29] compared ultrasound and CT in a prospective study of seventy-seven patients undergoing staging for SCLC. For liver metastases, the diagnostic sensitivity, specificity, and negative predictive value were not statistically different, although the positive predictive value was slightly lower for CT than for ultrasound (0.67 versus 0.86). Conversely, extrahepatic abdominal metastases were diagnosed more often by CT than by ultrasound, and in 14% of patients, extrahepatic metastases were diagnosed exclusively by CT. The median survival was 458 days for the 36 patients classified as having LD after both CT and ultrasound, compared to 242 days for the patients with ED. The median survival for the 10 patients with stage migration from LD to ED based on CT alone was intermediate at 242 days. In the subgroup of 22 good performance status patients with normal serum LDH and alkaline phosphatase levels, the two-year survival was 31%. Five of these patients were downgraded from limited to ED by CT scanning. When these five patients were removed from the good prognostic group, the two-year survival rose to 41%.

Some investigators[30] have also recommended liver biopsies performed either under ultrasound guidance or by peritoneoscopy. In the prospective study discussed earlier, sixty patients underwent peritoneoscopy and biopsy as well as CT and ultrasound. In only one patient was metastatic disease identified by biopsy that had not been previously identified by CT or ultrasound. This result would indicate that invasive biopsy procedures are probably not indicated as a routine staging procedure. Dearing and colleagues[31] assessed the prognostic impact of demonstrating liver metastases by biopsy as opposed to CT scan. They demonstrated that liver metastases were associated with shorter survival when diagnosed by CT scan compared to those identified microscopically by a routine liver biopsy. This finding again demonstrates the important impact that the sensitivity of individual staging procedures may have on the assessment of survival of cancer patients.

Bone Marrow Staging

A bone marrow aspirate and trephine biopsy reveal involvement of the marrow by SCLC in 20% or more of patients at the time of initial diagnosis,[15,32] but in less than 5% of patients is this the only site of extrathoracic spread. Single iliac crest aspirations and biopsies are usually carried out, but some investigators have recommended bilateral biopsies. In contrast, oncologists have been questioning whether the bone marrow needs to be investigated. Campling and associates[33] were the first to report that bone marrow examination changed the stage in less than 5% of patients. Since then, similar results have been reported by other investigators,[34,35] and there appears to be general agreement that bone marrow examination should be performed only when no metastatic sites have been found. In fact, outside the clinical trial setting, bone marrow examination can probably be abandoned

completely for patients who have normal peripheral blood counts. This point is emphasized in a review by Shepherd.[36]

When more sensitive techniques are employed, a higher incidence of bone marrow involvement may be detected. Stahel and colleagues[37] used a monoclonal antibody reactive with the surface membrane of SCLC cells, SM1, and tumor cells were detected in 69% of patients examined with this technique, compared to only 16% when the bone marrow was examined only by routine microscopy. Unexpected marrow involvement has also been detected using systemically administered monoclonal antibodies,[35] and SCLC colonies have been grown from apparently normal bone marrow in the tumor stem cell assay.[34] Another method of possibly improving on the diagnosis of bone marrow involvement is the use of monoclonal antibody to MLuC1. In a recently published study,[38] when the bone marrow was incubated with this antibody, positive cells were detected in 38% of 108 samples 60 patients compared to only 13% of the biopsies not incubated with the antibody (p < 0.001), and these patients also had a poorer survival. Although these latter approaches may be useful for the evaluation of patients being assessed for possible autologous bone marrow transplantation, they must be considered research tools at this time and are not part of the routine evaluation of patients with SCLC. Many studies using MRI to evaluate bone marrow involvement by SCLC have been carried out.[39,40,41] This technique does seem to pick up involvement more often than other approaches but does not help to predict prognosis in these patients and, therefore, is still considered experimental in the staging of SCLC.

Biomarkers

Many biomarkers have been identified in patients with SCLC. Although they may correlate to the disease stage and provide some degree of prognostic information, most biomarkers have not proved to be useful independent prognostic indicators. Although rising levels of biomarkers may antedate clinical evidence of tumor relapse by several weeks or months, changes in tumor markers are seldom used to guide therapy.[42] The consensus is that biomarkers are of little value for pretreatment prognosis or as early markers of relapse. They add only to the cost and should at this time be considered as research tools.

The single exception is the serum LDH level. Several investigators have found this simple biochemical test to be an extremely useful prognostic factor.[3,5,6,43] Other more recent studies confirm the value of serum LDH levels as a good independent prognostic factor in this disease. It is an independent prognostic variable, and serial measurements often mirror clinical response. Furthermore, Sagman and associates[44] reported that LDH levels were rarely normal in patients with bone marrow involvement. They recommended that patients with normal LDH levels need not be subjected to invasive bone marrow staging procedures.

Although still controversial, many European studies suggest that elevated serum levels of neuron specific enolase (NSE) may be a useful marker to predict for a worse prognosis[45,46,47] This marker may be especially important because a high proportion of patients (88% in one study) have an elevated level of this marker at presentation;[45] therefore it may be possible to identify the small group of patients with normal levels who may have a particularly good survival. This marker is still not accepted as a routine to be used in patients with this disease. None of the markers discussed have been found to be better than clinical examination or imaging to detect early recurrence.[48]

Monoclonal Antibodies

Several groups evaluated the usefulness of monoclonal antibodies in the detection of bone marrow metastases in patients with SCLC. Balban and colleagues reported their results with a technetium-99mm–labeled monoclonal antibody (NRLU-10 Fab) administered intravenously, followed by total-body scanning 14 to 17 hours after injection. Fifteen patients were studied, and metastases to the marrow compartment were identified in one patient who had known bone marrow involvement. Unexpected radioactive marrow uptake led to the reassessment of the bone marrow and histologic confirmation of metastatic disease in two patients.

Skov and associates[49] evaluated a panel of monoclonal antibodies using immunohistochemical techniques in the diagnosis of bone marrow infiltration. Although the monoclonal antibodies detected tumor deposits in patients with known involvement, they did not detect metastatic tumor in bone marrow sections from patients who did not have tumor identified by routine histologic examination.

Monoclonal antibody imaging techniques appear to be neither sensitive nor specific enough to replace any of the staging procedures more commonly in use. Nonetheless, monoclonal antibody staging of the bone marrow is potentially beneficial for the small proportion of patients who may be considered for high-dose chemotherapy and autologous bone marrow transplantation, should this type of treatment prove successful in future trials. Anti-Hu antibodies (HuAb) recognize antigens expressed by neurons and SCLC. In a recent study involving 196 patients, the presence of the antibody at diagnosis of patients with SCLC was found to be a strong and independent prognostic factor that predicted for complete response and hence prolonged survival.[50] This interesting data requires confirmation.

Many studies have been conducted to evaluate iii octreotide scans for staging patients with SCLC.[51,52,53,54,55] Although some of these studies are encouraging, many do not support its general use at the present time. It rarely detects disease not detected by other imaging techniques.

Other new markers, such as vascular endothelial growth factor, (VEG-F)[56] TPS and CYFRA-21-1,[57] look promising as possible future prognostic factors in patients with SCLC

based on the preliminary data from the quoted studies, whereas the presence or absence of anti-*p53* antibodies does not look encouraging in this regard.[58]

Restaging

Plain chest radiographs provide a simple and cost-effective way to follow patients and assess response during treatment for SCLC. However, as reported by Quoix and associates,[59] the ability to reliably assess tumor size on chest radiographs falls considerably after treatment. Nonetheless, it should not be necessary to repeat CT scans routinely unless a radiotherapy decision needs to be made. For patients with LD who have responded to chemotherapy, little is to be gained by routine restaging of extrathoracic sites. In a retrospective study reported by Feld and colleagues[60] for the National Cancer Institute of Canada, posttreatment bronchoscopy revealed residual disease in 9% of patients who had achieved complete clinical response based on radiologic assessment. A small survival benefit was demonstrated for the subgroup of patients who had a negative posttreatment bronchoscopy, but because all patients received radiotherapy, the results of this investigation did not alter treatment strategies for any patient. The investigators suggested, therefore, that posttreatment bronchoscopy should be undertaken only in clinical trials. An economic analysis that was also part of this study supported the concept of not undertaking extrathoracic restaging. In contrast, Stahel[14] still recommends restaging, including repeat bronchoscopy.

New Concepts for Staging

Although the simple LD and ED staging system for SCLC has provided worthwhile prognostic and therapeutic information for several decades, analyses of large patient databases from several cooperative groups have identified subgroups of patients within both the LD and ED categories who have significantly different prognoses. Shepherd and colleagues[11] reported significantly longer survival for patients with LD who had no evidence of mediastinal lymph node involvement, obstructive pneumonia, or pleural effusion. This subgroup of patients had a projected five-year survival of 25%, and because this group of patients represents most of the five-year survivors in this disease, an imbalance of this group in a clinical trial could have major consequences on the interpretation of outcome.

Albain and colleagues[5] for the Southwest Oncology Group, and Sagman and colleagues,[43] for the University of Toronto Group, have analyzed multiple prognostic variables using recursive partitioning and amalgamation techniques to refine the two-stage system.

PROGNOSTIC FACTORS

A general truism of both clinical and biologic aspects of SCLC is its remarkable heterogeneity. Studies of prognostic factors aim directly or indirectly to explain the nature of this heterogeneity. It has therefore become the goal of investigators to identify and assess prognostic factors as predictors of the natural history of the disease. Both practical and theoretic reasons for studying prognostic factors exist, particularly as they relate to SCLC. *A priori*, it should be possible to predict the outcome of patients with disease with a great degree of accuracy. The assessment of prognostic factors also allows for valid comparison in assessing the results of treatment. As such, prognostic factors are used to stratify patients into comparable prognostic groups. In the design of clinical studies, prognostic factors are used to define eligibility criteria or assignment of patients into specific risk groups. Prognostic factors therefore aid in the stratification of patients and aim to minimize confounding factors that may influence the results of treatment. Prognostic factors may also serve as a guide in the selection of alternative treatment for patients both in clinical studies and in the management of individual patients. Finally, prognostic factors may clarify the understanding of the natural history of the disease and hence may provide insight into further studies.

Relation to Staging

The primary role of staging investigations is to assess tumor bulk and its anatomic distribution. The extent of detectable tumor spread, however, has inherent limitations in predicting the natural history of the disease, and in fact measurable extent of disease may not necessarily reflect the aggressivity of the tumor. Staging, therefore, cannot be used in isolation in making accurate prognostication. The influence of other factors that may reflect tumor activity must complement clinical staging. The identification of prognostic attributes that reflect the biologic behavior of tumors have led to the realization that several factors provide separate and additional value in the prediction of disease outcome. In turn, efforts have been mounting to exploit the collective impact and influence of select prognostic factors in addition to disease extent.

Chronology

The most consistent prognostic attribute in SCLC in the past was extent of disease as determined by staging investigations. Disease extent partitions patients into those with disease confined to a hemithorax (LD) and those with disease outside those confines (ED). As demonstrated universally and by data from the Toronto group (Figure 34.1), the probability of survival for LD patients is significantly superior relative to that for patients with ED. Further progress in the identification and assessment of prognostic factors in SCLC has evolved along two principal paths. First, it has become apparent that the current staging system lacks stringency and, in fact, may not reflect tumor burden accurately, so that dissection of each stage by further assessment of

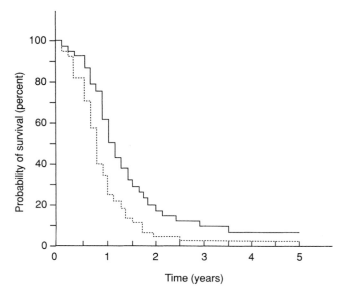

FIGURE 34.1. Overall survival curves from date of first treatment for patients grouped by extent of disease.

tumor bulk is essential. As illustrated in Figure 34.2, evidently, patients with LD can be further divided into those with and without mediastinal involvement, and the number of metastatic sites further segregates patients with ED. Consequently, four distinct prognostic groups are formed. Furthermore, the actual metastatic site bears prognostic significance in patients with ED, as illustrated by the uniformly grave outcome for those with brain involvement and the more favorable prognosis for those with bone metastasis relative to patients with liver spread (Figure 34.3). The amalgamation of patients into either disease category under the current system enshrines prognostic biases that may have deleterious bearing on treatment planning approaches and on the interpretation of response to treatment.

Second, it has become clear that clinical staging is an important prognostic factor but of a different nature from biologic factors. The influence of biologic prognostic factors are to be seen as a measure of tumor aggressivity and must complement clinical staging. As an example, in Figure 34.4, elevated levels of serum LDH in patients with LD predict poorer survival relative to patients with LDH in the normal range. Moreover, the survival of a subset of LD patients, those with markedly elevated levels of LDH, is not significantly different from that of patients with ED.

Emphasis on the further assessment of tumor bulk and the identification of substances that reflect the biologic behavior of tumors have led to the identification of numerous

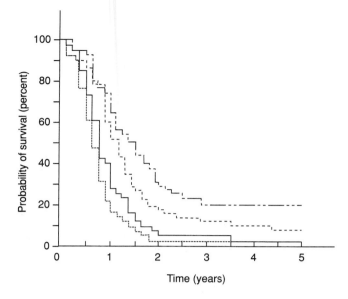

Disease Stage	Number of patients	Median survival time (weeks)	
– · – LD (-MED)	46	69	
– – – LD (+MED)	197	52	
——— ED (= 1 site)	172	38	p=0.0001
·········· ED (> 1 site)	139	31	

FIGURE 34.2. Overall survival curves from date of first treatment according to mediastinal involvement for patients with limited disease (LD) and according to number of metastatic sites for patients with extensive disease (ED).

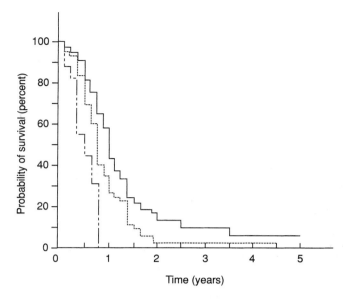

Extensive disease sites	Number of patients	Median survival time (weeks)	
——— A. bone other	(57)	49	
·········· B. liver bone marrow nodes	(104)	36	p=0.00005
– · – C. brain	(11)	22	

FIGURE 34.3. Overall survival curves from date of first treatment for patients with extensive disease according to specific sites of metastasis.

prognostic factors in SCLC. These factors encompass attributes of clinical determinants, tumor markers, routine laboratory parameters, biologic features, and host factors. Table 34.2 outlines the most important of these prognostic factors. The realization that several factors provide separate and additional value in the prediction of disease outcome forged the basis for analysis of multivariate prognostic models. These models, in turn, seek to exploit the collective impact and importance of select prognostic factors. Multivariate models inherently depend on the methodology used for their development. Traditional and novel methods have been used in the analysis of multivariate models. These methods are described in more detail before a discussion of multivariate prognostic models for SCLC.

STATISTICAL METHODS FOR PROGNOSTIC STRATIFICATION

Standard methods for forming prognostic strata are the familiar statistical tools used to explore censored survival data, such as the Kaplan-Meier estimator of the survival function,[61] the logrank test statistic for assessing differences in

survival between two or more groups,[62] and Cox's proportional hazards regression model.[63] These methods are well known and often used for developing prognostic stratifications. In addition, tree-based methods for exploring survival data have been developed and are particularly useful for forming prognostic groupings of patients.

Tree-Based Methods for Survival Data

Tree-based methods, often called *recursive partitioning methods*, have found applications in many scientific fields, including pattern recognition, artificial intelligence, and medicine. Tree-based methods have several advantages over traditional linear model methods such as linear regression, logistic regression, or the Cox regression models. Probably most important to clinicians, the decision tree representation of the model can yield easier interpretations than linear models, especially for classification and prognostic stratification. Although the tree-based methods have been in existence since the early 1960s,[64] advances in the methodology, as included in the Classification and Regression Tree (CART) algorithm of Breiman, Friedman, Olshen, and

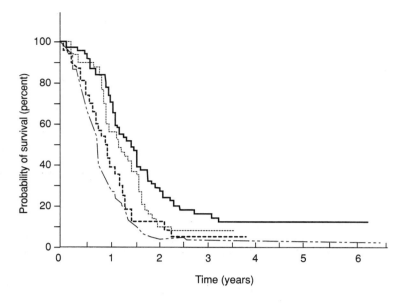

Extent of disease	LDH (IU/L)	Number of patients	Median survival time (weeks)	
—— LD	0-193	76	62	p<0.0042
········· LD	194-274	39	56	
- - - - LD	275-999	26	37	p≤0.3000
– · – ED	0-999	328	35	

FIGURE 34.4. Survival curves from date of first treatment for patients grouped by extent of disease and by different ranges of pretreatment serum lactate dehydrogenase (LDH) levels.

Stone,[65] and the availability of software have helped tree-based methods become popular tools for classification.

Tree-based methods as applied to prognostic classification models can be described as follows: A rule splits the initial patient population into two groups according to a splitting rule that maximizes their differences. This splitting rule is applied repeatedly until all the patient population has been split into prognostic groups, each containing only a few observations. The partition is represented as a binary tree. The data within each of the prognostic groups is assumed to be relatively homogenous. Therefore, for survival data, the simple Kaplan-Meier estimate of the survival function can be used to describe prognosis in each group. Typically, a large tree or model that overfits the data is formed to ensure that all possible distinct prognostic groups have been investigated, and the tree is then "pruned" back. This process is analogous to forward stepwise regression and backward stepwise regression methods that are available in many statistical packages. A schematic of the recursive partitioning approach is depicted in Figure 34.5.

Tree-based methods for survival data that adopt most aspects of the CART algorithm have been proposed by several authors.[66–70] Although differences exist in the algorithms, basic components of the tree-based methods for survival data include general rules. For the sake of brevity, these have been expounded on in the Appendix at the end of this chapter and are outlined under the headings.

Multivariate Models

During the past decade, at least nine groups reported on multivariate assessment of prognostic factors for SCLC. These models used different statistical methodologies, with most employing proportional hazard models (Table 34.3). Some conclusions could be drawn from the tabulation of factors incorporated into these models. The first is that each model uses a different permutation of prognostic factors; that is, no two models used identical factors. Second, most models used factors in addition to those employed in clinical practice, such as disease extent and performance status. For example, mediastinal status in LD and sites of disease in ED, and age and sex as attributes of disease bulk and patient characteristics, respectively, were predominant in most models. These same conclusions are further illustrated with the incorporation of biologic attributes in these same models. These attributes included serum LDH and alkaline phosphatase biochemically; aspartate transaminase, albumin, urate, sodium, and bicarbonate, serologically; and hematologic parameters, such as hemoglobin and total white blood cell count. Here, in fact, some models have not incorporated any of these biologic attributes, whereas others used them exclusively in their models.

Reasons for the analysis of multiple prognostic factors vary. The methods of analysis used may depend heavily on the reasons for doing the analysis. In considering assessment of multiple factors, interactions between prognostic factors

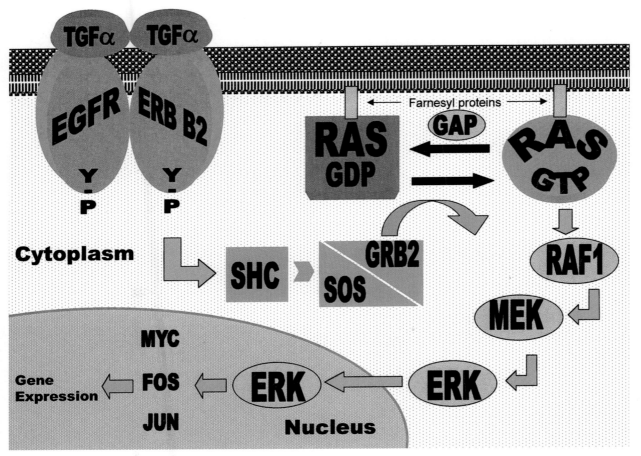

COLOR FIGURE 4.1. *Ras* signaling transduction pathway. *Ras* functions as a switch to relay extracellular ligand-stimulated signals from the inner cell membrane surface through the cytoplasm, and to the nucleus. The pathway places *RAS* downstream from a receptor tyrosine kinase, such as the epidermal growth factor receptor (EGFR)/ERB B2 heterodimer, and upstream of multiple serine/threonine kinases. A signal can be carried from outside the cell to the cell nucleus, where activated extracellular signal-regulated kinase (ERK) can be transported across the nuclear membrane and activate transcription factors known as *MYC*, JUN, and FOS. Tumor growth factor alpha (TGF-α), Src homologous complex (SHC), Son of Sevenless (SOS), growth factor response binding protein (GRB2), GTPase activating protein (GAP), guanosine diphosphate (GDP), guanosine triphosphate (GTP), MAPK/ERK kinase (MEK). (From Vojtek AB, Der CJ. Increasing complexity of the Ras signaling pathway. *J Biol Chem* 1998;273:19925, with permission.)

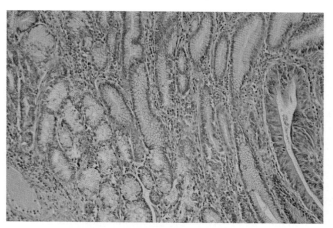

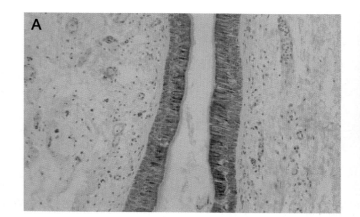

COLOR FIGURE 8.4. Immunohistochemistry of a gastric adeno-carcinoma for expression of Fhit protein. As shown in the figure, the normal gastric epithelial cells stain strongly positive for Fhit, whereas the adenocarcinoma cells are completely negative. (From Croce C, Sozzi G, Huebner K. Role of FHIT in human cancer. *J Clin Oncol* 1999;17:1618, with permission.)

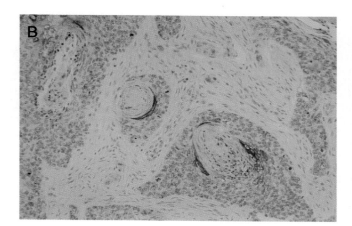

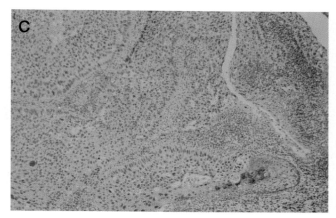

COLOR FIGURE 8.5. Loss of Fhit expression in human non–small cell lung carcinoma (hNSCLC). As shown in **(A)** all cells of the normal bronchus stain positively with the anti-Fhit antibody. On the contrary, NSCLCs are negative for Fhit expression **(B,C)**. (From Croce C, Sozzi G, Huebner K. Role of FHIT in human cancer. *J Clin Oncol* 1999;17:1618; Sozzi G, Pastorino U, Moiraghi L, et al. *Cancer Res* 1998;58:5032, both with permission.)

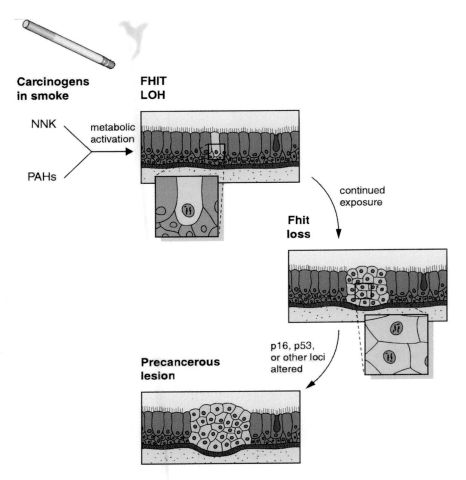

Carcinogens in smoke

NNK

PAHs

metabolic activation

FHIT LOH

continued exposure

Fhit loss

p16, p53, or other loci altered

Precancerous lesion

COLOR FIGURE 8.6. Tobacco smoking causes loss of function of the *FHIT* gene. Carcinogens present in tobacco smoke cause deletion in a *FHIT* allele. Continued exposure causes deletion in the second allele, leading to loss of Fhit expression. *FHIT* alterations and then mutations in p16, *p53,* and other loci cause precancerous lesions (bronchial dysplasia), some of which will later evolve into frank carcinomas (From Heubner K, Sozzi G, Brenner C, et al. *FHIT* loss in lung cancer: diagnostic and therapeutic implication. *Adv Oncology* 1999:15;3, with permission.)

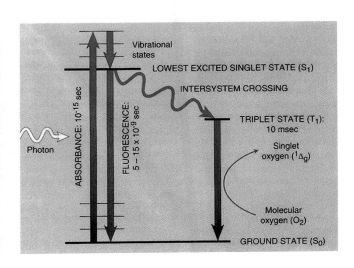

Photon

ABSORBANCE: 10⁻¹⁵ sec

FLUORESCENCE: 5 – 15 × 10⁻⁹ sec

Vibrational states

LOWEST EXCITED SINGLET STATE (S_1)

INTERSYSTEM CROSSING

TRIPLET STATE (T_1): 10 msec

Singlet oxygen ($^1\Delta_g$)

Molecular oxygen (O_2)

GROUND STATE (S_0)

COLOR FIGURE 24.1. Energy states and interaction of photosensitizing agents. Before exposure to light, a molecule of sensitizer is in the ground state. When a photon of the appropriate wavelength is absorbed, an electron is raised to a higher energy level. The molecule then rearranges to a stable excited state. At this point, there are two possibilities. The excited molecule can fluoresce, emitting a photon and dropping back to the ground state, or an intersystem crossing can change the spin of an electron. During the lifetime of the resulting triplet state, absorbed energy can be passed along to molecular oxygen in tissue, activating the oxygen molecule to the singlet state. Singlet oxygen can oxidize any oxidizable biologic molecule with which it is in contact. (From Kessel D. Photodynamic therapy. *Sci Med* 1998;5:46, with permission.)

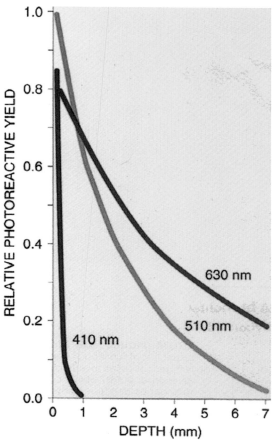

COLOR FIGURE 24.2. The relative phototoxic effect of a sensitizer is a function of irradiation wavelength. Longer wavelengths penetrate tissue to a greater depth. (From Kessel D. Photodynamic therapy. *Sci Med* 1998;5:46, with permission.)

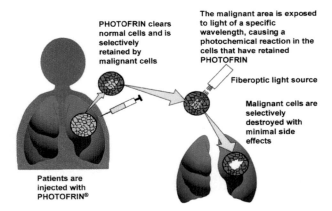

PHOTOFRIN clears normal cells and is selectively retained by malignant cells

The malignant area is exposed to light of a specific wavelength, causing a photochemical reaction in the cells that have retained PHOTOFRIN

Fiberoptic light source

Malignant cells are selectively destroyed with minimal side effects

Patients are injected with PHOTOFRIN®

COLOR FIGURE 24.4. Schema of photodynamic therapy for bronchial lesions. See text for details. (Courtesy of Dr. Jeffrey Wiemann, Louisville, Kentucky.)

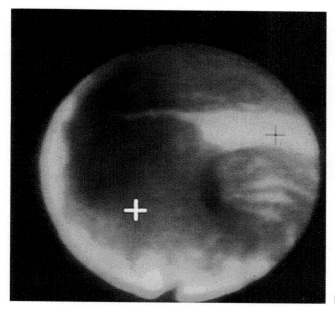

B

COLOR FIGURE 24.3. B: Reddish brown fluorescence of carcinoma *in situ* distinguished from the green fluorescence of normal bronchial mucosa. (Courtesy of XILLIX Technologies Corporation, British Columbia, Canada.)

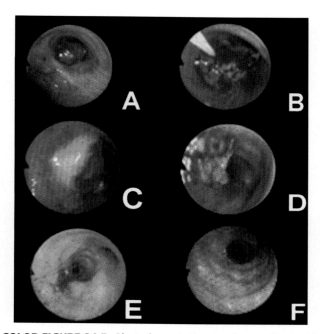

COLOR FIGURE 24.5. Photodynamic therapy for a patient with partial obstruction of the right mainstem bronchus. A: 90% obstructive non–small cell lung cancer 0.5 cm from the main carina. B: Laser fiber is positioned for interstitial treatment 48 hours after the patient received Photofrin II. C: Appearance of the lesion 48 hours after treatment before any debridement of the avascular base. D: Appearance of the lesion base after bronchoscopic debridement revealing the right upper lobe orifice to the right and the bronchus intermedius straight ahead. E: Appearance of the airway 2 months later. Only a superficial ulcer is present at the site of the original lesion F: Appearance of the airway 3 months after treatment. A histological complete response was documented.

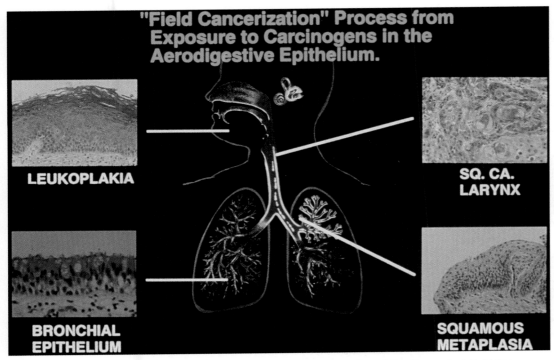

COLOR FIGURE 25.1. A Schematic and Pathologic Representation of the Concept of Field Cancerization: Epithelium throughout the respiratory tract is affected by similar toxins, hence the concern about second primary cancer prevention.

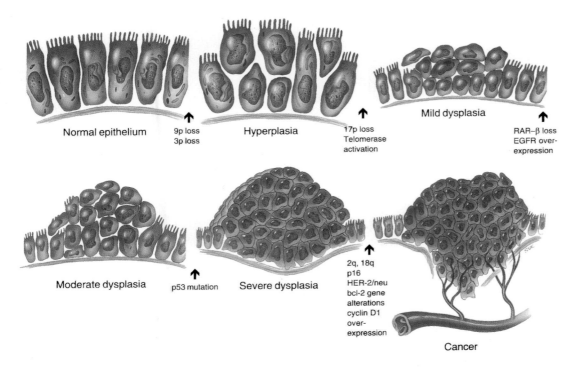

COLOR FIGURE 25.2. Multi-step Process of Lung Carcinogenesis: A schema of molecular changes that have been reported to occur during the multi-step lung carcinogenic process. While representing potential points for intervention (i.e., chemoprevention), these events could potentially (once available) serve as biomarkers of cancer risk and intermediate end points for clinical studies. (From Papadimitrakopoulou VA. New developments in the chemoprevention of lung cancer. *Prim Care Cancer* 1998;18[Suppl. 1]:52.)

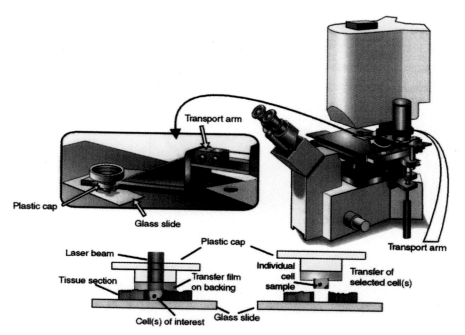

COLOR FIGURE 27.1. Laser capture microdissection (LCM) system showing the process of microdissection of cells from tissue. The laser beam activates the thermoplastic film embedding the underlying cells, which can then be separated from the tissue.

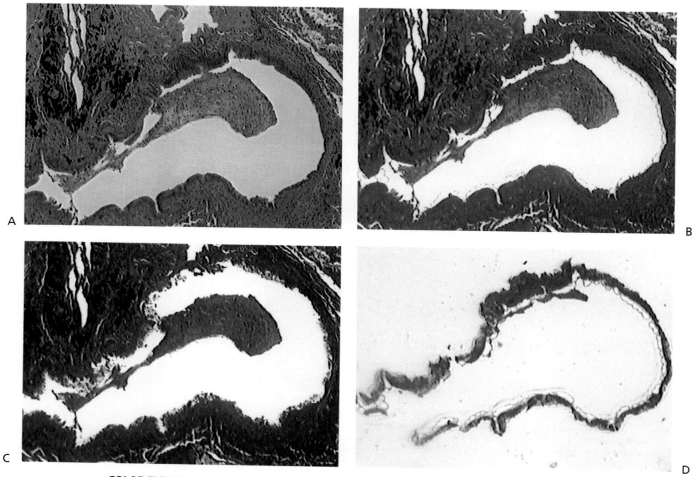

COLOR FIGURE 27.2. Microdissection of normal bronchiolar epithelium. **A:** roadmap, **(B)** before microdissection, **(C)** after microdissection, and **(D)** cap with dissected tissue (200X magnification).

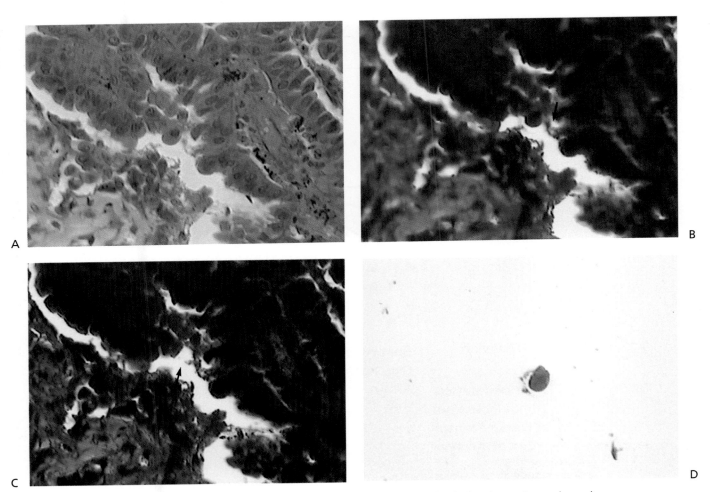

COLOR FIGURE 27.3. Microdissection of a single cell from bronchioloalveolar carcinoma (*arrow*); **A:** roadmap, **(B)** before microdissection, **(C)** after microdissection, and **(D)** cap demonstrating microdissected cell (1000X magnification).

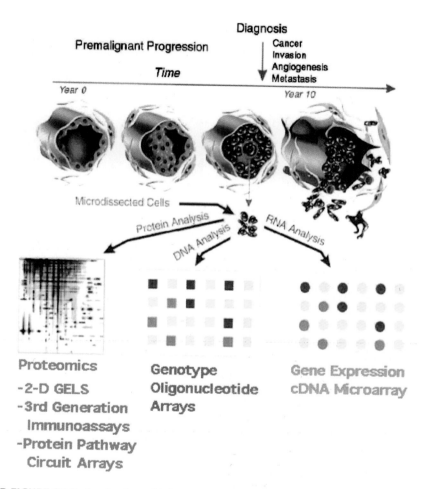

COLOR FIGURE 27.4. Application of LCM to study the molecular events associated with cancer progression. The expression pattern of proteins (two-dimensional gel electrophoresis or immunoassays), RNA (differential display, microarray hybridization, or cDNA libraries), and DNA genotype (mutational analysis, loss of heterozygosity, comparative genomic hybridization) can be compared within the same patient. In the tissue section, normal precursor epithelium, premalignant lesions, and invasive cancer foci can be microdissected and compared.

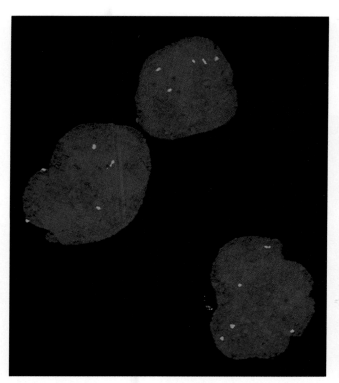

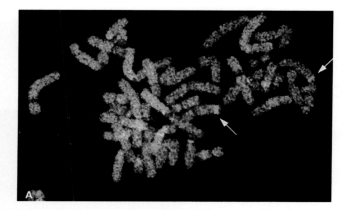

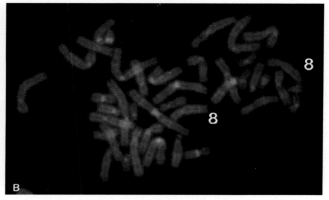

COLOR FIGURE 28.4. Fluorescence *in situ* hybridization of two chromosome-specific centromere repeat probes to interphase cell nuclei, counterstained blue with diamidino-2-phenylindole, from a human non–small cell lung cancer specimen. DNA probes labeled with biotin or digoxigenin hybridizing to complementary centromere sequences within the nuclei were detected by immunofluorescence using fluorophores emitting green (fluorescein isothiocyanate) or red (rhodamine). The nuclei exhibit abnormally high numbers of chromosome 7 (red spots) and chromosome 18 (green) fluorescent signals, indicative of gains of these chromosomes.

COLOR FIGURE 28.5. A: Computer-generated fluorescence ratio image of a normal human metaphase spread after comparative genome hybridization with biotin-labeled DNA, detected by fluorescein isothiocyanate (FITC), from a lung cancer cell line, and digoxigenin-labeled DNA, detected by rhodamine, from normal placenta. Yellow-green indicates balance between the FITC and rhodamine values. Bright green indicates overrepresentation of DNA in the tumor, and red represents underrepresentation of tumor DNA. Intense green fluorescence on chromosome 8q24 (*arrows*) suggests that the MYC protooncogene located in this band may be amplified in the lung cancer cells. **B:** The same metaphase spread, stained with diamidino-2-phenylindole, which permits the identification of each chromosome. The two copies of chromosome 8 are indicated by numbers.

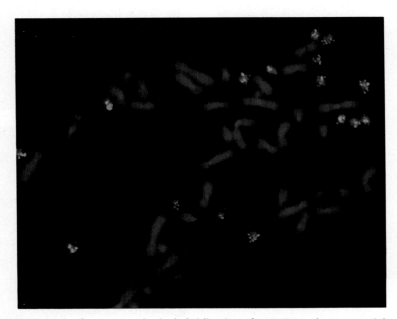

COLOR FIGURE 28.6. Fluorescence *in situ* hybridization of a MYCN probe to a partial metaphase spread from the small cell lung cancer cell line. Multiple fluorescent signals are observed on each of the double minutes, indicating that the amplified *MYCN* oncogene resides within these small chromatin bodies.

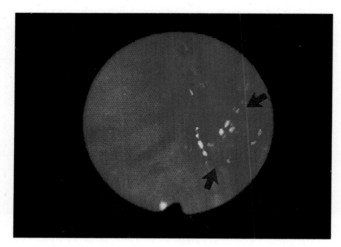

COLOR FIGURE 31.1. Endobronchial mass occluding a segmental bronchus.

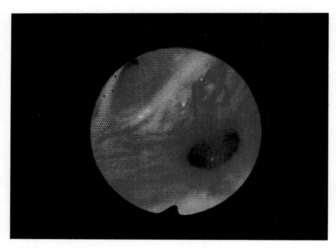

COLOR FIGURE 31.2. Submucosal infiltration of bronchogenic carcinoma. Normal bronchial markings are lost and engorged bronchial collateral vessels are prominent.

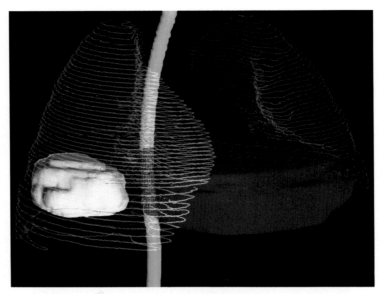

COLOR FIGURE 48.5. A: Lung cancer tumor target and normal organs displayed in "room view."
B: Multiple images of anteropostero (AP) beam from lung cancer treatment. Note in the upper-right image that the green contour CTV does not have an adequate margin around the red GTV contour. This is because a 3D margin tool to generate the CTV was not used, thus only 2D margins were generated.

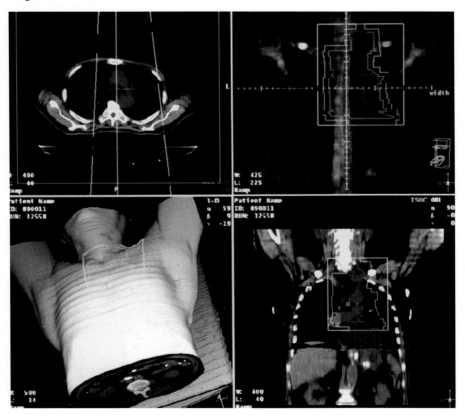

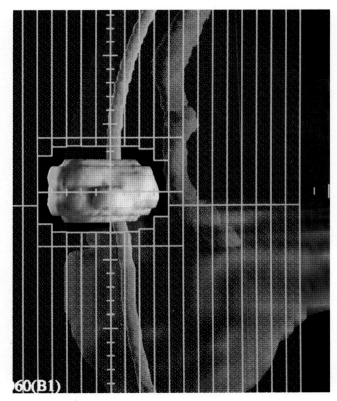

COLOR FIGURE 48.6. Beam's eye view of tumor with port defined by multileaf colimation.

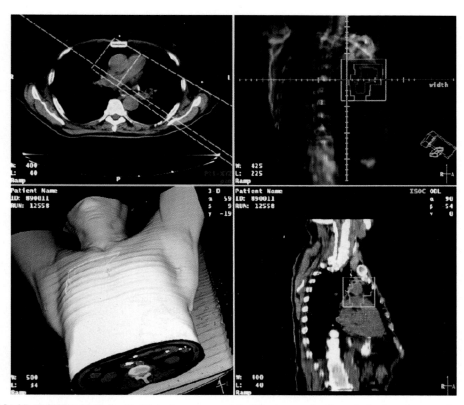

COLOR FIGURE 48.7 A: Multiple images used in 3D plan evaluation, including "room view," beam's eye view, axial, and saggital views.

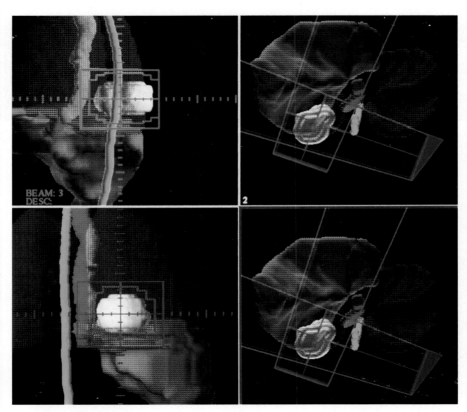

COLOR FIGURE 48.7 B: Multiple images used in 3D plan evaluation, including "room view," beam's eye view, axial, and saggital views.

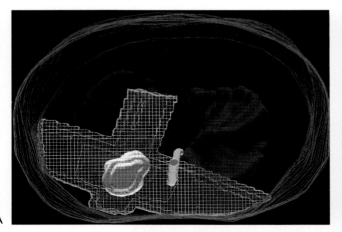

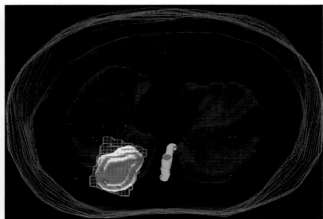

COLOR FIGURE 48.8 A,B,C: Various images depicting isodose coverage and various dose levels in 3D.

TABLE 34.2. SUMMARY OF PROGNOSTIC FACTORS IN SMALL CELL LUNG CANCER

Prognostic Factor	References
Clinical Features	
Age	7, 39, 54, 55, 56
Sex	39, 55
Performance status	39, 54, 55
Weight change	39, 55
Disease extent	39, 54, 55, 56
Mediastinal spread (limited disease)	11, 35, 39
Site of primary tumor	39
Number of metastasis	39
Liver metastasis	39, 55, 57
Brain metastasis	39, 55, 57
Bone marrow metastasis	39, 55, 57
Bone metastasis	39, 55, 57
Laboratory Parameters (Common)	
Serum lactate dehydrogenase	5, 33, 39
Alkaline phosphatase	5, 39
Albumin	58
Serum glutamic-oxaloacetic transaminase, serum glutamate pyruvate transaminase	58
Sodium	39, 55
Uric acid	55
Hemoglobin	39, 55
White blood cell count	39, 55
Platelets	39
Serologic Markers	
Carcinoembryonic antigen	37, 39, 59, 60
Neuron-specific enolase	59, 61, 62, 63, 64
Kinase	65
Calcitonin	59
Tissue polypeptide antigen	66
Ferritin	67
Protein-bound carbohydrates	68
Urinary polyamines	69
Paraneoplastic Syndromes	
Syndrome of inappropriate antidiuretic hormone	70, 71
Cushing syndrome	72
Biologic Factors	
Neuroendocrine features	73
Oncogene products	74
Oncogene abnormalities	74
Growth factors and receptors	75
Flow cytometry	76
Cell lines (*in vitro*)	77
Small cell lung cancer subtyping	78
Host Immune Factors	
Delayed skin hypersensitivity	79

are important and, in fact, not explored fully by the proportional hazard models. Therefore, other multivariate methods were evaluated in the analysis of prognostic factors in SCLC.

Tree Classification Approach

As a statistical tool, recursive partition and amalgamation algorithm have been developed in an effort to integrate clustering and amalgamation techniques into a biomedical context. The tree classification methodology and respective computer program have been detailed elsewhere.[67] In its application to data on SCLC, the aim of the analysis is to define homogeneous prognostic strata on the basis of censored survival times. At the University of Toronto Hospitals, we have accrued retrospective data on 614 patients with SCLC entered into four therapeutic studies during a ten-year interval (1976 to 1985). Twenty-one prognostic factors encompassing attributes of both clinical and biologic significance were evaluated by the tree classification method. Figure 34.6 illustrates the tree classification model for the patients with SCLC. Disease extent, the first split decision statement, partitions the initial population into those with LD and ED. Subsequent partitioning of those with LD ensues by knowledge of mediastinal status, white blood cell count, sex, and serum LDH. Patients with ED are further partitioned by the attributes, performance status, serum alkaline phosphatase, sex, and liver involvement. Ultimately, the amalgamation of eight terminal nodes elaborates four prognostic groups. The respective survival curves of the groups are illustrated in Figure 34.7.

Several features are important to emphasize regarding the tree classification model. First, in contrast to multivariate regression models, in which prognostic factors impart global influences, the tree classification model emphasizes interactions among prognostic factors and hence identifies the importance of specific prognostic factors to specific subpopulations of patients. Second, the assignment of patients by the tree classification model into four prognostic groups defies the conventional two-stage classification for SCLC and, hence, infers that the current staging system has inherent limitations. In fact, the intermediate prognostic groups (B and C; see Figure 34.6) are obtained by amalgamating nodes issuing from both the ED and LD categories. Finally, the model clearly shows that patients in each prognostic group are easily identified by a constellation of distinct prognostic attributes. A particular advantage of the tree classification model, then, is that the identification and definition of prognostic groups in clinical terms enable the application of complex prognostic analysis to direct clinical settings.

Consensus Model

As joint consideration of many prognostic factors led to development of diverse prognostic models, a need to establish a consensus model evolved. Ideal methodology to achieve this aim is being sought to enable applications both in clinical trials and in the management of individual patients. Toward this end, efforts have been mounting to develop a new prognostic classification for SCLC through an overview analysis of available collective data.

A working schema for the attainment of a consensus model through an overview analysis has been developed. The analysis was based on an aggregated pool of prognostic data from diverse international centers conducting studies

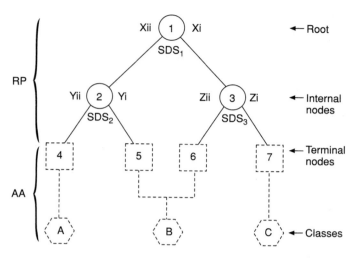

FIGURE 34.5. The first split decision statement (SDS) allocates patients into internal nodes 2 and 3 as stipulated by covariates Xii and Xi, respectively. Recursive splitting of nodes 2 and 3 by SDS$_2$ and SDS$_3$ culminates in four terminal nodes dictated by covariates Yi and Yii for nodes 4 and 5, respectively, and Zi and Zii for nodes 7 and 6, respectively. Terminal nodes 4 and 7 are distinctly different with regard to the outcome criteria, and hence by definition are designated as classes A and C, respectively. Terminal nodes 5 and 6, which originate from different internal nodes, are similar with regard to the outcome criteria and hence are amalgamated into a homogeneous class, B. Classes A, B, and C are homogeneous and by definition significantly different from each other. Recursive partitioning steps are outlined by solid lines, and the amalgamation algorithm by broken lines. Note that the root defines the initial patient population.

on lung cancer. The tree classification methodology was chosen for the analysis as a vehicle for use both in clinical trials and in the management of individual patients. The variables selected to define the resulting four prognostic groups allocated a pivotal role to serum LDH in addition to extent of disease and performance status.[71] The other prognostic variables chosen to define prognostic groups included age, sex, and the present of brain metastases. The consensus model was tested for each individual center participating in the overview analysis. Similar prognostic groups were obtained for each center.

The consensus model confirms the importance of select prognostic attributes that bear on disease outcome in addition to knowledge of disease extent, which traditionally is assessed by staging procedures. The impact of newer approaches to prognostication and staging in SCLC is yet to be fully realized in patient care. However, as more effective treatments evolve, it is hoped that staging strategies and disease prognostication will bear more extensively on direct patient management, clinical studies, and healthcare costs.

Recent Studies

A group of Danish investigators tried to identify a subset of SCLC patients at increased risk for early death due to treatment.[72] They looked at a population of 937 patients on recent randomized trials by this group. Poor performance status, high serum LDH at presentation, and initial therapy with epipodophyllotoxins (etoposide and tenoposide) and cisplatin during the first course of therapy predicted for a high risk of early toxic death. They produced an algorithm to remove the high-risk patients from clinical trials to minimize early deaths. The Medical Research Council in Great Britain also posed a similar question.[73] This kind of data could be very useful if it is confirmed by others.

A 408-patient study evaluated the prognostic significance

TABLE 34.3. MULTIVARIATE ASSESSMENT OF PROGNOSTIC FACTORS IN SMALL CELL LUNG CANCER

	Statistical Method	Disease Extent					Patient Characteristics			Biologic Attributes								
		DE	LD	ED	Med	STS	PS	Age	Sex	LDH	AP	AST	Alb	Urt	Sod	HCO	HG	WBC
Stanley et al, 1980[80]	ψ	X				X	X											
Souhami et al, 1985[81]	PH						X				X		X		X			X
Osterlind et al, 1986[55]	PH						X		X	X				X	X			
Sagman et al, 1986[39]	TC																	
Cerney et al, 1987[82]	PH	X					X			X	X				X	X		
Vincent et al, 1987[57]	PH						X					X	X					
Spiegelman et al, 1989[83]	PH	X			X	X	X		X									
Albain et al, 1989[5]	TC	X						X		X							X	
Shinkau et al, 1989[84]	PH	X				X	X	X	X									

ψ, ψ statistic; PH, proportional hazard model; TC, tree classification model; DE, disease extent; LD, limited disease; ED, extensive disease; Med, mediastinal disease; STS, number/site of metastasis; PS, performance status; LDH, lactate dehydrogenase; AP, alkaline phosphatase; AST, alanine transaminase; Alb, albumin; Urt, urate; Sod, sodium; HCO, bicarbonate; HG, hemoglobin; WBC, white blood cell count.

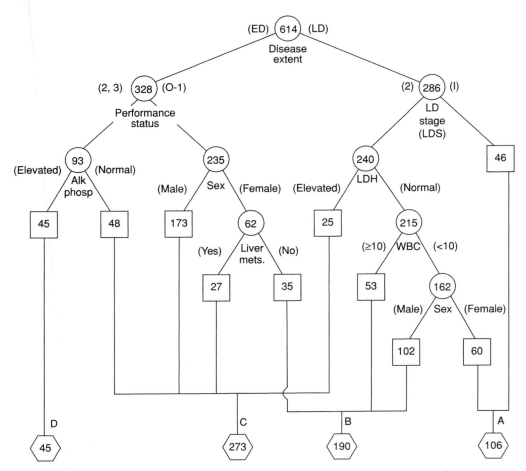

FIGURE 34.6. Tree classification model for patients with small cell lung cancer. Classes A, B, C, and D are homogeneous and significantly different from each other. By definition, leftward branchings and increasing class order denote poorer prognosis. LDH, lactate dehydrogenase; LD, limited disease stage; ED, extensive disease.

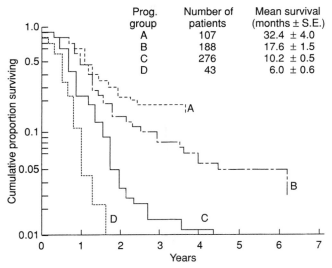

Prog. group	Number of patients	Mean survival (months ± S.E.)
A	107	32.4 ± 4.0
B	188	17.6 ± 1.5
C	276	10.2 ± 0.5
D	43	6.0 ± 0.6

FIGURE 34.7. Survival curves for the prognostic groups identified in the tree classification model.

of the presence or absence of superior vena cava syndrome as part of the initial presentation of SCLC patients.[74] They were surprised to find that the syndrome was not a negative prognostic factor. Rapid treatment with present-day active combination chemotherapy along with the high response rate usually makes this syndrome nonissue, but this data confirms our clinical impression and allows us to reassure patients regarding this common and somewhat terrible syndrome.

An English group looked at the value of other prognostic models in this disease and developed a prognostic index that included initial serum LDH, hypoalbuminemia, neutrophilia, disease extent, and performance status.[75] The index defined three different risk groups with quite different survivals, but this data was not very different from other published studies on this subject.

A Danish cooperative group published an important study looking at the characteristics of long-term survivors (5 and 10 + years) treated for SCLC.[76] Seventeen hundred and fourteen consecutive patients were included in the study. The characteristics of the patient's surviving 5 to 18 + years were analyzed. The five-year survival was 3.5% and the ten-year survival was 1.8%. Late relapses occurred in 15% of patients surviving longer than five years and secondary malignancies (including lung) occurred in 20% of these long-term survivors. Extensive disease, performance status more than 2, liver and bone metastases, and elevated serum LDH at presentation were all had prognostic factors. The authors concluded that long-term surviros were at high risk for continued relapses and death because disease but also were at high risk for aerodigestive second malignancies (mostly smoking associated). This high risk of second malignancies has been seen worldwide, particularly associated with continued smoking.[77,78]

A Swiss cooperative group looked at something a little different.[78] They used quality of life as an endpoint rather than survival in a group of patients treated for SCLC on a clinical trial. Patients with poor prognostic factors especially poor performance status, extensive disease, and significant weight loss reported a worse quality of life at baseline but improved on treatment. More data of this kind may be helpful in the care of these patients.

Staging and prognostic factor analysis evolved since the first edition of this book, and the changes and new data have been reviewed. Staging has changed the least, but many new potential prognostic factors have been identified. More models and indexes, are also available to consider for use in clinical trials. These new factors require more study, and then models need to be developed that select out which of the factors are truly independently significant and which ones can be substituted for by older and more well-established factors. This study required a worldwide effort perhaps best facilitated by IASLC. Our prime aim for the future is to develop a simple prognostic index that can be easily applied by clinicians all over the world to give their patients the best information on their prognosis and to help select appropriate patients for specific clinical trials.

APPENDIX

Growing a Tree-based Model

Tree-based methods for survival data split the covariate space on a rule that maximizes some measure of improvement. The simplest and most interpretable class of splits are those on a single covariate; they can be described by the following rules:

1. Each split depends on the value of one predictor Xj.
2. If Xj is an ordered variable, splits induced by questions of the form, "is Xj < c?" are allowed; for example, "is sodium < 136?" Note that if a variable has K distinct values, up to K − 1 different splits are possible.
3. If Xj is nominal, with values in B = {b₁, b₂, .., b'}, then splits induced by any question of the form, "is Xj

in S," where S is a subset of B, is allowed; for example "is smoking in (never, infrequently)."

Partitioning a node, h, involves finding the split, s, among all variables and values of the variables that maximize some measurement of improvement, G(s, h). In our case, G(s, h) is usually a standardized two-sample logrank test statistic between the resulting two groups of observations; however, G(s, h) could also be the reduction in the model deviance:

$$G(s, h) = R(h) - [R(1(h)) + R(r(h))], \qquad (1)$$

where R(h) is the deviance for node h being split, and R(1(h)) and R (r(h)) are the deviances for the left and right daughter nodes 1(h) and r(h).

The split, s, that corresponds to the variable and value that maximizes G(s, h) is chosen to partition the data. The procedure is then repeated on each of the resulting groups of data until a large tree that overfits the data is constructed.

It is important to determine if splits in the tree represent real structure in the survival times or if they are just caused by chance. This determination is not easily made because of the large number of possible splits that are evaluated before choosing a split. Simple calculations for approximate p-values that do not account for the multiple-comparison problem are not valid; therefore, better ways of helping to determine the tree size are needed.

Pruning and Selecting Tree Size

After growing a large tree, informal methods of removing branches (or terms) can be used to select a set of more parsimonious tree-based models. For instance, one could start removing the splits lowest in the tree that correspond to the smallest improvements G(s, h), or the smallest logrank test statistics or reductions in deviance. A more formal method of obtaining good trees can also be used. In the CART algorithm, the cost–complexity measure of tree performance is:

$$R_a (T) = \sum R(h) + a \text{ \# of terminal nodes in } T, \qquad (2)$$

where a is a penalty per terminal node, R(h) is within-node goodness-of-fit, and T are the terminal nodes in the tree.

Some authors have proposed using exponential model deviance for R(h), a full likelihood deviance based on the proportional hazards model or other measurements of goodness-of-fit. The parameter, a, controls the tradeoff between how well a tree fits the data and the simplicity of the tree. The advantage of using such a penalty is that a simple and efficient algorithm exists for finding the best pruned subtree (a tree obtained by removing splits or branches) for any parameter, a. This issue is important because a tree with only 32 terminal nodes can have almost 500,000 different pruned subtrees.

A measure of tree performance analogous to the cost

complexity of the CART algorithm can also be defined for recursive partitions based on two sample logrank tests statistics, when within node error is not used to grow or prune the tree. Let $S = T - T$ denote the set of internal nodes of T. Again, define $a \geq O$ as the complexity parameter, and define split complexity $G_a(T)$ as

$$G_a(T) = G(T) - a \text{ \# of splits in } T, \qquad (3)$$

where $G(T)$ is the sum over the standardized splitting statistics, $G(h)$, in the tree T:

$$G(T) = \sum_{hint} G(h). \qquad (4)$$

Just as with the cost–complexity measure, there is an efficient way to find the best pruned subtree for any complexity parameter, a.

Pruning algorithms based on the complexity measures described gives the best trees for various values of parameter *a*. Alternative, less formal methods can also be used to obtain a smaller number of potential tree-based models.

Finally, an important difficulty is picking the best tree objectively. The expected deviance or prediction error can be estimated by K-fold cross-validation.[47] Boot-strapping methods or permutation techniques can be used to select tree sizes for methods that only use two sample test statistics.[52]

Combining Nonadjacent Nodes and Missing Data

Until this point, we have only pruned the tree-based models or equivalently recombined adjacent nodes in the tree. However, only a few prognostic strata with widely different survival may be required, and some nonadjacent nodes in the tree may have similar prognoses. Therefore, methods have been developed for recombining nodes with the most similar prognoses.[49,52]

Tree-based methods can efficiently use data with missing values on some covariates. For some tree-based methods, if an observation is missing on a variable chosen for a split, then the observation stops at that branch of the tree. However, if an observation is not missing on the variable used in the split (but it can be missing values for other variables), then it can be used farther down in that branch. Note that this is different than for other regression methods, which require that all observations have complete data.

For example, consider a tree grown for SCLC. Suppose that a split is on LDH but that many of the observations are missing LDH, so those observations could not be used in branches below an LDH split. However, observations missing on another covariate, such as sodium, could still be used farther down the tree for modeling.

Other methods, such as CART, even use observations that are missing on the variable corresponding to the split by using surrogate variables (correlated to the missing variables with the missing values) to send those observations down the tree.

REFERENCES

1. Mountain CF. A new international staging system for lung cancer. *Chest* 1986;89(Suppl 4):2255.
2. Zelen M. Keynote address on biostatistics and data retrieval, part 3. *Cancer Chemo Rep* 1973;4(2):31.
3. Hansen HH, Dombernowsky P, Hirsch FR. Staging procedures and prognostic features in small cell anaplastic bronchogenic carcinoma. *Semin Oncol* 1982;5:280.
4. Abrams J, Doyle LA, Aisner J. Staging, prognostic features and special considerations in small cell lung cancer. *Semin Oncol* 1988;15:261.
5. Albain KS, Crowley JJ, LeBlanc M, et al. Determinants of improved outcome in small cell lung cancer: an analysis of the 2,580 patient Southwest Oncology Group data base. *J Clin Oncol* 1990; 8:1563.
6. Livingstone RB, McCraken JC, Trauth CJ, et al. Isolated pleural effusion in small cell lung carcinoma: favorable prognosis. *Chest* 1982;81:208.
7. Stahel R, Aisner J, Ginsberg R, et al. Staging and prognostic factors in small cell lung cancer. *Lung Cancer* 1989;5:119.
8. Mountain CF. Revisions in the International System for Staging Lung Cancer. *Chest* 1997;111:1710.
9. Shepherd FA, Ginsberg RJ, Feld F, et al. Surgical treatment for limited small-cell lung cancer. *J Thorac Cardiovasc Surg* 1991; 101:385.
9a. Naruke T, Goya T, Tsuchiya R, et al. Prognosis and survival in resected lung carcinoma-based on the new international staging system. *J Thorac Cardiovasc Surg* 1988;96:440.
10. Karrer K, Shields TW, Denck H, et al. The importance of surgical and multi-modality treatment for small cell bronchial carcinoma. *J Thorac Cardiovasc Surg* 1989;97:168.
11. Shepherd FA, Ginsberg RJ, Haddad R, et al. The importance of clinical staging in limited small cell lung cancer: a valuable system to separate prognostic subgroups. *J Clin Oncol* 1993;8:1592.
12. Feinstein AR, Sosin DM, Wells CK. The Will Rogers phenomenon: stage migration and new diagnostic techniques as a source of misleading statistics for survival in cancer. *N Engl J Med* 1985; 312:1604.
13. Darling GE. Staging of the patient with small cell lung cancer. [Review][54 refs]. *Chest Surgery Clinics of North America* 1997; 7:81.
14. Stahel RA. Diagnosis, staging and prognostic factors of small cell lung cancer. *Curr Opin Oncol* 1991;3:306.
15. Richardson G, Venzon D, Phelps R, et al. Application of an algorithm for staging small-cell lung cancer can save one third of the initial evaluation costs. *Arch Intern Med* 1993;153:329.
16. Batra P, Brown K, Aberle D, et al. Imaging techniques in the evaluation of pulmonary parenchymal neoplasms. *Chest* 1992; 101:329.
17. Heelan R. Lung cancer imaging: primary diagnosis, staging and local recurrence. *Semin Oncol* 1991;18:87.
18. Kerr KM, Lamb BD, Wathen CG, et al. Pathological assessment of mediastinal lymph nodes in cancer: implications for noninvasive mediastinal staging. *Thorax* 1992;47:337.
19. Harper PG, Houang M, Spiro SG, et al. Computerized tomography in the pretreatment assessments of small-cell lung carcinoma of the bronchus. *Cancer* 1981;47:1775.
20. Griffin CA, Lu C, Fishman EK, et al. The role of computed

tomography of the chest in the management of small-cell lung cancer. *J Clin Oncol* 1984;2:1359.

21. Jolly PC, Hutchinson CH, Detterbeck F, et al. Routine computed tomographic scans, selective mediastinoscopy and other factors in evaluation of lung cancer. *J Thorac Cardiovasc Surg* 1991;102:226.

22. Dales RE, Stark RM, Sankaranarayan AN. Computed tomography to stage lung cancer. *Rev Respir Dis* 1990;141:1096.

23. McLoud T, Bourgouin P, Greenberg R, et al. Bronchogenic carcinoma: analysis of staging in the mediastinum with CT by correlative lymph node mapping and sampling. *Radiology* 1992;182:319.

24. Webb, Gatsonis C, Zerhouni EA, et al. CT and MR imaging in staging non-small-cell bronchogenic carcinoma: report of the Radiologic Diagnostic Oncology Group. *Radiology* 1991;178:705.

25. Heelan R, Martini N, Westcot JW, et al. Carcinoma involving the hilum and mediastinum: computed tomographic and magnetic resonance evaluation. *Radiology* 1987;162:651.

26. Nakhosteen JA, Niederle N. Small cell lung cancer: serial bronchofibroscopy and photographic documentation. *Chest* 1983;83:12.

27. Giannone L, Johnson DH, Handle KR, et al. Favorable prognosis of brain metastasis in small cell lung cancer. *Ann Intern Med* 1987;106:386.

28. Hirsch FR, Osterlind K, Jensen LI, et al. The impact of abdominal computerized tomography on the pretreatment staging and prognosis of small cell lung cancer. *Ann Oncol* 1992;3:469.

29. Jensen LI, Hirsch FR, Peters K, et al. Diagnosis of abdominal metastasis in small cell carcinoma of the lung: a prospective study of computer tomography and ultrasonography. *Lung Cancer* 1992;8:37.

30. Hansen SW, Jensen F, Pedersen NT, et al. Detection of liver metastasis in small cell lung cancer: a comparison of peritoneoscopy with liver biopsy and ultrasonography with fine-needle aspiration. *J Clin Oncol* 1987;5:255.

31. Dearing M, Steinberg S, Phelps R, et al. Outcome of patients with small cell lung cancer: effect of changes in staging procedures and imaging technology on prognostic factors over 14 years. *J Clin Oncol* 1990;8:1042.

32. Feliu J, Gonzalez A, Baron M, et al. Bone marrow examination in small-cell lung cancer: when is it indicated? *Acta Oncol* 1986;30:587.

33. Campling B, Quirt I, DeBoer G, et al. Is bone marrow examination in small-cell lung cancer really necessary? *Ann Intern Med* 1986;105:508.

34. Humblet Y, Symann M. Detection of small-cell lung cancer bone marrow metastasis by tumour stem cell assay. *Pathol Biol* 1988;36:83.

35. Balban E, Walker B, Cox J, et al. Radionuclide imaging of bone marrow metastasis with a Tc-99m labelled monoclonal antibody to small cell lung carcinoma. *Clin Nuclear Med* 1991;16:732.

36. Shepherd FA. Screening diagnosis and staging of lung cancer. *Curr Opin Oncol* 1993;5:310.

37. Stahel RA, Mabry M, Skarin AT, et al. Detection of bone marrow metastasis in small-cell lung cancer by monoclonal antibodies. *J Clin Oncol* 1985;3:445.

38. Pasini F, Pelosi G, Verlato G, et al. Positive immunostaining with MLuC1 of bone marrow aspirate predicts poor outcome in patients with small-cell lung cancer. *Annals of Oncology* 1998;9(2):181–5.

39. Layer G, Steudel A, Schuller H, et al. Magnetic resonance imaging to detect bone marrow metastases in the initial staging of small cell lung carcinoma and breast carcinoma. *Cancer* 1999;85:1004.

40. Seto T, Imamura F, Kuriyama K, et al. Effect on prognosis of

41. Milleron BJ, Le Breton C, Carette MF, et al. Assessment of bone marrow involvement by magnetic resonance imaging in small cell lung cancer. No significant change of staging. *Chest* 1994;106:1030.

42. Biran H, Feld R, Malkin A, et al. Circulating arginine-vasopressin, calcitonin, carcinoembryonic antigen, neuron-specific enolase, and beta-2 microglobulin fluctuations during combined modality induction therapy for small cell bronchogenic carcinoma: association of post chemotherapy AVP surge with high tumour response rate and durable remission. *Tumour Biol* 1991;12:131.

43. Sagman U, Maki E, Evans WK, et al. Small-cell carcinoma of the lung: derivation of a prognostic staging system. *J Clin Oncol* 1991;9:1639.

44. Sagman U, Feld R, Evans WK, et al. The prognostic significance of pre-treatment serum lactate dehydrogenase in patients with small-cell lung cancer. *J Clin Oncol* 1991;9:945.

45. Fizazi K, Cojean I, Pignon JP, et al. Normal serum neuron specific enolase (NSE) value after the first cycle of chemotherapy: an early predictor of complete response and survival in patients with small cell lung carcinoma. *Cancer* 1998;82:1049.

46. Pinson P, Joos G, Watripont P, et al. Serum neuron-specific enolase as a tumor marker in the diagnosis and follow-up of small-cell lung cancer. *Respiration* 1997;64:102.

47. Jorgensen LG, Osterlind K, Genolla J, et al. Serum neuron-specific enolase (S-NSE) and the prognosis in small-cell lung cancer (SCLC): a combined multivariate analysis on data from nine centres [published erratum appears in Br J Cancer 1996 Dec;74:2043]. *Br J Cancer* 1996;74:463.

48. Perez EA, Loprinzi CL, Sloan JA, et al. Utility of screening procedures for detecting recurrence of disease after complete response in patients with small cell lung carcinoma. *Cancer* 1997;80:676.

49. Skov B, Hirsch P, Bobrow L. Monoclonal antibodies in the detection of bone marrow metastasis in small-cell lung cancer. *Br J Cancer* 1992;65:593.

50. Graus F, Dalmou J, Rene R, et al. Anti-Hu antibodies in patients with small-cell lung cancer: association with complete response to therapy and improved survival. *J Clin Oncol* 1997;15:2866.

51. Hochstenbag MM, Heidendal GA, Wouters EF, ten Velde GP. In-111 octreotide imaging in staging of of small cell lung cancer. *Clin Nucl Medicine* 1997;22:811.

52. Bombardieri E, Chiti A, Crippa F, et al. 111 in-DTPA-D-Phe-1-octreotide scintigraphy of small cell lung cancer. *Quar J Nucl Med* 1995;39(4 Suppl):4.

53. Berenger N, Moretti JL, Boaziz C, et al. Somatostatin receptor imaging in small cell lung cancer. *Eur J Cancer* 1996;32A:1429.

54. Semprebene A, Ferraironi A, Franciotti G, 111 in-octreotide scintigraphy in small cell lung cancer. *Quar J Nucl Medicine* 1995;39(4 Suppl 1):108.

55. Kwekkebbom DJ, Kho GS, Lamberts SW, et al. The value of octreotide scintigraphy in patients with lung cancer. *Eur J Nucl Med* 1994;21:1106.

56. Salven P, Ruotsalainen T, Matson K, et al. High pre-treatment serum level of vascular endothelial growth factor (VEGF) is associated with poor outcome in small-cell lung cancer. *Int J Cancer* 1998;79:144.

57. Boher JM, Pujol JL, Grenier J, et al. Markov model and markers of small cell lung cancer: assessing the influence of reversible serum NSE, CYFRA 21-1, and TPS levels on prognosis. *Br J Cancer* 1999;79:1419.

58. Rosenfeld MR, Malats N, Schramm L, et al. Serum anti-p53 antibodies and prognosis of patients with small-cell lung cancer. *J Natl Cancer Inst* 1997;89:381.

59. Quoix E, Wolkove N, Hanley J, et al. Problems in radiographic

estimation of response to chemotherapy and radiotherapy in small cell lung cancer. *Cancer* 1988;62:489.

60. Feld R, Pater J, Goodwin PJ, et al. The restaging of responding patients with limited small-cell lung cancer: is it really useful? *Chest* 1993;103:1010.

61. Kaplan E, Meier P. Nonparametric estimation from incomplete observations. *J Am Stat Assoc* 1958;53:457.

62. Davis R, Anderson J. Exponential survival trees. *Stat Med* 1989; 8:947.

63. Cox DR. Regression models and life tables. *J R Stat Soc B* 1972; 34:187.

64. Mantel N. Evaluation of survival data and two new rank order statistics arising in its consideration. *Cancer Chemother Rep* 1966; 50:163.

65. McCullagh P, Nelder J. *Generalized linear models.* New York: Chapman & Hall, 1989.

66. Butler J, Gilpin E, Gordon L, et al. *Tree-structured survival analysis. II. Technical report.* Stanford, CA: Stanford University Press, 1989.

67. Ciampi A, Hogg S, McKinney S, et al. RECPAM: a computer program for recursive partition and amalgamation for censored survival data. *Comp Meth Prog Biomed* 1988;26:239.

68. Segal M. Regression trees for censored data. *Biometrics* 1988;44: 35.

69. LeBlanc M, Crowley J. Relative risk regression trees for censored survival data. *Biometrics* 1992;48:411.

70. LeBlanc M, Crowley J. Survival trees by goodness of split. *J Am Stat Assoc* 1993;88:457.

71. Sagman U, Leblanc M, Maki E, et al. Verification of a multicenter prognostic model for small cell lung carcinoma: consensus group for prognostic factors. (Abstract 1125) *Proc ASCO* 1993;12:337.

72. Lassen UN, Osterlind K, Hirsch FR, et al. Early death during chemotherapy in patients with small-cell lung cancer: derivation of a prognostic index for toxic death and progression. *Br J Cancer* 1999:79:515.

73. Stephens RJ, Girling DJ, Machin D. Treatment-related deaths in small cell lung cancer trials: can patients at risk be identified? Medical Research Council Lung Cancer Working Party. *Lung Cancer* 1994;11:2559.

74. Wurschmidt F, Bunemann H, Heilmann HP. Small cell lung cancer with and without superior cava syndrome: a multivariate analysis of prognostic factors in 408 cases. *International Journal of Radiation Oncology, Biology, Physics* 1995;33:77.

75. Maestu I, Pastot M, Gomez-Codina J, et al. Pretreatment prognostic factors for survival in small-cell lung cancer: a new prognostic index and validation of three known prognostic indices on 341 patients. *Annals of Oncology* 1997;8:547.

76. Lassen U, Osterlind K, Hansen M, et al. Long-term survival in small-cell lung cancer: posttreatment characteristics in patients surviving 5 to 18 + years—an analysis of 1,714 consecutive patients. *J Clin Oncol* 1995;13:1215.

77. Janssen-Haijnen ML, Gatta G, Forman D, Capocaccia R, Coebergh JW. Variation in survival of patients with lung cancer in Europe, 1985–1989. EUROCARE Working Group. *Eur J Can* 1998;34(14 Spec No):2191–6.

78. Johnson BE, Linnoila RI, Williams JP, et al. Risk of second aerodigestive cancers increases in patients who survive free of small-cell lung cancer for more than 2 years. *J Clin Oncol* 1996; 13:101.

79. Bernhard J, Hurny C, Bacchi M, et al. Initial prognostic factors in small-cell lung cancer patients predicting quality of life during chemotherapy. Swiss Group for Clinical Cancer Research (SAKK). *Br J Cancer* 1996;74:1660.

35

SURGICAL STAGING OF THE MEDIASTINUM

AMIR ABOLHODA
STEVEN M. KELLER

MEDIASTINOSCOPY

Historical Perspectives

The first formal diagnostic technique for pathologic evaluation of mediastinal lymph nodes was described by Daniels in 1949[1] and consisted of digital exploration of the superior mediastinum following a scalene fat pad biopsy. In 1954, Harken[2] introduced a Jackson laryngoscope to visualize and explore paratracheal mediastinal lymph nodes via bilateral cervical incisions. He was the first to associate poor survival following surgical resection with the presence of tumor in mediastinal lymph nodes. Radner, in 1955, reported the value of a single suprasternal notch incision to provide bilateral access to the paratracheal nodes.[3] Carlens introduced the use of a cervical mediastinoscope under general anesthesia and named the procedure *mediastinoscopy*.[4] Although mediastinoscopy rapidly became popular in Europe, it was not until the mid 1960s that Pearson and colleagues in Toronto began performing mediastinoscopy routinely in the prethoracotomy staging of non–small cell lung cancer (NSCLC). They established systematic mediastinal lymph node evaluation as a reliable procedure for the appraisal of the regional extent of metastatic disease in NSCLC.[5,6]

Indications

Mediastinoscopy is utilized to demonstrate the presence or absence of metastatic disease in the ipsilateral or contralateral mediastinal lymph nodes. Similar to any test, it should be performed only if the results will alter the patient's future therapy. Biopsy of bulky, unresectable, mediastinal lymph nodes in a patient with a lung mass provides both a diagnosis and staging information. Biopsy of enlarged but potentially resectable lymph nodes may document evidence of metastatic disease in multiple levels, a finding that places the patient in a cohort with an extremely poor prognosis. Similarly, patients with T3 or T4 tumors should undergo mediastinoscopy regardless of lymph node size because these pa-

tients do not appear to benefit from pulmonary resection in the presence of mediastinal lymph node metastases.

Patients with synchronous bilateral pulmonary lesions may have either two primary lung cancers or a single tumor with a solitary metastases. By convention, if tumor is not present in the mediastinal lymph nodes, then the tumors are treated as independent neoplasms. Therefore, a mediastinoscopy is indicated to determine if the patient should be treated for two early-stage lung cancers or stage IV disease. Mediastinal lymph node biopsy may also be required to determine patient eligibility for participation in neoadjuvant therapy trials. Finally, the rare patient with documented small cell lung cancer (SCLC) that has presented as a solitary pulmonary mass should undergo mediastinoscopy prior to pulmonary resection.

The role of mediastinoscopy remains controversial in the absence of enlarged mediastinal lymph nodes. If the attending physicians believe that the presence of any tumor within the mediastinal lymph nodes, no matter how minute, renders the patient inoperable (at least initially), then mediastinoscopy should be performed routinely. If, however, the consensus is to recommend removal of completely resectable N2 disease (usually disease in a single nodal level), then mediastinoscopy is unnecessary. This approach is satisfactory for patients with right lung cancers in whom all the ipsilateral mediastinal lymph nodes are easily resected during a right thoracotomy. However, because of the aortic arch, the left paratracheal region is not readily accessible during a left thoracotomy; therefore, some surgeons believe that all patients with resectable tumors of the left upper lobe should undergo mediastinoscopy.[7]

Relative Contraindications

Few anatomic conditions preclude safe cervical mediastinoscopy. These include severe cervical arthritis (preventing adequate extension of the neck and physical insertion of the scope), the presence of a large cervical goiter, extensive calcification or aneurysmal dilatation of the aortic arch or innominate artery, and the presence of a tracheostomy. Repeat mediastinoscopy can be safely accomplished in most pa-

TABLE 35.1. CORRELATION OF PREOPERATIVE STAGING MODALITY WITH PATHOLOGIC NODAL STAGING

	CXR	CT	MRI	Mediastinoscopy
Sensitivity (%)	80	82	71	87
Specificity (%)	43	76	84	100
Accuracy (%)	57	81	83	95
Positive Predictive Value (%)	45	74	81	100
Negative Predictive Value (%)	79	91	84	93

CXR: chest roentgenography; CT: computed tomography; MRI: magnetic resonance imaging. (From Patterson GA, Ginsberg RJ, Poon PY, et al. A prospective evaluation of magnetic resonance imaging, computed tomography, and mediastinoscopy in the preoperative assessment of mediastinal node status in bronchogenic carcinoma. *J Thorac Cardiovasc Surg* 1987;94:679, with permission.)

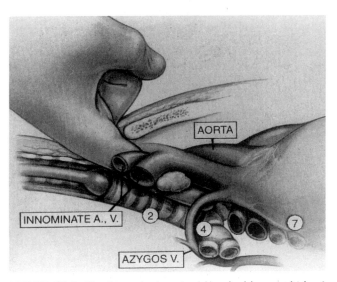

FIGURE 35.1. The innominate artery is palpable anteriorly. A gentle sweeping motion clears soft tissue from the anterior tracheal surface. (Reproduced with permission of WB Saunders from *Seminars in oncology*, 1993, Sugarbaker D and Strauss G.)

tients despite the peritracheal fibrosis and obliteration of cervical mediastinal fascial planes caused by prior mediastinoscopy.

STANDARD CERVICAL MEDIASTINOSCOPY

Mediastinoscopic examination of the mediastinum via the standard cervical approach allows assessment of the highest mediastinal and upper and lower paratracheal mediastinal lymph nodes (levels 1, 2R, 2L, 4R, and 4L) as well as anterior subcarinal lymph nodes (level 7). Standard cervical mediastinoscopy has a sensitivity of 85% to 90%, a specificity of 100%, and a negative predictive value of greater than 90%. Cervical mediastinoscopy remains the most accurate modality for preresectional mediastinal staging of patients with NSCLC[8] (Table 35.1).

Operative Technique

General endotracheal anesthesia is established, and the patient is placed supine with the occiput at the edge of the operating table. A right radial artery catheter and/or a digital pulse oximeter are utilized to monitor not only blood pressure and oxygen saturation, but also the duration and extent of inadvertent innominate artery compression that occurs during the procedure. A roll is placed beneath the shoulders, and the neck is hyperextended to draw the trachea upward from the mediastinum and to facilitate insertion of the mediastinoscope. The endotracheal tube is positioned in the mouth contralateral to the side from which the surgeon utilizes the dissecting instrument. The anterior chest is prepped and draped to the level of the xiphoid and a 3- to 4-cm transverse skin incision is made approximately 1 to 2 cm above and parallel to the sternal notch. The incision is carried through the platysma, the strap muscles are retracted

laterally, and a longitudinal dissection plane is developed down to the pretracheal fascia.

The pretracheal fascia is incised and elevated by insertion of the index finger into the pretracheal space (Figure 35.1). This important maneuver permits blunt digital dissection of the pretracheal space to the level of the carina and often allows palpation of abnormal lymph nodes. The mediastinoscope is introduced into the predissected tunnel and is gently advanced under direct vision (Figure 35.2). A blunt dissecting instrument equipped with suction and cautery is utilized to identify both the constant nonlymphatic structures and the mediastinal lymph nodes. The carina, proximal mainstem bronchi, innominate artery, main pulmonary artery, and azygous vein are commonly visualized. In order to avoid injury to the left recurrent laryngeal nerve, dissection in the left paratracheal region should be performed cautiously and the cautery used sparingly. After adequate hemostasis, the wound is closed in layers. A video-mediastinoscope is useful for demonstrating the operative technique.

Complications

Minor hemorrhage, most commonly related to the bronchial arterial supply to the mediastinal lymph nodes (particularly the subcarinal nodes), is the most common complication. This is usually controlled with electrocautery or gauze packing. Massive hemorrhage from injury to a major blood vessel is potentially life-threatening and requires prompt recognition, tamponade, and repair. Bleeding from the azygos vein can sometimes be controlled by packing the mediastinum. However, a right thoracotomy may be necessary

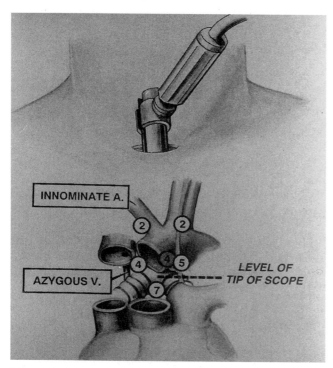

FIGURE 35.2. A small-gauge needle may be used to aspirate the "lymph node" prior to biopsy in order to avoid injury to vascular structures. No attempt is made to excise the entire lymph node. A twisting motion, rather than a direct pull, is used to remove the biopsy specimen. (Reproduced with permission of WB Saunders from *Seminars in oncology*, 1993, Sugarbaker D and Strauss G.)

to achieve hemostasis. Injury to the innominate artery, aortic arch, or pulmonary artery generally requires a sternotomy for repair. Another rare complication of mediastinoscopy potentially requiring thoracotomy is tracheobronchial tear.

Other structures at risk of injury during standard cervical mediastinoscopy are the left recurrent laryngeal nerve (vulnerable at the left tracheobronchial angle), the mediastinal pleura (right greater than left), and the esophagus (vulnerable in the posterior subcarinal region). Recurrent nerve palsy and pneumothoraces are generally treated observantly. Esophageal perforation is rare and may elude diagnosis until signs and symptoms of mediastinal sepsis develop.

Despite the potential complications, cervical mediastinoscopy is a safe procedure and is commonly performed in the ambulatory setting. Pearson reported minor complications in 1.6% of 432 patients who underwent mediastinoscopy (2 pneumothoraces, 3 recurrent nerve palsies, and 2 hemorrhages).[6] No patient required thoracotomy and no patient died following the procedure. Coughlin[9] documented 1,259 consecutive preresectional mediastinoscopies performed in patients with proven and operable lung cancer; no deaths occurred. Right pneumothorax was the most common complication, occurring in eight patients, and in every instance was the result of transmediastinal pleural bi-

opsy of the lung. Seven patients had left recurrent nerve injury, three of whom recovered with normal voice. Three patients (0.2%) required thoracotomy for a pulmonary artery branch avulsion, an esophageal tear, or a cautery burn of the right main bronchus. Complications occurred in 1.7% of patients. Luke reported[10] 1,000 cervical mediastinoscopies. Three patients (0.3%) sustained major complications that required thoracotomy two for hemorrhage, one for tracheal tear), and twenty patients (2%) sustained minor complications for a collective morbidity of 2.3%; no operative mortality occurred.

SCALENE LYMPH NODE BIOPSY WITH THE MEDIASTINOSCOPE

Scalene lymph nodes are no longer routinely biopsied as part of the preoperative evaluation of patients with NSCLC. However, investigators have reported that occult metastases may be found in nonpalpable lymph nodes[11-14] in 4% to 24% of patients with potentially resectable cancers. The presence of tumor in the supraclavicular lymph nodes (N3) drastically alters the prognosis and treatment recommendations. Therefore, evaluation of this region is appropriate.

Lee and Ginsburg[1] have described a modification of standard cervical mediastinoscopy that permits biopsy of the supraclavicular lymph nodes. Following completion of the mediastinal biopsies, the mediastinoscope is rotated behind the carotid sheath and into the supraclavicular fossa (Figure 35.3).

Results

The authors have reported their experience with a select group of 81 patients in whom N2 or N3 disease was suspected. Twenty-nine patients were proven N0 by standard mediastinoscopy, and none had supraclavicular lymph node metastases. However, of the 39 patients found to have metastases to the N2 lymph nodes, 15% also had tumor in the supraclavicular lymph nodes. Finally, 13 of 19 (68%) patients with contralateral N3 disease also had metastases to the supraclavicular lymph nodes. All of the tumor-containing supraclavicular lymph nodes were found in patients whose tumors were central (visible by fiberoptic bronchoscopy) and of nonsquamous histology.

EXTENDED CERVICAL MEDIASTINOSCOPY

Extended cervical mediastinoscopy (ECM), a procedure originally described by Kirchner in 1971,[16] has been popularized by Ginsberg and colleagues[17] as a single staging procedure for preoperative assessment of bronchogenic carcinomas of the left upper lobe. Considered as an alternative technique to circumvent the limitations and potential com-

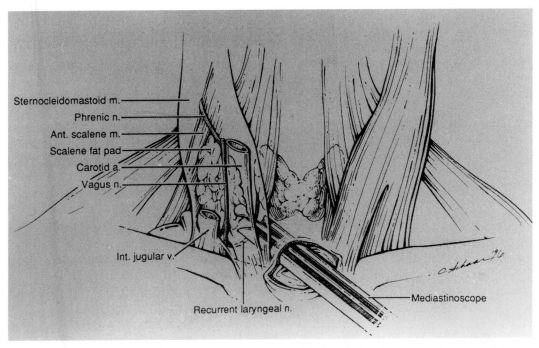

FIGURE 35.3. The medial aspect of the scalene fat pat is dissected and lymph nodes biopsied or removed. (Reproduced with permission of Elsevier Science LTD from *Annals of thoracic surgery*, 1996;62:338, Lee D and Ginsberg R.)

plications of anterior mediastinotomy, ECM has been designed to provide full invasive staging of the paratracheal and para-aortic mediastinal lymph nodes in patients with left upper lobe tumors. Indications are similar to those previously cited for mediastinoscopy.

Operative Technique

Following completion of a standard cervical mediastinoscopy, the mediastinoscope is withdrawn from the cervical incision. The fascia investing the aorto-innominate junction is opened with an index finger, and the innominate triangle along the anterolateral surface of the aortic arch posterior to the innominate vein is entered (Figure 35.4). The mediastinoscope is gently advanced through the previously created tunnel into the para-aortic mediastinal compartment. Utilizing blunt dissection, the loose fatty tissue encompassing the lymph nodes is cleared and node biopsies are obtained. Care is taken not to transgress the mediastinal pleura. After ensuring absence of significant bleeding, the mediastinoscope is withdrawn and the cervical incision is closed in the usual fashion.

Complications and Results

ECM has a steep learning curve and should be employed with caution. The first attempts with this technique should

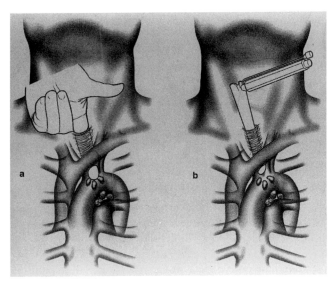

FIGURE 35.4. A: Finger dissection between the innominate artery and left carotid arteries. **B:** The mediastinoscope in place for anterior mediastinal and aortopulmonary node biopsy. (Reproduced with permission of Lippincott-Raven from *Mastery of cardiothoracic surgery*, pg. 23, Kaiser, ed.)

be performed with an anterior mediastinostomy counter-incision to allow bimanual palpation and to facilitate atraumatic advancement of the mediastinoscope into the innominate triangle.[17] Ginsberg and associates from Toronto reported the results of their first 100 consecutive patients with left upper lobe tumors who underwent ECM.[18] Twenty patients were found to have nodal spread to the superior or anterior mediastinum or both, with seven patients having sole involvement of the superior mediastinum. A total of 75 thoracotomies were performed, and 74 patients were able to have complete resection of their tumors. Eight false-negative ECM procedures were reported. In each, microscopic N2 disease in the level 5 or 6 lymph nodes was identified only following a final histologic examination. In all eight patients the tumors were completely resectable. In this series, the only reported complication was a superficial cervical wound infection.

Lopez and associates reported the use of ECM in 50 patients with bronchogenic carcinoma of the left upper (38) and left lower (12) lobes.[19] Mediastinoscopy was positive in nine patients, five via the extended approach. Resectability in the remaining 41 patients was 97.6%. This study identified a negative predictive value of 97.5% and a diagnostic accuracy of 97.8%.

A case report of a cerebrovascular accident following an ECM by Urschel et al. has questioned the safety of this staging procedure.[20] Indeed, presence of aortic arch calcification on CT scan or palpation of atheromatous plaques in the great vessels should constitute an absolute contraindication to ECM. However, with careful patient selection, the incidence of major complications including neurologic sequella should remain negligible.

ANTERIOR MEDIASTINOTOMY (CHAMBERLAIN PROCEDURE)

Left anterior parasternal mediastinostomy was introduced by McNeil and Chamberlain in 1966[21] as a method for establishing the diagnosis and resectability of tumors of the left upper lobe. Chamberlain believed that the procedure would enable the thoracic surgeon to not only biopsy the left hilar and aortopulmonary window lymph nodes, but also assess the degree of fixation of the left upper lobe tumor to the mediastinal structures and, therefore, would avoid unnecessary thoracotomy in patients with locally advanced unresectable bronchogenic carcinoma. Currently, the Chamberlain procedure is utilized as a staging technique for assessment of the mediastinal nodal levels inaccessible by standard cervical mediastinoscopy: aortopulmonary window and para-aortic (levels 5 and 6, respectively).[22] Indications are similar to those of mediastinoscopy.

In 1983, Deneffe[23] reported a series of 45 anterior mediastinotomies in patients with a presumed left lung cancer and a clinically negative mediastinum. Of the biopsies, 28.9% (13) demonstrated N2 metastatic disease, none of which were associated with lower lobe tumors. In this pre–computed tomography (CT) scan era report, the authors concluded that anterior mediastinostomy should be performed in patients with left upper lobe tumors to improve operability. Jolly[24] demonstrated that a negative anterior mediastinostomy in patients with primary tumors of the left lung predicted resectability in 25 of 26 (96%) cases.

More recently, Barendregt and colleagues[25] reported the results of parasternal mediastinotomy and mediastinoscopy in 37 clinically N0 patients with proven left upper lobe tumors. In conjunction with manual palpation, the mediastinoscope was inserted into the mediastinotomy incision. Lymph node tissue was identified in 16 patients, but only one patient was found to have N2 disease. The authors concluded that anterior medistinoscopy is not necessary in the absence of clinical N2 disease.

Surgical Technique

The patient is positioned supine under general anesthesia and is intubated with a single-lumen endotracheal tube. A 5- to 6-cm transverse skin incision is made lateral to the sternum, overlying the second or third costal cartilage and deepened through the pectoralis muscle. The perichondrium is incised and the costal cartilage is removed in a subperichondrial plane (Figure 35.5). Alternatively, the incision is placed over the intercostal space without removing the cartilage. The internal mammary artery and vein are within the operative field and should be retracted or ligated and divided. The mediastinal pleural reflection is bluntly separated from the posterior table of the sternum and reflected laterally to expose the para-aortic and aortopulmonary mediastinal space. Enlarged lymph nodes are sampled under direct vision by excision or biopsy. The mediastinoscope can be introduced via the incision to facilitate exploration of the mediastinum.

Anatomic definition and access may be improved by opening the pleura. If the pleural space is entered, then a chest tube is not required provided the lung is not injured. Evacuation of air is accomplished by positioning a catheter in the pleural space prior to closure of the incision and placing the opposite end under 2 cm of water. After hemostasis is ascertained, the wound is closed in layers and the catheter is withdrawn as the anesthesiologist fully inflates the lungs.

Complications and Results

Anterior mediastinostomy is associated with little morbidity and mortality and can be performed safely in an ambulatory setting. The main disadvantages of this procedure are the local pain and potential wound healing problems that follow

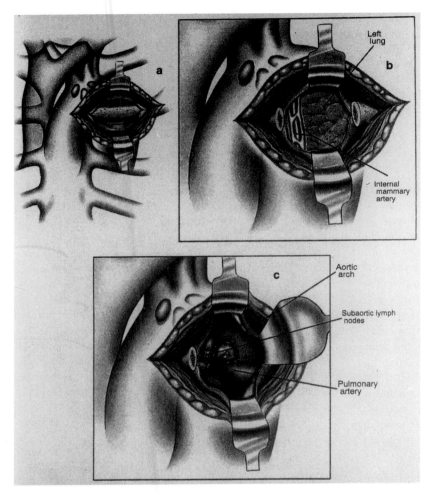

FIGURE 35.5. A: Incision over the second costal cartilage, **B:** After resection of the costal cartilage. **C:** View of enlarged subaortic nodes. (Reproduced with permission of Lippincott-Raven from *Mastery of cardiothoracic surgery,* pg. 24, Kaiser, ed.)

resection of the second costal cartilage, particularly if adjuvant radiation therapy is administered.[22] The major structures at risk for injury during the operation are the aorta, the internal mammary artery, the pulmonary artery, the superior pulmonary vein, the phrenic nerve, and the left recurrent laryngeal nerve. However, damage to these structures, aside from the internal mammary artery, are rare. The most commonly reported complications are superficial wound infections and pneumothoraces.

VIDEO-ASSISTED THORACOSCOPIC MEDIASTINAL LYMPH NODE SAMPLING

Video-assisted thoracoscopic mediastinal exploration and lymph node sampling has emerged as yet another invasive staging modality in the preresectional evaluation of patients with NSCLC. Video-assisted thoracoscopy (VATS) not only permits sampling of the mediastinal lymph node stations accessible by the standard cervical mediastinoscopy,

but also allows evaluation of mediastinal adenopathy in those N2 stations inaccessible by the traditional mediastinoscopic techniques (nodal levels 3, 5, 6, posterior subcarinal 7, 8, and 9). In addition, VATS may provide additional staging information by demonstrating unsuspected malignant pleural effusions or pleural carcinomatosis.

Operative Technique

Following intubation with a double-lumen endotracheal tube, the thoracoscope is inserted via an 11-mm trocar through the sixth intercostal space in the midaxillary line. Additional access sites for insertion of endoscopic dissecting instruments and clip appliers are created under direct thoracoscopic vision. A lung-retracting instrument is often useful to allow unimpeded thoracoscopic view of the periazygous region and aortopulmonary window. The pleura is opened and the appropriate nodal levels biopsied. Care is taken to avoid injury to the phrenic and vagus nerve trunks. A chest tube is place under direct vision and may be removed in the immediate perioperative period if no air leak and little drainage occur.

Results

Gossot et al.[26] reported the results of a prospective nonrandomized study of cervical mediastinoscopy versus VATS for assessment of mediastinal masses and lymph nodes. The diagnostic yield of VATS was 91.9% (versus 94.3% for the mediastinoscopy group). Four of the five failures in the VATS group were the result of insufficient mediastinal exposure because of the inability to completely collapse the ipsilateral lung. There were three complications in the VATS group: one injury to the internal thoracic artery, one small tear of the trachea during biopsy of a paratracheal lymph node, and one prolonged air leak. In addition, the mean length of hospital stay was 3.2 days in the VATS group and 1.1 days for the mediastinoscopy group. The authors noted that although thoracoscopy has a comparable diagnostic yield to conventional mediastinoscopy, the complication rate and duration of hospital stay of patients who underwent diagnostic VATS was greater than that of patients who had standard mediastinoscopy. They concluded that VATS should be reserved for those clinical situations in which the mediastinal lesions are not within the reach of the mediastinoscope or when prior biopsy and fibrosis make repeat mediastinoscopy difficult or unsafe.

Landreneau and colleagues reported their experience with thoracoscopic mediastinal exploration in 40 patients with NSCLC, in whom VATS was utilized as an adjunct to cervical mediastinoscopy.[27] All patients had CT scan evidence of enlarged (>1.5 cm) aortopulmonary window (n = 30) or right peri/subazygous or subcarinal (n = 10) lymph nodes. Thirty-four patients had undergone a prior negative cervical mediastinoscopy. In 18 patients, thoracoscopic sampling of the mediastinal adenopathy detected malignant tissue. Fourteen of these patients had mediastinal lymph node metastases from a lung primary. In this study, adjunctive thoracoscopic nodal sampling was 100% sensitive and 100% specific in diagnosing the nature of the mediastinal adenopathy. The sole postoperative complication was a chylous leak, which spontaneously resolved. The mean length of stay for the patients undergoing VATS without subsequent thoracotomy was 3 days.

Mediastinal lymph node dissection can be accomplished during a VATS lobectomy comparable to that achieved during thoracotomy. Kaseda[28] performed 36 VATS lobectomies and reported that all lymph node levels were accessible. The number of lymph nodes removed was comparable to that obtained with an open procedure. Similar results were documented by Iwasaki,[29] who performed 25 VATS lobectomies for stage I NSCLC.

INTRAOPERATIVE MEDIASTINAL LYMPH NODE DISSECTION

Mediastinal staging is an integral part of the surgical treatment of lung cancer. Just as a pulmonary resection involves transecting and ligating the appropriate pulmonary arterial branches, pulmonary venous branches, and bronchi, so too must the intrathoracic extent of the malignancy be determined. Histologic staging completely depends on the material submitted during the operative procedure, and hence the surgeon must *accurately identify* and *properly label* the requisite specimens.

The T category of the primary tumor is readily apparent to both surgeon and pathologist. However, the presence or absence of tumor within the intrathoracic lymph nodes is often not at all obvious. Indeed, the lymph nodes may not be apparent and must be diligently sought. Microscopic assessment is required to accurately determine the N status.

Appreciation for the rationale of lymph node dissection is gained through knowledge of the patterns of lung cancer metastases. The definitions of lymph node levels and the techniques of lymph node dissection are best understood in their anatomic and historic perspectives. Finally, the benefits of a mediastinal lymph node dissection can only be fully comprehended through a review of the attendant risks and benefits.

Purpose of Lymph Node Dissection

Accurate and thorough lymph node dissection is crucial for appropriate staging of lung cancer. Without precise staging, the comparison of results from different institutions is impossible, as is the conduct of multi-institutional trials. Most authors do not believe that even the most aggressive lymph node dissections have therapeutic value. However, some investigators (principally from Japan) believe that complete removal of all intrathoracic and supraclavicular lymph nodes in the likely drainage pathway results in improved survival.[30-33]

Critical assessment of the published literature relating survival to pathologic stage in patients with NSCLC requires knowledge of the intrathoracic staging technique. In general, *sampling* means that only those lymph nodes that were obviously abnormal were removed. *Systematic sampling* refers to routine biopsy of lymph nodes at levels specified by the author. *Complete mediastinal lymph node dissection* indicates that all lymph node–containing tissue was routinely removed at those levels indicated by the investigators.

Only one English-language publication directly compares intraoperative visual evaluation of lymph nodes with pathologic examination. Gaer and Goldstraw[34] reported on a series of 95 consecutive patients with NSCLC who underwent pulmonary resection and mediastinal lymph node dissection. Based on inspection and palpation of the lymph nodes after their dissection, the surgeon recorded his

TABLE 35.2. INTRAOPERATIVE ASSESSMENT OF LYMPH NODES

Assessment	No. of Node Stations	No. of Patients
True negative	238	88
True positive	25	16
False positive	14	11
False negative	10	9
Total number of resection	95	

Accuracy, 91.6%; predictive value: positive, 25/(25 + 14) = 64.1%; negative, 238/(238 + 10) = 96.0%.
From Gaer JAR, Goldstraw P. Intraoperative assessment of nodal staging at thoracotomy for carcinoma of the bronchus. *Eur J Cardiothorac Surg* 1990;4:207, with permission.

impression regarding the tumor status of the lymph nodes. Two hundred and eighty-seven nodal levels were removed; results appear in Table 35.2. Sensitivity was 1%, and the positive predictive value was 64%. These values would presumably have been even lower if only a tactile inspection of the nodal levels was made through unopened mediastinal pleura.

The need for some type of routine intraoperative systematic lymph node sampling was further demonstrated by Graham and colleagues,[35] who reported the results of systematic sampling of right levels 2–4 and 7–10 or left levels 4–10 in 240 patients with clinical T1-3N0 NSCLC. All patients had undergone mediastinoscopy prior to thoracotomy if the CT scan demonstrated mediastinoscope-accessible lymph nodes greater than 1.5 cm. No patient with known N2 disease underwent attempted resection. Mediastinal lymph node metastases were demonstrated in 20% of patients, the majority of whom had T1 or T2 tumors.

Haiderer and colleagues[36] reported on 83 patients who underwent routine mediastinal lymph node dissection as part of their operation for NSCLC. Enlarged mediastinal lymph nodes were found in 34 patients (41%); however, only 19 (56%) contained metastatic disease. Of the 49 patients with normal-appearing mediastinal lymph nodes, 2 were documented to have micrometastatic disease (4.1%). Supporting data are contained in a publication by Bollen and colleagues,[37] who found that the discovery ratio (calculated in a fashion similar to the more familiar relative risk ratio) of N2 disease in patients with NSCLC who underwent mediastinal lymph node dissection was 1.9 (confidence interval, 0.9–4) when compared to patients whose lymph nodes were removed only if they appeared or felt abnormal.

The extent of mediastinal biopsy necessary to obtain accurate staging information has been evaluated by several investigators. In a retrospective review, Bollen[37] found that systematic sampling of mediastinal lymph nodes was as successful as mediastinal lymph node dissection in identifying N2 disease (discovery ratio 2.7; confidence interval

1.04–4.2). Izbicki[38] compared systematic lymph node sampling to mediastinal lymph node dissection in a randomized prospective trial containing 182 patients. Although the percentage of patients found to have N1 or N2 disease was not significantly different between the two study arms, the number of N2 positive levels was greater in the patients who had full lymph node dissections. Sugi[39] conducted a similar study in 115 patients with clinical T1N0 tumors that were less than 2 cm in diameter. Mediastinal metastases were found in 13% of each study group. Thus it appears that systematic lymph node sampling is as efficient as mediastinal lymph node dissection for staging NSCLC. The survival advantage of mediastinal lymph node dissection, if any, has not been proven.

Identification of the sentinel lymph node has been proposed as a selective method for directing mediastinal lymph node biopsy. Following thoracotomy, Little[40] injected each quadrant of lung tissue surrounding the tumors of 36 clinically N0 patients with isosulfan blue dye. Systematic mediastinal lymph node sampling was performed following pulmonary resection. A sentinel lymph node was identified in 17 patients, 5 in the mediastinum and 12 within the pleural reflection. All of the former contained tumor, whereas only three of the latter harbored metastatic cancer. Among the 19 patients in whom no sentinel lymph node could be found, 5 patients proved to have N1 disease and 1 patient had N2 disease. Additional data are necessary to determine the role of this technique in intraoperative lung cancer staging.

N Category

The N of the TNM system is the stumbling block of accurate lung cancer staging because of competing definitions for a number of the N levels (levels 2 through 4) as well as disagreement about the stage to which they should be assigned (level 10).

The definitions of the N category grew from the realization that clinical outcome varied with the location of the tumor-containing lymph node. Although prosectors provided a detailed description of lymph nodes found within the thorax, the input of the clinicians was required to correlate the anatomic findings with treatment outcome. The lymph node mapping schema proposed by Naruke and colleagues[41] and accepted by the American Joint Committee for Cancer Staging and End Results Reporting (AJCC) achieved universal acceptance after publication in 1978 (Figure 35.6). Numbers were assigned to regional locations where lymph nodes were commonly found. However, the lack of precise anatomic definitions allowed wide interinstitutional as well as intrainstitutional interpretation of lymph node levels. For example, level 10 was given the vague term *hilar*. Were these lymph nodes within the pleural reflection, or were they located in the mediastinum? If they were located outside the pleural reflection, why were they included in the N1 category, and how could they be differentiated

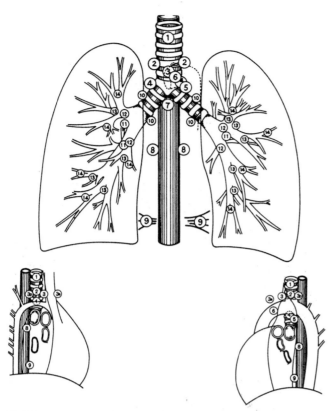

FIGURE 35.6. Lymph node map originally proposed by Naruke. *1,* Superior mediastinal or highest mediastinal; *2,* paratracheal; *3,* pretracheal, retrotracheal, or posterior mediastinal (3p), and anterior mediastinal (3a); *4,* tracheobronchial; *5,* subaortic or Botallo; *6,* para-aortic (ascending aorta); *7,* subcarinal; *8,* paraesophageal (below carina); *9,* pulmonary ligament; *10,* hilar; *11,* interlobar; *12,* lobar (upper lobe, middle lobe, and lower lobe); *13,* segmental; *14,* subsegmental. (From Naruke T, Suemasu K, Ishikawa S. Lymph node mapping and curability at various levels of metastasis in resected lung cancer. *J Thorac Cardiovasc Surg* 1978;76:832, with permission.)

from the contiguous level 4 lymph nodes? The exact limits of the *superior mediastinal lymph nodes* (levels 1 through 4) and *aortic lymph nodes* (levels 5 and 6) were similarly imprecise, allowing some investigators to report multilevel metastases, whereas others reported only single-level involvement.

The resultant confusion led the American Thoracic Society (ATS) to form a Committee on Lung Cancer, one of whose charges was to: "Develop a map of regional pulmonary lymph nodes that would be acceptable to all physicians who care for the patient with lung cancer."[42] This committee recommended that the vague terms "hilar" and "mediastinal" be discarded in favor of nodal level definitions based on constant anatomic structures. For instance, right level 4 lymph nodes were defined as those lymph nodes found ". . . to the right of the midline of the trachea between the cephalic border of the azygous vein and the intersection of the caudal margin of the brachiocephalic artery with the

right side of the trachea." This committee recognized the difficulty in deciding whether level 10 lymph nodes belonged in the N1 or N2 category and recommended that this determination be made after examination of survival data of patients who had accurate and thorough intraoperative lymph node dissections. The ATS nodal definitions have become widely used, although they were not officially accepted by the AJCC.

The former Lung Cancer Study Group initially used the AJCC lymph node definitions in their numerous prospective randomized trials but later adopted and modified the ATS definitions.[43,44] They firmly placed the level 10 lymph nodes in the N2 category. A revised international staging system for lung cancer was adopted by the AJCC and the Union Internationale Contre Cancer in 1986[45] and utilized by most investigators during the ensuing decade.

The staging system and lymph node level definitions were again significantly modified in 1997[46,47] and are discussed in detail in Chapter 32. The new mediastinal lymph node level definitions are based on constant anatomic structures that are readily identified by CT scans (Fig. 35.7 and 35.8, Table 35.3). This was done to enable accurate and reproducible preoperative clinical staging. Unfortunately, the revised definitions render the intraoperative identification of some of the lymph node levels more difficult (right

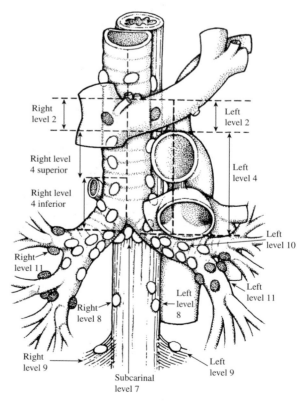

FIGURE 35.7. Graphic representation of current lymph node level definitions.

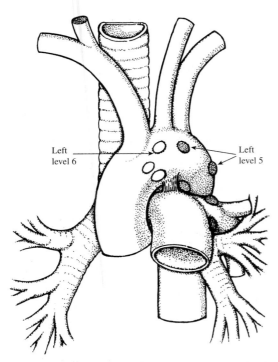

FIGURE 35.8. Details of the current lymph node definitions in the left hemithorax.

levels 2 and 4) because they utilize structures that are difficult to accurately identify during surgery. The uncertainty surrounding level 10 lymph nodes was eliminated by defining them as N1 lymph nodes found along the anterior surface of the mainstem bronchus distal to the pleural reflection. The importance of identifying the nodal and stage definitions used by different authors when interpreting and comparing their results has been emphasized by Mountain and colleagues.[48] Studies presently being conducted under the aegis of the various American national cooperative oncology groups utilize the new revised staging system.

Anatomy and Patterns of Metastatic Spread

The development of the pulmonary lymphatics within the human embryo has been documented by Harvey.[49] The definitive description of the locations of the extrapulmonary intrathoracic adult human lymph nodes was written by Rouviere.[50] Excellent summaries of the common intrapulmonary lymphatic anatomy and its interconnecting network were made by Borrie[51] and Weinberg.[52]

Borrie[51] investigated the patterns of lung cancer dissemination within the intrapulmonary lymphatics of resected specimens. Because a thorough mediastinal lymph node sampling or dissection was not routinely performed, the patterns of mediastinal spread were not as reliably deter-

mined. Borrie found that right upper lobe tumors spread to the lymph nodes surrounding the right upper lobe bronchus and to those lymph nodes "in the angle between the upper and middle lobe bronchus and also along the medial surface of the right main bronchus."[61] The latter region became known as the *lymphatic sump of Borrie*. Tumor from the right upper lobe did not spread below the level of the middle lobe bronchus.

Right middle lobe tumors spread to the lymph nodes surrounding the middle lobe bronchus and proximally to the previously described bronchial sump. Tumors within the right lower lobe metastasized not only to the peribronchial lymphatics but also to the lymph nodes contained within the inferior pulmonary ligament and sump of Borrie. The presence of endobronchial tumor in the middle or lower lobe orifices has been found to correlate with metastases to the lymphatic sump.[53]

Left upper lobe cancers metastasized to lymph nodes surrounding the left upper lobe bronchus and to those surrounding the apical and basilar segmental bronchi of the left lower lobe. Sites of lymphatic metastases of left lower lobe tumors included nodes surrounding the left lower lobe bronchus, the inferior pulmonary ligament, and the left upper lobe bronchus.

Nohl-Oser[54,55] confirmed these observations and extended them to include the patterns of mediastinal spread. He examined the locations of nodal specimens from 749 patients who underwent mediastinoscopy or scalene node biopsy. If patients underwent surgery, then the mediastinal lymph nodes removed during operation were included in the analysis. Histology was not stated. A summary of the results are presented in Table 35.4. Right upper lobe tumors spread rarely to the subcarinal region (1%) or to the contralateral scalene nodes or mediastinum (3%), but they commonly spread to the ipsilateral mediastinum (50%). Sufficient numbers of right middle lobe tumors were not present to allow analysis. Similarly, tumors within the right lower lobe metastasized to the contralateral scalene nodes or mediastinum infrequently (4%), but more commonly spread to the subcarinal region (13%) and ipsilateral mediastinum (29%).

Tumors originating in the left upper lobe metastasized to the subcarinal region (5%) and contralateral mediastinum (7%) more often. Tumors within the left lower lobe did metastasize to the subcarinal region (3%) and the contralateral mediastinum. Nohl-Oser[56] cites clinical data from Greschuchna obtained in a similar fashion that differed from his results. The latter documented a much higher prevalence of subcarinal lymph node metastases from upper lobe tumors and a greater occurrence of paratracheal disease from lower lobe neoplasms.

Watanabe and colleagues[57] reported the intrathoracic metastatic patterns of 124 patients with N2 NSCLC who underwent pulmonary resection and mediastinal lymph node dissection. In contradistinction to Nohl-Oser, he re-

TABLE 35.3. AMERICAN THORACIC LYMPH NODE LEVEL DEFINITIONS

Nodal Station	Anatomic Landmarks
N2 nodes—All N2 nodes lie within the mediastinal pleural envelope.	
1 Highest mediastinal	Nodes lying above a horizontal line at the upper rim of the bracheocephalic (left innominate) vein where it ascends to the left, crossing in front of the trachea at its midline.
2 Upper paratracheal	Nodes lying above a horizontal line drawn tangential to the upper margin of the aortic arch and below the inferior boundary of No. 1 nodes.
3 Prevascular and retrotracheal	Prevascular and retrotracheal nodes may be designated 3A and 3P; midline nodes are considered to be ipsilateral.
4 Lower paratracheal	The lower paratracheal nodes on the right lie to the right of the midline of the trachea between a horizontal line drawn tangential to the upper margin of the aortic arch and a line extending across the right main bronchus at the upper margin of the upper lobe bronchus, and contained within the mediastinal pleural envelope; the lower paratracheal nodes on the left lie to the left of the midline of the trachea between a horizontal line drawn tangential to the upper margin of the aortic arch and a line extending across the left main bronchus at the level of the upper margin of the left upper lobe bronchus, medial to the ligamentum arteriosum and contained within the mediastinal pleural envelope.
	Researchers may wish to designate the lower paratracheal nodes as No. 4s (superior) and No. 4l (inferior) subsets for study purposes; the No. 4s nodes may be defined by a horizontal line extending across the trachea and drawn tangential to the cephalic border of the azygos vein; the No. 4l nodes may be defined by the lower boundary of No. 4s and the lower boundary of No. 4 as described above.
5 Subaortic (aorto-pulmonary window)	Subaortic nodes are lateral to the ligamentum arteriosum or the aorta or left pulmonary artery and proximal to the first branch of the left pulmonary artery and lie with the mediastinal pleural envelope.
6 Para-aortic (ascending aorta or phrenic)	Nodes lying anterior and lateral to the ascending aorta and the aortic arch or the innominate artery, beneath a line tangential to the upper margin of the aortic arch.
7 Subcarinal	Nodes lying caudal to the carina of the trachea, but not associated with the lower lobe bronchi or arteries within the lung.
8 Paraesophageal	Nodes lying adjacent to the wall of the esophagus and to the right or left of the midline, excluding subcarinal nodes.
9 Pulmonary ligament	Nodes lying within the pulmonary ligament, including those in the posterior wall and lower part of the inferior vein.
N1 nodes—All N1 nodes lie distal to the mediastinal pleural reflection and within the visceral pleura.	
10 Hilar	The proximal lobar nodes, distal to the mediastinal pleural reflection and the nodes adjacent to the bronchus intermedius to the right; radiographically, the hilar shadow may be created by enlargement of both hilar and interlobar nodes.
11 Interlobar	Nodes lying between the lobar bronchi.
12 Lobar	Nodes adjacent to the distal lobar bronchi.
13 Segmental	Nodes adjacent to the segmental bronchi.
14 Subsegmental	Nodes around the subsegmental bronchi.

TABLE 35.4. PATTERN OF MEDIASTINAL METASTASES

Lymph Node Location	Right Upper Lobe (N = 230)	Right Lower Lobe (N = 108)	Left Upper Lobe (N = 202)	Left Lower Lobe (N = 68)
Ipsilateral				
Scalene	27	10	13	5
Levels 2–4	78	21	4	0
Level 10	36	9	46	15
Level 7	2	13	9	5
Contralateral				
Scalene	6	3	10	6
Levels 2–4	1	1	10	6
Level 10	0	0	3	5

From Nohl HC. An investigation into the lymphatic and vascular spread of carcinoma of the bronchus. *Ann Roy Coll Surg Engl* 1972;51:157, with permission.

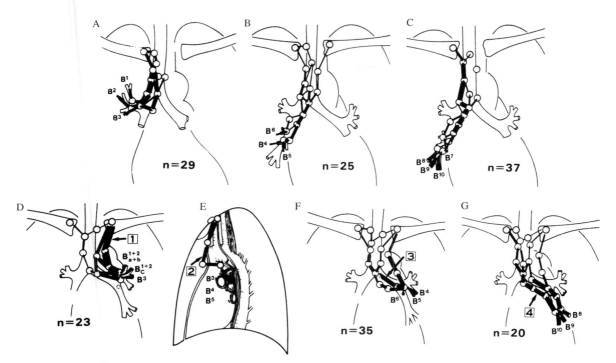

FIGURE 35.9. The width of each arrow corresponds to the relative frequency of lymphatic drainage. **A:** Apical and dorsal segments of the right upper lobe. **B:** Middle lobe and superior segment of the lower lobe. **C:** Basal segments of the lower lobe. **D–G:** Four routes of drainage were identified from the left lung: **(D)** through the subaortic lymph nodes and then divides to run proximally along either the vagus nerve to the scalene nodes or along the recurrent laryngeal nerve to the mediastinal nodes; **(E)** by way of the phrenic nerve to the scalene nodes; **(F)** along the mainstem bronchus to the paratracheal nodes; **(G)** under the mainstem bronchus to the subcarinal lymph nodes. (From Hata E, Hayakawa K, Miyamoto H, et al. Rationale for extended lymphadenectomy for lung cancer. *Theor Surg* 1990;5:19, with permission.)

ported frequent metastases from right upper lobe tumors to the subcarinal lymph nodes (36%). He also demonstrated that tumors originating in the right middle and lower lobes commonly (28%) spread to the ipsilateral paratracheal region (level 4). Metastases were commonly found in the subcarinal lymph nodes from tumors of the left upper (20%) and left lower (38%) lobes.

Hata and colleagues[31] provided experimental support for these results. They performed 192 lymphoscintigraphies in 179 patients without evidence of lymph node involvement by injection of antimony sulfide or rhenium colloid labeled with technetium-99m into the submucosa of each segmental bronchus using the flexible bronchoscope. Hourly anterior and lateral scanning with a gamma camera for up to 6 hours demonstrated patterns of lymphatic drainage that recapitulated the clinical findings of Greschuchna (cited in Nohl-Oser[56]) and Watanabe and colleagues[67] (Fig. 35.9).

Techniques of Lymph Node Sampling and Dissection

The earliest detailed description of a thorough intrathoracic lymph node dissection as part of an operation for lung can-

cer was given in 1951 by Cahan and colleagues,[58] although Brock[59] indicated that it was a routine part of his operative procedure for lung cancer several years earlier. Great emphasis was placed on the need for *en bloc* removal of the lymphatics and lung. Other authors[60–65] soon published their techniques, which were variations on the same theme. The lymph node locations were described only in general anatomic terms. Weinberg[60] was the first to assign numbers to the lymph node regions.

A more recent description was given by Martini,[66] who detailed their dissection of three mediastinal lymph node compartments: (a) the right paratracheal, (b) the subcarinal, and (c) the aorticopulmonary window. During a right thoracotomy, the right paratracheal and subcarinal regions were routinely cleared of all lymphatic tissue, whereas during a left thoracotomy, the subcarinal and aorticopulmonary window lymph nodes were removed in their entirely. Lymph nodes were not resected in continuity with the pulmonary specimen. Level numbers were assigned according to Naruke and colleagues.[41]

Those surgeons who believe that removal of regional lymphatics offers a survival advantage have devised more extensive lymphadenectomies. These have included contralateral mediastinal lymph nodes and, in some cases, supraclavicular lymph nodes. During a right thoracotomy, Watanabe and colleagues[30] transect the azygos vein to gain access to the upper mediastinal lymph nodes (Naruke levels 1 through 4). Nodes anterior to the superior vena cava with associated thymic tissue are also removed. In addition, left levels 2 through 4 have been resected by continuing the dissection to the contralateral aspect of the trachea. The subcarinal region is cleared of all lymph node–containing tissue. During this aspect of the procedure, both ipsilateral and contralateral levels 8 and 10 lymph nodes are removed.

An equally aggressive lymph node dissection is performed in the left hemithorax for patients with left lung cancers. However, because of the aortic arch, such an approach is of necessity more complicated. Watanabe's attempt at left mediastinal lymph node dissection involved mobilizing the arch of the aorta and a portion of the descending aorta. This was accomplished by transecting several intercostal arteries. In this fashion, left levels 3 and 4 as well as portions of level 2 could be resected.[30]

This group have modified their operative procedure to permit more thorough dissection of all left mediastinal lymph nodes. After completion of pulmonary resection by means of a standard posterolateral thoracotomy, a median-sternotomy is performed. This allows complete dissection of all left levels 1 through 4 as well as access to contralateral levels 1 through 4 and 10. This approach has been investigated by Mitsuoka and colleagues.[67]

Nakahara and colleagues[32] described a similar approach to right lung cancer. A mediansternotomy was not employed for left lung cancer. Rather, the ligamentum arteriosum was severed and the aorta encircled with a catheter. Traction was applied caudally, and the pleura between the left common carotid and subclavian arteries was opened to expose the trachea and left mainstem bronchus.

Hata and colleagues[31,33] have pursued an even more aggressive approach, extending the right lymphadenectomy performed during posterolateral thoracotomy to include ipsilateral scalene lymph nodes if the most cephalad right paratracheal lymph nodes (Naruke levels 1, 2, and 4) contain metastatic cancer. This group advocates broadening the supraclavicular dissection to include the left scalene lymph nodes if anterior mediastinal lymph node (Naruke level 3) involvement is suspected.

Their procedure for left lymphadenectomy was determined by tumor histology and stage. The mediastinal lymph nodes of patients with stage I squamous cell cancers were removed by means of a left posterolateral thoracotomy. Although the details of this approach are not specifically stated, they appear to include division of the ligamentum arteriosum and mobilization of the aortic arch. Patients with other stages and histologies undergo mediansternotomy followed by anterior and bilateral paratracheal lymphadenectomy (levels 1 through 4). Exposure is obtained by retracting the ascending aorta to the left and the superior vena

cava to the right. Access to the subcarinal nodes is obtained by caudal retraction of the right main pulmonary artery. The left lobe of the thymus is resected to uncover the aortopulmonary window lymph nodes. These are removed to the ligamentum arteriosum. Left upper lobectomy and pneumonectomy are performed by means of the sternotomy. Should a left lower lobectomy be necessary, an anteroaxillary thoracotomy is added.

Cervical dissection is performed if metastatic disease is found in the highest mediastinal, supraclavicular, or scalene lymph nodes. This procedure is accomplished using a cervical collar incision. The sternocleidomastoid muscles are retracted laterally and the strap muscles divided. The fascia over the internal jugular vein is opened and the vein is skeletonized. The cervical paraesophageal lymph nodes are removed while the recurrent laryngeal nerve is gently retracted forward.

COMPLETE DISSECTION

Right Hemithorax

Entry into the chest through the fifth interspace provides ready access to the mediastinal lymph nodes. A posterolateral thoracotomy or vertical muscle-sparing skin incision may be used with equal success. The authors usually perform the lymph node dissection at the completion of the pulmonary resection. However, if the presence of tumor within the lymph nodes changes the operative procedure, then the lymph node resection may be performed before lung removal. The mediastinal lymph node dissection is most easily accomplished if the lung is collapsed with either a double-lumen endotracheal tube or a bronchial blocker.

The lung is retracted anteriorly and inferiorly, exposing the superior mediastinum, which is bounded by the trachea, superior vena cava, and azygos vein (Figure 35.10). The phrenic nerve is visible, coursing over the superior vena cava. The vagus nerve traverses the superior mediastinum and is usually visible through the unopened mediastinal pleura. The mediastinal pleura is grasped with a forceps just cephalad to the azygos vein and opened with cautery between the trachea and superior vena cava. A right angle clamp is inserted, and the pleura is incised to the level of the innominate artery. The pleural edge over the trachea is grasped, and the mediastinal fat pad is dissected off the tracheal surface from the azygos vein to the innominate artery (Figure 35.11). A peanut sponge rolled tightly on a clamp is satisfactory for this portion of the operation. The pleural edge over the superior vena cava is similarly grasped, and the mediastinal fat pad is gently dissected from the junction of the superior vena cava and azygos vein to the level of the innominate artery. Not infrequently, a small vein drains from the mediastinal fat pad directly into the superior vena cava. If present, it must be identified and properly ligated to prevent unnecessary blood loss.

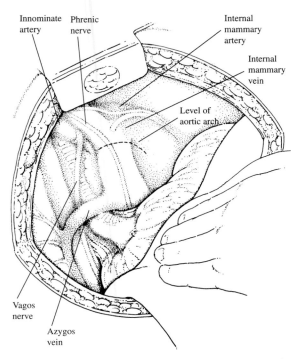

FIGURE 35.10. Exposure of right superior mediastinum with mediastinal pleura intact.

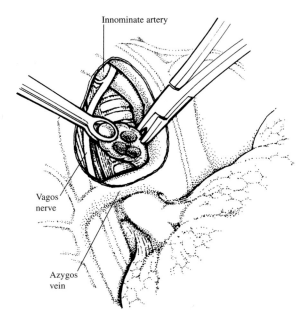

FIGURE 35.12. The lymphadenectomy may be extended to the contralateral lymph node levels. Care must be taken not to injure the left recurrent laryngeal nerve, which is found in the tracheoesophageal groove.

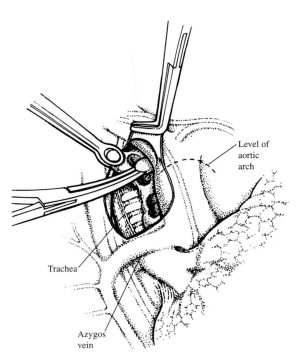

FIGURE 35.11. The internal mammary vein drains into the approximate juncture between the right and left innominate veins as they combine to form the superior vena cava and is a reliable structure with which to differentiate the division between *level 2* and *level 4* lymph nodes. The dashed line represents the aortic arch.

The mediastinal fat pad is grasped with an empty ring clamp and is removed from the superior vena cava anteriorly to the trachea posteriorly, and from the cephalic border of the azygos vein inferiorly to the cephalic border of the left innominate vein superiorly. Nonmagnetic clips (to avoid artifacts on future CT scans) are used liberally. Those lymph nodes between the cephalic border of the aortic arch and the cephalic border of the innominate vein are labeled *right level 2* (Figure 35.11). The lymph nodes distal to the aortic arch and proximal to the azygos vein are labeled *right level 4 superior* (Figure 35.12).

The azygos vein is elevated with a vein retractor, and all lymph nodes between its cephalad border and the origin of the right upper lobe bronchus are removed with sharp and blunt dissection (Figure 35.13). Care must be taken not to injure the pulmonary artery during dissection of these *level 4 inferior* lymph nodes.

Extension of the dissection behind the trachea reveals *level 3 posterior* nodes located between the esophagus and membranous portion of the trachea (Figure 35.14). Additional lymph nodes, *level 3 anterior,* are found anterior and medial to the superior vena cava at the insertion of the azygos vein.

Right level 10 lymph nodes are located along the anterior border of the bronchus intermedius distal to the pleural reflection (Figure 35.15). The interlobar, *level 11,* lymph nodes located in the sump of Borrie are dissected with the lung retracted anteriorly. The pulmonary artery is located anteriorly, and therefore clips must be placed under direct

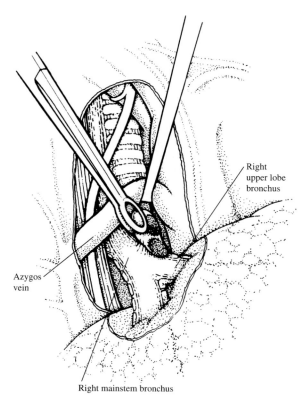

FIGURE 35.13. Division of the azygos vein is rarely necessary.

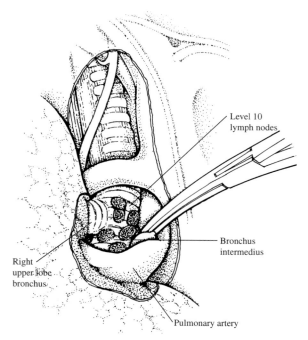

FIGURE 35.15. Exposure of the *level 10* lymph nodes is accomplished by retracting the pulmonary artery anteriorly.

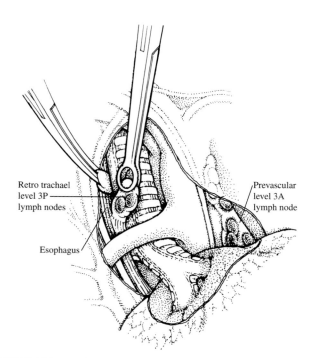

FIGURE 35.14. The location of the membranous portion of the trachea and the phrenic nerve must be determined prior to application of clips.

vision. *Level 12* nodes are adjacent to the distal lobar bronchus and are removed with the specimen (Figure 35.16).

Exposure of the *level 7* subcarinal region is obtained by retracting the lung directly anteriorly (Figure 35.17). The mediastinal pleura is opened, and the edge overlying the esophagus is grasped with a right-angle clamp. The esophagus is retracted posteriorly, and the subcarinal lymph node packet is swept anteriorly. Small vessels are coagulated or tied as necessary. The fat pad is grasped with a ring clamp and elevated off the pericardium. Attachments to the right and left mainstem bronchi are clipped before transection. The blood supply to this lymph node packet includes vessels that course along the anterior border of the trachea to enter the lymph nodes from the carina. Particular care must be taken to identify and control these vessels before they are transected because once they retract beneath the carina, they may be difficult to locate.

Level 9 lymph nodes are located within the inferior pulmonary ligament and are easily visualized. They can be grasped with a ring forceps and removed with cautery or clips. *Level 8,* paraesophageal lymph nodes, are not always present.

Left Hemithorax

Thoracotomy through the fifth interspace provides excellent exposure for dissection of the aortopulmonary (*levels 5* and *6*) and subcarinal (*level 7*) lymph nodes (Figure 35.18). The

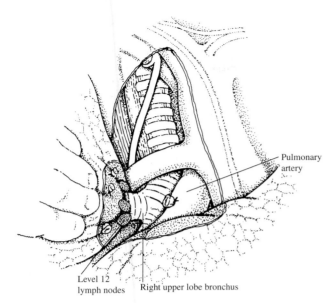

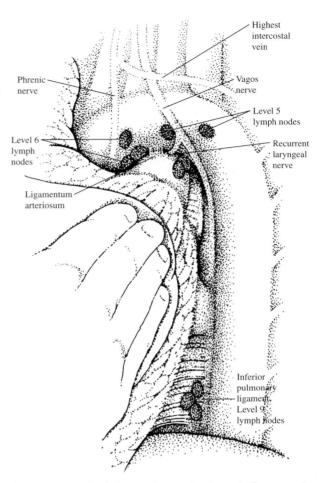

FIGURE 35.16. A peanut sponge is utilized to dissect the *level 12* lymph nodes and include them with the specimen. Cautery is employed to transect soft tissue because a clip may interfere with application of a stapling device.

lung is retracted inferiorly, and the pleura is incised in a cephalad direction midway between and parallel to the vagus and phrenic nerves, beginning at the level of the aortopulmonary window and extending above the aortic arch. The ligamentum arteriosum is readily palpated but less easily visualized. The *level 6* lymph nodes are exposed by grasp-

FIGURE 35.18. The left superior mediastinum before opening the mediastinal pleura. Exposure of *level 2* or *4* lymph nodes would require mobilization of the aortic arch.

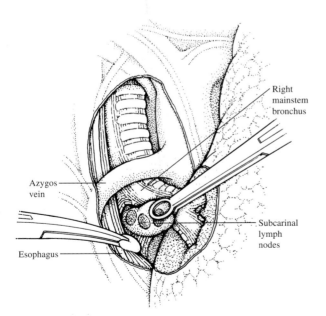

FIGURE 35.17. The esophagus and membranous portion of the bronchus must not be injured when applying clips.

ing the pleural edge closest to the phrenic nerve and dissecting away the lymph node–containing fat pad. This step is best accomplished with blunt dissection. Vessels should be controlled with clips or ties to avoid electrical injury to the nearby nerves. The location of the phrenic nerve must be constantly known to avoid iatrogenic diaphragm paralysis. *Level 5* lymph nodes are exposed by grasping the posterior pleural edge and bluntly dissecting the fat pad posterior to the ligamentum arteriosum. The recurrent laryngeal nerve and the proximal vagus nerve must be zealously protected because vocal cord paralysis is a potential complication.

The subcarinal lymph nodes, *level 7,* are approached with the lung retracted anteriorly (Figure 35.19). The pleura is opened anterior and parallel to the aorta at the level of the left mainstem bronchus. The lymph nodes are grasped with a ring clamp, and clips are liberally applied before excision of the nodal packet. An arterial vessel usually enters the lymph nodes at the carina. It must be identified and clipped to avoid postoperative hemorrhage.

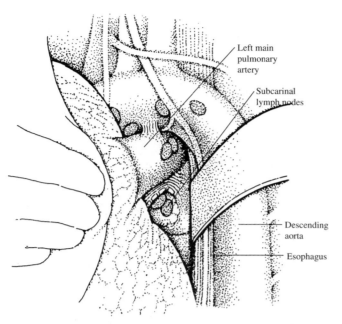

Left main pulmonary artery

Subcarinal lymph nodes

Descending aorta

Esophagus

FIGURE 35.19. The subcarinal lymph nodes are more difficult to expose in the left hemithorax than in the right hemithorax. A malleable retractor is used to retract the aorta and esophagus posteriorly.

Level 11 interlobar nodes are best approached with the lung retracted anteriorly. The pulmonary artery is immediately anterior and must be protected if clips are applied or cautery utilized. *Level 12* lymph nodes are located along the distal bronchus near its junction with the mainstem bronchus (Figure 35.20). The *level 9,* pulmonary ligament lymph nodes are identified within this structure and re-

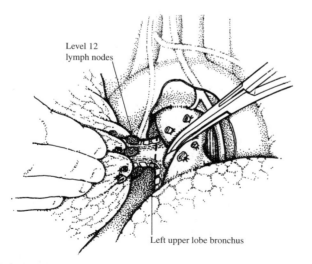

Level 12 lymph nodes

Left upper lobe bronchus

FIGURE 35.20. As the soft tissue is cleared to permit application of the stapling device, the nodes are pushed distally with a peanut sponge.

moved with cautery or clips. Esophageal injury must be avoided.

Even the most detailed lymph node dissection provides little information if the resected specimens are not correctly labeled. Many surgeons have not adopted the habit of routinely performing a lymph node dissection, and many pathologists do not report their histologic findings by individual lymph node level. To ensure that each level is reported separately and that levels are not lumped together as "mediastinal lymph nodes," they must be sent from the operating room as discrete specimens.

COMPLICATIONS OF MEDIASTINAL LYMPHADENECTOMY

Some surgeons are hesitant to perform a complete mediastinal lymph node dissection for fear of complications that might arise from either interrupting the blood supply to the bronchial stump or removing a large portion of the intrathoracic lymphatics. Bollen and colleagues[37] compared the postoperative complications of 155 patients with NSCLC who underwent no mediastinal lymph node dissection or sampling (n = 70), complete mediastinal lymph node dissection (n = 65), or systematic mediastinal lymph node sampling (n = 20). No significant difference among the groups was noted for intraoperative blood loss or the need for transfusion. Unintentional left recurrent laryngeal nerve injury occurred in three patients (5%) who underwent complete nodal dissection. Two additional patients developed chylothoraces. One patient who underwent node dissection required reoperation for bleeding not related to the lymphadenectomy. The two patients who developed bronchopleural fistulas had not undergone node dissection. Hata and colleagues[31] reported two left recurrent laryngeal nerve injuries and one phrenic nerve paralysis in 50 patients who underwent extensive mediastinal dissection. Reoperation or bronchopleural fistulas were not reported.

Izbicki and colleagues[68] compared the morbidity and mortality associated with systematic mediastinal sampling and mediastinal lymph node dissection in a randomized prospective study (n = 182). They found that although mediastinal lymph node dissection added approximately 20 minutes to the operative procedure, there was no increase in blood loss, mortality, or need for reoperation. One chylothorax occurred in each group. Recurrent laryngeal nerve injury was reported in six patients who underwent systematic sampling and in five patients who underwent mediastinal lymph node dissection. The duration of chest tube drainage and hospitalization were similar in both groups.

RESULTS OF LYMPH NODE SAMPLING AND DISSECTION

Five-year survival of patients with N2 disease after pulmonary resection and mediastinal lymph node dissection performed in a fashion similar to that described earlier is reported from 9% to 29%.[66,69–74] Most investigators make no therapeutic claim for nodal dissection but rather emphasize the benefits of accurate staging. The proponents of the more extensive nodal dissections, however, purport to demonstrate improved survival.

Hata and colleagues[33] reported five-year survival of 66% in 15 patients with N2 disease and 35% in 13 patients with N3 (contralateral mediastinal) disease who underwent bilateral mediastinal lymph node dissection by means of sternotomy. The five-year survival of 12 patients with scalene or supraclavicular N3 disease who underwent sternotomy and cervical dissection was 33%. Nakahara and colleagues[32] documented a three-year median survival for 13 patients with N2 disease who also underwent bilateral mediastinal lymph node dissection. No patient found to have N3 disease survived more than 14 months (n = 4). Watanabe and colleagues[30] claimed significantly improved survival of patients with left upper lobe tumors who underwent bilateral lymph node dissections when compared to patients who had only suspicious lymph nodes removed. These studies should be interpreted carefully because they contain small numbers of patients whose improved survival may result from factors unrelated to the extensive lymph node dissection. Indeed, Mitsuoka and colleagues[67] found no significant survival advantage for patients with pathologic stage IIIa left lung cancers who underwent sternotomy and nodal dissection when compared to patients who had thoracotomy only. In addition, no patients with N3 disease survived 3 years.

REFERENCES

1. Daniels AC. A method of biopsy useful in diagnosing certain intrathoracic diseases. *Dis Chest* 1949;16:360.
2. Harken DE, Black H, Clauss R, et al. A simple cervicomediastinal exploration for tissue diagnosis of intrathoracic disease. With comments on the recognition of inoperable carcinoma of the lung. *N Engl J Med* 1954;251:1041.
3. Radner S. Suprasternal node biopsy in lymph spreading intrathoracic disease. *Acta Med Scand* 1955;152:413.
4. Carlens E. Mediastinoscopy: a method for inspection and tissue biopsy in the superior mediastinum. *Dis Chest* 1959;36:343.
5. Pearson FG. Mediastinoscopy: a method of biopsy in the superior mediastinum. *J Thorac Cardiovasc Surg* 1965;49:11.
6. Pearson FG. An evaluation of mediastinoscopy in the management of presumably operable bronchial carcinoma. *J Thorac Cardiovasc Surg* 1968;55:617.
7. Ginsberg RJ. The role of preoperative surgical staging in left upper lobe tumors. *Ann Thorac Surg* 1994;57:526.
8. Patterson GA, Ginsberg RJ, Poon PY, et al. A prospective evaluation of magnetic resonance imaging, computed tomography, and mediastinoscopy in the preoperative assessment of mediastinal node status in bronchogenic carcinoma. *J Thorac Cardiovasc Surg* 1987;94:679.
9. Coughlin M, Deslauriers J, Beaulieu M, et al. Role of mediastinoscopy in pretreatment staging of patients with primary lung cancer. *Ann Thorac Surg* 1985;40:556.
10. Luke WP, Pearson FG, Todd TRJ, et al. Prospective evaluation of mediastinoscopy for assessment of carcinoma of the lung. *J Thorac Cardiovasc Surg* 1986;91:53.
11. Bernstein MP, Ferra JJ, Brown L. Effectiveness of scalene node biopsy for staging of lung cancer in the absence of palpable adenopathy. *J Surg Oncol* 1985;29:46.
12. Brantigan JW, Brantigan CO, Brantigan OC. Biopsy of nonpalpable scalene lymph nodes in carcinoma of the lung. *Am Rev Respir Dis* 1973;107:962.
13. Palumbo LT, Sharpe WS. Scalene node biopsy-correlation with other diagnostic procedures in 550 case. *Arch Surg* 1969;98:90.
14. Schatzlein MH, Mc Auliffe S, Orringer MB, et al. Scalene node biopsy in pulmonary carcinoma: when is it indicated? *Ann Thor Surg* 1981;31:322.
15. Lee JD, Ginsberg RJ. Lung cancer staging: the value of ipsilateral scalene lymph node biopsy performed at mediastinoscopy. *Ann Thorac Surg* 1996;62:338.
16. Kirschner P. "Extended" mediastinoscopy. In: Jepsson O, Ruhbek-Sorensen H, eds. *Mediastinoscopy*. Odense, Denmark: Odense University Press, 1971.
17. Ginsberg RJ. Extended cervical mediastinoscopy. *Chest Surg Clin NA* 1996;6:21.
18. Ginsberg RJ, Rice TW, Goldberg M, et al. Extended cervical mediastinoscopy. A single staging procedure for bronchogenic carcinoma of the left upper lobe. *J Thorac Cardiovasc Surg* 1987; 94:673.
19. Lopez L, Varela A, Freixinet J, et al. Extended cervical mediastinoscopy: prospective study of fifty cases. *Ann Thorac Surg* 1994; 57:555.
20. Urschel JD, Vretenar DF, Dickout WJ, et al. Cerebrovascular accident complicating extended cervical mediastinoscopy. *Ann Thorac Surg* 1994;57:740.
21. McNeill TM, Chamberlain JM. Diagnostic anterior mediastinotomy. *Ann Thorac Surg* 1966;2:532.
22. Olak J. Parasternal mediastinoscopy (chamberlain procedure). *Chest Surg Clin NA* 1996;6:31.
23. Denefee G, Lacquet LM, Gyselen A. Cervical mediastinoscopy in patients with lung cancer and radiologically normal mediastinum. *Eur J Respir Dis* 1983;64:613.
24. Jolly PC, Li W, Anderson RP. Anterior and cervical mediastinoscopy for determining operability and predicting resectability in lung cancer. *J Thorac Cardiovasc Surg* 1980;79:366.
25. Barendregt WB, Deleu HWO, Joosten HJM, et al. The value of parasternal mediastinoscopy in staging bronchial carcinoma. *Eur J Cardiothorac Surg* 1995;9:655.
26. Gossot D, Toledo L, Fritsch S, et al. Mediastinoscopy vs thoracoscopy for mediastinal biopsy. Results of a prospective nonrandomized study. *Chest* 1996;110:1328.
27. Landreneau RJ, Hazelrigg SR, Mack MJ, et al. Thoracoscopic mediastinal lymph node sampling: useful for mediastinal lymph node stations inaccessible by cervical mediastinoscopy. *J Thorac Cardiovasc Surg* 1993;106:554.
28. Kaseda S, Hangai N, Yamamoto S, et al. Lobectomy with extended lymph node dissection by video-assisted thoracic surgery for lung cancer. *Surg Endosc* 1997;11:703.
29. Iwasaki M, Nishiumi N, Maitani F, et al. Thoracoscopic surgery for lung cancer using the two small incisional method. Two windows method. *J Cardiovasc Surg* 1996;37:79.
30. Watanabe Y, Shimizu J, Oda M, et al. Improved survival in left non-small-cell N2 lung cancer after more extensive operative procedure. *Thorac Cardiovasc Surgeon* 1991;39:89.
31. Hata E, Hayakawa K, Miyamoto H, et al. Rationale for extended lymphadenectomy for lung cancer. *Theor Surg* 1990;5:19.
32. Nakahara K, Fujii Y, Matsumura A, et al. Role of systematic mediastinal dissection in N2 non-small cell lung cancer patients. *Ann Thorac Surg* 1993;56:331.
33. Hata E, Miyamoto H, Tanaka M, et al. Superradical operation

for lung cancer: bilateral mediastinal dissection (BMD) with or without cervical dissection (CD). *Lung Cancer* 1994;11(Suppl 2):41.

34. Gaer JAR, Goldstraw P. Intraoperative assessment of nodal staging at thoracotomy for carcinoma of the bronchus. *Eur J Cardiothorac Surg* 1990;4:207.

35. Graham ANJ, Chan KJM, Pastorino U, et al. Systematic nodal dissection in the intrathoracic staging of patients with non-small cell lung cancer. *J Thorac Cardiovasc Surg* 1999;117:246.

36. Haiderer O, Wustinger E, Lexer G, et al. Die mediastinale lymphadenektomie: anatomische grundlagen und ihre chirurgische relevanz beim zentralen bronchuskarzinom. *Wien Med Wochenschr* 1990;140:422.

37. Bollen ECM, van Duin CJ, Theunissen PHMH, et al. Mediastinal lymph node dissection in resected lung cancer: morbidity and accuracy of staging. *Ann Thorac Surg* 1993;55:961.

38. Izbicki JR, Passlick B, Karg O, et al. Impact of radical systematic mediastinal lymphadenectomy on tumor staging in lung cancer. *Ann Thorac Surg* 1995;59:209.

39. Sugi K, Nawata K, Fujita, et al. Systematic lymph node dissection for clinically diagnosed peripheral non-small-cell lung cancer less than 2 cm in diameter. *World J Surg* 1998;22:290.

40. Little AG, DeHoyos A, Kirgan DM, et al. Intraoperative lymphatic mapping for non-small cell lung cancer: the sentinel node technique. *J Thorac Cardiovasc Surg* 1999;117:220.

41. Naruke T, Suemasu K, Ishikawa S. Lymph node mapping and curability at various levels of metastasis in resected lung cancer. *J Thorac Cardiovasc Surg* 1978;76:832.

42. Tisi GM, Friedman PJ, Peters RM, et al. Clinical staging of primary lung cancer. *Am Rev Respir Dis* 1983;127:659.

43. Rusch VW, Ginsberg RJ, Holmes EC. *A thoracic surgery handbook for clinical trials.* New York: Memorial Sloan-Kettering Cancer Center, 1993.

44. Holmes EC. *Staging non-small cell lung cancer.* Evansville, IN: Bristol-Meyers Squibb, 1990.

45. Mountain CF. A new international staging system for lung cancer. *Chest* 1986;89(Suppl):225S.

46. Mountain CF. Revisions in the international system for staging lung. *Chest* 1997;111:1710.

47. Mountain CF, Dresler CM. Regional lymph node classification for lung cancer staging. *Chest* 1997;111:1718.

48. Mountain CF, Libshitz HI, Hermes KE. Lung cancer: a handbook for staging and imaging. Houston: Charles P Young, 1992.

49. Harvey DF, Zimmerman, HM. Studies on the development of the human lung. *Anat Rec* 1934–1935;61:203.

50. Rouviere H. Anatomy of the human lymphatic system. (Tobias MJ, transl. Anatomie des lymphatiques de l'homme.) Ann Harbor; Edward Brothers, 1938:83.

51. Borrie J. Primary carcinoma of the bronchus: prognosis following surgical resection. *Ann R Coll Surg Engl* 1952;10:165.

52. Weinberg JA. The intrathoracic lymphatics. In: Haagensen CD, Feind CR, Herter FP, eds. *The lymphatics in cancer.* Philadelphia: WB Saunders, 1972:231.

53. Murray GF, Mendes OC, Wilcox BR. Bronchial carcinoma and the lymphatic sump: the importance of bronchoscopic findings. *Ann Thorac Surg* 1982;34:634.

54. Nohl-Oser HC. An investigation of the anatomy of the lymphatic drainage of the lungs. *Ann R Coll Surg Engl* 1972;51:157.

55. Nohl HC. An investigation into the lymphatic and vascular spread of carcinoma of the bronchus. *Thorax* 1956;11:172.

56. Nohl-Oser HC. Lymphatics in the lung. In: Shields TW, ed. *General thoracic surgery,* 3rd ed. Philadelphia: Lea & Febiger, 1989:68.

57. Watanabe Y, Shimizu J, Tsubota M, et al. Mediastinal spread of metastatic lymph nodes in bronchogenic carcinoma. *Chest* 1990; 97:1059.

58. Cahan WG, Watson WL, Pool JL. Radical pneumonectomy. *J Thorac Surg* 1951;22:449.

59. Brock RD. Bronchial carcinoma. *Br Med J* 1948;2:737.

60. Weinberg JA. Identification of regional lymph nodes in the treatment of bronchogenic carcinoma. *J Thorac Surg.* 1951;22:517.

61. Brock R, Whytehead LL. Radical pneumonectomy for bronchial carcinoma. *Br J Surg* 1955;43:8.

62. Cahan WG. Radical lobectomy. *J Thorac Cardiovasc Surg* 1960; 39:555.

63. Kirsh MM, Kahn DR, Gago O, et al. Treatment of bronchogenic carcinoma with mediastinal metastases. *Ann Thorac Surg* 1971; 12:11.

64. Higginson JF. Block dissection in pneumonectomy for carcinoma. *J Thorac Surg* 1953;25:582.

65. Naruke T, Suemasu K, Ishikawa S. Surgical treatment for lung cancer with metastasis to mediastinal lymph nodes. *J Thorac Cardiovasc Surg.* 1976;71:279.

66. Martini N. Mediastinal lymph node dissection for lung cancer. *Chest Surg Clin N Am* 1995;5:189.

67. Mitsuoka M, Hayashi A, Takamori S, et al. The significance of lymph nodes (LN) dissection through median sternotomy for left lung cancer. *Lung Cancer* 1994;11(Suppl 1):149.

68. Izbicki JR, Thetter O, Habekost M, et al. Radical systematic mediastinal lymphadenectomy in non-small cell lung cancer: a randomized controlled trial. *Br J Surg* 1994;81:229.

69. Watanabe Y, Hayashi Y, Shimizu J, et al. Mediastinal nodal involvement and the prognosis of non-small cell lung cancer. *Chest* 1991;100:422.

70. Regnard JF, Magdeleinat P, Azoulay D, et al. Results of resection for bronchogenic carcinoma with mediastinal lymph node metastases in selected patients. *Eur J Cardiothorac Surg* 1991;5:583.

71. Naruke T, Goya T, Tsuchiya R, et al. The importance of surgery to non-small cell carcinoma of lung with mediastinal lymph node metastasis. *Ann Thorac Surg* 1988;46:603.

72. Watanabe Y, Shimizu J, Oda M, et al. Aggressive surgical intervention in N2 non-small cell cancer of the lung. *Ann Thorac Surg* 1991;51:253.

73. van Klaveren RJ, Festen J, Ottenn HJAM, et al. Prognosis of unsuspected but completely resectable N2 non-small cell lung cancer. *Ann Thorac Surg* 1993;56:300.

74. Maggi G, Casadio C, Mancuso M, et al. Resection and radical lymphadenectomy for lung cancer: prognostic significance of lymphatic metastases. *Int Surg* 1990;75:17.

SURGERY

36

MEDICAL EVALUATION AND MANAGEMENT OF THE LUNG CANCER PATIENT PRIOR TO SURGERY, RADIATION, OR CHEMOTHERAPY

FERNANDO J. MARTINEZ
MARK IANNETTONI
ROBERT PAINE, II

For the patient with non–small cell carcinoma of the lung (NSCLC), lung resection remains the best potentially curative therapy. Therefore, it behooves physicians who manage lung cancer to approach such patients as though surgery is possible and to tailor their evaluation with this goal in mind. However, surgery cannot benefit the patient if it results in early postoperative death or intractable respiratory failure. The determination that a given patient should undergo resectional surgery hinges on four factors: a resectable tumor (decided after a staging evaluation, which is described elsewhere in this text); adequate respiratory reserve to allow sufficient lung resection for cure; the absence of a major medical contraindication to surgery; and an agreeable patient. In those patients in whom surgery is not feasible because one or more of these requirements cannot be met, radiation therapy and/or chemotherapy are often utilized. We will describe our approach, based on available literature, to the patient to whom surgery, radiation therapy, and chemotherapy are offered to treat bronchogenic cancer. The goal of this evaluation is to identify patients at inordinate risk for posttreatment respiratory insufficiency and major perioperative morbidity.[1] Much of the earlier literature describes an approach to standard thoracic resection, while the later literature emphasizes improved methods of postoperative pain management and lung-conserving procedures.[2–5] These techniques are revolutionizing the preoperative evaluation of patients with suspected thoracic malignancies. We will also describe perioperative management strategies which can be used to decrease such complications.

CONSIDERATIONS FOR SURGICAL THERAPY
Physiology of Thoracotomy

The surgical invasion of the thorax to remove a portion of the lung is a major attack on the respiratory system. In addition to the resection of significant portions of functioning lung, there are major physiologic consequences of thoracotomy that are independent of actual lung resection. The major effects of entering the thorax appear to relate to a change in chest wall compliance and an increase in the work of breathing, due both to the direct influences of the surgical wound on the chest wall, including any chest wall resection, and to postoperative pain. Peters and colleagues[6] examined total chest compliance and work of breathing in 16 patients prior to, as well as one, three, and seven days after one of three different thoracic surgical procedures (thoracotomy only; thoracotomy with lung resection; or midline thoracotomy with open-heart surgery). Thoracotomy with or without lung resection decreased chest compliance to 47% of control values on postoperative day three. There were significant increases in work of breathing in the thoracotomy and thoracotomy plus resection groups (143% of control values on postoperative day three). Interestingly, these effects were much less prominent with "midline thoracotomy" (see below).

In part as a consequence of these changes in compliance, thoracotomy results in dramatic falls in the vital capacity that are sustained over the first three postoperative days.[7] This decrease in ventilatory capacity often results in alveolar hypoventilation with respiratory acidosis in the early postoperative period.[7] A drop in oxygen saturation is most marked two to three days postoperatively.[8] Cough is also frequently impaired after thoracotomy. Byrd and Burns[9] studied 24 adult patients undergoing thoracotomy. Cough pressures (measured using pleural pressures from intraesophageal catheters) dropped to 29% of preoperative values in the immediate postoperative period and had increased to only 50% of control one week after surgery. Since many patients with bronchogenic cancer are older and have underlying COPD, it is not surprising that thoracotomy and its resulting physiologic defects may be associated with significant postoperative cardiopulmonary complications.

Median sternotomy as described by Peters and colleagues[6] has been shown to preserve postoperative lung function better. Cooper and associates[10] examined the changes seen in pulmonary function after median sternotomy (n = 14 for coronary artery bypass surgery) and lateral thoracotomy (n = 14, left lateral thoracotomy for repair of hiatal hernia). Both groups showed a 50% reduction in peak expiratory flow rate and vital capacity by the second hospital day. Subsequent to that, however, the sternotomy group showed progressive improvements in pulmonary function. One week postoperatively, vital capacity had increased to 71% of control in the sternotomy group but only to 58% of control in the lateral thoracotomy group. As such, in marginal cases, this operative approach may be associated with better preservation of postoperative pulmonary function. There are limitations to this operative approach, however. In general, pulmonary anatomy may be more difficult to expose via sternotomy, particularly the left lower lobe.[7]

PREOPERATIVE PULMONARY EVALUATION

Overview of Physiologic Assessment of Operability

The benefit of surgical resection of a bronchogenic tumor can be manifest only if the patient survives the surgery and avoids chronic respiratory insufficiency due to the loss of resected pulmonary parenchyma. The normal adult has an enormous respiratory reserve that would allow removal of an entire lung with relatively little compromise. However, the vast majority of patients with lung cancer have smoked cigarettes and thus are at risk for chronic obstructive pulmonary disease (COPD). In some series, up to 90% of lung cancer patients have had signs and symptoms of COPD, and at least 20% of these patients have had severe respiratory dysfunction at initial evaluation.[11] A major goal of the preoperative evaluation of the patient with potentially resectable lung cancer is to predict the likelihood of severe postoperative respiratory insufficiency, based upon the patient's preoperative characteristics. It would be relatively easy to define criteria that would be sensitive predictors of postoperative respiratory difficulties (for example, prior cigarette use). However, this approach would lead to exclusion from potentially curative surgery of a significant number of patients. Ideally, it would be possible to exclude from surgery all patients who develop postoperative respiratory failure, while at the same time allowing surgery in the maximum number of individuals who could survive surgery without respiratory compromise. Thus over the last 45 years an extensive literature has been devoted to efforts to define preoperative characteristics that are both sensitive and specific predictors of postoperative respiratory insufficiency due to lost of resected lung. In addition, in some instances these

studies also have provided opportunities to predict overall perioperative complications based upon preoperative characteristics.

The history of efforts to define with ever-greater precision the subset of patients with potentially resectable carcinoma of the lung in whom surgery is feasible on physiologic grounds provides an instructive overview of our evolving understanding of the pathophysiology of chronic respiratory insufficiency. Investigators have attempted to define the limits of safe resection based upon traditional ventilatory parameters, measurements of gas transfer, techniques aimed at determining the contributions of specific portions of the lung to the patient's respiratory function, studies of pulmonary vascular reserve, and cardiopulmonary exercise testing (Tables 36.1, 36.2). While simple measures may suffice for patients with relatively well-preserved lung function, the use of multiple parameters is often necessary for patients with more significant impairment. The historical perspective presented in the discussion that follows is helpful for understanding the complimentary roles of the different parameters for the determination of operative risk. Recent series describe postoperative mortality that ranges from 0.9% to as high as 11.6% depending on the type of resection (higher for pneumonectomy).[12–15] Operative morbidity ranges from the teens to higher than 40%.[16] However, in comparing figures for morbidity and mortality from different surgical series, it is critical to recognize not only the differences in the patient characteristics but also differences in the accepted limits of operability in each study.

Spirometry/Lung Volumes

A spirometric study is one of the most widely used measures of ventilatory function. Well-accepted standards for measurement[17] and interpretation are available.[18] With a spirometer one can measure expired volumes such as the FVC, and the time components including the FEV_1. These studies are particularly valuable in assessing airflow obstruction.[18] Maximum breathing capacity (MBC), now named the maximum voluntary ventilation (MVV), can be measured as the total volume of air which can be rapidly inhaled and exhaled repetitively for up to 12 seconds. Using such measures (timed FVC and MBC), Gaensler and associates[19] studied 460 patients treated surgically for pulmonary tuberculosis. Those patients with an MBC of less than 50% predicted and a FVC of less than 70% predicted suffered a 40% postoperative mortality due to respiratory insufficiency.

Mittman[20] retrospectively reviewed various pulmonary function parameters in 196 patients undergoing thoracic surgical procedures (103 for thoracic malignancy). The best parameter in separating those with postoperative mortality was a MBC of less than 50% predicted. The addition of an elevated RV/TLC ratio (suggesting hyperinflation from underlying COPD) and an ECG with "nonspecific abnormalities" strengthened the ability to identify patients at high risk for thoracic surgery.

Boushy and colleagues[21] studied 142 patients with bronchogenic carcinoma using various pulmonary function studies, and followed for up to three years postoperatively. Those patients (n = 12) with severe postoperative respiratory difficulty including death had a lower FEV_1. These authors felt that an FEV_1 of less than 2 L and an FEV_1/FVC of less than 50% were poor prognostic signs in patients over the age of 60 undergoing pulmonary resection. These criteria have been widely accepted and often quoted.

Lockwood[22] measured multiple pulmonary function studies in 243 patients evaluated for thoracotomy for lung carcinoma. This author advocated using multiple parameters in identifying high-risk patients.[23] He found the following parameters to identify these high-risk patients: VC less than 1.85L, FVC less than 1.7L, RV more than 3.3L, TLC more than 7.9L, RV per TLC more than 47%, FEV_1 less than 1.2L, FEV_1/FVC less than 35% or MVV less than 28 L per minute. Note that these parameters were not indexed to a patient's age, sex, race, or weight, and as such their widespread applicability to all patients is limited.

Boysen and associates[24] prospectively studied 72 patients considered for thoracotomy. Postoperative respiratory complications (mainly pulmonary) were seen in 40 patients. FEV_1, FVC, and MVV were lower in these patients compared to those without postoperative complications. Miller,[25] using preoperative pulmonary function testing, split perfusion lung scans (see below), and Reichel exercise tests (see below) reported surgical results in 2,340 patients who underwent pulmonary resection over a 16-year period. Using the criteria shown in Table 36.1 (based in large part on predicted postoperative pulmonary function testing described later), the author reported an operative mortality, confined to the 30-day hospital period, of less than 1%.

The authors reported that 39 patients were denied the operation on the basis of preoperative pulmonary function.

These data suggest that simple pulmonary function testing has a role in identifying patients at particularly high risk for resection. Nevertheless, there is not uniform agreement in the literature. Larsen and Cliffton[26] retrospectively examined the results of 533 patients who underwent thoracic surgery at Memorial Sloan-Kettering Cancer Center from 1949 to 1960. Seventy-three of these patients did not tolerate surgery (died in hospital or developed severe respiratory failure). No difference was seen in VC or MBC between these patients and those who "tolerated" surgery. Of interest, is that "chronic lung disease" was present in only 33.7% of all patients but was more likely to be seen in those with respiratory insufficiency after surgery than in those without respiratory insufficiency. Furthermore, FEV_1 was not examined, nor were spirometric measures performed in a standard fashion throughout the course of the study period. Keagy and colleagues[27] studied 90 patients undergoing pneumonectomy for lung cancer with spirometry. The authors found no correlation between morbidity or mortality after surgery and preoperative spirometry. The authors, however, did not report the number of patients during the study period that had been evaluated for surgery but rejected on the basis of pulmonary function testing. This selection bias limits the conclusions reached by the authors. Kearney and colleagues prospectively studied 331 patients undergoing thoracic resections over a two-year period.[15] An FEV_1 below 1 L was not predictive of postoperative complications.

In summary, spirometry serves as a simple, cheap, and reproducible test of respiratory function that is a sensitive but not specific predictor of postoperative difficulty. Most studies have shown that parameters such as FEV_1, FVC, and FEV_1/FVC can identify patients who are likely to experience perioperative complications and/or postoperative re-

TABLE 36.1. PUBLISHED CRITERIA OF PULMONARY FUNCTION FOR PREDICTING HIGH RISK FOR LUNG RESECTION

Parameter	General Cutoff for Resection	Pneumonectomy	Lobectomy	Segmentectomy
FVC	under 2 L[19] under 1.7 L[23]			
FEV_1	under 1.2 L[23] under 2 L[21]	under 2 L[25,257]	under 1 L[25,257]	under 0.6 L[25,257]
FEV_1/FVC	under 35%[23] under 50%[21]			
MVV	under 50% pred[19] under 28 L per min[23] under 45 L per min[20]	under 55% pred[25,257]	under 40% pred[25,257]	under 35% to 45% pred[25,257]
RV	Increased[20] over 47% pred[23]			
DLCO	under 40% pred[34] under 50% pred[258] under 60% pred[32]			

spiratory insufficiency. However, as surgery is the only good curative alternative in patients with NSCLC, we must be sure to minimize the number of patients who are inappropriately denied surgery based on simple spirometric results. Therefore, we use spirometry to identify the highest-risk patients and exclude only those patients with severely abnormal pulmonary function (see Table 36.1) unresponsive to aggressive efforts to improve airflow obstruction (as will be described later) or unsuitable for lung sparing surgical resection. Further studies are usually required to define better the clinical situation.

Diffusion Capacity (DLCO)

The DLCO has been widely available for over 30 years.[28] The test measures the available alveolar-capillary surface area for gas diffusion, the alveolar membrane integrity, and the pulmonary capillary blood volume. It is thus a particularly sensitive, albeit nonspecific, test for pulmonary disease.[29] In patients with COPD, the DLCO is closely correlated with the extent of anatomic emphysema.[30,31] Limited study has been devoted to this test as a predictor of postthoracotomy outcome. Ferguson and colleagues[32] retrospectively studied the results of lung resection in 237 patients (lung cancer in 199). The DLCO (as a percent of predicted) was the most important predictor of mortality and the sole predictor of postoperative pulmonary complications. The same group confirmed these findings in a prospective study of 40 patients undergoing lung resection.[33] Those patients with a postoperative complication had a lower DLCO (65.3% of predicted) than those not experiencing such a complication (90.1% of predicted). In an excellent study, Markos and associates[34] prospectively studied 55 consecutive patients with suspected lung cancer. Patients were studied with spirometry, DLCO (expressed as a percent of predicted), pulmonary scintigraphy (described below), and exercise testing (discussed below). Among their findings, the DLCO was the best predictor of overall complications. In a retrospective study of 62 resections in 61 patients at high risk (FEV₁ less than 60% predicted or DLCO less than 50% predicted), a low DLCO identified patients at higher risk of respiratory complications and long-term respiratory morbidity.[35] In a prospective study of resection in 54 patients, Pierce and colleagues confirmed that preoperative DLCO as a percent of predicted was an excellent predictor of surgical complications, although not of cardiovascular or respiratory complications.[36] It is plausible that the DLCO, because of its sensitivity in identifying pulmonary parenchymal or vascular abnormality, may be particularly sensitive in identifying gas exchange difficulty after thoracotomy.[11]

Measure of DLCO may serve as an additional parameter which aids in identifying patients at high risk for perioperative complications and/or postoperative respiratory failure. The data are limited, however, and, as such, elimination of patients from curative resection solely on the basis of a decreased DLCO may not be appropriate. We use the DLCO to identify patients needing further testing and more intensive preoperative "tuning," as will be discussed later. In addition, DLCO data are used to strengthen our initial suspicion of unresectability as suggested by spirometric data.

Split Lung Function Studies

As we approach the question of resection of a portion of lung for treatment of carcinoma, it seems intuitively obvious to take into account that all portions of the lung may not contribute equally to the patient's ventilatory reserve. It is likely that a patient who is not experiencing respiratory compromise despite complete atelectasis of one lung will survive resection of that lung without postoperative respiratory insufficiency. Since the time of the height of the tuberculosis epidemic, investigators have attempted to estimate unilateral lung function in an effort to predict loss of function after aggressive surgical therapy in the individual case. More recently, additional efforts have focused on the ability to predict precisely postoperative lung function after lobectomy.

Bronchospirometry

Neuhaus and Cherniack[37] used the technique of bronchospirometry to predict postoperative VC and MBC. This technique involved the placement of a double-lumen endotracheal tube under local anesthesia, which allowed the isolation of each lung. In this way, during quiet breathing and maximal ventilation, the VC of each lung could be estimated. Furthermore, the oxygen uptake (VO₂) of each lung could be measured. These investigators[37] studied 80 patients who underwent pneumonectomy for tuberculosis and had undergone bronchospirometry preoperatively. They were able to predict postoperative VC and MBC with correlation coefficients between predicted and actual postoperative values of 0.86 and 0.67, respectively. An earlier study using bronchospirometry in 45 patients undergoing pneumonectomy and 97 patients after thoracoplasty allowed Snider and Shaw[38] to construct regression equations to predict the loss of VC and MVV resulting from surgery. The authors noted that the bronchospirometrically determined function of lung resected had little effect on postoperative lung function unless the preoperative pulmonary function was low. These data, in conjunction with the difficulty in performing the studies as well as the discomfort associated with the placement of the double-lumen endotracheal tube, have markedly limited the use of this study. The equipment to perform this test is now rarely available. We describe these studies to emphasize their historical role as the first accurate way to predict unilateral lung function.[11]

Lateral Position Test (LPT)

This study was first developed by Bergan in the late 1950s[39] and consists of a period of tidal breathing from an oxygen-filled spirometer containing a CO_2 absorber. A baseline VO_2 is obtained with the patient breathing supine from functional residual capacity (FRC). The patient is then asked to lie in a right or left lateral decubitus position while still breathing from the spirometer. After lying supine again to reestablish a baseline, the patient lies with the other lung superior. The difference in FRC owing to hyperinflation of the uppermost part of the superior lung as a percentage of the total volume change allows the unilateral lung function to be estimated.[11]

Marion and colleagues[40] and Walkup and colleagues[41] noted good correlations between predicted and actual pulmonary function (particularly FEV_1 and FVC; DLCO and lung volume estimates were less accurate) using LPT to predict postsurgical function. The limitations of the LPT quickly became evident however. Walkup and colleagues[41] correctly pointed out that lobar function could not be estimated using this technique. Furthermore, an earlier study[42] compared LPT, radionuclide studies, and bronchospirometry to determine unilateral lung function. There was an excellent correlation between values estimated using radionuclide studies and bronchospirometry (for FVC, r = 0.95). Values estimated by LPT were "statistically inferior" (for FVC, r = 0.87). A subsequent study by Jay and colleagues[43] revealed the major limitation of this study when they examined the variability of values obtained using this technique. In ten normal subjects, tests were performed in triplicate for five consecutive days. The variability of same-observer and different-observer measurements was minimal. However, there was significant variability in tests conducted in the same subject on the same day and in day-to-day measurements in any given subject. Finally, Schoonover and associates[44] examined the variability of the LPT in patients with COPD (24 patients with an FEV_1 of less than 2 L). A good correlation was found between estimated postpneumonectomy FEV_1 predicted from radionuclide scan and LPT (r = 0.72). There was however a more than 10% difference between these results in 59% of the patients. Furthermore, a subgroup of patients performed multiple LPTs. The variation was 14 times greater than in normal subjects, suggesting that as many as 37 tracings would be needed on each patient to obtain a value with an acceptably low measurement error. Because of these limitations, the LPT appears to have a limited applicability in the preoperative evaluation of patients being considered for lung resection. It is rarely used now and usually in centers without access to radionuclide studies.

Radionuclide Studies

Over the past 20 years, radionuclide techniques have become widely accepted for estimating postoperative function after lung resection. These techniques have been used predominantly to minimize postoperative respiratory failure by identifying particularly high-risk patients. The techniques available have recently been reviewed.[45] Kristersson and associates[46] first estimated unilateral lung function by measuring ^{133}Xe (^{133}Xe-ventilation radiospirometry). The estimated postpneumonectomy values for spirometry were compared with actual values measured one month to one year postsurgery. The correlations between these values were reasonably for FEV_1 (r = 0.63) and FVC (r = 0.73). The authors suggested that a postoperative FEV_1 of less than 1 L was the lower limit of operability.

Subsequently, Olsen et al[47] modified the technique by estimating unilateral lung *perfusion* by injecting ^{99m}technetium ferric hydroxide macroaggregates intravenously. This approach is designed to identify the extent of alveolar-capillary membrane that would remain following resection. The radioactivity emanating from each hemithorax was quantified and the predicted postoperative pulmonary function estimated using the formula:

Postsurgery PFT = (Preoperative PFT) × (% of total function contributed by the lung remaining).

In this way PFT parameters were compared to values measured three months following pneumonectomy. Thirteen patients in the study had moderately severe COPD preoperatively. The correlations between predicted and actual postpneumonectomy values were significant for FEV_1 (r = 0.72), FVC (r = 0.71), MVV (r = 0.75), and DLCO (r = 0.62). A significant error was present in the majority of cases. However, the predicted values were generally lower giving a "margin of safety." The authors suggested a postoperative FEV_1 of less than 0.8 L as being particularly high risk, although no specific evaluation of this cutoff was provided. Furthermore, pulmonary function was not corrected for age, sex, and height, particularly as the patients in this study were from an elderly, male, veteran population.

Ali and associates[48] prospectively studied 27 patients undergoing pneumonectomy for lung cancer using ^{133}Xe to study regional ventilation and perfusion. The correlation of percentage loss in FEV_1 and FVC as compared to predicted loss using estimated single lung function was in a range similar to prior studies (r = 0.63). These authors expressed postoperative function as a percent of predicted values, thereby normalizing function across all patients. The authors showed that seven of eight patients with an FEV_1 of less than 40% predicted had died, while ten of seventeen with an FEV_1 of more than 40% predicted remained alive. The causes of death were not provided, however. These same authors[49] in a subsequent study investigated the ability of ^{133}Xe radiospirometry to predict postoperative function after pneumonectomy (n = 97) or lobectomy (n = 44). They noted a good correlation between predicted FVC and FEV_1 and measured postoperative values for resections involving *more* than three segments (r = 0.83). Resections involving less than three segments (generally right upper lobectomies) were associated with less reliable predictions. Furthermore, the authors noted relatively stable function after pneumonectomy but a disproportionate early loss after lobectomy, which improved over time. This is quite significant, as patients with marginal pulmonary function may have very little reserve in the early postoperative period, leading to a greater likelihood of respiratory failure. More recently the same group[50] reported that a postoperative FEV_1 (ppoFEV_1) of less than 40% predicted was associated with a greater short-term mortality, but that long-term mortality was more closely related to tumor stage. Highest-risk individuals were noted to have estimated ppoFEV_1 values of less than 33% predicted with evidence of severe generalized airway obstruction (FEV_1/FVC less than 50%) and abnormal distribution of regional ventilation or perfusion within the non–tumor bearing lung. The importance of a predicted postoperative FEV_1 of more than 40% predicted is evident.

Boysen and colleagues[51] studied 33 patients felt to be at high risk for pneumonectomy on the basis of prior PFT criteria (similar to those shown in Table 36.1). Quantitative perfusion lung scans were used to predict postoperative FEV_1 (ppoFEV_1) as described earlier. If the ppoFEV_1 was more than 0.8 L, surgery was offered to the patient. Perioperative mortality before 30 days after surgery) was found to be an "acceptable" 15% (particularly given the high-risk nature of the patients). A subsequent study by the same group[52] of high-risk individuals (mean preoperative FEV_1 of 1.68 L prior to pneumonectomy) was published in 1981. These authors followed patients for a minimum of one year after surgery. A low incidence of deaths due to respiratory failure (17%) was noted, which was felt by the authors to related to the estimation of an adequate postoperative pulmonary reserve (FEV_1 of more than 0.8 L). The majority of deaths occurred from metastatic disease (69% of the deaths).

Wernly et al.[53] used a similar radionuclide technique (^{133}Xe ventilation and ^{99m}Te-macroaggregated albumin perfusion scans) prospectively in 85 patients (45 pneumonectomies, 40 lobectomies). Correlation of predicted postpneumonectomy pulmonary function was similar to the results of other investigators described earlier, whether ventilation or perfusion scans were used to estimate postsurgical lung function. The authors provided novel information in predicting ppoFEV_1 after lobectomy. They noted an excellent correlation (mean percent error less than 10%) using perfusion scans to estimate unilateral lung function and the following equation to estimate postlobectomy FEV_1:

$$\text{Expected loss of function} = \text{Preoperative } FEV_1$$
$$\times \ (\% \text{ function to affected lung})$$
$$\times \ \frac{(\text{number of segments in lobe to be resected})}{(\text{total number of segments in that lung})}$$

Similar correlations occurred if expected loss of function was estimated by regional function of the lobe to be resected (estimated from the perfusion scan) or by simply subtracting the number of segments to be removed as a fraction of all segments in both lungs. Using a ppoFEV_1 of over 1 L as the lower limit of operability the authors noted no postoperative deaths from respiratory failure in 22 patients with a preoperative FEV_1 of less than 2 L who underwent pneumonectomy. Forty patients with an FEV_1 of less than 1.5 L underwent lobectomy (again assuming a ppoFEV_1 of over 1.0 L) with no deaths or cases of postoperative respiratory insufficiency. A similar study by Egeblad and colleagues[54] estimated the loss of lung function expected by estimating the number of lung segments to be resected. No unilateral measure of lung function was performed; the authors estimated at the time of bronchoscopy the number of patent and nonventilated segments (occlusion defined as over 75% luminal narrowing) and estimated ppoFEV_1 using the following equation:

$$ppoFEV_1 = \text{Preoperative } FEV_1$$
$$\times \ \frac{\text{number of segments remaining postresection}}{20-\text{number of nonventilated segments preresection.}}$$

In studying 96 patients undergoing lung surgery, they found a correlation coefficient between ppoFEV_1 and actual FEV_1 six months postoperatively of $r = 0.83$; the correlation coefficient was $r = 0.85$ for FVC. The obvious limitations to this technique include the failure to account for differences in ventilation/perfusion ratios of the varying pulmonary regions (particularly in patients with COPD) and the failure to consider the differences in size between the two lungs. An overestimation in predicting functional loss has been measured at approximately 250 mL after lobectomy and 500 mL after pneumonectomy.[55] Furthermore, patients with severe atelectasis, endobronchial tumor involvement, and/or hilar disease may not have equal ventilation to each segment.[15] Nakahara and associates accounted for this in a nonscintigraphic estimate of postoperative pulmonary function which made a distinction between obstructed and nonobstructed airways.[56] Using this technique, ppoFEV_1 was predictive of postoperative complications. If a physician has no access to radionuclide studies, this crude method may be able to provide a rough estimate of ppoFEV_1.

Radionuclide scanning has also been reported to accurately predict postoperative exercise function. Corris et al[57] used ^{133}Xe ventilatory and ^{99m}Te perfusion scans in 28 patients before pneumonectomy. Estimates of ppoFEV_1 showed good correlation with measured values postsurgery. Fourteen patients performed exercise tests with measures of maximum ventilation (maxVE) and maximum oxygen uptake (maxVO$_2$) before and four months after pneumonectomy. A significant correlation was found between the change in maxVE and maxVO$_2$ after surgery and the percentage perfusion to the resected lung. Estimation of postoperative maxVE and maxVO$_2$ on the basis of ^{99m}Te perfusion scans showed good agreement with observed values. Similarly, Bolliger and colleagues were able to accurately estimate postsurgical aerobic capacity in 22 patients after thoracic resection.[58] These data suggest that estimates of unilateral lung function may serve to estimate exercise capacity after pneumonectomy.

Not all data have been consistently supportive of radionuclide scanning, however. Ladurie and Ranson-Bitker[59] recently reviewed their experience with 159 patients who had undergone pneumonectomy (131 for lung cancer). Unilateral functional determination was done with bronchospirometry in 47 patients and with radionuclide scanning in 112. The difference between the ppoFEV$_1$ and the actual postoperative FEV$_1$ was greater than one standard deviation in 37 patients (mean difference 415 mL). Overestimation of ppoFEV$_1$ was seen in 20 patients, while underestimation was seen in 17. In addition, Holden and colleagues found neither the ppoDLCO nor ppoFFEV$_1$ predictive of complications in a small study of 16 patients.[60]

Markos and associates[34] published an excellent prospective study of 55 consecutive patients with suspected lung cancer which places many of these issues into practical perspective. The patients were studied preoperatively with spirometry, lung volume measurements, DLCO measurements, radionuclide studies to predict postoperative function, and an exercise test (discussed later). Eighteen patients underwent pneumonectomy, while 29 underwent lobectomy. Predicted pulmonary function correlated well with measured postoperative values. The lower correlations seen with pneumonectomy in this study were felt to reflect the effects of postoperative radiation therapy. PpoFEV$_1$ was less than 0.8 L in 12 of 29 patients treated with lobectomy. However, expressing data as a percent of predicted allowed the authors to show that ppoFEV$_1$ of over 40% predicted was associated with no mortality, while ppoFEV$_1$ of less than 40% predicted was associated with a 50% mortality. Furthermore, predicted postoperative DLCO (ppoDLCO) of less than 40% predicted was also associated with a high mortality and morbidity. PpoFEV$_1$ and ppoDLCO were the best predictors of postoperative death and postoperative respiratory failure, respectively. It should be noted however, that 47% of the patients studied had a preoperative FEV$_1$ of over 2 L with only 6% having a preoperative FEV$_1$ of less than 50% predicted. These patients were thus generally "healthier" than those reported in most previous studies. Nevertheless, this study showed the value of predicting postoperative function in estimating not only postoperative mortality but complications as well. Furthermore, expressing data as a percent of normal predicted for a given patient had a clear, practical value.

Recent data have expanded the role of postsurgical prediction of lung function. Pierce and colleagues prospectively examined 54 patients undergoing thoracic resection.[36] Postoperative pulmonary function was estimated using quantitative perfusion scanning in those patients with a presurgical FEV$_1$ of over 55% predicted and by estimating the proportional loss of pulmonary segments in those patients with a presurgical FEV$_1$ of less than 55% predicted. They confirmed the value of ppoFEV$_1$ and ppoDLCO in predicting

surgical mortality, while ppoDLCO predicted surgical complications. A composite score generated by multiplying ppoFEV$_1$ and ppoDLCO, the PPP, or predicted postoperative product, was highly predictive of complications and the best single predictor of surgical mortality in contrast to baseline pulmonary function studies. A PPP over 1850 was seen in seven of eight patients dying but in only five of 44 survivors. Similarly, Ribas and colleagues prospectively examined 65 patients scheduled for thoracotomy by estimating postoperative pulmonary function.[61] They confirmed that ppoFEV$_1$ was the only value that differed between those patients experiencing postoperative respiratory complications and those that did not experience such complications. Filaire and associates prospectively defined predictive factors of postoperative hypoxemia and mechanical ventilation in 48 patients undergoing lung resection.[62] In lobectomy but not pneumonectomy the best predictor was ppoFEV$_1$. Similarly, Wang and colleagues retrospectively examined 410 patients undergoing lung resection over a 17-year period at the University of Chicago.[63] A low ppoDLCO was predictive of operative death but of long-term survival.

Wu and colleagues estimated postoperative pulmonary function using quantitative computed tomography (CT).[64] Excellent correlations were noted between CT estimates and actual measurements of postoperative FEV$_1$ (r = 0.93). As most patients with suspected bronchogenic cancer undergo preoperative CT scanning, this technique could prove particularly useful if prospective validation is provided in comparison to standard scintigraphic techniques.

Measurement of predicted pulmonary function after lobectomy or pneumonectomy is easily done with the use of radionuclide imaging (either perfusion or ventilation). Using a ppoFEV$_1$ of over 40% predicted likely minimizes postoperative respiratory failure and may identify those patients with lower perioperative complications. If radionuclide scanning is not available, then estimates of the number of segments to be resected can be made at the time of bronchoscopy. The data supporting this technique are limited, however. In most patients it is not necessary to estimate postoperative function. This approach is reserved for those patients in whom initial spirometric or DLCO measurements suggest a higher risk of postoperative respiratory insufficiency, as defined in Table 36.1. If one is unsure of the extent of resection, then estimates of ppoFEV$_1$ should be made for both limited and extensive resection (including pneumonectomy). In this way the surgeon carries all necessary information into the operating room, where the final decision will be made.

Vascular Studies

The role of pulmonary hypertension and cor pulmonale in respiratory disability became evident during the tuberculosis epidemics. In 1958, Harrison and colleagues[65] noted significant rises in pulmonary artery pressure with exercise in 28 patients after pneumonectomy. The authors also found a correlation between the degree of disability and abnormal pulmonary hemodynamics, confirming the importance of abnormal pulmonary vasculature in the postoperative morbidity after pulmonary resection. Subsequently, measures of preoperative pulmonary vascular function were felt to be useful in minimizing postoperative respiratory failure.

Temporary unilateral pulmonary artery occlusion (TUPAO) was felt to aid in assessing the pulmonary vascular response to planned pulmonary resection. TUPAO was first described with the use of a cardiac catheter with a large distal rubber cuff by Carlens and associates.[66] When passed into the pulmonary artery of the lung to be removed, inflation of the catheter occluded the blood flow to this lung. This occlusion was felt to result in a "physiologic pneumonectomy."[11] Measurement of pulmonary artery pressures and arterial hypoxemia was felt to identify patients at high risk for postoperative hemodynamics instability. Uggla[67] examined the role of TUPAO in 1956 in 109 patients with varying bilateral benign disease. The patients were separated into three groups, based on follow-up: "dead," "cardiorespiratory cripples," and "fit for work." There was a progressively larger VC and MBC across these groups although the differences were not striking. Resting pulmonary artery pressures were somewhat higher in the patients who had died, with a resting pressure of 22 mm Hg carrying a "very grave prognosis." With TUPAO, the pulmonary artery pressure in all patients rose approximately 50%. This was accentuated with activity. The authors reported that a pulmonary artery pressure of over 35 mm Hg and a systemic arterial oxygen level of less than 45 mm Hg during TUPAO was frequently associated with death.

Rams et al[68] incorporated intraoperative TUPAO as part of the routine evaluation of patients undergoing pneumonectomy. The authors reported results in 61 patients studied in such a fashion. The duration of pulmonary artery occlusion was not reported. The patients who survived the immediate 30-day postoperative period (n = 45) were compared to those who died within this 30-day period (n = 16). The former patients showed a resting pulmonary artery pressure of 22 increasing to 26 with TUPAO, while the latter group showed a resting pulmonary artery pressure of 26 mm Hg which rose to 30 with TUPAO. The authors could not define absolute criteria but felt that a patient with a resting pulmonary artery pressure of over 25 mm Hg with a further rise on TUPAO as well as low preoperative VC and MBC was at particularly high risk. Similar data were provided by Van Nostrand and associates,[69] who felt that a rise in pulmonary artery pressure to over 40 mm Hg with TUPAO during exercise may be a reasonable cutoff for operability, although this rarely happened in their patients.

Laros and Swierenga[70] studied 142 patients with TUPAO prior to lung cancer surgery. TUPAO was performed for ten minutes at rest and with 20 to 25 leg raises. No correlation was found between preoperative findings

and early postoperative mortality. In three patients right ventricular rupture complicated the procedure, with death resulting in two. In an often quoted study, Olsen and colleagues[71] prospectively studied 56 patients with abnormal screening pulmonary function studies using TUPAO and split lung function measured with radionuclide scanning. Surgery was offered to those patients with a ppoFEV$_1$ of over 0.8 L, pulmonary artery pressure with occlusion (at rest or exercise) of less than 35 mm Hg, and systemic paO$_2$ with TUPAO during exercise of over 45 mm Hg. Using these criteria, 42 patients underwent surgical exploration (resulting in 17 pneumonectomies and 13 lobectomies). The cardiopulmonary mortality was 17.6% for pneumonectomy and 7.7% for lobectomy, which the authors felt was acceptable particularly given the high-risk nature of the patients. Of interest is that TUPAO was not technically possible in 26% of the patients. Given the technical difficulties and risk of TUPAO, it is now rarely used and likely has a very limited role in the preoperative evaluation of a candidate for pulmonary resection.

More recently Lewis and colleagues performed detailed hemodynamic monitoring at rest and after pulmonary artery clamping in 20 patients with moderately severe COPD (FEV$_1$ of 66% predicted) undergoing pneumonectomy.[72] No relation was noted between any pulmonary function test or derived hemodynamic variable and length of hospital stay or the development of in-hospital complications. Late cardiopulmonary disability was more likely in those patients with a right ventricular ejection fraction less than 35%, pulmonary vascular resistance greater than or equal to 200 dyne-sec-cm^{-5}, and a pulmonary vascular resistance/right ventricular ejection fraction ratio greater than or equal to 5.0 after pulmonary artery clamping.

Given the technical difficulties and poorly defined thresholds for resection, pulmonary vascular measurements are rarely made. We reserve this for the rare patient in whom the studies described earlier (spirometry, DLCO, radionuclide testing) are contradictory but resection is felt feasible.

Exercise Testing

Exercise tests have become widely accepted in the evaluation of cardiovascular disease, dyspnea, and disability, and for the determination of exercise prescriptions. As they provide an objective assessment of a subject's exercise capacity, much interest has been devoted to examining their role in the evaluation of the lung resection candidate. The majority of studies use exercise capacity to predict postoperative morbidity. This has been elegantly reviewed by Olsen[73] and Bolliger and Perrucoud.[1] Olsen separated exercise tests in this setting into three categories: simple tests of exercise tolerance, tests of pulmonary vascular response to exercise, and tests of aerobic capacity utilizing expired gas analysis. We will discuss each of these in turn.

Simple Exercise Tolerance Tests

Tests of exercise tolerance were among the first used to assess "operability" in patients being considered for lung surgery for tuberculosis. Gaensler[19] in 1955 measured ventilation during walking 180 feet within one minute in a large group of patients undergoing surgical treatment of tuberculosis. There was no prognostic value to this measurement. Olsen[73] estimated this degree of exercise to translate to a VO_2 (see below) of approximately 12 mL per kg per minute in a 70 kg male, a moderate workload at best. Bagg[74] used a similar simple test of ambulation. Thirty patients with lung cancer walked for 12 minutes with a measure of the total distance walked (12-minute walk test). There was no significant ability of this 12-minute walking distance or the level of dyspnea experienced to discriminate the seven patients who suffered postoperative ventilatory complications. This level of stress was likely inadequate.

Van Nostrand and colleagues,[69] as part of their preoperative evaluation, assessed the ability of patients to climb one flight of stairs (19 steps) without severe dyspnea. The authors pointed to the death of two of the four patients who could not walk one flight of stairs without severe dyspnea. Only seven of 63 patients who were able to climb two flights with little dyspnea failed to survive pneumonectomy. The authors recommended rejection for pneumonectomy if: (a) patients were unable to climb one flight without severe dyspnea; (b) estimated postoperative FEV_1 was less than 0.7 L; or (c) pulmonary artery pressure rose to more than 40 mm Hg with intraoperative pulmonary artery clamping (see above). The importance of a single flight of stairs climbed without dyspnea is still widely used despite limited supporting data.

Recently stair climbing has received more rigorous investigation. Bolton and associates[75] related pulmonary function to a stair climb (performed at subject's own pace as far as possible to a maximum of 127 steps, five flights) in 70 male patients. There was a correlation between the number of steps climbed and FVC (r = 0.59), FEV_1 (r = 0.65), FEV_1/FVC (r = 0.56), and MVV (r = 0.55). The authors further noted that patients who climbed all five flights had an FEV_1 of over 1.75 L, while of those who climbed less than three flights the majority had an FEV_1 of less than 1.7 L.

A subsequent study by these same investigators[76] examined the ability of such a stair climb to serve as a preoperative study prior to thoracotomy. The ability to climb three flights was associated with a decreased complication rate, shorter mechanical ventilation time, and shorter hospital stay. Unfortunately, due to the small number of fatal complications, mortality could not be accurately predicted. The retrospective nature of data collection and inconsistent collection of data were obvious limitations to this study. Nevertheless, it suggested that this simple test of exercise endurance could serve as a predictor of outcome after thoracotomy.

In a recent prospective study of 16 patients with lung cancer, Holden and colleagues[60] studied all patients with spirometry, DLCO, cycle ergometry (with gas exchange measurements as described below), radionuclide scanning with prediction of $ppoFEV_1$, walking distance, and a symptom-limited stair climb (at the patient's own pace). Those patients who died within 90 days of surgery (n = 5) had a shorter six-minute walk distance and lower stair climb than those who had minor or no postoperative complications (n = 11). A six-minute walk distance greater than 1000 feet and stair climb greater than 44 steps (four flights) were predictive of a successful surgical outcome. This level of work is clearly greater than that of Gaensler and colleagues[19] and Van Nostrand and colleagues.[69]

Pollock and colleagues[77] studied 31 men with moderate COPD (mean FEV_1 52% predicted; range 21% to 89% predicted). All underwent cycle ergometry with gas exchange measures and a symptom-limited stair climb. During the latter, expired gases were collected and VO_2 and VE calculated during each of the last three flights. The VO_2, VE, and heart rate were greater during stair climbing than cycle ergometry, suggesting a greater metabolic load to the former. The number of steps climbed correlated well with VO_2 (see Figure 36.1). This study allows a reasonable estimation of aerobic capacity (VO_2) using a readily accessible method of testing exercise capacity (stair climbing). It also suggests that to achieve a significant metabolic load, a patient may need to climb more than one or two flights. In a recent, prospective study, Pate and colleagues compared spirometric and radionuclide techniques, stair climbing, and formal cardiopulmonary exercise testing in 12 patients at high risk based on routine spirometric criteria (FEV_1 over 2 L).[78] All patients underwent thoracic resection, with two experiencing major complications (one death) and five

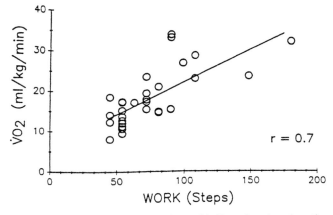

FIGURE 36.1. The peak VO_2 achieved is linearly related to the number of steps climbed by 31 men with moderately severe chronic airflow obstruction (FEV_1 52% predicted). (From Pollock M, Roa J, Benditt J et al. Estimation of ventilatory reserve by stair climbing. A study in patients with chronic airflow obstruction. *Chest* 1993;104:1378, with permission.)

minor complications. Ten of the 12 patients were able to climb more than three flights, which the authors felt was an appropriate threshold for considering thoracic resection.

Rao and colleagues reported a retrospective review of 396 consecutive patients of whom 299 underwent both preoperative spirometry and oximetry during a standard 150 meter walk.[79] Abnormal oxygen saturation during this limited exercise test was defined as an oxygen saturation below 90%, with subgroups experiencing a greater than 4% or 5% absolute drop in oxygen saturation. Compared with spirometric indices, abnormal oximetry more reliably predicted home oxygen requirements, the need for intensive care unit admission, prolonged hospital stay, and respiratory failure. Prospective validation in comparison with postoperative prediction of pulmonary function is required, however.

Several investigators have explored more formal exercise endurance tests in the preoperative assessment of patients prior to thoracotomy. Reichel[80] reported a retrospective study of 75 patients undergoing pneumonectomy. Thirty-one of these patients performed an incremental treadmill exercise test (performed in six stages of increasing grade, speed, and cumulative time). No patient who finished all six stages of the protocol experienced postoperative complications. Fifty-seven percent of those who did not complete the test experienced significant postoperative complications. Of the four unable to walk through stage 1, two died and one survived with severe complications. Apparently, other measures of pulmonary function could not predict mortality or morbidity in this study. Others have utilized this exercise protocol. Miller[25] reported a less than 1% operative mortality using a preoperative evaluation including the Reichel exercise test (performed in 217 of 2,340 patients). Of the 160 patients who passed the test, 84 underwent pneumonectomy (four died); 67 patients failed the test, with seven undergoing pneumonectomy and two dying.

Berggren and associates[81] reported the results of bicycle ergometry in 82 elderly patients performed as part of a preoperative evaluation prior to lung cancer surgery. Exercise was performed at 50 watts for six minutes, and the workload was increased at 10-watt increments to a maximal cardiac frequency of less than 170 beats per minute. The results for lobectomy (44 patients) were presented in detail. Postoperative mortality was 7.7% in those who completed more than 83 watts in six minutes, while it was 22% for those completing less than this. Mortality was also higher with lower pulmonary function (FEV$_1$ of less than 2.4 L, FVC below 3.7 L, FEV$_1$/FVC less than 68%).

Gerson and associates[82] reported the results of bicycle ergometer in predicting cardiac and pulmonary complication in 177 elderly patients (age over 65 years) undergoing abdominal or noncardiac thoracic surgery. Exercise was on a supine bicycle ergometer with an initial workload of 25 watts; load was increased by 12.5 watts per minute until limiting dyspnea, chest pain, or fatigue. "Inability to complete exercise" was defined as the inability to raise heart rate above 99 beats per minute for two minutes. The result of exercise testing was the best predictor of perioperative pulmonary, cardiac, or combined complications. In the 108 patients who were able to "complete the exercise" ten patients (9.8%) suffered a complication (with one death); in the 69 patients who were unable to complete the exercise protocol (as defined earlier) 29 suffered complications (with five deaths). As such, simple measures of exercise endurance (treadmill, bicycle ergometer, or stair climbing) may be appropriate in selected patients to aid in predicting postoperative mortality and morbidity. We do not use these routinely, but reserve them for those patients in whom preoperative screening studies suggest a higher risk (Table 36.1).

Vascular Response to Exercise

As described earlier, pulmonary hypertension was noted as a complication of thoracic resection in the tuberculosis era. The importance of assessing the pulmonary vascular bed was thereby recognized.[65,83] Such early studies of pulmonary vascular response were described above with use of TUPAO at rest and during exercise.[67,70,71,83] As noted earlier, the results of these studies were inconclusive.

Recently the pulmonary vascular response during exercise has again come under scrutiny as a predictor of postoperative complications in patients undergoing lung resection. Fee and associates[84] reported results of resting pulmonary function testing and pulmonary vascular resistance (PVR) measurements at rest and with exercise. Forty-five patients were separated on the basis of resting pulmonary function. Group A (n = 27) had a room air paO$_2$ of over 50 mm Hg and FEV$_1$ and FVC more than 50% predicted; Group B (n = 18) had paO$_2$ of less than 50 mm Hg and FEV$_1$ or FVC less than 50% predicted. All patients underwent right heart catheterization while sitting on a treadmill, allowing measurement of pulmonary artery pressure (PAP). Exercise was begun at a low level (two miles per hour and 4% grade) and PAP, cardiac output, and pulmonary capillary wedge pressure were measured. After a 45-minute rest period, patients exercised at four miles per hour and 4% grade with repeat measurement of pulmonary vascular response and cardiac output. Patients were separated on the basis of PVR: Group A had maximum exercise PVR of less than 190 dynes-sec-cm^{-5} and Group B had PVR of over 190 dynes-sec-cm.$^{-5}$ Thirty of the patients underwent lung resection. Five patients died (all with exercise PVR over 190 dynes-sec-cm^{-5}). Four of these were in the Group A, with better pulmonary function. The authors concluded that a PVR with exercise over 190 dynes-sec-cm^{-5} were at high risk for lung surgery. However, seven of the 25 *surviving* patients also had an exercise PVR over 190 dynes-sec-cm^{-5} and would have been denied surgery. This study confirms the limitation of simple measures of pulmonary function in predicting postthoracotomy outcome and suggests a possible role for the assessment of the pulmonary vasculature during exercise. An absolute criterion for rejecting a patient from lung resection remains unsettled.

Olsen and colleagues[85] studied 52 elderly men with COPD and a lung mass. Pulmonary function tests at rest and radionuclide scanning were performed and a high risk for lung resection confirmed (FEV_1 of under 2 L, MVV less than 50% predicted). All underwent exercise seated on a bicycle ergometer with a pulmonary artery catheter in place. Exercise was performed at 25 watts for two to four minutes while data (cardiac function, pulmonary vascular resistance and pressures, VO_2 and oxygen delivery) were collected. After a rest period, exercise was repeated at 40 watts, with similar data collected. Patients were approved for pneumonectomy or lobectomy if ppoFEV_1 was over 0.8 L and PVR at the highest workload was less than 190 dynes-sec-cm^{-5}. Twenty-nine patients underwent surgery (eight pneumonectomies, 13 lobectomies, seven wedge resections and one bronchoscopy), with seven dying within 60 days or needing prolonged (over 30 days) mechanical ventilation ("intolerant of surgery"). The parameters found to be predictive of "intolerance" included: low cardiac index, low oxygen delivery, and low VO_2 (see below). The study suggested that a deficit in oxygen transport may be predictive of surgical complications. Clearly, the invasiveness of this protocol limits widespread applicability of the technique. As with other cumbersome modalities, it may have a role in particularly difficult cases.

On the other hand, Bolliger and colleagues examined five patients with severe COPD using both maximal exercise testing (see below) and rest and exercise pulmonary hemodynamic measurements.[86] Using traditional exclusions based on hemodynamic measurements would have excluded four patients from surgery, although all patients were able to tolerate resection with little postoperative difficulty. Similarly, Ribas and colleagues were unable to find clinically useful hemodynamic measurements at rest or during exercise which predicted postoperative outcome in a group of 46 patients undergoing thoracotomy.[61]

Tests of Aerobic Capacity

The most recent exercise measurement to achieve some degree of popularity is the measure of aerobic capacity. The analysis of expired gases allows the calculation of aerobic capacity as defined by maximum achieved VO_2 (VO_{2max}). This is a sensitive parameter which can reflect limitation in any component involved in the response to exercise (cardiac, pulmonary, vascular, and peripheral muscles). Conflicting data have been published regarding the value of VO_{2max} measurements in the preoperative assessment of the lung resection candidate (Table 36.2).

Eugene and associates[87] reported the results of VO_{2max}

TABLE 36.2. STUDIES EXAMINING MEASURE OF AEROBIC CAPACITY IN THE PREOPERATIVE EVALUATION OF LUNG CANCER PATIENTS

Reference	Exercise Type	Number of Patients	Prediction Threshold		
			No Complication	Morbidity	Mortality
Eugene, et al.[87]	Maximal	19	over 1 L/min	NA	under 1 L/min
Colman, et al.[96]	Maximal	57	None	None	None
Smith, et al.[88]	Maximal	22	over 20 mL/kg/min	under 15 mL/kg/min	None
Bechard, et al.[89]	Maximal	50	over 20 mL/kg/min	under 10 mL/kg/min	under 10 mL/kg/min
Miyoshi, et al.[90]	Maximal (lactate 20 mg per dL)	33	None	None	under 400 mL/min/m^2
Olsen, et al.[85]	Submaximal	29	None	None	under 10 mL/kg/min*
Markos, et al.[34]	Maximal	55	None	None	None
Boysen, et al.[97]	Maximal	17	None	None	None
Morice, et al.[92]	Maximal	8	over 15 mL/kg/min	None	None
Olsen, et al.[76]	Maximal	12	over 10 mL/kg/min	None	under 10 mL/kg/min
Nagakawa, et al.[91]	Maximal (lactate 20 mg per dL)	31	over 300 mL/min/m^2	None	under 300 mL/min/m^2
Dales, et al.[259]	Maximal	117	over 1.25 L/min	None	None
Pierce, et al.[36]	Maximal	42	None	under 500 mL/m^2/min	None
Bolliger, et al.[86]	Maximal	5	≥ 69% predicted	None	None
Bolliger, et al.[94]	Maximal	80	over 75% predicted	under 60% predicted	under 60% predicted
Bolliger, et al.[58]	Maximal	25	None	None	under 10 mL/kg/min*
Torchio, et al.[95]	Maximal	54	AT over 14.5 mL/kg/min	under 20 mL/kg/min	None
Ribas, et al.[61]	Maximal	65	None	None	None
Wang, et al.[33]	Maximal	40	None	None	None

* postoperative predicted value; AT, anaerobic threshold.

measurement in 19 patients prior to pulmonary resection (six pneumonectomies, 12 lobectomies, one segmentectomy). Three patients died from cardiopulmonary failure. Pulmonary function studies did not identify this group preoperatively. Of patients who achieved a VO_{2max} of less than 1 L per minute, three died, while none who achieved a VO_{2max} of over 1 L per minute died (p = 0.004). Smith and colleagues[88] supported the use of VO_{2max} measurements in a study of 23 patients scheduled for thoracotomy who were prospectively evaluated with incremental exercise testing. Pulmonary function tests and radionuclide scanning were performed in all. Eleven of the patients had no cardiopulmonary complications postoperatively. The only preoperative value separating the 11 patients who suffered complications postoperatively from those who did not was VO_{2max} (22.4 mL per kg per minute in those without complications versus 14.9 mL per kg per minute in those with complications). Only one of ten with a VO_{2max} greater than 20 mL per kg per minute had a complication compared to all six with a VO_{2max} of less than 15 mL per kg per minute.

A similar study was published by Bechard and Wetstein in 1987[89] of 50 consecutive patients studied with pulmonary function testing and incremental exercise testing. A criterion for FEV_1 as shown in Table 36.1 was used to determine suitability for resection. There were ten pneumonectomies, 28 lobectomies, and 12 wedge resections. Seven patients suffered cardiopulmonary complications within 30 days of surgery. Pulmonary function tests did not separate these seven patients from the 43 who did not suffer cardiopulmonary complications. A significant difference was seen in VO_{2max} (17 mL per kg per minute for those without complications versus 9.95 mL per kg per minute for those with complications). This difference extended across all types of pulmonary resection. The authors reported no complications in those with a VO_{2max} of over 20 mL per kg per minute. There was a 71% complication rate in those with a VO_{2max} of less 10 mL per kg per minute. Those with a VO_{2max} between 10 and 20 mL per kg per minute had a complication rate of 10.3%. The study by Holden and colleagues[60] supports this conclusion. Both patients with a VO_{2max} under 10 mL per kg per minute died postoperatively, while only one of eight with a VO_{2max} over 10 mL per kg per minute died (this patient died of lung metastases after hospital discharge and not as a result of postoperative complications).

Miyoshi and colleagues[90] studied 33 lung cancer patients with spirometry, DLCO measurement, and an incremental exercise test. Cycle ergometry workload was increased at three-minute increments with arterial lactate level measured during the last 30 seconds of each workload. Complications occurred in 45% of the patients. FEV_1 corrected for body surface area (BSA), FEV_1/FVC, DLCO, and MVV/BSA were different between those with complications and those without. No difference was seen in those parameters between those surviving and those who died (n = 4). When VO_2/BSA was examined at a submaximal lactate level of 20 mg per dL, this parameter did differ between surviving and deceased patients. A follow-up study by the same group[91] of 31 lung cancer patients supported parameters during exercise testing as the best predictors of fatal versus nonfatal complications. Data relating to oxygen delivery (O_2D = blood O_2 content times cardiac output) per BSA showed that an O_2D per BSA of under 500 mL per minute per m^2 at a lactate of 20 mg per dL was seen in all patients who died, and greater than this value in all who survived. The authors suggested that: (a) an exercise test be considered in all those patients with borderline "performance status"; (b) if VO_2 per BSA_{lac20} is over 400 mL per minute per m^2, thoracotomy should be safe; and (c) if VO_2 per BSA_{lac20} is below this level, then O_2D per BSA_{lac20} should be measured and if it is over 560 mL per minute per m^2, thoracotomy should be safe. These results support the earlier data of Olsen and colleagues.[85] Confirmation of these data is required in a larger prospective study. Due to the expense and cumbersome nature of the testing, it would likely find applicability in a small, select group of patients felt to be at high risk for postoperative respiratory failure or perioperative morbidity on the basis of screening studies.

Morice and associates[92] reported results in 37 patients at high risk for resection due to an FEV_1 of less than or equal to 40% predicted, a $ppoFEV_1$ of less than or equal to 33% predicted or a $paCO_2$ of over or equal to 45 mm Hg. All underwent incremental exercise testing and surgery was offered if VO_{2max} was greater than 15 mL per kg per minute. Eight patients underwent resection (three lobectomy, one bilobectomy and four wedge resections). Six of these eight had an uncomplicated postoperative course. Two had complications but did not die as a result of surgery or postoperative complications. This small study suggests that VO_2 measurements may indeed have a role in the evaluation of those patients felt unresectable by standard pulmonary function criteria. This same group reported similar results in a prospective series of 66 patients felt to be at high risk for pulmonary complications.[93] Twenty patients achieved a maximal VO_2 of over 15 mL per kg per minute and underwent surgical resection with no mortality and a complication rate of 40%. Five patients with a maximal VO_2 of under 15 mL per kg per minute underwent resection, with one death. Thirty-four patients with a low maximal VO_2 and seven who declined surgery were treated with chemotherapy or radiation therapy. The median duration of survival was 48 months in the surgically treated patients and 17 months in the nonsurgical patients. The authors concluded that surgical resection is feasible in patients with severe pulmonary function abnormality, and that survival is improved with surgical therapy in this group. In a small series of five patients at high risk for resection, a VO_{2max} of over 69% predicted allowed a safe lobectomy.[86]

Bolliger and colleagues described a consecutive series of 80 patients undergoing preoperative exercise testing.[94]

These investigators confirmed that the VO_{2max} was the best predictor of postoperative complications. Furthermore, receiver operating characteristic analysis suggested that the percent predicted VO_{2max} was significantly more sensitive than absolute values in mL per kg per minute. The probability of suffering no postoperative complication was 90% if the VO_{2max} was greater than 75% predicted, and was 10% if the VO_{2max} was less than 43% predicted. A value of less than 60% predicted proved to be prohibitive in resections of more than one lobe. In a subsequent study by the same group, a 100% mortality was noted in those patients with a scintigraphically estimated $ppoVO_{2max}$ under 10 mL per kg per minute.[58] Pate and colleagues noted a threshold of over 10 mL per kg per minute as the best predictor of successful outcome in their prospective study of 12 patients at high risk for thoracic resection.[78] Torchio and associates examined maximal exercise testing in 54 patients with mild to moderate COPD before lung resection.[95] Only one patient with a maximal VO_2 of over 20 mL per kg per minute suffered severe complications, while 11 of 26 patients with a maximal VO_2 under 20 mL per kg per minute suffered such complications. Interestingly, all 11 of these latter patients had an anaerobic threshold of less than or equal to 14.5 mL per kg per minute. Further data are required to confirm the value of the anaerobic threshold as a predictor of postoperative complications.

Not all studies support these concepts, however. In 1982, Colman and colleagues[96] studied 59 consecutive patients with suspected lung cancer. All underwent pulmonary function testing, two-flight stair climb, and progressive, symptom-limited bicycle ergometry with measurement of VO_{2max}. A logistic regression model was used to test whether VO_{2max} could predict postoperative complications (*all* complications, including technical ones such as blood loss or wound infection). FEV_1 and FVC were weakly predictive, whereas VO_{2max} was not. It is unclear if physiologic assessment should be used to predict technical postoperative complications, however. As such, this negative conclusion should be interpreted with caution. Similarly the study by Markos and colleagues[34] described earlier showed no difference in VO_{2max} between those patients suffering and those not suffering postoperative complications. Boysen and associates[97] studied 17 patients preoperatively with incremental exercise testing. No significant difference was seen in exercise parameters between patients with and without cardiopulmonary complications after lung resection. The study was limited by only two patients experiencing such complications, however. Pierce and associates were unable to identify a clear threshold value of VO_{2max} which predicted postsurgical complications.[36] Most recently, Wang and colleagues examined preoperative pulmonary function testing and maximal exercise testing in 40 patients undergoing lung resection.[33] No difference was seen in maximal VO_2 between those patients experiencing postoperative complications (16.3 mL per kg per minute) and those not experiencing such complications (17.8 mL per kg per minute). The differences in the results of these studies include different patient groups, and widely varying definitions of postsurgical complications and exercise formats.

A study by Epstein and colleagues[98] adds an interesting twist. These investigators analyzed the findings in 42 patients considered for lung resection. All subjects had detailed analysis of cardiac risk factors (adapted from Goldman and colleagues[99]) as well as pulmonary factors (obesity, productive cough, wheezing, tobacco use, ratio of FEV_1/FVC of under 70%, $paCO2$ over 45 mm Hg). A cardiopulmonary risk index (CPRI) was generated, ranging from 1 to 10 points. All subjects had pulmonary function testing, radionuclide scanning when appropriate, DLCO measurement, and a symptom-limited exercise test with expired gas analysis. Fourteen patients suffered at least one postoperative cardiopulmonary complication. When stratified by VO_{2max} of over 15 mL per kg per minute, no significant difference was seen between those suffering complications and those not suffering a complication. When corrected for BSA (VO_2 per BSA), a VO_{2max} per BSA of under 500 mL per m^2 was predictive of pulmonary and total complications. Patients with a CPRI of more than or equal to 4 were 22 times more likely to develop a complication. This level of CPRI was also associated with a lower VO_{2max}. With multiple logistic regression analysis, VO_{2max} was *not* an independent predictor of postoperative complications. Although the study supports the value of VO_{2max} measurement, *clinical* assessment with generation of a CPRI was able to predict high-risk patients. In a subsequent study from the same group, the value of the CPRI was confirmed, although the inability to perform bicycle ergometry also predicted postoperative complications.[100]

A unique variation of this exercise format was described by Pierce and colleagues[101] in 1986. In six high-risk patients (based on parameters shown in Table 36.1) incremental exercise on a bicycle ergometer was performed with expired gas analysis. A subsequent steady-state exercise study was performed with bronchoscopic occlusion (during exercise) of the segments felt involved by tumor and likely needing resection. If the patient was able to tolerate exercise while the appropriate bronchus was occluded, he underwent pulmonary resection. Five of the six patients tolerated resection well, with the sixth suffering an early postoperative death (this patient had the lowest VO_{2max}, 13 mL per kg per minute). The format of this exercise study is creative but obviously limited by the level of complexity required.

SIMULTANEOUS LUNG VOLUME REDUCTION SURGERY AND CANCER RESECTION

The resurgence of lung volume reduction surgery (LVRS) has provided a potentially valuable surgical approach to improving short-term lung function and exercise capacity in

TABLE 36.3. REPORTS OF COMBINED LUNG VOLUME REDUCTION SURGERY (LVRS) AND RESECTION OF A PULMONARY NODULE

Reference	Sample Size (patients with nodules/all patients undergoing LVRS)	Preoperative FEV$_1$ (mean, % predicted)	Resections Performed	Pathologic Findings	Length of Stay (days)	Operative Mortality (%)
McKenna, et al.[4]	51/325	21	Lobectomy 4 Wedge 47	Benign 42 Malignant 11	11.1	3.5*
Pigula, et al.[105]	10/128	25	Wedge 10	Malignant 10	NA	0
Ojo, et al.[5]	11/75	26	Wedge 11	Benign 8 Malignant 3	7.6	0
Hazelrigg, et al.[106]	111/281	26*	Wedge 78	Benign 61 Malignant 17	NA	5*
DeRose, et al.[107]	14/NA	24	Lobectomy 3 Wedge 11	Benign 6 Malignant 8	14.4	7
DeMeester, et al.[108]	5/142	30	Lobectomy 5	Malignant 5	14	0

selected patients with advanced emphysema after unilateral[102] and bilateral[103] reduction procedures. Although controversial, patients with severe airflow obstruction, hyperinflation, and heterogeneous emphysema with surgical target areas appear to be better candidates for surgical volume reduction.[104] Several groups have reported short-term results of combined LVRS and resection of suspected lung cancer, as reviewed in Table 36.3.

McKenna and colleagues have reported the largest series, with 51 patients undergoing resection of 53 lung masses (11 NSCLC, and 42 benign lung masses).[4] Of the 11 lung cancers, three were specifically referred to this group for combined LVRS and cancer resection, while seven were found during evaluation for LVRS, and in one it represented an incidental pathologic finding. The mean preoperative FEV$_1$ was 21% of predicted, with all patients considered inoperable by all criteria described earlier. No operative deaths were reported despite lobectomy in four patients, while short-term improvement in lung function was reported in most patients.

Pigula and colleagues described ten patients undergoing simultaneous LVRS and wedge resections of malignant nodules.[105] As enumerated in Table 36.3, the mean FEV$_1$ of 25% predicted would have resulted in denial of standard thoracic resection procedures. Data from our center confirms these findings, as we have recently described successful combined LVRS and nodule resection in a group of 11 patients with severe emphysema (preoperative FEV$_1$ 26% of predicted).[5] All underwent successful wedge resection, with a mean length of stay (7.55 days) similar to a matched control group undergoing lobectomy (8.81 days). Minor postoperative complications occurred in two COPD patients and three control patients. Figure 36.2A illustrates the improvement noted in spirometry before and after surgery, while Figure 36.2B demonstrates significant baseline dyspnea in most patients, and improvements after surgery.

The importance of these findings is highlighted by the report of Hazelrigg and associates, who described the finding of at least on lung nodule in 39.5% of 281 patients prospectively evaluated for LVRS.[106] Of these 111 patients with nodules, 52 were felt to have benign lesions by radiographic imaging. Of the remaining nodules, 78 were resected, with 17 being cancerous lesions. Interestingly, of the neoplastic lesions, three were identified by CT only, five by both chest radiograph and CT, four in the operating room (not seen radiographically), and five incidentally by the pathologist. The overall incidence of cancer was 6.4%.

DeRose and colleagues confirmed these findings in 14 patients successfully undergoing combined LVRS and resection of solitary pulmonary nodules.[107] DeMeester and associates[108] extended these findings by performing an anatomic lobectomy in a small group (n = 5) of patients with severe emphysema (mean FEV$_1$ 30% of predicted). Importantly, all patients demonstrated short-term physiologic and functional improvement. As such, in some patients with otherwise prohibitive pulmonary function, consideration of simultaneous LVRS may be appropriate.

CONSIDERATIONS FOR SURGICAL THERAPY: A RATIONAL APPROACH

Since our approach to the patient with NSCLC emphasizes surgical therapy, much of the preoperative evaluation is

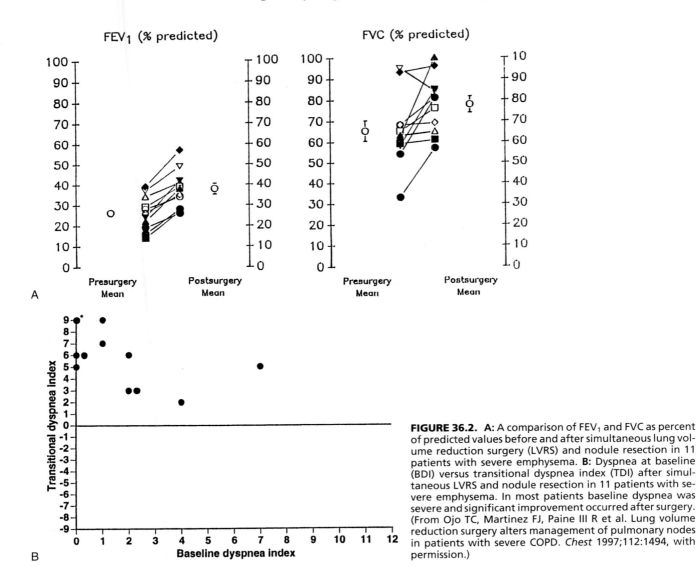

FIGURE 36.2. A: A comparison of FEV_1 and FVC as percent of predicted values before and after simultaneous lung volume reduction surgery (LVRS) and nodule resection in 11 patients with severe emphysema. **B:** Dyspnea at baseline (BDI) versus transitional dyspnea index (TDI) after simultaneous LVRS and nodule resection in 11 patients with severe emphysema. In most patients baseline dyspnea was severe and significant improvement occurred after surgery. (From Ojo TC, Martinez FJ, Paine III R et al. Lung volume reduction surgery alters management of pulmonary nodes in patients with severe COPD. *Chest* 1997;112:1494, with permission.)

aimed at identifying those patients in whom the risk of postoperative respiratory failure is excessive. The possibility of perioperative morbidity is considered as secondary. This is particularly so as most of the above studies did not incorporate recent advancements in postoperative care. For example, extrapleural intercostal blocks in a recent study[109] led to a marked improvement in immediate postoperative FEV_1 (an average of 40% higher) than with saline injection (as a placebo). Similarly, Richardson and colleagues noted improved pain relief and preservation of postoperative pulmonary function in a group treated with preincisional pain prophylaxis and postoperative, continuous, extrapleural, intercostal nerve block and nonsteroidal anti-inflammatory agents.[110] These approaches, among other recent innovations described by Boysen,[111] may allow a much more rapid improvement in pulmonary function and secretion clearance in the early postoperative period, which is the highest-risk period for cardiopulmonary complications.[11] As such,

current and future studies should show a lower cardiopulmonary complication rate. Nevertheless some patients will always have an increased risk from thoracotomy due to markedly abnormal pulmonary function. It is in identifying these patients that pulmonary function studies will retain a prominent role in the preoperative assessment of the lung resection candidate.

An algorithmic approach has recently been suggested by Marshall and Olsen[11] for an approach to the thoracic resection candidate. We have adapted these in our center, as illustrated in Figure 36.3. It is evident that all patients should have measures of FEV_1, FVC, and DLCO. Those with values greater than 60% predicted should tolerate resection, although if functional status is particularly low (as in unusually decreased exercise capacity) there may be an increased risk of complications and further testing, including exercise testing, may be required.[91] In those patients with screening studies showing function below 60%, pre-

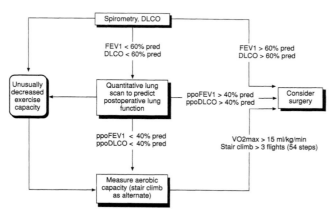

FIGURE 36.3. Algorithm of the physiologic assessment of the lung volume resection candidate. DLCO, diffusing capacity for carbon monoxide; FEV_1, forced expiratory volume in one second; ppo, predicted postoperative VO_2; pred, predicted; VO_{2max}, maximal oxygen uptake. (From Marshall MC, Olsen CN. The physiologic evaluation of the lung resection candidate. *Clin Chest Med* 1993; 14:305, with permission.)

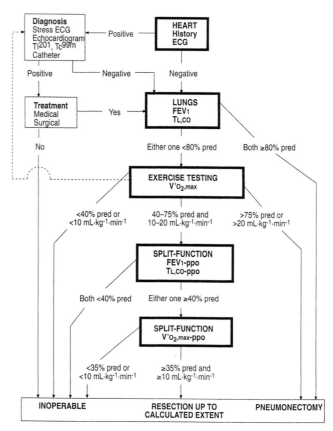

FIGURE 36.4. Alternate proposed algorithm for the assessment of cardiorespiratory reserve in patients evaluated for lung resection. (From Bolliger CT, Perrucoud AP. Functional evaluation of the lung resection candidate. *Eur Respir J* 1998;11:198, with permission.)

dicted radionuclide studies are used to estimate postoperative spirometric function and DLCO. Predicted postoperative function over 40% of predicted generally indicates acceptable risk with a similar caution as mentioned above. Predicted postoperative values below 40% of predicted certainly suggest a greater risk and warrant further evaluation. Exercise testing should be quite useful in this setting. A VO_{2max} greater than 15 mL per kg per minute is felt to reflect a lower risk, with VO_{2max} greater than 20 mL per kg per minute reflecting the lowest risk. If expired gas analysis is not available, then the data of Pollock and colleagues[77] suggests that a stair climb of over three flights (18 steps per flight) approximates this degree of metabolic load in patients with COPD. A cardiopulmonary exercise test provides more information than simple stair climbing, as it examines the ventilatory response (including gas exchange) and the cardiac response during exercise, and should be utilized first if available. Patients who cannot meet these criteria may still be candidates for resection but will require more complex study (exercise with bronchial occlusion or measurement of pulmonary vascular function with exercise). As further prospective information becomes available, the CPRI of Epstein and colleagues[98] may become more widely used during the initial evaluation of a lung cancer patient. Given the poor long-term prognosis in NSCLC without surgery, all patients should be considered for surgical treatment if at all possible. This should include consideration of simultaneous lung volume reduction surgery and cancer resection.

Bolliger and Perrucoud have proposed an alternate, although similar, algorithm which highlights the importance of cardiopulmonary exercise testing in the preoperative evaluation of patients considered for thoracic resection (see Fig-

ure 36.4). This group recently presented prospective application of this algorithm in 137 consecutive patients with clinically resectable lesions.[1] Five patients were deemed inoperable, while 132 underwent resection. The postoperative complication rate was reduced from 20% in a previous publication[94] to 11%, while the mortality decreased from 3.8% to 1.5%. Interestingly, the two patients who died achieved a maximal VO_2 of under 10 mL per kg per minute. As such, the authors suggested modifying the algorithm demonstrated in Figure 36.4 by excluding patients with a VO_{2max} under 10 mL per kg per minute regardless of the percent of predicted. These authors noted that an exercise test was easier to obtain and substantially cheaper than radionuclide imaging at their institution. Prospective comparison is required to define better the cost-effectiveness of routine exercise testing versus (or in addition to) estimation of postoperative pulmonary function. These algorithms will, it is hoped, minimize the risk of this approach and will continue to be modified as further data are published and simultaneous LVRS is incorporated into routine surgical practice.

GENERAL MEDICAL EVALUATION AND PREOPERATIVE RISK ASSESSMENT

There is considerable information available regarding the risk of medical morbidity and mortality after major surgical procedures.[112–114] Much of this literature has focused on the preoperative evaluation of patients prior to general surgical procedures such as laparotomy. However, it appears that much of this information is applicable to the patient undergoing pulmonary resection.

Obese patient have been felt to have an incidence of general, postoperative pulmonary complications ranging from 3.9% to 95%.[113] The increase in incidence of postoperative mortality is best established for abdominal surgery in morbidly obese patients (height to weight ratio in inches to pounds of less than or equal to 10.4). Data regarding risk in thoracotomy are scarce. Nevertheless, given the difficulties expected in intubating and mobilizing morbidly obese patients during operation,[115] it is intuitive that obesity should have a detrimental role on the postoperative course after thoracotomy.

Smoking clearly has an effect on postthoracotomy course, as it relates to underlying lung disease and will be discussed in great detail later. There are extensive data in coronary artery bypass grafting (CABG) that active smoking increases postoperative risk. Warner and colleagues[116] retrospectively reviewed the records of 500 CABG patients at the Mayo Clinic over a two-year period. The amount, duration, and most recent extent of cigarette smoking were recorded, as were details of the postoperative course. Those patients with an over 20-pack-year history of smoking had an increased risk of postoperative complications compared with nonsmokers. The authors also noted that a statistically significant decrement in postoperative complications occurred only in patients who had stopped smoking over eight weeks prior to surgery (see below). Similar findings were reported by Bluman and associates, who noted an odds ratio for developing postoperative pulmonary complications of 5.5 compared to never-smokers.[117] Reduction in smoking within one month of general surgery was not associated with a reduction in the risk of postoperative pulmonary complications. Although the data in these studies were not collected in patients undergoing pulmonary resection, it seems obvious that the results should be more impressive in this patient population, as the extent of postoperative physiologic abnormality is greater with lateral thoracotomy than other incisions.

Preexisting disease can certainly influence the postoperative course after any surgical procedure. Prior cardiac disease, in particular, has been investigated extensively. The screening for cardiac risk in the preoperative setting has been reviewed by Gerson.[118] Goldman and colleagues[99] prospectively evaluated 1,001 patients over the age of 40 undergoing noncardiac surgery (including 31 intrathoracic procedures). Using multivariate, discriminant analysis, they identified nine significant correlates of life-threatening or fatal cardiac complications. These included preoperative third heart sound or jugular venous distention; myocardial infarction within the six months prior to surgery; cardiac rhythm other than sinus or premature atrial complexes on the preoperative electrocardiogram; greater than five premature ventricular contractions at any time preoperatively; intraperitoneal, *intrathoracic,* or aortic operation; age of over 70 years; important aortic stenosis; emergency operation; or poor general medical condition. Using these criteria, a cardiac risk index was calculated which separated the patients into four risk classes. Ten of 19 postoperative cardiac deaths occurred in the 18 patients in the highest-risk group. This study has served as a foundation for many published subsequently. Of interest is that Mittman[20] identified an inordinate risk for patients with an "abnormal" electrocardiogram prior to thoracic surgery, suggesting that these criteria should be applicable to those patients being considered for lung resection.

Gerson[118] uses these criteria to separate patients by degree of cardiac risk. Those felt to be at highest risk should have objective documentation of cardiac function and aggressive preoperative and perioperative management. Those in the low-risk group should have little added cardiac risk. Those in the moderate-risk category (which includes all elderly patients undergoing thoracotomy) should be subjected to an exercise study, if possible (the format used by these authors will be described subsequently), or a dipyridamole thallium scan to assess functional coronary reserve. Although this approach has not been rigorously subjected to prospective evaluation in the lung resection candidate, it seems quite reasonable.

The American College of Cardiology has published an exhaustive guideline for perioperative cardiovascular evaluation and management of patients undergoing noncardiac surgery.[119] This recommendation is based on an algorithmic approach to establishing cardiac risk, the need for preoperative cardiac evaluation, and modification of risk.[120] The initial steps determine the urgency of the proposed surgical procedure and the history of previous coronary revascularization or coronary evaluation. In those patients undergoing nonurgent surgery with no recent cardiac evaluation, risk is initially established on the basis of clinical predictors. Major clinical predictors include unstable coronary syndromes, decompensated congestive heart failure (CHF), significant arrhythmias, or severe valvular disease. These patients require specific management of these clinical predictors. Intermediate clinical predictors include mild angina pectoris, prior myocardial infarction, compensated or prior CHF, or diabetes mellitus. Further stratification in this group is based on exercise capacity and the surgical risk, with intrathoracic operations invoking an intermediate risk. Minor clinical predictors include advanced age, an abnormal EKG, a cardiac rhythm other than sinus, low functional capacity, history of stroke, or uncontrolled systemic hypertension. Further evaluation in these individuals is based on functional capacity and surgical risk, as in the previous group. Validation of this algorithm in thoracic resection is not available, although the principles are remarkably similar to the functional evaluation suggested in the previous section.

Although age has been noted by some to be an independent risk factor for cardiopulmonary complications (as by Goldman and colleagues[99]) it is more controversial when examined in the thoracic surgery population.[115] Boushy and associates,[21] for example, found a high mortality in patients over the age of 60 and impaired pulmonary function after lung resection. Berggren and colleagues[81] found an increased mortality in 82 patients over the age of 70 subjected to thoracotomy for bronchogenic carcinoma. They also felt that an aggressive preoperative assessment for cardiopulmonary risk could minimize this risk, however. Djokovic and Hedley-Whyte[121] noted that 57% of elderly (over 80 years) patients undergoing thoracic surgery required controlled endotracheal ventilation for more than 24 hours postoperatively, compared with 2% of those undergoing surgery that did not enter the pleura or peritoneum. Contrary to these data, several authors have not found age to be an independent risk factor[121–124] and suggest that age should not be used in the absence of other contraindications to reject a patient from possible curative lung resection. With aggressive preoperative and perioperative management we do not routinely use age in excluding patients from surgical treatment.

Unfortunately, further data specifically addressing risk factors for thoracotomy are scant. Nagasaki and associates[126] reviewed the experience at the Memorial Sloan-Kettering Cancer Center from 1973 to 1980 (961 patients undergoing thoracotomy). They studied the effect of various preoperative factors including age, sex, cardiopulmonary status, and factors relating to the tumor and extent of surgery. They identified high risk factors as age (over 70 years), decreased cardiopulmonary function, and the need for more extensive pulmonary resection (pneumonectomy). In a similar review of 476 thoracotomies, Kohman and colleagues[127] examined 37 factors (including age, weight, pulmonary factors, cardiac factors, and characteristics of the tumor and the extent of lung resection) in predicting postoperative mortality. They noted that the risk of postoperative death could not be predicted from the patient's preoperative status. Most recently, Epstein and colleagues[98] formulated a cardiopulmonary risk index (CPRI) using the principles described by Goldman and associates.[99] In this fashion patients were assigned not only a cardiovascular risk index but also an index based on pulmonary risk factors (including obesity, smoking use, productive cough, wheezing, spirometric values, and an increase in $paCO_2$). By combining both these indices into a CPRI (scores ranging from 1 to 10), they noted that a combined score above 4 was associated with a 22-fold increase in the likelihood of pulmonary complications.

One can see that thoracotomy is associated with distinct physiologic changes in the postoperative pulmonary status. Cardiopulmonary complications can be commonly seen, particularly as many patients have underlying cardiac and/or pulmonary disease. Nevertheless, as surgery is the optimal treatment for NSCLCs, the physician should make every effort to consider a patient as resectable. In this context, a thorough preoperative medical evaluation may identify particular risk factors that can be modified (such as active smoking or heart disease). As most postoperative complications are pulmonary, detailed evaluation of pulmonary function is likely the most important aspect of the preoperative evaluation.

PERIOPERATIVE RESPIRATORY MANAGEMENT

Having determined that the patient with NSCLC is a candidate for potentially curative resectional surgery, based on a staging evaluation and a physiologic evaluation, the goal of pre- and postoperative respiratory management is to prevent postoperative respiratory morbidity. While these patients may succumb to a very wide variety of complications, many of these are independent of or only loosely related to the respiratory system. Wound dehiscence, perioperative myocardial infarction, and acute tubular necrosis are important sources of morbidity and mortality but are not respiratory complications that may be amenable to prevention by the application of appropriate pulmonary management. The focus of the current discussion is on the preventable respiratory complications that are common features of the postoperative course of patients who have undergone lung resection. These include clinically significant atelectasis, acute bronchitis, pneumonia, bronchospasm, respiratory failure, and pulmonary thromboemboli (Table 36.4).

Because long-term cigarette use is the most important risk factor for carcinoma of the lung and for chronic obstructive pulmonary disease (COPD), it would be anticipated that chronic airflow obstruction is the most common pulmonary physiologic abnormality in patients with lung cancer. In fact several series found that the vast majority of

TABLE 36.4. POSTOPERATIVE PULMONARY COMPLICATIONS

Atelectasis
Bronchitis
Bronchospasm
Pneumonia
Pulmonary thromboemboli
Respiratory failure (hypoxemic or hypercapnic)

patients presenting for resection of lung cancer had preoperative airflow obstruction.[11,128,129] Thus the focus of the discussion of respiratory management of patients undergoing pulmonary resection for carcinoma of the lung is on the patient with underlying COPD.

There is a strong physiologic relationship between COPD and most of the postoperative complications listed in Table 36.4. Individuals with chronic bronchitis produce increased quantities of respiratory secretions that are often colonized with pathogenic bacteria.[130] Diminished flow rates in patients with obstructive lung disease result in a less effective cough and impaired ability to expel secretions obstructing the airway lumen. These factors place the patient at risk for atelectasis with retained secretions, acute bronchitis, and pneumonia. Many individuals with COPD have nonspecific airway hyperactivity and may develop bronchospasm as a consequence of airways inflammation,[131,132] further worsening their ability to clear secretions in addition to direct effects on gas exchange. To reduce these risks of pulmonary complications in patients with underlying COPD, the interventions described in the discussion that follows largely are aimed specifically at (a) reversing or minimizing airflow obstruction, and (b) minimizing retained secretions.

Smoking Cessation

In the face of both carcinoma of the lung and COPD, many patients who present for resectional surgery still are smoking cigarettes at the time of initial assessment. It has long been recognized that current smoking increases the risk of postoperative complications for many different surgical procedures.[133] There is a tendency to assume that smoking cessation preoperatively is a significant benefit in reducing the risk of postoperative pulmonary complications. In fact, many thoracic surgeons view smoking cessation as a requirement before patients can be allowed to undergo resectional surgery for lung carcinoma. There are reasons for this view. Cigarette smoke is a constant irritant and may promote inflammatory changes in the airways and contribute to excess mucous secretion, chronic bronchitis, and airways hyperactivity.[134] At a cellular level, Chalon and associates found that cigarette smoking was correlated with airway epithelial injury and with increased risk of postoperative pulmonary complications.[135] Current cigarette smokers also maintain significantly elevated levels of carboxyhemoglobin as high as 10%, thereby reducing oxygen transport and increasing the risk of ischemic cardiovascular or cerebrovascular insults during surgery.[136] Finally, smoking cessation may serve as an important indicator of the patient's willingness to be responsible for and participate in his or her own health care.

However, despite these observations, there is surprisingly little data that directly support this assumption. Warner and colleagues compared the time since last cigarette to the risk of significant pulmonary complications.[116,137] As anticipated, current smokers were at significantly increased risk compared to lifelong nonsmokers or to individuals who had stopped smoking more than eight weeks prior to surgery. Unfortunately, the rate of complications was actually slightly higher for those who had stopped smoking less than four weeks prior to surgery than for current smokers. This was recently confirmed by Bluman and associates.[117] The apparent benefit of eight weeks without smoking prior to surgery may be a reflection of continued inflammatory changes in the airways or of the period required to repair the chronically injured airway epithelium. The degree to which these observations can be extended to patients undergoing pulmonary resection is not clear.

We routinely insist that patients stop smoking prior to surgery for the theoretical reasons described above. Physicians in general do a rather poor job of counseling patients to stop smoking. In some series, as few as 25% of smokers reported having discussed smoking cessation with their primary care physician.[138] Emphasizing to the patient that the use of cigarettes is a major source of morbidity and mortality is the first step in helping the patient to stop this habit. However, it is clear that encouragement by the physician often is not sufficient to induce even a temporary respite, much less long-term abstinence. Additional aids, including patient-directed literature, videotapes, support groups, and pharmacological interventions such as nicotine transdermal patches and gums are available and potentially very helpful in reducing or stopping the patient's use of tobacco.[139,140] The balance between the time required for a patient to stop smoking and the potential benefit of a longer cigarette-free period prior to surgery, on the one hand, and the potential progression of the patient's tumor, on the other, must be determined in each individual case.

Pharmacological Therapy for COPD

While it had long been assumed that individuals with COPD have fixed abnormalities in airway resistance leading to irreversible airflow obstruction, there is considerable evidence that many of these patients do have a component of reversible airflow obstruction over and above their underlying, fixed abnormality.[131,141] There are several pharmacological interventions that may potentially improve airflow obstruction by alleviating this reversible abnormality in patients undergoing pulmonary resection for bronchogenic carcinoma. While a detailed discussion of the pharmacology of each of these agents is beyond the scope of the present work, it will be useful to consider certain features related to the selection and use of agents in this group of patients.

Inhalation Therapy

Many of the drugs that are most useful for the treatment of airflow obstruction may be administered by the inhalation route. There are important advantages in taking this approach in contrast to systemic administration.[142] Specifically, there is excellent availability of the drug within the airways, with greatly decreased or no systemic side effects. Unfortunately, unless the drug is administered with proper technique, large amounts may be deposited in the oropharynx and upper airways, with a significant loss of therapeutic effect.[143] The most common means of delivering aerosolized drugs to the lungs is with a metered dose inhaler. With each activation, these canisters deliver a preset dose of drug as a stream of particles of uniform size optimal for deposition in the peripheral airways. For best effect, the patient must synchronize the activation of the canister with the initiation of a slow inspiration from functional residual capacity to total lung capacity, followed by a breath hold of up to ten seconds. Many authorities suggest that the metered dose inhaler be held several inches from the open mouth to decrease deposition in the oropharynx. This maneuver requires careful teaching with demonstrations to maximize patient compliance. There are a number of points at which many individuals, particularly those who are older or more dyspneic, may have difficulties. For this reason, devices such as tube spaces or chambers into which the cloud of drug is released prior to inhalation have been developed. These devices can significantly improve drug delivery and are of benefit for any individuals who have difficulty mastering the basic technique.[143] Furthermore, several alternative preparations of β-agonists have recently been developed that place less stringent requirements on patient coordination. These include breath actuated inhalers (Maxair Autohaler)[144] and finely powdered preparations of drug that are inhaled directly from a holder and require no actuation (Ventolin rotohaler).[145] Finally, it is possible to give both β-agonists and anticholinergic agents using updraft nebulizers powered by an external compressed gas source. Due to a larger particle size that results in considerable upper airway deposition and the delivery of drug during expiration as well as inspiration, the use of nebulizers is a relatively inefficient approach to inhalation therapy.[143] However, in patients who are unable to use metered dose inhalers due to difficulties with coordination or severe dyspnea, they provide an important modality.

Beta-Adrenergic Agonists

β-agonists have long been the first line drug for the treatment of reversible airflow obstruction in asthma (Table 36.5). They also have proven to be effective agents for many patients with increased airways resistance due to COPD.[142,146] Binding to β2 selective adrenergic receptors in the small airways, these agents raise intracellular cAMP levels within airway smooth muscle cells and induce relaxation with reduced airflow obstruction.[147] When administered by inhalation, they have an excellent therapeutic index. At standard doses, modern agents such as albuterol and pirbuterol induce limited increases in cardiac rate and with rare instances of cardiac arrhythmias, even in older individuals with underlying cardiac disease.[142,148]

In patients who demonstrate airflow obstruction by spirometry or who have had episodes of acute bronchitis with symptoms suggesting airflow obstruction, we institute therapy with a β2 selective agonist prior to pulmonary resectional surgery, even if the patient has not been using the drug previously. Therapy is then continued throughout the perioperative period. In selected individuals we then reassess the benefit of the β-agonist after the patient has recovered from surgery and returned home. We prefer to use metered dose inhalers (often with spacer devices) rather than updraft nebulizers for reasons of cost and convenience, even in the postoperative period, so long as the patient can manage to use the device with a technique adequate to insure delivery of the drug to the airways.

Anticholinergic agents

Anticholinergic drugs cause bronchodilation by blocking the bronchoconstricting effects of stimulation of parasympathetic nerves that are most abundant in the central and larger airways.[149] Thus it is likely that these agents influence bronchomotor tone at a more proximal anatomic site than do β-adrenergic agonists. Anticholinergic agents are generally less potent than β-agonists in individuals with asthma, but are of particular benefit in patients with chronic bronchitis.[150,151] Ipratropium bromide is a quaternary derivative of atropine that is a potent anticholinergic agent. It is very poorly absorbed into the circulation from the airways, and thus has very few systemic effects when administered via inhalation.[150,152] Recent data have confirmed that the combination of ipratropium and a β-agonist results in greater clinical and physiologic improvement than the β-agonist alone.[153] Furthermore, the addition of ipratropium to a regimen of β-agonists has been demonstrated to result in fewer exacerbations and an improved treatment cost and cost-effectiveness.[154] Although no data specific to the postoperative state exist, we encourage the use of ipratropium bromide at relatively high doses (such as three to four puffs four times daily) as well as a β-agonist beginning as soon as possible preoperatively in patients who have chronic airflow obstruction and are undergoing pulmonary resection. As with the β-agonists, the drug should be continued throughout the perioperative period, with emphasis on proper use of the metered dose inhaler. The potential benefits of long-term administration of ipratropium are then assessed after the patient has left the hospital, during outpatient follow-

TABLE 36.5. COMMERCIALLY AVAILABLE β-AGONISTS

Albuterol	Levalbuterol
Bitolterol	Metaproterenol
Epinephrine	Pirbuterol
Isoethane	Salmeterol
Isoproterenol	Terbutaline

up. The recent development of long-acting β-agonists has improved the ability to provide bronchodilation in patients with COPD. Salmeterol xinafoate has demonstrated prolonged bronchodilation and improved breathlessness in patients with COPD.[155] The relative safety and simplicity of administration may make this class of agents the optimal β-agonists for this patient population.

Anti-Inflammatory Agents

Many individuals with airflow obstruction due to chronic bronchitis and emphysema have chronic inflammation of the bronchial wall.[156] This inflammatory process can result in superimposed bronchoconstriction, exacerbating the fixed abnormality of the underlying process. Inhaled corticosteroids can be effective agents for the reduction of mucosal inflammation in patients with asthma and in selected individuals with COPD.[142,157] When administered by inhalation, these drugs have very few side effects. They can induce coughing, a problem that can be largely alleviated by administering a β-agonist prior to the anti-inflammatory drug. Inhaled steroids can cause oral thrust and modest changes in phonation.[158,159] Recent data suggest that inhaled fluticasone may improve pulmonary function and clinical symptoms and decrease the incidence of exacerbations in patients with COPD.[160] Similar results have been suggested with long-term use of this agent,[161] although inhaled budesonide does not appear to provide the same benefit.[162] This may reflect differences in the patient groups studied, however.[161] On the basis of these data, we opt to begin therapy preoperatively in selected individuals based on their clinical history and results of spirometry. In particular, individuals who have coughing or wheezing in response to specific allergens, cold air, or exercise may well benefit from the addition of inhaled steroids to their bronchodilator regimen. Similarly, patients with significant variability in their spirometry, especially those with over 10% improvement in FEV_1 after the administration of an inhaled β-agonist, are good candidates for a trial of inhaled corticosteroids or cromolyn.[163] For maximum benefit, inhaled steroids should be used at relatively high doses initially and tapered to lower maintenance doses after several weeks. We continue these agents in the postoperative period after the patient no longer requires mechanical ventilation, and we assess the potential benefit of continued therapy as an outpatient.

Approximately 10% of stable patients with airflow obstruction due to COPD will have a statistically significant improvement in spirometry after a course of systemic corticosteroids.[164] Patients who have evidence of significant reversible obstruction, as indicated by improvement in spirometry after the use of an inhaled β-agonist, may be more likely to show physiologic benefit from a trial of steroids than are patients whose spirometric abnormality appears to be fixed.[165] However, the chronic inflammatory changes that have developed over months to years may improve only

over a more extended period, with little initial response to a single dose of a bronchodilator. Therefore, in patients with marginal pulmonary function or in individuals with very labile pulmonary function despite aggressive therapy with bronchodilators and inhaled corticosteroids, we will often give a trial of prednisone therapy, 40 mg daily for up to two weeks, and then repeat spirometry. If this trial results in clinically significant improvement in FEV_1, the prednisone then is tapered, while inhaled corticosteroids are continued at high doses. The benefits of any improvement in pulmonary function must be weighed against the important risks of difficulties with wound healing and postoperative infection. In general, we hope to have patients on at most low-dose prednisone (approximately 10 mg per day) at the time of surgery. Occasional patients who develop acute exacerbation of bronchitis without pneumonia postoperatively may require short courses of systemic steroids as well.

Methylxanthines

While theophylline preparations were previously considered first-line agents for patients with airflow obstruction of all sorts, these drugs have largely fallen out of favor in recent years. They are less potent bronchodilators than inhaled β-agonists and have a very low therapeutic index.[142,147] Potentially life-threatening side effects, including cardiac arrhythmias and seizures, can occur at serum levels only modestly higher than the traditional therapeutic range.[166] This problem is worsened by the highly variable hepatic metabolism of theophylline, which can result in wide fluctuations in serum levels despite a constant daily dose. However, there are arguments to suggest that theophylline may yet have a role in selected patients.[166,167] In addition to the fact that occasional patients have impressive symptomatic improvement with the drug, especially those troubled by nocturnal awakenings due to dyspnea, theophylline has been shown to enhance both strength and endurance of diaphragmatic muscle.[168,169] If theophylline is used in the perioperative period for the patient undergoing pulmonary resection for lung carcinoma, serum levels must be monitored closely. The target level should be 10 μg per dL, and levels of greater than 15 μg per dL are to be carefully avoided. The physician must be aware of and adjust the dose accordingly in patients in whom hepatic metabolism of theophylline will be reduced, including those with hepatic dysfunction or congestive heart failure, and patients receiving drugs such as erythromycin, ciprofloxacin, or cimetidine that inhibit the hepatic P450 system.[147]

Antibiotics

All patients who are being assessed for thoracic surgery should be questioned regarding cough and sputum. Of particular importance are the volume and characteristics of the sputum.[169] Individuals who are producing sputum with any purulence should be treated with a seven to ten day course of oral antibiotics prior to surgery. In this circumstance, the therapy is generally empiric; there is no evidence to suggest that there is benefit from routine sputum culture to determine bacterial species and antibiotic resistance. Amoxicillin or ampicillin (250 mg three times daily or four times daily, respectively), trimethoprim/sulfamethoxazole (one double-strength tablet twice daily), or doxycycline have all been considered appropriate choices. These antibiotics cover the most common bacterial flora in patients with chronic bronchitis (*Streptococcus pneumoniae, Haemophilus influenzae, Moraxella catarrhalis*)[130,170] and are well tolerated and inexpensive.[171]

Recent data have suggested different bacterial flora in patients with more severe disease, however. In a prospective study of 211 patients admitted to the hospital with an exacerbation, Eller and colleagues performed detailed studies to identify pathogens[172] and characterized the patients by performing spirometry at the time of discharge. Those patients with more severe airflow obstruction (FEV_1 under 50% of predicted) were more likely to have infections caused by enteric gram-negative rods. In addition, in a prospective study of 471 patients with chronic obstructive pulmonary disease, Ball and associates examined the features which predicted a high likelihood of failure to recover during the treatment of an exacerbation.[173] The only factors predicting failure to recover from an exacerbation included coexisting cardiopulmonary disease and the number of chest infections during the preceding 12 months. As such, recent recommendations suggest treating younger individuals with less severe disease and infrequent exacerbations with first-line antibiotics (amoxicillin, trimethoprim/sulfamethoxazole, or doxycycline), while older patients with more severe disease or frequent exacerbations should be treated with a second-line agent (newer macrolide or fluoroquinolone).[174] Recent data support the above concepts as cost-effective. Grossman and colleagues randomized a total of 240 adult patients with a type I or II exacerbation and history of frequent exacerbations over the previous year.[175] Patients received the fluoroquinolone ciprofloxacin or non-fluoroquinolone antibiotics. Assessments included symptoms, all medications used, adverse events, hospitalizations, outpatient health care utilization, and health-related quality of life. Cost-effectiveness of ciprofloxacin use was demonstrated in older patients (age over 56), those with more severe or long-standing disease (over ten years), more frequent exacerbations (more than four per year) or more comorbid conditions (over three comorbidities). As such, the choice of antibiotic should be individualized to the patient.

Respiratory Physiotherapy

Following the induction of general anesthesia for a surgical procedure, there is a rapid decrease in functional residual capacity.[176] Even in individuals whose preoperative lung is normal, this decrement in lung volume results in atelectasis in dependent zones. These atelectatic regions can be detected on CT scans through the thorax performed within minutes after the induction of anesthesia, and result in significant increase in intrapulmonary shunting.[177,178] In the postoperative period, functional residual capacity is assaulted by many different factors, including pain that causes splinting and diminished inspiratory effort, diaphragmatic dysfunction, prolonged supine position, and clouded sensorium due to narcotics. In addition to these general considerations, patients who have undergone a thoracic surgical procedure may have an incision through accessory muscles of respiration, pain with respiration due to irritation of the pleura, and more severe atelectasis of portions of the dependent lung if a lateral incision has been used.[111] Together, these factors greatly diminish pulmonary compliance and promote atelectasis.[6,177] Atelectasis in turn places the patient at risk for bronchitis, pneumonia, or respiratory failure. A major goal in the perioperative management of patients undergoing pulmonary resection for bronchogenic carcinoma is the reversal of these physiologic derangements and the attendant reduction in the risk of postoperative respiratory complications.

Several different physiologic and mechanical techniques have been used in an attempt to prevent or correct alveolar collapse after surgery. Early approaches often emphasized forced expiratory maneuvers with the use of "blow bottles" or balloons. These devices encouraged the patient to make repeated and sustained forced expiratory efforts. In retrospect, it is clear that Valsalva maneuvers can cause compression of airways due to increased intrathoracic pressure and in fact may be counterproductive in the postoperative period.[179]

The recognition that general anesthesia and surgery consistently cause a reduction in functional residual capacity led to the use of methods that focused not on expiration, but on inspiration, in hopes of returning lung volumes towards normal. Available measures include supervised cough and deep-breathing exercises (CDB), incentive spirometry, intermittent positive pressure breathing (IPPB), and constant positive airway pressure (CPAP) delivered by face mask. In CDB and incentive spirometry the immediate goal is to encourage repeated and sustained maximal inspiratory efforts and thereby prevent alveolar collapse and recruit atelectatic lung units.[179-181] They thus require active participation on the part of the patient. IPPB and CPAP devices use positive airway pressure to increase functional residual capacity.[182-184] The patient may play a more passive role when using these devices than with CDB or incentive spirometry.

The benefits of these different approaches to lung expansion have not been assessed in trials using patients who have undergone pulmonary resection. However, several prospective studies have evaluated these measures in patients who have undergone upper abdominal surgery. Morran and colleagues evaluated the efficacy of routine postoperative chest physiotherapy compared to no prophylactic physiotherapy in 102 patients undergoing upper abdominal surgery.[185] In this randomized trial, the incidence of postoperative pulmonary infections was reduced significantly in the group that received prophylactic physiotherapy, compared to the control group (seven of 51 versus 19 of 51). Celli and colleagues[182] prospectively randomized 172 patients undergoing upper abdominal surgery into four treatment groups: CDB, incentive spirometry, IPPB, and control patients who received no specific prophylactic therapy. Pulmonary complications were significantly reduced for patients receiving any of the three prophylactic treatment regimens, compared to the controls. Of note was that the rate of complications was virtually identical for all three treatment groups. There was also a trend towards decreased length of stay in the prophylactically treated groups, although this achieved statistical significance only for the patients treated with incentive spirometry. These randomized studies support the widely held belief, shared by surgeons, anesthesiologists, and pulmonologists, that postoperative respiratory measures to promote lung expansion can reduce the risk of pulmonary complications.

Several studies have compared the relative benefits of specific approaches to prophylactic respiratory care. Celli and colleagues[182] found that IPPB was associated with increased patient discomfort and, as noted above, found no benefit of IPPB compared to either CDB or incentive spirometry. Similarly, Oikkonen and associates found no advantage to IPPB compared to incentive spirometry in a study involving 52 patients undergoing coronary artery bypass grafting.[186] In an early direct comparison of incentive spirometry with routine chest physiotherapy in 70 patients undergoing upper abdominal surgery, Craven and colleagues[187] found that use of the incentive spirometer was associated with a reduced rate of pulmonary complications and increased number of patients with no postoperative abnormality. However, in this study the intensity of treatment in the incentive spirometer group was considerably greater than for the chest physiotherapy group. More recently, Hall and associates[188] used a large prospective trial of 876 patients undergoing laparotomy to compare the prophylactic benefit of incentive spirometry to that of routine chest physiotherapy. The rate of overall pulmonary complications, of specific complications, and the length of stay were not different between the groups.

Both incentive spirometry and CDB techniques are very dependent upon patient cooperation for maximum benefit. Because CPAP has been used to increase functional residual capacity and improve gas exchange in patients with reduced pulmonary compliance due to lung injury,[189] it has been suggested that the application of this intervention prophylactically in the postoperative period might reduce pulmonary complications with diminished dependence on patient effort. When applied for 12 hours after extubation in patients who had undergone aortocoronary bypass surgery,

nasal CPAP improved gas exchange but did not affect the incidence of pulmonary complications, including atelectasis, throughout the postoperative course.[190] Stock and colleagues[184] directly compared CPAP, incentive spirometry, and CDB in a prospective, randomized study involving 65 patients undergoing upper abdominal surgery. CPAP was delivered by face mask at 7.5 cm H_2O for 15 minutes every two hours. Functional residual capacity decreased in all three groups postoperatively, compared to baseline values. The rate of recovery of functional residual capacity was faster in the CPAP group than with incentive spirometry or CDB; however, this difference was apparent only if values were normalized to the postoperative nadir, not the preoperative baseline. Furthermore, the rate of postoperative pulmonary complications was low in all three groups, with no differences between modalities. Based on this information, these authors concluded that CPAP may be of equal benefit to incentive spirometry or CDB. However, until more extensive controlled trials are performed to assess adequately the impact of CPAP on the rate of clinically significant complications, it is difficult to assess its proper role in the prevention of postoperative pulmonary complications.[191]

Bilevel positive airway pressure (BiPAP) is a recently developed technique that shows great promise in the treatment of acute respiratory failure during exacerbations of COPD. The BiPAP machine delivers gas at a set pressure throughout inspiration (providing an inspiratory assist), with a lower level of pressure during the expiratory phase of the ventilatory cycle. Unlike IPPB, the patient determines the flow rates, the duration of the respiratory cycle, and the tidal volume. BiPAP may be delivered by a variety of nasal masks or by a full face mask. In the patient with COPD who has significant respiratory muscle fatigue in the setting of an exacerbation of his or her underlying lung disease (but who does not emergently require intubation and mechanical ventilation), periods of BiPAP ventilation may reduce the work of breathing, improve gas exchange, and prevent the progression to more severe respiratory failure.[192] In a randomized study of 85 patients with acute exacerbations of COPD, patients treated with BiPAP had a lower rate of intubation (26% versus 74%) and lower in-hospital mortality (9% versus 29%) compared to patients who received standard therapy only. Patients who required emergent intubation in the emergency department were excluded from the study. This study suggests that elective BiPAP ventilation may improve respiratory muscle function and gas exchange in patients experiencing an acute exacerbation of COPD.[193] Patients with marginal respiratory reserve who undergo lobectomy for the treatment of lung carcinoma may have a disproportionate decline in pulmonary function during the early postoperative period, with increased work of breathing and limitation of ventilatory capacity. In selected patients, the early application of BiPAP therapy may avoid progression to respiratory failure and provide a temporary support to allow time for improvement in pulmonary mechanics.

Several important conclusions can be drawn regarding the use of respiratory therapy in the perioperative period. There are few data from randomized studies involving patients undergoing thoracotomy for pulmonary resection; however, physiologic considerations suggest that information derived from studies of patients undergoing upper abdominal surgery or coronary artery bypass grafting are quite likely to be applicable to patients undergoing pulmonary resection as well. It is clear that the use of some form of respiratory therapy is of benefit in reducing the incidence of postoperative pulmonary complications and, potentially, length of hospital stay. This principle is now almost universally accepted.[194] It also is likely that maximum benefit can be achieved if patient education is begun and respiratory care is initiated prior to surgery, before incisional pain and an impaired sensorium due to narcotics interfere with patient participation in the therapy.[195] As long ago as 1954, Thorens[195] presented information suggesting that therapy initiated prior to surgery was more effective in reducing pulmonary complications than therapy begun postoperatively.

There is little information to suggest that one particular modality is clearly superior to others in terms of the risk of postoperative complications. The critical factor appears to be the use of some form of therapy. Because IPPB is cumbersome, expensive, and has no advantages over simpler interventions, it has largely fallen out of favor. The choice between CDB and incentive spirometry is best made based upon a number of considerations, including local resource availability and costs, and the ability of the individual patient to participate with either modality. We initially use incentive spirometry in virtually all patients because, once taught, the patient can perform the therapy with little or no supervision multiple times throughout the day. In individuals who have difficulty using the incentive spirometer, who are having problems with postoperative atelectasis or hypoxemia, or who have remained in the intensive care setting, it is reasonable to use CDB under the supervision of a trained nurse or respiratory therapist. In selected patients with large volumes of sputum, postural drainage and chest percussion may play an adjunct role, although this intervention can cause transient deterioration in gas exchange and increase chest wall discomfort in individuals whose respiratory reserve may be already quite limited.[197] On physiologic grounds there is intuitive appeal to the use of CPAP to increase functional residual capacity in the postoperative period. However, further studies are required to define both the benefits and the relative costs of this more complex intervention.

Pain Control

Many of the adverse effects of thoracic surgery on pulmonary function are independent of pain.[110] However, the control of postoperative pain remains an issue of particularly great importance for the patient who has undergone pulmonary resection for bronchogenic carcinoma. The majority of patients will have lateral incisions that involve injury to respiratory muscles. Pain at the surgical wound may be a problem with each breath. Furthermore, many of these patients have significant underlying chronic obstructive pulmonary disease, rendering them susceptible to the hypoventilatory effects of injudiciously administered narcotics.

Traditionally, postoperative pain has been controlled with periodically administered narcotics. This approach gives significant variation in narcotic levels, with often inadequate pain control when the level is at a nadir and unacceptable effects on sensorium and respiratory drive when the level is at a peak.[111,198] Several recent innovations offer the promise of considerably improved the therapy of postoperative pain while lessening adverse side effects. Patient controlled analgesia (PCA) and epidural analgesia are approaches that may be of benefit following any surgical procedure in which postoperative pain is a major consideration.[199] Both methods can give improved analgesia with relatively easily controlled side effects. In PCA, the patient receives a low-dose continuous infusion of intravenous narcotic that he or she can supplement on demand with a controlled bolus of drug. This approach has been well accepted by patients, with improved patient comfort and perhaps fewer effects of peak narcotic levels on sensorium. If the limits on bolus doses are adjusted appropriately, there is little risk of significant overdose.[111]

Epidural analgesia is now an accepted method of pain control in this patient population. Narcotics are delivered in bolus fashion, controlled either by the patient or the nursing staff, via an epidural catheter for up to 24 hours after surgery. Pain control and patient acceptance are generally excellent.[200,201] Pruritis and urinary retention are problems that are easily treated with an antihistamine or short-term urinary catheterization, respectively. In general there are few problems with significant respiratory depression.[111] Of note is that, in a prospective study in which oxygen saturation was monitored continuously for 24 hours after lower abdominal surgery, Wheatley and colleagues[202] found more frequent episodes of mild arterial oxygen desaturation (over 94% for less than six minutes per hour) in patients receiving epidural analgesia than in groups receiving PCA or traditional intramuscular narcotics. These episodes occurred almost exclusively during sleep at night and were not predicted by decreases in respiratory rate. To prevent this complication, some authors have advocated concomitant therapy with an opiate antagonist given intravenously.[203]

An innovative approach to pain control after thoracotomy involves regional anesthesia with a long-acting local anesthetic agent such as bupivacaine used for extrapleural intercostal nerve block[109] or instilled into the pleural space at the end of the surgical procedure.[204,205] With either repeated administration or a continuous infusion of drug, there is excellent local control of thoracic pain with no evidence of respiratory depression or other major side effects. In theory, these uses of regional analgesia may significantly improve patient comfort, decrease the requirement for systemic narcotics, and improve pulmonary function in the postoperative period. For example, Berrisford and colleagues[109] showed that extrapleural intercostal nerve block with bupivocaine led to an immediate postoperative FEV_1 which was 40% higher than with saline placebo.

CONSIDERATIONS FOR RADIATION THERAPY

For those patients for whom surgery is not a therapeutic option, radiation therapy often serves as a good alternative. Similarly, for those patients with extensive local disease at the time of thoracotomy, postoperative radiation therapy is often employed. The clinical indications and techniques employed in this form of therapy will be discussed elsewhere in this volume. Pulmonary changes have been known to occur after pulmonary radiation for almost 100 years.[206] Recent work has clearly described two major clinical phases of lung injury from pulmonary radiation: an acute pneumonitis and a later-appearing fibrosis.[207–209] Because many patients with lung cancer have underlying lung disease, it would be expected that an additional effect of radiation-induced lung injury will occur. Furthermore, the effect of radiation injury would be expected to be different from the effect of surgical resection on lung function. The extent of functional loss should not be as well defined after radiation therapy, and the time course of functional loss will be different (immediate for resection versus delayed for radiation injury).[210] The risk of an early radiation pneumonitis seems to be strongly influenced by the dosage delivered and the field size.[211,212] The late effect may be quite important, as severe or fatal pulmonary complications were seen in 3% of patients receiving 4,000 cGy in four weeks through a Radiation Oncology Group (RTOG) study[213] and in 5% of patients receiving 6,960 cGy in another RTOG study.[214]

Brady and colleagues[206] monitored spirometry, lung volumes, MBC, DLCO, dynamic lung compliance, and arterial blood gases prior to and four weeks after thoracic radiation therapy in lung cancer patients. Little change was seen during this brief period of follow-up in most parameters. A decrease in DLCO was highly significant and appeared to correlate with the volume dosage delivered to the thorax. Mattson and colleagues[215] studied 34 patients treated with split-course radiation therapy for lung cancer in addition to chemotherapy. At regular intervals after radiation, pulmonary function was measured, as was regional pulmonary perfusion using ^{133}Xe (as described earlier for thoracic resection). Only decreases in DLCO were significant and seen six and nine months after finishing radiation. In a large prospective study, Choi and colleagues[216] measured pulmonary function (spirometry, lung volumes, MBC, and arterial blood gases) prior to initiation of postoperative (lobectomy in 49 and pneumonectomy in 22 patients) radiation and one year after finishing radiation (and every year thereafter). They noted very little change in pulmonary function regardless of the surgical procedure. In four of 137 patients there was symptomatic pulmonary toxicity.

Two groups have utilized similar techniques of split perfusion scans to estimate postradiation therapy pulmonary function as was described earlier for lung resection. Rubenstein and associates[217] prospectively examined 22 patients (six treated postoperatively and 16 treated with primary radiation therapy) using quantitative perfusion lung scanning. Careful estimates were made of the volume of lung exposed to radiation. Assuming this lung would no longer contribute to the patient's FEV_1, the authors predicted postradiation therapy pulmonary function by using the following equation:

Postradiation FEV_1 = Preradiation FEV_1
$\times$ (1-fraction of total lung perfusion in radiated portal)

After sequential follow-up, the authors noted that a latent period in FEV_1 was followed by a decline in FEV_1. Nevertheless in only two patients was postradiation FEV_1 below the predicted postradiation pulmonary function.

In a more ambitious study, Choi and coworkers[210,218,219] prospectively studied patients with unresectable lung cancer treated with radiation therapy. Using quantitative radionuclide lung scans to measure regional lung function, the authors estimated postradiation therapy FEV_1 using an equation similar to that of Rubenstein and colleagues.[217] The authors noted that the change in pulmonary function after radiation therapy depended on pretreatment lung function, the extent of bronchial or pulmonary vascular obstruction by tumor, and the location of treatment. In this way, group A patients, with preradiation-therapy FEV_1 of less than 50% predicted (and over 10% shift in ventilation or perfusion to the uninvolved side of the lung), showed the greatest decrement in lung function. In these patients, FEV_1, FVC, MBC, and PEFR decreased by 15% to 25%, TLC decreased by 12%, and DLCO by 6%. In group B patients, with preradiation FEV_1 of over 50% predicted (and over 10% shift in ventilation or perfusion to the uninvolved side of the lung), there was a small *increase* in pulmonary function 12 months after radiation therapy. The predictability of loss in pulmonary function was greater in group A patients (69% correlation between measured and predicted postradiation therapy pulmonary function). Only 10% of group B patients showed the decrease predicted (50% showed a small increase in pulmonary function, with 40% showing a small decrease). Choi suggested in an editorial[210] that the functional loss in pulmonary function after radiation therapy depends on the balance between direct tissue injury due to the radiation and possible improvement in pulmonary function by improved traction of adjacent lung caused by radiation. Axford and associates[220] suggested that radiation may actually relieve breathlessness in emphysema patients via a similar process. As such, in patients with relatively normal preradiation pulmonary function, there is likely to occur a predictable loss in pulmonary function with radiation therapy. Patients with markedly reduced pulmonary function may have some improvement. The extent of airway or vascular obstruction by tumor may also have an impact. Fazio and colleagues[221] noted an early improvement in ventilation (in 83% of patients) and perfusion (in 86% of patients) after radiation therapy for unresectable lung cancer. Of interest was that subsequent decrease in pulmonary function was seen and was felt to be due to delayed radiation fibrosis.

The value of pulmonary function testing and accurate estimation of dose-volume calculation was highlighted by Marks and colleagues, who prospectively studied 100 patients (67 with lung cancer) during the course of radiation therapy.[222] They utilized three-dimensional, CT-based estimates of dosage and pretherapy pulmonary function studies to predict the development of symptoms (which occurred in 21 of 100 patients) and decrements in pulmonary function. The authors noted that the extent of alteration in whole-lung function, as defined by symptoms or pulmonary function change, was best related to dose-volume and pretherapy pulmonary function. As such, most patients with pulmonary symptoms had either a high dose-volume parameter or low pretherapy pulmonary function. Interestingly, there was no quantitative relation between dose-volume parameters and the percent reduction in pulmonary function. Further data are required to develop more accurate predictive models.

In conclusion, radiation therapy results in clear-cut injury to normal lung. In most patients this should not prohibit treatment. In some patients prediction of postradiation therapy pulmonary function may be useful, particularly if one uses similar criteria established for postresection lung function. This is particularly true because the measured posttreatment pulmonary function is rarely lower than predicted function. This should provide a "cushion of error" which may quite clinically useful. In patients with severe pulmonary dysfunction, the resulting late decrement in pulmonary function with high-dose radiation must be taken into account when weighing therapeutic options.

CONSIDERATIONS FOR CHEMOTHERAPY

As with surgical treatment and radiation therapy, chemotherapeutic agents used to treat bronchogenic carcinoma have been shown adversely to affect pulmonary function. A comprehensive review of this topic is outside the range of this chapter. The reader is referred to several excellent reviews.[223–227] In this discussion we will primarily address issues of pretreatment assessment in an effort to minimize toxicity, and we will concentrate on agents commonly used to treat lung cancer.[228,229]

TABLE 36.6. INCIDENCE AND RISK FACTORS FOR CHEMOTHERAPY-ASSOCIATED PULMONARY TOXICITY

Drug	Incidence	Risk Factors
Bleomycin[226,260,261]	2% to 40%	Age over 70 years Cumulative dose over 400 to 450 units Radiotherapy to chest Supplemental oxygen therapy Renal dysfunction Bolus intravenous administration Concomitant use of other cytotoxic drugs
Cyclophosphamide[225,226]	less than 1%	Concomitant use of other cytotoxic drugs Radiotherapy to chest Dosage?
Mitomycin[223,225,226]	3% to 36%	Concomitant use of other cytotoxic drugs Frequency of dosing Total dose? Radiotherapy to chest? Supplemental oxygen therapy
Vinca alkaloids[223,225]	Unknown	Concomitant use of other cytotoxic drugs (mitomycin)
Doxorubicin[226]	Unknown	Radiotherapy to chest

The incidence and major risk factors associated with these chemotherapeutic agents are summarized in Table 36.6. Bleomycin is included because it is considered by many to be the prototypical agent of drug-induced lung damage.[226] Furthermore this agent has been the most extensively studied, with two major clinical scenarios described: a chronic, progressive fibrosis, and an acute hypersensitivity reaction.[223] The risk factors described in Table 36.6 are the best-defined in the literature. Mitomycin C has been shown to result in pulmonary toxicity 3% to 36% of the time.[226] Toxicity can occur after a single dose or several months after stopping therapy; clinical scenarios include pulmonary pneumonitis/fibrosis, hemolytic-uremic syndrome, and bronchospasm.[225] Risk factors for lung toxicity with this drug are less well defined; the major ones are shown in Table 36.6. Cyclophosphamide is the most common agent used in the treatment of lung cancer. Toxicity has been reported after a single dose or up to 13 years after discontinuing therapy.[223,226] The reports of cyclophosphamide toxicity are difficult to interpret as this drug has been usually administered with other agents. Fortunately, the incidence of lung toxicity is less than 1%.[223] Risk factors for development of pulmonary toxicity are also poorly defined. Vinca alkaloids administered alone rarely cause significant pulmonary toxicity but can when administered in conjunction with mitomycin. Several studies[230–232] have noted this association, with the unusual syndrome of acute bronchospasm described by some.[231,232]

Data have been published reporting an increased risk of pulmonary toxicity in the face of combined therapy with chemotherapeutic agents and thoracic radiation.[233] This relation is best established for bleomycin,[234–236] cyclophosphamide,[225,237,238] doxorubicin,[239–242] dactinomycin,[243] irinotecan,[244] and possibly vindesine.[245] This should be taken into account, as combined therapy is often considered for lung cancer patients, particularly if administered concurrently.[244,246] A review of series published before 1994 that used combined modality therapy suggested that, in multivariate analysis, radiation pneumonitis was most commonly seen in the setting of high dose per fraction.[247] These authors suggested the use of twice-daily radiation in this setting to minimize risks of pulmonary toxicity.

The role of pulmonary function testing in this setting remains unclear. Most data have been published regarding bleomycin. Many authors feel that DLCO is the most useful test to monitor for potential toxicity,[248,249] while others do not concur.[250–252] Most recently Wolkowicz and colleagues[253] prospectively studied 59 patients undergoing treatment for testicular cancer. DLCO dropped significantly with bleomycin but failed to differentiate patients with pneumonitis. The TLC was found to be a more specific indicator of significant pneumonitis. Van Barneveld and associates[254] studied 39 patients treated for testicular cancer by combining various parameters in a discriminant analysis to predict pulmonary toxicity. The combination of a low normal creatinine clearance, decrease in VC, and decrease in alveolar volume with no decrease in pulmonary capillary blood volume predicted an increased risk of pulmonary toxicity. Unfortunately, similar data are not available for other chemotherapeutic regimens. Limited information has been published during treatment for small cell cancer. Sorensen and colleagues[255] prospectively studied 30 patients treated with aggressive chemotherapy (six achieved a complete response and ten a partial response). In both of these groups VC, FEV$_1$, TLC, and PEFR increased three months after initiation of treatment. This improvement paralleled the roentgenographic improvement. As described earlier for radiation therapy, the treatment of lung cancer may lead to an initial improvement in pulmonary function as tumor bulk decreases along with associated airway involvement. In a preliminary communication, Valdivieso and associates[256] reported an increased incidence of pulmonary toxicity in patients with a lower FEF$_{25-75}$ who were treated for lung cancer with mitomycin, etoposide, platinum, and radiation therapy.

It is likely that the role of pulmonary function testing is limited in those patients undergoing chemotherapy for lung cancer. In those with multiple risk factors (Table 36.6), pretreatment spirometry, lung volume, and DLCO measurement as well as close monitoring during treatment are appropriate. Isolated abnormalities in pretreatment pulmonary function should not preclude chemotherapy. On the other hand, decreases in lung volumes or DLCO during therapy should lead one to reassess the benefits of further chemotherapy. In this fashion pulmonary toxicity should be minimized.

CONCLUSIONS

The treatment of bronchogenic cancer includes surgical resection, radiation therapy and chemotherapy; frequently combinations of these are used. Unfortunately, all of these modalities have associated deleterious effects on pulmonary function. In this chapter we have summarized the role of pretreatment evaluation in these patients. With aggressive testing and appropriate treatment the majority of patients should be able to undergo treatment while minimizing pulmonary side effects.

REFERENCES

1. Bolliger CT, Perrucoud AP. Functional evaluation of the lung resection candidate. *Eur Respir J* 1998;11:198.
2. Olsen GN. Lung cancer resection. Who's inoperable? *Chest* 1995;108:298.
3. Reilly JJ. Benefits of aggressive perioperative management in patients undergoing thoracotomy. *Chest* 1995;107:312S.
4. McKenna RJ, Fischel RJ, Brenner M, et al. Combined operations for lung volume reduction surgery and lung cancer. *Chest* 1996;110:885.
5. Ojo TC, Martinez FJ, Paine III R, et al. Lung volume reduction surgery alters management of pulmonary nodules in patients with severe COPD. *Chest* 1997;112:1494.
6. Peters RM, Wellons HA, Htwe TM. Total compliance and work of breathing after thoracotomy. *J Thorac Cardiovasc Surg* 1969;57:348.
7. Bolton JWR, Weiman DS. Physiology of lung resection. *Clin Chest Med* 1993;14:293.
8. Siebecker KL, Sadler PE, Mendenhall JT. Postoperative ear oximeter studies on patients who have undergone pulmonary resection. *J Thorac Surg* 1958;36:88.
9. Byrd RB, Burns JR. Cough dynamics in the post-thoracotomy state. *Chest* 1975;67:654.
10. Cooper JD, Nelems JM, Pearson FG. Extended indications for median sternotomy in patients requiring pulmonary resection. *Ann Thorac Surg* 1978;26:413.
11. Marshall MC, Olsen GN. The physiologic evaluation of the lung resection candidate. *Clin Chest Med* 1993;14:305.
12. Deslauriers J, Ginsberg RJ, Dubois P, et al. Current operative morbidity associated with elective surgical resection for lung cancer. *Can J Surg* 1989;32:335.

13. Romano PS, Mark DH. Patient and hospital characteristics related to in-hospital mortality after lung cancer resection. *Chest* 1992;101:1332.

14. Whittle J, Steinberg EP, GF Anderson, et al. Use of Medicare claims data to evaluate outcomes in elderly patients undergoing lung resection of lung cancer. *Chest* 1991;100:729.

15. Kearney DJ, Lee TH, Reilly JJ, et al. Assessment of operative risk in patients undergoing lung resection. Importance of predicted pulmonary function. *Chest* 1994;105:753.

16. Keagy BA, Lores ME, Starek PJ, et al. Elective pulmonary lobectomy: factors associated with morbidity and operative mortality. *Ann Thorac Surg* 1985;40:349.

17. American Thoracic Society. Standardization of spirometry 1987 update. ATS statement. *Am Rev Respir Dis* 1987;1987:

18. American Thoracic Society. Lung function testing: selection of reference values and interpretative strategies. *Am Rev Respir Dis* 1991;144:1202.

19. Gaensler EA, Cugell DW, Lindgren I, et al. The role of pulmonary insufficiency in mortality and invalidism following surgery for pulmonary tuberculosis. *J Thorac Cardiovasc Surg* 1955;29:163.

20. Mittman C. Assessment of operative risk in thoracic surgery. *Am Rev Respir Dis* 1961;84:197.

21. Boushy SF, Billig DM, North LB, et al. Clinical course related to preoperative and postoperative pulmonary function in patients with bronchogenic carcinoma. *Chest* 1971;59:383.

22. Lockwood P. The principles of predicting the risk of post-thoracotomy function-related complications in bronchial carcinoma. *Respiration* 1973;30:329.

23. Lockwood P. Lung function test results and the risk of post-thoracotomy complications. *Respiration* 1973;30:529.

24. Boysen PG, Block AJ, Moulder PV. Relationship between preoperative pulmonary function tests and complications after thoracotomy. *Surg Gynecol Obstet* 1981;152:813.

25. Miller JI. Physiologic evaluation of pulmonary function in the candidate for lung resection. *J Thorac Cardiovasc Surg* 1993;105:347.

26. Larsen MC, Cliffton EE. The prognostic value of preoperative evaluation of patients undergoing thoracic surgery. *Dis Chest* 1965;47:589.

27. Keagy BA, Schorlemmer GR, Murray GR, et al. Correlation of preoperative pulmonary function testing with clinical course in patients after pneumonectomy. *Ann Thorac Surg* 1983;36:253.

28. Ogilvie CM, Forster RE, Blakemore WS, et al. A standard breathholding technique for the clinical measurement of the diffusing capacity of the lung for carbon monoxide. *J Clin Invest* 1957;36:1.

29. Weinberger SE, Johnson TS, Weiss ST. Use and interpretation of the single-breath diffusing capacity. *Chest* 1980;78:483.

30. Morrison NJ, Abboud RT, Ramadan F, et al. Comparison of single breath carbon monoxide diffusing capacity and pressure-volume curves in detecting emphysema. *Am Rev Respir Dis* 1989;139:1179.

31. Cotton DJ, Soparkar GR, Graham BL. Diffusing capacity in the clinical assessment of chronic airflow obstruction. *Med Clin North Am* 1996;80:549.

32. Ferguson MK, Little L, Rizzo L, et al. Diffusion capacity predicts morbidity and mortality after pulmonary resection. *J Thorac Cardiovasc Surg* 1988;96:894.

33. Wang J, Olak J, Ultmann RE, et al. Assessment of pulmonary complications after lung resection. *Ann Thorac Surg* 1999;67:1444.

34. Markos J, Mullan BP, Hillman DR, et al. Preoperative assessment as a predictor of mortality and morbidity after lung resection. *Am Rev Respir Dis* 1989;139:902.

35. Bousamra II M, Presberg KW, Chammas JH, et al. Early and late morbidity in patients undergoing pulmonary resection with low diffusing capacity. *Ann Thorac Surg* 1996;62:968.

36. Pierce RJ, Copland JM, Sharpe K, et al. Preoperative risk evaluation for lung cancer resection: predicted postoperative product as a predictor of surgical mortality. *Am J Respir Crit Care Med* 1994;1994:

37. Neuhaus H, Cherniack NS. A bronchospirometric method of estimating the effect of pneumonectomy on the maximum breathing capacity. *J Thorac Cardiovasc Surg* 1968;55:144.

38. Snider GL, Shaw AR. A critical evaluation of bronchospirometric measurement in predictive loss of ventilatory function due to thoracic surgery. *J Lab Clin Med* 1964;64:321.

39. Bergan F. A simple method for determination of the relative function of the right and left lung. *Acta Chir Scand* 1960;253[Suppl]:58.

40. Marion JM, Alderson PO, Lefrak SS, et al. Unilateral lung function. Comparison of the lateral position test with radionuclide ventilation-perfusion studies. *Chest* 1976;69:5.

41. Walkup RH, Vossel LF, Griffin JP, et al. Prediction of postoperative pulmonary function with the lateral position test. *Chest* 1980;77:24.

42. DeMeester TR, Van Heertum RL, Karas JR, et al. Preoperative evaluation with differential pulmonary function. *Ann Thorac Surg* 1974;18:61.

43. Jay SJ, Stonehill RB, Kiblaw SO, et al. Variability of the lateral position test in normal subjects. *Am Rev Respir Dis* 1980;121:165.

44. Schoonover GA, Olsen GN, McLain WC, et al. Lateral position test and quantitative lung scan in the preoperative evaluation for lung resection. *Chest* 1984;86:854.

45. Ryo UY. Prediction of postoperative loss of lung function in patients with malignant lung mass. Quantitative regional ventilation-perfusion scanning. *Radiol Clin North Am* 1990;28:657.

46. Kristersson S, Lindell SE, Svanberg L. Prediction of pulmonary function loss due to pneumonectomy using ^{133}Xe-radiospirometry. 1972;62:694.

47. Olsen GN, Block AJ, Tobias JA. Prediction of postpneumonectomy pulmonary function using quantitative macroaggregate lung scanning. *Chest* 1974;66:13.

48. Ali MK, Mountain C, Miller JM, et al. Regional pulmonary function before and after pneumonectomy using 133Xenon. *Chest* 1975;68:288.

49. Ali MK, Mountain CF, Ewer MS, et al. Predicting loss of pulmonary function after pulmonary resection for bronchogenic carcinoma. *Chest* 1980;77:337.

50. Ali MK, Ewer MS, Atallah MR, et al. Regional and overall pulmonary function changes in lung cancer. Correlations with tumor stage, extent of pulmonary resection, and patient survival. *J Thorac Cardiovasc Surg* 1983;86:1.

51. Boysen PG, Block AJ, Olsen GN, et al. Prospective evaluation for pneumonectomy using the ^{99m}Technetium quantitative perfusion lung scan. *Chest* 1977;72:422.

52. Boysen PG, Harris JO, Block AJ, et al. Prospective evaluation for pneumonectomy using perfusion scanning. Follow-up beyond one year. *Chest* 1981;80:163.

53. Wernly JA, DeMeester TR, Kirchner PT, et al. Clinical value of quantitative ventilation-perfusion lung scans in the surgical management of bronchogenic carcinoma. *J Thorac Cardiovasc Surg* 1980;80:535.

54. Egeblad K, Aunsholt NA, Funder V, et al. A simple method for predicting pulmonary function after lung resection. *Scand J Thor Cardiovasc Surg* 1986;20:103.

55. Zeiher BJ, Gross TJ, Kern JA, et al. Predicting postoperative pulmonary function in patients undergoing lung resection. *Chest* 1995;208:68.

56. Nakahara K, Monden Y, Ohno K, et al. A method for predicting

postoperative lung function and its relation to postoperative complications in patients with lung cancer. *Ann Thorac Surg* 1985;39:260.

57. Corris PA, Ellis DA, Hawkins T, et al. Use of radionuclide scanning in the preoperative estimation of pulmonary function after pneumonectomy. *Thorax* 1987;42:285.

58. Bolliger CT, Wyser C, Roser J, et al. Lung scanning and exercise testing for the prediction of postoperative performance in lung resection candidates at increased risk for complications. *Chest* 1995;108:341.

59. Ladurie MLR, Ranson-Bitker B. Uncertainties in the expected value for forced expiratory volume in one second after surgery. *Chest* 1986;90:222.

60. Holden DA, Rice TW, Stelmach K, et al. Exercise testing, 6-min walk, and stair climb in the evaluation of patients at high risk for pulmonary resection. *Chest* 1992;102:1774.

61. Ribas J, Diaz O, Barbera JA, et al. Invasive exercise testing in the evaluation of patients at high risk for lung resection. *Eur Respir J* 1998;12:1429.

62. Filaire M, Bedu M, Naamee A, et al. Prediction of hypoxemia and mechanical ventilation after lung resection for cancer. *Ann Thorac Surg* 1999;67:1460.

63. Wang J, Olak J, Ferguson MK. Diffusing capacity predicts operative mortality but not long-term survival after resection for lung cancer. *J Thorac Cardiovasc Surg* 1999;117:581.

64. Wu MT, Chang JM, Chiang AA, et al. Use of quantitative CT to predict postoperative lung function in patients with lung cancer. *Radiology* 1994;191:257.

65. Harrison RW, Adams WE, Long ET, et al. The clinical significance of cor pulmonale in the reduction of cardiopulmonary reserve following extensive pulmonary resection. *J Thorac Surg* 1958;36:352.

66. Carlens E, Hanson HE, Nordenstrom B. Temporary unilateral occlusion of the pulmonary artery. A new method of determining separate lung function and of radiologic examinations. *J Thorac Surg* 1951;22:527.

67. Uggla LG. Indications for and results of thoracic surgery with regard to respiratory and circulatory function tests. *Acta Chir Scand* 1956;111:197.

68. Rams JJ, Harrison RW, Fry WA, et al. Operative pulmonary artery pressure measurements as a guide to postoperative management and prognosis following pneumonectomy. *Dis Chest* 1962;41:85.

69. Van Nostrand D, Kjelsberg MO, Humphrey EW. Preresectional evaluation of risk from pneumonectomy. *Surg Gynecol Obstet* 1968;127:306.

70. Laros CD, Swierenga J. Temporary unilateral pulmonary artery occlusion in the preoperative evaluation of patients with bronchial carcinoma. Comparison of pulmonary artery pressure measurements, pulmonary function tests and early postoperative mortality. *Med Thorac* 1967;24:269.

71. Olsen GN, Block AJ, Swenson EW, et al. Pulmonary function evaluation of the lung resection candidate: A prospective study. *Am Rev Respir Dis* 1975;111:379.

72. Lewis JW, Bastanfar M, Gabriel G, et al. Right heart function and prediction of respiratory morbidity in patients undergoing pneumonectomy with moderately severe cardiopulmonary dysfunction. *J Thorac Cardiovasc Surg* 1994;108:169.

73. Olsen GN. The evolving role of exercise testing prior to lung resection. *Chest* 1989;95:2118.

74. Bagg LR. The 12-min walking distance; its use in the preoperative assessment of patients with bronchial carcinoma before lung resection. *Respiration* 1984;46:342.

75. Bolton JW, Weiman DS, Haynes J, et al. Stair climbing as an indicator of pulmonary function. *Chest* 1987;92:783.

76. Olsen GN, Bolton JWR, Weiman DS, et al. Stair climbing as

77. Pollock M, Roa J, Benditt J, et al. Estimation of ventilatory reserve by stair climbing. A study in patients with chronic airflow obstruction. *Chest* 1993;104:1378.

78. Pate P, Tenholder MF, Griffin JP, et al. Preoperative assessment of the high-risk patient for lung resection. *Ann Thorac Surg* 1996;61:1494.

79. Rao V, Todd TRJ, Kuus A, et al. Exercise oximetry versus spirometry in the assessment of risk prior to lung resection. *Ann Thorac Surg* 1995;60:603.

80. Reichel J. Assessment of operative risk of pneumonectomy. *Chest* 1972;62:570.

81. Berggren H, Ekroth R, Malmberg R, et al. Hospital mortality and long-term survival in relation to preoperative function in elderly patients with bronchogenic carcinoma. *Ann Thorac Surg* 1984;38:633.

82. Gerson MC, Hurst JM, Hertzberg VS, et al. Prediction of cardiac and pulmonary complications related to elective abdominal and noncardiac thoracic surgery in geriatric patients. *Am J Med* 1990;88:101.

83. Soderholm B. The hemodynamic effects of the lesser circulation in pulmonary tuberculosis: Effect of exercise, temporary unilateral pulmonary artery occlusion, and operation. *Scand J Clin Lab Invest* 1957;[Suppl 26]:1.

84. Fee HJ, Holmes EC, Gewirtz HS, et al. Role of pulmonary vascular resistance measurements in preoperative evaluation of candidates for pulmonary resection. *J Thorac Cardiovasc Surg* 1978;75:519.

85. Olsen GN, Weiman DS, Bolton JWR, et al. Submaximal invasive exercise testing and quantitative lung scanning in the evaluation for tolerance of lung resection. *Chest* 1989;95:267.

86. Bolliger CT, Soler M, Stulz P, et al. Evaluation of high-risk lung resection candidates: pulmonary hemodynamics versus exercise testing. A series of five patients. *Respiration* 1994;61:181.

87. Eugene J, Brown SE, Light RW, et al. Maximum oxygen consumption: a physiologic guide to pulmonary resection. *Surg Forum* 1982;33:260.

88. Smith TP, Kinasewitz GT, Tucker WY, et al. Exercise capacity as a predictor of post-thoracotomy morbidity. *Am Rev Respir Dis* 1984;129:730.

89. Bechard D, Wetstein L. Assessment of exercise oxygen consumption as preoperative criterion for lung resection. *Ann Thorac Surg* 1987;44:344.

90. Miyoshi S, Nakahara K, Ohno K, et al. Exercise tolerance test in lung cancer patients: the relationship between exercise capacity and postthoracotomy hospital mortality. *Ann Thorac Surg* 1987;44:487.

91. Nagakawa K, Nakahara K, Miyoshi S, et al. Oxygen transport during incremental exercise load as a predictor of operative risk in lung cancer patients. *Chest* 1992;101:1369.

92. Morice RC, Peters EJ, Ryan MB, et al. Exercise testing in the evaluation of patients at high risk for complications from lung resection. *Chest* 1992;101:356.

93. Walsh GL, Morice RC, Putnam JB, et al. Resection of lung cancer is justified in high-risk patients selected by exercise oxygen consumption. *Ann Thorac Surg* 1994;58:704.

94. Bolliger CT, Jordan P, Soler M, et al. Exercise capacity as a predictor of postoperative complications in lung resection candidates. *Am J Respir Crit Care Med* 1995;151:1472.

95. Torchio R, Gulotta C, Parvis M, et al. Gas exchange threshold as a predictor of severe postoperative complications after lung resection in mild-to-moderate chronic obstructive pulmonary disease. *Monaldi Arch Chest Dis* 1998;53:127.

96. Colman NC, Schraufnagel DE, Rivington RN, et al. Exercise

testing in evaluation of patients for lung resection. *Am Rev Respir Dis* 1982;125:604.

97. Boysen PG, Clark CA, Block AJ. Graded exercise testing and postthoracotomy complications. *J Cardiothorac Anesth* 1990;4:68.

98. Epstein SK, Faling LJ, Daly BDT, et al. Predicting complications after pulmonary resection. Preoperative exercise testing vs a multifactorial cardiopulmonary risk index. *Chest* 1993;104:694.

99. Goldman L, Caldera D, Nussbaum SR, et al. Multifactorial index of cardiac risk in noncardiac surgical procedures. *N Engl J Med* 1977;297:845.

100. Epstein SK, Faling LJ, Daly BDT, et al. Inability to perform bicycle ergometry predicts increased morbidity and mortality after lung resection. *Chest* 1995;107:311.

101. Pierce RJ, Pretto JJ, Rochford PD, et al. Lobar occlusion in the preoperative assessment of patients with lung cancer. *Br J Dis Chest* 1986;80:27.

102. Sciurba F, Rogers R, Keenan R, et al. Improvement in pulmonary function and elastic recoil after lung-reduction surgery for diffuse emphysema. *N Engl J Med* 1996;334:1095.

103. Cooper J, E Trulock, Triantafillou A, et al. Bilateral pneumectomy (volume reduction) for chronic obstructive pulmonary disease. *J Thorac Cardiovasc Surg* 1995;109:106.

104. Martinez FJ. Surgical therapy for chronic obstructive pulmonary disease: conventional bullectomy and lung volume reduction surgery in the absence of giant bullae. *Semin Respir Crit Care Med* (in press).

105. Pigula FA, Keenan RJ, Ferson PF, et al. Unsuspected lung cancer found in work-up for lung reduction operation. *Ann Thorac Surg* 1996;61:174.

106. Hazelrigg SR, Boley TM, Weber D, et al. Incidence of lung nodules found in patients undergoing lung volume reduction. *Ann Thorac Surg* 1997;64:303.

107. DeRose JJ, Argenziano M, El-Amir N, et al. Lung reduction operation and resection of pulmonary nodules in patients with severe emphysema. *Ann Thorac Surg* 1998;65:314.

108. DeMeester SR, Patterson GA, Sundaresan RS, et al. Lobectomy combined with volume reduction for patients with lung cancer and advanced emphysema. *J Thorac Cardiovasc Surg* 1998;115:681.

109. Berrisford RG, Sabenathan SS, Mearns AJ, et al. Pulmonary complications of lung resection: the effect of continuous extrapleural intercostal nerve block. *Eur J Cardiothorac Surg* 1990;4:407.

110. Richardson J, Sabanathan S, Mearns AJ, et al. Efficacy of preemptive analgesia and continuous extrapleural intercostal nerve block on post-thoracotomy pain and pulmonary mechanics. *J Cardiovasc Surg* 1994;35:219.

111. Boysen PG. Perioperative management of the thoracotomy patient. *Clin Chest Med* 1993;14:321.

112. Tisi GM. Preoperative evaluation of pulmonary function. Validity, indications, and benefits. *Am Rev Respir Dis* 1979;119:293.

113. Jackson CV. Preoperative pulmonary evaluation. *Arch Intern Med* 1988;148:2120.

114. Kroenke K, Lawrence VA, Theroux JF, et al. Operative risk in patients with severe obstructive pulmonary disease. *Arch Intern Med* 1992;152:967.

115. Mohr DN, Jett JR. Preoperative evaluation of pulmonary risk factors. *J Gen Intern Med* 1988;3:277.

116. Warner MA, Divertie MB, Tinker JH. Preoperative cessation of smoking and pulmonary complications in coronary artery bypass patients. *Anesthesiology* 1984;60:380.

117. Bluman LG, Mosca L, Newman N, et al. Preoperative smoking habits and postoperative pulmonary complications. *Chest* 1998;113:883.

118. Gerson MC. Cardiac risk evaluation and management in noncardiac surgery. *Clin Chest Med* 1993;14:263.

119. Eagle KA, Brundage BH, Chaitman BR, et al. Guidelines for perioperative evaluation for noncardiac surgery. Report of the American College of Cardiology/American Heart Association Task Force on Practice Guidelines. Committee on Perioperative Cardiovascular Evaluation for Noncardiac Surgery. *J Am Coll Cardiol* 1996;27:910.

120. Mehta R, Eagle KA. How to assess cardiac risk before noncardiac surgery. *Intern Med* 1998;19:27.

121. Djokovic JL, Hedley-Whyte J. Prediction of outcome of surgery and anesthesia in patients over 80. *JAMA* 1979;242:2301.

122. Yellin A, Benfield JR. Surgery for bronchogenic carcinoma in the elderly. *Am Rev Respir Dis* 1985;131:197.

123. Sherman S, Guidot CE. The feasibility of thoracotomy for lung cancer in the elderly. *JAMA* 1987;258:927.

124. Ishida T, Yokoyama H, Kaneko S, et al. Long-term results of operation for non-small cell lung cancer in the elderly. *Ann Thorac Surg* 1990;50:919.

125. Jack C, Lye M, Lesley F, et al. Surgery for lung cancer: age alone is not a contraindication. *Int J Clin Pract* 1997;51:423.

126. Nagasaki F, Flehinger BJ, Martine N. Complications of surgery in the treatment of carcinoma of the lung. *Chest* 1982;82:25.

127. Kohman LJ, Meyer JA, Ikins PM, et al. Random versus predictable risks of mortality after thoracotomy for lung cancer. *J Thorac Cardiovasc Surg* 1986;91:551.

128. Legge JS, Palmer KN. Pulmonary function in bronchial carcinoma. *Thorax* 1973;28:588.

129. Boushy SF, Helgason AH, Billig DM, et al. Clinical, physiologic, and morphologic examination of the lung in patients with bronchogenic carcinoma and the relation of the findings to postoperative deaths. *Am Rev Respir Dis* 1970;101:685.

130. Reynolds HY, Swisher JW. Preoperative management of chronic bronchitis. *Infect Med* 1993;10:21.

131. Anthonisen NR, Wright EC, Group IPPB Trial. Bronchodilator response in chronic obstructive pulmonary disease. *Am Rev Respir Dis* 1986;133:814.

132. Ramsdell JW, Nachtwey FJ, Moser KM. Bronchial hyperreactivity in chronic obstructive bronchitis. *Am Rev Respir Dis* 1982;126:829.

133. Morton HJV. Tobacco smoking and pulmonary complications after operation. *Lancet* 1944;368:38.

134. Gerrard JW, Cockcroft DW, Mink JT, et al. Increased nonspecific bronchial reactivity in cigarette smokers with normal lung function. *Am Rev Respir Dis* 1980;122:577.

135. Chalon J, Tayyab MA, Ramanathan S. Cytology of respiratory epithelium as a predictor of respiratory complications after operations. *Chest* 1975;67:32.

136. Kaubam JR, Chen LH, Hyman SA. Effect of short term smoking halt on carboxyhemoglobin levels and P-50 values. *Anesth Analg* 1986;65:1186.

137. Warner MA, Offord KP, Warner ME, et al. Role of preoperative cessation of smoking and other factors in postoperative pulmonary complications: a blinded prospective study of coronary artery bypass patients. *Mayo Clin Proc* 1989;64:609.

138. Coultas DB. The physician's role in smoking cessation. *Clin Chest Med* 1991;12:755.

139. Sachs DPL, Leischow SJ. Pharmacologic approaches to smoking cessation. *Clin Chest Med* 1991;12:769.

140. Thompson B, Hopp HP. Community-based programs for smoking cessation. *Clin Chest Med* 1991;12:801.

141. Gross NJ. COPD: a disease of reversible airflow obstruction. *Am Rev Respir Dis* 1986;133:725.

142. Ziment I. Pharmacologic therapy of obstructive airway disease. *Clin Chest Med* 1990;11:461.

143. Newhouse MT, Dolovich MB. Control of asthma by aerosols. *N Engl J Med* 1986;315:870.

144. Chapman KR, Love L, Brubaker H. A comparison of breath-actuated and conventional metered-dose inhaler inhalation techniques in elderly subjects. *Chest* 1993;104:1332.

145. Pover GM, Dash CH. A new, modified form of inhaler ("Rotahaler") for patients with chronic obstructive lung disease. *Pharmatherapeutica* 1985;4:98.

146. Ferguson GT, Cherniack RM. Management of chronic obstructive pulmonary disease. *N Engl J Med* 1993;328:1017.

147. Barnes PJ. Airway pharmacology. In: J. Murray and J. Nadel, eds. *Textbook of respiratory medicine.* Philadelphia: W.B. Saunders Co., 1988.

148. Conradson T-B, Eklundh G, Olofsson B. Arrhythmogenicity from combined bronchodilator therapy in patients with obstructive lung disease and concomitant ischemic heart disease. *Chest* 1987;91:5.

149. Nadel JA, Barnes PJ. Autonomic regulation of the airways. *Annu Rev Med* 1984;35:451.

150. Gross NJ. Ipratropium bromide. *N Engl J Med* 1988;319:486.

151. Braun SR, McKenzie WN, Copeland C, et al. A comparison of the effect of ipratropium and albuterol in the treatment of chronic obstructive airway disease. *Arch Intern Med* 1989;149:544.

152. Gross NJ, Skorodin MS. Anticholinergic, antimuscarinic bronchodilators. *Am Rev Respir Dis* 1984;129:856.

153. Campbell S. For COPD a combination of ipratropium bromide and albuterol sulfate is more effective than albuterol alone. *Arch Intern Med* 1999;159:156.

154. Friedman M, Serby CW, Menjoge SS, et al. Pharmacoeconomic evaluation of a combination of ipratropium plus albuterol compared with ipratropium alone and albuterol alone in COPD. *Chest* 1999;115:635.

155. Mahler DA, Donohue JF, Barbee RA, et al. Efficacy of salmeterol xinafoate in the treatment of COPD. *Chest* 1999;115:957.

156. Thurlbeck WM. Pathophysiology of chronic airflow obstruction. *Clin Chest Med* 1990;11:389.

157. Weir DC, Burge PS. Effects of high dose inhaled beclomethasone dipropionate, 750 micrograms and 1500 micrograms twice daily, and 40 mg per day oral prednisolone on lung function, symptoms, and bronchial hyperresponsiveness in patients with non-asthmatic chronic airflow obstruction. *Thorax* 1993;48:309.

158. Vogt FC. The incidence of oral candidiasis with use of inhaled corticosteroids. *Ann Allergy* 1979;43:205.

159. Williams AJ, Baghat MS, Stableforth DE, et al. Dysphonia caused by inhaled steroids: recognition of a characteristic laryngeal abnormality. *Thorax* 1983;38:813.

160. Paggiaro PL, Dahle R, Bakran I, et al. Multicentre randomised placebo-controlled trial of inhaled fluticasone propionate in patients with chronic obstructive pulmonary disease. International COPD Study Group. *Lancet* 1998;351:773.

161. Burge PS. EUROSCOP, ISOLDE and the Copenhagen City Lung Study. *Thorax* 1999;54:287.

162. Vestbo J, Sorensen T, Lange P, et al. Long-term effect of inhaled budesonide in mild and moderate chronic obstructive pulmonary disease: a randomised controlled trial. *Lancet* 1999;353:1819.

163. Petty TL, Rollins DR, Christopher K, et al. Cromolyn sodium is effective in adult chronic asthmatics. *Am Rev Respir Dis* 1989;139:694.

164. Callahan CM, Dittus RS, Katz BP. Oral corticosteroid therapy for patients with stable chronic obstructive pulmonary disease. *Ann Intern Med* 1991;114:216.

165. Mendella LA, Manfreda J, Warren CP, et al. Steroid response in stable chronic obstructive pulmonary disease. *Ann Intern Med* 1982;96:17.

166. Snider GL. Theophylline in the ambulatory treatment of chronic obstructive lung disease: resolving a controversy. *Cleveland Clin J Med* 1993;60:197.

167. Vaz Fragoso CA, Miller MA. Review of the clinical efficacy of theophylline in the treatment of chronic obstructive pulmonary disease. *Am Rev Respir Dis* 1993;147:S40.

168. Aubier M, DeTroyer A, Sampson M, et al. Aminophylline improves diaphragmatic contractility. *N Engl J Med* 1981;305:249.

169. Murciano D, Auclair M-H, Pariente R, et al. A randomized, controlled trial of theophylline in patients with severe chronic obstructive pulmonary disease. *N Engl J Med* 1989;320:1521.

170. Anthonisen NR, Manfreda J, Warren CPW, et al. Antibiotic therapy in exacerbations of chronic obstructive pulmonary disease. *Ann Intern Med* 1987;106:196.

171. Chodosh S. Treatment of acute exacerbations of chronic bronchitis: state of the art. *Am J Med* 1991;91[Suppl 6A]:87S.

172. Eller J, Ede A, Schaberg T, et al. Infective exacerbations of chronic obstructive pulmonary disease. Relation between bacteriologic etiology and lung function. *Chest* 1998;113:1542.

173. Ball P, Harris JM, Lowson D, et al. Acute infective exacerbations of chronic bronchitis. *QJM* 1995;88:61.

174. Grossman RF. Guidelines for the treatment of acute exacerbations of chronic bronchitis. *Chest* 1997;112[Suppl 6]:311S.

175. Grossman R, Mukherjee J, Vaughan D, et al. A 1-year community-based health economic study of ciprofloxacin vs usual antibiotic treatment in acute exacerbations of chronic bronchitis. The Canadian Ciprofloxacin Health Economic Study Group. *Chest* 1998;113:131.

176. Sykes LA, Bowe EA. Cardiorespiratory effects of anesthesia. *Clin Chest Med* 1993;14:211.

177. Hedenstierna G, Tokics L, Strandberg A, et al. Correlation of gas exchange impairment to development of atelectasis during anaesthesia and muscle paralysis. *Acta Anaesthiol Scand* 1986;30:183.

178. Tokics L, Hedenstierna G, Strandberg A, et al. Lung collapse and gas exchange during general anesthesia: effects of spontaneous breathing, muscle paralysis, and positive end-expiratory pressure. *Anesthesiology* 1987;66:157.

179. Demers RR, Saklad M. The etiology, pathophysiology, and treatment of atelectasis. *Respir Care* 1976;21:234.

180. Bartlett R, Brennan ML, Gazzaniga AB, et al. Studies on the pathogenesis and prevention of postoperative pulmonary complications. *Surg Gynecol Obstet* 1973;137:925.

181. Bartlett RH, Gazzaniga AB, Geraghty TR. Respiratory maneuvers to prevent postoperative pulmonary complications: a critical review. *JAMA* 1973;224:1017.

182. Celli BR, Rodriguez KS, Snider GL. A controlled trial of intermittent positive pressure breathing, incentive spirometry, and deep breathing exercises in preventing pulmonary complications after abdominal surgery. *Am Rev Respir Dis* 1984;130:12.

183. Lindner KH, Lotz P, Ahnefeld FW. Continuous positive airway pressure effect on functional residual capacity, vital capacity, and its subdivisions. *Chest* 1987;92:66.

184. Stock MC, Downs JB, Gauer PK, et al. Prevention of postoperative pulmonary complications with CPAP, incentive spirometry, and conservative therapy. *Chest* 1985;87:151.

185. Morran CG, Finlay IG, Mathieson M, et al. Randomized controlled trial of physiotherapy for postoperative pulmonary complications. *Br J Anaesth* 1983;55:1113.

186. Oikkonen M, Karjalainen K, Veikko K, et al. Comparison of incentive spirometry and intermittent positive pressure breathing after coronary artery bypass graft. *Chest* 1991;99:60.

187. Craven JL, Evans GA, Davenport PJ, et al. The evaluation of

the incentive spirometer in the management of postoperative pulmonary complications. *Br J Surg* 1974;61:793.

188. Hall JC, Tarala R, Harris J, et al. Incentive spirometry versus routine chest physiotherapy for prevention of pulmonary complications after abdominal surgery. *Lancet* 1991;337:953.

189. Katz JA, Marks JD. Inspiratory work with and without continuous positive airway pressure in patients with acute respiratory failure. *Anesthesiology* 1985;63:598.

190. Pinilla JC, Oleniuk FH, Tan L, et al. Use of a nasal continuous positive airway pressure mask in the treatment of postoperative atelectasis in aortocoronary bypass surgery. *Crit Care Med* 1990; 18:836.

191. Forshag MS, Cooper AD. Postoperative care of the thoracotomy patient. *Clin Chest Med* 1992;13:33.

192. Brochard L, Isabey D, Piquet J, et al. Reversal of acute exacerbations of chronic obstructive lung disease by inspiratory assistance with a face mask. *N Eng J Med* 1990;323:1523.

193. Brochard L, Mancebo J, Wysocki M, et al. Noninvasive ventilation for acute exacerbations of chronic obstructive pulmonary disease [see comments]. *N Eng J Med* 1995;333:817.

194. O'Donohue WJ. National survey of the usage of lung expansion modalities for the prevention and treatment of postoperative atelectasis following abdominal and thoracic surgery. *Chest* 1985;87:76.

195. Gracey DR, Divertie MB, Didier EP. Preoperative pulmonary preparation of patients with chronic obstructive pulmonary disease. *Chest* 1979;76:123.

196. Thorens L. Postoperative pulmonary complications: observations on their prevention by means of physiotherapy. *Acta Chir Scand* 1954;107:194.

197. Faling LJ. Pulmonary rehabilitation—physical modalities. *Clin Chest Med* 1986;7:599.

198. Conacher ID. Pain relief after thoracotomy. *Br J Anaesth* 1990; 65:806.

199. Coleman DL. Control of postoperative pain. Nonnarcotic and narcotic alternatives and their effect on pulmonary function. *Chest* 1987;92:520.

200. Badner NH, Sandler AN, Koren G, et al. Lumbar epidural fentanyl infusions for post-thoracotomy patients: analgesic, respiratory, and pharmacokinetic effects. *J Cardiothorac Anesth* 1990;4:543.

201. Yeager MP, Glass DD, Neff RK, et al. Epidural anesthesia and analgesia in high-risk surgical patients. *Anesthesiology* 1987;66: 729.

202. Wheatley RG, Somerville ID, Sapsford DJ, et al. Postoperative hypoxemia: comparison of extradural, I.M. and patient-controlled opioid analgesia. *Br J Anaesth* 1990;64:267.

203. Baxter AD, Samson B, Doran R. Prevention of epidural morphine-induced respiratory depression with intravenous nalbuphine infusion in post-thoracotomy patients. *Can J Anaesth* 1989;36:503.

204. Ferrante FM, Chan VWS, Arthur GR, et al. Interpleural analgesia after thoracotomy. *Anesth Analg* 1991;72:105.

205. Mann LJ, Young GR, Williams JK, et al. Intrapleural bupivacaine in the control of postthoracotomy pain. *Ann Thorac Surg* 1992;53:449.

206. Brady LW, Germon PA, Cander L. The effects of radiation therapy on pulmonary function in carcinoma of the lung. *Radiology* 1965;85:130.

207. Gross NJ. Pulmonary effects of radiation therapy. *Ann Interm Med* 1977;86:81.

208. Maasilta P. Radiation-induced lung injury. From the chest physician's point of view. *Lung Cancer* 1991;7:367.

209. Movsas B, Raffin TA, Epstein AH, et al. Pulmonary radiation injury. *Chest* 1997;111:1061.

210. Choi NC. Prospective prediction of postradiotherapy pulmonary function with regional pulmonary function data: Promise and pitfalls. *Int J Radiat Oncol Biol Phys* 1988;15:245.

211. Byhardt RW, Martin L, Pajak TF, et al. The influence of field size and other treatment factors on pulmonary toxicity following hyperfractionated irradiation for inoperable non-small cell lung cancer (NSCLC)—analysis of a radiation therapy oncology group (RTOG) protocol. *Int J Radiat Oncol Biol Phys* 1993;27: 537.

212. Kwa SLS, Lebesque JV, Thews JCM, et al. Radiation pneumonitis as a function of mean lung dose: an analysis of pooled data of 540 patients. *Int J Radiat Oncol Biol Phys* 1998;42:1.

213. Perez CA, Stanley K, Rubin P, et al. A prospective randomized study of various irradiation doses and fractionation schedules in the treatment of inoperable non-oat-cell carcinoma of the lung. *Cancer* 1980;45:2744.

214. Simpson JR, Francis ME, Perez-Tamayo R, et al. Palliative radiotherapy for inoperable carcinoma of the lung: final report of a RTOG multi-institutional trial. *Int J Radiat Oncol Biol Phys* 1985;11:751.

215. Mattson K, Holsti LR, Poppius H, et al. Radiation pneumonitis and fibrosis following split-course radiation therapy for lung cancer. A radiologic and physiologic study. *Acta Oncol* 1987; 26:193–196.

216. Choi NC, Kanarek DJ, Grillo HC. Effect of postoperative radiotherapy on changes in pulmonary function in patients with Stage II and IIIA lung carcinoma. *Int J Radiat Oncol Biol Phys* 1990;18:95.

217. Rubenstein JH, Richter MP, Moldofsky PJ, et al. Prospective prediction of post-radiation therapy lung function using quantitative lung scans and pulmonary function testing. *Int J Radiat Oncol Biol Phys* 1988;15:83.

218. Choi NC, Kanarek DJ, Kazemi H. Physiologic changes in pulmonary function after thoracic radiotherapy for patients with lung cancer and role of regional pulmonary function studies in predicting postradiotherapy pulmonary function before radiotherapy. *Cancer Treat Symp* 1985;2:119.

219. Choi NC, Kanarek DJ, Kazemi H. Prospective study of pulmonary tolerance to radiotherapy or radiotherapy plus multidrug chemotherapy for loco-regional lung carcinoma. International association for the study of lung cancer workshop on combined radiotherapy and chemotherapy modalities in lung cancer, Basel, Switzerland: Karger, 1988.

220. Axford AT, Cotes JE, Deeley TJ, et al. Clinical improvement of patients with emphysema after radiotherapy. *Thorax* 1977; 32:35.

221. Fazio F, Pratt TA, McKenzie CG, et al. Improvement in regional ventilation and perfusion after radiotherapy for unresectable carcinoma of the bronchus. *AJR Am J Roentgenol* 1979; 133:191.

222. Marks LB, Munley MT, Bentel GC, et al. Physical and biological predictors of changes in whole-lung function following thoracic irradiation. *Int J Radiat Oncol Biol Phys* 1997;39:563.

223. Cooper J, White D, Matthay R. Drug-induced pulmonary disease. Part 1: cytotoxic drugs. *Am Rev Respir Dis* 1986;133:321.

224. Lehne G, Lote K. Pulmonary toxicity of cytotoxic and immunosuppressive agents. A review. *Acta Oncol* 1990;29:113.

225. Twohig K, Matthay R. Pulmonary effects of cytotoxic agents other than bleomycin. *Clin Chest Med* 1990;11:31.

226. Kreisman H, Wolkove N. Pulmonary toxicity of antineoplastic therapy. *Semin Oncol* 1992;19:508.

227. Rosenow E, Myers J, Swensen S, et al. Drug-induced pulmonary disease. An update. *Chest* 1992;102:239.

228. Murren J, Buzaid A. Chemotherapy and radiation for the treatment of non-small-cell lung cancer. A critical review. *Clin Chest Med* 1993;14:161.

229. Johnson B. Management of small-cell lung cancer. *Clin Chest Med* 1993;14:173.
230. Ozols R, Hogan W, Ostchega Y, et al. MVP 9mitomycin, vinblastine, and progesterone: a second-line regimen in ovarian cancer with a high incidence of pulmonary toxicity. *Cancer Treat Rep* 1983;67:721.
231. Kris M, Pablo D, Gralla J, et al. Dyspnea following vinblastine or vindesine administration in patients receiving mitomycin plus vinca alkaloid combination therapy. *Cancer Treat Rep* 1984;68:1029.
232. Luedke D, McLaughlin T, Daughaday C, et al. Mitomycin C and vindesine associated pulmonary toxicity with variable clinical expression. *Cancer* 1985;55:542.
233. Van Houtte P. Radiation and chemotherapy induced lung injury. *Int J Radiat Oncol Biol Phys* 1987;13:647.
234. Catane R, Schwade J, Turrisi A, et al. Pulmonary toxicity after radiation and bleomycin: a review. *Int J Radiat Biol* 1979;42:253.
235. Samuels M, Johnson D, Holoye P, et al. Large-dose bleomycin therapy and pulmonary toxicity: a possible role of prior radiotherapy. *JAMA* 1976;235:1117.
236. Einhorn L, Krause M, Hornback N, et al. Enhanced pulmonary toxicity with bleomycin and radiotherapy in oat cell lung cancer. *Cancer* 1976;37:2414.
237. Trask C, Joannides T, Harper P, et al. Radiation-induced lung fibrosis after treatment of small cell carcinoma of the lung with very high-dose cyclophosphamide. *Cancer* 1985;55:57.
238. Phillips TL, Fu KK. Quantification of combined radiation therapy and chemotherapy effects on critical normal tissues. *Cancer* 1976;37:1186.
239. Johnson R, Brereton H, Kent C. "Total" therapy for small cell carcinoma of the lung. *Ann Thorac Surg* 1978;25:510.
240. Veschoore J, Lagrange J, Boublil J, et al. Pulmonary toxicity of a combination of low-dose doxorubicin and irradiation for inoperable lung cancer. *Radiother Oncol* 1987;9:281.
241. Maurer H, Modeas C, Goutsou M, et al. Adult respiratory distress syndrome after combined modality chemotherapy and radiation therapy in limited small cell lung cancer. *Proc Am Soc Clin Oncol* 1990;9[abst]:229.
242. Mah K, Keane TJ, Van Dyk J, et al. Quantitative effect of combined chemotherapy and fractionated radiotherapy on the incidence of radiation-induced lung damage: a prospective clinical study. *Int J Radiat Oncol Biol Phys* 1994;28:563.
243. Wara WM, Phillips TL, Margolis LW, et al. Radiation pneumonitis: a new approach to the derivation of time-dose factors. *Cancer* 1973;32:547.
244. Yamada M, Kudoh S, Hirata K, et al. Risk factors of pneumonitis following chemoradiotherapy for lung cancer. *Eur J Cancer* 1998;34:71.
245. Bott S, Stewart F, Prince-Fiocco M. Interstitial lung disease associated with vindesine and radiation therapy for carcinoma of the lung. *South Med J* 1986;79:894.
246. Lingos TI, Recht A, Vicini F, et al. Radiation pneumonitis in breast cancer patients treated with conservative surgery and radiation therapy. *Int J Radiat Oncol Biol Phys* 1991;21:355.
247. Roach III M, Gandara DR, Yuo HS, et al. Radiation pneumonitis following combined modality therapy for lung cancer: analysis of prognostic factors. *J Clin Oncol* 1995;13:2606.
248. Sorensen P, Rossing N, Rorth M. Carbon monoxide diffusing capacity: a reliable indicator of bleomycin-induced pulmonary toxicity. *Eur J Respir Dis* 1985;66:333.
249. Comis R, Kuppinger M, Ginsberg S, et al. Role of single-breath carbon monoxide-diffusing capacity in monitoring the pulmonary effects of bleomycin in germ cell tumor patients. *Cancer Res* 1979;39:5076.
250. Lucraft H, Wilkinson P, Stretton T, et al. Role of pulmonary function test in the prevention of bleomycin pulmonary toxicity during chemotherapy for metastatic testicular teratoma. *Eur J Cancer Clin Oncol* 1982;18:133.
251. McKeage M, Evans B, Atkinson C, et al. Carbon monoxide diffusing capacity is a poor predictor of clinically significant bleomycin lung. *J Clin Oncol* 1990;8:779.
252. Bell M, Meredith D, Gill P. Role of carbon monoxide diffusing capacity in the early detection of major bleomycin-induced pulmonary toxicity. *Aust N Z J Med* 1985;15:235.
253. Wolkowicz J, Sturgeon J, Rawji M, et al. Bleomycin-induced pulmonary function abnormalities. *Chest* 1992;101:97.
254. Van Barneveld P, van der Mark T, Sleijfer D, et al. Predictive factors for bleomycin-induced pneumonitis. *Am Rev Respir Dis* 1984;130:1078.
255. Sorensen P, Osterlind K, Groth S, et al. Effects of intensive chemotherapy on respiratory function in patients with small cell carcinoma of the lung. *Eur J Cancer Clin Oncol* 1983;19:901.
256. Valdivieso M, Kraut M, Lattin P, et al. Pulmonary function tests predict pulmonary toxicity in non–small cell lung cancer patients receiving chemotherapy plus radiotherapy. *Proc Am Assoc Cancer Res* 1992;33:A1352.
257. Miller JI, Grossman GD, Hatcher CR. Pulmonary function test criteria for operability and pulmonary resection. *Surg Gynecol Obstet* 1981;153:893.
258. Candler L. Physiologic assessment and management of the preoperative patient with pulmonary emphysema. *Am J Cardiol* 1963;12:324.
259. Dales RE, Dionne G, Leech JA, et al. Preoperative prediction of pulmonary complications following thoracic surgery. *Chest* 1993;104:155.
260. Jules-Elysse K, White DA. Bleomycin-induced pulmonary toxicity. *Clin Chest Med* 1990;11:1.
261. Sleijfer S, van der Mark TW, Koops HS, et al. Enhanced effects of bleomycin on pulmonary function disturbances in patients with decreased renal function due to cisplatin. *Eur J Cancer* 1996;32A:550.

37

SURGICAL THERAPY OF STAGE I AND NON-T3N0 STAGE II NON-SMALL CELL LUNG CANCER

ROBERT J. GINSBERG
JEFFREY L. PORT

In North America, less than 25% of patients will present with stage I or II disease. Unfortunately, this early stage of disease is where potential for cure is greatest and where surgical resection is undoubtedly the treatment of choice.

In this chapter, we discuss the indications for surgery, principles of surgical oncologic therapy, and results of such treatment of patients deemed to have stage I or II (N1) lung cancer. The role of adjuvant and neoadjuvant therapies is discussed in Chapters 42–44.

HISTORICAL BACKGROUND

Surgery for lung cancer dates back to the mid-nineteenth century with multiple reports of nonanatomic partial resections for lung cancer. Davies in 1912 was first to describe a dissection lobectomy for lung carcinoma.[1] "The various structures at the pedicle of the lower lobe were ligated separately, and the lobe containing the growth was removed. The patient's condition was quite good for the first 6 days; he then developed an empyema and died on the eight day." The author concluded that lung carcinomas in their earliest forms were amenable to surgical resection and complete removal. He prophetically stated that it was incumbent upon the clinician to perform early radiologic diagnosis prior to tumor extension beyond the boundaries of potential resection.

The modern era of thoracic surgery was ushered in with the advent of underwater pleural drainage and improved x-ray technology, which could detect smaller, more resectable lesions. Brunn described a one-stage lobectomy in 1929, followed by Allan and Smith who described a two-stage lobectomy in which adhesions were first created by pleural abrasion followed by lobectomy 12 days later.[2,3] By 1931 there were only six reported cases of patients successfully treated for lung carcinomas by surgical resection. In 1933 Graham and Singer reported on the historic, successful removal of a lung carcinoma via left pneumonectomy.[4] This was the first one-stage pneumonectomy. They proposed that pneumonectomy for lung carcinoma was not only technically feasible but also offered the patient the greatest chance for complete cure. Radical pneumonectomy with *en bloc* removal of mediastinal nodes was proposed by Allison in 1946.[5] For the next 10 years, pneumonectomy became the standard of care for non–small cell lung cancer (NSCLC).

Over the ensuing several decades, the concept that the more radical a cancer resection the better was challenged. Several factors set the stage for a transition from radical pneumonectomy to less extensive operations. Surgical techniques improved and hilar dissection with lobectomy became practical. Improved x-ray technology allowed for earlier detection of smaller and more peripheral lesions. In addition, it became apparent that many of the surgical candidates suffered from chronic obstructive lung disease and would not tolerate a pneumonectomy. Lobectomy was no longer considered a compromise operation but rather the new standard of care for early-stage lung cancer. More recently, surgeons have questioned the need for lobectomy in early-stage disease. Jensik reported on the results of segmentectomy as an alternative to lobectomy for the treatment of lung cancer in 1973.[6] The technique was not widely adopted because of the increased technical difficulty. However, the more recent, widespread use of surgical stapling devices and thoracoscopy has rekindled the controversy over performing more limited resections, especially in T1N0 tumors.

This chapter discusses the management of those patients with relatively early-stage disease where, following clinical evaluation, a complete resection is anticipated. Although clinical staging underestimates final pathologic staging in at least 25% of cases, those patients with clinical stage I and II disease are usually offered surgical resection as the initial therapy.

DIAGNOSIS AND STAGING

The methods of diagnosing and staging lung cancer are well reviewed in Chapters 29–35. Many are asymptomatic and include patients who are smokers screened by their family physician, or who had a routine chest x-ray for employment medical clearance or preadmission testing prior to nonthoracic surgery. Surgical resection remains the mainstay of treatment for these patients, provided a complete resection can be performed and is warranted by a patient's functional status. Five-year survival following a complete resection of this early asymptomatic stage of disease (usually stage I) can approach 70%.[7-13]

The chest radiograph remains the most common and most inexpensive imaging modality to detect the pulmonary abnormalities related to early-stage disease. It must be remembered that early-stage lung cancers can often cause atelectasis or postobstructive pneumonias and may be mistaken for benign processes. One must be compulsive with follow-up before dismissing new x-ray abnormalities as benign processes, especially in smokers. The plain chest x-ray delineates the primary tumor and may also suggest mediastinal node involvement or direct tumor extension into the chest wall or mediastinum. A computed tomography (CT) scan of the chest remains the standard of care for further evaluation of a suspected lung cancer. This should include the entire chest and upper abdomen through the kidneys. We routinely use IV contrast to better delineate mediastinal structures. The diagnosis can be established by sputum cytology or bronchoscopy for more central lesions and percutaneous needle biopsy or thoracoscopy for peripheral abnormalities. Positron emission tomography (PET) scans have proven useful with an accuracy of up to 90%.

Whenever possible, we believe that a preoperative histologic or cytologic diagnosis of malignancy is worthwhile. If a diagnosis has not been reached prior to surgical resection, it is our practice to perform a wedge excision or intraoperative needle aspiration biopsy to obtain a diagnosis prior to the formal resection. Unfortunately, errors can occur with frozen section histology, usually the pathologist mistaking a malignant process for a more benign one. When the clinical suspicion of malignancy is great, and a frozen section analysis is unavailable, a formal resection (segmentectomy or lobectomy) is indicated for diagnosis and treatment. However, a pneumonectomy should never be performed without a preresection diagnosis of malignancy.

The minimum staging requirements include a complete history and physical examination, chest x-ray, and, whenever available, a CT scan of the chest and upper abdomen. Whether a search for distant metastases by other imaging techniques is warranted in these early stages of disease, is a moot point. The cost-effectiveness of this investigation, beyond a complete history and physical examination as well as screening blood chemistries, has never been substantiated. In our own practice, those patients with clinical stage Ib or II are usually screened for occult brain and bone metastases. With increasing frequency, we are employing PET scanning together with CT scanning as one-stop shopping.[14]

The role of invasive staging is even more debatable. Except for tiny peripheral tumors, occult mediastinal lymph node disease occurs in 10% to 25% of patients with stage I disease and an even greater percentage in clinical stage II disease. For this reason, we have employed mediastinoscopy liberally in our preoperative assessment. However, the standard of care in North America suggests that if mediastinal lymph nodes are clinically negative (<1 cm in transverse diameter), then mediastinoscopy is not required before offering surgical resection. In our own practice, if mediastinal lymph nodes are negative on CT scan but a patient has a 2 cm or greater peripheral nodule or has clinical evidence of stage Ib or II disease, we perform mediastinoscopy just before the formal thoracotomy, cautioning the patient that surgical resection will not proceed if the mediastinal lymph nodes prove to have N2 disease, believing that, in this group of patients, surgery alone is insufficient. With this approach, the likelihood of unresectability at the time of thoracotomy is lessened and, for patients harboring mediastinal lymph node involvement, the opportunity to be treated by multimodality therapy, including preoperative chemotherapy, is still available.

PREOPERATIVE ASSESSMENT

Although the preoperative assessment of the surgical patient has been discussed in Chapter 36, we believe that this assessment must be performed by the thoracic surgeon in every instance prior to surgical therapy and is useful to highlight again.

The thoracic surgeon must be compulsive in his or her initial assessment of the patient. Because the majority of postoperative complications and deaths are related to cardiopulmonary events, risk factors for these complications should be identified preoperatively. The surgeon must also ensure that the anticipated resection will leave the patient with a reasonable quality of life without chronic respiratory failure. A multitude of risk factors have been analyzed as predictors of postoperative morbidity and mortality.[15-23] The extent of resection, stage of disease, co-morbid medical disease, weight loss more than 10% and age over 70 appear to be most significant. Interestingly, a patient's attitude toward his or her disease has been confirmed in a prospective analysis as an important predictor of outcome.[24]

The history and physical examination are the most important tools in physiologically evaluating patients with lung cancer. Most patients with lung cancer are current or former smokers, which increases their risk for vascular, cardiac, and obstructive pulmonary disease. The history should focus on the patients' cardiopulmonary reserve, smoking status, and current sputum production. It is extremely important to also assess the patient's ability to cough. Marked preoperative improvement can occur by smoking cessation (minimum of 2 weeks preoperatively),

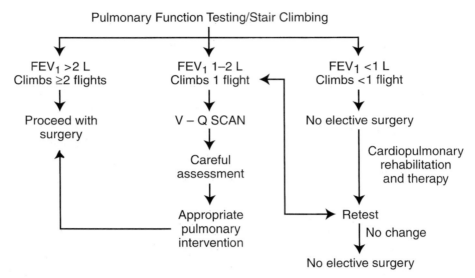

Pulmonary Function Testing/Stair Climbing

FEV$_1$ >2 L
Climbs ≥2 flights

FEV$_1$ 1–2 L
Climbs 1 flight

FEV$_1$ <1 L
Climbs <1 flight

Proceed with surgery

V – Q SCAN

No elective surgery

Careful assessment

Cardiopulmonary rehabilitation and therapy

Appropriate pulmonary intervention

Retest

No change

No elective surgery

FIGURE 37.1 The usual algorithm for assessing people with regard to suitability of pulmonary resection. The recent evidence suggests that even severely compromised patients can undergo thoracotomy and lobectomy. There is no absolute FEV1 value that contraindicates any surgical approach in selected patients.

antibiotics, bronchodilators, steroids, pulmonary rehabilitation, and patient education on how to cough effectively.[16,25]

Pulmonary function testing runs the gamut from simple physical examination with stair-climbing to sophisticated exercise testing. Stair-climbing with pulse oximetry has been well documented to accurately predict function.[26,27] However, the standard of practice requires preoperative spirometry with carbon monoxide diffusion capacity (DLCO) and an arterial blood gas in patients prior to resection.[28] Ventilation–perfusion scanning is usually reserved for patients requiring pneumonectomy or for those who have severely compromised function on spirometry. Although guidelines for predicting high risk for resection are not absolute, a predicted FEV$_1$ of less than .8 after any resection, an MVO$_2$ less than 10, hypercarbia, or cor pulmonale make surgery risky and pneumonectomy prohibitive (Figure 37.1). However, prior to denying any patient a potentially curative resection, aggressive pulmonary rehabilitation programs can be instituted for up to 2 months. Many patients subsequently show significant improvements and often qualify for resection. More recently, lung volume reduction surgery has been used in conjunction with pulmonary resection to improve lung function for patients with COPD.[29–31]

An accurate cardiac assessment is crucial in the thoracic patient. Hypertension, coronary artery disease, valvular disease, and arrhythmias are predictors of increased risk. A routine electrocardiogram is part of the preoperative assessment. More often, exercise stress testing and thallium imaging are being routinely utilized in patients over age 60 or with other risk factors to identify correctable defects.

STAGE I DISEASE (T1-2N0)

The Solitary Pulmonary Nodule

The solitary pulmonary nodule (SPN) deserves special attention because it often poses a diagnostic and therapeutic dilemma (Figure 37.2). More refined imaging and minimally invasive techniques have reduced the need for open thoracotomy for diagnosis. The SPN is defined as a round, 1 to 4 cm, well-circumscribed lesion surrounded by lung and without evidence of bronchial obstruction. Most often, these lesions present on routine chest x-ray as an unexpected finding in an asymptomatic patient. A thorough history, including questions regarding smoking history and previous malignancy, as well as a thorough physical examination may direct the clinician toward a diagnosis. A search for previous x-rays for comparison is imperative. If a lesion has not changed over 2 years, then one can ascribe a benign diagnosis with confidence.

If old x-rays are unavailable, initial attempts should be directed at characterizing the lesion. Features such as dense, central, "popcorn," or lamellar calcification suggest a benign lesion. CT scans have proven invaluable. High CT Hounsfield units indicating a dense lesion point toward a benign diagnosis. If doubt remains following these investigations, fluoroscopic or CT-guided percutaneous needle biopsy or transbronchial biopsy utilizing fluoroscopy can be performed. Recently, PET scans have been used to differentiate benign from malignant nodules with high accuracy.[32] This method appears highly accurate, approaching 95%. However, it has been shown that bronchoalveolar tumors

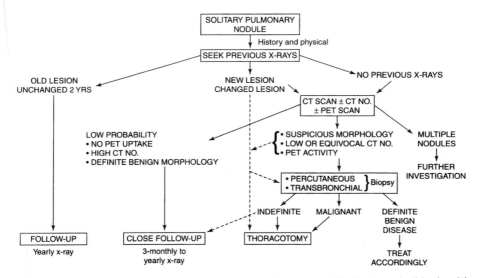

FIGURE 37.2 Algorithm for investigating a solitary pulmonary nodule. Not seen in this algorithm is the insertion of PET scanning. A high SUV number (greater than 7) would indicate malignancy. However, significant errors are seen with bronchoalveolar carcinomas.

are not well-suited for assessment by PET scanning (See also Chapter 30).

Several patients will remain whose lesions continue to elude tissue diagnosis. In these situations, tissue must be obtained either by open or video-assisted techniques, through which intraoperative aspiration cytology, core needle biopsy, wedge or segmental resection, and occasionally lobectomy can be performed for diagnosis.

Occult Lung Cancer

Patients with occult lung cancer (positive cytology, no lesion identified on x-ray) account for less than 1% of all lung cancer patients.[33–35] These patients usually include individuals who have participated in early lung cancer screening programs or who have developed hemoptysis without x-ray findings and have a positive sputum cytology documenting squamous cell cancer. Prior to any treatment, a thorough aerodigestive exam is required. One-third of these patients will actually have a head and neck cancer.[34] Following head and neck exam, bronchoscopy must be performed under local anesthesia to accurately examine the proximal and distal airway. A lesion that is easily visualized can be biopsied. When no endobronchial lesion is seen, brushings and washings from segmental bronchi must be obtained. Most recently, newer techniques have been established to assist in the detection of occult disease (see also chapters 22 and 24). These techniques include detection of early dysplasia and carcinoma with autofluorescence endoscopy (LIFE).[36] This technique has been reported to allow for almost 50% better detection of early carcinomas compared to ordinary flexible bronchoscopy.

Except for *in situ* carcinoma, or tiny superficially invasive tumors (less than 1 cm^2), the treatment of choice for even these early occult lesions is surgical resection. In such instances, lung-sparing operations are often indicated using bronchoplastic techniques because tumors often occur in major airways. The long-term survival following surgical resection for radiologically occult disease is excellent, approaching 100%. Although recurrences are rare, 45% of patients will develop new primary carcinomas of the aerodigestive tract. It is therefore imperative that surveillance endoscopy continue to be carried out.

SURGICAL ONCOLOGIC PRINCIPLES

Surgical resection remains the mainstay of treatment for early-stage lung carcinoma. However, an incomplete resection rarely benefits a patient. Several basic, yet important oncologic guidelines should be followed to provide an optimal and complete resection and complete the final TNM staging.

1. The tumor and its draining intrapulmonary lymphatic tributaries should be resected in their entirety whenever possible.
2. The tumor should be completely excised without spilling or traversing it.
3. The surgeon should resect *en bloc* any structure invaded by tumor in order to achieve negative margins.
4. A complete ipsilateral mediastinal lymph node dissection or sampling should be performed in all patients.

Lobectomy Versus Pneumonectomy

It has been clearly established that incomplete resections rarely lead to cure. Intraoperatively, the surgeon must determine if a lobectomy will suffice to provide a complete resection. All resection margins must be confirmed as negative by frozen section. In addition, lymph nodes lying on the pulmonary artery and straddling adjacent lobes must be examined by frozen section. If these nodes are positive, then a larger resection may be required to effect a complete resection (e.g., bilobectomy, sleeve resection, or pneumonectomy). Lymph node involvement of the airway or vessels proximal to the upper lobe takeoff involving the mainstem bronchus or the main pulmonary artery may necessitate a sleeve resection of the main bronchus or pneumonectomy.

Lymph Node Sampling Versus Mediastinal Lymph Node Dissection

During the conduct of surgical resection for lung cancer, surgeons must perform adequate nodal staging (see also Chapter 35). This process requires sampling of lymph nodes at the hilum and at all available mediastinal lymph node stations. If a mediastinoscopy has been done prior to the surgical resection, then those areas already sampled at mediastinoscopy need not be sampled again. If any sampled lymph nodes contain metastatic disease, then it is recommended that a complete ipsilateral mediastinal lymph node dissection be performed. Whether this latter procedure is required as routine (versus sampling) in all pulmonary resections for cancer is a debatable point. Advocates point out that in at least 10% of cases, occult mediastinal lymph node involvement occurs and may be missed unless an ipsilateral node dissection is carried out. On the other hand, the only randomized trial available to date suggests that although surgical staging is improved with regard to the number of mediastinal lymph node stations involved, the overall incidence of N2 disease discovered at the time of sampling is not improved with mediastinal lymph node dissection and, in this small randomized trial, no improvement in survival was demonstrated with the use of ipsilateral node dissection.[37] A North American trial was begun in 1999, comparing these two approaches in early-stage lung cancer.

Limited Resection Versus Lobectomy

The standard treatment for stage I disease is a complete removal of the primary tumor, usually lobectomy, and at minimum lymph node sampling of all available hilar and mediastinal nodes.

Advocates of limited (wedge or segmental) resections have argued that small peripheral T1N0 tumors can be removed safely by wedge resection with minimal risk of local residual lymphatic involvement. However, Ishida and colleagues reported that only for very small tumors (less than

1 cm in diameter) is the incidence of lymphatic permeation and nodal involvement near zero.[38,39] Tumors of 1.1 to 2 cm had intrapulmonary lymphatic spread in up to 17% of cases. Tumors greater than 2 cm had lymph channel or nodal spread in 38% of cases. This data suggests that to achieve complete resection in tumors greater than 1 cm in diameter, removal of local and regional nodes by standard lobectomy should be performed. Because less than 5% of lung cancers are discovered as peripheral tumors smaller than 1 cm, extensive data on these very small tumors is limited.

In a multivariate analysis of completely resected T1, N0, M0 tumors, Macchiarini and colleagues were unable to find a statistical correlation between tumor size and survival.[40] In their study, blood vessel invasion and mitotic index were more important factors in predicting survival. In a similar study by Ichinose and colleagues, tumor size alone was not a significant prognostic factor, and in multivariate analysis, only grade of differentiation and DNA ploidy patterns significantly impacted on survival in stage I disease.[41] Thus even very small peripheral tumors have the potential for local, regional, and systemic spread.

Types of Limited Resection

Limited resection can be defined as removal of a pulmonary tumor and surrounding lung by a technique designed to preserve lung parenchyma encompassing less than a lobectomy.

Segmentectomy

Segmental resection of the lung was originally described for the treatment of bronchiectasis by Churchill and Belsey.[42] The lymphatic drainage of each segment usually but not always follows the segmental anatomy without crossing into the adjacent segment. Segmentectomy has the theoretic advantage over other parenchyma-conserving operations of encompassing all or most of the local lymphatic drainage. Thus this operation can be considered the most reasonable compromise to lobectomy in the treatment of lung cancer.

The classic operation includes isolation and division of the segmental artery and bronchus centrally. The segment is manually stripped from surrounding segments along the plane delineated by the intersegmental veins. With the advent of stapling devices and the risk of entering tumor during the stripping procedure, in cancer surgery, stapling rather than stripping is often employed. Those segments abutting a single other segment, such as the lingula or superior segment, are the most appropriate for segmentectomy by virtue of technical simplicity (Figure 37.3).

Wedge Resection

Small peripheral tumors can be totally removed by a wedge excision. Complete local resection of the primary tumor is

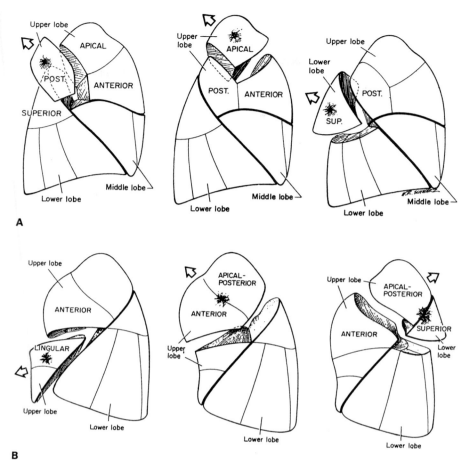

FIGURE 37.3 Various types of segmentectomies. **A:** Right lung. **B:** Left lung.

the goal of the operation, and no attempt is made to encompass the draining lymphatics. It is not known how much normal surrounding tissue should be resected as an adequate margin.

Precision-Cautery Dissection

When tumors cannot be excised by wedge excision and segmentectomy is not an option, precision-cautery dissection has been proven to be extremely useful.[43] This technique is done on the expanded lung and, using electrocautery or laser-cautery, the tumor and at least 2 cm of surrounding lung are dissected as deeply as necessary, usually ending up at the origin of a subsegmental bronchus and artery. This technique provides good hemostasis and, surprisingly, minimal air-leakage.

Video-Assisted Thoracoscopic Limited Resection

Video-assisted thoracoscopic (VAT) pulmonary resection has progressed substantially over the last several years.[44-52]

Initial thoracoscopic reports were aimed primarily at determining the technical feasibility and safety (mortality 0% to 3%) of thoracoscopic wedge resection. Shannib et al. recently studied the role of VAT wedge resection in 30 patients with T1 tumors and severe pulmonary compromise and found only a 3% mortality rate.[47] Further assessment of this technique combined with postoperative radiation therapy is the focus of an ongoing intergroup study.

Multiple reports have now emerged documenting the technical feasibility of thoracoscopic lobectomy and lymph node dissection.[48,49] To date, no long-term data has demonstrated equivalent survival in NSCLC patients resected by VAT compared to conventional open lobectomy. Despite the claims of improved cosmesis, acute and chronic postoperative pain relief, and reduced hospital stays, randomized studies to date have failed to demonstrate any advantages of video-assisted surgery other than improved cosmesis. As the role of thoracoscopy in lung cancer becomes better defined, surgeons must hold thoracoscopic procedures to the basic principles of cancer surgery and not compromise the resection for the sake of convenience.

TABLE 37.1. RESULTS OF REPORTED SERIES OF LIMITED RESECTIONS FOR EARLY-STAGE LUNG CANCER IN PAST 20 YEARS*

Investigators	No. of Patients	Type of Resection	Local Recurrence (%)	5-Year Survival (%)
Bennett & Smith, 1978	44	Segmental	40	36
McCormack et al., 1980	53	Wedge/segmentectomy	19.3	35
Errett et al., 1985	100	Wedge	NS	69
Jensik, 1986	193	Segmental	NS	15 (est.)
Miller & Hatcher, 1987*	32	Wedge/segmental + radiotherapy	6.25	31 (5 y)
Temeck et al., 1992	61	Wedge	4–9	29 (est.)
Read et al., 1990**	107	Segmentectomy	4.4	70
Wain et al., 1991	164	Wedge/segmentectomy	5	<50
Ginsberg & Rubenstein, 1994	123	Segmentectomy	17.5	70
Warren & Faber, 1993	74	Segmentectomy	21.6	50

* A wedge reaction was utilized; postoperative radiotherapy appeared to improve survival and approached that of segmentectomy.
** Stage T1, N0, M0 cancer.
NS, not significant; est., estimated.

Results of Limited Resection for Early-Stage Lung Cancer

Segmentectomy

The results of segmentectomy were the first and most widely reported limited resections for lung cancer. Two broad categories have been reported: (a) compromise operations when pulmonary function would not permit standard lobectomy, and (b) intentional segmentectomies for T1-2 N0 lung cancers when the surgeon considered this to be an adequate resection.[53–58] In pulmonary compromise situations, patients with both N1 and N2 disease were often included in studies, thus five-year survival ranges from 15% to 30%. Although local recurrence rates were not reported, limited data suggested they were high (Table 37.1).[6,59–63]

In the few series that reported on patients resected with curative intent, the five-year survival rate ranged from 50% to 70% for T1, N0 tumors, which is comparable to the results of lobectomy. Local recurrence rates in these series ranged from 5% to 17.5%, higher than the 5% seen after lobectomy (Table 37.1).[55,64–66]

The Rush-Presbyterian group has continued to report their extensive retrospective experience with segmentectomy as a curative treatment option for early lung cancer.[6,67] Most recently, they reported on 169 patients who underwent either a standard lobectomy (n = 103) or a segmental resection (n = 66) for pathologic stage I (T1, N0; T2N0) primary NSCLC. Patients in the segmentectomy group fared worse in terms of local recurrence, which was 22.7% compared to 4.9% after lobectomy. Five-year survival in the segmentectomy group was 45%, compared to 63% in the lobectomy group (p≤0.035).

The North American Lung Cancer Study Group (LCSG) confirmed previous retrospective studies with a prospective, randomized trial.[41] Patients with T1, N0 NSCLC were randomized to lobectomy (n = 125) or limited resection (n = 122: seg. = 82, wedge = 40). In this prospective study, the locoregional recurrence rate for lobectomy was 5%. There was a 2.4-fold increase in locoregional recurrence with limited resection (17%). There was a 30% increase in the overall death rate and a 50% increase in death with cancer for the limited resection group. There was no late functional advantage or decrease in perioperative morbidity for the limited resection group.

Wedge Resection

The reported series of wedge resections in the management of NSCLC have primarily involved compromise resections in patients with limited pulmonary reserve. However, there have been recent reports of intentional limited resections for small peripheral tumors after open and thoracoscopic procedures.[68] Little data exist to support the widespread use of wedge resection even for small peripheral tumors, except in the setting of pulmonary compromise. In the previously mentioned study of limited resection reported by the LCSG, 40 patients underwent wedge resection as a curative procedure. Even worse than segmentectomy, the locoregional recurrence rate was four-fold higher than the lobectomy group. No data on the results of precision-cautery dissection is available.

In summary, based on the available data, lobectomy and adequate nodal sampling or dissection should remain the mainstay of treatment for early-stage lung cancer. In compromise situations, limited resection can be performed, but with an expected increase in locoregional recurrence and decreased five-year survival. Only rarely is a bilobectomy or pneumonectomy required for stage I tumors. Occasionally, proximal T1N0 or large T2N0 lesions require this enlarged resection to effect complete removal.

STAGE II (N1) DISEASE

When intrapulmonary lymph nodes either within the lung or at the hilum are involved with metastases, the overall survival following surgical resection for lung cancer decreases considerably. Also, to effect a complete resection, pneumonectomy is required with increasing frequency. In our experience, approximately 25% of stage II lung cancers require pneumonectomy for complete tumor extirpation by virtue of the size or portion of the primary tumor or involvement of hilar lymph nodes.[69]

In this group of patients, lung-preserving procedures may indeed allow less than a pneumonectomy to be performed. When lymph nodes involve the main bronchus or invade the adjacent pulmonary artery, sleeve resection of the bronchus with or without a vascular sleeve resection of the pulmonary artery can be employed to preserve lung function, allowing a lobectomy to occur. Although no randomized trial has ever been performed to assess the value of this vis-à-vis complete pneumonectomy, most studies do indicate that the survival rate, stage for stage, of a sleeve lobectomy or combined vascular sleeve resection is identical to that seen with pneumonectomy.[70] With right lower lobe tumors, involved lymph nodes at the origin of the lower lobe bronchus or near the middle lobe take-off necessitate that a bilobectomy be performed. Similarly, upper or lower lobe tumors invading the middle lobe often require bilobectomy for complete excision.

In this stage of disease, especially with hilar lymph node involvement, we believe that concomitant mediastinal lymph node dissection (versus sampling) should be carried out because the incidence of occult mediastinal lymph node involvement in presumed stage II disease is much greater than with presumed stage I and approaches 25% of all cases.

POSTOPERATIVE COMPLICATIONS

Major complications occur in 10% of patients operated on with stage I and II disease.[71-74] (See also Chapter 41.) In a review of 961 patients who underwent major pulmonary resection, there was a 2% mortality and a 17% morbidity: 9% had major complications, which included pneumonia, pulmonary embolus, bronchopleural fistula, empyema, arrhythmia, and respiratory failure, and 8% had minor complications. The morbidity and mortality following resection for stage I and II tumors is less than that seen in stage III disease.

In a 1983 LCSG study, 2,220 patients undergoing resection for lung cancer were analyzed. Eighty-one postoperative deaths occurred (3.7%). The mortality was 6.2% for pneumonectomy and 2.9% for lobectomy. Most recently, morbidity and mortality were prospectively analyzed in 783 patients.[75] This study may reflect current trends toward aggressive neoadjuvant chemotherapy. Mortality was 3.9%,

and the major complication rate was a startling 27%. Complications occurred more often in men, in patients greater than 60 years of age, and in patients with a Karnofsky index of less than 9. The high incidence of morbidity in surgically resected lung cancer patients makes careful preoperative assessment and meticulous perioperative care mandatory. In our own center, postoperative mortality in stage I lung cancer resection approaches zero (1 death in the most recent 300 cases).

SURVIVAL

In the literature, survival following surgical treatment of stage I and II NSCLC varies considerably.[7-13,76-85] These differences may be related to the heterogeneity of the patient population, criteria for surgical resection, the proportion of patients in a subset (i.e., T1N0 versus T2N0), the extent of the staging process (mediastinoscopy versus mediastinal lymph node dissection versus sampling), and length of follow-up. Significant differences in survival exist even among patients with early-stage lung cancer. The best predictor of survival within each stage is in the comparison of the TNM subsets.

The overall survival for pathologic stage I and stage II disease was recently analyzed (Figure 37.4).[77] These results confirm that nodal involvement has the strongest adverse influence on survival, and results also demonstrate that a significant number of patients are clinically understaged. In our experience, overall survival for stage II is not only affected by the presence of N1 disease but also by the number of involved N1 nodes.[86] Furthermore, improved survival has also been noted in stage II patients with tumors less than 5 cm in size.[8] Several studies have also shown that histology may impact on survival. The LCSG reported an improved survival for squamous carcinomas versus nonsquamous lesions.[83,87] However, this difference has not been borne out in all series. It is important to note that within a given TNM category, it is impossible to predict which patients will experience a relapse of their disease.

Other prognostic factors, including gender, age, performance status, weight loss, and tumor location, have been analyzed.[15,17,18,36,41,86,88-91] None of these factors to date has clearly been proven to impact on survival. Numerous molecular and biologic markers are currently being investigated as predictors of survival in patients with NSCLC. They include tumor-associated antigens, aberrantly expressed genes, enzymes, hormones, or other biologic markers. The recognition and development of molecular markers has given new insight into our understanding of the biology of NSCLC. These markers may soon provide a more accurate method for predicting patient survival (See also Chapter 33).

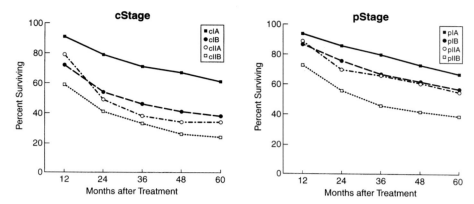

FIGURE 37.4 Survival following clinical staging versus pathologic staging. (From Mountain CF. Revisions in the international system for staging lung cancer. *Chest* 1997;111:1710, with permission.)

PATTERNS OF FAILURE AND RECURRENCE

The majority of patients who are resected for stage I NSCLC will enjoy long-term, disease-free survival.[8,12,13,80–83,92,93] However, approximately one-third of resected patients will relapse. The majority of these relapses will be distant metastases, with the risk of a local recurrence after complete resection being less than 10%. The brain is the most common site of metastatic recurrence, followed closely by bone, ipsilateral and contralateral lung, liver, and adrenal. More than 80% of recurrences occur within 2 years.

The rate of recurrence for patients with stage II disease is high despite surgical treatment. More than 50% of resected stage II patients can be expected to relapse. Similar to all stages of lung cancer, most recurrences are distant and suggest a need for effective systemic therapy once nodal metastases have occurred. However, the role of induction and/or adjuvant chemotherapy with or without radiotherapy has not been well defined. The patterns of recurrence may differ by histology with more local recurrences seen for patients with squamous carcinoma and more distant metastases seen in patients with adenocarcinoma.

ADJUVANT THERAPIES

Although discussed elsewhere (see Chapters 42, 43, 44), adjuvant therapies following complete resection of stage I and stage II lung cancer have failed to make a significant impact. Neither chemotherapy, radiotherapy nor both modalities used in an adjuvant setting have improved survival significantly following complete resection. This has been borne out in two recent metaanalyses of adjuvant chemotherapy and adjuvant radiotherapy. Also, a recent North American trial comparing postoperative adjuvant radiotherapy to adjuvant chemoradiotherapy in stage II and III lung cancer has failed to demonstrate an impact of the combined treatment.[94]

Because of the failures of adjuvant treatments and the apparent success of induction therapies in more advanced disease, studies are now being conducted to assess the value of induction chemotherapy followed by surgery in patients with clinically staged Ib and II disease.[95,96]

FOLLOW-UP

Resected NSCLC patients must be followed closely, not only for recurrences but also for new lung as well as nonthoracic primary malignancies. Patients with early-stage lung cancer were followed in a study by the LCSG for more than 5 years and were found to develop a significant number of new lung, breast, prostate, and colon cancers. In a recent analysis of 598 patients resected with stage I disease followed at Memorial Sloan-Kettering Cancer Center, 206 patients or 34% developed second cancers. One-third of these new primaries were lung cancers. This finding underscores the need to follow lung cancer patients closely postoperatively. We recommend that surgeons see their patients every 3 months for the first postoperative year, followed by every 6 months for 2 years, and then annually. Follow-up visits should include repeat chest x-rays and thorough physical examinations monitoring weight loss and respiratory and performance status. Screening blood work plays no role in routine follow-up of the postoperative patient. The value of CT scanning in follow-up is currently being investigated. The recommendations for close follow-up in general have recently been questioned in regards to cost-effectiveness.[97] In a small percentage of patients, disease relapse is confined to one local site without distant spread. These patients should be extensively reinvestigated. If no metastatic or mediastinal disease is discovered, such patients should be considered for re-resection and possible completion pneumonectomy. A recent analysis of patients undergoing completion pneumonectomy demonstrated a slightly higher mortality (10%) than patients undergoing pneumonectomy as their initial operation (6.2%), but a considerable number of patients were salvaged by this approach.[45]

FUTURE DIRECTIONS

Future directions in the surgical treatment of early-stage lung cancer await a variety of ongoing clinical trials. Currently, studies are evaluating the role of PET scanning in preoperative staging, whether complete ipsilateral mediastinal lymphadenectomy improves cure rates over lymph node sampling in stage I and II disease, and the role of genetic markers, immunohistochemical staining, bone marrow evaluation, PET scan activity (SUV), and pleural lavage as prognostic indicators. Also ongoing are trials analyzing the efficacy of 13-*cis*-retinoic acid as a chemoprevention agent for second primaries and the role of thoracoscopic wedge resection followed by radiation therapy for patients with severely compromised pulmonary function.

Although adjuvant and neoadjuvant therapies have yet to prove valuable following complete resection in these early stages of disease, trials are continuing to explore these treatments.

CONCLUSIONS

Surgical resection remains the gold standard for treatment of patients with stage I and II NSCLC who have potentially completely resectable lesions and adequate pulmonary reserve. Lobectomy and pneumonectomy afford the greatest chance for complete resection with the lowest recurrence rates and longest durable survival. Limited resections, either conventional or via video-assisted thoracoscopy have been advocated by some as an alternative to standard resections for patients with limited disease. These lesser resections have demonstrated alarmingly high local recurrence rates and shorter survival and should be considered compromise operations for patients who might not tolerate larger resections or who have synchronous disease necessitating more than one resection.

There is an increasing need for more accurate preoperative staging techniques for NSCLC. The current TNM staging system provides a method of standardization, improves our ability to determine ultimate prognosis, and allows us to identify groups that might benefit from trials of neoadjuvant and adjuvant therapy. As we push the treatment envelope further with investigational preoperative therapy, meticulous preoperative assessment becomes even more important if we are to reduce perioperative morbidity and mortality.

REFERENCES

1. Davies HM. Recent advances in the surgery of the lung and pleura. *BJS* 1913;1:228.
2. Brunn H. Surgical principles underlying one-stage lobectomy. *Arch Surg* 1929;18:490.
3. Allen CI, Smith J. Primary carcinoma of the lung. *Surg Gynecol Obstet* 1932;55:151.
4. Graham EA, Singer JJ. Successful removal of an entire lung for carcinoma of the bronchus. *JAMA* 1933;101:1371.
5. Allison PR. Intrapericardial approach to the lung root in the treatment of bronchial carcinoma by dissection pneumonectomy. *J Thorac Surg* 1946;15:99.
6. Jensik RJ, Faber LP, Milloy FJ, et al. Segmental resection for lung cancer, a fifteen year experience. *J Thorac Cardiovasc Surg* 1973;66:563.
7. Nesbitt JC, Putnam, Jr, Garrett LW, et al. Survival in early-stage non-small cell lung cancer. *Ann Thorac Surg* 1995;60:466.
8. Martini N, Burt M, Bains MS, et al. Survival after resection of stage II non-small cell lung cancer. *Ann Thorac Surg* 1992;54:460.
9. Williams DE, Pairolero PC, Davis CS, et al. Survival of patients surgically treated for stage I lung cancer. *J Thorac Cardiovasc Surg* 1981;82:70.
10. Moores DWO, McKneally MF. Treatment of stage I lung cancer (T1NOMO, T2NOMO). *Surg Clin North Am* 1987;67:937.
11. Holmes EC. Treatment of stage II lung cancer (T1N and T2N1). *Surg Clin North Am* 1987;67:945.
12. Martini N, Beattie EJ. Results of surgical treatment of stage I lung cancer. *J Thorac Cardiovasc Surg* 1977;74:499.
13. Harpole DH, Herndon, II, Young, Jr, et al. Stage I nonsmall cell lung cancer. *Cancer* 1995;76:787.
14. Scott WJ, Gobar LS, Terry JD. Mediastinal lymph node staging of NSCLC. A prospective comparison of CT and PET scanning. *J Thor Cardiovasc Surg* 1996;111:642.
15. Gail MH, Eagan RT, Feld R, et al. Prognostic factors in patients with resected stage I non-small cell lung cancer. *Cancer* 1984;54:1802.
16. Reilly JJ, Jr. Benefits of aggressive perioperative management in patients undergoing thoracotomy. *Chest* 1995;107:312S.
17. Nugent WC, Edney MT, Hammerness PG, et al. Non-small cell lung cancer at the extremes of age: impact on diagnosis and treatment. *Ann Thorac Surg* 1997;63:193.
18. Reilly JJ. Preparing for pulmonary resection. *Chest* 1997;112:206S.
19. Markos J, Mullan BP, Hillman DR, et al. Preoperative assessment as a predictor of mortality and morbidity after lung resection. *Am Rev Resp Dis* 1989;139:902.
20. Epstein SK, Faling JL, Daly B. Predicting complications after pulmonary resection. *Chest* 1993;104:694.
21. Julio ER, Persson AV. Preoperative evaluation of high risk patient. *Surg Clin North Am* 1985;65:3.
22. Miller JL. Preoperative evaluation. *Chest Surg Clin North Am* 1992;4:701.
23. Ginsberg RJ, Hill LD, Eagan RT. Modern 30 day operative mortality for surgical resections in lung cancer. *J Thorac Cardiovasc Surg* 1983;86:654.
24. Ruckdeschel J, Piantadori S. Quality of life assessment in lung surgery for bronchogenic carcinoma. *J Theorac Cardiovasc Surg* 1991;6:201.
25. Weiner P, Man A, Weiner M, et al. The effect of incentive spirometry and inspiratory muscle training on pulmonary function after lung resection. *J Thorac Cardiovasc Surg* 1997;113:552.
26. Bolton JWR, Weiman DS, Haynes JL. Stair climbing is an indicator of pulmonary function. *Chest* 1987;82:783.
27. Olsen GN, Bolton JWR, Weunab DS. Stair climbing as an exer-

cise test predicts the postoperative complications of lung cancer. *Chest* 1991;99:587.

28. Bousamra M II, Presberg KW, Chammas JH, et al. Early and late morbidity in patients undergoing pulmonary resection with low diffusion capacity. *Ann Thorac Surg* 1996;62:968.

29. Korst RJ, Ginsberg RJ, Ailawadi M, et al. Lobectomy improves ventilatory function in selected patients with severe COPD. *Ann Thorac Surg* 1998;66:898.

30. McKenna RJ, Jr, Brenner M, Fischel RJ, et al. Should lung volume reduction for emphysema be unilateral or bilateral? *J Thorac Cardiovasc Surg* 1996;112:1331.

31. Cooper JD, Patterson GA, Sundaresan RS, et al. Results of 150 consecutive bilateral lung volume reduction procedures in patients with severe emphysema. *J Thorac Cardiovasc Surg* 1996;112:1319.

32. Coleman RE. Clinical PET in oncology. *Clin Pos Imag* 1998;1:15.

33. Cortese DA, Pairolero PC, Bergstralh EJ, et al. Roentgenographically occult lung cancer. *J Thorac Cardiovasc Surg* 1983;86:373.

34. Martini N, Melamed M. Occult carcinomas of the lung. *Ann Thorac Surg* 1980;30:215.

35. Melamed M, Flehinger B, Zaman M. Impact of early detection on the clinical course of lung cancer. *Surg Clin North Am* 1998;67:909.

36. Lam S, MacAulay C, Hung J, et al. Detection of dysplasia and carcinoma in situ with a lung imaging fluoresence endoscope device. *J Thorac Cardiovasc Surg* 1993;105:1035.

37. Izbicki JR, Thetter O, Habekost M, et al. Radical systematic mediastinal lymphadenectomy in non-small cell lung cancer: a randomized controlled trial. *BJS* 1994;81:229.

38. Ishida T, Yano T, Maeda K. Strategy for lymphadenenopathy in lung cancer 3 cm or less in diameter. *J Thorac Cardiovasc Surg* 1991;50:708.

39. Riquet M, Hidden G, Debesse B. Direct lymphatic drainage of lung segments to the mediastinal nodes, an anatomic study of 260 adults. *J Thorac Cardiovasc Surg* 1989;97:623.

40. Jensik RJ, Faber LP, Kittle CF, et al. Survival following resection for second primary bronchogenic carcinoma. *J Thorac Cardiovasc Surg* 1981;82:658.

41. Ichinose Y, Hara N, Ohta M, et al. Is T factor of the TNM staging system a predominant prognostic factor in pathologic stage I non-small-cell lung cancer? *J Thorac Cardiovasc Surg* 1993;106:90.

42. Churchill ED, Belsey HR. Segmental pneumonectomy in bronchiectasis. *Ann Surg* 1939;109:481.

43. Cooper JD, Perelman M, Todd TRJ, et al. Precision cautery excision of pulmonary lesions. *Ann Thorac Surg* 1986;41:51.

44. Kirby TJ, Mack MJ, Landreneau RJ, et al. Lobectomy-video-assisted thoracic surgery versus muscle-sparing thoracotomy. *J Thorac Cardiovasc Surg* 1995;109:997.

45. Kittle CF. Which way in?—The thoracotomy incision. *Ann Thorac Surg* 1988;45:234.

46. Mentzer SJ, DeCamp MM, Harpole DH, et al. Thoracoscopy and video-assisted thoracic surgery in the treatment of lung cancer. *Chest* 1995;107:298S.

47. Shennib HAF, Landreneau RJ, Mulder DS, et al. Video-assisted thoracoscopic wedge resection of T1 lung cancer in high-risk patients. *Ann Surg* 1993;218:555.

48. McKenna R, Jr. Lobectomy by video-assisted thoracic surgery with mediastinal node sampling for lung cancer. *J Thorac Cardiovasc Surg* 1994;107:879.

49. Lewis RJ, Caccavale RJ, Sisler GE, et al. One hundred video-assisted thoracic surgical simultaneously stapled lobectomies without rib spreading. *Ann Thorac Surg* 1997;63:1415.

50. Lewis RJ, Caccavale RJ, Sisler GE, et al. Video-assisted thoracic

51. Craig SR, Walker WS. Potential complications of vascular stapling in thoracoscopic pulmonary resection. *Ann Thorac Surg* 1995;59:736.

52. Ginsberg RJ. Resection of non-small cell lung cancer, how much and by what route. *Chest* 1997;112:203S.

53. Ginsberg RJ, Rubinstein LV. Randomized trial of lobectomy versus limited resection for T1 N0 non-small cell lung cancer. *Ann Thorac Surg* 1995;60:615.

54. Miller JI, Hatcher CR. Limited resection of bronchogenic carcinoma in the patient with marked impairment of pulmonary function. *Ann Thorac Surg* 1987;44:340.

55. Warren WH, Faber LP. Segmentectomy versus lobectomy in patients with stage I pulmonary carcinoma. *J Thorac Cardiovasc Surg* 1994;107:1087.

56. Jensik RJ. Miniresection of small peripheral carcinomas of the lung. *Surg Clin North Am* 1987;67:951.

57. Kodama K, Doi O, Higshiyama M, et al. Intentional limited resection for selected patients with T1 N0 M0 non-small-cell lung cancer: a single institution study. *J Thorac Cardiovasc Surg* 1997;114:347.

58. Benner SE, Lippman SM, Hong WK. Chemoprevention of lung cancer. *Chest* 1995;107:316S.

59. Bennet WF, Smith RA. Segmental resection for bronchogenic carcinoma. *Ann Thorac Surg* 1978;27:169.

60. McCormack PM, Martini N. Primary lung carcinoma: results with conservative resection in treatment. *NY State J Med* 1980;80:612.

61. Errett LE, Wilson J, Chiu RC. Wedge resection as an alternative for the compromised patient. *J Thorac Cardiovasc Surg* 1985;90:656.

62. Miller JL, Hatcher CR. Limited resection of bronchogenic carcinoma in the patient with marked impairment of pulmonary function. *Ann Thorac Surg* 1987;44:340.

63. Temeck BK, Schafer PW, Saini N. Wedge resection for bronchogenic carcinoma. *South J Med* 1992;85:1081.

64. Read RC, Yoder G, Schaeffer RC. Survival after conservative resection for T1N0 non-small cell lung cancer. *Ann Thorac Surg* 1990;49:391.

65. Pastorino U, Valente M, Bedini V. Limited resection for stage I lung cancer. *Eur J Onc* 1991;17:42.

66. Wain JC, Mathisen DJ, Hilgenberg AD. Wedge and segmental resection for primary lung carcinoma. *Proc Am Assoc Thorac Surg* 1991;71:abstract.

67. Jensik RJ. The extent of resection for localized lung cancer. In: Kittle CF, editor. *Current controversies in thoracic surgery.* WB Saunders, 1986.

68. Landreneau RJ, Sugarbaker DJ, Mack MJ, et al. Wedge resection versus lobectomy for stage I (T1 N0 M0) non-small-cell lung cancer. *J Thorac Cardiovasc Surg* 1997;113:691.

69. Martini N, Burt ME, Bains MS, et al. Survival after resection of stage II non-small cell lung cancer. *Ann Thorac Surg* 1992;54:460.

70. Rendina EA, Venuta F, DeGiacomo T, et al. Safety and efficacy of bronchovascular reconstruction after induction chemotherapy for lung cancer. *J Thorac Cardiovasc Surg* 1997;114:830.

71. Deslauriers J, Ginsberg RJ, Piantadosi S, et al. Prospective assessment of 30-day operative morbidity for surgical resections in lung cancer. *Chest* 1994;106:329S.

72. Amar D, Burt M, Reinsel R, et al. Relationship of early postoperative dysrhythmias and long-term outcome after resection of non-small cell lung cancer. *Chest* 1996;110:437.

73. Nagasaki F, Flehinger BJ, Martini N. Complications of surgery in the treatment of carcinoma of the lung. *Chest* 1982;82:25.

74. Ginsberg RJ, Hill LD, Eagan RT. Modern 30-day operative mor-

tality for surgical resection in lung cancer. *J Thorac Cardiovasc Surg* 1983;86:654.

75. Deslauriers J, Ginsberg RJ, Dubois P, et al. Modern operative morbidity for elective surgical resection in lung carcinoma. *CJS* 1989;32:335.

76. Mountain CF, Dressler CM. Regional lymph node classification for lung cancer staging. *Chest* 1997;111:1718.

77. Mountain CF. Revisions in the international system for staging lung cancer. *Chest* 1997;111:1710.

78. Ginsberg RJ. Lymph node involvement, recurrence, and prognosis in resected small, peripheral, non-small-cell lung carcinomas. *J Thorac Cardiovasc Surg* 1996;111:1123.

79. Feins RH. Surgery for early stage non-small cell lung cancer. *Semin Oncol* 1997;24:419.

80. Thomas PA, Jr, Rubinstein L. Malignant disease appearing late after operation for T1N0 non-small-cell lung cancer. *J Thorac Cardiovasc Surg* 1993;106:1053.

81. The Ludwig Lung Cancer Study Group. Patterns of failure in patients with resected stage I and II non-small-cell carcinoma of the lung. *Ann Surg* 1987;305:67.

82. Yano T, Yokoyama H, Inoue T, et al. Surgical results and prognostic factors of pathologic N1 disease in non-small-cell carcinoma of the lung. *J Thorac Cardiovasc Surg* 1994;107:1398.

83. Thomas PA, Piantadosi S. Postoperative T1 N0 non-small cell lung cancer. *J Thorac Cardiovasc Surg* 1987;94:349.

84. Sagawa M, Saito Y, Takahashi S, et al. Clinical and prognostic assessment of patients with resected small peripheral lung cancer lesions. *Cancer* 1990;66:2653.

85. Pairolero PC, Williams DE, Bergstralh EJ, et al. Postsurgical stage I bronchogenic carcinoma: morbid implications of recurrent disease. *Ann Thorac Surg* 1984;38:331.

86. Izbicki JR, Passlick B, Hosch SB, et al. Mode of spread in the early phase of lymphatic metastasis in non-small-cell lung cancer: significance of nodal micrometastasis. *J Thorac Cardiovasc Surg* 1996;112:623.

87. Weisenburger TH, Gail M. The effects of postoperative mediastinal radiation in complete resected stage II epidermoid cancer of the lung. *N Engl J Med* 1986;315:1377.

88. Johnson BE. Biologic and molecular prognostic factors—impact on treatment of patients with non-small cell lung cancer. *Chest* 1995;107:287S.

89. Mulshine JL, Scott F. Molecular markers in early cancer detection. *Chest* 1995;107:280S.

90. Harpole D, Jr. Prognostic issues in non-small cell lung cancer. *Chest* 1995;107:267S.

91. Padilla J, Calvo V, Penalver JC, et al. Surgical results and prognostic factors in early non-small cell lung cancer. *Ann Thorac Surg* 1997;63:324.

92. Thomas P, Rubinstein L. Cancer recurrence after resection: T1 NO non-small cell lung cancer. *Ann Thorac Surg* 1990;49:242.

93. Martini N, Bains MS, Burt M, et al. Incidence of local recurrence and second primary tumors in resected stage I lung cancer. *J Thorac Cardiovasc Surg* 1995;109:120.

94. Keller SM, Adak S, Wagner H, et al. Prospective randomized trial of postoperative adjuvant therapy in patients with completely resected stage II and IIIa non-small cell lung cancer: an intergroup trial (E3590). *Proc ASCO* 1999;18:465.

95. Depierre A, Milleron B, Moro D, et al. Phase III trial of non-adjuvant chemotherapy (NCT) in resectable stage I (except T1N0), II, IIIa, non-small cell lung cancer (NSCLC): the French experience. *Proc ASCO* 1999;18:465.

96. Pisters KMW and Gissberg RJ on behalf of the Bimodality Lung Oncology Team (BLOT). Phase II trial of induction Paclitaxel & Carboplatin (PC) in early stage (T2N0, T1-2N1), & selected T3N0-1 non-small cell lung cancer (NSCLC). *Proc ASCO* 1998: 17(Abs. 1738):451a.

97. Virgo KS, Naunheim KS, McKirgan LW, et al. Cost of patient follow-up after potentially curative lung cancer treatment. *J Thorac Cardiovasc Surg* 1996;112:356.

38

EXTENDED RESECTIONS FOR LOCALLY ADVANCED NON-SMALL CELL LUNG CANCER

WILLIAM H. WARREN
L. PENFIELD FABER

For half a century, complete surgical resection has been recognized as the cornerstone of curative management of carcinoma of the lung. Despite advances in chemotherapy and radiotherapy, a complete surgical resection, whenever possible, continues to be the best therapeutic option for most patients with locally advanced primary pulmonary carcinoma, either alone or in conjunction with adjuvant therapy.

The first complete, one-stage resection for a primary pulmonary carcinoma was performed more than 60 years ago.[1] The success of this operation and the long-term survival of the patient encouraged thoracic surgeons to further develop the field of pulmonary surgery. In the years that followed, it became evident that long-term survival for pulmonary carcinoma could be achieved, but only in the setting of complete surgical resection.[2]

This perspective emboldened thoracic surgeons to develop surgical techniques to resect tumors considered initially to be unresectable on the basis of local invasion of chest wall, mediastinal structures, or the diaphragm. In 1959, Chamberlain[3] proposed the term *extended resections* to distinguish these aggressive procedures from the *standard resections* of extrapericardial pneumonectomy and lobectomy. Analysis of the surgical experience that followed is, at best, problematic. Incomplete, "palliative" resections were sometimes combined with those that were "curative" (i.e., tumor completely resected). Results from resecting various mediastinal structures were often grouped together. Adjuvant radiotherapy, when given, was used sporadically. Even among complete resections, however, it is clear that initial perioperative morbidity was high, and long-term survival was poor.[4]

At least three factors contributed to these disappointing early results. First, there was only limited understanding of intraoperative and postoperative pathophysiology. The development of newer anesthesia techniques and agents, the availability of better monitoring, and improved surgical techniques have minimized perioperative complications. Second, much of this early experience with extended resections was performed before a clinicopathologic staging system was accepted. The adoption of an international staging classification for lung carcinoma and the development of sophisticated scanning techniques to detect extrathoracic metastases and to assess intrathoracic structures before operation have enabled surgeons to select cases more appropriately for these aggressive surgical resections. Third, we have come to recognize that the biologic behavior of certain tumors, such as poorly differentiated neuroendocrine carcinomas, precludes surgical cure even in the face of an apparently complete resection. In a retrospective histologic reevaluation of neoplasms resected as "small cell carcinoma," it was found that, among patients who survived beyond 3 years, in most cases the tumors would now be reclassified as *well-differentiated neuroendocrine carcinomas*.[5] Most believe that patients with poorly differentiated neuroendocrine carcinomas should not be considered for these extended surgical resections, despite the development of adjuvant chemotherapy and radiotherapy protocols. The exclusion of these latter cases has no doubt led to overall improved results.

During the past three decades, adjuvant radiotherapy protocols (see also Chapter 43) have been devised to improve the resectability rate and to reduce the incidence of postoperative locoregional recurrence. The results of these clinical trials suggest that, although the resectability rate may be improved, the five-year survival is not affected, with the exception of that for superior sulcus tumors[6–10] and possibly a subset of patients with N2 nodal involvement.[11–13] Because most patients with locally advanced disease die from distant metastases, the role of adjuvant multiagent concurrent chemotherapy and radiotherapy is being assessed (see also Chapter 44).

Despite these developments, some of these extended resections have not been widely accepted. In some cases, clinical experience has been limited, and many reports simply describe surgical technique without long-term follow-up. The purpose of this chapter is to review the development of these extended surgical operations, to present the technical aspects of these resections, and, when possible, to discuss their applicability in the modern surgery.

INTRAPERICARDIAL PNEUMONECTOMY

Radical pneumonectomy was first described by Allison[14] as an approach to performing *en bloc* complete mediastinal node dissection with intrapericardial ligation of the pulmonary vessels. Some surgeons adopted intrapericardial dissection as the approach of choice in performing a pneumonectomy,[15,16] although the advantages and logic of this approach were challenged by many.[17–20] Although few now use an intrapericardial approach as a matter of routine, it remains a useful technique when the tumor has directly involved the pericardium, foreshortened the pulmonary veins, or invaded the left atrium. The intrapericardial approach also provides access to the proximal pulmonary artery and the superior vena cava (SVC) when the tumor involves the pericardium over the hilum.

Preoperative computed tomographic (CT) scans and magnetic resonance imaging (MRI) are of limited value in distinguishing involvement of the pericardium and intrapericardial pulmonary veins from involvement of the left atrium.[21–25] Two-dimensional echocardiography, transesophageal ultrasound endoscopy, and intraoperative ultrasonography may be more valuable in this regard.[26,27]

Technical Considerations

An incision is made in the pericardium anterior to the superior pulmonary vein but sparing, if possible, the phrenic nerve, which is often drawn up into the field of dissection. After entering the pericardium, the incision is carried superiorly and inferiorly to identify the pulmonary artery and to identify the inferior pulmonary vein. The intrapericardial extent of tumor must be carefully assessed. If the intrapericardial length of vein is free, then it can be stapled or divided and oversewn.

On occasion, a tumor directly invades the wall of the left atrium. Under these circumstances, a vascular clamp can be placed on the left atrium (Figure 38.1), taking care not to compromise the pulmonary venous drainage from the contralateral lung. The left atrium should be closed in a running double layer of 3-0 monofilament nonabsorbable suture. Bailey and colleagues[28] described three patients who underwent cardiopulmonary bypass to resect larger portions of the left atrial wall with reconstruction using a pericardial patch to avoid a restrictive left atrium.

The intrapericardial approach also allows proximal dissection of the pulmonary artery. On the right side, the pericardium is opened anterior to the phrenic nerve, and the pulmonary artery can be dissected out at the bifurcation. The pulmonary artery can be secured either by stapling or by clamping and oversewing. Simple or double ligation is not sufficient.

Care must be taken to assess whether the tumor directly involves the posterior wall of the SVC. If the SVC is involved, resection and reconstruction can be performed (see also Chapter 62 and later in this chapter).

On the left side, the division of the ligamentum arteriosum provides optimal exposure to the proximal left pulmonary artery, which can be managed in a fashion similar to the right. Ricci and colleagues[29] reported on three cases of resection and reconstruction of the proximal left main pulmonary artery in conjunction with a left pneumonectomy under cardiopulmonary bypass using a median sternotomy.

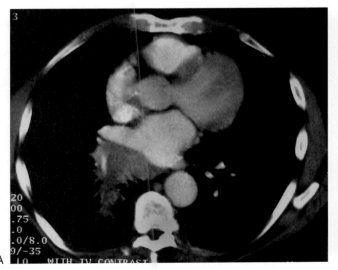
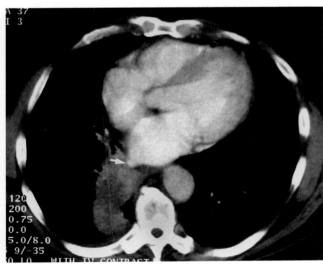

FIGURE 38.1. **A:** CT scan demonstrating right lower lobe tumor abutting the posterior pericardium and the superior pulmonary vein. **B:** Same patient as **(A)** with tumor obstructing inferior pulmonary vein but not invading left atrium.

Results

Although thoracic surgeons are familiar with intrapericardial dissection, it is associated with an increased incidence of supraventricular arrhythmia, and few occasions exist when it is necessary. However, when tumors directly invade the pericardium or foreshorten the pulmonary vessels, intrapericardial dissection is successfully performed with acceptable perioperative morbidity and mortality.

One of the most dramatic complications of intrapericardial dissection is cardiac torsion, whereby the heart herniates through the defect, resulting in diminished cardiac return.[30–36] This complication almost always occurs within the first three days of surgery and is often precipitated by a change in position or forceful coughing. With right-sided herniation, kinking of the SVC, inferior vena cava, and pulmonary artery causes sudden hypotension, tachycardia, cyanosis, and venous congestion. Therefore, a right-sided pericardium defect must be closed, either primarily or with a patch. Parietal pleura, fascia lata, pedicle flap of diaphragm, and prosthetic material (e.g., Gore-Tex, Dacron, Vicryl mesh) have all been used.[35–37]

On the left side, similar attempts must be made to close the defect primarily whenever possible. Herniation of the heart through a restricting left-sided defect can present as myocardial ischemia from compression of the coronary arteries at the edge of the defect.[35,38] There have also been reports of tearing of the inferior vena cava, right ventricle, or coronary vessels.[35,39] Therefore, when a moderate-size defect persists on the left side, the pericardium should either be widely resected (to allow free mobility of the heart out of the pericardial sac into the pleural space) or closed with a patch, as on the right side. Even when the defect is patched, there has been a report of the patch tearing free, resulting in cardiac herniation.[36] There have also been isolated reports of this complication occurring 14 weeks after a left upper lobectomy with intrapericardial dissection[40] and after a pericardiotomy for trauma without pulmonary resection.[38] Therefore, the surgeon must be alert to this complication whenever the pericardium has been opened.

Because intrapericardial dissection is usually performed in conjunction with the resection of mediastinal structures (including pericardium, phrenic nerve, SVC, left atrium, carina, and aorta) and for tumors with and without mediastinal node involvement, interpretation of the results of this approach is problematic. According to Pitz and associates, tumors found to involve the mainstem bronchus but sparing surrounding mediastinal structures (especially T3 N0) have a better prognosis than tumors with invasion of mediastinal pleura, pericardium, and/or phrenic nerve.[41] Predictably, the best results have been reported when invasion is limited to the pericardium and in the absence of mediastinal nodal metastases.

Patients have survived longer than 5 years when this approach was used to dissect out pulmonary veins.[42,43] In contrast, when the tumor involves the wall of the left atrium, the results are much more discouraging. Of 29 patients undergoing complete resection by pneumonectomy or lobectomy with resection of a portion of the left atrium, the longest survivor is 36 months.[28,44–50] None of the three patients who underwent *en bloc* resection of left atrial wall in the Rush-Presbyterian-St. Luke's (RPSL) experience survived beyond 2 years, despite the use of adjuvant chemotherapy and radiotherapy. Clearly, tumors that invade the wall of the atrium have a worse prognosis than tumors limited to the pulmonary veins or the pericardium. Preoperatively and even intraoperatively, however, such a distinction may be difficult. Two-dimensional echocardiography may be valuable in this regard.[26]

Levett and colleagues[51] reported their experience resecting eight patients with intrapericardial left pneumonectomies with bulky disease in the aortopulmonary window; no patients survived beyond 2 years despite adjuvant chemotherapy. Ricci and colleagues[29] reported their experience with three patients who underwent left pneumonectomy with *en bloc* resection of the origin of the left main pulmonary artery on cardiopulmonary bypass; one patient survived beyond 2 years.

Survival beyond 5 years has been reported when intrapericardial dissections were performed for major pulmonary resections with *en bloc* resection of the carina, a portion of the SVC, and the muscular wall of the esophagus (see following).

SLEEVE PNEUMONECTOMY

Carinal involvement by tumor occurs either primarily from spread through the mucosa or submucosa, or from peribronchial tissues, or secondarily from tumor invasion from metastatic nodes at the tracheobronchial angle or subcarinal space.

Tumor involvement of the carina was initially considered to be a contraindication for complete resection; however, endeavors to resect at least portions of the carina can be traced as far back as 1950.[52] Such early attempts were limited by anesthetic techniques and were limited to resection of the tracheobronchial angle using an atrial clamp. This technique not only provided only a minimal resection margin but also tended to narrow the left mainstem bronchus. The first successful carinal resection for carcinoma, with reconstruction using an end-to-end anastomosis, was reported by Mathey and colleagues in 1966.[53] Other reports ensued as surgical and anesthetic techniques evolved.[54–62] Although cardiopulmonary bypass has been used successfully to accomplish complicated tracheal and carinal resections, it has been surpassed by the use of small endotracheal tubes and the jet ventilation catheter, which provides better exposure and safer control of the airway. Intraoperatively, transesophageal ultrasonic endoscopy and intraoperative ultrasonography have both been used with superior results.[27]

Sleeve pneumonectomy should be considered for patients with large, central carcinomas that are otherwise resectable, with limited involvement of the carina as assessed by bronchoscopy or CT findings. At bronchoscopy, thickening and corrugation of the mucosa at the tracheobronchial angle indicates submucosal infiltration of tumor. Narrowing of the orifice of the proximal mainstem bronchus also should alert the surgeon that the patient may require a more extended resection than a standard pneumonectomy. Involvement of the trachea should be limited to less than 3 cm in length because resections of the trachea and left mainstem bronchus of 4 cm or longer tend to put excessive tension on the anastomosis.[63]

Mediastinal nodes assessed to be larger than 1 cm by CT should undergo biopsy by mediastinoscopy. The presence of positive mediastinal nodes above the tracheobronchial angle indicates a poor prognosis and has led some[63,64] to consider these cases to be inoperable. However, others[61] believe that if metastatic disease is confined to the ipsilateral tracheobronchial angle or subcarinal nodes, the patient should be considered for preoperative adjuvant chemotherapy and radiotherapy, and the surgeon should proceed with the appropriate resection (Figures 38.2 through 38.5).

Patients older than 65 years are not good candidates for sleeve pneumonectomy because they tolerate this procedure poorly, and their long-term survival is lower than in younger patients. Each patient, however, must be considered individually. A careful physiologic assessment is mandatory, including complete pulmonary function tests and quantitative

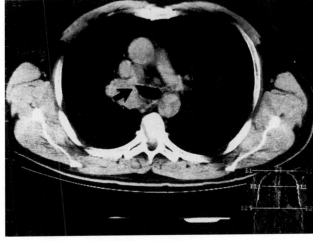

FIGURE 38.3. CT scan showing extensive involvement of the right tracheobronchial angle in the same case as in Figure 38.2. Note the compression of the right mainstem bronchus (*arrow*).

ventilation–perfusion lung scans if the FEV_1 is less than 1.8 L or less than 50% of predicted.

Technical Considerations

Careful anesthetic planning is mandatory when sleeve resection is contemplated. The anesthesiologist must be prepared to ventilate the remaining lung for 30 to 45 minutes through an open trachea while the anastomosis is being

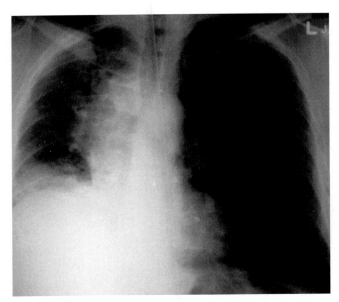

FIGURE 38.2. Posterior radiograph demonstrating a bulky, squamous carcinoma extensively involving the hilum with associated marked volume loss of the right lung.

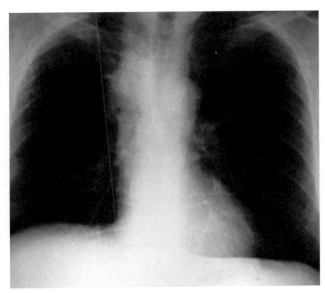

FIGURE 38.4. Posteroanterior radiograph of same patient as in Figure 38.2 after four cycles of preoperative combined chemotherapy and radiotherapy. Note that the mass is significantly smaller and that the right lung is fully reinflated.

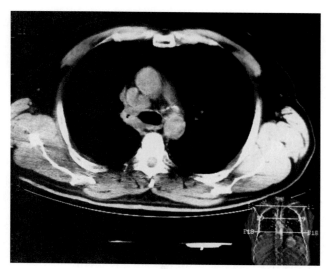

FIGURE 38.5. CT scan of same patient as in Figure 38.2 after four cycles of preoperative combined chemotherapy and radiotherapy. Involvement of the right tracheobronchial angle is still evident but more limited.

performed. High-frequency ventilation can be achieved through a 2-mm catheter passed through an 8-mm standard endotracheal tube. The advantages of this technique are that it allows for adequate ventilation and oxygenation and provides excellent exposure during the anastomosis. Intraoperative bronchoscopy is performed as indicated.

Alternative techniques include the use of an uncut single-lumen endotracheal tube, which can be intermittently passed down the left mainstem bronchus, or a sterile second endotracheal tube, intermittently passed over the surgical field and down the distal bronchus during the anastomosis. Double-lumen tubes offer no advantage over these techniques and make the exposure for the anastomosis considerably more difficult. Limited experience with cardiopulmonary bypass for complex carinal resections has been fraught with complication of parenchymal hemorrhage into the remaining lung and should be avoided at all costs.[64]

The technique of sleeve pneumonectomy has been well described elsewhere.[56,60,61] The preferred approach at RPSL for a right sleeve pneumonectomy is a posterolateral thoracotomy through the fourth intercostal space. The patient is not positioned to allow for a laryngeal release, but could be repositioned for an anterior cervical approach if this became necessary. The azygos vein is ligated and divided, and resectability is assessed. If necessary, portions of the SVC or the muscular wall of the esophagus can be resected (see also Chapter 62. Care is taken to preserve blood supply of the distal trachea and the left mainstem bronchus. Dissection is begun along the anterior and posterior aspects of the trachea, preserving the lateral blood supply above and below the levels of transection; mediastinal lymphadenectomy is performed, with care taken not to injure the small arterial

branches. During this part of the procedure, the endotracheal tube can be advanced down the left mainstem bronchus to optimize exposure. If any question exists about carinal involvement, a pneumonectomy can be performed and a frozen section obtained of the bronchial resection margin.

Once the need for carinal resection is confirmed, the distal trachea and left mainstem bronchus are dissected out. The left recurrent laryngeal nerve is sometimes seen at the left tracheobronchial angle. If necessary, it may be divided because the right laryngeal nerve should be out of the field of dissection. The thoracic duct or one of its branches is sometimes injured at this point, and a chylous leak should be carefully sought. Major lymphatic channels should be oversewn; metal clips should be avoided because they tend to sever the walls of these fragile vessels. The trachea is then transected 1 to 3 cm above the carina, and the left mainstem bronchus is transected as close to the carina as possible. No attempt is made to compensate for lumen disparity. The jet ventilation catheter is advanced down the left mainstem bronchus under direct control (Figure 38.6).

Frozen sections of the proximal and distal tracheobronchial resection margins are obtained. A positive resection margin is an indication for additional resection, if this action will not place undue tension on the anastomosis. The anastomosis is performed using interrupted 3-0 polyglycolic sutures. Traction sutures of 2-0 polyglycolic acid are placed at the lateral resection margins of the trachea and the mainstem bronchus to relieve tension while the anastomotic sutures are being tied. If necessary, the traction sutures can be tied for additional support. The anastomosis should be covered with viable tissue to seal minute leaks and to minimize complications of a small anastomotic separation. A

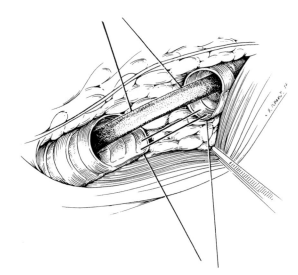

FIGURE 38.6. Operative view of the anastomosis of the left mainstem bronchus to the distal trachea. Note the use of a jet ventilation catheter to facilitate placement of the sutures while maintaining ventilation to the left lung.

mediastinal fat pad obtained from the anterior mediastinum draping over the pericardium, a pleural flap, or an intercostal muscle bundle can be used.

Although there has been some experience performing a left sleeve pneumonectomy through a left posterolateral thoracotomy with mobilization of the aortic arch,[57,65] in most cases, this was performed for low-grade tumors with little or no extension into the peribronchial tissues. In bulky, central tumors, a left posterolateral thoracotomy usually does not provide adequate exposure for a carinal resection and reconstruction. If a positive bronchial resection margin is encountered in the course of a left pneumonectomy (such that a carinal resection is necessary), then the bronchus should be closed despite a positive resection margin, deferring the carinal resection through a right thoracotomy for 4 weeks, as described by Gilbert and colleagues.[66] The obvious morbidity and mortality of these two major procedures must be weighed against the technical difficulties of approaching the dissection and the anastomosis of the right mainstem bronchus through the aortopulmonary window. An alternative approach to left sleeve pneumonectomies is to perform a right thoracotomy first, resecting the carina and performing the anastomosis of the right mainstem bronchus to the trachea, stapling the left mainstem bronchus, and dividing the left pulmonary artery to minimize shunting. A left thoracotomy is subsequently performed to complete the resection.[63]

Experience using a median sternotomy to perform a left sleeve pneumonectomy has been limited to low-grade tumors (such as adenoid cystic carcinoma) and is unlikely to provide adequate exposure in the case of a central bronchopulmonary carcinoma. Another approach that has been used is the clamshell incision through the fourth intercostal space; however, this procedure comes at great physiologic cost to the patient, according to Mitchell.[64]

Results

According to the surgical literature, most sleeve pneumonectomies are performed for squamous carcinoma. Most patients are male, with an average age of 55 years. Most of these resections are performed for central carcinomas of the right lung.

Anastomotic complications are frequent. Stenosis of the anastomosis can occur, leading to retained secretions and respiratory failure. Dilation and placement of endobronchial stents have been successfully used in this setting. In cases with exuberant granulation tissue, YAG laser photoablation should be considered.

Adult respiratory distress syndrome complicating sleeve pneumonectomy continues to be a major problem and has been reported in all series.[56,58,59,63,65] Restriction of intraoperative and postoperative fluid intake, prompt clearance of retained secretions, and institution of broadspectrum antibiotics at the first sign of a pulmonary infiltrate are important measures to minimize this risk.

The operative mortality, even in this select group of patients, is significant, ranging from 11% to 25%[64,65,67,68,69]; the RPSL overall operative mortality is 23% (10/43) for sleeve pneumonectomy, 20.5% (8/39) for right sleeve pneumonectomy.[61] Candidates for this procedure should therefore be carefully chosen, and surgeons should know the many aspects of the postoperative care and management of complications as well as the technique of the procedure.

In the largest published series, Dartevelle and colleagues[69] reported a 23% (6/55) five-year survival. In their series, there was a difference in survival in patients with involved subcarinal nodes (mean survival, 33 months) compared to those with involved paratracheal nodes (mean survival, 11 months). In the RPSL series of 43 sleeve pneumonectomies (including patients with positive mediastinal nodes), the five-year survival was 19%.[60,61]

The largest experience with left sleeve pneumonectomy for carcinomas was reported by Gilbert and colleagues.[66] Of the five cases reported, three patients had staged thoracotomies and an additional two had a local recurrence in the left mainstem bronchial stump. There were no operative deaths; three patients lived for at least 2 years; and one patient lived for at least 4½ years.

Local recurrence is a well-recognized late complication if adjuvant radiotherapy has not been used. Some have advocated postoperative radiotherapy. The most common cause of death is systemic recurrence. To minimize the risk of local recurrence, the risk of distant metastases, and the incidence of incomplete resections, preoperative chemotherapy and radiotherapy should be used in these T4 carcinomas.[60] Preliminary experience in the RPSL protocol indicates that, in most cases, significant tumor shrinkage occurs with little or no deleterious effect on anastomotic healing. These resections, however, require considerable clinical judgment and should only be performed by experienced thoracic surgeons who are able to recognize and manage the various intraoperative and postoperative complications.

RESECTION OF PORTIONS OF THE SUPERIOR VENA CAVA (SEE ALSO CHAPTER 62)

The SVC may be invaded directly by a carcinoma arising in the anterior segment of the right upper lobe or secondarily by tumor metastatic to the right paratracheal or right tracheobronchial angle nodes (Figure 38.7). Traditionally, involvement of the SVC has been a criterion of unresectability. Early attempts to resect a portion of the SVC involved clamping and direct repair and provided discouraging results, in part attributed to cerebral venous congestion and hypoxic injury.[70] Therefore, both external bypass and internal shunts have been devised to maintain cerebral drainage while resection and reconstruction is being performed.[71–73]

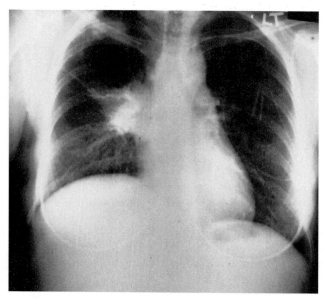

FIGURE 38.7. Posteroanterior radiograph demonstrating a large, central adenocarcinoma with associated mediastinal adenopathy involving the superior vena cava. Note the volume loss of the right lung.

During the past 15 years, there has been considerable experience using these techniques for the resection of bulky mediastinal tumors and selected primary lung carcinomas, particularly in patients who underwent adjuvant therapy. Accumulating laboratory and clinical evidence suggests that simple clamping of the SVC can be tolerated in most patients for periods longer than 30 minutes without neurologic deficiency,[73–77,79,80] provided no associated hypotension is present. Nakahara and colleagues[74] advocated selecting patients for shunting on the basis of subclavian venous pressure greater than 40 cm H_2O. Based on its experience, however, RPSL continues to advocate an SVC bypass whenever technically possible to minimize the risk of cerebral venous congestion.[78,81]

The indication for resection and reconstruction of the SVC is restricted to tumors confined to the thorax otherwise considered to be resectable, with involvement of the SVC that is technically resectable. In most cases, resection of a portion of the SVC wall is all that is necessary, and this can be reconstructed with a patch. When the tumor encases the SVC, complete resection and reconstruction with a tube graft of 18 or 20 mm polytetrafluoroethylene (PTFE) is necessary.[76,77] The superior anastomosis is performed first, and the graft is flushed of air prior to completing the anastomosis at the cardiac end of the graft. When the SVC is obstructed from mediastinal involvement of carcinoma of the lung, however, most agree that resection is contraindicated.

Technical Considerations

Whenever involvement of the SVC is suspected, central venous catheters should be avoided because this compromises venous control. Through a posterolateral thoracotomy, the involvement of the SVC is assessed before committing to a major pulmonary resection. The azygos vein is routinely divided. Umbilical tapes are passed around the innominate veins or the SVC above the tumor. The pericardium is opened close to the hilum, sparing the phrenic nerve if possible. The surgeon must then assess the intrapericardial extent of the tumor, including the proximal right pulmonary artery and involvement of the carina. A Rumel tourniquet should be placed proximal to the atriocaval junction to avoid potential injury of the sinoatrial node.

The pulmonary resection is performed first. Although an *en bloc* resection is ideal, if the tumor is bulky, the specimen may be transected, leaving tumor on the SVC. With the pulmonary specimen out of the surgical field, the resection of the SVC is greatly facilitated.

If the planned resection is limited to a portion of the SVC wall, a 20F thoracostomy tube is prepared to serve as an internal venous shunt (Figure 38.8). The distal end of the tube must be trimmed so that only two or three side holes remain and are beyond the proximal innominate tourniquet. The tube is then measured against the length of the SVC and the right atrium. A proximal side hole is then cut in the tube to allow the shunted venous blood to drain into the atrium.

The patient is then anticoagulated with 5000 U sodium heparin, and a pursestring suture is placed in the side wall of the right atrium. A small incision is made in the right atrium, and the clamped chest tube is advanced through the right atrium and up the SVC. Once the tourniquets are at the atriocaval junction and the innominate veins are tightened, the SVC should be effectively isolated and can be opened. The affected portion of the SVC can then be safely resected, in most cases, retaining a portion of the medial wall to allow a patch closure (Figure 38.9). Although some surgeons have experience using prosthetic material,[74–76,80–83] others prefer using autologous pericardium, primarily because of the decreased thrombogenicity (Figure 38.10). Bypass of the SVC for SVC syndrome is covered in detail in Chapter 43.

Results

On reviewing the surgical literature, fewer than 50 cases of SVC resection for pulmonary carcinoma have been reported, many with limited follow-up.

Long-term patency of the SVC after reconstruction has been documented by venography[79] and clinical follow-up, including autopsy.[75] However, thrombosis is a recognized complication of spiral vein grafts when used in benign dis-

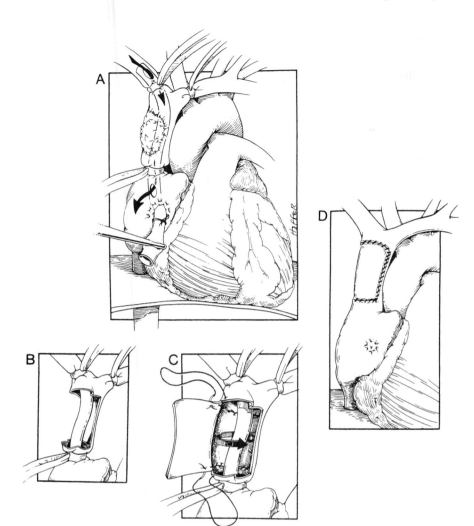

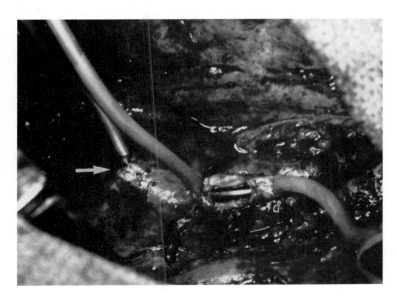

FIGURE 38.8. Operative views of **(A)** placement of an internal shunt and isolation of the superior vena cava (SVC) with tumor invasion of the wall; **(B)** resection of the wall of the SVC, leaving the uninvolved medial wall intact; **(C)** closure of the defect with a patch of pericardium; and **(D)** removal of the shunt with distension of the SVC without narrowing.

FIGURE 38.9. Operative photograph showing wall of superior vena cava resected and tourniquets in place. Note the placement of the shunt through the right atrium at the left of the photograph, with tourniquet in place (*arrow*).

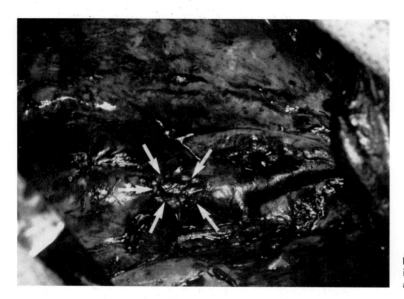

FIGURE 38.10. Operative photograph in same patient as in Figure 38.9 after placement of pericardial patch (*arrows*) and removal of shunt.

ease to shunt the SVC[82,84] and in SVC reconstruction for bulky mediastinal malignancies.[76] On the basis of this experience, most surgeons choose to anticoagulate patients with sodium warfarin (Coumadin) for at least 3 months.

Analysis of the survival of patients undergoing resection of the SVC is, at best, limited. The largest series consist of six or fewer cases. In many cases, the SVC resection was part of a larger procedure. In two of three patients in Nakahara's series,[74] one of six patients in Dartevelle's series,[75,76] and one of six in the RPSL series,[78,81] the SVC resection was combined with a right sleeve pneumonectomy.

The prognosis for these patients is guarded. In the experience of the Memorial Sloan-Kettering Cancer Center,[46] no five-year survivors were among 18 patients undergoing *en bloc* resections of the SVC. In the experience of Dartevelle and colleagues,[75] three of six patients survived beyond 1 year, and the 3-year survival was 33% (2/6). In the RPSL series,[78,81] three of nine patients presently with lung carcinoma are alive and free of disease more than 5 1/2 years after resection; Inoue and colleagues[79] and Dartevelle and colleagues[75,76,85] have each reported five-year, disease-free survivors after SVC resection. Most of these five-year survivors had adjuvant chemotherapy and radiotherapy.[78,79,81]

Although SVC resection and reconstruction are technically possible in patients presenting with SVC occlusion, Dartevelle and colleagues[75,76] believe that the presence of extensive thrombosis and collateral venous drainage are contraindications to reconstruction. Mori and colleagues[83] reported on two patients with primary pulmonary tumors presenting as SVC obstruction who underwent resection and reconstruction with ringed PTFE grafts. Neither patient developed recurrence of the SVC obstruction; one was alive at 7 months, and the other died 22 months after resection from massive hemoptysis. Certainly, the presence of

an SVC syndrome carries a poor prognosis, and SVC resection and reconstruction should be performed in only select cases.

Most of these patients die from distant metastases. According to Dartevelle and colleagues,[75] neither of the two patients who presented with N2 nodal metastases survived beyond 8 months. One of three patients reported on by Nakahara and colleagues[74] presented with N2 nodal involvement and died 5 months later with systemic metastases. Yoshimura and colleagues[3] reported on one patient with N2 nodal metastases who died with a cerebral metastasis 3 months later. The survival is better for patients with N1 or N0 disease. For these reasons, adjuvant chemotherapy and radiotherapy should be instituted preoperatively in these T4 carcinomas,[86] and every attempt should be made to exclude distant metastases before resection.

EXTENDED RESECTIONS FOR SUPERIOR SULCUS TUMORS

Since the early 1960s, the role of surgical resection of superior sulcus tumors has been established (see also Chapter 39). Contraindications to surgery have been the presence of distant metastases, extensive involvement of the brachial plexus, and extensive involvement of the paraspinal extension, including involvement of the intervertebral foramina or the bodies or laminae of the thoracic vertebrae. Likewise, the involvement of the subclavian artery or vein, while distinctly uncommon among these tumors, has been traditionally regarded as a criterion of unresectability. Resections "extended" beyond those classically performed for superior sulcus tumor have included carcinomas involving the transverse process, or up to one-fourth of the vertebral body, and anterior tumors involving the subclavian vessels. Although experience with these resections is still limited, the techniques involved and the preliminary results merit review.

Similar to all other extended surgical procedures, careful preoperative planning is of the utmost importance. Involvement of the head of the rib, the transverse process, and the vertebral body should be assessed by CT scan or MRI. Extension into the spinal canal, with or without cord compression, is a sign of unresectability. If the tumor extensively destroys the body, then it is considered inoperable, but a tumor that simply abuts the vertebral body should be considered for resection. Extension into the intervertebral foramen must be anticipated to avoid excessive traction on the nerve root or bleeding in this region.

Anteriorly, tumor metastatic to the scalene node is a criterion of inoperability. Extensive involvement of the brachial plexus is a relative contraindication to surgical resection. Although some consider the involvement of N2 nodes to be a contraindication to surgery, others believe that these cases should be entered in a trial of preoperative combination chemotherapy and radiotherapy, and restaged before resection.[86]

Technical Considerations

Extended Posterior Resections

The operative approach in patients with extensive posterior disease is through a high posterolateral thoracotomy, dividing the trapezius and rhomboid muscles as well as the latissimus dorsi and the serratus anterior to provide optimal exposure. The pleural space is entered early in the procedure to assess the pulmonary component of the tumor. The chest wall resection is performed before the pulmonary resection because exposure of the hilum is limited. The superior and posterior components of the dissection are determined by the extent of the tumor mass. The scalenus anterior and medius are divided either at the insertion onto the first rib or higher if necessary. The affected ribs, intercostal muscles, and vessels are divided anterior to the tumor mass, and the first rib is pulled inferiorly to expose the superior extent of the tumor. The subclavian vessels are identified and dissected off the first rib. Dissection of the subclavian artery off the tumor mass may be tedious but can usually be accomplished through an adventitial plane. Occasionally, branches of the subclavian artery have to be sacrificed, including, on occasion, the vertebral artery.[87] The lower trunk of the brachial plexus must then be identified and examined for tumor involvement. If any question exists about the ability to save the T1 or C8 nerve root, division may be deferred until further dissection of the posterior elements.

Division of the posterior elements begins inferiorly by rotating the chest wall anteriorly and retracting the erector spini complex posteriorly. If the transverse process is not involved in the tumor mass, then the costotransverse junc-

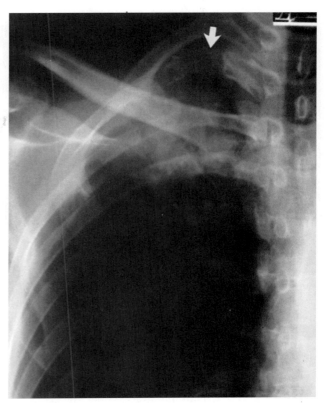

FIGURE 38.11. Posteroanterior radiograph illustrating a squamous carcinoma with extensive involvement of the posterior chest wall. Note destruction of the posterior aspect of the second rib (*arrow*).

tion is opened using a periosteal elevator, and the rib is rotated anteriorly. The intercostal nerves and vessels are then ligated and divided. Bipolar cautery should be used near the intervertebral foramina. The tumor is then elevated off the thoracic spine. The transverse process can be resected using rib shears. If the transverse process or the vertebral body is involved, an osteotome is used to complete the resection, approaching the body tangentially from the posterolateral aspect (Figures 38.11 and 38.12). Up to 25% of the vertebral body can be removed without compromising spinal support. Walsh, et al. reported four cases of Pancoast tumor with extensive involvement of the thoracic spine, necessitating resection up to one-half of the vertebral body at several levels.[88] The spine was reconstructed for stability. In the Walsh experience, complete resection was accomplished; however, patients had poor outcome secondary to ventilator dependence and radiation pneumonitis. Dartevelle has resected seven such patients with spinal reconstruction, and six are alive without recurrence with a median follow-up of 1 year.[69]

The sympathetic chain is divided. As the head of the first rib is approached, the serratus posterior is divided, and the status of the C8 and the T1 nerve roots can be further

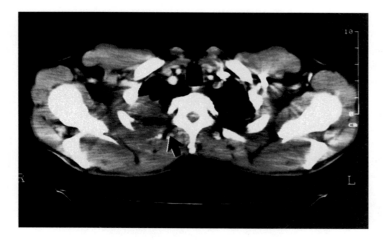

FIGURE 38.12. CT scan of same patient as in Figure 38.11 demonstrating destruction of the rib and the transverse process (*arrow*), but without involvement of the vertebral body.

assessed. If one or both are involved, they should be divided at this point. Division of the C8 nerve root causes some loss of sensation over the inner aspect of the arm to involve the fifth finger and part of the fourth finger.

Extended Anterior Resections

If, clinically or radiologically, the carcinoma is assessed to involve the subclavian vessels extensively and predominantly, an anterior approach is indicated. The anterior approach should be reserved for those cases in which the posterior chest wall is largely spared.

The patient is placed in the supine position, with the neck extended and the head turned to the uninvolved side. An L-shaped incision is made, with the vertical limb over the anterior border of the sternocleidomastoid muscle and the horizontal limb over the inferior aspect of the medial end of the clavicle. The sternocleidomastoid is dissected off the clavicle. The scalene fat pad is dissected out and examined microscopically to assess for metastatic disease. If the tumor is deemed resectable and the scalene node is free of metastasis, then the medial third of the clavicle is resected to provide excellent exposure of the subclavian vessels, according to the Dartevelle technique. Nazari et al. and Spaggiari have performed this resection by disarticulating the clavicle, dividing and reconstructing the clavicle at the completion of the case or dividing the manubrium[89–91] (Figure 38.13). On the left side, dissection of the subclavian vein is begun with ligation of the thoracic duct. Ligation and division of the internal jugular vein affords excellent exposure of the innominate and the distal subclavian veins. Direct tumor invasion of the subclavian vein does not preclude resection; a segment of the subclavian vein can be resected *en bloc* with the specimen after proximal and distal control is achieved. Reconstruction of the vein is not necessary.

Attention is then turned to the subclavian artery and its branches. After proximal and distal control is achieved,

branches, including the internal thoracic artery, the thyrocervical trunk, and, if necessary, the vertebral artery, can be ligated and divided. Often, the subclavian artery can be dissected off the tumor mass using a subadventitial plane. If the tumor mass invades the wall of the subclavian artery, then a segment of the artery can be resected with the specimen; revascularization is usually accomplished by end-to-end anastomosis without prosthetic material, but in some cases, an arterial graft is necessary. Most experience has been with PTFE.[87]

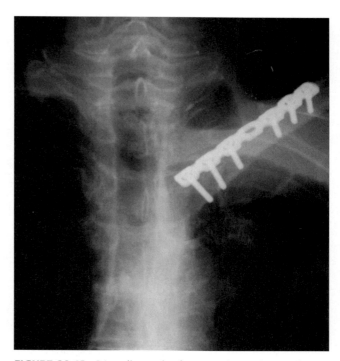

FIGURE 38.13. PA radiograph after anterior and posterior approaches to a Pancoast tumor with reconstruction of the left clavicle.

The scalenus medius is divided remote from the tumor mass. The branches of the brachial plexus are then dissected from the distal branches back to the spinal foramina, depending on the level of tumor involvement. The sympathetic chain, the heads of the ribs, and the vertebral bodies are then exposed; the first and second ribs can often be divided behind the mass.

Improved exposure to the posterior aspect of the tumor can be achieved if the incision is extended into the deltopectoral groove, according to Dartevelle and colleagues.[87] If both anterior and posterior exposure is necessary, then the anterior dissection is performed first, and the resection is completed using a posterolateral thoracotomy.

Results

Reported surgical experience with these extended posterior surgical resections has been limited. According to Shaw and colleagues,[6] DeMeester and associates,[92] Wright and colleagues,[93] and Paulson and coworkers,[94] minimal additional operative morbidity or mortality occurred in patients who underwent extended posterior resections (including resections of the transverse process or a portion of the vertebral body) when compared to the more traditional resections.

Despite the extent of disease, according to DeMeester and colleagues,[91] only 3 of 12 patients with tumor adherent to the vertebral column developed local recurrence, and the overall five-year survival was 42%.

Most patients die from distant metastatic disease. According to Paulson and colleagues,[94] few patients survive beyond 2 years with an extended posterior resection. This view is shared by Santori and colleagues,[95] who reported that none of eight patients with vertebral body erosion survived beyond 1 year. According to Wright and associates,[93] vertebral body involvement does not preclude long-term survival, but none of their five patients demonstrated bony destruction by CT scan preoperatively. In that series, one of five patients was alive 36 months after resection of a portion of the vertebral body. DeMeester and colleagues[92] reported experience with 12 patients with tumors abutting the spine. The resected specimens were decalcified and assessed regarding the level of invasion; neither of the two patients who had cortical bone destruction survived beyond 3 months, whereas of six patients with tumor confined to the vertebral periosteum, two patients survived beyond 5 years, and two others were alive 1 to 5 years after resection. Accordingly, the most favorable results are seen in tumors without obvious destruction of the vertebral body. Although CT scans are sometimes helpful in identifying bony destruction, they are not entirely reliable in ruling it out. MRI may be marginally superior to CT in demonstrating bony destruction.[96]

Combined radiotherapy and surgery provides better palliation of pain in these patients than irradiation alone. Moreover, these survival statistics are a vast improvement over the results of radiotherapy alone with a local recurrence rate of more than 50% among which there are no two-year survivals.[97,98]

The largest experience with extended anterior transcervical–thoracic resections has been reported by Dartevelle and colleagues.[87] These authors reported no significant operative morbidity and no mortality in 29 patients, 20 of whom also underwent a posterolateral thoracotomy to complete the posterior part of the resection. Twelve of the 29 patients had involvement of the subclavian artery or its branches, and nine of these patients required reconstruction. The branches of the subclavian artery, including the vertebral artery, have been successfully ligated without cerebrovascular insufficiency, provided the patient has good collateral flow.[87] Revascularization of the subclavian artery, however, is imperative because radiotherapy and division of the upper intercostal vessels compromise collateral flow to the arm. Without vascular reconstruction, there have been several reports of ischemic gangrene of the forearm.[93,94] Dartevelle and associates[87] reported on one of nine patients reconstructed with an unringed PTFE graft who developed a late graft occlusion, and therefore they recommend using a 6- or 8-mm externally supported PTFE graft when an end-to-end anastomosis cannot be safely performed.

Similar to the experience of extended posterior resections, long-term pain control is better after an extended anterior resection (with or without a posterolateral thoracotomy) than with irradiation alone. The incidence of local recurrence was reported by Dartevelle and associates[87] to be 7% (2/29), and the survival ranged from 4 to 137 months.

The two- and five-year survival statistics were 50% and 31%, respectively, as reported by Dartevelle and colleagues.[87] According to Wright and colleagues,[93] one of four patients with documented invasion of the subclavian artery was alive 29 months after complete resection and reconstruction. The most common cause of death is metastatic disease, the most common site being the brain.

Most believe that 3,000 to 4,500 cGy radiation delivered preoperatively shrinks the tumor, providing a wider margin of resection and decreasing the number of incomplete resections. Several authors have emphasized the prognostic significance of achieving a complete resection. Shahian has examined the value of providing additional postoperative radiation therapy in patients who were found to have incomplete resections and/or positive mediastinal nodes. Hilaris et al. have examined the value of providing brachytherapy at the time of surgery to improve local regional control.[99] More recently, Ginsberg et al. were unable to show any improvement in five-year survival by providing brachytherapy in patients undergoing incomplete resection.[100]

In the absence of mediastinal adenopathy, some[6,90,94,97] believe that 3,000 to 4,500 cGy preoperative radiotherapy shrinks the tumor and provides a wider resection margin; Shahian and colleagues[101] suggested that there may be an

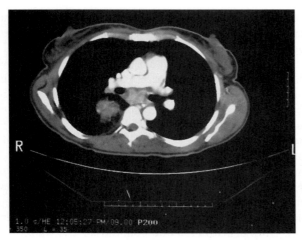

FIGURE 38.14. CT scan illustrating an adenocarcinoma of the right lower lobe with extensive subcarinal adenopathy.

advantage to giving additional postoperative radiotherapy if the resection is incomplete, or if positive mediastinal nodes are discovered at the time of resection. Trials of combined preoperative chemotherapy and radiotherapy are being conducted to improve the incidence of local control, distant recurrence, and five-year survival in these T3 and T4 tumors.

Most consider the presence of mediastinal lymph node metastases as a contraindication for these extended resections. RPSLMC advocates treating these patients with preoperative adjuvant chemotherapy and radiotherapy. Preliminary results using this combined modality are encouraging.[86]

Miscellaneous Extended Pulmonary Resections

Although the early literature alludes to the practicality of extending pulmonary resections to include portions of the muscular wall of the esophagus, the diaphragm, and the aorta, no operative mortality and long-term survival statistics could be provided.[3,19,20] During the years that followed, occasional cases involving resections of the muscular wall of the esophagus appeared without a long-term survivor[45,102,103] (Figures 38.14 and 38.15). Burt and colleagues[47] reported the only five-year survival in a patient with pulmonary carcinoma involving the esophageal wall.

Experience with tumors fixed to the aorta has been more limited but equally discouraging. The two largest series[47,50,51] reported on a combined experience with 27 patients who underwent *en bloc* resection of the aorta; no patient survived beyond 2 years. Nakahara and colleagues[74] reported that one of three patients who underwent *en bloc* resection of the aortic arch survived disease-free for 17 months. If such resections are to be undertaken, the surgeon must be prepared to perform cardiopulmonary bypass in order to resect and graft the aorta because resections limited to the subadventitial plane are often found to be incomplete.[50,74,104,105] Clearly, such aggressive resections should be reserved for exceptional cases.

In contrast to the incidence of chest wall involvement, pulmonary tumors rarely directly invade the diaphragm. Although the option to resect portions of the diaphragm was acknowledged as far back as 1959,[3] only a few case reports have appeared[44,45,103] (Figures 38.16 through 38.18). Others[106–110] have explored the option of extrapleural pneumonectomy and hemidiaphragmectomy in the

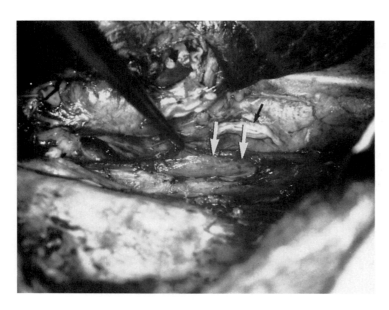

FIGURE 38.15. Operative photograph of same patient as in Figure 38.14 demonstrating *en bloc* resection of the muscular wall of the esophagus with the subcarinal mass after preoperative chemotherapy and radiotherapy. White arrows identify the edge of the muscular wall; black arrow indicates bronchial stump.

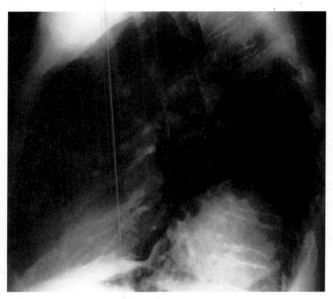

FIGURE 38.16. Lateral radiograph demonstrating a carcinosarcoma of the left lower lobe and obscuring the diaphragm.

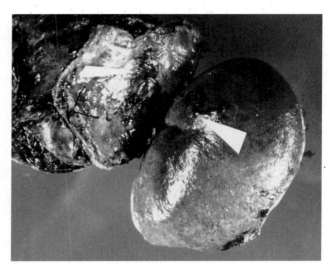

FIGURE 38.18. Operative photograph of same patient as in Figure 38.16 showing tumor invasion across the diaphragm and directly invading the spleen, removed *en bloc.*

presence of an associated malignant pleural effusion, with predictably poor results.

BRONCHIAL SLEEVE LOBECTOMY

A sleeve resection of the bronchus is indicated when tumor approximates or involves the lobar orifice so that a standard lobectomy leaves a positive bronchial resection margin.

Bronchoscopy is often the first examination that alerts

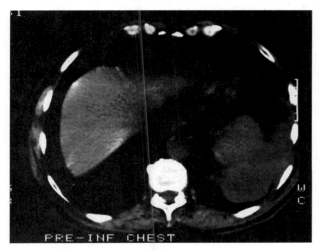

FIGURE 38.17. CT scan of same patient as in Figure 38.16 showing tumor obscuring tissue planes between diaphragm and spleen.

the surgeon that the tumor may not be completely resected using a standard lobectomy. Pertinent findings include mucosal changes of corrugation, erythema, and dilated submucosal vessels at the lobar orifice, which are all indications of submucosal infiltration of tumor. More obvious findings include gross extension of polypoid endobronchial tumor to or beyond the lobar orifice and thickening of the lobar spur. Compression or distortion of the bronchial orifice indicates extrinsic disease. The thoracic surgeon is obliged to perform a repeat bronchoscopy, possibly at the time of thoracotomy, if the same surgeon did not perform the initial bronchoscopy. This is especially true in patients with compromised cardiopulmonary reserve, who require a lung-sparing operation.

Patients with central tumors should have a CT scan, which often alerts the surgeon to the need for a resection beyond a standard lobectomy. The tumor mass may be seen extending to the mainstem bronchus or obliterating the normal tissue plane of the main pulmonary artery. Correlating the bronchoscopic and CT or MRI findings is important in planning the resection.[111]

In addition, mediastinal nodes greater than 1.5 cm indicate the need for mediastinoscopy. Involved contralateral mediastinal nodes and extension of tumor beyond the capsule of superior mediastinal nodes contraindicate resection. If the tumor is limited to ipsilateral or subcarinal nodes, the patient should be considered for a program of adjuvant chemotherapy and radiotherapy.

Patients older than 65 years and those with compromised cardiopulmonary reserve are ideal candidates for sleeve lobectomies. The elderly do not tolerate a pneumonectomy well, and every attempt should be made to perform a lesser resection whenever technically possible. A predicted postoperative FEV_1 of less than 1 L is a good predictor of complications after a pneumonectomy, and preservation of lung tissue in this setting is of paramount importance. Preoperative pulmonary function studies, quantitative ventilation–perfusion lung scans, and a full cardiac evaluation are necessary in the compromised patient.

Despite the preoperative assessment, the patient and the family must be made aware that, for technical or anatomic reasons, a pneumonectomy may become necessary, with its attendant increased morbidity and mortality. There are too many instances in which a sleeve lobectomy is planned when a pneumonectomy is required.

Technical Considerations

The performance of a bronchoplastic procedure requires one-lung ventilation. The surgeon should be able to perform preoperative or intraoperative bronchoscopy, and the choice of endotracheal tube should be discussed with the anesthesiologist. An uncut, single-lumen endotracheal tube can be advanced down the contralateral mainstem bronchus. For left thoracotomies, the tube is easily passed down the right mainstem bronchus. Under bronchoscopic control, the side hole is positioned at the right upper lobe to ensure that the entire right lung is ventilated. For procedures on the right side, the endotracheal tube is advanced down the left mainstem bronchus intraoperatively. This technique allows the surgeon to use a standard flexible bronchoscope, with excellent optics to visualize the anastomosis, and a 2.2-mm instrument channel to aspirate blood and secretions from the distal airway. Increased minute ventilation minimizes hypercarbia, and oxygenation is well maintained despite shunting through the nonventilated lung. Occlusion of the pulmonary artery is not required. High-frequency ventilation is usually not necessary.

A double-lumen endotracheal tube also permits satisfactory one-lung anesthesia and is preferred by many. The anesthesiologist must be experienced in placing these tubes, and it is necessary to have a pediatric bronchoscope available to confirm proper positioning. Although this instrument can be used to inspect the anastomosis, secretions and clots cannot be easily aspirated. Furthermore, patients who need continued ventilation in the recovery room require replacement of the double-lumen tube with a standard single-lumen tube.

The Univent tube is often unsatisfactory for a right-sided sleeve resection because the blocker is positioned too close to the upper lobe orifice. Furthermore, the blocker has a tendency to migrate proximally and can act as a ball valve at the tip of the endotracheal tube.

Through a posterolateral or a muscle-sparing lateral thoracotomy, the hilum is explored. Operative dissection of the bronchus is performed with careful attention to the bronchial arteries. The thoracic surgeon must be aware of the normal and variant locations of the bronchial arterial

supply of the right and left mainstem bronchi. To safeguard this blood supply, the bronchus must not be denuded or skeletonized. When dissecting level 5 and 6 lymph nodes, it is important not to injure the left bronchial artery, which arises under the transverse aortic arch. Careful dissection of the subcarinal nodes is required because branches of the bronchial arteries are always located in this area. When dissecting out level 7 nodes on the right side, care must be taken not to injure a branch of the bronchial artery that passes through the subcarinal area posterior and lateral to the right mainstem bronchus.

The branches of the pulmonary artery are isolated with care. The primary tumor or hilar nodes often abut the lobar arterial branches. On occasion, however, tumor may invade or encase the artery, which may require arterioplasty or a pneumonectomy (see later). If difficulty is encountered in this part of the dissection, it is wise to obtain proximal control of the artery. Some have advocated reconstruction of the bronchial defect using a bronchial flap to avoid complete transsection of the bronchus. However, an unacceptably high incidence of kinking and distortion of the bronchus has occurred using this method.[112,113]

Once one-lung ventilation is obtained, the bronchus is transected using a #15 blade to ensure a clean, straight margin. No attempt is made to bevel the distal bronchus to accommodate the larger mainstem bronchial orifice. Immediately after removal of the specimen, frozen sections of the proximal and distal bronchial margins are obtained. If a positive resection margin is discovered, the surgeon must decide whether an additional bronchial margin can be safely obtained or whether a pneumonectomy is necessary. The resection of additional bronchus may put undue tension on the anastomosis. Care must be taken that resection of additional distal margin does not compromise a segmental bronchus of the remaining lung. Under these circumstances, it may be prudent to perform the pneumonectomy rather than risk anastomotic complications.

The bronchial anastomosis is performed using simple sutures of 3-0 or 4-0 polyglycolic acid. The anastomosis is started by placing two or three simple sutures at the medial junction of the cartilaginous and membranous portions of the bronchus. These sutures are tied, placing the knots on the outside of the bronchus and bringing the cartilaginous rings together. These sutures are placed to minimize tension and to allow accurate placement of the remaining sutures. The remaining sutures are then serially tied as they are placed to approximate the cartilaginous rings. Luminal disparity is addressed when closing the membranous bronchus, as illustrated in Figure 38.19. No attempt should be made to compensate for lumen disparity by oblique placement of the sutures because this causes bronchial distortion and risks tearing of the tissue from uneven tension. Not infrequently, the distal bronchus "telescopes" into the proximal bronchus, causing some compromise of the lumen size, but this

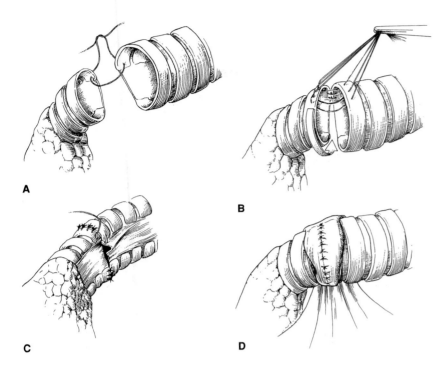

FIGURE 38.19. Operative drawings illustrating the technique of bronchial anastomosis. **A:** The first suture is placed at the corner of the bronchus to provide orientation. **B:** The cartilaginous rings are approximated using simple sutures and avoiding telescoping. **C:** Discrepancy in the lumen size is addressed when closing the membranous bronchus. **D:** A pleural wrap is performed to seal the anastomosis and cover the knots, protecting the adjacent pulmonary artery.

technique may provide additional security of the anastomosis.

The practice at RPSL is to encircle the bronchial anastomosis with a broad-based pleural flap or with a pedicled anterior mediastinal fat pad. This tissue protects the pulmonary artery from erosion by the knots of the anastomotic sutures and minimizes the complications of a minor anastomotic leak. Others,[112–114] however, have provided experimental evidence that a pleural flap actually impedes revascularization of the anastomosis. More recently, Kutlu and Goldstraw have reported their series of 100 patients undergoing a bronchial anastomosis using a continuous suture technique with an acceptable incidence of airway stenosis.[115]

Results

According to several large series, the mean age of patients undergoing sleeve lobectomies is 60 to 65 years, with a strong male predominance. Approximately 75% of tumors are classified as squamous carcinoma. The most common site is the right upper lobe, followed in frequency by the left upper lobe and the left lower lobe. Other bronchial sleeve resections have been described, including right upper and middle lobe, right middle and lower lobe, right middle lobe and superior segment, and even right upper, middle, and superior segment resections, anastomosing the basal segments to the mainstem bronchus.[116]

Postoperative complications are mainly related to the anastomosis. Accumulations of clot and secretions at the anastomosis may lead to atelectasis. For this reason, blood and secretions should be routinely aspirated from the distal airway in the operating room, and the anastomosis should be inspected. If the distal airway is compromised (especially the superior segment of the lower lobe or the middle lobe bronchus), part or all of the anastomosis is refashioned.[117] Tedder and associates[118] reported the incidence of postoperative atelectasis to be 5.2%. Retained, inspissated secretions may be managed with a minitracheostomy or a daily bronchoscopy.

Persistent air leak for greater than 7 days may be evidence of an anastomotic leak. Under these circumstances, the anastomosis must be carefully inspected with a fiberoptic bronchoscope. Dehiscence appears as an area of pale discoloration of the bronchial margins, and careful inspection may disclose to-and-fro movement of secretions through the bronchial wall. Careful judgment must be used to determine the next course of action. If the leak is small and more than half of the anastomosis is intact, then judicial observation, leaving the chest tubes in place, may be the best option, particularly if the anastomosis was wrapped with a pleural flap. An empyema can usually be avoided. If more than half of the anastomosis is in jeopardy, or if a large leak is evident with an air space around the anastomosis, a completion pneumonectomy should be performed. An abscess at the anastomosis can erode into the pulmonary artery; therefore, proximal control of the pulmonary artery must be achieved early on reoperation. When close attention is paid to the details of the anastomotic closure, including the preservation of the bronchial arterial supply and wrapping of the bronchial anastomosis, only about 6% of patients require completion pneumonectomy for complications relating to the bronchial anastomosis.[117]

The operative mortality rates vary widely in reported series, in part because of controversy over indications for the procedure.[116–125] The mortality rates are as low as 2%.[117] The mortality rate has been reported to be as low as 2%.[117] The long-term survival is primarily determined by the nodal status. Excellent long-term functional results have been reported by Gaissert et al. and Van Schil et al.[119,120]

PULMONARY ARTERIOPLASTY WITH PULMONARY RESECTION

Some patients considered to be candidates for pulmonary resection are found to have tumor invading or encasing the pulmonary artery or its branches. This finding may be on the basis of direct invasion by the pulmonary tumor, or the artery may be invaded by tumor metastatic to the lobar or mediastinal nodes. Occasionally, involvement of the wall of the pulmonary artery can be suspected on the basis of preoperative pulmonary arteriography or CT scan.[29] In most cases, however, involvement of the artery is first discovered intraoperatively.

When a sufficiently long segment of artery is available, a segment of the artery can be resected along with the lung and reconstructed using a variety of techniques. Such reconstructive operations on the pulmonary artery were first discussed by Allison in 1954.[126] In 1959, Johnston and Jones[127] reported their experience with sleeve resections, including eight resections of the pulmonary artery. Wurning,[128] Pichlmaier and Spelsberg,[129] and Vogt-Moykopf and colleagues[130–132] further explored the techniques of pulmonary angioplastic reconstruction. Other reports have further popularized pulmonary arterioplasty.[133–137]

Because a much longer segment of pulmonary artery is available for reconstruction on the left side, most experience has been with carcinomas arising from the left upper lobe. However, right-sided resections and reconstructions have also been performed.[127–130,133,136,137]

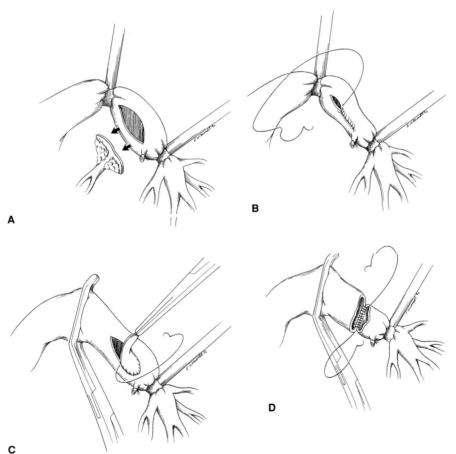

FIGURE 38.20. Operative drawings depicting several techniques of pulmonary arterioplasty. **A:** Proximal and distal control of the pulmonary artery is achieved, and the wall is resected. **B:** If less than one-third of the wall circumference is resected, then the defect may be closed primarily without stenosis. **C:** If more than one-third of the wall is resected, then the defect may be patched. In this case, proximal control is achieved using a vascular clamp to minimize distortion. **D:** If a short length of pulmonary artery is resected, then an end-to-end anastomosis is performed.

Technical Considerations

When exposing the hilum, the pulmonary artery is explored proximal and distal to the area of suspected involvement. On the left side, an adequate length can usually be obtained by dividing the ligamentum arteriosum. On the right side, the pulmonary artery may have to be dissected out behind the SVC, or using the intrapericardial approach.

The artery is encircled proximally and distally. If only a small portion of the arterial wall is involved, umbilical tapes are passed around the artery distal to the involved segment and secured with a Rumel tourniquet. In this setting, tapes are preferred because they are less likely to traumatize the pulmonary arterial wall. If greater portions of the artery are involved, vascular clamps should be used because they are less likely to distort the artery during reconstruction. Great care must be taken when applying even a soft atraumatic clamp to the proximal pulmonary artery because these vessels are often sclerotic and the intima is easily torn. If sufficient length of pulmonary artery is not available to achieve distal control of the artery, then the lower lobe vein can be secured with a Rumel tourniquet or a vascular clamp. Collateral bronchial flow, however, may still compromise exposure.

Uninvolved upper lobar branches of the pulmonary artery are ligated and divided to facilitate mobilization and exposure. The pulmonary vein draining the involved lobe is dissected out and ligated to minimize back-bleeding. The bronchial dissection is then completed.

Then, 5000 U of heparin is given, and vascular control is achieved. If a bronchial sleeve resection is indicated, then the mainstem bronchus is divided, resecting a portion of the wall of the pulmonary artery. If the artery is more extensively involved, then it may be transected, dividing the distal pulmonary artery tangentially to minimize any discrepancy in the lumen size. The bronchial anastomosis is performed first to avoid placing undue tension on a completed vascular suture line.

If only a segment of the arterial wall is resected, then care must be taken that simple oversewing does not leave the artery significantly narrowed. If more than one-third circumference of the wall is resected, then the defect should be closed using a patch of pericardium[29,61,136,137] (Figures 38.20 and 38.21).

If a resection of a short length of artery is indicated, then it should be reconstructed using an end-to-end anastomosis. Care must be taken that the artery is not twisted or kinked at the closure and that no tension exists. Continuous-stitch 4-0 or 5-0 polypropylene suture is used for the arterial closure or anastomosis. A flap of pleura can be used to encircle and separate the bronchial anastomosis from the vascular suture line.

If a length of pulmonary artery is resected so that an end-to-end anastomosis cannot be performed without ten-

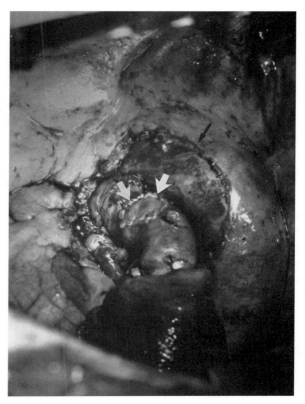

FIGURE 38.21. Operative photograph showing a pericardial patch (*white arrows*) on the proximal left pulmonary artery under the aortic arch (*black arrow*).

sion, then an interposition graft may be necessary. Saphenous vein, Dacron, and PTFE grafts have been used successfully.[134,135] Alternatively, a bronchial sleeve can be resected to minimize tension on the vascular anastomosis, as proposed by Vogt-Moykopf.[130–132]

The tip of the chest tube should be directed away from the field of dissection. The heparin is not reversed at the conclusion of surgery, but the patient is not anticoagulated further.

Results

Although the technique of pulmonary arterioplasty was described more than 40 years ago, clinical experience has been limited to a few centers with a total reported experience of less than 250 patients. Technically, it is much simpler to perform a pneumonectomy, but this procedure carries greater attendant morbidity and mortality and greater pulmonary compromise.

The pulmonary artery remains patent in most cases, as determined by routine postoperative pulmonary angiograms or nuclear perfusion scans.[130,134,136] However, thrombosis of the pulmonary artery has been reported, presenting as pulmonary consolidation and fever without bronchial obstruction. At least four cases have been reported,[127,133,138,139] and in most cases, this is an indication for a completion pneumonectomy. One case, however, was discovered 6 months after surgery in an asymptomatic patient who went on to survive for 11 years.[138]

Vogt-Moykopf and colleagues[130] reported a 5% operative mortality for patients undergoing combined bronchial and vascular sleeve resections. The median survival for 29 patients undergoing bronchial and vascular sleeve resections was 625 days.

Read and colleagues[138] performed six interposition grafts (three saphenous vein, three PTFE) of the left pulmonary artery without thrombosis or infection; four of six patients were alive and disease free an average of 17 months after resection.[134] Rendina et al. have reported a series of 68 patients who have undergone Cisplatin-based induction chemotherapy and underwent bronchial and/or pulmonary artery reconstruction with excellent results.[136,137,140]

SUMMARY

The surgical experience of the last four decades has supported the contention that a complete surgical resection provides the best chance of cure for pulmonary carcinomas, even in most of those cases that are locally advanced by virtue of direct extension to mediastinal structures and the chest wall. Perioperative care has been vastly improved, resulting in lower morbidity and mortality when compared with earlier results.

The best prognostic factors in these cases are the stage of the tumor and the completeness of the resection. Among stage IIIA carcinomas, T3, N0-1 tumors have a better prognosis than T1-2, N2 tumors, according to several reports.[86,141,142] This has also been the experience with sleeve pneumonectomies, for which patients with T4, N0-1 tumors have a more favorable prognosis than patients with N2 metastases. The importance of careful staging in these cases is paramount when it comes to predicting the outcomes.[143] Overall, squamous cell carcinomas and adenocarcinomas appear to have a better prognosis than large cell carcinomas.[144] The risk of local recurrence has been minimized by the use of adjuvant external radiotherapy, administered either preoperatively or postoperatively. Intraoperative or postoperative brachytherapy has also been employed[145–147] (see also Chapters 43, 49).

The long-term survival statistics, however, are still disappointing. The most common cause of death continues to be distant metastatic disease. The assumption that microscopic metastases are present at the time of presentation has been the main rationale for including chemotherapy in the adjuvant setting. In addition, some chemotherapeutic agents are known to act as radiosensitizing agents.

REFERENCES

1. Graham EA, Singer JJ. Successful removal of an entire lung for carcinoma of the bronchus. *JAMA* 1933;101:1371.
2. Smith RA. The results of raising the resectability rate in operations for lung carcinoma. *Thorax* 1957;12:79.
3. Chamberlain JM, McNeill TM, Parnassa P, et al. Bronchogenic carcinoma: an aggressive surgical attitude. *J Thorac Cardiovasc Surg* 1959;38:727.
4. Watson WL. Radical surgery for lung cancer: evolution of the operation of radical pneumonectomy and five-year end results. *Cancer* 1956;9:1167.
5. Warren WH, Memoli VA, Jordan AG, et al. Reevaluation of pulmonary neoplasms resected as small cell carcinomas: significance of distinguishing between well-differentiated neuroendocrine carcinoma and small cell neuroendocrine carcinoma. *Cancer* 1990;65:1003.
6. Shaw RR, Paulson DL, Kee JL. Treatment of the superior sulcus tumor by irradiation followed by resection. *Ann Surg* 1961;154:29.
7. Baker NH, Cowley RA, Linberg E. A follow-up in patients with bronchogenic carcinoma "locally cured" by preoperative irradiation. *J Thorac Cardiovasc Surg* 1963;46:298.
8. Linberg EJ, Cowley RA, Bloedorn F, et al. Bronchogenic carcinoma: further experience with preoperative irradiation. *Ann Thorac Surg* 1965;1:371.
9. Sherman DM, Neptune W, Weichslebaum R, et al. An aggressive approach to marginally resectable lung cancer. *Cancer* 1978;41:2040.
10. Patterson GA, Ilves R, Ginsberg RJ, et al. The value of adjuvant radiotherapy in pulmonary and chest wall resection for bronchogenic carcinoma. *Ann Thorac Surg* 1982;34:692.
11. Warram J. Preoperative irradiation of cancer of the lung: final report of a therapeutic trial. A collaborative study. *Cancer* 1975;36:914.
12. Shields TW, Higgins GA, Lawton R, et al. Preoperative x-ray therapy as an adjuvant in the treatment of bronchogenic carcinoma. *J Thorac Cardiovasc Surg* 1970;59:49.
13. Pearson FG, Nelems JM, Henderson RD, et al. The role of mediastinoscopy in the selection of treatment for bronchial carcinoma with involvement of the superior mediastinal nodes. *J Thorac Cardiovasc Surg* 1972;64:382.
14. Allison PR. Discussion. *J Thorac Surg* 1950;20:362.
15. Cahan WG, Watson WL, Pool JL. Radical pneumonectomy. *J Thorac Surg* 1951;22:449.
16. Aylwin AJ. Avoidable vascular spread in resection for bronchial carcinoma. *Thorax* 1951;6:250.
17. Johnson J, Kirby CK, Blakemore WS. Should we insist on "radical pneumonectomy" as a routine procedure in the treatment of carcinoma of the lung? *J Thorac Surg* 1958;36:309.
18. Burford TH, Center S, Ferguson TB. Results in the treatment of bronchogenic carcinoma: an analysis of 1,008 cases. *J Thorac Surg* 1958;36:316.
19. Churchill ED, Sweet RH, Soutter L, et al. The surgical management of carcinoma of the lung: a study of the cases treated at the Massachusetts General Hospital 1930–1950. *J Thorac Surg* 1950;20:349.
20. Churchill ED, Sweet RH, Scannell JG, et al. Further studies in the surgical management of carcinoma of the lung: a further study of the cases treated at the Massachusetts General Hospital from 1950 to 1957. *J Thorac Surg* 1958;36:301.
21. Amparo EG, Higgins CB, Farmer D, et al. Gated MRI of cardiac and paracardiac masses: initial experience. *AJR* 1984;143:1151.
22. McMurdo KK, de Geer G, Webb WR, et al. Normal and occluded mediastinal veins: MR imaging. *Radiology* 1986;159:33.

23. Barakos JA, Brown JJ, Higgins CB. MR imaging of secondary cardiac and paracardiac lesions. *AJR* 1989;153:47.

24. Levitt RG, Glazer HS, Roper CL, et al. Magnetic resonance imaging of mediastinal and hilar masses: comparison with CT. *AJR* 1985;145:9.

25. Martini N, Heelan R, Westcott J, et al. Comparative merits of conventional, computed tomographic, and magnetic resonance imaging in assessing mediastinal involvement in surgically confirmed lung carcinoma. *J Thorac Cardiovasc Surg* 1985;90:639.

26. Lestuzzi C, Biasi S, Nicolosi GL, et al. Secondary neoplastic infiltration of the myocardium diagnosed by two-dimensional echocardiography in seven cases with anatomic confirmation. *J Am Coll Cardiol* 1987;9:439.

27. Tatsumura T. Preoperative and intraoperative ultrasonographic examination as an aid in lung cancer operations. *J Thorac Cardiovasc Surg* 1995;110:606.

28. Bailey CP, Schechter DC, Folk FS. Extending operability in lung cancer involving the heart and great vessels. *Ann Thorac Surg* 1971;11:140.

29. Ricci C, Rendina EA, Venuta F et al. Reconstruction of the pulmonary artery in patients with lung cancer. *Ann Thorac Surg* 1994;57:627.

30. Levin PD, Faber LP, Carleton RA. Cardiac herniation after pneumonectomy. *J Thorac Cardiovasc Surg* 1971;61:104.

31. Bettman RB, Tannenbaum WJ. Herniation of the heart through a pericardial incision. *Ann Surg* 1948;128:1012.

32. Gates GF, Sette RS, Cope JA. Acute cardiac herniation with incarceration following pneumonectomy. *Radiology* 1970;94:561.

33. Dippel WF, Ehrenhaft JL. Herniation of the heart after pneumonectomy. *J Thorac Cardiovasc Surg* 1973;65:207.

34. Takita H, Mijares WS. Herniation of the heart following intrapericardial pneumonectomy: report of a case and review. *J Thorac Cardiovasc Surg* 1970;59:443.

35. Deiraniya AK. Cardiac herniation following intrapericardial pneumonectomy. *Thorax* 1974;29:545.

36. Yacoub MH, Williams WG, Ahmad A. Strangulation of the heart following intrapericardial pneumonectomy. *Thorax* 1968;23:261.

37. Goldstraw P, Jiao X. Pericardial repair after extensive resection: another use for the pedicled diaphragmatic flap. *Ann Thorac Surg* 1996;61:1112.

38. Glass JD, McQuillen EN, Hardin NJ. Iatrogenic cardiac herniation: post mortem case. *J Trauma* 1984;24:632.

39. Papsin BC, Gorenstein LA, Goldberg M. Delayed myocardial laceration after intrapericardial pneumonectomy. *Ann Thorac Surg* 1993;55:756.

40. Ohri SI, Siddiqui AA, Townsend ER. Cardiac torsion after lobectomy with partial pericardectomy. *Ann Thorac Surg* 1992;53:703.

41. Pitz CCM, Brutel de la Riviere A, Elbers HRJ, et al. Results of resection of T3 non-small cell lung cancer invading the mediastinum or main bronchus. *Ann Thorac Surg* 1996;62:1016.

42. Smith RA, Nigam BK. Resection of proximal left main bronchus carcinoma. *Thorax* 1979;34:616.

43. Smith RA. Surgery in the treatment of locally advanced lung carcinoma. *Thorax* 1963;18:21.

44. Lawrence GH, Walker JH, Pinkers L. Extended resection of bronchogenic carcinoma: a reappraisal and suggested plan of management. *N Engl J Med* 1960;263:615.

45. Trastek VF, Pairolero PC, Piehler JM, et al. En bloc (non-chest wall) resection for bronchogenic carcinoma with parietal fixation: factors affecting survival. *J Thorac Cardiovasc Surg* 1984;87:352.

46. Burt ME, Pomerantz AM, Bains MS, et al. Results of surgical treatment of stage III lung cancer invading the mediastinum. *Surg Clin North Am* 1987;67:987.

47. Shuhtsu A, Inoue H, Ogawa J, et al. Resection of lung cancer involving the heart and great vessels. *Tokai J Exp Clin Med* 1981;6:373.

48. Kodama K, Doi O, Tatsuta M. Unusual extension of lung cancer into the left atrium via the pulmonary vein. *Int Surg* 1990;75:22.

49. Fukuse T, Wada H, Hitomi S. Extended operation for non-small cell lung cancer invading great vessels and left atrium. *Eur J Cardiothorac Surg* 1997;11:664.

50. Tsuchiya R, Asamura H, Kondo H, et al. Extended resection of the left atrium, great vessels, or both for lung cancer. *Ann Thorac Surg* 1994;57:960.

51. Levett JM, Darakjian HE, DeMeester TR, et al. Bronchogenic carcinoma located in the aortic window: the importance of the primary lesion as a determinant of survival. *J Thorac Cardiovasc Surg* 1982;83:551.

52. Abbott OA. Experiences with the surgical resection of the human carina, tracheal wall and contralateral bronchial wall in cases of right total pneumonectomy. *J Thorac Cardiovasc Surg* 1950;19:906.

53. Mathey J, Binet JP, Galey JJ, et al. Tracheal and tracheobronchial resections: technique and results in 20 cases. *J Thorac Cardiovasc Surg* 1966;51:1.

54. Jensik RJ, Faber LP, Milloy FJ, et al. Tracheal sleeve pneumonectomy for advanced carcinoma of the lung. *Surg Gynecol Obstet* 1972;134:231.

55. Naef AP. Extensive tracheal resection and tracheobronchial reconstruction. *Ann Thorac Surg* 1969;8:391.

56. Jensik RJ, Faber LP, Kittle CF, et al. Survival in patients undergoing tracheal sleeve pneumonectomy for bronchogenic carcinoma. *J Thorac Cardiovasc Surg* 1982;84:489.

57. Grillo HC. Carcinoma of the lung: what can be done if the carina is involved? *Am J Surg* 1982;143:694.

58. Mathisen DJ, Grillo HC. Carinal resection for bronchogenic carcinoma. *J Thorac Cardiovasc Surg* 1991;102:16.

59. Tsuchiya R, Goya T, Naruke T, et al. Resection of tracheal carina for lung cancer: procedure, complications, and mortality. *J Thorac Cardiovasc Surg* 1990;99:779.

60. Faber LP. Results of surgical treatment of stage III lung carcinoma with carinal proximity: the role of sleeve lobectomy versus pneumonectomy and the role of sleeve pneumonectomy. *Surg Clin North Am* 1987;67:1001.

61. Faber LP. Sleeve resections in lung cancer. *Semin Thorac Cardiovasc Surg* 1993;5:238.

62. Roviaro GC, Varoli F, Rebuffat C, et al. Tracheal sleeve pneumonectomy for bronchogenic carcinoma. *J Thorac Cardiovasc Surg* 1994;107:13.

63. Deslauriers J, Beaulieu M, Benazera A, et al. Sleeve pneumonectomy for bronchogenic carcinoma. *Ann Thorac Surg* 1979;28:465.

64. Mitchell JD, Mathisen DJ, Wright CD, et al. Clinical experience with carinal resection. *J Thorac Cardiovasc Surg* 1999;117:39.

65. Dartevelle PG, Khalife J, Chapelier A, et al. Tracheal sleeve pneumonectomy for bronchogenic carcinoma: report of 55 cases. *Ann Thorac Surg* 1988;46:68.

66. Gilbert A, Deslauriers J, McClish A, et al. Tracheal sleeve pneumonectomy for carcinomas of the proximal left main bronchus. *Can J Surg* 1984;27:583.

67. Dartevelle PG, Khalife J, Chapelier A, et al. Tracheal sleeve pneumonectomy for bronchogenic carcinoma: report of 55 cases. An update. *Ann Thorac Surg* 1995;60:1854.

68. Dartevelle PG, Macchiarini P. Carinal resection for bronchogenic cancer. *Semin Thorac Cardiovasc Surg* 1996;8:414.

69. Dartevelle PG. Extended operations for the treatment of lung cancer. *Ann Thorac Surg* 1997;63:12.
70. Price Thomas C. Conservative and extensive resection for carcinoma of the lung. *Ann R Coll Surg Engl* 1959;24:345.
71. Salsali M. A safe technique for resection of the nonobstructed superior vena cava. *Surg Gynecol Obstet* 1966;123:91.
72. Gomes MN, Hufnagel CA. Superior vena cava obstruction. *Ann Thorac Surg* 1975;20:344.
73. Yoshimura H, Kazama S, Asari H, et al. Lung cancer involving the superior vena cava: pneumonectomy with concomitant partial resection of superior vena cava. *J Thorac Cardiovasc Surg* 1979;77:83.
74. Nakahara K, Ohno K, Mastumura A, et al. Extended operation for lung cancer invading the aortic arch and superior vena cava. *J Thorac Cardiovasc Surg* 1989;97:428.
75. Dartevelle P, Chapelier A, Navajas M, et al. Replacement of the superior vena cava with polytetrafluoroethylene grafts combined with resection of mediastinal-pulmonary malignant tumors: report of thirteen cases. *J Thorac Cardiovasc Surg* 1987;94:361.
76. Dartevelle PG, Chapelier AR, Pastorino U, et al. Long-term follow-up after prosthetic replacement of the superior vena cava combined with resection of mediastinal-pulmonary malignant tumors. *J Thorac Cardiovasc Surg* 1991;102:259.
77. Masuda H, Ogawa T, Kikuchi K, et al. Total replacement of superior vena cava because of invasive thymoma: seven years' survival. *J Thorac Cardiovasc Surg* 1988;95:1083.
78. Piccione W, Faber LP, Warren WH. Superior vena caval reconstruction using autologous pericardium. *Ann Thorac Surg* 1990;50:417.
79. Inoue H, Shohtsu A, Koide S, et al. Resection of the superior vena cava for primary lung cancer: 5 years' survival. *Ann Thorac Surg* 1990;50:661.
80. Marshall WG, Kouchoukos NT. Management of recurrent superior vena caval syndrome with an externally supported femoral vein bypass graft. *Ann Thorac Surg* 1988;46:239.
81. Warren WH, Piccione WJ, Faber LP. Update: superior vena caval reconstruction using autologous pericardium. *Ann Thorac Surg* 1998;66:291.
82. Doty DB, Doty JR, Jones KW. Bypass of superior vena cava: fifteen years' experience with spiral vein graft for obstruction of superior vena cava caused by benign disease. *J Thorac Cardiovasc Surg* 1990;99:889.
83. Mori Y, Hadama T, Takasaki H, et al. Reconstruction of the superior vena cava with externally stented Gore-Tex graft for malignant diseases. *Thai J Surg* 1987;8:53.
84. Magnan PE, Thomas P, Giudicelli R, et al. Surgical reconstruction of the superior vena cava. *Cardiovasc Surg* 1994;2:598.
85. Dartevelle P, et al. Technique of superior vena cava resection and reconstruction. *Chest Surg Clin North Am* 1995;5:345.
86. Faber LP, Kittle CF, Warren WH. Preoperative chemotherapy and radiation for stage III non-small cell lung cancer. *Ann Thorac Surg* 1989;47:669.
87. Dartevelle PG, Chapelier AR, Macchiarini P, et al. Anterior transcervical-thoracic approach for radical resection of lung tumors invading the thoracic inlet. *J Thorac Cardiovasc Surg* 1993;105:1025.
88. Walsh GL, Gokaslan ZL, McCutcheon IE, et al. Anterior approaches to the thoracic spine in patients with cancer: indications and results. *Ann Thorac Surg* 1997;64:1611.
89. Nazari S. Transcervical approach (Dartevelle technique) for resection of lung tumors invading the thoracic inlet, sparing the clavicle. *J Thorac Cardiovasc Surg* 1996;112:558.
90. Onuki T, Murasugi M, Mae M, et al. Modification of anterior approach to superior sulcus tumors. *J Thorac Cardiovasc Surg* 1998;116:663.
91. Spaggiari L, Pastorino U. Anterior approach to the superior sulcus tumors: The transmanubrial osteomuscular sparing approach. Letters to the Editor. *J Thorac Cardiovasc Surg* 1999;117:1042.
92. DeMeester T, Albertucci M, Dawson P, et al. Management of tumor adherent to the vertebral column. *J Thorac Cardiovasc Surg* 1989;97:373.
93. Wright CD, Moncure AC, Shepard JAO, et al. Superior sulcus lung tumors: results of combined treatment (irradiation and radical resection). *J Thorac Cardiovasc Surg* 1987;94:69.
94. Paulson DL. Superior sulcus carcinomas. In: Baue A, ed. *Glenn's thoracic and cardiovascular surgery,* 5th ed. Norwalk, CT: Appleton & Lange, 1991.
95. Sartori F, Rea F, Calabro F, et al. Carcinoma of the superior pulmonary sulcus: results of irradiation and radical resection. *J Thorac Cardiovasc Surg* 1992;104:679.
96. Gefter WB. Magnetic resonance imaging in the evaluation of lung cancer. *Semin Roentgenol* 1990;25:73.
97. Komaki R. Preoperative radiation therapy for superior sulcus lesions. *Chest Surg Clin North Am* 1991;1:13.
98. Van Houtte L, MacLennan I, Poulter C, et al. External radiation in the management of superior sulcus tumors. *Cancer* 1984;54:223.
99. Hilaris BS, Nori D, Beattie EJ, et al. Value of perioperative brachytherapy in the management of non-oat cell carcinoma of the lung. *Int J Radiat Oncol Biol Phys* 1983;9:1161.
100. Ginsberg RJ. Surgery for higher-stage lung cancer. *Chest Surg Clin North Am* 1991;1:61.
101. Shahian DM, Neptune WB, Ellis FH. Pancoast tumors: improved survival with preoperative and postoperative radiotherapy. *Ann Thorac Surg* 1987;43:32.
102. Higginson JF. Discussion. *J Thorac Surg* 1951;22:471.
103. Weissberg D. Extended resections of locally advanced stage III lung cancer. *J Thorac Cardiovasc Surg* 1981;29:238.
104. Klepetko W, Wisser W, Birsan T, et al. T4 lung tumors with infiltration of the thoracic aorta: is an operation reasonable? *J Ann Thorac Surg* 1999;67:340.
105. Okubo K, Yagi K, Yokomise H, et al. Extensive resection with selective cerebral perfusion for a lung cancer invading the aortic arch. *Eur J Cardiothorac Surg* 1996;10:389.
106. Cotton B, Penido JRF. Pleuropulmonary resection with hemidiaphragmectomy. *J Thorac Surg* 1951;2:474.
107. Wu S-F, Huang O-L, Wu H-S, et al. Critical evaluation of results of extension of indication for surgery for primary bronchogenic carcinoma. *Semin Surg Oncol* 1985;1:23.
108. Weksler B, Bains M, Burt M, et al. Resection of lung cancer invading the diaphragm. *J Thorac Cardiovasc Surg* 1997;114:500.
109. Yokoi K, Miyazawa N. Pleuropneumonectomy and postoperative adjuvant chemotherapy for carcinomatous pleuritis in primary lung cancer: a case report of long-term survival. *J Cardiothorac Surg* 1996;10:141.
110. Shimizu J, Oda M, Morita K, et al. Comparison of pleuropneumonctomy and limited surgery for lung cancer for pleural dissemination. *J Surg Oncol* 1996;61:1.
111. Kesler KA, Conces DJ, Heimansohn DA, et al. Assessing the feasibility of bronchoplastic surgery with magnetic resonance imaging. *Ann Thorac Surg* 1991;52:145.
112. Khargi K, Duurkens VAM, Versteegh MMI, et al. Pulmonary function and postoperative complications after wedge and flap reconstructions of the main bronchus. *J Thorac Cardiovasc Surg* 1996;112:117.
113. Ishihara T, Nemoto E, Kikuchi K, et al. Does pleural bronchial wrapping improve wound healing in right sleeve pneumonectomy? *J Thorac Cardiovasc Surg* 1985;89:665.
114. LoCicero J III, Massad M, Oba J, et al. Short-term and long-

term results of experimental wrapping techniques for bronchial anastomosis. *J Thorac Cardiovasc Surg* 1992;103:763.

115. Kutlu CA, Goldstraw P. Tracheobronchial sleeve resection with the use of a continuous anastomosis: results of one hundred consecutive cases. *Thorac Cardiovasc Surg* 1999;117:1112.

116. Kittle CF. Atypical resections of the lung: bronchoplasties, sleeve resections and segmentectomies—their evolution and present status. *Curr Probl Surg* 1989;26:57.

117. Faber LP, Jensik RJ, Kittle CF. Results of sleeve lobectomy for bronchogenic carcinoma in 101 patients. *Ann Thor Surg* 1984; 37:279.

118. Tedder M, Anstadt MP, Tedder SD, et al. Current morbidity, mortality, and survival after bronchoplastic procedures for malignancy. *Ann Thorac Surg* 1992;54:387.

119. Gaissert HA, Mathisen DJ, Moncure AC, et al. Survival and function after sleeve lobectomy for lung cancer. *J Thorac Cardiovasc Surg* 1996;111:948.

120. Van Schil PE, Brutel de la Riviere A, Knaepen PJ, et al. Long-term survival after bronchial sleeve resection: Univariate and multivariate analyses. *Ann Thorac Surg* 1996;61:1087.

121. Paulson DL, Urschel HC, McNamara JJ, et al. Bronchoplastic procedures for bronchogenic carcinoma. *J Thorac Cardiovasc Surg* 1970;59:38.

122. Keszler P. Sleeve resection and other bronchoplasties in the surgery of bronchogenic carcinomas. *Int Surg* 1986;71:229.

123. Deslauriers J, Gaulin P, Beaulieu M, et al. Long-term clinical and functional results of sleeve lobectomy for primary lung cancer. *J Thorac Cardiovasc Surg* 1986;92:871.

124. Van den Bosch JMM, Bergstein PGM, Laros CD, et al. Lobectomy with sleeve resection in the treatment of tumors of the bronchus. *Chest* 1981;80:154.

125. Weisel RD, Cooper JD, Delarue NC, et al. Sleeve lobectomy for carcinoma of the lung. *J Thorac Cardiovasc Surg* 1979;78: 839.

126. Allison PR. Quoted by Jones PW. Course of thoracic surgery in Groningen. *Ann R Coll Surg* 1954;25:20.

127. Johnston JB, Jones PH. The treatment of bronchial carcinoma by lobectomy and sleeve resection of the main bronchus. *Thorax* 1959;14:48.

128. Wurning P. Technische Vorteile bei der Hauptbronchusresektion rechts und links. *Thoraxchirurgie* 1967;15:16.

129. Pichlmaier H, Spelsberg F. Organerhaltende Operation des Bronchuskarzinoms. *Langenbecks Arch Chir* 1971;328:221.

130. Vogt-Moykopf I, Toomes H, Heinrich ST. Sleeve resection of the bronchus and the pulmonary artery for pulmonary lesions. *Jpn J Surg* 1982;12:311.

131. Vogt-Moykopf I, Fritz Th, Meyer G, et al. Bronchoplastic and angioplastic operation in bronchial carcinoma: long-term results

of a retrospective analysis from 1973 to 1983. *Int Surg* 1986; 71:211.

132. Vogt-Moykopf I, Meyer G, Naunheim KS, et al. Bronchoplastic techniques for lung resection. In: Baue AE, ed. *Glenn's thoracic and cardiovascular surgery,* 5th ed. Norwalk, CT: Appleton & Lange, 1991.

133. Maggi G, Casadio C, Pischedda F, et al. Bronchoplastic and angioplastic techniques in the treatment of bronchogenic carcinoma. *Ann Thorac Surg* 1993;55:1501.

134. Read RC, Ziomek S, Ranval TJ, et al. Pulmonary artery sleeve resection for abutting left upper lobe lesions. *Ann Thorac Surg* 1993;55:850.

135. Belli L, Meroni A, Rondinara G, et al. Bronchoplastic procedures and pulmonary artery reconstruction in the treatment of bronchogenic cancer. *J Thorac Cardiovasc Surg* 1985;90:167.

136. Rendina EA, Venuta F, Ciriaco P, et al. Bronchovascular sleeve resection: Technique, perioperative management, prevention, and treatment of complications. *J Thorac Cardiovasc Surg* 1993; 106:73.

137. Rendina EA, Venuta F, DeGiacomo T, et al. Sleeve resection and prosthetic reconstruction of the pulmonary artery for lung cancer: functional and long-term results. *Ann Thorac Surg* 1999; 68:995.

138. Bennett WF, Abbey Smith R. A twenty-year analysis of the results of sleeve resection for primary bronchogenic carcinoma. *J Thorac Cardiovasc Surg* 1978;76:840.

139. Naruke T. Bronchoplastic and bronchovascular procedures of the tracheobronchial tree in the management of primary lung cancer. *Chest* 1989;96(Suppl):53SS.

140. Rendina EA, Venuta F, DeGiacomo T, et al. Safety and efficacy of bronchovascular reconstruction after induction chemotherapy for lung cancer. *J Thorac Cardiovasc Surg* 1997;114:830.

141. Rusch VW. Neoadjuvant therapy for stage III lung cancer. *Semin Thorac Cardiovasc Surg* 1993;5:258.

142. Bonomi P. Treatment of locally advanced non-small cell lung cancer. *Lung Cancer* 1993;9:S49.

143. Miller JD, Gorenstein LA, Patterson GA. Staging: the key to rational management of lung cancer. *Ann Thorac Surg* 1992; 53:170.

144. Kotlyarov EV, Rukosuyev AA. Long-term results and patterns of disease recurrence after radical operations for lung cancer. *J Thorac Cardiovasc Surg* 1991;102:24.

145. Aye RW, Mate TP, Anderson HN, et al. Extending the limits of lung cancer resection. *Am J Surg* 1993;165:572.

146. Ginsberg RJ, Martini N, Zaman BS et al. Influence of surgical resection and brachytherapy in the management of superior sulcus tumor. *J Thorac Cardiovasc Surg* 1994;57:1440.

147. Van Raemdonck DE, Schneider A, Ginsberg RJ. Surgical treatment for high stage non-small cell lung cancer. *Ann Thorac Surg* 1992;54:999.

39

CHEST WALL INVOLVEMENT INCLUDING PANCOAST TUMORS

WILLIAM H. WARREN

In 1959, Chamberlain proposed the term "extended resections" to describe operative procedures that were intended to completely resect locally advanced lung cancers, and in so doing, distinguish them from the "standard resections," a term reserved for lobectomies and pneumonectomies.[1] These so-called "extended resections" included the resection of lung cancers involving the chest wall. The physiologic consequences and operative techniques involved in resecting and reconstructing a portion of the chest wall were, at that time, largely unknown, and the therapeutic value of doing so was controversial. Over the last 40 years, the operative techniques of chest wall resection and reconstruction have evolved and become incorporated into the thoracic surgeon's armamentarium. Moreover, the prognosis of patients undergoing a complete extirpation by pulmonary and *en bloc* chest wall resection is so vastly superior to those undergoing nonsurgical therapy or incomplete resection that the value of chest wall resections is no longer controversial.

This chapter is devoted to resections of the lung involving the chest wall, including the conventional approach to resecting superior sulcus tumors. The topic of alternative operative approaches, including anterior approaches to locally advanced superior sulcus tumors and tumors involving the thoracic spine, is discussed in a separate chapter (see also Chapter 38).

PRIMARY LUNG CARCINOMA INVOLVING THE CHEST WALL (EXCLUDING APICAL TUMORS)

Historical Perspective

In 1947, Coleman reported his experience of five patients undergoing pulmonary and *en bloc* chest wall resections with only one mortality.[2] It was subsequently reported that two of these patients survived 8 and 13 years after the procedure.[3,4] This was the first study documenting the feasibility and survival advantage of patients undergoing this type of resection. Over the following years, the techniques of resec-

tion and materials available for reconstruction improved to the degree that the resection of lung cancer involving the chest wall is no longer considered to be an "extended" resection.

It is estimated that 5% of all primary tumors of the lung have, at the time of presentation, involvement of the chest wall. Most of these tumors are classified as T3, and thus represent at least stage III disease according to the International Staging System.[5] T4 tumors of the chest wall are distinguished by involvement of the vertebral body, involvement of the great vessels (including the aorta, subclavian artery, and vein), or association with a malignant pleural effusion (Figures 39.1, 39.2).

Preoperative Assessment

Chest wall discomfort ranging from a vague ache to a discrete localized pain is a presenting symptom in 37% to 88% of patients.[6–18] On occasion, the pain may be referred to the shoulder or anterior to the area of involvement, presumably referred from intercostal nerve involvement. Almost invariably, if the patient presents with any chest wall symptom, some degree of chest wall involvement can be anticipated. On the other hand, there are reported cases where a patient can present without any chest wall complaint and be found to have periosteal involvement at the time of surgery.

By definition, these tumors are peripheral. Patients who present with a cough, with or without hemoptysis, predictably have large tumors and/or metastases to mediastinal lymph nodes. However, presenting symptoms have not been demonstrated to have prognostic significance with respect to resectability or long-term survival.

In most patients, a plain posterior-anterior assessment and lateral chest radiograph demonstrates a solitary, peripheral lung mass. In the absence of chest wall symptoms, the computed tomography (CT) scan may provide the first evidence that the tumor may involve the chest wall because this relationship may be difficult to appreciate on plain films, and the physical examination is seldom revealing. Although CT scans are generally poor in distinguishing pul-

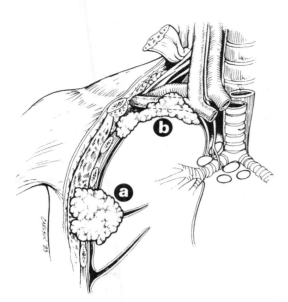

FIGURE 39.1. Schematic of International Staging System definitions for T3 disease involving the chest wall. Diagram shows chest wall invasion in a nonsulcus position **(A)** and with the superior sulcus presentation **(B)**. (From Mountain CF. A new international staging system for lung cancer. *Chest* 1986;89:225S, with permission.)

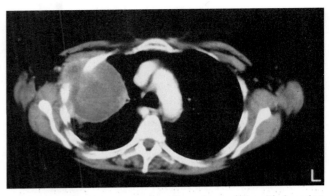

FIGURE 39.3. Lung cancer invading chest wall, with invasion through the intercostal bundles into the external chest wall musculature. This patient was completely resected after mediastinoscopy revealed the absence of N2 involvement.

monary tumors that are simply abutting the chest wall from true chest wall invasion, certain features have been proposed to aid in interpretation. These include contact of tumor against the chest wall over a distance of greater than 3 cm, the ratio of pleural tumor contact/tumor diameter, and obliteration of the extrapleural fat plane[19,20] (Figures 39.3, 39.4). CT with artificial pneumothorax and expiratory dynamic CT have both been used with some success to increase the diagnostic accuracy, but these techniques are rarely justifiable.[21–23]

Thoracic ultrasound has been utilized to detect movement of the tumor against the chest wall.[24] Magnetic resonance imaging may demonstrate a disruption in the normal extrapleural fat plane on the T2-weighted images, although distinction between tumor invasion and associated inflammatory changes may be impossible.[25–29] In the final analysis, these tests are not able to reliably predict the degree of involvement of the chest wall, and therefore the surgeon must be prepared to make intraoperative decisions about chest wall involvement, and consequently, the best technique of resection.

Ideally, a diagnosis is established prior to embarking on a major chest wall resection. Bronchoscopic examination is usually normal but may reveal extrinsic compression of segmental bronchi, and diagnostic material is occasionally provided using this technique. Postbronchoscopy sputum cytology, transbronchial biopsies, and brushings have all

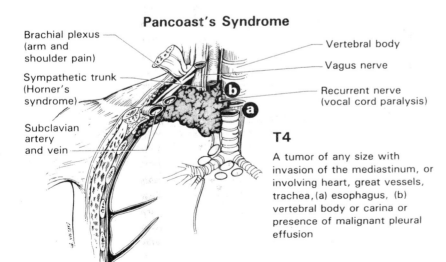

Pancoast's Syndrome

Brachial plexus (arm and shoulder pain)

Sympathetic trunk (Horner's syndrome)

Subclavian artery and vein

Vertebral body

Vagus nerve

Recurrent nerve (vocal cord paralysis)

T4

A tumor of any size with invasion of the mediastinum, or involving heart, great vessels, trachea, (a) esophagus, (b) vertebral body or carina or presence of malignant pleural effusion

FIGURE 39.2. Schematic of International Staging System definitions for superior sulcus tumors, including the Pancoast syndrome. (From Mountain CF. A new international staging system for lung cancer. *Chest* 1986;89:225S, with permission.)

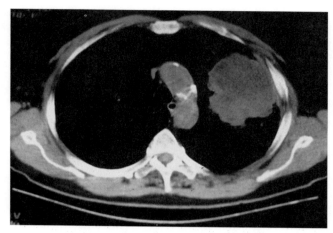

FIGURE 39.4. Lung cancer with abutment of the pleura and partial obliteration of the fat stripe. Patient was found to have chest wall invasion, requiring *en bloc* chest wall resection.

yielded diagnostic material. Many surgeons prefer to perform the bronchoscopy at the time of resection and establish the diagnosis preoperatively by percutaneous fine-needle aspiration.

Percutaneous transthoracic needle aspiration can be performed under fluoroscopic, ultrasound, or CT-directing techniques depending on the size and location of the lesion. With fine-needle (21-gauge) aspiration, a diagnostic accuracy of more than 80% has been reported.[30] Implantation of tumor into the subcutaneous tissue of the chest wall has been documented but is exceedingly rare.[31] Some surgeons have advocated using 14-gauge needle biopsies to establish a histologic diagnosis with lower false-negative and false-positive rates than seen in fine-needle aspiration.[32]

Controversy continues over the issue of performing mediastinoscopy to assess the status of the mediastinal nodes. While some surgeons continue to advocate routine mediastinoscopy,[33–35] most reserve this study for patients with nodes larger than 1.5 cm, tumors greater than 5 cm, or patients with systemic complaints in the absence of extrathoracic metastases.[36–39] Similarly, controversy exists about the role of nuclear bone scans and serum alkaline phosphatase. According to one study, among patients who were found to have carcinomas with chest wall involvement, only 21% had a positive bone scan and 43% had an elevated serum alkaline phosphatase.[10] The value of a CT brain scan is also controversial. These tests should be performed in patients with tumors greater than 5 cm, with radiologic evidence of mediastinal nodal invovement, complaints consistent with distant metastases, or with a weight loss of greater than 5%.

Preoperative Neoadjuvant Therapy

The role of preoperative radiotherapy has been debated for decades without any clear consensus. Several single-institu-

tional series have been published advocating 3,000–3,700 cGy to the chest wall. However, most of these reports did not randomize patients, instead selecting those patients with large tumors for preoperative therapy in the hopes that a wider margin could be achieved.[15,40]

The leading cause of death in these patients is tumor recurrence at distant sites. Therefore, preoperative adjuvant therapy protocols have been modified to incorporate chemotherapy in an attempt to improve the long-term survival.[41,42] The preliminary results have been encouraging, especially in cases without mediastinal nodal involvement. However, the results of preoperative chemo- and radiotherapy in cases of T3N2 carcinomas have been predictably disappointing.[42] Controlled, prospective, and randomized trials are underway to further explore the role of neoadjuvant therapy.

Operative Strategies

The goal of surgery is complete resection of the carcinoma with resection of the involved chest wall and regional nodes with reconstruction, when necessary, to minimally compromise respiration.

Most tumors are approached through a standard posterolateral thoracotomy. Occasionally, when the sternum or apex of the chest is involved (superior sulcus tumors), the incision has to be modified. The chest wall must be opened so that the surgeon can assess the tumor involvement without compromising the resection. Usually, this means entering the chest one interspace below the lowest rib assessed radiologically to be involved by the carcinoma. Once the pleural space has been opened, a finger is inserted to confirm the location of the tumor. The muscles of the appropriate intercostal space are then divided. With greater exposure of the mass, the degree of chest wall invasion can be assessed. Inflammatory adhesions are usually thin and friable, whereas maligant adhesions are usually broad and firm. If the tumor is adherent to the chest wall by only inflammatory adhesions and is completely mobile, then an extrapleural plane is developed 3 to 4 cm from the tumor mass and mobilization is begun. By gentle blunt dissection, the tumor can often be dissected completely free of the chest wall, avoiding a formal chest wall resection and reconstruction. If resistance is met or if any doubt about the adequacy of the margin exists/then a chest wall resection should be performed. Although the technique of extrapleural dissection is widely practiced and studies have supported its use,[10,11,14] some centers have warned about the overuse or inadequacy of this technique, impacting on both the incidence of local/regional recurrence and the five-year survival.[34,38]

In most cases, the chest wall resection is performed first to allow optimal exposure of the hilar structures. However, when the lung mass is 10 cm or greater, it may be easier to perform the pulmonary resection first. Some surgeons have advocated stapling through the lung remote from the tumor and completing the lobectomy after the specimen is out.[15,43] Others, however, have warned that survival is significantly compromised after discontinuous resection.[19,37]

Controversy also exists regarding the margins of the chest wall resection when a formal chest wall resection is necessary. Some surgeons advocate complete resection of all involved ribs, plus one rib above and below providing at least a 5 cm margin whenever possible.[9,43] Others have shown that complete resection of an involved rib is not necessary, and that a 3 cm margin without resection of adjacent but clearly uninvolved ribs above and below the tumor mass is adequate.[35,36] Excising overlying chest wall muscles or subcutaneous tissue is rarely necessary.

Recent studies have documented that the incidence of local/regional recurrence in the setting of stage I carcinoma is much lower with a lobectomy than a segmental resection.[44] Furthermore, some studies have suggested that the postoperative pulmonary function tests performed 3 months after resection are not significantly different when comparing patients undergoing segmentectomy versus lobectomy. Whether or not these observations apply specifically in the setting of lung carcinomas invading the chest wall has not been addressed, but in most series, lobectomy is preferred in low-risk patients. Pneumonectomy with chest wall resection can be performed with acceptable perioperative morbidity and mortality, but the long-term results have been disappointing chiefly because of the development of distant metastases.[16,33]

A mediastinal lymph node dissection must be performed to properly and completely stage the carcinoma.[5,35] The involvement of mediastinal nodes has been widely recognized as an important prognostic factor.[37,39,40]

Reconstruction of the chest wall defect can be avoided if the defect is smaller than 5 cm in greatest diameter unless the patient has marginal pulmonary reserve. Defects between 5 and 10 cm warrant reconstruction, especially if the defect is anterior, lateral, or posterior below the scapula. Higher posterior defects of this size lie under the scapula and reconstruction can be avoided. Defects larger than 10 cm should be reconstructed but rarely occur in this clinical setting.

Although reconstruction using autogenous tissue, such as rib grafts and fascia lata, has been described, the advent of synthetic material such as Marlex, Prolene, and Gore-Tex has largely relegated these techniques to historical reference only.[43] Marlex has the advantage of tissue ingrowth into the interstices, presumably limiting the potential for long-term infections. In addition, a "Marlex sandwich" technique has been developed, whereby even large defects can be patched using a contoured prosthetic patch. This technique is particularly valuable in reconstructing very large defects after the resection of large primary chest wall tumors but is seldom necessary in this setting. Gore-Tex is water-proof and therefore preferable after pneumonectomy. This material is more pliable than Marlex and handles easily. Sutures should be passed through the folded edge of the Dualmesh (reinforced Gore-Tex) patch to minimize the risk of tearing the material. Intrapleural chest tubes are positioned, and the soft tissues of the chest wall are closed in the usual fashion. Chest wall drains are best avoided.

Postoperative Care

Prior to the widespread use of prosthetic patches, the major postoperative complication was pulmonary insufficiency manifest by either inability to clear secretions, or in some cases, ventilatory insufficiency. Vigorous chest physiotherapy and optimal pain management are the cornerstones of postoperative care. Aspiration bronchoscopy is often necessary to clear secretions but in exceptional circumstances, should postoperative ventilatory support may be necessary.

Seromas often form over the prosthesis, but the temptation to aspirate them to avoid an infection should be avoided. Antibiotic coverage is usually provided for only 48 hours unless a seroma is detected, in which case a 7-day course is indicated. If infection of the prosthesis is established, then management depends on the prosthetic material used and the size of the defect. Marlex mesh infections can be eradicated by antibiotics and drainage, providing time for tissue ingrowth. Prosthetic infections tend to wall off early, protecting the adjacent structures. The temptation to remove an infected prosthesis should be balanced against the potential consequences of a flail defect. If the defect is large and the patient is not toxic, a delay of 6 weeks before the removal of the prosthesis allows a fibrous capsule to form, providing an element of chest wall stability.

Prognosis

The overall five-year survival among patients undergoing a complete resection of a primary lung carcinoma invading the chest wall ranges from 15% to 40%.[7–9,11–13] Several reports have appeared about the importance of obtaining a complete resection. Patients undergoing "incomplete" resections rarely survive beyond 5 years despite the use of adjuvant therapy, including brachytherapy. Patients undergoing incomplete resections (including tumors adherent to the aorta or invading the vertebral bodies) should be analyzed separately from those undergoing complete resections.

Among those cases that underwent a complete resection, by far the single most important prognostic factor is the status of the regional and mediastinal nodes. In patients with T3N0 carcinomas, the five-year survival ranges from 22% to 56%. Patients with T3N1 tumors have a five-year survival of 0% to 33%. Predictably, the worst survival is seen in patients with T3N2 carcinomas, with a five-year survival of only 0% to 16%.[9,19,33]

Several other factors have been assessed for their prognostic value. Conflicting data exist regarding the depth of invasion of the chest wall, histology of the tumor, and the extent of the resection without a clear consensus. One study concluded that the depth of invasion into the chest wall had prognostic significance. It is generally recognized that tumors peripheral enough to require a chest wall resection yet involving central structures necessitating a pneumonectomy have a poor prognosis, regardless of their nodal status. Generally speaking, larger tumors have a worse prognosis. Age, gender, presenting symptom, and histologic classification have not been shown to affect survival.

Postoperative Adjuvant Therapy (see also Chapter 43)

In order to decrease the incidence of local recurrence, some surgeons have advocated the use of routine postoperative radiotherapy.[15] Several reports concluded that postoperative radiotherapy did not improve survival in those patients who had a complete resection.[7,16,39] Most centers, however, continue to advocate radiotherapy for patients in whom wide margins of resection are impossible (e.g., tumor abutting the spine), or in whom the margins of resection were microscopically positive.

The value of combination chemoradiotherapy delivered postoperatively is still debated. One large trial found that no apparent survival advantage was achieved by administering postoperative chemoradiotherapy to patients with T3N1 completely resected carcinomas.[33] When patients are found to have mediastinal nodal involvement (N2 nodes), additional therapy is often given, but without evidence that this treatment improves their long-term survival.

PANCOAST TUMORS

Introduction and Historical Perspective

Lung carcinomas that invade the apex of the thoracic cage merit consideration beyond those tumors invading the chest wall but sparing the apex for several reasons. First, the apex of the chest is difficult to assess using conventional chest radiographs, and carcinomas arising in this location are often overlooked. Second, proximity to the brachial plexus, the subclavian vessels, and the vertebral column make complete resection difficult, and wide margins of resection are seldom achieved, presenting certain technical challenges. Finally, because of the proximity of these structures, patients with these locally advanced tumors are almost always candidates for some form of adjuvant therapy.

The earliest reference to tumors invading the apex of the chest was made by Hare in 1838.[46] Although several other authors offered case histories of such an entity,[47,48] this entity gained much wider recognition with the publications of Pancoast,[49,50] wherein seven cases were discussed. The

degree of invasion of the chest wall can so overshadow the pulmonary component that this tumor was initially considered to be a new entity, arising from an embryonal epithelial rest—possibly arising from the fifth brachial pouch. In keeping with the belief that this entity was new (and specifically to distinguish it from the more common tumors arising in the lung and the chest wall), Pancoast initially offered the term "superior pulmonary sulcus" tumor. The superior sulcus is not a recognized anatomic feature of the lung or the chest wall.[51] Even though Tobias published data to the effect that these tumors were locally advanced pulmonary carcinomas, as early as 1932,[48] the view that these tumors represented a new entity was held for more than a decade. By 1946, several authors had presented additional data supporting the conclusion that at least some of these cases were lung carcinomas.[52,53] For these reasons, the term "superior sulcus tumor" has been rejected by some authorities.[54]

Until 1950, these tumors were considered to be unresectable for cure and palliated with external-beam radiotherapy. In 1954, Haas and colleagues reported on the experience of radiotherapy on "hopeless" cases with significant palliation of arm and shoulder pain and prolonged survival.[55] The radiosensitivity of these tumors was further documented by five-year survivors with external-beam radiotherapy alone.[56]

In 1950, Chardack and MacCallum performed the first successful resection of a Pancoast tumor, followed by 6,500 Gy of irradiation. The patient survived for more than 5 years, renewing interest in the role of surgical resection.[57] The use of such a combination of radiotherapy and surgery however, was accepted as standard only after the report of Shaw and colleagues in 1961.[58]

Clinical Presentation

Although not all patients with an apical tumor involving the chest wall present with a full-blown Pancoast clinical syndrome, most patients present with some clinical complaints. Detection of small, asymptomatic tumors in this region is hampered by difficulty in visualizing the apices by plain chest radiographs.

The most common presenting symptom is shoulder pain, which is often present for 6 months or more before the diagnosis is suspected. The pain is initially located along the vertebral border of the scapula. Headache is also common. The pain becomes constant and progressive as the T1 and the C8 nerve roots become entrapped. Pain and numbness now extends down the arm in the ulnar distribution affecting the forearm and the fourth and fifth fingers. The progression of the pain and the shift in pain distribution often leads the clinician to obtain the diagnostic chest radiograph.

In time, the patient may develop a Horner's syndrome, with ptosis and miosis. This clinical finding carries a poor prognosis because it usually signifies involvement of the vertebral column. In the latter stages, as the pain progressively worsens, the patient may characteristically support the affected elbow with the opposite arm to minimize traction on the brachial plexus. At this time, atrophy of the hypothenar muscles and weakness of the hand is easily appreciated. Weight loss and insomnia from pain are common findings, but cough and dyspnea are rare. Somewhat surprisingly, hemoptysis is not uncommon. Because of the location of the tumor, the primary tumor is rarely palpable. In latter stages, metastatic spread to a scalene node may render it palpable.

Preoperative Assessment

By plain chest radiograph, Pancoast tumors appear as a homogeneous density at the extreme apex of the chest. Apical lordotic views can be helpful,[59] but if clinical symptoms are present, a chest CT scan should be performed.[20,60] Classically, Pancoast tumors are located in the posterior aspect of the apex and usually spare the subclavian vessels until late in their course. However, tumors located more anteriorly have been identified with early involvement of the subclavian vessels. Arteriograms and venograms are occasionally indicated (Figures 39.5–39.6).

In several studies, magnetic resonance imaging (MRI) has been shown to have advantages over CT scan in the assessment of tumor invasion through the apical chest wall, with improved imaging of the subclavian vessels, the brachial plexus, the ribs, and the vertebral bodies.[27,28,60–62]

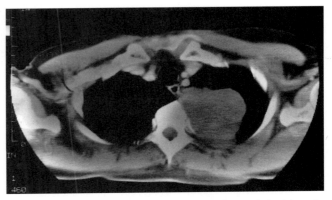

FIGURE 39.6. CT of the patient whose radiograph is shown in Figure 39.5. Note the absence of transverse process or vertebral body destruction.

The diagnosis should be established before embarking on therapy because several neoplasms and non-neoplastic masses can mimic apical lung carcinoma.[59] Neurogenic tumors of the posterior mediastinum or the brachial plexus,[63] thyroid masses, lymphoma,[64] and an aneurysm of the axillary or subclavian artery all must be considered in the differential diagnosis. Small cell carcinoma of the lung has been described in this location,[65] but its diagnosis must be accepted with caution because it may be confused with peripheral neuroectodermal tumors of the chest wall (Askin tumor), lymphoma, or plasmacytoma of the first or second ribs.[66,67] Staphylococcus aureus,[68] cryptococcsis,[69,70] aspergillus,[71] and actinomyces[72] apical pulmonary abscesses have all been reported to cause symptoms simulating Pancoast's syndrome.

Because the diagnosis can be established by flexible bronchoscopy in only 10% to 30% of cases, even when fluoroscopy is used, most surgeons have adopted percutaneous needle biopsy as the diagnostic procedure of choice.[73–77] Although this procedure can be performed using ultrasonography or biplane fluoroscopy, most lesions are biopsied under CT guidance.[75,78] A posterior approach is most popular,[76] but shallow or small lesions are sometimes approached using a transcervical route.

Similar to all lung cancers, accurate staging has been the cornerstone for rational therapeutic protocols.[79–83] Although the distinction between T3 and T4 is not clearly defined in the current classification system,[5] T3 describes tumors where invasion is limited to the parietal pleura, the ribs, and the intercostal muscles. Sensory changes limited to the T1 nerve root alone do not require that these be considered T4 tumors, especially if these symptoms resolve with preoperative radiotherapy and/or the nerve root can be spared at the time of resection. A tumor is classified as T4 by evidence of direct invasion of the vertebral bodies (including the presence of a Horner's syndrome), the presence of any motor dysfunction of the brachial plexus or any

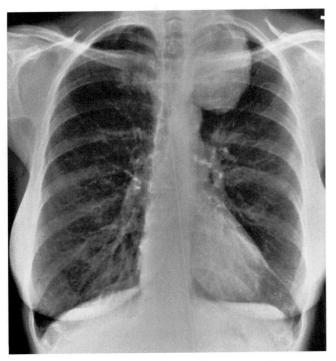

FIGURE 39.5. Chest radiograph revealing tumor in the superior sulcus. Patient presented with arm and shoulder pain.

of its branches, or involvement of the subclavian vessels. Because most patients who undergo surgical resection undergo some form of preoperative therapy (to which they can respond dramatically), the initial staging is based only on clinical judgement.

Many surgeons advocate nodal staging by routine preoperative mediastinoscopy in cases of superior sulcus lesions, whereas a few surgeons advocate mediastinoscopy only if the nodes are measured to be greater than 1.5 cm as measured by CT scan. CT scans of the chest are routinely performed to visualize the liver and the adrenal glands. A CT scan of the brain and nuclear bone scan are often performed to complete the staging protocol.

The presence of Horner's syndrome has clearly been recognized as a poor prognostic indicator. Nevertheless, long-term survival has been reported with aggressive surgical management. Although surgical resection of neoplasms invading the vertebral bodies or laminae has been described, this procedure is usually performed for palliation, and five-year survivors are rarely reported. Long-term survival has been reported in patients undergoing resections, including division of the T1 nerve root. However, tumors requiring a more extensive sacrifice of the brachial plexus carry a worse prognosis. Extended resections (utilizing an anterior approach) have been described for tumors abutting or with limited involvement of the subclavian vessels, with encouraging early follow-up results. However, encasement of the subclavian vessels or involvement of the subclavian artery at its origin from the aortic arch should still be approached with caution (see also Chapter 38).

Patients with metastatic disease limited to the ipsilateral mediastinal nodes (N2) should be considered for a protocol of preoperative chemo- and radiotherapy. Involvement of the contralateral nodes or supraclavicular nodal disease (N3) or the presence of metastatic disease preclude curative resection.

Role of Preoperative Therapy: Preoperative Radiotherapy versus Neoadjuvant Therapy

The early results of surgical resection alone were sufficiently discouraging that some surgeons believed that Pancoast tumors were categorically unresectable for cure. The natural history of this tumor was limited, with Herbut reporting that none of eight untreated patients survived beyond 8 months from the time of diagnosis.[53] Because all patients eventually become very symptomatic, most patients (even those with limited disease) were submitted for radiotherapy. In 1954, Haas et al.[55] reported significant palliation with occasional prolonged survival with external-beam radiation. Subsequently, five-year survivors were reported with radiotherapy alone.[55,84-87]

However, the first reported five-year survivor was documented in 1956 by Chardack and MacCallum in a patient who underwent surgical resection followed with 65 Gy irra-

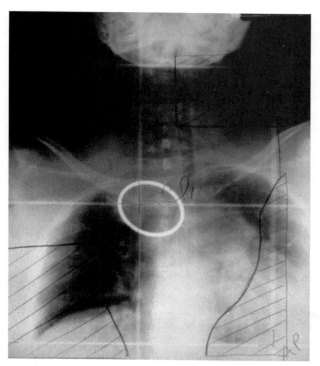

FIGURE 39.7. Typical radiation portal for a superior sulcus tumor. See text for details.

diation.[57] Subsequently, Shaw et al. reported their results with preoperative radiotherapy, followed by complete surgical resection.[58,88] Their aggressive surgical approach was based, in fact, on the observation that some patients (including those initially considered to have "unresectable" disease), can have a remarkable clinical response and diminution of the tumor mass with limited doses of preoperative radiotherapy. Their initial preoperative radiotherapy protocol was 3,000 cGy given in 10 consecutive days. Most current protocols give 200 cGy 5 days/week for each of 4 weeks, which is better tolerated. This treatment is followed by a four-week period to allow the patient to recover with respect to their nutritional status, as well as to heal their radiation-induced burn, which can occasionally cause ulceration of the skin (Figures 39.5–39.9). Also, additional time may be necessary to allow the erythema to subside prior to surgery.

In a review of the literature on the results of preoperative radiotherapy followed by surgical resection with intent to cure, complete resection was achieved in 70% of cases and was the most important prognostic factor.[89,90,92,94,95,98] Five-year survival ranges from 15% to 50%. The range in results can be attributed to the degree of preoperative selection. The most common cause of death was the development of distant metastatic disease, and the most common site was the brain, with bony metastases being the second most common.[82,85,96,97]

Because distant metastatic disease is an important cause

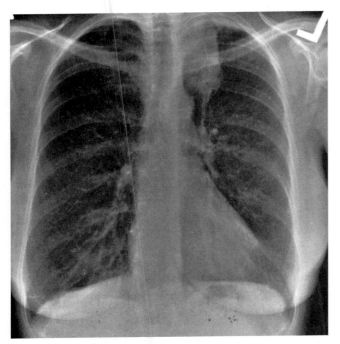

FIGURE 39.8. Chest radiograph before resection in the patient seen in Figures 39.5 and 39.6. Patient received preoperative external-beam radiotherapy.

from these protocols should help to define the role of neoadjuvant therapy.

Technical Considerations

A high posterolateral thoracotomy is performed, providing access to the chest wall by dividing the latissimus dorsi. The posterior aspect of the serratus anterior is also divided. Generally, the chest is opened though the fourth or fifth intercostal space, between the highest ribs not invaded by the tumor as judged by the preoperative chest radiograph and CT scan. The intercostal muscles are divided, and the pleural space is entered to allow for intraoperative assessment of resectability and the extent of resection with respect to the number of ribs and/or involvement of the vertebral bodies and subclavian vessels.

Once resectability has been assured, the skin incision is extended into the parascapular region. Division of the lower portion of the trapezius and rhomboid major and minor provides wider exposure to the upper thoracic spine and the posterior aspect of the upper ribs. The ribs judged to be invaded by the tumor are divided anteriorly. The subclavian vessels are identified and preserved, as are the phrenic and vagus nerves. Posterior dissection is started by dividing the rib where necessary to accomplish a complete resection. Often, the lowest rib can be divided at the costovertebral angle, sparing mobilization of the head of the rib off the vertebral column. The posterior dissection of higher ribs, however, is accomplished by mobilizing the neck of the rib off the transverse process utilizing a periosteal elevator. The head of the rib can then be elevated off the vertebral body (Figures 39.10–39.12).

of death in these patients after an apparent complete surgical resection, many surgeons have looked to chemotherapy to control micrometastatic disease, on the assumption that these patients have subclinical metastatic deposits at the time of presentation.[98–103] Another rationale for the introduction of chemotherapy into the preoperative radiotherapy regime has been the recognition that some chemotherapy drugs are radiosensitizing agents. Most notable on this list are cisplatin and VP-16, on which many protocols are based. Such a neoadjuvant preoperative combination approach has been the basis of current neoadjuvant protocols. The data

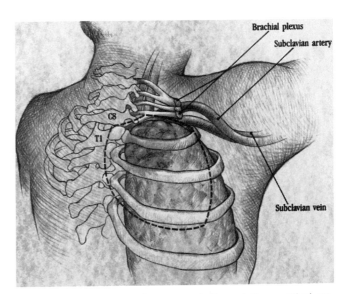

FIGURE 39.10. Schematic representation of the surgical approach to the superior sulcus tumor resection. (From McKneally MF. Cardiothoracic techniques. In: Burde PE, ed. *A pictorial review of surgical procedures.* Albany, NY: Learning Technology Incorporated, 1982, with permission.)

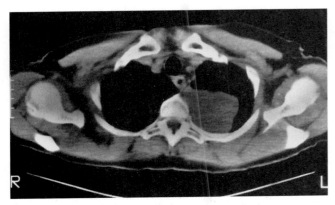

FIGURE 39.9. CT corresponding to the preoperative chest radiograph seen in Figure 39.8.

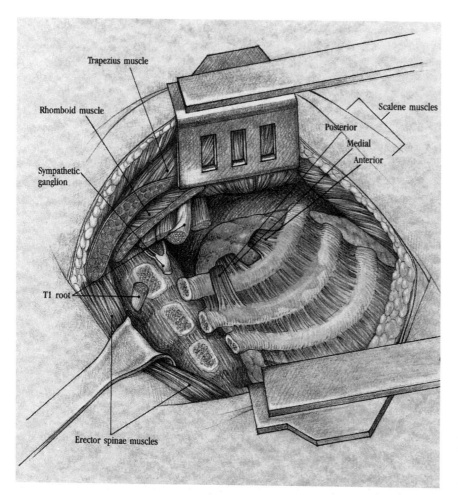

FIGURE 39.11. Schematic representation of *en bloc* resection of superior sulcus tumor. See text for details. (From McKneally MF. Cardiothoracic techniques. In: Burde PE, ed. *A pictorial review of surgical procedures.* Albany, NY: Learning Technology Incorporated, 1982, with permission.)

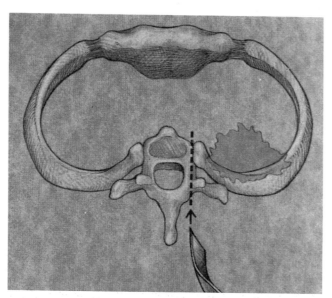

FIGURE 39.12. Use of the osteotome for the posterior margin. (From McKneally MF. Cardiothoracic techniques. In: Burde PE, ed. *A pictorial review of surgical procedures.* Albany, NY: Learning Technology Incorporated, 1982, with permission.)

If tumor is found to invade the vertebral column, then the transverse process (and even a portion of the vertebral body) can be resected at this stage using an osteotome (see also Chapter 38). Sparing the transverse process, and even the neck of the ribs posteriorly (provided it does not compromise the margin of resection), helps to minimize the risk of scoliosis. This is especially true when more than three ribs are resected. Once the posterior aspect of the first rib is divided, the specimen is considerably more mobile. At this point, the T1 nerve root is optimally exposed and spared or divided as necessary to accomplish a complete resection. The C8 nerve root may occasionally also have to be sacrificed. Care must be taken to secure the nerve roots with ligatures at the neural foramina to avoid troublesome leaks of cerebrospinal fluid. If such a leak is caused, it is best managed by patching the neural foramen with a piece of free muscle or erector spinae muscle tacked to the lateral aspect of the vertebral bodies. Opening the neural foramen in an attempt to directly oversew the dural tear is fraught with difficulty and is often unsuccessful. Care must also be taken to identify and ligate branches of the intercostal vessels, especially in the region of the neural foramina to avoid troublesome bleeding. If bleeding is encountered from the neural foramen, it is best controlled with bipolar electrocautery. Occasionally, the neural foramen has to be opened to visualize the vessel. The surgeon must resist the temptation to leave pledgets of Gelfoam in this region because there are case reports of paraplegia resulting from migration into the spinal canal.[104]

The hilar dissection is then performed, resulting in an *en bloc* specimen of lung and chest wall. When the chest wall involvement is bulky, it may occasionally be advantageous to perform the hilar dissection first to facilitate exposure to the posterior aspect of the first and second ribs. If the tumor cannot be dissected off the subclavian vessels, then it may be necessary to complete the resection and/or arterial reconstruction using an anterior approach (see also Chapter 38).

Some controversy exists regarding the optimal pulmonary resection. Some authors believe that limited resections (either wedge or segmental resections) are adequate.[105] In fact, at least two studies suggest that no statistically significant survival advantage is achieved by performing a lobectomy when compared to a more limited pulmonary resection.[44,106] However, Ginsberg et al. found a lower local/regional recurrence rate and a survival advantage in those patients who underwent a lobectomy.[107] All patients undergoing a curative resection should have a mediastinal node dissection.

Because the resulting chest wall defect lies under the scapula, reconstruction is not necessary unless more than three ribs are resected. When a chest wall mesh is used, care must be taken to avoid compromise of the subclavian vessels and the brachial plexus. This goal is best accomplished by avoiding sutures along the superior margin of the patch. The incision is closed in the usual fashion.

Prognostic Factors after Resection with Preoperative Irradiation

Over the last 25 years, many potential prognostic factors have been assessed, including completeness of resection, TNM stage, and histologic evaluation. Overall, approximately 75% of patients in whom a curative operation is intended were found to have a "complete resection," the rest being found to have a microscopically positive margin. This statistic is not surprising given the technical difficulties facing the surgeon. The most common sites for positive margins are the brachial plexus, vertebral bodies, neural foramina, and the subclavian vessels. In this setting, some surgeons have advocated the use of brachytherapy to improve local control.[108,109] However, according to Ginsberg et al., there appears to be little difference in the survival of patients undergoing incomplete resections compared to those patients having no resection even with the use of brachytherapy.[110] Two other studies also report a significantly worse two-year survival in patients undergoing incomplete resections.[96,111] The completeness of the resection is a statistically significant and independent prognostic factor for five-year survival, and every attempt should be made to achieve negative microscopic margins.

Not surprisingly, the stage of the carcinoma has also been found to carry prognostic significance. Factors that determine that the tumor is T4 (i.e., subclavian vessel involvement, Horner's syndrome, and vertebral body involvement) have all been found to negatively impact the five-year survival. Limited involvement of the vertebral bodies (with or without Horner's syndrome) and/or the subclavian vessels does not preclude a complete resection, however, and long-term survivors have been reported.[94,105,112–114] The size of the tumor and presence or absence of bony destruction of the ribs by the tumor have not been clearly identified to be significant prognostic factors, but one study found that the depth of invasion into the chest wall did correlate with prognosis.[45]

Involvement of the mediastinal nodes has also been identified as a poor prognostic factor.[35,94,95,108,110,112,115] According to Ginsberg et al., the five-year survival in patients undergoing complete resection with N0,N1 disease is 46% compared to 15% in a carefully selected cohort of patients found to have N2,N3 disease and offered combined preoperative radiotherapy followed by complete resection.[110] In other series, patients with N2 or N3 disease either were not offered surgery or underwent resections that were determined to be incomplete. Somewhat ironically, experience at Memorial Sloan-Kettering cancer center suggests that patients with metastatic disease limited to the ipsilateral supraclavicular (N3) node (in the absence of any other nodal metastases) have a better survival than patients found to have mediastinal (N2) nodal metastases.[108,110] Further refinements of the TNM staging classification may be necessary to address this special issue. The mere presence of N2 or N3 nodal disease, however, does not preclude a complete resection, and five-year survivors have been reported.

Survival and Patterns of Recurrence After Curative Resection

The overall five-year survival statistics from various centers reporting over the last 15 years range from 21% to 68%.[82,96,116] In 1987, Shahian et al. reported a 68.6% five-year survival in a highly selected subgroup of patients, who underwent a complete resection of T3N0 tumor and both preoperative and postoperative radiotherapy.[115] Most report a five-year survival, even in the most favorable subset of patients, of 30% to 40%.

Several studies have documented the patterns of recurrence and the survival of patients undergoing curative resections. Local/regional recurrence has been documented to occur in as many as 60% to 70% of cases according to Ginsberg et al.[110] The apical chest wall is often the first site of recurrence. Although this pattern is a reflection of the limitation of the chest wall resection margins, and is an important cause of morbidity, patients are more likely to die from systemic metastases. The most common site of distant metastasis is the brain, accounting for 40% to 80% of systemic recurrences.[83,87,90,96,108,110] According to several authors, bony metastases are the second most common site.[82,90,108]

Alternative Radiotherapy Strategies

In view of the disappointingly high local/regional recurrence rate after preoperative irradiation, alternative radiotherapy strategies have been investigated. Attar et al. reported that increasing the preoperative radiation dose to 55 Gy was associated with wound healing problems (including a 23% incidence of bronchopleural fistula) and a 15% operative mortality.[103] Although Fuller et al. had far fewer complications, higher doses of external-beam irradiation do not seem to improve resectability or survival.[82] Brachytherapy has also been used in an attempt to decrease the incidence of local/regional recurrence after complete resection while minimizing the risk of wound healing problems.[108,109] However, upon reviewing the data, Ginsberg et al. concluded that there was no apparent benefit either with respect to local/regional control or long-term survival after a complete resection.[110] Brachytherapy should be considered, however, if the patient had been explored, anticipating a complete resection, but an incomplete resection had to be performed. If an incomplete resection is inevitable, the patient should not undergo a surgical procedure simply to debulk the tumor and implant brachytherapy sources because this strategy does not provide the patient with better local control or long-term survival when compared to the results of external-beam radiotherapy alone.[110]

Postoperative radiation has been given usually in conjunction with preoperative irradiation.[115,117,118] Interpretation of the results is difficult at best. Most surgeons believe that giving additional postoperative radiotherapy has not been shown to provide better local/regional control or survival advantage after a complete resection. A somewhat atypical but encouraging report was issued by Hagan et al., who gave 14 patients with close or even positive resection margins postoperative radiotherapy. Eleven had no evidence of local/regional recurrence and seven were five-year survivors.[119]

Sundaresean et al. have explored the value of attempting resection prior to radiotherapy in patients with locally advanced tumors, including patients with spinal cord involvement and extensive brachial plexopathy. Although brachytherapy was used, as well as postoperative radiotherapy, predictably poor results were reported because most patients underwent an incomplete palliative resection, in some cases with gross residual and/or metastatic tumor.[118]

Even if the patient is found to have undergone an incomplete resection, with only a microscopically positive margin, the prognosis is not statistically different from those patients who do not undergo a resection, with a two-year survival of 15%. Analysis of this population of patients is poor, but the value of postoperative radiotherapy and/or brachytherapy is questionable. Few believe that additional radiotherapy after an incomplete resection offers any benefit.

The role of radiotherapy alone in doses of 50 to 70 Gy has been studied by some, with two-year survival reported to be high as 29%. Few consider the results to rival those of combined radiation therapy and surgery. Some surgeons have reported on the results of combining hyperthermia and radiotherapy, in an attempt to improve local control.[120] Others have investigated the role of hyperfractionated radiotherapy, but the results have been inconclusive.[121]

SUMMARY

Management of lung carcinoma invading the chest wall has undergone slow but steady improvement over the last 25 years. This advance has been due, in part, to improved materials available for reconstruction, as well as experience in using them. The treatment of apical carcinomas invading the chest wall presents special technical challenges and remains one of the few clinical scenarios where preoperative irradiation impacted on the resectability and the long-term survival. New techniques have been forged to allow resection of apical carcinomas involving the subclavian vessels, and preliminary long-term survival statistics are encouraging. The current limits of resectability continue to be extensive involvement of the thoracic spine, the subclavian vessels, or the brachial plexus. Current protocols continue to explore the role of adjuvant preoperative chemoradiotherapy.

REFERENCES

1. Chamberlain M, McNeill TM, Parnassa P, et al. Bronchogenic carcinoma: an aggressive surgical attitude. *J Thorac Cardiovasc Surg* 1959;38:727.
2. Coleman FP. Primary carcinoma of the lung with invasion of the ribs. Pneumonectomy and simultaneous resection of the chest wall. *Ann Surg* 1947;126:156.
3. Meade RH. Palliative resection for cancer of the lung. In: *Proceedings of the Second National Cancer Conference.* Chicago, American Cancer Society. 1952;2:935.
4. Gronqvist YKJ, Clagett OT, McDonald JR. Involvement of the thoracic wall in bronchogenic carcinoma. *J Thorac Surg* 1957; 33:487.
5. Mountain CF. A new international staging system for lung cancer. *Chest* 1986;89:225S.
6. Jamieson MPG, Walbaum PR, McCormack RJM. Surgical management of bronchial carcinoma invading the chest wall. *Thorax* 1979;34:612.
7. Paone JF, Spees EK, Newton CG, et al. An appraisal of en bloc resection of peripheral bronchogenic carcinoma involving the thoracic wall. *Chest* 1982;81:203.
8. Janni A, Santini P, Mussi A, et al. Results of en bloc resections for lung cancer. *Tumori* 1984;70:245.

9. Allen MS, Mathisen DJ, Grillo HC, et al. Bronchogenic carcinoma with chest wall invasion. *Ann Thorac Surg* 1991;51:948.

10. McCaughan BC, Martini N, Bains MS, et al. Chest wall invasion in carcinoma of the lung. Therapeutic and prognostic implications. *J Thorac Cardiovasc Surg* 1985;89:836.

11. Casillas M, Paris F, Tarrazona V, et al. Surgical treatment of lung carcinoma involving chest wall. *Eur J Cardiothorac Surg* 1989;3:425.

12. Ricci C, Rendina EA, Venuta F. En bloc resection for T3 bronchogenic carcinoma with chest wall invasion. *Eur J Cardiothorac Surg* 1987;1:23.

13. Burnard RJ, Martini N, Beattie EJ. The value of resection in tumors involving the chest wall. *J Thorac Cardiovasc Surg* 1974;68:530.

14. Lopez L, Pujol JL, Varela A, et al. Surgical treatment of stage III non-small cell bronchogenic carcinoma involving the chest wall. *Scand J Thorac Cardiovasc Surg* 1992;26:129.

15. Patterson GA, Ilves R, Ginsberg RJ, et al. The value of adjuvant radiotherapy in pulmonary and chest wall resection for bronchogenic carcinoma. *Ann Thorac Surg* 1982;34:692.

16. Geha AS, Bernatz PE, Woolner LB. Bronchogenic carcinoma involving the thoracic wall. Surgical treatment and prognostic significance. *J Thorac Cardiovas Surg* 1967;54:394.

17. Ramsay HE, Cliffton EE. Chest wall resection for primary carcinoma of the lung. *Ann Surg* 1968;167:342.

18. Grillo HC, Greenberg JJ, Wilkins EW. Resection of bronchogenic carcinoma involving the thoracic wall. *J Thorac Cardiovasc Surg* 1966;51:417.

19. Ratto GB, Piacenza G, Frola C, et al. Chest wall involvement by lung cancer: computed tomographic detection and results of operation. *Ann Thorac Surg* 1991;51:182.

20. Glazer HHS, Duncan-Meyer J, Aronberg DJ, et al. Pleural and chest wall invasion in bronchogenic carcinoma: CT evaluation. *Radiology* 1985;157:191.

21. Yokoi K, Mori K, Miyazawa N, et al. Tumor invasion of the chest wall and mediastinum in lung cancer: evaluation with pneumothorax CT. *Radiology* 1991;181:147.

22. Watanabe A, Shimokata K, Saka H, et al. Chest CT combined with artificial pneumothorax: value in determining origin and extent of tumor. *AJR* 1991;156:707.

23. Murata K, Takahashi M, Mori M, et al. Chest wall and mediastinal invasion by lung cancer: evaluation with multisection expiratory dynamic CT. *Radiology* 1994;191:251.

24. Suzuki N, Saitoh T, Kitamura S. Tumor invasion of the chest wall in lung cancer: diagnosis with US. *Radiology* 1993;187:39.

25. Webb WR. The role of magnetic resonance imaging in the assessment of patients with lung cancer: a comparison with computed tomography. *J Thorac Imaging* 1989;4:65.

26. Padovani BP, Mouroux J, Seksik L, et al. Chest wall invasion by bronchogenic carcinoma: evaluation with MR imaging. *Radiology* 1993;187:33.

27. Haggar AM, Pearlberg JL, Froelich JW, et al. Chest-wall invasion by carcinoma of the lung: detection by MR imaging. *AJR* 1987;148:1075.

28. Musset D, Grenier P, Carette MF, et al. Primary lung cancer staging: prospective comparative study of MR imaging with CT. *Radiology* 1986;160:607.

29. Swensen SJ, Ehman RL, Brown LR. Magnetic resonance imaging of the thorax. *J Thorac Imag* 1989;4:19.

30. Sinner WN. Pulmonary neoplasms diagnosed with transthoracic needle biopsy. *Cancer* 1979;43:1533.

31. Fry W. Needle biopsy for the diagnosis of intrathoracic lesion: transthoracic needle biopsy. In: Grillo H and Eschapasse H, eds. *Controversies in thoracic surgery.* Philadelphia: WB Saunders, 1986;87.

32. Nakano N, Yasumitsu T, Kotake Y, et al. Preoperative histologic diagnosis of chest wall invasion by lung cancer using ultrasonically guided biopsy. *J Thorac Cardiovasc Surg* 1994;107:891.

33. Van Velzen E, de la Riviere AB, Elbers HJ, et al. Type of lymph node involvement and survival in pathologic N1 stage III non-small cell lung carcinoma. *Ann Thorac Surg* 1999;76:903.

34. Albertucci M, DeMeester TR, Rothberg M, et al. Surgery and the management of peripheral lung tumors adherent to the pleura. *J Thorac Cardiovasc Surg* 1992;103:8.

35. Miller JD, Gorenstein LA, Patterson GA. Staging: the key to rational management of lung cancer. *Ann Thorac Surg* 1992;53:170.

36. Pairolero PC, Trastek VF, Payne WS. Treatment of bronchogenic carcinoma with chest wall invasion. *Surg Clin N Am* 1987;67:959.

37. McCaughan BC. Primary lung cancer invading the chest wall. *Curr Prosp Thorac Oncol* 1994;4:17.

38. Trastek VF, Pairolero PC, Piehler JM, et al. En bloc (non-chest wall) resection for bronchogenic carcinoma with parietal fixation. *J Thorac Cardiovasc Surg* 1984;87:352.

39. Piehler JM, Pairlero PC, Weiland LH, et al. Bronchogenic carcinoma with chest wall invasion: factors affecting survival following en bloc resection. *Ann Thorac Surg* 1982;34:684.

40. Carrel T, Nachhbur B, Veraguth P. En bloc resection for bronchogenic carcinoma with chest wall invasion. Value of pre-operative radiotherapy. *Eur J Cardiothorac Surg* 1990;4:534.

41. Eagan RT, Lee RE, Frytak S, et al. Thoracic radiation therapy and qadriamycin/cisplatin containing chemotherapy for locally advanced non-small-cell bronchogenic carcinoma. *Cancer Clin Trials* 1981;2:381.

42. Albain K, Hoffman PC, Little AG, et al. Pleural involvement in stage III M0 non-small-cell bronchogenic carcinoma. A need to differentiate subtypes. *Am J Clin Oncol* 1986;9:255.

43. McCormack PM, Bains MS, Martini N, et al. Methods of skeletal reconstruction following resection of lung carcinoma invading the chest wall. *Surg Clin N Am* 1987;67:979.

44. Warren WH, Faber LP. Segmentectomy versus lobectomy in patients with stage I pulmonary carcinoma. Five-year survival and patterns of intrathoracic recurrence. *J Thorac Cardiovasc Surg* 1994;107:1087.

45. Mishina H, Suemasu K, Yoneyama T, et al. Surgical pathology and prognosis of the combined resection of chest wall and lung in lung cancer. *Jap J Clin Oncol* 1978;8:161.

46. Hare ES. Tumor involving certain nerves. (Letter) *London Med Gaz* 1838;1:16.

47. Rialdoni A. An Fac Med Montevideo 1918 as quoted by Carneiro JF. Manifestacoes clinicas do cancer bronquico. *An Fac Med Porto Alegre* 1099;19:77.

48. Tobias JW. Sindrome apico-costo-vertebral dolorosa por tumor apexiano: su valor diagnostico en el cancer promitivo del pulmonar. *Rev Med Lat Am* 1932;17:1522.

49. Pancoast HK. Importance of careful roentgen-ray investigations of apical chest tumors. *JAMA* 1924;83:1407.

50. Pancoast HK. Superior pulmonary sulcus tumor: tumor characterized by pain, Horner's syndrome, destruction of bone and atrophy of the hand muscles. *JAMA* 1932;99:1391.

51. Teixeira JP. Concerning the Pancoast tumor: where is the superior sulcus? *Ann Thorac Surg* 1938;35:577.

52. James I, Pagel W. Miniature scar-carcinoma of the lung and "upper sulcus tumous" of Pancoast. *Br J Surg* 1944;32:85.

53. Herbut PA, Watson JS. Tumor of the thoracic inlet producing the Pancoast syndrome. A report of seventeen cases and a review of the literature. *Arch Pathol* 1946;42:88.

54. Spencer H. *Pathology of the lung (excluding pulmonary tuberculosis),* 2nd ed. Oxford: Pergamon, 1968;2:849.

55. Haas LL, Harvey RA, Langer SS. Radiation management of otherwise hopeless thoracic neoplasms. *JAMA* 1954;154:323.

56. Fry WA, Carpenter JWJ, Adams WE. Superior sulcus tumor with 14-year survival. *Arch Surg* 1967;94:142.
57. Chardack WM, MacCallum JD. Pancoast tumor: five-year survival without recurrence or metastases following radical resection and postoperative irradiation. *J Thorac Cardiovasc Surg* 1956;31:535.
58. Shaw RR, Paulson DL, Kee JL, Jr. Treatment of the superior sulcus tumor by irradiation followed by resection. *Ann Surg* 1961;154:29.
59. Simon H, Moon AC. Pitfalls in the diagnosis of Pancoast tumors. *Radiology* 1982;82:235.
60. Heelan RT, Demas BE, Caravelli JF, et al. Superior sulcus tumors: CT and MR imaging. *Radiology* 1989;170:637.
61. Pennes DR, Glazer GM, Wimbish KJ, et al. Chest wall invasion by lung cancer: limitations of CT evaluation. *AJR* 1985;144:507.
62. McCloud TC, Filion RB, Edelman RR, et al. MR imaging of superior sulcus carcinoma. *J Comput Assist Tomogr* 1989;13:233.
63. Horowitz J, Kline DG, Keller SM. Schwannoma of the brachial plexus mimicking an apical lung tumor. *Ann Thorac Surg* 1991;52:555.
64. Mills PR, Han LY, Dick R, et al. Pancoast syndrome caused by a high grade B cell lymphoma. *Thorax* 1994;49:92.
65. Johnson DH, Hainsworth JD, Greco FA. Pancoast's syndrome and small cell lung cancer. *Chest* 1982;82:602.
66. Warren WH, Gould VE. Differential diagnosis of small cell neuroendocrine carcinoma of the lung. *Chest Surg Clinics N Am* 1997;7:49.
67. Chen KT, Padmanbhan A. Pancoast syndrome caused by extramedullary plasmacytoma. *J Surg Oncol* 1983;24:117.
68. Gallagher KJ, Jeffrey RR, Kerr KM, et al. Pancoast syndrome: an unusual complication of pulmonary infection by Staphylococcus aureus. *Ann Thorac Surg* 1992;53:903.
69. Ziomek S, Weinstein W, Margulies, et al. Primary pulmonary cryptococcus presenting as a superior sulcus tumor. *Ann Thorac Surg* 1992;53:892.
70. Mitchell DH, Sorrell TC. Pancoast's syndrome due to pulmonary infection with Cryptococcus neoformans variety gattii. *Clin Infect Dis* 1992;14:1142.
71. Simpson FG, Morgan M, Cooke NJ. Pancoast's syndrome associated with invasive aspergillosis. *Thorax* 1986;41:156.
72. Stanaley SL, Jr, Lusk RH. Thoracic actinomycosis presenting as a brachial plexus syndrome. *Thorax* 1985;40:1985.
73. Maxfield RA, Aranda CP. The role of fiberoptic bronchoscopy and transbronchial biopsy in the diagnosis of Pancoast's tumor. *NY State J Med* 1987;87:326.
74. Krumpe PE. Diagnostic approaches to Pancoast's syndrome. *NY State J Med* 1987;87:326.
75. Siderys H, Pittman JN. Percutaneous needle biopsy of the lung in cases of superior sulcus tumors. *J Thorac Cardiovasc Surg* 1967;53:716.
76. Walls WJ, Thornbury JR, Naylor B. Pulmonary needle aspiration biopsy in the diagnosis of Pancoast tumors. *Radiology* 1974;111:99.
77. Paulson DL, Weed TE, Rian RL. Cervical approach for percutaneous needle biopsy of Pancoast tumors. *Ann Thorac Surg* 1985;39:586.
78. Yang P-C, Lee L-N, Luh K-T, et al. Ultrasonography of Pancoast tumor. *Chest* 1988;94:124.
79. Stanford W, Barnes RP, Tucker AR. Influence of staging in superior sulcus (Pancoast) tumors of the lung. *Ann Thorac Surg* 1980;29:406.
80. Paulson DL. The importance of defining location and staging of superior pulmonary sulcus tumors. *Ann Thorac Surg* 1973;15:549.
81. Attar S, Miller JE, Satterfield J, et al. Pancoast's tumor: irradiation or surgery? *Ann Thorac Surg* 1979;28:578.
82. Fuller DB, Chambers JS. Superior sulcus tumors: combined modality. *Ann Thorac Surg* 1994;57:1133.
83. Miller JI, Mansour KA, Hatcher CR, et al. Carcinoma of the superior pulmonary sulcus. *Ann Thorac Surg* 1979;28:44.
84. Hepper NGG, Herskovic T, Witten DM, et al. Thoracic inlet tumors. *Ann Intern Med* 1966;64:979.
85. Hilaris BS, Martini N, Wong GY, et al. Treatment of superior sulcus tumor (Pancoast tumor). *Surg Clin N Am* 1987;67:965.
86. van Houtte P, MacLennan I, Poulter C, et al. External radiation in the management of superior sulcus tumor. *Cancer* 1984;54:223.
87. Komaki R, Mountain CF, Holbert JM, et al. Superior sulcus tumors: treatment selection and results for 85 patients without metastasis (M0) at presentation. *Int J Radiat Oncol Biol Phys* 1990;19:31.
88. Shaw RR. Pancoast's tumor. *Ann Thorac Surg* 1984;37:343.
89. Wright CD, Moncure AC, Shepard JO, et al. Superior sulcus lung tumors: results of combined treatment (irradiation and radical resection). *J Thorac Cardiovasc Surg* 1987;94:69.
90. Komaki R, Roh J, Cox JD, et al. Superior sulcus tumors: results of irradiation of 36 patients. *Cancer* 1981;48:1563.
91. Komaki R. Preoperative radiation therapy for superior sulcus lesions. *Chest Surg Clin North Am* 1991;1:13.
92. Okubo K, Wada H, Fukuse, et al. Treatment of Pancoast tumors. Combined irradiation and radical resection. *Thorac Cardiovasc Surg* 1995;43:284.
93. Muscolino G, Valente M, Andreani S. Pancoast tumors: clinical assessment and long term results of combined radiosurgical treatment. *Thorax* 1997;52:284.
94. Sartori F, Rea F, Calabro F, et al. Carcinoma of the superior pulmonary sulcus. Results of irradiation and radical resection. *J Cardiovasc Thorac Surg* 1992;104:679.
95. Paulson DL. Carcinomas in the superior pulmonary sulcus. *J Thorac Cardiovasc Surg* 1975;70:1095.
96. Maggi G, Casadio C, Pischedda F, et al. Combined radiosurgical treatment of Pancoast tumor. *Ann Thorac Surg* 1994;57:198.
97. Komaki R, Derus SB, Perez-Tamayo C, et al. Brain metastasis in patients with superior sulcus tumors. *Cancer* 1987;59:1649.
98. Roth JA, Fossella F, Komaki R, et al. A randomized trial comparing perioperative chemotherapy and surgery with surgery alone in resectable stage IIIA non-small-cell lung cancer. *J Natl Cancer Inst* 1994;86:673.
99. Rosell R, Gomez-Codina J, Camps C, et al. A randomized trial comparing preoperative chemotherapy plus surgery with surgery alone in patients with non-small-cell lung cancer. *N Engl J Med* 1994;330:153.
100. Rusch VW, Albain KS, Crowley JJ, et al. Surgical resection of Stage IIIA and Stage IIIB non-small-cell lung cancer after concurrent induction chemoradiotherapy: a Southwest Oncology Group trial. *J Thorac Cardiovasc Surg* 1993;105:97.
101. Macchiarini P, Chapelier AR, Monnet I, et al. Extended operations after induction therapy for stage IIIb (T4) non-small cell lung cancer. *Ann Thorac Surg* 1994;57:966.
102. Faber LP, Kittle CF, Warren WH, et al. Preoperative chemotherapy and irradiation for stage III non-small cell lung cancer. *Ann Thorac Surg* 1989;47:669.
103. Attar S, Krasna MJ, Sonett JR, et al. Superior sulcus (Pancoast) tumor: experience with 105 patients. *Ann Thorac Surg* 1998;66:193.
104. Short HD. Paraplegia associated with the use of oxidized cellulose in posterolateral thoracotomy incisions. *Ann Thorac Surg* 1990;50:178.
105. Dartevelle PG, Chapelier AR, Macchiarini P, et al. Anterior transcervical-thoracic approach for radical resection of tumors

invading the thoracic inlet. *J Thorac Cardiovasc Surg* 1993;105: 1025.

106. Read RC, Yoder G, Schaeffer RC. Survival after conservative resection for T1N0M0 non-small cell lung cancer. *Ann Thorac Surg* 1990;49:391.

107. Ginsberg RJ, Rubenstein LV for the Lung Cancer Study Group. Randomized trial of lobectomy versus limited resection for T1N0 non-small cell lung cancer. *Ann Thorac Surg* 1995;60: 615.

108. Hilaris BS, Nori D, Beattie E, et al. Value of perioperative brachytherapy in the management of non-small cell carcinoma of the lung. *Int J Radiation Oncology Biol Phys* 1983;9:1161.

109. Nori D, Sundaresan N, Bains M, et al. Bronchogenic carcinoma with invasion of the spine. *JAMA* 1982;248:2491.

110. Ginsberg RJ, Martini N, Zaman M, et al. Influence of surgical resection and brachytherapy in the management of superior sulcus tumor. *Ann Thorac Surg* 1994;57:1440.

111. Niwa H, Masaoka A, Yamakawa Y, et al. Surgical therapy for apical invasive lung cancer: different approaches according to tumor location. *Lung Cancer* 1993;10:63.

112. Anderson TM, Moy PM, Holmes EC. Factors affecting survival in superior sulcus tumors. *J Clin Oncol* 1986;4:1598.

113. Ginsberg RJ. Surgery for higher stage lung cancer. *Chest Surg Clinics North Am* 1991;1:61.

114. Dartevelle PG. Extended operations for the treatment of lung cancer. *Ann Thorac Surg* 1997;63:12.

115. Shahian DM, Neptune WB, Ellis FH, Jr. Pancoast tumors: improved survival with preoperative and postoperative radiotherapy. *Ann Thorac Surg* 1987;43:32.

116. Neal CR, Amdur RJ, Mendenhall WM, et al. Pancoast tumor: radiation therapy alone versus preoperative radiation therapy and surgery. *Int J Radiation Oncology Biol Phy* 1991;21:651.

117. Ricci C, Rendina EA, Venuta F, et al. Superior pulmonary sulcus tumors: radical resection and palliative treatment. *Int Surg* 1989;74:175.

118. Sundaresan N, Hilaris BS, Martini N. The combined neuro-surgical-thoracic management of superior sulcus tumors. *J Clin Oncol* 1987;5:1739.

119. Hagan MP, Choi NC, Mathisen DJ, et al. Superior sulcus lung tumors: impact of local control on survival. *J Thorac Cardiovasc Surg* 1999;117:1086.

120. Terashima H, Nakata H, Yamashita S, et al. Pancoast tumor treated with radiotherapy and hyperthermia: a preliminary study. *Int J Hypertherm* 1991;7:417.

121. Jeremic B, Shibanmoto Y, Acimovic L, et al. Randomized trial of hyperfractionated radiation therapy with or without concurrent chemotherapy for stage III non-small-cell lung cancer. *J Clin Oncol* 1995;13:452.

40

SURGICAL MANAGEMENT OF SECOND PRIMARY AND METASTATIC LUNG CANCER

JEMI OLAK
MARK K. FERGUSON

Surgical management of lung cancer that has metastasized to other sites has for the most part been confined to selected patients with metastasis to other pulmonary segments or lobes, or to the brain. Patterns of failure for patients with surgically treated lung cancer are changing due to earlier detection, the use of more rigorous staging procedures, and the use of induction and adjuvant therapies. Reports of surgical management of metastatic disease to the liver, pleura, or bone from primary lung cancer are scarce, whereas reports of surgical management of metastatic adrenal disease are increasing.[1–4] This chapter reviews the surgical treatment of multiple primary lung cancer (both synchronous and metachronous) as well as lung cancer which has metastasized to distant sites. The chapter also provides guidelines to the approach and management of these problems.

OTHER PULMONARY LESIONS

Introduction

The incidence of multiple primary lung cancers has been estimated to be between 0.8% and 7.6%.[5–10] A review of English literature published between 1931 and 1983 identified 382 cases of multiple primary lung cancers from a total of 12,685 patients with lung cancer, an incidence of 1.7%.[10] Subsequent reports have identified 229 additional cases from among 10,791 lung cancer patients, increasing the overall incidence to 2.1% (Table 40.1). An autopsy study of 255 patients who died of bronchogenic carcinoma, however, revealed multiple primary lung cancers in 3.5% using strict criteria and 14% using less strict criteria.[11] The true incidence of multiple primary lung cancers has been hard to estimate because the criteria used to establish this diagnosis have been difficult to agree upon. In addition, the incidence varies depending upon the rigor with which a second primary carcinoma is sought during both the initial clinical staging and the assessment of the pathological specimen.

The efficacy of therapy and the length of patient survival also impact on the incidence of multiple primary lung cancer.[5]

Synchronous Pulmonary Tumors

The incidence of synchronous primary lung cancer is sufficiently low that the simultaneous discovery of two pulmonary tumors mandates careful consideration of the diagnostic possibilities listed in Table 40.2. Distinguishing among synchronous primary lung cancers, a primary lung cancer with a metastasis, and two metastases from an extrathoracic carcinoma can be difficult.

Synchronous Primary Carcinomas of Lung
The incidence of synchronous primary carcinomas of the lung is reported to be between 0.26 and 1.33% (Table 40.3).[6,7,9,11,12] The average incidence among 17,567 patients with lung cancer was 0.52%, although slightly different criteria were used to determine the incidence in individual reports. Synchronous carcinomas of the lung (Figure 40.1) are diagnosed less commonly than metachronous carcinomas, the former comprising between 11% and 45% of all cases of multiple bronchogenic carcinomas (Table 40.4).[6,7,9,13–15]

In 1889 Billroth suggested that a diagnosis of two primary tumors could be made only if they were anatomically or temporally separate, of different histologic type, and if each produced its own metastasis.[16] Beyreuther reported the first case of synchronous bilateral primary lung cancers in 1924.[17]

Controversy continues to be associated with the definition of synchronous primary lung cancer. Chaudhuri suggested that the tumors needed to be of different cell types.[18] This definition clearly underestimates the true incidence of synchronous primary lung cancer and incorrectly labels some patients as having stage IV disease. Warren and Gates,

TABLE 40.1. INCIDENCE OF MULTIPLE PRIMARY LUNG CANCERS

Author (Year)	Patients with Lung Cancer	Patients with Multiple Primaries (%)
Bewtra (1984)[10]	12,685	382 (1.7)
Mathisen (1984)[6]	341	26 (7.6)
Wu (1987)[7]	3,815	30 (0.8)
Verhagen (1989)[8]	1,004	32 (3.2)
Deschamps (1990)[9]	9,611	117 (1.2)
Okunaka (1991)[5]	1,180	24 (2.0)
Total	28,636	611 (2.1)

TABLE 40.3. INCIDENCE OF SYNCHRONOUS PRIMARY LUNG CANCER

Author (Year)	Lung Cancer Patients	Synchronous Lung Cancer Patients (%)
Mathisen (1984)[6]	2,041	10 (0.48)
Ferguson (1985)[12]	2,100	28 (1.33)
Wu (1987)[7]	3,815	10 (0.26)
Deschamps (1990)[9]	9,611	44 (0.46)
Total	17,567	92 (0.52)

on the other hand, suggested that synchronous lesions should be bilateral.[19] This definition also underestimates the true incidence of synchronous disease. In an effort to standardize the reporting of synchronous primary lung cancers, Martini and Melamed proposed criteria for their classification in 1975 (Table 40.5).[20] These criteria have been adapted with minor modifications by several authors in publications since that time.[6–9,12]

One Primary Lung Carcinoma and One Metastasis

This category includes patients with a primary lung cancer and a metastasis to a different lobe. According to the 1997 lung cancer staging revision of the American Joint Commission on Cancer (AJCC) and the Union Internationale Contre Cancer (UICC), these patients are considered to have M1 disease. Also included in this category are patients with a primary lung cancer and a satellite nodule(s). The AJCC-UICC considers these patients to have T4 disease.[21]

The diagnosis of a primary lung cancer with an ipsilateral metastasis can often be difficult to make. A retrospective report of 53 patients with lung cancer and another lesion in the same lung revealed that the second lesion was an intrapulmonary metastasis in 16 patients (30%) and a synchronous primary lung cancer in seven (13%).[19] When the cell type, DNA indices, and ploidy studies are identical, an intrapulmonary metastasis is probable. In a second series of 42 patients with intrapulmonary metastasis detected at the time of thoracotomy, the five-year survival was 25.7%. Patients with T1 or N0 status had a better prognosis.[22]

A satellite nodule has been defined as a well-circum-

scribed accessory focus of carcinoma clearly separate from the main tumor but within the same lobe and with identical histologic characteristics.[23] In 1989, Deslauriers and colleagues reported that the prognosis in 84 resected lung cancer patients found to have satellite nodules was worse at one, three, and five years (61%, 33%, 22%) than in 1,021 resected lung cancer patients without satellite nodules (78%, 54%, 44%). They suggested that patients with a primary carcinoma and a satellite nodule(s) be classified as having stage IIIa disease in view of their relatively poor prognosis.[23] The 1997 revision of the TNM staging system takes into account the poor prognosis of patients with satellite nodule(s) and considers them to be of T4 status and thus at least stage IIIb.[21]

Lung cancer does not appear to metastasize to the contralateral lung as commonly as to other distant sites. In two necropsy studies of patients who died of bronchogenic carcinoma, a metastasis to the contralateral lung was found in 20% and 22%, respectively.[24,25] Establishing the cell type of a contralateral tumor prior to finalizing the surgical plan, by transbronchial biopsy, CT-guided fine-needle aspiration biopsy (FNAB), or thoracoscopic excision, is recommended.

Two Metastases from an Extrathoracic Primary

This diagnostic scenario should be considered when any of the following apply: (a) the patient's history and physical

TABLE 40.2. SYNCHRONOUS PULMONARY TUMORS—DIAGNOSTIC POSSIBILITIES

i. Synchronous primary carcinomas of lung
ii. One primary carcinoma, one metastasis
iii. Two metastases from an extrathoracic primary
iv. One primary carcinoma, one benign lesion
v. Two benign lesions

TABLE 40.4. INCIDENCE OF SYNCHRONOUS AND METACHRONOUS LUNG CANCER IN PATIENTS WITH MULTIPLE PRIMARY TUMORS

Author (Year)	Patients	Synchronous (%)	Metachronous (%)
Razzuk (1974)[14]	34	5 (15)	29 (85)
Abbey-Smith (1976)[15]	55	10 (18)	45 (72)
Mathisen (1984)[6]	90	10 (11)	80 (89)
Wu (1987)[7]	30	10 (33)	20 (67)
Deschamps (1990)[9]	80	36 (45)	44 (55)
Rosengart (1991)[13]	111	33 (30)	78 (70)
Total	400	104 (26)	167 (74)

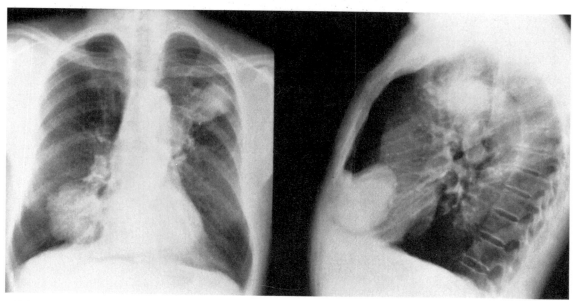

FIGURE 40.1. Synchronous lung cancer.

exam suggest an extrathoracic primary site; (b) the radiological characteristics of the tumors are not suggestive of a primary lung cancer (Figure 40.2); or (c) the patient is a nonsmoker without a history of exposure to a known environmental pulmonary carcinogen. When more than two tumors are identified on chest roentgenogram, the suspicion that they represent metastatic disease is heightened. Factors favoring metastatic disease from an extrathoracic primary include a history of extrapulmonary carcinoma, the absence of bronchial wall invasion, a lack of pulmonary or mediastinal lymph node metastases, and histologic features of a nonbronchogenic cell type.[26]

One Primary Carcinoma, One Benign Lesion
In Kunitoh's study of 53 patients with two ipsilateral lung nodules, one of which was a carcinoma of the lung, the other nodule was found to be benign in 30 cases (56.7%). Foci of pulmonary infarction, inflammation, and fibrosis were found in addition to intrapulmonary lymph nodes,

hamartomas, granulomas, and adenomatous hyperplasia (Figure 40.3).[27] In the setting of one known carcinoma of the lung and one indeterminate tumor, a search for evidence of extrathoracic metastases should be conducted. If extrathoracic metastases are found, surgical therapy is not recommended. If no evidence of extrathoracic disease is found, then further evaluation of the second tumor should be left to the discretion of the surgeon. If it is felt to be a granuloma, for example, observation is appropriate, but if there is any question with regard to the diagnosis, further workup

TABLE 40.5. CRITERIA FOR THE DIAGNOSIS OF SYNCHRONOUS LUNG CANCER

A. Tumors physically distinct and separate
B. Histology
  1. Different
  2. Same, but in different segment, lobe or lung, and
    a. origin from carcinoma *in situ*
    b. no carcinoma in lymphatics common to both
    c. no extrapulmonary metastases at time of diagnosis

From Martini N and Melamed MR. Multiple primary lung cancers. *J Thorac Cardiovasc Surg* 1975, 20:610, with permission.

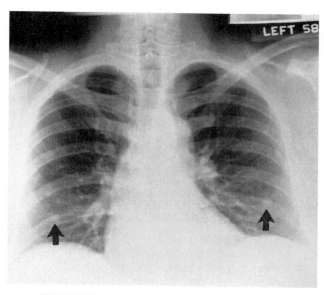

FIGURE 40.2. Two metastatic pulmonary tumors.

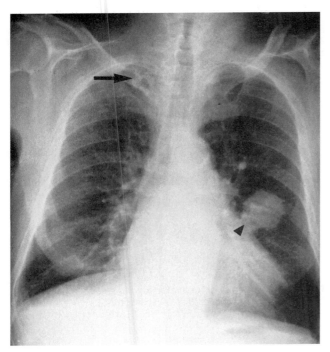

FIGURE 40.3. Primary lung cancer and a benign pulmonary tumor.

is recommended. Ipsilateral lesions can be evaluated and treated at the time of a planned thoracotomy, whereas contralateral lesions might require transbronchial biopsy, transthoracic biopsy, or thoracoscopic resection.

Two Benign Lesions

When the history and physical examination are inconsistent with carcinoma of the lung or carcinoma metastatic to the lung, and when confirmation of the nature of pulmonary nodules is indicated, then bronchoscopy with transbronchial biopsy, FNAB, or thoracoscopic excision are possible diagnostic modalities. Because either nodule might represent a primary lung cancer, however, consideration should be given to performing a biopsy on both nodules.

Evaluation

Before the advent of computed tomography, second pulmonary tumors were most often detected either at the time of pulmonary resection or at autopsy. Presently, however, a second pulmonary tumor is most commonly discovered during noninvasive preoperative assessment, less commonly at the time of bronchoscopy, and least commonly at the time of thoracotomy.[28] Deschamps and colleagues reported that 21 of 36 synchronous lesions were first discovered during preoperative evaluation, while the remaining tumors were identified at thoracotomy.[9] Only three of 28 patients were found to have a second lesion during preoperative

bronchoscopy in a report by Ferguson[28] and only one of ten was found by this means in a report by Mathisen and associates.[6]

When two pulmonary tumors are discovered on a chest roentgenogram, a computed tomogram of the chest is performed to evaluate the rest of the lung parenchyma for evidence of other lesions. The liver and adrenal glands are imaged in this study to exclude the possibility of metastatic disease to these sites. If multiple nodules are found, either metastatic disease or benign (granulomatous) disease should be suspected, depending upon the clinical scenario. PET scanning in the alveolar is becoming increasingly popular (see also Chapter 30).

Bronchoscopy is performed to be certain that there are no asymptomatic foci of endobronchial disease. McElvaney and colleagues found additional synchronous foci of adenocarcinoma on close examination of the pathological specimens of 12 of 62 patients who underwent resection. These additional foci were identified preoperatively in only two of 12 patients and led the authors to conclude that the incidence of multiple primaries might be even higher than currently estimated, but that they are clinically inapparent due to their slow growth and asymptomatic nature.[29] The role that lung imaged fluorescence endoscopic (LIFE) devices will have in detecting additional foci of carcinoma *in situ* or invasive carcinoma in lung cancer patients is currently being investigated[30] (see also Chapter 24).

Mediastinoscopy is an essential component of the prethoracotomy evaluation for patients with possible synchronous primaries. While some surgeons believe that completely resected mediastinal disease does not preclude a contralateral thoracotomy if the patient is free of recurrence or progressive disease at three months, others do not agree.[28] An algorithm for the evaluation of a patient with synchronous masses on chest roentgenogram is presented in Figure 40.4.[12]

Treatment

Patients who are believed to have synchronous tumors are offered surgery if clinical staging indicates that each lesion is stage I.[12] Patients with stage II disease are often treated with surgery, with the knowledge that survival is substantially diminished when N1 lymph nodes are involved. This occurs in part because the status of N1 lymph nodes is often difficult to determine preoperatively. Klingman and DeMeester advise that the intraoperative finding of positive hilar or mediastinal lymph nodes should preclude further surgery in patients with bilateral primaries because of their poor prognosis (median survival 11 months) compared to those with negative lymph nodes (median survival 26 months).[31] Similarly, Deschamps and associates do not recommend additional surgery for patients with bilateral primaries found to have positive mediastinal lymph nodes during initial resection.[9]

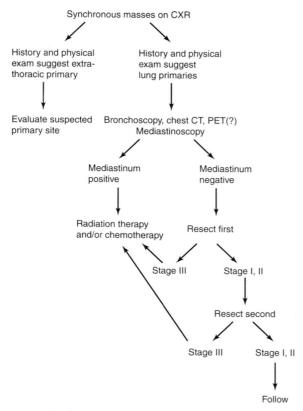

FIGURE 40.4. Algorithm for evaluation of synchronous lung tumors.

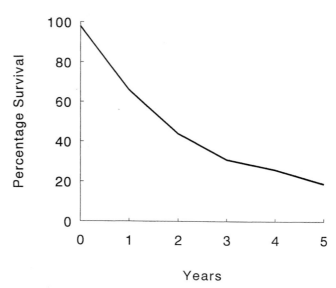

FIGURE 40.5. Actuarial survival following resection of synchronous primary lung cancers. (From Ferguson MK. Synchronous primary lung cancers. *Chest* 1993;103s:399, with permission.)

When carcinomas are bilateral, resection of the lesion that is felt on clinical grounds to be more advanced is advocated first.[5,8,13,14,31] Further resection is dependent upon (a) the pathological stage of the first tumor, (b) the extent of the second tumor, (c) the anticipated magnitude of the second resection when compared with the first, and (d) the patient's pulmonary reserve.[8,14] Parenchyma-sparing procedures (for example, wedge resection, segmentectomy, sleeve lobectomy) should be considered when a contralateral lesion is present, as long as it does not jeopardize the chance for a curative resection.[13,14] While resection of bilateral carcinomas is approached most often using staged thoracotomies, in selected situations a median sternotomy or bilateral sternothoracotomy is appropriate, the latter made easier by the use of thoracic epidural analgesia.[32]

In patients with ipsilateral lesions confined to one lobe of the lung, a lobectomy is sufficient. When the tumors are ipsilateral and are in different lobes, however, a pneumonectomy is the operation of choice. Conservation of pulmonary tissue is advised (for example, lobectomy and wedge resection or two wedge resections) only when pulmonary function precludes performance of a pneumonectomy.[3] Mediastinal and hilar lymph node sampling are necessary in all cases to complete pathological staging.

Prognosis

Survival after resection of synchronous primary lung carinomas is worse, stage for stage, than after resection of solitary bronchogenic carcinomas, as illustrated in Figure 40.5. Pairolero and others suggest that these patients should be considered to have stage IV disease.[33] Their poor prognosis might be explained by the more aggressive nature of their disease, by an increased risk of developing cancer, by the fact that the second lesion really was a metastasis all along, or by the fact that both lesions were metastatic from an extrathoracic primary.[9,13] A final possible explanation for the poor prognosis of synchronous tumors is the fact that the second tumor is treated more often by wedge or segmental resection, procedures associated with increased risk of local recurrence.[34,35]

Metachronous Tumors

In 1975 Martini and Melamed developed criteria for the classification of metachronous tumors (Table 40.6).[20] They

TABLE 40.6. CRITERIA FOR THE DIAGNOSIS OF METACHRONOUS LUNG CANCER

A. Histology different
B. Histology same if:
   1. free interval between cancers at least two years, or
   2. origin from carcinoma *in situ,* or
   3. second cancer in different lobe or lung, and
      a. no carcinoma in lymphatics common to both
      b. no extrapulmonary metastases at time of diagnosis

From Martini N and Melamed MR. Multiple primary lung cancers. *J Thorac Cardiovasc Surg* 1975, 20:610, with permission.

TABLE 40.7. INCIDENCE OF METACHRONOUS LUNG CANCER IN RESECTED LUNG CANCER PATIENTS

Author (Year)	Resected Lung Cancer Patients	Metachronous Lung Cancer Patients (%)
Abbey-Smith (1976)[15]	1,400	45 (3.2)
Wu (1987)[7]	3,815	20 (0.5)
Verhagen (1989)[8]	1,004	25 (2.5)
Total	6,219	90 (1.5)

proposed a tumor-free interval of at least two years as one of their criteria for the diagnosis of metachronous primary lung cancers. Others have stated that an interval of 30 to 36 months is necessary between tumor occurrences in order to call the second lesion a metachronous primary cancer. At least five series have reported the median interval between treatment of the first and second primary lung cancer to be in excess of 48 months.[6–8,15,36] Three other series, however, have reported median intervals between 24 and 48 months,[9,37,38] while a fourth reported two peaks at two and five years.[8] There is no consistent evidence that the interval varies among different cell types or for different initial resections.

Metachronous tumors are estimated to occur in 0.5% of all lung cancer patients overall, in 2% of lung cancer patients who undergo resection, and in 10% to 32% of long-term survivors of lung cancer surgery (Table 40.7).[18,30,32,33] This percentage increases as patient survival improves. The risk of developing a second primary lung cancer is between 0.65% and 5% per year for patients following resection of a lung cancer.[9,14,32,39,40] Shields and associates reported that the incidence of a second primary was 7.6% at 5 years and 10% at ten years in a Veteran's Administration study of 535 patients with resected lung cancer.[36] The Mayo Clinic reported a 10% incidence of second primary lung cancers in their group of 346 patients with resected stage I non–small cell lung cancer (NSCLC).[33] The incidence may be rising in part as a result of its being looked for with increasing vigor. A Lung Cancer Study Group trial reported by Feld and co-workers revealed the contralateral lung to be the site of first relapse in 13% (20 of 158) of 390 patients with resected stage I and II NSCLC, whereas ipsilateral relapse occurred in 26% (41 of 158). Nonsquamous or mixed tumors were twice as likely to recur as squamous cell cancer.[41] DNA flow cytometry and DNA index can help to differentiate between a recurrence and a new primary.

Evaluation

Approximately 80% of patients who develop second primary lung cancers are asymptomatic, and the diagnosis is based upon finding an abnormality on a surveillance chest roentgenogram.[6,8,14,15,20,42] This reinforces the need for continued long-term follow-up of all lung cancer patients. Patients who continue to smoke may be at increased risk for developing a second primary lung cancer.[15] Symptoms, if present, include cough, hemoptysis, and dyspnea.[6–9,42] The second tumor is evaluated and treated in a manner similar to the initial lesion.[14,41] This includes assessment of the locoregional extent of disease and a search for sites of extrathoracic spread. A positive mediastinoscopy contraindicates a thoracotomy in most cases.

Treatment

It has been stated that it makes no difference whether or not a new lung tumor is a primary or recurrent carcinoma. If the new lesion appears localized and is amenable to surgical excision, then this should be the procedure of choice.[43] There is no doubt that resection offers the best chance of cure and should be attempted in appropriately selected patients.[14] Distinguishing between a stump recurrence or a recurrence at the site of a previous resection might not be critical if the disease is otherwise localized and the patient is a candidate for resection.[6,15,20]

Only one third of patients with a second primary lung cancer are candidates for surgery despite the fact that their second tumor is clinically resectable.[5,14,15,32,38] For example, only 17 of 55 patients in Abbey-Smith's series[15] were surgical candidates, compared to ten of 41 in Shields's series[36] and 12 of 34 in the series by Razzuk and others.[14] Inadequate pulmonary reserve is the reason most commonly given for inoperability. When the metachronous tumor is ipsilateral and in a different lobe from the first tumor, and when the patient's pulmonary reserve is adequate, a completion pneumonectomy is advised. If, however, pulmonary reserve is limited, a segmentectomy or wedge resection with lymph node sampling is appropriate.

When the metachronous tumor is contralateral and the patient has not had a previous pneumonectomy, a lobectomy is the preferred procedure. If, however, the patient underwent pneumonectomy in the first instance, a segmentectomy or wedge resection is performed most often, with lobectomy reserved for highly selected patients with adequate pulmonary reserve.[40,44]

Survival/Prognosis

Morbidity and 30-day mortality after resection of metachronous lung cancer is higher than after initial lung resection.[32] Morbidity in one series was 39%, which is similar to that reported after completion pneumonectomy. Mortality rates range from 4.5% to 9.3%.[6,9,38]

Five- and ten-year survival after resection of metachronous primary lung cancer are 30% and 20%, respectively (Figure 40.6).[6–9,13,42] The poorest survival is seen in patients who undergo limited resection (segmentectomy, wedge) of their second lung cancer.[42] This might be explained by inadequate margins, underlying pulmonary dys-

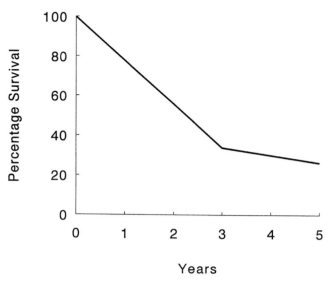

FIGURE 40.6. Survival after resection of metachronous lung cancer.

function, advanced age at the time of the second resection, misdiagnosis of metastatic disease, and/or increased operative mortality. Sleeve lobectomy is also associated with decreased survival when compared to lobectomy, which might be due to an increase in the rate of local recurrence.[6] The increased risk of local recurrence must be weighed against the benefit of preserving pulmonary parenchyma in anticipation of metachronous disease when advocating conservative resection of lung cancer. Survival is not inferior when the cell type of the second tumor is the same as the first.[12] Verhagen and associates also felt that survival was better if three as opposed to two pulmonary lobes remained after the second resection.[8] Many series report improved survival when the interval between treatment of the lung cancers is greater than two years,[6,8,13] although this has not been a universal finding.[38] This is most likely due to the fact that the longer a patient survives after initial surgery, the more likely a second tumor represents a second primary as opposed to either a metastasis or a missed synchronous tumor.

All authors conclude that the follow-up of a lung cancer patient should continue indefinitely. It is recommended that patients be followed quarterly for the first two years, biannually for the next three years, and yearly thereafter.[6] This regimen is currently under review by investigators of cost-effective health management strategies but does not take into account the psychological impact of not having continued follow-up care by their surgeon.

BRAIN METASTASIS

Introduction

Bronchogenic carcinoma is the neoplasm that most commonly metastasizes to brain.[45] It is estimated that in 1998,

170,000 persons were diagnosed with bronchogenic carcinoma and that 51,000 will develop brain metastasis during the course of their disease.[46] Unfortunately a brain metastasis is usually a manifestation of widely disseminated disease. Arbit and Wronski reported that only 38 of 201 patients had brain metastases as the only site of distant disease. Among patients diagnosed with a solitary brain metastasis, 28% to 68% are found to have a primary carcinoma in the lung and between 4% to 20% have no evidence of a primary carcinoma.[45,47,48] An estimated 40% of lung cancer patients develop brain metastases during the course of their disease.[49-53] The incidence of brain metastases in lung cancer patients at autopsy is approximately 20% higher owing to their sometimes asymptomatic nature.[54-56] In one report of 259 patients with inoperable adenocarcinoma of the lung, 24% had or developed clinical evidence of brain metastases during the course of their illness, but brain metastases were found in 44% of the 87 patients autopsied.[57]

In early-stage NSCLC, first recurrences involve distant sites in 50% of patients, and the brain is the site of first recurrence in 20%. The relative risk of recurrence in the brain is higher among patients with T1N1 and T2N0 disease when compared to those with T1N0 tumors. Patients with non–squamous cell or mixed-histology tumors are at an increased risk of developing brain metastasis.[41,58,59]

Without treatment, the median survival after discovery of brain metastases is one month.[60-61] Treatment with steroids both palliates symptoms and prolongs median survival to approximately two months.[62,63] Radiation therapy is associated with symptomatic improvement and an increase in the median survival to between three and six months.[64,65] Stereotactic radiosurgery has been applied to lesions under three centimeters, with a median survival of 9.4 months. The exact role of this treatment modality has yet to be defined, and to date no randomized trial data are available for review.[48]

Results of early surgical efforts were not favorable owing to a lack of availability of steroids and modern-day neuroanesthetic and neurosurgical techniques.[66] The availability of steroids, coupled with the development of cortical mapping, laser technology, and the ultrasonic aspirator, has resulted in the development of surgical resection of brain metastasis from bronchogenic carcinoma as an important therapeutic option in selected patients.[47,67,68] The median survival of 583 patients treated by surgical resection at a major cancer center was 9.4 months, and their operative mortality was 5.3%.[48]

Evaluation

The first step in the assessment of a lung cancer patient with a lesion in the brain (Figure 40.7) is to determine whether or not it represents a metastasis.[69] In Patchell's randomized trial of cancer patients with solitary brain lesions, 10% (6 of 59) did not represent metastatic disease,

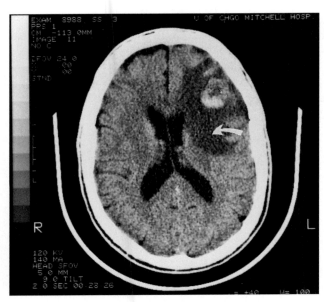

FIGURE 40.7. Brain metastasis from carcinoma of the lung.

TABLE 40.8. PERCENTAGE OF NSCLC PATIENTS WITH SOLITARY BRAIN METASTASIS-AUTOPSY SERIES

Author (Year)	Patients Autopsied	Patients with Solitary Metastasis (%)
Flavell (1949)[101]	85	26 (31)
Galuzzi (1955)[55]	741	103 (14)
Richards (1963)[60]	127	24 (19)
Deeley (1968)[64]	63	30 (48)
Total	1,016	183 (18)

illustrating the importance of establishing the diagnosis before developing a treatment plan.[70] Overall, approximately 3% of NSCLC patients develop an operable solitary brain metastasis during the course of their disease. The goal of the evaluation, therefore, is to select patients most likely to benefit from surgical treatment of their brain metastasis.

Neurologic symptoms precede lung cancer symptoms in about 80% of patients found to have synchronous disease.[71-73] Headache is the symptom most commonly associated with brain metastasis and occurs in approximately 50% of patients.[74] Focal weakness or hemiparesis occurs in about 40%, and dysphasia, seizure, or visual changes occur less frequently.[51,74] Patients with adenocarcinoma have an increased incidence of asymptomatic brain metastases compared to those with other non–small cell types.[74]

Computed tomography (CT) and magnetic resonance imaging (MRI) are the primary radiographic modalities used to evaluate patients suspected of having brain metastasis.[73,75,76] CTs are more sensitive in detecting small tumors and in assessing the effect of steroids, whereas MRI allows for improved visualization of the brainstem.[74,75] Since it has been estimated that CT of the head may reveal silent brain metastases in only 3% of lung cancer patients at the time of initial staging, it is not cost-effective to include a head CT as part of routine staging in patients who are early-stage by clinical criteria and have no neurologic symptoms.

At presentation, between 30% to 50% of brain metastases are solitary, 20% of patients have two metastases, and 13% have three metastases. Local therapy can thus be offered to up to 70% of patients. Only 30% to 50% of patients with brain metastases are candidates for resection

(Table 40.8).[45,48,52,55,71,74,77-79] Reasons for inoperability are: (a) location of metastasis in a surgically inaccessible area, (b) other distant sites of failure detected concurrently, (c) poor general medical condition, and (d) anticipated life expectancy of less than three months.[80]

One percent of patients diagnosed with lung cancer are found to have a synchronous solitary brain metastasis. A metachronous presentation is more common, and the median interval between resection of the lung primary and the diagnosis of a metachronous brain metastasis is 12 months (Table 40.9).[81]

Supratentorial metastases develop in 66% to 84% of patients. The frontal and parietal regions of the brain are affected most often. Cerebellar metastases account for approximately 25% of brain metastases, are solitary about 25% of the time, and may cause symptoms earlier than lesions in other regions.[45,47,73] The distribution of brain metastasis reflects a vascular pattern of dissemination, most commonly via the middle cerebral artery.[71]

Treatment

When deciding upon the most appropriate treatment option for an individual patient, the following need to be taken into consideration: (a) symptoms, (b) general condition of the patient, (c) extent and status of cerebral disease, and (d) extent and status of extracranial disease. Modalities include external beam radiotherapy, brachytherapy, surgical resection, stereotactic radiosurgery, and combinations thereof.

TABLE 40.9. INCIDENCE OF SYNCHRONOUS AND METACHRONOUS BRAIN METASTASIS

Author (Year)	Patients	Synchronous Disease (%)	Metachronous Disease (%)
Read (1989)[83]	92	28 (30)	64 (70)
Macchiarini (1991)[87]	37	10 (27)	27 (73)
Burt (1992)[81]	185	65 (35)	120 (65)
Total	314	103 (33)	211 (64)

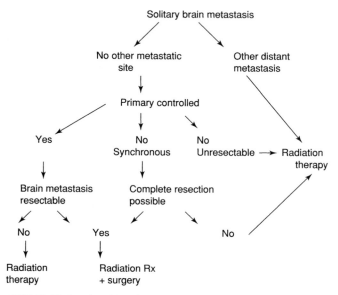

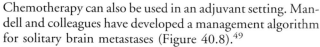

FIGURE 40.8. Algorithm for management of solitary brain metastasis.

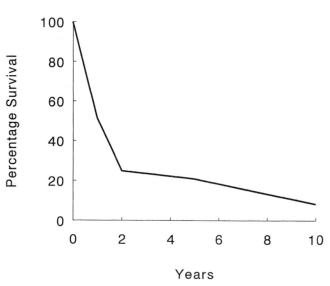

FIGURE 40.9. Survival after resection of solitary brain metastasis from non–small cell lung cancer.

Chemotherapy can also be used in an adjuvant setting. Mandell and colleagues have developed a management algorithm for solitary brain metastases (Figure 40.8).[49]

Surgery is preferred for (a) solitary lesions associated with significant edema, (b) large lesions, (c) superficial lesions, (d) patients with symptoms requiring immediate relief, and (e) lesions associated with hemorrhage.[69] Radiosurgery is recommended if the lesion is deep but less than 3 cm in diameter, if there are medical contraindications to surgery, or, in some cases, when the tumor is recurrent.

In the metachronous setting, resection of the intracranial metastasis follows the guidelines above. In the synchronous setting, craniotomy is generally completed first, because patients are more often symptomatic from their brain metastasis. If the radiographic appearance of the lung primary suggests it to be unresectable, however, thoracosopy may be used to assess this prior to proceeding with craniotomy, if the lung primary is resectable, or other palliative treatment, if it is not.[82]

Operative mortality following craniotomy is between 0% to 11.1% in recent series.[70,73,79,81,83–86] Complete resection was accomplished in 90% of the 583 patients treated at one major cancer center.[48] Morbidity averages 20% and is primarily neurological in nature. Improvement in neurological status is reported in between 57% and 84% of patients, while 13% to 33% of patients have either stable or worsening neurological status.[47,70,73,77,78,83,86,87] The median duration of neurological improvement is 15 months.[73,86]

Five-year survival after resection of solitary brain metastasis is approximately 20% (Figure 40.9). Median disease-free survival after resection is between six and 20 months. A randomized trial comparing surgery plus radiation to ra-

diation alone in patients with solitary brain metastases from solid tumors revealed a decreased incidence of local recurrence, increased survival, and prolonged improvement in functional status in the group treated with surgery plus radiation compared to the radiation-alone group (20% versus 52%, 40 weeks versus 15 weeks, and 38 weeks versus 8 weeks, respectively).[70]

Recurrent cranial disease develops in approximately 50% of patients following surgical management of brain metastasis, and in some series as many as half of these recurrences involve the site of original disease.[51,78,81] Craniotomy has been recommended for recurrence only if the disease continues to be limited to the brain. This approach can be expected to result in an improvement in neurological status in two thirds of patients and a two-year survival rate of 25%. Despite these modest results, most reports caution that the uniformly dismal prognosis of recurrent brain metastases should preclude surgery, and that radiosurgery or a boost of external beam radiation therapy is appropriate for most patients. The roles of brachytherapy and chemotherapy have not been assessed. The cause of death in patients with brain metastasis from any cancer is due most commonly to either the brain metastasis (25% to 50%), diffuse systemic disease (20% to 25%), or both (10%).[74,78,83]

Prognosis

Among patients with lung cancer metastatic to the brain, the most favorable prognosis is associated with a completely resected primary lung tumor.[84–88] Control of the primary site of cancer is mandatory for long-term survival.[52,80] Multivariate analysis revealed that wedge resection of the primary lung cancer was the only significant prognostic factor, implying that patients with tumors amenable to wedge resection were more likely to survive.[78] The completeness of resection of the lung primary was found to impact significantly on the survival of a group of 256 patients with brain metastases from NSCLC.[89] Solitary metastases have a better prognosis than multiple metastases,[81,88] and surgical management of multiple metastases is rarely indicated.[88] An improved prognosis is associated with brain metastases less than 3 cm in diameter.[47,80] The prognosis may also be better if the metastasis is either asymptomatic or mildly symptomatic.[74] Whether a brain metastasis is metachronous or synchronous has not generally been found to influence survival.[50,78,81,83,87–89] It has been reported that both disease-free survival and actuarial survival were better among the 35 patients with metachronous disease compared to 15 with synchronous disease (actuarial survival 31% versus 6%).[90] In the metachronous setting, however, a prolonged interval between resection of the lung primary and diagnosis of the brain metastasis is associated with improved prognosis,[90,91] but this has not been a universal finding.[81] While age has not been found to affect prognosis in most reports, a univariate analysis by Hankins and associates found that age younger than 55 years was a favorable sign.[47,57,59,61,81,85,90,92] It is unclear whether or not the lymph node status of the primary tumor is of prognostic significance in patients who undergo resection of a solitary brain metastasis.[50,78] Similarly, whether or not a supratentorial metastasis is more favorable than an infratentorial one is uncertain.[45,51,81,85,87] A recent abstract reported that 31 of 256 patients with cerebellar metastasis had a decreased survival when compared to patients with a supratentorial metastasis.[89] Salvati's review of eighteen ten-year survivors, however, revealed that none had had a posterior fossa metastasis.[76]

METASTASIS TO OTHER SITES

Sporadic reports have addressed the role of surgery with curative intent in settings where lung cancer has metastasized to sites other than those discussed in the preceding sections.[1,2,93] Surgical management of lung cancer that has metastasized to bone is palliative and is aimed at restoring functional status. The bone represents an isolated site of first recurrence in approximately 5% of lung cancer patients. The prognosis is similar to that of patients who develop brain metastases and is worse than in patients who recur in either the ipsilateral or contralateral lung.[58] Bone biopsy is indicated when a solitary focus of suspected metastasis is discovered in a patient who is otherwise operable.

Adrenal metastases are found at autopsy in 10% to 59% of NSCLC patients.[94,95,96] Unilateral adrenal masses are discovered in approximately 4% of patients with otherwise operable NSCLC but only 40% represent metastatic disease.[3,97] In one series of 598 patients with operable or oper-

ated NSCLC, 39 had adrenal masses (18 benign, 21 malignant) and 11 of the patients had their adrenal metastasis resected.[4] Patient age, lung cancer stage, or mass size did not help to distinguish benign from malignant lesions.[99] Proper treatment planning, therefore, mandates cytologic or histologic confirmation of the true nature of a unilateral adrenal mass in a patient with NSCLC. In one series, the specificity of needle aspiration biopsy in detecting metastatic disease was 100%; however, nondiagnostic results necessitated adrenalectomy in five of ten patients, all of whom had benign glands.[99] The report that 12% of adrenal glands that appeared normal on CT scan harbored metastatic disease in a group of 32 NSCLC patients needs to be confirmed.[98] A series of 14 patients found to have isolated adrenal metastasis associated with NSCLC revealed a median survival of 22 months for the eight patients treated surgically, compared to 8.5 months for the six patients treated with platinum-based chemotherapy.[99]

Pleurectomy for metastatic lung cancer has been attempted in a handful of patients, either alone or with concomitant lung resection, in the hope of improving quality and duration of survival. Disease status was reported in five patients, one of whom had died ten months after lobectomy and pleurectomy. The remaining four patients were alive between 15 and 35 months postoperatively; however, only one patient was free of disease.[93] The presence of pleural metastases precludes surgery with curative intent.[100]

REFERENCES

1. Ettinghausen SE, Burt ME. Prospective evaluation of unilateral adrenal masses in patients with operable non-small-cell lung cancer. *J Clin Oncol* 1991;9:1462.
2. Twomey P, Montgomery C, Clark O. Successful treatment of adrenal metastases from large cell carcinoma of the lung. *JAMA* 1982;248:581.
3. Luketich JD, Van Raemdonck DE, Ginsberg RJ. Extended resection for higher-stage non–small cell lung cancer. *World J Surg* 1993;17:719.
4. Porte HL, Roumilhac D, Graziana JP, et al. Adrenalectomy for a solitary adrenal metastasis from lung cancer. *Ann Thorac Surg* 1998;65:331.
5. Okunaka T, Kato H, Konaka C, et al. Photodynamic therapy for multiple primary bronchogenic carcinoma. *Cancer* 1991;68:253.
6. Mathisen DJ, Jensik RJ, Faber LP, et al. Survival following resection for second and third primary lung cancers. *J Thorac Cardiovasc Surg* 1984;88:502.
7. Wu S-C, Lin Z-Q, Xu C-W, et al. Multiple primary lung cancers. *Chest* 1987;92:892.
8. Verhagen AF, van de Wal HJ, Cox AL, et al. Surgical treatment of multiple primary lung cancers. *J Thorac Cardiovasc Surg* 1989;37:107.
9. Deschamps C, Pairlero PC, Trastek VF, et al. Multiple primary lung cancers. *J Thorac Cardiovasc Surg* 1990;99:769.
10. Bewtra C. Multiple primary bronchiogenic carcinomas with a review of the literature. *J Surg Oncol* 1984;25:207.
11. Auerbach O, Stout AP, Hammond EC, et al. Multiple primary bronchochial carcinomas. *Cancer* 1967;20:699.

12. Ferguson MK, DeMeester TR, Deslauriers J, et al. Diagnosis and management of synchronous lung cancers. *J Thorac Cardiovasc Surg* 1985;89:378.
13. Rosengart TK, Martini N, Ghosn P, et al. Multiple primary lung carcinoma: prognosis and treatment. *Ann Thorac Surg* 1991;52:773.
14. Razzuk MA, Pockey M, Urschel HC Jr., et al. Dual primary bronchogenic carcinoma. *Ann Thorac Surg* 1974;17:425.
15. Abbey-Smith R, Nigam BK, Thompson JM. Second primary lung carcinoma. *Thorax* 1976;31:507.
16. Billroth T. [Die allgemeine chirugische pathologie und therapie in 51 vorlesungen; ein handbuch fur studierende und arzte.] 14:908, Berlin 1889, aufl. G. Reimer.
17. Beyreuther H. Multiplicatat von Carcinomen bei einem Fall von sog. "Schneeberger" Lungenkregs mit tuberkulose. *Virchows Arch Path Anat* 1924;250:230.
18. Chaudhuri MR. Independent bilateral primary bronchial carcinoma. *Thorax* 1971;26:476.
19. Warren S, Gates O. Multiple primary malignant tumors: a survey of the literature and a statistical study. *Am J Cancer* 1932; 16:1358.
20. Martini N, Melamed MR. Multiple primary lung cancers. *J Thorac Cardiovasc Surg* 1975;70:606.
21. Mountain CF. Revisions in the international system for staging lung cancer. *Chest* 1997;111:1710.
22. Shimizu N, Ando A, Moriyama S, et al. Outcome of patients with undetected intrapulmonary metastases in resected lung cancer [Abstract]. *Lung Cancer* 1994;10:160.
23. Deslauriers J, Brisson J, Cartier R, et al. Carcinoma of the lung. *J Thorac Cardiovasc Surg* 1989;97:504.
24. Onuigbo WIB. Contralateral pulmonary metastases in lung cancer. *Thorax* 1974;29:132.
25. Muir CS. Cancer of the lung, trachea and larynx in Singapore. *Br J Cancer* 1960;14:1.
26. Payne WS, Clagett OT, Harrison EG. Surgical management of bilateral malignant lesions of the lung. *J Thorac Cardiovasc Surg* 1962;43:279.
27. Kunitoh H, Eguchi K, Yamada K, et al. Intrapulmonary sublesions detected before surgery in patients with lung cancer. *Cancer* 1992;70:1876.
28. Ferguson MK. Synchronous primary lung cancers. *Chest* 1993; 103:S398.
29. McElvaney G, Miller RR, Muller NL, et al. Multicentricity of adenocarcinoma of the lung. *Chest* 1989;95:151.
30. Lam S, MacAulay C, LeRiche JC, et al. Fluorescence imaging of pre-malignant and malignant tissue with and without photosensitizers. *SPIE* 1993;1881:160.
31. Klingman RR, DeMeester TR. Surgical approach to non–small cell lung cancer stage I and II. *Hematol Oncol Clin N Am* 1990; 4:1079.
32. Shields TW. Multiple primary bronchial carcinoma. *Ann Thorac Surg* 1979;27:1.
33. Pairolero PC, Williams DE, Bergstrahl EJ, et al. Postsurgical stage I bronchogenic carcinoma: morbid implications of recurrent disease. *Ann Thorac Surg* 1984;38:331.
34. Ginsberg RJ. personal communication, 1992.
35. Darteville P, Khalife J. Surgical approach to local recurrence and the second primary lesion. In: Delarue NC, Eschapasse H, eds. *International trends in general thoracic surgery*. Philadelphia: W.B. Saunders, 1985:156.
36. Shields TW, Drake CT, Sherrick JC. Bilateral primary bronchogenic carcinoma. *J Thorac Cardiovasc Surg* 1964;48:401.
37. Salerno TA, Munro DD, Blundell PE, et al: Second primary bronchogenic carcinoma: life-table analysis of surgical treatment. *Ann Thorac Surg* 1979;27:3.
38. Rohwedder JJ, Weatherbee L. Multiple primary bronchogenic

39. carcinoma with a review of the literature. *Am Rev Resp Dis* 1974; 109:435.
39. Bower SL, Choplin RH, Muss HB. Multiple primary bronchogenic carcinomas of the lung. *AJR* 1983;140:253.
40. Spaggiari L, Grunewald D, Girard P, et al. Cancer resection on the residual lung after pneumonectomy for bronchogenic carcinoma. *Ann Thorac Surg* 1996;62:1598.
41. Feld R, Rubinstein LV, Weisenberger TH. Sites of recurrence in resected stage I non–small cell lung cancer: a guide for future studies. *J Clin Oncol* 1984;2:1352.
42. Jensik RJ, Faber LP, Kittle CF. Survival following resection for second primary bronchogenic carcinoma. *J Thorac Cardiovasc Surg* 1981;82:658.
43. Neptune WB, Woods FM, Overholt RH. Reoperation for bronchogenic carcinoma. *J Thorac Cardiovasc Surg* 1966;52:507.
44. Vaaler AK, Hosanah HO, Wagner RB. Pneumonectomy after contralateral lobectomy: is it reasonable? *Ann Thorac Surg* 1995; 59:178.
45. Merchut MP. Brain metastases from undiagnosed systemic neoplasms. *Arch Int Med* 1989;149:1076.
46. *Cancer facts and figures 1998* Atlanta GA: American Cancer Society.
47. Winston KR, Walsh JW, Fischer EG. Results of operative treatment of intracranial metastatic tumors. *Cancer* 1980;45:2639.
48. Arbit E, Wronski M. Clinical decision making in brain metastases. *Neurosurg Clin North Am* 1996;7:447.
49. Mandell L, Hilaris B, Sullivan M, et al. The treatment of single brain metastasis from non–oat cell lung carcinoma. *Cancer* 1986;58:641.
50. Sundaresan N, Galicich JH, Beattie EJ. Surgical treatment of brain metastases from lung cancer. *J Neurosurg* 1983;58:666.
51. Torre M, Quaini E, Chiesa G, et al. Synchronous brain metastasis from lung cancer: result of surgical treatment in combined resection. *J Thorac Cardiovasc Surg* 1988;95:994.
52. Rizzi A, Tondini M, Rocco G, et al. Lung cancer with a single brain metastasis: therapeutic options. *Tumori* 1990;76:579.
53. Cox JD, Yesner R. Adenocarcinoma of the lung: recent results from VA lung group. *Am Rev Resp Dis* 1979;120:1025.
54. Mussi A, Janni A, Pistolesi M, et al. Surgical treatment of primary lung cancer and solitary brain metastasis. *Thorax* 1985; 40:191.
55. Galuzzi S, Payne MM. Bronchial carcinoma. A statistical study of 741 necropsies with special reference to the distribution of blood born metastases. *Br J Cancer* 1955;9:511.
56. Halpert B, Fields WS, DeBakey ME. Intracranial metastasis from carcinoma of the lung. *Surgery* 1954;35:346.
57. Sorensen JB, Hansen HH, Hansen M, et al. Brain metastases in adenocarcinoma of the lung: frequency, risk groups, and prognosis. *J Clin Oncol* 1988;6:1474.
58. Figlin RA, Piantadosi S, Feld R, et al. Intracranial recurrence of carcinoma after complete surgical resection of stage I, II, and III non-small-cell lung cancer. *N Engl J Med* 1988;318:1300.
59. Chang DB, Yang PC, Luh KT, et al. Late survival of non–small cell lung cancer patients with brain metastases. *Chest* 1992;101: 1293.
60. Richards P, McKissock W. Intracranial metastases. *Br Med J* 1963;1:15.
61. Stoier M. Metastatic tumors of the brain. *Acta Neurol Scand* 1965;41:262.
62. Galicich JH, French LA, Melby J. Use of dexamethasone in treatment of cerebral edema associated with brain tumors. *Lancet* 1961;1:46.
63. Posner JB. Brain tumor; current status of treatment and its complications. *Arch Neurol* 1975;32:781.
64. Deeley TJ, Birm MB, Rice-Edwards JM, et al. Radiotherapy in

the management of cerebral secondaries from bronchial carcinoma. *Lancet* 1968;1:1209.

65. Cairncross JG, Kim JH, Posner JB. Radiation therapy for brain metastases. *Ann Neurol* 1980;7:529.

66. Cushing H. *Intracranial tumors: notes upon a series of two thousand verified cases with surgical mortality percentages pertaining thereto.* Springfield: Charles C Thomas, 1932.

67. Galicich JH, Sundaresan N, Thaler HT. Surgical treatment of single brain metastasis: evaluation of results by computerized tomography scanning. *J Neurosurg* 1980;53:63.

68. Sundaresan N, Galicich JH. Surgical treatment of brain metastases: clinical and computerized tomography evaluation of the results of treatment. *Cancer* 1985;55:1382.

69. Black PMcL. Solitary brain metastases. Radiation, resection or radiosurgery. *Chest* 1993;4:367s.

70. Patchell RA, Tibbs PA, Walsh JW, et al. A randomized trial of surgery in the treatment of single metastases to the brain. *N Engl J Med* 1990;322:494.

71. Veith RG, Odom GL. Intracranial metastases and their neurosurgical treatment. *J Neurosurg* 1965;23:375.

72. Simionescu MD. Metastatic tumors of the brain: follow-up study of 195 patients with neurosurgical considerations. *J Neurosurg* 1960;17:361.

73. Dubois F, Lafitte JJ, Rousseaux M, et al. Brain metastases revealing lung cancer. The effect of combined surgery on quality and duration of survival. In: Chatel M, Darcel F, Pecker J, eds. *Brain oncology.* Dordrecht: Martinus Nijhoff Publishers, 1987: 288.

74. Pladdet I, Boven E, Nauta J, et al. Palliative care for brain metastasis of solid tumour types. *Neth J Med* 1989;34:10.

75. Tarver RD, Richmond BD, Klatte EC. Cerebral metastases from lung carcinoma: neurological and CT correlation. *Radiology* 1984;153:689.

76. Salvati M, Artico M, Carlioa S, et al. Solitary cerebral metastasis from lung cancer with very long survival: report of two cases and review of the literature. *Surg Neurol* 1991;36:458.

77. Magilligan DJ Jr., Rogers JS, Knighton RS, et al. Pulmonary neoplasm with solitary cerebral metastasis: results of combined excision. *J Thorac Cardiovasc Surg* 1976;76:690.

78. Magilligan DJ Jr. Duvernoy C, Malik G, et al. Surgical approach to lung cancer with solitary cerebral metastasis: twenty-five years' experience. *Ann Thorac Surg* 1986;42:360.

79. Deviri E, Schachner A, Levy MJ. Carcinoma of lung with a solitary cerebral metastasis: surgical management and review of the literature. *Cancer* 1983;52:1507.

80. Patchell RA, Cirrincione C, Thaler HT, et al. Single brain metastases: surgery plus radiation or radiation alone. *Neurology* 1986;36:447.

81. Burt M, Wronski M, Arbit E, et al. Resection of brain metastases from non–small cell lung carcinoma: results of therapy. *J Thorac Cardiovasc Surg* 1992;103:399.

82. Catinella FP, Kittle CF, Faber LP, et al. Surgical treatment of primary lung cancer and solitary intracranial metastasis. *Chest* 1989;95:972.

83. Read RC, Boop WC, Yoder G, et al. Management of non–small cell lung carcinoma with solitary brain metastasis. *J Thorac Cardiovasc Surg* 1989;98:884.

84. Salerno TA, Munro DD, Little JR. Surgical treatment of bronchogenic carcinoma with a brain metastasis. *J Neurosurg* 1978; 48:350.

85. Yardeni D, Reichenthal E, Zucker G, et al. Neurosurgical management of single brain metastasis. *Surg Neurol* 1984;21:377.

86. Tummarello D, Porfiri E, Rychlicki F, et al. Non–small cell lung cancer: neuroresection of the solitary intracranial metastasis followed by radiochemotherapy. *Cancer* 1972;56:2569.

87. Macchiarini P, Buonaguidi R, Hardin M, et al. Results and prognostic factors of surgery in the management of non–small cell lung cancer with solitary brain metastasis. *Cancer* 1991;68: 300.

88. Ide Y, Oka K, Tsuchimochi H, et al. Surgical results of brain metastasis from lung cancer: prognostic factors. *Neurol Med Chir (Tokyo)* 1991;31:18.

89. Wronski M, Burt M, Arbit E, et al. Craniotomy and thoracotomy in 206 patients with non–small cell lung cancer (NSCLC) metastatic to brain [Abstract]. *Lung Cancer* 1994;10:160.

90. Hankins JR, Miller JE, Salcman M, et al. Surgical management of lung cancer with solitary cerebral metastasis. *Ann Thorac Surg* 1988;46:24.

91. Mussi A, Chella A, Ribechini A, et al. Lung cancer and solitary brain metastasis: surgical therapy [Abstract]. *Lung Cancer* 1944; 10:165.

92. Noterman J, Hilderbrand J, Rocmans P, et al. Survie a long terme apres ablation d'une metastase cerebrale solitaire d'un cancer pulmonaire. *Neurochir* 1990;36:308.

93. Hasse J. Surgery in bronchial carcinoma with metastasis. *Lung* 1990;168 [Suppl]:1145.

94. Abrams HL, Sprio R, Goldstein N. Metastases in carcinoma: analysis of 1000 autopsied cases. *Cancer* 1950;3:74.

95. Englemen RM, McNamara WL. Bronchgenic carcinoma: a statistical review of two hundred twenty-four autopsies. *J Thorac Surg* 1954;27:227.

96. Matthews MJ. Problems in morphology and behavior of bronchopulmonary malignant disease. In: Israel L, Chahinian AL, eds. *Lung cancer: natural history, prognosis, and therapy.* San Diego: Academic Press, 1976:23.

97. Sandler MA, Paerberg JL, Madrazo BL, et al. Computed tomographic evaluation of the adrenal gland in the preoperative assessment of bronchogenic carcinoma. *Radiology* 1982;145:733.

98. Pagnani JJ: Non–small cell carcinoma adrenal metastases: computed tomography and percutaneous needle biopsy in their diagnosis. *Cancer* 1984;53:1058.

99. Luketich JD, Burt ME. Does resection of isolated adrenal metastases in non–small cell lung cancer (NSCLC) improve survival? [Abstract]. *Lung Cancer* 1994;10:153.

100. Lynch TJ Jr. Management of malignant pleural effusions. *Chest* 1993;103:s385.

101. Flavell G. Solitary cerebral metastasis from bronchial carcinomata: their incidence and a case of successful removal. *BMJ* 1949:2:736.

41

COMPLICATIONS OF SURGERY

L. PENFIELD FABER
WILLIAM PICCIONE

Surgical resection remains a mainstay of therapy for patients with carcinoma of the lung. Unfortunately, any surgical intervention carries with it the potential of morbidity and mortality. Although many advances have occurred in the preoperative, intraoperative, and postoperative care of these patients to minimize the risk of surgery, complications still occur.[1] Complications after surgery can never be totally eliminated, but they can be minimized by careful attention to the many details of prevention. When complications do occur, proper management usually yields a satisfactory result. Prevention includes accurate preoperative assessment, meticulous surgical technique, and a knowledge of surgical maneuvers to minimize potential problems.

PREOPERATIVE ASSESSMENT

Traditional attempts to assess surgical morbidity and mortality after pulmonary resection have primarily focused on clinical assessment and static pulmonary function testing, such as spirometry, radionuclide scans, and temporary unilateral pulmonary artery balloon occlusion. Nagasaki and associates[2] studied 961 patients undergoing surgical treatment for carcinoma of the lung. Variables including age, gender, cell type, extent of resection, cardiopulmonary status, and stage of disease were evaluated. The authors found that certain high-risk groups could be identified:

1. patients older than 70 years of age in whom a major resection is necessary;
2. patients with a positive cardiac history;
3. patients with severely restricted pulmonary reserve, regardless of age.

Gender, stage of disease, and cell type were found to have little influence on the frequency of postoperative complications. Kohman and colleagues[3] studied 476 patients undergoing thoracotomy more thoroughly by analyzing 37 preoperative risk factors, including the forced-expiratory volume at 1 second (FEV1) and arterial blood gases, and their effects on morbidity and mortality. Only three of these factors were found to have a significant association with

mortality. These consisted of age 60 years or older, need for pneumonectomy, and premature ventricular contractions on admission electrocardiogram. However, all these preoperative risk factors together were found to account for only 12% of the risk of mortality observed. The authors speculated that most deaths after pulmonary resection might therefore be random, unpredictable events. Clearly then, increased accuracy in preoperative assessment necessitates measure of more physiologic parameters.

Boysen and colleagues[4] studied the predictive value of simple spirometric testing with and without more specific testing, and concluded that additional testing over spirometry did not appear to add any predictive value. In contrast, most investigators believe that static pulmonary function tests lack the specificity and sensitivity to predict postoperative cardiopulmonary complications accurately.[5,6] The dilemmas are to define which additional patient parameters will add to the predictive value and to accomplish this task in a minimally invasive, cost-effective manner. Keagy and associates[7] sought to increase the predictive value of preoperative spirometry in 90 patients undergoing pneumonectomy. All patients had forced vital capacity (FVC), FEV_1, and FEV_1/FVC ratio measured. The results demonstrated no correlation between postoperative morbidity and mortality with FVC, FEV_1, and FEV_1/FVC ratio. A further limitation of standard spirometric measurements is that they do not compensate for variations in body surface area. This reduces the usefulness of such measures when applied to either very large or very small patients.

The diffusing capacity of the lung for carbon monoxide (DLCO) was included in the preoperative assessment of 165 pulmonary resection patients by Ferguson and colleagues.[6] Using logistic regression analysis, the authors found that the most important single predictor of postoperative complications or death was the preoperative DLCO. The DLCO estimates pulmonary capillary surface area and can reveal diffusion defects and emphysematous changes even with acceptable spirometric values. This increase in sensitivity and predictive value appears to justify measurement of diffusion capacity as part of the preoperative assessment. In a retrospective review of 376 patients, Ferguson[8] noted that the most reliable predictor of postoperative complications was the percent predicted postoperative diffusing capacity. Predicted postoperative FEV_1 percent was also analyzed in this review, and statistical analysis determined that there was no correlation between PPO FEV_1 percent and PPO DLCO percent in predicting morbidity or mortality after major lung resection. Each value should be analyzed separately and correlated with the planned amount of lung tissue to be removed. Ferguson[9] concludes that a preoperative diffusing capacity under 60% of predicted indicates an increased risk for complications following pneumonectomy. This increase in sensitivity and predicted value appears to justify measurement of diffusion capacity as part of the preoperative assessment.

Several investigators have sought a more accurate measurement of functional cardiopulmonary reserve. The measurement of maximum oxygen consumption during exercise (VO_{2max}) has been used to predict postoperative complications. A postulate is that oxygen consumption is directly related to cardiac output and that a reduced peak oxygen consumption may correlate with increased postoperative complications. Bechard and Wetstein[10] reported minimal risk of postoperative complications in 50 consecutive patients in whom the VO_{2max} was greater than 20 mL per kg per minute. Patients with a VO_{2max} of less than 50 mL per kg per minute accounted for 75% of all postoperative complications observed. Bolliger[11] concluded that a VO_{2max} under 10 mL per kg per min is predictive of a high risk of complications following any pulmonary resection and could even be considered prohibitive. A value greater than 20 mL per kg per min or greater than 75% of predicted normal is safe for major pulmonary resection, including pneumonectomy.

Recent studies have evaluated exercise oximetry to predict operative risk. Rao[12] carried out a retrospective analysis of 299 patients who underwent both exercise oximetry and spirometry. Sensitivity of oximetry was low, but compared with spirometry it more reliably predicted prolonged hospital stay and respiratory failure. Ninin and colleagues[13] evaluated 46 consecutive patients undergoing pneumonectomy with exercise oximetry and concluded that exercise oximetry was predictive of morbidity and prolonged intensive care stay following pneumonectomy. Prospective randomized trials are needed to confirm the reliability of this test.

Although much effort has been expended to define high-risk patient populations for pulmonary resection, the dilemma of choosing appropriate therapy for such patients remains. Postoperative deaths are dreaded by all involved. However, a more conservative approach might deny a patient a potentially curative resection. Vigorous preoperative respiratory therapy, cessation of smoking, bronchodilator therapy, and even short-term corticose steroid therapy have been shown to improve the operability of lung cancer patients with marginal pulmonary reserve.[14] Finally, tailoring the procedure to the patient, such as a segmentectomy ver-

sus a lobectomy or sleeve lobectomy versus a pneumonectomy, might also offer an otherwise marginal patient the chance of a curative procedure. For more discussion of preoperative risks see Chapter 36.

TABLE 41.1. POTENTIAL FACTORS RELATING TO POSTOPERATIVE ARRHYTHMIAS

Pericardial irritation
Increased sympathetic discharge
Atrial damage
Electrolyte disturbance
Atrial distention
Underlying coronary or valvular heart disease
Postoperative myocardial ischemia
Hypoxia
Preoperative theophylline use

ARRHYTHMIAS

Atrial and ventricular arrhythmias can occur after pulmonary resection. Many factors may contribute to the development of arrhythmias postoperatively (Table 41.1), with potentially serious complications. As early as the 1940s, several investigators noted the increased incidence of arrhythmias after pulmonary resection.[15,16] The incidence of arrhythmias after pulmonary resection has been cited as 3.4% to 30%. Atrial arrhythmias are far more common, consisting of fibrillation, flutter, and supraventricular tachycardia.[17–19] Loss of sinus rhythm adversely affects cardiac output, with resultant decrease in coronary, renal, and cerebral blood flow. When arrhythmias do occur, it is usually during the first few days after surgery and most commonly on the second or third postoperative day. Shields and Ujiki[18] studied 125 consecutive patients and reported a 22% mortality in those patients who developed a postoperative arrhythmia, as compared with a 7% mortality in patients who remained in normal sinus rhythm. These findings are consistent with a series of 236 pneumonectomy patients studied retrospectively by the Mayo Clinic.[15] In this study, the authors observed a 25% 30-day mortality in patients developing tachyarrhythmias after surgery.

The relation of age to the development of postoperative arrhythmias is somewhat conflicting in the literature. Although some authors[17] have reported a near linear relationship between the incidence of arrhythmias with increasing age, Krowka and associates[20] studied 236 pneumonectomy patients and failed to demonstrate any significant association between the patient age and development of arrhythmias. It seems intuitive, however, that age should be a strong predictor of postoperative arrhythmias, because the conduction system also ages, as reflected by a decreasing number of functional sinus node pacemaker cells.[21] In addition, patients of advanced age are more likely to also have coexisting predisposing factors. This is consistent with the findings of Wheat and Burford[19] of a 50% incidence of postoperative arrhythmias in patients 70 years and older who underwent pulmonary resection.

Several series have confirmed a direct relationship between the magnitude of resection and the incidence of postoperative arrhythmias. Mowry and Reynolds[17] reported an overall incidence of 19.4% after pneumonectomy as opposed to 3.1% after lobectomy in their series of 301 patients. Other series[18,19] have observed a less dramatic disparity and have suggested that the relationship between the incidence of arrhythmias and the magnitude of resection is less pronounced in the older population. Krowka and associates[20] studied the relationship between preoperative pulmonary function and the incidence of postoperative arrhythmias. Although they did not demonstrate a firm correlation, they did report an increased incidence in patients with radiographic evidence of fluid overload after a pneumonectomy. This would follow, because right heart distention is felt to be an important factor in the development of postoperative arrhythmias. Wittnich and associates[22] pointed out that Swan-Ganz measurements of pulmonary artery pressures may not be accurate after pneumonectomy. In this situation, the inflation of the balloon tip catheter to measure pulmonary wedge pressure may in fact increase right ventricular afterload, with resultant decreased cardiac output and therefore decreased left atrial pressure. The authors suggest that in this situation, central venous pressure measurements may in fact be a more accurate measure of true cardiac output.

Although many known factors contribute to postoperative arrhythmias, we still cannot accurately identify patients that are of the greatest risk of developing them. In addition, while may studies have used preoperative digoxin or low-dose beta-blockage in the prevention of postoperative arrhythmias, the data are conflicting. Digoxin has long been the drug of choice for the prevention of arrhythmias following thoracic surgery. However, potential side effects and the development of newer pharmacologic agents have diminished its popularity. Digoxin's predominant action is thought to be a slowing of conduction through the AV node, mediated by enhanced vagal tone. This is consistent with the known effect of digoxin in slowing the ventricular response to a rapid supraventricular rate while at the same time being relatively ineffective in converting to a sinus rhythm. This mechanism is also consistent with the observation of a reduced efficacy of digoxin in the immediate postoperative period, when andrologic influences are more pronounced.

There is some evidence that low-dose beta-blockage may have a beneficial prophylactic effect. However, many of the patients presenting for pulmonary resection have underlying pulmonary disease or reduced ventricular function and are therefore not ideal candidates for the administration of beta-blocking agents.[23,24]

The prophylactic administration of the calcium-channel-blocking agent verapamil has been shown to reduced significantly the occurrence of postoperative arrhythmias following thoracotomy.[25] In addition, verapamil was found to lower right ventricular systolic and diastolic pressures, an important action because elevated right-sided pressures are felt to predispose to atrial arrhythmias.[26] A recent study by Van Mieghem and associates[27] demonstrated that a relatively large dose of intravenous verapamil (10 mg bolus) following pulmonary resection effectively reduced the incidence of atrial arrhythmias by 50%. However, side effects such as bradycardia and hypotension seen with this dosage led to discontinuation of the drug in many patients.

Diltiazem, also a calcium-channel-blocking agent, has been shown to be equally efficacious to verapamil in treating atrial arrhythmias, but with fewer side effects. This has led to the greater acceptance of this agent in the postthoracotomy patient.[28,29] Amar[30] recently reported on a comparison of diltiazem and digoxin for the prevention of postoperative atrial arrhythmias in pneumonectomy patients. They found that when compared to digoxin, diltiazem was safe and more effective in preventing atrial arrhythmias in these patients. In addition, the observed incidence of postoperative arrhythmias in digoxin treated patients was similar to that observed in the untreated controls. Amiodarone has also been used in the treatment of postoperative atrial arrhythmias; however, its association with the development of pulmonary infiltrates and dysfunction has prevented its widespread acceptance in pulmonary resection patients.

Once postoperative arrhythmias such as atrial fibrillation occur, there are several therapeutic guidelines that should be followed. First, the heart rate should be acutely controlled. Rapid atrial fibrillation results in poor cardiac filling and therefore reduced cardiac output. Digoxin can be administered intravenously over several hours to a total loading dose of 1 mg in the adult patient. However, digoxin does not slow the ventricular rate acutely and often requires several hours to produce an effect. In addition, digoxin does not reliably convert the patient to a sinus rhythm nor maintain the sinus rhythm. Postoperative atrial fibrillation with a rapid ventricular response requires prompt intervention and generally responds to intravenous calcium-channel-blocking agents such as diltiazem, as previously discussed. In addition, underlying predisposing conditions such as metabolic derangements or hypoxia should be accurately sought and corrected. Digoxin may be used as an initial drug in patients with compromised ventricular function and in patients not hemodynamically compromised by the increased ventricular rate, which would require a more rapidly acting agent. Conversion to normal sinus rhythm in patients with refractory atrial fibrillation or flutter generally requires administration of other pharmacologic agents such as quinidine or procainamide. Rarely do patients become so refractory that they require electrocardioversion unless they have a long history of preoperative atrial fibrillation. Patients who require pharmacologic conversion should generally be kept on these medications for at least three months after surgery.

Patients undergoing lobectomy are generally not prophylactically digitalized. If postoperative atrial arrhythmias occur, the patient is treated pharmacologically. In contrast, pneumonectomy patients are generally prophylactically digitalized and maintained on a daily dose postoperatively. As previously mentioned, there are no data indicating that this prevents the patient from experiencing atrial fibrillation, but it should prevent a rapid ventricular response should atrial fibrillation occur. Occasionally a planned lesser resection results in a pneumonectomy secondary to intraoperative findings. In these situations, the patient is loaded with digoxin postoperatively and maintained on a daily dose. All pulmonary resection patients should have cardiac monitoring for at least 24 hours postoperatively. We generally extend the observation period in pneumonectomy patients and in older patients with other comorbid conditions that might predispose them to arrhythmias.

POSTRESECTION PULMONARY EDEMA

Noncardiogenic pulmonary edema following lung resection was first discussed by Gibbon and Gibbon[31,32] in 1942. At that time, they reported on two patients who had undergone bilateral lobectomies and succumbed within 12 hours of surgery. This clinical experience as well as experimental studies conducted in a feline model led the authors to conclude that edema occurs because of increased capillary blood pressure following acute reduction of the pulmonary vascular bed. More recently Zeldin and associates[33] compiled ten cases from several institutions and retrospectively compared them with controls. After comparison, the authors identified three significant risk factors for postresection pulmonary edema (PPE); right pneumonectomy, increased administration of perioperative fluid, and high urine output as a sign of relative overhydration. In conclusion, it was recommended that "the anesthesiologist must not boldly load the patients up with fluids prior to induction." Since then, several more recent studies have confirmed and expanded upon this earlier work. Verheijen-Breemhaar[34] and associates reviewed 243 pneumonectomy patients in the Netherlands and found that postoperative pulmonary edema occurred in 4.5% of patients, with a mortality rate of 27% in affected patients. As in Zeldin's[33] report, the authors found an increased incidence of PPE in right versus left pneumonectomy patients and in those who had a more positive fluid balance as well as in patients who required reoperation for bleeding. Patel and associates[35] retrospectively studied 197 pneumonectomy patients in England and found a 15% inci-

TABLE 41.2. POSTPNEUMONECTOMY EDEMA

Incidence of 2% to 5% after pneumonectomy
Appears two to three days after otherwise uncomplicated postoperative period
Radiologic onset may precede symptoms by 12 to 24 hours
Radiologic image of interstitial pulmonary edema
Unresponsive to conventional therapies
Mortality of 50% to 100%
Histology compatible with ARDS
Occurs despite a normal pulmonary wedge pressure

From Deslauriers J, Aucoin A, Gregoire J. Postpneumonectomy pulmonary edema. *Chest Surg Clin N Am* 1998;8(3):611, with permission.

dence of postoperative pulmonary edema and a mortality rate of 43%.

A larger series involving 402 lung resection patients from Leeds, England, was reported by Waller and associates.[36] In this series, PPE occurred in 5.1% of right pneumonectomies, 4.0% of left pneumonectomies, and 1% of all lobectomies. The mortality rate was 55% in patients who developed this complication. Interestingly, these authors did not observe a correlation between perioperative fluid administration and postresection pulmonary edema, which prompted discussion regarding other possible mechanisms. Turnage and Lunn[37] retrospectively reviewed charts on 806 pneumonectomy patients at the Mayo Clinic and found 21 cases (2.6%) who experienced postresection pulmonary edema. Affected patients had a 100% mortality rate and histologic evidence of adult respiratory distress syndrome (ARDS) at autopsy. Patients who had a right-sided resection had a threefold higher incidence of PPE as compared to left pneumonectomy patients. Interestingly, no significant difference was found between the affected patients and age- and sex-matched control groups with regard to administration of perioperative fluids. The authors concluded that while postresection pulmonary edema is more common following right pneumonectomy, the etiology was still uncertain. Shapira and Shahian[38] reviewed the literature in their report and confirmed that pulmonary edema developed in approximately 4% of patients following a major lung resection. They further concluded that several factors were involved in the pathogenesis of interstitial pulmonary edema. Finally, in a recent review by Deslauriers and colleagues,[39] current understanding of factors associated with the development of postresection pulmonary edema was presented and summarized in Table 41.2.

Pathogenesis

Slinger[40] pointed out in his review that the cause of PPE was probably multifactorial since no single factor could adequately explain the clinical experience. He further character-

746 *Surgery*

TABLE 41.3. CAUSES OF THE POSTPNEUMONECTOMY PULMONARY EDEMA

1. Probable:	Fluid overload
	Interrupted lung lymphatics
	Increased pulmonary capillary pressure
	Pulmonary endothelial damage
2. Possible:	Hyperinflation
	Right ventricular dysfunction
	Cytokine release
	Oxygen toxicity

From Slinger PD. Perioperative fluid management for thoracic surgery: the puzzle of postpneumonectomy pulmonary edema. *J Cardiothorac Vasc Anesth* 1995;9:442, with permission.

ized the causes of PPE into probable, possible or of questionable influence (Table 41.3).

Fluid overload has been implicated in the pathogenesis of PPE since the early work of Gibbon and Gibbon,[31,32] and almost certainly plays a major role. Forty years later, Zeldin and associates[33] confirmed the role of overhydration in the canine model. In their study, dogs were randomized to receive lactated Ringers at 100 mL per kg before or during a right pneumonectomy, and compared to a control group that received lactated Ringers but no resection. Six of the 12 pneumonectomy dogs developed PPE, while none of the controls did [p = less than 0.05]. The authors concluded that following pneumonectomy, the entire cardiac output is directed to the remaining lung with resultant increase in the intracapillary pressure, which predisposes to edema formation. Increased cardiac output from catecholamine release secondary to pain or from excessive fluid administration will exacerbate this situation.

Interruption of mediastinal lymphatics probably also plays a role in the formation of PPE. In normal lungs, it has been estimated that lymph flow can increase seven- to tenfold without leading to pulmonary edema. Following pneumonectomy, a proportional amount of lymphatic channels is removed with the specimen. In addition, mediastinal and subcarinal dissection can effectively compromise the lymphatic drainage from the remaining lung. Little and colleagues[41] studied the effect of pneumonectomy and mediastinal lymphatic interruption in a canine model. Their findings suggested that following pneumonectomy, the contralateral lung was more prone to extravascular fluid development secondary to the loss of parenchymal and hilar lymphatic drainage routes. Nohl-Oser[42] has further described the lymphatic drainage of the lung and mediastinum and reported that the lymphatics from the right and left lungs are notably different. The majority of lymphatic channels from the left lung cross the midline. Therefore a right pneumonectomy is more likely also to disrupt lymphatic drainage from the remaining left lung, possibly contributing to edema formation.

Other possible factors implicated in the formation of

PPE include increased capillary pressure and endothelial cell damage producing a "leaky capillary" situation. This is consistent with an ARDS histology previously described in these patients.

Preventative Maneuvers

As previously described, following pneumonectomy the entire cardiac output is directed to the remaining lung, with resultant elevation in pulmonary capillary pressure. Because of this, efforts should be made to restrict fluid administration during the intraoperative and early postoperative periods. Total positive fluid balance in the first 24 hours perioperatively should not exceed 20 mL per kg, typically, less than 2 liters intraoperatively followed by less than 50 mL per hour postoperatively for an average adult. Urine output greater than 0.5 mL per kg is unnecessary in the early postoperative period unless renal insufficiency exists. Placement of a central venous pressure monitoring line is often useful in assessing intravascular volume and will aid in the decision to administer diuretic or inotropic therapy.

Adequate pain control is essential to minimize catecholamine release with resultant increase in cardiac output. Recently, lumbar or thoracic epidural anesthesia has proved extremely useful in this situation by providing adequate pain control without oversedation of the patient.

Avoidance of mediastinal shift and overdistention of the remaining lung is also essential. Experimental work by Raffensperger and colleagues[43] in dogs confirmed that overdistention of the contralateral lung following pneumonectomy led to deterioration in lung function. These changes were reflected by an increase in the alveolar-arterial gradient. It is now believed that acute hyperinflation of the remaining lung is probably a significant factor in the development of PPE.

Treatment

As previously stated, the development of PPE is associated with a mortality rate in excess of 50%. Current therapy advocated is supportive and essentially the same as for ARDS. This generally consists of fluid restriction, diuretic therapy, and maintenance of adequate oxygenation and nutritional support. Most patients will require intubation and mechanical ventilation. Unfortunately, prolonged ventilation may increase barotrauma and bronchial stump dehiscence. Inspired oxygen concentrations of 80% to 100% may be required to maintain adequate arterial saturation. Peak inspiratory pressures greater than 30 mm of mercury should be avoided if possible. Empiric administration of antibiotics is probably of little benefit because the underlying process is not infectious in nature.

Mathisen and colleagues[44] have recently reported on the use of inhaled nitric oxide in a series of ten PPE patients with reasonable success. In their series affected patients were treated with standard supportive measures plus inhaled nitric oxide at 10 to 20 parts per million. Overall mortality for this limited series was 30%. Finally, in refractory cases, extracorporeal membrane oxygenation (ECMO) may improve survival, but its role is not yet fully defined.

CARDIAC HERNIATION

Cardiac herniation is a rare but potentially lethal complication that can occur after pulmonary resection when a pericardial defect is created. The mechanism is simply anatomic displacement of the heart through the pericardial defect, which results in entrapment of the heart, thereby effectively obstructing both venous inflow and arterial outflow. This results in elevation of central venous pressure and resultant diminished cardiac output.[45] This complication was first reported in 1948 after a left intrapericardial pneumonectomy with resultant pericardial defect.[46] Since then, about 30 additional cases of cardiac herniation have been reported after both left and right pneumonectomies. Patients who develop cardiac herniation typically experience cardiovascular collapse, and if not promptly reoperated to reposition the heart within the pericardial space, death ensues. Most series in the literature have reported about a 50% mortality rate with this complication.[47,48] Physical findings include cardiovascular collapse with tachycardia, hypotension, and jugular venous distention. This complication usually occurs either during the procedure or in the immediate postoperative period. Beyond that time, intrapericardial adhesions usually form, thereby preventing gross displacement of the heart. The precipitating event is often a change in the patient's position, coughing, positive pressure ventilation, or excessive negative pressure in a pneumonectomy space. A chest radiograph often diagnoses right-sided herniation (Figure 41.1), but left-sided herniation can be somewhat more difficult to appreciate on a standard posteroanterior film. A lateral chest radiograph may help to demonstrate posterior displacement of the heart. Fluoroscopy has also been suggested as a diagnostic aid in this condition, but this may needlessly postpone timely reexploration to reduce the herniation. Any patient suspected of having cardiac herniation should undergo prompt reexploration and repositioning of the heart into the pericardial space. The pericardial defect should then be closed to prevent reoccurrence.

To prevent cardiac herniation, some authors have advocated wide excision of the pericardium to prevent entrapment and strangulation of the heart through a small defect. Others have documented the inability of partial pericardiectomy to prevent hemodynamic embarrassment when cardiac displacement does occur.[49] Closure of the pericardial defect after a resection is the more widely held method of prevention. Many authors have advocated closure of pericardial defects with a variety of materials, including pleura, Vicryl mesh,[24] fascia, and even a latticework of catgut.[48] Dippel and Ehrenhaft[50] have advocated a technique of suturing the pericardial defect edge to the adjacent atrial and ventricular myocardium.

We believe that all small pericardial defects should be closed. On the right side, large pericardial defects must be

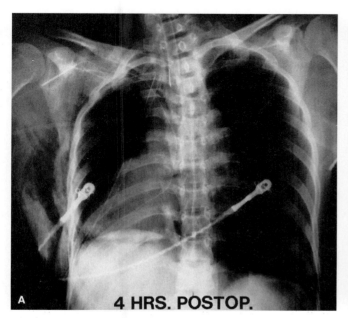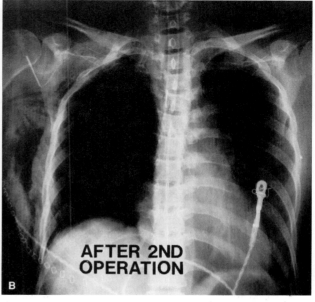

A: 4 HRS. POSTOP.

B: AFTER 2ND OPERATION

FIGURE 41.1. **A:** Cardiac herniation after radical right pneumonectomy. **B:** Chest radiograph after repair with prosthetic patch to close the defect in the pericardium.

closed, owing to the fact that right-sided displacement of the heart, even without entrapment, causes hemodynamic compromise. In contrast, large left-sided defects do not necessarily have to be patched because the heart normally resides in the left thorax, and further displacement will not result in hemodynamic compromise unless the heart is strangulated through a small defect. We generally do not attempt primary closure of pericardial defects but rather place a material such as Gore-Tex, which is durable and easy to suture. Suturing of the edge of the pericardial defect directly to the myocardium should be discouraged because of unwarranted risk to the coronary vessels.[51]

LOBAR TORSION

Postresection lobar torsion has been most commonly described involving the right middle lobe after a right upper lobectomy.[52] If the middle lobe is not secured by either an incomplete transverse fissure or by direct suturing to the remaining lower lobe, the middle lobe can rotate on its bronchovascular pedicle, with resultant circulatory embarrassment of the involved lung parenchyma. Schuler[53] reviewed this complication and reported a 16% mortality rate in a series of 31 patients. Less commonly, lobar torsion can occur on the left side, either in the left upper lobe after lower lobectomy (Figure 41.2) or in the lower lobe after upper lobectomy.[54,55,56] Pulmonary lobar torsion involves rotation of the lung parenchyma on its bronchovascular pedicle. This results in occlusion of the pulmonary veins, with resultant infarction and eventual gangrene of the parenchyma involved. Angulation of the bronchus also compromises the bronchial circulation, which further endangers remaining lung parenchyma. Pulmonary infarction can also

occur postoperatively in the absence of lobar torsion. Pulmonary vein thrombosis, pulmonary artery occlusion, and intraoperative damage to the bronchial circulation have all been implicated in postoperative pulmonary infarction.[57]

Early recognition of this complication is essential to prevent irreversible damage to the involved lobe. A baseline chest radiograph should be obtained shortly after the completion of any pulmonary resection. This is done to ascertain that all remaining lung tissue is fully expanded, with proper positioning of chest tubes. Radiographic findings consistent with torsion include hilar displacement, bronchial cutoff, and lobar consolidation. Nuclear perfusion scans and pulmonary angiography can support the diagnosis by demonstrating lack of arterial blood flow to the affected lobe. However, pulmonary artery blood flow is also decreased in patients with large areas of atelectasis or postoperative parenchymal hematomas. Urgent flexible bronchoscopy should be considered to examine the bronchus and remove any retained secretions, thereby facilitating reexpansion of the pulmonary parenchyma. A bronchus with a "fishmouth" occlusion generally indicates that torsion has taken place. The bronchoscope can be manipulated through the narrowed area, only to have the bronchus reobstruct after removal of the bronchoscope, which is a diagnostic finding. Clinically, the patient may lack any significant symptoms early in the postoperative period. However, once the parenchyma has infarcted with ensuing gangrene, patients commonly develop foul-smelling or blood-tinged sputum, fever, and malodorous chest drainage.[58,59] If left untreated, these patients can progress to frank sepsis with hemodynamic instability and even death. Treatment consists of early recognition of this condition in the postoperative period and a low threshold for performing flexible bronchoscopy in any patient suspected of having this condition. Reexploration

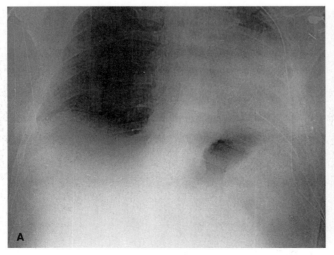
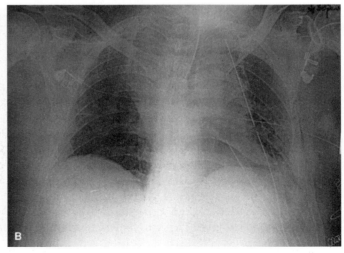

FIGURE 41.2. A: Torsion of the left upper lobe after left lower lobectomy. **B:** Chest radiograph after repositioning of the left upper lobe and fixation with a pleural flap.

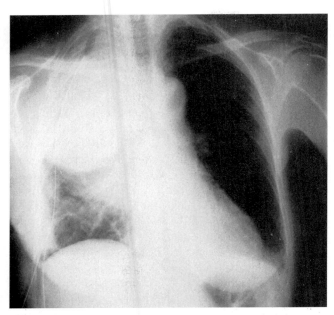

FIGURE 41.3. Pulmonary infarction caused by obstructive venous drainage of the right upper lobe.

is required with repositioning of the affected lobe, securing it to the adjacent lobe to prevent recurrence. If the affected lobe is clearly infarcted at the time of reexploration, resection is mandatory.

Prevention of lobar torsion is essential and begins in the operating room after pulmonary resection. Careful inspection of the remaining lung tissue should be performed while the lung is carefully reexpanded. Complete interlobar fissures permit rotation of a remaining lobe and should be prevented by placement of sutures to the adjacent lobe. Avoidance of unnecessary dissection of a fissure also minimizes this complication. Finally, any inadvertent compromise of lobar venous drainage results in pulmonary infarction (Figure 41.3). When recognized intraoperatively, the affected lobe should be resected if the venous injury is not easily repaired. Accidental ligation of the middle lobe vein requires middle lobectomy.

ATELECTASIS

Atelectasis after thoracotomy is probably the most common postoperative complication. The reported incidence varies widely in the literature as a result of an inability adequately to define significant atelectasis. An incidence as high as 70% has been reported, but other large series of patients generally agree on an overall incidence of 20% to 30% after thoracotomy.[2,60,61]

Atelectasis was previously believed to result from mucus plugging of small airways, with resultant distal gas absorption and alveolar collapse.[62] Although airway occlusion from retained secretions, blood, foreign bodies, or bronchospasm can lead to atelectasis, the etiology is far more complex. Other causes of atelectasis include prolonged shallow breathing or splinting secondary to pain, absorption atelectasis with high inspired oxygen concentration, and parenchymal compression from retraction, hemothorax, pneumothorax, or other space-occupying lesions.

At least two mechanisms normally prevent alveolar collapse. The first is a periodic sigh breath, which is generally twice the usual resting tidal volume and serves to recruit collapsed alveolar. Patients who have shallow breathing secondary to pain and ventilated patients with inadequate tidal volumes may experience progressive alveolar closure with resultant atelectasis.[63,64]

The second preventive physiologic mechanism involves surfactant, a normally occurring wetting agent in the alveoli. LaPlace's theorem states that the surface tension of a distensible sphere increases proportionately as the radius decreases. This relation alone would favor collapse of smaller alveoli into larger units. Surfactant, however, acts to reduce the surface tension within alveoli and thereby prevent preferential collapse of smaller alveoli. Conditions such as malnutrition, sepsis, parenchymal injury, and prolonged collapse can adversely affect production of surfactant and predispose to alveolar collapse.

A condition known as absorption atelectasis merits comment. Normally, the sum of the partial pressures of gases in the alveoli exceeds the partial pressure in mixed venous blood. It follows that, with proximal airway occlusion, distal gases in the alveoli are absorbed, resulting in alveolar collapse. In addition, a higher concentration of oxygen in the trapped or anesthetic gases is more readily absorbed, thereby hastening the process.

Physiologically significant atelectasis results in decreased lung compliance, functional residual capacity, and vital capacity. This results clinically in increased work of breathing and impaired gas exchange.[65,66] Patients typically manifest with varying degrees of fever, tachycardia, tachypnea, and impaired gas exchange. Atelectasis may also render the lung more susceptible to infection.[67] Physical findings usually include crackles over the affected area. More extensive atelectasis results in tubular breath sounds, indicating involvement of entire segments or lobes. Sudden stoppage of an air leak frequently occurs with atelectasis. The radiologic appearance of atelectasis varies depending on the extent of involvement. Linear horizontal densities in the basilar segments are typical of small areas of atelectasis and usually occur near the diaphragm. Larger areas can usually be visualized if entire segments are involved, and this can progress to collapse of an entire lobe.

Several maneuvers can be extremely valuable in the prevention of postoperative atelectasis. Patients must refrain from smoking for as long as possible before thoracotomy. In addition, any bronchospasm detected either clinically or on preoperative pulmonary function testing should be minimized with medical therapy. Patient training and use of incentive spirometry should be initiated in the preoperative period and continued postoperatively. Adequate analgesia is essential to prevent splinting and to allow adequate pulmonary hygiene. We continue to use epidural analgesics routinely for three to five days postoperatively because they provide excellent pain relief with minimal adverse effects.[68]

Treatment of postoperative atelectasis involves many of the principles used in its prevention. Airways must remain free of retained secretions, and collapsed lung tissue must be reexpanded. Adequate postoperative analgesia is essential to allow for deep breathing, effective cough, and therapeutic physiotherapy. Epidural analgesia is an effective means of obtaining adequate analgesia without significant sedation. Local analgesics or opiates are injected into the epidural space continuously to achieve the proper level of analgesia. Contraindications to placement of an epidural catheter include bleeding diathesis, spinal deformity, neurologic deficit, or local infection in the area of catheter placement. Side effects and symptoms of overdosing include respiratory depression, nausea, pruritus, urinary retention, and hypotension secondary to peripheral vasodilatation. We routinely leave epidural catheters in place for 72 hours postoperatively but have maintained selected patients for up to five days.

Patient positioning in the early postoperative period is also important. Functional residual capacity declines by about 40% in the supine position as compared with upright. Routine elevation of the head of the bed to 45 degrees and early ambulation promote effective inspiration. Incentive spirometry is inexpensive and effective in preventing atelectasis. Patients are best trained in this technique preoperatively.

Intermittent positive-pressure breathing may be of some benefit in selected patients but has generally not been effective in treating postoperative atelectasis.[60,65] These results, along with increased cost, have persuaded many to abandon this technique.

Patients with thick or copious secretions require a more aggressive approach. Nasotracheal aspiration is effective when performed by personnel experienced in passing the catheter into the trachea. Passing a catheter through a nasal trumpet may facilitate the process while decreasing patient discomfort. Caution should be exercised when passing the catheter blindly into a patient's airway after pneumonectomy or a bronchoplastic procedure. Also, prolonged suctioning can precipitate hypoxia and should therefore be performed only intermittently for short periods following administration of supplemental oxygen.

A technique of percutaneous cricothyroidotomy, or "minitracheostomy," has been developed. A 20F tracheostomy tube is inserted into the trachea through the cricothyroid membrane under local anesthesia. Au and colleagues[69] reported using this technique in 144 postthoracotomy patients. The minitracheostomy tract was found to be a relatively safe and effective means to prevent postoperative sputum retention. Others[70,71,72] have confirmed the efficacy of this technique for pulmonary hygiene and treatment of atelectasis secondary to retained secretions. Complications with this technique are uncommon and consist mostly of bleeding at the insertion site. Catheter aspiration, pneumothorax, and vocal cord dysfunction from hematoma have also been reported.[73,74]

Patients who require more aggressive treatment of secretions should undergo flexible bronchoscopy (Figure 41.4). Routine use of flexible bronchoscopy for the prevention of postoperative atelectasis has been studied prospectively and found to offer no advantage over other less invasive tech-

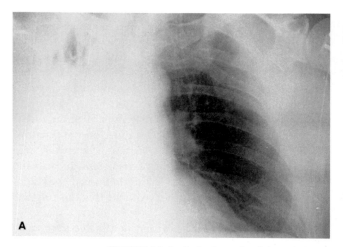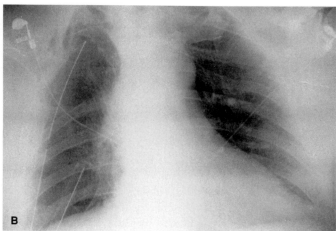

FIGURE 41.4. **A:** Atelectasis of the residual right middle and lower lobes after right upper lobectomy and chest wall resection. **B:** Full expansion after aspiration of retained secretions by flexible fiberoptic bronchoscopy.

niques.[63,75] However, in the setting of significant pulmonary collapse or after bronchoplastic procedures, fiber-optic bronchoscopy is a safe and effective method to aspirate secretions under direct vision. Bronchoscopy can be easily performed at the bedside using local analgesia and, if necessary, can be repeated often.[76] Treatment of postoperative atelectasis should be graded according to the patient's clinical status and risk factors as described by Massard.[77]

BRONCHIAL FISTULA

The incidence of bronchopleural fistula after pulmonary resection is reported to be under 5%.[78,79,80] Both systemic and local factors are associated with the development of a bronchopleural fistula, and a lung cancer patient may be particularly prone to this complication. Systemic factors include the patient's general nutrition status and the presence of sepsis. Lung cancer patients frequently lose weight, and the ability of tissues to heal is decreased. Sepsis can also retard bronchial healing, and many patients with an obstructive endobronchial neoplasm have distal pneumonitis producing chronic low-grade infection. Neoadjuvant protocols for the treatment of clinically advanced lung cancer include chemotherapy and radiation. Effects of chemotherapy can be debilitating to the patient, and depleted nutritional status can be a significant factor in the development of a bronchial fistula. Radiation destroys small blood vessels, creates fibrous tissue, and is associated with an increased incidence of bronchial fistula.[81] Vester and colleagues[78] reported that, of 33 patients who developed a bronchopleural fistula after resection for bronchogenic carcinoma, 20 had received radiation or chemoradiation. It is mandatory that special care be given to the bronchial stump in all patients who have received neoadjuvant therapy.

Numerous studies indicate that the causes of bronchial fistula include devitalization and devascularization by excessive dissection, parabronchial infection related to nonabsorbable suture, residual bronchial disease, poor approximation of the mucosa, the length of the stump, and the surgeon's lack of experience.[82] The avoidance of the complication of a bronchial fistula implies prevention, and several technical factors can minimize this complication.

Preoperative bronchoscopy is an important step in evaluating the status of the bronchial mucosa at the site of the planned resection. If inflammation is present, specific attention is made to the stump closure along with coverage by flaps of tissue for reinforcement and added blood supply. If surgery for the cancer is semielective, then it can be delayed for additional supportive therapy and antibiotics.

In a patient with lung cancer, the bronchial tissues must be cleared with care and precise sharp dissection. It is important for the surgeon to have knowledge of the anatomic location of the bronchial arteries and to preserve as many as possible despite the necessity for a radical procedure. This is particularly true when carrying out mediastinal lymphadenectomy in the lung cancer patient. The subcarinal area is traversed by feeding bronchial arteries, and this dissection must be done as carefully as possible to preserve some of these nutrient vessels. The right mainstem bronchus receives its blood supply from vessels posterior to the trachea and bronchus, and it is appropriate to not dissect this area if at all possible. The lymphadenectomy between the vena cava and trachea is done carefully to minimize damage to the blood supply to the lateral walls of the trachea. On the left side, a large bronchial artery has its origin from the distal transverse aorta and, on occasion, can be preserved despite removal of lymph nodes in the aorticopulmonary window. An excessively long bronchial stump accumulates excessive secretions, and its distal margin has a limited blood supply; both factors predisposing to poor healing. The bronchus should always be divided as proximally as possible, but closure must not compromise the adjacent trachea or bronchial lumen.

The method of bronchial stump closure is generally the surgeon's preference. In 1980, Forrester-Wood[83] reported results of 450 pneumonectomies. Bronchial closure was carried out by using stapling techniques in half of the patients, and the other half had bronchial closure with nonabsorbable suture or stainless steel. The incidence of fistula formation was 11% in the suture group and 2.6% in the staple group. Vester and colleagues[78] reported on 30 bronchial fistulas in 1773 pulmonary resections (1.7%) after staple closure of the bronchus. There were 23 fistulas in 506 pneumonectomy patients (4.5%). Al-Kattan and associates[84] reviewed the incidence of bronchopleural fistula in 530 consecutive pneumonectomies after hand-suture closure of the bronchus. Polypropylene suture was used for the closure, and there were seven fistulas (1.3%). In 1982, Lawrence and colleagues[79] studied 378 patients undergoing pulmonary resection and found no significant difference between the hand-sewn and stapled bronchial closure. The surgeon must be aware of contraindications to close the bronchus by stapling techniques. If the cancer is close to the bronchial orifice, as observed by bronchoscopy or identified during hilar dissection, the stapling techniques should not be used. In this instance, the bronchus is transected by a knife, and both the proximal and distal margins are inspected. Whenever there is a question about the proximal extent of the cancer, the bronchus is transected by knife dissection, and suture closure of the bronchus is carried out. After neoadjuvant therapy, the bronchial tissues can be particularly thick and fibrotic. In this instance, careful judgment is required to determine the appropriate type of bronchial closure. A thickened bronchus does not hold the staples, and excessive tension permits edges of the bronchus to separate. In this instance, it is recommended that the hand-suture technique be carried out with either nonabsorbable or absorbable monofilament suture (see also Chapter 38).

The same principles used in dissecting and closing the

bronchus for a pneumonectomy apply to the bronchus after lobectomy. If the tissues are too thick or the cancer is too close to the margin of resection, stapling techniques are not used. We prefer to use a 4.8-leg-length staple for the lobar bronchus because there is less compression of the tissue and distal blood supply is preserved through the B shape of the staple. Special attention must be given to the bronchial stump of a bilobectomy. Vester and colleagues[78] reported ten bronchial fistulas in 965 patients receiving either bilobectomy or lobectomy, and there were nine fistulas after bilobectomy for primary cancer of the lung (right upper lobe and right middle lobe, four; right middle lobe and right lower lobe, five). The increased incidence of fistula after a bilobectomy undoubtedly relates to the extensive dissection of the bronchus, with a probable decrease in blood supply to the surrounding tissues. It is important to consider tissue coverage of the bronchial stump after bilobectomy to minimize this complication. This is particularly true if the patient has received neoadjuvant therapy.

Tissue coverage of the pneumonectomy stump can minimize the complication of a small bronchial fistula and can also bring additional blood supply to the bronchus to promote healing. All right pneumonectomy stumps should be covered with some form of tissue. The left pneumonectomy stump, if done correctly, retracts deeply into the mediastinum, and the decision for tissue coverage requires careful judgment. All pneumonectomy patients who have received neoadjuvant therapy should have both the right and left pneumonectomy stumps covered with tissue.

Several methods are available for tissue coverage of a pneumonectomy stump. Al-Kattan and colleagues[84] recommend burying the bronchial stump beneath the mediastinal tissues. Azygos vein, adjacent pleura, pericardium, and esophageal wall can all be used for this technique. It was noted that this maneuver is important to decrease the incidence of bronchial fistula in patients older than 60 years and in those who underwent resection for lung cancer. A broad-based pleural flap can also be used to cover the bronchial stump. The pleura is tacked to both sides of the bronchus with a 4–0 absorbable suture. Only the parabronchial tissues are sutured to the pleura, and every attempt is made to avoid placing the needle through the entire thickness of the bronchial wall. This only distorts the bronchus and decreases its blood supply. However, the pleura contains few blood vessels and does not enhance the healing process with additional blood supply. For this reason, other tissue coverage is generally recommended. The intercostal muscle pedicle flap provides good reinforcement of a bronchial closure. It has also been demonstrated to deliver increased blood supply to the bronchial tissue.[85] It is helpful to have made the decision to use the intercostal muscle flap before opening the chest, because the flap can be developed with a portion of parietal pleura, ensuring its viability and blood supply. This flap is best created through a posterolateral thoracotomy. When the flap is used after completion of the

resection, it is not as suitable. The rib spreader can traumatize the intercostal muscle, and the vessel can be damaged by retraction or extension of the thoracotomy incision posteriorly. Rendina and associates[85] clearly described the construction of the intercostal pedicle flap. It was used in 59 patients, and postoperative angiographic studies of the intercostal artery in 14 patients demonstrated full patency of this vessel.

The serratus anterior muscle provides excellent coverage to the bronchial stump and is the muscle flap of choice for some thoracic surgeons.[86,87] The serratus anterior muscle is mobilized at the time of the posterolateral thoracotomy, and its insertion is detached from the ribs with a cautery technique. The lateral thoracic artery is preserved, and the muscle is not separated from its scapular attachments until a final decision is made to use it as a tissue flap. Muscle is easily brought through the incised third intercostal space or through a defect made by a subperiosteal excision of a small portion of the third rib. The muscle is then sutured in place with 4–0 absorbable sutures and amply covers the stump and areas of mediastinal dissection. Care must be taken that the muscle flap is not under tension and that its vascularity is not compromised by compression of tissues in the intercostal space. Regnard and colleagues[87] used this technique in seven patients who underwent pneumonectomy after 6,000 to 6,500 cGy of radiation. There were four empyemas in this group of patients, but only one recurrent fistula, which was successfully treated by antibiotics and additional tissue placed into the pneumonectomy space.

The use of this flap for bronchial coverage is reserved for patients who have received an excessive amount of radiation or when there is concern about the viability of the bronchial stump closure. In patients who have received neoadjuvant therapy, the serratus anterior muscle can be preserved during a posterolateral thoracotomy. Added exposure is obtained by detaching it from several ribs. If the surgeon decides to use this muscle flap to cover the bronchus, the construction of the flap can be completed at the end of the procedure. If this muscle flap is not used to cover the bronchus, then it can be resutured to the tissue adjacent to the ribs, with the incision closed in the standard fashion. One problem associated with the serratus flap is that the patient may complain of a winged scapula due to detachment of the fibers from the inferior portion of the scapula. We use a broad-based mediastinal fat pad for coverage of both the right and left pneumonectomy stumps (Figure 41.5). Most patients have an adequate amount of fat that extends down to the cardiophrenic angle, and dissection frequently encompasses the lateral wall of the thymus gland. The fat pad is sharply dissected from the pericardium and freed to the upper mediastinum; it is easily brought over to the bronchial stump. Its blood supply is not as generous as that of a serratus anterior muscle or intercostal muscle flap, but secure tissue coverage is obtained (see Figure 41.5). Again, it is important to place fixation sutures in the peri-

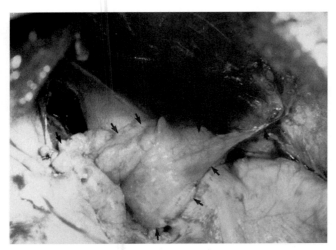

FIGURE 41.5. Large mediastinal fat pad covers the right pneumonectomy stump. Arrows depict the superior vena cava, and the head of the patient is to the left.

bronchial wall, both anteriorly and posteriorly, to secure the coverage. It is not appropriate just to place the fat pad over the bronchus and suture to the adjacent pleura, because this does not provide an adequate seal.

Use of the omentum is not recommended for routine coverage of pneumonectomy stump. It requires the placement of additional incision in the abdomen and a longer operating time than the flaps described earlier. The omentum is reserved for closure of a bronchial fistula if the complication does develop.[88]

Patients who develop a bronchial fistula three to four weeks after pneumonectomy expectorate varying amounts of serosanguineous fluid, may become dyspneic, and frequently develop subcutaneous emphysema. Chest radiograph illustrates a decreasing amount of fluid in the pneumonectomy space and the presence of subcutaneous air. In the hospital, the patient should be positioned with the operated side down to prevent spillage of the pleural fluid into the contralateral lung. Without delay or diagnostic studies, a chest tube is inserted into the pleural space to remove all of the fluid. Balanced pleural drainage is preferable, but a standard underwater-seal drainage system can also be adequate. The drainage system must not be connected to suction, because detrimental physiologic mediastinal shift can occur. Flexible fiber-optic bronchoscopy should be done to evaluate the status of the pneumonectomy stump and clear the airway of any secretions or fluid. With the development of vascular tissue flaps for stump coverage, new antibiotics, and the success of antibiotic irrigation in combating empyema, reoperation and bronchial stump reclosure can be considered up to 14 days after the initial operation.

If the patient undergoes reoperation, a long single-lumen endotracheal tube is placed into the contralateral bronchus with the aid of the flexible fiber-optic bronchoscope under local anesthesia. Precise placement of the endotracheal tube is achieved under direct bronchoscopic visualization and eliminates any possibility of contamination of the dependent lung during positioning of the patient. A double-lumen catheter can be used, but it can be difficult to position in the presence of a mainstem bronchial fistula, and excessive manipulation of the tube may only make the fistula larger. Proper position of the double-lumen tube must be documented with the small-diameter flexible bronchoscope.

The necrotic edges of the bronchial stump are carefully debrided back to viable tissue, and the stump is closed with an interrupted suture technique using nonabsorbable monofilament suture. Omentum provides excellent coverage and blood supply to a dehisced bronchial stump, and the pedicle would have been prepared before opening the chest.[88] If the serratus anterior muscle was preserved at the time of the original thoracotomy, it is also an excellent flap to provide coverage for the bronchial fistula. Intercostal muscle and mediastinal fat can also be used, but their blood supply is not as generous as the previously mentioned flaps.

The pleural space is cultured to determine whether infection is present and also to obtain antibiotic sensitivities for postoperative antibiotic irrigation. Antibiotic irrigations are begun in the first postoperative 48 hours through a previously placed intercostal catheter, and the pleural space is filled twice daily with an appropriate concentration of antibiotics and 1,000 mL of sterile saline. The tube is clamped, and the chest is emptied every ten hours. Serum levels of the antibiotics are obtained to be certain that toxic blood levels are not present. After ten days of antibiotic irrigation, cultures of the draining fluid are obtained to be certain that the effluent fluid is sterile, and the chest tube is then removed. Before removal, the space is filled with the antibiotic solution. If an empyema develops at a later date, it is treated by adequate dependent drainage, and the space eventually closed by thoracoplasty or myoplasty or both. The antibiotic sterilization can again be attempted if a fistula is not present, as described by Claggett and Gerace.[89]

A two-stage procedure is advocated by Deschamps et al.[90] for fistula closure and sterilization of the empyema space. The first stage consists of opening of the thoracotomy incision with debridement and closure of the bronchial fistula and coverage with viable tissue. The empyema cavity is thoroughly debrided and the cavity is packed open with gauze soaked in povidone-iodine solution diluted 20 to 1. The packing is changed daily, and when healthy granulation tissue appears in the pleural space, the cavity is filled with antibiotic solution and a watertight chest wall closure is obtained.

The management of a bronchopleural fistula that occurs several weeks or months after pneumonectomy requires that the space be clean and dependently drained. This is best accomplished with the open-window thoracostomy or Eloesser flap.[91] The presence of a chronic bronchopleural fistula requires direct closure because it will not heal on its own, and the pneumonectomy space cannot be closed or sterilized until the fistula has healed. Puskas and colleagues[91] described successful closure of chronic bronchopleural fistulas in 40 of 47 patients (85%) using direct suture closure of the bronchial stump in 37 patients and suturing of omental or tissue flaps over the fistula in ten patients. All of these closures were buttressed with vascularized pedicle flaps of omentum, muscle, or pleura. At the time of the bronchial fistula closure, the empyema cavity can be obliterated using myoplasty and thoracoplasty techniques. Any residual cavity that remains can be successfully sterilized using the Claggett[89] technique.

Failure of sterilization of the residual space can be successfully managed with packing and daily dressing change, with expected obliteration of the space by granulation tissue over several months. Pairolero and colleagues[86] used muscle grafts of pectoralis, serratus anterior, latissimus dorsi, and rectus abdominis, along with the omentum, and achieved an 88% success rate in closing fistulas and controlling intrathoracic sepsis. Extrathoracic muscle transpositions, along with omentum, are now the accepted standard of therapy for treatment of the chronic bronchopleural fistula and empyema. These techniques have significantly decreased the need for a disfiguring thoracoplasty, which is the alternative method of treating postpneumonectomy empyema and fistula.

If a pneumonectomy fistula occurs in a long bronchial stump, consideration can be given to the transsternal approach for reamputation of the stump. This is a technically demanding procedure, and the surgeon must thoroughly review the literature before embarking on this repair.[93] After successful transsternal closure of the fistula, antibiotic sterilization of the pneumonectomy space is done.

Fibrin glue can successfully close a small fistula up to 4 mm in size, and its use should be considered when a small fistula has been identified. Tissue glue in the United States can be made from cryoprecipitate and thrombin, and the European version with a stronger tensile strength is now available. Closure of small fistulas in both pneumonectomy and lobar stumps has been achieved. The cryoprecipitate and thrombin are instilled through catheters passed through the channel of a fiber-optic bronchoscope. This technique is associated with low morbidity and can be the initial therapeutic maneuver if the fistula is small.[94,95]

Bronchial fistula after lobectomy is a rare occurrence, and it is more common for a lobar bronchial fistula to occur after a bilobectomy than a standard lobectomy. A cancer resection requires an extensive dissection when carrying out a bilobectomy, and bronchial blood supply is jeopardized. The surgeon must pay particular attention to closure and coverage of bilobectomy stumps.

Early dehiscence of a bronchial stump after lobectomy is evidenced by a persistent and moderate air leak, a sudden increase in the size of an air leak, or the development of a space after chest tubes have been removed. Other symptoms include fever and a cough productive of serosanguineous fluid or purulent material from a developing empyema. If a fistula is suspected, bronchoscopy should be carried out. Complete separation of a bronchial closure is obvious, but small defects in a lobar bronchus may be difficult to identify. A to-and-fro motion of secretions at the stump, necrotic tissue, and granulations are all indicators of a fistula. If the chest tubes have been removed, a new chest tube must be inserted into the developing space as soon as the diagnosis of a lobar stump fistula is made. A decision is then made about appropriate therapy.

In general, it is better to treat lobar bronchial fistula in a long-term conservative manner, for several reasons. First, acute debridement of a dehisced lobar stump may result in little remaining bronchus to reapproximate, and closure would compromise a mainstem bronchus. Second, to achieve closure of viable bronchial tissue, a completion pneumonectomy may be required, with increased morbidity and mortality. Third, the probable infected space may predispose the fistula closure to failure, resulting in an increase in morbidity and mortality.

If reoperation for a lobar fistula is decided on, the surgeon has several options. The bronchus can be resected to obtain more healthy tissue, and the stump is reapproximated with a fine, nonabsorbable, monofilament suture. If the bronchial tissues are necrotic, the amputation of the bronchus at a higher level must be considered. This technique is applicable when a right lower lobectomy stump has developed a fistula, and the middle lobe can be resected with bronchial closure at the proximal bronchus intermedius. Sleeve lobectomy can be considered after an upper-lobe bronchial fistula, but the surgeon must be aware of possible anastomotic failure along with probable difficulty in reexpansion of the residual lung tissue. All reoperative bronchial closures must be covered by a viable tissue flap.

Despite the fact that adequate tube drainage after lobar bronchial fistula may result in a more protracted course, a successful long-term result can usually be achieved. Myoplasty or thoracoplasty, or both, may be necessary to close the fistula and obliterate the associated space, but they are accomplished at less risk when the patient's condition is able to withstand a second operation. Tube drainage is maintained until the residual lung tissue is adherent to the parietal pleura, and the fistula is then treated as a chronic problem. A small fistula may eventually close with fibrotic resolution of the space, but most remain open. Basic criteria to be carried out include control of the underlying disease process and a clean, dependently drained space.[96]

SPACES AND AIR LEAKS

A decrease in the incidence of the development of the postoperative space and prolonged air leak directly results in a decreased incidence of postoperative complications. The lung cancer patient is particularly prone to the development of these complications. The normal mechanisms of compensation for the loss of lung tissue are (a) expansion of the residual lung, (b) mediastinal shift, (c) narrowing of the intercostal spaces, and (d) elevation of the diaphragm. Frequently, lung cancer patients have had neoadjuvant irradiation and chemotherapy, and there is fibrosis in the mediastinum that limits its ability to shift its position. The lung tissue, if fibrotic from irradiation, does not fully expand, and parenchymal air leaks fail to heal. The elderly lung cancer patient is prone to prolonged air leaks from emphysematous lung tissue.

Most persistent air leaks originate from small bronchi or disrupted alveoli and can be termed alveolo-pleural fistulas. Most air leaks close within seven days of the operative procedure, but some require special maneuvers in an attempt to stop the leak. Alveolo-pleural fistulas originate from lung tissue that has been denuded of its visceral pleura, incomplete lung fissures, the raw surface of a segmentectomy, and nonanatomic resections for neoplasms. These leaks can be minimized at the time of resection by careful attention to technical detail, and prevention is the best method of treatment.

The use of the stapler can minimize air leaks from a divided minor or major fissure and helps to separate the upper lobe from the middle lobe. The stapling device can also minimize air leaks when carrying out wedge resection or segmental resection, depending on the surgeon's technique. The staple line should be reinforced with a bovine pericardium or Gore-Tex when the lung tissue is emphysematous. At the close of the operation, the anesthetist fully expands the lung to 20 to 25 cm of airway pressure with the lung and bronchus submerged in saline, and the bronchial stump and lung parenchyma are carefully observed. Air leaks from staple lines and disrupted parenchyma are closed with fine, interrupted absorbable sutures. Small air leaks near the hilum can be approximated with carefully placed sutures to avoid damage to major arteries or veins. A defect in the bronchial stump is repaired.

A pedicle flap of pleura can be used to cover air leaks from tissue just as well as it can cover a bronchial stump. Absorbable sutures can be placed through the pleura and then through the lung tissue to anchor the pleura flap securely over the leaking area of lung. On occasion, a free graft of pleura can be used to reinforce sutures. If a segmentectomy has not been done by the stapling technique, the residual segmental lung surface can be approximated to the adjacent lobe. This technique is particularly applicable to posterior, superior, anterior, and medial basal and lingular segmentectomies.

If an air leak persists at seven days, there are several therapeutic maneuvers that can be attempted. Suction can be discontinued, because it is possible that the increased negative intrapleural pressure is maintaining the air leak, and discontinuing the suction will cause the leak to close. A

chest radiograph is obtained in 24 hours, and if a space is developing, the suction is restarted. Chest-tube suction is maintained for the initial postoperative seven days because it has been our experience that if the lung collapses in the early postoperative period, reexpansion can be difficult, with a resultant residual space. A second maneuver is to withdraw the anterior chest tube by 1 or 2 inches. A chest-tube hole may be directly adjacent to a small air leak; repositioning the tube allows the lung to expand, and the leaking lung surface adheres to the parietal pleura. Suction is never increased if the residual lung is fully expanded because increased suction may potentiate the air leak.

If the lung remains expanded after discontinuation of suction, consideration can be given to removing the chest tubes, despite the presence of a small air leak. This technique can be successful, but if a space does develop, a chest tube must be reinserted. Suction is maintained until the air leak stops or the patient is discharged with a Heimlich valve attached to the leaking chest tube. The patient is seen at weekly intervals in the office. The leak usually stops by the time of the first office visit, and the tube is then removed. It may be necessary to leave the tube in place for an additional two to three weeks until the air leak stops. If the air leak persists four weeks after hospital discharge, the patient is considered to have an empyema, and open drainage is instituted. The tube is then shortened by 1 or 2 inches at weekly intervals until it is removed. This method of tube management is predicated on the fact that the patient does not have an infected space and the lung is expanded.

There are no specific guidelines for the indications of reoperation of a patient with a persistent air leak at seven to 14 days. Factors that play a role in this decision include the general condition of the patient, the emphysematous nature of the remaining lung, the speculated cause of the persistent air leak, and the presence and magnitude of an intrapleural space. Reoperation and necessary decortication can create new air leaks, and careful judgment is required to reoperate for a persistent air leak. A large and increasing air leak may make reoperation necessary. The management of a persistent air leak is noted in Figure 41.6.

The development of a postoperative space is commonly related to a persistent and large air leak, but other causes include resection of two lobes on the right side, only the basal segments of either lobe remaining, fibrosis in the remaining lung that limits expansion, and incomplete decortication from prior pleural effusion or infection. Postoperative atelectasis and a fixed mediastinum due to irradiation or prior inflammation also contribute to the development of a space. All of these factors are seen in patients undergoing resection for lung cancer. Kirsch and colleagues[97] reported on the natural history of the pleural space and noted that 74% undergo spontaneous resolution, 13% require temporary drainage, 7% are persistently sterile, and only 6% become infected. Despite the relatively low incidence of major complications associated with a persistent space, the tho-

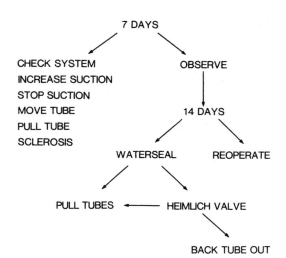

```
                    7 DAYS
                   ↙      ↘
CHECK SYSTEM              OBSERVE
INCREASE SUCTION            |
STOP SUCTION                |
MOVE TUBE                14 DAYS
PULL TUBE                ↙      ↘
SCLEROSIS         WATERSEAL      REOPERATE
                   ↙      ↘
        PULL TUBES ← HEIMLICH VALVE
                            ↘
                        BACK TUBE OUT
```

FIGURE 41.6. Suggested management of prolonged air leak. (From Piccione W Jr, Faber LP. Management of complications related to pulmonary resection. In: Waldhausen JA, Orringer MB, eds. *Complications in cardiothoracic surgery.* St. Louis: Mosby Year Book, 1991:336, with permission.)

racic surgeon must make every attempt to minimize it because an infected space is a problem for both the patient and the thoracic surgeon.

Practical steps can be carried out in the management of a postoperative space. The first is to be certain that the residual lung tissue is clear of all secretions and that postoperative atelectasis is aggressively treated. Early postoperative

consideration must be given to increasing the amount of chest-tube suction. We routinely start with 20 cm of water suction immediately after the operation and recommend increasing suction to 30 or 40 cm of water pressure if there is a space in association with an air leak. Evacuation of the air permits the raw lung surface to reach the parietal pleura, and small air leaks close. The patient can be dyspneic owing to a decrease in tidal volume as inspired air is removed by increasing suction. Significant pleural pain can also be troublesome. Suction should be increased in increments of only 10 cm of water to evaluate the patient's ability to tolerate it. We do not use suction set at more than 40 cm of water pressure because of patient discomfort.

Certain intraoperaive maneuvers can also minimize the possible complications of the postoperative space. One method is to use a pleural tent (Figure 41.7). If an extrapleural dissection was required to resect an upper-lobe lesion, then a pleural tent is obviously not available. Even if a constructed pleural tent is not airtight, the large pleural flap can cover residual lung tissue and expedite the closure of parenchymal air leaks, which effectively eliminates a space problem. Transplantation of the diaphragm and crushing of the phrenic nerve have been advocated to minimize the postoperative space, but have not been used in our experience. Disadvantages include the time involved to transplant the diaphragm and the loss of diaphragmatic motion, which decreases the patient's ability to cough as well as long-term pulmonary function. The most extensive intraoperative procedure is to bring the chest wall to the lung tissue. This is accomplished by either a tailoring or an osteoplastic thora-

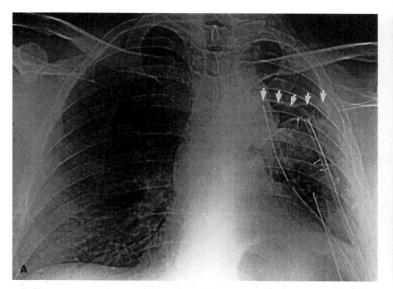
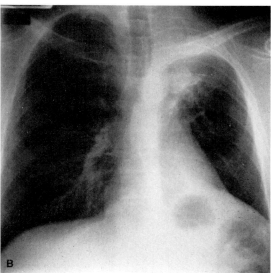

FIGURE 41.7. A: Pleural tent constructed to minimize air leak and pleural space after left upper lobectomy and resection of a portion of the superior segment of the left lower lobe. Arrows depict the location of the pleural tent. One chest tube drains the space above the pleural tent, and two chest tubes drain the normal pleural space. **B:** Chest radiograph six months later in the same patient.

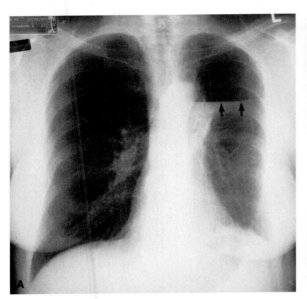
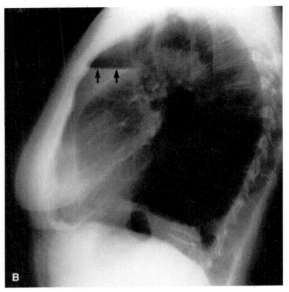

FIGURE 41.8. Frontal **(A)** and lateral **(B)** views of a sterile space after left upper lobectomy. Space will obliterate in several weeks with no postoperative sequela.

coplasty. A tailoring thoracoplasty entails subperiosteal resection of the first and second ribs along with a portion of the third rib to decrease the size of the apex. An osteoplastic thoracoplasty is a subperiosteal resection of the posterior portions of ribs 2, 3, 4, and 5, with wire fixation of these ribs to the posterior sixth rib. A standard five- or seven-rib thoracoplasty in association with an extended pulmonary resection is not recommended, because it will result in inadequate postoperative ventilation owing to paradoxical chest wall motion.

If the air leak stops and there is a persistent space, the chest tube is removed, and the space is treated as if it were sterile. The patient can be safely discharged without antibiotic therapy and is followed with periodic chest radiographs (Figure 41.8). The sterile space obliterates with fibrous tissue over time.

If an empyema does develop in a postoperative space, tube drainage is mandatory. If the space is small, it is managed with open-tube drainage, and the tube is slowly backed out as the space obliterates. If closure of an infected space does not occur after several weeks, or if the space is large, there remain two surgical options. The first is thoracoplasty, and the space must be located so that the appropriate type of thoracoplasty obliterates it. A large space necessitates a standard posterior seven-rib thoracoplasty.

The pedicle muscle flap is the most effective method of obliterating almost any infected residual space, and the muscle can be used to close any residual bronchial fistula.[98] The pectoralis major is particularly well suited for placement into the apex of the chest and avoids the deformity of a thoracoplasty. Other tissues that can be used include the omentum, serratus anterior muscle, and latissimus dorsi

muscle if it has not been transected by the previous thoracotomy.

Careful attention to all the preoperative and postoperative details in managing the lung cancer patient minimizes the complications of the postoperative space. Space management is detailed in Figure 41.9.

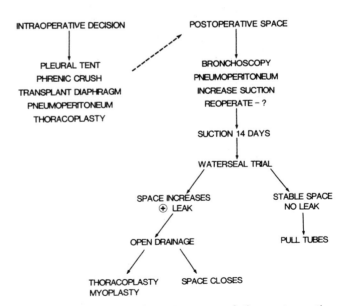

FIGURE 41.9. Suggested management of the postoperative space. (From Piccione W Jr, Faber LP. Management of complications related to pulmonary resection. In: Waldhausen JA, Orringer MB, eds. *Complications in cardiothoracic surgery.* St. Louis: Mosby Year Book, 1991:336, with permission.)

INTRAOPERATIVE HEMORRHAGE

Hilar dissection can be extremely difficult when central lung cancers are removed, because they often invade major vascular structures, and the avoidance of damage to these vessels is difficult. Neoadjuvant therapy for a clinically advanced lung cancer frequently obliterates tissue planes and makes the hilar dissection extremely difficult. The normal tissue plane of the pulmonary artery and its branches can be totally obliterated, and meticulous sharp dissection is necessary to remove the cancer from these structures. Neoadjuvant therapy, coupled with prior mediastinoscopy, also renders the paratracheal tissues fibrotic and further complicates mediastinal lymphadenectomy. The thoracic surgeon must be prepared to handle intraoperative hemorrhage, and there are various technical maneuvers that can be undertaken to minimize its occurrence.

Right Hilum

The primary cancer or involved regional lymph nodes may render approach to the pulmonary artery or its branches technically difficult. In this instance, it is appropriate to obtain provisional control of the more proximal pulmonary artery. Also, in many instances, the cancer obliterates the standard approach to the main pulmonary artery, and other maneuvers must be undertaken to ligate it more proximally.[99]

An approach to the right main pulmonary artery is to open the pericardium at the level of the superior pulmonary vein and extend this opening to a level onto the superior vena cava above the azygos vein. If the azygos vein can be encircled, it is ligated proximally and distally and transected to provide added exposure. The right main pulmonary artery can then be isolated medial to the superior vena cava (Figure 41.10). If a difficult lobectomy is to be attempted, a provisional Rumel tourniquet can be applied to control the main pulmonary artery if bleeding does occur during the dissection. This approach can also be used to transect the pulmonary artery either by using the stapling technique with vascular staples or by placing a vascular clamp proximal and then suturing the transected pulmonary artery stump.

A second approach to the right pulmonary artery is more medial, and it is necessary to open the pericardium widely to provide exposure to the pulmonary artery between the ascending aorta and superior vena cava (Figure 41.11). A significant portion of this dissection must be done by blunt finger dissection, and care must taken not to disrupt the main artery with this maneuver. It is rare that a tumor extends to this level of the main pulmonary artery, and provisional proximal control can usually be obtained by this technique. If a pneumonectomy is being done, the artery is usually ligated at this level with a heavy permanent suture. Transection of the main artery is then done on the other side of the superior vena cava. The vascular stapling tech-

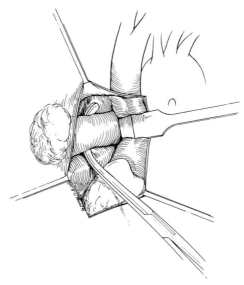

FIGURE 41.10. The right main pulmonary artery is isolated medial to the superior vena cava after the pericardium is widely opened.

nique can also be used to divide the main artery, but the instrument can be difficult to position.

An upper-lobe tumor may totally occlude the anterior approach to the pulmonary artery, but the mainstem bronchus remains free of cancer involvement. In this instance, the posterior aspect of the pulmonary artery is readily accessible and it can be isolated by initially dissecting the right mainstem bronchus so that it can be transected. The pneumonectomy stump is closed by the staple technique (Figure

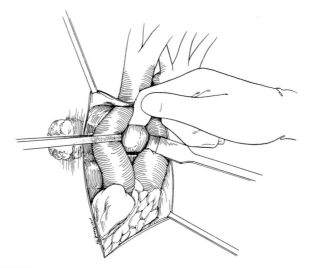

FIGURE 41.11. The proximal right main pulmonary artery is isolated between the aortic arch to the right and the superior vena cava. The pericardium has been widely opened, and the technique of isolation is by both sharp and blunt finger dissection.

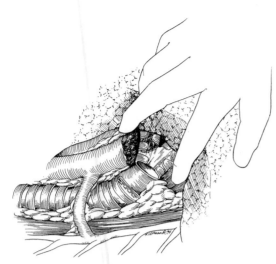

FIGURE 41.12. The right main pulmonary artery is approached posteriorly after transection and closure of the right mainstem bronchus. Tumor obliterates the customary anterior approach to the right main pulmonary artery.

41.12). To avoid contamination of the space during continued aspects of the dissection, the stapler can also be used to close the distal bronchus. After transection of the bronchus, the posterior aspect of the pulmonary artery becomes readily available, and a more proximal dissection with ligation and transection of the right main pulmonary artery can be carried out. This approach is predicated on the finding that the proximal right mainstem bronchus can be freed for transection and closure. Despite proximal control of the main pulmonary artery, a defect in a large lobar branch can bleed profusely from atrial back bleeding and large bronchial arteries supplying the tumor. In this instance, distal control of the pulmonary artery must be obtained, or vascular clamps can be placed on both the superior and inferior pulmonary veins to minimize blood loss while the arterial defect is closed.

Involvement of either the superior or inferior pulmonary vein by the cancer necessitates opening of the pericardium to obtain more proximal control. The vascular stapling device can be placed on the atrium to obtain an adequate margin of resection beyond the tumor, and proximal control is achieved. On occasion, both the superior and inferior pulmonary veins are involved by the tumor, and the stapling instrument is not long enough to close a single atrial cuff. In this situation, a large vascular clamp is placed to occlude the atrium, and it is transected. The atrial tissues are then reapproximated by a running monofilament suture.

The primary tumor or involved lymph nodes may invade the superior vena cava. If the invasion is minimal, a partially occluding vascular clamp can be placed, and a portion of the vena cava wall is transected. The defect is closed with a running monofilament suture. In other instances, a por-

tion of the wall of the vena cava may require resection to remove all of the tumor. The right and left innominate veins must be isolated, and provisional ligatures are placed. The pericardium is opened, and a provisional tourniquet is placed at the level of the caval-atrial junction. The vena cava can be bypassed by a catheter technique, as described by Piccione and colleagues,[100] and the defect in the vena cava is repaired by a patch graft of pericardium. The vena cava can also be replaced or bypassed by Gore-Tex grafts, as described by Dartevelle and associates.[101] For more on these techniques, see Chapter 62.

Left Hilum

Left-sided lung cancer frequently invades the aorticopulmonary window, and the pulmonary artery cannot be dissected safely outside the pericardium. The pericardium is then opened medial or lateral to the phrenic nerve, and this opening is extended up above the aortic arch. The main pulmonary artery is identified, and the proximal left main pulmonary artery is dissected free (Figure 41.13). It is usually necessary to isolate and transect the ligamentum arteriosum to provide exposure for proximal transection and closure. It is also necessary to identify the proximal portion of the right pulmonary artery to ensure that the main pulmonary artery is not ligated or compromised. Staple closure of the artery with the vascular stapling technique is effective in this instance. Provisional proximal left pulmonary artery control can also be obtained with a Rumel tourniquet after the pericardium is opened during a difficult lobar dissection.

The left main pulmonary artery can also be approached

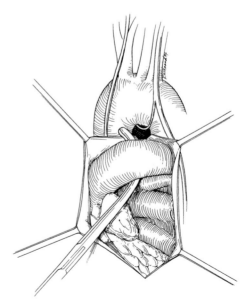

FIGURE 41.13. The left main pulmonary artery is isolated after the pericardium is opened. The right main pulmonary artery must be clearly identified before transection.

posteriorly after dissection and transection of the left mainstem bronchus. This approach provides additional exposure if the anterior, intrapericardial approach is particularly difficult. The atrium is handled in similar fashion as described for the right side.

The primary tumor or involved lymph nodes frequently are densely adherent to the transverse aortic arch. This is particularly true when a large hilar tumor has been treated with neoadjuvant therapy and the fibrotic tissues are difficult to dissect. In this instance, careful sharp dissection is necessary to free the tumor from the aorta. It is important to avoid development of a plane of dissection between the adventitia of the aorta, because this defect can rupture during the dissection or in the postoperative course. It is rarely indicated to resect a portion of the transverse or descending thoracic aorta *en bloc* with a primary lung cancer. This type of invasion usually precludes long-term survival of the patient, and aortic graft replacement with its attendant morbidity is not indicated.

POSTOPERATIVE HEMORRHAGE

Postoperative bleeding usually occurs from the site of the pulmonary resection or from an intercostal vessel in the thoracic incision. Lung cancers invade the mediastinum, chest wall, and diaphragm, and blood vessels, both large and small, are transected during the resection. Frequently, it is necessary to carry out an extrapleural dissection, and the persistent oozing of blood from the chest wall can be difficult to control. A ligature can roll off a previously tied branch of the pulmonary artery or pulmonary vein, and blood loss in the recovery unit can be sudden and precipitous. The second major cause of postoperative bleeding is a coagulation defect related to transfusion of several units of stored bank blood during the operative procedure.

Many elderly patients who undergo resection for lung cancer take aspirin as a prophylactic measure to avoid vascular problems. This is particularly true in patients who have had either transient ischemic attacks or coronary bypass surgery for atherosclerotic heart disease. Others may take aspirin for chest pain, arthritis, or prophylaxis to avoid a stroke because of a prior family history. This information should be obtained in the patient's history, and all aspirin-related products must be stopped before the surgical procedure. It is appropriate to stop aspirin two weeks before the operation. Aspirin affects platelet function, and if generalized oozing persists during an extended difficult dissection for lung cancer, then platelets can be administered to the patient who did not stop aspirin before the thoracotomy.

Symptoms of postoperative hemorrhage include tachycardia and hypotension. The usual evidence of significant postoperative bleeding is the drainage of about 200 mL or more of blood per hour through the chest tubes into the drainage system. A portable chest radiograph should be obtained to ensure that blood is not accumulating in the thorax, because the quantity of chest-tube drainage is not a reliable indicator. It is important to obtain the chest radiograph in the upright position to quantitate better the amount of retained blood in the chest cavity.

Blood replacement is carried out dependent on measured blood loss during the operative procedure, the patient's physiologic status, and the measured blood loss through the chest tubes. Continued blood loss at a rate of 200 mL per hour for four hours is generally an indication for reoperation to identify and control the source of bleeding. In this situation, continued observation can be carried out if the surgeon thinks that the trend of blood loss is slowing and the patient's condition is stable. This decision must be carefully correlated with the operative findings and the speculative cause for the postoperative bleeding. Coagulation studies are obtained, and when defects are identified, they are corrected. Agents used include fresh frozen plasma, cryoprecipitate, or platelets as indicated.

A sudden rush of blood into the chest drainage system approximating several hundred milliliters mandates immediate reexploration. A ligature may have slipped from a large vessel, or a vascular repair may have partially separated.

Prevention is the key to the avoidance of the postoperative complication of bleeding. Meticulous hemostasis is carried out during and after the resection. Cautery is used generously on the chest wall or pleural surface to stop the ooze from the many disrupted small vessels after pleurectomy. The mediastinum is carefully explored for a large bronchial artery that may have clotted off but that will start bleeding after the clot moves or the patient has an episode of postoperative hypertension. The main pulmonary artery and veins are carefully inspected for any defects in the closure, and persistent bleeding is controlled with fine interrupted sutures. Lobar branches from the pulmonary artery must be securely tied, and the operator can feel a break in the intima as the initial knot is placed. Large vessels require suture ligation, including the more proximal ligature, to prevent slippage. The anterior and posterior portions of a thoracotomy are always carefully inspected to ensure that there is no bleeding from a traumatized intercostal artery.

POSTOPERATIVE CHYLOTHORAX

Chylothorax after pulmonary resection is a rare complication and occurs more frequently after pneumonectomy than after lobectomy or segmentectomy. The thoracic duct enters the chest through the aortic hiatus at the level of T-12 and is adjacent to the aorta. It remains on the right side of the vertebral bodies until it crosses to the left at the level of the fifth or sixth thoracic vertebra. It then passes behind the aortic arch to an area adjacent to the esophagus and exits the mediastinum to drain into the left subclavian vein. The duct can be multichanneled and have many tributaries in the area of the subcarinal space. Damage to the main duct or tributaries can occur anywhere along the mediastinum. Subcarinal lymphadenectomy requires exposure of the esophagus, and the removal of these lymph nodes may result in unrecognized thoracic duct injury. Damage can also occur on the left side when the proximal left mainstem bronchus is freed for transection, and lymph nodes involved by a tumor are removed along the descending thoracic esophagus.

Frequently, damage to the duct or its tributaries is clearly identified during the dissection. Whenever a small flow of milky fluid is identified, it is mandatory that the defect in the main duct or one of its branches be closed with interrupted permanent sutures. If the patient has not eaten for several hours before the surgical procedure, the chyle can appear more golden-yellow than milky, and this is a clue to the fact that a defect has been created.

Often, patients do not eat solid food after a major pulmonary resection, and the chest-tube drainage is not the characteristic milky color. However, the continued drainage of serous fluid measuring more than 1,000 mL in 24 hours alerts the surgeon to the possibility of a thoracic duct fistula. As soon as the patient begins to eat solid food, the classic milky appearance of the fluid appears. Analysis of the pleural fluid shows chylomicrons with lipoprotein electrophoresis, and the triglyceride level is more than 100 mg per dL if the fluid is chyle.

After pneumonectomy, the development of a chylothorax is indicated by rapid filling of the pneumonectomy space with deviation of the mediastinum away from the operated side.[102] The initial treatment of a postresection chylothorax is conservative. Chest-tube drainage is maintained to provide expansion of the remaining lung or mediastinum stabilization, and total parental nutrition is carried out. All oral feedings are discontinued, and meticulous observation of the amount of daily drainage is recorded. Miller[103] reported that spontaneous closure after an operative injury may be expected in only about half of patients. The maximal amount of time for observation is two weeks, but if fluid loss is persistent at seven days, operation for closure of the fistula is undertaken. Sarsam and colleagues[102] reported postpneumonectomy chylothorax in nine patients; in five patients, conservative therapy managed the problem, and in four, reoperation was required. The pneumonectomy space must be drained by tube thoracostomy, and central hyperalimentation is carried out. Although two weeks can again be used as a time limit for conservative management, a persistent loss of fluid at seven days indicates the need for reoperation in our experience.

At reoperation, the chest should be opened on the side of the fistula. The patient can be given cream or olive oil two to three hours before the thoracotomy, and this will enhance recognition of the site of the fistula. Frequently, the area of the fistula is edematous, and tissues do not hold sutures well. Further dissection to visualize the fistula better can result in bleeding, and secure closure of the boggy tissues is not obtained. We recommend that in reoperation for a thoracic duct fistula after pulmonary resection, supradiaphragmatic ligation of the main duct should be carried out, as reported by Lampson.[104] Just above the diaphragm, the tissue between the aorta and the azygos vein is bluntly freed with an angled clamp, and mass ligation of this tissue is carried out with a heavy silk suture. Clips should be avoided because they damage the duct and a new fistula will occur where the duct is clipped. This ligation can be accomplished through either a right or left thoracotomy. However, it is more easily accomplished through a limited lower right thoracotomy, and on occasion, this approach has been used despite a left-sided chylous fistula.

Other surgical options include pleurectomy, placement of a pleural peritoneal shunt, application of fibrin glue, and thorascopic ligation of the thoracic duct. However, the gold standard to which all other techniques must be compared is direct ligation of the duct.

Long-term conservative management of the postoperative chylous fistula is to be avoided, because the patient's condition will only deteriorate and nutritional depletion will cause further complications and possible mortality.

ESOPHAGOPLEURAL FISTULA

The anatomic pathway of the esophagus is in close proximity to the lower trachea and right mainstem bronchus, and its muscular wall can be directly invaded by a large hilar cancer. Pneumonectomy and resection of the neoplasm may result in an unrecognized defect in the wall of the esophagus, with a resultant esophagopleural fistula. The esophagus is also directly posterior to the subcarinal space, and it can be damaged during subcarinal lymphadenectomy from either the right or left side. The performance of a left pneumonectomy requires exposure of the carina and the medial aspect of the proximal right mainstem bronchus, and during this aspect of the dissection, the esophagus must be freed from the adjacent tissues to permit a high amputation of the left mainstem bronchus. Damage to the esophagus can also occur during this phase of the dissection.

A careful review of the preoperative computed tomographic scan usually reveals the presence of the tumor in close proximity to the esophageal wall. This finding alerts the surgeon to the need for clear anatomic definition of the esophageal wall during the dissection, and the placement of a nasogastric tube before the procedure assists in early definition of the entire thoracic esophagus. If a defect is made in both the muscular and mucosal layers of the esophagus, a two-layer repair is accomplished with a fine absorbable monofilament suture. Interrupted sutures are evenly placed to achieve a watertight seal. An adjacent pleural flap is easily constructed to buttress the repair. If it is determined during the resection that only the muscularis of the esophagus has been removed and that the mucosa is intact, the muscularis is reapproximated with similar suture material.

Several bronchial arteries traverse the subcarinal space and are in close proximity to the esophageal wall because they originate from the aorta. These arteries can be large because they have nourished the cancer or involved subcarinal lymph nodes. These vessels should be individually ligated as they are encountered; on occasion, bleeding can be significant if the vessels are not seen and cut. In this instance, vigorous cautery should be avoided because unrecognized damage and subsequent necrosis of the esophageal wall can occur. Cautious use of cautery in the subcarinal space is directly applicable to subcarinal lymphadenectomy from both the right and left sides.

An esophagopleural fistula after a pulmonary resection can occur either in the early or late postoperative period. The signs and symptoms are those of an empyema, with fever, chest discomfort, loss of appetite, a falling air fluid level in the pneumonectomy space, and the appearance of an air fluid level in a previously opacified hemithorax. The placement of a chest tube may reveal food particles, but a diagnosis of empyema is obvious. Bronchoscopy is usually carried out to detect the presence of a bronchial fistula, and an immediate esophagogram confirms the presence of the clinically suspected esophageal fistula (Figure 41.14). Massard and associates[105] recommend the routine use of a barium swallow whenever a postpneumonectomy empyema develops. This diagnostic study is particularly important after the development of a late empyema.

In the early postoperative period, therapy is directed toward direct repair of the fistula. The previous thoracotomy space is opened, and careful debridement of the pneumonectomy space is carried out. The esophageal fistula is identified and repaired in two layers. It must be buttressed with a vascularized tissue flap that includes intercostal muscle, serratus anterior muscle, and omentum. A gastrostomy for drainage and jejunostomy for feeding and postoperative alimentation are also recommended. The pneumonectomy space is lavaged with antibiotic solution, and if sterilized, the chest tube can be removed. However, this is a difficult empyema to sterilize, and it may be necessary to provide long-term open drainage with attempted later sterilization by the Claggett technique. An alternative approach is to exclude the esophagus by a proximal cutaneous fistula and perform a distal ligation with a second-stage reconstruction. However, the one-stage repair is generally recommended.[106] The development of an esophagopleural fistula in the late postoperative period requires rib resection and adequate drainage of the pleural space. Gastrostomy and jejunostomy are required for alimentation and drainage of gastric con-

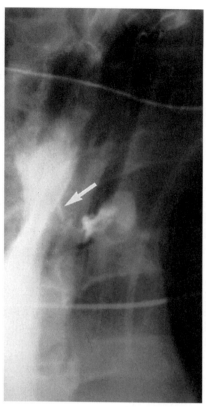

FIGURE 41.14. Bronchoscopy is usually carried out to detect the presence of a bronchial fistula, and an immediate esophagogram confirms the presence of the clinically suspected esophageal fistula.

tents. When the patient's condition is stabilized and the pleural space is clean, thoracotomy and direct repair of the esophageal defect are carried out. The fistula must be buttressed with tissue, and in this instance, omentum is an excellent choice because of its vascularity and adhesive qualities. The pneumonectomy space must be obliterated; this is accomplished by thoracoplasty in association with thoracoplasty and myoplasty. A small pneumonectomy space can be obliterated by myoplasty alone. The development of an esophageal pleural fistula after pulmonary resection is associated with high mortality and morbidity. The fistula must be treated aggressively because it will not close spontaneously.

REFERENCES

1. Ginsberg RJ, Hill LD, Eagan RT, et al. Modern thirty-day operative mortality for surgical resections in lung cancer. *J Thorac Cardiovasc Surg* 1983;86:654.
2. Nagasaki F, Flehinger BJ, Martini N. Complications of surgery in the treatment of carcinoma of the lung. *Chest* 1982;82:25.

3. Kohman LJ, Meyer JA, Ikins PM, et al. Random versus predictable risks of mortality after thoracotomy for lung cancer. *J Thorac Cardiovasc Surg* 1986;91:551.

4. Boysen PG, Block AJ, Moulder PV. Relationship between preoperative pulmonary function tests and complications after thoracotomy. *Surg Gynecol Obstet* 1981;152:813.

5. Epstein SK, Faling LJ, Daly BDT, et al. Predicting complications after pulmonary resection: preoperative exercise testing vs a multifactorial cardiopulmonary risk index. *Chest* 1993;104:694.

6. Ferguson MK, Little L, Rizzo L, et al. Diffusing capacity predicts morbidity and mortality after pulmonary resection. *J Thorac Cardiovasc Surg* 1988;96:894.

7. Keagy BA, Schorlemmer GR, Murray GF, et al. Correlation of preoperative pulmonary function testing with clinical course in patients after pneumonectomy. *Ann Thorac Surg* 1983;36:253.

8. Ferguson MK, Reeder LB, Mich R. Optimizing selection of patients for major lung resection. *J Thorac Cardiovasc Surg* 1995;109:275.

9. Ferguson MK. Assessment of operative risk for pneumonectomy. *Chest Surg Clin Am* 1999;9:339.

10. Bechard D, Wetstein L. Assessment of exercise oxygen consumption as preoperative criterion for lung resection. *Ann Thorac Surg* 1987;44:344.

11. Bollinger CT, Perruchoud AP. Functional evaluation of lung resection candidate. *Eur Respir J* 1998;11:198.

12. Rao V, Todd TRV, Kuus A, et al. Exercise oximetry versus spirometry in the assessment of risk prior to lung resection. *Ann Thorac Surg* 1995;60:603.

13. Ninin M, Somers E, Landreneau RJ. Standardized exercise oximetry predicts post pneumonectomy outcome. *Ann Thorac Surg* 1997;64:328.

14. Peters RM, Clausen JL, Tisi GM. Extending resectability for carcinoma of the lung in patients with impaired pulmonary function. *Ann Thorac Surg* 1978;26:250.

15. Bailey CC, Betts RH. Cardiac arrhythmias following pneumonectomy. *N Engl J Med* 1943;229:356.

16. Currens JH, White PD, Churchill ED. Cardiac arrhythmias following thoracic surgery. *N Engl J Med* 1943;229:360.

17. Mowry FM, Reynolds EW. Cardiac rhythm disturbances complicating resection surgery of the lung. *Ann Intern Med* 1964;61:688.

18. Shields TW, Ujiki GT. Digitalization for prevention of arrhythmias following pulmonary surgery. *Surg Gynecol Obstet* 1968;126:743.

19. Wheat MW, Burford THE. Digitalis in surgery: extension of classical indications. *J Thorac Cardiovasc Surg* 1961;41:162.

20. Krowka MJ, Pairolero PC, Trastek VE, et al. Cardiac dysrhythmia following pneumonectomy. *Chest* 1987;91:490.

21. Wei JY. Age and the cardiovascular system. *N Engl J Med* 1992;327:1735.

22. Wittnich C, Trudel H, Zidulka A, et al. Misleading "pulmonary wedge pressure" after pneumonectomy: its importance in postoperative fluid therapy. *Ann Thorac Surg* 1986;42:192.

23. Simpson RJ, Foster WL Jr, Woelfel AK, et al. Management of atrial fibrillation and flutter. *Postgrad Med* 1986;79:241.

24. Smith TW. Digitalis: mechanisms of action and clinical use. *N Engl J Med* 1988;318:358.

25. Lindgren L, Lepantalo M, Von Knorring J, et al. Effect of verapamil on right ventricular pressure and atrial tachyarrhythmia after thoracotomy. *Br J Anaesth* 1991;66:205.

26. Amar D, Roistacher N, Burt M, et al. Effects of diltiazem versus digoxin on dysrhythmias and cardiac function after pneumonectomy. *Ann Thorac Surg* 1997;63:1374.

27. Van Mieghem W, Coolen L, Malysse I, et al. Amiodarone and the development of ARDS after lung surgery. *Chest* 1994;105:1642.

28. Salerno DM, Dias VC, Kleiger RE, et al. Efficacy and safety of intravenous diltiazem for treatment of atrial fibrillation and atrial flutter. *Am J Cardiol* 1989;63:1046.

29. Ellenbogen KA, Dias VC, Plumb VJ, et al. A placebo-controlled trial of continuous intravenous diltiazem infusion for 24-hour heart rate control during atrial fibrillation and atrial flutter: A multi center study. *J Am Coll Cardiol* 1991;18:891.

30. Amar D. Cardiac arrhythmias. *Chest Surg Clin N Am* 1998;8:479.

31. Gibbon Jr, JR, Gibbon MH, Kraul CW. Experimental pulmonary edema following lobectomy and blood transfusion. *J Thorac Surg* 1942;12:60.

32. Gibbon Jr, JR, Gibbon MH. Experimental pulmonary edema following lobectomy and plasma infusion. *Surgery* 1942;12:694.

33. Zeldin RA, Normandin D, Landtwing D, et al. Postpneumonectomy pulmonary edema. *J Thorac Cardiovasc Surg* 1984;87:359.

34. Verheijen-Breemhaar L, Bogaard JM, Van Den Berg B, et al. Postpneumonectomy pulmonary edema. *Thorax* 1988;43:323.

35. Patel RL, Townsend ER, Fountain SW. Elective pneumonectomy: factors associated with morbidity and mortality. *Ann Thorac Surg* 1992;54:840.

36. Waller DA, Gebitekin C, Saunders NR, et al. Noncardiogenic pulmonary edema complicating lung resection. *Ann Thorac Surg* 1993;55:140.

37. Turnage WS, Lunn JJ. Postpneumonectomy pulmonary edema: A retrospective analysis of associated variables. *Chest* 1993;103(6):1646.

38. Shapira OM, Shahian DM. Postpneumonectomy pulmonary edema. *Ann Thorac Surg* 1993;56:190.

39. Deslauriers J, Aucoin A, Gregoire J. Postpneumonectomy pulmonary edema. *Chest Surg Clin N Am* 1998;8(3):611.

40. Slinger PD. Perioperative fluid management for thoracic surgery: the puzzle of postpneumonectomy pulmonary edema. *J Cardiothorac Vasc Anesth* 1995;9(4):442.

41. Little AG, Langmuir VK, Singer AH, et al. Hemodynamic pulmonary edema in dog lungs after contralateral pneumonectomy and mediastinal lymphatic interruption. *Lung* 1984;162:139.

42. Nohl-Oser HC. An investigation of the anatomy of the lymphatic drainage of the lungs as shown by the lymphatic spread of bronchial carcinoma. *Ann R Coll Surg Engl* 1972;51:157.

43. Raffensperger JG, Luck SR, Inwood RJ, et al. The effect of overdistention of the lung on pulmonary function in beagle puppies. *J Pediatr Surg* 1979;14(6):757.

44. Mathisen DJ, Kuo EY, Hahn C, et al. Inhaled nitric oxide for adult respiratory distress syndrome after pulmonary resection. *Ann Thorac Surg* 1998;65:1894.

45. Patel DR, Shrivastav R, Sabety AM. Cardiac torsion following intrapericardial pneumonectomy. *J Thorac Cardiovasc Surg* 1972;65:626.

46. Bettman RB, Tannenbaum WJ. Herniation of the heart. *Ann Surg* 1948;128:1012.

47. Rodgers BM, Moulder PV, DeLaney A. Thoracoscopy: new method of early diagnosis of cardiac herniation. *J Thorac Cardiovasc Surg* 1979;78:623.

48. Deiraniya AK. Cardiac herniation following intra-pericardial pneumonectomy. *Thorax* 1974;29:545.

49. Levin PD, Faber LP, Carleton RA. Cardiac herniation after pneumonectomy. *J Thorac Cardiovasc Surg* 1971;61:104.

50. Dippel WF, Ehrenhaft JL. Herniation of the heart after pneumonectomy. *J Thorac Cardiovasc Surg* 1973;65:207.

51. Papsin BC, Gorenstein LA, Goldberg M. Delayed myocardial laceration after intrapericardial pneumonectomy. *Ann Thorac Surg* 1993;55:766.

52. Wong PS, Goldstraw P. Pulmonary torsion: a questionnaire survey and a survey of the literature. *Ann Thorac Surg* 1992; 54:286.

53. Schuler JG. Intraoperative lobar torsion producing pulmonary infarction. *J Thorac Cardiovasc Surg* 1973;65:951.

54. Kucich VA, Villarreal JR, Schwartz DB. Left upper lobe torsion following lower lobe resection. *Chest* 1989;95:1146.

55. Kelly MV, Kygere R, Miller WC. Postoperative lobar torsion and gangrene. *Thorax* 1977;32:501.

56. Linaudais W, Cavanaugh DG, Geer TM. Rapid post-operative thoracotomy for torsion of the left lower lobe: case report. *Mil Med* 1980;145:698.

57. Kim H, Roldan CA, Shively BK. Pulmonary vein thrombosis. *Chest* 1993;104:624.

58. Mullin MJ, Zumbro GL, Fishback ME, et al. Pulmonary lobar gangrene complicating lobectomy. *Ann Surg* 1972;175:62.

59. Kirsh MM, Rotman H, Behrendt DM, et al. Complications of pulmonary resection. *Ann Thorac Surg* 1975;20:215.

60. Iverson LIG, Ecker RR, Fox HE, et al. A comparative study of IPPB, the incentive spirometer, and blow bottles: the prevention of atelectasis following cardiac surgery. *Ann Thorac Surg* 1978; 25:197.

61. O'Donohue WJ. National survey of the usage of lung expansion modalities for the prevention and treatment of postoperative atelectasis following abdominal and thoracic surgery. *Chest* 1985;87:76.

62. Lewis FR. Management of atelectasis and pneumonia. *Surg Clin North Am* 1980;67:1391.

63. Bartlett RH. Pulmonary pathophysiology in surgical patients. *Surg Clin North Am* 1980;60:1323.

64. Marini JJ. Postoperative atelectasis: pathophysiology, clinical importance, and principles of management. *Respir Care* 1984; 29:516.

65. Ali J, Serrette C, Wood LDH, et al. Effect of post-operative intermittent positive pressure breathing on lung function. *Chest* 1984;85:192.

66. Stock MC, Downs JB, Gauer PK, et al. Prevention of postoperative pulmonary complications with CPAP, incentive spirometry, and conservative therapy. *Chest* 1985;87:151.

67. Nguyem DM, Mulder DS, Shennib H. Altered cellular immune functioning of the atelectatic lung. *Ann Thorac Surg* 1981;51: 76.

68. Lubenow TR, Faber LP, McCarthy RJ, et al. Postthoracotomy pain management using continuous epidural analgesia in 1,324 patients. *Ann Thorac Surg* 1994;58:924.

69. Au J, Walker WS, Iinglis D, et al. Percutaneous cricothyroidostomy (minitracheostomy) for bronchial toilet: results of therapeutic and prophylactic use. *Ann Thorac Surg* 1989;48:850.

70. Wain JC, Wilson DJ, Mathisen DJ. Clinical experience with minitracheostomy. *Ann Thorac Surg* 1990;49:881.

71. Randell TT, Tierala EK, Lepantalo MJ, et al. Prophylactic minitracheostomy after thoracotomy: a prospective, random control, clinical trial. *Eur J Surg* 1991;157:501.

72. Mastboom WJ, Wobbes T, van den Dries A, et al. Bronchial suction by minitracheostomy as an effective measure against sputum retention. *Surg Gynecol Obstet* 1991;173:187.

73. Beenhakkers JC, Stoutenbeek CP. Inhalation of a mini-tracheostomy tube [Letter]. *Intensive Care Med* 1993;19:123.

74. Randell T, Kalli I. Position of minitracheostomy tube verified fiberoptically: a report of 2 cases. *Acta Anaesthesiol Scand* 1990; 34:455.

75. Jawroski A, Goldberg SK, Walkenstein MD, et al. Utility of immediate postlobectomy fiberoptic bronchoscopy in preventing atelectasis. *Chest* 1988;94:38.

76. Mahajan VK, Catron PW, Huber GL. The value of fiber-optic bronchoscopy in the management of pulmonary collapse. *Chest* 1978;73:817.

77. Massard G, Wihlm JM. Postoperative atelectasis. *Chest Surg Clin North Am* 1998;8:503.

78. Vester SR, Faber LP, Kittle CF, et al. Bronchopleural fistula after stapled closure of bronchus. *Ann Thorac Surg* 1991;52: 1253.

79. Lawrence GH, Ristroph R, Wood JA, et al. Methods for avoiding dire surgical complications: bronchopleural fistula after pulmonary resection. *Am J Surg* 1982;144:136.

80. Williams NS, Lewis CT. Bronchopleural fistula: a review of 86 cases. *Br J Surg* 1976;63:530.

81. A collaborate study. Preoperative irradiation of cancer of the lung: final report of a therapeutic trial. *Cancer* 1975;36:914.

82. Kaplan DK, Whyte RJ, Donnelly RD. Pulmonary resection using automatic stapling devices. *Eur J Cardiothorac Surg* 1987; 1:152.

83. Forrester-Wood CP. Bronchopleural fistula following pneumonectomy for carcinoma of the bronchus. *J Thorac Cardiovasc Surg* 1980;80:406.

84. Al-Kattan K, Cattalani L, Goldstraw T. Bronchopleural fistula after pneumonectomy with a hand suture technique. *Ann Thorac Surg* 1994;58:1433.

85. Rendina EA, Venuta F, Ricci P, et al. Protection of revascularization of bronchial anastomoses by the intercostal pedicle flap. *J Thorac Cardiovasc Surg* 1994;107:1251.

86. Pairolero PC, Arnold PG, Piehler JM. Intrathoracic transposition of extrathoracic skeletal muscle. *J Thorac Cardiovasc Surg* 1983;86:809.

87. Regnard JF, Icard P, Deneuville M, et al. Lung resection after high doses of mediastinal radiotherapy (sixty grays or more). *J Thorac Cardiovasc Surg* 1994;106:607.

88. Mathisen DJ, Grillo HC, Vlahakes GJ, et al. The omentum in the management of complicated cardiothoracic problems. *J Thorac Cardiovasc Surg* 1988;95:677.

89. Claggett OT, Gerace JE. A procedure for the management of post-pneumonectomy empyema. *J Thorac Cardiovasc Surg* 1963;45:141.

90. Deschamps C, Pairolero PC, Allen MS, et al. Management of post-pneumonectomy empyema and bronchopleural fistula. *Chest Surg Clin N Am* 1996;6:519.

91. Eloesser L. An operation for tuberculosis empyema. *Surg Gynecol Obstet* 1935;60:1096.

92. Puskas JD, Mathisen DJ, Grillo HC et al. Treatment strategies for bronchopleural fistula. *J Thorac Cardiovasc Surg* 1995;109: 989.

93. Baldwin JC, Mark JBD. Treatment of bronchopleural fistula after pneumonectomy. *J Thorac Cardiovasc Surg* 1985;90:813.

94. Spotnitz WD, Dalton MS, Baker JW, et al. Successful use of fibrin glue during 2 years of surgery at a university medical center. *Am Surg* 1989;55:1660.

95. Torre M, Chiesa G, Ravini M, et al. Endoscopic gluing of bronchopleural fistula. *Ann Thorac Surg* 1994;58:901.

96. Horrigan TP, Snow NJ. Thoracoplasty: current application to the infected pleural space. *Ann Thorac Surg* 1990;50:695.

97. Kirsch MM, Rotman H, Behrendt DM, et al. Complications of pulmonary resection. *Ann Thorac Surg* 1975;20:215.

98. Arnold PG, Pairolero PC. Intrathoracic muscle flaps: an account of their use in the management of 100 consecutive patients. *Ann Surg* 1990;211:656.

99. Mansour KA, Downey RS. Managing the difficult pulmonary artery during completion pneumonectomy. *Surg Gynecol Obstet* 1989;169:161.

100. Piccione W, Faber LP, Warren WH. Superior vena caval reconstruction using autologous pericardium. *Ann Thorac Surg* 1990; 50:417.

101. Dartevelle F, Chapelier A, Pastorino U, et al. Long-term follow-

up after prosthetic replacement of the superior vena cava combined with resection of mediastinal-pulmonary malignant tumors. *J Thorac Cardiovasc Surg* 1991;102:259.

102. Sarsam MAI, Rahman AN, Deiraniya AK. Postpneumonectomy chylothorax. *Ann Thorac Surg* 1994;57:689.

103. Miller JI. Chylothorax. In: Shields TW, ed. *General thoracic surgery,* 4th ed. Baltimore: Williams & Wilkins, 1994:714.

104. Lampson RS. Traumatic chylothorax: a review of the literature and report of a case treated by mediastinal ligation of the thoracic duct. *J Thorac Surg* 1948;17:778.

105. Massard G, Ducrocq X, Hentz JG, et al. Esophagopleural fistula: an early and long-term complication after pneumonectomy. *Ann Thorac Surg* 1994;58:1437.

106. Asaoka U, Imaizumi M, Kajita M, et al. One stage repair for an oesophageal fistula after pneumonectomy using an omental pedicle flap. *Thorax* 1988;43:943.

SURGERY AND ADJUVANT THERAPY

42

SURGERY AND CHEMOTHERAPY

KATHERINE M.W. PISTERS

Surgery remains the best treatment modality for potential cure for patients with non–small cell lung cancer (NSCLC). However, at the time of initial presentation, only about half of all patients will have localized disease and less than a third are actually candidates for surgical exploration.[1] Survival following surgical resection is best predicted by pathologic stage at surgery[2] (see also Chapter 32).

The major prognostic determinants for patients with early stage disease are the size of the primary tumor and the presence or absence of lymph node metastases.[2] Therefore, precise information concerning staging, both with respect to the primary tumor and lymph node involvement is critical to ensure proper balance in randomized clinical trials. This requires thorough intraoperative staging with at least lymph node sampling if not dissection. The staging system gives general guidelines for expected survival within each T and N classification. Survival also varies by the number and extent of nodal involvement. Although potentially resectable, once ipsilateral mediastinal and subcarinal lymph nodes are involved, the prognosis is much worse. When diagnosed preoperatively by imaging or invasive techniques, less than 10% of all patients treated with surgery survive five years. Adverse prognostic factors include multiple levels of N2 disease, multiple lymph nodes at one level involved with tumor, adenocarcinoma, and extranodal extension of disease. More than 75% of patients with N2 disease present with involvement extending beyond one lymph node station.[3] The presence of N2 disease is not a contraindication to surgery as a single modality therapy, because it may be curative in very select patients. However, the survival of the N2 patients as a whole is poor, and effective combined modality treatment strategies need to be identified.

Histology has also been found to impact on survival in surgically resected patients. The former North American Lung Cancer Study Group (LCSG) has carefully analyzed approximately 1,000 resected patients and found a survival of 83% for T1N0 squamous cell carcinoma patients, compared to 69% for T1N0 adenocarcinomas.[4] Similarly, the survival of resected stage IB or II adenocarcinoma patients was significantly worse than those of identical stage with squamous cell carcinomas. Others have reported that the outcomes for large cell carcinoma are possibly different from those for resected squamous or adenocarcinomas.[5]

The identification of biologic markers, which may influence prognosis, is an active area of research. Growth factor production (epidermal growth factor or transforming growth factor alpha), surface epitopes (blood group antigen expression), oncogenes (*RAS* mutations) and tumor-suppressor genes (*p53* or *RB*) have been reported to influence prognosis.[6] Further research is necessary to validate the prognostic importance of these markers and identify other markers of importance (see also Chapter 33).

Recognition of prognostic and surgical factors that predict for specific anatomic failure patterns can allow selection of patients for local, systemic, or combined therapy.[3] After surgical resection, patients with pathologic stage I disease have survival rates in excess of 50%. Isolated mediastinal or local recurrence is unusual, and postoperative radiotherapy should not be employed. For patients with T1N1 or T2N1 disease, local recurrence is uncommon (12% to 14%), while distant failures occur in roughly one third of patients.[3] Survival decreases for patients with N2 disease discovered intraoperatively. When no adjuvant therapy is used, thoracic recurrence rates approach 20% and distant metastases become even more common.[7] Further evidence of occult metastatic disease comes from an autopsy series of patients who died within 30 days of "curative" surgical resection. In that series, one third of squamous carcinomas had locally persistent disease, and 17% had distant metastases. Adenocarcinoma patients had a 40% incidence of persistent local disease, and a similar percentage had metastatic disease.[8] Given that death in the majority of resected patients is cancer-related and follows systemic recurrence, efforts at improving survival following surgical resection have focused on the use of postoperative chemotherapy and irradiation.

EARLY TRIALS

Randomized, prospective studies examining postoperative adjuvant chemotherapy in bronchogenic carcinoma were initiated in the 1960s and 1970s. The University Surgical Adjuvant Lung Project Cooperative Group reported its experience with over 1,100 patients randomized to receive nitrogen mustard intrapleurally and intravenously in the perioperative period, or placebo.[9] No difference in disease-free survival or overall survival was seen. Moreover, a significantly higher postoperative complication rate was found in those patients treated with chemotherapy. The investigators concluded that nitrogen mustard, as administered in this study, was not beneficial.

The Veterans Administration Surgical Adjuvant Group conducted a series of adjuvant chemotherapy studies in resected lung cancer patients.[10] Its first trial examined the effect of intrapleural and intravenous nitrogen mustard administered in the perioperative period. Similar to the University Surgical Adjuvant Lung Project, no difference in disease-free survival or overall survival was found. The next adjuvant trial examined cyclophosphamide. Well over 800 patients were randomly assigned to receive cyclophosphamide (6 mg per kg), daily for five days following surgery. A second course, administered in the fifth postoperative week, consisted of cyclophosphamide (8 mg per kg) for five days. Only 65% of the patients assigned to receive adjuvant chemotherapy were able to begin the second cyclophosphamide course, and an increased complication rate in the chemotherapy-treated patients was seen. Again, long-term follow-up revealed no benefit in overall survival for those patients treated with adjuvant chemotherapy versus surgery alone. The third Veterans Administration Surgical Adjuvant Group trial was a three-arm randomized study comparing no adjuvant therapy versus adjuvant cyclophosphamide versus adjuvant cyclophosphamide alternating with methotrexate. Chemotherapy was administered daily for five days every five weeks for a total of eighteen months, beginning two to four weeks postoperatively. Over 130 patients were enrolled into each arm of the study, and again the results were disappointing, with no significant difference in overall survival detected at five years. The fourth trial examined the combination of lomustine (CCNU) and hydroxyurea given orally for one year following surgery, versus no further treatment.[11] Again, no significant difference in disease-free or overall survival was found.

Data from the Swiss Group for Clinical Cancer Research was reported by Brunner and colleagues.[12] The group conducted a randomized, long-term adjuvant chemotherapy trial of cyclophosphamide versus placebo following radical resection of bronchogenic carcinoma. The study assigned 172 patients to receive no further treatment or intravenous cyclophosphamide administered as eight to nine weekly injections every four months for two years. At follow-up ranging between 3.5 to 5.5 years, 68% of the patients treated with adjuvant cyclophosphamide had experienced recurrences and 63% had died. In contrast, of the untreated control group, only 49% had recurred and 39% had died. Moreover, the median times to recurrence and death were eight months earlier in the cyclophosphamide arm. The authors concluded that treatment with intermittent courses of cyclophosphamide over a two-year period seemed to in-

crease the recurrence and death rates significantly over that observed in the untreated control group. Despite a careful analysis, no factor other than the cyclophosphamide itself was found to explain these observations.

In 1985, Girling reported the 15-year follow-up of 726 bronchogenic carcinoma patients entered into a double-blind, randomized trial.[13] Patients received oral adjuvant cytotoxic chemotherapy with either busulfan or cyclophosphamide for two years, or placebo. At 15 years, 8% of the busulfan-treated patients, 9% of the cyclophosphamide-treated patients, and 10% of the placebo-treated patients were alive. The authors concluded that prolonged oral cytotoxic chemotherapy with cyclophosphamide or busulfan did not improve survival over surgery alone.

None of the prospective trials reviewed above demonstrated improvement in disease-free or overall survival for adjuvant chemotherapy in bronchogenic carcinoma. However, these trials have been criticized, as factors such as histology, nodal involvement, performance status, age, or intraoperative staging were not considered in the design of these trials. In addition, the chemotherapeutic agents studied have minimal activity in NSCLC. Other trials have examined the potential benefit of adjuvant immunotherapy in resected bronchogenic carcinoma. BCG (bacillus Callmette-Guerin) has been studied extensively. It has been given intrapleurally[14] or subcutaneously.[15] Intrapleural BCG has been associated with increased postoperative complications, and neither route of administration has yielded improved survival.

In the late 1970s cisplatin-based combination chemotherapy regimens were developed and found to have activity in NSCLC patients with metastatic disease. This led to renewed interest in adjuvant chemotherapy in the mid 1980s. In addition, improved pre- and intraoperative staging of patients with NSCLC and the identification of important prognostic factors allowed better selection of those patients who could potentially benefit from this approach, and allowed for proper stratification of patients on study.

CISPLATIN-BASED REGIMENS

The Lung Cancer Study Group (LCSG) has conducted a series of prospective, randomized trials evaluating combination chemotherapy in the surgical adjuvant setting.[16] In LCSG trial 772, completely resected stage II and stage III (AJCC criteria) adenocarcinoma and large cell undifferentiated carcinoma patients were randomized to receive postoperative chemotherapy or immunotherapy (see Table 42.1). Chemotherapy consisted of cyclophosphamide 400 mg per m^2, doxorubicin 40 mg per m^2, and cisplatin 40 mg per m^2 (CAP) monthly for six months. Immunotherapy was comprised of intrapleural BCG and 18 months of oral levamisole. Careful intraoperative nodal sampling of all patients was performed to insure adequate staging. Before randomization, patients were stratified by stage, weight loss,

TABLE 42.1. SELECTED ADJUVANT CHEMOTHERAPY TRIALS

Trial	Adjuvant Treatment	Eligible Pts	Median (mo)	Overall Survival (%)			p value
				2 yr	5 yr	10 yr	
LCSG 772	CAP × 6	62	*23.5*	*40*	—	—	0.078
	BCG, levamisole	68	*16*	*30*	—	—	
LCSG 791	CAP × 6 + RT	78	*20*	*40*	—	—	0.113
	RT	86	*13*	*32*	—	—	
LCSG 801	CAP × 4	136	*76*	*73*	*56*	—	0.915
	Control	133	*76*	*80*	*52*	—	
Niiranen	CAP × 6	54	—	—	67	61	0.05*
	Control	56	—	—	56	48	
Ohta	VP × 3	90	31	—	35	—	0.86
	Control	91	37	—	41	—	
MSKCC	VP × 4 + RT	36	16	31	17	—	0.35
	RT	36	19	44	30	—	
Intergroup 0115	EP × 4 + RT	351	39	—	—	—	0.99
	RT	(total)	41	—	—	—	
Imaizumi	CAUFT	155	—	—	62	—	0.35†
	Control	154	—	—	58	—	
Wada	CVUFT	109	—	—	61	—	0.05
	UFT	103	—	—	64	—	
	Control	98	—	—	49	—	

Pts, patients; mo, months; CAP, cyclophosphamide, doxorubicin, cisplatin; RT, radiation therapy; VP, vindesine, cisplatin; EP, etoposide, cisplatin; CAUFT, cyclophosphamide, doxorubicin, uracil + tegafur; CVUFT, cyclophosphamide, vindesine, uracil + tegafur; —, not reported.
Data in italics are estimated from published survival curves.
* Reanalysis for imbalance in randomization found no significant difference.
† Reanalysis for imbalance in randomization yielded significant results favoring CAUFT, p = 0.44.

history of cardiac arrhythmia and institution. Of the 130 eligible patients, 23 did not receive the assigned treatment but were included in the final analysis. Disease-free survival was significantly prolonged in the treatment arm receiving adjuvant CAP chemotherapy (p = 0.018). Median survival was also increased by seven to eight months on the CAP arm, but this difference was not statistically significant. Follow-up of both treatment groups revealed systemic recurrence to be the most frequent type of relapse.

The next LCSG trial examined the use of postoperative CAP chemotherapy plus thoracic irradiation versus adjuvant radiation therapy alone.[17] Eligible patients had incomplete resection, defined as the presence of residual tumor in the resection margin or tumor in the highest lymph node sampled. Radiation therapy was administered on a split-course schedule with 20 Gy delivered in five fractions over five days as two courses separated by three weeks. In the group randomized to receive chemotherapy, cyclophosphamide, doxorubicin, and cisplatin were administered every four weeks for six cycles, with the first two cycles administered on the first day of each radiation course. Patients were stratified according to histology, extent of residual disease and performance status. The study accrued 172 patients of whom 164 were eligible. The distribution of nodal disease was significantly imbalanced in favor of the CAP-treated patients. A significant difference in disease-free survival was found in favor of combined postoperative therapy (14 versus eight months), and a nonsignificant improvement in median survival was noted (20 versus 13

months). Analyses adjusted for nodal status yielded similar results. With further follow-up, the survival curves converged at about 2.5 years.

The final adjuvant trial from the LCSG enrolled patients with completely resected T2N1 and T2N0 NSCLC.[18] This trial randomized eligible patients to receive or not to receive four courses of postoperative CAP (same doses as above except for cisplatin 60 mg per m²) chemotherapy beginning 30 days after surgery. Stratification by prognostic factors included histology (squamous versus nonsquamous), white blood cell count before surgery (more than or equal to 9,100 per mm³ versus less than 9,100 per mm³), and Karnofsky performance status before surgery (100% versus less than 100%). A total of 269 eligible patients were entered into the study. Only 53% of the eligible patients received all four courses of CAP, and only 57% of such patients received all four cycles on time. In 74% of the patients, the site of recurrence was distant. No difference in time to recurrence or overall survival was found.

A study from Finland reported in 1992 randomized 110 completely resected T1-3N0 NSCLC patients to postoperative CAP chemotherapy for six cycles or no further treatment.[19] The doses of chemotherapy employed were cyclophosphamide 400 mg per m², doxorubicin 40 mg per m², and cisplatin 40 mg per m². Eligible patients had a good performance status (over 60%) and were less than 70 years of age. After ten years of follow-up, survival in the chemotherapy arm was significantly better than control (61% versus 48%, p = 0.050). Disease free survival also favored the use of chemotherapy (69% versus 52%, p = 0.01). Although time to recurrence and death was significantly delayed, a major imbalance in randomization resulted in the assignment of twice as many patients who underwent pneumonectomy (and therefore likely to have more advanced disease) to the control arm. After adjustment for this imbalance, results were no longer significant. In addition, only 57% of patients received all their cycles of chemotherapy.

Two published trials have examined the use of postoperative vindesine and cisplatin.[20,21] A trial conducted in Japan[20] randomized 181 eligible patients with completely resected stage III NSCLC to receive postoperative cisplatin 80 mg per m^2 and vindesine 3 mg per m^2 on day 1 and 8 for three months or no further treatment. Patients were stratified by histology (squamous versus nonsquamous), and prognostic variables such as histology, performance status, extent of operation, tumor and nodal status were equally distributed among the two study arms. There was no difference in disease-free survival (18 versus 23 months, p = 0.5954), with the majority of recurrences being distant in both groups. Moreover, there was no difference in survival between the two groups, with a median survival time and five-year survival of 31 months and 35% in the chemotherapy arm versus 37 months and 41% in the control arm (p = 0.8606). The average cumulative dose of chemotherapy received was only 68% of the full protocol dosage.

The second study using adjuvant vindesine-cisplatin was conducted at Memorial Sloan-Kettering Cancer Center.[21] This study entered 72 patients with histologically confirmed T1-3N2 NSCLC. Patients were stratified by extent of resection (complete versus incomplete) and histology (squamous versus nonsquamous). Thirty-six were randomized to receive postoperative vindesine 3 mg per m^2 weekly for five weeks, then every two weeks eight times and cisplatin 120 mg per m^2 every four weeks four times plus thoracic irradiation (40 Gy beginning six to seven weeks postthoracotomy). Incompletely resected patients had intraoperative I^{125} and/or Ir^{192} implantation. There was no difference in time to progression (9.2 months for radiation and chemotherapy versus nine months for radiation alone, p = 0.35), with the majority of recurrences being distant in both groups. Overall survival was slightly better for the patients treated with postoperative radiotherapy alone (16.3 months for radiation and chemotherapy versus 19.1 months for radiation, p = 0.42). Similar to the findings in the Japanese trial above, only two-thirds of patients received the fully planned dosages of chemotherapy.

The results of Intergroup trial E3590 were recently presented.[22] This study was designed to determine if concomitant chemoradiotherapy was superior to radiotherapy alone in prolonging survival and preventing local tumor recurrence in completely resected stage II and IIIA NSCLC patients. The study randomized 488 patients between April 1991 and February 1997 to receive either four cycles of cisplatin (60 mg per m^2, day 1) and VP-16 (120 mg per m^2, days 1 to 3) administered concurrently with thoracic radiotherapy (5,040 cGy) or radiotherapy alone. Patients were stratified by weight loss (less than 5% versus more than 5%), histology (squamous versus other), nodal biopsy technique (sampling versus complete lymph node dissection), and stage (II versus IIIA), and 351 patients were eligible for analysis with a median follow-up of 37 months. Similar to the two vindesine-cisplatin adjuvant studies presented above,[20,21] only two-thirds of the chemoradiotherapy patients received all four planned cycles of chemotherapy, while 76% of these patients received the entire planned course of radiation. Slightly more (83%) patients in the radiation-alone arm completed the radiation as prescribed. Grades 3 and 4 toxicity, consisting largely of leukopenia and esophagitis, occurred in 8.8% and 1.3% of patients who received radiotherapy only, and 25% and 65% of patients who received the combined treatment. Treatment-associated mortality was roughly 2% in both arms of the study. Median survival overall was 38.6 months for the combined postoperative treatment and 41.1 months for patients treated with adjuvant radiation (p = 0.99). Three- and five-year survival rates were approximately 50% and 35%, and did not differ between the two arms. No difference was detected in disease-free survival or local recurrence rates. The authors concluded that postoperative chemoradiotherapy with etoposide and cisplatin does not prolong survival or alter local recurrence rates in patients with completely resected stages II and IIIa NSCLC when compared to postoperative radiation alone.

NON-CISPLATIN-BASED REGIMENS

Several interesting studies have been conducted in Japan. These trials have examined the use of tegafur (FT), a fluorouracil (5-FU) derivative, or UFT (a combination of tegafur and uracil at a molar ratio of 1 to 4). These agents can be administered orally.[23] FT has good absorption following oral administration and is gradually converted to 5-FU *in vivo*.[24] Degradation of 5-FU is inhibited by uracil; therefore the oral combination of UFT results in sustained levels of 5FU in tumor tissue.[25] The first two studies reported were conducted by the Chuba Branch of the Japan Society of Lung Cancer. In the first study, postoperative mitomycin, cyclophosphamide, and tegafur were compared to surgery alone.[26] After 2.5 years of follow-up, no significant difference in survival was seen between the two arms. The second Chuba study examined the effect of postoperative cisplatin, doxorubicin, and tegafur plus uracil (UFT) on completely resected stage I to III NSCLC.[27] The study randomized 309 eligible cases: 155 to surgery and chemotherapy, and 154 to surgery alone. The majority of patients entered had stage I disease (n = 118), while a few patients had stage II (n = 13), and the remainder, stage III (n = 78). In the combined modality arm, chemotherapy consisted of cisplatin 66 mg per m2 and doxorubicin 26 mg per m^2 within two weeks of surgery, followed by UFT orally at a dose of 8 mg per kg per day for six months or more. Chemotherapy was interrupted because of side effects of postoperative complications in only 14.9% of cases (in contrast to the cisplatin-based adjuvant studies discussed above, where usually only two-thirds of the planned chemotherapy is actually administered). Despite no planned stratification for known prognostic factors, gender, age, pathologic T-stage, histology, surgical procedure, and performance status were equally distributed between the two groups. There was an imbalance with respect to pathologic N stage, with more advanced cases assigned to the combined modality arm (p = 0.018). The overall five-year survival rate was 62% for surgery and chemotherapy versus 58% for surgery alone (not significant). Because a significant difference was observed between the two groups regarding pathological lymph node metastasis, a reanalysis incorporating prognostic factors using the Cox proportional hazard model was performed. With this prognostic-factor-adjusted analysis, a significant difference in overall and disease-free survival rates favoring the use of adjuvant chemotherapy was found (p = 0.044 and p = 0.036, respectively).

A third trial from Japan also evaluated the use of UFT in the postoperative setting.[28] In this trial, 310 eligible completely resected NSCLC (stages I to III) patients were enrolled. After surgery, patients were randomly assigned using the envelope method to one of three treatment groups. The first group (CVUFT) received cisplatin 50 mg per m^2 and vindesine 2 to 3 mg per kg, one to three weeks after surgery. In addition, vindesine 2 to 3 mg per kg was administered twice at intervals of one to two weeks. Two weeks later, a one-year period of oral administration of UFT 400 mg per day was started. The second group received one year of oral UFT 400 mg per day beginning one to three weeks after surgery. The control group received no postoperative adjuvant chemotherapy. Of the eligible patients, 109 received CVUFT, 103 got UFT, and 98 received no further therapy; 210 patients had stage I disease, 36 had stage II and 62 had stage III (including seven patients with stage IIIB disease). Although there was no planned stratification, no significant differences between the three groups with respect to gender, age, histology, pathologic T, N, or stage were observed. Compliance with the UFT was better than seen in other adjuvant trials, with the mean total dose being approximately 70% and 80% on the CVUFT and UFT arms, respectively. The five-year survival rates were 61% for CVUFT, 64% for UFT and 49% for the control group (differences among the three groups: p = 0.053 by logrank and p = 0.044 by Wilcoxon). In addition, a significant difference was observed between the UFT group and the control group (p = 0.022 by log-rank and p = 0.019 by Wilcoxon). Postoperative adjuvant chemotherapy was also found to be a significant prognostic factor for survival, with

hazards ratios (against control) of 0.64 (95% confidence intervals (CI): 0.42 to 0.97) in the CVUFT group and 0.55 (95% CI: 0.36 to 0.86) in the UFT group. Adverse effects were generally mild. Hematologic toxicity above or at grade 1 occurred in 29% of the CVUFT group versus 12% of the UFT group. A lower incidence of fatigue, anorexia, and nausea/vomiting were seen in the UFT group. Hepatic dysfunction was more common in the UFT group (13% versus 9% in the CVUFT). However, adverse reactions were tolerable and generally did not require interruption of UFT administration. Overall recurrence rates were 39% (29% distant) for the CVUFT group, 40% (28% distant) for the UFT-alone group, and 43% (33% distant) for the control group. Death from primary lung cancer occurred in 31%, 28%, and 39% of CVUFT, UFT, and control patients respectively. Deaths attributable to nonrecurrent second primary lung cancers occurred in 2.8%, 1.9% and 5.1% of CVUFT, UFT, and control patients respectively.

UFT administered in these studies was well tolerated and appeared to inhibit recurrences and prolong survival when administered over a long time period after complete resection. There is little data about the use of UFT in metastatic NSCLC. However, the results of these trials are compelling. Further study of this agent in randomized trials entering a more homogeneous patient population is warranted to confirm the effects of UFT therapy on survival following complete resection of NSCLC.

THE METAANALYSIS

The role of chemotherapy in NSCLC was extensively examined in a metaanalysis published in 1995.[29] This analysis was undertaken to determine the effect of cytotoxic chemotherapy on survival in patients with NSCLC. The vast majority of randomized trials conducted in NSCLC have been too small to detect a moderate treatment effect. Consequently, although a few trials have reported significant results, most have been inconclusive. In order to assess the evidence and establish the size of any possible treatment effect, a metaanalysis was conducted. Updated data on individual patients from all available randomized trials, both published and unpublished, were gathered, and 9,387 patients (7,151 deaths) from 52 randomized trials were analyzed. Patients with NSCLC were classified into three broad categories according to the primary treatment they received: surgery, radical or potentially curative radiotherapy, and supportive care. The main objective was to investigate the effect of chemotherapy on survival in these treatment settings. Trials were eligible if recruitment started after January 1, 1965 and was completed by December 31, 1991. For the purposes of this chapter, only the data regarding the use of postoperative chemotherapy will be presented here. Only adjuvant trials where patients had undergone a potentially curative resection and had no prior history of treatment for other malignancy were analyzed.

Surgery versus Surgery plus Chemotherapy

Data were available from 14 trials (4,357 patients and 2,574 deaths). Five trials used long-term alkylating agents (mainly cyclophosphamide and nitrosourea); eight employed cisplatin-based regimens, three trials had CAP chemotherapy (cyclophosphamide, doxorubicin, and cisplatin), and the remaining three employed cisplatin/vindesine. The intended dose of cisplatin ranged from 40 mg per m^2 to 80 mg per m2 per cycle and total dose from 50 mg per m2 to 240 mg per m2. A further three trials used other drug regimens, all of which included tegafur or UFT (tegafur plus uracil). In all the trials, chemotherapy was scheduled to start no later than six weeks after surgery.[29]

The results showed considerable diversity and evidence of a difference in direction of effect between the predefined categories of chemotherapy (see Table 42.2). The results for long-term alkylating agents were consistent. The hazard ratio estimates all favored surgery alone with a combined hazard ratio of 1.15 (p = 0.005). This 15% increase in the risk of death translated to an absolute detriment of chemotherapy of 4% at two years and 5% at five years.[29] For regimens containing cisplatin, the pattern of results was consistent with most trials favoring chemotherapy. An overall hazard ratio of 0.87 (p = 0.08) or a 13% reduction in the risk of death was found. The absolute benefit from cisplatin-based chemotherapy was 3% at two years and 5% at five years (95% CI: −1% to 10%). The trials that were classified as using "other" regimens were found to have an estimated hazard ratio of 0.89 in favor of chemotherapy (p = 0.30), but there was insufficient information to draw reliable conclusions (see Table 42.2).

Surgery plus Radiotherapy versus Surgery plus Radiotherapy plus Chemotherapy

Data were available from seven trials (807 patients, 619 deaths). Six trials used a cisplatin-based regimen, with intended doses of cisplatin ranging from 40 mg per m2 to 100 mg per m2 per cycle and total dose from 80 mg per m2 to 400 mg per m2. Total planned doses of radiotherapy ranged from 40 Gy in ten fractions to 65 Gy in 33 fractions, and the delay between surgery and the first adjuvant treatment was scheduled to be no longer than seven weeks.[29]

The overall hazard ratio of 0.98 (p = 0.76) was marginally in favor of chemotherapy (see Table 42.2). For the cisplatin-based trials, a hazard ratio of 0.94 (p = 0.46) or a 6% reduction in the risk of death favored chemotherapy, suggesting a 2% absolute benefit at both two and five years.

This metaanalysis suggests that cisplatin-based chemotherapy regimens may provide an absolute benefit of about 5% in the surgical adjuvant setting. The confidence intervals are such, however, that the results are consistent with benefits of as much as 10%, or as little as a 1% detriment. The authors concluded that although the effects of postoperative cisplatin-based chemotherapy were modest, these improvements, given the high incidence of lung cancer, could be important in public health terms. In addition, studies of patients' opinions of treatments for cancer have shown that many patients accept considerable toxicity in return for small improvements in survival.[30]

ONGOING TRIALS

Currently, there are several ongoing international trials evaluating the use of postoperative chemotherapy. The International Adjuvant Lung Cancer Trial (IALT) should determine the impact on survival of three to four cycles of cisplatin-based chemotherapy in completely resected stage

TABLE 42.2. RESULTS OF METAANALYSIS FOR ADJUVANT CHEMOTHERAPY IN NSCLC

Chemotherapy	Surgery				Surgery and Radiotherapy			
	Hazard Ratio (95% CI)	p Value	% Absolute Benefit		Hazard Ratio (95% CI)	p Value	% Absolute Benefit	
			2 yr	5 yr			2 yr	5 yr
Alkylating agents	1.15 (1.04 to 1.27)	0.005	−4	−5	1.35 (0.83 to 2.20)	0.023	−11	−7
"Other" drugs	0.89 (0.72 TO 1.11)	0.30	3	4	NA	NA	NA	NA
Cisplatin-based	0.87 (0.74 to 1.02)	0.08	3	5	0.94 (0.79 to 1.11)	0.46	2	2

CI, confidence intervals
From Non–Small Cell Lung Cancer Collaborative Group. Chemotherapy in non–small cell lung cancer: a meta-analysis using updated data on individual patients from 52 randomized clinical trials. *Br Med J* 1995;311:899, with permission.

I, II, or III NSCLC. Eligible patients receive cisplatin (80 to 120 mg per m^2 per cycle) and either a vinca alkaloid (vinblastine, vindesine, or vinorelbine) or etoposide, or no further therapy.[31] Chemotherapy must begin within 30 to 60 days of surgery. In the first 3.5 years since the study was opened, approximately 1,300 patients have accrued. The trial was designed to show a reduction in mortality of 5% to 10% with the use of adjuvant cisplatin-based chemotherapy. No results are available to date.

The ALPI trial (Adjuvant Lung Project Italy) is another large study evaluating the role of postoperative cisplatin chemotherapy. This trial, being conducted in Italy with participation from the EORTC, randomizes completely resected stage I, II, and IIIA NSCLC patients to receive either MVP (mitomycin 8 mg per m^2 on day 1, vindesine 3 mg per m2 on day 1 and 8, cisplatin 100 mg per m2 on day 1) every three weeks for three cycles, or control.[32] Chemotherapy must begin within 14 to 42 days after surgery. Radiotherapy can be given at the discretion of the participating center, beginning three to five weeks after completion of chemotherapy or four to six weeks following surgery (control group). Patients are stratified by center, T- and N-stage, and use of radiotherapy. The study was designed to detect a 20% relative reduction in five-year mortality rate, with 80% power at the 5% level of statistical significance. Since the trial opened in 1994, accrual has been relatively constant at about 250 patients per year. Approximately 1,200 patients have been enrolled as of October 1998. Analysis of survival and recurrence will occur when a predefined number of events (635) have occurred.

The results of these two large, randomized, prospective adjuvant trials will likely shed light on the controversial issue of the efficacy of cisplatin-based adjuvant chemotherapy in the treatment of stage I, II, and IIIA NSCLC. These results are anxiously awaited.

Cisplatin plus vinorelbine as a surgical adjuvant is currently undergoing evaluation in North America in the NCIC BR10 trial. This trial, chaired by the National Cancer Institute of Canada with participation by several cooperative groups in the United States, randomizes completely resected stage IB and II NSCLC to observation or cisplatin plus vinorelbine. Patients are stratified based on the presence or absence of *RAS* mutations. Another North American cooperative group (Cancer and Leukemia Group B) is using carboplatin plus paclitaxel postoperatively in patients with resected stage IB NSCLC. This regimen is being compared to observation. These two studies will help define the role of "newer" drug combinations in the adjuvant setting.

FUTURE STRATEGIES

When designing future trials of adjuvant therapy in NSCLC, it is important to keep in mind a number of guid-

TABLE 42.3. ISSUES IN ADJUVANT CHEMOTHERAPY TRIAL DESIGN AND REPORTING

Trial Design:
Appropriate preoperative evaluation to exclude metastases
Complete surgical resection, negative pathologic margins
Careful intraoperative staging, extensive nodal sampling or dissection
Tissue banking for analysis of biologic markers
Untreated control arm
Stratification for known major prognostic factors
Randomization after pathologic staging and clinical recovery from surgery
Optimal chemotherapy regimen
Trial Reporting
Intention to treat analysis
Compliance and toxicity of adjuvant therapy
Disease-free and overall survival rates
Recurrence patterns—local, distant, or both
Second primary tumor rates

ing principles.[1,33] Table 42.3 outlines various issues relevant in the design and reporting of adjuvant chemotherapy trials. Appropriate preoperative evaluation to exclude metastatic disease should be performed in all patients. An exciting new modality, whole-body positron emission tomographic (PET) scanning, appears to add to the precision of preoperative staging accomplished by CT and mediastinoscopy.[3] More experience with this technique is required fully to define its role in the staging of NSCLC, but it may play a central role in identifying resectable patients in the near future. Trials should enter patients of similar prognosis who have undergone a complete surgical resection with negative pathologic margins. In order to insure accurate staging, all patients should have extensive nodal sampling or dissection performed intraoperatively. At present, an untreated control arm is best to most accurately assess the impact of the experimental adjuvant therapy. Patients should be stratified for known major prognostic factors. Randomization should occur after pathologic staging is known and following clinical recovery from surgery. Efforts should be made to collect tumor specimens prospectively to facilitate biologic studies that might lead to the identification of new biologic prognostic factors. The adjuvant chemotherapy regimen chosen for study should be the most active one known for metastatic disease at the time of the trial design. Analysis of adjuvant trials should be done on an intent-to-treat basis. Compliance with adjuvant therapy should be noted, because trials to date have often found a significant number of patients not completing the adjuvant therapy as planned. Disease-free and overall survival rates as well as site of initial recurrence—local, distant, or both—should be reported. The occurrence of second primary tumors should also be noted.

Despite what appears to be a complete resection of

NSCLC, death follows in the majority of patients after developing recurrent disease. Therapy aimed at eradicating micrometastatic disease has been the primary goal of adjuvant chemotherapy. The majority of clinical trials performed have not found unequivocal, reproducible evidence of efficacy for adjuvant therapy. The chemotherapy regimens tested to date have been marginally effective, if at all. This may in part be due to the frequent discontinuation of chemotherapy in most of the adjuvant studies preventing demonstration of a benefit that might otherwise have been proven.[34]

The past few years have witnessed the identification of new chemotherapeutic agents with improved activity against metastatic NSCLC (taxanes, camptothecins, vinorelbine, and gemcitabine). Incorporation of these new agents into the adjuvant setting may improve survival for resected patients. Trials confirming the efficacy of postoperative UFT are clearly warranted. In addition, the role of even newer classes of antineoplastic therapies, such as the antiangiogenesis inhibitors, matrix metalloproteinase inhibitors, farnesyl transferase inhibitors, tyrosine kinase inhibitors or other biologic therapies, should be defined in the upcoming years.

REFERENCES

1. Evans WK. Adjuvant chemotherapy: results and perspectives. *Lung Cancer* 1995;12[Suppl 1]:S35.
2. Mountain CF. Revisions in the international system for staging lung cancer. *Chest* 1997;111:1710.
3. Ginsberg RJ, Vokes EE, Raben A. Cancer of the lung. In: Devita VT, Jr. Hellman S, Rosenberg SA, eds. *Cancer: principles and practice of oncology.* 5th ed. Philadelphia: Lippincott-Raven, 1997: 858.
4. Mountain CF, Lukeman JM, Hammar SP, et al. Lung cancer classification: the relationship of disease extent and cell type to survival in a clinical trials population. *J Surg Oncol* 1987;35(3): 147.
5. Kayser K, Bulzebrck H, Probst G, et al. Retrospective and prospective tumor staging evaluating prognostic factors in operated bronchus carcinoma patients. *Cancer* 1987;59:355.
6. Minna JD, Sekedo Y, Fong KM, et al. Cancer of the lung. In: Devita VT, Jr. Hellman S, Rosenberg SA, eds. *Cancer: principles and practice of oncology.* 5th ed. Philadelphia: Lippincott-Raven, 1997:849.
7. Feld R, Rubinstein LV, Weisenburger TH. Lung Cancer Study Group. Sites of recurrence in resected stage I non–small cell lung cancer: a guide for future studies. *J Clin Oncol* 1984;2:1352.
8. Matthews MJ, Kanhouwa S, Pickren J, et al. Frequency of residual and metastatic tumor in patients undergoing curative surgical resection for lung cancer. *Cancer Chemother Rep* 1973;4:63.
9. Slack NH. Bronchogenic carcinoma. Nitrogen mustard as a surgical adjuvant and factors influencing survival. University surgical adjuvant lung project. *Cancer* 1970;25:987.
10. Higgins GA, Shields TW. Experience of the Veterans Administration surgical adjuvant group. In: Muggia F and Rozencweig M, eds. *Lung cancer: progress in therapeutic research.* New York: Raven Press, 1979:433.
11. Shields TW, Higgins Jr GA, Humphrey EW, et al. Prolonged intermittent adjuvant chemotherapy with CCNU and hydroxy-urea after resection of carcinoma of the lung. *Cancer* 1982;50: 1713.
12. Brunner KW, Marthaler T, Muller W. Effects of long-term adjuvant chemotherapy with cyclophosphamide (NSC-2627,2) for radically resected bronchogenic carcinoma. *Cancer Chemother Rep* 1973;4:125.
13. Girling DJ, Stott H, Stephens RJ, et al. Fifteen-year follow-up of all patients in a study of postoperative chemotherapy for bronchial carcinoma. *Br J Cancer* 1985;52:867.
14. The Ludwig Lung Cancer Study Group (LLCSG). Immunostimulation with intrapleural BCG as adjuvant therapy in resected non–small cell lung cancer. *Cancer* 1986;58:2411.
15. Millar JW, Roscoe P, Pearce SJ, et al. Five-year results of a controlled study of BCG immunotherapy after surgical resection in bronchogenic carcinoma. *Thorax* 1982;37:57.
16. Holmes EC, Gail M, for the Lung Cancer Study Group. Surgical adjuvant therapy for stage II and stage III adenocarcinoma and large-cell undifferentiated carcinoma. *J Clin Oncol* 1986;4:710.
17. Lad T, Rubinstein L, Sadeghi A. The benefit of adjuvant treatment for resected locally advanced non–small cell lung cancer. *J Clin Oncol* 1988;6:9.
18. Feld R, Rubinstein L, Thomas PA, and the Lung Cancer Study Group. Adjuvant chemotherapy with cyclophosphamide, doxorubicin, and cisplatin in patients with completely resected stage I NSCLC. *J Natl Cancer Inst* 1993;85:299.
19. Niiranen A, Niitamo-Korhonen S, Kouri M, et al. Adjuvant chemotherapy after radical surgery for non–small cell lung cancer: a randomized study. *J Clin Oncol* 1992;10:1927.
20. Ohta M, Tsuchiya R, Shimoyama M, et al. Adjuvant chemotherapy for completely resected stage III non–small cell lung cancer. *J Thorac Cardiovasc Surg* 1993;106:703.
21. Pisters KMW, Kris MG, Gralla RJ, et al. Randomized trial comparing postoperative chemotherapy with vindesine and cisplatin plus thoracic irradiation with irradiation alone in stage III (N2) NSCLC. *J Surg Oncol* 1994;56:236.
22. Keller SM, Adak S, Wagner H, et al. Prospective randomized trial of postoperative adjuvant therapy in patients with completely resected stages II and IIIa non–small cell lung cancer: an intergroup trial (E3590) [Abstract]. *Proc ASCO* 1999;465a.
23. Fujii S, Kitano S, Ikenaka K, et al. Studies on coadministration of uracil or cytosine on antitumor activity of FT-207 or 5-FU derivative. *Jpn J Cancer Chemother* 1979;6:377.
24. Ansfield FJ, Kallas GJ, Singson JP. Phase I–II studies of oral tegafur. *J Clin Oncol* 1983;1:107.
25. Fujii S, Ikenaka M, Fukushima M, et al. Effect of coadministration of uracil or cytosine on the antitumor activity of clinical doses of 1-(2-tetrahydro-furyl)-5-fluorouracil and level of 5-fluorouracil in rodents. *Gann* 1979;70:209.
26. Kunishima K, Karasawa K, Imaizumi M, et al. A randomized controlled trial of postoperative adjuvant chemotherapy in non–small cell lung cancer. [In Japanese]. *Haigan* 1992;32:481.
27. Imaizumi M and The Study Group of Adjuvant Chemotherapy for Lung Cancer (Chuba, Japan). A randomized trial of postoperative adjuvant chemotherapy in non–small cell lung cancer (the second cooperative study). *Eur J Surg Oncol* 1995;21:69.
28. Wada H, Hitomi S, Teramatsu T, et al. Adjuvant chemotherapy after complete resection in non–small cell lung cancer. *J Clin Oncol* 1996;14:1048.
29. Non–Small Cell Lung Cancer Collaborative Group. Chemotherapy in non–small cell lung cancer: a meta-analysis using updated data on individual patients from 52 randomized clinical trials. *Br Med J* 1995;311:899.
30. Slevin ML, Stubbs L, Plant JF, et al. Attitudes to chemotherapy: comparing views of patients with cancer with those of doctors, nurses, and general public. *Br Med J* 1990;300:1458.
31. LeChevalier T, Auquier A, Tarayre M, et al. The international

adjuvant lung cancer trial (IALT) [Abstract]. In: Proceedings of the Perugia International Cancer Conference VI. *Chemotherapy of non–small cell lung cancer: ten years later.* October 1998.

32. Torri V, Flann M, Tinazzi A, et al. Randomized study of adjuvant chemotherapy for stage I–I–IIA NSCLC: report on the ALPI trial. The International Adjuvant Lung Cancer Trial (IALT) [Abstract]. In: Proceedings of the Perugia International Cancer Con-ference VI. *Chemotherapy of non–small cell lung cancer: ten years later.* October 1998.

33. Ihde D, Ball D, Arriagada R, et al. Postoperative adjuvant therapy for non–small cell lung cancer: a consensus report. *Lung Cancer* 1994;11[Suppl 3]:S15.

34. Ihde DC. Is there a place for classical adjuvant treatment? *Lung Cancer* 1994;11[Suppl 3]:S111.

43

POSTOPERATIVE IRRADIATION IN NON–SMALL CELL LUNG CANCER

TIMOTHY E. SAWYER
JAMES A. BONNER

Surgical resection is the cornerstone of management for non-small cell lung cancer (NSCLC). Postoperative irradiation likely has no benefit for patients with pathologic T1N0 or T2N0 lesions, which have low rates of local failure. Moreover, the role of adjuvant therapy after complete resection and modal dissections of tumors that are found to involve hilar (N1) or mediastinal (N2 or N3) lymph nodes, as defined by the American Joint Committee on Cancer (AJCC), is controversial.[1]

Attempts to define the potential benefits of postoperative therapy have been reported from a large number of retrospective and prospective studies (see Table 43.1). Several retrospective studies suggest benefit from mediastinal postoperative irradiation for various groups of patients; however, survival benefit has not been corroborated by any randomized study. Each retrospective study is limited by selection bias inherent in all retrospective analyses. However, the randomized studies that have considered this question have also been limited, to various extents, by substantial design flaws. The majority of them have more than one limitation.

First, several published randomized trials include some patients who have low risk for local-regional recurrence. So any potential benefit of postoperative radiation therapy, in terms of survival, may be diluted by the low-risk patients in these local trials, which did not stratify or analyze patients according to level of risk. Emerging information about prognostic factors has recently become available, and imbalances of these factors in the randomized studies may influence the results of randomized studies. Some trials have analyzed patients of varying risk groups independently. However, these subgroup analyses are essentially retrospective reanalyses that were not initially planned and do not possess statistical validity that is significantly superior to that of retrospective studies.

Second, many of the randomized trials took place in the 1960s and 1970s, a period during which the technical quality of radiation therapy was significantly inferior to current techniques. Many of these trials occurred before the regular use of linear accelerators. Linear accelerators have significantly enhanced the ability to deliver high doses to target tissues while reducing the dose to superficial tissues and structures. Most of these trials occurred before the availability of computed tomography, which allows better staging radiographically and definition of the target volume, and also facilitates more sophisticated radiation treatment planning and beam directing. All the trials were limited to varying extents by other limitations, including the use of spinal cord blocks (which potentially block mediastinal disease), poor quality control relating to both irradiated volume and target volume dose, and split-course and hypofractionation regimens.

Third, the majority of randomized trials included a very small number of patients, with little or no statistical hope of demonstrating even a moderate-sized difference in outcome. Had these trials demonstrated a radiation-related improvement in outcome (assuming a difference actually exists), it would have to have been due to a statistical fluke. The absence of a statistically significant difference in outcome in these trials should be considered as nothing more than a self-fulfilling prophecy. Possibly, trials that are extremely limited in power do more harm than good in improving our therapeutic knowledge.

There are nine published randomized trials considering postoperative irradiation.[2–10] Some of the technical and methodologic limitations of these trials are given in Table 43.1. (Two other trials are not listed in Table 43.1 because the results have not been published except in abstract form.[11,12])

The Ideal Patient

Despite the popularity of neoadjuvant (preoperative) chemotherapy and radiation therapy in lung cancer, surgery has a significant advantage as the initial therapeutic modality: the undisturbed pathologic features. The findings can be used to categorize patients as to ultimate risk for death, systemic failure, and local failure. The best patient category to investigate benefit of postoperative radiotherapy probably

TABLE 43.1. TRIALS EVALUATING THE EFFICACY OF POSTOPERATIVE RADIATION THERAPY FOR NON–SMALL CELL LUNG CANCER

Study	Tumor	Stratification	No. of Patients	Survival	Comments
Paterson, 1962[7]	All histologies Node +, node −	None	202	No difference	Full mediastinum not treated. 77% of patients received full dose (45 Gy)—according to authors, dosimetry was "tentative" Inclusion of low-risk patients, with no attempt to distinguish between low and high risk, makes results nonapplicable to high-risk patients
Bangma, 1971[5]	All histologies Node +, node −	None	73	No difference	Orthovoltage Included only hilum and homolateral mediastinum Low power and inclusion of low-risk groups means little hope of demonstrating benefit Not truly randomized (patients were assigned alternately to 1 of 2 groups)
EORTC, 1979[6]	Squamous only Node +, node −	N0 All patients	142 88 230	No difference No difference No difference	Exclusion of 162 of 392 patients, with significant imbalances between groups, makes these results essentially uninterpretable Results never published in a peer-reviewed journal A trend toward improved rate of local-regional recurrence in the irradiated group (p = 0.09)
Van Houtte et al., 1980[2]	All histologies Node −	None	175	No difference	A nonsignificant trend toward lower survival rate in irradiated patients may be related to treatment toxicity caused by high dose (60 Gy in 6 weeks) and low energy (^{60}Co) Suggestion of a decreased local recurrence rate among irradiated patients
LCSG, 1986[8]	Squamous only Stage II and III	*	230	No difference	Supervoltage (^{60}Co) and megavoltage Several technical limitations have been previously suggested[77] Irradiated group had reduced rate of first local recurrence (p less than 0.001) On subgroup analysis for N2 patients, irradiated group had improved DFS (p = 0.03) Too little power to provide realistic hope of demonstrating survival benefit in N2 or stage III patients
Debevec et al., 1996[10]	All histologies N2 only	None	74	No difference	A nonstatistically significant trend toward improved survival 3,000 cGy in 10 fractions means dose significantly below that needed to permanently sterilize microscopic disease Too little power to provide realistic hope of demonstrating statistically significant benefit
Lafitte et al., 1996[3]	All histologies T2N0 only	None	132	Superior in control arm, p = 0.049	19% of patients excluded postrandomization, resulting in 10 fewer patients in radiation therapy arm Few technical details given, although the lower mediastinum was excluded from the treatment field
MRC, 1996[9]	All histologies T1–2, N1–2	N1 N2 All patients	183† 106† 308†	No difference No difference No difference	The strongest published trial to date 40 Gy in 15 fractions roughly equivalent to only 42 Gy in 2 Gy fractions; however, posterior cord block placed to limit spinal cord dose to less than or equal to 35 Gy Only 36% of patients allocated to radiotherapy had radiotherapy given precisely as specified in protocol For all patients, radiotherapy led to improved rate of definite‡ local recurrence (p = 0.04) For N2 patients, radiotherapy led to improved survival rate but p = 0.18 (see text) For N2 patients, radiotherapy led to improved local recurrence rate but p = 0.07

(continued)

TABLE 43.1. *Continued.*

Study	Tumor	Stratification	No. of Patients	Survival	Comments
Dautzenberg et al., 1999[4]	All histologies Node +, node —	§	728	Superior in control arm, p = 0.002	Patients treated at 32 centers in Europe and South America 60 Gy, with large (up to 2.5 Gy) fractions Very limited quality assurance for surgery or radiation therapy, e.g., no central film review, unknown what percentage of patients received fractions over 2 Gy per fraction Most patients not stratified by risk, separate analyses for individual stages performed via regression analysis, but not performed for patients as randomized Analysis of patients as randomized grouped patients of disparate risk levels Excess mortality rate in irradiated patients due to excess of intercurrent deaths (in all nodal subgroups), the rate of which increased with dose per fraction Trend toward decreased local recurrence rate in N2 patients

* Stratified by clinical center, stage (II or III), previous weight loss, and age, but subgroup analysis performed according to nodal status.
† The first two numbers do not add up to 308 because 19 patients were of unknown stage.
‡ Recurrences were defined as suspected or definite at the discretion of the individual clinicians.
§ The majority of patients were stratified in accordance with treating institution, but not according to risk.
DFS, Disease-free survival; EORTC, European Organization for the Research and Treatment of Cancer; LCSG, Lung Cancer Study Group; MRC, Medical Research Council Lung Cancer Working Party.

has a higher frequency of local failure, but the precise factors need clearer definition. Multiple series do suggest which patients are at highest risk. Matthews and colleagues'[13] autopsy study assessed 202 patients who died within 30 days after purportedly curative resection for NSCLC. The pattern of documented residual disease was telling. Cancer recurrence was found within the chest of 24 of these patients. Subsequent data have suggested that conventional histologic techniques underestimate the true incidence of subclinical disease.[14,15]

If adjuvant irradiation confers a survival advantage, it most likely would rise in conjunction with the risk for local-regional recurrence. However, there may be a "leveling off" effect. This "leveling off" hypothesis suggests that the risk for distant metastasis increases in conjunction with the risk for local-regional recurrence. Thus, patients with an extremely high risk for local-regional recurrence may possibly be less likely to benefit from local therapy than patients with a lower risk, because their distant metastasis risk would diminish the chance of cure.

Many studies have attempted to define outcome-related prognostic factors in cases of completely resected NSCLC. The majority have focused on survival as the only end point. The data evaluating prognostic factors with respect to local-regional recurrence have allowed one to assess the efficacy of radiation therapy within risk-related subgroups, with possibly one exception. A Mayo Clinic study of patients with

completely resected N2 disease attempted to evaluate the role of postoperative irradiation in relation to local-regional recurrence risk. The analysis suggested that as local-regional recurrence and mortality risks increase, the benefit from postoperative irradiation also appears to increase[16] (Figure 43.1). The "leveling off" effect was not seen, but it may be that the patients with a very high risk of developing distant metastases were not included in the population of patients who were able to undergo complete resection or who were selected for postoperative therapy.

The Ideal End Point

The theoretic "leveling off" effect (the disappearance of a survival benefit with increasing local-regional recurrence risk) mentioned above may become irrelevant depending on the end point used as justification for the use of adjuvant therapy. This effect would apply primarily to the use of survival as an end point. Many have cited a decreased rate of local-regional recurrence as sufficient justification for recommending adjuvant radiotherapy. In this case, the absence of a survival benefit would not, in itself, be enough to dissuade one from recommending irradiation. However, if the justification for a potentially toxic therapy is improvement in local control with or without an associated survival advantage, it becomes particularly important to ensure that the

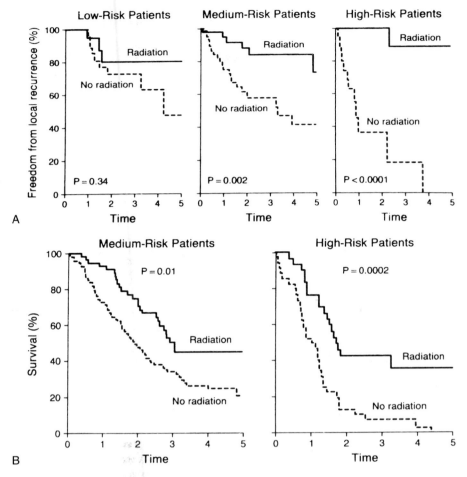

FIGURE 43.1. In a cohort of 224 consecutive patients undergoing complete resection for pathologic N2 non–small cell lung cancer, the radiation-related improvement in outcome appeared to increase with increasing risk for local recurrence **(A)**, and death **(B)**. (From Sawyer TE, Bonner JA, Gould PM, et al. Effectiveness of postoperative irradiation in stage IIIA non-small cell lung cancer according to regression tree analyses of recurrence risks. *Ann Thorac Surg* 1997;64:1402. By permission of the Society of Thoracic Surgeons.)

benefits of postoperative therapy are not outweighed by the toxicity.)

Radiation therapy to the mediastinum is associated with numerous potential side effects, and at least three randomized studies and one metaanalysis showed a *decreased* survival rate with the use of adjuvant irradiation for patients at relatively low risk for local-regional recurrence.[2–4,17] Two of these trials used 60 Gy as a standard postoperative dose[2,4] and one trial allowed doses of up to 60 Gy.[3] Treatment-related mortality was not reported from the Mayo Clinic series, which used 50 Gy.[16] However, because of the potential for irradiation-associated mortality, postoperative irradiation should be considered only in patients for whom a reasonable improvement in the chance of survival is expected (that is, patients for whom the absolute magnitude of an improved survival rate is likely to outweigh a small potential incidence of radiation-induced fatality). Another argument against the administration of postoperative irradiation only for local control after complete resection is that 50 Gy to the mediastinum is associated with several acute side effects, including fatigue, malaise, odynophagia, dysphagia, anorexia, and others. It is unclear whether the prevention of a symptomatic local progression (which can often be palliated effectively) justifies the delivery of therapy that has these associated side effects.

Still unanswered is the question: For whom should adjuvant irradiation be recommended? Despite much evidence, no survival benefit has been proved for any subgroup of patients. Despite this absence of proof, there are patients for whom radiation therapy may be justified on the basis of a large body of evidence that is not conclusive. Specific recommendations are given and supported in the following sections.

AJCC STAGE I (T1N0, T2N0)

Efficacy Data

Multiple randomized trials of postoperative irradiation have included patients with AJCC stage I (T1N0, T2N0) disease. Two trials included only patients with node-negative disease.[2,3] The findings from these trials, as well as a randomized trial[4] that analyzed but did not stratify according to nodal status, and a recent metaanalysis[17] are the basis for current treatment recommendations for node-negative disease.

The first trial, published in 1980 by Van Houtte and colleagues,[2] included 224 patients with node-negative disease (175 evaluable). Three patients in each arm had T3 disease; all other patients were found at surgery to have either T1 or T2 tumors. After complete resection, patients were randomly assigned to either 60 Gy delivered in 2 Gy fractions via a three-field technique using ^{60}Co or to no adjuvant treatment. Local-regional recurrences, defined as recurrences within the treatment field, were slightly less common in irradiated patients. The incidence of local recurrence was 8% for the irradiated group compared with 13% for the control group (this difference did not reach statistical significance). However, there was a high frequency of radiation-associated late tissue effects in the study arm, and patients in the irradiated group had an inferior rate of survival (but this difference did not reach statistical significance).[2]

In 1996, Lafitte and colleagues[3] reported the results of a study that used megavoltage radiation therapy. Only patients with T2 tumors were included. In this study, 132 evaluable patients were randomly assigned either to postoperative irradiation or to no further treatment. The five-year survival rate for all patients in the study was 44.2%. There was no difference between the two groups in the pattern of recurrence. The difference in survival between the two groups was of borderline significance in favor of the nonirradiated group (p = 0.049). However, the report contained few technical details about the radiation therapy, other than that the total radiation doses were between 45 and 60 Gy and that treatment was centered on the hilum and upper mediastinum. The inferior mediastinum was not routinely treated.

In a recently reported trial by Dautzenberg and colleagues,[4] 728 patients with stage I, II, or III NSCLC were randomly assigned, after complete resection, either to postoperative radiation therapy (60 Gy at 2 to 2.5 Gy per fraction) or to no further therapy. The trial included 221 patients with stage I disease. Although the first 189 patients in the trial were stratified by stage, the next 539 were not. For all patients, the five-year overall survival rate was 43% for the control group, and 30% for the irradiated group (log-rank p = 0.002). The excess mortality rate in the irradiated group was due to an excess of intercurrent deaths, the rate of which increased with increasing dose per fraction. The excess overall (log-rank p = 0.07) and radiation therapy-related (p value not available) death rates were also present for stage I patients. As discussed below in AJCC Stage III—Perspectives, this trial had several methodologic flaws.

A recently reported metaanalysis from the Medical Research Council Lung Cancer Working Party (MRC) organized and updated the results from these and other trials. This analysis included nine randomized trials (2,128 patients) comparing surgery alone versus surgery plus postoperative radiation therapy. For patients with all stages of disease,

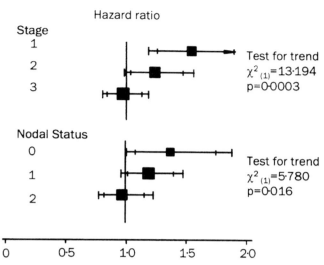

FIGURE 43.2. Stage- and lymph node status-based hazard ratios for PORT (postoperative radiation therapy) versus no PORT. (From PORT Meta-analysis Trialists Group. Postoperative radiotherapy in non-small-cell lung cancer: systemic review and metaanalysis of individual patient data from nine randomised controlled trials. *Lancet* 1998;352:257. By permission of the Lancet Ltd.)

postoperative irradiation was associated with an absolute survival rate decrement of 7% at two years. This hazard was most pronounced for patients with early-stage disease (N0, N1)[17] (Figure 43.2).

Patterns of Recurrence

Although randomized studies have not demonstrated a benefit for the addition of postoperative irradiation for stage I disease, the concept of adjuvant local treatment may still be worth exploring if subgroups of patients with stage I disease with particularly high risks of local failure were identified. It would be reasonable to continue to study the efficacy of postoperative irradiation in patients at high risk for local-regional recurrence, especially if ongoing trials reveal that adjuvant chemotherapy is helpful in reducing systemic failure (which would then bring local control more relevance and prominence).

Several recently published studies have used multivariate analyses to determine which patients with stage I disease are at highest risk for local recurrence after complete resection.[18–22] Factors influencing prognosis in this setting had included the preoperative presence of cancer-related symptoms,[22] tumor size,[21,22] T stage,[18] tumor grade,[19] tumor histology,[21] presence of satellite nodules,[21] blood vessel invasion,[20,22] pleural invasion,[22] high mitotic index,[20,22] DNA ploidy pattern,[23] and extent of surgery (wedge resection versus lobectomy).[22] However, all of these studies used overall survival or disease-free survival as the end points for their multivariate analyses. None considered local-regional recurrence; thus these studies are silent on issues pertaining to local recuirrence and control.

Two recent studies have identified factors that appear to independently predict the rate of local-regional recurrence. A randomized trial from the Lung Cancer Study Group (LCSG) indicated that a lobectomy, instead of a wedge or segment resection, leads to a lower local-regional recurrence rate (local-regional recurrence, two-sided p = 0.008; survival, one-sided p = 0.08).[24] In addition, a recent study considered 13 potential prognostic factors for independent prognostic significance and, with the use of multivariate analyses, evaluated freedom from local recurrence, freedom from distant metastasis, and survival. The study included 370 consecutive patients with stage I disease who, over a four-year period, had complete resection at the Mayo Clinic. The five-year actuarial local recurrence risk for all 370 patients (defined as a recurrence in N1, N2, or N3 lymph nodes or at the bronchial stump) was 15%. Factors that independently predicted a lower rate of local recurrence included the presence of a T2 lesion (as opposed to T1, p = 0.04) and less than 15 lymph nodes resected (p = 0.001). The adverse outcome associated with fewer removed lymph nodes was possibly simply a function of staging (the fewer the number of nodes removed, the greater the likelihood of not accurately detecting stage II or III disease). Alternatively, a full lymph node dissection may be therapeutic. The analysis of survival revealed that greater tumor size and the removal and/or pathologic evaluation of fewer lymph nodes were independent predictors for an inferior survival rate (p = 0.001).[25]

Perspectives

Presently, in the setting of completely resected stage I NSCLC for which mediastinal lymph nodes have been dissected or at least sampled, there appears to be no established role for postoperative irradiation. Postoperative radiation therapy does not improve the rates of local control or survival, and may increase noncancer deaths in patients with stage 1 disease.

Efforts continue to identify patients at particularly high risk for local-regional recurrence. Recent data from the Mayo Clinic, outlined above, represent an attempt to identify such prognostic factors and to use a regression tree analysis to assign patients to risk groups[26] (Figure 43.3). These results, from a retrospective review from a single referral institution,[25] cannot be considered definitive, and corroboration from other institutions or within cooperative groups is needed. If these results are confirmed, they may establish the ideal patient group for future study in a large randomized trial.

Another clinical situation deserves discussion. Although it is believed that mediastinal nodes should be dissected or at least sampled whenever possible, the radiation oncologist may occasionally be asked to consult postoperatively on a patient with stage I disease from whom no mediastinal lymph nodes were removed or evaluated. No definitive recommendations can be made about the role of postoperative mediastinal irradiation in this setting.

The most relevant data that can be used to address this question are related to the early-stage (radiographically uninvolved mediastinum) medically inoperable setting when the primary tumor is irradiated to definitive doses. Although several retrospective series imply no adverse outcome associated with omission of irradiation to clinically uninvolved nodes,[27–30] other series suggest that both local control and survival rates decrease when the mediastinum is not treated.[31,32] Factors associated with subclinical nodal involvement have been assessed.[33–37] Recently, Sawyer and colleagues[33] employed regression tree analysis in an attempt to use clinical (preoperative) factors to predict the incidence of subclinical N1 or N2 involvement in the clinical N0 setting. In relatively rare patients with low-grade (grade 1 or 2) and peripheral tumors, the incidence of subclinical involvement was approximately 15%. In all other patients, the incidence of subclinical involvement depended on the status of the preoperative bronchoscopy and maximal tumor diameter, but it was at least 35% (Table 43.2). It was also found that the risk of skip metastases (positive mediastinal nodes with negative N1 nodes) was 15% when a group of more than 300 consecutive patients who had thoracotomy for any stage NSCLC was considered.[38] The incidence of skip metastasis was higher when patients without nodal involvement were excluded. In summary, whereas irradiation to the mediastinum cannot be definitively recommended in the clinical N0 setting when no mediastinal lymph nodes have been removed, it may be of some benefit, and it cannot be considered inappropriate when the risk of subclinical involvement is considered. Postoperative pulmonary function and the volume of lung irridated to high dose should be considered in attempting to determine the therapeutic ratio associated with mediastinal treatment.

AJCC STAGE II (T1N1, T2N1, EXCLUDING T3N0)

Efficacy Data

Several retrospective studies have examined the efficacy of postoperative irradiation after complete resection of NSCLC.[39–42] However, most studies contain few patients with N1 disease[39,40,42] and consider patients with N1 and N2 tumors together as a group without providing statistical comparisons for the N1 group separately.[39,40] These studies demonstrate radiation-associated benefits only within narrow subgroups[40] or no benefit at all.[41,42] The retrospective study with the greatest number of patients, by Martini and colleagues,[41] suggests an independent radiation-associated survival decrement. However, these studies do not provide definitive, or even strong, evidence that adjuvant irradiation

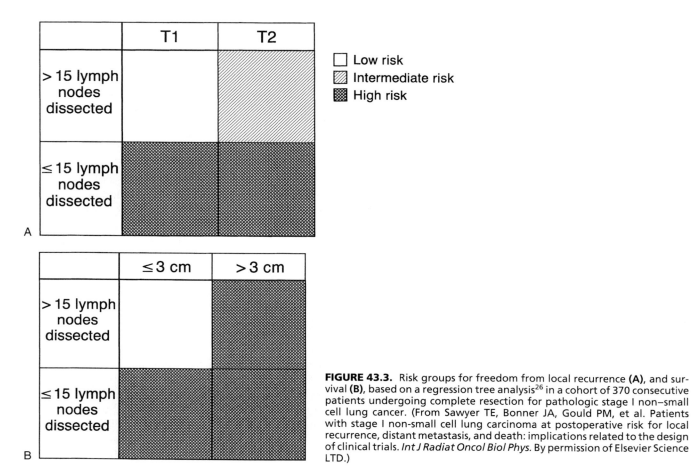

FIGURE 43.3. Risk groups for freedom from local recurrence **(A)**, and survival **(B)**, based on a regression tree analysis[26] in a cohort of 370 consecutive patients undergoing complete resection for pathologic stage I non–small cell lung cancer. (From Sawyer TE, Bonner JA, Gould PM, et al. Patients with stage I non-small cell lung carcinoma at postoperative risk for local recurrence, distant metastasis, and death: implications related to the design of clinical trials. *Int J Radiat Oncol Biol Phys.* By permission of Elsevier Science LTD.)

TABLE 43.2. RISK GROUPS FOR SUBCLINICAL NODAL INVOLVEMENT IN PATIENTS WHO ARE N0 OR N1 BASED ON THE PREOPERATIVE CT SCAN

Risk for Subclinical Nodal Involvement		Incidence (%)
Low (n = 32)	Negative bronchoscopy* Tumor grade 1/2	15.6
Low-intermediate (n = 227)	Negative bronchoscopy* Tumor grade 3/4	35.2
High-intermediate (n = 24)	Positive bronchoscopy CT tumor size 3 cm or less	41.7
High (n = 44)	Positive bronchoscopy CT tumor size over 3 cm	68.2

* Includes patients with no preoperative bronchoscopy performed.
CT, computed tomography.

leads to an improved outcome in patients with N1 tumors, with respect to either local-regional recurrence or survival.

Several published randomized trials have studied the issue of postoperative irradiation and have included patients with N1 tumors.[4–9] However, the majority of studies grouped patients with N1 tumors together with other patients and thus provided few meaningful conclusions related exclusively to N1 disease. Two studies used stratification techniques and provided important information for patients with stage II disease or N1 tumors.[8,9]

In the Lung Cancer Study Group (LCSG 773), 230 patients with stage II or III squamous cell carcinoma were randomly assigned, after complete resection, to either 50 Gy or no further treatment.[8] Patients were stratified by stage, and approximately two thirds of them had stage II disease. Approximately 75% of the patients had N1 tumors. For the entire group of 230 patients, adjuvant irradiation produced a significant reduction in local recurrence (defined as a first recurrence in the ipsilateral lung or mediastinum) (p less than 0.001), with only one documented local recurrence in the irradiated group. However, a local recurrence analysis was not performed in the separately stratified group of patients with stage II disease. Although patients were stratified by overall stage, separate overall recurrence or survival analyses were performed according to nodal status; therefore the results for patients with N1 tumors represent a retrospective subgroup analysis. Patients with N1 disease did not experience even a trend toward improvement in outcome due to radiation therapy, either for overall recurrence (p = 0.92) or for survival (p = 0.95).

In a more recent effort from the MRC, 308 patients with T1 or T2, N1 or N2 lesions were randomly assigned postoperatively to 40 Gy in three weeks or to no further therapy.[9] Patients were stratified by the TNM classification, and 183 patients had N1 disease. Postoperative radiation therapy did not improve survival (p = 0.99) or local control (p = 0.24) when the entire population was analyzed. However, the rate of definite local recurrence was lower in the irradiated group (p = 0.04). (Whether a recurrence was considered definite or suspected was at the discretion of the individual clinician.) Specifically for patients with N1 tumors, radiation therapy was not associated with improved rates of survival (p = 0.26), local recurrence (p = 0.96), or distant metastasis.

Although the majority of patients were not stratified with respect to nodal status, one other trial deserves special mention. In the trial of Dautzenberg and colleagues,[4] subgroup analysis suggests that the patients with stage II disease receiving adjuvant irradiation had an inferior survival rate compared with patients observed without treatment (log-rank p = 0.003). This difference in patients with stage II disease appeared to be related to radiation-induced toxicity.[4]

The postoperative radiotherapy (PORT) metaanalysis suggests a radiation-related hazard for patients with N1 disease, although the risk was less than for patients with N0 disease[17] (Figure 43.2).

Patterns of Recurrence

Several prognostic factors have been identified in completely resected N1 NSCLC, including T stage,[43–46] size,[41–46] extent of N1 nodal dissection,[25] findings on the preoperative bronchoscopy,[46] specific site of N1 node involvement,[42,44] and histologic features.[21,41,42] However, the majority of studies have not focused on local-regional recurrence as an important end point and/or have not used multivariate analyses to assess for independent local-regional recurrence-prognostic factor relationships. Thus they provide limited information about predicting which patients might most likely benefit from adjuvant irradiation and thus which patients might be most appropriate for inclusion in future studies.

Recently, the Mayo Clinic group[46] examined retrospectively the potential prognostic significance of multiple patient-, treatment-, and tumor-related factors in a series of 107 patients with completely resected N1 tumors who did not receive therapy other than surgery. Separate multivariate

analyses were performed with respect to freedom from local recurrence (defined as a recurrence in N1, N2, or N3 nodes or at the bronchial stump), freedom from distant metastasis, and survival. The main factor that independently predicted a higher freedom from local recurrence rate was the presence of a central tumor (positive preoperative bronchoscopic findings, p = 0.005). The main factors that independently predicted higher freedom from distant metastases and improved survival rates were removal of more than ten N1 nodes (p = 0.02) and the presence of a T1 tumor (p = 0.01), respectively. Regression tree analyses were performed for each end point (by the method of Breiman and associates[26]). The results for the local recurrence regression tree are shown in Figure 43.4.[46] The results of this study await corroboration by others and should be considered preliminary.

Perspectives

At many institutions, the administration of adjuvant thoracic irradiation after complete resection of pathologic N1 NSCLC has long been the standard of care. A local-regional recurrence benefit is frequently cited as justification for this, along with a possible, yet unproven, survival benefit. Currently, however, the data do not support any survival benefit in this setting, nor has a local-regional recurrence benefit been proven definitively or even strongly suggested. Although improvements in local-regional recurrence rate have been reported in some of the retrospective studies, these studies generally considered patients with N1 or N2 tumors as a single group. Few if any retrospective data have demonstrated a statistically significant benefit in the local-regional recurrence rate for a cohort consisting entirely of patients with N1 tumors. In addition, in the randomized studies in which patients were stratified so that those with N1 tumors or stage II disease could be considered independently, neither local-regional recurrence nor survival benefits were demonstrated.[8,9] Moreover, the randomized trial of Dautzenberg and colleagues[4] and the MRC metaanalysis[17] have suggested a radiation-related survival decrement for patients with N1 tumors.

The potential shortcomings of the LCSG study, which are related to both study design and radiation technique, have been cited frequently.[47] Analysis of the MRC study also reveals certain issues that may call into question the validity of using the results of the study to determine treatment. The MRC study design recommended use of a posterior spinal cord block at 35 Gy, which could potentially block mediastinal disease. Also, the MRC study used doses of radiation that may be suboptimal: 40 Gy in 2.67 Gy fractions, which is equivalent to a dose of 42 Gy in 2 Gy fractions, for an alpha to beta ratio of 10. This dose is well below the currently accepted "adjuvant dose" of 50 Gy. Furthermore, both the LCSG and MRC studies lacked the

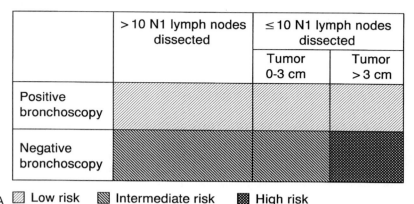

	> 10 N1 lymph nodes dissected	≤ 10 N1 lymph nodes dissected	
		Tumor 0-3 cm	Tumor > 3 cm
Positive bronchoscopy			
Negative bronchoscopy			

A ▨ Low risk   ▨ Intermediate risk   ▨ High risk

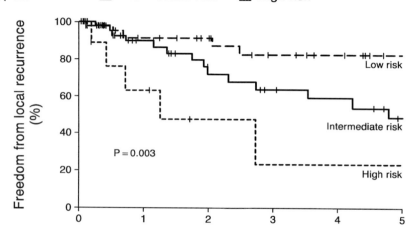

B

FIGURE 43.4. Risk groups for freedom from local recurrence based on a regression tree analysis[26] in a cohort of 107 patients undergoing complete resection and receiving no adjuvant therapy for pathologic N1 non–small cell lung cancer **(A)**. Patients in each risk group were well separated for outcome (log-rank p = 0.003) **(B)**. (From Sawyer TE, Bonner JA, Gould PJ, et al. Identification of risk groups in patients with completely resected N1 non–small cell lung carcinoma (*abstr*). *Int J Radiat Oncol Biol Phys* 1997;39:317, with permission.)

statistical power needed to detect small differences in outcome.

Currently, in the setting of completely resected (negative pathologic margins) AJCC stage II NSCLC for which mediastinal lymph nodes are dissected or at least sampled, there is not a definite role for postoperative irradiation. As for stage I NSCLC, the ideal study should evaluate this topic with appropriate stratification, state-of-the-art radiation therapy techniques, and the statistical power to identify small improvements in survival.

The local-regional recurrence risk for patients with N1 tumors who have had a complete resection is in the range of 21% to 44%.[9,41,45,46] With the potential for distant metastasis, it is unknown whether a treatment that effectively and considerably reduces this risk will lead to an improvement in survival. More work is needed to define the factors that place a patient at high risk for local-regional recurrence; these factors should aid in decisions related to the selection of patients for inclusion in future randomized trials and to the selection of stratification factors within the N1 patient population.

One clinical scenario is occasionally encountered and deserves special mention: the patient with N1 disease who has undergone complete resection but has not had surgical-pathologic staging of the mediastinum. In this setting, there are no data. Today, some institutions will have PET scans available to aid in decision making. Some prefer to irradiate the mediastinum postoperatively when lung function is not prohibitive.

AJCC N2, N3

Efficacy Data

Several randomized trials have investigated patients with completely resected N2 NSCLC, but have considered these patients together with patients having N1 and even N0 tumors.[5–7] These are all negative trials and little can be concluded about the role of adjuvant radiation therapy specifically for patients with N2 tumors. Several trials, however, have considered patients with N2 tumors by themselves, either by limiting the trial to such patients[10] or by considering stage or nodal status as a stratification factor during the randomization process.[8,9]

In the LCSG 773 study mentioned above, 230 patients with stage II or III squamous cell carcinoma were randomly assigned, after complete resection of disease, to either 50 Gy or no further treatment. Although patients were stratified by stage, only 74 of the 210 eligible patients had stage III disease. The results for the entire group of patients have been discussed above (see Stage II—Efficacy Data). Of the 74 patients with stage III disease, only 43 had N2 tumors; thus the results for patients with N2 tumors represent a subgroup analysis rather than an analysis of patients as randomized. Local recurrence rates were given only for the entire group of patients with stage II or stage III disease; however, the overall recurrence rate was reduced for those with N2 tumors (p = 0.03). However, this did not translate to improved survival (p = 0.81).[8]

A recently published randomized study by Debevec and colleagues[10] had only slightly more statistical power for patients with N2 disease than did the LCSG study. Over a five-year period, 74 patients who had complete resection for N2 NSCLC were randomly assigned to 3,000 cGy in ten fractions or no further therapy. Although postoperative therapy was associated with a trend toward improved survival, the difference was not statistically significant.

The randomized study with the most statistical power for evaluating the efficacy of radiation therapy after complete resection of N2 NSCLC was performed by the MRC and published in 1996.[9] This trial stratified 106 patients with N2 tumors and randomly assigned them to 40 Gy in 15 fractions or no postoperative treatment. The results for the entire group have been presented above (see Stage II—Efficacy Data). For patients with N2 tumors, there was a trend toward a lower local recurrence rate with the addition of irradiation (p = 0.07). The three-year survival rates for irradiated and nonirradiated patients were 36% and 21%, respectively. A slight trend toward statistical significance was noted, but the log-rank p-value was only 0.18 (Figure 43.5). The patients in the irradiated group also experienced a superior rate of freedom from distant metastasis (p = 0.03).[9]

Although the majority of patients were not stratified according to stage or nodal status before randomization, the trial conducted by Dautzenberg and colleagues[4] warrants specific mention. Details of the trial and the results for all patients as randomized (including those with stage I, stage II, or stage III disease) have been presented above (see Stage I—Efficacy Data). Of the 728 patients in this analysis, 327 had stage III disease and 190 were classified as N2. The subgroup analysis of patients with stage III disease revealed that postoperative radiation therapy was associated with a statistically significant increase in the rate of non-cancer-related deaths (specific log-rank P values, relative risks, and confidence intervals not given, except as shown), a nonstatistically significant trend toward an increased rate of death from any cause (log-rank p = 0.30; relative risk, 1.14; 95% confidence interval, 0.97 to 2.03), and essentially no difference in the cancer-related survival rates. Similar results were seen for patients with N2 tumors. The radiation-related survival decrement was more pronounced for patients who

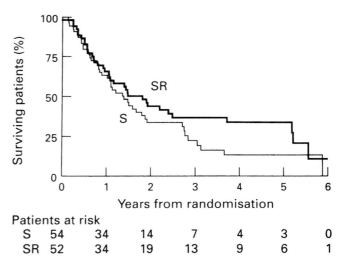

FIGURE 43.5. Results of the Medical Research Clinical Lung Cancer Working Party randomized study for patients with completely resected N2 disease. Patients receiving postoperative radiation therapy (SR) had survival rates superior to those of patients receiving surgery alone (S), but the difference was not statistically significant (log-rank p = 0.18). (From Stephens RJ, Girling DJ, Bleehen NM, et al. The role of post-operative radiotherapy in non-small-cell lung cancer: a multicentre randomised trial in patients with pathologically staged T1–2, N1–2, M0 disease. *Br J Cancer* 1996;74:632. By permission of Cancer Research Campaign.)

received higher doses per fraction. In the overall study, 22% of all irradiated patients received more than 2 Gy per fraction; however, it was unclear what the corresponding percentage rates were specifically for patients with stage III disease or N2 tumors.

In the N2 setting, perhaps the strongest evidence for the efficacy of postoperative irradiation in patients who have had complete resection is found in the retrospective studies. Several early studies suggested a radiation-associated benefit but provided statistical comparisons only for larger groups of patients, including patients with N2 tumors together with those with other nodal stages.[39,40] These studies often did not use statistical comparison methods at all[48] and showed benefits only in specific N2 subgroups.[40] Most importantly, they did not use regression analyses to attempt to determine whether the administration of radiation therapy was actually an independent prognostic factor.[39,40,48]

In a retrospective series by Miller and colleagues[49] from the Mayo Clinic, postoperative radiation therapy was found on multivariate analysis to be one of several factors independently associated with an improved survival rate. A later study from the same institution included a more contemporary group of 224 consecutive patients with N2 tumors who had surgical resection from 1987 to 1993, and regression analysis revealed that postoperative irradiation was the dominant independent prognostic factor in predicting both a lower rate of local-regional recurrence (p = 0.0001) (Figure 43.6A) and a higher rate of survival (p = 0.0001) (Figure

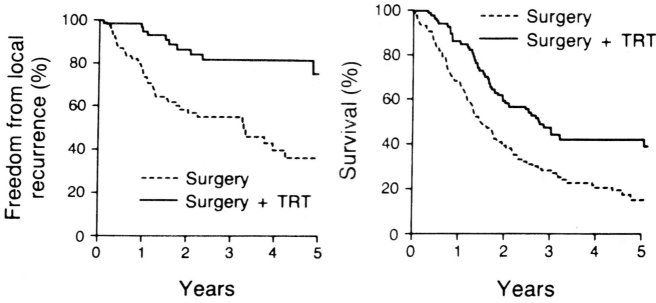

A

B

FIGURE 43.6. Freedom from local recurrence (log-rank P = 0.0001) **(A)** and survival (log-rank p = 0.0001), **(B)** outcomes for 136 patients with completely resected N2 disease receiving no postoperative thoracic radiation therapy (TRT), compared with 88 patients receiving adjuvant TRT. On multivariate analysis, TRT was the dominant factor in predicting superior local recurrence and survival outcomes. (From Sawyer TE, Bonner JA, Gould PM, et al. The impact of surgical adjuvant thoracic radiation therapy for patients with nonsmall cell lung carcinoma with ipsilateral mediastinal lymph node involvement. *Cancer* 1997;80:1399. By permission of the American Cancer Society.)

43.6B). The actuarial four-year freedom from local-regional recurrence and survival rates with the administration of postoperative radiation therapy were 83% and 43%, respectively, compared with 40% and 22% with surgery alone. During the period of this study, there was controversy among Mayo Clinic radiation oncologists about the benefits of adjuvant radiation therapy, and the views of the particular consulting radiation oncologist were thought to be one of the most important determinants of whether adjuvant therapy was recommended. A χ^2 analysis revealed that the 88 patients who had irradiation and the 136 who did not were well balanced with respect to multiple potential prognostic factors, including gender, age, histology, tumor grade, T stage, number of dissected N2 lymph node stations, number of involved N2 lymph node stations, number of involved N1 lymph nodes, level of mediastinal involvement (superior versus inferior versus both), and margin status. Imbalances included the tendency for patients with right lower lobe tumors to receive surgery alone, the tendency for those with multiple (versus solitary) involved N2 lymph nodes to receive postoperative irradiation (suggesting that the patients receiving irradiation were actually a higher-risk group), and the use of adjuvant chemotherapy in 24 of the 88 patients who received radiation therapy (compared with two of the 136 in the nonirradiated group).[50]

The MRC metaanalysis, described above, suggested neither survival decrement nor survival improvement with the administration of postoperative radiation therapy in the N2 setting[17] (Figure 43.2).

Patterns of Recurrence

For patients with completely resected N2 disease, multiple tumor-related prognostic factors have been identified. A lengthy list includes the number of involved N1 nodes,[25] the number of involved N2 nodes,[10,51] the number of involved mediastinal stations,[49,52,53] the location of nodal involvement within the mediastinum,[48,49,51–55] the presence versus absence of extracapsular extension,[56] the pathologic margin status,[50] the AJCC T stage,[51,54] the status of the mediastinum on preoperative chest computed tomography,[54,57] and the status of the mediastinum on preoperative mediastinoscopy.[58]

These studies focused largely on survival and either did not attempt to identify prognostic factors related to local-regional recurrence or did not use regression analyses to evaluate for potential independent prognostic significance. Therefore, none of these studies was specifically designed to assess the role of a local modality such as postoperative irradiation in the context of multiple potential confounding prognostic factors.

A 1997 study by Sawyer and colleagues[16] evaluated multiple potential prognostic factors and their ability to independently predict local-regional recurrence in 136 consecu-

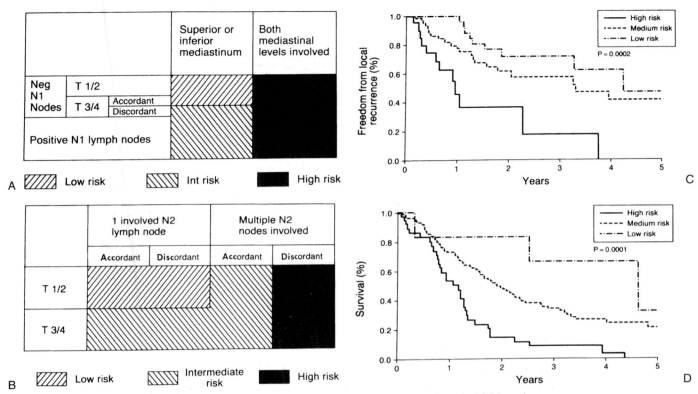

FIGURE 43.7. Risk groups for freedom from local recurrence **(A)** and survival **(B)** based on regression tree analyses[26] in a cohort of 136 patients undergoing complete resection and receiving no adjuvant therapy for pathologic N2 non–small cell lung cancer. Patients in each risk group were well separated for freedom from local recurrence **(C,** log-rank p = 0.0002) and survival **(D,** log-rank p = 0.0001). ("Accordant" tumors included upper lobe tumors with superior-only mediastinal nodal involvement or lower lobe tumors with inferior-only mediastinal nodal involvement; "discordant" tumors were those that did not fit "accordant" criteria.) (From Sawyer TE, Bonner JA, Gould PM, et al. Effectiveness of postoperative irradiation in stage IIIA non–small cell lung cancer according to regression tree analyses of recurrence risks. *Ann Thorac Surg* 1997;64:1402. By permission of the Society of Thoracic Surgeons.)

tive patients with N2 disease who, over a seven-year period at the Mayo Clinic, had complete resection and no adjuvant radiation therapy. This study used regression analyses with respect to both freedom from local recurrence and survival in an attempt to determine independent prognostic factors. Subsequently, regression tree analyses were used to categorize these prognostic factors further and to divide patients into groups according to risk. The actuarial four-year local-regional recurrence risk for the entire group of patients who received no adjuvant therapy was 60%. The results of the regression tree analyses are shown in Figure 43.7. It remains to be seen whether future studies will corroborate these regression tree findings. In particular, other studies have suggested that lower mediastinal involvement (as opposed to superior involvement) is associated with decreased survival.[48,49,53,54] Still other studies have supported the findings of Sawyer and colleagues that superior mediastinal lymph node involvement is a more ominous finding.[51,58]

Perspectives

In contrast to the N1 and node-negative scenarios, for which neither prospective nor retrospective data support the use of postoperative irradiation, the data as a whole suggest that postoperative thoracic irradiation may lead to both local control and survival benefit after complete resection of N2 NSCLC. However, these data are not conclusive, and further study with adequately powered investigations is warranted in this patient population.

In the Mayo Clinic analysis, patients were selected for radiotherapy or observation predominantly based on the bias of the radiation oncologist. There appeared to be little "referral" bias in terms of directing patients at particularly high risk or low risk toward or away from radiation therapy.[50] However, this study is retrospective; hence, the potential for undetected selection bias is possible. Although these data can be considered strong evidence, they cannot be considered conclusive.

The strongest support in the randomized literature is found in the MRC study. The p-value associated with the absolute 16% survival rate difference at three years favoring patients who had irradiation was only 0.18, and because of this, the study is termed "negative." However, a p-value of 0.18 means that if the null hypothesis (namely that there is no outcome difference between the two groups) is true, there would be only an 18% chance of finding a difference of the magnitude seen in this study (or of a greater magnitude). An 18% chance is relatively small—were it less than 5%, the majority of the medical community would probably be willing to accept postoperative irradiation as a contributor to improved survival for patients with completely resected N2 disease. Although these results should be considered suggestive evidence that postoperative irradiation leads to survival benefit after complete resection of N2 NSCLC, they cannot be considered conclusive. However, it is possible that the lack of statistical power in this study is related to the negative results.

The trial of Dautzenberg and colleagues,[4] which suggested a radiation therapy–associated survival decrement that appeared in patients with stage III disease to be solely related to radiation-induced toxicity, possesses considerably more power than the MRC trial, with 327 patients with stage III and 190 with N2 tumors. No stratification was performed (with respect to either stage or nodal status) for the majority of patients during the randomization process. The results for stage III disease and/or N2 tumors specifically are thus essentially a retrospective reanalysis of a stage-specific patient subgroup within a large randomized trial. The absence of stratification, the lack of central randomization (patients were randomly assigned separately within each of the 31 treating institutions), the lack of stated quality assurance with respect to either field design or total dose, and the presence of a radiation-associated survival decrement in the setting of total doses (60 Gy) and doses per fraction (up to 2.5 Gy) (which are higher than conventional doses delivered in the United States) make the results of this trial difficult to interpret.

The results of the retrospective studies that examined the issue of postoperative irradiation after complete resection of stage III or N2 NSCLC are frequently discounted, and significantly more weight is placed on randomized trials. In general, this policy is appropriate if the randomized trials are well designed, well conducted, and statistically powerful. In general, retrospective results are limited by the potential for undetected selection bias. It is often forgotten that a reference standard randomized trial has not been performed in this setting. Thus each randomized and retrospective study must be interpreted in the context of its quality. Quality should be assessed by the study's statistical power, appropriateness and uniformity of both surgical and radiation treatment, and the potential for selection or design-related bias. Randomized or retrospective studies that are limited by quality—so that the lack of a radiation-related improvement in outcome is essentially a self-fulfilling prophecy—cannot be considered strong evidence of the lack of a radiation-related benefit.

The discussion above suggests that the potential for a radiation-related benefit exists in patients with completely resected N2 NSCLC. However, it is important to elaborate upon the results of the recently completed MRC metaanalysis, which demonstrated neither survival decrement nor survival benefit associated with the use of postoperative irradiation for patients with N2 tumors.[17] All the trials included in this metaanalysis had one or more flaws (see above and Table 43.1), ranging from the use of sub-megavoltage energies to inadequate treatment volumes, inadequate doses, complete lack of quality assurance, and use of posterior spinal cord blocks that may block tumor. A metaanalysis made up almost entirely of flawed studies must itself be considered flawed. Therefore, it is not unexpected that the metaanalysis did not demonstrate survival benefit. Although proper consideration should be given to these metaanalysis results, they cannot be considered the final word.

On the basis of the above discussion, the recommendation for postoperative irradiation in the setting of completely resected N2 disease must balance the risks of treatment versus the potential of benefit. The benefit has not been glaringly obvious in any trial. This treatment remains controversial.

Currently, a randomized study that considers the issue of adjuvant irradiation for patients with N2 disease is being performed by the Cancer and Leukemia Group B (CALGB).

SPECIAL SITUATIONS

Completely Resected T3 Tumors with Chest Wall Involvement

The relatively favorable prognosis of T3N0 NSCLC, compared with T3 lesions with nodal involvement, is well established. This prognostic finding is reflected in the recent decision by the AJCC to reclassify T3N0 tumors to stage IIB from their previous stage IIIA designation.[1] After either extrapleural dissection or *en bloc* resection (the controversy about which one is the procedure of choice is discussed elsewhere in this textbook) for either node-negative or node-positive T3 lesions, the role of radiation therapy is less clear. This is especially true when the surgical margins are uninvolved. Margin-negative peripheral T3 tumors have the potential to recur either locally (at the chest wall) or regionally (within N1, N2, or N3 lymph nodes), and it is useful to consider these sites separately.

Local (Chest Wall) Issues

Several series have suggested that after either a margin-negative *en bloc* chest wall resection or an extrapleural dissection, the chance of recurrence in the primary tumor bed is low.[59,60] Postoperative irradiation to the chest wall is not recommended in this setting. Although few data exist to suggest that postoperative irradiation is effective when margins are microscopically positive, our recommendation is to consider postoperative radiation therapy to the tumor bed in this setting. Situations such as diffuse chest wall involvement and very close but negative margins are considered on a case-by-case basis.

Ipsilateral Hilum and Mediastinum

Several series, all retrospective and most with very limited power, have attempted to evaluate the efficacy of postoperative irradiation to regional (hilar and mediastinal) lymph nodes after resection of lesions that are T3 because of chest wall/parietal pleural involvement.

When the status of the hilar and mediastinal lymph nodes has been determined pathologically and these nodes are uninvolved, the majority of series have suggested that radiation therapy to the mediastinum (with or without hilar irradiation) is of no benefit.[61–63] However, an often quoted series by Patterson and colleagues,[55] in which eight of 35 patients received preoperative irradiation and nine of 35 received postoperative irradiation, demonstrated a 56% five-year survival rate for the irradiated group, compared with 30% for the group receiving no neoadjuvant or adjuvant therapy. This difference in survival was not statistically significant, possibly because of the small number of patients in the series. It is of interest that nine of the patients who received irradiation had curative resections for T3N0 lesions. Of these patients, seven (78%) were alive and disease-free at the time of publication, compared with three of the 14 (21%) patients with curatively resected T3N0 disease who did not receive postoperative irradiation. In a larger series by Gould and colleagues,[60] which compared 74 patients with completely resected T3N0 disease and no irradiation with 18 patients who received adjuvant (postoperative) irradiation, special attention was given to the patterns of postoperative recurrence. The actuarial four-year regional recurrence rate (defined as recurrence in N1, N2, or N3 lymph nodes) was 0% with radiation therapy, compared with 32% without radiation therapy (p = 0.05). There was only a slight suggestion of improved survival in favor of the irradiated group (p = 0.10). Of note was that patients with medial tumors (mediastinal pleural involvement) had a four-year nodal recurrence risk of 50% without postoperative irradiation.

No definitive conclusions can be drawn about the role of radiation therapy after complete resection of T3N0 NSCLC. The majority of the studies contained very few patients and often examined the role of radiation therapy as a minor topic. Two of the studies specifically oriented toward examining the efficacy of radiation therapy were inconclusive. The series of Patterson and associates[55] sug-

gested a radiation-related survival benefit; however, the more modern series of Gould and colleagues,[60] with a greater number of patients than the series of Patterson and associates, showed only a statistically insignificant trend. Currently, in the setting of a T3N0 lesion that has been resected with wide negative margins and for which an extensive hilar and mediastinal lymph node dissection or sampling has been performed, postoperative irradiation is not recommended.

The majority of studies that have explored the issue of adjuvant irradiation after complete resection of NSCLC that is designated T3 because of parietal pleural involvement or chest wall invasion contained very few patients with pathologic N1 and N2 tumors. Therefore, little insight can be gained into the efficacy of radiation therapy in the node-positive setting. For T3 node-positive disease, it is reasonable to consider the same data and the same rationale regarding nodal irradiation after complete resection of T1 and T2 and N1 and N2 tumors (explained in preceding sections).

Incomplete Resection

Although the setting of postthoracotomy residual disease is ominous, studies have suggested that the presence of a microscopically positive margin is associated with a better prognosis than the presence of gross residual disease.[64–66] Therefore, these scenarios should be considered separately.

Incomplete Resection, Microscopic Residual Disease

In the presence of microscopic residual disease, some authors have reported long-term survivors after surgical resection alone.[64,67] It is assumed that when long-term survival occurs any tumor cells that were left behind must not have been viable. However, the potential exists for viable tumor regrowth in this situation, and the recommendation herein is to consider postoperative irradiation for microscopic residual disease.

Reinfuss and colleagues[66] reported on 22 patients with NSCLC who had microscopic residual disease after thoracotomy, all of whom received postoperative radiation therapy. Seven of these patients (five without nodal disease) were alive five years after treatment. In a series of 124 patients with stage III disease, Minet and colleagues[68] reported that the median and five-year survival rates with no postoperative irradiation were 163 days and 3%, respectively, compared with 304 days and 7% for patients who received postoperative radiation therapy. Machtay and colleagues at the University of Pennsylvania have found that the prognosis for patients with microscopically positive margins who received postoperative irradiation is not different from that for patients with margin-negative resections who did not receive irradiation. However, both groups of patients were at high risk for distant metastasis (64% at three years). On the basis of studies such as these, the recommendation herein is to offer postoperative irradiation in the setting of microscopic residual disease.

Few data are available with which to make firm recommendations about the appropriate dose and/or treatment volume in this setting; however, the recent data of Emami and colleagues[69] are useful. In their series of 173 patients who received postoperative irradiation, 32 were treated because of the presence of positive margins. For these 32 patients, local control was greatest if at least 50 Gy was administered and survival was best if at least 60 Gy was given. These and dose response studies for related malignancies of the head and neck[70] suggest that a dose of 50 Gy at 2 Gy per fraction should be delivered to the tumor bed, with a dose of at least 60 Gy delivered to an area encompassing the site of microscopic residual disease. It is recommended that treatment include the tumor bed plus appropriate margin, without an attempt to treat electively regional nodal sites, when the following conditions are met: (a) the involved margin is located within the far lateral parietal pleura or chest wall; (b) in the opinion of the radiation oncologist, the field needed to encompass the tumor bed with margin would not compromise the ability to treat hilar and mediastinal nodes if necessary at a later date; and (c) the patient has had a complete mediastinal and hilar lymph node dissection (or extensive sampling) that revealed no evidence of N1, N2, or N3 disease. In all other patients, provided there is no medical contraindication, we prefer to include regional nodes in the treatment field.

Incomplete Resection, Gross Residual Disease

As mentioned above, several series have suggested that the presence of gross residual disease after thoracotomy is a more ominous finding than the presence of microscopically positive margins,[64–66] and local control and survival rates are poor regardless of further postoperative therapy.[23,58,64,66,71]

In 1988, the LCSG reported the results of a phase III trial that randomly assigned patients with incompletely resected disease to either radiation therapy alone or radiation therapy with six cycles of cyclophosphamide, doxorubicin (Adriamycin), and cisplatin (CAP) chemotherapy.[71] Incomplete resection was defined as the presence of microscopic residual disease, macroscopic residual disease, or disease in the highest resected paratracheal lymph node. Because patients in both arms of the study were treated with adjuvant irradiation, the magnitude of the radiation therapy–associated benefit could not be ascertained. However, the addition of chemotherapy led to a significantly longer progression-free survival (p = 0.004), with only a marginally improved median survival (p = 0.13). In the setting of macroscopic residual cancer, it is reasonable to institute therapy that would be considered for unresectable disease; combined chemotherapy and radiation therapy are discussed elsewhere in this volume.

TECHNIQUES

In the process of administering radiation therapy after complete resection of NSCLC, the importance of proper technique cannot be overstated. The majority of randomized trials that have been performed are routinely criticized for the use of inadequate techniques or for failing to pay close enough attention to the degree to which proper doses were administered to proper volumes (see Table 43.1). At least one series specifically demonstrated a statistically significantly decreased rate of local-regional control when inferior techniques were used (inferior techniques were defined as the failure to cover at least 90% of the target volume with at least 90% of the prescribed radiation dose).[72] In this series, technical inadequacies were thought to be the reason a majority of patients had local-regional recurrence.

Target Volume

Few data demonstrate the specific pattern of local-regional recurrence after complete resection of NSCLC. Therefore, recommendations for target volume are based largely on what is known about the pattern of nodal involvement at the time of surgery, the risk factors for and patterns of recurrence, and pulmonary tolerance issues.

Many patients with lung cancer have reduced lung function. Furthermore, lung capacity may be compromised after a surgical procedure. Therefore, every attempt should be made to limit the fields to areas at greatest risk for harboring residual subclinical disease.

In the setting of a T1 or T2 tumor or a tumor that is T3 based on other than chest wall or parietal pleural involvement, the following areas are included in the target volume: bronchial resection line, ipsilateral hilum, paratracheal and tracheobronchial angle lymph nodes (stations 1, 2, 3, and 4, as defined by Naruke and associates[44]), and subcarinal lymph nodes (station 7). In the setting of either subaortic or ascending aorta involvement (stations 5 and 6, respectively) or in the setting of left upper lobe tumors, stations 5 and 6 are also included in the field. Stations 8 and 9 (paraesophageal and inferior pulmonary ligament nodes, respectively) are treated only when nodes in these sites are specifically found to be involved, because elective treatment of these regions significantly increases the size of the irradiated field and any benefits of elective treatment are unproved. Supraclavicular regions are included in the setting of upper lobe tumors or when upper paratracheal nodes are found to be involved pathologically, although the need to treat supraclavicular regions in these settings has not been proved.

Additional details about target volume in the setting of chest wall involvement or microscopically positive margins are presented above (see Special Situations—Completely Resected T3 Tumors with Chest Wall Involvement, and Special Situations—Incomplete Resection).

Fields and Energy

To find the appropriate balance between maximizing postoperative healing and minimizing the ability for residual tumor cells to repopulate, postoperative irradiation is generally begun three or four weeks after the thoracotomy. Patients are treated in the supine position, with strict immobilization techniques. We prefer to use a two-field (AP:PA) approach, followed by opposed off-cord oblique fields (right-anterior and left-posterior obliques for left-sided tumors, and left-anterior and right-posterior obliques for right-sided tumors). The oblique fields are begun when the area of the spinal cord that is receiving the greatest dose (generally near the superior aspect of the field) reaches a dose of 43 to 45 Gy, provided that the isocenter is being treated at 2 Gy per day. Therefore, because of the oblique-field scatter dose to the spinal cord, portions of the spinal cord may receive total doses slightly greater than 45 Gy, although this additional dose is delivered at only a few cGy per day. The oblique fields are generally 30 to 45 degrees off vertical. Miller and associates[73] have demonstrated that when the posterior border of the oblique field is placed at the anterior border of the vertebral pedicles, 30-degree fields place slightly more margin on the spinal cord (mean field edge to spinal cord distance, 8.7 mm) than do 45-degree fields (mean field edge to spinal cord distance, 8.0 mm). However, CT planning is routinely used, and oblique angles are adjusted on a patient-by-patient basis to maximize coverage of the above target areas while minimizing the dose to the heart, lung tissue, and spinal cord.

CT-based treatment planning also facilitates the ability to correct for lung inhomogeneities with appropriate software. A case can be made against the use of lung correction in the "gross disease setting," because treatment is based on dose-response studies that did not use lung correction calculations; however, similar dose-response data are much more sparse in the postoperative setting. Therefore, lung correction calculations are routinely used in the postoperative setting to ensure that all at-risk areas are brought to the desired dose. Generally, lower megavoltage energies (6 or 10 MV) are recommended over higher energies such as 18 MV. The data from Miller and associates[74] have demonstrated that 18 MV beams have a wider penumbra in lung tissue than do 10 or 15 MV beams, requiring the use of a greater margin of normal lung tissue.

Field Borders

Because of the above recommendation to include the ipsilateral hilum and bronchial resection line in the field, the fields are almost never perfectly rectangular; shaped fields with custom blocks are used. The following dimensions can be used as general guidelines because these dimensions are similar to those used in recent trials in the United States (it should be noted that these dimensions will vary on a case-by-case basis with CT planning): for the anterior : posterior fields, the superior border is generally placed 2 cm superior to the suprasternal notch (this border is adjusted further superiorly when the supraclavicular fossae are treated). The inferior border is placed 5 cm below the level of the carina but may extend as inferiorly as the diaphragm when, at the time of surgery, station 8 and/or 9 lymph nodes are found to be involved. The lateral borders are placed either 2 cm lateral to the vertebral bodies or 2 cm lateral to the tracheal edge, whichever is more lateral. For subaortic or aortopulmonary window involvement (stations 5 or 6) or for left upper lobe tumors, a 1 cm margin is placed on the most lateral portion of the shadow of the aortic arch. A 2 cm margin is placed on the ipsilateral hilum and on the bronchial resection line. If CT performed preoperatively showed gross hilar or mediastinal adenopathy, these nodes are transposed to the simulation film and the borders are widened or lengthened as necessary to ensure a 2 cm margin on these preoperative volumes.

The goal of the oblique fields is to include the entire volume at risk to full microscopic tumoricidal doses (see below). The oblique field is not a reduced boost field. Therefore, the superior and inferior borders remain the same in the oblique treatment as in the anterior/posterior treatment. The posterolateral border is placed at the anterior borders of the vertebral pedicles. The anterolateral border is placed so that all the hilar and mediastinal nodes along with the bronchial resection line are treated. Generally, this border is placed at least 3 cm anterolateral to the anteriormost portion of the trachea, although these borders are adjusted in accordance with the preoperative CT hilar and mediastinal nodal volumes.

Additional details about field borders in the setting of chest wall involvement are mentioned above (see Special Situations—Completely Resected T3 Tumors with Chest Wall Involvement).

Dose

Few data are available about the optimal radiation therapy dose in the postoperative NSCLC setting. Therefore, recommendations are based on small retrospective series, on the potential for radiation-induced toxicity with higher doses, and on data from other tumor sites.

In the series of Choi and colleagues,[40] no patient who received at least 50 Gy after complete resection of NSCLC had local recurrence. Similarly, although data from Emami and colleagues[69] demonstrated no statistically significant difference in local-regional control with increasing dose, they did show a trend toward inferior control with mediastinal doses of less than 50 Gy. In an earlier series by Emami and colleagues,[72] none of the patients who received a dose of at least 60 Gy had local-regional recurrence. These data must be considered in the context of the several randomized trials outlined above in this chapter that suggested a decrease

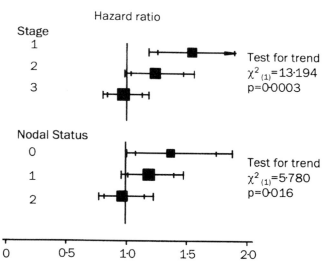

FIGURE 43.2. Stage- and lymph node status-based hazard ratios for PORT (postoperative radiation therapy) versus no PORT. (From PORT Meta-analysis Trialists Group. Postoperative radiotherapy in non-small-cell lung cancer: systemic review and metaanalysis of individual patient data from nine randomised controlled trials. *Lancet* 1998;352:257. By permission of the Lancet Ltd.)

in survival rate in patients with early-stage disease treated with doses of 60 Gy[2-4] (this suggests that radiation therapy doses in the 60 Gy range may be associated with life-threatening toxicity in a percentage of patients) and in the context of the recently reported metaanalysis that demonstrated a radiation therapy–associated inferior outcome in early-stage (N0 and N1) disease[17] (Figure 43.2).

In considering all these data and the subclinical dose-response data from tumors at other sites,[70,75,76] we recommend a postoperative irradiation dose of 50 Gy using 2 Gy fractions. When margins are microscopically positive, similar doses are used, with a boost to bring the site of residual disease to at least 60 Gy (see Special Situations—Incomplete Resection).

CONCLUSIONS

Although the effectiveness of postoperative irradiation for a patient with NSCLC who is found to have positive margins is not of proven benefit, most experts continue to recommend its use, despite a lack of data. Considerably more controversy exists regarding NSCLC that has been resected and has negative margins. Currently, the data do not support the use of adjuvant irradiation for pathologic N0 and N1 disease for the improvement of either local-regional control or survival rates. Although certain data sets suggest that local control and even survival rates improve with the addition of postoperative radiation therapy for patients with completely resected N2 disease, conclusive information is

lacking. Therefore, the use of postoperative irradiation is a reasonable treatment option in the N2 setting; however, the importance of informed consent cannot be overstated, considering the suggestion in at least three randomized studies,[2-4] one metaanalysis,[17] and one retrospective study[41] that this treatment may be associated with a decreased survival rate for low-risk (N0, N1) patients.

The majority of both retrospective and randomized trials have not adequately considered which patients are truly at high risk for either local-regional recurrence or death and instead have examined the efficacy of postoperative irradiation in mixed groups consisting of both low- and high-risk patients. Further research should focus strongly on the development of more effective adjuvant therapies, but it will also be important to identify factors that place patients at high risk for postoperative cancer-related events.

Previously, the majority of retrospective studies attempted to identify prognostic factors in resected NSCLC based on conventional pathologic and histologic techniques. Recently, a growing body of literature has focused on the use of chromosomal, genetic, and nongenetic molecular markers[77-93] (see also Chapter 33). Some of the genetic markers currently demonstrating the most promising prognostic significance in the postoperative setting include K-*ras* (point mutations of the K-*ras* oncogene[88] or overexpression of the protein product of the K-*ras* oncogene, p21),[79,89,91] particularly in adenocarcinomas; *p53* (gene mutations, or p53 protein overexpression as determined by immunostaining[77,81,83]); C-*erbB-2* (overexpression of the C-ErbB-2 protein product, p185[80]), again mainly in adenocarcinoma; bcl-2 protein;[78,87] and retinoblastoma (RB protein expression.[92]

In addition to these genetic markers, nongenetic molecular markers are being investigated for correlation with the propensity for local recurrence or metastasis. The studies of Chen and colleagues[14] and Passlick and colleagues[15] both demonstrated that immunochemical techniques can frequently detect the presence of cancer in lymph nodes that is not detectable by conventional histologic techniques, and also suggested an adverse outcome for patients with immunohistochemically detected nodal disease, as compared with patients with truly lymph node–negative tumors.[14,15] Another recent study used similar techniques to detect the presence of tumor cells in the bone marrow of patients with completely resected NSCLC,[94] and work of this nature may allow physicians to stage disease in patients more accurately before instituting therapy.

The presence or absence of other tumor-related markers may also be associated with increased risk of recurrence after complete resection. A representative sample includes the expression of cathepsin B (a proteinase that may facilitate invasion and/or metastasis[90]) and the presence of cell membrane proteins such as ABH blood group[82] and Lewis-related antigens.[85] Techniques used to assess the potential for proliferation have been shown to be of prognostic significance and include immunohistochemical analysis for KI-67 antigen[86] and flow cytometry[91,93] (although it is not clear that assessments of either DNA content or the percentage of cells in the synthetic phase of the cell cycle are any more useful than routine histopathologic assessment of mitotic index).

It is hoped that one or more of these markers may be found to predict reliably and consistently the chance of cancer recurrence after surgical resection; such factors will prove to be instrumental in deciding which patients are most appropriate for inclusion in studies examining the efficacy of both adjuvant radiation therapy and adjuvant chemotherapy.

Studies examining the usefulness of these potential prognostic markers frequently have conflicting results. Although some studies may demonstrate the prognostic significance of a particular factor, other studies frequently fail to support this significance or even suggest that the marker is associated with the opposite prognosis. Currently, none of these markers can be considered to be of definitive prognostic significance. Furthermore, many studies have assessed the relationship of various factors with end points such as overall recurrence and survival, but few have specifically evaluated the ability of these factors to predict the risk of local-regional recurrence (an end point that is most likely of great importance in determining which patients are likely to have survival benefit with the addition of postoperative radiation therapy).

Considerable work in the identification of patients at high postoperative risk is ongoing. Recently, an Intergroup study has been initiated to evaluate multiple genetic and nongenetic molecular factors in resected NSCLC. It remains to be seen whether any of these new markers are truly more efficacious than such factors as the size of the primary tumor and the status of the N1 and N2 lymph nodes in predicting the risk of recurrence. Also, it is possible that genetic and nongenetic molecular factors may be found to be independent predictors of outcome in the nonoperative or preoperative setting, while their independent prognostic significance may be lost postoperatively, when the precise status of the primary tumor and regional lymph nodes has been defined. At least two studies, with multivariate analysis, have suggested that factors such as DNA ploidy pattern[23] and mitotic count[20] are better predictors of outcome than T stage in completely resected stage I disease. However, other investigators have suggested that T stage is extremely important. For example, a study by Giatromanolaki and colleagues[95] suggested that C-ErbB-2 protein expression was not as useful as T and N stage in predicting postoperative prognosis. In addition, a recent analysis of 20 potential prognostic factors in 250 consecutive patients with completely resected NSCLC with stage I disease suggested that traditional pathologic features such as lymphatic invasion and adenocarcinoma subtype were more useful in predicting prognosis than contemporary molecular studies such as p185neu im-

munostaining, K-*ras* oncogene mutations, RB immunostaining, and bcl-2 immunostaining.[96] It is hoped that the Intergroup study, which is seeking correlations between six separate molecular factors and histology, TNM stage, and clinical outcome, will begin to help bridge the relationship between conventional prognostic factors and molecular factors.

REFERENCES

1. American Joint Committee on Cancer. Fleming ID, Cooper JS, Henson DE, et al., eds. *AJCC cancer staging manual.* 5th ed. Philadelphia: Lippincott-Raven Publishers, 1997:127.
2. Van Houtte P, Rocmans P, Smets P, et al. Postoperative radiation therapy in lung cancer: a controlled trial after resection of curative design. *Int J Radiat Oncol Biol Phys* 1980;6:983.
3. Lafitte JJ, Ribet ME, Prevost BM, et al. Postresection irradiation for T2 N0 M0 non–small cell carcinoma: a prospective, randomized study. *Ann Thorac Surg* 1996;62:830.
4. Dautzenberg B, Arriagada R, Chammard AB, et al. A controlled study of postoperative radiotherapy for patients with completely resected non-small cell lung carcinoma. Groupe d'etude et de traitement des cancers bronchiques. *Cancer* 1999;86:195.
5. Bangma PJ. Postoperative radiotherapy. In: Deeley TJ, ed. *Carcinoma of the bronchus: modern radiotherapy.* New York: Appleton-Century-Crofts, 1971:163.
6. Israel L, Bonadonna G, Sylvester R. Controlled study with adjuvant radiotherapy, chemotherapy, immunotherapy, and chemoimmunotherapy in operable squamous carcinoma of the lung. In: Muggia FM, Rozencweig M, eds. *Lung cancer: progress in therapeutic research.* New York: Raven Press, 1979:443.
7. Paterson R, Russell MH. Clinical trials in malignant disease. IV—Lung cancer. Value of post-operative radiotherapy. *Clin Radiol (Lond)* 1962;13:141.
8. Weisenburger TH, Gail M, The Lung Cancer Study Group. Effects of postoperative mediastinal radiation on completely resected stage II and stage III epidermoid cancer of the lung. *N Engl J Med* 1986;315:1377.
9. Stephens RJ, Girling DJ, Bleehen NM, et al. The role of postoperative radiotherapy in non-small-cell lung cancer: a multicentre randomised trial in patients with pathologically staged T1-2, N1-2, M0 disease. *Br J Cancer* 1996;74:632.
10. Debevec M, Bitenc M, Vidmar S, et al. Postoperative radiotherapy for radically resected N2 non-small-cell lung cancer (NSCLC): randomised clinical study 1988–1992. *Lung Cancer* 1996;14:99
11. Ricci SB, Milani F, Gramaglia A, et al. Surgery (S) vs surgery + radiotherapy (S + RT) in T2-N1-2 non small cell lung carcinoma (NSCLC). An analysis of mean term data (abstract). *Lung Cancer* 1991;7[Suppl]:99.
12. Mei W, Xianzhi G, Weibo Y, et al. Randomized clinical trial of post-operative irradiation after surgery for non-small cell lung carcinoma (NSCLC) [Abstract]. *Lung Cancer* 1994;10:386.
13. Matthews MJ, Kanhouwa S, Pickren J, et al. Frequency of residual and metastatic tumor in patients undergoing curative surgical resection for lung cancer. *Cancer Chemother Rep* 1973;4:63.
14. Chen ZL, Perez S, Holmes EC, et al. Frequency and distribution of occult micrometastases in lymph nodes of patients with non-small-cell lung carcinoma. *J Natl Cancer Inst* 1993;85:493.
15. Passlick B, Izbicki JR, Kubuschok B, et al. Detection of disseminated lung cancer cells in lymph nodes: impact on staging and prognosis. *Ann Thorac Surg* 1996;61:177.
16. Sawyer TE, Bonner JA, Gould PM, et al. Effectiveness of postop-

erative irradiation in stage IIIA non–small cell lung cancer according to regression tree analyses of recurrence risks. *Ann Thorac Surg* 1997;64:1402.

17. PORT Meta-analysis Trialists Group. Postoperative radiotherapy in non-small-cell lung cancer: systematic review and meta-analysis of individual patient data from nine randomised controlled trials. *Lancet* 1998;352:257.

18. Pairolero PC, Williams DE, Bergstralh EJ, et al. Postsurgical stage I bronchogenic carcinoma: morbid implications of recurrent disease. *Ann Thorac Surg* 1984;38:331.

19. Ichinose Y, Hara N, Ohta M, et al. Is T factor of the TNM staging system a predominant prognostic factor in pathologic stage I non-small-cell lung cancer? A multivariate prognostic factor analysis of 151 patients. *J Thorac Cardiovasc Surg* 1993;106:90.

20. Macchiarini P, Fontanini G, Hardin MJ, et al. Blood vessel invasion by tumor cells predicts recurrence in completely resected T1 N0 M0 non-small-cell lung cancer. *J Thorac Cardiovasc Surg* 1993;106:80.

21. Cangemi V, Volpino P, D'Andrea N, et al. Local and/or distant recurrences in T1–2/N0–1 non–small cell lung cancer. *Eur J Cardiothorac Surg* 1995;9:473.

22. Harpole DH Jr, Herndon JE II, Young WG Jr, et al. Stage I nonsmall cell lung cancer. A multivariate analysis of treatment methods and patterns of recurrence. *Cancer* 1995;76:787.

23. Ichinose Y, Hara N, Ohta M, et al. Survival of patients with non–small cell lung cancer undergoing incomplete resection or exploratory thoracotomy with no resection. *Lung Cancer* 1993;8:265.

24. Ginsberg RJ, Rubinstein LV. Randomized trial of lobectomy versus limited resection for T1 N0 non–small cell lung cancer. Lung Cancer Study Group. *Ann Thorac Surg* 1995;60:615.

25. Sawyer TE, Bonner JA, Gould PM, et al. Patients with stage I non–small cell lung carcinoma at postoperative risk for local recurrence, distant metastasis, and death: implications related to the design of clinical trials. *Int J Radiat Oncol Biol Phys* 1999;45:315.

26. Breiman LI, Friedman JH, Olshen R, et al. *Classification and regression trees*. Belmont, CA: Wadsworth International Group, 1984.

27. Dosoretz DE, Galmarini D, Rubenstein JH, et al. Local control in medically inoperable lung cancer: an analysis of its importance in outcome and factors determining the probability of tumor eradication. *Int J Radiat Oncol Biol Phys* 1993;27:507.

28. Slotman BJ, Njo KH, Karim AB. Curative radiotherapy for technically operable stage I nonsmall cell lung cancer. *Int J Radiat Oncol Biol Phys* 1994;29:33.

29. Krol AD, Aussems P, Noordijk EM, et al. Local irradiation alone for peripheral stage I lung cancer: could we omit the elective regional nodal irradiation? *Int J Radiat Oncol Biol Phys* 1996;34:297.

30. Kupelian PA, Komaki R, Allen P. Prognostic factors in the treatment of node-negative nonsmall cell lung carcinoma with radiotherapy alone. *Int J Radiat Oncol Biol Phys* 1996;36:607.

31. Morita K, Fuwa N, Suzuki Y, et al. Radical radiotherapy for medically inoperable non–small cell lung cancer in clinical stage I: a retrospective analysis of 149 patients. *Radiother Oncol* 1997;42:31.

32. Sibley GS, Jamieson TA, Marks LB, et al. Radiotherapy alone for medically inoperable stage I non-small-cell lung cancer: the Duke experience. *Int J Radiat Oncol Biol Phys* 1998;40:149.

33. Sawyer TE, Bonner JA, Gould PM, et al. Predictors of subclinical nodal involvement in clinical stages I and II non–small cell lung cancer: implications in the inoperable and three-dimensional dose-escalation settings. *Int J Radiat Oncol Biol Phys* 1999;43:965.

34. Borrie J. Primary carcinoma of bronchus: prognosis following surgical resection (clinico-pathological study of 200 patients); Hunterian lecture. *Ann Roy Coll Surg Engl* 1952;10:165.

35. Weinberg JA. The intrathoracic lymphatics. In: Haagensen CD, Feind CR, Herter FP, et al., eds. *The lymphatics in cancer*. Philadelphia: WB Saunders Company, 1972:231.

36. Nohl-Oser HC. An investigation of the anatomy of the lymphatic drainage of the lungs as shown by the lymphatic spread of bronchial carcinoma. *Ann R Coll Surg Engl* 1972;51:157.

37. Watanabe Y, Shimizu J, Tsubota M, et al. Mediastinal spread of metastatic lymph nodes in bronchogenic carcinoma. Mediastinal nodal metastases in lung cancer. *Chest* 1990;97:1059.

38. Garces YI, Bonner JA, Sawyer TE, et al. The frequency of noncontiguous lymph node involvement in patients with resectable non–small cell lung cancer. *Int J Radiat Oncol Biol Phys* 1997;39[Suppl]:317.

39. Green N, Kurohara SS, George FW III, et al. Postresection irradiation for primary lung cancer. *Radiology* 1975;116:405.

40. Choi NC, Grillo HC, Gardiello M, et al. Basis for new strategies in postoperative radiotherapy of bronchogenic carcinoma. *Int J Radiat Oncol Biol Phys* 1980;6:31.

41. Martini N, Burt ME, Bains MS, et al. Survival after resection of stage II non–small cell lung cancer. *Ann Thorac Surg* 1992;54:460.

42. Yano T, Yokoyama H, Inoue T, et al. Surgical results and prognostic factors of pathologic N1 disease in non-small-cell carcinoma of the lung. Significance of N1 level: lobar or hilar nodes. *J Thorac Cardiovasc Surg* 1994;107:1398.

43. Mountain CF. A new international staging system for lung cancer. *Chest* 1986;89[Suppl 4]:225S.

44. Naruke T, Goya T, Tsuchiya R, et al. Prognosis and survival in resected lung carcinoma based on the new international staging system. *J Thorac Cardiovasc Surg* 1988;96:440.

45. Ramacciato G, Paolini A, Volpino P, et al. Modality of failure following resection of stage I and stage II non–small cell lung cancer. *Int Surg* 1995;80:156.

46. Sawyer TE, Bonner JA, Gould PJ, et al. Identification of risk groups in patients with completely resected N1 non–small cell lung carcinoma (abstract). *Int J Radiat Oncol Biol Phys* 1997;39:317.

47. Emami B, Graham MB. Lung. In: Perez CA, Brady LW, eds. *Principles and practice of radiation oncology*. 3rd ed. Philadelphia: Lippincott-Raven Publishers, 1998:1193.

48. Kirsh MM, Sloan H. Mediastinal metastases in bronchogenic carcinoma: influence of postoperative irradiation, cell type, and location. *Ann Thorac Surg* 1982;33:459.

49. Miller DL, McManus KG, Allen MS, et al. Results of surgical resection in patients with N2 non–small cell lung cancer. *Ann Thorac Surg* 1994;57:1095.

50. Sawyer TE, Bonner JA, Gould PM, et al. The impact of surgical adjuvant thoracic radiation therapy for patients with nonsmall cell lung carcinoma with ipsilateral mediastinal lymph node involvement. *Cancer* 1997;80:1399.

51. Mountain CF. Surgery for stage IIIa–N2 non–small cell lung cancer. *Cancer* 1994;73:2589.

52. Naruke T, Suemasu K, Ishikawa S. Lymph node mapping and curability at various levels of metastasis in resected lung cancer. *J Thorac Cardiovasc Surg* 1978;76:832.

53. Regnard JF, Magdeleinat P, Azoulay D, et al. Results of resection for bronchogenic carcinoma with mediastinal lymph node metastases in selected patients. *Eur J Cardiothorac Surg* 1991;5:583.

54. Martini N, Flehinger BJ, Zaman MB, et al. Results of resection in non–oat cell carcinoma of the lung with mediastinal lymph node metastases. *Ann Surg* 1983;198:386.

55. Patterson GA, Piazza D, Pearson FG, et al. Significance of meta-

static disease in subaortic lymph nodes. *Ann Thorac Surg* 1987; 43:155.

56. Mountain CF. Expanded possibilities for surgical treatment of lung cancer. Survival in stage IIIa disease. *Chest* 1990;97:1045.

57. Daly BD, Mueller JD, Faling LJ, et al. N2 lung cancer: outcome in patients with false-negative computed tomographic scans of the chest. *J Thorac Cardiovasc Surg* 1993;105:904.

58. Pearson FG, DeLarue NC, Ilves R, et al. Significance of positive superior mediastinal nodes identified at mediastinoscopy in patients with resectable cancer of the lung. *J Thorac Cardiovasc Surg* 1982;83:1.

59. Trastek VF, Pairolero PC, Piehler JM, et al. En bloc (non–chest wall) resection for bronchogenic carcinoma with parietal fixation. Factors affecting survival. *J Thorac Cardiovasc Surg* 1984;87:352.

60. Gould PJ, Bonner JA, Sawyer TE, et al. Patterns of failure and overall survival in patients with completely resected T3N0M0 non small cell lung cancer. *Int J Radiat Oncol Biol Phys* 1997; 39[Suppl]:319.

61. McCaughan BC, Martini N, Bains MS, et al. Chest wall invasion in carcinoma of the lung. Therapeutic and prognostic implications. *J Thorac Cardiovasc Surg* 1985;89:836.

62. Mishina H, Suemasu K, Yoneyama T, et al. Surgical pathology and prognosis of the combined resection of chest wall and lung in lung cancer. *Jpn J Clin Oncol* 1978;8:161.

63. Piehler JM, Pairolero PC, Weiland LH, et al. Bronchogenic carcinoma with chest wall invasion: factors affecting survival following en bloc resection. *Ann Thorac Surg* 1982;34:684.

64. Shields TW. The fate of patients after incomplete resection of bronchial carcinoma. *Surg Gynecol Obstet* 1974;139:569.

65. Hara N, Ohta M, Tanaka K, et al. Assessment of the role of surgery for stage III bronchogenic carcinoma. *J Surg Oncol* 1984; 25:153.

66. Reinfuss M, Glinski B, Mitus J. Postoperative radiotherapy for non-small cell lung cancer: a report in 75 cases. *Bull Cancer Radiother* 1993;80:163.

67. Soorae AS, Stevenson HM. Survival with residual tumor on the bronchial margin after resection for bronchogenic carcinoma. *J Thorac Cardiovasc Surg* 1979;78:175.

68. Minet P, Limet R, Chevalier P. Non small cell carcinoma of the lung. A progress report of 14 years experience. In: Motta G, ed. *Lung cancer: advanced concepts and present status.* Genoa: Grafica LP, 1989:216.

69. Machtay M (*in preparation*).

70. Emami B, Kaiser L, Simpson J, et al. Postoperative radiation therapy in non–small cell lung cancer. *Am J Clin Oncol* 1997; 20:441.

71. Peters LJ, Goepfert H, Ang KK, et al. Evaluation of the dose for postoperative radiation therapy of head and neck cancer: first report of a prospective randomized trial. *Int J Radiat Oncol Biol Phys* 1993;26:3.

72. The Lung Cancer Study Group. The benefit of adjuvant treatment for resected locally advanced non-small-cell lung cancer. *J Clin Oncol* 1988;6:9.

73. Emami B, Kim T, Roper C, et al. Postoperative radiation therapy in the management of lung cancer. *Radiology* 1987;164:251.

74. Miller RC, Bonner JA, Wenger DE, et al. Spinal cord localization in the treatment of lung cancer: use of radiographic landmarks. *Int J Radiat Oncol Biol Phys* 1998;40:347.

75. Miller RC, Bonner JA, Kline RW. Impact of beam energy and field margin on penumbra at lung tumor-lung parenchyma interfaces. *Int J Radiat Oncol Biol Phys* 1998;41:707.

76. Mendenhall WM, Million RR, Cassisi NJ. Elective neck irradiation in squamous-cell carcinoma of the head and neck. *Head Neck Surg* 1980;3:15.

77. Fletcher GH. Keynote address: the scientific basis of the present

and future practice of clinical radiotherapy. *Int J Radiat Oncol Biol Phys* 1983;9:1073.

78. Carbone DP, Mina JD. Molecular biology of lung cancer. In: Broder S, ed. *Molecular foundations of oncology.* Baltimore: Williams & Wilkins, 1991:339.

79. Fontanini G, Vignati S, Bigini D, et al. Bcl-2 protein: a prognostic factor inversely correlated to p53 in non-small-cell lung cancer. *Br J Cancer* 1995;71:1003.

80. Harada M, Dosaka-Akita H, Miyamoto H, et al. Prognostic significance of the expression of ras oncogene product in non-small cell lung cancer. *Cancer* 1992;69:72.

81. Harpole DH Jr, Herndon JE II, Wolfe WG, et al. A prognostic model of recurrence and death in stage I non–small cell lung cancer utilizing presentation, histopathology, and oncoprotein expression. *Cancer Res* 1995;55:51.

82. Horio Y, Takahashi T, Kuroishi T, et al. Prognostic significance of p53 mutations and 3p deletions in primary resected non–small cell lung cancer. *Cancer Res* 1993;53:1.

83. Matsumoto H, Muramatsu H, Shimotakahara T, et al. Correlation of expression of ABH blood group carbohydrate antigens with metastatic potential in human lung carcinomas. *Cancer* 1993;72:75.

84. Mitsudomi T, Oyama T, Kusano T, et al. Mutations of the p53 gene as a predictor of poor prognosis in patients with non-small-cell lung cancer. *J Natl Cancer Inst* 1993;85:2018.

85. Mitsudomi T, Steinberg SM, Oie HK, et al. Ras gene mutations in non–small cell lung cancers are associated with shortened survival irrespective of treatment intent. *Cancer Res* 1991;51:4999.

86. Ogawa J, Sano A, Inoue H, Koide S. Expression of Lewis-related antigen and prognosis in stage I non–small cell lung cancer. *Ann Thorac Surg* 1995;59:412.

87. Pence JC, Kerns BJ, Dodge RK, et al. Prognostic significance of the proliferation index in surgically resected non-small-cell lung cancer. *Arch Surg* 1993;128:1382.

88. Pezzella F, Turley H, Kuzu I, et al. bcl-2 protein in non-small-cell lung carcinoma. *N Engl J Med* 1993;329:690.

89. Rosell R, Li S, Skacel Z, et al. Prognostic impact of mutated K-ras gene in surgically resected non-small cell lung cancer patients. *Oncogene* 1993;8:2407.

90. Slebos RJ, Kibbelaar RE, Dalesio O, et al. K-ras oncogene activation as a prognostic marker in adenocarcinoma of the lung. *N Engl J Med* 1990;323:561.

91. Sukoh N, Abe S, Ogura S, et al. Immunohistochemical study of cathepsin B. Prognostic significance in human lung cancer. *Cancer* 1994;74:46.

92. Volm M, Hahn EW, Mattern J, et al. Five-year follow-up study of independent clinical and flow cytometric prognostic factors for the survival of patients with non–small cell lung carcinoma. *Cancer Res* 1988;48:2923.

93. Xu HJ, Quinlan DC, Davidson AG, et al. Altered retinoblastoma protein expression and prognosis in early-stage non-small-cell lung carcinoma. *J Natl Cancer Inst* 1994;86:695.

94. Zimmerman PV, Hawson GA, Bint MH, et al. Ploidy as a prognostic determinant in surgically treated lung cancer. *Lancet* 1987; 2:530.

95. Pantel K, Izbicki J, Passlick B, et al. Frequency and prognostic significance of isolated tumour cells in bone marrow of patients with non-small-cell lung cancer without overt metastases. *Lancet* 1996;347:649.

96. Giatromanolaki A, Gorgoulis V, Chetty R, et al. C-erbB-2 oncoprotein expression in operable non–small cell lung cancer. *Anticancer Res* 1996;16:987.

97. Kwiatkowski DJ, Harpole DH, Godleski J, et al. Prognostic factor analysis of 250 stage I NSCLC patients: pathologic features are more important than molecular analysis [Abstract]. *J Clin Oncol* 1997;16:457.

44

INDUCTION THERAPY FOR LOCALLY ADVANCED NON-SMALL CELL LUNG CANCER

KATHY S. ALBAIN
HARVEY I. PASS

A MAJOR CONTROVERSY IN LUNG CANCER THERAPY

Changing Rationale for Induction Therapy over Time

The proper role for chemotherapy with or without radiotherapy (RT) applied as induction therapy before surgical resection in non–small cell lung cancer (NSCLC) is greatly debated.[1–7] The paradigm has changed over time. Initially, the rationale for "neoadjuvant" or induction treatment was to render unresectable disease resectable. However, more recently it was recognized that early eradication of systemic micrometastases was critical to the success of any local approach. The goal in current studies is to optimize control of local bulk disease and distant micrometastases simultaneously through use of systemic chemotherapy, with or without RT. Surgical resection is then utilized for definitive local control, followed by variable postoperative therapy directed at residual local and/or distant disease.

Therefore, the theoretical advantages of a successful presurgery induction program include concurrent cytoreduction of distant and local disease, improvement in resection rates for technically difficult cases, potential sparing of normal lung tissue, an *in vivo* test of chemosensitivity, and, ultimately, improved survival. These benefits must be weighed against the potential risks of increased morbidity and mortality from combined modality induction regimens. Induction programs may result in postoperative pulmonary complications and treatment-related deaths, technical challenges during thoracotomy due to radiation fibrosis, prolonged recovery from surgery, and an altered immune system from the induction treatment.

Two Current Debates

Numerous small trials and, more recently, larger phase II and phase III studies were conducted over the course of the changing paradigm. These trials yielded a broad spectrum of outcomes that set the stage for two ongoing debates. The controversy is defined by two major questions based upon the disease burden and substage (see Table 44.1).

The first group for which there is controversy regarding induction therapy and surgery are patients with advanced stage subsets who present with bulky disease. These scenarios include bulky N2 disease on CT scan or chest radiograph, T4 (no effusion) primaries, or N3 disease. The standard of care is one of several published programs of chemotherapy plus RT (chemoRT), given either concurrently or sequentially, that have demonstrated significant benefit over RT alone[1,5,8] (see also Chapter 52). The debate in this group is whether surgical resection after induction chemoRT improves outcome over chemoRT alone.

The second controversy involves the group of patients with either early-stage or nonbulky N2 disease (Table 44.1). These stage subsets include T2 or T3N0; T1, T2, or T3N1; and T1, T2, or T3N2 ("minimal"), defined as either nonenlarged N2 nodes on computerized tomography (CT) scan or unexpected microscopic N2 nodal involvement after a normal preoperative CT scan of the mediastinum. Initial surgical resection has been the standard of care for this group, and the amount of mediastinal disease is critical in determining potential for cure after the surgical resection.[9–11] However, the majority of these patients die of metastatic disease despite a successful complete surgical resection of known disease. Thus the debate on this group is whether induction chemotherapy with or without RT improves survival over the standard approach of surgery alone.

Caveats

Several caveats merit emphasis when considering this debate. The controversy regarding optimal management within both categories of disease burden exists in part because the published pilot studies, and now several small randomized trials, addressed a wide range of stage III and stage IIB(T3N0) subsets. Recent trials included even earlier-stage subsets (IB, IIA). Collectively, only a few studies have attempted to answer one of the questions posed in Table

TABLE 44.1. INDUCTION THERAPY BEFORE SURGERY IN NSCLC: TWO CURRENT DEBATES

Disease Burden	Subsets	Standard of Care	Debate
Advanced stage or bulky	• N2 nodal enlargement on CT scan or chest x-ray •T4 (no effusion) • N3 disease	Chemotherapy and RT combined or sequenced	Does subsequent resection improve survival?
Early stage or nonbulky	• T2 or 3N0 • 1, 2, 3N1 • Nonenlarged N2 nodes on CT scan • Normal CT scan with microscopic N2	Initial surgical resection	Should preoperative chemotherapy with or without RT be given routinely?

RT, radiotherapy; CT, computerized tomography.
(From Albain KS. Induction chemotherapy with or without radiation followed by surgery in stage III non–small cell lung cancer: update and perspectives. *Oncology* 1997;11[Suppl 9]:51, with permission.)

44.1 within the context of strictly defined and narrow substage categories. In many of the trials there was inconsistent pathologic documentation of nodal status, and variable staging criteria were utilized. Interpretation of bi- and trimodality trials that include surgery requires close attention to the definition of eligible stage subsets and the required method for documentation (radiographic versus biopsy proof of N2, N3, or T4 status).

Furthermore, these trials varied in the definition of "bulky" disease, such as different size criteria for clinically involved nodes on CT scan, the number of positive nodes, the presence of extranodal extension of tumors, and various combinations of these criteria. The published studies utilized different protocol mandates for resection after induction therapy (resection of stable disease also or only resection of the responding tumors). The definition of a complete resection was also variable in that most studies required resection of gross disease, whereas a few mandated negative margins and/or a negative "highest" node. Other factors that may influence survival were variably available in these reports, such as single intranodal N2 disease, involvement of nodal stations N5 or N6 only, or positive N7 nodes.[11] Not all trials properly provided resection rates and overall survival rates for the entire denominator of patients accrued, in addition to those same outcomes for patients eventually eligible for thoracotomy. Other important data only sporadically available in published trials are local and distant relapse rates, postoperative morbidity and mortality, late causes of death, and predictors of long-term survival (optimally addressed in multivariate models).

Chapter Objectives

The objectives of this overview are to provide a perspective on these two critical questions (Table 44.1) via a review of early studies, second- and third-generation trials, and ongoing approaches. Wherever possible, the disease bulk and stage subsets contained within a given study, along with the other caveats emphasized above, will be stated.

Throughout, stage classifications will be those in use at the time of the particular study, but with the current modifications of the International Staging System mentioned where appropriate (usually a change in classification of the T3N0 subset from stage IIIA to IIB).[12,13] Other important aspects of the induction controversy will be surveyed, including whether RT is a necessary component of programs that give induction chemotherapy before surgery; if so, should RT be sequenced or given concurrently with chemotherapy; whether surgery is needed after induction therapy; and if there is a defined role for the newer chemotherapeutic agents with or without RT prior to surgery.

Morbidity and mortality considerations unique to multimodality therapy that includes surgery, the importance of multidisciplinary collaboration and comprehensive patient evaluation, and special surgical and radiotherapeutic issues will be outlined. The chapter concludes by addressing whether safety and outcome data are sufficiently mature to recommend new standards of care for the two groups of patients defined by disease burden and if so, are the answers to the questions posed in Table 44.1 "yes"?

FIRST-GENERATION INDUCTION TRIALS

Radiation Therapy as the Sole Induction Modality

The earliest induction therapy studies used preoperative RT alone in an attempt to convert unresectable disease to resectable.[14–17] These initial trials were conducted from the 1950s to the early 1970s without the benefit of modern staging technologies. Nevertheless, initial results were provocative. Pathologic complete responses were reported in up to 15% of patients, but operative morbidity rates rose with RT doses greater than 40 Gy. The consensus was that the resections were technically easier, although in retrospect most cases were probably initially resectable in terms of bulk and extent of disease by modern standards.

This early enthusiasm for preoperative RT alone dimin-

TABLE 44.2. DESIGNS OF FIRST-GENERATION PHASE II INDUCTION TRIALS FOR NSCLC

Investigators	Stage Subsets	Treatment Program	Number of Patients	Biopsy-Proven N2/N3 Disease (%)
Dana Farber I[20]	T3 or low-bulk stage III(N2)	CAP × 2 → RT → surgery→RT→CAP × 3	41	68
LCSG 831[21]	T3 or low-bulk stage III(N2)	CAP × 3 with split RT → surgery	39	51
U. of Chicago[22]	Bulky T3 or T4N2 or N3	VdEP × 2 → surgery → RT	21	100
Dana Farber II[23]	T1–3N2 (mixed bulk)	CAP × 4 ± RT → surgery → RT	54	94
Perugia[24]	T1–3N2 (clinically bulky)	EP × 2–3 → surgery → variable RT	42	0

LCSG, Lung Cancer Study Group; C, cyclophosphamide; A, doxorubicin; P, cisplatin; RT, radiotherapy; Vd, vindesine; E, etoposide; RT, radiotherapy.

ished when subsequent randomized trials demonstrated no survival benefit.[18] The most recent cooperative group study was one arm of a randomized phase II trial of the Lung Cancer Study Group, LCSG 881.[19] Patients who had pathologic stage IIIA(N2) disease were given 44 Gy before surgery. The results were disappointing, with only one pathologic complete response and a median survival of 12 months. Thus, based on more recent studies, RT is no longer recommended as the sole induction modality prior to surgery.

Early Phase II Studies of Induction Chemotherapy with or without RT

The next series of trials, conducted mostly in the 1980s, was of phase II tests of first-generation cisplatin-based chemotherapy with or without sequential RT prior to surgery.[20–24] The study designs are described in Table 44.2. These were small trials that accrued a wide mix of stage subsets with broad variability in both the amount of minimal versus bulky disease and in the percentage of biopsy-proven N2 disease. Three trials employed the CAP regimen (cyclophosphamide, doxorubicin, and low-dose cisplatin), whereas two studies used cisplatin plus etoposide-based preoperative chemotherapy.

The outcomes of these trials are outlined in Table 44.3. Response rates from the induction therapy were 39% to 82%, resection rates (percent of original number accrued)

were 14% to 88%, and the survivals were highly variable. The stage and bulk mix within these trials precludes conclusions about efficacy or comparisons across trials. However, these were pivotal studies that demonstrated the general safety of surgery after induction therapy and, in some instances, provided intriguing survival data.

Therefore, second-generation trials were designed. These studies were larger, in general enrolled more restricted stage subsets, and required in most instances pathologic documentation of nodal disease. The following three sections review the major categories of second-generation studies and long-term survival from selected trials.

SECOND-GENERATION PHASE II STUDIES OF INDUCTION CHEMOTHERAPY AS THE SOLE INDUCTION MODALITY

Trial Designs

Five phase II second-generation studies of induction therapy tested preoperative chemotherapy. These trials are described in Table 44.4.[19,25–29] Although all studies required pathologic documentation of N2 disease, tumors with a wide range of disease bulk were accrued. Four of the studies utilized preoperative vinblastine and cisplatin with or without mitomycin C (MVP, VP) and the fifth trial tested continuous infusion cisplatin and 5-fluorouracil with leucovorin rescue. The RT was variably given (intraoperative, postoper-

TABLE 44.3. RESULTS FROM FIRST-GENERATION PHASE II INDUCTION TRIALS FOR NSCLC

Investigators	Response Rate (%)	Resection Rate (% original n)	Median Survival (months)	Long-Term Survival
Dana Farber I[20]	43	88	32	31%, 3-year
LCSG 831[21]	51	33	11	8%, 2-year
U. of Chicago[22]	70	14	8	34%, 1-year
Dana Farber II[23]	39	56	18	22%, 5-year
Perugia[24]	82	72	24	24%, 3-year

LCSG, Lung Cancer Study Group.

TABLE 44.4. DESIGN OF SECOND-GENERATION TRIALS OF INDUCTION CHEMOTHERAPY FOR PATHOLOGIC STAGE IIIA (N2) NSCLC

Investigators	Disease Burden	Chemotherapy	Radiotherapy
LCSG 881[19]	Most bulky	MVP	None
Memorial[25,26]	Majority 1 nodal station positive; mixed bulk	MVP	Variable, either intra- or postoperative
Toronto[27]	Mixed bulk	MVP	Postoperative
Dana Farber III[28]	Mixed bulk	PFL (continuous infusion)	Postoperative
CALGB II[29]	Most bulky	VP	Postoperative

LCSG, Lung Cancer Study Group; CALGB, Cancer and Leukemia Group B; M, mitomycin C; V, vinblastine; P, cisplatin; F, 5-fluorouracil; L, leucovoran.

ative, or not at all), and information on why RT was either given or withheld was not provided in detail for some of the studies. Thus lack of concordance on the disease bulk and RT utilization variables makes comparison of results among the studies difficult.

Results

The outcomes reported in these five trials of preoperative chemotherapy in N2 disease are shown in Table 44.5. Response rates were 46% to 78% and resection rates (of the entire denominator) were 51% to 68%. Pathologic complete response rates (pCR) of 0%, 5%, and 11% were observed in the CALGB, Toronto, and Memorial Sloan-Kettering Cancer Center studies, respectively.[25–27,29]

Postoperative mortality rates were 0% to 17% and were predominantly pulmonary or cardiopulmonary events. Significant pulmonary morbidity was also observed in some of these studies, usually in the postoperative time period. Thirteen percent of patients treated with MVP in the Memorial Sloan-Kettering Cancer Center study and 12% of those who received VP on the Cancer and Leukemia Group B (CALGB) trial experienced major pulmonary events.[25,29] It was difficult to complete the planned RT in the "posterior" or postoperative time period, especially when all RT was to be given postoperatively. For instance, only 42% of patients received the prescribed dose in the CALGB study.[29]

Survival outcomes were also variable, with median survivals reported from 12 to 21 months (Table 44.5). Sites of first failure were included in three of the reports: local-regional disease as the only site of first relapse occurred in 26%, 24%, and 25% of patients.[25,28,29] These "local-only" recurrences occurred in the subgroup with residual disease at surgery in the Memorial Sloan-Kettering Cancer Center trial.[25] The Dana Farber investigators noted that 15% of first relapses were solely in the brain.[28]

SECOND-GENERATION PHASE II STUDIES OF INDUCTION CHEMORADIOTHERAPY BEFORE SURGERY

Trial Designs

The other major category within the second-generation studies utilized concurrent chemoRT induction therapy in which the RT began on day 1 of the chemotherapy. These phase II trials are described in Table 44.6.[30–34] The RT varied in schedule across trials from continuous to split-course and in total dose (single fractionation) from 30 Gy to 59 Gy. All induction chemotherapy was cisplatin-based, with the addition of either etoposide, 5-fluorouracil, vinblastine, or some combination of these drugs. The treatment prescribed after surgical resection was highly variable among these five studies. There was no therapy after surgery in

TABLE 44.5. RESULTS OF SECOND-GENERATION TRIALS OF INDUCTION CHEMOTHERAPY FOR PATHOLOGIC STAGE IIIA(N2) NSCLC

Investigators	No. of Patients (n)	Response Rates (%)	Complete Resection Rates (% initial n)	Operative Mortality (%)	Median Survival (months)
LCSG 881[19]	28	46	68	17.0	12
Memorial[25,26]	136	78	65	4.4	19
Toronto[27]	55	71	51	8.0	21
Dana Farber III[28]	34	65	62	0	18
CALGB II[29]	74	64*	62	3.1	15

LCSG, Lung Cancer Study Group; CALGB, Cancer and Leukemia Group B.
* Includes stable disease.

TABLE 44.6. DESIGN OF SECOND-GENERATION TRIALS OF CONCURRENT INDUCTION CHEMORADIOTHERAPY (STANDARD FRACTIONATION) IN NSCLC

Investigators	Disease Burden	IIIA(N2) (%)	T3N0–1/T4 or N3 (%)	Biopsy of Mediastinal Nodes or T4 Required?	Induction Chemotherapy	Induction RT	Postoperative Treatment
SWOG 8805[30]	Bulky	60	0/40	Yes	EP	Continuous, 45 Gy	Chemo × 2 + RT 14 Gy if positive nodes or margins or if unresectable
LCSG 852[31]	Mixed bulk	87	0/13	Yes	PF	Continuous, 30 Gy	None
Rush-Presbyterian[32]	Mixed bulk	73	21/6	Yes	PF/PEF	Split, 40 Gy	None
CALGB I[33]	Mixed bulk	80	20/0	Yes	PVF	Continuous, 30 Gy	Chemo × 1 + RT 30 Gy
Tufts[34]	Bulky	47	0/53	No	EP	Continuous, 59 Gy	PE or Carbo T

SWOG, Southwest Oncology Group; LCSG, Lung Cancer Study Group; CALGB, Cancer and Leukemia Group B; E, etoposide; P, cisplatin; F, 5-fluorouracil; V, vinblastine; Carbo, carboplatin; T, paclitaxel; Gy, gray.

the Rush Presbyterian and LCSG 852 trials; two cycles of additional chemotherapy plus 14 Gy of RT were given in the Southwest Oncology Group (SWOG) 8805 study (if residual disease in chest or mediastinum); and one cycle of chemotherapy plus 30 Gy of RT was used in the CALGB trial (all patients). The Tufts investigators initially gave etoposide plus cisplatin postoperatively, but later in the trial allowed use of the carboplatin-plus-paclitaxel regimen.

Eligibility criteria for the five second-generation chemoRT induction trials (Table 44.6) were more varied than for the studies of induction chemotherapy alone (Table 44.4). Biopsy documentation of N2 disease or T4 status was not always required. The SWOG trial was unique in this regard, because pathologic proof of N2, T3, or N3 disease was mandated. A broad range of stage subsets was included across trials, so that stage IIIA(N2) accounted for 47% to 87% of patients per trial. Two studies included T3N0 or T3N1 (21% and 20% in the Rush Presbyterian and CALGB studies, respectively), whereas all patients with stage IIIA disease in the SWOG 8805, LCSG 852, and Tufts trials had N2 nodal involvement (Table 44.6). The stage IIIB subsets of T4 and/or N3 were allowed in all trials except the CALGB study and accounted for 6% to 53% of patients per trial. The SWOG 8805 and Tufts trials were designed for bulky disease, whereas the others allowed a mix of minimal and bulky presentations.

Results

The outcomes of the second-generation concurrent chemoRT induction trials are summarized in Table 44.7. Response or "response plus stable" (one study) rates were 56% to 92%, and 52% to 76% of the total number of patients accrued to each study had a complete resection at thoracotomy. Of the 30 patients with stable disease as the "best" response to induction chemoRT, 26 underwent a complete resection of tumor in the SWOG 8805 trial.[30] The pCR rates were 16%, 21%, and 27% in the LCSG, SWOG, and Rush Presbyterian trials, respectively.[30–32] An additional 37% had rare microscopic foci of tumor cells as the sole residual disease in the SWOG trial. Of the 26 patients with resectable stable disease in the SWOG study, 46% had pCR or only rare microscopic foci.[30] Thus postinduction assessment of nonresponse by CT scan is often misleading.

The operative mortality rates were 4% to 15% in these trials (Table 44.7). These events were predominantly pulmonary-related, as observed in the induction chemotherapy trials. The cause of death often resembled the adult respira-

TABLE 44.7. RESULTS OF SECOND-GENERATION TRIALS OF INDUCTION CHEMORADIOTHERAPY IN NSCLC

Investigators	No. of Patients	Response Rate (%)	Complete Resection Rate (% initial n)	Operative Mortality (%)	Median Survival (months)
SWOG 8805[30]	126	59	71	8	15
LCSG 852[31]	85	56	52	7	13
Rush-Presbyterian[32]	85	92*	71	4	22
CALGB I[33]	41	64*	61	15	16
Tufts[34]	55	69*	76	5	20

SWOG, Southwest Oncology Group; LCSG, Lung Cancer Study Group; CALGB, Cancer and Leukemia Group B.
* Includes stable disease.

tory distress syndrome (ARDS), to be considered in more detail in the morbidity and mortality section of this chapter. The Tufts trial was unique in that postoperative ARDS was not observed, despite the high total dose of induction RT.[34] A rigid protocol to minimize fluids, transfusions, and the FiO2 was employed in this study. Finally, it is uncertain whether "posterior" treatment, in particular the additional relatively small doses of "boost" RT given after surgery, added anything to the efficacy of the program or only contributed to late morbidity.

Overall survival results for the second-generation studies of concurrent chemoRT are shown in Table 44.7. The median survival for the two studies that excluded T3N0–1 tumors and required pathologic staging were 15 and 13 months.[30,31] In contrast, the other three trials included this better prognostic subset and did not require biopsy proof of the T and N substages. For these studies, the median survivals were 22, 16, and 20 months.[32–34] Patterns of first recurrence in the SWOG 8805 trial were 11%, locoregional only and 61% distant alone.[30] There was no difference in the sites of relapse between those patients with negative mediastinal nodes at the time of operation (but originally positive) versus those who had persistent involvement of the mediastinal nodes. A significant number of the distant first relapses (and in many cases, the only relapse or the sole cause of mortality) occurred in the brain.[30] The Tufts investigators also reported a very high rate of isolated brain metastases, all of which occurred within the first 32 months of follow-up.[34]

The Stage IIIB Subgroup in Second-Generation ChemoRT Induction Trials

Some data are available regarding the role of induction therapy followed by surgery in selected stage IIIB subsets. Patients enrolled in the second-generation trials of induction chemotherapy alone all had stage IIIA(N2) disease. However, all but one of the chemoRT induction trials allowed inclusion of patients with stage IIIB tumors. The LCSG 852 trial and the Rush Presbyterian study (Table 44.6) included 13% "minimal T4" and 6% "selected T4" lesions (clinically staged), respectively.[31,32] Separate survival data for this subset were not provided. Of note was that two groups of investigators had reported equivalence in outcome of clinical stage IIIA and IIIB disease in combined modality trials *with no surgery*.[35,36] However, these authors suggested that the clinical T4N0 subset may have a better outcome than the other subsets and perhaps should be removed from the IIIB category, just as the T3N0 subset was recently reassigned to stage IIB instead of its former designation of IIIA.[13] Based on this observation in chemoRT-alone trials, the SWOG 8805 study was designed prospectively to include a sufficient sample of the stage IIIB subgroup to allow independent assessment of outcome.

The SWOG 8805 trial stands alone among the other

chemoRT trials that included stage IIIB disease. Pathologic documentation of T4 or N3 disease was required and outcome was analyzed separately for this subset.[30,37] The Tufts investigators also reported outcome separately for the IIIB group, but the staging requirements were radiographic rather than pathologic.[34] The resection rates in these two studies for stage IIIA(N2) were 76% and 76%, and for stage IIIB, 63% and 50%, respectively.

The median two-year and three-year survivals were identical for the IIIA(N2) versus the IIIB group in the SWOG 8805 study (27%, 24%).[30] The three-year survivals were 73% and 32% for the clinical IIIA(N2) and IIIB subsets, respectively, in the Tufts trial. Of note was that in the SWOG 8805 study, the T4N0-1 subset had an outcome identical to the T1N2 substage and achieved a two-year survival of 64%. This substage variable was the only independent predictor of favorable outcome from the time of registration to the study in a multivariate analysis.[30] Exploratory survival analyses were conducted within the N3 subset of the SWOG trial, in which 27 patients were accrued. The two-year survival for the contralateral nodal N3 subgroup was zero, whereas it was 35% for the supraclavicular N3 subset. However, the resection rate in this latter group was only 39%. An update of SWOG 8805 provided six-year survival statistics: IIIA(N2), 20%; T4N0-1, 49%; and N2 or N3, 18%.[38]

A follow-up trial to SWOG 8805 for pathologic stage IIIB disease was conducted by the SWOG (SWOG 9019). Identical induction chemoRT was utilized as in SWOG 8805, but no surgery was given; instead, the RT was continued without a break to 61 Gy, and two additional cycles of EP were given.[39] The overall survival rate in this study was identical to that observed for the stage IIIB group in SWOG 8805. This suggested that in an identically staged patient population, chemoRT with definitive-dose RT may achieve the same benefit as surgical resection after induction chemoRT (and lower RT total dose). However, in the SWOG 9019 trial (chemoRT alone), the two-year survival rate was only 33% for the T4N0-1 subset, compared to 64% for two years and 49% for six years in the surgical study, SWOG 8805.[38,39] This historical comparison of these two consecutive trials in pathologically staged IIIB disease provides a hint that surgery for stage IIIB tumors might be beneficial only in the select substage of T4N0-1. However, a prospective randomized study is needed to validate this observation.

SECOND-GENERATION INDUCTION TRIALS: LONG-TERM SURVIVAL AND PREDICTORS OF OUTCOME

Mature Survival Data

Long-term survival data were reported in several of the trials of induction chemotherapy and induction chemoRT that

TABLE 44.8. SECOND-GENERATION PHASE II INDUCTION TRIALS IN NSCLC: LONG-TERM SURVIVAL AND PREDICTORS OF FAVORABLE OUTCOME

Investigators	Bulky Disease Only?	T3N0 or N1 Included?	Biopsy Proof of N2 Status Required?	Selected Stage IIIB Included?	Long-Term Survival	Predictors of Favorable Outcome
Memorial[25,26]	No	No	Yes	No	17%, 5-year	Pathologic CR
Toronto[27]	No	No	Yes	No	34%, 5-year	Complete resection
SWOG 8805[30,38]	Yes	No	Yes	Yes	N2: 20%, 6-year IIIB: 22%, 6-year	N2/3 → N0 at resection; T4N0 or 1 Complete resection
CALGB I[33,40]	No	Yes	No	No	22%, 7(+)-year	No survival advantage for complete resection or pathologic CR
CALGB II[29]	Yes	No	Yes	No	23%, 3-year	Complete resection
Rush-Presbyterian[32]	No	Yes	No	Yes	31%, 3-year	T3N0 or T3N1
Tufts[34]	Yes	No	No	Yes	N2: 73%, 3-year IIIB: 32%, 3-year	CR to induction

CR, complete response; SWOG, Southwest Oncology Group; CALGB, Cancer and Leukemia Group B.

were reviewed in the preceding two sections (Tables 44.4, 44.6). Selected studies with a minimum of three years of long-term survival data are summarized in Table 44.8.[25–27,29,30,32–34,38,40] These studies differed in several critical aspects, including disease bulk, the inclusion of T3N0 or N1 subsets, whether or not pathologic documentation of N2 disease was required, and the inclusion of stage IIIB subsets. The variation in disease bulk and stage subsets as well as potential inaccuracies from staging solely on clinical grounds may to a major degree explain the wide range of three-to-seven-year survivals shown in Table 44.8.

Long-term follow-up of several of the trials suggested that a plateau emerged on the tails of the survival curves. As shown in Table 44.8, five-to-seven-year survivals of 17% to 34% were recently reported. The SWOG 8805 study suggested a plateau between years 4 and 6,[38] the Toronto study between years 3 and 5,[27] and the CALGB I study from years 5 to 7 and over.[40] However, indefinite plateaus are not expected, because of competing causes of death in a patient population with a high incidence of comorbid diseases.

Factors that Predict Favorable Outcome

The seven phase II trials of induction chemotherapy or chemoRT depicted in Table 44.8 analyzed predictors of long-term survival. Methods of analysis varied: univariate versus multivariate and predictors of overall survival either from registration or from time of thoracotomy. Favorable outcome predictors included postinduction pCR, complete resection, T3N0 or T3N1 disease, T4N0 or N1 disease, and pathologic clearance of initial N2 or N3 involvement (nodal downstaging). The significance of these predictive factors varied across trials, but all factors were not uniformly assessed in each study. Nevertheless, a factor related to the

efficacy of the induction therapy was important in most trials. It was suggested that the inclusion of RT in the induction removes the possible importance of pCR as a predictor observed in chemotherapy-only induction programs. However, the Memorial Sloan-Kettering Cancer Center trial of MVP alone did not report statistical significance to pCR.[25,26] Response to induction therapy was not an important predictive factor in some trials, most likely because of the mandate in those studies to resect disease even if "stable" was the best response.[30] This observation underscores the inability of standard CT scanning to detect those patients with major postinduction responses.

The SWOG 8805 trial analysis that described an independent favorable prognostic impact of nodal downstaging on intermediate (two-to-three-year) survival is of interest, given that it was the only significant factor in a multivariate model that included complete resection rate, pCR, and multiple other factors.[30] This variable was also the most important univariate discriminant of six-year survival, although complete resection emerged as a long-term survival predictor as well.[38] The survivals three and six years after thoracotomy for patients with uninvolved nodes at surgery were 41% and 33%, respectively, versus only 11% and 11% if there was persistent mediastinal disease. The prognostic variable of nodal downstaging was not assessed in multivariate models for any other study with second-generation therapy.

Implications of the nodal downstaging observation are that lack of residual disease in the mediastinum may be a surrogate marker for eradication of distant chemotherapy-sensitive micrometastases. These patients may be the optimal candidates for additional postoperative chemotherapy. Conversely, persistent N2 or N3 disease may predict the presence of distant resistant disease. Thus the question must be asked whether surgery was necessary for those cases with nodal downstaging, or were these patients the best candidates for maximal local control with surgery? If postinduction mediastinal status is clearly of prognostic value, then there would be a critical role for a second mediastinal assessment after induction, even though in some cases this would be technically difficult. The question of whether molecular correlates such as proliferative rate, *p53* or K-*ras* status obtained on biopsy material pre- and/or postinduction might improve identification of the optimal patients for surgical resection awaits the results of ongoing ancillary projects within several of these trials and current phase III studies outlined later in this chapter.

THIRD-GENERATION PHASE II STUDIES OF INDUCTION CHEMOTHERAPY PLUS CONCURRENT HYPERFRACTIONATED RADIOTHERAPY

The outcomes of two important phase II pilot studies of concurrent induction chemoRT, in which the RT was given as twice-daily fractions, were recently reported.[41,42]

Trial Designs

The eligibility criteria and treatment programs are described in Table 44.9. Forty-two patients with mixed-bulk, biopsy-proven stage III(N2) disease were treated in the Massachusetts General Hospital (MGH) trial. The West German Cancer Center (WGCC) study required mediastinoscopy, and all 94 patients had advanced disease: either bulky, central T3 (six patients), two or more positive N2 nodes (n = 46), or stage IIIB (n = 42, either T4 or contralateral N3 nodes).

The MGH group used split-course twice-daily RT, split before the surgery as well as after, when it was given with one additional cycle of chemotherapy. In contrast, the WGCC

investigators employed continuous hyperfractionated RT concurrent with the third cycle of induction chemotherapy, and all treatment was completed before the surgery. This trial was amended midway to require prophylactic cranial irradiation (PCI). Surgical resections were not performed in the WGCC study if there was evidence on postinduction radiographs or biopsy of T4, N2, or N3 disease, whereas the MGH trial required resection of stable disease.

Response, Survival, and Predictors of Favorable Outcome

The results of the two studies of induction therapy with concurrent chemoRT (twice daily) are summarized in Table 44.10. Complete resections were accomplished in 93% of 42 patients in the MGH study.[41] Significant nodal downstaging was noted: 10%, T0N0 (pCR); 24%, N0; 33%, N1. The WGCC investigators reported that 60% of 52 patients with stage IIIA disease and 45% of 42 patients with stage IIIB had complete resections.[42] The pCR rate was 26%. The difference in resection rates between the two studies is due in part to a large percentage of cases with nonbulky disease in the MGH study, as well as the mandate to withhold surgery in the WGCC trial if there was residual T4, N2, or N3 disease. Postoperative death rates in both studies (5%, 7%) were no greater than reported in trials that tested either induction chemotherapy alone or induction chemoRT with standard single daily fractionation of RT. No cases of postoperative ARDS were observed in either study, but complex stump insufficiency was a problem in the WGCC trial. Completion of the planned "posterior" chemoRT in the MGH trial was feasible in 60% of patients.

Sites of initial failure in the MGH study were analyzed in detail. Only locoregional relapse occurred in 15% of those with a recurrence, only brain in 30%, other distant site in 45%, and both local and systemic in 10%. The WGCC investigators also reported a high rate of initial brain relapses that occurred relatively early in the follow-up period. This

TABLE 44.9. THIRD-GENERATION PHASE II TRIALS OF CONCURRENT INDUCTION CHEMORADIOTHERAPY WITH HYPERFRACTIONATION IN NSCLC

Investigators	Stage Subset(s)/ No. Patients	Disease Burden	Chemotherapy	Radiotherapy
MGH[41]	Biopsy-proven stage IIIA(N2), n = 42	Mixed bulk	PVF × 2 concurrent with RT → surgery → PVF × 1 concurrent with RT	42 Gy split (1.5 bid × 7 → 10 day rest → 1.5 bid × 7); postoperative 12–18 Gy (1.5 bid)
West German Cancer Center[42]	Mediastinoscopy required: 6, advanced T3; 46, 2 or more N2 nodes; 42, IIIB (T4 or contralateral N3)	Bulky	EP × 3 → reduced dose EP × 1 with RT → surgery	45 Gy (1–5 Gy bid over 3 weeks); PCI later in trial

MGH, Massachusetts General Hospital; P, cisplatin; V, vinblastine; F, 5-fluorouracil; E, etoposide; Gy, gray; PCI, prophylactic cranial irradiation.

TABLE 44.10.   RESULTS FROM THIRD-GENERATION TRIALS OF INDUCTION CHEMORADIOTHERAPY WITH HYPERFRACTIONATION IN NSCLC

Investigators	No. of Patients	Resection Rate (of initial n)	Postoperative Deaths	Survival	Predictors of Favorable Outcome	
MGH[41]	42	93%	5%	37%, 5-year	5-year survival from downstaging at thoracotomy: pStage 0 or I 79%, pStage II 42%, pStage III 18%	
West German Cancer Center[42,43]	94	53%* (60% IIIA, 45% (IIIB)	7%	28%, 4-year (32% IIIA 26% IIIB)	4-year survival from registration: • complete resection* • N2/3 → N0 • LDH ≤ 240 or not • PCI	46% vs 11%, p=0.0001 38% vs 15%, p=0.11 37% vs 0%, p=0.003 Decrease in first brain metastases, p=0.005

MGH, Massachusetts General Hospital; CR, complete response; p, pathologic; PCI, prophylactic cranial irradiation.
* Resection not mandated if persistent T4 or N2/N3 disease.

is a recurring theme of all induction trials for NSCLC. The PCI that was mandated in the latter half of the WGCC trial significantly reduced first and overall brain relapses and prolonged survival for those patients who had a complete or partial response.[43]

Long-term survivals were reported for both pilot studies (Table 44.10). The five-year survival of 37% in the MGH trial was identical to that reported by the Toronto group for their study of induction chemotherapy alone in pN2 disease (Table 44.8). However, it is not possible to determine if the hyperfractionated RT, as given in the third-generation induction trials, might result in a greater benefit than induction chemoRT with a single daily fraction or chemotherapy alone. For example, it is not clear if the percentage of patients with high disease bulk was the same in the MGH and Toronto studies. The WGCC trial clearly accrued more patients with bulky disease, which may in part explain the slightly lower survival (28% overall at four years, with 32% of IIIA and 26% of IIIB alive at four years). Therefore the intriguing results of the MGH and WGCC trials support the conduct of a randomized study of single versus twice-daily fractionation within the context of identical concurrent chemotherapy in patients with pathologically staged tumors with uniform disease bulk.

The analysis of predictors of survival from the MGH investigators (Table 44.10) provides independent validation of the SWOG observation that mediastinal nodal downstaging at time of surgery is a critical favorable determinant for long-term survival.[30,38,41] Patients with stage 0 or I tumors at surgery had a 79% five-year survival after thoracotomy in the MGH trial, and those with N0 or N1 downstaging had a 33% six-year survival in SWOG 8805. These two trials cannot be directly compared due to major differences in disease bulk (higher in SWOG 8805).

Nodal downstaging was also noted in the WGCS study—80% for the subset with N2 or N3 disease.[42] A

complete resection predicted statistically favorable four-year survival from time of registration (46% versus 11% if resection or not; Table 44.10). However, survival by this variable should have been reported from time of surgery for those eligible for thoracotomy. Also, a resection was not performed for all patients with nonprogression. Thus it is not surprising that there was no difference in survival by the variable of pCR. The critical group with radiographically stable disease postinduction, some of whom might have had pCRs, were perhaps erroneously included in the group "no pathologic CR." An important observation was that the lactic dehydrogenase (LDH) cutpoint of less than 240 was a strong univariate discriminant of favorable survival at four years (37% versus 0%). A multivariate analysis was not conducted.

COMPLETED RANDOMIZED TRIALS OF SURGERY ALONE VERSUS INDUCTION THERAPY FOLLOWED BY SURGERY IN RESECTABLE DISEASE

This section addresses the second debate outlined on Table 44.1 regarding the role of induction therapy for patients with either early-stage or minimal N2 disease (negative CT scans of mediastinum with either no or microscopic N2 involvement on mediastinoscopy). Up-front surgical resection is the standard treatment for this group of patients. The disease burden in patients enrolled in these trials was generally smaller than trials described in Tables 44.4, 44.6, and 44.9.

Eligibility Criteria and Trial Design

Four small randomized studies and one large phase III trial were conducted for NSCLC in which the control arms were

TABLE 44.11. REPORTED PHASE III TRIALS OF SURGERY WITH OR WITHOUT INDUCTION THERAPY IN RESECTABLE NSCLC

Investigators	Stage Subset(s)	Disease Burden	Chemotherapy	Radiotherapy	No. of Patients	2–3-Year Survival		
						No ChT	ChT	P-value
NCI[44]	IIIA(N2) by biopsy	Bulky	EP pre- and postoperative	Postoperative in no-ChT arm only	28	21%	46%	0.12
Japan[45]	Clinical IIIA and IIIB	Bulky	VdP preoperative	Concurrent with CT	83	40%	37%	NS
M.D. Anderson[46]	IIIA(N2) not required; node biopsy not required; some IIIB	Minimal bulk	CEP pre- and postoperative	Postoperative only if residual disease	60	15%	56%	<0.05
Spain[47]	IIIA(N2) not required; node biopsy not required	Minimal bulk	PIM preoperative	Postoperative for both arms	60	0%	30%	<0.05
French Thoracic Cooperative Group[48]	Clinical T2N0, II, IIIA	Minimal bulk	MIP × 2 preoperative; also postoperative, if objective response	Postoperative, if pT3 or pN2 for both arms	355	41%	52%	p=0.09*

E, etoposide; P, cisplatin; V, vinblastine; I, ifosfamide; Vd, vindesine; M, mitomycin C; C, cyclophosphamide; NS, not significant; NCI, National Cancer Institute; ChT, chemotherapy.
* Cox model adjusted for stage and N status: p=0.053 for preoperative chemotherapy.
(From Albain KS. Induction chemotherapy with or without radiation followed by surgery in stage III non–small cell lung cancer: update and perspectives. *Oncology* 1997;11:51, with permission.)

surgery alone, as described in Table 44.11.[44–48] The comparator arms were induction chemotherapy with or without variably timed RT. The first two studies are rarely discussed, the second two are debated frequently, and the last was presented at the 1999 meeting of the American Society of Clinical Oncology.

Although surgery alone (with or without some RT) was deemed acceptable for the control arms of these trials, the eligibility criteria for bulk of disease varied among the five studies. Patients with more advanced disease were enrolled in the NCI (multiple N2 nodes on mediastinoscopy) and Japanese (clinically bulky) trials.[44,45] The NCI trial was the most homogeneous in the stage subsets accrued. However, neither the M.D. Anderson nor the Spanish studies required microscopic N2 disease, and mediastinal node biopsy was not mandated if the CT scan was negative.[46,47] In fact, in the surgical control arm of the M.D. Anderson trial, 40% of cases were actually stage IIIB or IV at time of operation. Thus the treatment groups of the small M.D. Anderson and Spanish studies had heterogeneous stage subset distributions. The same stage-mix issues exist in the large French Thoracic Cooperative Group (FTCG) trial, with some imbalance of stage subsets between the two arms (p = 0.07).[48] Furthermore, clinical staging alone was accepted and documentation of N2 status was not required in the FTCG study.

The induction chemotherapy regimens for the five trials were cisplatin-based and were also variably given after surgery depending on the study design (Table 44.11). The use of RT was also different in each trial, so these were not "pure" trials of induction chemotherapy followed by surgery versus surgery alone. For example, RT was employed either postoperatively only in the nonchemotherapy arm, concurrent with the induction chemotherapy, postoperatively only if residual disease in both arms, or postoperatively for all patients.

Outcome of the Five Phase III Trials with a Noninduction Control Arm

Three of the five trials closed before the target accrual goal was met. The NCI trial was halted due to slow accrual, whereas the M.D. Anderson and Spanish studies were stopped early by data monitoring committees due to large survival differences (Table 44.11). The NCI investigators found no statistical difference between the two arms, but the p-value decreased with longer follow-up to 0.11 in favor of the chemotherapy arm.[44] There were differences in recurrence patterns by arm in the NCI trial, in that less distant but more local disease was observed in the induction chemotherapy group. The group with preoperative chemoRT had a survival rate identical to the surgery-alone arm in the Japanese study.[45] However, only clinical staging was required in this small phase III trial, resulting in stage and disease bulk imbalances.

The two small randomized trials were stopped early due to strongly positive results in favor of the induction chemotherapy arms, as shown in Table 44.11.[46,47] With additional follow-up of the M.D. Anderson trial cohort (median follow-up, 81 months), 32% of patients were alive in the induction chemotherapy group versus 16% in the surgery-alone arm (p = 0.06).[49] The p-value became significant if only deaths due to cancer were considered. The Spanish trial was updated in a meeting presentation at the 1997 World Lung Cancer Congress. No patients survived in the surgery group, whereas 16% were long-term survivors in the induction chemotherapy arm.

These M.D. Anderson and Spanish trials continue to generate discussion and debate. The consensus is that these results were provocative but not definitive. There are aspects of the design and outcome of the studies that call for confirmatory trials. The major concern is the marked substage heterogeneity within these two trials. It is not clear if early-stopping rules for these very small trials accounted for the strong potential influence of even slight substage or molecular prognostic factor imbalances between the two arms. Minor shifts of these factors between arms would have a major impact on the survival differences due to the small sample sizes. Furthermore, the surgical control arms fared poorly, possibly due to substage imbalances. There was a large number of unexpected stage IIIB/IV disease at time of surgery in the control arm of the M.D. Anderson trial. The Spanish trial control arm had 37% patients with N0 or N1 disease, but this arm contained more tumors with K-*ras* mutations and aneuploid DNA, both potential adverse prognostic factors. Small differences in unstratified prognostic factors such as K-*ras* could potentially affect the results.

The results of the FTCG trial in 355 eligible patients were presented at the 1999 meeting of the American Society of Clinical Oncology.[48] There were two treatment-related deaths during induction chemotherapy. Eight postoperative deaths (4.5%), six due to pneumonia, occurred in the surgical control arm. There were 14 postoperative deaths (8%) following induction chemotherapy, six due to fistula or empyema and seven from pneumonia. The overall survival rate favored the induction chemotherapy arm but did not reach statistical significance at a median follow-up of 59 months (p = 0.09). The hazards were not proportional over time, with later emergence of superiority in the cohort that received induction chemotherapy. The median survivals were 37 and 26 months, and the three-year survivals were 52% and 41% in the induction and surgery-alone arms, respectively. The lack of pathologic staging and wide range of stage subsets were problematic, but a Cox multivariate model adjusted for stage and N status revealed a p-value of 0.053 in favor of induction chemotherapy. The benefit of induction chemotherapy was statistically significant for those patients with N0 or N1 disease, but not for N2, although this is a subset analysis. Induction therapy also significantly decreased distant relapses (p = 0.009), but there was no difference between arms in the local relapse rates.

Despite the specific concerns regarding each of them raised in the preceding discussion, these five trials, provide encouragement regarding the potential role of induction therapy in earlier-stage disease. The large ongoing phase III

trials worldwide (discussed later in this chapter) that are designed to minimize stage-mix and bulk-of-disease biases will definitively address the value of induction therapy in resectable disease. These trials also include ancillary biomarker and PET imaging substudies that will analyze characteristics to predict the best candidates for induction therapy approaches and those who will derive the most benefit from postinduction surgery.

PHASE III INDUCTION TRIALS THAT ADDRESSED OTHER IMPORTANT QUESTIONS

Radiotherapy as a Component of the Induction Regimen

The only randomized trial to date that addressed the need for RT in the induction regimen was conducted in Brazil and published as a meeting abstract.[50] Ninety-six patients with either clinically bulky or biopsy-proven stage IIIA(N2) and T4 IIIB disease were randomized between chemoRT followed by surgery versus chemotherapy alone followed by surgery (Table 44.12). Two programs commonly employed at the time were compared: cisplatin and 5-fluorouracil plus RT versus the MVP regimen. At the 1994 abstract presentation, survival was significantly better in the chemoRT arm. More neutropenia and neurologic toxicity were observed in the MVP arm, whereas there was a higher rate of mucositis in the chemoRT group. Updated results were provided during a 1997 meeting presentation but are not published at this writing. The five-year survival was 31% in the chemoRT arm but only 15% in the MVP arm (p = 0.05). However, this study enrolled mixed bulk disease with some but not all cases pathologically staged.

To determine definitively the worth of induction RT, additional study is needed in a homogeneously staged population with identical induction chemotherapy on both arms. A major concern for the group of patients with advanced stage disease is that induction chemotherapy alone may not be enough to deal with bulky local disease. One other lead regarding the necessity of RT was provided in a Japanese trial that did not include surgery.[51] Patients with stage III disease without progression after two cycles of cisplatin-containing chemotherapy were randomized to RT with 60 Gy (2 Gy per day) or to no additional therapy. The three-year survival rate was 29% versus 3% in favor of the addition of RT. An ongoing phase III trial in Germany tests the contribution of hyperfractionated RT to induction chemotherapy versus induction chemotherapy alone.[52] Radiotherapy is given after surgery in the arm without induction RT, so it is not a pure test of the question. However, this study will determine if induction chemoRT yields a higher rate of pCR, complete resection, and nodal downstaging (all important variables for long-term survival, as discussed above) than induction chemotherapy alone. Japanese investigators plan to conduct a phase III trial of induction chem-

TABLE 44.12. COMPLETED PHASE III INDUCTION TRIALS FOR NSCLC THAT ASKED OTHER QUESTIONS

Investigators	Stage Subset	Question	Study Design	No. of Patients	Outcome/Comment
Brazil[50]	Stage IIIA(N2) and T4 IIIB; N2 nodes bulky on CT or biopsy-proven	Role of RT in the induction?	PF + RT vs MVP ↓ Surgery ↓ RT vs MVP (if residual disease)	96	5-yr survival 31% vs 15% in favor of PF + RT (p = 0.05)*
NCI Canada[54]	Biopsy-proven stage IIIA(N2)	Postinduction surgery vs RT?	PV ↓ Surgery vs RT	31	Closed early due to slow accrual; survival cuves superimposed at 2 years
RTOG 89–01[55]	Biopsy-proven stage IIIA(N2)	Postinduction surgery vs RT?	MVP or VP ↓ Surgery vs RT ↓ MVP or VP	71	Closed early due to slow accrual; p = 0.62 for overall survival; 4-year: 13% for surgery vs 20% for RT
CALGB[56]	Biopsy-proven stage IIIA(N2)	Induction RT or chemo?	RT → Surgery → RT vs PE → Surgery → PE → RT	47	Closed early due to slow accrual; survival curves identical

P, cisplatin; F, 5-fluorouracil; M, mitomycin C; V, vinblastine; RTOG, Radiation Therapy Oncology Group; CALGB, Cancer and Leukemia Group B.
* Update provided by Fleck J, during a 1997 meeting presentation.

oRT versus induction chemotherapy. But for now, the role of RT as an induction modality is still debated, especially questioned in the subset with low-bulk, early-stage disease.

Radiotherapy Timing and Fractionation in Induction Trials

If the added value of RT is accepted in multimodality trials that include surgical resection, controversy also exists regarding the optimal timing of RT with respect to chemotherapy and surgery. The debate has been that concurrent induction chemoRT is more toxic than sequential and that no data exist to support its use over sequential therapy for unresectable disease.[8] No trials have been completed with postinduction surgery to address the question of concurrent versus sequential chemoRT. However, a Japanese study without surgery was conducted regarding this issue in unresectable, stage III disease.[53] There was a significant long-term survival advantage to the concurrent over the sequenced regimen. An ongoing RTOG trial directly tests this question in locally advanced disease (but without surgical resection). The phase III German trial compares induction chemotherapy followed by concurrent chemoRT (hyperfractionated) followed by surgery with induction chemotherapy followed by surgery followed by standard RT. This is the only induction trial planned at this writing to address the "position" of RT in the multimodality treatment program, although the RT fractionation is different in each arm.

Because there are no completed studies that directly address the radiation timing question, it is difficult to determine if there is added excessive morbidity from concurrent

chemoRT induction compared with chemotherapy alone. The toxicity profiles reported in the various second- and third-generation phase II studies reviewed herein were similar regardless of when the RT was given, although concurrent chemoRT regimens perhaps resulted in a higher rate of esophagitis. The overall operative mortality and pulmonary complication rates were not significantly different between the two approaches, even when hyperfractionated RT regimens were employed (discussed later in this chapter). The CALGB investigators had difficulty completing the planned RT that was prescribed in the trial "posterior" to the surgery because of patient compliance and dropout because of toxicity.[29]

Whether induction chemoRT with hyperfractionation is better than standard, once-daily dosing is another important question. The safety profile and efficacy of preoperative hyperfractionated RT combined with chemotherapy followed by surgery were defined in two recent trials.[41,42] A randomized study of single versus twice-daily fractionation combined with chemotherapy (but with no subsequent surgery) is ongoing by the RTOG, but no trial that compares the type of induction fractionation with the addition of surgery is in progress at this writing.

Surgery versus Radiation after Induction Chemotherapy

Which modality—surgery or RT—provides optimal local control after induction chemotherapy is another critical question. Prior study results were mixed regarding whether achievement of a complete resection was a favorable predictor of long-term survival. For example, the CALGB I study update reported that many of the long-term survivors did not undergo a complete resection, and the Memorial Sloan-Kettering Cancer Center investigators did not find this to be a major discriminant like pCR.[25,40] However, the SWOG and Toronto investigators found prolonged five to six-year survival if complete resection was accomplished.[27,38]

Two randomized studies were designed directly to address the worth of postinduction surgery versus postinduction RT: one by the NCI Canada (n = 31) and the other by the RTOG (n = 71).[54,55] These phase III trials are described in Table 44.12. Both protocols randomized the study population to induction chemotherapy followed by either surgical resection or definitive RT. The studies required biopsy proof of mediastinal nodal involvement, and only patients with stage IIIA(N2) disease were eligible. Both studies closed prematurely because of impaired accrual but were recently reported with mature follow-up. The survival curves overlap in both studies. The four-year survival was 13% in the surgery arm and 20% for the RT group in the RTOG study. These findings are intriguing, but do not answer the question due to lack of statistical power. Large, ongoing phase III studies by the North American Intergroup and the European Organization for the Research and Treatment of Cancer (EORTC) are designed to answer the question regarding definitive RT versus surgical resection, and both should meet their accrual goals (described later in this chapter).

Chemotherapy or Radiation as the Sole Induction Modality

Only one phase III trial has been designed directly to compare induction chemotherapy with induction RT.[56] This trial of the CALGB in patients with biopsy-proven N2 disease is described in Table 44.12. One arm had both induction and posterior RT ("best local-regional therapy"), whereas the other arm had induction chemotherapy and adjuvant chemotherapy followed by posterior RT. The study closed prematurely because of poor accrual, with only 47 patients enrolled. At last report, the survival curves were identical. However, this one incomplete study should not be used to argue against proceeding with other randomized trials of induction chemotherapy.

OLDER VERSUS NEWER CHEMOTHERAPY REGIMENS WITHIN INDUCTION PROGRAMS

Many chemotherapy regimens are effective in the induction setting, and response rates in general are higher than observed with the same combinations in stage IV disease. However, no one regimen can currently be recommended as superior to the others, and no phase III trials asked or plan to address this question. All protocols with published

safety data and long-term follow-up employed second-generation cisplatin-based combinations, either alone as induction therapy or in sequence or concurrent with RT. Mature data are lacking on trimodality approaches that incorporate new agents, and only a few pilot studies in early stage disease assessed the role of new agent-based induction chemotherapy. It is too early to determine if these programs will be at least as safe and effective as the studies reviewed in this chapter. Prior to recommending new agent combinations for presurgery induction programs, the feasibility and superiority (either in terms of survival or patient tolerance or both) of adding new agents within a chemoRT approach with no surgery in locally advanced disease must first be proven.

Pilot studies of induction chemotherapy or induction chemoRT that used one of the newer agents, such as a taxane, gemcitabine, or vinorelbine, in combination with cisplatin or carboplatin, or as doublets without a platin, have been initiated. To date these are reported in meeting summaries or in abstract form only, and follow-up is short. One example is the phase II study of the Bimodality Lung Oncology Team (BLOT).[57] Ninety-eight patients with early stage, minimal disease burden and a negative mediastinoscopy (T2N0, T3N0, T1–3N1) were treated with two to three cycles of carboplatin plus paclitaxel, followed by surgery and an additional two to three cycles of chemotherapy. Patients with unresectable disease, positive margins, or N2 nodes were taken off the study. The response rate was 54%, the complete resection rate was 82%, and there were four pCRs. There were two postoperative deaths. This was a well-tolerated induction regimen, but so far, with short follow-up, the results are not superior to the standard second-generation induction regimens. Thus ongoing phase III trials in early-stage disease that employ second-generation induction chemotherapy regimens should not be critiqued on this issue.

Many of these ongoing studies incorporate etoposide in the induction regimen, but its role is often questioned. The Avignon, France, group conducted two successive phase II trials for patients with mixed stage III disease, with identical staging criteria in each trial, in which the addition of etoposide was the only difference between studies. Superior five-year survival was achieved with concurrent cisplatin, etoposide, and RT (26%), compared with cisplatin and RT (12%, p = 0.008).[58] The addition of etoposide was an independent favorable predictor of survival in a multivariate analysis, and local control was significantly improved.

Another concern regarding ongoing studies with second-generation induction chemotherapy or chemoRT is that, based on current practice patterns in stage IV NSCLC, new drug combinations should replace the old. This recommendation is premature for several reasons. So far, no regimen has emerged as superior to second-generation regimens in the stage IV setting.[59,60] Furthermore, numerous phase II pilot studies of a taxane, or a platin plus a taxane, (usually paclitaxel) in combination with RT but without subsequent surgery were recently reported in stage III disease, with encouraging early results.[61-64] However, none of these newer programs tested in carefully staged subsets have to date reported superior efficacy or long-term survival over second-generation programs. Response rates in four successive trials of paclitaxel and RT with or without carboplatin were 73% to 77%, very similar to the response rates of the second- and third-generation induction chemoRT programs reviewed herein.[62,65] The three-year survivals of 15.5% and 19% reported in two of these trials and the two-year survival of 38% from a third study are comparable to those reported in the past for second-generation cisplatin-containing chemoRT bimodality regimens without surgery. For example, the two- and three-year survivals after the combination of cisplatin, etoposide, and concurrent RT without surgical resection in the SWOG 9019 stage IIIB study were 33% and 26%, respectively.[39] Overall response and one-year survival rates were also no different from the SWOG 9019 findings in a recent randomized phase II study conducted by the CALGB.[66] This bimodality study for patients with clinical stage III disease tested chemoRT with cisplatin plus either paclitaxel, gemcitabine, or vinorelbine. Longer follow-up is needed to determine if the "tail" on the survival curves is better than seen to date with second-generation chemotherapy plus RT. Until then, completion of ongoing phase III randomized studies that employ second-generation chemotherapy in combination with RT prior to surgery can be justified.

Safety and tolerability data reported to date from new agent-based approaches with bimodality chemoRT regimens (either sequenced or concurrent with no surgery) and trimodality studies (with surgery) raise concern. Severe esophagitis, neutropenic fever, hospital admissions, stump insufficiency, and other serious problems were reported at rates as high as 49%.[62,64,66-68] Given these early observations of significant toxicity, more data is needed before routine use of new agents as part of induction regimens can be recommended. Ideally, ongoing trials of chemoRT alone should mature with complete safety analyses before making the leap to incorporate surgery. With all new trials involving new agents, it will be critical to monitor the stage subset mix and methods of substage documentation in order to determine if the anticipated reports of superiority can be attributed solely to the change in chemotherapy.

TREATMENT-RELATED MORBIDITY AND MORTALITY IN COMBINED MODALITY INDUCTION TRIALS

The morbidity from combined modality therapy that includes surgery is not insignificant. It is often difficult to attribute a particular toxicity to just one modality, because the entire "package" effects patient tolerance and the treat-

ment-related mortality. All combined modality induction programs were tested in the "fittest" patients, who were fully ambulatory and had general medical conditions that permitted the rigors of this therapy. Eligibility criteria were of necessity quite strict in these trials. It may be dangerous to offer this type of treatment outside a clinical trial, especially to patients who have a poor performance status and/or major comorbidities, because the literature will underestimate the extent of morbidity and mortality in this group. Clinical trials designed for the large group of patients ineligible for these aggressive approaches are needed. But for patients who match the eligibility criteria of published studies, the literature provides some information on the expected morbidity and mortality during induction therapy, the postoperative period, the late or posterior chemotherapy and/or RT, and after all treatment is completed.

During Induction Therapy

The most common toxicity reported among all trials during the presurgery induction phase is myelosuppression from chemotherapy. This is usually short-lived and in most studies did not result in admissions for neutropenic fever. Other drug-specific side effects, such as nausea and emesis, diarrhea, mucositis, and cisplatin-related malaise, are variably reported. In fact, nausea and emesis are now quite infrequent compared to the rates reported in the initial trials because of the expanded number of compounds effective against this toxicity. Esophagitis is more often observed after induction chemoRT than chemotherapy alone, although severe events occurred in less than 10% of patients in most series with single fractionation RT.[30-34] The two third-generation trials with hyperfractionated RT reported severe esophagitis rates of 6% and 14%.[41,42] Pneumonitis during induction therapy is quite rare, except that the risk of septic deaths from postobstructive pneumonia may have been greater with the MVP regimen in one large series.[27] Overall, most second-generation induction regimens were fully managed in an outpatient setting. A significant proportion of patients who enter induction therapy with symptoms related to bulk disease in the chest report a gradual improvement in sense of well-being and performance status as treatment is ongoing. However, formal quality-of-life studies have not been conducted for this group of patients.

During the 30-Day Postoperative Time Period

Despite the wealth of clinical trials that follow algorithms leading to eventual exploration and resection after induction therapy, there is no consensus as to what constitutes expected or acceptable postinduction surgical morbidity and mortality. This lack of consensus is due to the marked heterogeneity of induction regimens (as reviewed in preceding sections); the lack of consistency across trials in the adequate reporting of surgical complications; different criteria for pre-operative eligibility regarding pulmonary function, comorbidities and conditioning (see section to follow); and variable experience of the surgeon in dealing with postinduction surgical scenarios at the time of thoracotomy and in providing the required supportive care during the postoperative time period.

A number of publications document the risk of pulmonary resection in the noninduction situation. The modern 30-day mortality for pneumonectomy is 3% to 6.2% and the mortality of a standard lobectomy is 1% to 2%.[69–71] As detailed in Chapter 41, the most frequent complications after pulmonary resection include supraventricular arrhythmias (16% to 18%), atelectasis (7%) and air leak lasting longer than seven days (5%). These rates are rarely provided in the induction therapy literature. However, in a large series involving multiple institutions, the SWOG investigators observed a similar spectrum of perioperative complications.[30,37] Acute surgical morbidities appear to be similar regardless of the type of induction, unless RT is given and too much time is allowed to elapse so that extensive fibrosis is encountered. Whether drugs that rarely cause pulmonary reactions during induction therapy increase the rates of these types of postoperative complications is not clear. However, the incorporation of drugs such as mitomycin C in the induction regimen often leads to higher rates of major pulmonary morbidity (13% in the Memorial Sloan-Kettering Cancer Center series).[25]

Pulmonary complications and deaths due to pulmonary causes during the postoperative time period are the greatest concern after induction therapy, and collectively rates are probably greater than reported in the literature after surgery alone. In particular, events such as extensive pneumonitis (usually culture-negative), ARDS, and bronchopleural fistula have a high mortality in the postoperative period. Pulmonary morbidity and mortality rates are often quoted to be greater after induction regimens with chemoRT than after induction chemotherapy alone. However, a careful review of all the literature available (detailed in preceding sections) discloses great variability. Postoperative mortality rates from 3.1% to 17% (including some cases of ARDS) were reported after MVP- or VP-containing induction chemotherapy, from 4% to 15% after second-generation induction chemoRT, and from 5% to 7% after induction chemoRT with hyperfractionation.

The specific type of mortal postoperative event may differ according to whether RT was included with induction chemotherapy or not, although this issue is not fully resolved. For example, complicated stump insufficiency was the most common cause of postoperative death in the WGCC experience with twice-daily RT in the induction[42], whereas ARDS may be the most common cause of postoperative deaths after single fractionation chemoRT in multiple series. The presence of RT in the induction regimen, however, may not be the sole explanation for greater pulmonary-

related mortality, especially ARDS, after certain induction regimens. For the most part, many of the patients treated with concurrent chemoRT induction approaches had advanced, central disease that required a pneumonectomy after induction. Pulmonary-related postoperative mortality rates are expected to be much higher in this population with advanced disease.[30,32,42] So far, there has been no difference in overall postoperative mortality rates compared to the surgery-alone control arms in trials with induction chemotherapy for early, more minimal bulk disease.[46–48] Complete data regarding pulmonary-related complications after pneumonectomy is needed from these three trials.

It is too soon to know the true mortality rates and cause after incorporation of the newer chemotherapy agents into the induction regimen. The BLOT investigators reported a reassuringly low postoperative mortality rate after induction carboplatin plus paclitaxel.[57] However, other reports are worrisome. The Vanderbilt investigators observed life-threatening complications after induction carboplatin plus paclitaxel in 32% of 25 patients, with an 8% postoperative mortality.[68] The Rush Presbyterian St. Lukes group reported an increased incidence of ARDS and bronchopleural fistulae using preoperative paclitaxel-containing chemotherapy with concurrent RT.[67]

Serious pulmonary complications in the postoperative period clearly result from a combination of causes in addition to the type of induction therapy.[72–75] Although doses of RT higher than 45 Gy have been implicated,[74] the occurrence of ARDS in trials with no induction RT and the lack of an excess rate of ARDS in other trials with higher-dose RT or altered fraction RT[34,41,42] underscore that the tolerance of lymphatic sump disruption and postpneumonectomy shunts is variable after both induction chemotherapy and induction chemoRT. The type of complication may also vary based on the schedule of the RT, with perhaps more events of serious stump insufficiency but less ARDS after hyperfractionated versus single-fraction RT. The preoperative DLCO may be the most important screen for the risk of serious postoperative pulmonary complications, an hypothesis that is being studied prospectively in the current North American Intergroup phase III trial in N2 disease (see Table 44.13).

After the Postoperative Time Period

Many induction program algorithms recommend additional chemotherapy with or without RT after the patient has recovered from surgery. Usually the spectrum of toxicities from posterior chemotherapy are similar to those observed during induction,[30] although it may be more difficult to complete a boost dose of RT.[29] Patients are at greater risk for pneumonitis, either from prior RT or due to infectious causes, beyond the postoperative time period, especially if the prior surgery was a pneumonectomy. Data on this issue are rarely reported in the induction therapy literature.[30]

TABLE 44.13. ONGOING OR PLANNED PHASE III STUDIES THAT ADDRESS THE ROLE OF SURGERY FOR BIOPSY-PROVEN STAGE IIIA(N2) NSCLC

Investigators	Projected Number of Patients	Trial Design
North American Intergroup[76] (Chair: RTOG)	510	EP × 2 + concurrent single fx RT to 45 Gy
		⟨
		Complete RT Surgery
		to 61 Gy without ↓
		break concurrent with EP × 2
		↓
		EP × 2
EORTC Intergroup[77]	480	Any cisplatin-containing regimen × 3
		⟨
		Surgery Single fx RT
West German Consortium*	400	PT × 3 → hyperfx RT to 45 Gy + concurrent EP
		⟨
		Surgery Continue to 66–75 Gy (conformal)

Fx, fraction; Gy, gray, E, etoposide; P, cisplatin; T, paclitaxel; RTOG, Radiation Therapy Oncology Group; EORTC, European Organization for Research and Treatment of Cancer.
* Planned; also includes stage IIIB subsets T4 (noneffusion) and contralateral (N3) nodes.

Prompt attention to symptoms of infection with broad-spectrum antibiotic coverage is critical to minimize the risk of mortality.

The other major morbidity experienced by many patients after induction therapy followed by surgery is a posttreatment constitutional syndrome. This consists of a constellation of symptoms including thoracotomy pain, malaise, anorexia, and poor pulmonary reserve. This syndrome probably occurs at a greater frequency than with radiation or surgery alone, but its rate is grossly underreported.[30] It often resolves within a year after treatment, although its lingering presence is clearly discouraging to the patient and caregiver. Prospective quality-of-life analyses and active rehabilitation protocols for this population are needed. Patients also continue to experience problems from their comorbid diseases long after treatment is completed, especially cardiovascular disease and noncancer pulmonary events. Competing cause-of-death reporting is rare, and death certificates often attribute cause to "lung cancer" even when the disease has never recurred. The SWOG investigators categorized cause of death via a review of flow sheets for the patients without disease progression, rather than assume all were cancer-related. Although cancer accounted for 64% of all deaths, 20% were due to various other causes, such as late pneumonia long after the end of treatment, myocardial infarction, pulmonary embolus, cerebrovascular accidents, trauma, ulcer, or second primaries.[30]

OTHER IMPORTANT CONSIDERATIONS REGARDING THE INDUCTION THERAPY APPROACH

Several areas more relevant to the treatment of patients with induction therapy followed by surgery than other aspects of lung cancer care merit special mention. These include the importance of a multidisciplinary patient evaluation, management, and follow-up; assessment of the functional status of the patient before and after induction; various radiotherapy issues; and special surgical considerations such as the extent of resection, the timing of surgery, and technical issues during the operation.

Evaluation and Management by a Multidisciplinary Team

A multidisciplinary team approach is mandatory from the time of diagnosis. This team should include a thoracic surgeon with expertise in the technical demands of postinduction surgery and postoperative care, medical and radiation oncologists, a pulmonologist, a pathologist and a radiologist. The team discusses details of both the anatomic and functional workup, the patient's performance status and comorbid illnesses, the extent of staging workup needed, and whether the patient is eligible for a clinical trial (or if not, whether he or she fits the eligibility criteria for a published trial that reported a favorable risk-benefit ratio). The role for special staging procedures is also reviewed, including whether MRI or PET scanning would add to the information provided by the standard CT-scan-based approach.

During this initial multidisciplinary case review, the surgeon must specifically address issues related to the chest wall and mediastinum, including nodal status and the presence of chest wall or mediastinal invasion (T3 or T4 descriptors from the radiology review). This thoracic surgical evaluation will determine if a simple mediastinoscopy or mediastinotomy can provide all the necessary nodal sampling to establish fully the substage designation, or whether thoracoscopy or thoracotomy is needed to provide more data regarding N2 or T3–4 status. This comprehensive evaluation will also enable proper planning for the extent of operation that might be needed after induction therapy is complete. The pathologist's contribution regarding histologic subtype may influence the use of additional invasive staging of the mediastinum in the absence of suspicion on the CT scan (for example, undifferentiated tumors or large, central adenocarcinomas).

Airway assessment is also critical and can be obtained jointly by the pulmonary and thoracic surgery components of the team. A proximal obstruction might be cleared by laser or nonlaser techniques to provide better assessment of the airway for special surgical approaches such as bronchial sleeve resection. Moreover, as a patient enters an induction program, establishment of an adequate, nonobstructed airway lessens the chance for obstructive pneumonia or other airway complications such as hemoptysis during the hematologic nadir from chemotherapy. If the patient presents with a *de novo* pleural effusion that is large enough to access at the bedside or under radiographic guidance, cytologic examination of the fluid is mandatory to rule out pleural metastases that would make the patient ineligible for an induction approach.

Multidisciplinary team management is also necessary during induction and at the reevaluation point after induction therapy is completed. All specialists involved should see the patient at this time and discuss results of the restaging tests. New pleural or pericardial effusions are most often due to the intervening induction therapy if small, but should not be dismissed without evaluation if large enough to access. The functional status of the patient and degree of recovery from the induction therapy, along with any serious complications experienced up to that point, should also be reviewed jointly. A decision about whether to proceed to surgery is made, and if so, the optimal time for surgery is determined. The degree of radiographic response, together with anatomic location, functional evaluation (see below), and type and tolerance of induction therapy, will dictate the extent of resection needed and whether it is feasible and safe. The role of the nonsurgical members of the team is also important during the postoperative period to assist in the management of treatment-related morbidity.

Functional Evaluation of the Patient

In parallel with the important pretherapy anatomic evaluation of disease reviewed above, a thorough assessment of the patient's physiologic and functional status is critical before an induction approach is selected. This evaluation must be repeated after induction is completed but before surgery is attempted. The treatment of comorbid illnesses should be optimized, and a full cardiovascular and pulmonary assessment must be conducted. If there is a history of angina, hypertension, arrhythmia, or congestive heart failure, active

medical therapy should be optimized, and prior catheterization or echocardiographic data should be retrieved and reviewed. A stress test to evaluate myocardial reserve is often indicated, along with other invasive cardiac testing as necessary. Right heart function must be considered, especially if a pneumonectomy is planned or possible.

Complete pulmonary function testing (PFT) that includes spirometry and lung volumes, an arterial blood gas measurement, and a DLCO is mandatory before induction and also before surgery. Special attention should be paid to the DLCO, since it may be the most important predictor of risk of subsequent serious pulmonary morbidity or mortality. Quantitative (split-function) perfusion studies should be added to the standard PFTs if the FEV1 is marginal for the planned lobectomy or pneumonectomy. Active pulmonary rehabilitation and general reconditioning directed by the pulmonologist and others is often needed during the entire course of the induction program. The latter includes nutritional support, functional conditioning, smoking cessation assistance, and application of appropriate bronchodilator, antibiotic, and steroid therapy as needed (see also Chapter 36).

Radiotherapy Considerations

If RT is given as part of the induction, careful joint evaluation of the patient by the radiation and medical oncologists is necessary. Close attention to the granulocyte count and hemoglobin as well as early indicators of esophagitis will minimize serious complications. This careful follow-up must be tailored to the regimen and the patient's specific needs, and requires experience on the part of both disciplines. For most chemoRT induction regimens, there is a clear "learning curve," so the expertise of those familiar with a given approach should be tapped when embarking upon a program for the first time. When to hold the RT in the face of emerging toxicity versus the importance of continuing with full supportive care to maximize benefit is an important issue to balance in most chemoRT induction programs.

In addition to these practical matters, a number of theoretical concerns remain unresolved regarding the role of RT. One issue is the definition of the proper margin of normal lung. Radiation oncologists with experience in concurrent chemoRT induction recommend closer margins than usually employed in regimens without surgery. Tightening of the margin may decrease the risk of postoperative pulmonary complications.[30] Another important outstanding issue is the need to define the optimal target volume and dose within induction regimens. Clinical trials must be conducted to address how conformal RT approaches could be applied to minimize toxicity and fibrosis and to maximize the dose to the tumor.

Special Surgical Issues after Induction Therapy

An attempt at surgical resection is recommended even if disease remains stable on postinduction radiographic evaluation. Thus, mandating a formal response assessment beyond documentation of lack of progression may not be necessary. Patients with stable disease on CT scans of the chest after the induction is completed are often found to have either minimal or no tumor in the pathology specimen, and should also be offered resection. For example, in the SWOG 8805 study, there were 37 patients who had stable disease after induction. Thirty of these underwent thoracotomy, of whom 26 were resected. Of these, 12 (46%) had no residual tumor or only rare microscopic foci of disease.[30]

The timing of the resection after induction therapy will be defined in the clinical trial if a patient is enrolled in one. If not, the usual recommendation is to proceed with surgery three to six weeks after completion of the induction. A delay longer than six weeks may result in greater fibrosis if RT was used as part of induction. This finding adds major technical difficulty and risk of complications to the often already-complex resection. Even when the timing of surgery is optimal, the technical aspects of pulmonary resection after induction therapy can be quite demanding. Vascular planes may be obliterated by fibrosis, and the scarring at sites of previous tumor invasion can be unyielding to the standard maneuvers of pulmonary resection. The degree of fibrosis cannot be predicted, so operative time must be planned accordingly.

Guidelines for intraoperative assessment of resectability have not been standardized for the patient who has received an induction regimen. Bronchoscopy just before the resection often yields valuable information on the extent of the proximal margin and should be compared with the preinduction results, if one was done. General principles of operative conduct include the use of double-lumen endotracheal intubation, fluid restriction, and low concentration of inspired oxygen. The use of right-heart (Swan Ganz) monitoring should be selective, and pulmonary embolism prophylaxis should be considered.

The type of surgical resection required is to a large degree determined by the initial extent and bulk of disease, together with the predicted functional reserve of the patient. At least for approaches delivered to patients with advanced stage III disease, complex operations were often found to be necessary and the technical experience of the thoracic surgeon in postinduction surgery was critical to a favorable outcome.[2] Of the resections performed in the SWOG 8805 trimodality trial, 43% were standard lobectomies, 15% were complex lobectomies (extrapleural, spine, chest wall or sleeve resections), 13% were pneumonectomies, and 29% were intrapericardial pneumonectomies.[30,37] Resection criteria may also extend to atrial and caval resections, which is justified if the T4N0–1 designation remains true during intraoperative assessment of the mediastinal nodes.[38] However, there is no data yet to support similar extensive resections when N2 or N3 involvement persists.

The thoracic surgeon is often forced to deal with theoretical issues as induction regimens become more innovative and aggressive. In particular, what should define a "complete resection" after a major response to induction therapy? Should the margins of resection encompass the original extent of disease, or only what remains? Should a complete assessment be made of potential contralateral nodal disease, or should only the initially involved stations be resampled? Is a complete resection contraindicated if there is viable tumor in the nodes and lung, or is this the situation for which surgery would have the greatest impact on long-term survival? If the most aggressive course is favored, then extended approaches using median sternotomy or the clamshell incision to allow for bilateral dissection may be justified. The ultimate question, however, that will dictate replies to all these other issues is whether the surgery is needed "simply" for optimal local control, or if it truly impacts on long-term survival. Fortunately, ongoing phase III trials that address the role of surgery, with careful assessment of pathology variables in the chest and mediastinum at time of surgery and a full analysis of patterns of recurrence, will provide answers to these questions.

ONGOING PHASE III TRIALS WORLDWIDE

It is clear that an optimal induction approach cannot be recommended, since none has emerged as superior to date. Lack of consensus exists because: (a) no large randomized trial addressed a single question in a homogeneously staged, subset-restricted group of patients; (b) inconsistent application of careful staging methods resulted in marked variability in T and N subset groupings; (c) there was often a mix of extent of disease bulk within trials; and (d) many trials lacked a reproducible definition of what constituted "resectable" versus "unresectable" disease upfront. Therefore the ongoing phase III trials around the world are most welcome, in that most of these problems are addressed in the study protocols. These trials are designed to either address the role of postinduction surgery or induction radiation in more advanced disease or question the value of induction chemotherapy in early stage disease.

Phase III Trials for Advanced Stage IIIA(N2) Disease

There are two large phase III trials ongoing worldwide to address the role of surgery and a third study is planned for patients with biopsy-proven stage IIIA(N2) disease (and selected IIIB in the third study). The trial designs are shown in Table 44.13. The current High Priority North American Intergroup Trial 0139 (RTOG, SWOG, ECOG, CALGB,

NCCTG, and NCI Canada) compares the trimodality program developed by the SWOG[30] with the same induction chemoRT with full-dose RT but no surgery in pathologically documented, bulky, N2 disease.[76] Two cycles of posterior chemotherapy are given to all patients, but no posterior "boost" RT is used in the surgical arm. The trial is accruing well and planned analyses of toxicity and outcome by the Data and Safety Monitoring Committee permit completion of accrual. No unexpected toxicities or excess postoperative mortality were observed in the first 200 patients accrued by this broad North American consortium. The second trial is ongoing within the European Intergroup (Table 44.13). It asks whether surgical resection or RT is the optimal local control after three cycles of induction chemotherapy with any cisplatin-containing regimen.[77] At the point of accrual of 179 patients, an interim analysis showed a resection rate of 89%, three treatment-related deaths, and downstaging in 42%. Patients were able to complete the postchemotherapy RT. The third phase III trial also addresses the role of surgery after induction therapy and is planned at this writing. It is a follow-up study to the phase II West German Cancer Center trial[42] and will also include the stage IIIB subsets of T4 and N3 (contralateral mediastinal nodes only). This study will test the worth of surgery after induction chemotherapy plus concurrent, hyperfractionated RT versus, instead of surgery, continuing the RT to 66 to 75 Gy using a conformal approach.

Phase III Trials that Ask a Radiotherapy Question in Stage III Disease

An ongoing study in Germany for patients with stage IIIA and IIIB disease is designed to test whether hyperfractionated RT as part of induction is better than induction chemotherapy alone. Its design is outlined in Table 44.14, and so far, this approach appears feasible and safe.[52] However, this study does not provide a pure test of the RT question, because those patients assigned to induction chemotherapy alone will receive single daily fraction RT after surgery. But this trial will provide important information regarding the contribution of RT to the achievement of pCR, complete resection, and nodal downstaging. A planned trial by Japanese investigators for patients with IIIA(N2) disease will test the important RT question. The only variable is the presence or absence of RT in the induction regimen (Table 44.14).

Phase III Trials that Address the Role of Chemotherapy in Early-Stage Disease

The remainder of the trials described in Table 44.14 consider whether or not chemotherapy is indicated before surgery in patients with early-stage, nonbulky disease. These trials are all large enough, with careful restriction of the eligible stage subsets, that the critiques of the completed trials discussed previously will be addressed.[46–48] The Ger-

TABLE 44.14. ONGOING PHASE III TRIALS THAT QUESTION THE ROLE FOR INDUCTION CHEMOTHERAPY OR RADIOTHERAPY

Investigators	Stage Subsets	Design
North American Intergroup (Chair: SWOG)	IB, IIA, IIB	CarboT × 3 → surgery vs surgery alone
Germany[52]	IIIA and IIIB	PE × 3 → HfRT + Carbo Vd → surgery* vs PE × 3 → surgery → RT
German Krebshilfe	Central T3N0/1 Minimal N2 (1 or 2 nodes)	PE × 3 → HfRT + PE → surgery vs surgery → RT
Netherlands	T2N0, N1, T3N0	EP × 2–4 (to maximum response) → surgery vs surgery alone
England	"Early stage"	Cisplatin-containing ChT × 3 → surgery vs surgery alone
EORTC**	IB, II	CarboT, PG or PN × 3 (choice) → surgery vs surgery alone
Japan**	IIIA(N2)	MNP × 2 + RT 45Gy (split) → surgery vs MNP × 2 → surgery

SWOG, Southwest Oncology Group; EORTC, European Organization for Research and Treatment of Cancer; E, etoposide; P, cisplatin; Carbo, carboplatin; T, paclitaxel; Vd, vindesine; G, gemcitabine; N, navelbine; ChT, chemotherapy; HfRT, twice-daily radiotherapy.
* Additional HfRT after surgery if no complete resection.
** Planned to open at this writing.

man Krebshilfe trial is ongoing for patients with central T3N0–1 or very minimal N2 disease (one or two positive nodes only). The designs of the trials from the North American Intergroup (follow-up of the BLOT phase II study, at this writing soon to open), EORTC (planned), Netherlands, and England are similar, differing primarily in the use or not of newer chemotherapy regimens.

INDUCTION THERAPY BEFORE SURGERY: THE TWO DEBATES, REVISITED

The questions posed in Table 44.1 can now be revisited, informed by the worldwide data reviewed herein on induction therapy followed by surgery. Can standard-of-care recommendations be made at this time in both categories of disease burden? That is, for patients with advanced stage or bulky disease, does subsequent resection improve survival, and if so, for which subsets? And should preoperative chemotherapy with or without RT be given routinely in patients with early stage or nonbulky disease who are candidates for resection? Many practitioners, especially in North America, have concluded "yes" to both debates and routinely prescribe such treatments outside a clinical trial setting for many stage subsets. However, the majority Consensus Statement of the International Association for the Study of Lung Cancer (IASLC) emphasized that the data argue it is premature to reach these conclusions in either disease group and that completion of the ongoing trials is needed to establish new practice guidelines.[7] Trials completed since this consensus statement do little to change this position.

The First Debate in Advanced, Bulky Disease Subsets

The IASLC Consensus Statement pointed out that feasibility and safety were demonstrated for postinduction surgery and that some provocative outcome data were reported for patients with advanced stage III disease. But postinduction surgery has not yet been proven to be superior to chemoRT or chemotherapy alone in this subgroup, even when phase II trials reported since publication of the position paper are considered. Thus this approach should not be routinely applied to initially unresectable or marginally resectable, bulky, N2 or stage IIIB disease, for which chemoRT remains the standard of care. Outside a clinical trial, exceptions might be considered for the special circumstances of either T4N0–1 disease or if all initial N2 and N3 disease is eradicated by the induction therapy. However, practice guidelines cannot be based solely on these subset analyses of phase II trials, so validation of the observations in the ongoing phase III trials is needed.

The Second Debate in Early, Nonbulky Disease Subsets

At the time of the IASLC Consensus Statement, data was available from four small randomized trials regarding the role of induction chemotherapy in early-stage, resectable disease. The position paper concluded that surgery alone was still the standard (versus preoperative chemoRT or chemotherapy) for these patients. This issue was unsettled at that time because of the concern over stage subset biases in the two randomized trials with positive results.[46,47] Since then, the superimposition of survival curves was reported in the two other (albeit incomplete) trials that tested surgery versus RT after induction chemotherapy,[54,55] thus keeping the debate alive. However, 1999 brought the first presentation of the results of the first large phase III trial, the French Thoracic Cooperative Group Study. The results were in favor of induction CT but as yet do not reach statistical significance.[48] Stage subset imbalances and the use of only clinical staging contribute to the uncertainty regarding the findings, but longer follow-up is needed. Thus there is justification to continue trials with surgery-alone control arms and complete accrual.

Resolution of the Debates

It is hoped that the two debates will be resolved with definitive answers via completion of the phase III trials outlined in Tables 44.13 and 44.14. Yet there are growing trends to attempt resection of disease in all patients following chemotherapy with or without RT, to add new agents to induction RT ahead of published pilot safety and efficacy data in clearly defined subsets, and routinely to give third-generation chemotherapy prior to resection in those patients with early-stage disease. These practice trends may jeopardize the worldwide accrual to the randomized trials, and if so, this debate will remain the most controversial area in the management of NSCLC. All medical and radiation oncologists and thoracic surgeons involved in the care of these patients must support these studies, which in turn will resolve these two debates and establish new practice standards for a large subset of patients with NSCLC.

CURRENT AND FUTURE CHALLENGES

Apart from the critical questions addressed by the ongoing clinical trials (Tables 44.13 and 44.14), a number of other areas must be addressed in parallel to achieve the next level of improvement in survival for these patients. Perhaps the most critical area for study is novel approaches for the treatment of residual distant microscopic disease after completion of a standard induction program. Even the newer chemotherapy regimens, when merged into induction programs, are not expected to result in "quantum" improvements in long-term survival. Many types of approaches are available for testing as "consolidation," including matrix metalloproteinases, angiogenesis inhibitors, antibodies to growth factor receptors, gene therapy, and vaccines. At the same time, however, new approaches to achieve better local control are needed. The role for the PET scan and functional imaging approaches within induction therapy programs must be defined, as well as optimal use of molecular markers and other variables to predict better which patients benefit from surgery after induction therapy.

Concurrent with this research, studies are needed on how to maximize quality of life and functional reserve (especially pulmonary, via active rehabilitation programs) during combined modality induction therapy, and how to minimize treatment-related pulmonary morbidity and mortality. Brain metastases must be prevented, since they are the major site of first distant relapse in this population. Chemoprevention of second primary cancers, smoking cessation initiatives, and aggressive treatment of comorbid conditions will lengthen the survival time of the patients who are free of recurrence after completion of combined modality induction programs.

REFERENCES

1. Strauss GM, Langer MP, Elias AD, et al. Multimodality treatment of stage IIIA non-small cell lung carcinoma: a critical review of the literature and strategies for future research. *J Clin Oncol* 1992;10:829.
2. Rusch VW, Benfield JR. Neoadjuvant therapy for lung cancer: a note of caution. *Ann Thorac Surg* 1993;55:820.
3. Green M, Brodin O, Choi N, et al. Pre-operative and postoperative treatments in stage III NSCLC. *Lung Cancer* 1994; 10[Suppl]:S15.
4. Johnson DH, Piantadosi S. Chemotherapy for resectable stage III non-small cell lung cancer—can that dog hunt? *J Natl Cancer Inst* 1994;86:650.
5. Edelman MJ, Gandara DR, Roach M III, et al. Multimodality therapy in stage III non-small cell lung cancer. *Ann Thorac Surg* 1996;61:1564.
6. Albain KS. Induction chemotherapy with or without radiation followed by surgery in stage III non-small cell lung cancer: update and perspectives. *Oncology* 1997;11:51.
7. Perry MC, Deslauriers J, Albain KS, et al. Induction treatment for resectable non-small-cell lung cancer: a consensus report. *Lung Cancer* 1997;17[Suppl 1]:15.
8. Gordon GS, Vokes EE. Chemoradiation for locally advanced, unresectable NSCLC: new standard of care, emerging strategies. *Oncology* 1999;13:1075.
9. Martini N, Flehinger BJ, Zaman M, et al. Results of resection in non-oat cell carcinoma of the lung with mediastinal lymph node metastases. *Ann Surg* 1983;198:386.
10. Martini N, Flehinger BJ. The role of surgery in N2 lung cancer. *Surg Clin North Am* 1987;67:1037.
11. Vansteenkiste JF, De Leyn PR, Deneffe GJ, et al. Clinical prognostic factors in surgically treated stage IIIAN2 non-small cell lung cancer: analysis of the literature. *Lung Cancer* 1998;19:3.
12. Mountain CF. Prognostic implications of the international staging system for lung cancer. *Semin Oncol* 1988;3:236.
13. Mountain CF. Revisions in the international system for staging lung cancer. *Chest* 1997;111:1710.
14. Bromley LL, Szur L. Combined radiotherapy and resection for carcinoma of the bronchus: experience with 66 patients. *Lancet* 1955;2:937.
15. Bloedorn FG, Cowley RA, Cuccia CA, et al. Combined therapy with irradiation and surgery in the treatment of bronchogenic carcinoma. *Am J Roentgenol* 1961;85:875.
16. Shields T, Higgins G, Lawton KR, et al. Preoperative x-ray therapy as an adjuvant in the treatment of bronchogenic carcinoma. *J Thorac Cardiovasc Surg* 1970;59:49.
17. Warram J. Preoperative irradiation of cancer of the lung: final report of a therapeutic trial. A collaborative study. *Cancer* 1975; 36:914.
18. Payne DG. Pre-operative radiation therapy in non-small cell cancer of the lung. *Lung Cancer* 1991;7:47.
19. Lad T, Wagner H, Piantadosi S for the Lung Cancer Study Group. Randomized phase II evaluation of pre-operative chemotherapy alone and radiotherapy alone in stage IIIA non-small cell lung cancer. *Proc Am Soc Clin Oncol* 1991;10:258.
20. Skarin A, Jochelson M, Sheldon T, et al. Neoadjuvant chemotherapy in marginally resectable stage III M0 non-small cell lung cancer: long-term follow-up in 41 patients. *J Surg Oncol* 1989; 40:266.
21. Eagan RT, Ruud C, Lee RE, et al. for the Lung Cancer Study Group. Pilot study of induction therapy with cyclophosphamide, doxorubicin and cisplatin (CAP) and chest irradiation prior to thoracotomy in initially inoperable stage III M0 non-small cell lung cancer. *Cancer Treat Rep* 1987;71:895.
22. Bitran JD, Golomb HM, Hoffman PC, et al. Protochemotherapy in non-small cell lung carcinoma. An attempt to increase surgical resectability and survival. A preliminary report. *Cancer* 1986;57: 44.
23. Elias AD, Skarin AT, Gonin R, et al. Neoadjuvant treatment of stage IIIA non-small cell lung cancer. *Am J Clin Oncol (CCT)* 1994;17:26.
24. Darwish S, Minotti V, Crino L, et al. Neoadjuvant cisplatin and etoposide for stage IIIA (clinical N2) non-small cell lung cancer. *Am J Clin Oncol (CCT)* 1994;17:64.
25. Martini N, Kris MG, Flehinger BJ, et al. Preoperative chemotherapy for stage IIIA(N2) lung cancer: the Sloan-Kettering experience with 136 patients. *Ann Thorac Surg* 1993;55:1365.
26. Pisters KMW, Kris MG, Gralla RJ, et al. Pathologic complete response in advanced non-small-cell lung cancer following preoperative chemotherapy: implications for the design of future non-small-cell lung cancer combined modality trials. *J Clin Oncol* 1993;11:1757.
27. Burkes RL, Shepherd FA, Ginsberg RJ, et al. Induction chemotherapy with MVP in patients with stage IIIA(N2) unresectable non-small cell lung cancer: the Toronto experience. *Proc Am Soc Clin Oncol* 1994;13:327.
28. Elias AD, Skarin AT, Leong T, et al. Neoadjuvant therapy for surgically staged IIIAN2 non-small cell lung cancer. *Lung Cancer* 1997;17:147.
29. Sugarbaker DJ, Herndon J, Kohman LJ, et al. Results of Cancer and Leukemia Group B Protocol 8935: a multi-institutional phase II trimodality trial for stage IIIA(N2) non-small-cell lung cancer. *J Thorac Cardiovasc Surg* 1995;109:473.
30. Albain KS, Rusch VW, Crowley JJ, et al. Concurrent cisplatin/etoposide plus chest radiotherapy followed by surgery for stages IIIA(N2) and IIIB non-small cell lung cancer: mature results of Southwest Oncology Group Phase II Study 8805. *J Clin Oncol* 1995;13:1880.
31. Weiden PL, Piantadosi S, for the Lung Cancer Study Group. Preoperative chemotherapy (cisplatin and fluorouracil) and radia-

tion therapy in stage III non–small cell lung cancer: a phase II study of the LCSG. *J Natl Cancer Inst* 1991;83:266.

32. Faber LP, Kittle CK, Warren WH, et al. Preoperative chemotherapy and irradiation for stage III non–small cell lung cancer. *Ann Thorac Surg* 1989;47:669.

33. Strauss GM, Herndon JE, Sherman DD, et al. Neoadjuvant chemotherapy and radiotherapy followed by surgery in stage IIIA non-small-cell lung carcinoma of the lung: report of a Cancer and Leukemia Group B phase II study. *J Clin Oncol* 1992;10:1237.

34. Law A, Daly B, Madsen M, et al. High incidence of isolated brain metastases following complete response in advanced non–small cell lung cancer: a new challenge. *Lung Cancer* 1997;18[Suppl 1]:65.

35. Bonomi P, Gale M, Faber LP, et al. Is clinical stage III non–small cell lung cancer a homogeneous group? *Proc Am Soc Clin Oncol* 1992;11:292.

36. Curran WJ, Stafford PM. Lack of apparent difference in outcome between clinically staged IIIA and IIIB non–small cell lung cancer treated with radiotherapy. *J Clin Oncol* 1995;8:409.

37. Rusch VW, Albain KS, Crowley JJ, et al. Neoadjuvant therapy: a novel and effective treatment for stage IIIB non–small cell lung cancer. *Ann Thorac Surg* 1994;58:290.

38. Albain K, Rusch V, Crowley J, et al. Long-term survival after concurrent cisplatin/etoposide plus chest radiotherapy followed by surgery in bulky, stages IIIA(N2) and IIIB non–small cell lung cancer: 6-year outcomes from Southwest Oncology Group Study 8805. *Proc ASCO* 1999;18:467a.

39. Albain KS, Crowley JJ, Turrisi AT, et al. Concurrent cisplatin/etoposide plus radiotherapy for pathologic stage IIIB non–small cell lung cancer: a Southwest Oncology Group phase II study (S9019). *Proc Am Soc Clin Oncol* 1997;16:128a.

40. Strauss GM. Author update on neoadjuvant chemotherapy and radiotherapy followed by surgery in stage IIIA non-small-cell lung carcinoma of the lung: report of a Cancer and Leukemia Group B phase II study. *Classic Papers and Current Comments* 1997;2:159.

41. Choi NC, Carey R, Daly W, et al. Potential impact on survival of improved tumor downstaging and resection rate by preoperative twice-daily radiation and concurrent chemotherapy in stage IIIA non-small-cell lung cancer. *J Clin Oncol* 1997;15:712.

42. Eberhardt W, Wilke H, Stamatis G, et al. Preoperative chemotherapy followed by concurrent chemoradiation therapy based on hyperfractionated accelerated radiotherapy and definitive surgery in locally advanced non–small cell lung cancer: mature results of a phase II trial. *J Clin Oncol* 1998;16:622.

43. Stuschke M, Eberhardt W, Pottkgen C, et al. Prophylactic cranial irradiation in locally advanced non-small-cell lung cancer after multimodality treatment: long-term follow-up and investigations of late neuropsychologic effects. *J Clin Oncol* 1999;17:2700.

44. Pass HI, Pogrebniak H, Steinberg SM, et al. Randomized trial of neoadjuvant therapy for lung cancer: interim analysis. *Ann Thorac Surg* 1992;53:992.

45. Yoneda S, Hibino S, Gotoh I, et al. A comparative trial on induction chemoradiotherapy followed by surgery or immediate surgery for stage III NSCLC. *Proc Am Soc Clin Oncol* 1995;14:367.

46. Roth J, Fossella F, Komaki R, et al. A randomized trial comparing perioperative chemotherapy and surgery with surgery alone in resectable stage III non–small cell lung cancer. *J Natl Cancer Inst* 1994;86:673.

47. Rosell R, Gomez-Codina J, Camps C, et al. A randomized trial comparing preoperative chemotherapy plus surgery with surgery alone in patients with non-small-cell lung cancer. *N Engl J Med* 1994;330:153.

48. Depierre A, Milleron B, Moro D, et al. Phase III trial of neoadjuvant chemotherapy in resectable stage I (except T1N0), II,

49. Roth JA, Atkinson EN, Fossella F, et al. Long-term follow-up of patients enrolled in a randomized trial comparing perioperative chemotherapy and surgery with surgery alone in resectable stage IIIA non-small-cell lung cancer. *Lung Cancer* 1998;21:1.

50. Fleck J, Camargo J, Godoy D, et al. Chemoradiation therapy versus chemotherapy alone as a neo-adjuvant treatment for stage III non–small cell lung cancer. Preliminary report of a phase III prospective randomized trial. *Proc Am Soc Clin Oncol* 1994;12:333.

51. Kubota K, Furuse K, Kawahara M, et al. Role of radiotherapy in combined modality treatment of locally advanced non–small cell lung cancer. *J Clin Oncol* 1994;12:1547.

52. Thomas M, Rube Ch, Semik M, et al. Randomized trial of chemotherapy and twice-daily chemoradiation versus chemotherapy alone before surgery in stage III non–small cell lung cancer: interim analysis of toxicity. *Proc Am Soc Clin Oncol* 1999;18:458a.

53. Furuse K, Fukuoka M, Kawahara M, et al., for the West Japan Lung Cancer Group. Phase III study of concurrent versus sequential thoracic radiotherapy in combination with mitomycin, vindesine and cisplatin in unresectable stage III non-small-cell lung cancer. *J Clin Oncol* 1999;17:2692.

54. Shepherd FA, Johnston MR, Payne D, et al. Randomized study of chemotherapy and surgery versus radiotherapy for stage IIIA non-small-cell lung cancer: a National Cancer Institute of Canada Clinical Trials Group Study. *Br J Cancer* 1998;78:683.

55. Inculet R, Scott C, Dar AR, et al. Phase III study comparing chemotherapy and radiation therapy with preoperative chemotherapy and surgical resection in patients with non–small cell lung cancer with spread to mediastinal lymph nodes: a Radiation Therapy Oncology Group study (RTOG 89–01). *Lung Cancer* 1997;18[Suppl 1]:65.

56. Elias ED, Herndon J, Kumar P, et al., for the Cancer and Leukemia Group B. A phase III comparison of "best local-regional therapy" with or without chemotherapy for stage IIIA T1–3N2 non–small cell lung cancer. *Proc Am Soc Clin Oncol* 1997;16:448a.

57. Pisters KMW, Ginsberg RJ, Putnam JB, et al., on behalf of the Bimodality Lung Oncology Team (BLOT). Induction paclitaxel and carboplatin in early stage non–small cell lung cancer: early results of a completed phase II trial. *Proc Am Soc Clin Oncol* 1999;18:467.

58. Reboul F, Vincent P, Chauvet B, et al. Concurrent chemoradiotherapy for stage III non–small cell lung cancer with cisplatin alone or cisplatin-etoposide: five year results. *Proc Perugia Int Cancer Conf* 1998;6:143.

59. Belani CP, Natale RB, Lee JS, et al. Randomized phase III trial comparing cisplatin/etoposide versus carboplatin/paclitaxel in advanced and metastatic non–small cell lung cancer. *Proc Am Soc Clin Oncol* 1998;17:455a.

60. Giaccone G, Splinter TAW, Dubruyne C, et al., for the European Organization for Research and Treatment of Cancer Lung Cancer Cooperative Group. Randomized study of cisplatin plus paclitaxel versus cisplatin plus teniposide in patients with advanced non-small-cell lung cancer. *J Clin Oncol* 1998;16:2133.

61. Choy H, Akerley W, Safran H, et al. Phase I trial of outpatient weekly paclitaxel and concurrent radiation therapy for advanced non-small-cell lung cancer. *J Clin Oncol* 1994;12:2682.

62. Choy H, Akerley W, Safran H, et al. Multiinstitutional phase II trial of paclitaxel, carboplatin and concurrent radiation therapy for locally advanced non-small-cell lung cancer. *J Clin Oncol* 1998;16:3316.

63. Frasci G, Comella P, Scoppa G, et al. Weekly paclitaxel and cisplatin with concurrent radiotherapy in locally advanced

non–small cell lung cancer. A phase I study. *J Clin Oncol* 1997; 15:1409.

64. Langer CJ, Movsas B, Hudes R, et al. Induction paclitaxel and carboplatin followed by concurrent chemoradiotherapy in patients with unresectable, locally advanced non–small cell lung carcinoma: report of Fox Chase Cancer Center Study 94–001. *Semin Oncol* 1997;24:S12–89.

65. Choy H. Author update on: phase I trial of outpatient weekly paclitaxel and concurrent radiation therapy for advanced non-small-cell lung cancer. *Classic Papers and Current Comments* 1997; 2:167.

66. Vokes EE, Leopold KA, Herndon JE II, et al. A randomized phase II study of gemcitabine or paclitaxel or vinorelbine with cisplatin as induction chemotherapy and concomitant chemoradiotherapy for unresectable stage III non–small cell lung cancer. *Proc Am Soc Clin Oncol* 1999;18:459a.

67. Bonomi P, Faber LP, Warren W, et al. Postoperative bronchopulmonary complications in stage III lung cancer patients treated with preoperative paclitaxel-containing chemotherapy and concurrent radiation. *Semin Oncol* 1997;24:S12–123.

68. Roberts JR, DeVore RF, Carbone P, et al. Neoadjuvant chemotherapy increases perioperative complications in patients undergoing resection for NSCLC. *Proc Am Soc Clin Oncol* 1999; 18:465a.

69. Harpole DH, Liptay MJ, DeCamp MM, et al. Prospective analysis of pneumonectomy: risk factors for major morbidity and cardiac dysrhythmias. *Ann Thorac Surg* 1996;61:977.

70. Ginsberg RJ, Hill LD, Eagen RT, et al. Modern thirty-day operative mortality for surgical resections in lung cancer. *J Thorac Cardiovasc Surg* 1983;86:654.

71. Mitsudomi T, Mizoue T, Yoshimatsu T, et al. Postoperative complications after pneumonectomy for treatment of lung cancer: multivariate analysis. *J Surg Oncol* 1996;61:218.

72. Zeldin RA, Normandin D, Landtwing D, et al. Post-pneumonectomy pulmonary edema. *J Thorac Cardiovasc Surg* 1984;87:359.

73. Mathru M, Blakeman B, Dries DJ, et al. Permeability pulmonary edema following lung resection. *Chest* 1990;98:1216.

74. Fowler WC, Langer CJ, Curran WJ, et al. Postoperative complications after combined neoadjuvant treatment of lung cancer. *Ann Thorac Surg* 1993;55:986.

75. Roach M, Gandara DR, Yuo H-S, et al. Radiation pneumonitis following combined modality therapy for lung cancer: analysis of prognostic factors. *J Clin Oncol* 1995;13:2606.

76. Albain K, Rusch V, Turrisi A, et al., for the Lung Cancer Intergroup. Interim update of the National Cancer Institute High Priority North American Intergroup Trial 0139(RTOG 9309) for stage IIIA(N2) non–small cell lung cancer: a phase III comparison of concurrent chemotherapy plus standard radiotherapy versus concurrent chemotherapy plus radiotherapy followed by surgical resection. *Proc Perugia Int Cancer Conf* 1998;6:35.

77. Splinter TAW, Kirkpatrick A, van Meerbeeck J, et al., for the EORTC Lung Cancer Cooperative Group and VKSL. (1997a) Randomized trial of surgery versus radiotherapy in patients with stage IIIA non–small cell lung cancer after a response to induction chemotherapy. Intergroup Study 08941. *Proc Am Soc Clin Oncol* 1998;17:453a.

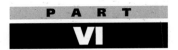

RADIATION THERAPY

45

RADIOTHERAPY FOR LOCALLY ADVANCED LUNG CANCER: AN OVERVIEW

WALTER J. CURRAN, Jr

WHAT IS LOCALLY ADVANCED NON–SMALL CELL LUNG CANCER?

The term locally advanced non–small cell lung cancer (LA-NSCLC) is used to describe disease that is too extensive for primary surgical resection, is limited to the thorax, and technically allows the inclusion of the entire tumor within a reasonable radiation field. This definition typically includes patients with bulky inoperable stage IIIA and stage IIIB lesions, usually with the exclusion of patients with a malignant pleural effusion. In the most recent revision of the staging system for lung cancer,[1] T3N0 tumors were assigned to stage IIB because of their distinctively more favorable prognosis when compared to lymph node–positive subgroups of stage IIIA. Although controversy exists regarding the selection of clinically stage IIIA patients for surgery as a component of their initial management, the following discussion addresses issues related to the management of patients whose treatment excludes surgery.

EFFECT OF THORACIC RT ON LOCAL CONTROL

Patients with LA-NSCLC comprised 25% to 40% of 178,100 new lung cancer patients diagnosed in 1997 in the United States.[2] Until recently, the standard treatment administered to those patients has been a six-week course of fractionated external beam thoracic radiation therapy (RT) to 60.0 Gray (Gy). The dose of photon irradiation has been investigated by trials conducted by the Radiation Therapy Oncology Group (RTOG). RTOG 73-01[3] randomized 551 patients to four arms of thoracic RT: 40.0 Gy delivered in a continuous fashion (2.0 Gy daily, 5 days a week, for 4 weeks) versus 40.0 Gy in a split course, versus 50.0 Gy continuous versus 60.0 Gy continuous. The highest treatment response rate (55%), the lowest rate of local tumor failures at 3 years (36% versus 63%), and the best three-year survival rate (20% versus 10%) were observed among patients assigned to the 60.0 Gy arm. Unfortunately,

these tumor control and survival advantages were lost by 5 years, with identical estimated local failures and survival rates in the 60.0 and 40.0 Gy arms of 70% and 7%, respectively. The dose 60.0 Gy over 6 weeks was adopted as the standard dose for definitive RT of patients with LA-NSCLC despite a six-year survival of only 5%. Lack of benefit of standard thoracic RT on survival was the main conclusion of a randomized Southeastern Cancer Study Group trial,[4] where 319 patients with LA-NSCLC received either thoracic RT, or single-agent vindesine, or both combined. The overall response rate was superior in both RT arms (30% versus 10%, p = 0.001), but median survival time (MST) was 8.4 months for patients receiving RT alone, 9.4 months for those receiving RT + vindesine and 10.1 months for those receiving vindesine (p = 0.58). The study reported a large (37%) proportion of patients on the vindesine arm receiving delayed RT, therefore making it a study of immediate versus delayed thoracic RT.

Reports on the ability of any nonoperative therapy to locally control LA-NSCLC vary markedly, depending on the nature of the assessment and the time interval since therapy. Furthermore, short survival and varying methods of assessing for local and distant failure compounds this problem. When posterior-anterior and lateral chest radiographs were used in RTOG 73-01[5] and a cross-section of the tumor or the pulmonary shadow is recorded, a complete response was reported in 24% of patients treated to 60.0 Gy, and a partial response in 32%. Another 35% had stable disease, and only 9% progressive disease. One has to note that those two-dimensional data may not reflect the true volumetric responses. When a complete response was defined rigorously as absence of tumor by the clinical, radiographic, and bronchoscopic examinations, with a negative endoscopic biopsy,[6] and the evaluation of a response repeated every 6 months, only 16% to 20% of patients had a complete response, 15% a partial response, 16% to 20% stable disease, and 45% to 53% progressive disease at 3 months after the completion of radiotherapy; however, at 3 years local control was only 7% to 8%. More recently, an impressive bronchoscopically verified local control of

71% at 2 years has been reported by King et al.,[7] with a higher dose, chemotherapy-assisted novel hyperfractionated accelerated RT to a total dose of 73.6 Gy, directed to the primary tumor and adjacent enlarged lymph nodes.

The tumor control probability for bronchogenic carcinoma can be estimated to be 10% for tumors of more than 4 cm at a dose of 80.0 Gy, with an assumption that an average sized lung cancer may require doses beyond 100.0 Gy to control tumor with a 50% to 80% probability.[8] Therefore, if the local tumor control is a prerequisite for improved survival, one may expect to start seeing the impact of a local control on survival only, when eradication of the tumor will be possible in more than 50% of treated patients.

MEDICALLY INOPERABLE STAGE I NSCLC AND LOCAL CONTROL

Radiotherapy can effectively control small lung tumors. There are several reports of a durable intrathoracic control achieved in patients with clinical stage I (T1 or T2) tumors.[9–15] Precise data on the relationship between tumor size (or volume) and the degree of local control are lacking in the radiotherapy literature, but it appears that the rate of local failure with standard thoracic RT increases sharply with the largest tumor diameter exceeding 3 or 4 cm. For example, the intrathoracic failure rate at 3 years was only 4% (1/24) in medically inoperable stage I patients whose tumors measured no more than 4 cm, but increased to 47.8% (11/23) in patients with larger tumors, treated with a hypofractionated course of RT to a dose of 48 or 56 Gy.[9] Similarly, Kupelian et al.[15] quote a local failure at 3 years of 11% for T1 lesions and 39% for T2 tumors, with significant favorable prognostic factors for local control being tumor size of less than or equal to 4 cm, no chest wall invasion, a radiation dose of at least 60 Gy, and a complete response at 6 months after RT. It appears, however, that with longer follow-up, local failure rates increase significantly, even for those small tumors.[11] Nevertheless, definitive RT can provide three-year cause-specific survivals of 30% to 49%[11,13,15] for patients with small tumors and no radiographic evidence of lymph node involvement, and serve as a noninvasive equivalent of wedge resection. A clear-cut dependence of local control and disease-free survival (DFS) of T1 tumors on RT dose is evident in several reports,[10,11,15] with DFS of 90% at 3 years when doses of 65 Gy or higher are used, compared to 29% if doses between 60–65 Gy are delivered (p = 0.0611).[10] Overall, it appears that the dose-response relationship in NSCLC is evident only for tumors 3 cm or smaller, at least within the range of doses of 60–65 Gy. In those patients with larger tumors, doses much higher than 65 Gy would likely have to be delivered to expect local control. This dose is difficult to achieve with larger tumors because of the constraints of toxicity to the surrounding normal tissues, mostly lung, spinal cord and heart.

Results of definitive RT cannot be directly compared to those of surgical resection because the pathologic status of regional lymph nodes is not routinely investigated prior to initiating RT, and patients often do not undergo as rigorous of a systemic staging before RT as they would before surgery.[13]

ALTERED FRACTIONATION RT IN THE TREATMENT OF LOCALLY ADVANCED NSCLC (SEE ALSO CHAPTER 47)

The realization that local control of lung cancer with conventional RT (2.0 Gy daily, 5 days per week) remains unsatisfactory has led to various efforts at optimizing RT, including the altering RT fractionation schedule. One such alteration, called *hyperfractionation* (HF), or delivery of a larger number of smaller fractions, may potentially allow a higher total dose to be delivered to the tumor and result in improved local control, with the same probability of late effects to surrounding normal tissues. Although the MST (13 months) and two-year survival rates (29%) in the 69.6 Gy arm appeared superior to the benchmark standard fractionation results, there was no apparent improvement in five-year survival results, ranging between 6% to 8% in all dose levels.[16] In a phase III study coordinated by the RTOG (RTOG 88-08/Eastern Cooperative Oncology Group [ECOG] 4588) (discussed in detail in the following section), the 69.6 Gy hyperfractionated dose was tested against two other arms, standard once-daily RT or induction chemotherapy/standard RT,[17] with HF RT producing an early survival result intermediate between the combined modality arm and standard RT, with one-year survival rates of 59% versus 51% versus 46%, respectively.

Continuous hyperfractionated accelerated radiation therapy (CHART) is a regimen that tested the hypothesis that tumor cell repopulation is an important cause of failure in conventional RT. To counteract repopulation, a continuous treatment regimen was designed, delivering 1.5 Gy three times per day on every day, including Saturday and Sunday, to a total dose of 54.0 Gy. An interval of at least 6 hours was maintained between RT fractions to avoid late toxicity in slowly repairing tissue, such as spinal cord. Preliminary results of a randomized trial[18] comparing CHART versus standard RT to 66.0 Gy in 563 patients with good performance LA-NSCLC has been published recently. With a minimum potential follow-up of 2 years, there was a significant improvement in survival for the CHART-treated patients over conventionally treated patients (30% versus 20%, p = 0.006). The incidence of acute esophagitis was higher in the CHART arm (49% versus 19%), but it subsided quickly in both arms and without apparent chronic sequelae. Although these results are exciting, longer observation is necessary before drawing final conclusions.

In the United States, thrice-daily RT was tested in the

RTOG 92-05 trial (1.1 Gy TID, 5 days a week, to 79.2 Gy). Results of this study are pending. An ECOG pilot study was also completed,[19] in which 1.5 Gy was delivered three times daily to a total dose of 57.6 Gy in 30 patients, with a one-year survival rate of 63%, which has provided the basis for a larger trial to assess the true efficacy of such a regimen.

ROLE OF RT IN SYMPTOMATIC CONTROL

For patients with known extrathoracic metastases, poor performance status, or intrathoracic disease not amenable to aggressive, full-dose irradiation, thoracic RT can still provide rapid and durable relief of several life-threatening or distressing symptoms. Intrathoracic symptoms palliated by thoracic RT in more than 80% of patients include hemoptysis, tumor-related pain, and superior vena cava obstruction. Cough and dyspnea are palliated in about two-thirds of patients, and atelectasis and vocal cord paralysis are improved in a smaller number of cases (23% and 6%, respectively).[20–22] A total symptomatic relief can be accomplished in 61% of patients.[20] It is important to note that comparative information regarding the ability of multiagent chemotherapy to palliate these symptoms is limited.

The optimal RT dose/fractionation schedule for palliation of intrathoracic symptoms is unsettled. Although most practicing radiation oncologists would agree that a six-week course of treatment is unnecessarily protracted for patients with known distant metastases, there is also concern that more accelerated courses may produce more severe treatment-related esophagitis. A randomized trial conducted by the Medical Research Council compared two RT fractionation schemes for 509 such patients: 39 Gy in thirteen daily fractions versus 17 Gy in two weekly 8.5 Gy fractions.[23] The symptoms were more rapidly palliated by the shorter regimen, and esophagitis was shorter lasting (6.5 days) in the two-fraction regimen than in the 13-fraction regimen (14 days).

PATIENT SELECTION

One of the observations derived from the RTOG 73-01[3] was a better treatment outcome (at 2 years) for patients with a favorable performance status (Karnofsky index of more than 70). Since then a body of evidence has been accumulated, attesting to the need to identify different prognostic groups within all patients with LA-NSCLC. A large group of patients (1,052) with locally advanced or metastatic NSCLC treated with cisplatinum-based chemotherapy by the European Lung Cancer Working Party was analyzed with regard to the prognostic factors for survival, using univariate and multivariate methods.[24] Among 16 pretreatment variables, a limited disease extent, good Karnofsky

performance status, normal leukocyte and neutrophil counts, normal serum calcium, absence of skin metastases, age less than 60, and female gender were all associated with a significantly improved survival. After application of recursive partitioning algorithm and amalgation algorithm, four subgroups of patients were identified, heterogeneous for survival. The best group included limited-disease females with Karnofsky index of at least 80, and these women had an MST of 14.1 months. The least favorable group were those patients with disseminated disease, abnormal leukocyte count, and poor Karnofsky index, and they had an MST of 3.3 months. A thorough knowledge of differences in outcome is essential for the proper design of therapeutic trials because an effective treatment applied to the *a priori* unfavorable group of patients may result in an erronous conclusion regarding the likelihood of treatment benefit.

COMBINED MODALITY STUDIES: CHEMOTHERAPY AND STANDARD FRACTIONATED RT

Because most patients with LA-NSCLC have metastatic disease at the time of their death,[3] the testing of systemic therapy in their management was a logical step. Several prospective randomized trials have been conducted to examine the role of chemotherapy in NSCLC, in addition to thoracic RT, with varying conclusions. Dillman et al. [Cancer and Leukemia Group B (CALGB) 8433][25] reported an MST of 13.7 months for patients receiving sequential treatment: induction chemotherapy with vinblastine/cisplatin for two cycles followed by 60.0 Gy standard fractionated RT, in comparison to 9.6 months for those receiving 60.0 Gy alone (p = 0.012). A seven-year follow-up report[26] confirmed a long-term improved survival rate for chemotherapy/RT-treated patients. It is crucial to emphasize that only favorable prognosis patients were eligible for the CALGB study; that is, those with minimal, if any, weight loss (maximum of 5%) and a Karnofsky score of at least 70.

Schaake-Koning et al. [European Organization of Research in the Treatment of Cancer (EORTC) 08844][27] reported that concurrent chemoradiation provides a statistically significant survival benefit over RT alone using a schedule of low-dose daily cisplatin or weekly cisplatin during RT. Although a survival benefit over TRT alone was observed in the low-dose daily cisplatin arm advantage (three-year survival rate of 16% versus 2%; p = 0.009), the weekly schedule did not provide a statistically significant benefit. The survival benefit of daily combined treatment appeared to be caused by improved control of local disease (p = 0.003).

LeChevalier et al. [French Multicenter Trial, CEBI 138][6] reported results similar to those of the Dillman trial but in 353 patients: 12-months MST for chemoradiotherapy versus 10 months for TRT alone. The relative risk of death was 1.2 for the radiotherapy arm compared to that of the chemoradiation arm. The metastasis rate was significantly lower in the combined modality arm (p < 0.001). Despite employing an RT dose of 65.0 Gy in both treatment arms, local tumor control rates, as evaluated at 3 months, were disappointingly low (15% to 17%). Complete remission was indicated in this study by the complete disappearance of all objective tumor shown by chest radiograph, and no evidence of new disease shown by optical and histologic examination during fiberoptic bronchoscopy.

In RTOG 88-04,[17] 30 patients received both induction vinblastine and cisplatin as well as concomitant cisplatin during a standard RT course. Although nearly 30% of enrolled patients did not meet the good performance status and minimal weight loss criteria, the survival results were encouraging, with an MST of 16.1 months and two-year survival rate of 34%.

Two metaanalyses using data extracted from all published randomized trials comparing RT to RT and cisplatin-based chemotherapy in LA-NSCLC were performed.[28,29] Although they differ with regard to the methodology used[30] (analysis based on published data versus based on the updated individual patient data), they both report a small improvement in survival (absolute benefit of 4% at 2 years and 2% at 5 years, or a lengthening of life by 4 months, or a 13% reduction in the risk of death).

In summary, although the observed benefits of chemotherapy in addition to thoracic RT are modest, they offer hope for progress and demonstrate that the role of chemotherapy should be further investigated.

COMBINED MODALITY STUDIES: CHEMOTHERAPY AND ALTERED FRACTIONATION RT

The RTOG has completed three phase II trials evaluating concomitant delivery of high-dose cisplatin-based chemotherapy and HF thoracic RT for LA-NSCLC. RTOG 90-15 enrolled 42 patients to receive immediate hyperfractionated RT (69.6 Gy) and cisplatin/vinblastine.[16] Toxic reactions were primarily hematologic, and MST was 12.1 months in this unfavorable patient population. Among the 10 most favorable patients in this protocol, the MST was 16 months. In RTOG 91-06,[31] 76 patients received immediate HF thoracic RT and concomitant cisplatin and oral etoposide. As recently analyzed, the estimated one-year survival rate is 67%, and MST is 19 months. Grade 4 hematologic toxic reactions in RTOG 91-06 were 43% and 57%, respectively, and were comparable to the 48% rate seen in the induction chemotherapy arm of RTOG 88-08; however, grade 3 or worse esophagitis was substantially worse, with a rate of 36% versus 4% in RTOG 88-08. A third phase II trial (RTOG 92-04) confirmed the encouraging results of RTOG 91-06 and RTOG 88-04.

Further evidence in support of improved survival with the addition of chemotherapy to HF RT came from the randomized Yugoslavian/Japanese study[32] of 131 patients, reporting an MST of 14 months for HF RT alone (69.6 Gy) versus 22 months for HF RT and carboplatinum/etoposide chemotherapy, with four-year survival rates of 9% versus 23%, respectively. Survival was probably improved as a result of improved local control, which may suggest a radiosensitizing effect of daily chemotherapy dosing in that study.

An ongoing RTOG study (94-10) attempts to define the optimal sequencing of chemotherapy in those patients, comparing sequential chemotherapy/RT to concurrent chemotherapy/RT and concurrent chemotherapy with HF RT. Using the MST of 13–14 months seen in both the RTOG and CALGB trials with sequential cisplatin-based chemoradiation, this trial is powered to detect a 43% improvement in MST based on the 19-month MST in the phase II RTOG trial of concurrent oral etoposide, cisplatin, and hyperfractionated RT.

CONFORMAL RADIOTHERAPY

Because the established pathways of the primary lung tumor spread follow the lymphatic flow from the tumor to the hilum, mediastinum, and supraclavicular lymph nodes, traditional radiation volumes include the primary lesion, ipsilateral hilum, bilateral mediastinum, and often ipsilateral supraclavicular region. Elective nodal irradiation has been commonplace since it was demonstrated that survival of patients treated on RTOG 73-01 who did not receive elective nodal RT was inferior to those who did.[33] However, there is a recent movement to limit the size of the RT fields to include gross primary and only known nodal disease, as defined by thoracic computerized tomography (CT) scans. Because larger RT field sizes have limited total dose and have been related to increased acute and late toxicity,[34–36] several investigators have delivered thoracic RT to the gross tumor only, reporting no compromise in locoregional control or survival.[15,37–39] Although there is interest in treating smaller RT volumes in lung cancer, this concept remains a project without firmly established benefits and risks (see also Chapter 48).

Tumor volume definition is improved with three-dimensional (3-D) planning, and doses to critical structures can often be reduced, especially if multiple noncoplanar beams are used.[40] An ongoing RTOG study is evaluating the feasibility of dose escalation for patients with LA-NSCLC, treated with 3D conformal RT to the gross tumor only, without elective nodal irradiation. Maximum doses as high as 77.4–90.3 Gy are being planned, depending on the percentage of the total lung receiving more than 20.0 Gy. Such dose escalation is based on pilot experience,[41] correlating the incidence of grade 3 or higher radiation pneumonitis with the percentage volume of normal lung to doses exceeding 20.0 Gy. There is also a prospective trial ongoing at the University of Michigan in which total RT doses are also partitioned according to the percentage of the entire lung volume receiving 20.0 Gy. Among patients with the lowest percentage of lung receiving 20.0 Gy, the current prescribed doses are more than 100.0 Gy.[39]

FUTURE DIRECTIONS

The prognosis of the vast majority of patients with LA-NSCLC remains poor, and more effective therapeutic approaches need to be investigated, including RT dose escalation and novel chemotherapy agents. Identification of prognostic factors may facilitate the design of clinical trials, allowing physicians to limit more aggressive and more toxic approaches to the subgroups of patients who may derive benefit from them.

Development of improved staging methods, based not only on radiographic evidence of anatomic organ enlargements (CXR, CT), but also on functional and immunologic or molecular techniques, such as immunohistochemical assessment of individual tumor cells in lymph nodes,[42] functional scans (labeled monoclonal antibodies; thallium-201 or PET scans),[43–45] may allow definition of more uniform patient populations with predictable treatment outcomes.

Finally, an international effort to increase participation of adult patients in clinical trials from the current 2% of all patients with cancer to larger percentages would allow for a more effective investigation of new therapeutic modalities and a faster establishment of new standards of care.

REFERENCES

1. Mountain CF. Revisions in the international system for staging lung cancer [see comments]. *Chest* 1997;111(6):1710.
2. Parker SL, Tong T, Bolden S, et al. Cancer statistics, 1997 [published erratum appears in *CA Cancer J Clin* 1997;47(2):68]. *CA Cancer J Clin* 1997;47(1):5.
3. Perez CA, Pajak TF, Rubin P, et al. Long-term observations of the patterns of failure in patients with unresectable non-oat cell carcinoma of the lung treated with definitive radiotherapy. *Cancer* 1987;59:1874.
4. Johnson DH, Einhorn LH, Bartolucci A, et al. Thoracic radiotherapy does not prolong survival in patients with locally advanced, unresectable non-small cell lung cancer [see comments]. *Ann Intern Med* 1990;113(1):33.
5. Perez CA, Stanley K, Rubin P, et al. A prospective randomized study of various irradiation doses and fractionation schedules in the treatment of inoperable non-oat-cell carcinoma of the lung. *Cancer* 1980;45:2744.
6. Le Chevalier T, Arriagada R, Quoix E, et al. Radiotherapy alone versus combined chemotherapy and radiotherapy in nonresectable non-small-cell lung cancer: first analysis of a randomized trial in 353 patients. *J Natl Cancer Inst* 1991;83:417.
7. King SC, Acker JC, Kussin PS, et al. High-dose, hyperfractionated, accelerated radiotherapy using a concurrent boost for the treatment of nonsmall cell lung cancer: unusual toxicity and

promising early results. *Int J Radiat Oncol Biol Phys* 1996;36: 593.
8. Emami B. Three-dimensional conformal radiation therapy in bronchogenic carcinoma. *Semin Radiation Oncol* 1996;6:92.
9. Slotman BJ, Njo KH, Karim A BMF. Curative radiotherapy for technically operable stage I nonsmall cell lung cancer. *Int J Radiat Oncol Biol Phys* 1994;29:33.
10. Dosoretz DE, Galmanini D, Rubenstein JH, et al. Local control in medically inoperable lung cancer: an analysis of its importance in outcome and factors determining the probability of tumor eradication. *Int J Radiat Oncol Biol Phys* 1993;27:507.
11. Kaskowitz L, Graham MV, Emami B, et al. Radiation therapy alone for stage I non-small cell lung cancer. *Int J Radiat Oncol Biol Phys* 1993;27:517.
12. Graham PH, Gebski VJ, Stat M, et al. Radical radiotherapy for early nonsmall cell lung cancer. *Int J Radiat Oncol Biol Phys* 1995; 31:261.
13. Sandler HM, Curran WJ, Turrisi AT. The influence of tumor size and pre-treatment staging on outcome following radiation therapy alone for stage I non-small cell lung cancer. *Int J Radiat Oncol Biol Phys* 1990;19:9.
14. Noordijk EM, Poest Clement, Evd Wever AMJ, et al. Radiotherapy as an alternative to surgery in elderly patients with resectable lung cancer. *Radiother Oncol* 1988;13:83.
15. Kupelian PA, Komaki R, Allen P. Prognostic factors in the treatment of node-negative nonsmall cell lung carcinoma with radiotherapy alone. *Int J Radiat Oncol Biol Phys* 1996;36:607.
16. Byhardt RW, Scott CB, Ettinger DS, et al. Concurrent hyperfractionated irradiation and chemotherapy for unresectable nonsmall cell lung cancer. *Cancer* 1995;75:2337.
17. Sause W, Scott C, Taylor S, et al. Radiation Therapy Oncology Group (RTOG) 88-08 and Eastern Cooperative Oncology Group (ECOG) 4588: preliminary results of a phase III trial in regionally advanced, unresectable non-small-cell lung cancer. *J Natl Cancer Inst* 1995;87:198.
18. Saunders MI, Dische S, Barrett A, et al. Randomized multicentre trials of CHART vs. conventional radiotherapy in head and neck and non-small cell lung cancer: an interim report. *Br J Cancer* 1996;73:1455.
19. Tannehill SP, Froseth C, Wagner H, et al. A multi-institutional Phase II study of hyperfractionated accelerated radiation therapy for unresectable non-small cell lung cancer: initial report of ECOG 4593. *Int J Radiation Oncol Biol Phys* 1996;36:207.
20. Slawson RG, Scott RM. Radiation therapy in bronchogenic carcinoma. *Radiology* 1979;132:175.
21. Stanley KE. Prognostic factors for survival in patients with inoperable lung cancer. *J Natl Cancer Inst* 1980;65:25.
22. Lutz ST, Huang DT, Ferguson CL, et al. A retrospective quality of life analysis using the lung cancer symptom scale in patients treated with palliative radiotherapy for advanced nonsmall cell lung cancer. *Int J Radiat Oncol Biol Phys* 1997;37:117.
23. Macbeth FR, Bolger JJ, Hopwood P, et al. Randomized trial of palliative two fraction versus more intensive 13-fraction radiotherapy for patients with inoperable non-small cell lung cancer and good performance status. Medical Research Council Lung Cancer Working Party. *Clin Oncol* 1996;8:167.
24. Paesmans M, Sculier JP, Libert G, et al. J. Prognostic factors for survival in advanced non-small-cell lung cancer: univariate and multivariate analyses including recursive partitioning and amalgamation algorithms in 1,052 patients. *J Clin Oncol* 1995;13: 1221.
25. Dillman RO, Seagren SL, Herndon J, et al. A randomized trial of induction chemotherapy plus high-dose radiation versus radiation alone in stage III non-small-cell lung cancer. *N Engl J Med* 1990;323:940.
26. Dillman RO, Herndon J, Seagren SL, et al. Improved survival

in stage III non-small cell lung cancer: seven-year follow-up of Cancer and Leukemia Group B (CALGB) 8433 trial. *J Natl Cancer Inst* 1996;88:1210.

27. Schaake-Koning C, Van Den Bogert W, Dalesio O, et al. Effects of concomitant cisplatin and radiotherapy in inoperable non-small cell lung cancer. *N Engl J Med* 1992;326:524.

28. Marino P, Preatoni A, Cantoni A. Randomized trials of radiotherapy alone vs. combined chemotherapy and radiotherapy in stages IIIa and IIIb nonsmall cell lung cancer: a meta-analysis. *Cancer* 1995;76:593.

29. Non-Small Cell Lung Cancer Collaborative Group. Chemotherapy in non-small cell lung cancer: a meta-analysis using updated individual patients data from 52 randomized clinical trials. *Br Med J* 1995;311:899.

30. Pignon JP. Randomized trials of radiotherapy alone versus combined chemotherapy and radiotherapy in stages IIIa and IIIb non-small cell lung cancer: a meta-analysis. *Cancer* 1996;77:2413.

31. Lee JS, Scott C, Komaki R, et al. Concurrent chemoradiation therapy with oral etoposide and cisplatin for locally advanced inoperable non-small-cell lung cancer: radiation therapy oncology group protocol 91-06. *J Clin Oncol* 1996;14(4):1055.

32. Jeremic B, Shibamoto Y, Acimovic L, et al. Hyperfractionated radiation therapy with or without concurrent low-dose daily carboplatin/etoposide for stage III non-small-cell lung cancer: a randomized study. *J Clin Oncol* 1996;14:1065.

33. Perez CA, Stanley K, Grundy G. Impact of irradiation technique and tumor extent in tumor control and survival of patients with unresectable non-oat cell carcinoma of the lung. *Cancer* 1982; 48:101.

34. Curran WJ, Moldofsky PH, Solin LJ. Analysis of the influence of elective nodal irradiation on postirradiation pulmonary function. *Cancer* 1990;65:2488.

35. Byhardt RW, Martin L, Pajak TF, et al. The influence of field size and other treatment factors on pulmonary toxicity following hyperfractionated irradiation for inoperable non-small cell lung cancer (NSCLC)—analysis of a radiation therapy oncology group (RTOG) protocol. *Int J Radiat Oncol Biol Phys* 1993;27: 537.

36. Oetzel D, Schraube P, Hensley F, et al. Estimation of pneumonitis risk in three-dimensional treatment planning using dose-volume histogram analysis. *Int J Radiat Oncol Biol Phys* 1995;33: 455.

37. Krol A, Aussems P, Noordijk EM, et al. Local irradiation alone for peripheral stage I lung cancer: could we omit the elective regional nodal irradiation? *Int J Radiat Oncol Biol Phys* 1996;34: 297.

38. Emami B, Scott C, Byhardt R, et al. The value of regional nodal radiotherapy (dose/volume) in the treatment of unresectable non-small cell lung cancer: an RTOG analysis. *Int J Radiat Oncol Biol Phys* 1996;36:209.

39. Hayman J, Martel M, Ten Haken R, et al. Dose escalation in non small cell lung cancer: using conformal 3-dimensional radiotherapy. Update of a phase I trial. *Proc Am Soc Clin Oncol* 1999; 18:459a.

40. Graham MV, Matthews JW, Harms WB, et al. Three-dimensional radiation treatment planning study for patients with carcinoma of the lung. *Int J Radiat Oncol Biol Phys* 1994;29:1105.

41. Graham MV, Shiue K, Emami B, et al. Dose-volume correlations with early pneumonitis for #D treatment planning for non-small cell lung cancer patients. *Int J Radiat Oncol Biol Phys* (in press).

42. Passlick B, Izbicki JR, Kubuschok B, et al. Immunohistochemical assessment of individual tumor cells in lymph nodes of patients with non-small-cell lung cancer. *J Clin Oncol* 1994;12:1827.

43. Vansant JP, Johnson DH, O'Donnell DM, et al. Staging lung carcinoma with a Tc-99m labeled monoclonal antibody. *Clin Nucl Med* 1992;17:431.

44. Takekawa H, Takaoka K, Tsukamoto E, et al. Thallium 201 single photon emission computed tomography as an indicator of prognosis for patients with lung carcinoma. *Cancer* 1997;80:198.

45. Frank A, Lefkowitz D, Jaeger S, et al. Decision logic for retreatment of asymptomatic lung cancer recurrence based on positron emission tomography findings. *Int J Radiat Oncol Biol Phys* 1995;32(5):1495.

46

RESECTABLE NON—SMALL CELL LUNG CANCER IN THE MEDICALLY INOPERABLE PATIENT: CURATIVE MANAGEMENT WITH RADIATION THERAPY

HENRY WAGNER, Jr

Surgery produces better survival than radiotherapy. In 1963, Morrison and colleagues published the results of a prospective trial, conducted between 1954 and 1958 by the Medical Research Council (MRC), which randomized 58 patients with clinically operable carcinoma of the lung to surgery or radical radiation therapy.[1] Survival at four years was seven of 30 (23%) for the surgery patients versus two of 28 (7%) for the radiation therapy patients, which was "almost significant" at the 5% level. When only patients with squamous cell carcinoma were considered, excluding cases with anaplastic carcinoma (ten surgery, nine radiation therapy) and two otherwise unclassified cases in the radiation therapy group, the survival differences were more pronounced (30% versus 6% at four years) and significant at the $p = 0.05$ level. These superior results for surgery were obtained despite the fact that only 17 of the 30 cases randomized to surgery were able to undergo potentially curative resections and there were three postoperative deaths in this group, very low resectability, and high postoperative mortality by present standards. "Under the conditions in which this trial has been conducted it appears that surgery is the better method for treatment for operable cases of squamous carcinoma of the lung." Some incorrectly assume that radical radiation therapy was of little if any value in the treatment of patients with lung cancer. Equally unsupported is the assertion that unresected disease was incurable disease.

Not all patients with resectable tumors, however, are fit candidates for surgery. Other patients adamantly refuse surgery despite its appropriateness as the treatment most likely to cure them. Since chronic tobacco abuse ravages the physiologic function of the cardiopulmonary system, and the median age for lung cancer in the United States is about 65, many patients with early-stage lung cancers, whose tumors are suitable for resection, are poor operative candidates. Despite marked improvements in operative and postoperative management of patients with limited cardio-

pulmonary reserve, some patients pose too high a risk of immediate postoperative complications or chronic respiratory insufficiency for surgery to be feasible.

Over the past several decades many institutions have reported their results using radical radiation therapy for patients with clinically operable non–small cell lung cancer (NSCLC). Generally these conclude that radiotherapy represents a valid treatment option for patients medically inoperable or refusing surgery. Some results have been sufficiently positive to suggest that thoracic radiotherapy might equal surgery for lung cancer, particularly for elderly patients, warranting a modern direct prospective comparative trial. This chapter reviews these series and discusses several points critical to assessment of the proper role of radical radiation therapy for patients with stage I-II NSCLC. These include patient selection, patterns of failure, radiation therapy technique, treatment volumes, treatment dose and fractionation, and investigational approaches to improved local and systemic control appropriate for this population.

While surgical resection remains the present standard of care for these patients, all standards shift. At the time of the original MRC trial, pneumonectomy was considered the appropriate operation for most patients, even those with early-stage disease. Now most of these patients would be treated with lobectomy and even less aggressive resections, such as segmentectomy or wedge resection, particularly for patients with compromised cardiopulmonary function. However, a prospective trial by the Lung Cancer Study Group, which randomized patients with T1N0M0 NSCLC to lobectomy or lung conserving resection (segmentectomy or nonanatomic wedge resection), showed that the more conservative resections were associated with significantly higher rates of overall and local recurrence, and a 50% increase in the rate of death with cancer ($p = 0.10$).[2] The conservative resections did not reduce acute or late pulmonary morbidity, and thus could not be recommended.

TABLE 46.1. MORBIDITY OF RESECTION IN PATIENTS WITH LUNG CANCER

Type of Resection and Age of Patient	Number of Resections	30-Day Mortality (%)
All resections	2,220	3.7
Pneumonectomy	569	6.2
Lobectomy	1,508	2.9
Segmentectomy or wedge resection	143	1.4
<50	230	1.3
50–59	617	1.3
60–69 years	920	4.1
70–79	416	7.0
≥80	37	8.1

From Ginsberg R, Hill L, Eagan R, et al. Modern day operative mortality for surgical resection in lung cancer. *J Thorac Cardiovasc Surg* 1983;86:654, with permission.

SURGICAL MORTALITY

As shown in Table 46.1, operative mortality rises with both the age of the patient and the extent of resection performed, from 1.3% for patients less than 60 years old to 8.1% for patients over 80, and from 1.4% for limited resections to 6.2% for pneumonectomy.[3] The greater mortality for older patients, particularly since these were selected as fit for surgery, must be weighed with other factors in the choice of their optimal treatment (see also Chapter 41). Furthermore, these data represent results obtained by thoracic surgeons with particular interest and expertise in the management of lung cancer. One might anticipate poorer results for either general or cardiothoracic surgeons without special training or experience in lung surgery. In one series, 1,538 resections were analyzed; one half of lobectomies and nearly 60% of pneumonectomies were performed by general surgeons. Mortality was significantly higher for lobectomies performed by general surgeons rather than thoracic surgeons (5.3% versus 3.0%; p less than 0.05), in patients with major comorbidity (43.6% versus 25.4%; p = 0.03) or age over 65 years (7.4% versus 3.5% p less than 0.05). The number of resections performed differed strikingly, with 70% of general surgeons performing fewer than ten resections per year and 75% of thoracic surgeons performing more than ten cases per year.[4,5]

Several strategies may be effective in reducing postoperative pulmonary complications in patients at risk.[6] Preoperatively patients should undergo optimization of lung function, including smoking cessation for several weeks, treatment of airflow obstruction and infection, when present, and education regarding postoperative lung expansion maneuvers. Good postoperative pain control and vigorous attention to lung expansion by methods including deep breathing exercises, incentive spirometry, or continuous positive airway pressure are also important. Attention to such details may make the difference between an uncompli-

cated resection and a complicated one, or a patient deemed medically inoperable and one at acceptable risk for resection.

RESULTS OF SURGICAL THERAPY: STAGING BIAS

In comparing the results of surgical and nonsurgical therapy, it is essential to be aware of the potential biases in comparing clinically versus surgically staged patients. Patients who receive nonsurgical therapy for stage I-II disease have clinical rather than surgical staging. Ideally, we would want to compare the results of radical radiation therapy with the results of radical surgery in a population of similar age, and compare clinical stage to clinical stage rather than clinical stage to pathological stage. Such a direct comparison cannot be made without accurate assessment of mediastinal nodes.

Mountain, in his 1986 article describing the data for 3,753 patients on which the International Staging System was based, reported five-year survivals by both clinical and surgical stage. The results were markedly better for the surgically staged patients in most TNM subgroups.[7] Despite detailed imaging of the hila and mediastinum by CT or MRI, the ability to distinguish between reactively enlarged and metastatic nodes is imperfect, as is the ability to detect metastatic disease in nodes of normal size. Inaccuracy results in false-positive and -negative rates of 20% to 30%. While radiographic upstaging does occur, more commonly occult microscopic N1 or N2 disease occurs, resulting in the surgical upstaging of patients clinically classified as N0. Oda and colleagues have reported a series of patients with peripheral T1 NSCLC and normal mediastinal nodes by CT.[8] However, microscopic involvement of N1 or N2 nodes occurred in about 15% of patients with squamous cell carcinoma and about 25% with adenocarcinoma. These frequencies of occult nodal involvement and surgical upstaging have implications both for attempts to compare surgically and nonsurgically staged and treated patients and in determining appropriate target volumes for radiation therapy.

Positron emission tomography (PET) with [18]fluorodeoxyglucose (FDG) has been reported to improve the sensitivity and specificity when combined with CT scanning, with some investigators reporting better than 90% for these parameters.[9–14] It remains to be seen how well these results will stand up with more general availability of this technology outside of specialized centers. If its accuracy is corroborated, FDG scanning may provide comparability of surgical and nonsurgical staging and may obviate the benefit of invasive staging procedures for some patients.

In choosing treatment, it is important to consider both the physician's and the patient's assessment of relative risk and evaluation of short-term and long-term survival. McNeil and associates reported a study of 14 patients with operable (stage I-II) NSCLC who had recently undergone treatment (surgery in six, radiation therapy in eight).[15] Through a structured interview technique, they attempted to elicit preferences for a guarantee of survival at an early date as compared with the likelihood of survival at some later time. Their survival model, based on surgical data and the radiation therapy data of Hilton and Smart,[16] was that radiation therapy would yield a greater probability of short-term survival, while surgery was more likely to obtain long-term survival. The actual probabilities of survival with surgical and nonsurgical therapy, as well as the perioperative mortality used in this study are based on series from the 1950s through the 1970s, and do not reflect results of current treatment. Within the limitations of these data, however, the analysis suggested that, while surgery was more likely to be curative for almost all age groups of patients, the preference of most patients for early versus later survival probability would lead them to favor radiation therapy. The authors speculated that the phenomenon of patients being more risk-averse than their (generally younger and healthier) physicians may be common. The concept that patients may well have different preferences regarding early versus late utilities of differing modes of therapy is probably valid, and should be taken into account in making recommendations for the individual patient. An updated study using prospective rather than retrospective interviews and using modern estimates of operative mortality and survival with surgery or radiation therapy would provide useful information. As lung cancer becomes increasingly a disease of former rather than active smokers and with an increasing incidence in women, there may well be shifts in patient preferences for more or less aggressive risks of treatments balanced against potentials for long-term survival. In practice, it is essential to introduce the concept of early versus late risks to the patient and help them to make an individually appropriate decision.

OVERVIEW OF TREATMENT RESULTS

Table 46.2 summarizes the results of published series describing results of radical radiation therapy for patients with early-stage NSCLC. There is considerable variation in the clinical stages of the patients treated (as well as the techniques used for ascertaining stage), characteristics of the patients (Table 46.3), and details of radiation therapy technique (Table 46.4). With these cautions, however, several clear conclusions may be reached from these data, which span four decades.

1. Radiation therapy can produce long-term survival in a proportion of these patients, ranging from 6% for ill-staged patients to 42% for patients with T1N0M0 disease. The variability of staging and treatment technique limit confidence about the exact five-year survival rates.
2. Survival of patients treated with radical radiation therapy

is inferior to that of patients with similar clinical stage selected for surgical resection by either open thoracotomy or thoracoscopy.
3. Local failure within the irradiated volume is frequent, with the best series reporting 30% local failure for T1 lesions, and rising to 70% for T2 lesions. Local failure rates following surgery, even with limited resections, are less than 20%. These high local failure rates suggest that the difference in survival between the surgical and radiotherapeutic series is not due solely to stage imbalance but reflects in part the inferior local control achieved with the technique and doses of radiation therapy used. Improved radiation therapy techniques for target volume delineation, dose delivery, and fractionation may improve local control and survival.

PATTERNS OF FAILURE

Determining patterns of failure in patients with lung cancer treated with radiation therapy is essential to improvement of treatment, but these data are frustratingly difficult to obtain. Accurate distinction between tumor recurrence and postradiation can be difficult. Patients who develop systemic disease will usually die rapidly, often before local recurrence can become apparent. Differing statistical methodologies for reporting failure rates (crude ratio, actuarial risk, competing risk models) can produce different apparent rates for the same data. With these caveats in mind, Table 46.5 summarizes the reported patterns of failure for published series treating patients with clinical stage I-II NSCLC with irradiation alone. It must be cautioned that these series did not generally specify either how (clinical, radiographic for symptomatic sites only, thorough restaging) or when (first failure, site of any failure during the patient's life, autopsy distribution of disease) these failure patterns were reported. In the following sections we consider treatment and patient factors that relate to treatment outcome.

OPTIMAL DOSE AND FRACTIONATION

A detailed analysis of failure patterns as a function of both stage and radiation dose is found in the series reported by Dosoretz and colleagues.[17] These are valuable data, but note that the series was retrospective, spanned a period of eight years, and a wide range of radiation doses was used (from less than 50 to over 70 Gy, although the majority of patients (91 of 152) received doses between 60 and 69 Gy). They reported a decrease in local failure with increasing dose; however, this decrease is seen only at the highest dose level (over 70 Gy), which was given to fewer than ten patients. Considering all patients in the series, the actuarial risk of local failure was 50% for patients receiving under 50 Gy, 57.8% for 50 to 59 Gy, 60.2% for 60 to 69 Gy, and 33.3%

TABLE 46.2. RADIATION THERAPY FOR PATIENTS WITH CLINICALLY RESECTABLE NSCLC

Author	Patients	Stage (Clinical)	Dose (Gy)	Median Survival	Two-Year Survival	Five-Year Survival	Local Failure (%)
Morrison[1]	28	operable	45/4 wks	n/a	14%	6% 4yr	n/a
Smart[68*]	40	operable	50–55 (250kV)	~30 mo	~50%	22%	n/a
Coy[69*α]	141	T1–3Nx	50–57.5 Gy	n/a	31%	11%	45#
Cooper[70]	72	T1–3N0–1	variable	9 mo	n/a	6%	n/a
Hafty[24]	43	T1–2N0–1	54–59	28 mo	60%	21%	39
Noordijk[25]	50	T1–2N0	60	25 mo	56%	16%	70
Zhang[19]	44	T1–2N0–2 (80% T1–2N0)	55–70	>36 mo	~55%	32%	27% for those with data
Talton[71]	77	T1–3N0	60	17 mo	36%	17%	n/a
Sandler[72]	77	T1–2	60	20 mo	30%	~10%	56+
Ono[20]	38	T1N0	60–70	~40 mo	68%	42%	–n/a
Dosoretz[17]	152	T1–3N0–1	50–70	17 mo	40%	10%	70%
	44	T1	"	not reached	~60%	~60%	30%
	63	T2	"	~12 mo	~30%	~10%	80%
	41	T3	"	~12 mo	~30%	~10%	86%
Hayakawa[21]	17	Stage I	60–80β		75%	31%	n/a
	47	Stage II	60–80β		44%	22%	n/a
Rosenthal[73]	62	T1–2N1	18–65 (median 60)	17.9 mo	33%	12%	60%
Kaskowitz[27]	53	T1–2N0	50–70 (median 63)	20.9 mo	43%	6%	55%
Graham[74]	103	Stage I–II	median 60, mean 56.8	16.1	35%	14%	n/a
Gauden[75]	347	T1–2N0M0	50Gy/20Fx/4 wks	27.9 mo	~50%	27% / 32% T1 / 21% T2	n/a
Kupelian[76]	71	T1–4N0	median 62.2	16 mo	~30%	12%	11% T1 / 39% T2 / 58% T3 / 45% T4
Morita[27]	149	I	55–75 (mean 64.7)	27.3 mo	34.2% 3yr	22.2	57% of 116 patients dying within 5 years
Sibley[77]	156	I	50–80 (median 64)	18 mo	39%	13%	42% local only

* Includes some patients with small cell carcinoma.
α Includes some patients with unresectable proximal T3 lesions.
Data from autopsies of 31 patients (22% of entire series), of whom 14 had locoregional disease, 17 disseminated disease, and 6 with no evidence of disease.
β Dose received by "majority of patients." Some received lower doses, and 13 patients showing a good response at 70 Gy were boosted to 80 Gy or higher.

for over 70 Gy (p = 0.13).[18] However, only four patients were in each of the highest and lowest dose groups. Disease-free survival at 30 months was better for patients receiving doses under 65 Gy, compared with 60 to 65 Gy both for patients with tumors over 3 cm (90% versus 29%, p = 0.06) and under 5 cm (39% versus 20%, p = 0.02), but not for tumors of intermediate size (p = 0.35). With the multiple analyses performed in this study, the likelihood of finding some reasonable correlations by chance is high. In any case, the arguments made regarding dose-control relations are more desired than established by the data.

Zhang and associates also reported improved local control and survival with higher radiation doses.[19] Patients receiving 55 to 61 Gy had five-year survival of 27% (six of 22) versus 36% (eight of 22) for those receiving 69 to 70 Gy (significance not stated). Local recurrence was seen in

eight of 22 (36%) of the low-dose group versus four of 22 (18%) of the high-dose group. While the trends are in line with expectation, these numbers are very small. In Ono's and colleagues' series, the number of five-year survivors was three of five (60%) for doses over 60 Gy, four of 11 (36%) for 60 to 69 Gy, and ten of 22 (45%) for 70 Gy.[20] Both series are too small for establishing either reliable survival or local control rates.

Hayakawa reported slightly better two-year survival for patients receiving ≥80 Gy (54%) than for those receiving doses of ≥70 Gy (37%) or ≥60 Gy, but this apparent advantage was lost over the next several years, and the best five-year survival was seen for the 60 to 69 Gy group, which had a five-year survival of 24% versus 8% for the ≥80 Gy group.[21] There was no suggestion of superiority of the 70 to 79 Gy group over the 60 to 69 Gy group at any time

TABLE 46.3. RADIATION THERAPY FOR PATIENTS WITH CLINICALLY RESECTABLE NSCLC: CLINICAL CHARACTERISTICS

Author	Patients	Stage (clinical)	Median Age	% with KPS <70 or ECOG (2–3)	% with Weight Loss >5%	Squamous Cell (%)	Exclusions
Morrison[1]	28	operable	n/a	n/a	n/a	60.7	included 25% with anaplastic cancer. Excluded patients unable to undergo pneumonectomy
Smart[68]*	40	operable	57.7 (average)	n/a	n/a	63.1	included 25% with SCLC
Coy[69]*[a]	141	T1-T3 "localized"	60–69	0	n/a	68.1	KPS <70
Cooper[70]	72	T1-T3	66	n/a	n/a	72	N2 nodes on mediastinoscopy
Hafty[24]	43	T1, T2	64 (mean)	n/a	n/a	53	any attempt at surgery before or after RT
Noordijk[25]	50	T1, T2	74 (mean)	0	n/a	n/a	KPS <80
Zhang[19]	44	T1–2N0–2 (only 2 N2 Pts.)	57.1	n/a	n/a	63.6	n/a
Talton[71]	77	T1–3N0	n/a	n/a	n/a	84.0	<60 Gy
Sandler[76]	77	T1, T2	70+	18.2	n/a	57.1	prior malignancy
Ono[20]	38	T1N0	n/a	n/a	n/a	50	n/a
Dosoretz[17]	152	T1-T3	74	<17	n/a	n/a	noncurati ve intent
Hayakawa[21]	17	Stage I-III	70+	39.5	n/a	100	n/a
Rosenthal[73]	62	T1–2N1	68	33.8	40.2	64.5	patients receiving chemo. or altered fractionation
Kaskowitz[23]	53	T1–2N0	73	9.4	32.1	60.4	failure to complete RT
Graham[74]	103	Stage I-II	67	13%	less than 33%	48*	From 150 cases referred for radiotherapy, 18 received no treatment, 21 palliative RT, and 8 surgery
Gauden[75]	347	T1–2N0M0	70	13%	n/a	61%	noncurative intent
Kupelian[76]	71	T1–4N0	n/a	43%	n/a	47%	
Morita[27]	149	Stage I	74.6	n/a	n/a	50	patients who received over 55 Gy
Sibley[77]	156	T1–2N0	70	n/a	26%	52	n/s or n/a

* Includes some patients with small cell carcinoma.
[a] Includes some patients with unresectable proximal T3 legions.

interval. The poor late results for the high-dose group were attributed to a high incidence (four of 13) of fatal bronchial stenoses in this group.[22] These results correlating dose and survival were for all patients in the series, about half of whom had stage IIIA or IIIB disease, and were not reported separately for the stage I and II patients. Kaskowitz and associates reported trends favoring improved local control and survival for patients receiving doses ≥65 Gy, but these did not reach statistical significance.[23]

Hafty and colleagues reported that, in their series of 43 patients, local control and survival was superior for the 11 patients receiving continuous-course RT than for the 32 receiving split-course treatment.[24] Overall five-year survival for the entire patient group was 21%, while it was 45% for the patients receiving continuous-course RT versus 12%

for those treated with split course. There was, however, an imbalance in prognostic factors between the two groups, with a higher percentage of patients with T1 tumors (36% versus 25%) in the group receiving continuous course radiation therapy. Several other series which have reported excellent survival, including those of Noordijk and colleagues and Ono and colleagues, have used split-course treatment for all patients.[20,25] In the U.S., the bias against split-course treatment may have resulted in assignment of this technique for patients with poorer expected outcome.

TREATMENT VOLUME

Hayakawa and associates noted a strong inverse correlation between portal size and survival.[21] For patients treated to

TABLE 46.4. RADIATION THERAPY FOR PATIENTS WITH CLINICALLY RESECTABLE NSCLC: TECHNICAL DETAILS

Author	Dose Range (Gy)	Average	Continuous (C) vs. Split-Course (SC)	Field Size (cm)	Hilum Treated?	Mediastinum Treated?
Morrison[1]	45/4 wk (planned)	n/a	C	120 cm² average	yes	yes
Smart[68]*	40–45 or undifferentiated 50–55 for squamous cell*	n/a	C	n/a	yes for undifferentiated; ? for squamous cell	yes for undifferentiated; no for squamous cell
Coy[69]*[a]	50–57.5/4 wk	n/a	C	6 × 7 to 10 × 15	n/a	n/a
Cooper[70]	26% <30 21% 30–40 53% 40	n/a	n/a	n/a	n/a	n/a
Hafty[24]	n/a	59 C 54 SC	C 25%; SC 75%	n/a	yes	88% of patients
Noordijk[25]	60	59	SC	n/a	no	no
Zhang[19]	55–70	n/a	C	64–216 cm²	yes	yes
Talton[71]	60	60	C	n/a	yes	yes
Sandler[72]	16% < 55 27% 55–60 57% < 60	60	C	n/a	90%	90%
Ono[20]	39–70 8% < 59 29% 60–69 63% 70	n/a	SC 50 Gy/25fx 1–2 wk rest 20 Gy/10 fx	n/a	32% of patients	32% of patients
Dosoretz[17]	<50 − >70 most had 60–69	n/a	C	n/a	most patients	most patients
Hayakawa[21]	60–74 for the majority of patients; as high as 80	n/a	C 72% SC 28%	n/a	yes	yes
Rosenthal[73]	18–65	60	C?	n/a	yes	n/a
Kaskowitz[23]	39.9–79.2	63	C	196 cm²	83% of patients	85% of patients
Graham[74]	18–06	Median 60 Mean 58.6	C	varied	80%	80%
Gauden[75]	50Gy/20F x/4 wk	50Gy	C	n/a	100%	100%
Kupelian[76]	80% > 60Gy	Median 63.2	C	n/a	72%	72%
Morita[27]	55–75	Mean 64.7	C	n/a	44%	44%
Sibley[77]	50–80	64	C	varied	73%	58%

* Orthovoltage.
[a] C, continuous; SC, split-course.

portals 100 cm² or less, five-year survival was 22%, compared to 6% for those with larger portals. These data, however, include patients with stage III disease (78 of the 142) and it is entirely possible that this negative correlation simply reflects the use of larger portals for patients with higher-stage disease. Review of other series, however, also shows that some of the most favorable results have been obtained with the use of small fields, with the intent to treat the primary tumor but not electively irradiate regional nodes.

In Hafty's and colleagues' series of patients with clinical stage I disease, the mediastinum was treated in about 90% of patients, and the five-year survival was 21%.[24] By contrast, in Noordijk's and colleagues' series, the mediastinum was not treated, and the five-year survival was 16%.[25] This clinical experience was expanded and reported with longer follow-up by Krols and associates, with a similar conclusion questioning the value of elective nodal irradiation.[26] Ono and associates used a policy of only local treatment for patients with peripheral tumors, but inclusion of the hilum and mediastinum for patients with "hilar type lung cancer."[20] The five-year survivals for these two groups were five of 12 (42%) for the hilar lesions and 12 of 26 (46%) for the peripheral ones. This may be interpreted as showing either a lack of need for elective nodal irradiation or its appropriate benefit for that subgroup requiring it. Of concern, however, was a five of 12 (41%) incidence of fatal

TABLE 46.5. RADIATION THERAPY FOR PATIENTS WITH CLINICALLY RESECTABLE NSCLC: PATTERNS OF FAILURE

Author	Patients	Stage	No Failure	Local Component	Distant Component	Local Only	Distant Only
Morrison[1]	28	operable	n/a				
Smart[68]*	40	operable	n/a				
Coy[69]*[α]	141	T1–T3	n/a	45% of 31 autopsied patients	n/a	n/a	n/a
Cooper[70]	72	T1–T3	n/a	62%	n/a	n/a	n/a
Hafty[24]	43	T1, T2	n/a	39% 18% for C 46% for SC	n/a	n/a	n/a
Noordijk[25]	50	T1, T2	n/a	70%			
Zhang[19]	44	T1	n/a	27% as cause of death	6% as cause of death		
Talton[71]	77	T2, T3	n/a	n/a	n/a	n/a	n/a
Sandler[72]	77	T1–2N0	n/a	56%			
Ono[20]	38	T1, T2	n/a	n/a	n/a	n/a	n/a
Dosoretz[17]	152	T1–T3	34%	70%		55%	15%
	44	T1	n/a	30%	9	28	6
	63	T2	n/a	80%	40	77	33
	41	T3	n/a	86%	40	81	20
Hayakawa[21]	59	Stage I–III					
Rosenthal[73]	62	T1–2N1	15%	55%	30%		
Kaskowitz[23]	53	T1–2N0		49% local only 55% including mediastinum			
Graham[74]	103	Stage I–II	n/a	n/a	n/a	n/a	n/a
Gauden[75]							
Kupelian[76]	71	T1–4N0		44%	n/a	n/a	n/a
Morita[27]	149	Stage I		44%	n/a	n/a	12%
Sibley[78]	122	T1–2N0	67	27%	28%	23%	21%

* Includes some patients with small cell carcinoma.
α Includes some patients with unresectable proximal T3 lesions.
Data from autopsies of 31 patients (22% of entire series), of whom 14 had locoregional disease, 17 had disseminated disease, and 6 had no evidence of disease.
β The percentage of patients not failing is based on the entire population of 152 patients. The distribution of sites of failure is based only on the 67 patients (out of 101 who failed) on whom there were data on sites of failure.

radiation pneumonitis in the patients treated to the larger fields.

Morita and colleagues reported results somewhat at variance with the other authors, noting a significantly superior rate of complete response and five-year survival for patients who received elective hilar/mediastinal irradiation (five-year survival 31.3% versus 14.9%; p = 0.022).[27] The choice of whether or not to give elective irradiation was dictated by the patient's cardiopulmonary status and location of the tumor, with elective irradiation more commonly given for upper lobe tumors. The authors do not comment whether there was an correlation between tumor size and elective nodal treatment. If elective nodal radiation were more commonly given to smaller upper lobe tumors, it could well correlate with better outcome without being its cause.

Sibley has recently reviewed nine published series through 1996 as well as his own data from 1998.[28] Beneficial outcomes, either local control or survival, correlated with tumor dose but *not* with volume treated in the majority of these series. He observed that although treatment only to local fields might be predicted to miss disease in about 25% of cases, the observed rate of regional progression after local-only treatment is only about 3% to 7%, suggesting that distant failure, local failure, and intercurrent death reduce the clinical magnitude of regional failure and need for regional treatment.

In summary, there are now reasons to suggest that treatment of patients with T1–2N0 lesions to small volumes encompassing the primary tumor without elective nodal irradiation may be an appropriate option. It should be recognized that this represents a choice between leaving possible microscopic nodal disease rather than undertreating known disease at the primary site. Success of such a strategy will rely on there being a steep dose-control relation in the range of dose escalation facilitated by elimination of nodal irradiation. So long as local failure rates are high, the survival benefits to be gained by increasing the treatment volume to include suspected subclinical mediastinal disease are likely to be small. The ability of 3D treatment planning to devise effective plans for the delivery of high doses to the target volume is hampered as the target volume increases, and a reasonable research strategy will be to escalate doses to a limited target volume.[29–31] For patients with clinical T1–2N1 disease, there are no good data supporting treatment of restricted volumes, and the mediastinum should probably be irradiated in these patients.

CONFOUNDING OF SELECTION AND TREATMENT EFFECTS IN CORRELATING DOSE, TREATMENT VOLUME, AND OUTCOME, PARTICULARLY LOCAL CONTROL

The attempt to correlate radiation dose and volume with treatment outcomes, particularly local control, must be viewed critically. On basic physics and radiobiologic principles, one would expect several correlations:

1. For a tumor of given size, local control will increase with total radiation dose, at least for most of the dose-control curve. There will be little change in control with dose at very high or very low rates of local control.
2. For a given tumor dose, control should decrease as tumor size increases.
3. Local control requires adequate margins around the tumor volume to account for errors in planned tumor volume, microscopic extensions of tumor, daily variation in patient positioning, changes in tumor position with respiration, and patient movement during treatment.

There are, however a number of nonradiobiologic factors which will tend to skew the distribution of tumor doses in patients not randomly assigned to dose, which may result in similar apparent correlations without requiring a radiobiologic mechanism:

1. For a tumor of given size, higher doses will tend to be given to patients appearing to have a favorable response to treatment and tolerating treatment well, rather than to those who clinically deteriorate during the initial weeks of treatment. Such a policy of higher doses for "good" patients was explicit in the series of Hayakawa and may also have been operative in others.[21]
2. In clinically similar patients with tumors of varying size, it is expected that the most aggressive treatment would be given to the patients expected to have a chance at a good outcome. With a bias favoring a good outcome for patients with smaller tumors (perhaps also because of their better performance status), they would be more likely to receive higher doses.
3. In this group of patients, selected in part because of their poor pulmonary function, there is a natural desire to spare as much normal lung as possible. Treating a small

tumor (e.g., a 2 by 2 cm T1 lesion) with a reasonable margin may still result in a tolerable overall field size. As the lesion increases, so does the volume of normal lung treated, and, with the lower expectation of control of the large lesion, there may be a tendency to skimp on margins. Thus even for similar nominal central axis or 100% isodose line prescribed doses, it is more likely that there will be underdose at the margins of larger rather than smaller tumors.

It is not clear to what extent any of these potential biases occurred in any of these trials, but it is likely that some of the apparent variation in dose-control and treatment volume–survival correlations is due to differences in such decisions about treatment. This in no way negates the importance of the radiobiologic principles that have been well substantiated in other tumor sites better suited for dose-control analysis (e.g., head and neck).

Martel and colleagues have reviewed the effects of tumor volume on local control and survival in patients with NSCLC treated with definitive radiotherapy using three-dimensional treatment planning in a dose escalation trial.[30] For patients with positive lymph nodes, there was no clear correlation between tumor size and outcome. For node-negative patients, however, there was a significant survival advantage for patients with tumor volumes less than 200 cc. This volume corresponds to a sphere of radius 3.6 cm, that is, a T2 tumor. However T staging poorly reflects the tumor volume, as demonstrated in this study. Within a given T-stage, there were wide (more than tenfold) variations in tumor volume. For example, a 2 cm diameter tumor (volume 4.2 cc) involving visceral pleura and a 8 cm tumor (volume 268 cc) in the lower lobe, without chest wall or mediastinal invasion, would both be considered T2 lesions by the TNM classification, including its most recent modifications.[7,32,33] For nonsurgical treatments (radiation alone or combined with chemotherapy), a staging system based more explicitly on volume might well be superior to the present system, based primarily on surgical therapy.[34] Sculier and associates have analyzed results of a trial, conducted by the European Lung Cancer Working Party, of induction chemotherapy followed by either irradiation or further chemotherapy for patients with stage III NSCLC, and found that patients with several subgroups of stage group IIIB (T1–2N3 and T4N0–1) had survival similar to that of patients with stage IIIA disease.[35] Their best discriminant of survival came from classifying patients as stage IIIB (T3–4N3) or IIIA (all other subgroups of stages IIIA and IIIB), with median survivals of 29 versus 45 weeks (p less than 0.0001). These results are intriguing but will require prospective validation in other trials. The major importance of clinical factors other than anatomic stage, such as age, weight loss, and performance status must also be kept in mind in comparing series from different institutions.[36]

THE MYTH OF ORGAN PRESERVATION—OR, WHY THE LUNG IS NOT LIKE THE BREAST

It has been suggested that the efficacy of radiation therapy in controlling microscopic disease in NSCLC should prompt attempts to conduct lung-conserving therapy which would consist of a local excision, by wedge or bronchopulmonary segment, followed by radiation therapy (interstitial or external beam) to the tumor bed. Such conservative local surgery would be combined with surgical staging of hilar and mediastinal nodes. The Cancer and Leukemia Group B (CALGB), with the participation of the Eastern Cooperative Oncology Group (ECOG), has instituted a phase I-II evaluation of the feasibility of such an approach in patients with T1–2N0 NSCLC whose cardiac and/or pulmonary function is so poor as to contraindicate lobectomy. If it is shown that such an approach is feasible, the plan is to compare this strategy with lung-conserving surgery alone, omitting radiotherapy to the tumor bed (L. Kohman, 1993, personal communication). Such considerations fail to take into account that the success of organ conservation therapy, whether of the breast or of the rectum, lies in the ability of the organ in question to tolerate the doses of radiation needed to control the suspected microscopic residual disease while maintaining organ function. There is no strong reason to expect that this will hold true for the lung. The portion of the lung treated to doses of 50 Gy or so expected to be required to control microscopic residual disease will lose function. Even with careful treatment planning and the use of multiple non-coplanar beams, it is not possible to avoid treating some volume of entirely normal lung to doses well above the 30 Gy or so which is the limit of lung tolerance.

COMPLICATIONS

Most series have reported good tolerance to radiation therapy in this population (Table 46.6). The report by Ono and colleagues is an exception.[20] They note that, of 38 patients, seven developed radiation pneumonitis (diagnostic criteria not specified) which was fatal. This complication was seen in five of 12 (42%) of patients whose fields included the primary tumor, hilum, and mediastinum but in only two of 26 (8%) of patients whose treatment volume

TABLE 46.6. RADIATION THERAPY FOR PATIENTS WITH CLINICALLY RESECTABLE NSCLC: COMPLICATIONS

Author	Complications
Morrison[1]	7% fatal late fibroses (1 lung, 1 esophageal stricture, patient died after attempted dilation)
Smart[68]*	n/a; patients were seen daily during radiation therapy and dose and fractionation adjusted according to acute toxicity
Coy[69]ᵃ	not reported
Cooper[70]	not reported
Hafty[28]	9% worsening pulmonary symptoms; 2% worsening CHF
Noordijk[25]	no serious early or late complications; radiation fibrosis was seen radiographically but was asymptomatic
Zhang[19]	2% radiation myelitis
Talton[71]	frequent transient symptoms of radiation pneumonitis; occasional symptomatic radiation fibrosis
Sandler[72]	"rarely reported"; none fatal
Ono[20]	7/38 (18%) fatal radiation pneumonitis; 5/12 in patients with mediastinal and hilar RT; 2/26 in patients treated to primary tumor only
Dosoretz[17]	No major complications; no mortality associated with radiation
Hayakawa[21]	2.5% fatal bronchial stenosis (all 4 patients received <80 Gy); includes data on patients with stage II disease
Rosenthal[73]	not reported
Kaskowitz[23]	6% chronic pneumonitis; 4% pericarditis
Graham[74]	1% grade 3 pneumonitis; 2% grade 2 pneumonitis
Gauden[75]	none requiring hospitalization or causing death
Kupelian[76]	no treatment-related deaths; symptomatic pneumonitis in 7%; no different in complications between patients treated to primary tumor only or with regional nodes
Morita[27]	no major complications reported
Sibley[77]	1.5% grade 3–5 complications, both pneumonitis

* Includes some patients with small cell carcinoma.
ᵃ Includes some patients with unresectable proximal T3 lesions.

encompassed only the primary tumor. Other series have reported occasional problems with late pulmonary fibrosis, pericarditis, or esophageal stricture, but these have occurred in only about 5% of cases. As with surgery, improvements in radiation therapy technique over the years should lead to a reduction in such complications. One review of the toxicity of postoperative radiation therapy following pneumonectomy has noted a reduction in complication rates from 18% to 4% and of lethal complications from 12% to 4% with a shift from treatment planning with orthogonal radiographs and treatment with ^{60}Co beams to CT based treatment planning and treatment on linear accelerators.[37]

In planning radiation therapy for these patients, it is important to recognize some of the present deficiencies in our database on dose and volume effects on lung tolerance to radiation. Tolerance values derived from data on younger patients treated to partial lung volumes for Hodgkin's disease are not likely to be very applicable to this population. The presence of substantial chronic obstructive lung disease in these patients, often with loss of much functioning lung parenchyma, will perturb dose distributions. Most reported series have reported dose calculations without correction for lung density, even by a nominal "healthy" lung tissue density value such as 0.23 to 0.33. When one considers the often lower actual lung density in these patients, the doses reported, based on no density correction, are likely 10% to 20% lower than the actual received dose to the tumor. Institutions routinely doing planning using either nominal or individualized lung density corrections should keep this in mind and increase their prescribed doses appropriately.

Recent clinical data also suggest that, even when treatment technique and dose are standardized, there is considerable individual variation in the susceptibility to radiation-induced lung damage which may have a genetic basis.[38] In animal systems, such genetic differences between strains of mice with low or high incidences of fibrosis following radiation or drugs such as bleomycin have been well described and appear to be mediated by different levels of induction of fibrogenic cytokines such as TGFβ.[39,40] (see also Chapter 13).

Another theoretic technical physical consideration comes from the lack of electronic equilibrium in the transition region between low-density tissue such as emphysematous lung and a solid tumor nodule or mediastinal lymph node. The result of such disequilibrium is underdosing of the first several millimeters of the tumor mass. Attention to this theoretic problem, with phantom modeling studies, has led to the suggestion that high-energy photons (e.g. over 12 MV) should be avoided in treatment plans where there will be lung-tumor interfaces. The clinical impact of this factor is that treating patients with bulky stage IIIA and IIIB disease has been difficult to measure, and the one study which has examined survival as a function of beam energy has failed to find such a relation.[41] One would not expect this review of patients with advanced-stage disease to be a partic-

ularly sensitive test, however, and the impact of such dose inhomogeneity would likely be greater in the scenario of treating small peripheral lesions surrounded by low-density lung parenchyma. While a general recommendation is difficult to make, it would seem wise to use multiple-beam techniques with lower- or moderate-energy photons, if these are available, rather than parallel opposed treatments with higher-energy beams.

Radiation toxicity to the lung depends on the dose and the volume of lung treated. Clinical and radiographic changes appear at doses of 18 to 20 Gy (with 1.8 to 2.0 Gy fractions) to the whole lung. Higher doses to smaller volumes will produce more severe changes, which appear earlier with higher doses. The precise shape of the curve relating irradiated volume, dose, and complication probability is not presently known. Attempts to model this, as well as the more complex yet realistic situation wherein differing lung volumes receive differing doses, are essential to the practical implementation of 3D treatment planning systems.[31]

In conjunction with the development of more accurate models of dose-volume-complication effects, we need better understanding of the effects of various "standard" treatment volumes (e.g. tumor only, tumor plus hilar and/or mediastinal nodes, etc.) on pulmonary function. (see also Chapter 36.) Several groups have attempted to do this by measuring baseline pulmonary function by routine flow and volume measurements, and in the case of the Fox Chase group, lung perfusion scans. Curran and colleagues reported on measurements made of 165 nonoperative patients (of unspecified stage) and reported that the percent of functioning lung irradiated increased from 11.3% ± 4.9% for treatment of the primary tumor plus a 2 cm margin to 31.2% ± 10.2% when the ipsilateral hilum and mediastinum were irradiated as well.[42] Choi and associates noted relatively small and transient changes in pulmonary function in patients receiving postoperative radiation therapy to the mediastinum; however, this may not predict the effects of treatment of parenchymal lesions in patients with marginal pulmonary function.[43] Marks and colleagues have developed image correlation methods for combining nuclear medicine delineation of lung function by ventilation and perfusion and CT delineation of lung anatomy, and thus quantitate predicted functional loss for various treatment plans.[44,45] Such techniques have not been widely used in choosing beam arrangements for patients with stage I and II lesions but have the potential to maximize sparing of functional lung on an individualized basis.

AVENUES FOR IMPROVEMENT

It is unrealistic to expect that randomized trials will be conducted to define the role of altered radiation fractionation or the addition of chemotherapy to radiation therapy in patients with clinical stage I–II NSCLC who are treated with radical radiation therapy. Use of such techniques must be guided by reasonable extrapolation from their results in other tumor sites and an understanding of patterns of failure for patients with stage I–II treated with present conventional irradiation.

While systemic failure due to occult metastatic disease is a major problem even in patients with clinical stage I NSCLC, as it is in all of lung cancer, local control has also been frustratingly difficult to achieve in these patients. They, more than patients with more advanced disease, are most likely to have a good correlation between local control and survival.[46]

Altered Fractionation

The RTOG conducted several phase II trials in patients with unresectable NSCLC, investigating both dose response and the role of altered fraction—either BID treatment with small fractions and escalating the total dose, or accelerated fractionation with a concomitant boost. The most promising development of these was a regimen of 1.2 Gy fractions given twice a day to a total dose of 69.5 Gy (see also Chapter 47). In a sequential phase II trial, this gave a survival which was significantly better than standard fractionation for patients with favorable clinical characteristics of minimal weight loss and good performance status.[47] A confirmatory phase III trial conducted by the RTOG and ECOG directly compared this regimen with standard daily fractionation to a dose of 60 Gy in 30 fractions over six weeks.[48,49] The hyperfractionated regimen appeared slightly better than the standard one, but this difference did not reach statistical significance. When local control was analyzed, a significant benefit was seen only for peripheral T3 tumors without nodal involvement. A metaanalysis of three randomized trials of hyperfractionated RT for NSCLC has suggested a significant improvement in survival, although the total number of patients in these trials was relatively small.[50]

In the UK, Saunders and associates have reported promising results with a regimen incorporating TID fractionation and treatment without weekend interruptions (continuous hyperfractionated accelerated radiation therapy or CHART) to a dose of 54 Gy in two weeks.[51] On the basis of favorable phase II data, patients with unresectable NSCLC, of whom about 80% had squamous histology and about one quarter had early-stage but medically inoperable disease (criteria not specified) were randomized to either CHART or conventional once-daily radiation therapy to 60 Gy in six weeks. Results have shown statistically significant improvements in local control and survival, at least to four years, favoring the CHART regimen.[52,53]

It is likely that further improvement in local control and survival can be achieved by strict attention to completing treatment without undue interruptions. Cox and colleagues have analyzed data from three separate RTOG trials and reported that, for the favorable subset of patients described above, survival was significantly compromised by delays of overall treatment time.[54] No effect was seen in less-favorable patients or in patients receiving total doses less than 69.6 Gy. While it is difficult to separate treatment interruption as a cause of bad outcome from treatment interruption as an index of poor patient performance status and underlying tumor burden, the results are in line with radiobiologic prediction that even short treatment interruptions may allow significant proliferation of remaining tumor and greatly reduce local control. The use of agents which are cytostatic but not particularly cytotoxic (e.g., DMFO or inhibitors of *ras* prenylation) may be of use in ameliorating the harmful effects of treatment protraction.

Combining Radiation and Chemotherapy

The addition of chemotherapy to radiation therapy for patients with NSCLC could improve survival through improvement in local control or reduction in distant metastases. While the series which have reported improved survival for patients with stage III disease by treating with induction chemotherapy followed by radiation have reported a reduction in distant failure but no improvement in local control, the use of concurrent daily cisplatin during radiation therapy has been reported to improve local control and survival in one study, although another study of similar design showed no benefit.[55] The effectiveness of present chemotherapy appears restricted to prognostically favorable patients with excellent performance status and minimal weight loss,[56] so its role in the treatment of elderly patients, or patients with significant medical problems other than cancer, with medically inoperable stage I–II NSCLC should be explored with some caution. However, several newer, less-toxic agents such as vinorelbine can be used even in older and sicker patients, and one recent trial in such a group, the ELVIS (Elderly Lung Vinorelbine Italian Study) trial, showed a survival benefit for single-agent chemotherapy when compared with best supportive care. Several trials combining weekly or daily chemotherapy with BID radiation for patients with stage III NSCLC have shown significant improvements in local control and survival not limited to favorable performance status patients[57,58] (see also Chapter 52).

To date, the role of induction chemotherapy has only been tested in some studies in patients with resectable stage I–II NSCLC. However, based on favorable results of induction chemotherapy for patients with resectable stage III NSCLC,[59-61] trials have recently been conducted to demonstrate the feasibility of such management of patients with stage Ib, IIa, IIb, and selected IIIa (T3N0) NSCLC prior to a phase III trial which will compare immediate surgery to surgery following induction chemotherapy. Based on the results of trials of radiation therapy alone or preceded by induction chemotherapy for patients with stage IIIA/B

NSCLC showing survival benefits for the combined modality approach,[49,62–64] it is reasonable (though of unproven benefit) to consider such a sequence in patients with medically inoperable stage I and II disease so long as they able to tolerate chemotherapy.

CONCLUSIONS

Surgery remains the preferred treatment for patients with clinical stage I-II NSCLC who are or can be made to be of reasonable operative risk. The role of radiation therapy in the management of patients with clinical stage I and II NSCLC is a secondary one. There is little reason to expect radiation alone, or a combination of limited surgery and radiation, to replace surgical management for the patient without significant contraindications to surgery. Based on current data, there is little reason to consider mounting a trial comparing lobectomy versus limited resection plus radiation for the good-risk patient.

The situation is quite different when we consider the patient whose physiologic age, concurrent medical problems, or preference make him or her a poor surgical candidate. Present data lead to the following recommendations:

1. Radical radiation therapy is curative in a worthwhile proportion of these patients, with five-year survivals as high as 40% for patients with clinical stage I disease, and should be offered as the present standard of care for patients with medically inoperable stage I-II NSCLC.
2. While there are no prospective trials that address issues of optimal radiation dose, fractionation, and volume, data would suggest the following guidelines:
2.1 The primary tumor should receive a dose of at least 65 Gy (as calculated without correction for lung density; make appropriate adjustments if lung corrections are used) if conventional fractionation of one daily fraction of 1.8 to 2.0 Gy is used. Exploration of higher total doses and alternatives to once-daily fractionation has shown promise and should be continued.
2.2 Good results have been reported with both split-course and continuous-fractionation schemes. Some retrospective comparisons have suggested superiority of continuous regimens, but such analysis is confounded by the frequent practice of selecting better patients for continuous treatment. In either case, undue protraction of treatment time, either by a long-planned split or by frequent or long treatment interruptions for bothersome but not life-threatening acute toxicities such as esophagitis is likely to decrease local control. Reduction of target volumes to the known tumor without elective nodal radiation should largely prevent significant acute esophagitis and other toxicities, and thus remove the impetus for split-course treatment.
2.3 The appropriate treatment volume remains undefined.

Data from the LCSG surgical trial comparing wedge or segmental resection to lobectomy in *surgical* stage I NSCLC suggests that local control and probably survival are decreased by the more conservative resection without any gain in preservation of pulmonary function. It is not clear, however, that such a conclusion should be extended to patients with *clinical* stage I disease, or to those in whom poor pulmonary function is a major reason for their avoiding surgical therapy in the first place. Several of the series with the best survival results have used small treatment volumes encompassing only areas of known macroscopic disease, with a margin but without elective irradiation of nodal regions of suspect drainage. There is also a suggestion, although not universal agreement, that such reduction of target volume will reduce the incidence of pulmonary toxicity. It may well be that, for this patient population, such restricted target volumes are most appropriate. The introduction of three-dimensional treatment planning techniques will allow dose escalation and normal tissue sparing to a greater degree as the target volume is kept limited.[65,66] At the present time, it seems quite reasonable to treat these patients to restricted target volumes without routine prophylactic irradiation of hilar or mediastinal lymph nodes.

3. With current treatment techniques, both local and systemic failure are major causes of treatment failure, and both need to be addressed in order to improve treatment outcomes. The advanced age and frequent multiorgan disease in these patients may limit their suitability for treatment with many current chemotherapeutic agents, although recent development of less-toxic drug analogues (e.g., carboplatin versus cisplatin) and improvement in management of treatment toxicities (e.g., ondansetron for management of nausea and vomiting, hematopoetic growth factors such as G-CSF for amelioration of myelosuppression) may make such therapy reasonable for some patients. The frequency of local failure, as well as the possibility of treating limited-target volumes for this patient population, make them good potential candidates for applications of altered radiation fractionation schemes, such as dose escalation with hyperfractionation, accelerated fractionation, or concurrent boost approaches.

These broad conclusions are fairly consistently reached by the authors of most of the recent treatment series as well as reviews.[28,67] Radical radiation therapy has an established position as a potentially curative modality for those patients with stage I and II NSCLC who are medically inoperable and/or refuse surgery, and should be offered to them rather than relegating such patients to observation or treatment without curative potential. As both local and systemic failure are common with radiation therapy techniques, continued clinical research to improve both components of therapy is needed.

REFERENCES

1. Morrison R, Deeley T, Cleland W. The treatment of carcinoma of the bronchus: a clinical trial to compare surgery and supervoltage radiotherapy. *Lancet* 1963;1:683.
2. Ginsberg R, Rubenstein L. Randomized trial of lobectomy versus limited resection for T1N0 non–small cell lung cancer. Lung Cancer Study Group. *Ann Thorac Surg* 1995;60:615.
3. Sawyer T, Bonner J, Gould P, et al. Effectiveness of postoperative irradiation in stage IIIA non–small cell lung cancer according to regression tree analysis of recurrence risks. *Ann Thorac Surg* 1997;64:1402.
4. Silvestri G, Handy J, Lackland D, et al. Specialists achieve better outcomes than generalists for lung cancer surgery. *Chest* 1998;114:675.
5. Kohman L. What constitutes success in cancer surgery? Measuring the value of specialist care. *Chest* 1998;114:663.
6. Smetana G. Preoperative pulmonary evaluation. *N Engl J Med* 1999;340:937.
7. Mountain C. A new international staging system for lung cancer. *Chest* 1986;89[suppl]:225.
8. Oda M, Watanabe Y, Shimizu J, et al. Extent of mediastinal node metastasis in clinical stage I non-small-cell lung cancer: the role of systematic nodal dissection. *Lung Cancer* 1998;22:23.
9. Schiepers C. Role of positron emission tomography in the staging of lung cancer. *Lung Cancer* 1997;17:S29.
10. Vansteenkiste J, Stroobants S, De Leyn P, et al. Mediastinal lymph node staging with FDG-PET scan in patients with potentially operable non—small cell lung cancer: a prospective analysis of 50 cases. *Chest* 1997;112:1480.
11. Steinert H, Hauser M, Allemann F, et al. Non–small cell lung cancer: nodal staging with FDG PET versus CT with correlative lymph node mapping and sampling. *Radiology* 1997;202:441.
12. Bury T, Paulius P, Dowlati A, et al. Staging of the mediastinum: value of positron emission tomography imaging in non–small cell lung cancer. *Eur Respir J* 1996;9:2560.
13. Hebert M, Lowe V, Hoffman J, et al. Positron emission tomography in the pretreatment evaluation and follow-up of non–small cell lung cancer patients treated with radiotherapy: preliminary findings. *Am J Clin Oncol* 1996;19:416.
14. Patz E, Lowe V, Goodman P, et al. Thoracic nodal staging with PET imaging with 18FDG in patients with bronchogenic carcinoma. *Chest* 1995;108:1617.
15. McNeil B, Weichselbaum R, Pauker S. Fallacy of the five year survival in lung cancer. *N Engl J Med* 1978;299:1397.
16. Hilton G. Present position relating to cancer of the lung: results with radiotherapy alone. *Thorax* 1960;15:17.
17. Dosoretz D, Katin M, Blitzer P, et al. Radiation therapy in the management of medically inoperable carcinoma of the lung: results and implications for future treatment strategies. *Int J Radiat Oncol Biol Phys* 1992;24:3.
18. Dosoretz D, DG, Rubenstein J, et al. Local control in medically inoperable lung cancer: an analysis of its importance in outcome and factors determining the probability of tumor eradication. *Int J Radiat Oncol Biol Phys* 1993;27:507.
19. Zhang H, Yin W, Yang Z. Curative radiotherapy of early operable non-small-cell lung cancer. *Radiother Oncol* 1989;14:89.
20. Ono R, Egawa S, Suemasu K, et al. Radiotherapy in inoperable stage I lung cancer. *Jpn J Clin Oncol* 1991;21:125.
21. Hayakawa K, Mitsuhashi N, Nakajima N, et al. Radiation therapy for stage I-II epidermoid carcinoma of the lung. *Lung Cancer* 1992;8:213.
22. Hayakawa K, Mitsuhashi N, Furuta M, et al. High-dose radiation therapy for inoperable non–small cell lung cancer without mediastinal involvement (clinical stage N0, N1). *Strahlenther Onkol* 1996;172:489.
23. Kaskowitz B, Graham M, Emami B, et al. Radiation therapy alone for stage I non–small cell lung cancer. *Int J Radiat Oncol Biol Phys* 1993;27:517.
24. Hafty B, Goldberg N, Gerstley J, et al. Results of radical radiation therapy in clinical stage I, technically operable non–small cell lung cancer. *Int J Radiat Oncol Biol Phys* 1988;15:69.
25. Noordijk E, Poest C, Hermans J, et al. Radiotherapy as an alternative to surgery in elderly patients with resectable lung cancer. *Radiother Oncol* 1988;13:83.
26. Krol A, Aussems P, Noordijk E, et al. Local irradiation alone for peripheral stage I lung cancer: could we omit the elective regional nodal irradiation? *Int J Radiat Oncol Biol Phys* 1996;34:297.
27. Morita K, Fuwa N, Suzuli Y, et al. Radical radiotherapy for medically inoperable nonsmall cell lung cance in clinical stage I: a retrospective analysis of 149 patients. *Radiother Oncol* 1997;42:31.
28. Sibley G. Radiotherapy for patients with medically inoperable stage I nonsmall cell lung carcinoma: smaller volumes and higher doses—a review. *Cancer* 1998;82:433.
29. Graham M, Purdy J, Emami B, et al. 3-D conformal radiotherapy for lung cancer. The Washington University experience. *Front Radiat Ther Oncol* 1996;29:188–98.
30. Martel M, Strawdeman M, Hazuka M, et al. Volume and dose parameters for survival of non–small cell lung cancer patients. *Radiother Oncol* 1997;44:23.
31. Ten Haken R, Martel M, Kessler M, et al. Use of Veff and iso-NTCP in the implementation of dose escalation protocols. *Int J Radiat Oncol Biol Phys* 1993;27:689.
32. Mountain C. Revisions in the international system for staging lung cancer. *Chest* 1997;111:1710.
33. Mountain C, Dresler C. Regional lymph node classification for lung cancer staging. *Chest* 1997;111:1718.
34. Ginsberg R. Continuing controversies in staging NSCLC: an analysis of the revised 1997 staging system. *Oncology (Huntingt)* 1998;12:51.
35. Sculier J, Paesmans M, Ninane V, et al. Evaluation of the TN substaging in patients with initially unresectable stage III non–small cell lung cancer treated by induction chemotherapy. *Lung Cancer* 1998;22:201.
36. Sause W, Scott C, Byhardt R, et al. Recursive partitioning analysis of 1,592 patients on four RTOG studies in non–small cell lung cancer. *Proc ASCO* 1993;12:336.
37. Phlips P, Rocmans P, Vanderhoef P, et al. Postoperative radiotherapy after pneumonectomy: impact of modern treatment facilities. *Int J Radiat Oncol Biol Phys* 1993;27:525.
38. Geara F, Komaki R, Tucker S, et al. Factors influencing the development of lung fibrosis after chemo-radiation for small cell carcinoma of the lung: evidence for inherent interindividual variation. In: Mornex F, van Houte P, eds. *Treatment optimization for lung cancer: from classical to innovative procedures.* Paris, Elsevier, 1998:139.
39. Franko A, Sharplin J, Ward W, et al. The genetic basis of strain dependant differences in the early phase of radiation injury in mouse lung. *Radiat Res* 1991;126:349.
40. Johnson C, Piedboeuf B, Baggs R, et al. Differences in correlation of mRNA gene expression in mice sensitive and resistant to radiation-induced pulmonary fibrosis. *Radiat Res* 1995;142:197.
41. Foote R, Robinow J, Shaw E, et al. Low- versus high-energy photon beams in radiotherapy for lung cancer. *Med Dosim* 1993;18:65.
42. Curran W, Moldofsky P, Solin L. Quantitative analysis of the

impact of adiation therapy field selection on post-RT pulmonary function [Abstract]. *Int J Radiat Oncol Biol Phys* 1988;15:12.

43. Choi N, Kanarek D, Grillo H. Effect of postoperative radiotherapy on changes in pulmonary function in patients with stage II and IIIA lung carcinoma. *Int J Radiat Oncol Biol Phys* 1990;18:95.

44. Marks L, Spencer D, Sherouse G, et al. The role of three-dimensional functional lung imaging in radiation treatment planning: the functional dose-volume histogram. *Int J Radiat Oncol Biol Phys* 1995;33:65.

45. Marks L, Munley M, Spencer D, et al. Quantification of radiation-induced regional lung injury with perfusion imaging. *Int J Radiat Oncol Biol Phys* 1997;38:399.

46. Komaki R, Scott C, Byhardt R, et al. Failure patterns by prognostic group determined by recurvise partitioning analysis (RPA) of 1547 patients on four adiation Therapy Oncology Group (RTOG) studies in inoperable nonsmall–cell lung cancer (NSCLC). *Int J Radiat Oncol Biol Phys* 1998;42:263.

47. Cox J, Azarnia N, Byhardt R, et al. A randomized phase I/II trial of hyperfractionated radiation therapy with total doses of 60.0 Gy to 79.2 Gy: Possible survival benefits with >69.6 Gy in favorable patients with stage III radiation therapy oncology group non-small-cell lung carcinoma: report of the radiation therapy oncology group 83–11. *J Clin Oncol* 1990;8:1543.

48. Sause W, Scott C, Taylor S, et al. Radiation Therapy Oncology Group (RTOG) 88–08 and Eastern Cooperative Oncology Group (ECOG) 4588; preliminary results of a phase III trial in regionally advanced, unresectable, non–small cell lung cancer. *J Natl Cancer Inst* 1995;87:198.

49. Sause W, Kolesar P, Taylor S, et al. Five-year results; phase III trial of regionally advanced unresectable non–small cell lung cancer, RTOG 8808, ECOG 4588, SWOG 8992 [Abstract 1743]. *Proc ASCO* 1998;17:453.

50. Stuschke M, Thames H. Hyperfractionated radiotherapy of human tumors: overview of the randomized clinical trials. *Int J Radiat Oncol Biol Phys* 1997;37:259.

51. Saunders M, Dische S: Continuous, hyperfractionated, accelerated radiation therapy (CHART) in non-small-cell carcinoma of the bronchus. *Int J Radiat Oncol Biol Phys* 1990;19:1211.

52. Saunders M, Dische S, Barrett A, et al. Randomised multicentre trials of CHART vs conventional radiotherapy in head and neck and non-small-cell lung cancer: an interim report. CHART Steering Committee. *Br J Cancer* 1996;73:1455.

53. Saunders M, Dische S, Barrett A, et al. Continuous hyperfractionated accelerated radiotherapy (CHART) versus conventional radiotherapy in non-small-cell lung cancer: a randomised multicentre trial. *Lancet* 1997;350:161.

54. Cox J, Pajak T, Asbell S, et al. Interruptions of high-dose radiation therapy decrease long-term survival of favorable patients with unresectable non–small cell carcinoma of the lung: analysis of 1244 cases from 3 radiation therapy oncology group (RTOG) trials. *Int J Radiat Oncol Biol Phys* 1993;27:493.

55. Trovo M, Zanelli G, Minatel E, et al. Radiotherapy versus radiotherapy enhanced by cisplatin in stage III non–small cell lung cancer. *Int J Radiat Oncol Biol Phys* 1992;24:573.

56. Ruckdeschel J, Findelstein D, Ettinger D, et al. A randomized trial of the four most active regimens for metastatic non–small cell lung cancer. *J Clin Oncol* 1986;4:14.

57. Jeremic B, Jevremovic S, Mijatovic L, et al. Hyperfractionated radiation therapy with and without concurrent chemotherapy for advanced non–small cell lung cancer. *Cancer* 1993;71:3732.

58. Jeremic B, Shibamoto Y, Acimovic L, et al. Hyperfractionated radiation therapy with or without concurrent low-dose daily carboplatin/etoposide for stage III non-small-cell lung cancer: a randomized study. *J Clin Oncol* 1996;14:1065.

59. Pass H, Pohrebnia H, Steinberg S, et al. Randomized trial of neoadjuvant therapy for lung cancer: Interim analysis. *Ann Thorac Surg* 1992;53:992.

60. Rossell R, Codina J, Camps C, et al. A randomized trial comparing preoperative chemotherapy plus surgery with surgery alone in patients with non–small cell lung cancer. *N Engl J Med* 1994;330:23.

61. Roth J, Fossella F, Komaki R, et al. A randomized trial comparing preoperative chemotherapy and surgery with surgery alone in resectable stage III non–small cell lung cancer. *J Natl Cancer Inst* 1994;86:673.

62. Dillman R, Seagren S, Herndon J, et al. Randomized trial of induction chemotherapy plus radiation therapy vs RT alone in stage III non–small cell lung cancer (NSCLC): five year follow up of CALGB. *Proc ASCO* 1993;12:329.

63. Dillman R, Herndon J, Seagren S, et al. Improved survival in stage III non–small cell lung cancer: seven year follow-up of Cancer and Leukemia Group B (CALGB) 8433 trial. *J Natl Cancer Inst* 1996;88:1210.

64. Le Chevalier T, Arriagada R, Quoix E, et al. Radiotherapy alone versus combined chemotherapy and radiotherapy in unresectable non–small cell lung carcinoma. *Lung Cancer* 1994;10:S239.

65. McGibney C, Holmberg O, McClean B, et al. The potential impact of 3-D conformal radiotherap (3DCRT) on continuous hyperfractionated accelerated radiotherapy (CHART) for NSCLC [Abstract 486]. *Lung Cancer* 1997;18:

66. Saunders M, Lyn E, Pigott K, et al. Experience of a dose escalation study using CHARTWEL (continuous hyperfractionated acelerated radiotherapy weekendless) in non–small cell lung cancer [Abstract 482]. *Lung Cancer* 1997;18:

67. Armstrong J, Minsky B. Primary radiation therapy for stage I and II medically inoperable non–small cell lung cancer. *Cancer Treat Rev* 1989;16:247.

68. Smart J. Can lung cancer be cured by irradiation alone? *JAMA* 1966;195:158.

69. Coy P, Kennelly G. The role of curative radiotherapy in the treatment of lung cancer. *Cancer* 1980;45:698.

70. Cooper J, Pearson F, Todd T, et al. Radiotherapy alone for patients with operable carcinoma of the lung. *Chest* 1985;87:289.

71. Talton B, Constable W, Kersh C. Curative radiotherapy in non–small cell carcinoma of the lung. *Int J Radiat Oncol Biol Phys* 1990;19:15.

72. Sandler H, Curran W, Turrisi A. The influence of tumor size and pre-treatment staging on outcome following radiation therapy alone for stage I non–small cell lung cancer. *Int J Radiat Oncol Biol Phys* 1991;19:9.

73. Rosenthal S, Curran WJ, Herbert S, et al. Clinical stage II non–small cell lung cancer treated with radiation therapy alone. The significance of clinically staged ipsilateral hilar adenopathy. *Cancer* 1992;70:2410.

74. Graham P, Gebski V, Langlands A. Radical radiotherapy for early nonsmall cell lung cancer. *Int J Radiat Oncol Biol Phys* 1995;31:261.

75. Gauden S, Ramsay J, Tripcony L. The curative treatment by radiotherapy alone of stage I non-small-cell carcinoma of the lung. *Chest* 1995;108:1278.

76. Kupelian P, Komaki R, Allen P. Prognostic factors in the treatment of node-negative nonsmall cell lung carcinoma with radiotherapy alone. *Int J Radiat Oncol Biol Phys* 1996;36:607.

77. Sibley G, Jamieson T, Marks L, et al. Radiotherapy alone for medically inoperable stage I non-small-cell lung cancer: the Duke experience. *Int J Radiat Oncol Biol Phys* 1998;40:149.

47

ALTERED FRACTIONATION SCHEDULES FOR LUNG CANCER

MINESH P. MEHTA
PAUL M. HARARI

Of the 170,000 to 180,000 lung cancer cases, approximately 50,000 patients present with locoregionally advanced, non-metastatic, non-small cell lung cancer (NSCLC). This group generally receives definitive radiation therapy.[1] Unfortunately, with standard radiation therapy alone, the overall cure rate is less than 5%.[2] With a survival advantage demonstrated from recent sequential chemoradiation trials for these patients, the standard therapy for these patients is two cycles of vinblastine-cisplatin chemotherapy followed by 60 Gy external-beam radiation therapy.[3] Despite the small survival gains achieved through this strategy, the overall long-term survival remains poor because of an unacceptably high frequency of local and distant failure. The role of radiotherapy is to improve local control. One change would be to alter the conventional 1 fraction per day, 5 days per week given over 6 weeks to shorten overall time and deliver multiple daily treatment. We address the biologic rationale for such altered fractionation schedules and assess the various manipulations of standard fractionation. Subsequently, we discuss the clinical data supporting the role of altered fractionation in the management of locoregionally advanced nonmetastatic NSCLC.

Standard schedules preclude high local failure rate.[3] Data from the Institut Gustave Roussy in Paris indicated that distant metastasis was achieved with combination therapy, but local control remained only 8% at 5 years.[4] Improving the control of local disease remains a very high priority. Several clinical trials are currently undertaking this mission, either by incorporating surgery into the regimen or by altering the radiotherapeutic strategy by escalating or intensifying the radiation with strategies such as hyperfractionation, acceleration, brachytherapy boost, three-dimensional (3-D) conformal techniques, and the use of radiosensitizers.

FRACTIONATION

Biologic Basis for Fractionation

Manipulation of fractionation, or doses per session, for radiation therapy has received considerable attention in recent years. The original observations regarding the advantages of fractionating radiation into multiple doses over single doses date back to the early 1900s.[5,6] Current understanding of radiobiologic principles focus on tumor division times versus acute and late effects in normal tumors. Indeed, work published in the early 1980s postulated that the more specific modifications of dose/fractionation parameters might improve tumor control rates.[7–10] These reports clarified a differential radiation repair response between early-responding and late-responding tissues. Early-responding tissues, including epithelium of the aerodigestive tract and some tumor types, are not as efficient at repairing damage from small radiation doses compared to late-responding normal tissues. The late-responding tissues, such as kidney and spinal cord, efficiently repair radiation damage between individual small fractions. Fractionation modifications must recognize this differential tissue repair capacity to radiation, and that late-tissue damage is not time-critical but more dependent on size of fractions and interval between fractions. The more common of these altered fractionation strategies are further defined.

Fractionation Factors

The four primary fractionation factors are:

- Dose per fraction
- Total dose
- Overall treatment time (for completing the entire radiation schedule)
- Interfraction treatment interval

Each of the altered fractionation methods exploits manipulations of one or more of these four primary fractionation factors in an attempt to provide a therapeutic advantage. The two most common strategies are referred to as "hyperfractionation" and "acceleration," and the differences between these are illustrated in Table 47.1.

TABLE 47.1. COMMON STRATEGIES FOR ALTERED FRACTIONATION

Hyperfractionation
  ↓ fraction size
  ↑ fraction number
  ↑ total dose
  Maintain overall treatment time
Rationale: Allows safe delivery of slightly higher tumor dose without increase in late normal tissue toxicity.
Acceleration
  ↓ Overall treatment time
  Maintain or slightly reduce:
    Fraction size
    Fraction number
    Total dose
Rationale: Counteracts tumor cell proliferation in tumors with short T_{pm} by decreasing overall treatment time.

Hyperfractionation

Hyperfractionation requires a reduced fraction size (below 1.4–1.5 Gy per exposure), an increased fraction number, and a modest increase in total dose with minimal extension of the overall treatment time. The main benefit of hyperfractionation rests in the sparing of late normal tissue complications. By using an increased number of smaller doses (1.0–1.2 Gy) per fraction, late-effect injury is reduced. The increased total dose is safely accomplished by the use of smaller doses per fraction that "spare" the late-reacting normal tissues from increased complication rates. The most important predictor of enhanced late radiation morbidity is an increase in the size of the radiation fraction. An example of hyperfractionation is provided in Table 47.2.

Acceleration/Accelerated Fractionation

The primary rationale for accelerated fractionation in radiation therapy is to deliver radiotherapy to a tumor cell population dividing more than once in 24 hours and to reduce the overall treatment time. This approach limits the surviving tumor cells' repopulation during the radiation treatment course. Tumor cell repopulation during treatment increases clonogenic cell number, thereby decreasing tumor control for a given radiation dose. Flow cytometry techniques allow more understanding of human tumor kinetics. Cytometric data support the concept of the tumor potential doubling time (T_{pot}). T_{pot} represents the minimum time it takes for a tumor to double. Because cell loss occurs, cell-doubling and volume-doubling are independent, but *in situ* measurements of T_{pot} from human biopsy estimate (T_{pot}) values of 3 to 6 days. Volume-doubling times (T_{vol}) for human tumors are commonly on the order of several months (cell loss factor includes processes such as necrosis, exfoliation, apoptosis, etc.). Acceleration provides a reduction in the overall treatment time, fraction number, and total dose. An example of treatment acceleration is provided in Table 47.2.

Growth Kinetics of Lung Cancer

The data for volume-doubling time of lung cancer comes from patients with solitary lung nodules followed or observed. Two such follow-up trials conducted in the late 1960s and reported in the early 1970s suggest that radiographic doubling times of asymptomatic solitary nodules range from 30 to 490 days with an approximate median volume-doubling time of 120 days.[11,12] Unfortunately, the identification of such long volume-doubling times led to the

TABLE 47.2. FRACTIONATION SCHEMES

Clinical Examples of Altered Fractionation*		Comments
Hyperfractionation		
60 fx × 1.1 Gy twice daily = 66 Gy (6 wks)		↑ No. of small fractions
[*30 fx × 2.0 Gy per day = 60 Gy (6 wks)*]		↑ Total dose, same overall time
Acceleration		
25 fx × 2.0 Gy per day = 50 Gy (3.5 wks, Mon–Sun)		↓ Overall time
[*25 fx × 2.0 Gy per day = 50 Gy (5 wks, Mon–Fri)*]		
Accelerated Hyperfractionation		
55 fx × 1.2 Gy twice daily = 66 Gy (<6 wks)		Combination of features above
[*30 fx × 2.0 Gy per day = 60 Gy (6 wks)*]		
Dose Escalation		
Large Field	25 fx × 2.0 Gy per day = 50 Gy (5 wks)	↑ Dose per fraction at time of field reduction
Boost Field	5 fx × 2.5 Gy per day = 12.5 (Gy (1 wk)	
	Total = 62.5 Gy (6 wks)	
Hypofractionation/Split Course		
Part I	5 fx × 4 Gy = 20 Gy (1 wk)	Simple and effective regimen for palliation
	Two-week break	
Part II	5 fx × 4 Gy = 20 Gy (1 wk)	
	Total = 40 Gy (4 wks)	

* Schedules in *italics* represent comparable conventional schedules.

clinical belief that lung cancers do not proliferate rapidly. Despite the time measured to double volume, active cell division, cell loss, and opportunities to metastasize occur. Therefore, prolonged courses of radiation therapy theoretically would not be detrimental in the management of these patients. As alluded to previously, recent biologic advances have allowed us to identify the concept of the tumor potential doubling time, which is a more appealing measure of cellular proliferative activity. Recent studies have confirmed that NSCLC proliferates rapidly, with relatively short potential doubling times, with a median of 7 days.[13]

Accelerated Hyperfractionation

This common altered fractionation strategy incorporates components of both hyperfractionation and acceleration as defined previously. This amalgamation of features from the two primary altered fractionation themes (hyperfractionation and acceleration) exploits both the concept of reduced fraction size to minimize normal tissue effects and reduced overall treatment time to diminish the adverse impact of tumor cell repopulation during therapy. Many examples of accelerated hyperfractionation exist in clinical cancer therapy, and a representative example is provided in Table 47.2.

Dose Escalation

Dose escalation can be accomplished by altered fractionation that simply employs an increase in the individual fraction size during a course of radiotherapy. A patient receiving 2.0 Gy fractions in the initial phase of a treatment course might escalate to 2.5 Gy fractions during the reduced volume boost segment of his or her radiotherapy treatment course. An example of this dose escalation concept is provided in Table 47.2. The rationale is to enhance the "dose intensity" during the latter segment of treatment, while exposing only the smallest target volume to these higher doses.

Hypofractionation

Despite the sound radiobiologic rationale and promising clinical results with intensified fractionation schedules that exploit the concepts of hyperfractionation and acceleration, there remains an important clinical role for hypofractionation in radiation therapy. With this method, significantly fewer radiation fractions are employed, with higher doses per fraction, such as 4 Gy times 5 = 20 Gy. Hypofractionation may provide advantages for palliation. For the symptomatic patient with limited overall life expectancy, concern about late normal tissue toxicities many months after radiation therapy may be misplaced. Because the late normal tissue effects of radiation generally require 9 to 24 months to emerge, the use of hypofractionation may facilitate rapid and efficient treatment completion with effective doses with lesser concern over long-term side effects. Daily fractions

of between 3 and 8 Gy, depending on the particular setting and anatomic treatment site, may provide rapid, cost-effective palliation of pain, bleeding, obstruction, or tumor progression using a brief delivery schedule, which inconveniences the patient less. In some settings, a single fraction of 8 Gy may control the symptom complaint for the remainder of the patient's life. For larger treatment volumes, schedules employing 3 to 7 Gy fractions over 1- to 3-week schedules may be used to deliver radiation doses with a high biologic effect in light of the large dose per fraction (See example in Table 47.2.)

Split-Course Fractionation

Although split-course radiation fractionation is uncommonly used in the context of curative radiation therapy because of the current understanding of the importance of repopulation and tumor proliferation, this method remains a useful method for palliation.* The main disadvantage of split-course radiation is the treatment break between two components of the treatment schedule. This break enables accelerated tumor repopulation. The original basis for this strategy was to allow adequate repair to be completed in acutely responding normal tissues, reoxygenation of the tumor, and thereby reducing the toxicity of the radiation schedule. Biologically, however, this philosophy is not sound because the therapeutic ratio could actually deteriorate as a consequence of tumor repopulation. The strategy is characterized by splitting the total radiation course into halves with an interdigitated break lasting several days. The clinical rationale allowed for a field reduction in the second portion of the radiation course. It also selected patients who would either progress or deteriorate during the break. These would then not be treated further. The biologic rationale for split-course radiation included the expectation that a several-day break would enhance reoxygenation by allowing neovascularization and angiogenesis, permit an improvement in the therapeutic ratio by allowing greater normal tissue repair in comparison to tumor repair, and cause redistribution of cells from G_0 to more sensitive phases in the cell cycle. This method is particularly valuable for bulky, locoregional solid tumors involving the head and neck or lung, for which palliation is the primary treatment objective. The brief hypofractionated initial course allows delivery of a moderate radiation dose in large fractions to initiate tumor shrinkage. The split-course break is then introduced to prevent brisk acute toxicity and to provide several weeks for

---

* A few intensified fractionation regimens, which incorporate a split-course design, are delivered with curative intent. The most well studied is the CC Wang accelerated hyperfractionation split-course schedule for head and neck cancer, which uses a 1.6 Gy twice-daily fractionation and provides a 10 to 14-day mid-course break to allow healing of the intense mucosal reactions.[14]

tumor shrinkage. The second hypofractionated treatment course can thereby be delivered to a smaller treatment volume to maximize the effectiveness and durability of the palliative regimen. (See example in Table 47.2.)

Advantages and Disadvantages of Altered Fractionation Strategies

Although the potential radiobiologic advantages of altered fractionation strategies have been well formulated and confirmed in a variety of clinical treatment settings, several potential disadvantages are worth considering. The primary advantage for intensified fractionation strategies involves the potential for higher tumor control rates, particularly for rapidly proliferating tumors in which radiation therapy plays a dominant treatment role.[15–17] The most well-studied histology and anatomic site for such altered fractionation approaches involves squamous cell carcinoma of the head and neck.[18] Randomized trials have revealed a reproducible improvement in locoregional disease control rates with the use of both hyperfractionation and treatment acceleration strategies. However, one clear consequence of these intensified fractionation approaches includes increased acute toxicities that occur with this more rapid accumulation of total dose. Accelerated hyperfractionation schedules provide an increased total dose delivered in smaller fractions over a reduced overall treatment time compared to standard therapy. The enhancement of acute mucosal toxicity can influence not only the patient's tolerance to therapy, but also the degree of medical assistance that must be provided during and after therapy with regard to pain control, nutrition, and subsequent healing processes. For slower growing tumors for which radiation therapy does not play a dominant therapy role, the potential advantages of intensified fractionation schedules may be outweighed by the increase in acute toxicity.

Today, split-course radiation is less used in the context of curative radiation because of the concern that treatment interruption may allow tumor proliferation. Although significant data regarding the negative impact of treatment interruptions are available from a variety of other epithelial neoplasms such as head and neck carcinoma and cancer of the cervix, limited data exist for NSCLC. The best evidence for such a negative outcome results from an analysis of three Radiation Therapy Oncology Group (RTOG) studies (8311, 8321 and 8403), where the impact of treatment delay was evaluated.[19] Whereas only 3% of patients in protocols 8321 and 8403 had any significant treatment interruptions, 11% of patients on RTOG 8311, a protocol that evaluated hyperfractionation, experienced treatment interruptions. The proportion of patients experiencing delay in timely completion increased with total dose. Survival was significantly shortened in those patients whose treatment duration was prolonged compared to those treated per protocol. Estimated two- and five-year survival rates were 24%

and 10%, respectively, for patients treated without interruptions, compared to 13% and 3% for those experiencing treatment interruptions. These data, although possibly influenced by other variables, provide a suggestion that prolongation of the treatment schedule may result in accelerated tumor repopulation with subsequent negative impact on survival.

CLINICAL APPLICATION OF ALTERED FRACTIONATION REGIMENS

Split-Course Radiation

Split-course radiotherapy for lung cancer was standard during the 1960s and 1970s. At least five clinical trials tested the split-course concept.[20–24] None of these randomized clinical trials proved a survival benefit from split-course radiation therapy. Although Holsti and Mattson[20] concluded that split-course was better tolerated, and Lee and colleagues[21] suggested that this regimen was "more practical," Levitt's study[22] found that more side effects occurred in the group receiving split-course radiation therapy than in the group receiving continuous fractionated radiotherapy. In addition, Perez's study[23] reported that local control was superior in the 60 Gy continuous arm compared to the 40 Gy split-course arm. In that particular study (RTOG 7301), the intrathoracic failure rate with split-course radiation therapy was 44% compared to 33% with the continuous fractionated course. In a more recent trial, Routh and colleagues also could find no survival advantage from the split-course schedule, but like Lee suggested that it was associated with lower morbidity.[24] As a consequence of these trials, split-course therapy cannot be substituted as standard for NSCLC.

Hypofractionation

This method utilizes fewer radiation fractions but a higher dose per fraction. It has the advantage of efficiency and cost-effectiveness by less use of radiation therapy equipment. Additionally, the reduced total number of clinic visits may potentially have a bearing on patient convenience and quality-of-life issues. However, the use of large fraction radiation typically has a higher frequency of late toxicity. This method has been less widely utilized in curative lung cancer treatment. In fact, in a trial by Pritoli and colleagues,[25] 86 patients with NSCLC were randomized to receive weekly fractions of 5.57 or 8.8 Gy to a total dose ranging from 42 to 44 Gy. These patients experienced an unusually high rate of late pulmonary (56%) and connective tissue (40%) toxicity. In two other studies,[26,27] no significant increase in late toxicity was identified. This outcome however, may be influenced by the paucity of patients alive after 2 to 3 years. Despite toxicity, neither of these two latter studies found a survival difference. Slawson and colleagues reported on 120 patients randomized to 60 Gy given by a once-a-week schedule with a single fraction of 5 Gy for 12 weeks.[27] These patients were compared to patients receiving standard fractionated radiation therapy to a total of 60 Gy in 30 fractions over 6 weeks. No statistically significant differences in toxicity, response rates, or two-year survival were reported. Although not widely accepted or used, this study raises some interesting considerations. Particularly in patients who can be selected on the basis of poor prognostic factors and identified as having very short expected survival, it may be reasonable to consider hypofractionated radiation therapy.

Hyperfractionated Radiation Therapy

Hyperfractionation represents a plan that uses multiple daily radiation fractions with smaller than usual radiation doses per fraction within a treatment time of 6 to 7 weeks. The advantages of this strategy include a potential reduction in long-term tissue toxicity and the possibility of improving the therapeutic ratio by reduced injury to late-effect tissues, improving reoxygenation between radiation fractions, and redistributing cells into a more radiosensitive phase (G_2-M-phase).

Pure accelerated fractionation strategies have been extensively tested by the RTOG. Between 1983 and 1987, the RTOG enrolled 848 patients in a phase I/II trial where patients were randomized to receive 60, 64.8, 69.6, 74.4, or 79.2 Gy minimum total dose.[28] Two daily fractions of 1.2 Gy each were utilized with a minimum four-hour interfraction interval. Overall, no significant differences in either acute or late toxicities were identified in the five arms of the study. In order to evaluate possible survival benefit, a subgroup analysis was performed on 350 patients who met the criteria utilized by the Cancer and Leukemia Group B (CALGB) Protocol 8433. These criteria included a Karnofsky score of $\geq$70 and <6% body weight loss. In this subset analysis from a phase I/II study, those receiving 69.6 Gy had significantly improved median (13 months) and two-year survival (29%) (p = 0.02) compared to patients receiving lower total doses. Subsequent to these suggestive data, a three-arm prospective randomized trial included a 69.6 hyperfractionated treatment arm. Patients were randomized to the then "standard" radiotherapy, 60 Gy in 30 fractions of 2 Gy each, or two cycles of vinblastine-cisplatin chemotherapy preceding 60 Gy, or the hyperfractionated 1.2 Gy twice daily to a total of 69.6 Gy in 6 weeks. In the initial analysis of this trial,[29] the combination therapy arm verified the principle that chemotherapy improved survival regardless of the radiotherapy-alone schedule used. Median survival was 11.4 months for 60 Gy, 12.3 months for hyperfractionated radiotherapy 69.6 Gy, and 13.8 months for the combined modality arm. The one-year survival rates for the three arms were 46%, 51%, and 60%. The report by Sause et al. on five-year results shows long-term results poorer than long-term results for CALGB[3]—qualitatively similar but quantitatively different.[29]

Accelerated Radiation Therapy

The distinguishing hallmark of accelerated radiotherapeutic regimens is an overall reduction in treatment time with the expectation that this change will overcome accelerated tumor repopulation. From a practical perspective, this goal can be achieved and has been tested in patients with NSCLC using two different strategies; concomitant boost (field within a field technique) and a combination of multiple daily fractions with increased total daily dose (accelerated hyperfractionation).

Concomitant Boost

The technique of accelerating radiotherapy dose delivery reduces the overall treatment time by 1 to 2 weeks by giving the boost as a second fraction during the normal course of standard radiotherapy. Phase I and II studies have been carried out by the RTOG. In the largest such report, 355 patients received 1.8 Gy fractions to standard large fields, followed 4 to 6 hours later by a 1.8 Gy boost, given two to three times each week.[30] The total dose was escalated from 63 to 70.2 Gy in 5 weeks. Although some increase in acute toxicity occurred in the higher dose arm, late toxicities were not enhanced. Median survival remained at 9 months for the various cohorts, but in the high-dose arm, one- and two-year survival rates were 44 and 22%, respectively, comparable to what is contemporarily achieved with combination therapy. This approach has recently been tested in a randomized fashion by investigators from Taiwan. In a preliminary analysis of their data, they have identified improved response rates in the concomitant boost arm compared to the standard radiotherapy arm. Because of limited follow-up, survival data have not been analyzed thus far (Sun et al. personal communication, 1999).

Accelerated Hyperfractionation

The second major radiotherapeutic altered fractionation technique that permits an overall decrease in total treatment time is referred to as *accelerated hyperfractionation* and has recently been extensively tested clinically. The biologic basis for this technique stems from the recognition that the potential doubling time of lung cancer is relatively short (5 to 7 days).[13] The rapid repopulation from these tumor cells implies loss of effectiveness within a couple weeks of initiation of therapy. In order to overcome this loss it would be necessary to considerably shorten the overall treatment time. From a practical standpoint, the easiest way to accelerate is to use multiple daily fractions, less than 1.8 to 2.0 Gy each, but with a daily cumulative dose greater than 2.8 to 3.0 Gy, a biologically comparable total dose, and a significantly shortened overall treatment duration. This concept, therefore, marries acceleration with hyperfractionation and is known as *hyperfractionated accelerated radiation therapy* (HART). When weekend breaks are eliminated so that no interruption occurs the word "continuous" is added, resulting in the well-known acronym CHART.

Clinical trials of CHART in NSCLC were first reported from England by Saunders and Dische. Based on their encouraging preliminary data, a large multicenter randomized European trial has been completed.[31] A total dose of 54 Gy was delivered over 12 continuous treatment days at 1.5 Gy twice daily, separated by intervals of 6 hours, resulting in an 18-hour treatment day, weekends included. The initial results of this randomized trial demonstrate a significant 10% survival benefit at 2 years compared to a standard 60 Gy schedule. The odds ratio in favor of the CHART regimen was 0.75, suggesting a 25% decline in the risk of death.

The CHART regimen has not gained popularity in the U.S. because of personnel and logistic constraints demanded by three treatments per day. An alternative, more practical regimen, spaced over 15 days, including two weekend breaks, has been piloted by the Eastern Cooperative Oncology Group (ECOG 4593) with a median and one-year survival of 13.5 months and 57% respectively.[32] Although a direct comparison of these various trials is not valid, a simple comparison of the various combination therapy trials and altered fractionation trials is presented in Table 47.3. These data suggest that the more aggressive treatment, including combination therapy and altered fractionation, yield results superior to conventional, once-daily radiotherapy.

The ECOG HART experience differs from the European CHART trial in that weekend treatment was omitted from the ECOG regimen, resulting in a small prolongation in overall treatment time. This prolongation in treatment theoretically predicts a modest loss in local control because of accelerated repopulation. Investigators at Wisconsin derived the dose and fractionation regimen for the current trial using the linear-quadratic formula and increased the total dose to compensate for the treatment prolongation resulting from weekend breaks.[33] Table 47.4 compares various characteristics and endpoints between the ECOG HART trial and the European CHART trial. The ECOG HART trial has a higher percentage of patients with more advanced primary tumors and a greater proportion of N3 patients. The survival from both trials warrants further comparative trials. Moreover, the one-year survival in the ECOG trial is comparable to that achieved in several contemporary trials using sequential chemotherapy and once-daily radiation therapy. It is also accomplished in a much shorter time frame without the toxicities associated with chemotherapy.[3,29,34]

Chemotherapy Plus Altered Fractionation

Based on the principles and results outlined thus far, the logical next step is to test a combination of chemotherapy and altered fractionation. Several such phase I/II trials have now been reported and are summarized in Table 47.5. Results with these methods were reported in a North Central Cancer Treatment Group (NCCTG) study reported by Shaw et al.[35] These investigators treated 23 patients in a pilot of split-course hyperfractionated radiotherapy using 1.5 Gy bid to a total of 30 Gy, followed by a two-week break and an additional 30 Gy using a similar schedule.

TABLE 47.3. SURVIVAL COMPARISON OF SELECTED RADIOTHERAPY, CHEMORADIOTHERAPY, AND ALTERED FRACTIONATION TRIALS

Author	Study	Arm	Survival: median, % 1–3 years			
			M	1	2	3
Dillman	CALGB 8433	qd RT	9.6	40	13	10
Sause	RTOG 8808	qd RT	11.4	46	19	6
Schaake-Konig	EORTC	qd RT	—	46	13	2
Le Chevalier	IGR	qd RT	10	41	14	4
Saunders	CHART	qd RT	≅12	≅50	20	≅10
Cox	RTOG 8311	bid RT	13	56	29	≅20
Sause	RTOG 8808	bid RT	12.3	51	24	13
Saunders	CHART pilot	tid RT	≅15	64	34	≅18
Saunders	CHART	tid RT	≅15	≅61	30	≅20
Tannehill	ECOG 4593	tid RT	13.3	57	—	—
Dillman	CALGB 8433	CT + RT	13.7	54	26	24
Sause	RTOG 8808	CT + RT	13.8	60	32	15
Schaake-Konig	EORTC	RT + qwk CT	—	44	19	13
Schaake-Konig	EORTC	RT + qd CT	—	54	26	16
Le Chevalier	IGR	CT + RT	12	51	21	12

Qd, Once daily; bid, twice daily; tid, thrice daily; qwk, once weekly; RT, radiotherapy; CT, chemotherapy; ≅, estimated from survival curves; M, median survival in months.

TABLE 47.4. COMPARISON BETWEEN ECOG 4593 AND CHART

Characteristic	ECOG 4593	CHART
Tumor and nodal stages, %		
T1	17	9
T2	10	44
T3	37	25
T4	37	22
N0	20	49
N1	3	13
N2	37	36
N3	40	3
Prognostic factors, %		
Performance status of 0	27	40
Weight loss	40	NS
Squamous cell histology	47	81
Outcome end points		
1-year survival rate	57	~61*
Median survival, months	13	~15*
Toxicities, %		
Death from other causes	24	13
Esophagitis ≥ grade 3	22	NA†
Dysphagia, moderate to severe	NA†	49

Abbreviations: NS, not significant; NA, not applicable.
* One-year and median survival percentages are estimated from survival curve.
† Esophagitis grading systems differed among studies.

Two cycles of etoposide and cisplatin were given, one with commencement of the first radiation session, and the other when the second half of the radiotherapy course was commenced. Although toxicities were considerable, with 26% grade 3 or greater acute pneumonitis, the overall median and one- and two-year survival figures were an impressive 26 months and 74% and 51%.[35]

The RTOG has tested the 1.2 Gy twice-daily regimen to 69.6 Gy with vinblastine (5 mg/m^2 weekly × 5) and cisplatin (75 mg/m^2 on days 1, 29, and 50) in their trial 90–15. Enhanced acute toxicities were substantial, with 45% grade 4 or greater hematologic and 24% grade 3 or greater esophagitis. The median and one- and two-year survival rates were 12.2 months, 54% and 28%. In a subgroup with prognostic features similar to CALGB 8433, these survival figures were 17.5 months and 60% and 30%.[36]

These rather excessive toxicities led the RTOG to substitute etoposide for vinblastine because this regimen had previously been tested and better tolerated in SCLC. Seventy-nine patients received two cycles of oral etoposide 100 mg/d, intravenous cisplatin 50 mg/m^2 on days 1 and 8 and hyperfractionated radiation therapy to 69.6 Gy. The median survival for patients comparable to CALGB 8433 was 21 months, with one- and two-year survival figures of 70% and 42% (these values for CALGB 8433 were 13.7 months and 54% and 26%). Unfortunately, the associated toxicities from this regimen were also substantial, with 57% grade 4 hematologic toxicity, 53% ≥ grade 3 esophagitis, and 25% ≥ grade 3 pulmonary toxicity.[37]

In a 34-patient phase II trial, the feasibility of combined concurrent hyperfractionated radiotherapy (60 Gy in 48 fractions of 1.25 Gy, twice-daily) and chemotherapy consisting of cisplatin (6 mg/m^2 every day of radiotherapy) and vindesine (2.5 mg/m^2 once weekly) was tested. After a three-week rest period, two full cycles of cisplatin (120 mg/m^2 on weeks 10 and 14) and vindesine (2.5 mg/m^2 on weeks 11, 12, and 13) were given. Treatment evaluation with thoracic computed scan, bronchoscopy, and bronchial biopsies was performed 3 months after completion of radiation therapy. Failure rates were estimated using a competing risk approach. The complete response rate was 50%. Local failure

TABLE 47.5. CHEMORADIOTHERAPY TRIALS WITH ALTERED FRACTIONATION

Study	N	RT (Gy)	All Bid	CT	Seq	Toxicity (%) Bm	Eso	Lu	Survival Other	M	1	2
Shaw	23	60 S	1.5	PE	C			26		26	74	51
R 9015	42	69.6	1.2	PV	C	45	24			12	54	28
R 9106	79	69.6	1.2	PE	C	57	53	25		19	67	35
Jeremic	61	64.8	1.2	—	—				G4 = 2	8	39	25
Jeremic	52	64.8	1.2	CbE	C				G4 = 4	18	73	35
Jeremic	56	64.8	1.2	CbE	C alt				G4 = 1	13	50	27
Pechoux	34	60	1.25	P Vd	C Con				G5 = 2		53	33
Jeremic	66	69.6	1.2	—						14		
Jeremic	65	69.6	1.2	CbE	D					22		

N, Number of patients in each arm or study; RT (Gy), total radiation dose in Gy; bid, twice daily (the numbers in this column represent fraction size in Gy); CT, chemotherapy; P, cisplatin; V, vinblastine; E, etoposide; Vd, vindesine; Cl, carboplatin; Sec, sequencing of chemotherapy and radiotherapy; C, concurrent; con, conslidation; D, daily with radiation; qwk, weekly; alt, every other week; Toxicity (%), percentage of patients experiencing severe toxicity; bm, heatologic toxicity; eso, acute esophagitis; lu, acute pneumonitis; other, other toxicity; G5, death; G4, grade 4 toxicity; M, median survival in months; 1 and 2, percent survival at 1 and 2 years.

rates at 1 and 3 years were 53% and 56%, respectively. Distant metastases rates at 1 and 3 years were 27% and 29%. Overall survival rates at 1, 2, and 3 years were 53%, 33%, and 12%, respectively. Severe esophagitis was observed in three patients (9%). Lethal toxicity was observed in two patients. This phase II trial confirmed the feasibility of this type of approach and suggested that it may improve local control compared to conventional approaches.[38]

The excess toxicity from combining chemotherapy with altered fractionation has been investigated in a multicenter randomized trial using accelerated radiotherapy with or without concurrent carboplatin. One hundred patients with NSCLC were randomized to receive one of four treatments: (arm 1) radiotherapy 60 Gy (2 Gy daily) in 30 fractions in 6 weeks; (arm 2) accelerated radiotherapy (2 Gy twice-daily) 60 Gy in 30 fractions in 3 weeks; (arm 3) radiotherapy as in arm 1, plus carboplatin 350 mg/m^2 during weeks 1 and 5 of radiotherapy; (arm 4) radiotherapy as in arm 2, plus carboplatin 350 mg/m^2 during week 1. The median survival for all patients was 17.1 months, with 33% survival at 2 years. The major toxicities were hematologic and esophageal. Patients receiving carboplatin had more neutropenia ($p < 0.0001$) and thrombocytopenia ($p = 0.002$) than patients receiving radiotherapy alone, and this reaction was most marked in patients on arm 3. Both carboplatin and accelerated radiotherapy caused more severe esophagitis when compared to conventional radiotherapy alone ($p = 0.011$ and $p = 0.0017$, respectively). Esophagitis was more prolonged in patients having accelerated radiotherapy ($p < 0.0001$, median duration 3.2 months compared to 1.4 months for patients receiving conventional fractionation). Six patients (23%) treated on arm 2 required dilatation of esophageal stricture, one dying with a laryngoesophageal fistula.[39]

The first statistically significant survival advantage (median survival 34 versus 77 weeks; $p = 0.003$) from chemo-hyperfractionated radiotherapy was reported by Jeremic in a three-arm randomized trial in the group receiving 100 mg/d carboplatin on days 1 and 2 with 100 mg etoposide on days 1 to 3 of each week during the course of radiotherapy (64.8 Gy; 1.2 Gy twice-daily) compared to the same radiation alone.[40] However, both acute and late toxicities were increased with this approach. Grade 4 acute toxicities were seen in 2%, 4%, and 11% of patients receiving radiation alone, radiation with weekly chemotherapy, and radiation with chemotherapy on alternate weeks, respectively; the late toxicity values were 2%, 4%, and 9%.

Jeremic's group then conducted a subsequent phase III follow-up study with a design change. To investigate the efficacy of concurrent hyperfractionated radiation therapy and low-dose daily chemotherapy in stage III NSCLC, 131 patients were randomly treated as follows: group I, 1.2 Gy twice-daily to 69.6 Gy; group II, same radiation with 50 mg of carboplatin and 50 mg of etoposide given on each day of radiotherapy. Group II patients had a significantly

longer survival time than group I patients, with a median survival of 22 versus 14 months and four-year survival rates of 23% versus 9% ($p = .021$). The median time to local recurrence and four-year local recurrence-free survival rate were also significantly higher in group II than in group I (25 versus 20 months and 42% versus 19%, respectively, $p = .015$). In contrast, the distant metastasis-free survival rate did not significantly differ in the two groups. The two groups showed similar incidence of acute and late high grade toxicity.[40]

Further detailed analysis of response, toxicity, and failure patterns in trials combining chemotherapy with radiation either sequentially or concurrently was recently conducted and published by Byhardt and colleagues.[40] In this analysis, five completed RTOG trials utilizing either sequential chemotherapy followed by standard radiotherapy or sequential and concurrent chemotherapy with standard radiation, or concurrent chemotherapy and hyperfractionated radiation were evaluated. Both acute and late toxicities were compared. Patients were divided into three groups. All patients had a Karnofsky score of $\geq 70\%$ and a weight loss of $< 5\%$. Group 1 included patients receiving sequential chemotherapy followed by standard radiation therapy to 60 Gy in 6 weeks; group 2 included patients who received both sequential and concurrent chemotherapy followed by a standard 60 Gy radiation therapy; and group 3 included patients who received concurrent chemotherapy and hyperfractionated radiotherapy to a total of 69.6 Gy in 6 weeks. The chemotherapy in all five of the trials utilized cisplatin with either vinblastine or oral etoposide. Overall, life-threatening acute toxicities (grade 4/5) were equivalent among the three groups. However, the severe nonhematologic acute toxicities were significantly different based on the treatment regimen. Specifically, group 3 patients had a significantly greater incidence of severe acute nonhematologic toxicity (55%) compared to group 1 (27%) or group 2 (34%). This result was accounted for in large measure by the severe acute esophagitis rate of 34% in group 3 compared to 1.3% in group 1 and 6% in group 2 ($p < 0.0001$). Similarly, although the overall incidence of life-threatening (grade 4/5) late toxicities did not differ by treatment group, the incidence of severe late nonhematologic toxicity was higher in both groups 2 (26%) and 3 (28%) compared to group 1 (14%). In large measure, this outcome was accounted for not by severe late esophagitis but by severe late lung toxicity, the incidence for which was 10% for group 1, 21% for group 2, and 20% for group 3 ($p = 0.033$). These data therefore provide a substantial database, suggesting that concurrent chemotherapy and hyperfractionated radiotherapy carry a significantly higher incidence of not only acute esophageal toxicity but also enhanced late pulmonary toxicity.

Despite the encouraging aspects of the results from Jeremic's trials, further supportive evidence is necessary before combination chemo-altered fractionation radiotherapy can

TABLE 47.6. ACUTE SEVERE ESOPHAGITIS IN LUNG CANCER TRIALS

Study	Radiation		Chemotherapy			% Esophagitis
	Standard	Hyperfractionated	Pre-XRT	W/XRT	Post XRT	(Grade 3 and 4)
RTOG 9015[28]	N	Y	N	Y	N	24
RTOG 9106[37]	N	Y	N	Y	N	53
Le Pechoux[38]	N	Y	N	Y	Y	9 (Grade 4)
Byhardt[30]	Y	N	Y	N	N	1–3
Byhardt[36]	Y	N	Y	Y	N	6
Byhardt[40]	N	Y	N	Y	N	34

be recommended outside a protocol context. The RTOG has initiated an important three-arm randomized trial (RTOG 94-10) comparing sequential chemoradiotherapy to concurrent chemoradiotherapy in one experimental arm and concurrent chemoradiotherapy with twice-daily radiation in the other arm; results of this trial are eagerly awaited.

CONCLUSIONS

Early therapeutic strategies assumed that local control was of paramount significance in leading to cure of lung cancer. High rates of local control could be achieved with conventional fractionation radiotherapy to 60 Gy. Chemotherapy of the 1970s was minimally active, without impact on micrometastatic disease or survival. However, randomized induction chemoradiotherapy trials demonstrated a small but measurable survival gain, resulting from increased control of metastatic disease and some improvement in locoregional control. Contemporaneously, better assessment of local control by bronchoscopy indicated that radiographic evaluation overestimated local control rates, which really were only 8%. This realization leads to renewed efforts at controlling the disease locally. Altered fractionation, which has effects on local disease and normal tissues within the target volume, demonstrates statistically significant and meaningful survival benefit. Combinations of chemotherapy and altered fractionation therefore represent a "new frontier," and although it is too soon to judge its overall impact, this strategy has certainly resulted both in increased toxicity as well as improved survival in preliminary reports. The formidable toxicity needs to be addressed, perhaps with volume reduction or chemotherapy choices.

Are we reaching a therapeutic ceiling? Table 47.6 provides the acute grade 3 and 4 esophagitis rates from various aggressive combination chemotherapy plus hyperfractionated radiotherapy trials. With conventional sequential chemoradiotherapy strategies, the rate of severe esophagitis is usually below 5%, but with the aggressive strategies, the incidence rises to 24% to 53%. Future progress in this disease must balance toxicities with outcome, measured not just in survival terms, but also as it pertains to quality-of-

life. The societal impact, particularly cost-effectiveness, will become a critical question. For example, how justifiable is it to treat the majority of advanced, nonmetastatic lung cancer patients with poor prognostic features with aggressive therapies when they have been excluded from the randomized trials? Even if the hyperfractionation results hold up as being equivalent to survival with combination therapy, it may not be useful if toxicity is too high. The provocative benefits of altered fraction schemes require proof from randomized phase III trials. One such study is the prospective randomized phase III ECOG trial (ECOG E2597), in which patients receive two cycles of carboplatin and taxol followed by a randomization to once-daily radiation therapy to 64 Gy, or thrice-daily radiation therapy to 57.6 Gy as piloted in the ECOG HART regimen. Collective and collaborative clinical trial effort will answer such questions.

REFERENCES

1. Bonomi P. Combined modality treatment for stage III non-small cell lung cancer. *Lung Cancer* 1995;12(suppl 2):41.
2. Perez CA, Pajak TF, Rubin P, et al. Long-term observations of the patterns-of-failure in patients with unresectable non-oat cell carcinoma of the lung treated with definitive radiotherapy. Report by the Radiation Therapy Oncology Group. *Cancer* 1987;59:1874.
3. Dillman RO, Herndon J, Seagren SL, et al. Improved survival in stage III non-small cell lung cancer: 7-yr follow-up of cancer and leukemia group B (CALGB) 8433 Trial. *J Natl Cancer Inst* 1996;88:1210.
4. Lechevalier T, Arriagada R, Quoix E, et al. Radiotherapy alone vs. combined chemotherapy and radiotherapy in nonresectable, non-small cell lung cancer: first analysis of a randomized trial in 353 patients. *J Natl Cancer Inst* 1991;83:417.
5. Thames HD, Hendry JH. *Fractionation in radiotherapy.* London; Taylor and Francis, 1987:137.
6. Thames HD. On the origin of dose fractionation regimens in radiotherapy. *Sem Radiat Oncol* 1992;2:3.
7. Fowler JF. Non-standard fractionation in radiotherapy. *Int J Radiat Oncol Biol Phys* 1984;10:755.
8. Thames HD, Peters LJ, Withers HR, et al. Accelerated fractionation vs. hyperfractionation: rationales for several treatments per day. *Int J Radiat Oncol Biol Phys* 1983;9:127.
9. Withers HR, Peters LJ, Thames HD. Hyperfractionation (editorial). *Int J Radiat Oncol Biol Phys* 1982;8:1807.

10. Withers HR. Biologic basis for altered fractionation schemes. *Cancer* 1985;55:2086.

11. Weiss W. Proliferation measures of brochogenic carcinoma. *Am Rev of Resp Dis* 1971;103:198.

12. Steele JD, Buell P. Asymptomatic solitary pulmonary nodules: host survival, tumor site and growth rate. *J Thorac Cardiovasc Surg* 1971;65:140.

13. Wilson GD, Saunders MI, Dische S, et al. Direct comparison of bromodeoxyuridine and Ki-67 labeling indices in human tumors. *Cell Prolif* 1996;29:141.

14. Wang CC, Blitzer PH, Suit H. Twice-a-day radiation therapy for cancer of the head and neck. *Cancer* 1985;55:2100.

15. Ang KK, Peters LJ. Altered fractionation in radiation oncology. In: Devita VT, Hellman S, Rosenberg SA, eds. *Cancer: principles and practice of oncology (PPO Updates)*. Philadelphia: JB Lippincott, 1994;8(4):1.

16. Fowler JF. Brief summary of radiological principles in fractionated radiotherapy. *Sem Radiat Oncol.* 1992;2:16.

17. Fowler JF, Harari PM. Hyperfractionation's promise in cancer treatment: rationales for treating patients twice a day. *Contemp Oncol* 1993;3:14.

18. Harari PM. Altered fractionation strategies in radiation oncology for the head and neck cancer patient. In: Williams TP, ed. *Oral and maxillofacial surgery clinics of North America.* Philadelphia: WB Saunders, 1997.

19. Cox JD, Pajakt F, Aspell S, et al. Interruptions of high dose radiation therapy decrease long-term survival of favorable patients with unresectable non-small cell carcinoma of the lung: analysis of 1,244 cases from three radiation therapy oncology group (RTOG) trials. *Int J Radiat Oncol Biol Phys* 1993;27:493.

20. Holsti LR, Mattson K. A randomized study of split-course radiotherapy of lung cancer: long-term results. *Int J of Radiat Oncol Biol Phys* 1980;6:977.

21. Lee RE, Carr DT, Childs D. Comparison of split-course radiation therapy and continuous radiation therapy for unresectable bronchogenic carcinoma: 5-year results. *Am J Roentgenol Radiat Thera Nucl Med* 1976;126:116.

22. Levitt SH, Bogrdus CR, Ladd G. Split-dose intensive radiation therapy in the treatment of advanced lung cancer: a randomized study. *Radiology* 1967;88:1159.

23. Perez CA, Stanley K, Grundy G, et al. Impact of irradiation technique and tumor extent in tumor control and survival of patients with unresectable non-small cell carcinoma of the lung: report of the Radiation Therapy Oncology Group. *Cancer* 1982; 50:1091.

24. Routh A, Hickman BT, Khansur T. Report of a prospective trial—split-course versus conventional radiotherapy in the treatment of non-small cell lung cancer. *Radiat Med* 1995;13:115.

25. Pritoli L, Bindi M, Belezza A, et al. Unfavorable experience with hypofractionated radiotherapy in unresectable lung cancer. *Tumori* 1992;78:305.

26. Deely T. *The chest: monographs in oncology.* London: Butterworth, 1973.

27. Slawson R, Salazer O, Poussin-Rosilloh, et al. Once-a-week vs. conventional daily radiation treatment for lung cancer; final report. *Intel J Radiat Oncol Biol Phys* 1998;15:61.

28. Cox JD, Azarnia N, Byhardt RW, et al. A randomized phase I/II trials of hyperfractionated radiation therapy with total doses of 60.0 Gy–79.2 Gy: possible survival benefit with ≥69.6 Gy in favorable patients with Radiation Therapy Oncology Group's stage III non-small cell lung carcinoma: report of Radiation Therapy Oncology Group 83-11. *J Clin Oncol* 1990;8:1543.

29. Sause W, Scott C, Taylor S, et al. Radiation Therapy Oncology Group (RTOG) 88-08 and Eastern Cooperative Oncology Group (ECOG) 4588: preliminary results of a phase III trial in regionally advanced unresectable non-small cell lung cancer. *J Natl Cancer Inst* 1995;87:198.

29a. Sause W, Kolesar P, Taylor S, et al. Five-year results; phase III trial of regionally advanced unresectable non-small cell lung cancer, RTOG 8808, ECOG 4588, SWOG 8992. *Proc ASCO* 1998; 17:453A.

30. Byhardt RW, Pajak F, Emami B, et al. A phase I/II study to evaluate accelerated fractionation via concomitant boost for squamous, adenol and large cell carcinoma of the lung: report of Radiation Therapy Oncology Group 8407. *Intl J Radiat Oncol Biol Phys* 1993;26:459.

31. Saunders MI, Dische S, Barrett A, et al. Randomized multi-center trials of CHART vs. conventional radiotherapy in head and neck and non-small cell lung cancer: an interim report. *Br J Cancer* 1996;73:1455.

32. Mehta MP, Tannehill SP, Adak S, et al. Phase II trial of hyperfractionated accelerated radiation therapy (HART) for nonresectable non-small cell lung cancer: results of ECOG 4593. *J Clin Oncol* 1998;16(11):3518.

33. Fowler JF. The linear quadratic formula and progress in fractionated radiotherapy. *Br J Radiol* 1989;162:679.

34. Schaake-Konig C, VanDen Bogaert W, Dalesio O, et al. Effects of concomitant cisplatin and radiotherapy in inoperable non-small cell lung cancer. *N Eng J Med* 1992;326:524.

35. Shaw EG, McGinnis WL, Jett JR, et al. Pilot study of accelerated hyperfractionated thoracic radiation therapy plus concomitant etopside and cisplatin chemotherapy in patients with unresectable stage III non-small cell carcinoma of the lung. *J Natl Cancer Inst* 1993;85:321.

36. Byhardt RW, Scott CB, Ettinger DS, et al. Concurrent hyperfractionated irradiation and chemotherapy for unresectable non-small cell lung cancer: results of Radiation Therapy Oncology Group (RTOG) 90-15. *Cancer* 1995;75:2337.

37. Lee JS, Scott C, Komaki R, et al. Concurrent chemoradiation therapy with oral etoposide and cisplatin for locally advanced inoperable non-small cell lung cancer: Radiation Therapy Oncology Group Protocol 91-06. *J Clin Oncol* 1996;14:1055.

38. Le Pechoux C, Arriagada R, Le Chevalier T, et al. Concurrent cisplatin-vindesine and hyperfractionated thoracic radiotherapy in locally advanced non-small cell lung cancer. *Int J Radiat Oncol Biol Phys* 1996;35:519.

39. Ball D, Bishop J, Smith J, et al. A phase III study of accelerated radiotherapy with and without carboplatin in non-small cell lung cancer: an interim toxicity analysis of the first 100 patients. *Int J Radiat Oncol Biol Phys* 1995;31:267.

40. Byhardt RW, Scott C, Sause WT, et al. Response toxicity failure patterns and survival in five Radiation Therapy Oncology Group (RTOG) trials of sequential and/or concurrent chemotherapy and radiotherapy for locally advanced non-small cell carcinoma of the lung. *Int J Radiat Oncol Biol Phys* 1998;42:469.

41. Jeremic B, Shibamoto Y. Pre-treatment prognostic factors in patients with stage III non-small cell lung cancer treated with hyperfractionated radiation therapy with or without concurrent chemotherapy. *Lung* 1995;13:21.

48

THREE-DIMENSIONAL RADIATION THERAPY

MARY V. GRAHAM
WILLIAM B. HARMS

Radiation therapy remains a cornerstone of therapy for lung cancer. With the emergence of specialized volumetric three-dimensional radiation therapy planning and treatment systems (3DRTP), the potential benefits for lung cancer were quickly realized.[1] These benefits included (a) better localization of the tumor target(s), (b) improved ability to assess and potentially reduce normal tissue toxicity, and (c) increased tumoricidal doses of radiation to the tumor target(s). This chapter reviews the progress that has been made in the last decade in achieving these goals and the emerging issues in 3D radiation therapy for lung cancer.

BACKGROUND

The "standard of care" for the dose, volume, and beam arrangements for the treatment of non–small cell lung cancer (NSCLC) was established by the Radiation Therapy Oncology Group (RTOG) dose-escalation trial 7301.[2] In this study, 375 patients were randomly assigned to receive either 40 Gy in 4 weeks with a 2-week break (split-course), 40 Gy in 4 weeks, 50 Gy in 5 weeks, or 60 Gy in 6 weeks. The complete and partial response rates (as assessed clinically and radiographically) were 48% in patients treated with 40 Gy, 53% in those treated with 50 Gy, and 56% in those receiving 60 Gy. The incidence of local failure (also evaluated clinically) was lower in patients treated with 60 Gy (33%) than in those receiving 50 Gy (39%) or 40 Gy (44% to 49%). Perez and co-workers[3] reported that irradiation technique clearly affected results. Patients with major deviation from protocol compliance had poorer response rates and decreased survival. In this protocol, large volumes of the chest and regional lymphatics were included in the treatment volume. The electively irradiated areas included both hila, bilateral regions of the mediastinum, bilateral supraclavicular areas, and 5 to 8 cm below the carina of the inferior mediastinum. Despite a modest improvement at 3 years, by 5 years the overall survival was approximately 5%.

In the early 1990s the results of several large randomized trials reported increased survival with the addition of cisplatin-based chemotherapy.[4–6] Each of these trials utilized conventional radiation therapy and delivered 40 to 50 Gy to the elective nodal regions and 60 to 65 Gy to the gross disease. Despite the modest improvement demonstrated in these trials, there remains much room for improvement. Long-term survival is still only 8% to 14%.[4,6] LeChevalier and co-workers[5] reported a decreased metastatic incidence, but both arms had a local control rate of only 15% to 17% when evaluated by bronchoscopy and biopsy at 3 months and 10% at 2 years after completion of therapy. These results are considerably lower than the local control rates of 40% to 60% reported by soft clinical evaluation.[2,3] Perhaps contributing to poor local control was the uncertainty of target delineation and localization. Dillman and associates reported that a retrospective quality control review identified 23% of cases in which portal films failed to completely encompass the tumor.[4] In addition, lung cancers are usually quite large at presentation. It is the norm to have bulky tumors measuring greater than 2 to 5 cm. From basic principles advocated by Fletcher, it is thought that doses up to 100 Gy may be necessary to sterilize the size of tumors often treated in bronchogenic carcinoma.[7]

Further attempts at dose escalation were carried out in the RTOG prospective hyperfractionation trial 8301.[8] Fractions of 1.2 Gy were administered twice daily, and patients were dose-escalated through 60 Gy, 64.8 Gy, 69.6 Gy, 74.4 Gy, and 79.2 Gy. Among the 519 patients, 248 were considered favorable (absence of weight loss and a Karnofsky performance status of 70 to 100). Although no significant difference in disease-free survival was found in the unfavorable patients among the five arms, among the favorable patients a survival benefit was seen at the 69.6 Gy dose level but not higher. The reasons for this outcome have never been fully elucidated, although a higher incidence of high-grade pneumonitis was seen in the higher dose arms of the study.

This result suggested that indiscriminate dose escalation, without knowledge of dose and volume effects to the surrounding lungs may have a deleterious effect on survival.

It is well known that the lungs are exquisitely sensitive to the damaging effects of radiation, resulting in a significant chance for injury, including acute pneumonitis and symptomatic pulmonary fibrosis.[9,10] What is less well understood or quantitated is the impact of radiation lung damage on long-term survival.

From the previous discussion, it is apparent that efficacy and toxicity are significantly impacted by volume of tumors treated. 3DRTP may impact on these issues. Thus the primary goals of 3DRTP have been as follows: (a) evaluation and reduction of pulmonary (and possibly other) sequelae, and (b) improved precision and targeting of tumor with dose escalation to improve local control and subsequently overall survival.

THREE-DIMENSIONAL RADIATION THERAPY PLANNING FOR NSCLC

In order to realize the full potential of 3DRTP, all components of such planning must be utilized. Using specific components (i.e., beam's-eye view or limited cuts of computed tomography [CT] data solely) does not constitute 3D therapy. Tumor and target definition using full 3D volume techniques, virtual simulation, 3D dose calculation, and dose-volume histogram plan evaluation are all critical components to successful 3D therapy for NSCLC.

Defining the Target: Aquisition, Immobilization, Views, and Displays

The initiation of 3D radiotherapy is accomplished with the aquisition of the CT data set. The thoracic data set must include not only the entire volume of the tumor but also the complete lung volume. Many institutions have found it important to also included the entire volumes of the brachial plexi (base of neck), the heart, and the liver. If organs are not included in their entirety, then they are potentially inadvertently treated (when noncoplanar beams are utilized and regions not scanned or contoured are irradiated through the entrance or exit of beams), and/or the volumetric analysis and dose-volume histograms (DVHs) are meaningless because of lack of the full volume information of the organ.

At Washington University, patients are "immobilized" in the supine position using an alpha cradle device with the arms comfortably and securely positioned above the head (Figure 48.1). Multiple laser markings on the anterior and lateral aspect of the patient's thorax, arms, and hips help reproducibly set up the patient on a day-to-day basis and move the patient from scanner to simulator to treatment machine. CT slices of 2 to 5 mm thickness are obtained from the level of the patient's larynx through the entire liver (Figure 48.2). This results, on average, in 70 to 120 CT slices, each of which usually requires approximately 0.5 GByte of storage. Although such thin CT slices through

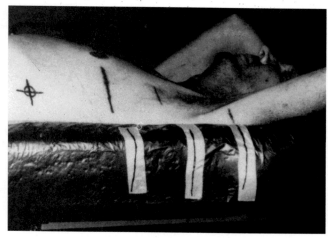

FIGURE 48.1. Lung cancer patient, immobilized using alpha cradle. Note multiple laser setup points to ensure reproducible setup.

regions not harboring tumor are rarely needed, the quality of the digitally reconstructed images (DRRs) is much enhanced by thinner cut and greater number of CT slices. At Washington University, radio-opaque markers are placed on the patient's skin anteriorly and laterally at the time of CT scanning to establish the coordinate system (initial isocenter), which is also used as a reference for the CT and verification simulation. To facilitate the registration of the CT and verification simulation, as well as in some cases the verification port films, DRRs with bony anatomy enhanced are printed out in the anteropostero and lateral beam orien-

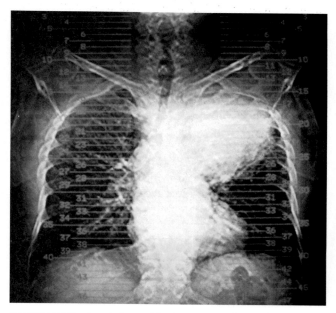

FIGURE 48.2. Scout view of lung cancer patient's three-dimensional (3D) computerized tomography (CT) data set.

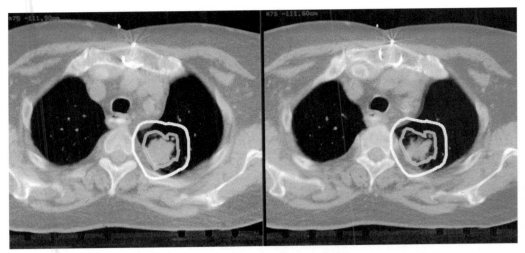

FIGURE 48.3. Representative gross tumor volume (GTV) on selected CT slices.

tations at isocenter. All movements of the isocenter during planning are made relative to the original isocenter, which is directly translated to the patient's reference marks.

The next step in treatment planning is to identify targets and normal anatomy on the CT data set. This step, called *image segmentation,* "divides" the CT data set into parts so that anatomic objects of interest and tumor volumes are identified. The skin or external contour is easily identified automatically by threshholding and edge-detection algorithms. Delineation of the skin-air boundary is the 3D analogue of the traditional 2D skin contour measurement and is necessary for dose calculation. Normal anatomy that should be contoured includes the brachial plexi (labeled ipsilateral and contralateral), the total lung volume (the volume of both lungs together), the heart (from its base to the level of the base of the aorta), the esophagus (in its entirety from larynx to gastroesophageal junction), and the liver.

International Commission on Radiation Units (ICRU) 50 defined tumor and treatment targets.[11] The gross tumor volume (GTV) includes all identifiable gross tumor (Figure 48.3). It should include the primary tumor as identified by CT. However, CT data are not perfectly accurate in the identification of lung cancer and staging.[12–15] Other imaging modalities such as magnetic resonance imaging (MRI), endoscopic ultrasound, and/or positron emission tomography (PET) may be important in identifying the GTV. It also includes the grossly identifiable regional lymph nodes, such as those abnormally enlarged on CT (short axis greater than 1 cm),[15] those that are mediastinoscopically positive, and possibly those with abnormal metabolic activity identified on PET scanning. Some institutions have found useful to designate the primary disease as GTV1 and the nodal disease as GTV2 (or vice versa). We have not found utility in this approach because all GTV is treated to the same dose level at Washington University and on the RTOG

dose-escalation trial. However, if in the future different gross disease is treated to different dose levels, then it would be helpful to subdivide these categories at the time of target delineation. The clinical target volume (CTV) is that anatomic region(s) thought to harbor subclinical or microscopic disease (Figure 48.4). Institutions have done this in different ways also. Some define a specific 3D margin around the gross disease and call this CTV2. Elective nodal regions are called CTV1. Both of these could be lumped together. Because of failure to reach consensus of where the CTV is exactly, the RTOG elected not to have a separate CTV and defined the CTV as equal to the GTV.

Planning target volumes (PTVs) are 3D growth margins around the GTV and/or CTV to account for daily setup variations and patient motion. Because of physiologic motion in the chest, the volume of the PTV may be significantly larger than the GTV. Recently, Wong and co-workers demonstrated that breath holding can reproducibly

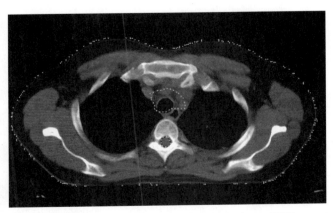

FIGURE 48.4. Representative clinical target volume (CTV) on selected CT slices.

"immobilize" targets and lungs between CT scans and presumably treatment sessions.[16] Theoretically, the volume of irradiated lung could be reduced, PTV margins could be reduced, and targets could be better localized during treatment with such a device. Such clinical experience and the measured therapeutic gain from such an approach is expected to be forthcoming.

After the CT data are segmented, a 3D model of the patient is produced and displayed for treatment planning. Organs and targets may be displayed as wire frames, solid surfaces, or with various degrees of opacification (Fig. 48.5A). The 3D images must be reviewed prior to planning or treatment plan acceptance to ensure that organs were contoured correctly, in their entirety, and without image

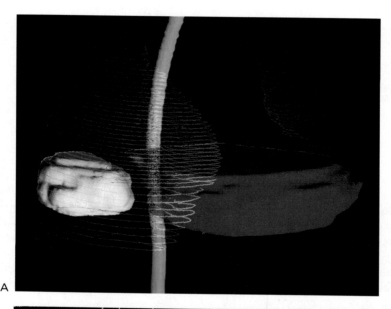

A

FIGURE 48.5. **A:** Lung cancer tumor target and normal organs displayed in "room view." **B:** Multiple images of anteropostero (AP) beam for lung cancer treatment. Note in the upper-right image that the green contour CTV does not have an adequate margin around the red GTV contour. This is because a 3D margin tool to generate the CTV was not used, thus only 2D margins were generated. (See Color Figure 48.5.)

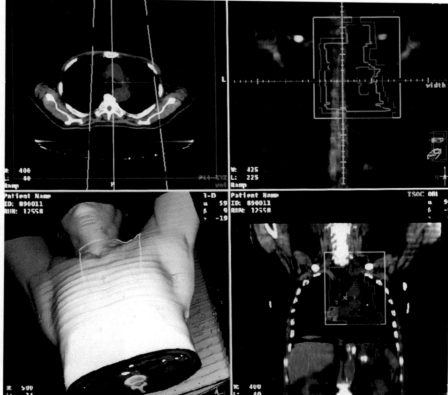

B

corruption. We have also found it important to ensure at this time that margins for CTV and/or PTV are fully 3D. Figure 48.5B actually shows an example where a 3D margin tool was *not* used, and one can see areas where PTV does not cover the GTV in superior 3D.

Virtual Simulation

Virtual simulation begins after all targets and normal anatomy are contoured and treatment planning begins.[12–20] In essence, the concept of virtual simulation is that the functions of the physical simulator are emulated by the treatment planning software. The patient in reality goes home, but the planning and "simulation" of the patient model proceed. Quite complex and difficult simulations can be planned without the patient present. This method is ultimately more comfortable for the patient and often more efficient. The objectives of virtual simulation are to design the treatment apertures (portals) and the beam directions (gantry, collimator, and table angles). In most 3D systems, the simulation of the beam arrangement is performed on the 3D model of the patient. At most institutions, one of two approaches is taken. The first is the development of "class solutions" (i.e., a four- or five-field approach with beams AP/PA to spinal cord tolerance and then off cord oblique fields to the desired tumor dose). This approach is often a good starting point and allows the planner to assess target coverage and irradiation to the lungs and other organs to assess the acceptability of this initial plan.

The second approach is for an experienced planner or dosimetrist to utilize the beam's-eye view and develop a unique beam arrangement for any one individual patient by avoiding specific normal organs. For example, noncoplanar, non–AP/PA beams may be particularly desirable for a plan specifically designed to avoid the heart and minimize the treated lung volume. Beam placement is particularly facilitated with the beam's-eye view.[21] Ideally, treatment angles are found that "separate" the tumor from surrounding normal structures (i.e., the beam is angled to treat just the target volume and miss the normal structures). Figure 48.6 shows a beam's-eye view of a field defined with multileaf collimation around a target volume.

A feature called "autoblocking" is a time-saving tool that allows the planner to choose a specific margin desired around a target and have the block automatically conform to the target and the leaf position numerically and positionally specified. The virtual simulator records and reports all the necessary simulation data, including beam names, energy of beams, table, gantry and collimator positions, isocenter location, and any beam modifiers. The display of such data is often facilitated by multiple images and views of the plan (Figure 48.7). Axial, coronal, and saggital displays, as well as room view display and an opaque view of the patient's skin and the surface appearance of the entrance portal are all often useful in evaluating the virtual simulation process.

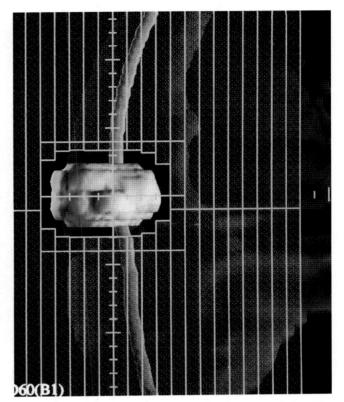

FIGURE 48.6. Beam's eye view of tumor with port defined by multileaf colimation. (See Color Figure 48.6.)

Most systems also have an icon that displays the position of the gantry and the table to conceptually show their position. Some systems have implemented formal collision prevention components into their software to avoid the development of plans that are not implementable or dangerous to the patient or the equipment.

Dose Calculation

Technically, in some systems it may be difficult to separate the process of virtual simulation and dose calculation, so the process of dose calculation and subsequent beam angle and shape readjustment is usually an integral part of the 3D treatment planning. The dose is calculated and displayed on the 3D model. Isodose displays are usually color-coded and can be isodose "nets" or wireframes or color wash displays of dose (Figure 48.8ABC). Dose may be calculated with a variety of algorithms. It is imperative for the planners and evaluators to understand the strengths and weaknesses of their particular system's dose calculation algorithm. In the near past, the dose calculation methods used in planning systems were based on parameterizing dose distributions measured in water phantoms under standard conditions and applying correction factors to the beam representations for the nonuniform surface contour of the patient or the obliq-

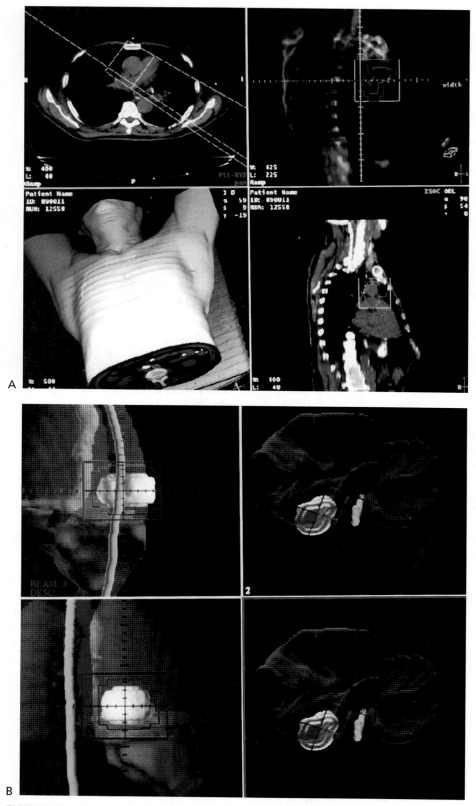

FIGURES 48.7 A, B: Multiple images used in 3D plan evaluation, including "room view," beam's eye view, axial, and saggital views. (See Color Figures 48.7 A,B.)

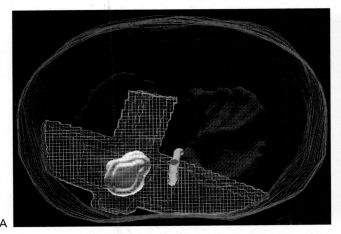

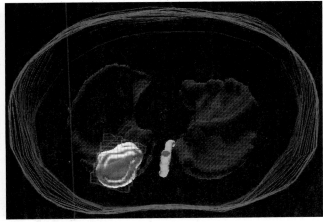

A

B

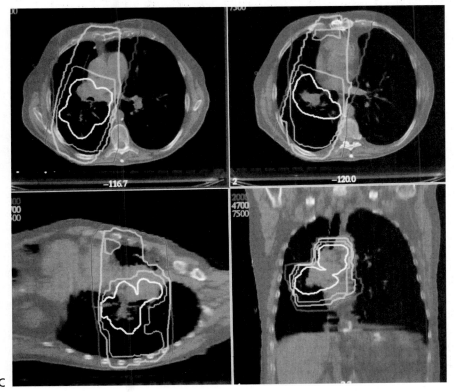

C

FIGURE 48.8 A,B,C: Various images depicting isodose coverage and various dose levels in 3D. (See Color Figures 48.8 A,B,C.)

uity of the beam, tissue heterogeneities, and beam modifiers such as blocks, wedges, and compensator. However, more advanced models have now been developed that compute the dose more from first principles and that use only a limited set of measurements to obtain a better fit of the model.[22] These 3DRTP methods utilize convolution energy deposition kernels that describe the distribution of dose about a single primary photon interaction site.

In addition to describing how scattered photons contribute to dose absorbed at some distance away from the interaction site of primary photons, the convolution kernels take into account charged particle transport. This information

can be used to compute dose in electronic disequilibrium situations such as in the buildup regions and in the beam penumbra. Therefore, depending on the user's age and development of their treatment planning system, dose may be calculated with simple pencil beam algorithms, with or without heterogeneity, with Clarkson-type irregular field calculations, and/or with scatter effects of blocks and other beam modifiers. A simple example of how this ability may affect planning is that if scatter of penumbra effects are not taken into account in dose calculation algorithm, then the planner must realize that block edges must be wider than the target by approximately 7 to 10 mm or greater. This will not necessarily be appropriately displayed in the target DVHs. There may be significant differences in target coverage and normal organ partial volume irradiation depending on whether heterogeneity corrections are applied or not. The reader is cautioned to be thoroughly acquainted with their own 3D system dose calculation engine.

In the future, Monte Carlo simulations are expected to be the preferred method for 3DRTP dose computation. As the price/performance ratio of computer workstations continues to decrease, this type of dose calculation may be practical in the near future.

Plan Optimization and Evaluation

The optimization of a treatment plan currently involves an expert planner and allows for modification of the beam direction, beam shape, beam weights, and beam modifiers. Rapid calculation and recalculation and display of dose distributions allow the planner to make incremental improvements in plans.

The "optimal" plan must achieve the following goals:

1. The tumor target(s) treated to sufficiently high (prescription) dose. For most 3D institutions this is 70 Gy or greater. Although in the past the uniformity of dose across the tumor was thought to be a desirable goal, this theory has recently been called into question. Theoretical models suggest that even partial target volume irradiation may result in improved outcome.[23] Prior to 3D treatment systems and accurate dose calculation algorithms, there was little way to test this hypothesis. Graham and co-workers presented preliminary clinical data for NSCLC patients suggesting that maximum tumor target doses of greater than 79 Gy resulted in improved survival for patients with low-volume tumors (GTV less than 113 cc).[24]

2. The volume of irradiated lung must be kept sufficiently low. Experience with what constituted acceptable levels of lung irradiation is presented later in this chapter.

3. Radiation dose to other nearby organs, such as esophagus, heart, and brachial plexi, must also be kept minimal. There are few clinical data on what the partial volume tolerance doses for these organs are using 3D data.

The development of dose volume histograms (DVHs) has greatly facilitated the objective plan evaluation and the consolidation of vast amounts of data depicted in the isodose displays.[25] At present, nothing has replaced the isodose display and "room view" displays for the spatial dose information regarding, but DVHs allow a planner to rapidly assess the adequacy, uniformity, and target dose coverage as well as the potential tolerability of nonuniform normal organ radiation treatment. Each contoured target and organ have a separate DVH. Many systems automatically report specific dose statistics from the DVH, such as minimum, mean, and maximum doses with the structure and the percent of the organ exceeding various threshold dose levels.

Typical DVHs depict dose on the x-axis and volume (in absolute or percentage) on the y-axis (Figure 48.9). Traditionally, DVHs of normal organs and targets are depicted in a cumulative fashion. See Figure 48.9, or a DVH showing the 22% of the total lung volume received in excess of 20 Gy.

It is anticipated that in the future, optimization of plans will be more automated. This goal will require a greater amount of clinical outcomes to be related to DVH data. But as this data becomes more available, specific parameters upon which to optimize a plan are utilized. Computerized optimization utilizing normal tissue complication probabilities (NTCPs), tumor control probabilities (TCPs), and DVHs and "inverse" planning is used in intensity modulated radiation therapy (IMRT). At the time of this writing, little information on IMRT for lung cancer has been published. This lack is probably because of two reasons: (a) concern about the respiratory movement during treatment and resultant intensity modulated calculations not reproducibly produced during treatment, and (b) heterogeneity factors (most important in the lungs) not reproducibly accounted for in some intensity modulated systems. Pilot planning studies have been reported by Derycke and co-workers.[26] The authors reported that certain class solutions utilizing specific TCP and NTCP parameters could be used to optimize lung plans using IMRT for stage III NSCLC patients.

Other approaches to optimization of treatment planning include (a) a database of previously designed successful (or acceptable) treatment plans could be used to establish a rule-based computer system and used as a template to match the current needs of a given plan. This type of artificial intelligence has not been used very much thus far;[27] (b) utilization of radiation beams that avoid specific normal structures;[28] or (c) various algebraic methods or objective functions for treatment plan optimization.[29–36]

A common mathematic design for an objective function is to minimize the sum of the squares of the errors between the dose desired in each volume element (voxel) of the target and normal structures from the dose that would be delivered by a treatment plan condition. The "cost" of not meeting the goal would rise slowly as the solution varied from the goal and would then have a more rapid increase in cost as the deviation increased. In this approach the best solution has the minimum "cost." In fact, this quadratic formulation is common in the literature and was utilized in the first release of the NOMOS planning system for IMRT. However, the only restriction on objective functions is that they can be characterized mathematically, which means that one is not limited to dose as the only parameterization of outcome. Systems using biologic models that incorporate knowledge of dose-volume effects and dose-fractionation effects have been described.[37–41] Specific attempts to relate such to lung clinical outcomes are discussed later in this chapter.

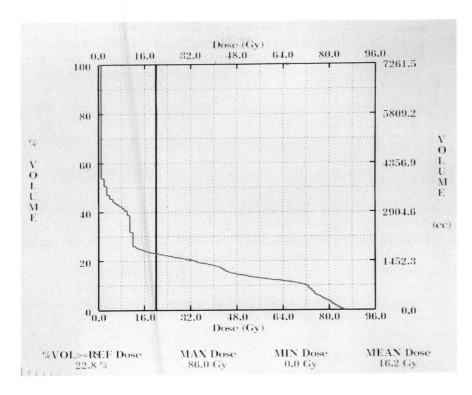

FIGURE 48.9. Dose volume histogram (DVH) of total lung volume. In this case, 22% of the total lung volume exceeded 20 Gy. Thus the V20 was 22%.

Unfortunately, each of these approaches suffers from serious drawbacks. There is a significant lack of correlation of 3D dose-volume data to clinical outcomes. Even if good dose-volume data become available, it is unclear how to combine all the DVH data from the various targets and normal organs into a single "goodness" of plan. Jain and co-workers attempted to develop a figure of merit (FOM) approach to the evaluation of plans.[42–44] Unfortunately, neither the FOM approach nor the inverse calculation techniques can consider such factors as patient preferences, patient desire to minimize complications or maintain quality of life, institutional standards or practices, or specific physician beliefs and opinions regarding goals and desired outcomes of a given patient.

CLINICAL EXPERIENCE WITH 3DRTP FOR NSCLC

Treatment Planning Studies

Early studies with 3DRTP were computer-simulated studies comparing 3D with conventional 2D treatment plans for lung cancer.[28,45–47] In each of these studies, the authors demonstrated the improvement in treatment planning by either dose escalation, reduction in dose to surrounding organs, or both. The authors concluded that 3D planning potentially improved tumor target delineation and target volume coverage.[28,47] It appeared that traditional beam arrangements were inadequate or potentially harmful (in terms of normal lung irradiation effects) in the delivery of target doses of greater than 70 Gy.[46,47]

Assessment of Normal Tissue Toxicity

The development of acute pneumonitis is an undesirable and potentially very debilitating or even fatal complication after radiation therapy to the chest (Chapter 13). The doses of radiation that cause either acute radiation pneumonitis or chronic radiation fibrosis have only been partially characterized.

Emami and co-workers gathered data of available literature and published initial estimates of partial volume lung tolerance.[45] The data published normal tissue tolerance doses for a 5% (TD5/5) and 50% (TD50/5) chance of a complication occurring by 5 years of uniform irradiation of one-third, two-thirds, and whole lung. The TD50/5 for whole lung was 17.5 Gy, for two-thirds of the lung was 30 Gy, and for one-third of the lung was 45 Gy.

Martel and co-workers retrospectively reviewed the 3D DVHs for the lungs of 21 patients with Hodgkin's disease and 42 lung cancer patients with the development of acute pneumonitis.[48] The authors reported a reasonable prediction for low versus high risk for the development of pneumonitis by dividing the patients into risk groups based on the calculation of the effective volume (Veff) of the total lung volume (both lungs together). There were differences in the mean lung dose between patients with complications versus no complications for both groups of patients. Patients without the development of acute pneumonitis had mean lung doses of 18 to 21 Gy (average doses) versus 24 to 26.1 Gy (average doses) for patients with acute pneumonitis.

A study by Oetzel and coworkers showed good correlation for the pneumonitis risk estimations with observed complication rates for ipsilateral lung DVHs but not paired lungs (or total lung volume).[49] Mean lung dose differed somewhat for patients with and without complications (23.8 Gy versus 20.1 Gy). Marks and co-workers found that the total lung NTCP was the single best predictor for pulmonary symptoms after irradiation.[50] The V30 (volume receiving $\geq$ 30 Gy) was also a strong predictor. Graham et al. reported that the single best predictor of acute pneumonitis was the V20 (volume of total lung receiving $\geq$ 20 Gy), although on univariate analysis both Veff and total lung mean dose were also correlated with acute pneumonitis.[51] Kwa et al. pooled the data from five institutions (University of Michigan, University of Heidelberg, Washington University, Duke University, and Netherlands Cancer Institute) for a total of 540 patients.[52] Mean lung dose was the only dosimetric parameter collected. Increasing mean lung dose correlated well with the increasing pneumonitis rate.

Others have attempted to evaluate local radiation damage and dose-response relationship to the overall volumetric function of the lung.[53,56] Changes in perfusion and ventilation pre- and postirradiation was examined, and a dose-effect for local changes were determined. Boersma reported that "overall response parameter" as a mean reduction in perfusion over the total lung correlated to the incidence of pneumonitis.[55] Marks investigated whether functional DVHs (fDVHs) resulted in better predictions of pneumonitis.[46] These fDVHs were based on pretreatment SPECT perfusion data, and were used to consider local lung function in the design of the optimal treatment plan. Unfortunately, there appeared to be too many confounding factors, such as patients with very severe PFTs improving after radiation therapy, and the functional DVHs did not result in an improved ability to predict pneumonitis. Further studies at Duke University with biochemical markers such as TGF-β showed elevated levels related to increased pulmonary symptoms, although this could not be related to dose or volume dependence, nor when compared with NTCPs or V30 was it a strong predictive factor for the development of pneumonitis.[46,56] Another factor not accounted for in the models is the indication that the lower lobes of the lungs, or dependent lung bases, are more radiosensitive than the upper lobes.[51,52] However, these may simply be a volume effect, and that irradiation of lower lobe tumors results in greater volume of lung irradiation.[51]

Graham and co-workers reported the correlation between the V20 and actuarial incidence of $\leq$ grade 2 pneumonitis to be very strong (p = 0.001).[61] When the V20 was less than 22%, the incidence of pneumonitis was 0.

When the V20 was 22% to 31%, 32% to 40%, and more than 40% the actuarial incidence of pneumonitis was 7%, 13%, and 36%, respectively. Graham reported the severity of pneumonitis to also be related to the V20.[61]

V20(%)	Grade 2(%)	Grade 3–5(%)
<22	0	0
22–31	8	0
32–40	13	5 (1 fatal)
>40	19	23 (3 fatal)

Graham also reported the very close relationship between the V20, Veff, and mean lung dose (Figure 48.10). She reported that from the Washington University data, upon multivariate analysis the V20 was the single best predictor of acute pneumonitis.[51]

Results of Clinical Trials

The results of single-institution 3D clinical trials for NSCLC are shown in Table 48.1. Because these early trials were before significant dose escalation, the doses treated ranged from 60 to 74 Gy. These reports thus represent the results of more standard doses but with the technical support such as BEV and 3D dose calculation. One can see that the results appear somewhat better than those from the large chemoradiation trials of the early 1990s. Of course one must be cautious about any significant conclusions because these are single-institution trials.

Dose-Escalation Trials

The University of Michigan began its dose-escalation trial in 1992. The trial was designed to dose-escalated different patient populations based on their calculated risk of pneumonitis. The Veff parameter was chosen to stratify the patients for their risk of pneumonitis. The risk groups were as follows: (a) the lowest risk group had a Veff of less than 0.20 Gy; (b) the intermediate risk groups had Veffs of 0.20 to 0.25 Gy, 0.25 to 0.31 Gy, and 0.31 to 0.40 Gy; (c) the highest risk group had a Veff of more than 0.40 Gy. As of August 1995, 48 patients had been accrued to the study.[62] Since that time the addition of chemotherapy has been allowed prior to entering the study, and in the lowest risk group the administered doses have been as high as 100.8 Gy. To date no acute radiation pneumonitis has been observed in any volume or dose group. Other encountered toxicity has been the development of two patients with $\geq$ grade 3 esophagitis. Two patients developed exsanguinating hemorrhages (both patients had tumors surrounding the main pulmonary artery). Biopsy-proven radiographic local failures were documented in two patients having received 84 Gy tumor dose. Of the 10 patients treated to $\geq$84 Gy, biopsy-proven residual disease or locally recurrent disease

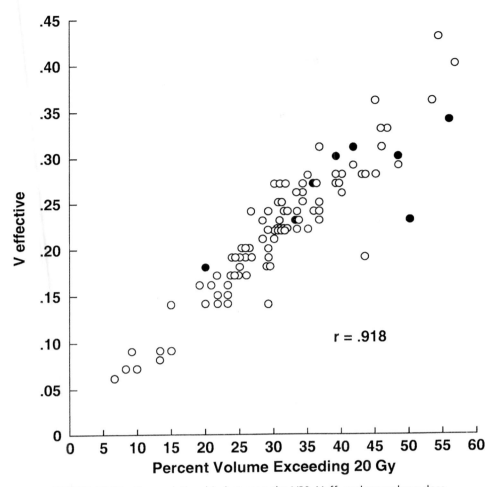

FIGURE 48.10. Close relationship between the V20, Veff, and mean lung dose.

occurred in three patients, and three patients had complete histologic response on follow-up bronchoscopy.[62]

The Memorial Sloan Kettering Cancer Center reported using dose-volume histogram analysis, grade 3 or higher toxicity occurred in 38% of patients receiving greater than 30% of their lung volume ≥25 Gy versus 4% of patients with less that or equal to 30% of their lung volume ≥25 Gy. Pneumonitis was also correlated with the NTCP. Their dose-escalation protocol proceeds based on a single-dose es-

calation schema but limits who may enter the protocol to an NTCP of ≤20%.[60]

The RTOG dose-escalation trial for NSCLC patients stratifies the patients for risk of pneumonitis based on the pretreatment plan V20. The risk groups are less than 25%, 25% to 37%, and more than 37%.[63] Patients have been successfully dose escalated to 83.8 Gy without the development of high-grade acute pneumonitis.

Each of the aforementioned trials has eliminated elective

TABLE 48.1. RESULTS OF CLINICAL TRIALS FOR NSCLC USING 3DCRT

Institution	Number of Patients	Dose	Survival			
			Median	1 yr (%)	2 yr (%)	3 yr (%)
University of Michigan[58]	88	>60 Gy	15 mo	—	37	15
University of Chicago[59]	37	60–70 Gy	19.5 mo	75	37	—
Memorial Sloan Kettering[60]	45	64–72 Gy	16 mo	—	33	—
Washington University[61]	126	60–74 Gy	21.5 mo	57	43	29

nodal irradiation in an attempt to reduce pulmonary toxicity. This decision was based on the recognition that most failures in lung cancer are at the site of gross disease. It is hoped that in this era of combined modality therapy, chemotherapy will reduce the recurrence of microscopic disease in the regional lymphatics. It is also recognized that even though the mediastinum is not targeted for the prescription dose, it receives some dose. Clearly, portions of the mediastinum and ipsilateral hilum receive varying doses of the entry or exit or scatter dose, depending on their proximity to the gross tumor. However, it has been very difficult to quantitate this dose. The issue of elective nodal irradiation is extremely controversial, and the results of the ongoing trials are imperative to establish the practice as a standard of care or not. In addition, after the maximum tolerated dose or doses for NSCLC are established, further trials comparing 3D therapy to conventional doses and volumes may be necessary to establish a therapeutic advantage. Only in this way will the true value and efficacy of 3D therapy for lung cancer be confirmed.

SUMMARY

3D radiotherapy for lung cancer has emerged as an important component of therapy for lung cancer. Results of single institutions have given us parameters on which to evaluate the risk of acute pneumonitis and thereby stratify patients for dose-escalation studies. Individual planners using 3D planning for NSCLC can use these parameters to assess and reduce (by interactive planning) the lung complication rates in patients. Further clinical data correlated for esophagus, heart, soft tissue, and late pulmonary sequelae are needed. The value of dose-escalation with combined modality therapy remains to be established. It is anticipated that more sophisticated, user-friendly computer-assisted or optimized treatment radiation treatment plans will be used for the treatment of lung cancer in the future.

REFERENCES

1. Lichter AS. Three-dimensional conformal radiation therapy: a testable hypothesis. *Int J Radiat Oncolo Biol Phys* 1991;21:853.
2. Perez CA, Pajak TF, Rubin P, et al. Long-term observations of the patterns of failure in patients with unresectable non-oat cell carcinoma of the lung treated with definitive radiotherapy. Report by the Radiation Therapy Oncology Group. *Cancer* 1987;59:1874.
3. Perez CA, Stanley K, Rubin P, et al. Impact of irradiation technique and tumor extent in tumor control and survival of patients with unresectable non-oat cell carcinoma of the lung. Report by the Radiation Therapy Oncology Group. *Cancer* 1982;50:1091.
4. Dillman RO, Seagren SL, Propert KJ, et al. A randomized trial of injection chemotherapy plus high-dose radiation versus radiation alone in stage III non-small-cell lung cancer *N Engl J Med* 1090;323:940.
5. Le Chevalier T, Arriagada R, Quoix E, et al. Radiotherapy alone versus combined chemotherapy and radiotherapy in nonresectable non-small-cell lung cancer: first analysis of a randomized trial in 353 patients. *J Natl Cancer Inst* 1991;83:417.
6. Sause W, Scott C, Taylor S, et al. Radiation Therapy Oncology Group (RTOG) 8808 and Eastern Cooperative Oncology Group (ECOG) 4588: preliminary results of a phase III trial in regionally advanced unresectable non-small-cell lung cancer. *J Natl Cancer Inst* 1995;87:198.
7. Fletcher G. Clinical dose-response curves of human malignant epithelial tumours. *Br J Radiol* 1973;46:1.
8. Cox J, Axarnia N, Byhardt R, et al. A randomized phaseI/II trial of hyperfractionated radiation therapy with total doses of 60.0 Gy to 79.2 Gy. Possible survival benefit with ≥69.6 Gy in favorable patients with Radiation Therapy Oncology Group stage III non-small-cell lung carcinoma. Report of Radiation Therapy Oncology Group 8311. *J Clin Oncol* 1990;8:1543.
9. Maasilta P. Radiation-induced lung injury. From the chest physician's point of view. *Lung Cancer* 1991;7:367.
10. Roberts CM, Foulcher E, Saunders JJ, et al. Radiation pneumonitis: a possible lymphocyte-mediated hypersensitivity reaction. *Ann Intern Med* 1993;118(9):696.
11. International Commission on Radiation Units and Measurements. *Report no. 50: prescribing, recording, and reporting photon beam therapy.* Bethesda, MD: International Commission on Radiation Units and Measurements, 1993.
12. Venuta F, Rendina EA, Ciriaca P, et al. Computed tomography to stage for preoperative assessment of T3 and T4 bronchogenic carcinoma. *Eur J Cardiothoracic Surg* 1992;6(5):238.
13. Dales RE, Stark RM, Raman S. Computed tomography to stage lung cancer, approaching a controversy using meta-analysis. *Am Rev Respir Dis* 1990;141(5):1096.
14. Platt JF, Glazer GM, Orringer MB, et al. Radiologic evaluation of the subcarinal lymph nodes: a comparative study. *AJR* 1988;151(2):279.
15. McCloud TC, Bourgouin PM, Breeberg RW, et al. Bronchogenic carcinoma: analysis of staging in the mediastinum with CT by correlative lymph node mapping and sampling. *Radiology* 1992;182:319.
16. Wong J, Sharpe M, Jaffray D. The use of active breathing control (ABC) to minimize breathing motion in conformal therapy. *Int J Radiol Oncol Biol Phys* 1999:44;911.
17. Lichter AS, Sandler HM, Robertson JM, et al. Clinical experience with three-dimensional treatment planning. *Semin Radiat Oncol* 1992;2:257.
18. Sailer SL, Chaney EL, Rosenman JG, et al. Treatment planning at the University of North Carolina at Chapel Hill. *Semin Radiat Oncol* 1992;2:267.
19. Sherouse GW, Chaney EL. The portable virtual simulator. *Int J Radiat Oncol Biol Phys* 1991;21:475.
20. Cullip TJ, Symon JR, Rosenman JG, et al. Digitally reconstructed fluoroscopy and other interactive volume visualizations in 3-D treatment planning. *Int J Radiat Oncol Biol Phys* 1993;27:145.
21. Fraass BA, McShan DL, Weeks KJ. 3-D treatment planning III: complete beam's-eye-view planning capabilities. In: Bruinvis IAD, van Kleffens F, Wittkamper FW, eds. *The use of computers in radiotherapy.* Amsterdam: North-Holland, 1987;193.
22. Mackie TR, Reckwerdt P, McNutt T, et al. Photon beam dose

computations. In: Palta J, Mackie TR, eds. *Teletherapy: present and future.* College Park, MD: Advanced Medical Publishing, 1996:103.

23. Deasey TO. *Tumor control probability models for nonuniform dose distributions,* Madison, Wisconsin: 5th International Conference on Dose, Time and Fractionation in Radiation Oncology, 1997: 65.

24. Graham MV, Purdy JA, Harms W, et al. Survival and prognostic factors of non-small cell lung cancer (NSCLC) patients treated with definitive three-dimensional (3D) radiation therapy. *Int J Radiat Oncol Biol Phys* 1998;42:166.

25. Drzymala RE, Mohan R, Brewster L, et al. Dose-volume histograms. *Int J Radiat Oncol Biol Phys* 1991;21:71.

26. Derycke S, DeGersem WRT, VanDuyse BB, et al. Conformal radiotherapy of stage III non-small cell lung cancer: a class solution involving non-coplanar intensity-modulated beams. *Int J Radiat Oncol Biol Phys* 1998;41:771.

27. Kalet IJ, Jacky JP. Knowledge-based computer simulation for radiation therapy planning. In: Bruinvis AD, vander Biessen PH, van Kleffens HF, eds. *Proceedings of the 19th International Conference on the Use of Computers in Radiation Therapy.* Amsterdam: Elsevier Science, 1987;553.

28. Chen GTY, Spelbring DR, Pelizzari CA, et al. The use of beams eye view volumetrics in the selection of non-coplanar ports. *Int J Radiat Oncol Biol Phys* 1992;23:153.

29. Rosen IJ, Lane RG, Morrill SM, et al. Treatment plan optimization using linear programming. *Med Phys* 1991;18:141.

30. Gokhale P, Hussein E. Determination of beam orientation in radiotherapy planning. *Med Phys* 1994;21(3):393.

31. Starkschall G. A constrained least-squares optimization method for external beam radiation therapy treatment planning. *Med Phys* 1984;11:659.

32. Bortfield TR, Boyer AL. The exponential radon transform and projection filtering in radiotherapy planning. *Int J Imaging Syst Technol* 1995;6:62.

33. Gustafsson A, Lind BK, Brahme A. A generalized pencil beams algorithm for optimization of radiation therapy. *Med Phys* 1994; 21:343.

34. Powlis D, Altschuler MD, Censor Y, et al. Semi-automated radiotherapy treatment planning with a mathematical model to satisfy treatment goals. *Int J Radiat Oncol Biol Phys* 1989;16:271.

35. Llacer J. Inverse radiation treatment planning using the dynamically penalized likelihood method. *Med Phys* 1997;24:1751.

36. Cho PS, Lee S, Marks RJ, et al. Optimization of intensity modulated beams for volume constraints using two methods: cost function minimization and projections onto convex sets. *Med Phys* 1998;25:435.

37. Lyman JT, Wolbarst AB. Optimization of radiation therapy III: a method of assessing complication probabilities from dose-volume histograms. *Int J Radiat Oncol Biol Phys* 1987;13:103.

38. Kutcher GI, Burman C. Calculation of complication probability factors for non-uniform normal tissue radiation: the effective volume method. *Int J Radiat Oncol Biol Phys* 1989;1:1623.

39. Mohan R, Mageras GS, Baldwin B, et al. Clinically relevant optimization of 3D conformal treatments. *Med Phys* 1992;19: 933.

40. Kallman P, Lind BK, Brahme A. An algorithm for maximizing the probability of complication-free tumour control in radiation therapy. *Phys Med Biol* 1992;37:871.

41. Niemierko A, Urie M, Goitein M. Optimization of 3D radiation therapy with both physical and biological end points and constraints. *Int J Radiat Oncol Biol Phys* 1992;23:99.

42. Jain NL, Kahn MG, Drzymala RE, et al. Objective evaluation of 3D radiation treatment plans: a decision-analytic tool incorporating treatment preferences of radiation oncologists. *Int J Radiat Oncol Biol Phys* 1993;26:321.

43. Graham MV, Jain NJ, Kahn MG, et al. Evaluation of an objective plan-evaluation model in the three dimensional treatment of non-small cell lung cancer. *Int J Radiat Oncol Biol Phys* 1996;34: 469.

44. Graham MV, Jain NJ, Kahn MG, et al. Objective plan evaluation using a score function tool. *Front Radiat Ther Oncol* 1996;29: 81.

45. Emami BE, Lyman J, Brown A, et al. Tolerance of normal tissues to therapeutic irradiation. *Int J Radiat Oncol Biol Phys* 1991;21: 109.

46. Armstrong JG, Burman C, Leibel S, et al. Three-dimensional conformal radiation therapy may improve the therapeutic ratio of high dose radiation therapy for lung cancer. *Int J Radiat Oncol Biol Phys* 1993;26:685.

47. Graham MV, Mathews JW Harms WB, et al. 3-dimensional radiation treatment planning study for patients with carcinoma of the lung. *Int J Radiat Oncol Biol Phys* 1994;29:1105.

48. Martel MK, Ten Haken RK, Hazuka MB, et al. Dose-volume histogram and 3-D treatment planning evaluation of patients with pneumonitis. *Int J Radiat Oncol Biol Phys* 1994;28(3): 575.

49. Oetzel D, Schraube P, Hensley F, et al. Estimation of pneumonitis risk in three-dimensional treatment planning using dose-volume histogram analysis. *Int J Radiat Oncol Biol Phys* 1995;33: 455.

50. Marks LB, Munley M, Bentel G, et al. Physical and biological predictors of changes in whole-lung function following thoracic irradiation. *Int J Radiat Oncol Biol Phys* 1997;39:563.

51. Graham MV, Purdy JA, Emami BE, et al. Clinical dose volume histogram analysis for pneumonitis after 3D treatment for non-small cell lung cancer (NSCLC). *Int J Radiat Oncol Biol Phys* 1999;45:323.

52. Kwa S, Lebesque J, Theuws J, et al. Radiation pneumonitis as a function of mean dose: an analysis of pooled data of 540 patients. *Int J Radiat Oncol Biol Phys* 1998;42:1.

53. Boersma LJ, Damen EMF, de Boer RW, et al. A new method to determine dose-effect relations for local lung-function changes using correlated SPECT and CT data. *Radiother Oncol* 1993; 29(2):110.

54. Marks LB, Munley MT, Spencer DP, et al. Quantification of radiation-induced regional lung injury with perfusion imaging. *Int J Radiat Oncol Biol Phys* 1997;38(2):399.

55. Boersma LJ, Damen EM, deBoer RW, et al. Estimation of overall pulmonary function after irradiation using dose-effect relations for local functional injury. *Radiother Oncol* 1995;36:15.

56. Anscher MS, Kong FM, Andrews K, et al. Plasma transforming growth factor betal as a predictor of radiation pneumonitis. *Int J Radiat Oncol Biol Phys* 1998;41:1029.

57. Liao ZX, Travis EL, Tucker SL. Damage and morbidity from pneumonitis after irradiation of partial volumes of mouse lung. *Int J Radiat Oncol Biol Phys* 1995;32:1359.

58. Hazuka MB, Turrisi AT, Lutz ST, et al. Results of high-dose thoracic irradiation incorporating beam's eye view display in non-small cell lung carcinoma: a retrospective multivariate analysis. *Int J Radiat Oncol Biol Phys* 1993;27:273.

59. Sibley GS, Mundt AJ, Shapiro C, et al. The treatment of stage III nonsmall cell lung cancer using high dose conformal radiotherapy. *Int J Radiat Oncol Biol Phys* 1995;33:1001.

60. Armstrong J, Zelefsky M, Burt M, et al. Promising survival with

3-dimensional conformal radiation therapy for non-small cell lung cancer. *Proc Am Soc Clin Oncol* 1994;13:651.

61. Graham MV, Purdy JA, Harms WB, et al. Survival and prognostic factors of non-small cell lung cancer (NSCLC) patients treated with definitive three-dimensional (3D) radiation therapy. *Int J Radiat Oncol Biol Phys* 1999 (*submitted*).

62. Robertson JM, Ten Haken RK, Hazuka MB, et al. Dose escala-

tion for non-small cell lung cancer using conformal radiation therapy. *Int J Radiat Oncol Biol Phys* 1997;37:1079.

63. Graham MV. Predicting radiation response (editorial). *Int J Radiat Oncol Biol Phys* 1997;39:561.

64. Graham MV, Purdy JA, Emami BE, et al. Preliminary results of a prospective trial using three dimensional radiotherapy for lung cancer. *Int J Radiat Oncol Biol Phys* 1995;33:993.

49

ENDOBRONCHIAL AND INTERSTITIAL BRACHYTHERAPY

BURTON L. SPEISER
JOHN J. KRESL

BRACHYTHERAPY FOR LUNG CANCER

The treatment of lung cancer by radiation has consisted primarily of the use of external-beam radiation. The use of brachytherapy in the form of manually arranged, low-dose-rate afterloaded sources emerged in the early to mid-1980s. It was not until the mid- and late 1980s that high-dose-rate, remote afterloading brachytherapy began to be utilized in increasing numbers. At the present time it is the most prevalent means of treating endobronchial disease with brachytherapy in the world. Endobronchial brachytherapy, however, has been used primarily for palliation, for new or recurrent disease. The use for curative intent treatment, while performed occasionally, is not as prevalent. Even less common is the use of radiation for occult carcinomas of the lung.

Brachytherapy for carcinoma of the lung, for ease of discussion, is categorized into endobronchial/intralumenal (within a lumen) and interstitial (in tissue) techniques. Endobronchial/intralumenal treatment is divided into low-, intermediate-, and high-dose-rate applications and refers to the temporary placement of the isotope into the tracheobronchial tree. Generally, interstitial implantation most commonly applies to the use of Iodine-125 implanted permanently at the time of surgical resection.

Brachytherapy was probably first used at the close of the nineteenth century when the Curies gave a small radium tube to Danlos for insertion into a malignancy. During the next 20 years, Kernan,[1] using a rigid bronchoscope, reported the implantation of Radon-222 seeds into carcinomas of the tracheas and bronchus. He reported 10 cases treated with Radon-222 seed implantation and diathermy treatment. He commented that, "It was possible to destroy the tumors with diathermy and Radon implantation, and there have been no local recurrences as yet, although one case has been followed for 5 years." During this time, and for the next 10 years, work was being performed on standardization of dose calculation and prescription for brachytherapy. The publication of the Manchester System of Patterson, Parker,

and Meredith (1934) set the foundation for brachytherapy dosimetry. This system was expanded by the manual, *Radium Dosage*.[2] Pool[3] reported on Radon-222 used at Memorial Hospital in 42 patients implanted between 1936–1960. The implanted seeds were sealed gold capillary tubes filled with Radon-222 gas. The technique reported by Pool "proved to benefit patients with primary tracheal tumors, and patients with bronchial stump recurrences following pulmonary resection." Radon-222 seed implantation was also used during thoracotomy with the first reported case by Graham and Singer.[4]

To decrease the radiation safety problems (potential leakage) with Radon-222, radioactive isotopes of shorter half-life and lower decay energies were sought. Afterloading techniques, reducing medical personnel's and patient's exposures, inserted catheters or tubes later filled with live, radiation-emitting sources. Henschke[5] introduced standardized afterloading techniques with Gold-198 and, subsequently, Iridium-192. With the shorter half-life of Iridium-192 and afterloading techniques, interstitial implantation became commonplace in medical use. However, despite this general rapid increase, there were few changes and limited use of brachytherapy for carcinoma of the lung. Early transbronchial implantation techniques initially utilizing Radon-222 and then Iodine-125 through the rigid bronchoscope were difficult and associated with a considerable expenditure of physician time and effort. By their nature, these were less commonly afterloaded situations, so this fostered lack of development and acceptance. With the advent of the flexible bronchoscope, a new flexible applicator system was designed and reported on by Martinez and colleagues.[6] In addition, Farber and colleagues in an unpublished study in 1986 described a system using Gold-198 with a flexible bronchoscope system.

The use of intraluminal brachytherapy, the placement of an afterloading flexible applicator bronchoscopically, was first reported in the American literature by Mendiondo.[7] About 1984 the neodymium-YAG laser was introduced into clinical use for treatment of tracheal and endobronchial obstructions for both primary and metastatic lung malignancies. This caused a renaissance of interest in intraluminal brachytherapy, now utilizing the afterloading techniques after YAG laser photoresection.

Most patients with lung malignancies present with locally advanced or metastatic disease. Unresectable patients, whether or not they undergo an attempted resection, have a high risk of subsequent local recurrence. Despite treatment with external beam radiation therapy, doses have been inadequate due to normal tissue limitation, so local recurrence remains a problem. In addition, with improved overall survival and local control for inoperable patients treated with combined radiochemotherapy, local tumor recurrence remains a problem. This component of local recurrence spurred many clinicians to employ brachytherapy to deliver additional ionizing radiation therapy, which concentrates dose to tumor regions and limits dose to sensitive adjacent normal tissue structures.

Brachytherapy provides direct application of radioactive sources to an anatomic site, such as a surgical tumor bed or within a tumor mass. Brachytherapy can be performed by implantation of radioactive sources, such as seeds within the tumor mass (interstitial brachytherapy), or by insertion of the radioactive source within the lumen of a catheter placed within the surgical bed or tumor mass (intraluminal or endobronchial brachytherapy). Brachytherapy offers the potential advantage of providing a high-dose gradient of ionizing radiation that delivers a high dose to the seeded tumor-bearing area and a rapid decrement in dose to the surrounding normal structures. This occurs because of the inverse square law of ionizing radiation, which states that the dose of radiation decreases by one divided by the square of the distance $[R_2 = R_1/D_2]$.

Brachytherapy for lung malignancies may be placed most commonly as a permanent interstitial or temporary endobronchial radiation source, with remote or manual afterloading. Permanent implants are typically low-dose-rate sources of radiation delivered over an infinite period of time (for 1–125 the dose is calculated for 90 days) and for placement of individual radioactive sources/seeds within the target (surgical bed) or tumor (mass) volume. Step one is placement of afterloaded catheters at the target (surgical bed) or within the tumor site. Temporary or afterloaded implants are placed within the lumen of these catheters. Afterloaded implants can deliver either low-intermediate-, or high-dose-rate ionizing radiation at less than 2 Gy per hour (low-dose-rate LDR), 2-12 Gy per hour (intermediate dose rate IDR), or greater 2 Gy per minute (high dose rate HDR). A typical afterloading system utilizes hollow catheters and Iridium-192 seeds embedded in nylon ribbon for low dose rate, or Iridium-192 sources (10 curie) to be placed within the lumen of the treatment catheters.

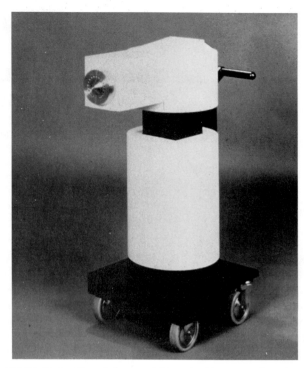

FIGURE 49.1. Micro-Selectron-HDR unit. (Courtesy of Nucletron Corporation, Columbia, MD.)

TECHNICAL ASPECTS OF REMOTE AFTERLOADING UNITS

Most remote afterloading units utilize high-activity radioactive sources of a small physical size, usually Iridium-192, whose initial activity is 10 curie (Fig. 49.1). The radioactive source is securely attached to the end of a wire cable. This is mechanically driven by a high-precision mechanism that allows for positioning of the radioactive source at specific stations within the catheter for specific dwell periods. The translocation of the source between these preassigned stops and times, as well as removal of the source out of the catheter into the shielded unit's compartment is rapid to minimize transit time exposure. The treatment sequence for each cable/catheter, which defines the various dwell times and dwell positions, is calculated by treatment-planning computers. The plan is executed under the control of an external computer, which drives the remote afterloading unit.

TREATMENT-PLANNING COMPUTER

The basics of dose-calculation techniques require orthogonal radiographs taken after catheter placement with dummy seeds in place to determine catheter position. On the simulator radiographs, the seed positions are digitized from the first dwell position at the end of the catheter to the most proximal dwell position in the catheter along the dummy source seed line. Next, the treatment target volume is defined by the treating physician. A treatment plan is then formulated, optimizing treatment points (dwell positions) and treatment time (dwell times position). This treatment plan is evaluated in the four cardinal directions utilizing isodose lines as well as evaluation of the patient's individual anatomy to calculate the final prescription dose and point. New techniques use CAT scans for a better three-dimensional picture.

ENDOBRONCHIAL CATHETERS

A variety of commercial catheters are available for use. Basically, physical characteristics of each catheter must allow for easy placement and removal from the endobronchial tree and immobilization within place. The catheters must fit through the biopsy channel of the endoscope and the source-compatible (most commonly used 5 or 6 French with a 1.7 or 2 mm internal diameter, respectively) and must be navigable through the scope. Finally, the catheter has a closed end to prevent loss of dummy seeds or the active sources.

The patient must be able to satisfactorily tolerate an endobronchial procedure. Then, with a pulmonologist, the catheter can be placed in an endoscopy suite. The procedure requires vital sign monitoring, topical anesthesia, and intravenous sedation. By bronchoscopy, the malignant lesion is identified by the pulmonologist and radiation oncologist. Photographic documentation and anatomical characteristics of the malignancy are noted, including distance from anatomical landmarks, such as bronchial segment branch points and carinae. The extent of the malignant lesion can be further localized utilizing radioopaque markers placed externally on the patient's thorax corresponding to the most distal and proximal extent of the malignancy as identified by the bronchoscope and correlated under fluoroscopy. After this visual inspection and fluoroscopic confirmation, a guidewire in a catheter is placed through the biopsy channel. Its placement is confirmed visually and fluoroscopically. The bronchoscope is removed and, when the catheter is positioned so that the tip is several centimeters distal to the most distal point of the malignancy, the proximal end of the catheter is then secured to the nose (Figure 49.2). The guidewire is removed and replaced by a set of dummy seed sources to identify source location for treatment planning and orthogonal simulation films (Figure 49.3).

TREATMENT FOR DOSE PRESCRIPTION

The prescription depth is measured for the three-dimensional volume by multiple points perpendicular to the axis

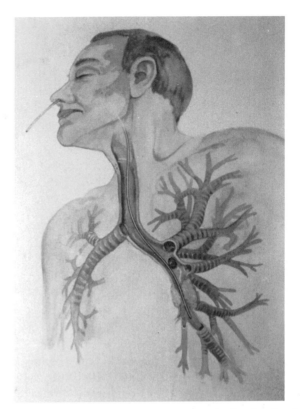

FIGURE 49.2. Clinical setting depicting an afterloading brachytherapy catheter. (Courtesy of Nucletron Corporation, Columbia, MD.)

of the catheter or source train to which the minimum target dose is prescribed. The prescriptions that are suggested in the literature range from 0.5–2 cm. To ensure treatment of the entire tumor volume, accommodating possible source or tumor movement due to cardiorespiratory, swallowing, and patient movement, the maximal distance from source center to the edge of the malignancy or target must be considered as part of three-dimensional brachytherapy planning. A longitudinal margin of approximately 2 cm proximal and distal to the malignant margins is commonly used. This margin allows for an effective dose distribution that encompasses the tumor volume without overdosing the tolerance dose to bronchial mucosa. The prescription point should be documented for comparative purposes.

Strategies for Treatment of Occult Carcinomas of the Endobronchus

Occult carcinomas of the lung are defined as carcinomas diagnosed by sputum cytology and bronchoscopy using brushings, washings, and/or biopsy. Frequently, fewer patients undergo bronchoscopy for cough and/or hemoptysis.

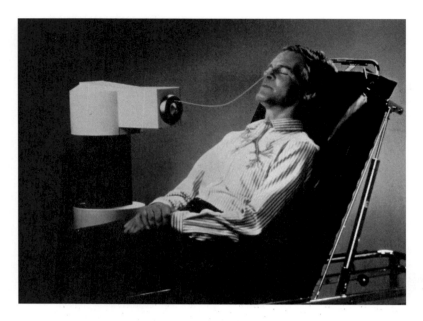

FIGURE 49.3. Patient with an endobronchial afterloading catheter and endobronchial malignancy. (Courtesy of Nucletron Corporation, Columbia, MD.)

These cannot be detected by conventional radiographic means before or immediately after the initial diagnosis.

In 1974, Sanderson et al.[8] published "Bronchoscopic Localization of Radiographically Occult Lung Cancer." In 1980, Cortese et al.[9] published their study, "Roentgenographically Occult Lung Cancer." In the same year, Martini and Melamed[10] published "Occult Carcinoma of the Lung." Initially, the treatment of choice was surgery, either lobectomy or pneumonectomy; however, as photodynamic therapy (PDT) and then endobronchial brachytherapy (EBBT) increased, the "menu" of treatment modalities increased.

This subpopulation of roentgenographically occult carcinomas of the lung is associated with interesting attributes. First, the time interval from the initial abnormal sputum cytology to bronchoscopic confirmation, as reported by the Mayo Lung Project,[9] ranged from 1 to 1,014 days (median, 70 days; 75[10] percentile, 169 days). Second, the disease is most often Tis, T1, and N0 (Saito et al[11] found that of 94 patients, 17% were Tis and 77% were T1.) Third, most cases are squamous cell carcinomas; in a significant number dysplasia initially had been the only finding.[9] Fourth, no findings are apparent on plain radiography or, when available, on computerized axial tomography. Fifth, no adverse prognostic factors (i.e., weight loss) that predict lower cure or survival rates exist, and rarely are symptoms present.[2–15] Finally, synchronicity and metachronicity are significant. In a surgical series, Nagamoto et al.[6] reported a rate of 1.09 lesions per patient; Kato et al.[17] found 1.21 lesions per patient; and Saito et al.[11] found 1.2 lesions per patient. In the Mayo Lung Project Study,[9] a metachronous rate of 5% per year was reported, and in a study by Saito et al.[18] a rate of 0.022 lesions per patient-year was documented. In the latter study, the rate was 0.041 lesions per patient-year when synchronous and metachronous tumors were combined.

In this study of Saito et al.[18] if a patient had a second lesion, there was a 47% probability that within 5 years, a third lesion would be identified, at a rate of 0.11 lesions per patient-year. The five-year survival rate for patients with a single lesion and no evidence of synchronous or metachronous lesions was 90%. If, however, there was more than one other metachronous or synchronous lesion, the five-year survival rate was 59%. Survival is inversely related to probability of multiple lesions.

Other factors associated with successful outcomes include the size of the lesion. Many studies have found that lesions (10 mm in size are associated with the most favorable outcomes). In a surgical study of 127 patients,[19] 55 patients had lesions of this size, and no metastatic lymph nodes were identified. Of 46 patients with lesions more than 10 mm but less than 20 mm, 4 patients (9%) had nodal metastasis. Of 26 patients with lesions that were more than 20 mm but less than 55 mm, four patients (15%) had metastatic disease. In summary, there was no documentation of nodal metastasis with lesions less than 10 mm. For lesions more than 10 mm, however, the frequency was 11%. Thus lesion size may determine which patients have probability of nodule metastasis.

In an earlier study by Saito,[11] deep bronchial invasion was documented by pathologic analysis in 16 (17%) of 94 patients. Five (31%) of these 16 patients had nodule disease. Only 1 (1%) of 78 patients had nodal disease without evidence of extrabronchial invasion. No recurrences were identified in 75 patients who had intrabronchial disease, had no lymphatic spread, and who underwent a complete resection.

Overall, the cause-specific five-year survival rate was 93.5% and 80.4% for all causes combined.

In 108 patients who underwent surgical resection for occult carcinoma. Nagamato et al.[6] identified 10 patients (9.2%) who had additional squamous cell carcinomas less than 1 mm in size. In turn, these lesions were associated with either dysplasia or marked atypia.

Kato et al.[17] treated 45 lesions fulfilling the criteria for occult carcinomas in 40 patients (1.13 lesions per patient). PDT was the only treatment used for 30 lesions in 20 patients, and the complete response rate was 100%. Three patients (15%) had recurrences, one (5%) of whom later died of the disease. An additional nine patients (45%) died of unrelated causes.

Considerably fewer patients with occult carcinomas were treated with endobronchial brachytherapy (EBBT) than with photodynamic therapy (PDT) or surgery (see also Chapter 24). Sutedja et al.[20] reported two patients with T1 squamous cell carcinoma who were treated with high-dose-rate EBBT. Three fractions of 10 Gy were delivered at a 1 cm depth. Both patients were alive without disease at follow-up examinations, at 54 and 25 months, respectively.

Tredaniel et al.[21] treated 29 patients with a variety of lesions, whose common denominator was that their carcinomas were limited to the bronchus, and were therefore radiographically occult. Consequently, the disease could be encompassed by intraluminal brachytherapy. In contrast to all other reported series, however, these patients had undergone prior treatment, which included surgery, external radiation, and/or chemotherapy. The patients were treated with high-dose-rate EBBT using a dose of 7 Gy calculated at a 1 cm depth for 6 fractions (42 Gy). The median actuarial survival of these patients had not been reached after 23 months of follow-up.

Saito et al.[11] treated 49 occult carcinomas in 41 patients (1.2 lesions per patient) with external-beam radiation using 40 Gy in 20 fractions, and with EBBT of 25 Gy in 5 fractions. Doses were customized, and the prescription point varied between 3 to 9 mm depth, based principally on the average diameter of the airway being treated. With a median follow-up of 24.5 months, only two patients (5%) had experienced recurrences.

A prospective study reported by Perol and coworkers,[22] had the following selection criteria in the treatment of occult lung cancer with EBBT: All cases were proximal non–small cell lung carcinomas from an area not previously irradiated, with a size of less than 1 cm. All lesions were roentgenographically occult, and the patients all had severe chronic respiratory failure or had already had surgery or external radiation for previous lung carcinoma to other sites. An escalating dose protocol was used, and all doses were prescribed at 1 cm.

The first two patients received three fractions of 7 Gy each, the next four patients received four fractions of 7 Gy each, and the last 13 patients received five fractions of 7 Gy each. Two months after the completion of treatment, 15 (83%) of the 18 evaluable patients' cases were locally controlled with negative biopsies. At one year, 12 (75%) of 16 evaluable patients revealed no evidence of disease. Actuarial one- and two-year survival rates were 78% and 58%, respectively, with a median survival of 28 months. Of 13 patients who received five fractions of 7 Gy, two developed necrosis of the bronchial wall. These patients died of hemoptysis, one with no evidence of carcinoma.

This group of patients was selected for minimal disease but also for their common co-morbid conditions: a history of prior lung cancer and moderate to severe medical problems precluding surgery. Ten patients had undergone surgical treatment for a previous lung carcinoma. Six patients had pneumonectomy, and five of these had mediastinal irradiation. Two were treated for previous carcinoma of the lung by radiation therapy alone. One patient was in cardiac failure at the time of treatment, and another patient had HIV infection with severe immunodepression. Of four patients with previous carcinoma of the lung, two were treated before the EBBT, one with cryotherapy and the other with chemotherapy, but without affecting the endobronchial lesion. Thus this group of patients, with their adverse medical history of either prior lung carcinoma (treated by surgery and/or radiation) or severe medical problems, had respectable one- and two-year actuarial survival rates.

The substantial synchronous and metachronous rate and the findings of additional small carcinomas with dysplasia and marked atypia all lead to the concept of a "field defect" (see also Chapter 23). Thus it is likely that the entire bronchial mucosa is at risk with a high probability of more than one lesion developing, either as a synchronous or metachronous lesion, in this select group of patients. If this is the case, then the strategy of treatment must include this as a basic assumption. Although lobectomy and/or pneumonectomy cure a certain percentage of patients, the remaining lung will continue to be at risk.

Therefore, selected lesions, that is, those less than 10 mm, with no evidence of extrabronchial extension, and squamous cell histology can be considered for therapies designed to preserve pulmonary function (PDT or EBBT). Lesions more than 10 mm or with evidence or suggestion of extrabronchial extension or nonsquamous histologies are less optimal candidates because they have higher risks of morbid disease. A suggested strategy is outlined in Fig. 49.4. We propose to randomize lesions less than 10 mm with squamous cell histology to the two therapeutic modalities most conserving of pulmonary function.

We have treated more than 600 patients on protocols using EBBT. Of these patients, only 19% were treated for curative intent, and of these, only five (4%) met the criteria to be classified as radiographically occult carcinomas and are summarized in Table 49.1. The symptom index score used to classify each patient is listed in Table 49.2. This is a semiquantitative symptom index described later in the

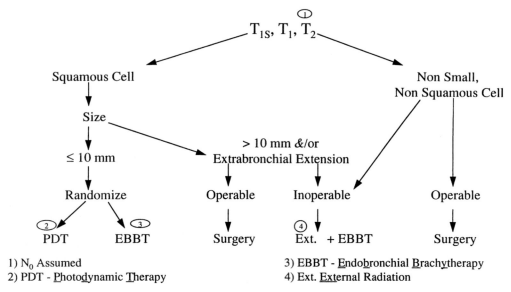

FIGURE 49.4. Algorithm for the management of an occult lung carcinoma.

chapter, which allows for description and scoring of the symptoms of the patients during their medical course. Five patients are included, with a total of six lesions treated, for a rate of 1.2 lesions per patient. The rate of death from intercurrent disease was high, with two of five patients (40%) dying from intercurrent disease. One patient died of recurrence at 676 days. At the time of analysis, two of the patients were alive and with no evidence of disease (NED) at 1,228 and 650 days, respectively. In contrast to other reported studies, these patients were treated with a more conventional approach utilizing the current curative intent protocol described later in detail, which allowed for the delivery of 60 or 64 Gy, with external radiation therapy given concurrently with their EBBT. In this group of five patients treated with the combination of external beam radiation and EBBT, no complications occurred.

A frequently asked question is "what percentage of patients with lung cancer will benefit from intraluminal brachytherapy?" To attempt to answer this question, the total number of patients diagnosed with lung cancer within the referral area was approximated. For the greater Phoenix/Maricopa county area, the cases of lung cancer for 1986 through 1996 were estimated to be 9,000 cases. Of these, only 19% received radiation, and 16% of that group, or 3% of all patients, were treated on protocol, whereas an additional 11% of patients receiving radiation, or 2% of all patients, were treated with brachytherapy off protocol. Thus 27% of all patients receiving radiation, or 5% of all diagnosed patients, received brachytherapy. For patients on the curative protocol, these figures were 3% and 0.5%, respectively.

Results of Endobronchial Brachytherapy for Stages I, II, and III$_A$ or Recurrent Lung Cancer

Bronchogenic carcinoma often leads to symptoms indicating airway involvement, including obstructive pneumonia,

TABLE 49.1. BRACHYTHERAPY FOR RADIOGRAPHICALLY OCCULT CARCINOMA

Patient	Disease	Symptoms	Prior Rx or Med. Prob	Brachy/Ext.	Survival/ days	Status	Complications
1	T1s RUL T1 RLL	Dyspnea-1 Cough-1	PDT × 4	7.5 Gy × 3 60 Gy	202	Died-Intercurrent	None
2	T1 LUL	Hemoptysis-2 Dyspnea-3 Cough-1	COPD-Severe	7.5 Gy × 3 60 Gy	1,228	Alive NED	None
3	T1 RUL	Hemoptysis-1 Dyspnea-4 Cough-1	COPD-Severe	5 Gy × 4 60 Gy	676	Died Loc. Rec.	None
4	T2 RLL	Cough-2	COPD-Severe	5 Gy × 3 64 Gy	650	Alive NED	None
5	T2 RMS	Hemoptysis-1 Dyspnea-3 Cough-4	COPD-Severe	5 Gy × 3 64 Gy	104	Died-Intercurrent	None

TABLE 49.2. SYMPTOM INDEX SCORING SYSTEM

Score	Definition
	Dyspnea
0	None
1	Dyspnea on moderate exertion
2	Dyspnea with normal activity, walking on level ground
3	Dyspnea at rest
4	Requires supplemental oxygen
	Cough
0	None
1	Intermittent, no medication necessary
2	Intermittent, non-narcotic medication
3	Constant or requiring narcotic medication
4	Constant, requiring narcotic medication but without relief
	Hemoptysis
0	None
1	Less than 2/week
2	Less than daily but greater than 2/week
3	Daily, bright red blood or clots
4	Decrease of Hb and/or Hct > 10%; greater than 150cm, requiring hospitalization or transfusion
	Pneumonia/Elevated Temperature
0	Normal temperature, no infiltrates, WBC less than 10,000
1	Temperature greater than 38.5°C and infiltrate, WBC less than 10,000
2	Temperature greater than 38.5°C and infiltrate and/or WBC greater than 10,000
3	Lobar consolidation on radiograph
4	Pneumonia or elevated temperature requiring hospitalization

atelectasis, hemorrhage, cough, and interference with airflow. YAG laser photo resection has immediate results but is restricted to central airways and to use by highly experienced operators. Unfortunately, conservative photo resection of the tumor without other interventions usually results in a fairly rapid reobstruction of the airway. The principle of endobronchial brachytherapy is that a high dose of radiation is delivered in a short period to the tumor and much less to normal tissues, in contradistinction to external radiation which, because of its inability to avoid considerable amounts of normal tissue, must be given in much lower doses per day to prevent undue complications.

Historically, it is always of interest to note that as early as 1922, Yankauer[23] placed radium capsules into the region of bronchogenic carcinoma for two patients with airway obstruction. In 1933, Kernan[1] used radon seed implantation. With the advent of fiberoptic bronchoscopy, new techniques became possible. The first reported use for transbronchial implantation was by Moylan[24] in 1983, using Gold-198 seeds. Also in 1983, Mendiondo[2] used an afterloading tube placed with the aid of the fiberoptic bronchoscope and then placed an Iridium-192 source into the tube. A total of 3,000 cGy delivered at a 5 mm depth was prescribed, with an average treatment time of 10 hours. From this it was noted that all patients had "significant improvement" in bronchial obstruction. Schray et al.[6,25] reported on afterloading with Iridium-192 in 1985 and

again in 1988. A single catheter was used in 65 patients. Fifty-nine of his patients had either prior or concurrent external radiation, and forty of the patients underwent YAG laser photo resection. Roughly 60% of the patients showed a response, 20% were stable, and 20% had progression at follow-up bronchoscopy. In his second report in 1988, 11 patients had developed either fistulas or massive hemorrhage, 7 of which he felt were secondary to treatment. He also noted that six of the seven patients had undergone YAG photoresection and that this may have contributed to the complications.

High-dose-rate (HDR) remote afterloading was first reported in the American literature by Seagren et al.[26] in 1985. All patients in this reported series had endobronchial carcinoma and had previously received a minimum external-beam radiation therapy dose equivalent to 5,000 cGy prior to brachytherapy. Each patient had bronchoscopically documented disease with local symptoms and a Karnofsky performance status of 50 or greater. The HDR remote afterloading unit was a Brachyton using a 3 mm diameter Cobalt-60 source with an average strength of 0.7 Ci. The unit had the ability to oscillate the source up to a maximum of 16 cm. A single catheter was used, and a dose of 1,000 cGy in a single fraction was delivered at a prescription depth of 10 mm. The total time for treatment ranged between 12 and 27 minutes. They reported on a total of 20 patients treated between 1982 and 1983. Four patients had first received YAG laser photoresection prior to the brachytherapy procedure. Complete palliation of symptoms was seen in 25% of the patients, and a partial or complete palliation of symptoms was seen in 94% of the patients. In six of these patients, palliation was long-lasting with no recurrence of symptoms. In 12 patients, these symptoms recurred or progressed, with a mean time to recurrence of 4.3 months.

Joyner and colleagues (1985)[27] first reported on the use of Iridium-192 solid wire afterloading for endobronchial treatment. They treated 14 patients with stage III non–small cell lung cancer with a combination of neodymium-YAG laser photoresection followed by endobronchial radiation and external-beam radiation therapy treatments. Brachytherapy treatment times were approximately 8–20 hours to deliver 3,000 cGy at a prescription depth of 5 mm. Rooney and colleagues (1984)[28] presented their information on the use of HDR endobronchial treatment utilizing a Gamma Med unit with an Iridium-192 source. This technique allowed for the stepping sequence of the source in up to 12 dwell positions spaced at either 0.5 or 1.0 cm. The patients were treated on a weekly basis receiving 600 cGy per week at a prescription depth of 1 cm with a maximum of five treatments.

Macha et al.[29] published a report in 1987 in which they utilized HDR afterloading with an Iridium-192 source in which the treatment was fractionated into three treatments through a single catheter. The dose was 1,500 cGy at a 5 mm prescription depth. Patients had laser, external radiation, and/or chemotherapy and had a high complication rate.

In all of the studies cited, the procedure consisted of using a single catheter for intraluminal brachytherapy. This is one of the few circumstances in the use of brachytherapy that a single-line linear source is the preferred method of treatment delivery. Volume implants from a dosimetric perspective are almost always preferred over a single-line source. Thus the ability to use more than one catheter allows for better dosimetry as well as better coverage of the disease process, which is rarely limited to a single tubular structure. An ideal system would allow more than one catheter to be used simultaneously. In addition, based on radiobiologic principles, fractionation becomes an important factor when variables of total dose and dose rate are considered. However, the ideal number of fractions for HDR quickly reaches a point that it is not feasible clinically and, thus, compromises must be made. Other physics factors have to be taken into account, including the choice of radioactive isotope, the dose at the prescription depth relative to the radius and inverse square law, as well as correction factors for the attenuation in water equivalent tissue versus air. Iridium-192 has the ability to be fabricated in small physical sizes of high activity, allowing passage through catheters with an internal diameter of 1.5 mm or less. In addition, Iridium-192 has virtually no significant correction for attenuation in water versus air up to a distance of 5 cm from the source.

This makes Iridium-192 the preferred radioactive isotope to be used within tissues with a mixed air/water density interfaces such as intraluminal brachytherapy. The major drawback of Iridium-192 is its short half-life of 74 days, such that over a period of months, the activity and, thus, the dose rate changes considerably and the source needs replacement frequently. However, this disadvantage can be moderated by the frequent replacement of the sources and keeping the source strength well within the high-dose-rate range.

Table 49.3 is a compilation of most, but not all, of the studies published on high-dose-rate remote afterloading endobronchial brachytherapy. It covers the years 1985 to 1997 for a total of 2,842 patients. As the reader can see in the tabulation, there are different doses used per fraction, number of fractions, as well as the dose prescriptions point. Although the variation for fatal hemoptysis is extremely large, ranging from 0% to 50% of patients, the mean is 10.3%. Fatal hemoptysis depends on multiple factors, including total number of patients studied, extensiveness of follow-up, and level of aggressiveness of treatment. For a small series, such as that of Khanavkar,[30] where they reported 12 patients in their series and at 50% incidence of fatal hemoptysis, it is felt that this is not representative of what one may anticipate for the level of fatal hemoptysis. Likewise, there are reports of no fatal hemoptysis, such as that of Burt[31] reporting on 50 patients; however, when the same medical group updated their series and reported on a total of 406 patients,[32] their rate of fatal hemoptysis was 8%. Lastly is the question of level of aggressiveness. Some authors have attributed fatal hemoptysis to treatment, such as Bedwinel,[33] who reported a 32% rate of hemoptysis, whereas Macha[34] and Speiser[35] reporting on 365 and 485 patients, respectively, in 1995 reported rates of 21% and 8%, respectively, and had adequate information to indicate that many, if not all, of the cases were secondary to carcinoma, and thus, it can be construed that the treatment was not aggressive enough.

In 1986, Speiser and Spratling developed a series of scoring systems (see Table 49.2, Tables 49.4–49.6) for selecting patients for treatment as well as for outcome analysis. Their initial report[36] was based on experience with an intermediate-dose-rate unit, which was a modification of a low-dose-rate unit, to allow a much higher specific activity of Iridium-192 for rapid delivery of dose. In some of the low-dose experiences, delivery of radiation took as long as 60 hours. The increase of Iridium-192 activity allowed the treatment time to be decreased to 1.5 to 4 hours. The range is based on (a) shorter times when the sources were new, (b) longer times as the sources decayed, and (c) the use for the first time of multiple catheters to deliver treatment. All treatments were performed in an outpatient setting and followed a protocol, which is outlined in the next section. As mentioned earlier, entry into the protocol and analysis of out-

TABLE 49.3. COMPILATION OF ENDOBRONCHIAL HDR STUDIES

Author	Year	No. of Patients	Dose (Gy)	No. of Fractions	Symptoms Improved (%)	X-Ray Improved (%)	Bronchoscopy Improved (%)	Fatal Hemoptysis (%)
Seagren et al. (1B)[26]	1985	20	10 at 10 mm	1	94	NA	100	28
Macha et al. (2B)[29]	1987	56	7.5 at 10 mm	3	74	88	75	7
Norl et al. (3B)[47]	1987	15	20 at 10 mm	3	80	88	NA	0
Burt* et al. (4B)[32]	1990	50	15–20 at 10 mm	1	50–86	46	88	0
Fass et al. (5B)[48]	1990	15	5–36 at 10 mm	1–6	75	NA	NA	0
Miller et al. (6B)[49]	1990	88	10 at 10 mm	3	NA	NA	80	0
Stout* et al. (7B)[50]	1990	100	15–20 at 10 mm	1	50–86	46	NA	0
Khanavker et al. (8B)[30]	1991	12	8 at 5 mm	2–8	67	NA	100	50
Aygun et al. (9B)[51]	1992	62	5 at 10 mm	3–5	NA	36	76	15
Bedwinek et al. (10B)[33]	1992	38	6 at 10 mm	3	76	64	82	32
Gauwitz et al. (11B)[52]	1992	24	15 at 10 mm	2	88	83	100	4
Mehta et al.(12B)[53]	1992	31	4 at 20 mm	4†	88	71–100	85	3
Sutedja et al. (13B)[54]	1992	31	10 at 10 mm	3	82	NA	NA	32
Spelser et al. (14B)[55]	1993	144	10 at 10 mm	3	85–99	NA	80	7
		151	7.5 at 10 mm	3				8
Zajac et al. (15B)[56]	1993	82	10–47 at 10 mm	1–5	82	NA	74	0
Tredanlal et al. (16B)[21]	1994	51	7 at 10 mm	2–8	55–85	NA	84	10
Chang et al. (17B)[57]	1994	76	7 at 10 mm	3	79–95	NA	87	4
Gollins* et al. (18B)[39]	1994	406	10–20 at 10 mm	1 (94%) 2 (6%)	88 (H), 62 (C) 60 (D), 92 (S)	46	NA	8
Cotter et al. (19B)[58]	1993	65 (17 IDR, 48 HDR)	2.7–10 at 10 mm	2–4	66 (PS)	46	63	2
Goldman et al. (20B)[42]	1993	20	15 at 10 mm	1	37 (C), 89 (D), 100 (H)	58	55	0
Marsh et al. (21B)[59]	1993	12	26–53 at 10 mm; high activity[125]	1	92 (tumor response)			8
Nori et al. (22B)[60]	1993	32	4–5 at 10 mm	3–4	100 (H), 86 (C), 100 (P)	Local control	83	0
Pisch et al. (23B)[61]	1993	39	10 at 10 mm	1–2	93 (H), 80 (C), 20 (P)	NA	NA	3
Macha et al. (24B)[34]	1995	365	5–7.5 at 10 mm	1–6	69	NA	NA	21
Huber et al. (25B)[62]	1995	93	3.8 at 10 mm or 7.2 at 10 mm	4 2	Improved local control			21
Gustafson et al. (26B)[63]	1995	46	7 at 10 mm	3	74	69	92	7
Sur et al. (27B)[64]	1995	14	10 at 10 mm	1–2	100 (H)	NA	NA	7
Speiser‡ et al. (28B)[37]	1995	485 total				NA		
		47 IDR	10 at 5 mm	3	99 (H)		53 (CR)	4.4 (CUR)
		144 HDR	10 at 10 mm	3	99 (P)		29 (PR) 82 (TR)	7.3 (PAL)
		151 HDR	7.5 at 10 mm	3	86 (D)			9.1 (REC)
		143 HDR	7.5 at 10 mm or 5 at 10 mm	3 4	85 (C)			7.3 (ALL)
Saito et al. (29B)[65]	1996	40	5 at 3–9 mm	5	NA	NA	100	0
Delclos et al.[66]	1996	81	15 at 6 mm	2	32% excellent 31% moderate 21% minimal 84% Total median survival	NA	NA	0
Huber et al.[67]	1997	98						
		42	Ext only 60Gy#	22–30	30 wk			14
		56	Ext + Int Int 4.6 at 5 mm	2	43 wk			19
Total	1985–1997	2,842			20–100	36–88	55–100	0–50 Mean 10.3

P, Pneumonia; H, hemoptysis; C, cough; D, dyspnea; S, stridor; PS, performance status; CUR, curative; PAL, paliative; REC, recurrent; CR, complete response; PR, more than 50% response; TR, CR and PR; IDR, intermediate dose rate.
Patients in more than one publication were counted once.
* Same institution.
† Four treatments in 2 days.
‡ Spelser reporting different protocols.
# Mean dose ~50Gy +/− 13Gy.

TABLE 49.4. INFLUENCE OF PERFORMANCE STATUS ON PATIENTS WITH INOPERABLE LUNG CANCER

ECOG (Zubrod) (Host) (WHO)	Kamofsky	Definitions
0	100	Asymptomatic
1	80–90	Symptomatic: fully ambulatory
2	60–70	Symptomatic: in bed less than 50% of the day
3	40–50	Symptomatic: in bed more than 50% of the day but not bedridden
4	20–30	Bedridden

TABLE 49.6. OBSTRUCTION SCORE

Location	Percent Obstruction >50	10–50	<10
Trachea	10	5	2
Main stem	6	3	1
Lobar bronchi	2	1	
Atelectasis/pneumonia received additional 2 points per lobe			

come utilized semiquantitative measures, which will be discussed within the protocol area.

PROTOCOL

Our protocol was initiated in 1986 when EBBT was transformed from low-dose-rate manual afterloading to medium-dose-rate remote afterloading procedures. This was a transitory step of short duration, lasting for 9 months. The high-dose-rate remote afterloader was, in fact, a Nucletron Selectron low-dose-rate remote afterloader that was modified to accept a longer source train and a much higher level of radioactivity. The activity was usually maintained at greater than 20 mc per cm. Dose rates initially were calculated at a 5 mm depth perpendicular to the source train, and were in the range of 5 to 10 cGy per minute.

Eligibility

Eligibility for the protocol includes the following: (a) Disease must involve the trachea, mainstem, or lobar bronchi. (Involvement of the segmental bronchi without involvement more proximal was not considered to be sufficient for entry into the protocol.) (b) The central airway disease must be intraluminal, visualized, and biopsied via bronchoscopy. (Patients requiring transbronchial biopsy were ineligible for

TABLE 49.5. WEIGHT LOSS SCORE BASED ON PERCENTAGE OF LOSS OF BODY WEIGHT WITHIN 6 MONTHS PRECEDING DIAGNOSIS

Weight Loss Score (WLS)	Weight Loss (% of body weight)
0	0
1	1–4.9
2	5–9.9
3	10–19.9
4	>20.0

the protocol.) (c) Patients must have significant symptomatology within the four symptom groups consisting of cough, dyspnea, signs and symptoms of obstructive pneumonia, and hemoptysis.

Evaluation of the patients meeting eligibility criteria to be placed on the EBBT protocol schedule were reviewed within the context of all patients diagnosed with lung cancer within the referral area from 1986 through 1996. This involved the greater Phoenix/Maricopa county area and utilized a reconstruction of the Tumor Registry to calculate an incidence rate of approximately 9,000 cases of lung cancer during the ten-year period. Of these, only 19% received radiation, and 16% of that group, or 3% of all patients, were treated on protocol, while an additional 11% of patients receiving radiation, or 2% of all patients, were treated with brachytherapy off protocol. Thus 27% of all patients receiving radiation, or 5% of all diagnosed lung cancer patients, received brachytherapy. For patients on the curative protocol, these figures were 3% and 0.5%, respectively.

Indications

Indications for treatment are given in Table 49.7. The first three are those used in the protocol presented later in this chapter. The fourth is presently being used, and the fifth is an indication used occasionally.

Protocol 1.0 Curative Intent

To be eligible for this protocol, patients must not have had prior radiation within the thoracic area, which would preclude the adequate delivery of a full dose of external radiation. Patients must be inoperable and have a primary lung carcinoma with a non–small cell histology. Stages accepted were $T_{1,2,3} N_{1,2} M_3$. These stages correspond to stage groupings I, II, and IIIa. Performance status using the four-tiered weight loss system, likewise, must be 0, 1, or 2 and correspond to weight losses of 0, less than 5%, or less than 10%, respectively, of the patients weight in the 6 months prior to diagnosis. The rationale for selection of this level of weight loss is described in *Oncologic Assessment Using the Four Tiered Scoring System.*[37] Patients were treated within the group characterized by dose as described in Table 49.8.

TABLE 49.7. INDICATIONS FOR TREATMENT WITH ENDOBRONCHIAL BRACHYTHERAPY

Indications	Exclusions	Rationale
1. Tumors must be seen and biopsied by bronchoscopy (intraluminal).	Tumors presenting with extrinsic compression of the airway as seen by bronchoscopy, and the biopsy must be performed transbronchially (extraluminal).	Intraluminal brachytherapy delivers a very high dose to tumor close to the source axis. Extraluminal disease due to its much greater distance from the axis would lead to unacceptable doses to the bronchial mucosa and surrounding structures.
2. Tumors must be in the central airways, which are defined as the trachea, mainstem, and lobar bronchi.	Tumors in peripheral airways, which are defined as segmental bronchi or beyond.	Significant illness most often caused by disease in central airways. Treatment of small peripheral airways leads to stenosis of those airways.
3. Tumors in central airways causing significant illness.	Patients with significant preexisting dyspnea unrelated to carcinoma. Patients with dyspnea secondary to effusion, or large extrinsic masses.	Patients with symptoms second to disease other than central airway disease are not expected to improve with intraluminal brachytherapy.
4. *In situ* carcinoma for inoperable patients.	Patients entered into national protocols using other modes of treatment, i.e., photodynamic.	Preserves lung and pulmonary function. Excellent treatment for multifocal disease.
5. Preop for submucosal spread from a peripheral/central lesion.	Patients should be good candidates for lobectomy or pneumonectomy.	Treatment provides a clear margin for surgery.

Protocol 2.0 Palliative Intent

Protocol 2.1

Eligibility for these patients includes primary lung cancer with non–small cell histology, and stage T_1N_3 and/or M_1 disease. These stages correspond to stage groupings IIIb and

TABLE 49.8. MODIFICATION OF DOSES BY YEAR FOR THE CURATIVE, PALLIATIVE, AND RECURRENT PROTOCOLS

Group	Year	External cGy Dose	FXS	Internal cGy Dose	Depth	FXS	Unit
Curative Protocol							
1	1986–1988	6,000	30	1,000	5 mm	3	MDR
2	1988–1990	6,000	30	1,000	10 mm	3	HDR
3	1990–1992	6,000	30	750	10 mm	3	HDR
4	1992–1994	6,400	32	500	10 mm	3	HDR
Palliative Protocol							
1	1986–1988	3,750	15	1,000	5 mm	3	MDR
				1,000	5 mm	3	MDR
2	1988–1990	3,750	15	1,000	10 mm	3	HDR
				1,000	10 mm	3	HDR
3	1990–1992	3,750	15	750	10 mm	3	HDR
				750	10 mm	3	HDR
4	1992–1994	3,750	15	500	10 mm	3	HDR
				500	10 mm	4	HDR
				750	10 mm	3	HDR
Recurrent Protocol							
1	1986–1988			1,000	5 mm	3	MDR
2	1988–1990			1,000	10 mm	3	HDR
3	1990–1992			750	10 mm	3	HDR
4	1992–1994			500	10 mm	4	HDR

IV. In addition, the patients ineligible for protocol 1.0 because of performance scores of 3 or 4 or a weight loss of 3 or 4 (>10%) were reallocated to this protocol. Patients were treated within the group characterized by dose as described in Table 49.8.

Protocol 2.2

Primary lung cancer consisting of small cell histology, both limited and extensive, primary lung cancer with contralateral metastatic disease involving the endobronchial mucosa, and nonlung primaries with metastases primarily to the mucosa were treated within this category. Patients were treated within the group characterized by dose as described in Table 49.8.

Protocol 3.0 Recurrent Patients

All patients who had received prior radiation for a curative intent for carcinoma of the lung were included within this category. Patients were treated within the group characterized by dose as described in Table 49.8. Group I patients were treated with medium dose rate. In the palliative protocol, brachytherapy was constant and the use of external radiation was optional at the discretion of the treating oncologist. Its use was restricted to patients with extrinsic disease that caused a significant contribution to the level of obstruction and/or symptomatology.

Results

The following results incorporate 600 patients treated in the curative, palliative, and recurrent protocols outlined previously. In each of the successive periods of the operation of the protocol, the eligibility factors for the curative, palliative, and recurrent protocols have remained constant.

All patients treated in curative protocols with external radiation received 2 Gy per fraction, and in palliative protocols, 2.5 Gy per fraction. If patients received concurrent brachytherapy and external radiation, both treatments were not given on the same day. For the curative protocol, brachytherapy was delivered during weeks 1, 3, and 5. For palliative and recurrent protocols, brachytherapy was delivered weekly for three or four fractions, depending on the protocol.

The distribution of patients into the protocol groups was as follows: curative 19%, palliative 48%, and recurrent 33%. The age distribution of the patients had a median of 68 years and a mean of 67.1 years. Most of the patients fell within the range of 60–80 years old. The gender distribution was 62% male and 38% female. The percentage of female patients increased from 28% in group 1 to 41% in group 3 and 4. The breakdown for male/female patients was similar to that of all patients presenting with carcinoma of the lung within the geographic treatment area.

Squamous cell carcinoma is by far the most common cell type, overall, in the study (49%), and even to a greater extent for those treated in the curative protocol (70%). This percentage is considerably higher than is currently being seen in newly diagnosed outpatients with lung cancer (27%). This finding corresponds to long-held observations that squamous cell carcinomas tend to be more central and adenocarcinomas more peripheral.

The use of laser photoresection predated the wide use of high-dose-rate brachytherapy for airway carcinoma. In this study there was a gradual decrease in its use from an initial 32% to 16% in the latter part of the study. It is currently estimated that less than 5% of patients with central airway disease will require laser photoresection in the future.

The protocol required that patients must have one or more of the four primary symptom complexes in order to be included in this study. The incidence of the symptoms in the study were cough greater than 99%, dyspnea 97%, hemoptysis 64%, and the signs and symptoms of obstructive pneumonia 49%. Using the four-tiered symptom index as outlined in Table 49.2, the severity of the symptoms were weighted and the total weighted scores were subsequently normalized to 100%. Response for each symptom score is related to each brachytherapy procedure and the first follow-up bronchoscopy (Figure 49.5).

Hemoptysis had the most dramatic and rapid of the responses with improvements of 70%, 90% and more than 99% at each intervention point. Pneumonia improvement was only slightly less dramatic with responses of 57%, 85%, and more than 99%. Improvement in dyspnea occurred in 36%, 54%, and 86%, respectively. Lastly was cough, with improvements of 32%, 52%, and 85%, respectively. The improvements in hemoptysis and pneumonia were commonly seen within the first 24 hours following the first brachytherapy procedure. Thus patients who were admitted to the hospital with obstructive pneumonia and/or sepsis, or with severe bleeding requiring transfusion, have a prompt response allowing them to be moved from an area of intensive care to one of normal care or to be discharged from the hospital.

In the palliative protocol, the use of concurrent external radiation with brachytherapy was optional. When the weighted responses were measured for brachytherapy only, versus brachytherapy and external radiation, the results in

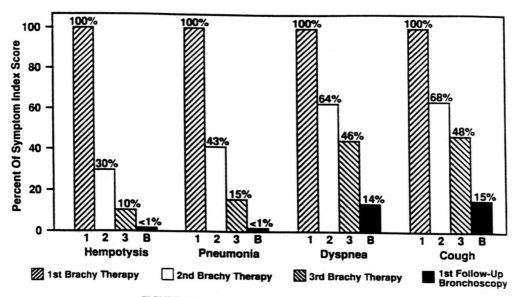

FIGURE 49.5. Percent of symptom index score.

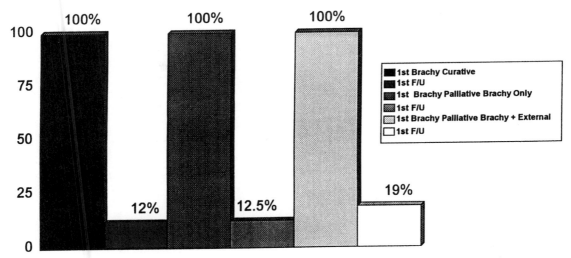

FIGURE 49.6. Obstruction score response. Obstruction score (mean) normalized to 100% (score obtained at bronchoscopy at first brachytherapy treatment) and compared to residual obstruction score at first follow-up bronchoscopy. Palliative Group combined result 17%.

terms of improvement at follow-up were as follows: hemoptysis 94% and 97%, pneumonia 86% and 82%, dyspnea 54% and 48%, and cough 51% and 57%, respectively. There was no statistical difference in response for each symptom group for each of these two therapies. The use of brachytherapy only was sufficient in itself to provide palliation without the need to add supplemental external radiation.

The obstruction scores, as seen in Figure 49.6, were analyzed in a different fashion. All of the scores were converted into median scores, which were normalized to 100%. These were obtained for each brachytherapy procedure and at the first follow-up bronchoscopy. The median score was normalized to 100%, and the residual level of obstruction is expressed as a percentage. (Any tissue including inflammatory tissue was included as part of the obstruction score.) The curative patients and the palliative groups fared better than the recurrent group, with scores of 12%, 12.5%, and 19%, respectively (Figure 49.6). This outcome is not unexpected considering that patients with recurrent carcinoma have had previous external radiation, which may select for a slightly more radioresistant, slower growing carcinoma and thus would be anticipated to be less sensitive to radiation. It is interesting that neither the use of concurrent external radiation or of laser photoresection led to improved clearing of obstruction. Thus, as in the symptom index results, the addition of external radiation or laser resection did not add to clearing endobronchial disease.

The survival of patients by protocol group was 10% for the curative patients and 5% for the palliative-recurrent patients years. The palliative-recurrent patients had disease that was most often recurrent, advanced, and/or metastatic at or shortly after presentation, leading to low survival rates.

The cause of death shows a significant failure rate for local disease in all categories. These rates were 31% and 30%, respectively, for the curative and palliative-recurrent protocols. As has been seen in numerous other studies, despite gradual increasing doses of radiation over the last several decades, local disease continues to be a significant problem.

Survival curves for the curative versus the palliative-recurrent patient illustrated in Figure 49.7 and are calculated from the date of diagnosis and date of the first brachytherapy procedure. There was no statistically different result between these two groups when analyzed from the date of diagnosis (p = 0.1); however, from the date of the first brachytherapy treatment, the p-value was less than 0.0001 comparing the curative versus the palliative-recurrent patients. (The recurrent patients are self-selected by the fact that they lived long enough to develop a symptomatic recurrence. This bias was eliminated when analyzing survival by date of treatment.)

COMPLICATIONS

The complication most often mentioned when discussing endobronchial carcinoma and its treatment is that of fatal hemoptysis. This complication is defined as bleeding that is most often caused by erosion into the right or left pulmonary artery with subsequent exsanguination within the tracheal bronchial tree. This is a known complication of progression of untreated or inadequately treated carcinoma involving the tracheal bronchial tree, most often in the region of the upper lobe bronchi, due to their proximity to the pulmonary arteries. With the advent of intraluminal

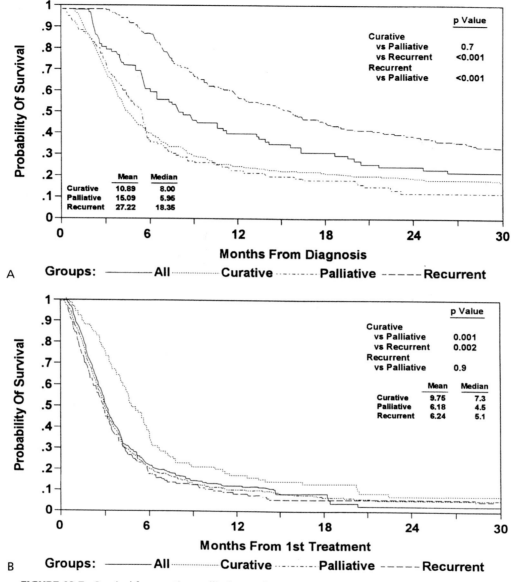

FIGURE 49.7. Survival for curative, palliative, and recurrent groups from initial diagnosis **(A)** and from first day of treatment **(B)**.

treatment, it must be considered as a possible complication of this modality.

In this study, the overall rate is 6% with the median time from diagnosis until death of 14 months; however, when measured from the date of the first brachytherapy until death, the median for the entire group is 5 months. Recurrent patients, as would be anticipated, have the highest rate of fatal hemoptysis at 9%, whereas the curative and palliative patients have rates of 5%. Of interest is that, in the different dose groups, there was an increase in fatal hemoptysis as the dose was increased from group 1 to 2; however, there was a slight further increase in the rate of hemop-

tysis as the dose was reduced and then a decrease in the rate of fatal hemoptysis (2%) with further dose reduction. Thus no dose-response relationship could be identified. In addition, the curative patients who had the greatest radiobiologic effect, in that all treatment was within a short period that is, external and internal radiation, had a rate of 5% versus the recurrent patients who had their treatment over a prolonged period, with a rate of 9%, and the palliative group of patients, who had the lowest doses delivered, had a rate of 5%. Fatal hemoptysis was measured in the palliative protocol patients where 41% of the patients were treated with brachytherapy only, and 59% with brachytherapy and exter-

TABLE 49.9. GRADES OF RADIATION BRONCHITIS AND STENOSIS (RBS)

Grade	Definition
1	Fibrinoid membrane without significant luminal obstruction: no symptoms
2	Increase of exudation and fibrous membrane with mild obstructive symptoms requiring therapeutic intervention, such as simple debridement or medical treatment
3	Characterized by severe inflammatory response with marked membranous exudate including fibrosis requiring multiple debridements
4	A greater degree of fibrosis resulting in stenosis with decreased luminal diameter requiring laser photo resection, balloon or bougie dilation, and/or stent placement

nal radiation. The rate of fatal hemoptysis was 5.5% in the brachytherapy-only group, and the combined group receiving higher doses of radiation had a rate of 4%. Once again, there was no evidence of a dose response.

The most common side effect seen that is definitively related to the intraluminal treatment was radiation bronchitis and stenosis. This was not an entity previously described until the initial description by Speiser and Spratling.[36] Table 49.9 is a definition of the grades of radiation bronchitis and stenosis utilized. The incidence of radiation bronchitis and stenosis by group are 9%, 12%, 14%, and 14%, respectively. By protocol, they were 23%, 12%, and 8%, respectively, for the curative, palliative, and recurrent protocols. The rate is clearly highest in the curative patients. When this rate was further analyzed, it was noted that the only significant factor predicting for this response was length of follow-up. Although the true incidence of this complication is not known for patients receiving external radiation only, it is still felt that this complication results primarily from intraluminal brachytherapy with its very high mucosal doses.

For palliative patients, this complication was studied in those patients receiving brachytherapy only versus those receiving brachytherapy along with concurrent external radiation, and the incidence was 17% and 10%, respectively. Although the incidence was slightly higher in the brachytherapy-only group, the median time to occurrence was slightly longer in this group at 3.6 months versus 2.5 months for the patients receiving combined treatment.

MANAGEMENT OF COMPLICATIONS

The treatment of brachytherapy-related hemoptysis is the same as hemoptysis from other causes. This includes bed rest, codeine, transfusion for hemodynamic stability, avoidance or reversal of anticoagulants, vascular embolization, electrocautery, or lasocautery to reduce bleeding volume.

One of the largest reported series of patients treated with palliative brachytherapy alone is from the Christy Hospital in Manchester, England.[38] Three hundred twenty-two patients with inoperable non–small cell lung cancers were treated with a single fraction of HDR with a total dose of 15–20 Gy delivered intraluminally with the dose prescription 1 cm from the central axis of the catheter. Patients were evaluated 6 weeks after completing the HDR treatment with regard to their symptoms, including stridor, hemoptysis, cough, dyspnea, pain, and pulmonary collapse. In addition, at various times following the brachytherapy procedure, 83 bronchoscopies were conducted on 55 patients. Massive hemoptysis leading to death occurred in 32 patients (8%). Cox multivariate analysis revealed that treatment-related factors associated with subsequent massive hemoptysis were brachytherapy dose more than 15 Gy, prior laser therapy, second brachytherapy treatment, and concurrent external-beam radiation therapy. Twenty of the 25 assessable deaths related to hemoptysis had recurrent and/or residual tumor suspected at the hemoptysis site. The chronology of the massive hemoptysis leading to death occurred between 9 and 12 months after completion of the HDR procedure. This was in stark contrast to deaths from all other causes, which usually occurred 3 to 6 months after completion of the HDR procedures.[39]

Brachytherapy-related bronchitis and stenosis are managed based on the level of severity of the reaction and/or stenosis. This can include observation for mild treatment-related bronchitis for the least symptomatic presentation, and can be actively treated in a more debilitating form with oral and/or aerosol administration of steroids, aerosol-administrated bronchodilators, codeine- or narcotic-based cough suppressants, and antifungal or antibiotic therapies for symptomatic management, as well as correction of the underlying cause. More aggressive interventional management for debilitating and/or life-threatening levels of bronchitis and/or stenosis may be managed with balloon and/or bougie dilation, laser photoresection, bronchoscopic debridement, and/or placement of intraluminal stents.

Although lung brachytherapy has been advocated by radiation oncologists for the past 20 years, recent technologic developments in the area of high-dose-rate brachytherapy, such as the design of high-activity, physically small Iridium-192 sources and remote afterloading machines have prompted renewed interest in lung endobronchial high-dose-rate brachytherapy. The specific role of lung EBBT is not clearly defined at this time to be instituted within the standard and/or uniform community practice. There is an ongoing evolution for the tumor selection criteria to identify those patients most likely to benefit from EBBT with regard to local control, which may translate ultimately to improved survival. The American Brachytherapy Society (ABS) HDR

Consensus Guidelines[40] currently state that, although endobronchial brachytherapy has demonstrated efficacy for symptomatic relief of bronchial obstructions and hemoptysis, either alone or in combination with external-beam radiation therapy, the curative benefit of brachytherapy in additional to conventional external-beam radiation therapy and/or chemotherapy has not been proven. The ABS recommends that brachytherapy for the definitive treatment of lung cancer be done within the context of a controlled clinical trial, if possible. Outside of clinical trials, the ABS suggests that brachytherapy be reserved for palliative treatments alone. Although the guidelines do not clearly state the indications for additional external beam radiation in newly diagnosed lung cancer patients, EBBT alone is recommended for recurrences after full-dose external-beam radiation therapy treatments have been administered. No single-dose fractionation scheme has been identified that provides for superior therapeutic ratio. Dose specifications have been recommended to be prescribed to a depth of 1 cm from the source center for uniform prescription dosimetry comparisons.

A study by the Radiation Therapy Oncology Group (RTOG) evaluated the palliation provided by external beam radiation to patients with newly diagnosed nonmetastatic, non–small cell lung cancers.[41] This study by Simpson et al. demonstrated that a short course of external-beam radiation therapy delivering 30 Gy in 10 fractions provided relief of hemoptysis in 74% of patients, cough in 55% of patients, and dyspnia in 43% of patients. Median survival was in the range of 6 months. Compared to this RTOG study, brachytherapy alone appears to provide equivalent palliation as external-beam radiation, with a similar survival outcome. Given this fact, brachytherapy may give more prompt symptomatic relief of obstructive symptoms in a more cost-effective manner.

In a small group of 19 patients treated with HDR to a total dose of 15 Gy,[42] in which a detailed assessment with rigorous testing was performed before and after administration of the HDR brachytherapy, and chest x-rays, CT scan of the thorax, direct bronchoscopic evaluation, objective obstruction index scoring, five-minute walking stress tests, isotope ventilation and profusion lung scanning, and formal pulmonary function tests with maximum inspiratory and expiratory full-volume measurements were conducted. Symptomatic relief was reported in 17 of the 19 patients. Atelectasis of a collapsed lobe or lung reported in 13 patients was demonstrated to have reinstituted ventilation in nine cases by radiographic imaging. Bronchoscopic evaluation of luminal patency had demonstrated improvement in 18 of the 19 patients. Isotope lung scans showed significant increase in the percentage of total lung ventilation and profusion in the abnormal lung. This rigorous study demonstrated the high correlation between objective and subjective improvement of the presenting symptomatology in these patients. In addition, it confirmed the palliative benefit of brachytherapy, which has been described in larger groups

of patients. A prospective randomized study of brachytherapy and external-beam radiation therapy are clearly needed to directly compare treatment efficacy and toxicity, as well as a cost-benefit analysis and quality-of-life analysis in this setting.

CONCLUSIONS

Endobronchial brachytherapy is an excellent means of treatment for palliation of symptoms for patients with lung cancer, with a low probability of cure; that is, the palliative protocol group and patients with lung cancer previously irradiated. This treatment does not require concurrent treatments for most of these patients as long as the disease process involves central airway disease secondary to intrinsic involvement.

For curative intent patients, it provides rapid relief of obstruction and the signs and symptoms of obstruction. In the survey of literature, as well as this study, survival advantage is not shown. This group of patients must, in the future, be randomized to external-beam radiation therapy versus external-beam plus intraluminal radiation to evaluate a possible survival benefit prospectively.

For the future, further studies will be necessary to determine the most optimal dose and number of fractions that will provide the greatest patient benefit, the lowest morbidity, and the lowest cost of treatment. In addition to randomized protocols of external-beam versus external plus internal radiation, it will be necessary to test the hypothesis that chemotherapy adds to the benefit obtained by radiation as the sole therapy. All proposed protocols for lung cancer should include the comorbid features and/or biologic markers that have been shown to be strong predictors for the probability of survival for lung cancer.

INTERSTITIAL

Interstitial brachytherapy began with Radon-222, and later Gold-198 and Iridium-192. Radon and gold in the form of seeds had been used because of their short half-life and rapid deposition of energy within the target area. Iridium-192 was most often used as individual seed sources sealed within polyethylene ribbons or strands, later to be placed in hollow nylon afterloaded tubes. However, it was not until the introduction of Iodine-125 with its low-energy gamma-ray emission primarily in the 30 KeV range (27–32 KeV) and a long half-life of 60 days (59.4) that the sources could be kept within the hospital and available in a standby mode. The newest isotope in use is Palladium-103, seeds that are, like the Iodine seeds, a low-energy gamma emitter (23 KeV), but with a shorter half-life (17 days). This isotope provides an increased dose rate, which is preferred for more rapidly growing tumors. The permanent seed implant with Iodine-125 or Palladium-103 is best used in those patients undergoing surgical resection when the margins are close or positive; the implant provides a high dose to a small volume aiming at improved local control.

The three primary methods of placement of seeds are (a) the use of loose seeds that are placed through a hollow stainless steel needle. The needles are placed within the target volume in an array usually with 1 cm spacings to accomplish a good dose distribution in two planes. The third plane is then set by deposition of seeds at either 5 or 10 mm increments along the needle length. The needles are placed at the maximum depth of interest, and then an applicator is attached to the needles such that the operator has the ability of depositing seeds at intervals of 5 mm or greater. Thus the three-dimensional array is first accomplished by placing the needles in a two-plane or more array and completing the third dimension by depositing the seeds along the needle track, slowly withdrawing the needle, and depositing the seeds. Placing hollow stainless steel needles into vital structures, bones, nerves, and vessels is not possible. (b) The needles or sources can also be placed within gelfoam or dacron sheets, the seeds deposited, and then the implanted material placed sheetlike over an area where implantation might not otherwise be possible. To stabilize the friable gelfoam, a Vicryl mesh or mobilization of tissue is needed to cover the implant to ensure that the gelfoam and seeds do not migrate. (c) A current technique uses Iodine seeds embedded within Vicryl suture. Standard Vicryl suture is modified by placing and spacing the seeds at 1 cm within the mesh suture. The Vicryl suture is supplied attached to a large-caliber needle to allow the operator to sew the strand. The size of the needle precludes its use in most clinical situations but allows the operator to remove the needle and to drape the suture using a needle of more appropriate size. The suture is sewn through an area, allowing excellent placement for spacing and fixation of the seeds. However, more often than not, the tissues in question (such as the major vascular structures and bronchial margins) will not allow this procedure to be performed in this manner, in which case, the needle is removed and the operator can then "implant the suture" by applying it to the critical structure by using vascular clips. The vascular clip should not crimp a seed but should be placed on the suture between the Iodine seeds. The doses judged sufficient to eradicate macroscopic disease are 160 Gy for Iodine-125 and 125 Gy for Palladium-103 (prior to TG-43).

RESULTS

Because of the varying shapes of the sites in the thoracic cavity, which attempted to be implanted, a reasonable way to assess the benefit of implantation is to look at local control rates as an end point. Clinical groups may have different outcomes. These are seen in Table 49.10: Stage I or higher

TABLE 49.10. RESULTS OF INTERSTITIAL BRACHYTHERAPY IN NON–SMALL CELL LUNG CARCINOMA

Author	Patient Category	No. of Patients	Brachytherapy Technique	Results of Treatment %	
				Local Control	Survival (Yrs)
Hilaris[44–47]	Early stage Stage I	55	Permanent interstitial	85	33 (5 yrs)
	Locally advanced Unresectable tumors with negative nodes	322	Permanent interstitial	71	20 (2 yrs)
	Locally advanced Unresectable tumors with positive nodes	152	Permanent interstitial	63	9 (2 yrs)
	Locally advanced Unresectable tumors with positive nodes	88	Permanent implant of primary + temporary implant (Ir-192) of Mediastinum (3,000 cGy/3 days)	76	51 (2 yrs)
	Superior sulcus tumors	127	Pre-op RT, partial resection + permanent and/or temporary implant	70	20 (10 yrs)
Burt[32,33]	Locally advanced Chest wall tumors (T.N.)	225	Permanent interstitial and/or temporary implants	70	≈30 (2 yrs) for a. Complete resection b. Incomplete resection + brachytherapy 21 (2 yrs) Brachytherapy only
TOTAL		969		71%	

stage disease as locally advanced, unresectable with negative nodes, unresectable with positive nodes, superior Sulcus tumors and T_3N_0 chest wall disease. Table 49.10 shows the results for these subgroupings in terms of technique used (including if external radiation was used), and whether local control and survival were influenced. Overall local control is 71%, which, in conjunction with (a) good surgical resection and (b) adjuvant radiation and/or chemotherapy, can lead to an improved five-year survival.

What will not be found in the literature is that this technique requires extensive individual experience and expertise to obtain results similar to those reported by Hilaris[43-46] and Burt[31,32] without having an excessive complication rate. A good example would be the last intraoperative consultation I performed on a patient who underwent a left upper lobectomy with tumor peeled off the left pulmonary artery. The consultation was to determine if I would "implant" the pulmonary artery. Surgery involved stripping the carcinoma off the pulmonary artery. The recommendation was that implantation was not advisable due to an extremely high risk of pulmonary artery rupture. One week postop, the patient's left pulmonary artery ruptured and carcinoma was found in the artery wall at autopsy.

DISCUSSION

Interstitial lung brachytherapy is used infrequently in the United States. This may be due to the difficulty in gaining expertise with interstitial implant procedures, as compared to external-beam treatment planning or even endobronchial brachytherapy procedures. The recent introduction of Iodine-125 with its 60-day half-life and low-energy ionizing photon emissions have made interstitial brachytherapy more practical for consideration and implementation in the clinical practice. However, at this time, there is no proven role for interstitial brachytherapy alone or in combination with other treatment modalities, such as surgery, chemotherapy, or external-beam radiation therapy. The decision to use interstitial brachytherapy modality in concert with other treatment modalities must consider not only possible local control and survival benefits, but also its ability to improve the final outcome of the patient's medical care by symptomatic relief duration and rapidity, treatment costs for acute and chronic toxicity, and the ability to preserve a pulmonary cardiac musculoskeletal and neurological function.

REFERENCES

1. Kernan JD. Carcinoma of the lung and bronchus. Treatment with radon implantation and diathermy. *Arch Otolaryngol* 1933; 17:457.
2. Paterson R, Spiers FW, Stephenson SK, et al. *Radium dosage.* The Manchester System; 1967.
3. Pool JL. Bronchoscopy in the treatment of lung cancer. *Trans Am Bronchoesoph Assoc* 1961;41:128.
4. Graham EA, Singer JJ. Successful removal of an entire lung for carcinoma of the bronchus. *JAMA* 1933;101:1371.
5. Henschke UK. Interstitial implantation in the treatment of primary bronchogenic carcinoma. *Am J Roentgenol Radium Ther Nucl Med* 1959;79:981.
6. Schray MF, McDougall JC, Martinez A, et al. Management of malignant airway obstruction: clinical and dosimetric considerations using an iridium-192 afterloading technique in conjunction with the neodymium-yag laser. *Int J Radiat Oncol Biol Phys* 1985; 11:403.
7. Mendiondo OA, Dillon M, Beach LJ. Endobronchial brachytherapy in the treatment of recurrent bronchogenic carcinoma. *Int J Radiat Oncol Biol Phys* 1983;9:579.
8. Sanderson D, Fontana R, Woolner L, et al. Bronchoscopic localization of radiographically occult lung cancer. *Chest* 1974;65:608.
9. Cortese DA, Pairolero PC, Bergstraih EJ, et al. Roentgenographically occult lung cancer. *J Thorac Cardiovasc Surg* 1980;86:373.
10. Martini N, Melamed MR. Occult carcinoma of the lung. *Ann Thorac Surg* 1980;30:215.
11. Saito Y, Nagamoto N, Ota S, et al. Results of surgical treatment for roentgenographically occult bronchogenic squamous cell carcinoma. *J Thorac Cardiovasc Surg* 1992;104:401.
12. Durci M, Komaki R, Oswald MJ, et al. Comparison of surgery and radiation therapy for non-small cell carcinoma of the lung with mediastinal metastasis. *Int J Radiat Oncol Biol Phys* 1991; 21:629.
13. Feinstein A, Wells C. A clinical-severity staging system for patients with lung cancer. *Lung Medicine* 1990;69:1.
14. Maki E, Feld R. Prognostic factors in patients with non-small cell lung cancer: a critique of the world literature. *Lung Cancer* 1991;7:27.
15. Pater J, Loeb M. Nonanatomic prognostic factors in carcinoma of the lung. *Cancer* 1982;50:326.
16. Nagamoto N, Saito Y, Sato M, et al. Lesions preceding squamous cell carcinoma of the bronchus and multicentricity of canceration—serial slicing of minute lung cancers smaller than 1 mm. *Tohoku J Exp Med* 1993;170:11.
17. Kato H, Kawate N, Kinoshita K, et al. Photodynamic therapy of early-stage lung cancer: a critique of the world literature. *Lung Cancer* 1991;7:27.
18. Saito Y, Sato M, Sagawa M, et al. Multicentricity in resected occult bronchogenic squamous cell carcinoma. *Ann Thorac Surg* 1994;57:1200.
19. Usuda K, Saito Y, Kanma K, et al. Resected roentgenographically occult bronchogenic squamous cell carcinoma tumor size, survival, and recurrence. *Nippon Geka Gakkai Zasshi* 1993;94:631.
20. Sutedja G, Baris G, van Zandwijk N, et al. High-dose rate brachytherapy has a curative potential in patients with intraluminal squamous cell lung cancer. *Respiration* 1993;61:167.
21. Tredanial J, Hennequin C, Zalcman G, et al. Prolonged survival after high-dose rate endobronchial radiation for malignant airway obstruction. *Chest* 1994;105:767.
22. Perol M, Caliandro R, Pommier P, et al. Curative irradiation of Limited endobronchial carcinomas with high-dose rate brachytherapy. *Chest* 1997;11:5:1417.
23. Yankauer S. Two cases of lung tumor treated bronchoscopically. *NY Med J* 1922;21:741.
24. Moylan D, Strubler K, Unal A, et al. Work in progress. Transbronchial brachytherapy of recurrent bronchogenic carcinoma: a new approach using the flexible fiberoptic bronchoscope. *Radiology* 1983;147:253.
25. Schray MF, McDougall JC, Martinez A, et al. Management of

malignant airway compromise with laser and low dose rate brachytherapy. *Chest* 1988;93:264.

26. Seagren SL, Harrell JH, Horn RA. High dose rate intraluminal irradiation in recurrent endobronchial carcinoma. *Chest* 1985; 88:810.

27. Joyner LR JR, Maran AG, Sarama R, et al. Neodymium-YAG laser treatment of intrabronchial lesions. *Chest Apr* 1985;87:4: 418.

28. Rooney SM, Goldiner PL, Bains MS, et al. Anesthesia for the application of endotracheal and endobronchial radiation therapy. *J Thorac Cardiovasc Surg* 1984;87:5:693.

29. Macha HN, Kock K, Stadler M, et al. New technique for treating occlusive and stenosing tumors of the trachea and main bronchi: endobronchial irradiation by high dose iridium-192 combined with laser canalization. *Thorax* 1987;42:511.

30. Khanavker B, Stern P, Alberti W, et al. Complications associated with brachytherapy alone or with laser in lung cancer. *Chest* 1991; 99:1062.

31. Burt ME, Pomerantz AH, Bains MS, et al. Results of surgical treatment of stage III lung cancer invading mediastinum. *Surg Clin North Am* 1987;67:997.

32. Burt PA, O'Driscoll BR, Notley HM, et al. Intraluminal irradiation for the palliation of lung cancer with the high dose rate microselectron. *Thorax* 1990;45:765.

33. Bedwinek J, Bruton C, Petty A, et al. High dose rate endobronchial brachytherapy and fatal pulmonary hemorrhage. *Int J Radiat Oncol Biol Phys* 1991;22:23.

34. Macha HN, Wahlers B, Reichle C, et al. Endobronchial radiation therapy for obstructing malignancies: ten years' experience with iridium-192 high dose radiation brachytherapy afterloading technique in 365 patients. *Lung* 1995;173:271.

35. Speiser B. The role of endobronchial brachytherapy in patients with lung cancer. *Clin Pulm Med* 1995;2:6:344.

36. Speiser B, Spratling L. Intermediate dose rate remote after loading brachytherapy for intraluminal control of bronchogenic carcinoma. *Int J Radiat Oncol Biol Phys* 1990;18:1443.

37. Speiser B. Oncological assessment using the four-tiered scoring system. *Curr Oncol* 1995;2:54.

38. Gollins S, Burt P, Barber P, et al. High dose rate intraluminal radiotherapy for carcinoma of the bronchus: outcome of treatment of 406 patients. *Radiotherapy* 1994;33:31.

39. Gollins SW, Ryder WJ, Burt PA, et al. Massive haemoptysis death and other morbidity associated with high dose rate intraluminal radiotherapy for carcinoma of the bronchus. *Radiation Oncology* 1996;39:105.

40. Nag S, Abitbol AA, Anderson LL, et al. Consensus guidelines for high dose rate remote brachytherapy in cervical, endometrial, and endobronchial tumors. *Int J Radiat Oncol Biol Phys* 1993; 27:124.

41. Simpson JR. Palliative radiotherapy for inoperable carcinoma of the lung: final report of a RTOG multi-institutional trial. *Int J Radiat Oncol Biol Physics* 1985;11:751.

42. Goldman J, Bulman A, Rathmell A, et al. Physiological effect of endobronchial radiotherapy in patients with major airway obstruction. *Thorax* 1993;48:110.

43. Hilaris BS, Martini N, Wong GY, et al. Treatment of superior sulcus tumor (Pancoast tumor). *Surg Clin North Am* 1987;67: 965.

44. Hilaris BS, Martini N. Interstitial brachytherapy in cancer of the lung: 20 year experience. *Int J Radiat Oncol Biol Phys* 1979;5: 1956.

45. Hilaris BS, Nori D, Beattie EJ Jr, et al. Value of perioperative brachytherapy in the management of non-oat cell carcinoma of the lung. *Int J Radiat Oncol Biol Phys* 1983;9:1161.

46. Hilaris BS, Nori D, Martini N. Results of radiation therapy in stage I and II unresectable non-small cell lung cancer. *Endocuri Hypertherm Oncol* 1986;2:15.

47. Nori D, Hilaris BS, Martini N. Intraluminal irradiation in bronchogenic carcinoma. *Surg Clin North Am* 1987;67(5):1093.

48. Fass DE, Armstrong J, Harrison LB. Fractionated high dose rate endobronchial treatment for recurrent lung cancer. *Endocurie/Hypertherm Oncol* 1990;6:211.

49. Miller JI, Phillips TW. Neodymium: YAG laser and brachytherapy in the management of inoperable bronchogenic carcinoma. *Ann Thorac Surg* 1990;50:190.

50. Stout R. Endobronchial brachytherapy. *Lung Cancer* 1998;9: 295.

51. Aygun C, Weiner S, Scariato A, et al. Treatment of non-small cell lung cancer with external beam radiotherapy and high dose rate brachytherapy. *Int J Radiat Oncol Biol Phys* 1992;23:127.

52. Gauwitz M, Ellerbroek N, Komaki R, et al. High dose endobronchial irradiation in recurrent bronchogenic carcinoma. *Int J Radiat Oncol Biol Phys* 1992;23:397.

53. Mehta MP, Petereit D, Shosy L, et al. Sequential comparison of low dose rate and hyperfractionated high dose rate endobronchial radiation for malignant airway occlusion. *Int J Radiat Oncol Biol Phys* 1992;23:133.

54. Sutedja G, Baris G, Schaake-Konig C, et al. High dose rate brachytherapy in patient with local recurrences after radiotherapy of non-small cell lung cancer. *Int J Radiat Oncol Biol Phys* 1992; 24:551.

55. Speiser B, Spratling L. High dose rate brachytherapy for local control of endobronchial carcinoma. *Int J Radiat Oncol Biol Phys* 1993;25:4:579.

56. Zajac AJ, Kohn ML, Heiser D, et al. High-dose rate intraluminal brachytherapy in the treatment of endobronchial malignancy. *Radiology* 1993;187(2):571.

57. Chang LFL, Horvath J, Peyton W, et al. High dose rate afterloading brachytherapy in malignant airway obstruction of lung cancer. *Int J Radiat Oncol Biol Phys* 1994;28:589.

58. Cotter GW, Larisey C, Ellingwood KE, et al. Inoperable endobronchial obstructing lung cancer treated with combined endobronchial and external beam irradiation; a dosimetric analysis. *Int J Radiat Oncol Biol Phys* 1993;27:531.

59. Marsh BR, Colvin DP, Zinreich ES, et al. Clinical experience with an endobronchial implant. *Radiology* 1993;89:147.

60. Nori D, Allison R, Kaplan B, et al. High dose rate intraluminal irradiation in broncogenic carcinoma. *Chest* 1993;104:1006.

61. Pisch J, Villamena P, Harvey J, et al. High dose rate endobronchial irradiation in malignant airway obstruction. *Chest* 1993; 104(3):721.

62. Huber R, Fischer R, Hautmann H, et al. Palliative endobronchial brachytherapy for central lung tumors. *Chest* 1995;107(2): 463.

63. Gustafson G, Vicini F, Freedman L, et al. High dose rate endobronchial brachytherapy in management of primary and recurrent broncogenic malignancies. *Cancer* 1995;75(9):2345.

64. Sur R, Mahomed G, Pacella J, et al. Initial report on the effectiveness of high dose rate brachytherapy in the treatment of hemoptysis in lung cancer. *Endocurie/Hypertherm Oncol* 1995;11:101.

65. Saito M, Yokoyama A, Kurita Y, et al. Treatment of roentgenographically occult endobronchial carcinoma with external beam radiotherapy and intraluminal low dose rate brachytherapy. *Int J Radiat Oncol Biol Phys* 1996;34:5:1029.

66. Delclos ME, Komali R, Morice RC, et al. Endobronchial brachytherapy with high-dose-remote after loading for recurrent endobronchial lesions. *Radiology*, 201;279.

67. Huber RM, Fischer R, Hautmann H, et al. Does additional brachytherapy improve the effect of external radiation? A prospective, randomized study in central lung tumors. *Int J Radiat Oncol Biol Phys* 1997;38:533.

FURTHER READINGS

Earlam R, Cunha-Melo Jr. Oesophageal squamous cell carcinoma II: a critical review of radiotherapy. *Br J Surg* 1980;67:456.

Landis S, Murray T, Bolden S, et al. Cancer statistics. *CA: A Cancer Journal for Clinicians* 1998;48:6.

Mehta MP. Endobronchial radiotherapy for lung cancer. Pass, Mitchell, Johnson, Turrisi, eds. *Lung Cancer: Principles and Practice.* Lippincott-Raven, Philadelphia, 1996;74.

Rider WD, Mendoza RD. Some opinions on the treatment of cancer of the esophagus. *Am J Roentgenol* 1969;105:514.

Spratling L, Speiser B. Endoscopic brachytherapy, thoracic endoscopy. *Chest Surg Clin N Am* 1996;6(2):293.

Yin W. Brachytherapy of carcinoma of the oesophagus in China. *Brachytherapy* 1989;2:439.

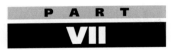

PART
VII

CHEMOTHERAPY

50

CHEMOTHERAPY FOR ADVANCED NON–SMALL CELL LUNG CANCER

JOAN H. SCHILLER

Lung cancer is a common and lethal disease, killing more than 160,000 Americans in 1997—more people than breast cancer, prostate cancer, and colon cancer combined.[1] Despite recent advances in locoregional therapy, approximately one-third of patients will present with disseminated disease at the time of diagnosis, and thousands more will ultimately die of disease that is amenable to neither surgery or radiation therapy. Clearly, strategies aimed at systemic control are crucial.

Despite the widespread use of chemotherapy for other neoplasms, there has been pessimism on the part of many physicians to prescribe chemotherapy for advanced non–small cell lung cancer (NSCLC). This reluctance arises in part from early studies in which chemotherapy had limited success, and no clear survival benefit could be shown for its use. Over the past 5 years, however, several newer agents have been developed that have resulted in modest improvements in survival. Furthermore, additional studies have demonstrated that chemotherapy can improve the quality of life and control symptoms in many patients with advanced NSCLC. The purpose of this chapter is to review some of the newer chemotherapeutic agents in the treatment of advanced NSCLC.

CHEMOTHERAPY IN THE 1980s

The natural history of metastatic NSCLC is poor at best. The median survival is approximately 5 to 6 months, and only 10% of patients can be expected to be alive at one year.[2,3] Several randomized studies have compared different chemotherapy regimens to best supportive care with mixed results.[3–10] The differences in magnitude of benefit caused by chemotherapy may be explained by differences in study size, patient population, and chemotherapeutic regimens, with some of the regimens being alkaloid, rather than cisplatin, based. Recently, metaanalyses have demonstrated a significant benefit in survival with older chemotherapy regimens compared to best supportive care, although this benefit was modest at best. The mean potential gain in survival

was only approximately 6 weeks, or 10% improvement in one-year survival.[2,11–13]

Until recently, no clear advantage to one chemotherapeutic regimen had been demonstrated. Randomized studies showed no significant benefit of cyclophosphamide, doxorubicin, methotrexate, and procarbazine (CAMP) vs. mitomycin, vinblastine, and cisplatin (MVP), etoposide and cisplatin (EP), or vindesine and cisplatin.[14] Indeed, in one randomized trial, first-line MVP resulted in a significantly higher response rate but poorer overall survival compared to single-agent carboplatin, which was associated with an overall response rate of 9% but a significantly longer median survival of 32 weeks.[15]

In one metaanalysis, the only chemotherapy drug that was associated with an improved survival compared to best supportive care was cisplatin.[2] Older trials using alkylating agents actually tend to show a detrimental effect with chemotherapy.[2] Furthermore, an analysis of survival determinants in more than 2,500 patients with advanced NSCLC by the Southwest Oncology Group (SWOG) found that the use of cisplatin was an independent predictor of improved outcome.[16] Hence, most of the newer agents have tended to be utilized in platin combinations.

Four randomized trials have compared single-agent cisplatin to combination therapy with "newer" agents (Table 50.1), which will be discussed in more detail following. All of the trials showed an improved response rate with the combination regimen, and three of the four showed an improvement in survival. Based on the results of the metaanalyses demonstrating an improved survival with chemotherapy over supportive care, and the randomized studies demonstrating an improvement in combination chemotherapy over single-agent cisplatin, the American Society of Clinical Oncology's clinical guidelines recognize that chemotherapy can prolong the survival of advanced NSCLC patients.[17]

Although cisplatin is the only agent that has been associated with improved survival, it has not been associated with a dose-response relationship. The European Organization for Research on Treatment of Cancer (EORTC) performed

TABLE 50.1. RANDOMIZED TRIALS OF SINGLE AGENT CISPLATIN VERSUS COMBINATION THERAPY

	Cisplatin: Median Survival (One-Year Survival)	Chemotherapy Combined with Cisplatin	Combination Chemotherapy: Median Survival (One-Year Survival)	P
Wozniak[23,24]	6 mos (20%)	+Vinorelbine	8 mos (36%)	0.0018
Sandler[55]	32 wks (28%)	+Gemcitabine	39 wks (39%)	0.008
Gatzemeier[29]	35 wks	+Paclitaxel	37 wks	>0.05
Von Pawel[60]	28 wks (21%)	+Tiripazamine	35 wks (33%)	0.008

a randomized study comparing a high dose of cisplatin (120 mg/m^2) to a standard dose (60 mg/m^2) in combination with etoposide in advanced NSCLC.[18] No difference in response rate or survival was noted between the two arms. The SWOG also randomized patients between standard-dose cisplatin (50 mg/m^2 days 1 and 8 on a 28-day cycle), high-dose cisplatin (100 mg/m^2 days 1 and 8 for four cycles), and high-dose cisplatin plus mitomycin (8 mg/m^2 day 1). No significant difference in response rates or median survival existed among the arms, and the high-dose arms were associated with an increased incidence of ototoxicity, emesis, and myelosuppression.[19]

Since the metaanalyses have been conducted, several new agents have become available which have continued to have a small but significant impact on advanced NSCLC. These agents are discussed in the following sections.

VINORELBINE

Vinorelbine is a newly developed semisynthetic vinca alkaloid that has been shown to have antitumor activity against advanced NSCLC in phase II studies. Recent randomized studies have compared vinorelbine with best supportive care, or with single-agent chemotherapy with fluorouracil plus leucovorin.[20–21] In a study comparing vinorelbine to best supportive care in elderly patients (≥70 years old) with advanced NSCLC, a median survival of 27 weeks and a 6-month survival of 54% was observed with vinorelbine compared to 21 weeks and 39% for best supportive care.[20] The one-year survival of 27% for vinorelbine was superior to the 5% one-year survival observed with best supportive care (p = 0.04), resulting in early closure of the trial. In a randomized phase III study comparing single-agent vinorelbine with fluorouracil plus leucovorin in patients with metastatic NSCLC, vinorelbine was associated with a higher response rate, median survival, and one-year survival (12%, 30 weeks, and 25%, respectively) compared to fluorouracil plus leucovorin (3%, 22 weeks, and 16%, respectively) (Table 50.2).[21]

Subsequent phase III trials comparing vinorelbine plus cisplatin to other combination regimens have also confirmed increased activity and prolonged survival with the vinorelbine-containing regimens. A French study involving 612 patients compared single-agent vinorelbine to vinorelbine plus cisplatin versus the control arm of vindesine plus cisplatin. The one-year survival of 35% in the vinorelbine/cisplatin arm was superior to the one-year survival of 30% in the vinorelbine-alone arm, and the 27% one-year survival in the control arm.[22] Finally, the SWOG confirmed the benefit of vinorelbine by comparing single-agent cisplatin with vinorelbine plus cisplatin in patients with stage IIIB and IV disease.[23,24] Not only was the response rate and median survival higher in the vinorelbine/cisplatin arm, but the trial also confirmed the long-term survival advantage for the combination compared to cisplatin alone. Thirty-six percent of patients treated with vinorelbine/cisplatin were alive at one year compared to 20% of patients treated with cisplatin alone; moreover, the two-year survival doubled on the vinorelbine/cisplatin arm.

One French study failed to observe a survival benefit with the combination of vinorelbine and cisplatin over cisplatin alone.[25] Two hundred thirty-one stage III or IV patients were randomized to receive either 30 mg/m^2 per week of vinorelbine or vinorelbine plus cisplatin (80 mg/m^2 every 3 weeks). Although a significant improvement in response rates and time to progression was observed, the median survival between the two groups was nearly identical (32 weeks versus 33 weeks). Furthermore, the addition of cisplatin resulted in a significant increase in toxicity, so that 21% of patients on the combined modality arm discontinued therapy early, compared to 8% of the patients on the vinorelbine arm.

PACLITAXEL

The taxanes, paclitaxel (Taxol) and docetaxel (Taxotere), have generated considerable enthusiasm because of their broad-spectrum activity against a variety of tumor types both preclinically and clinically. Derived from the western yew tree, *Taxus brevifolia,* and the European yew tree, *Taxus baccata,* respectively, these agents enhance tubulin assembly into microtubuoles and inhibit depolymerization of microtubuoles. Their activity as first- and second-line agents in ovarian and breast cancer is well established, prompting evaluation in other tumor types.

TABLE 50.2. RANDOMIZED PHASE III TRIALS OF VINORELBINE IN ADVANCED NON–SMALL CELL LUNG CANCER

		N (%IIIA/IIIB/IV)	Response Rate	Median Survival	Survival	
					One-Year	Two-Year
Perrone[20]						
Stage (%IIIA/IIIB/IV)						
IIIB/IV	Vinorelbine		20%	27 wks	27%	
(0/27%/73%)	vs.					
(N = 161)	Best Supportive Care		—	21 wks (S)	5% (S)	
Crawford[21]						
Stage						
IV	5FU + leukovorin	70 (0/0/100%)	3%	22 wks	16%	
	vs.					
	Vinorelbine	143 (0/0/100%)	12% (NS)	30 wks (S)	25% (S)	
LeChevalier[22]						
Stage						
IIIA/IIIB/IV	Vinorelbine	206 (10%/32%/59%)	14%	31 wks	30%	
	vs.					
	Vindesine + cisplatin	200 (11%/25%/65%)	19% (S**)	32 wks (S**)	27%	
	vs.					
	Vinorelbine + cisplatin	206 (13%/28%/61%)	30% (S*)	40 wks (S*)	35% (S)	
Wozniak[23,24]						
Stage						
IIIB/IV	Cisplatin	209 (0/8%/92%)	12%	6 mos	20%	6%
	vs.					
	Vinorelbine + cisplatin	206 (0/8%/92%)	26% (S)	8 mos (S)	36% (S)	12% (S)
Depierre[25]						
Stage						
IIIA/IIIB/IV	Vinorelbine	119 (38%/62%)	16%	32 wks		
	vs.					
	Vinorelbine + cisplatin	121 (41%/59%)	43% (S)	33 wks (NS)		

* vinorelbine/cisplatin compared to vinorelbine   (S), p ≤ 0.05.
** vinorelbine/cisplatin compared to vindesine/cisplatin   (NS), p > 0.05.

Based on phase I studies that suggested activity in advanced NSCLC, the Eastern Cooperative Oncology Group (ECOG) conducted a randomized phase II study of paclitaxel, merbarone, and pirozantrone in advanced NSCLC.[26] Twenty-four patients were randomized to receive 250 mg/m^2 of taxol as a 24-hour infusion; although the overall response rate was only 21%, the one-year survival was 40%, among the highest ECOG has observed in a multi-institutional trial in this disease. Although the trial design was such that a formal comparison of survival rates was not statistically possible, the one-year survival on the other two arms was 23% and 22%, respectively. These encouraging results with paclitaxel were confirmed by a group at MD Anderson, who also reported a 24% response rate and 38.5% one-year survival rate.[27]

Based on these results, ECOG compared standard therapy with cisplatin and etoposide versus cisplatin plus 135 mg/m^2 of paclitaxel, versus cisplatin plus 250 mg/m^2 of paclitaxel plus granulocyte colony-stimulating-factor (G-CSF) in E5592.[28] See Table 50.3 Five hundred ninety-nine patients were entered on the trial; 194 eligible patients on the control arm, and 190 eligible patients and 187 eligible patients on the low-dose paclitaxel/cisplatin and high-dose paclitaxel/cisplatin/G-CSF arms, respectively. The response rates for the high-dose paclitaxel/cisplatin/G-CSF, low-dose paclitaxel/cisplatin and etoposide/cisplatin arms were 31%, 26%, and 12%, respectively (p < 0.05). Median survival was 10 months, 9.5 months, and 7.6 months, respectively. The one-year survival was slightly higher in the high-dose paclitaxel and low-dose paclitaxel arms compared to the cisplatin/etoposide arm (40% and 37% versus 31%) (p < 0.05 for combined paclitaxel arms compared to cisplatin/etoposide). Neuropathy and myalgias were dose-dependent in the paclitaxel arms. There was increased gra-

TABLE 50.3. RANDOMIZED PHASE III STUDIES OF PACLITAXEL/PLATIN IN ADVANCED NSCLC

		N (% IIIB/IV)	Response Rates	Median Survival	One-Year Survival
Bonomi[28]					
Stage (% IIIB/IV)					
IIIB/IV	Etoposide/cisplatin	194 (19%/81%)	12%	7.6 mos	31%
	vs.				
	Cisplatin/high-dose Paclitaxel/G-CSF	190 (19%/81%)	31%	10 mos	40%
	vs.				
	Cisplatin/low-dose/paclitaxel	187 (19%/81%)	26% (S*)	9.5 mos (S*)	37% (S*)
Gatzemeier[29]					
Stage (% IIIB/IV)					
IIIB/IV	Cisplatin	206	17%	8.6 mos	
(30%/70%)	vs.				
	Paclitaxel/cisplatin	202	26% (S)	8.1 mos (NS)	
Glaccone[30]					
Stage					
IIIB/IV	Teniposide/cisplatin	162 (40%/60%)	28%	9.9 mos	41%
	vs.				
	Paclitaxel/cisplatin	155 (37%/63%)	4% (S)	9.7 mos (NS)	43% (NS)
Belani[39]					
Stage					
IIIB/IV	Etoposide/cisplatin	179 (21%/79%)	14%	9.1 mos	37%
	vs.				
	Carboplatin/paclitaxel	190 (23%/77%)	22% (NS)	7.7 mos (NS)	32% (NS)

* EP vs. two paclitaxel arms.
(S), $p < 0.05$.
(NS), $p > 0.05$.

nulocytopenia on the taxol arms, particularly the non–G-CSF-containing arm (55% on the cisplatin/etoposide, 65% for paclitaxel/cisplatin/G-CSF, and 74% for low-dose paclitaxel/cisplatin). However, the incidence of infections and deaths caused by infections was relatively low and was similar across all three arms. No significant differences in cardiac toxicities were observed. Because no significant differences in survival were observed between the two paclitaxel arms, ECOG has chosen the 135 mg/m^2 dose without G-CSF as the control arm for the next randomized phase III study (Table 50.4).

Two European trials, however, failed to confirm a survival advantage of paclitaxel plus cisplatin compared to cisplatin alone, or cisplatin combined with teniposide.[29,30] One trial compared 175 mg/m^2 of taxol over 3 hours plus 80 mg/m^2 of cisplatin with 100 mg/m^2 of cisplatin alone. Although the response rate was higher in the combination arm (26% versus 17%; p = 0.028), the median survival was not different (8.1 months for paclitaxel/cisplatin versus 8.6 months for high-dose cisplatin; p = 0.86). In a second study, patients were randomized to 80 mg/m^2 of cisplatin with either 175 mg/m^2 of paclitaxel over 3 hours, or with 100 mg/m^2 of teniposide.[30] Although responses were again higher on the paclitaxel/cisplatin arm, the median survivals were not different (9.9 months versus 9.7 months). With

the exception of increased myalgias and neuropathies on the paclitaxel arms, the treatments on both studies were well tolerated. Despite the lack of survival difference, patients on the paclitaxel/cisplatin arms of both studies reported a better quality of life.

These data suggest that the combination of paclitaxel and cisplatin is active in metastatic NSCLC. It is unclear, however, why a survival benefit has not been consistently observed, raising several questions regarding the optimal use of paclitaxel, including: What is the optimal duration of infusion? Would the substitution of other drugs result in enhanced efficacy?

Carboplatin is a platin analogue with a different toxicity profile than cisplatin. Unlike cisplatin, the primary toxicity is myelosuppression, with considerably less ototoxicity, renal toxicity, and neurotoxicity. Although the response rate to single-agent carboplatin is relatively low, it produced the best median survival time (31.4 weeks versus 25.8 weeks or less) in a randomized, five-arm ECOG trial.[15] Because of the single-agent activity of carboplatin and the neurotoxicity of the cisplatin/paclitaxel combination, several phase II trials have been conducted of carboplatin and paclitaxel with encouraging results.

With several exceptions,[31,32] these trials have been phase I/II trials or have been reported only in abstract form. The

TABLE 50.4. ONGOING OR RECENTLY COMPLETED COOPERATIVE GROUP RANDOMIZED STUDIES IN ADVANCED NSCLC

Group	Arms
ECOG	Paclitaxel (135 mg/m² IV over 24 hours) Cisplatin (75 mg/m² IV) vs. Gemcitabine (1,000 mg/m² IV days 1, 8, and 15 of a 28-day cycle)* Cisplatin (100 mg/m² IV) vs. Docetaxel (75 mg/m² IV) Cisplatin (75 mg/m² IV) vs. Paclitaxel (225 mg/m² over 3 hours) Carboplatin (AUC = 6)
SWOG	Vinorelbine (25 mg/m² weekly)* Cisplatin (100 mg/m²)* vs. Paclitaxel (225 mg/m² over 3 hrs) Carboplatin (AUC = 6)
CALGB	Paclitaxel (225 mg/m² over 3 hrs) vs. Paclitaxel (225 mg/m² over 3 hrs) Carboplatin (AUC = 6)

Each cycle repeated every 3 weeks.
* Four-week cycle.

starting doses of paclitaxel range from 135 mg/m² to 175 mg/m², and the duration of infusion from 3 hours to 24 hours.[31–36] Various doses of carboplatin have been utilized, including area under the curve (AUC) between 6 and 11[31,34,37] or doses calculated on body size (300 mg/m²–400 mg/m²).[32,33,35,36] Despite these differences in study design, preliminary results have been encouraging. Reported response rates range from 20% to 62%. Median survival on the two phase II trials were 38 weeks and 54 weeks, with one-year survivals of 32% and 54%.[31,32] Because of the tolerability of the regimen and ease of outpatient administration, as well as these early reports of efficacy, carboplatin/paclitaxel has become one of the most widely used regimens in the United States.

Preliminary results from a recent randomized study, however, failed to confirm the superiority of paclitaxel/carboplatin[38] (Table 50.3). Three hundred sixty-nine patients were randomized to receive carboplatin at an AUC of 6 and paclitaxel (225 mg/m² over a three-hour infusion), versus 75 mg/m² of cisplatin and etoposide (100 mg/m² days 1–3).[38] Although the response rate was higher for carboplatin/paclitaxel (14% versus 22%, respectively), the one-year and median survival were not significantly different between the two (37% and 9.1 months for cisplatin/etoposide and 32% and 7.7 months for carbo/paclitaxel, respectively) (results presented at ASCO, 1998). However, carboplatin paclitaxel was reported to be more tolerable than cisplatin/etoposide, with significantly less febrile neutropenia and vomiting.

A second randomized multicenter trial comparing paclitaxel/carboplatin to paclitaxel/cisplatin in advanced NSCLC is currently ongoing. Patients are randomized to receive paclitaxel (200 mg/m² over 3 hours) plus carboplatin (AUC of 6 by the Calvert formula) or 80 mg/m² of cisplatin every 3 weeks.[39] Six hundred eighteen patients from 16 different countries have been randomized. A planned interim analysis on the first 289 patients showed no unexpected toxicity or any large response difference, and the trial is continuing.

The encouraging phase II data have resulted in carboplatin and paclitaxel being incorporated as one of the study arms in three different cooperative group trials (Table 50.4). ECOG is comparing carboplatin/paclitaxel to the control arm of cisplatin and paclitaxel, as well as cisplatin and gemcitabine, and cisplatin plus docetaxel. The SWOG recently completed a trial comparing carboplatin and paclitaxel to the "standard" of cisplatin and vinorelbine. The Cancer and Leukemia Group B (CALGB) is comparing single agent paclitaxel to carboplatin/paclitaxel.

DOCETAXEL

Docetaxel has been explored as a single agent in phase II trials in patients with advanced NSCLC. Phase II trials have used 60 mg/m², 75 mg/m², and 100 mg/m² of docetaxel as a one-hour infusion every 3 weeks (Table 50.5).[40–45] Responses in previously untreated patients range from 18% to 38%, with median survivals of 6 to 11 months. Interestingly, a 20% response rate as a second-line agent has been reported in phase II trials.[46–48]

In a phase I study when combined with 75 mg/m² of cisplatin, 75 mg/m² of docetaxel induced responses in 7 of 14 patients.[49] This combination of 75 mg/m² of docetaxel and 75–100 mg/m² of cisplatin has been evaluated in several phase II studies.[50–52] Febrile neutropenia was the dose-limiting toxicity in all three studies. Other grade 3 or worse toxicities include hypersensitivity reaction, diarrhea, nausea/vomiting, cardiac abnormalities, fluid retention, and infection. Response rates varied from 25% to 53%.

GEMCITABINE

Gemcitabine is a nucleoside analogue that has several potent actions on cancer cells at both the DNA and RNA levels. The relatively mild toxicity profile and activity in metastatic pancreatic cancer have prompted investigation in advanced NSCLC. Following a series of phase II studies that showed activity of gemcitabine in NSCLC, two randomized phase II studies were conducted in Europe and Taiwan comparing single-agent gemcitabine with cisplatin and etoposide pa-

TABLE 50.5. PHASE II TRIALS OF DOCETAXEL IN NONSMALL CELL LUNG CANCER

	Dose (mg/m²)	N	Overall Response Rate	Median Survival	1-Year Survival
Single Agent					
Cerny[40]	100	35	23%	11 mos	
Francis[41]	100	29	38%	6.3 mos	
Fosella[42]	100	39	33%	11 mos	
Burris[43]	100	14	21%		
Miller[44]	75	20	25%		
Watanabe[45]	60	68	18%		
With Cisplatin					
Cole[50]	75	26	46%		
Cisplatin 75–100 mg/m²					
Le Chevalier[51]	75	24	25%		
Cisplatin 100 mg/m²					
Zalcberg[52]	75	36	39%	9.6 mos	33%
Cisplatin 75 mg/m²					

tients.[53,54] Both studies involved randomization between weekly gemcitabine (days 1, 8, and 15 on a 28-day schedule), versus cisplatin administered on day 1 and etoposide administered days 1, 2, and 3 on a 28-day schedule. Although the doses of the drugs were slightly different between the two studies (the European study used 1,000 mg/m² of gemcitabine, whereas the Taiwanese study used 800 mg/m² and the European study utilized 100 mg/m² of both cisplatin and etoposide compared to 80 mg/m² of both cisplatin and etoposide in the Taiwanese study), both studies confirmed that single-agent gemcitabine was probably as efficacious as etoposide/cisplatin (Table 50.6). It should be noted, however, that these were randomized phase II trials, and thus not powered to detect small differences between the arms.

Three randomized phase III studies have been conducted with cisplatin and gemcitabine (Table 50.6). A multicenter randomized study involving previously untreated patients with advanced NSCLC compared cisplatin (100 mg/m² day 1) with and without gemcitabine (1,000 mg/m² days 1, 8, and 15 of a 28-day cycle). An interim analysis of the results reported a 31% response rate on the gemcitabine/cisplatin arm compared to a 9% response rate on the cisplatin alone arm (p = 0.0001).[55] Updated results presented at the American Society of Clinical Oncology (ASCO) meeting in 1998 confirmed an improvement in median and one-year survival with cisplatin and gemcitabine (9.0 months and 39%, respectively) compared to cisplatin alone (7.6 months and 28%, respectively).[56]

A phase III European study randomized patients with advanced NSCLC to either gemcitabine/cisplatin (1000 mg/m² of gemcitabine on days 1, 8, and 15 of a 28-day cycle plus 100 mg/m² of cisplatin on day 2) or to mitomycin (6 mg/m² day 1), ifosfamide (3 gm/m² day 1), and cisplatin (MIC) (100 mg/m² on day 2 of a 28-day cycle).[57] A signifi-

cant improvement in overall response rate was observed (40% for the gemcitabine/cisplatin arm compared to 28% in the MIC arm; p = 0.03). Median survival was not different between the two arms (35 weeks in the gemcitabine/cisplatin arm and 38 weeks in the MIC arm).

A randomized study comparing gemcitabine/cisplatin to etoposide/cisplatin was conducted by the Spanish Lung Cancer Group.[58,59] Results demonstrate a significantly higher overall response rate in the gemcitabine/cisplatin arm (40.6%) compared to the cisplatin/etoposide arm (21.9%).[60] Overall survival was 8.7 months for the gemcitabine/cisplatin arm compared to 7.0 months in the cisplatin/etoposide arm (p = 0.18) One year survival was 32% from gem/CIS versus 26% from CIS/etop.

TIRAPAZAMINE

Tirapazamine is a novel bioreductive agent with selective cytotoxicity against hypoxic cells in preclinical models. The drug is converted to the biologically active, free-oxidizing radical in a reversible reaction driven by low oxygen concentration and catalyzed by cytochrome P450. The oxidizing radical abstracts hydrogen from DNA, resulting in single- and double-strand breaks. In *in vitro* and *in vivo* models, tirapazamine synergizes with cisplatin.

A randomized trial involving 446 patients with stage IIIB disease with pleural effusion or stage IV disease randomized patients to receive tirapazamine plus 75 mg/m² of cisplatin versus cisplatin alone.[61] The combination resulted in a 27% response compared to a 14% response rate observed with cisplatin alone (p < 0.001) and a superior median survival of 35 weeks versus 28 weeks, respectively (p = 0.0078). The one-year survival with tirapazamine/cisplatin was 33% compared to 21% with cisplatin alone (p = 0.042).

TABLE 50.6. RANDOMIZED PHASE II/III STUDIES OF GEMCITABINE IN ADVANCED NSCLC

		N (%IIIA/IIIB/IV)	Response Rate (%)	Median Survival	One-Year Survival
Manegold (Phase II)[54]					
Stage					
IIIA/IIIB/IV	Gemcitabine	71 (6%/18%/76%)	18%	6.6 mos	
	vs.				
	Cisplatin/etoposide	75 (8%/17%/75%)	15% (NS)	7.6 mos (NS)	
Perng (Phase II)[53]					
Stage					
IIIA/IIIB/IV	Gemcitabine	27 (3%/30%/67%)	19%	9 mos	
	vs.				
	Cisplatin/etoposide	26 (4%/15%/81%)	21% (NS)	12 mos (NS)	
Sandler (Phase III)[55]					
Stage					
IIIA/IIIB/IV	Cisplatin	262 (7%/23%/70%)	9%	7.6 mos	28%
	vs.				
	Gemcitabine/cisplatin	260 (7%/26%/67%)	31% (S)	9.0 mos (S)	39%
Crino (Phase III)[56]					
Stage					
IIIB/IV	Gemcitabine/cisplatin	154 (20%/80%)	40%	8.5 mos	53%
(21%/79%)	vs.				
	Mitomycin/ifosfamide/cisplatin	152 (21%/79%)	28% (S)	9.3 mos (NS)	34%
Lopez Cebrerizo (Phase III)[58,59]					
Stage					
IIIB/IV	Gemcitabine/cisplatin	69 (−/48%/52%)	40.6%	8.7 mos	32%
	vs.				
	Cisplatin/etoposide	65 (−/52%/49%)	21.9% (S)	7.0 mos (NS)	26%

(S), $p < 0.05$.
(NS), $p > 0.05$.

STANDARD OF CARE IN 2000?

These data regarding the different new possible combinations should be interpreted with caution. First, significant differences in patient populations (performance status and stage) can be found among different trials. For example, although administration of cisplatin on days 2 or 15 has been reported to be more efficacious than administration on day 1 in phase II studies with gemcitabine,[62] the day 2 and 15 studies tended to have more patients with stage IIIA and IIIB disease. Secondly, stage IIIB patients tend to be a heterogeneous group, with some trials allowing any clinical stage IIIB patients, whereas other trials restrict patients to stage IIIB with plueral effusion or pathologically confirmed stage IIIB. Differences in performance status are also critically important. Finally, retreatment of patients on clinical trials with second-line therapy (or in many cases, the crossover drugs) has complicated interpretation of these studies. Thus no definitive statement can be made as to which of these many combinations is "best." Because not all studies are positive, the need for confirmatory, controlled studies is crucial.[25,38] Randomized cooperative group studies comparing these different combinations are ongoing or planned (Table 50.6).

SYMPTOM CONTROL

Numerous studies have shown that chemotherapy improves symptom control.[63] For example, in a Canadian study, bleomycin, etoposide, and cisplatin controlled cough, hemoptysis, and pain in two-thirds of advanced NSCLC patients; one-half of the patients experienced an improvement in fatigue, and more than 40% of patients experienced a reversal of weight loss.[64] A Spanish study reported that 17 of 19 patients with stage III and IV NSCLC (89%) treated with combination chemotherapy with high-dose cisplatin gained weight; 10 of 20 patients (50%) who presented with anorexia improved; 7 of 15 patients (47%) had an improvement in pain; hemoptysis disappeared in 10 of 11 patients (91%); 7 of 9 patients had an improvement in dyspnea (78%); and asthenia was attenuated in 8 of 16 patients (50%).[65] Similarly, a trial conducted by Memorial Sloan Kettering, in which 85 patients with stage III or IV were treated with EDAM, mitomycin, and vinblastine, also reported a significant improvement in symptoms. Sixty-two percent gained weight with treatment, and performance status improved in 44% of patients.[66] In a European study involving 161 patients with stage IIIB or IV NSCLC treated with gemcitabine, improvements in performance status, weight, analgesic requirement, pain, and other disease-related symptoms such as cough, dyspnea, hemoptysis, anorexia, and somnolence were also noted.[67] A second European study evaluated vinorelbine in elderly patients (>70 years old) with advanced NSCLC; performance status improved in 26% of patients, cough and pain improved in more than 49% of patients symptomatic at entry, dyspnea improved in 28%, and approximately one-half of the patients had stabilization of their symptoms.[68]

Fewer studies have carried out formal quality-of-life (QOL) analysis in NSCLC. The ECOG analyzed (QOL) in patients on E1594, a randomized study comparing cisplatin/etoposide to cisplatin/high-dose taxol/G-CSF to cisplatin and low-dose paclitaxel.[69] QOL was measured using the Functional Assessment of Cancer Therapy-Lung (FACT-L) at baseline, 6 weeks, 12 weeks, and 6 months. No difference existed between treatment arms on QOL scores, suggesting that QOL was not adversely affected by myalgias and neurotoxicities. A trial outcome index (TOI) was calculated, which combined the physical, functional, and lung cancer scores. TOI correlated with survival, but change from baseline to assessment had an even higher correlation, suggesting that baseline QOL may be used to stratify patients entering clinical trials, and that QOL change may be a predictor of survival.

An EORTC randomized study comparing paclitaxel/cisplatin to teniposide/cisplatin evaluated QOL with the EORTC QLQ-C30 and LC-13 instruments at baseline and every 6 weeks thereafter.[30] Patients receiving paclitaxel/cisplatin achieved a better score at week 6 for emotional, cognitive, and social function, global health status, fatigue, and appetite loss, although this improvement was lost at 12 weeks. Peripheral neuropathy was higher in the paclitaxel arm. Similarly, a second European study comparing high-dose cisplatin to paclitaxel and cisplatin found that patients in the paclitaxel/cisplatin arm reported a better QOL using the EORTC QLQ-C30 and LC-13 scale.[29] Despite more neutropenia, peripheral neuropathy, and arthralgia/myalgia, patients receiving paclitaxel/cisplatin reported better physical functioning and significantly less nausea and vomiting, anorexia, and constipation than patients receiving high-dose cisplatin.

Two randomized studies from the United Kingdom evaluated mitomycin, cisplatin, and ifosfamide with thoracic radiotherapy in stage III NSCLC, and with best supportive care in stage IV disease. In both stages combination chemotherapy improved QOL and survival.[70]

POOR PERFORMANCE STATUS PATIENTS

Patients with poor performance status (PS ≥ 2) have traditionally done poorly on cooperative group clinical trials. ECOG retrospectively analyzed data from 1,960 evaluable patients with advanced NSCLC treated on five ECOG pro-

tocols between 1981 and 1994.[71] Performance status was a significant prognostic factor in predicting survival with patients with a PS of 0 having a median survival of 9.4 months compared to 3.3 months with a PS of 2. SWOG analyzed more than 2,500 patients with advanced NSCLC entered on clinical trials from 1974 to 1988.[16] Performance status was an independent prognostic predictor; patients with a PS of 0 or 1 had a median survival of 6.4 months and a 20% one-year survival, compared to a 3.4 months median survival and 9% one-year survival for patients with a performance status of more than 2.

Patients with a PS of 2 or greater not only are less likely to respond to chemotherapy and have an improvement in survival, but they are also more likely to experience toxicity. The four-arm ECOG trial by Ruckdeschel et al. discussed earlier, reported that PS 2 patients did significantly worse, with a 10% rate of treatment-related deaths.[14] Although their response rate did not differ significantly (PS0 = 26%, PS1 = 25%, PS2 = 20%), the median survival of PS 2 patients was significantly worse (median survival PS0 = 36 weeks; PS1 = 26 weeks, and PS2 = 10 weeks; p = 0.001). The current ECOG study, E1592, originally allowed patients with a PS of 0–2 to be entered. However, based on preliminary data suggesting a higher number of grade 3–5 adverse reactions in patients with performance status of 2, ECOG subsequently revised the study to limit it to patients with a PS of 0 or 1. Thus treatment of poor performance status patients cannot be recommended as because these patients tend to experience increased toxicity and decreased survival, and are unlikely to derive any clinical benefit.

SECOND-LINE THERAPY

Given the activity of some of the new compounds as first-line treatment for advanced NSCLC, it is reasonable to consider whether these drugs have activity as second-line agents.

Somewhat surprisingly, however, relatively few trials have rigorously examined the activity of second-line chemotherapy in NSCLC. Furthermore, these trials in general have not been well controlled for performance status, time to recurrence, and initial sensitivity or refractoriness to first-line chemotherapy. The greatest experience with second-line chemotherapy is with docetaxel. Two identical studies were conducted at the MD Anderson Cancer Center and the University of Texas at San Antonio, in which patients with locally advanced or metastatic disease whose disease was refractory to at least one prior cisplatin-containing regimen received 100 mg/m² of docetaxel every 3 weeks.[47] Patients were defined as platinum-resistant if they showed an initial response or stable disease to a platinum-containing regimen but then subsequently progressed, and platinum-refractory if they progressed during a platinum-containing regimen. Seventy-six of eighty-eight patients had a performance status of 0 or 1; 16% had stage III disease and 84% had stage IV. Fifty-eight percent were platinum-resistant and 42% were platinum-refractory. Fourteen of seventy-one evaluable patients (19.7%) achieved a partial response to treatment; the median survival was 9 months and one-year survival rate was 40%. Outcome results were not broken down by whether patients were platinum-resistant or platinum-refractory.

The authors subsequently retrospectively compared their data to a cohort of 36 NSCLC patients who would have met the entry criteria of advanced disease failing one platinum-based regimen and other similar patient criteria.[72] Both groups were balanced in stage, age, gender, histology, amount of prior chemotherapy, and response to first-line therapy, although more patients in the historical control arm (7/36) had a performance status of 2 compared to the docetaxel arm (2/44). Median survival was 42 weeks for the docetaxel-treated patients compared to 16 weeks in the historical control group, with one-year survivals of 39% and 16%, respectively (p = 0.003). An analysis of performance status of 0 or 1 only patients also showed a higher median survival and one-year survival in the docetaxel arm (42 weeks and 42%; n = 42) compared to the historical control patients (16 weeks and 16%; n = 29); (p = 0.018).

A multicenter phase II trial of docetaxel was recently conducted in platinum-treated NSCLC.[48] The results of this trial are somewhat lower than the MD Anderson and San Antonio trials; 12 of 80 patients responded (15%), with a median survival of 7 months and one-year survival of 25%. Confirmation of the activity of docetaxel as second-line treatment for NSCLC awaits the results of two phase III trials comparing docetaxel to best supportive care or a "control arm" of vinorelbine or ifosfamide.

The second-line activity of the related taxane, paclitaxel, has also been evaluated as a single agent. In a phase II study of 40 patients with metastatic NSCLC who had failed one prior platinum-containing regimen, only one partial response was observed out of 35 patients.[73] Median time from last treatment was 2 months; 68% of patients had a performance status of 0 or 1 and 32% had a performance status of 2. A second trial observed two responses out of 14 patients (14%) and a median survival of 120 days, although 5 patients were alive at 202 to 320 days.[74] A phase I dose-seeking study of paclitaxel reported that 6 of 16 patients who had received prior chemotherapy responded to 200 mg/m^2 of paclitaxel given over a one-hour infusion, whereas 0 of 10 patients responded to 135 mg/m^2.[75]

Despite the reported phase II activity of paclitaxel and carboplatin as a first-line treatment for advanced NSCLC,[31,32] no responses were observed in 17 previously treated patients who received paclitaxel (200 mg/m^2 administered over 1 to 3 hours) and carboplatin at an AUC of 6.[76] However, 7 of 18 partial responses were observed in previously treated patients receiving ifosfamide and 250–300 mg/m^2 of paclitaxel.[77] Twelve responses were observed in 17 previously treated patients treated on a phase I/II trial of mitomycin-C, 150 mg/m^2 of paclitaxel, and metronidazole.[74,78]

Vinorelbine has been shown to have modest activity as a single agent for the first-line treatment of advanced NSCLC.[21,22] However, no responses were observed in two phase II trials involving 15 and 18 pretreated patients.[79,80] When combined with 175 mg/m^2 of paclitaxel, three partial responses were observed in 17 patients with refractory disease, with a median survival of 179 days.[81] A randomized trial comparing vinorelbine to docetaxel has recently been completed.

Gemcitabine has also been evaluated in several phase II trials in previously pretreated patients with relapsed or recurrent NSCLC. A phase II study of single-agent gemcitabine (1,000 mg/m^2 weekly for 3 weeks out of 4) in 86 patients with advanced NSCLC previously treated with a platinum-containing regimen was recently reported.[82] Sixty-seven patients had received one prior chemotherapy; 13 patients had received two or three prior regimens, and two had received prior adjuvant therapy. Twenty-four of the eighty-three patients had initially responded to cisplatin-based chemotherapy. Sixteen partial responses (19%) were noted. Median duration of response was 29 weeks, median survival was 34 weeks, and one-year survival was 45%.

1,000 mg/m^2–1,250 mg/m^2 of gemcitabine was administered to 28 patients with a PS of 0–2 and advanced NSCLC who had progressed after prior carboplatin/paclitaxel, including 22 patients with refractory disease (had not responded to prior carboplatin/paclitaxel), six who had progressed within 3 months of treatment (resistant), and 6 who had progressed more than 3 months of prior response to carboplatin paclitaxel (sensitive).[83] Five of twenty-four evaluable patients (21%) responded, including two patients who were refractory to prior carboplatin/paclitaxel. Median time to progression was 86 days, and median survival had not been reached at more than 4 months.

The Greek Lung Cancer Cooperative Group conducted a phase II trial of gemcitabine (900 mg/m^2 on days 1 and 8) and paclitaxel (175 mg/m^2 on day 8 over 3 hours) with G-CSF.[84] Forty-nine patients with a PS of 0–2 who had failed prior cisplatin-based therapy were treated; 27 had also received docetaxel. Two patients (4%) achieved a complete response and eight patients (14%) achieved a partial response for an overall response rate of 18%. The median survival was 11 months.

In conclusion, the results of these studies suggest that single-agent docetaxel or gemcitabine may have activity as second-line agents in this disease, as might higher doses of paclitaxel in combination with vinorelbine, ifosfamide, or mitomycin C. These results, however, should be interpreted with caution until they can be confirmed in larger, multi-institutional, randomized studies. The patient populations that are included in most of these trials generally include good performance status patients. Furthermore, response to prior therapy and time to relapse has clearly been shown to be a significant prognostic factor in second-line therapy of small cell lung cancer (SCLC)[85]; this has not been rigorously reported or controlled for in many of these trials.

FUTURE DIRECTIONS

Several different chemotherapy regimens are currently being explored for metastatic NSCLC. These include the evaluation of non–cisplatin-based therapies involving combinations of gemcitabine, one of the taxanes, or vinorelbine. Another approach that is being considered includes combining three drugs (triplets), and some of these combinations have been reported to be well tolerated with somewhat attenuated doses of the drugs.[86] An alternative approach under investigation includes the utilization of "alternating doublets," in which cycles of a two-drug combination are alternated with a different, non–cross-resistant two-drug combination. Yet another approach involves sequential therapy, such as four cycles of one combination followed by two to four cycles of another regimen.

As these trials near completion, it is appropriate to consider additional prospects that may be available for the treatment of this disease. Many of these new approaches involve exploration of new treatments with a biologic basis. Although many of these treatments are in the earliest stage of development, some examples are worth mentioning to demonstrate the future potential of these approaches.

One of the most exciting areas currently being explored is in the area of antiangiogenesis and inhibition of the metastatic process. Continued growth and spread of tumors involves several different cellular processes regulating extracellular matrix (ECM) remodeling, tumor cell invasion and migration, and tumor neovascularization. Tumor neovascularization is a complex process that includes the activation, proliferation, and migration of endothelial cells, disruption of vascular basement membranes, and development of vascular tubes and linkage to preexisting vascular networks.[87]

All these tightly regulated processes involve the interaction of a variety of molecules, including adhesion molecules such as integrins, which modulate cell/extracellular matrix interactions. By regulating binding with such ECM components as collagen, fibronectin, and laminin, these proteins may play a role in cell adhesion, migration, blood vessel morphogenesis, and structural integrity.[88] Matrix metalloproteinases (MMPs) are a family of at least 11 proteolytic enzymes that degrade components of the ECM, including collagen and proteoglycan. Two MMPs in particular (MMP-2, or gelatinase A; and MMP-9, or gelatinase B) have been found to be expressed in human NSCLC cells, and their expression is correlated with pathologic invasiveness, suggesting an important role for these enzymes in tumor cell and endothelial cell invasion.[89–91] Angiogenesis itself is regulated by such positive growth factors as vascular

endothelial growth factor (VEGF) and basic fibroblastic growth factor (bFGF); it can be inhibited by endogenous growth factors such as angiostatin or transforming growth factor beta (TGF-β).

All of these processes, therefore, would appear to play critical roles in the growth and spread of cancer cells, and are being investigated as targets for anticancer therapy. Thus anti-integrins, MMP inhibitors, and angiogenesis inhibitors and antibodies are currently in phase I, phase II, and in some cases, phase III trials. For example, an antiangiogenic humanized monoclonal antibody to the vascular integrin $\alpha v \beta 3$ is undergoing clinical study in a phase I trial; one partial response has been reported.[93] Several MMP inhibitors are completing phase I and II studies, and are either in, or about to begin, phase III testing in SCLC or NSCLC. These compounds include products by Bayer (Bayer 12-9566),[94] Agaroun (AG3340),[95] and British Biotech.[96] A phase I trial of recombinant humanized monoclonal antivascular endothelial growth factor (anti-VEGF) was recently completed, in which anti-VEGF was reported to be well tolerated.[97] Direct endothelial inhibitors under investigation include TNP-470, a synthetic analog of fumagillin[98]; squalamine, an aminosterol derived from the soft tissues of sharks[99]; and thalidomide.[100] Thalidomide is an oral agent that was originally introduced as a sedative and antimetic but was quickly taken off the market when it was found to induce catastrophic fetal abnormalities. It has since been postulated that limb defects seen with the drug were secondary to an inhibition of blood vessel growth in the developing fetal limb bud, and its antiangiogenesis properties have been demonstrated in a rabbit cornea micropocket assay.[101] Clinical trials are underway in hormone-refractory prostate cancer, metastatic breast cancer, Kaposi's sarcoma, glioma, melanoma, renal cell, and ovarian cancer.[100,102] Thus many of these compounds are about to enter phase III testing in combination with standard cytotoxic drugs in the cooperative group setting for locally advanced or metastatic SCLC or NSCLC.

Another major area of research in the biologic treatment of NSCLC involves manipulation of the molecular biology of the disease. The *p53* tumor-suppressor gene is the most commonly mutated gene in human cancers, and is mutated in approximately 50% of NSCLCs. A retroviral vector and adenoviral vector containing the wild-type *p53* gene have been directly injected into human NSCLC and head and neck squamous cell carcinomas.[103,104] (see also Chapter 6). No clinically significant vector-related toxicities have been observed, and vector-p53 expression and increased apoptosis has been detected in posttreatment tumor biopsies. These approaches are about to be tested in bronchoalveolar carcinomas and in combination with radiation therapy within the ECOG.

The HER-2*neu* gene encodes for a growth factor receptor that signals the cell to enhance growth and has been associated with a poor outcome in metastatic breast cancer. A humanized anti-HER2*neu* antibody increases anticancer activity to first-line chemotherapy in women with HER2*neu* overexpressing breast cancer.[105] Approximately one-fourth of lung cancers also overexpress the HER2*neu* protein, although probably not to the same intensity as breast cancer; studies are being planned to determine the prognostic significance of HER2*neu* overexpression in NSCLC and the possible therapeutic benefit of the anti-HER2*neu* antibody (see also Chapter 4).

Thus the new treatments that are likely to be employed at the turn of the century will probably include agents other than traditional cytotoxic agents that attack normal and tumor cells alike. Instead, agents that specifically target abnormal cancer cells will continue to be developed, hopefully with increased specificity and decreased toxicity. A challenge will be how to incorporate these newer biologic agents with standard chemotherapeutic agents. The optimal clinical setting for their use will need to be identified—for example, immediately following surgery in patients with micrometastatic disease? In the setting of locally advanced, inoperable disease? To prevent the progression of metastatic disease? Following primary therapy, or in conjunction with chemoradiation therapy? Appropriate end points for clinical trials will need to be rethought: survival, time to progression, or response rates? The classic pathway of drug development from phase I to phase II to phase II trials will also need to be examined if survival is the primary end point, but the difficulties associated with conducting numerous large, randomized phase III trials with limited resources will need to be addressed. These challenges and others will provide continued interest in the development of new approaches to the treatment of advanced NSCLC, and hopefully ultimately result in better therapies for patients.

REFERENCES

1. Parker SL, Tong T, Bolden S, et al. Cancer statistics, 1997. *Cancer J Clin* 1997;47:5.
2. Group, N-sclcc. Chemotherapy in non-small cell lung cancer: meta-analysis using updated data on individual patients from 52 randomized clinical trials. *Br Med J* 1995;311:899.
3. Rapp E, Pater J, Willan A. et al. Chemotherapy can prolong survival in patients with advanced non-small-cell lung cancer—report of a Canadian multicenter randomized trial. *J Clin Oncol* 1988;6:633.
4. Woods RL, Williams CJ, Levi J, et al. A randomised trial of cisplatin and vindesine versus supportive care only in advanced non-small cell lung cancer. *Br J Cancer* 1990;61(4):608.
5. Cormier Y, Bergeron D, La Forge J, et al. Benefits of polychemotherapy in advanced non-small-cell bronchogenic carcinoma. *Cancer* 1982;50(5):845.
6. Buccheri GF, Ferrigno D, Curcio A, et al. Continuation of chemotherapy versus supportive care alone in patients with inoperable non-small cell lung cancer and stable disease after two or three cycles of MACC. Results of a randomized prospective study. *Cancer* 1989;63(3):428.
7. Cellerino R, Tummarello D, Guidi F, et al. A randomized trial of alternating chemotherapy versus best supportive care in advanced non-small-cell lung cancer. *J Clin Oncol* 1991;9(8):1453.
8. Ganz PA, Figlin RA, Haskell CM, et al. Supportive care versus supportive care and combination chemotherapy in metastatic non-small cell lung cancer. Does chemotherapy make a difference? *Cancer* 1989;63(7):1271.
9. Kaasa S, Lund E, Thorud E, et al. Symptomatic treatment versus combination chemotherapy for patients with extensive non-small cell lung cancer. *Cancer* 1991;67(10):2443.
10. Quoix E, Dietemann A, Charbonneau J, et al. [Is chemotherapy with cisplatin useful in non small cell bronchial cancer at staging IV? Results of a randomized study]. *Bull Cancer* 1991;78(4):341.
11. Grilli R, Oxman A, Julian J. Chemotherapy for advanced non-small-cell lung cancer: how much benefit is enough? *J Clin Oncol* 1993;11(10):1866.
12. Soquet PJ, Chauvin F, Boissel JP, et al. Polychemotherapy in advanced non-small cell lung cancer: a meta-analysis. *Lancet* 1993;342:19.
13. Marino P, Pampallona S, Preatoni A, et al. Chemotherapy vs. supportive care in advanced non-small cell lung cancer: results of a meta-analysis of the literature. *Chest* 1994;106:861.
14. Ruckdeschel J, Finkelstein D, Ettinger D, et al. A randomized trial of the four most active regimens for metastatic non-small cell lung cancer. *J Clin Oncol* 1986;4:14.
15. Bonomi PD, Finkelstein D, Ruckdeschel J, et al. Combination chemotherapy versus single agents followed by combination chemotherapy in stage IV non-small-cell lung cancer: a study of the Eastern Cooperative Oncology Group. *J Clin Oncol* 1989;7:1602.
16. Albain KS, Crowley JJ, LeBlanc M, et al. Survival determinants in extensive-stage non-small-cell lung cancer: the Southwest Oncology Group experience. *J Clin Oncol* 1991;9(9):1618.
17. Clinical practice guidelines for the treatment of unresectable non-small-cell lung cancer. Adopted on May 16, 1997 by the American Society of Clinical Oncology. *J Clin Oncol* 1997;15(8):2996.
18. Klastersky J, Sculier J, Ravez P, et al. A randomized study comparing a high and a standard dose of cisplatin in combination with etoposide in the treatment of advanced non-small-cell lung carcinoma. *J Clin Oncol* 1986;4(12):1780.
19. Gandara D, Crowley J, Livingston R, et al. Evaluation of cisplatin intensity in metastatic non-small-cell lung cancer: a phase III study of the southwest oncology group. *J Clin Oncol* 1993;11(9):873.
20. Perrone F, Rossi A, Ianniello GP, et al. Vinorelbine (VNR) plus best supportive care (BSC) vs. BSC in the treatment of advanced non-small cell lung cancer (NSCLC) elderly patients (PTS). Results of a phase III randomized trial. *Proc Am Soc Clin Oncol* 1998;17:455a.
21. Crawford J, O'Rourke M, Schiller JH, et al. A randomized trial of vinorelbine compared with 5-fluorouracil plus leucovorin in patients with stage IV nonsmall cell lung cancer. *J Clin Oncol* 1996;14:2774.
22. Le Chevalier T, Brisgand D, Douillard J, et al. Randomized study of vinorelbine and cisplatin versus vindesine and cisplatin versus vinorelbine alone in advanced non-small-cell lung cancer: results of a European multicenter trial including 612 patients. *J Clin Oncol* 1994;12:360.
23. Wozniak AJ, Crowley JJ, Balcerzak SP, et al. Randomized trial comparing cisplatin with cisplatin plus vinorelbine in the treatment of advanced non-small-cell lung cancer: a Southwest Oncology Group study. *J Clin Oncol* 1998;16(7):2459.
24. Wozniak AJ, Crowley JJ, Balcerzak SP, et al. Randomized phase III trial of cisplatin (CDDP) vs. CDDP plus navelbine (NVB) in treatment of advanced non-small cell lung cancer (NSCLC):

an update of a southwest oncology group study (SWOG-9308). *Proc Amer Soc Clin Onc* 1998;17:453a.

25. Depierre A, Chastang C, Quoix E, et al. Vinorelbine versus vinorelbine plus cisplatin in advanced non-small cell lung cancer: a randomized trial. *Ann Oncol* 1994;5(1):37.

26. Chang A, Kim K, Glick J, et al. Phase II study of taxol, merbarone, and piroxantrone in stage IV non-small-cell lung cancer: the Eastern Cooperative Oncology Group results. *J Natl Cancer Inst* 1993;85:388.

27. Murphy W, Fossella F, Winn R, et al. Phase II study of taxol in patients with untreated advanced non-small-cell lung cancer. *J Natl Cancer Inst* 1993;85:384.

28. Bonomi P, Kim K, Chang A, et al. Phase III trial comparing etoposide (E) cisplatin (C) versus taxol (T) with cisplatin-G-CSF(G) versus taxol-cisplatin in advanced non-small cell lung cancer: an ECOG trial. *Proc Am Soc Clin Onc* 1996;15:382.

29. Gatzemeier U, von Pawel J, Gottfried M, et al. Phase III comparative study of high-dose cisplatin (HD-CIS) versus a combination of paclitaxel (TAX) and cisplatin (CIS) in patients with advanced non-small cell lung cancer (NSCLC). *Proc Am Soc Clin Onc* 1998;17:454a.

30. Giaccone G, Splinter TA, Debruyne C, et al. Randomized study of paclitaxel-cisplatin versus cisplatin-teniposide in patients with advanced non-small-cell lung cancer. The European Organization for Research and Treatment of Cancer Lung Cancer Cooperative Group. *J Clin Oncol* 1998;16(6):2133.

31. Langer C, Leighton J, Comis R, et al. Paclitaxel and carboplatin in combination in the treatment of advanced non-small-cell lung cancer: a phase II toxicity, response, and survival analysis. *J Clin Oncol* 1995;13(8):1860.

32. Johnson D, Paul D, Hande K, et al. Paclitaxel plus carboplatin in advanced non-small-cell lung cancer: a phase II trial. *J Clin Oncol* 1996;14(7):2054.

33. Bunn PJ, Kelly K. A phase I study of carboplatin and paclitaxel in small-cell lung cancer: a University of Colorado Cancer Center study. *Sem Oncol* 1995;22(5):54.

34. Belani C, Hiponia D, Engstrom C, et al. Phase I study of paclitaxel and carboplatin (CBDCA) in advanced and metastatic non-small-cell lung cancer (NSCLC). *Proc Am Soc Clin Onc* 1995;14:174.

35. Giaccone G, Huizing M, Postmus PE, et al. Dose-finding and sequencing study of paclitaxel and carboplatin in non-small cell lung cancer. *Semin Oncol* 1995;22(4):78.

36. Rowinsky EK, Flood WA, Sartorius SE, et al. Phase I study of paclitaxel as a 3-hour infusion followed by carboplatin in untreated patients with stage IV non-small cell lung cancer. *Semin Oncol* 1995;22(4):48.

37. Muggia F, Vafai D, Natale R, et al. Paclitaxel 3-hour infusion given alone and combined with carboplatin: Preliminary results of dose escalation trials. *Sem Oncol* 1995;22:63.

38. Belani CP, Natale RB, Lee JS, et al. Randomized phase III trial comparing cisplatin/etoposide versus carboplatin/paclitaxel in advanced and metastatic non-small cell lung cancer (NSCLC). *Proc Am Soc Clin Onc* 1998;17:455a.

39. Macha HN, Gatzemeier U, Betticher DC, et al. Randomized multicenter trial comparing paclitaxel/carboplatin versus paclitaxel/cisplatin in advanced non-small cell lung cancer: results of a planned interim analysis. *Proc Am Soc Clin Onc* 1998; 17:465a.

40. Cerny T, Kaplan S, Pavlidis N, et al. Docetaxel (taxotere) is active in non-small-cell lung cancer: a phase II trial of the EORTC early clinical trials group (ECTG). *Br J Cancer* 1994; 70:384.

41. Francis PA, Rigas JR, Kris MG, et al. Phase II trial of docetaxel in patients with stage III and IV non-small-cell lung cancer. *J Clin Oncol* 1994;12(6):1232.

42. Fossella F, Lee J, Murphy W, et al. Phase II study of docetaxel for recurrent or metastatic non-small-cell lung cancer. *J Clin Oncol* 1994;12:1238.

43. Burris H, Eckardt J, Fields S, et al. Phase II trials of taxotere in patients with nonsmall cell lung cancer. *Proc Am Soc Clin Onc* 1993;12:335.

44. Miller VA, Rigas JR, Kile MG, et al. Phase II trial of docetaxel given at a dose of 75 mg/m^2 with prednisone premedication in nonsmall cell lung cancer (NSCLC). *Proc Am Soc Clin Onc* 1994;13:364.

45. Watanabe K, Yokoyama A, Furusel K, et al. Phase II trial of docetaxel in previously untreated nonsmall cell lung cancer (NSCLC). *Proc Am Soc Clin Onc* 1994;13:331.

46. Fossella FV, Lee JS, Shin DM, et al. Phase II study of docetaxel for advanced or metastatic platinum-refractory non-small-cell lung cancer. *J Clin Oncol* 1995;13(3):645.

47. Fossella FV, Lee JS, Berille J, et al. Summary of phase II data of docetaxel (Taxotere), an active agent in the first- and second-line treatment of advanced non-small cell lung cancer. *Semin Oncol* 1995;22(2):22.

48. Gandara DR, Vokes E, Green M, et al. Docetaxel (Taxotere) in platinum-treated non-small cell lung cancer (NSCLC): confirmation of prolonged survival in a multicenter trial. *Proc Am Soc Clin Onc* 1997;16:454a.

49. Bishop J, Zalcberg J, Webster L, et al. A phase I trial of the combination taxotere (docetaxel) and cisplatin in patients with advanced non-small cell lung cancer. *Lung Cancer* 1994;11:124.

50. Cole JT, Gralla RJ, Marques CB, et al. Phase II study of cisplatin + docetaxel (taxotere) in nonsmall cell lung cancer (NSCLC). *Proc Am Soc Clin Onc* 1995;14:1087.

51. Le Chevalier T, Belli L, Monnier A, et al. Phase II study of docetaxel (taxotere) and cisplatin in advanced nonsmall cell lung cancer (NSCLC): an interim analysis. *Proc Am Soc Clin Onc* 1995;14:1059.

52. Zalcberg JR, Bishop JF, Milward MJ, et al. Preliminary results of the first phase II trial of docetaxel in combination with cisplatin in patients with metastatic or locally advanced nonsmall cell lung cancer (NSCLC). *Proc Am Soc Clin Onc* 1995;14: 1062.

53. Perng RP, Chen YM, Ming-Liu J, et al. Gemcitabine versus the combination of cisplatin and etoposide in patients with inoperable non-small-cell lung cancer in a phase II randomized study. *J Clin Oncol* 1997;15(5):2097.

54. Manegold C. Single-agent gemcitabine versus cisplatin/etoposide in patients with inoperable, locally advanced, or metastatic non-small cell lung cancer. *Semin Oncol* 1998; 25(4):18.

55. Sandler A, Nemunaitis J, Dehnam C, et al. Phase III study of cisplatin (C) with or without gemcitabine (G) patients with advanced nonsmall cell lung cancer (NSCLC). *Proc Am Soc Clin Onc* 1998;17:454a.

56. Sandler AB, Nemunaitis J, Durham C, et al. Phase III trial of gemcitabine plus cisplatin alone in patients with locally advanced or metastatic non-small cell lung cancer. *J Clin Oncol* 2000;18:122.

57. Crino L, Conte P, De Marinis F, et al. A randomized trial of gemcitabine cisplatin (GP) versus mitomycin, ifosamide and cisplatin (MIC) in advanced non-small cell lung cancer (NSCLC). A multicenter phase III study. *Proc Am Soc Clin Onc* 1998;17:455a.

58. Lopez-Cabrerizo MP, Cardenal F, Artal A. Gemcitabine plus cisplatin versus etoposide plus cisplatin in advanced non-small cell lung cancer: a randomized trial by the Spanish Lung Cancer Group. *Lung Cancer* 1997;18:10.

59. Cardenal F, Rosell R, Anton A, et al. Gemcitabine + cisplatin versus etoposide + cisplatin in advanced non-small cell lung

cancer patients: preliminary randomized phase III results. *Proc Am Soc Clin Onc* 1997;16:458a.

60. Rosell R, Tonato M, Sandler A. The activity of gemcitabine plus cisplatin in randomized trials in untreated patients with advanced non-small cell lung cancer. *J Clin Oncol* 1999:17;12.

61. von Pawell I, von Roemeling R. Survival benefit from tirazone (tirapazamine) and cisplatin advanced non-small cell lung cancer (NSCLC) patients: final results from the international phase III catapult I trial. *Proc Am Soc Clin Onc* 1998;17:454a.

62. Shepherd FA, Anglin G, Abratt R, et al. Influence of gemcitabine (GEM) and cisplatin (CP) schedule on response and survival in advanced non-small cell lung cancer (NSCLC). *Proc Am Soc Clin Onc* 1998;17:472a.

63. Ellis PA, Smith IE, Hardy JR, et al. Symptom relief with MVP (mitomycin C, vinblastine and cisplatin) chemotherapy in advanced non-small-cell lung cancer. *Br J Cancer* 1995;71(2):366.

64. Osoba D, Rusthoven JJ, Turnbull KA, et al. Combination chemotherapy with bleomycin, etoposide, and cisplatin in metastatic non-small-cell lung cancer. *J Clin Oncol* 1985;3(11):1478.

65. Fernandez C, Rosell R, Abad-Esteve A, et al. Quality of life during chemotherapy in non-small cell lung cancer patients [see comments]. *Acta Oncol* 1989;28(1):29.

66. Kris MG, Grallia RJ, Potanovich LM, et al. Assessment of pretreatment symptoms and improvement after edam + mitomycin + vinblastin (EMV) in patients (PTS with inoperable non-small cell lung cancer (NSCLC). *Proc Am Soc Clin Onc* 1990; 9:229.

67. Gatzemeier U, Shepherd FA, Le Chevalier T, et al. Activity of gemcitabine in patients with non-small cell lung cancer: a multicentre, extended phase II study. *Eur J Cancer* 1996;32A(2): 243.

68. Gridelli C, Perrone F, Gallo C, et al. Vinorelbine is well tolerated and active in the treatment of elderly patients with advanced non-small cell lung cancer. A two-stage phase II study. *Eur J Cancer* 1997;33(3):392.

69. Cella D, Fairclough DL, Bonomi PB, et al. Quality of life in advanced non-small cell lung cancer: results from eastern cooperative oncology group. *Proc Am Soc Clin Onc* 1997;16:2a.

70. Billingham LJ, Cullen MH, Woods J, et al. Mitomycin, ifosfamide and cisplatin in non-small cell lung cancer: results of a randomized trial evaluating palliation and quality of life. *Lung Cancer* 1997;18:9.

71. Jiroutek M, Johnson D, Blum R, et al. Prognostic factors in advanced non-small cell lung cancer (NSCLC): analysis of eastern cooperative oncology group (ECOG) trials form 1981–1992. *Proc Am Soc Clin Onc* 1998;17:461a.

72. Fossella FV, Lee JS, Kau SW, et al. Docetaxel (D) for platinum-refractory non-small cell lung cancer (NSCLC): comparison of phase II results to historical controls (HC). *Proc Am Soc Clin Onc* 1997;16:468a.

73. Murphy WK, Winn RJ, Huber M, Phase II study of taxol (T) in patients (PT) with non-small cell lung cancer (NSCLC) who have failed platinum (P) containing chemotherapy (CTX). *Proc Am Soc Clin Onc* 1994;13:363.

74. Ruckdeschel L, Wagner HJ, Williams C, et al. Second-line chemotherapy for resistant metastatic, non-small cell lung cancer (NSCLC): the role of taxol (TAX). *Proc Am Soc Clin Onc* 1994;13:357.

75. Hainsworth JD, Thompson DS, Greco FA. Paclitaxel by 1-hour infusion: an active drug in metastatic non-small-cell lung cancer. *J Clin Oncol* 1995;13(7):1609.

76. Roa V, Conner A, Mitchell RB. Carboplatin and paclitaxel for advanced non-small-cell lung cancer in previously treated patients. *Proc Am Soc Clin Onc* 1996;15:403.

77. Hoffman PC, Masters GA, Drinkard LC, et al. Ifosamide plus

paclitaxel in advanced non-small-cell lung cancer: a phase I study. *Ann Oncol* 1996;7(3):314.

78. Haas CD, Gallardo RL, Moore B, et al. Effective salvage chemotherapy (CT) for relapsed or refractory non-small cell lung cancer (NSCLC) with mitomycin-c + paclitaxel + metronidazole (MMC + T + MNZ). *Proc Am Soc Clin Onc* 1996;15:391.

79. Pronzato P, Landucci M, Vaira F, et al. Failure of vinorelbine to produce responses in pretreated non-small cell lung cancer patients. *Anticancer Res* 1994;14(3B):1413.

80. Rinaldi M, Della GiuliVenturo I, Del Medico P, et al. Vinorelbine (VNB) as single agent in the treatment of advanced non small cell lung cancer (NSCLC). *Proc Am Soc Clin Onc* 1994; 13:360.

81. Chang AY, DeVore R, Johnson D. Pilot study of vinorelbine (navelbine) and paclitaxel in patients with refractory non-small cell lung cancer. *J Clin Oncol* 1999;17:2081.

82. Crino L, Mosconi AM, Scagliotti GV, et al. Gemcitabine as second-line treatment for relapsing or refractory advanced non-small cell lung cancer: a phase II trial. *J Clin Oncol* 1999;17: 2081.

83. Rosvold E, Langer CJ, Schilder R, et al. Salvage therapy with gemcitabine in advanced non-small cell lung cancer (NSCLC) progressing after prior carboplatin-paclitaxel (C-P). *Proc Am Soc Clin Onc* 1998;17:467a.

84. Georgoulias V, Androulakis N, Couroussis C, et al. Second-line treatment with paclitaxel (P) and gemcitabine (G) in patients with non-small cell lung cancer (NSCLC) who failed cisplatin-based chemotherapy. *Proc Am Soc Clin Onc* 1998;17: 468a.

85. Ardizzoni A, Hansen H, Wanders J, et al. Topotecan (T), a new active agent in the second-line treatment of "refractory" and "sensitive" small-cell lung cancer (SCLC). *Ann Oncol* 1996; 7:106.

86. Bunn PA, Jr. Triplet chemotherapy with gemcitabine, a platinum, and a third agent in the treatment of advanced non-small cell lung cancer. *Semin Oncol* 1999;26:25.

87. Gasparini G. Angiogenesis research up to 1996. A commentary on the state of art and suggestions for future studies. *Euro J Cancer* 1996;32A(14):237.

88. Brooks P. Role of integrins in angiogenesis. *Eur J Cancer* 1996; 32A:2423.

89. Liotta L, Kohn E. Grand rounds at the clinical center of the National Institutes of Health. *JAMA* 1990;263:1123.

90. Brown PD, Bloxidge RE, Stuart NS, et al. Association between expression of activated 72-kilodalton gelatinase and tumor spread in non-small-cell lung carcinoma. *J Natl Cancer Inst* 1993;85(7):574.

91. Anderson IC, Shipp MA, Docherty AJ, et al. Combination therapy including a gelatinase inhibitor and cytotoxic agent reduces local invasion and metastasis of murine Lewis lung carcinoma. *Cancer Res* 1996;56(4):715.

92. Folkman J. Clinical applications of research on angiogenesis. *N Engl J Med* 1995;333:1757.

93. Gutheil JC, Campbell TN, Pierce PR, et al. Phase I study of vitzxin, an anti-angiogenic humanized monoclonal antibody to vascular integrin åanb3. *Proc Am Soc Clin Onc* 1998;17:215a.

94. Goel R, Hirte H, Shah A, et al. Phase I study of the metalloproteinase inhibitor Bayer 12-9566. *Proc Amer Soc Clin Onc* 1998; 17:217a.

95. Johnston MR, Mullen JBM, Pagura M, et al. AG3340, a novel matrix metalloproteinase inhibitor, decreases growth and metastases of orthotopic human lung cancer in a nude rat preclinical model system. *Proc Am Soc Clin Onc* 1998;39:302.

96. Adams M, Thomas H. A phase I study of the matrix metalloproteinase inhibitor, marimastat, administered concurrently with

carboplatin, to patients with relapsed ovarian cancer. *Proc Am Soc Clin Onc* 1998;17:217a.

97. Gordon MS, Talpaz M, Margolin K, et al. Phase I trial of recombinant humanized monoclonal anti-vascular endothelial growth factor (RHUMABVEGF) in patients with metastatic cancer. *Proc Am Soc Clin Onc* 1998;17:210a.

98. Stadler WM, Shapiro CL, Sosmann J, et al. A multi-institutional study of the angiogenesis inhibitor TNP-470 in metastatic renal cell carcinoma. *Proc Am Soc Clin Onc* 1998;17:310a.

99. Schiller JH, Bittner GN, Williams JI, et al. Antitumor effects of squalamine, a novel antiangiogenic agent, plus cisplatin in human lung cancer xenografts. *Am Assoc Cancer Res* 1998;39:45.

100. Eisen T, Boshoff C, Vaughan MM, et al. Anti-angiogenic treatment of metastatic melanoma, renal cell, ovarian and breast cancers with thalidomide: a phase II study. *Proc Am Soc Clin Onc* 1998;17:441a.

101. D'Amato RJ, Loughnan MS, Flynn E, et al. Thalidomide is an inhibitor of angiogenesis. *Proc Natl Acad Science* 1994;91:4082.

102. Figg WD, Raymond B, Brawley O, et al. Randomized phase II study of thalidomide in androgen-independent prostate cancer (AIPC). *Proc Am Soc Clin Onc* 1997;16:333a.

103. Roth JA, Dguyen D, Lawrence DD, et al. Retrovirus-mediated wild-type p53 gene transfer to tumors of patients with lung cancer. *Nat Med* 1996;2(9):985.

104. Clayman GL, El-Naggar AK, Lippman SM, et al. Adenovirus-mediated p53 gene transfer in patients with advanced recurrent head and neck squamous cell carcinoma. *J Clin Oncol* 1998;16(6):2221.

105. Slamon D, Leyland-Jones B, Shak S, et al. Addition of herceptin (humanized anti-HER2 antibody) to first line chemotherapy for HER2 overexpressing metastatic breast cancer (HER2 +/MBC) markedly increases anticancer activity: a randomized, multinational controlled phase III trial. *Proc Am Soc Clin Onc* 1998;17:98a.

51

SECOND-LINE CHEMOTHERAPY FOR NON-SMALL CELL LUNG CANCER

FRANK V. FOSSELLA

In order to gain an appropriate perspective regarding second-line chemotherapy for relapsed non–small cell lung cancer (NSCLC), one must first consider the relative benefits of chemotherapy in the first-line setting. A metaanalysis of the eight randomized studies comparing cisplatin-based combination chemotherapy to best supportive care for advanced NSCLC has shown a modest, although statistically significant, impact on survival; median survival improved from 17 weeks to 27 weeks, and one-year survival increased from 5% to 15% in patients who received chemotherapy.[1,2] In one of those studies, the cost of the outpatient chemotherapy arm was actually less than best supportive care.[3–5] Experience with some of the newer agents such as paclitaxel, docetaxel, gemcitabine, vinorelbine, and CPT-11 has been encouraging, with more favorable median survivals in the range of 40 weeks. Although this success may be due, in part, to the effects of stage migration and better supportive care measures, certainly improvements in survival also reflect more active agents for NSCLC.

Despite the marginal benefit of chemotherapy for this disease, it has become customary to at least offer a trial of front-line systemic chemotherapy, usually with a platinum-based combination regimen, to patients with advanced NSCLC who have an acceptable performance status (i.e., 0 or 1, and possibly 2), and who are otherwise in good health. This practice is reasonable provided that the patient is fully aware of the risks of treatment and understands that the positive impact of therapy on quality of life and/or survival may be marginal.

Because the benefits of first-line platinum-based chemotherapy for advanced NSCLC are modest, the indications for second-line treatment of the patient who has failed initial chemotherapy are equally debatable. Nonetheless, many such patients do request of their medical oncologist a trial of second-line therapy, and we need to develop rational and cost-effective guidelines to follow in this setting.

DOCETAXEL

Docetaxel (Taxotere) is a taxane that, as a first-line agent for good performance status patients with advanced

NSCLC, has shown consistent activity for NSCLC. Response rates have ranged from 24% to 34% at a dose of 100 mg/m^2 over 1 hour every 3 weeks.[6–15] Average median survival in chemotherapy-naive patients is 39 weeks and one-year survival is 34%.

Docetaxel has also been systematically evaluated in the second-line setting for patients with NSCLC whose disease has progressed or failed to respond to first-line platinum-based chemotherapy. Four phase II studies that were designed specifically to evaluate the efficacy of docetaxel in the second-line setting have consistently demonstrated its activity as a second-line treatment (Table 51.1). Eligibility requirements for these trials included unresectable or stage IV disease and a performance status of 0–2. Patients must have received and failed at least one prior platinum-containing chemotherapy regimen (cisplatin and/or carboplatin). Docetaxel was administered at 100 mg/m^2 as a one-hour infusion every 21 days.

A total of 166 patients were treated in these four phase II studies. Most patients had a very good performance status (0 or 1) despite their advanced disease and extensive prior therapy. Most patients had stage IV disease, and the predominant histology was adenocarcinoma. Response rates were consistent and ranged from 15% to 22%. Median survival ranged from 5.8 to 11 months, and estimated one-year survival ranged from 25% to 40%.

The survival outcome of these trials compares favorably to that of historical controls as determined in a retrospective review done at M.D. Anderson Cancer Center (MDACC).[20] For that analysis we identified a cohort of 36 patients with advanced NSCLC who were enrolled in a variety of phase I studies at M. D. Anderson after having failed standard front-line combination chemotherapy. Both the docetaxel group (N = 44) and the historical controls (N = 36) were well balanced with regard to age, gender, stage, histology, number of prior chemotherapy cycles, and response to front-line combination chemotherapy. Median survival (all patients) was 42 weeks for the docetaxel patients versus 16 weeks for the historical control group, and one-year survival was 41% (docetaxel) versus 16% (controls);

TABLE 51.1. AN OVERVIEW OF PHASE II TRIALS OF SINGLE-AGENT DOCETAXEL IN PREVIOUSLY TREATED NSCLC[16–19]

Trial	Docetaxel Dose (mg/m²)	Number of Patients	Response Rate	Median Survival	One-Year Survival
Fossella[16]	100	37	22%	42 wks	44%
Burris[17]	100	35	17%	42 wks	NR
Gandara[18]	100	77	16%	30 wks	25%
Robinet[19]	100	18	22%	NR	NR

NR, not reported.

this difference was statistically significant (p = 0.003). Because the control group had more patients of performance status 2 (which might have skewed the survival in favor of the docetaxel arm), we calculated survival for the good performance status (i.e., 0 or 1) patients only. That analysis also showed a statistically significant improvement in survival for the docetaxel patients: median and one-year survivals were 43 weeks and 42% (N = 42) versus 16 weeks and 16% for the 29 historical controls (p = 0.018).

The most compelling evidence to support the activity of docetaxel in the second-line setting comes from two recently completed large, randomized phase III trials that compared docetaxel to either a comparator regimen of chemotherapy[21] or to best supportive care.[22] (Table 51.2).

The first of these phase III trials[21] was a multicenter U.S. trial. Eligible patients had locally advanced or metastatic NSCLC, which had progressed on or after at least one prior platinum-based chemotherapy regimen. There was no re-

striction on the number of prior cycles or regimens of chemotherapy, and, in particular, patients treated with prior paclitaxel were eligible for the study. Prior XRT was allowed. Patients must have had a performance status of 0–2. Patients with treated brain metastases were included.

Patients were stratified by their best response to prior platinum-based chemotherapy and performance status, and then randomized to either docetaxel 100 mg/m² every 3 weeks, docetaxel 75 mg/m² every 3 weeks, or a comparator arm of either vinorelbine 30 mg/m² per week or ifosfamide 2 gm/m² for 3 days every 3 weeks. Responses were assessed every two cycles. A total of 373 patients were enrolled, and their key patient characteristics are summarized in Table 51.2. Note that, despite being heavily pretreated, less than 20% of patients had performance status 2, and this was equally distributed across the three arms. The predominant histology was adenocarcinoma. Approximately 90% of patients across the three groups had stage IV disease. Approxi-

TABLE 51.2. PHASE III TRIALS OF DOCETAXEL IN THE SECOND-LINE TREATMENT OF NON–SMALL CELL LUNG CANCER[21,22]

	Fossella[21]			Shepherd[22]	
	Doc 100*	Doc 75*	V/I	Doc 100*/75*	BSC
Patient Characteristics					
N	125	125	123	49/55	100
PS 2	17%	18%	15%	24%	24%
Adenoca	41%	56%	52%	55%	57%
Stage IV	86%	90%	91%	77%	81%
Activity					
PR	12%**	8%**	1%	6%	n/a
26-wk PFS	19%**	17%**	8%	nr	nr
med surv	5.5 mos	5.7 mos	5.6 mos	7.2 mos**	4.7 mos
1-yr surv (ITT)					
uncensored	21%	32%**	19%	40%**	16%
censored	32%**	32%**	10%	n/a	n/a

* Docetaxel doses in mg/m² intravenous infusion every 3 weeks.
** Indicates statistically significant difference between docetaxel arm and comparator arm.
Doc, docetaxel; V/I, vinorelbine or ifosfamide; BSC, best supportive care; N, number of patients enrolled; PS, Zubrod performance status; adenoca, adenocarcinoma; PR, partial response rate; PFS, progression-free survival; med surv, median survival; 1-yr surv, 1-year survival; ITT, intent-to-treat.

mately 30% of patients had received two or more prior chemotherapy regimens, and prior treatment included paclitaxel in 30% to 40% of patients.

Results of the trial are summarized in Table 51.2. Partial response rate was 11.9% with docetaxel 100 mg and 7.5% with docetaxel 75 mg, both significantly greater than the 1% response noted in the control group. Median response duration was over 7 months. Interestingly, prior exposure to paclitaxel had no bearing on the likelihood of response to docetaxel.

Overall time-to-progression analysis (TTP) for the intent-to-treat (ITT) population favored treatment with docetaxel 100, and 26-week progression-free survival favored treatment with either docetaxel arm. The 26-week progression-free survivals were 19% with docetaxel 100 mg and 17% with docetaxel 75 mg, each being significantly greater than the 8% 26-week progression-free survival seen in the control group.

Survival analysis (ITT) showed no difference in overall survival by log-rank analysis, with median survival of approximately 5.6 months in the three groups. However, the one-year survival favored treatment with docetaxel 75 mg/m^2. The one-year survival was 32% for the docetaxel 75 mg group compared to 21% with docetaxel 100 mg and 19% in the control group. The difference in survival favoring docetaxel 75 mg was statistically significant. More than one-third of patients in each group received subsequent chemotherapy upon removal from this trial (including taxane therapy in 21% of patients in the control group). Because of the potential impact on survival such subsequent therapy may have had, we therefore generated an ITT survival curve in which survival observations were censored at the point at which patients received subsequent chemotherapy treatment. We observed in this ITT analysis that one-year survival significantly favored treatment with either docetaxel arm. The one-year survival was 32% with either docetaxel 100 mg or docetaxel 75 mg, compared to 10% one-year survival in the comparator group; these differences were highly statistically significant.

Quality-of-life analysis, which was evaluated prospectively using the LCSS, showed a trend favoring docetaxel 100 mg over the control treatment in all parameters considered, and favoring docetaxel 75 mg in all but two parameters. Several of these parameters reached statistical significance.

Grade 4 neutropenia and febrile neutropenia occurred with greater frequency in both docetaxel arms compared to the control group; documented infection and grade 4 thrombocytopenia, however, were equivalent across all three arms. G-CSF use was greatest with docetaxel 100 mg, at 28% of cycles, but was comparable between docetaxel 75 mg and the control group. Severe nonhematologic side effects, including treatment-related death, were equivalent across the three groups.

The second of these phase III trials was reported by Shepherd.[22] In this multicenter international trial, patients with advanced NSCLC, which had progressed on or after at least one prior platinum-containing chemotherapy regimen, were randomly assigned to receive either docetaxel or best supportive care. The initial dose of docetaxel was 100 mg/m^2, but this dose was changed midway into the trial because of toxicity to 75 mg/m^2.

A total of 204 patients were enrolled in this trial: 49 received docetaxel 100 mg/m^2, 55 received docetaxel 75 mg/m^2, and 100 received best supportive care. Patient characteristics are summarized in Table 51.2. Twenty-four percent of patients had a performance status of 2, and approximately 80% had stage IV disease. One-quarter of patients had received two or more prior chemotherapy regimens. The median number of cycles of treatment received was two and four for patients receiving 100 mg/m^2 and 75 mg/m^2, respectively.

Results are shown in Table 51.2. Partial response was observed in 6% of patients treated with docetaxel, and median response duration was 26 weeks. Overall survival favored treatment with docetaxel 75 mg/m^2. Median survival was 9.0 versus 4.6 months (p = 0.016), and one-year survival was 40% versus 16% (p = 0.016). The incidence of grade 3 or 4 neutropenia and febrile neutropenia were highest with docetaxel 100 mg/m^2. With docetaxel 75 mg/m^2, grade 3 or 4 neutropenia was higher than with best supportive care (43% versus 0%); however, no other significant differences in side effects were seen between the docetaxel 75 mg/m^2 arm compared to best supportive care. Quality-of-life analysis also showed statistically significant improvement in disease-related symptoms as compared to best supportive care.

In conclusion, two large randomized phase III trials of second-line chemotherapy for NSCLC have shown significant differences favoring docetaxel for response rate, TTP and one-year survival as compared to either a comparator chemotherapy regimen or best supportive care. Quality-of-life analysis also showed a strong trend favoring docetaxel. Interestingly, prior exposure to paclitaxel did not decrease the likelihood of response to docetaxel (in the one trial where this was looked at), suggesting a lack of complete cross-resistance between these two taxanes. Docetaxel appears to offer clinically meaningful benefit in this setting, with manageable toxicity. Based on the observed response rates, survival, impact on quality of life, and toxicity profile, the optimal dose of docetaxel in this heavily pre-treated population is 75 mg/m^2 every 3 weeks.

PACLITAXEL

The related taxane, paclitaxel (Taxol), has a single-agent response rate of 10% to 36% in good performance status chemotherapy-naïve patients with advanced NSCLC when given at doses of 200 to 250 mg/m^2 over 24 hours[23,24] or at 135 to 225 mg/m^2 over 1 to 3 hours.[25–28] Median and one-year survivals in the front-line setting average approximately 29 weeks and 40%.

The seven studies that report on paclitaxel's activity as second-line therapy for NSCLC show conflicting results: four are negative, two equivocal, and one positive.[25,29–34] However, interpretation of these data is somewhat hampered by the fact that the trials used varying doses and schedules of paclitaxel, patient numbers are small, some of the trials include both chemotherapy-naïve as well as pretreated patients so that the data regarding second-line activity must be teased out, and most are reported in abstract form only with limited details.

In a study done at MDACC through the Community Clinical Oncology Program (CCOP).[29] 40 NSCLC patients who had failed one prior platinum-containing chemotherapy regimen were treated with paclitaxel 175 mg/m^2 over 24 hours every 3 weeks. One-third of patients had a performance status of 2. Only 1 of 37 evaluable patients (3%) had a partial response (as compared to a response rate of 24% in a chemotherapy-naïve population reported by the same group). Median survival was 17.5 weeks and one-year survival was 16%.

In a trial reported by Socinski,[30] 13 patients with NSCLC, which had recurred after prior platinum-based chemotherapy, were treated with paclitaxel 140 mg/m^2 as a 96-hour infusion every 3 weeks. No objective responses were noted, although eight patients had stabilization of disease. Overall survival data were not reported.

Roa[31] reported on 18 NSCLC patients who received as second-line treatment paclitaxel 200 mg/m[32] over 1 to 3 hours plus carboplatin at area under the curve (AUC) 5 every 21 days (a regimen with which this group reported a 50% response rate in chemotherapy-naïve patients). All but two patients had received prior platinum-containing combination therapy (the other two had received a phase II drug). This abstract provided no details regarding performance status and survival. None of the 18 patients had response to the regimen in this second-line setting.

In Stewart's abstract.[32] 26 patients whose NSCLC had failed prior platinum-containing chemotherapy received paclitaxel at a starting dose of 135 mg/m^2 over 1 hour, which was escalated in approximately one-third of courses to 175 to 200 mg/m^2 over 1 hour; paclitaxel was given with hydroxyurea 500 mg orally three times per week. Nineteen percent of patients were of performance status 2. None of the first 20 evaluable patients showed response to this regimen. Survival was not reported.

Two studies have reported a possible marginal response to paclitaxel given as second-line therapy for advanced NSCLC. Tan[13] reported 38 patients who received first- or second-line paclitaxel at either 175 mg/m^2 over 3 hours (five patients) or 135 to 400 mg/m^2 over 24 hours (33 patients).

Eleven patients received this treatment as second-line therapy after having failed front-line platinum-based chemotherapy (10 patients) or mitomycin/VP-16 (1 patient). Performance status and survival data are not reported, nor does this abstract provide sufficient detail about which patients received which dose of paclitaxel. Nonetheless, one of the eleven second-line patients (9%) responded to therapy. Ruckdeschel[24] treated 14 patients who had failed prior chemotherapy (the details of which are not reported in this abstract) with paclitaxel at 200 or 250 mg/m^2 (depending on whether the subject had received prior radiotherapy) over 24 hours. Forty-three percent of these patients had a performance status of 2. Two of fourteen patients (14%) achieved a partial response; median survival was 17 weeks.

These five negative or equivocal studies are countered by Hainsworth's trial[25] of 30 NSCLC patients receiving treatment in a second-line setting, having failed one or two prior chemotherapy regimens (26 with platinum-based chemotherapy, and 4 with other regimens of known front-line activity). Patients were randomly assigned to either paclitaxel 135 mg/m^2 over 1 hour (10 patients) or 200 mg/m^2 over 1 hour (20 patients); the calculated dose was given either on 1 day or divided over 3 consecutive days. Neither performance status nor survival data is reported. None of the 10 patients treated at the 135 mg/m^2 dose level had response, but 6 of 16 evaluable patients at the 200 mg/m^2 dose (38%; 30% of ITT population) had a partial response to the second-line paclitaxel.

Given these conflicting data and varying study designs, it is difficult to draw definite conclusions regarding the role of paclitaxel in the second-line treatment of NSCLC. Larger trials using a consistent and effective dose and schedule of paclitaxel in a well-defined patient population are needed to clarify this issue. These studies ideally should randomize patients between paclitaxel versus either best supportive care or some other meaningful control arm to document not only response rate but also the drug's impact on survival and quality of life in these heavily poor prognosis patients.

VINORELBINE

Vinorelbine (Navelbine) is a novel vinca alkaloid. In chemotherapy-naïve patients with advanced NSCLC, the response rate to vinorelbine is in the range of 12% to 30%; median survival is about 30 weeks and one-year survival is 25% to 30%.[35]

Three European studies have been reported evaluating vinorelbine's activity against NSCLC in the second-line setting. Pronzato[36] studied 15 NSCLC patients who failed previous treatment with platinum-based (13 patients) or mitomycin-based (2 patients) combination chemotherapy. Performance status was not reported. None of the 14 evaluable patients responded to second-line treatment with vinorelbine at 25 mg/m^2 per week. Median survival for the group was 13 weeks.

Rinaldi[37] studied 18 NSCLC patients who had progressed while receiving platinum-based combination chemotherapy. These patients received second-line vinorelbine at 20 mg/m^2 per week. None of the 18 patients had a response to treatment (as compared to 2 of 9 chemotherapy-naïve patients enrolled in the same study). Neither performance status nor survival data were reported in this abstract.

Finally, in a small study reported by Santoro[38] 2 of 10 NSCLC patients, all with a performance status of 1, had a partial response to vinorelbine 30 mg/m^2 per week given as second-line treatment after prior chemotherapy. The relevance of this finding is difficult to ascertain, however, because this abstract provides no details about the prior chemotherapy the patients received.

GEMCITABINE

The nucleoside analog, gemcitabine (Gemzar), is an active drug for NSCLC. Several phase II trials show single-agent activity for advanced disease consistently in the range of 20% to 25% when used as a first-line treatment.[39] The experience with gemcitabine in the second-line setting has been mixed.

Crino[40] reported a trial of 32 patients previously treated with platinum-containing chemotherapy who were subsequently treated with gemcitabine 1,000 mg/m^2 per week for 3 weeks every 4 weeks (see also Chapter 50). Most patients had a performance status of 0–1, and 56% had stage IIIb disease. The drug was noted to have activity, with a 25% partial response rate (survival data were not reported). Similarly, Rosvold[41] reported on 24 evaluable patients with NSCLC whose disease progressed after initial therapy with carboplatin/paclitaxel, and who were subsequently treated with gemcitabine 1,000–1,250 mg/m^2 per week for 3 weeks every 4 weeks. Partial responses were noted in 21% of patients (survival data pending).

Three other phase II trials show a significantly lower response rate of gemcitabine in the second-line setting. In a small study reported by Guerra,[42] 11 evaluable patients with NSCLC previously treated with cisplatin-based chemotherapy were treated with gemcitabine 1,250 mg/m^2 per week for 3 weeks every 4 weeks. Only 1 of 11 patients (9%) showed partial response, and overall median survival was only 17 weeks. Garfield[43] reported a trial in which 36 patients received second-line gemcitabine at one of two dose levels: 1,000 mg/m^2 per week for 3 weeks every 4 weeks or 3,500 mg/m^2 every other week. Only 1 of 36 patients (3%) had a partial response (survival not reported). Finally, Fukuoka[44] conducted a phase II trial of gemcitabine 800–1,000 mg/m^2 per week for 3 weeks every 4 weeks for patients with advanced NSCLC who were both chemotherapy-naïve (42 evaluable patients) and previously treated (17 patients). This group reported no responses in the 17 patients treated in the second-line setting, whereas a response rate of 17% was noted in the 42 chemotherapy-naïve patients (survival was not reported).

CAMPTOTHECINS

Approximately one-third of chemotherapy-naïve patients with advanced NSCLC respond to single-agent CPT-11 (irinotecan).[45] Although CPT-11 also shows good second-line activity against small cell lung cancer (SCLC), two Japanese studies evaluating its second-line efficacy for NSCLC are conflicting.

Negoro[46] treated 26 "previously treated" (details of which are not reported) NSCLC patients with CPT-11 100 mg/m^2 per week, and observed no responses (versus a 34% response rate in chemotherapy-naïve patients in the same study). In contrast, Nakai[47,48] has reported that 3 of 22 (14%) "previously treated" (again, the details are not available) NSCLC patients responded to second-line therapy with CPT-11 at 200 mg/m^2 every 3 to 4 weeks (with first-line response in the same study of 31%). The data on second-line activity of the related camptothecin, topotecan (Hycamtin), is limited to a single anecdotal report of a patient with NSCLC progressive on cisplatin/VP-16 who had a complete response to second-line topotecan.[49]

CONCLUSIONS

In conclusion, phase II experience has shown consistent activity of docetaxel for NSCLC that has progressed after first-line platinum-based chemotherapy; this activity has been confirmed in two follow-up randomized phase III trials. These large multicenter phase III trials of almost 600 patients suggest that docetaxel does offer clinically meaningful benefit in good performance status patients. A statistically significant benefit of docetaxel over the control (vinorelbine or ifosfamide in one trial, and best supportive care in the other) was noted with respect to response rate, TTP, survival, and quality of life. Based on the observed activity and toxicity profile, the recommended dose of docetaxel in this heavily treated group of patients is 75 mg/m^2 every 3 weeks.

The related taxane, paclitaxel, has not been as systematically studied in the second-line setting, and available data are conflicting. Although one trial suggests that paclitaxel at 200 mg/m^2 over 1 hour produces a respectable response rate in platinum-resistant patients, the cohort of patients studied was small and survival data are unavailable. In contrast, six other small studies have reported no or minimal second-line activity with paclitaxel (although a greater proportion of performance status 2 patients were enrolled in

TABLE 51.3. PHASE II TRIALS OF SECOND-LINE CHEMOTHERAPY FOR STAGE IIIB/IV NSCLC: SINGLE-AGENT ACTIVITY[16–19,25,29–34,36–38,40–44,46–49]

Agent (Phase II Studies)	N	Overall Response Rate	Median Survival
Docetaxel (100 mg/m^2)[16–19]	166	15%–22%	6–11 mos
Paclitaxel (140–250 mg/m^2/24–96h)[25,29–34]	78	0%–14%	4 mos
Vinorelbine (20–35 mg/m^2)[35–39]	43	0%–20%	NR
Gemcitabine (800–3,500 mg/m^2)[40–44]	124	0%–25%	17 wks (1 trial)
CPT-11[46–49]	48	0%–14%	NR

NR, not reported.

these trials as compared to the docetaxel studies discussed, which may have affected the results).

Similarly, results of gemcitabine in the second-line setting have been conflicting. Two phase II trials have documented response rates as high as 25% in patients with advanced NSCLC whose cancer had progressed after first-line therapy. However, three other trials would suggest that activity of gemcitabine in the second-line setting may be minimal (at least as measured by objective response rate). The available data for second-line activity of vinorelbine and CPT-11 has been similarly disappointing (Table 51.3).

Given these data, a reasonable practice at this time would be to offer a trial of second-line chemotherapy with docetaxel 75 mg/m^2 every 3 weeks to patients with NSCLC who have failed first-line chemotherapy. However, because most of the subjects enrolled in the positive trials were in very good condition, the use of second-line therapy should probably be limited as well to good performance status patients (i.e., 0 or 1).

REFERENCES

1. Non-small Cell Lung Cancer Collaborative Group. Chemotherapy in non-small cell lung cancer: a meta-analysis using updated data on individual patients from 52 randomised clinical trials. *Br Med J* 1995;311:899.
2. Grilli R, Oxman AD, Julian JA. Chemotherapy for advanced non-small cell lung cancer: how much benefit is enough? *J Clin Oncol* 1993;11:1866.
3. Jaakkimainen L, Goodwin PJ, Pater J, et al. Counting the costs of chemotherapy in a National Cancer Institute of Canada randomized trial in nonsmall cell lung cancer. *J Clin Oncol* 1990; 8:1301.
4. Ruckdeschel JC. Is chemotherapy for metastatic nonsmall cell lung cancer "worth it"? *J Clin Oncol* 1990;8:1293.
5. Rapp E, Pater JL, Willan A, et al. Chemotherapy can prolong survival in patients with advanced non-small cell lung cancer—report of a Canadian multicenter randomized trial. *J Clin Oncol* 1988;6:633.
6. Fossella FV, Lee JS, Murphy WK, et al. Phase II study of docetaxel for recurrent or metastatic non-small cell lung cancer. *J Clin Oncol* 1994;12:1238.
7. Francis PA, Rigas JR, Kris MG, et al. Phase II trial of docetaxel in patients with stage III and IV non-small cell lung cancer. *J Clin Oncol* 1994;12:1232.
8. Cemy T, Kaplan S, Pavlidis N, et al. Docetaxel (Taxotere) is active in non-small cell lung cancer: a phase II trial of the EORTC early clinical trials group (ECTG). *Br J Cancer* 1994;70:384.
9. Burris HA, Eckardt J, Fields S, et al. Phase II trials of Taxotere in patients with non-small cell lung cancer. [Abstract] *Proc Am Soc Clin Oncol* 1993;12:335.
10. Fossella FV, Lee JS, Berille J, et al. Summary of phase II data of docetaxel (Taxotere), an active agent in the first- and second-line treatment of advanced non-small cell lung cancer. *Semin Oncol* 1995;22 (suppl 4):22.
11. Goh BC, Wang TL, Wong J, et al. Phase II trial of docetaxel (Taxotere) in inoperable stage III non-small cell lung cancer. [Abstract] *Proc Am Soc Clin Oncol* 1997;16:469a.
12. Robinet G, Kleisbauer JP, Thomas P, et al. Phase II study of docetaxel (Taxotere) in first- and second-line NSCLC. [Abstract] *Proc Am Soc Clin Oncol* 1997;16:480.
13. Lira-Puerto V, Zepeda G, Mohar A, et al. Phase II trial of Taxotere (docetaxel) in advanced non-small cell lung cancer. [Abstract] *Proc Am Soc Clin Oncol* 1995;14:382.
14. Latreille J, Laberge F, Gelmon K, et al. Docetaxel has moderate activity in patients with non small cell lung cancer. [Abstract] *6th International Congress on Anticancer Treatment* 1996;6:76.
15. Mattson K, Le Chevalier T, Bosquee L, et al. Interim results of a phase II study of docetaxel (Taxotere) in unresectable non-small cell lung cancer on 204 chemotherapy naïve or retreated patients. [Abstract] *Eur J Cancer* 1997;33 (suppl 8):S229.
16. Fossella FV, Lee JS, Shin DM, et al. Phase II study of docetaxel for advanced or metastatic platinum refractory non-small cell lung cancer. *J Clin Oncol* 1995;1:645.
17. Burris H, Eckardt J, Fields S, et al. Phase II trials of Taxotere with non-small cell lung cancer. [Abstract] *Proc Am Soc Clin Oncol* 1993;12:335.
18. Gandara DR, Vokes E, Green M, et al. Docetaxel (Taxotere) in platinum-treated non-small cell lung cancer: a confirmation of prolonged survival in a multicenter trial. [Abstract] *Proc Am Soc Clin Oncol* 1997;16:454a.
19. Robinet G, Kleisbauer JP, Thomas P, et al. Phase II study of docetaxel (Taxotere) in first- and second-line NSCLC. [Abstract] *Proc Am Soc Clin Oncol* 1997;16:480.
20. Fossella FV, Lee JS, Kau SW, et al. Docetaxel for platinum-refractory non-small cell lung cancer: comparison of phase II results to historical controls. [Abstract] *Proc Am Soc Clin Oncol* 1997;16:468a.
21. Fossella FV, DeVore R, Kerr R, et al. Phase III trial of docetaxel 100 mg/m^2 or 75 mg/m^2 versus vinorelbine/ifosfamide for non-small cell lung cancer previously treated with platinum-based chemotherapy. [Abstract] *Proc Am Soc Clin Oncol* 1999;18:460a.
22. Shepherd F, Ramlau R, Mattson K, et al. Randomized study of Taxotere versus best supportive care in non-small cell lung cancer

patients previously treated with platinum-based chemotherapy. [Abstract] *Proc Am Soc Clin Oncol* 1999;18:463a.

23. Murphy WK, Fossella FV, Winn RJ, et al. Phase II study of taxol in patients with untreated advanced non-small cell lung cancer. *J Natl Cancer Inst* 1993;85:384.

24. Chang AY, Kim K, Glick J, et al. Phase II study of taxol, merbarone, and piroxantrone in stage IV non-small cell lung cancer: the Eastern Cooperative Oncology Group results. *J Natl Cancer Inst* 1993;85:388.

25. Hainsworth JD, Thompson DA, Greco FA. Paclitaxel by 1-hour infusion: an active drug in metastatic non-small cell lung cancer. *J Clin Oncol* 1995;13:1609.

26. Gatzemeier U, Heckmayr M, Neuhauss R, et al. Phase II study with paclitaxel for the treatment of advanced inoperable non-small cell lung cancer. *Lung Cancer* 1995;12 (suppl 2): S101–S106.

27. Millward MJ, Bishop JF, Friedlander M, et al. Phase II trial of a 3-hour infusion of paclitaxel in previously untreated patients with advanced non-small cell lung cancer. *J Clin Oncol* 1996;14: 142.

28. Alberola V, Rosell R, Gonzalez-Larriba JL, et al. Single-agent Taxol, 3-hour infusion, in untreated advanced non-small cell lung cancer. *Ann Oncol* 1995;6 (suppl 3):S49.

29. Murphy WK, Winn RJ, Huber M, et al. Phase II study of Taxol in patients with non-small cell lung cancer who have failed platinum containing chemotherapy. [Abstract] *Proc Am Soc Clin Oncol* 1994;13:363.

30. Socinski MA, Steagall A, and Gillenwater H. Second-line chemotherapy with 96-hour infusional paclitaxel in refractory non-small cell lung cancer: report of a phase II trial. *Cancer Investigation* 1999;17:181.

31. Roa V, Conner A, Mitchell RB. Carboplatin and paclitaxel for advanced non-small cell lung cancer in previously treated patients. [Abstract] *Proc Am Soc Clin Oncol* 1996;15:403.

32. Stewart DJ, Tomiak E, Goss G, et al. Paclitaxel plus low dose hydroxyurea as second line therapy in non-small cell lung cancer. [Abstract] *Proc Am Soc Clin Oncol* 1995;14:367.

33. Tan V, Herrera C, Einzig AI, et al. Taxol is active as a 3 hour or 24 hour infusion in non-small cell lung cancer. [Abstract] *Proc Am Soc Clin Oncol* 1995;14:366.

34. Ruckdeschel J, Wagner H, Williams C, et al. Second-line chemotherapy for resistant metastatic non-small cell lung cancer: the role of Taxol. [Abstract] *Proc Am Soc Clin Oncol* 1994;13:357.

35. Crawford J. Update: vinorelbine (Navelbine) in non-small cell lung cancer. *Semin Oncol* 1996;23 (suppl 5):2.

36. Pronzato P, Landucci M, Vaira F, et al. Failure of vinorelbine to produce responses in pretreated non-small cell lung cancer patients. *Anticancer Res* 1994;14:1413.

37. Rinaldi M, Della Giulia M, Venturo I, et al. Vinorelbine as single agent in the treatment of advanced non-small cell lung cancer. [Abstract] *Proc Am Soc Clin Oncol* 1994;3:360.

38. Santoro A, Maiorino L, Santoro M. Second-line with vinorelbine in the weekly monochemotherapy for the treatment of advanced non-small cell lung cancer. [Abstract] *Lung Cancer* 1994;11 (suppl 1):130.

39. Hansen HH, Sorensen JB. Efficacy of single-agent gemcitabine in advanced non-small cell lung cancer: a review. *Semin Oncol* 1997;24 (suppl 7):S7.38.

40. Crino L, Mosconi AM, Scagliotti F, et al. Salvage therapy with gemcitabine (GEM) in pretreated advanced non-small cell lung cancer (NSCLC). [Abstract] *Proc Am Soc Clin Oncol* 1997;16: 446a.

41. Rosvold E, Langer CJ, Schilder R, et al. Salvage therapy with gemcitabine in advanced non-small cell lung cancer (NSCLC) progressing after prior carboplatin-paclitaxel (C-P). [Abstract] *Proc Am Soc Clin Oncol* 1998;17:467a.

42. Guerra JA, Lianes P, Paz-Ares L, et al. Efficacy and toxicity profile of gemcitabine in previously treated patients with non-small cell lung cancer (NSCLC). [Abstract] *Lung Cancer* 1997;18 (suppl 1):28.

43. Garfield DH, Dakhil SR, Whittaker TL, et al. Phase II randomized multicenter trial of two dose schedules of gemcitabine as second line therapy in patients with advanced non-small cell lung cancer. [Abstract] *Proc Am Soc Clin Oncol* 1998;17:484a.

44. Fukuoka M, Takada M, Yokoyama A, et al. Phase II studies of gemcitabine for non-small cell lung cancer in Japan. *Semin Oncol* 1997;24 (suppl 7):S7.42.

45. Rothenberg ML. CPT-11: an original spectrum of clinical activity. *Semin Oncol* 1996;23 (suppl 3):21.

46. CPT-11 Cooperative Study Group: A phase II study of CPT-11, a camptothecin derivative, in patients with primary lung cancer. *Jpn J Cancer Chemother* 1991;18:1013.

47. Nakai H, Fukuoka M, Furuse K, et al. An early phase II study of CPT-11 for primary lung cancer. *Jpn J Cancer Chemother* 1991;18:607.

48. Niitani H, Fukuoka M, Nagao K. Clinical development of irinotecan (CPT-11) in lung cancers. *Lung Cancer* 1994;11 (suppl 2): 30.

49. Rowinsky EK, Grochow LB, Hendricks CB, et al. Phase I and pharmacologic study of topotecan: a novel topoisomerase I inhibitor. *J Clin Oncol* 1992;10:647.

52

COMBINED MODALITY TREATMENT FOR LOCALLY ADVANCED, UNRESECTABLE NON–SMALL CELL LUNG CANCER

DAVID H. JOHNSON
ANDREW T. TURRISI

Locally advanced, unresectable non–small cell lung cancer (NSCLC) represents approximately 35% to 40% of all newly diagnosed cases of NSCLC.[1] During the past two decades, the management of these patients has undergone considerable change. Whereas radiotherapy as a sole treatment modality was the norm prior to 1980, current management commonly entails the combination of radiotherapy with chemotherapy in selected patients with good performance status.[2] On rare occasion, surgical resection also is appropriate. Candidates for surgery and this approach are discussed in more detail in Chapter 44. Progress in the management of locally advanced NSCLC came about in part because of the recognition that cisplatin-based chemotherapy imparts a modest but real survival benefit even in patients with far advanced disease[3,4] (reviewed in Chapter 50). With newer combination chemotherapy regimens containing vinorelbine, gemcitabine, or paclitaxel, additional albeit modest survival gains have been realized in recent years.[5–9] Thus the survival of individuals with locally advanced, unresectable NSCLC has improved in part because of more active chemotherapy regimens. However, improving local tumor control also is a key factor in optimizing survival.[10] The concepts and controversies surrounding the current management of locally advanced, unresectable NSCLC are reviewed in this chapter.

RADIOTHERAPY IN LOCALLY ADVANCED, UNRESECTABLE NSCLC

Historically, patients with locally advanced, unresectable NSCLC were treated with thoracic irradiation alone with a resultant five-year survival rate of 5% to 7%.[11] This narrow approach was based principally on the assumption that a small percentage of patients with localized tumor can be "cured" with thoracic radiotherapy (TRT). While radiotherapy can sterilize NSCLC within the irradiated field, and numerous retrospective single institutional studies indicate

"curative" radiotherapy is associated with a five-year survival rate of 5% or more, it remains unclear if radiotherapy actually cures localized NSCLC. Indeed, it is entirely possible that the biology of certain tumors is such that a five-year survival is possible without any treatment, calling into question the curative potential of radiotherapy.[1,12]

In support of a curative role for radiotherapy are the results of a randomized trial conducted by the Veterans Administration Study Group in the 1960s.[13] These investigators administered TRT (40–50 Gy in 4–6 weeks) or a placebo (lactose tablets) to NSCLC patients with unresectable, locally advanced tumors. Of note, patients with a Karnofsky performance status of less than 50% were included, as were some patients with small cell lung carcinomas (SCLCs). However, only 15% of participants had SCLC, and they were evenly distributed between the two arms. Patients with palpable supraclavicular lymph nodes were excluded. All patients received supportive care consisting of blood transfusions and antibiotics. A statistically significant survival advantage was demonstrated in the irradiated group, although the actual differences in median (142 days and 112 days) and one-year (18.2% and 13.9%) survivals were small and of questionable clinical relevance. This modest survival advantage prompted some experts to question the need for routine irradiation in asymptomatic patients.[14]

Because the Veterans Administration study was carried out in an era prior to the widespread availability of megavoltage equipment and at a time when treatment planning was considerably less sophisticated, the results have been justifiably criticized as not being reflective of present-day radiotherapeutic capabilities.[15] In an effort to address some of these shortcomings, the Southeastern Cancer Study Group (SECSG) undertook a prospective trial employing megavoltage equipment.[12] The study was planned and executed in the early 1980s. Patients were randomized to receive standard radiotherapy (60 Gy in 6 weeks) or no irradiation. The radiotherapy dose was based on the results of a landmark Radiation Therapy Oncology Group trial (RTOG 73-01) in which superior local control was achieved with high-dose irradiation administered without interruption over 5 to 6 weeks.[16] Given the strong prejudicial feelings regarding the curative potential of irradiation that existed at that time, it proved impossible to employ a placebo arm in the SECSG trial. Instead, patients randomized to the no radiotherapy arm received single-agent vindesine, which was believed to be one of the most active single chemotherapy drugs available at the time the study was undertaken. A third treatment arm consisted of standard TRT plus vindesine. Approximately 25% of the patients entered had stage I or II disease and were inoperable because of medical reasons or refusal to undergo thoracotomy. Patients were required to have a Karnofsky PS ≥50%, and those with supraclavicular node involvement were included but represented less than 5% of all cases entered. Patients who progressed on the vindesine arm were permitted to cross over to radiotherapy, and those who progressed after radiotherapy were allowed to receive vindesine. However, only one-third of the patients treated with vindesine actually crossed over to radiotherapy. There were no differences in the median survivals of the three treatment arms (TRT alone = 8.6 months, vindesine alone = 10.1 months; TRT + vindesine = 9.4 months), nor were long-term survival differences noted; five-year survivals = 3%, 1%, and 3%, respectively).[12] Other investigators have reported similar results.[17]

Although the SECSG trial results came under sharp criticism from some experts,[18,19] the results nevertheless indicate that modern TRT, when used alone, is rarely curative in patients with locally advanced unresectable NSCLC. Undoubtedly, some would counter that present day radiotherapy with its improved technology and better treatment planning is likely to improve survival. However, one only has to review the results of several recent randomized trials employing a TRT-alone arm to dispel these beliefs. Even in highly selected patient subsets, median survival remains in the 9- to 11-month range, and long-term survival rarely exceeds 5% to 6%.[20,21] Thus it appears the use of *conven-*

tional fractionation and scheduling of TRT is unlikely to yield substantial further improvements in survival without some additional therapeutic measures or technologic advances.

Analysis of treatment failure patterns provides clues as to how one might overcome the shortcomings of a treatment program and permit the development of new therapeutic strategies and protocols. Based on older literature, the principal cause of treatment failure in locally advanced NSCLC is typically presumed to be extrathoracic metastases. In RTOG 73-01, for example, between 40% and 65% of patients had recurrent disease identified first in extrathoracic sites.[22] Common sites of failure include the skeleton, liver, and central nervous system. Furthermore, as control of the intrathoracic tumor improves, the incidence of recurrence in extrathoracic sites increases.[22–24] However, local relapse remains a significant problem even when modern planning technology is employed. For example, French investigators found that more than 85% of patients had persistent local tumor when examined by bronchoscopy following a radiotherapy dose of 65 Gy.[25–27] Others have identified similar high rates of local failure.[22,28]

RTOG investigators have recently reviewed their patterns of treatment failure data derived from radiotherapy trials largely conducted during the 1980s[24] (Table 52.1). With radiotherapy alone, intrathoracic failure was documented as the initial site of failure in up to 60% of cases depending on the original histology of the primary tumor. Distant metastases as the initial failure site occurred in 40% to 70% of patients. Squamous carcinomas were found to have a higher incidence of local recurrence compared to adenocarcinomas and large cell carcinomas, whereas adenocarcinoma and large cell carcinomas were more likely to progress in the brain.[24]

Based on the aforementioned data, one might predict that chemotherapy would have a greater survival impact on nonsquamous histologies, whereas strategies designed to increase local control might have a greater impact on squamous carcinomas. Regardless, given these failure patterns, it is apparent that improved systemic and local therapies

TABLE 52.1. INITIAL SITES OF RECURRENCE FOLLOWING TRT OR TRT PLUS CHEMOTHERAPY

	Squamous Carcinoma		Adenocarcinoma		Large Cell Carcinoma	
	RT Alone (n = 778)	CT + TRT (n = 168)	RT Alone (n = 395)	CT + TRT (n = 137)	RT Alone (n = 242)	CT + TRT (n = 45)
Primary	26%	23%	20%	34%	23%	40%
Thorax	36%	39%	33%	26%	28%	22%
Brain	11%	20%	18%	8%	16%	16%
Distant	33%	48%	42%	14%	26%	16%
Dead-NP	35%	22%	24%	30%	15%	14%

NP, progression. From Cox JD, Scott CB, Byhardt RW, et al. Addition of chemotherapy to radiation therapy atters failure patterns by cell type within non-small cell carcinoma of lung (NSCCL); analysis of radiation therapy oncology group (RTOG) trials. *Int J Radiat Oncol Biol Phys* 1999;43:505, with permission.

are required to improve survival in locally advanced NSCLC.[29,30]

CHEMOTHERAPY IN LOCALLY ADVANCED, UNRESECTABLE NSCLC

Only a few antineoplastic agents have recognized activity against NSCLC.[9] In fact, much of what is known about the activity of chemotherapy in NSCLC has been derived from studies involving patients with metastatic disease (i.e., stage IV). In this setting, single agents seldom effect objective response rates greater than 15% to 20%, and complete responses are exceedingly rare. Although combining multiple active agents improves overall response rates (20% to 40%), the impact of the higher response rates on survival in patients with stage IV NSCLC is at best modest and controversial.[31]

Despite the relatively modest benefits seen in advanced NSCLC, good rationale for administering chemotherapy in less advanced disease still exists.[2,32–35] Tumor volume is a well-recognized prognostic factor in most chemosensitive tumors. Less bulky tumors demonstrate higher objective response rates and improved survival presumably because they possess fewer drug-resistant cells and have a higher growth fraction, and possibly a better blood supply, all of which contribute to a greater sensitivity to chemotherapy agents.[32] This phenomenon appears to hold true for NSCLC as well. Indeed, agents with only modest activity in advanced tumors are observed to effect much higher objective response rates in patients with stage III lesions.[2,33] Likewise, combination chemotherapy regimens appear to be more effective in locoregional NSCLC.[2,35–37] This relationship is perhaps best illustrated using data from an older study conducted by the European Oncology Radiation Therapy Council (EORTC).[38] In the latter trial, 94 NSCLC patients received cisplatin (60 mg/m^2) and etoposide (120 mg/m^2 per day for 3 days) and achieved an overall objective response rate of 38%. However, among the 40 eligible patients with previously untreated locoregional disease, the objective response rate was nearly twice that observed in patients with stage IV lesions (56% versus 32%, p = 0.038). Similar trends have been documented with newer chemotherapy regimens such as cisplatin and paclitaxel or cisplatin plus gemcitabine.[39,40]

Although the higher objective response rates in locally advanced NSCLC cannot be assumed *a priori* to result in a survival benefit,[41] good circumstantial evidence suggests that the higher objective response rates observed in stage III disease are beneficial. To illustrate, Elliott and colleagues treated a group of patients with unresectable NSCLC with either vindesine alone or cisplatin plus vindesine.[42] Nearly 70% of the patients entered into the trial had locally advanced lesions; these patients were evenly divided between the two treatment arms. Patients given the combination chemotherapy regimen experienced a higher objective response rate and marked improvement in median survival compared to individuals given vindesine alone. The survival benefit was most apparent in patients with locoregional disease. Similar observations were made by ECOG investigators using paclitaxel-based therapy in patients with stage IIIB disease.[39] Although the numbers of patients with locally advanced disease entered in the ECOG trial were relatively modest, a clear trend evolved toward improved response rates and survival with paclitaxel-cisplatin compared to etoposide-cisplatin therapy. Similarly, Woods and colleagues compared cisplatin plus vindesine to best supportive care in a large group of patients with unresectable NSCLC.[43] Included among the study population were patients with locoregional lesions. Similar to the aforementioned ECOG trial, too, few patients with locoregional disease were available to make a valid statistical comparison. However, in a subset analysis, an apparent survival benefit was observed for the chemotherapy-treated group (44 weeks versus 22 weeks). Collectively, these data strongly suggest that chemotherapy may be more effective in the setting of localized NSCLC.

COMBINED MODALITY TREATMENT IN LOCALLY ADVANCED, UNRESECTABLE NSCLC

The combined use of TRT and chemotherapy in locally advanced NSCLC is theoretically appealing because it addresses the need to control the primary lesion while attempting to eradicate occult distant micrometastases.[33,35] The possible advantages for combining chemotherapy and radiotherapy have been summarized by Fu and include: (a) changes in the slope of the radiotherapy dose-response curve; (b) decreased accumulation of inhibition of repair or sublethal repair; (c) decreased recovery from potentially lethal damage; (d) perturbation in cell kinetics, with an increase in proportion of cells in a sensitive phase of the cell cycle and proliferative state; (e) decreased tumor bulk and improved blood supply, leading to reoxygenation and recruitment, and increased sensitivity to irradiation and chemotherapy; and (f) increased drug delivery and uptake.[44]

Neoadjuvant Chemotherapy plus Radiotherapy

Pilot studies employing primary or neoadjuvant chemotherapy plus radiotherapy have yielded median survivals ranging from 9.6 months to more than 16 months and two-year survival rates between 20% and 40%.[45–51] These results appear better than those achieved with radiotherapy alone.[10] To validate the results of these pilot studies, randomized trials have been performed, the results of which are summa-

TABLE 52.2. RANDOMIZED TRIALS OF RADIOTHERAPY VERSUS RADIOTHERAPY PLUS CHEMOTHERAPY

Author	Radiotherapy Dose	Chemotherapy Regimen	Patient Number	Median Survival	One-Year Survival	Two-Year Survival
Mattson[52]	55 Gy	–	119	10.3 mos	41%	15%
		CAP	119	11.0 mos	41%	20%
Dillman[20]	60 Gy	–	77	9.6 mos	40%	13%
		PVlb	78	13.6 mos	54%	26%
Trovo[54]	45 Gy	–	62	11.7 mos	–	–
		CAMPr	49	10.0 mos	–	–
Morton[55]	60 Gy	–	58	10.3 mos	45%	16%
		MACCe	56	10.4 mos	46%	21%
LeChevalier[26]	65 Gy	–	177	10.0 mos	41%	14%
		VCPCe	176	12.0 mos	51%	21%
Sause[56]	60 Gy	–	149	11.4 mos	46%	19%
		PVlb	151	13.8 mos	60%	32%
Cullen[57]	≥40 Gy	–	224	9.9 mos	44%	18%
		MIC	223	13.0 mos	53%	24%

C, cyclophosphamide; A, doxorubicin (Adriamycin); M, methotrexate; Pr, procarbazine; V, vindesine; Ce, lomustine; P, cisplatin; E, etoposide; Vlb, vinblastine; I, ifosfamide.

rized in Table 52.2.[26,52–57] The studies yielded both negative[52,54,55] and positive results.[26,53,56,57]

The first cooperative group randomized trial to demonstrate a clear survival benefit with combined modality therapy was performed by the Cancer and Leukemia Group B (CALGB),[53] (Table 52.3). These investigators compared standard TRT (60 Gy in 6 weeks) to the same radiotherapy preceded by two cycles of cisplatin (100 mg/m² on days 1 and 29) plus weekly vinblastine (5 mg/m² per week for 5 weeks). Because of marked differences in survival detected during a planned interim analysis, the trial was closed early. Median (13.7 months and 9.6 months) and long-term survival rates were significantly improved in the combined modality arm. An update of this trial demonstrated a continued survival benefit with combined modality therapy even out to 7 years (13% and 6%).[20]

The CALGB trial differed from the negative studies listed in Table 52.2 in several ways. First, eligibility was limited to patients with a relatively favorable prognosis defined as low-bulk disease (i.e., supraclavicular nodal involvement excluded), good performance status (0 or 1), and minimal weight loss (5% or less of body weight). These selection criteria are fairly restrictive and exclude many stage III patients seen in daily practice. Second, the CALGB trial used cisplatin-based chemotherapy, which is not the case for most of the negative trials. Although no specific regimen can be recommended for all patients, the composition of chemotherapy is likely to be important.[3] Third, the sequence of chemotherapy and radiotherapy administration may have played a role in the positive outcome of this trial not so much because there is a biological rationale for its use but rather, simply because maximum dosages of both modalities were possible with the schedule used. It is a basic maxim of cancer therapy that delivery of maximum intended therapy is theoretically important to achieve optimal outcome.[58–60] It also should be noted that patients were not stratified according to subcategory of stage III (i.e., IIIA versus IIIB). Accordingly, one cannot easily discern the true relevance of clinical substaging in the CALGB study even though a retrospective analysis was performed to assess this issue.[61] Given these factors, the results of this trial are not clearly applicable to all stage III patients, nor can one assume that ad hoc modifications of the treatment regimen will effect similar results.[62]

The provocative but uncertain nature of the CALGB data, coupled with the statistical concerns raised by some experts,[63] prompted the RTOG and the Eastern Cooperative Oncology Group (ECOG) to undertake a confirmatory trial.[56] Using selection criteria that were essentially identical to that employed by the CALGB, 485 stage III NSCLC patients were randomized to receive standard TRT (60 Gy in 6 weeks), TRT preceded by cisplatin and vinblastine, or hyperfractionated radiotherapy (69.6 Gy given as 120 cGy fractions twice daily). In a small pilot study, RTOG investigators had shown that hyperfractionated irradiation could

TABLE 52.3. CHEMOTHERAPY PLUS TRT VERSUS RADIOTHERAPY ALONE

Survival	CT + TRT	TRT Alone
Median	13.7 mo	9.6 mo
2-year	26%	13%
5-year	17%	6%
7-year	13%	6%

From Dillman RO, Herndon J, Scagren SL, et al. Improved survival in stage III non-small cell lung cancer—seven-year follow-up of cancer and leukemia group B (CALGB) 8433 trial. *J Natl Canc Inst* 1996;88: 1210, with permission.

TABLE 52.4. CHEMOTHERAPY PLUS TRT VERSUS CHEMOTHERAPY ALONE

Survival	CT + TRT	CT Alone
Median	15.2 mos	14.7 mos
2-yrs	35.5%	9.4%
5-yrs	9.7%	3.1%

From Kubota K, Furuse K, Kawahara M, et al. Role of radiotherapy in combined modality treatment of locally advanced non-small cell lung cancer. *J Clin Oncol* 1994;12:1547, with permission.

produce excellent survival in patients meeting the aforementioned selection criteria established by the CALGB.[64] Both median and long-term survivals were superior in the group receiving combined modality treatment, confirming the results of the CALGB study (Table 52.2). A metaanalysis of the available data also affirms the survival advantage of combined modality therapy over radiotherapy alone in this patient population.[65] Lastly, when subset analyses are conducted on the data from some of the negative trials using the same restrictive entry criteria employed by CALGB, a small survival advantage emerges for combined modality therapy.

The observation that chemotherapy plus radiotherapy is superior to radiotherapy alone has led some to speculate that improved local control might be possible with chemotherapy alone and that radiotherapy might be unnecessary. This argument is reminiscent of the polemics that plagued development of combined modality treatment in SCLC almost two decades ago.[66,67] Japanese investigators attempted to address this issue in a prospective trial in which patients with locally advanced disease were randomized to chemotherapy with or without radiotherapy.[68] Median survival was similar in the two cohorts of patients, but long-term survival was clearly superior in the patients who received both chemotherapy and radiotherapy (Table 52.4). Local relapse was greater in the patients given chemotherapy alone. Although the design of this trial was not ideal, the results strongly indicate the need for both chemotherapy and radiotherapy to achieve optimal outcome in localized NSCLC—*chemotherapy alone results in excess local failures; radiotherapy alone results in excess systemic failures.*

Sequence of Chemotherapy and Radiotherapy

Most of the aforementioned combined modality studies administered chemotherapy and radiotherapy in a sequential manner (i.e., chemotherapy followed by radiotherapy) rather than concurrently. This approach was used to avoid anticipated greater toxicity with the concurrent treatment. However, in SCLC, concurrent administration of chemotherapy and radiotherapy is the norm and is generally well tolerated.[69–71] Furthermore, concomitant administration of

these modalities appears to be superior to their sequential administration.[72,73] Presumably, a similar relationship might apply in locally advanced NSCLC. To test this hypothesis, Japanese investigators compared concurrent and sequential chemotherapy and radiotherapy in a prospective trial.[74,75] The chemotherapy employed consisted of mitomycin (8 mg/m^2 on days 1 and 8), vindesin (3 mg/m^2 on days 1, 8, 29, and 36), and cisplatin (80 mg/m^2 on days 1 and 29) (MVP). In the concurrent TRT arm, radiotherapy was initiated starting on day 2 of MVP at 2 Gy fractions to a total dose of 56 Gy. However, TRT was administered as a split course with a ten-day rest period interposed between the first 28 Gy and the remaining TRT dose. In the sequential TRT arm, radiotherapy was initiated upon completion of the MVP, with the 56 Gy being administered in a conventional manner. Eligibility criteria included unresectable stage III NSCLC with supraclavicular lymph node involvement, age ≤75 years, and ECOG PS of 0–2. T3NOMO patients and those with pleural effusions were excluded. A total of 320 patients were enrolled, of whom 314 were eligible. The two groups were well balanced for standard prognostic factors. Overall response rate was higher in the group given concurrent chemotherapy and TRT (84% versus 66.4%). With a median follow-up of 5 years, there is also a survival advantage for the group given concurrent treatment (median survival = 16.5 months versus 13.3 months and five-year survival = 15.8% versus 8.9%) (Table 52.5). Of note, median survival for the sequential arm is similar to that reported from the CALGB and RTOG/ECOG trials employing sequential chemotherapy and radiotherapy.[20,56] These data suggest that concurrent chemotherapy and radiotherapy is superior to their sequential administration; however, additional ongoing trials are assessing this issue. Furthermore, the added toxicities of concurrent chemoradiotherapy are such that caution is appropriate, especially when altered fractionation schemas are also used.[76,77] Not all patients are necessarily candidates for concurrent treatment. Some patients may fare better

TABLE 52.5. CONCURRENT VERSUS SEQUENTIAL CHEMOTHERAPY AND RADIOTHERAPY IN LOCALLY ADVANCED NSCLC

Survival	Concurrent CT + TRT	Sequential CT + TRT
Median	16.5 mos	13.3 mos
1-yr	64.1%	54.8%
2-yrs	34.6%	27.4%
3-yrs	22.3%	14.7%
5-yrs	15.8%	8.9%

From Furuse K, Fukuoka M, Takada Y, et al. Phase III study of concurrent vs. sequential thoracic radiotherapy (TRT) in combination with mitomycin (M), vindesine (V) and cisplatin (P) in unresectable stage III non-small cell lung cancer (NSCLC): five-year follow-up results. *Proc Am Soc Clin Oncol* 1999:18:458a, with permission, and personal communication.

with and prefer a sequential approach, even though the survival may be slightly less than that achieved with a more aggressive treatment.[78]

New Strategies to Address Local Tumor Control

Although an obvious need exists for improved systemic therapy in locally advanced NSCLC, there also is a need for better local control of the tumor. Based erroneously on results from studies conducted more than 20 years ago, it is often assumed that standard daily fractionated radiotherapy alone can control intrathoracic disease in up to 50% of cases when 60 Gy or higher radiotherapy is employed.[22,79] These studies typically accepted stabilized tumor masses as evidence of local control. Based on more recent data, we know this is a gross overestimate of radiotherapy's ability to control bulk disease. Using more stringent means of assessing local control (e.g., bronchoscopy), fewer than 10% of patients are found to have good tumor control at 5 years post-treatment.[27] Patients who relapse with symptomatic distant metastases or die of intercurrent illness may never develop *clinical* evidence of local recurrence simply because they die before manifesting evidence of local recurrence. In addition, physicians do not usually document the exact pattern of disease recurrence upon recognition of relapse in part because formal restaging is not standard practice even in study settings. Furthermore, there is not an agreed-upon standard approach for restaging studies, and very few patients undergo an invasive procedure to confirm the recurrence histologically. Even if extensive radiographic restaging of the thorax is performed at the time of suspected relapse, the results may be misleading because changes in tumor size as determined radiographically only loosely correlate with actual pathologic findings and long-term survival.[80]

In the rare circumstance where a more extensive reevaluation has been performed, the frequency of local control is surprisingly low. For example, using bronchoscopy to visualize the local tumor site, LeChevalier and colleagues found that local tumor control was present in fewer than 20% of patients given thoracic radiotherapy to a dose of 65 Gy.[25] Thus efforts to improve local tumor control are apparently worthwhile because enhanced local control can translate into improved survival even in the absence of improved control of extrathoracic metastases.[28,81–83] For example, despite limitations in assessing local control in older trials such as the RTOG 73-01 study, it is noteworthy that patients who achieved a complete response locally enjoyed a longer survival even though no systemic therapy was administered.[28]

Strategies designed to improve local control include (a) the use of radiation-sensitizing drugs,[84] (b) escalated radiotherapy doses,[10] perhaps with three-dimensional (3-D) treatment planning,[85,86] and (c) through the use of altered fractionations of irradiation.[87] Surgical resection may be the ultimate in local tumor control and is discussed in greater detail in Chapters 37–41. To date, however, no study has yet demonstrated that surgery is superior to radiotherapy in maintaining local control in patients with *clinically unresectable* or so-called *"marginally" resectable* disease.[35] An ongoing United States intergroup trial is prospectively comparing these two modalities.

Radiation-Sensitizing Drugs

Several common antineoplastic agents such as cisplatin, etoposide, paclitaxel, and gemcitabine among others have the potential to act as radiation-sensitizing agents.[84,88–90] These preclinical observations have prompted several investigators to undertake studies combining radiation-sensitizing drugs and radiotherapy. European investigators performed a well-designed randomized trial in which split-course radiotherapy alone was prospectively compared to radiotherapy plus concomitant cisplatin given daily or weekly.[91] The combined administration of cisplatin and irradiation resulted in improved local tumor control and improved survival (Table 52.6). The improved survival was clearly attributable to improvement in the local failure rate because the rate of distant failure was not affected with the addition of the relatively low doses of cisplatin. Similar results have been noted by other investigators,[92] although this finding has not been universal.[93] One precautionary note—the simultaneous use of radiation and drugs can be a double-edged sword because increased host toxicities may ensue, resulting in dose reductions of one or both treatment modalities. Esophagitis and pulmonary toxicities are particularly worrisome in this regard.[76,94–96] Accordingly, strategies that permit concurrent administration of chemotherapy and radiotherapy and that minimize the likelihood of host toxicity need further exploration.

Increased Radiotherapy Dose and Altered Fractionation

The importance of radiotherapy dose and its relationship to the intrathoracic control of NSCLC is well established.[10,11]

TABLE 52.6. CHEMOSENSITIZATION WITH CISPLATIN PLUS TRT SURVIVAL WITHOUT LOCAL PROGRESSION

Treatment	1-Year	2-Year
TRT Alone	41 ± 5.6%	19 ± 5.1%
TRT + Weekly Cisplatin	42 ± 5.7%	30 ± 6.0%
TRT + Daily Cisplatin	59 ± 5.8%	31 ± 6.3%

From Schaake-Koning C, Maat B, Houtte PV, et al. Radiotherapy combined with low-dose cis-diamminedichloroplatinum (II) (CDDP) in inoperable nonmetastatic non-small cell lung-cancer (NSCLC): a randomized three arm phase II study of the EORTC lung cancer and radiotherapy cooperative groups. *Intl J Radiat Oncol Biol Phys* 1998; 42:487, with permission.

However, escalating the dose of thoracic irradiation beyond 60–66 Gy in lung cancer has been difficult largely because of the toxic effect on normal tissues, especially the lungs and esophagus. One potential means of increasing total radiation dose without engendering excessive host toxicity is the use of multiple daily fractions of irradiation.[87,97] In theory, giving radiotherapy in many small doses reduces the long-term adverse effects observed in normal tissues with little reduction in effect on most tumors because tumor cell repopulation is minimized.[98] Altered fractionation schemas attempt to exploit the differences in early-responding and late-responding tissues to repair radiation-induced DNA damage. Pilot studies indicate that this approach is feasible in locally advanced NSCLC.[64,99,100]

British investigators recently completed a randomized comparison of *continuous hyperfractionated accelerated radiotherapy* (CHART) and standard once-daily fractionated radiotherapy in NSCLC patients with locally advanced disease.[83] CHART consists of three daily fractions (1.5 Gy) of irradiation given over 12 consecutive days to a total dose of 54 Gy. CHART yielded a statistically significant improvement in overall survival compared to individuals treated with traditional once-daily radiotherapy (Table 52.7). Improved survival appears to have resulted from increased local tumor control because no systemic therapy was administered. Lending support to this conjecture is the observation that CHART imparted its greatest benefit in patients with squamous carcinoma. Squamous carcinomas tend to be localized more commonly than nonsquamous histologies, and because of this tendency, would presumably benefit more from improved local tumor control imparted by CHART. This relationship appears to be the case because squamous histology patients enjoyed a 34% reduction in the relative risk of death with CHART, which translates into an absolute two-year survival benefit of 14% (from 19% to 33%). The principal toxicities of CHART were esophagitis and dysphagia. However, pulmonary fibrosis also was more common among patients receiving CHART (16% versus 4%) compared to once-daily irradiation. Radiation morbidity accounted for a total of six deaths, three in each treatment arm.

The CHART data are extremely encouraging and correlate with other data derived from randomized trials in which multiple daily fractions of irradiation proved advantageous in NSCLCs and SCLCs.[56,101] However, the administration of 12 consecutive days of radiotherapy is logistically problematic. Fortunately, both the British group and ECOG investigators have reported equally encouraging results using a less burdensome schedule that avoids weekend radiotherapy treatments.[100,102] The British investigators refer to their regimen as "CHARTWEL" for "CHART—weekendless,"[102] whereas the ECOG investigators refer to their regimen as "HART," indicating noncontinuous hyperfractionated accelerated radiotherapy.

3-D Treatment Planning

3-D treatment planning provides an ability to increase radiotherapy dose while minimizing normal tissue toxicity.[86,103] 3-D capabilities are fully discussed in Chapter 48. However, the salient features employ computed tomographic images to better define the target (tumor and perhaps regional nodes), register normal tissues and record doses that they receive, and plan beam directions to optimize dose to the target while minimizing exposure to the adjacent normal organs and tissues. Preliminary studies indicate that this technique permits radiotherapy dose-escalation to levels as high as 85–103 Gy.[85,104–106] Dose-escalation trials have more sharply defined target volumes and even eliminate treatment of mediastinal nodes. In the recent Ann Arbor trial results,[107] 104 patients were treated, none with elective mediastinal irradiation. Toxicity has been moderate; moreover, no grade 3 pneumonitis has been observed despite high doses, and no patient failed exclusively in the untreated mediastinum. If radiotherapy ports can be reduced, and tumor doses increased, then TRT may be a better partner with surgery and chemotherapy in the treatment of NSCLC. Large tumors with multilevel mediastinal nodes may not benefit from these approaches. One study found that prognosis was adversely influenced if more than 20 percent of normal lung volume was included.[106] It remains to be seen if such approaches will prove beneficial in terms of improved local control and enhanced survival.

SUMMARY

The results of the CALGB trial prompted a clear paradigm shift in the management of locally advanced NSCLC.[2,105] Selected patients are now preferentially treated with combined modality approaches. The optimal means by which these two modalities are combined, however, as well as issues pertaining to optimal radiotherapy and chemotherapy, all require additional study. Newer chemotherapy drugs with higher response rates raise expectations for improved survival, although appropriate clinical studies are needed to validate these expectations.[9] Some of the newer agents—the taxanes, the topoisomerase-targeting drugs, and gemcitab-

TABLE 52.7. CHART IN LOCALLY ADVANCED NSCLC

Survival	CHART	Standard RT
1-yr	63%	55%
2-yrs	29%	20%

From Saunders M, Dische S, Barrett A, et al. Continuous hyperfractionated accelerated radiotherapy (CHART) versus conventional radiotherapy in non-small-cell lung cancer: a randomised multicentre trial. CHART Steering-Committee [see comments]. *Lancet* 1997;350:161, with permission.

ine—also hold promise as radiosensitizers as well as good systemic agents. The methods of improving local control are varied as described previously and each merits continued investigation. Potentially, these techniques will lead to additional modest improvement in the survival of NSCLC patients with locally advanced disease.

REFERENCES

1. Ginsberg RJ, Vokes EE, Raben A. Non-small cell lung cancer. In: DeVita VT, Hellman S, Rosenberg SA, eds. *Cancer: Principles & Practice of Oncology*, 4th ed. Philadelphia: JB Lippincott, 1997:858.
2. Livingston RB. Combined modality therapy of lung cancer. [Review]. *Clin Canc Res* 1997;3(12 Pt 2):2638.
3. Non-small Cell Lung Cancer Collaborative Group. Chemotherapy in non-small cell lung cancer: a meta-analysis using updated data on individual patients from 52 randomised clinical trials. *Br Med J* 1995;311(7010):899.
4. Ellis PA, Smith JE, Hardy JR, et al. Symptom relief with MVP (mitomycin C, vinblastine and cisplatin) chemotherapy in advanced non-small-cell lung cancer. *Br J Canc* 1995;71(2):366.
5. LeChevalier T, Brisgand D, Douillard JY, et al. Randomized study of vinorelbine and cisplatin versus vindesine and cisplatin versus vinorelbine alone in advanced non-small-cell lung cancer: results of a European multicenter trial including 612 patients [see comments]. *J Clin Oncol* 1994;12(2):360.
6. Bonomi P, Kim K, Chang A, et al. Phase III trial comparing etoposide (E) cisplatin (C) versus Taxol (T) with cisplatin-G-CSF (G) versus Taxol-cisplatin in advanced non-small cell lung cancer. An Eastern Cooperative Oncology Group (ECOG) trial. *Proc Am Soc Clin Oncol* 1996;15:382.
7. Sandler A, Nemunaitis J, Dehnam C, et al. Phase III study of cisplatin (C) with or without gemcitabine (G) in patients with advanced nonsmall cell lung cancer (NSCLC). *Proc Am Soc Clin Oncol* 1998;17:454a.
8. Wozniak AJ, Crowley JJ, Balcerzak SP, et al. Randomized trial comparing cisplatin with cisplatin plus vinorelbine in the treatment of advanced non-small-cell lung cancer: a Southwest Oncology Group study. *J Clin Oncol* 1998;16(7):2459.
9. Bunn PA, Jr, Kelly K. New chemotherapeutic agents prolong survival and improve quality of life in non-small cell lung cancer: a review of the literature and future directions. [Review]. *Clin Canc Res* 1998;4(5):1087.
10. Wagner H. Enhancing the role of radiotherapy in non-small cell lung cancer. [Review]. *Curr Opin Oncol* 1998;10(2):139.
11. Sause WT, Turrisi AT. Principles and application of preoperative and standard radiotherapy for regionally advanced non-small cell lung cancer. In: Pass HI, Mitchell JB, Johnson DH, et al., eds. *Lung Cancer: Principles and Practice*. Philadelphia: Lippincott-Raven, 1996:697.
12. Johnson DH, Einhorn LH, Bartolucci A, et al. Thoracic radiotherapy does not prolong survival in patients with locally advanced, unresectable non-small cell lung cancer. *Ann Intern Med* 1990;113:33.
13. Roswit B, Patno ME, Rapp R, et al. The survival of patients with inoperable lung cancer: a large scale randomized study of radiation therapy versus placebo. *Radiology* 1968;90:688.
14. Cohen MH. Is immediate radiation therapy indicated for patients with unresectable non-small cell lung cancer? No. *Canc Treat Rep* 1983;67:333.
15. Cox JD, Komaki R, Byhardt RW. Is immediate radiotherapy obligatory for any or all patients with limited-stage non-small cell lung cancer? Yes. *Cancer Treat Rep* 1983;67:327.

16. Perez CA, Stanley K, Rubin P, et al. A prospective randomized study of various irradiation doses and fractionation schedules in the treatment of inoperable non-oat-cell carcinoma of the lung. Preliminary report by the Radiation Therapy Oncology Group. *Cancer* 1980;45(11):2744.
17. Kaasa S, Thorud E, Host H, et al. A randomized study evaluating radiotherapy versus chemotherapy in patients with inoperable non-small cell lung cancer. *Radiother Oncol* 1988;11:7.
18. Curran WJ. Effectiveness of treatment for non-small cell lung cancer [letter; comment]. *Ann Intern Med* 1990;113(8):637.
19. Prosnitz LR. Radiotherapy for lung cancer [letter; comment]. *Ann Intern Med* 1991;114(1):95.
20. Dillman RO, Herndon J, Seagren SL, et al. Improved survival in stage III non-small-cell lung cancer—seven-year follow-up of Cancer and Leukemia Group B (CALGB) 8433 trial. *J Natl Canc Inst* 1996;88(17):1210.
21. Sause WT, Scott C, Taylor S, et al. RTOG 8808 ECOG 4588, preliminary analysis of a phase III trial in regionally advanced unresectable non-small cell lung cancer with minimum three year follow-up. *Intl J Radiat Oncol Biol Phys* 1995;32(Suppl 1):109.
22. Perez CA, Pajak TF, Rubin P, et al. Long-term observations of the patterns of failure in patients with unresectable non-oat cell carcinoma of the lung treated with definitive radiotherapy. Report by the Radiation Oncology Therapy Oncology Group. *Cancer* 1987;59:1874.
23. Komaki R, Scott CB, Byhardt R, et al. Failure patterns by prognostic group determined by recursive partitioning analysis (RPA) of 1547 patients on four Radiation Therapy Oncology Group (RTOG) studies in inoperable nonsmall-cell lung cancer (NSCLC). *Intl J Radiat Oncol Biol Phys* 1998;42(2):263.
24. Cox JD, Scott CB, Byhardt RW, et al. Addition of chemotherapy to radiation therapy alters failure patterns by cell type within non-small cell carcinoma of lung (NSCCL): analysis of radiation therapy oncology group (RTOG) trials. *Intl J Radiat Oncol Biol Phys* 1999;43(3):505.
25. LeChevalier T, Arriagada R, Quoix E, et al. Radiotherapy alone versus combined chemotherapy and radiotherapy in nonresectable non-small cell lung cancer: first analysis of a randomized trial in 353 patients. *J Natl Cancer Inst* 1991;83:417.
26. LeChevalier T, Arriagada R, Tarayre M, et al. Significant effect of adjuvant chemotherapy on survival in locally advanced non-small cell lung cancer. *J Natl Canc Inst* 1992;84:58.
27. Arriagada R, LeChevalier T, Rekacewicz C, et al. Cisplatin-based chemotherapy (CT) in patients with locally advanced non-small cell lung cancer (NSCLC): late analysis of a French randomized trial. *Proc Am Soc Clin Oncol* 1997;16:446a.
28. Perez CA, Bauer M, Edelstein S, et al. Impact of tumor control on survival in carcinoma of the lung treated with irradiation [published erratum appears in *Intl J Radiat Oncol Biol Phys* 1986 Nov;12(11):2057]. *Intl J Radiat Oncol Biol Phys* 1986;12(4):539.
29. Arriagada R. Current strategies for radiation therapy in non-small cell lung cancer. [Review]. *Chest* 1997;112(4 Suppl):209S.
30. Trodella L, Mantini G, Fontana A, et al. Radiotherapy, local control and survival in lung cancer. [Review]. *Rays* 1998;23(3):572.
31. Lilenbaum RC, Langenberg P, Dickersin K. Single agent versus combination chemotherapy in patients with advanced nonsmall cell lung carcinoma: a meta-analysis of response, toxicity, and survival. *Cancer* 1998;82(1):116.
32. Goldie JH. Scientific basis for adjuvant and primary (neoadjuvant) chemotherapy. *Semin Oncol* 1987;14:1.
33. Shepherd FA. Induction chemotherapy for locally advanced non-small cell lung cancer. [Review] [34 refs]. *Ann Thorac Surg* 1993;55(6):1585.

34. Edelman MJ, Gandara DR, Roach M, III, et al. Multimodality therapy in stage III non-small cell lung cancer [published erratum appears in *Ann Thorac Surg* 1996;62(6):1892]. [Review] [60 refs]. *Ann Thorac Surg* 1996;61(5):1564.

35. Einhorn LH. Neoadjuvant and adjuvant trials in non-small cell lung cancer. [Review] [22 refs] *Ann Thorac Surg* 1998;65(1):208.

36. Curran WJ, Jr, Werner-Wasik M. Issues in nonoperative management of locally advanced non-small-cell lung cancer. [Review]. *Oncology* 1998;12(1 Suppl 2):60

37. Vokes EE, Green MR. Clinical studies in non-small cell lung cancer: the CALGB experience. [Review] [48 refs]. *Canc Invest* 1998;16(2):72.

38. Longeval E, Klastersky J. Combination chemotherapy with cisplatin and etoposide in bronchogenic squamous cell carcinoma and adenocarcinoma. A study by the EORTC lung cancer working party (Belgium). *Cancer* 1982;50:2751.

39. Bonomi PB, Kim K, Kugler J, et al. Comparison of survival for stage IIIB versus stage IV non-small cell lung cancer (NSCLC) patients treated with etoposide-cisplatin versus Taxol-cisplatin: an Eastern Cooperative Group (ECOG) trial. *Proc Am Soc Clin Oncol* 1997:16:454a.

40. van Zandwijk N, Crino L, Kramer GW, et al. Phase II study of gemcitabine (GEM) plus cisplatin (CIS) as induction regimen for patients with stage IIIA non-small cell lung cancer (NSCLC) by the EORTC Lung Cancer Cooperative Group (EORTC 08955). *Proc Am Soc Clin Oncol* 1998;17:468a.

41. Markman M. Why does a higher response rate to chemotherapy correlate poorly with improved survival? [editorial]. *J Canc Res Clin Oncol* 1993;119(12):700.

42. Elliott JA, Ahmedozcie S, Hole D, et al. Vindesine and cisplatin combination chemotherapy compared to vindesine as a single agent in the management of non-small cell lung cancer. *Eur J Canc* 1984;20:1025.

43. Woods RL, Williams CJ, Levi J, et al. A randomized trial of cisplatin and vindesine versus supportive care only in advanced non-small cell lung cancer. *Br J Canc* 1990;66:608.

44. Fu KK. Biological basis for the interaction of chemotherapeutic agents and radiation therapy. *Cancer* 1985;55:2123.

45. Bitran JD, Desser RK, DeMeester T, et al. Combined modality therapy for stage IIIMO non-oat cell bronchogenic carcinoma. *Cancer* 1978;62:327.

46. LeChevalier T, Arriagada R, Baldeyrou P, et al. Combined chemotherapy (vindesine, lomustine, cisplatin, and cyclophosphamide) and radical radiotherapy in inoperable nonmetastatic squamous cell carcinoma of the lung. *Canc Treat Rep* 1985;69:469.

47. Cox JD, Samson MK, Herskovic AM, et al. Cisplatin and etoposide before definitive radiation therapy for inoperable squamous carcinoma, adenocarcinoma, and large cell carcinoma of the lung: A phase I-II study of the Radiation Therapy Oncology Group. *Canc Treat Rep* 1986;70:1219.

48. Freiss GG, Baikadi M, Harvey WH. Concurrent cisplatin and etoposide with radiotherapy in locally advanced non-small cell lung cancer. *Can Treat Rep* 1987;71:681.

49. Eagan RT, Ruud C, Lee RE, et al. Pilot study of induction therapy with cyclophosphamide, doxorubicin, and cisplatin (CAP) and chest irradiation prior to thoracotomy in initially inoperable stage III M non-small cell lung cancer. *Canc Treat Rep* 1987;71:895.

50. Rabinow JS, Shaw EG, Eagan RT, et al. Results of combination chemotherapy and thoracic radiation therapy for unresectable non-small cell carcinoma of the lung. *Intl J Radiat Oncol Biol Phys* 1989;17:1203.

51. Johnson DH, Strupp J, Greco FA, et al. Neoadjuvant cisplatin plus vinblastine chemotherapy in locally advanced non-small cell lung cancer. *Cancer* 1991;68(6):1216.

52. Mattson K, Holsti L, Holsti P, et al. Inoperable non-small cell lung cancer: radiation with or without chemotherapy. *Eur J Canc* 1988;24:477.

53. Diliman R, Seagren S, Propert K, et al. A randomized trial of induction chemotherapy plus high-dose radiation versus radiation alone in stage III non-small cell lung cancer. *N Engl J Med* 1990;323:940.

54. Trovo M, Minatel E, Veronesi A, et al. Combined radiotherapy and chemotherapy versus radiotherapy alone in locally advanced epidermoid bronchogenic carcinoma. A randomized study. *Cancer* 1990;65:400.

55. Morton R, Jett J, Mcginnis W, et al. Thoracic radiation therapy alone compared with combined chemoradiotherapy for locally unresectable non-small cell lung cancer. A randomized, phase III trial. *Ann Intern Med* 1991;115:681.

56. Sause WT, Scott C, Taylor S, et al. Radiation Therapy Oncology Group (RTOG) 88-08 and Eastern Cooperative Oncology Group (ECOG) 4588: preliminary results of a phase III trial in regionally advanced, unresectable non-small-cell lung cancer. *J Natl Canc Inst* 1995;87(3):198.

57. Cullen MH, Billingham LJ, Woodroffe CM, et al. Mitomycin, ifosfamide and cisplatin (MIC) in non-small cell lung cancer (NSCLC): 1. Results of a randomised trial in patients with localised, inoperable disease. *Lung Cancer* 1997;18(suppl 1):5.

58. Goldie JH, Coldman AJ. The genetic origin of drug resistance in neoplasms: implications for systemic therapy. *Canc Res* 1984;44:3643.

59. DeVita VT. The James Ewing Lecture: the relationship between tumor mass and resistance to chemotherapy. Implications for surgical adjuvant treatment of cancer. *Cancer* 1983;51:1207.

60. DeVita VT. Principles of cancer management: chemotherapy. In: DeVita VT, Hellman S, Rosenberg SA, eds. *Cancer: Principles & Practice of Oncology,* 5th ed. Philadelphia: Lippincott-Raven, 1997:333.

61. Kreisman H, Lisbona A, Olson L, et al. Effect of radiologic stage III substage on nonsurgical therapy of non-small cell lung cancer. *Cancer* 1993;72:1588.

62. Johnson DH. Combined-modality therapy for unresectable, stage III non-small-cell lung cancer—caveat emptor or caveat venditor. *J Natl Canc Inst* 1996;88(17):1175.

63. Souhami RL, Spiro SG, Cullen M. Chemotherapy and radiation therapy as compared with radiation therapy in stage III non-small cell lung cancer. *N Engl J Med* 1991;324:1136.

64. Cox JD, Azarnia N, Byhardt RW, et al. A randomized phase I/II trial of hyperfractionated radiation therapy with total doses of 60.0 Gy to 79.2 Gy: possible survival benefit with >69.6 Gy in favorable patients with Radiation Therapy Oncology Group stage III non-small cell lung carcinoma: report of Radiation Therapy Oncology Group 83-11. *J Clin Oncol* 1990;8:1543.

65. Pritchard RS, Anthony SP. Chemotherapy plus radiotherapy compared with radiotherapy alone in the treatment of locally advanced, unresectable, non-small-cell lung cancer—a meta-analysis. *Ann Intern Med* 1996;125(9):723 ff.

66. Cohen MH. Is thoracic radiation therapy necessary for patients with limited-stage small cell lung cancer? No. *Canc Treat Rep* 1983;67:217.

67. Byhardt RW, Cox JD. Is thoracic radiation therapy necessary for patients with limited-stage small cell lung cancer? Yes. *Canc Treat Rep* 1983;67:209.

68. Kubota K, Furuse K, Kawahara M, et al. Role of radiotherapy in combined modality treatment of locally advanced non-small cell lung cancer. *J Clin Oncol* 1994;12:1547.

69. Kumar P. The role of thoracic radiotherapy in the management of limited-stage small cell lung cancer: past, present, and future. [Review]. *Chest* 1997;112(4 Suppl):259S.

70. Wagner H, Jr. Radiation therapy in the management of limited small cell lung cancer: when, where, and how much?. [Review]. *Chest* 1998;113(1 Suppl):92S.

71. Sorensen M, Lassen U, Hansen HH. Current therapy of small cell lung cancer. [Review]. *Curr Opin Oncol* 1998;10(2):133.

72. Kies MS, Mira JG, Crowley JJ, et al. Multimodal therapy for limited small-cell lung cancer: a randomized study of induction combination chemotherapy with or without thoracic radiation in complete responders; and with wide-field versus reduced-field radiation in partial responders: a Southwest Oncology Group Study. *J Clin Oncol* 1987;5(4):592.

73. Takada M, Fukuoka M, Furuse K, et al. Phase III study of concurrent versus sequential thoracic radiotherapy (TRT) in combination with cisplatin (C) and etoposide (E) for limited-stage (LS) small cell lung cancer (SCLC): preliminary results of the Japan Clinical Oncology Group (JCOG) (meeting abstract). *Proc Am Soc Clin Oncol* 1996;15:A1103.

74. Furuse K, Fukuoka M, Takada Y, et al. A randomized phase III study of concurrent versus sequential thoracic radiotherapy (TRT) in combination with mitomycin (M), vindesine (V), and cisplatin (P) in unresectable stage III non-small cell lung cancer (NSCLC): preliminary analysis. *Proc Am Soc Clin Oncol* 1997; 16:459a.

75. Furuse K, Fukuoka M, Takada Y, et al. Phase III study of concurrent vs. sequential thoracic radiotherapy (TRT) in combination with mitomycin (M), vindesine (V) and cisplatin (P) in unresectable stage III non-small cell lung cancer (NSCLC): five-year median follow-up results. *Proc Am Soc Clin Oncol* 1999;18:458a.

76. Blanke C, DeVore RD, Shyr Y, et al. A pilot study of protracted low-dose cisplatin and etoposide with concurrent thoracic radiotherapy in unresectable stage III non-small cell lung cancer. *Intl J Radiat Oncol Biol Phys* 1996;15:35.

77. Komaki R, Scott C, Lee JS, et al. Impact of adding concurrent chemotherapy to hyperfractionated radiotherapy for locally advanced non-small cell lung cancer (NSCLC): comparison of RTOG 83-11 and RTOG 91-06. *Am J Clin Oncol* 1997;20(5): 435.

78. Brundage MD, Davidson JR, Mackillop WJ. Trading treatment toxicity for survival in locally advanced non-small cell lung cancer. *J Clin Oncol* 1997;15(1):330.

79. Perez CA, Stanley K, Rubin P, et al. Patterns of tumor recurrence after definitive irradiation for inoperable non-oat cell carcinoma of the lung. *Intl J Radiat Oncol Biol Phys* 1980;6: 987.

80. Mirimanoff RO, Moro D, Bolla M, et al. Alternating radiotherapy and chemotherapy for inoperable Stage III non-small-cell lung cancer: long-term results of two Phase II GOTHA trials. Groupe d'Oncologie Thoracique Alpine. *Intl J Radiat Oncol Biol Phys* 1998;42(3):487.

81. Schaake-Koning C, Maat B, Houtte PV, et al. Radiotherapy combined with low-dose cis-diamminedichloroplatinum (II) (CDDP) in inoperable nonmetastatic non-small cell lung cancer (NSCLC): a randomized three arm phase II study of the EORTC lung cancer and radiotherapy cooperative groups. *Intl J Radiat Oncol Biol Phys* 1990;19:967.

82. Jeremic B, Shibamoto Y, Acimovic L, et al. Hyperfractionated radiation therapy with or without concurrent low-dose daily carboplatin/etoposide for stage III non-small-cell lung cancer: a randomized study. *J Clin Oncol* 1996;14(4):1065.

83. Saunders M, Dische S, Barrett A, et al. Continuous hyperfrac-

tionated accelerated radiotherapy (CHART) versus conventional radiotherapy in non-small cell lung cancer: a randomised multicentre trial. CHART Steering Committee [see comments]. *Lancet* 1997;350:161.

84. Dewit N. Combined treatment of radiation and cisdiamminedichloroplatinum (II): A review of experimental and clinical data. *Int J Radiat Oncol Biol Phys* 1987;13:403.

85. Armstrong JG. Three-dimensional conformal radiotherapy. Precision treatment of lung cancer. [Review]. *Chest Surg Clin N Am* 1994;4(1):29.

86. Armstrong JG. Target volume definition for three-dimensional conformal radiation therapy of lung cancer. [Review] [24 refs]. *Br J Radiol* 1998;71(846):587.

87. Peters LJ, Ang KK. Unconventional fractionation schemes in radiotherapy. In: DeVite VT, Hellman S, Rosenberg SA, eds. *Important Advances in Oncology 1986* Philadelphia: JB Lippincott, 1986:269.

88. Chang AYC, Gu Z, Keng P, et al. Radiation sensitizing effects of topoisomerase I and II inhibitors. *Proc Am Assoc Canc Res* 1991;32:389.

89. Liebmann J, Cook JA, Fisher J, et al. In vitro studies of taxol as a radiation sensitizer in human tumor cells. *J Natl Canc Inst* 1994;86:441.

90. Lawrence TS, Eisbruch A, Shewach DS. Gemcitabine-mediated radiosensitization. [Review]. *Semin Oncol* 1997;24(2 Suppl 7): S7.

91. Schaake-Koning C, van den Bogaert W, Dalesio O, et al. Effects of concomitant cisplatin and radiotherapy on inoperable non-small cell lung cancer. *N Engl J Med* 1992;326:524.

92. Jeremic B, Shibamoto Y, Acimovic L, et al. Randomized trial of hyperfractionated radiation therapy with or without concurrent chemotherapy for stage III non-small cell lung cancer. *J Clin Oncol* 1995;13(2):452.

93. Trovo MG, Minatel E, Franchin G, et al. Radiotherapy versus radiotherapy enhanced by cisplatin in stage III non-small cell lung cancer. *Int J Radiat Oncol Biol Phys* 1992;24:11.

94. Choy H, Akerley W, Safran H, et al. Phase I trial of outpatient weekly paclitaxel and concurrent radiation therapy for advanced non-small-cell lung cancer. *J Clin Oncol* 1994;12(12):2682.

95. Reckzeh B, Merte H, Pfluger K-H, et al. Severe lymphocytopenia and interstitial pneumonia in patients treated with paclitaxel and simultaneous radiotherapy for non-small cell lung cancer. *J Clin Oncol* 1996;14:1071.

96. Byhardt RW, Scott C, Sause WT, et al. Response, toxicity, failure patterns, and survival in five Radiation Therapy Oncology Group (RTOG) trials of sequential and/or concurrent chemotherapy and radiotherapy for locally advanced non-small-cell carcinoma of the lung. *Int J Radiat Oncol Biol Phys* 1998; 42(3):469.

97. Thames HD, Ang KK. Altered fractionation: radiobiological principles, clinical results, and potential for dose escalation. [Review] [139 refs]. *Canc Treat Res* 1998;93:101.

98. Withers HR. Biological basis of radiation therapy for cancer. [Review] [19 refs]. *Lancet* 1992;339(8786):156.

99. Saunders MI, Dische S. Continuous hyperfractionated, accelerated radiotherapy (CHART) in non-small cell lung carcinoma of the bronchus. *Intl J Radiat Oncol Biol Phys* 1990;19:1211.

100. Mehta MP, Tannehill SP, Adak S, et al. Phase II trial of hyperfractionated accelerated radiation therapy for nonresectable non-small cell lung cancer: results of Eastern Cooperative Oncology Group 4593. *J Clin Oncol* 1998;16(11):3518.

101. Turrisi AT, Kim K, Blum R, et al. Twice-daily compared with once-daily thoracic radiotherapy in limited small cell lung cancer treated concurrently with cisplatin-etoposide chemotherapy. *N Engl J Med* 1999;340:265.

102. Saunders MI, Rojas A, Lyn BE, et al. Experience with dose escalation using CHARTWEL (continuous hyperfractionated accelerated radiotherapy weekend less) in non-small cell lung cancer. *Br J Canc* 1998;78(10):1323.

103. Lichter AS, Ten Haken RK. Three-dimensional treatment planning and conformal radiation dose delivery. [Review]. In: DeVita V, Hellman S, Rosenberg S, eds. *Cancer: Principles and Practice of Oncology.* Philadelphia: Lippincott-Raven, 1995, p. 95.

104. Hazuka MB, Turrisi AT, Martel MK, et al. Dose-escalation in non-small cell lung cancer (NSCLC) using conformal 3-dimensional radiation treatment planning (3DRTP): preliminary results of Phase I study (meeting abstract). *Proc Am Soc Clin Oncol* 1994;13:A1119.

105. Lichter AS, Lawrence TS. Recent advances in radiation oncology [see comments]. [Review]. *N Engl J Med* 1995;332(6):371.

106. Graham MV, Jain NL, Kahn MG, et al. Evaluation of an objective plan-evaluation model in the three dimensional treatment of nonsmall cell lung cancer. *Int J Radiat Oncol Biol Phys* 1996;34(2):469.

107. Hayman JA, Martel MK, Ten Haken RK, et al. Dose escalation in non-small cell lung cancer (NSCLC) using conformal 3-dimensional radiation therapy (C3DRT): update of a phase I trial. *Proc Am Soc Clin Oncol* 1999;18:459a.

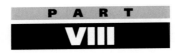

PART
VIII

TREATMENT OF SMALL CELL LUNG CANCER

53

CHEMOTHERAPY FOR SMALL CELL LUNG CANCER

RUSSELL F. DeVORE III
DAVID H. JOHNSON

Small cell lung cancer (SCLC) represents the sixth most commonly diagnosed cancer in the United States each year.[1] In comparison to non–small cell lung cancer (NSCLC), small cell carcinoma tends to disseminate earlier in the course of its natural history and displays a more aggressive clinical behavior.[2,3] Untreated patients rarely survive beyond a few months, and local treatment modalities such as radiotherapy or surgery are not effective in prolonging survival beyond a few weeks.[4,5] The cause of death in most instances is systemic disease. The propensity for SCLC to disseminate early is illustrated by a classic study conducted by Matthews and colleagues.[6] These investigators were able to perform a series of autopsies on a group of SCLC patients who had died within one month of an attempted curative surgical resection. In all but a few cases, systemic metastases were identified even though the patients had undergone a preoperative evaluation demonstrating no distant metastases. Given the systemic nature of SCLC, it is not surprising that chemotherapy has become the cornerstone of management. Current chemotherapy approaches are reviewed in this chapter, whereas surgical management and specific details pertaining to radiotherapy for SCLC are covered in Chapters 54 and 56.

SINGLE-AGENT CHEMOTHERAPY

Small cell carcinoma exhibits sensitivity to a variety of chemotherapy agents (Table 53.1).[7] The chemosensitivity of SCLC was first identified 50 years ago with the recognition that methyl-bis-β-chloroethyl) amine hydrochloride could effect tumor regression in more than 50% of patients.[8] It is now well recognized that numerous antineoplastic agents are capable of effecting objective responses of $\geq$30% in previously untreated patients.[9] Active agents include nitrogen mustard, doxorubicin, methotrexate, ifosfamide, etoposide, teniposide, vincristine, vindesine, nitrosoureas, cisplatin, and its analog carboplatin.[10] In the past decade, several new agents have been found to possess activ-

ity against SCLC, including paclitaxel, docetaxel, two topoisomerase I targeting agents topotecan and irinotecan (CPT-11), vinorelbine, and gemcitabine.[11] These newer agents are appealing because of their unique mechanisms of action.

COMBINATION CHEMOTHERAPY

Despite a plethora of active agents, SCLC is rarely treated with single agents largely because complete remissions are relatively infrequent and remission durations tend to be brief with single agents. Furthermore, in randomized trials conducted in the 1970s, combination therapy was shown to produce superior survival compared to single-agent treatment.[12,13,14] In addition, the simultaneous administration of multiple agents has been shown to be more efficacious than the sequential administration of the same agents.[13] Consequently, for more than 20 years, combination chemotherapy has been the mainstay of SCLC management.

Several chemotherapy combination regimens have demonstrated acceptable activity against SCLC.[7,15] In general, active regimens yield objective response rates in the range of 80% to 90% with complete remissions occurring in up to 50% of patients, depending on stage at presentation. Median survival averages 7 to 9 months in extensive-stage patients and up to 20 months in patients with limited disease.[7,16,17] The best survival is achieved in good performance status patients who present with limited-stage disease and who receive combined modality therapy with chemotherapy plus thoracic radiotherapy.[16,17]

No single induction combination chemotherapy regimen has been found to be ideal for all patients. During the late 1970s and early 1980s, cyclophosphamide-based regimens were most commonly employed, particularly the combination consisting of cyclophosphamide, doxorubicin, and vincristine (CAV). More recently, induction regimens have tended to be built around etoposide either as a substitution for one of the components of the CAV regimen or in combination with cisplatin (with or without additional agents).[7,18]

TABLE 53.1. ACTIVE SINGLE AGENTS AGAINST SCLC

Established Agents	New Agents
nitrogen mustard	paclitaxel
methotrexate	docetaxel
ifosfamide	topotecan
teniposide	irinotecan (CPT-11)
etoposide	vinorelbine
vincristine	gemcitabine
vindesine	
nitrosoureas	
cisplatin	
carboplatin	

In some randomized trials, induction chemotherapy regimens containing etoposide yielded slightly superior survival compared to regimens without etoposide.[19,20] In direct comparisons to CAV, however, cisplatin and etoposide (EP) failed to demonstrate a clear survival advantage in patients with extensive-stage disease.[21,22] Thus the choice of induction therapy is usually dictated by a patient's coexisting medical problems. For example, even though the EP regimen has a favorable therapeutic index, it may be contraindicated in an individual with renal dysfunction or a preexisting neuropathy (e.g., diabetic neuropathy). Preexisting heart disease also may make it impossible to administer cisplatin because of the requirement for intravenous hydration. In such circumstances, carboplatin represents an acceptable alternative to cisplatin because it is not nephrotoxic nor is it considered cardiotoxic.[23–26] Likewise, doxorubicin may be contraindicated in a patient with preexisting heart disease. In such circumstances, a combination regimen such as cyclophosphamide, etoposide, and vincristine may be preferable.

Toxicity to Combination Chemotherapy

All chemotherapy regimens used to treat SCLC are associated with host toxicities.[7,27] The most common complication of combination chemotherapy is severe myelosuppression, which occurs in 25% to 30% of patients treated with chemotherapy alone and in up to 75% of patients receiving combined modality treatment.[28,29] Culture-positive infections, however, develop in fewer than 5% of patients and fatal infections occur in less than 2%.[29] Other lethal side effects are extremely uncommon. Cyclophosphamide-based therapy is usually associated with the highest incidence of neutropenia, whereas cisplatin plus etoposide generally represents the least myelosuppressive regimen.[2,30,31] With moderate-dose cisplatin (80 mg/m^2) and etoposide (80 mg/m^2 per day for 3 days), life-threatening neutropenia develops in fewer than 5% of patients.[31]

The recent availability of hematopoietic growth factors (discussed following) has tended to make physicians more sanguine about myelosuppression. However, hematopoietic growth factors must be used judiciously because in selected circumstances, such as when given concomitantly with irradiation, they have proved detrimental.[32] Also, prophylactic antibiotics have not been adequately studied but appear to be effective for the prevention of fever during neutropenia and are considerably less costly.[33–36]

The incidence of gastrointestinal side effects varies, although nausea, emesis, esophagitis, and mucositis are relatively common, especially with cisplatin-based therapy or with combined modality programs. The availability of 5-HT, blocking agents can minimize or ameliorate many of the latter complications.[37] Late-developing complications related to chemotherapy also occur and include pulmonary fibrosis, cardiac toxicity, and second malignancies.[29,38] Second malignancies that are treatment related need to be distinguished from second primary malignancies, which are extremely common in long-term survivors of SCLC.[39–41] Neurotoxicities including mild dementia, ataxia, memory loss, and other neurologic abnormalities have been reported in patients who received prophylactic cranial irradiation, although the exact relationship to this therapeutic intervention has not been well characterized.[42–45]

Although considerable progress has been achieved in the overall management of SCLC, cure remains elusive for the most patients. Considering that fewer than 10% of extensive-stage patients survive beyond 2 years and no more than 15% to 25% of limited-stage patients are alive 5 years after diagnosis, new therapeutic approaches are clearly needed. The discovery of new agents with novel mechanisms of action is important in this regard but so is maximizing the benefits of currently available agents. The lack of curative potential of existing chemotherapy regimens is primarily related to the presence of drug resistance *ab initio* or possibly due to the emergence of drug resistance during chemotherapy administration. Treatment strategies employed to overcome drug resistance have dominated clinical research in SCLC for the past decade and include the following approaches: dose intensification, weekly chemotherapy, and alternating non–cross-resistant chemotherapy.

Dose Intensification

In preclinical tumor models, one of the simplest methods used to overcome drug resistance is drug dose escalation. This approach has been successfully used in a wide variety of murine malignancies, including leukemias and solid tumors.[46] With this knowledge, Cohen and colleagues undertook a randomized trial in the late 1970s, in which SCLC patients were randomized to receive standard dosages of cyclophosphamide, methotrexate, and lomustine or higher dose cyclophosphamide, lomustine, and standard-dose methotrexate.[47] These investigators observed both a higher overall response rate and a prolonged survival in the high-dose chemotherapy group. Furthermore, long-term survivors were observed only among those patients given high-dose chemotherapy. By today's standards, the high-dose regimen used by Cohen and his colleagues would be considered relatively modest. Nevertheless, this trial spawned a series of studies aimed at overcoming drug resistance through dose escalation.

High-Dose Induction Chemotherapy

Several randomized trials have tested the concept of high-dose induction therapy in SCLC (Table 53.2).[9,30,31,48–50] Based on pilot data demonstrating the feasibility of high-dose induction therapy,[51] the Southeast Cancer Study Group (SECSG) undertook a prospective study in which patients with extensive-stage SCLC were randomized to receive either high-dose CAV for the initial three cycles of therapy or standard-dose CAV.[30] No dose attenuation was allowed during the initial three cycles of therapy. Patients received a mean of ≥95% of the planned dosages of cyclophosphamide and doxorubicin during the first three treatment cycles, resulting in a 15% and 67% dose escalation of each drug, respectively. Although the complete remission rate was higher in the high-dose arm (22% and 12%; P < 0.05), overall response rates (63% and 53%) and median survival duration (29.3 weeks and 34.7 weeks) were not significantly different between the two treatment groups. Moreover, the high-dose CAV regimen was substantially more toxic, with a large percentage of patients experiencing life-threatening toxicities (grade 4 neutropenia: 79% and 40%; P < 0.05). Virtually identical results were reported by Figueredo et al. in a Canadian trial.[49]

Hong and associates randomized both limited and extensive-stage SCLC patients to high-dose cyclophosphamide (2,000 mg/m^2) plus vincristine (CV), standard-dose CAV, or standard-dose etoposide plus cyclophosphamide and vin-

cristine (CEV).[19] A total of 353 patients were studied. In limited-stage patients the complete response rates and median survivals for dose-intensive CV, standard-dose CAV, and standard-dose CEV were 31% and 41 weeks, 42% and 55 weeks, and 38% and 58 weeks, respectively. The median survival duration for all patients was superior in the standard-dose CEV arm (P = 0.01). The inclusion of etoposide in the CEV regimen may have been more important for efficacy than the strategy aimed at overcoming drug resistance.

More recently, Ihde et al. compared standard-dose etoposide (80 mg/m^2 per day for 3 days) plus cisplatin (80 mg/m^2 day 1) to high-dose etoposide (80 mg/m^2 per day for 5 days) plus cisplatin (27 mg/m^2 per day for 5 days).[31] Both regimens were administered every 21 days. The degree of myelosuppression with high-dose therapy was approximately twice that observed with the standard-dose regimen. However, there was no difference in response rates (85% and 81%), median survival (12 months and 11 months) or one-year survival rates (50% and 46%). It is particularly noteworthy that the incidence of grade 4 myelosuppression was just 2% in the standard-dose arm and more than 25% in the high-dose arm. These figures are considerably less than that generally reported for cyclophosphamide-based chemotherapy regimens.

Preclinical studies indicate that a survival benefit may not be observed until the dose of an active agent is increased two-fold or more.[46] Furthermore, the most convincing evidence for a survival benefit to dose intensification in animal model experiments comes from models with curative potential.[52] A two-fold dose intensity increase is not easily achieved in clinical oncology without some type of stem cell support. However, limited-stage SCLC is a curable entity, and efforts to exploit any biological or clinical advantage to dose intensification might better be pursued in this

TABLE 53.2. RANDOMIZED TRIALS OF HIGH-DOSE VERSUS CONVENTIONAL-DOSE CHEMOTHERAPY

Reference	Regimen[a]	Patient Number	Overall Response	Median Survival	One-Year Survival
Hande[48]	cd MCDVEH	21	67%	9 mos	10%[b]
	hd MCDVEH	21	74%	9 mos	7%[b]
Figuerdo[49]	cd CDV	51	61%	7 mos[c]	–
	hd CDV	52	71%	9 mos[c]	–
Johnson[20]	cd CDV	174	53%	34.7 wks	20%
	hd CDV	124	63%	29.3 wks	20%
Ihde[31]	cd PE	46	83%	10.7 mos	48%
	hd PE	44	86%	11.4 mos	45%
Arriagada[50]	cd PCDE	50[d]	54%[e]	14 mos	26%[f]
	hd PCDE	55[d]	67%[e]	18 mos	43%[f]

M, Methotrexate; C, cyclophospamide; D, doxorubibin; V, vincristine; E, etoposide; H, hexamethylmelamine; P, cisplatin.
[a] cd, Conventional-dose; hd, high-dose.
[b] Survival at 18 months.
[c] Median duration of response.
[d] All patients limited stage.
[e] Complete remission rate.
[f] Survival at 24 months.

patient subset. Arriagada and colleagues did a retrospective analysis of 131 consecutively treated limited-stage SCLC patients and observed a survival benefit for patients who received higher initial doses of cyclophosphamide and cisplatin.[53,54] Based on this observation, they undertook a phase III trial, in which limited-stage patients were randomly assigned to receive either conventional-dose cisplatin, cyclophosphamide, etoposide, and doxorubicin alternating with thoracic radiotherapy, or the identical treatment regimen except 20% higher doses of cyclophosphamide and cisplatin were given in the first treatment cycle only.[50] The complete response rate (67% versus 54%, p = 0.16) and two-year survival (43% versus 26%, p = 0.02) were superior in the dose-intensive group.

A more recent report by Stewart and colleagues also suggests that dose intensification might effect superior survival outcomes in early-stage patients.[55] These investigators enrolled patients with "good- or intermediate-prognosis" SCLC to a prospective multicenter study that involved a 2 × 2 factorial design, randomizing patients to conventional versus dose-intensified V-ICE chemotherapy (vincristine, ifosfamide, carboplatin, etoposide). Patients were randomly assigned to receive identical doses of all four drugs on either an every-three-week or every-four-week schedule. Both treatment groups were then randomized to receive either granulocyte-macrophage colony-stimulating factor (GM-CSF) or no growth factor support. Eligibility required that patients be classified as good- or intermediate-prognosis as defined by Cerny and colleagues.[50] One hundred and seventy eight of three hundred patients (59%) had limited-stage disease. Although there were greater proportions of limited-stage patients and patients with more favorable prognostic scores in the dose-intensive group, these differences were not statistically significant. The addition of GM-CSF neither reduced the incidence of complications from myelosuppression nor improved survival. However, patients in the three-week treatment arm experienced statistically superior median and two-year survivals (443 versus 351 days and 33% versus 18%, respectively).

The dose-intensive patients from the Arriagada and Steward trials experienced two-year survival rates of 43% and 33%, respectively. Although the treatment regimens varied significantly between the two trials, an indirect estimate of the relative dose intensity of the two regimens can be made by comparing the incidence of dose-limiting toxicity, that being grade IV neutropenia—59% and 65%, respectively. Turrisi and colleagues recently described the highest long-term survival rates ever observed in a multicenter phase III trial in limited-stage SCLC.[17] Patients were treated with etoposide and cisplatin and concurrent thoracic radiotherapy either by a conventional once-daily or a twice-daily schedule. For the entire patient group, the two-year survival rate was 44% and the grade IV neutropenia rate was 63%, results almost identical to those observed in the dose-intensive patients from the Arriagada and Steward trials.

The control regimens used in the latter trials effected grade IV neutropenia rates of only 23% (cycle 1 only) and 49%, respectively. The dose intensity of these regimens might better be considered suboptimal rather than standard. Therefore, dosing initial chemotherapy below the maximally tolerated dose of a given regimen might be detrimental in limited-stage SCLC.

It is safe to conclude that dose intensification of induction therapy is not beneficial to patients with extensive-stage disease. Optimal therapy for limited-stage disease should include doses at or near the maximal tolerated doses of the induction regimen. Compromising dose intensity in these patients may negatively impact long-term survival rates. Whether a survival benefit can be derived by intensifying induction therapy beyond the maximally tolerated doses of conventional outpatient therapy is unknown at this time and is a reasonable area for continued investigation in limited-stage patients.

Weekly Chemotherapy

As described in the preceding section, Steward and colleagues were able to effect a significant improvement in median survival in good- or immediate-prognosis SCLC patients by decreasing the treatment interval from 4 to 3 weeks. This success suggests that increasing dose intensity by more frequent dosing might be beneficial. This may be even better achieved with weekly chemotherapy using standard chemotherapy doses but alternating between myelosuppressive and nonmyelosuppressive agents. Early pilot trials testing this approach have produced promising results, leading to several phase III trials comparing weekly chemotherapy to conventional regimens (Table 53.3).[57–60] The European Organization for Research and Treatment of Lung Cancer (EORTC) conducted a large phase III study comparing a weekly multidrug chemotherapy regimen (doxorubicin, etoposide, cyclophosphamide, cisplatin, vindesine, vincristine, and methotrexate) to a standard chemotherapy regimen (cyclophosphamide, doxorubicin, and etoposide) administered every three weeks.[57] Both limited- and extensive-stage patients were enrolled. Although the response rate in the weekly regimen was higher in limited-stage patients, there was no difference in overall response rate, median survival, and two-year survival. The total relative dose-intensity for the drugs common to both regimens was significantly less in the weekly chemotherapy arm due to frequent treatment delays.

Souhami et al. reporting for the Cancer Research Campaign of the United Kingdom, also found no survival benefit when they compared a weekly multidrug regimen to a standard every-three-week approach.[58] In the U.K. trial, 438 patients with either limited disease or "good prognosis" extensive disease were randomized to receive 12 weekly cycles of ifosfamide and doxorubicin alternating weekly with cisplatin and etoposide or 6 cycles of CAV alternating every

TABLE 53.3. RANDOMIZED TRIALS OF WEEKLY VERSUS EVERY-THREE-WEEK CHEMOTHERAPY

Reference	Regimen	Patient Number	Overall Response %	Median Survival	Two-Year Survival %
Sculier[57]	Weekly[a]	98	69	49 wks	8.5
	Every 3 weeks[b]	101	62	43 wks	7.9
Souhami[59]	Weekly[c]	221	82.3	10.8 mos	11.8
	Every 3 weeks[d]	217	81.1	10.6 mos	11.7
Murray[59]	CODE	110	87	0.98 yrs	10[e]
	CAV/EP	109	70	0.91 yrs	10[e]
Furuse[60]	CODE, GCSF	114	84	11.6 mos	8.5
	CAV/EP	113	77	10.9 mos	12

[a] Doxorubicin, etoposide, cyclophosphamide, cisplatin, vindesine, vincristine, methotrexate.
[b] Cyclophosphamide, doxorubicin, etoposide.
[c] Ifosfamide, doxorubicin alternating with cisplatin, etoposide.
[d] Cyclophosphamide, doxorubicin, vincristine alternating with cisplatin and etoposide.
[e] Progression-free survival.

3 weeks with EP. Thoracic irradiation was administered only to limited-stage patients in complete or partial response. There were no reported differences in overall response rates (82.3% and 81.1%), median survival (10.8 months and 10.6 months) or two-year survival rates (11.8% and 11.7%). Hematologic toxicity was greater in the weekly chemotherapy arm and the ratio of intended-to-delivered dose intensity was greater in the standard arm. In both trials the chemotherapeutic agents differed between the two treatment arms. Although the ability to deliver full intended doses was superior in the standard regimens, it was not possible to directly compare dose intensity between the regimens.

Canadian investigators reported promising results from a pilot study of a weekly regimen referred to as CODE: cisplatin (25 mg/m^2 for 9 consecutive weeks); vincristine (1 mg/m^2 weeks 1, 2, 4, 6, 8); doxorubicin (40 mg/m^2 weeks 1, 3, 5, 7, 9); and etoposide (80 mg/m^2 days 1–3, weeks 1, 3, 5, 7, 9).[61] Excluding cyclophosphamide, the CODE regimen contained the same agents and same total cumulative doses as the conventional alternating CAV/EP regimen, but therapy was completed in 9 rather than 18 weeks. Thoracic and prophylactic cranial radiation therapy were also given to selected patients. These investigators were able to deliver close to full intended doses, thus effecting an increase in dose intensity of approximately twofold for the four drugs common to the two regimens. A two-year survival rate of 30% was observed, far superior to the historical rate of less than 10% in extensive-stage patients.

National Cancer Institute (NCI) Canada and Southwest Oncology Group (SWOG) collaborated on a phase III trial comparing CODE to conventional alternating CAV/EP in patients with extensive-stage SCLC.[59] Greater than 70% of intended doses were delivered for both regimens. CODE patients received slightly higher cumulative doses of each of the four common agents but completed their therapy in just 9 weeks rather than the 18 weeks received by the control

patients. Therefore, a twofold increase in the dose intensity of the four common agents was achieved. Although rates of neutropenia and fever were similar, 10 of 110 CODE patients versus 1 of 109 CAV/EP patients died during chemotherapy. Response rates were higher for the CODE patients, but progression-free and overall survival were not statistically different. In view of the increased mortality and similar efficacy, CODE was not recommended.

In the Canadian pilot and intergroup phase III trials, CODE patients received aggressive supportive care but were not routinely treated with prophylactic colony stimulating factor. Japanese investigators conducted a small randomized trial of CODE with or without G-CSF in patients with extensive-stage SCLC.[62] Use of G-CSF resulted in increased mean total received dose intensity for all drugs, reduced neutropenia and neutropenic fever, and a significant improvement in survival. This finding led to a phase III trial designed almost identical to that of the NCI Canada/SWOG trial.[60] Two hundred and twenty-seven patients with extensive-stage SCLC were randomized to receive either CODE plus G-CSF or conventional alternating CAV/EP. CODE patients received G-CSF on nontreatment days. The achieved dose intensity for CODE plus G-CSF was twice that of the CAV/EP regimen. The incidence of leukopenia was not different, but anemia and thrombocytopenia were significantly increased in the CODE plus G-CSF patients. The incidence of neutropenic fever was 18.8% versus 8.8% of patients in the CODE plus G-CSF and CAV/EP arms, respectively, and 4/114 (3.5%) of CODE plus G-CSF patients died from therapy-related causes. The response rate was slightly higher (77% versus 84%) in the CODE plus G-CSF arm, but there was no survival difference. Although dose-intensive weekly therapy has not been well tested in limited-stage patients, this approach has failed to effect any benefit for patients with extensive-stage disease.

Colony-Stimulating Factors

As outlined in the preceding sections, the addition of a colony-stimulating factor (CSF) allowed for dose intensification of the V-ICE and CODE regimens.[55,62] Decreasing the dosing interval of V-ICE improved survival, but the addition of GM-CSF had no independent impact on this outcome. The initial Japanese CODE plus G-CSF trial reported by Fukuoka and colleagues was designed to address dose intensity as the primary end point rather than survival. Therefore, only 63 patients were accrued, but median survival was superior for patients who received G-CSF (59 versus 32 weeks, p = 0.0004). Several phase III trials have investigated the impact of CSFs on SCLC chemotherapy (Table 53.4).[32,55,62–68] The primary end point of most trials was the incidence of neutropenia and associated sequelae. Most were not designed to directly address the relationship between dose intensity and therapeutic outcomes. As described previously, Steward and colleagues were able to increase dose intensity by adding GM-CSF to the dosing regimen.[55] Likewise, when Woll and colleagues added G-CSF to the V-ICE regimen, they were able to increase dose intensity, but the trial was not powered to accurately address survival end points.[67] Pujol and colleagues treated 125 patients with extensive-stage SCLC with either a dose-intensive regimen containing high doses of cyclophosphamide, epidoxorubicin, etoposide, and cisplatin plus GM-CSF or the same chemotherapy at conventional doses without GM-CSF.[63] In this attempt to improve survival by increasing dose intensity with the aid of GM-CSF, these investigators reported decreased dose intensity, worse hematologic toxicities, and inferior median survival (10.8 versus 8.9 months, p = 0.0005) for the high-dose chemotherapy/GM-CSF treated patients.

The Pujol data further corroborate the overwhelming evidence that attempting to intensify chemotherapy for extensive-stage patients is not beneficial and may be harmful.

However, the Arriagada and V-ICE data suggest that dose intensification might be beneficial in limited-stage patients. Although the previously cited trial by Woll and colleagues was not designed to address a primary survival end point, they did demonstrate a statistically significant increase in two-year survival (32% versus 15%) in primarily limited-stage patients receiving dose-intensified V-ICE plus G-CSF. Median survival was not improved (69 versus 65 weeks). Bunn and colleagues conducted a phase III trial in 230 limited-stage SCLC patients to determine whether GM-CSF could be used to reduce the incidence of neutropenic fever and hematologic toxicities of combined chemoradiotherapy.[32] All patients initially received etoposide 80 mg/m^2 and cisplatin 40 mg/m^2 days 1–3. Thoracic radiotherapy consisted of 45 Gy total delivered in 25 daily fractions of 1.8 Gy, 5 days per week given simultaneously with the chemotherapy over the first 5 weeks. GM-CSF was dosed at 250 μg/m^2 subcutaneously twice daily on days 4–18 of each cycle of therapy. There was a statistically significant increase in the frequency and duration of life-threatening thrombocytopenia (p < 0.001), more nonhematologic toxicity, more days of hospitalization, a higher incidence of intravenous antibiotic usage, more transfusions, and more toxic deaths in the patients receiving GM-CSF. There was no significant difference in median survival.

In summary, the addition of CSFs to chemotherapy in patients with SCLC can reduce the incidence of hematologic side effects if chemotherapy is given at conventional doses. Chemotherapy dose escalation or the addition of concurrent radiotherapy to CSFs has resulted in increased toxicity and death rates in some studies. Considering the expense and inconveniences of CSFs, the apparent lack of benefit from dose intensification, and the intolerability of concurrent use with radiotherapy, the routine use of these agents in the management of SCLC cannot be recommended. Indeed, recent pharmacoeconomic analyses have concluded

TABLE 53.4. RANDOMIZED TRIALS OF CHEMOTHERAPY WITH AND WITHOUT COLONY STIMULATING FACTORS (CSF) IN SCLC

Reference	CSF	LD/ED	Attempt ↑ DI*	Effect on DI	Effect on Toxicity	Effect on Median Survival
Pujol[53]	GM	ED	yes	decreased	increased	decreased
Steward[55]	GM	59% LD	yes	increased	none	none
Fukuoka[62]	G	ED	no	increased	decreased	increased
Bunn[32]	GM	LD	no	decreased	increased	none
Hamm[64]	GM	both	no	increased	↓ neutropenia ↑ thrombocytopenia	none
Miles[65]	G	both	no	none	decreased	none
Crawford[66]	G	both	no	N.A.	decreased	none
Trillet-Lenoir[68]	G	both	no	increased	decreased	none
Woll[67]	G	92% LD	yes	increased	increased deaths	none

DI, Dose intensity; G, granulocyte colony stimulating factor; GM, granulocyte macrophage stimulating factor; LD, limited disease; ED, extensive disease.
* An attempt was made to either increase doses or dose frequency in the CSF patients.
N.A., not available.

that despite a decrease in hematologic toxicity in most trials, the routine use of CSFs in SCLC is not justified by clinical benefits, improved patient comfort, or economic considerations.[34-36]

Late-Intensification Chemotherapy

Of the dose-intensification strategies discussed thus far, only the CODE regimen effects a ≥ two-fold increase in dose intensity. Some type of hematopoeitic stem cell support is needed to intensify therapy further. Late intensification has both scientific and clinical appeal.[69,70] Because SCLC patients are often ill at the time of presentation, they are often poor candidates for highly aggressive approaches. Patients are generally in better medical condition to be considered for high-dose therapy following induction. Consolidating with high-dose therapy also allows for the prospective identification and selection of patients who are most likely to benefit—those with limited-stage disease, good performance status, and those who obtained a major remission with induction chemoradiotherapy.[70] This approach has been studied by several investigators albeit rarely in a randomized trial. Humblet and colleagues reported the results of the only published multicenter randomized study testing late-intensification chemotherapy in patients responding well to induction therapy.[71] Autologous bone marrow transplantation was used to rescue patients from hematologic toxicities. Of 101 patients receiving standard induction chemotherapy, 45 patients with chemotherapy-sensitive disease were randomized to receive one additional cycle of either high-dose cyclophosphamide, carmustine (BCNU), and etoposide or conventional doses of the same drugs. In this highly selected group of patients, median overall survival after induction therapy was 68 weeks for the intensified group compared to 55 weeks for the conventional therapy group, a difference that is not statistically significant (P = 0.13).

In a large phase II study, SWOG treated 58 limited-stage SCLC patients with induction chemoradiotherapy followed by high-dose cyclophosphamide (150 mg/kg) intensification and autologous bone marrow rescue.[72] Only 21 patients completed the entire course of therapy, and seven treatment-related deaths occurred, four of which occurred during late-intensification chemotherapy. Median survival for all patients was 11.1 months. Nine of the twenty-one patients receiving late intensification were alive in complete remission with a median survival of 27 months.

Dana Farber Cancer Center investigators employed high-dose consolidation chemotherapy in patients with limited-stage SCLC in partial or complete remission following conventional first-line chemotherapy.[73] Patients received cumulative doses of 5,625 mg/m^2 cyclophosphamide, 165 mg/m^2 cisplatin, and 480 mg/m^2 carmustine followed by thoracic and prophylactic cranial irradiation. Of the 36 patients treated in this phase II trial, 29 of whom were in

complete or near complete remission before high-dose therapy, 14 remained disease free at a median of 21 months (range: 40–139) after treatment. Actuarial two- and five-year disease-free survival rates were 53% and 41%, respectively. Morbidity was relatively low and most patients were able to return to full-time work. Although the results of this trial are provocative, patients were highly selected and were accrued over a nine-year period. Furthermore, the median age of patients entered into this trial was 49 years, which is several years below the typical average age of SCLC patients. There are few reports of similarly selected patients from which historical control data can be derived and compared. However, the SECSG reported a phase III trial involving a similar subset of selected patients.[74] Patients with limited-stage SCLC were randomly assigned to receive either six cycles of induction chemotherapy with CAV or the same therapy with concurrent radiotherapy. Good performance status patients who had achieved an objective remission at the end of induction therapy were randomized to receive two cycles of consolidation etoposide and cisplatin or no further therapy. Twenty-six patients had received induction chemotherapy and radiotherapy and consolidation with etoposide and cisplatin. From the time of consolidation therapy initiation, these patients achieved a two-year survival rate of 55%, almost identical to the results reported by the Dana Farber group. There are too few data to draw any conclusions about the utility of high-dose consolidation therapy in limited-disease SCLC, but this approach should be considered experimental at this time. The Cancer and Leukemia Group B (CALGB) is now testing the Dana Farber regimen in a multicenter setting.

Dose-intensive induction therapy, weekly chemotherapy, attempts to intensify with CSFs, and high-dose consolidation therapy have all failed to show a convincing survival benefit for patients with SCLC. Intensification of therapy beyond that of conventional regimens has been mostly harmful to patients with extensive-stage disease, and there are no indications that dose intensification in these patients will be beneficial even if advances in supportive care are achieved. The available data suggest that limited-stage patients might benefit from dose intensification. Two randomized trials suggest that administration of combined modality therapy below the maximum tolerated dose (MTD) of conventional outpatient regimens might be detrimental, but no data suggest that intensifying beyond this level is beneficial. The utility of early- and late-intensification therapy for limited-stage SCLC is still not well addressed and remains an area of important research, especially as active new mechanism agents are identified and supportive care is improved.

ALTERNATING NON–CROSS-RESISTANT CHEMOTHERAPY

Theoretically, to obtain optimal antitumor effects, multiple active agents should be administered simultaneously at their optimal single-agent dose. However, because drug toxicities often overlap, strict adherence to this approach is often not possible in the clinical setting. Using mathematical modeling, Goldie and Coldman suggested that alternating two non–cross-resistant chemotherapy regimens of relatively comparable efficacy could potentially minimize the development of drug resistance while avoiding excessive host toxicity. The strategy of alternating two comparably effective chemotherapy regimens was empirically tested in SCLC in the late 1970s and was more rigorously studied in the 1980s following the publications of Goldie and Coldman (Table 53.5).[21,22,75–80] Most of the more recently conducted trials compared CAV to CAV alternating with EP. Because CAV and EP are both highly active against SCLC and contain compounds from divergent drug classes, integrating both combinations into an alternating non–cross-resistant regimen is appealing. Unfortunately, CAV and EP are not entirely non–cross-resistant. In CAV failures, EP generally effects response rates between 40% to 50%. Conversely, CAV is generally ineffective in EP failures, typically inducing objective remissions in less than 15% of patients.[21,22,81,82]

The National Cancer Institute in Canada (NCIC) reported the results of a prospective randomized study in patients with extensive-disease SCLC comparing conventional cyclophosphamide (1,000mg/m^2), doxorubicin (50 mg/m^2), and vincristine (2 mg) (CAV) given every 3 weeks for six cycles to CAV alternating with etoposide (100 mg/m^2 per day for 3 days) and cisplatin (25 mg/m^2 per day for 3 days) (EP) every 3 weeks for a total of six cycles (Table 53.5).[80] The overall response rate was modestly superior for the alternating regimen (80% versus 63%; p < 0.002), as was the overall survival (9.6 versus 8.0 months; p = 0.03). Although alternating therapy was statistically superior in this trial, this outcome might have been more related to the inclusion of EP in the regimen rather than the alternating design. In a similar study, the SECSG compared EP, CAV, and alternating EP and CAV in extensive-disease patients.[22] Response rates and survival were virtually identical for all

three regimens. The NCI tested this approach in patients with limited-disease SCLC.[79] Patients were randomized between two induction regimens—either alternating CAV/EP or sequential therapy with three cycles of CAV followed by the same number of cycles of EP. Chemotherapy was followed by radiotherapy in responding patients. Again, no significant differences in therapeutic outcomes were observed between the two arms. The authors concluded that either the differences between the two schedules were too small to detect an advantage for the alternating regimen, or EP is actually a superior regimen and any schedule that includes these drugs produces superior results.

Recently, the EORTC reported a trial testing two relatively non–cross-resistant regimens: CDE (cyclophosphamide, doxorubicin, etoposide) and VIMP (vincristine, carboplatin, ifosfamide, mesna).[83] Previously, they demonstrated that treatment of patients failing therapy with one regimen experienced response rates ≥50% when treated with the other.[84] Patients with extensive-stage SCLC were randomly assigned to receive either a maximum of five courses of CDE or five courses of alternating therapy, in which they received CDE cycles 1, 3, and 5 and VIMP cycles 2 and 4. The trial was designed to detect an increase in median survival from 9.2 months to 12 months. Although 360 patients were required to address the planned survival end point with a power of 80% and a significance level of 5%, only 148 patients were accrued. Median survival was 7.6 and 8.7 months for the standard versus the alternating arms, respectively (p = 0.243). Although an inadequate number of patients were accrued to this trial to accurately detect a small median survival advantage, these results suggest there is no major benefit to alternating therapy with conventional agents even when a significant lack of cross-resistance has been demonstrated.

Although the previous EORTC experience demonstrated a relative lack of cross-resistance between the CDE and VIMP regimens, there are no highly active salvage therapies for patients with resistant SCLC (discussed following). A better testing of the Goldie Coldman hypothesis awaits identification of truly active and more significantly non–cross-resistant agents and regimens.

TABLE 53.5. ALTERNATING NON–CROSS-RESISTANT CHEMOTHERAPY PHASE III TRIALS

Reference	Pt. No.	Chemo.	MS (Mos)	P-Value
Evans[20]	289	CAV	8.0	
		CAV/PE	9.6	0.03
Fukuoka[21]	142	CAV	8.7	
		EP	8.3	
		CAV/EP	9.0	0.898
Roth[22]	437	CAV	8.6	
		EP	8.3	
		CAV/EP	8.1	0.425
Postmus[83]	143	CDE	7.6	
		CDE/VIMP*	8.7	0.243

C, Cytoxan; A, doxorubicin; V, vincristine; E, etoposide; P, cisplatin; I, ifosfamide; M, MESNA; P*, carboplatin.

SINGLE-AGENT AND CHRONIC ORAL ETOPOSIDE

Ever since large cooperative group studies conducted in the 1970s demonstrated the superiority of combination chemotherapy over single-agent cyclophosphamide, research efforts have concentrated on combination regimens. Unfortunately, most strategies for improving combination chemotherapy have been unfruitful. Coincident with the conduction of the numerous trials focusing on dose-intensification of combination therapy, single-agent etoposide trials were yielding response rates and survival durations rivaling those of the most active combination regimens. Furthermore, these favorable results were often obtained in patients with advanced age or who were considered medically unfit for combination regimens. When etoposide became available as a soft gelatin capsule, chronic oral regimens were studied and yielded surprising activity in chemotherapy-naïve and recurrent patients alike.[85-87]

Slevin and colleagues treated chemotherapy-naïve extensive-disease SCLC patients with single-agent etoposide either as a single 500 mg/m^2 24-hour infusion or by a 100 mg/m^2 2-hour infusion for 5 consecutive days.[88] In this randomized study in which the etoposide schedule was the only variable, 89% of patients in the five-day treatment arm versus 10% of patients in the one-day treatment arm achieved an objective response to therapy. Pharmacokinetic measurements were performed, and the total exposure to etoposide, as expressed by area under the concentration versus time curve, was equivalent for both regimens. However, patients receiving the five-day schedule maintained a plasma etoposide level greater than 1 μg/ml for approximately twice the duration as did patients receiving the one-day treatment. The authors concluded that the prolonged maintenance of very low drug concentrations (1 μg/ml) was more important than achieving high peak concentrations. Furthermore, the prolonged maintenance of high drug concentrations was inversely related to antitumor effect; the duration of etoposide blood concentrations greater than 10 μg/ml was greater in the less effective one-day treatment arm. The correlation between the key drug levels characterized in this pharmacokinetic study and those determined in the preclinical cellular studies is remarkable.[89]

In the late 1980s etoposide became available as a 50 mg soft gelatin capsule. A phase I study conducted by investigators at Vanderbilt University led to a recommended phase II regimen of 50 mg/m^2 per day for 21 days of oral etoposide.[90] These same investigators then treated 22 patients with recurrent or refractory SCLC with this regimen.[85] All patients had received at least one prior combination regimen and 18 had received previous intravenous etoposide in combination with other agents. There were two complete and eight partial antitumor responses for an overall response rate of 46%. Prior etoposide exposure did not appear to influence response. However, patients who responded well to induction chemotherapy and those who had been off chemotherapy for more than 90 days prior to disease progression were more likely to respond. Median duration of response was 4 months and median survival was 5 months (range: 1–15 months). The activity of this regimen in recurrent SCLC was confirmed by a group from Indiana University in an even more heavily pretreated patient cohort.[86] Although modest, these results rival those of the most active, multiagent "salvage" regimens used in relapsed SCLC.

Clark and colleagues employed a different regimen of chronic oral etoposide (50 mg total dose, twice daily for 14 consecutive days) in chemotherapy-naïve patients who were

$\geq$70 years old and/or who were considered medically unfit for standard combination regimens.[87] An objective response rate of 80% and median survival duration of 8.0 months were observed. Despite the advanced age of the patients and a mean Karnofsky performance status of only 60%, these therapeutic outcomes rival those of the most active combination regimens, the activity of which is generally determined in patients with more favorable prognoses. Not only was this regimen highly active, but it also appeared less toxic than the 50 mg/m^2 per day given for 21 days and substantially less toxic than standard combination regimens such as EP and CAV. Similar results have been obtained in chemotherapy-naïve SCLC patients treated with five-day administration of intravenous or oral etoposide.[91,92]

The early trials of single-agent and chronic oral etoposide indicated that activity was similar to and perhaps even superior to conventional combination chemotherapy. It also appeared to have a more favorable toxicity profile and a lack of cross-resistance with conventional chemotherapy, including the three-day etoposide and cisplatin regimen. It appeared to be superior therapy for elderly and medically unfit patients, and there was reason to believe that integration of chronic low-dose etoposide into combination regimens might lead to therapeutic gains. Unfortunately, none of these characteristics has been confirmed in phase III trials (Table 53.6).[93-95]

The first randomized trial testing the efficacy of chronic oral etoposide in SCLC was reported by SWOG in 1995.[93] Patients with chemotherapy-naïve extensive-stage SCLC were randomized to receive conventional etoposide 130 mg/m^2 per day and cisplatin 25 mg/m^2 per day on days 1–3 versus oral etoposide 50 mg/m^2 per day for 21 days plus cisplatin 33 mg/m^2 days 1–3. The intravenous regimen was given every 3 weeks for eight cycles and the oral regimen was given every 4 weeks for a total of six cycles. Three hundred six patients were accrued. There were no differences in response rates and median survival, but hematologic toxicity was greater in the patients receiving chronic oral etoposide. Although the SWOG investigators may have been using the more toxic of the chronic oral etoposide regimens, the complete lack of any therapeutic advantage makes further development of this approach undesirable.

The SWOG chose to test oral etoposide in combination with cisplatin, but phase II trial results suggested that oral etoposide alone might be as active as conventional combination regimens and substantially less toxic. The Medical Research Council Lung Cancer Working Party conducted a randomized phase III trial comparing single-agent etoposide, 50 mg twice daily for 10 consecutive days on a three-week schedule, to a standard intravenous regimen of etoposide and vincristine or cyclophosphamide, doxorubicin, and vincristine.[94] Three hundred thirty-nine chemotherapy-naïve patients with poor performance status (World Health Organization grade 2–4) were accrued. The primary end point was palliation of major symptoms at 3 months after

TABLE 53.6. RANDOMIZED TRIALS TESTING ORAL ETOPOSIDE IN SCLC

Reference	Patient No.	Toxicity/QOL	Patient Selection	Treatment Arms*	Median Survival
Miller[93]	306	hematological toxicity	PS 0–2	Oral E + P	no diff.
				EP	greater ES
MRCLC[94]	339	greater hematological toxicity	PS 2–4	Oral E	130 dys
				EV or CAV	183 dys
Souham[95]	155	inferior symptom control	PS 2–3	Oral E	4.8 mos
				CAV/EP	5.9 mos

* Regimens are described in the text.
E, Etoposide; P, cisplatin; V, vincristine; C, cyclophosphamide; A, doxorubicin; PS, performance status; ES, extensive stage; QOL, quality of life.

randomization. The palliative effects of treatment were similar in the etoposide and control groups with 41% and 46% of patients, respectively, experiencing an improvement in their palliation score. Grade 2 or worse hematologic toxicity occurred in 29% of etoposide-treated patients and 21% of controls. Controls had a superior overall response rate (51% versus 45%) and a median survival advantage (130 versus 183 days, p = 0.03). These authors concluded that oral etoposide therapy was inferior to standard intravenous multidrug chemotherapy in the palliative setting and that oral etoposide should no longer be used in such patients. Souhami and colleagues reported similar results when they randomly assigned chemotherapy-naïve patients with performance status 2 or 3 to receive either five-day oral etoposide or conventional alternating CAV/EP.[95] After 155 patients were accrued, a planned interim analysis led to early study closure because the one-year survival rate, progression-free survival, overall response rate, symptom control, and quality of life were all inferior in the oral etoposide arm.

The experience with single-agent etoposide exemplifies the importance of randomized multicenter trials in the testing of new therapies in cancer patients. Single-agent therapy has no role in the management of chemotherapy-naïve patients. Chronic oral etoposide has not been extensively studied in the salvage setting and may still have a role in selected patients.

TREATMENT DURATION AND MAINTENANCE THERAPY

The optimal duration of induction chemotherapy for SCLC is not well defined. However, prolonged treatment is generally considered unnecessary because a survival advantage has not been demonstrated in randomized trials (Table 53.7).[96–103] In one randomized trial, 687 SCLC patients were treated with five cycles of cyclophosphamide, doxorubicin, and etoposide followed by randomization to seven additional cycles of the same chemotherapy or close follow-up alone.[98] No difference in overall survival or five-year survival was detected between the two treatment arms. Although progression-free survival duration was longer for patients given maintenance chemotherapy, patients not receiving maintenance therapy were more likely to respond to salvage chemotherapy, accounting for the similar survival outcome. Spiro and colleagues compared 4 versus 8 cycles of chemotherapy.[96] Within each treatment group, patients were also randomized to receive salvage chemotherapy at the time of disease progression or to receive no further therapy. Patients who received eight cycles of therapy with or without salvage chemotherapy did no better than patients who received four cycles of induction therapy and salvage therapy at the time of relapse. However, patients who received four cycles of induction therapy and no salvage therapy had an inferior median survival.

The Medical Research Council Lung Cancer Working Party has conducted sequential phase III trials addressing therapy duration. In the first trial, 497 SCLC patients received six courses of cyclophosphamide, methotrexate, etoposide, and vincristine.[97] Patients still in complete or partial remission at the end of six cycles were then randomized to an additional six cycles of the same regimen or to no further chemotherapy. No survival advantage was achieved with the longer duration of treatment, but maintenance therapy was associated with more toxicity and poorer quality of life. Their second trial attempted to reduce treatment duration even further and compared three to six treatment cycles. Patients were randomized at the beginning of therapy.[99,100] Three hundred six patients were accrued and no difference in overall survival, toxicity, or quality of life was observed. The authors concluded that a small advantage in median survival for the six-cycle regimen could not be ruled out, but there was no apparent advantage to treating patients beyond three cycles of therapy.

The results of the trials described in the previous paragraph along with the results obtained in other randomized trials indicate that an appropriate duration of induction treatment for SCLC is three to six cycles of a standard chemotherapy regimen (Table 53.7). A recently completed Eastern Cooperative Oncology Group/Research Treatment Oncology Group (ECOG/RTOG) trial in patients with limited disease conclusively demonstrates that prolonged

TABLE 53.7. PHASE III TRIALS ADDRESSING TREATMENT DURATION AND MAINTENANCE THERAPY

Reference	Pt. Number	ED/LD	Treatment	MS
Shevlin[103]	225	N.A.	EIMV × 3	307 dys
			EIMV × 6	313 dys
Bleehen[99]	265	both	ECMV × 3	39 wks
			ECMV × 6	(p = 0.27, log rank)
Bleehen[97]	306	both	ECMV × 6	7.4 mos
			ECMV × 12	8.6 mos
Spiro[96]	289	both	CEV × 4	38 wks
			CEV × 8	38–42 wks
Beith[101]	129	both	EP/RT × 4	52 wks
			EP/RT, VAC × 10	54 wks
Sculier[102]	84	both	induct × 6	38 wks
			same, EVds × 12	48 wks
				(p = 0.10)
Giaccone[98]**	434	both	CAE × 5	9.3 mos
			CAE × 12	9.3 mos

* Only patients with objective response to induction therapy were randomized to +/− maintenance therapy.
** Only patients with stable disease or better were randomized to +/− maintenance therapy.
E, Etoposide; I, ifosfamide; M, methotrexate; V, vincristine; C, cyclophosphamide; RT, radiotherapy; A, doxorubicin; Vds, vindesine; ED, extensive disease; LD, limited disease.

therapy duration is not necessary to achieve optimal therapeutic results.[17] Patients with limited-stage disease received just four cycles of cisplatin plus etoposide plus concomitant thoracic radiotherapy and achieved a median survival of more than 20 months and a two-year survival of more than 40%.

In extensive-stage patients, any of several different regimens administered for three to six courses represents adequate induction therapy. Maintenance chemotherapy or continuation of treatment beyond three to six cycles is unnecessary and more likely to produce toxicity than to extend survival or benefit quality of life provided treatment is reinstituted at the time of relapse.[96]

SALVAGE CHEMOTHERAPY

A majority of chemotherapy-treated SCLC patients eventually develop recurrent disease. Although many patients are in excellent physical condition at the time of relapse, few drugs or drug combinations are capable of effecting tumor regression in this setting. Ebi and colleagues from Japan studied 159 patients with SCLC who received first-line chemotherapy, of whom 123 (77%) were responders.[104] Of the responding patients, 88 relapsed and were eligible for salvage therapy. Forty-eight of the relapsed patients received salvage therapy, of whom sixteen (33%) achieved an objective response. These investigators found the following characteristics to be predictive of response to salvage therapy: (a) more than 90 days since completion of induction ther-

apy; (b) an induction therapy response duration of more than 270 days; (c) and a previous completed response (CR) to induction therapy. Performance status and extent of disease at presentation were not predictive of response to salvage therapy.

Several trials have demonstrated a correlation between the likelihood of response to salvage therapy and the treatment-free interval following induction therapy. Chute and colleagues reported a response rate of 56% in 20 patients treated with salvage therapy after surviving cancer free for ≥2 years after initial therapy.[105] In the Vanderbilt phase II chronic oral etoposide study, one of eight patients less than 90 days out from their previous therapy responded to oral etoposide, whereas 9 of 14 patients greater than 90 days since previous therapy responded.[85] Likewise, Giaccone and colleagues administered teniposide to 38 previously treated patients, most of whom had received previous cyclophosphamide, etoposide, and doxorubicin in various regimens.[106] Only 2 of 16 patients who had received chemotherapy ≤2.6 months prior to starting salvage therapy achieved an objective remission. On the other hand, of the 17 patients who were more than 2.6 months from previous therapy, 9 achieved an objective response. This same study demonstrated the importance of responsiveness to induction therapy in predicting the efficacy of salvage therapy. Ten of twenty-four patients who responded to induction therapy also responded to salvage teniposide, whereas none of the seven patients who failed induction chemotherapy responded to salvage therapy. The same observation was made in the chronic oral etoposide study, in which 10 of

18 patients who were initially chemotherapy-sensitive achieved an objective response to salvage chronic oral etoposide, whereas none of 4 initially resistant patients responded. Finally, some patients can be reinduced with the same regimen if a durable response was achieved from induction therapy.[107,108] Although not well studied, the likelihood of achieving a durable remission with salvage chemotherapy appears to be proportional to the remission duration following induction.

There is no established salvage chemotherapy standard. EP is a reasonable choice in CAV failures, and a likelihood of response of 40% to 50% can be expected.[81,82] Conversely, CAV is often inactive in EP failures.[21,22,109] Chronic oral etoposide induces responses in about 50% of patients recurring following treatment, with regimens that included conventional intravenous administration of the same agent.[85] Even in patients failing both CAV and EP, approximately 25% of patients respond to chronic low-dose etoposide.[86] Unfortunately, remissions with salvage therapy are usually short-lived.

Ifosfamide has been active in the salvage setting when used in combination with chronic oral etoposide and cisplatin.[110] A response rate of greater than 50% has been reported. Unfortunately, this level of efficacy is achieved at the cost of a considerably high incidence of life-threatening toxicities. Kubota and colleagues treated 17 patients with relapsed SCLC with the CODE regimen.[111] Fifteen patients (88%) experienced an objective response, but 76% of patients developed grade IV leukopenia. The median survival was 245 days for the five patients with CR and 156 days for the ten patients with partial response (PR). Although promising, this trial was small and confirmation is needed before such an aggressive approach can be recommended.

Topotecan is perhaps the most carefully studied single agent in SCLC. Activity has been demonstrated in both chemotherapy-naïve and previously treated patients.[112–115] Similar to other active chemotherapies, topotecan is relatively inactive in patients with refractory relapse (those relapsing less than 90 days since induction therapy and those not responding to induction therapy). Ardizzoni and colleagues demonstrated response rates of 6.4% in 47 refractory relapse patients and 37.8% in 45 patients with sensitive relapse.[113] The median survival for sensitive relapsed patients was 6.9 months. These promising results led to a recently completed phase III trial, in which 211 patients who relapsed more than 60 days after completion of induction therapy were randomized to receive either single-agent topotecan (1.5 mg/m^2 per day for 5 days, every 21 days) or conventional CAV.[114] The overall response rates and median survivals were not statistically different: 24.3% versus 18.3% and 25 weeks versus 24.7 weeks for topotecan and CAV, respectively. The proportion of patients who experienced symptom improvement was greater for the topotecan-treated patients. Grade III and IV hematologic toxicities were greater in the topotecan patients, whereas there was no significant difference in nonhematologic toxicities.

Irinotecan (CPT-11) and paclitaxel have also recently been evaluated in previously treated SCLC patients and demonstrated activity.[116–118] In patients with sensitive-relapse SCLC, irinotecan effects similar response rates and survivals to those of topotecan. Also similar to topotecan, irinotecan has no significant activity in patients with refractory relapse. Paclitaxel is the first agent demonstrating significant activity in patients with refractory relapse. Smit and colleagues treated 24 heavily pretreated SCLC patients relapsing within 3 months of cytotoxic therapy with paclitaxel 175 mg/m^2 intravenously over 3 hours on a three-week interval.[117] Seven partial responses (29%, 95% CI 12 to 51%) were observed, and a median survival of 100 days was reported. This trial was small and requires confirmation. However, a second report of activity in resistant relapse was recently published. Groen and colleagues conducted a phase II trial of paclitaxel and carboplatin in 35 patients relapsing within 3 months of receiving induction therapy with cyclophosphamide, doxorubicin, and etoposide.[118] The median time off treatment was 6 weeks. All patients had an ECOG performance status ≤1. Of 34 assessable patients, 2 complete and 23 partial responses were observed for an overall response rate of 73.5%. The median survival was 31 weeks. These results are encouraging and suggest that paclitaxel may be a non–cross-resistant regimen with CDE.

In summary, only a few patients benefit from salvage chemotherapy. The choice of therapy and likelihood of response can be accurately predicted based on the timing of disease recurrence and sensitivity to induction therapy. Topotecan is the most extensively studied drug in patients with sensitive relapse and should be considered for these patients. Historically, no therapy has been active in patients with refractory relapse, but paclitaxel-based therapy may offer these patients some chance of another tumor regression. None of the available salvage therapies are adequate, and these patients should always be considered for clinical trials of new therapeutic approaches.

IDENTIFICATION OF NEW AGENTS

Despite the large number of drugs available for treating SCLC, there is an ongoing need to identify additional active drugs, especially agents with unique mechanisms of action. The appropriate setting for new agent testing, however, is controversial.[119,120] Some investigators advocate evaluation of new agents in previously untreated patients arguing that chemotherapy-naïve patients represent the optimal setting.[121–123] Several new agents have been tested in this setting, including topotecan, paclitaxel, gemcitabine, docetaxel, and vinorelbine.[112,124–127] All but docetaxel were active. Such testing is conducted almost exclusively in patients with extensive-stage disease largely because these patients are rarely cured with conventional treatment. Experience with this approach has demonstrated that if patients are properly selected, those failing to respond to the new investigational agent can be salvaged with cisplatin and etoposide chemotherapy.[112,123,124] Even inactive agents tested in this manner have not resulted in adverse outcome.[122]

In contrast to the aforementioned approach, a cogent argument can be made for continuing the practice of testing new agents only in SCLC patients who have failed a standard induction therapy.[128] Based on a review of the SCLC phase II literature published between 1970 to 1990, investigators at Memorial Sloan Kettering Cancer Center concluded that a response rate greater than 10% in previously treated SCLC patients was adequate evidence that an agent was potentially active against SCLC.[129] They proposed a two-stage sequential design for phase II trials in SCLC using a response rate of 10% as an end point. A target enrollment of 20 patients in the initial phase of the study would allow for early termination of the trial if four or more patients responded because the agent under investigation would be expected to effect an objective response rate of at least 10%. On the other hand, if none of the initial 20 patients responded, the agent in question would not be subjected to further analysis because a true response rate greater than 10.9% would be excluded at the 90% confidence level. If one to three of the first 20 patients respond, an additional 15 patients would be entered to better estimate the agent's activity level. A maximum of 35 previously treated patients would be required to adequately assess the activity of a phase II agent against SCLC. This strategy maximizes the likelihood of identifying truly active agents and only slightly increases the possibility of mislabeling an inactive agent as active.

A compromise approach might be to test new agents in *selected* relapsed SCLC patients.[85,106,130] Topotecan, irinotecan, and vinorelbine have been tested and demonstrated activity in this setting.[116,131,130] Ideal candidates might include patients who maintained a good performance status, who do not have significant visceral metastases necessitating a rapid response, and who had not been treated for some interval prior to receiving the investigational agent. How long an interval should have transpired is not known with certainty but should probably be at least 90 days. Using these carefully defined guidelines, it would appear that new agent activity can be assessed in either previously treated or untreated SCLC patients without putting patients at increased risk.

CONCLUSIONS

Chemotherapy for SCLC is rarely curative except in limited-stage patients who are candidates for bimodality therapy with chemotherapy and thoracic radiotherapy. Although survival is significantly improved with chemotherapy, most patients succumb to their disease within one year of diagnosis. Thus, in SCLC, chemotherapy should be considered primarily a palliative treatment. The optimal induction regimens are either EP- or CAV-based. Multiple strategies designed to improve treatment with these agents have not yielded significant breakthroughs. Fortunately, several new drugs have recently been identified and given the exquisite chemosensitivity of this neoplasm, there is reason to expect improvements in therapy in the coming years. Furthermore, SCLC expresses a unique biology, thus making it an excellent disease in which to test emerging biologic and targeted therapies. Large strides forward will depend on our ability to translate new breakthroughs in our understanding of the biology of this neoplasm into clinically feasible therapeutic strategies.

REFERENCES

1. Parker SL, Tong T, Bolden S, et al. Cancer statistics, 1997. *CA Cancer J Clin* 1997;47:5.
2. Johnson DH, Greco FA. Small cell carcinoma of the lung. *Crit Rev Oncol Hematol* 1986;4:303.
3. Viallet J, Ihde DC. Small cell carcinoma of the lung: clinical and biological aspects. *Crit Rev Oncol Hematol* 1991;11:109.
4. Miller AB, Fox W, Tall R. Five-year follow-up of the Medical Research Council comparative trial of surgery and radiotherapy for the primary treatment of small-celled or oat-celled carcinoma of the bronchus. *Lancet* 1969;2:501.
5. Party MRCLCW. Radiotherapy alone or with chemotherapy in the treatment of small cell carcinoma of the lung: the results at 36 months. *Br J Cancer* 1981;44:611.
6. Matthews MJ, Kanhouwa S, Pickren J, et al. Frequency of residual and metastatic tumor in patients undergoing curative resection for lung cancer. *Cancer Chemother Rep* 1973;4(Part 3):63.
7. Ihde DC. Chemotherapy of lung cancer. *N Engl J Med* 1992;327:1434.
8. Karnofsky DA, Abelmann WH, Craver LF, et al. The use of nitrogen mustards in the palliative treatment of carcinoma. *Cancer* 1948;1:634.
9. Joss RA, Cavalli F, Goldhirsch A, et al. New drugs in small cell lung cancer. *Cancer Treat Rev* 1986;13:157.
10. Johnson DH. New drugs in the management of small cell lung cancer. *Lung Cancer* 1989;5:221.
11. Ettinger DS. New drugs for treating small cell lung cancer. [Review]. *Lung Cancer* 1995;12 Suppl 3:S53.
12. Bleehen NM, Fayers PM, Girling DJ, et al. Survival, adverse reactions and quality of life during combination chemotherapy compared with selective palliative treatment for small cell lung cancer. Report to the Medical Research Council by its Lung Cancer Working Party. *Resp Med* 1989;83:51.
13. Lowenbraun S, Bartolucci A, Smalley RV, et al. The superiority of combination chemotherapy over single agent chemotherapy in small cell lung carcinoma. *Cancer* 1979;44:406.
14. Alberto P, Brunner KW, Martz G, et al. Treatment of bronchogenic carcinoma with simultaneous or sequential combination chemotherapy, including methotrexate, cyclophosphamide, procarbazine and vincristine. *Cancer* 1976;38:2208.
15. Ihde DC. Small cell lung cancer: state-of-the-art therapy 1994. *Chest* 1995;435:107.
16. Murray N, Coy P, Pater JL, et al. Importance of timing for thoracic irradiation in the combined modality treatment of limited-stage small-cell lung cancer. The National Cancer Institute of Canada Clinical Trials Group. *J Clin Oncol* 1993;11:336.
17. Turrisi AT, 3rd, Kim K, Blum R, et al. Twice-daily compared

with once-daily thoracic radiotherapy in limited small-cell lung cancer treated concurrently with cisplatin and etoposide. *N Engl J Med* 1999;340:265.

18. Johnson DH, Hainsworth JD, Hande KR, et al. Current status of etoposide in the management of small cell lung cancer. *Cancer* 1991;67:231.
19. Hong WK, Nicaise C, Lawson R, et al. Etoposide combined with cyclophosphamide plus vincristine compared with doxorubicin plus cyclophosphamide plus vincristine and with high-dose cyclophosphamide plus vincristine in the treatment of small cell carcinoma of the lung: a randomized trial of the Bristol Lung Cancer Study Group. *J Clin Oncol* 1989;7:450.
20. Jackson DV, Case LD, Zekan PJ, et al. Improvement of long-term survival in extensive small cell lung cancer. *J Clin Oncol* 1988;6:1161.
21. Fukuoka M, Furuse K, Saijo N, et al. Randomized trial of cyclophosphamide, doxorubicin, and vincristine versus cisplatin and etoposide versus alternation of these regimens in small cell lung cancer. *J Natl Can Inst* 1991;83:855.
22. Roth BJ, Johnson DH, Einhorn LH, et al. Randomized study of cyclophosphamide, doxorubicin, and vincristine versus etoposide and cisplatin versus alternation of these two regimens in extensive stage small cell lung cancer: A phase III trial of the Southeastern Cancer Study Group. *J Clin Oncol* 1992;10:282.
23. Bunn PA. Clinical experiences with carboplatin (Paraplatin) in lung cancer. *Semin Oncol* 1992;19(suppl 2):1.
24. Bishop JF, Raghaven D, Stuart-Harris R, et al. Carboplatin (CBDCA, JM-8) and VP-16-213 in previously untreated patients with small cell lung cancer. *J Clin Oncol* 1987;5:1574.
25. Evans WK, Eisenhauser E, Hughes P, et al. VP-16 and carboplatin in previously untreated patients with extensive small cell lung cancer: a study of the National Cancer Institute of Canada Clinical Trials Group. *Br J Cancer* 1988;58:464.
26. Skarlos DV, Samantas E, Kosmidis P, et al. Randomized comparison of etoposide-cisplatin vs. etoposide-carboplatin and irradiation in small-cell lung cancer. A Hellenic Co-operative Oncology Group study. *Ann Oncol* 1994;5:601.
27. Johnson DH. Recent developments in chemotherapy treatment of small cell lung cancer. *Semin Oncol* 1993;20:315.
28. Feld R. Complications in the treatment of small cell carcinoma of the lung. *Cancer Treat Rev* 1981;8:5.
29. Abeloff MD, Klastersky J, Drings PD, et al. Complications of treatment of small cell carcinoma of the lung. *Cancer Treat Rep* 1983;67:21.
30. Johnson DH, Einhorn LH, Birch R, et al. A randomized comparison of high-dose versus conventional-dose cyclophosphamide, doxorubicin, and vincristine for extensive-stage small cell lung cancer: a phase III trial of the Southeastern Cancer Study Group. *J Clin Oncol* 1987;5:1731.
31. Ihde DC, Mulshine JL, Kramer BS, et al. Prospective randomized comparison of high-dose and standard-dose etoposide and cisplatin chemotherapy in patients with extensive-stage small-cell lung cancer. *J Clin Oncol* 1994;12:2022.
32. Bunn PA, Jr, Crowley J, Kelly K, et al. Chemoradiotherapy with or without granulocyte-macrophage colony-stimulating factor in the treatment of limited-stage small-cell lung cancer: a prospective phase III randomized study of the Southwest Oncology Group. *J Clin Oncol* 1995;13:1632.
33. de Jongh CA, Wade JC, Finley R, et al. Trimethoprim/sulfamethoxazole versus placebo: A double-blind comparison of infection prophylaxis in patients with small cell carcinoma of the lung. *J Clin Oncol* 1983;1:302.
34. Nichols CR, Fox EP, Roth BJ, et al. Incidence of neutropenic fever in patients treated with standard-dose combination chemotherapy for small-cell lung cancer and the cost impact of

treatment with granulocyte colony-stimulating factor. *J Clin Oncol* 1994;12:1245.
35. Chouaid C BL, Fuhrman C, Monnet I, et al. Routine use of granulocyte colony-stimulating factor is not cost-effective and does not increase patient comfort in the treatment of small-cell lung cancer: an analysis using a markov model. *J Clin Oncol* 1998;16:2700.
36. Messori A TS, Tnendi E. G-CSF for the prophylaxis of neutropenic fever in patients with small cell lung cancer receiving myelosuppressive antineoplastic chemotherapy: meta-analysis and pharmacoeconomic evaluation. *J Clin Phar Ther* 1996;21:57.
37. Cubeddu LX, Hoffmann IS, Fuenmayor NT, et al. Efficacy of ondansetron (GR-38032F) and the role of seratonin in cisplatin-induced nausea and vomiting. *N Engl J Med* 1990;322:810.
38. Johnson DH, Porter LL, List AF, et al. Acute non-lymphocytic leukemia following treatment of small cell lung cancer. *Am J Med* 1986;81:962.
39. Heyne KH, Lippman SM, Lee JJ, et al. The incidence of second primary tumors in long-term survivors of small cell lung cancer. *J Clin Oncol* 1992;10:1519.
40. Sagman U, Lishner M, Maki E, et al. Second primary malignancies following diagnosis of small cell lung cancer. *J Clin Oncol* 1992;10:1525.
41. Richardson GE, Tucker MA, Venzon DJ, et al. Smoking cessation after successful treatment of small-cell lung cancer is associated with fewer smoking-related second primary cancers. *Ann Intern Med* 1993;19:383.
42. Johnson BE, Patronas N, Hayes W, et al. Neurologic, computed cranial tomographic, and magnetic resonance imaging abnormalities in patients with small cell lung cancer: further follow-up of 6- to 13-year survivors. *J Clin Oncol* 1990;8:48.
43. Turrisi AT. Brain irradiation and systemic chemotherapy for small cell lung cancer: dangerous liaisons? *J Clin Oncol* 1990;8:196.
44. Arriagada R, Auperin A, Pignon JP, et al. Prophylactic cranial irradiation overview (PICO) in patients with small cell lung cancer in complete remission (CR). *Proc Annu Meet Am Soc Clin Oncol* 1998;17:112.
45. Arriagada R, Le Chevalier T, Borie F, et al. Prophylactic cranial irradiation for patients with small-cell lung cancer in complete remission [see comments]. *J Natl Cancer Inst* 1995;87:183.
46. Schabel FM, Griswold DP, Corbett TH, et al. Testing therapeutic hypotheses in mice and man: observations on the therapeutic activity against advanced solid tumors of mice treated with anticancer drugs that have demonstrated or potential clinical utility for treatment of advanced solid tumors in man. In: DeVita VT, Busch H, eds. *Methods in cancer research: Cancer drug development Part B*, Vol. XVII. New York: Academic Press, 1979:4.
47. Cohen MH, Creaven PJ, Fossieck BE, et al. Intensive chemotherapy of small cell bronchogenic carcinoma. *Cancer Treat Rep* 1977;61:349.
48. Hande KR, Oldham RK, Fer MF, et al. Randomized study of high-dose versus low-dose methotrexate in the treatment of extensive small cell lung cancer. *Am J Med* 1982;73:413.
49. Figueredo AT, Hryniuk WM, Strautmanis I, et al. Co-trimoxazole prophylaxis during high-dose chemotherapy of small cell lung cancer. *J Clin Oncol* 1985;3:54.
50. Arriagada R, Le Chevalier T, Pignon JP, et al. Initial chemotherapeutic doses and survival in patients with limited small-cell lung cancer. *N Engl J Med* 1993;329:1848.
51. Lowenbraun S, Birch R, Buchanan R, et al. Combination chemotherapy in small cell lung carcinoma: a randomized study of two intensive regimens. *Cancer* 1984;54:2344.
52. Murray N. Importance of dose and dose intensity in the treat-

ment of small-cell lung cancer. *Cancer Chemotherapy Pharmacol* 1997;40(suppl):S58.

53. Arriagada R, de The H, Le Chevalier T, et al. Limited small cell lung cancer: possible prognostic impact of initial chemotherapy doses. *Bull Cancer* 1989;76:604.

54. De Vathaire F AR, de The H. Dose intensity of initial chemotherapy may have an impact on survival in limited small cell lung carcinoma. *Lung Cancer* 1993;8:301.

55. Steward WP, von Pawel J, Gatzemeier U, et al. Effects of granulocyte-macrophage colony-stimulating factor and dose intensification of V-ICE chemotherapy in small-cell lung cancer: a prospective randomized study of 300 patients. *J Clin Oncol* 1998; 16:642.

56. Cerny T BV, Anderson H, Bramwell V, et al. Pretreatment prognostic factors and scoring system in 407 small-cell lung cancer patients. *Intl J Cancer* 1987;39:146.

57. Sculier JP, Paesmans M, Bureau G, et al. Multiple drug weekly chemotherapy versus combination regimen in small cell lung cancer: a phase III randomized study conducted by the European Lung Cancer Working Party. *J Clin Oncol* 1993;11:1858.

58. Souhami RL, Rudd R, Ruiz de Elvira M-C, et al. Randomized trial comparing weekly versus 3-week chemotherapy in small cell lung cancer: a Cancer Research Campaign trial. *J Clin Oncol* 1994;12:1806.

59. Murray N LR, Shepherd F, James K, et al. A randomized study of CODE versus alternating CAV/EP for extensive stage small cell lung cancer: an intergroup study of the National Cancer Institute of Canada Clinical Trials Group and the Southwest Oncology Group. *J Clin Oncol* 1999;17:2300.

60. Furuse K, Fukuoka M, Nishiwaki Y, et al. Phase III study of intensive weekly chemotherapy with recombinant human granulocyte colony-stimulating factor versus standard chemotherapy in extensive-disease small-cell lung cancer. The Japan Clinical Oncology Group. *J Clin Oncol* 1998;16:2126.

61. Murray N, Shah A, Osoba D, et al. Intensive weekly chemotherapy for the treatment of extensive-stage small cell lung cancer. *J Clin Oncol* 1991;9:1632.

62. Fukuoka M, Masuda N, Negoro S, et al. CODE chemotherapy with and without granulocyte colony-stimulating factor in small-cell lung cancer. *Br J Cancer* 1997;75:306.

63. Pujol JL, Douillard JY, Riviere A, et al. Dose-intensity of a four-drug chemotherapy regimen with or without recombinant human granulocyte-macrophage colony-stimulating factor in extensive-stage small-cell lung cancer: a multicenter randomized phase III study. *J Clin Oncol* 1997;15:2082.

64. Hamm J SJ, Cuffie C, Oken M, et al. Dose-ranging study of recombinant human granulocyte-macrophage colony-stimulating factor in small-cell lung carcinoma. *J Clin Oncol* 1994;12: 2667.

65. Miles DW, Fogarty O, Ash CM, et al. Received dose-intensity: a randomized trial of weekly chemotherapy with and without granulocyte colony-stimulating factor in small-cell lung cancer. *J Clin Oncol* 1994;12:77.

66. Crawford J, Ozer H, Stoller R, et al. Reduction by granulocyte colony-stimulating factor of fever and neutropenia induced by chemotherapy in patients with small cell lung cancer. *N Engl J Med* 1991;325:164.

67. Woll PJ, Hodgetts J, Lomax L, et al. Can cytotoxic dose-intensity be increased by using granulocyte colony-stimulating factor? A randomized controlled trial of lenograstim in small-cell lung cancer. *J Clin Oncol* 1995;13:652.

68. Trillet-Lenoir GJ, Manegold C, Von Pawel J, et al. Recombinant granulocyte colony stimulating factor reduces the infectious complications of cytotoxic chemotherapy. *Eur J Cancer* 1993;29A:319.

69. Norton L, Simon R. Tumor size, sensitivity to therapy, and design of treatment schedules. *Cancer Treat Rep* 1977;61:1307.

70. Elias A CB. Dose-intensive therapy in lung cancer. In: Armitage J AK, ed. *High-dose cancer therapy.* Baltimore: Williams & Wilkins, 1995:824.

71. Humblet Y, Symann M, Bosly A, et al. Late intensification chemotherapy with autologous bone marrow transplantation in selected small cell carcinoma of the lung: a randomized study. *J Clin Oncol* 1987;5:1864.

72. Goodman GE, Crowley J, Livingston RB, et al. Treatment of limited small cell lung cancer with concurrent etoposide/cisplatin and radiotherapy followed by intensification with high-dose cyclophosphamide: A Southwest Oncology Group study. *J Clin Oncol* 1991;9:453.

73. Elias A IJ, Skarin A, Wheeler C, et al. Dose-intensive therapy for limited-stage small-cell lung cancer: Long-term outcome. *J Clin Oncol* 1999;17:1175.

74. Johnson DH, Bass D, Einhorn LH, et al. Combination chemotherapy with or without thoracic radiotherapy in limited-stage small-cell lung cancer: a randomized trial of the Southeastern Cancer Study Group [see comments]. *J Clin Oncol* 1993;11: 1223.

75. Alberto A, Berchtold W, Sonntag R, et al. Chemotherapy of small cell carcinoma of the lung: comparison of a cyclic alternative combination with simultaneous combinations of four and seven agents. *Eur J Cancer* 1981;17:1027.

76. Krauss S, Lowenbraun S, Bartolucci A, et al. Alternating non-cross-resistant drug combinations in the treatment of metastatic small cell carcinoma of the lung. *Cancer Clin Trials* 1981;4: 147.

77. Goldie JH, Coldman AJ, Gudauskas GA. Rationale for the use of alternating non-cross-resistant chemotherapy. *Cancer Treat Rep* 1982;66:439.

78. Goldie JH, Coldman AJ. The genetic origin of drug resistance in neoplasms: implications for systemic therapy. *Cancer Res* 1984;44:3643.

79. Feld R, Evans WK, Coy P, et al. Canadian multicenter randomized trial comparing sequential and alternating administration of two non-cross-resistant chemotherapy combinations in patients with limited small cell carcinoma of the lung. *J Clin Oncol* 1987; 5:1401.

80. Evans WK, Feld R, Murray N, et al. Superiority of alternating non-cross-resistant chemotherapy in extensive small cell lung cancer. *Ann Intern Med* 1987;107:451.

81. Evans WK, Feld R, Osoba D, et al. VP-16 alone and in combination with cisplatin in previously treated patients with small cell lung cancer. *Cancer* 1984;53:1461.

82. Porter LL, Johnson DH, Hainsworth JD, et al. Cisplatinum and VP-16-213 combination chemotherapy for refractory small cell carcinoma of the lung. *Cancer Treat Rep* 1985;69:479.

83. Postmus P SG, Groen H, Gozzelino F, et al. Standard versus alternating non-cross-resistant chemotherapy in extensive small cell lung cancer: an EORTC phase III trial. *Eur J Cancer* 1996; 32A:1498.

84. Postmus P SE, Kirkpatrick A. Testing the possible non-cross resistance of two equipotent combination chemotherapy regimens against small cell lung cancer: a phase II study of the EORTC Lung Cancer Cooperative Group. *Eur J Cancer* 1993; 29A:204.

85. Johnson DH, Greco FA, Strupp J, et al. Prolonged administration of oral etoposide in patients with relapsed or refractory small cell lung cancer: a phase II trial. *J Clin Oncol* 1990;8: 1613.

86. Einhorn LH, Bond WH, Hornback N, et al. Phase II trial of oral VP-16 in refractory small cell lung cancer: a Hoosier Oncology Group study. *Semin Oncol* 1990;17:32.

87. Clark PI, Cottier B. The activity of 10-, 14-, and 21-day schedules of single-agent etoposide in previously untreated patients with extensive small cell lung cancer. *Semin Oncol* 1992; 19(Suppl 14):36.

88. Slevin ML, Clark PI, Joel SP, et al. A randomized trial to evaluate the effect of schedule on the activity of etoposide in small cell lung cancer. *J Clin Oncol* 1989;7:1333.

89. Drewinko B, Barlogie B. Survival and cycle-progression delay of human lymphoma cells in-vitro exposed to VP-16-213. *Cancer Treat Rep* 1976;60:1295.

90. Hainsworth JD, Johnson DH, Frazier SR, et al. A phase I trial of oral etoposide administered for twenty-one consecutive days. *J Clin Oncol* 1989;7:396.

91. Bork E, Ersboll J, Dombernowsky P, et al. Teniposide and etoposide in previously untreated small cell lung cancer: a randomized study. *J Clin Oncol* 1991;9:1627.

92. Carney DN, Grogan L, Smit EF, et al. Single-agent oral etoposide for elderly small cell lung cancer patients. *Semin Oncol* 1990;17(Suppl 2):49.

93. Miller AA, Herndon JE, Hollis DR, et al. Schedule dependency of 21-day oral versus 3-day intravenous etoposide in combination with intravenous cisplatin in extensive stage small cell lung cancer: a randomized phase III study of the Cancer and Leukemia Group B (CALGB 9033). *J Clin Oncol* 1995;13;1871.

94. Girling DJ, Thatcher N, Clark PI, et al. Comparison of oral etoposide and standard intravenous multidrug chemotherapy for small-cell lung cancer—a stopped multicentre randomised trial. *Lancet* 1996;348:563.

95. Souhami RL, Spiro SG, Rudd RM, et al. Five-day oral etoposide treatment for advanced small-cell lung cancer: randomized comparison with intravenous chemotherapy. *J Natl Canc Inst* 1997; 89:577.

96. Spiro SG, Souhami RL, Geddes DM, et al. Duration of chemotherapy in small cell lung cancer: a Cancer Research Campaign trial. *Br J Cancer* 1989;59:578.

97. Bleehen NM, Fayers PM, Girling DJ, et al. Controlled trial of twelve versus six courses of chemotherapy in the treatment of small cell lung cancer. *Br J Cancer* 1989;59:584.

98. Giaccone G, Dalesio O, McVie G, et al. Maintenance chemotherapy in small cell lung cancer: long-term results of a randomized trial. *J Clin Oncol* 1993;11:1230.

99. Bleehen N GD, Machin D, Stephens R. A randomized trial of three or six courses of etoposide cyclophosphamide methotrexate and vincristine or six courses of etoposide and ifosfamide in small cell lung cancer (SCLC) I: survival and prognostic factors. *Br J Cancer* 1993;68:1150.

100. Bleehen NM, Girling DJ, Machin D, et al. A randomised trial of three or six courses of etoposide cyclophosphamide methotrexate and vincristine or six courses of etoposide and ifosfamide in small cell lung cancer (SCLC). II: quality of life. Medical Research Council Lung Cancer Working Party. *Br J Cancer* 1993;68:1157.

101. Beith J CS, Woods R, Bell D, et al: Long-term follow-up of a randomised trial of combined chemoradiotherapy induction treatment, with and without maintenance chemotherapy in patients with small cell carcinoma of the lung. *Eur J Cancer* 1996; 32A:438.

102. Sculier JP, Paesmans M, Bureau G, et al. Randomized trial comparing induction chemotherapy versus induction chemotherapy followed by maintenance vhemotherapy in small cell lung cancer. *J Clin Oncol* 1996;14:2337.

103. Shevlin P SM, Brown I, Muers M, et al. A randomised trial of three versus six courses of etoposide, ifosfamide, mesna and vincristine in small cell lung cancer. [abstract]. *Lung Cancer* 1997;18(suppl 1):8.

104. Ebi N KK, Nishiwaki Y, Hojo F, et al. Second-line chemotherapy for relapsed small cell lung cancer. *Jap J Clin Oncol* 1997; 27:166.

105. Chute JP, Kelley MJ, Venzon D, et al. Retreatment of patients surviving cancer-free 2 or more years after initial treatment of small cell lung cancer. *Chest* 1996;110:165.

106. Giaccone G, Donadio M, Bonardi G, et al. Teniposide in the treatment of small cell lung cancer: the influence of prior chemotherapy. *J Clin Oncol* 1988;6:1264.

107. Batist G, Ihde DC, Zabell A, et al. Small cell carcinoma of the lung: Reinduction therapy after late relapse. *Ann Intern Med* 1983;98:472.

108. Giaccone G, Ferrati P, Donadio M, et al. Reinduction chemotherapy in small cell lung cancer. *Eur J Cancer* 1987;23:1697.

109. Shepherd FA, Evans WK, MacCormick R, et al. Cyclophosphamide, doxorubicin, and vincristine in etoposide- and cisplatin-resistant small cell lung cancer. *Cancer Treat Rep* 1987;71:941.

110. Faylona EA, Loehrer PJ, Ansari R, et al. Phase II study of daily oral etoposide plus ifosfamide plus cisplatin for previously treated recurrent small-cell lung cancer: a Hoosier Oncology Group Trial. *J Clin Oncol* 1995;13:1209.

111. Kubota KNY, Kakinuma R, Hojo F, et al. Dose-intensive weekly chemotherapy for treatment of relapsed small-cell lung cancer. *J Clin Oncol* 1997;15:292.

112. Schiller JH, Kim KM, Hutson P, et al. Phase II study of topotecan in patients with extensive-stage small-cell carcinoma of the lung—an Eastern Cooperative Oncology Group trial. *J Clin Oncol* 1996;14:2345.

113. Ardizzoni A HH, Dombernowsky P, Gamucci T, et al. Topotecan, a new active drug in the second-line treatment of small-cell lung cancer: a phase II study in patients with refractory and sensitive disease. *J Clin Oncol* 1997;15:2090.

114. von Pawel J SJ, Shepherd F, Fields S, et al. Topotecan versus cyclophosphamide, doxorubicin and vincristine for the treatment of recurrent small-cell lung cancer. *J Clin Oncol* 1999;17: 658.

115. Perez-Soler R, Glisson BS, Lee JS, et al. Treatment of patients with small-cell lung cancer refractory to etoposide and cisplatin with the topoisomerase I poison topotecan. *J Clin Oncol* 1996; 14:2785.

116. DeVore R BC, Denham C, Hainsworth J, et al. Phase II study of irinotecan (CPT-11) in patients with previously treated small cell lung cancer [abstract]. *Proc Am Soc Clin Oncol* 1998;17: 451a.

117. Smit EF, Fokkema E, Biesma B. A phase II study of paclitaxel in heavily pretreated patients with small-cell lung cancer. *Br J Cancer* 1998;77:347.

118. Groen H FE, Biesma B, Kwa B, et al. Paclitaxel and carboplatin in the treatment of small cell lung cancer patients resistant to cyclophosphamide, doxorubicin and etoposide: a non-cross-resistant schedule. *J Clin Oncol* 1999;17:927.

119. Aisner J. Identification of new drugs in small cell lung cancer: phase II agents first? *Cancer Treat Rep* 1987;71:1131.

120. Johnson DH. Investigation of new agents in small cell lung cancer. *Chest* 1993;103:423S.

121. Ettinger DS. Evaluation of new drugs in untreated patients with small cell lung cancer: Its time has come. *J Clin Oncol* 1990;8: 374.

122. Ettinger DS, Finkelstein DM, Abeloff DM, et al. Justification for evaluating new anticancer agents in selected untreated patients with extensive-stage small cell lung cancer: an Eastern Cooperative Oncology Group randomized study. *J Nat Canc Inst* 1992;84:1077.

123. Blackstein M, Eisenhauer EA, Wierzbicki R, et al. Epirubicin in extensive small cell lung cancer: a phase II study in previously untreated patients: a National Cancer Institute of Canada Clinical Trials Group study. *J Clin Oncol* 1990;8:385.

124. Ettinger DS, Finkelstein DM, Sarma RP, et al. Phase II study of paclitaxel in patients with extensive-disease small-cell lung cancer: an Eastern Cooperative Oncology Group study. *J Clin Oncol* 1995;13:1430.

125. Depierre A, LeChevalier T, Quoix E, et al. Phase II study of navelbine in small cell lung cancer. *Proc Am Soc Clin Oncol* 1995;14:348.

126. Latreille J CY, Martins H, Fisher B, et al. Phase II study of docetaxel in patients with previously untreated extensive small cell lung cancer. *Invest New Drugs* 1996;13:343.

127. Cormier Y, Eisenhauer E, Muldal A, et al. Gemcitabine is an active new agent in previously untreated extensive small cell lung cancer (SCLC). A study of the National Cancer Institute of Canada Clinical Trials Group. *Ann Oncol* 1994;5:283.

128. Grant SC, Kris MG. Phase II trials in small cell lung cancer: shouldn't we be doing better? *J Natl Canc Inst* 1992;84:1058.

129. Grant SC, Gralla RJ, Kris MG, et al. Single-agent chemotherapy trials in small cell lung cancer, 1970 to 1990: the case for studies in previously treated patients. *J Clin Oncol* 1992;10:484.

130. Ardizzoni A, Hansen H, Dombernowsky P, et al. Phase II study of topotecan in pretreated small cell lung cancer. *Proc Am Soc Clin Oncol* 1994;13:336.

131. Jassem J, Karnicka-Modkowska H, van Pottelsberghe C, et al. Phase II study of vinorelbine (Navelbine) in previously treated small cell lung cancer patients. EORTC Lung Cancer Cooperative Group. *Eur J Cancer* 1993;29A:1720.

54

MULTIMODALITY THERAPY FOR LIMITED-STAGE SMALL CELL LUNG CANCER: COMBINING CHEMOTHERAPY AND THORACIC IRRADIATION

NEVIN MURRAY
DAVID G. PAYNE
ANDREW J. COLDMAN

Within less than one month of starting treatment, relief of symptoms and improvement in the chest radiographs of small cell lung cancer (SCLC) patients are usually obvious and often dramatic. For the patient, this miraculous development understandably nurtures hope that the probability of curing this malignancy is high. Indeed, reviewing the x-rays with the patient and family is an effective way to enhance their morale and encourage them to soldier on through a vigorous treatment program. Frank oncologists must acknowledge that it is easy to make the chest x-ray look better with chemotherapy or thoracic irradiation. The unpleasant reality of the situation is that despite a satisfactory regression of the tumor, most patients harbor persistent elements of disease and are destined to experience the disappointment of an incurable recurrence. The challenge in the treatment of limited-stage small cell lung cancer (LSCLC) is to combine chemotherapy and thoracic irradiation in a more efficacious fashion so that the proportion of long-term survivors is increased.

The Veterans Administration Lung Group system[1] that divided patients into either limited or extensive stages has persisted for SCLC because of its simplicity, reliable prognostic value, and practical utility.[2-6] SCLC is defined as tumor confined to one hemithorax and the regional lymph nodes, whereas extensive-stage disease (ESCLC) is defined as disease beyond these bounds. The original operational definition of limited disease was tumor quantity and configuration that could be encompassed by a "reasonable" radiotherapy treatment volume. Because long-term survival is uncommon (7% to 9%) when chemotherapy alone is used to treat LSCLC,[7,8] the "reasonable" radiotherapy port rule continues to be of practical importance in the design of combined modality therapy.

The term "reasonable" lacks precision in this heterogeneous patient group. Using simple staging techniques, the University of Toronto Lung Oncology Group[9] identified a subgroup of patients with "very limited" SCLC without mediastinal node involvement who had a significantly better prognosis and a five-year survival of 18% with combined modality therapies used between 1976 and 1985. The five-year survival for patients with evidence of involved mediastinal nodes was 6%. Only 2% survived 5 years when pneumonic consolidation, atelectasis, pleural effusion, or involved supraclavicular nodes were present. The utility of a refined staging system may be greater with integrated chemotherapy and thoracic irradiation that generates a larger proportion of long-term survivors. The toxicity of thoracic irradiation volumes including all known disease may not be "reasonable" for patients with peripheral primary tumors or bulky mediastinal lymphadenopathy.

The necessity for accurate staging may be influenced by the sequence of chemotherapy and thoracic irradiation. Because expensive staging procedures delay symptom-relieving treatment and because chemotherapy is recommended for all fit patients anyway, some clinicians prefer not to bother with standard staging procedures outside the context of clinical trials. This pattern of practice may not be associated with negative consequences if the best model of treatment consisted of initial treatment with multiple chemotherapy cycles followed sequentially by administration of consolidative thoracic irradiation after drug treatment was finished. However, if patients with bona fide LSCLC benefit from early delivery of thoracic irradiation concurrent with combination chemotherapy, then careful staging determines the structure and intent (curative versus palliative) of the treatment program.[10] LSCLC patients have curative potential, which justifies the complexity and toxicity of integrated thoracic irradiation and combination chemotherapy. Such hopeful expectations cannot be entertained for palliation of extensive SCLC patients, and the vigor of noninvestigational therapy should be adjusted accordingly. Despite modern technology, the stage of some patients remains equivocal and clinicians must use their judgment.

Although the limited versus extensive stage system was created for practical purposes, its utility clearly reflects important biologic characteristics of the disease. When SCLC is overtly metastatic (ESCLC), we observe an underlying aggressiveness in the tumor that transcends the importance of the simple physical distribution of cancer cells within the body. Potentially curable LSCLC is quantitatively and qualitatively different from incurable ESCLC.

Therapeutic endeavors must contend with bulk concentrations of locoregional disease and a smaller metastatic population in widely different sites. These tissues vary in their tolerance of therapeutic interventions, just as the various tumor populations vary in their ability to resist the agents sent to destroy them. These clinical considerations and the biologic factors underlying them have led directly to modern concepts of multiple modality therapy for this disease.

HISTORY OF THE EVOLUTION OF COMBINED MODALITY THERAPY

The evolution of treatment for LSCLC can be described as a series of treatment paradigms.[11] The sequence of the paradigms did not always follow the chronologic order of the publication of important hypotheses or pilot studies. The evolution of treatment was determined by controlled trials of crucial issues of therapy and consensus by lung cancer investigators.

Paradigm 1: Surgery as Standard Treatment

World Wars I and II have had a large influence on the history of lung cancer. The stressful circumstances of wars, availability of tobacco products, and permissive attitude toward tobacco consumption during both wars were associated with a large increase in smoking among servicemen. The prevalence of smoking among women increased greatly during World War II. Surgical treatment of penetrating wounds to the chest during World War II resulted in advances in thoracic surgery, and the cadre of expert chest surgeons trained during the war had to contend with the increasing numbers of lung cancer casualties among veterans in the 1950s and 1960s.[12-14] In the post–World War II era, surgery was the treatment of choice for patients with all types of lung cancer, including SCLC.

Paradigm 2: Thoracic Irradiation Better than Surgery

The epithelial origin of SCLC was described in 1926,[15] and the separation of this virulent pathologic subtype on morphologic grounds was established in 1959.[16] From the earliest reports,[17] impressive regressions of SCLC induced by radiotherapy suggested an integral role of this modality in definitive management.

The median survival in surgically unresectable LSCLC patients randomized to supportive care alone in a trial conducted in the 1960s was 12 weeks.[18] A randomized trial comparing surgery alone to thoracic irradiation alone for SCLC patients was carried out by the Medical Research Council in the United Kingdom.[19,20] Eligibility criteria included (a) SCLC on bronchial biopsy; (b) no evidence of extrathoracic metastasis; (c) the tumor was regarded as operable on clinical examination and chest radiograph; (d) the patient was considered fit enough for resection; and (e) the patient was considered fit enough for radical radiotherapy. Although this study was done in an era before the availability of modern staging techniques, the intrathoracic extent of tumor was probably less than in most contemporary LSCLC trials. Of the 144 patients included in the main analysis, 71 were allocated to surgery and 73 to radical radiotherapy. A complete resection of all visible growth was performed in 48% of the surgical group, all of whom had a pneumonectomy. Thirty-four percent were unresectable and 18% had no operation because of preoperative deterioration or refusal of surgery. In the radiotherapy group, 85% had radical thoracic irradiation, 11% had palliative radiotherapy, and 4% had no radiotherapy because of deterioration or refusal. The median survival was 28.5 weeks for surgery and 43 weeks for radiotherapy (p = 0.04). Five-year survival was 1% for the surgical arm (the sole survivor refused surgery and was given radiotherapy) and 4% for radiotherapy. Outcome for both groups was poor, but treatment feasibility, toxicity, and survival all favored thoracic irradiation. The standard of treatment for LSCLC shifted from surgery to thoracic irradiation. The main aim was to give patients relief of local symptoms until their death from metastatic disease.

Paradigm 3: Thoracic Irradiation With Adjuvant Chemotherapy

The systemic nature of SCLC was emphasized by the rapid tempo of systemic relapse and low probability of long-term survival in patients with apparently localized disease given definitive local therapy only. In a classic study[21] of 19 patients subjected to potentially curative surgical resection who died within 30 days of operation of non–cancer-related causes, 13 were found to have persistent disease at autopsy. Moreover, metastases were distant in 12 of 13 cases. Although not all LSCLC patients have subclinical metastatic disease, the actual proportion is so high that the assumption of metastases is suitable for treatment planning.

A major step in the systemic treatment of SCLC was reported in 1969.[1] This randomized study[1] compared alkylating agents at several dose schedules to an inert compound in approximately 2,000 lung cancer patients at a group of

Veterans Administration hospitals. Antitumor effects of chemotherapy were analyzed according to cell type, and improvement in survival was the sole criterion of drug activity. The four-month median survival for SCLC patients treated with high intermittent doses of cyclophosphamide was only somewhat better than the 1.5-month median survival of placebo-treated patients (p = 0.0005). Nevertheless, the documentation of a survival improvement with chemotherapy for lung cancer patients was a notable development in cancer medicine, and cyclophosphamide became the cornerstone in SCLC chemotherapy regimens for decades. The credibility of cyclophosphamide efficacy in SCLC was augmented by randomized trials that showed prolonged survival for that agent as adjuvant chemotherapy compared to no further treatment after surgical resection.[12,13,22] Curiously, the lack of survival benefit for cyclophosphamide and other alkylating agents for non–small cell lung cancer (NSCLC) in these and other lung cancer trials[23–27] did not prevent them from being incorporated into combination chemotherapy regimens over the next 20 years.

The prescient observations of Watson and Berg[17] suggested thoracic irradiation coupled with chemotherapy as a model for treatment of SCLC. This hypothesis was first tested in a randomized trial by Bergsagel and colleagues from Toronto, Canada.[28] Patients with nonresectable lung cancer confined to the central area of the thorax were randomly assigned treatment with radiotherapy to the primary lesion and mediastinum or radiotherapy plus two schedules of intermittent intravenous cyclophosphamide. One-third of 123 patients in the study had SCLC, and both progression-free survival (29 weeks versus 16 weeks) and overall survival (42 weeks versus 21 weeks) were significantly superior for patients receiving combined modality therapy.

Two other randomized trials[29,30] showed significantly superior survival for thoracic irradiation and adjuvant chemotherapy versus radiotherapy alone. Median survival for LSCLC patients treated by radiotherapy alone was consistently about 5 to 6 months. Two additional controlled trials[31,32] showed some advantage for combined modality therapy, but survival differences between the groups were not statistically significant, probably because many patients on the radiotherapy arms received chemotherapy at the time of disease progression.

Paradigm 4: Combination Chemotherapy with Adjuvant Thoracic Irradiation

The success of combination chemotherapy in leukemia and lymphoma and the recognition of SCLC as a type of lung cancer with unique chemosensitivity stimulated exploration of multidrug regimens. The first published study of combination chemotherapy for lung cancer was published by Hansen and associates[33] using a regimen including cyclophosphamide, methotrexate, dactinomycin, and vincristine. All

eight patients with SCLC subtype responded; combination chemotherapy for SCLC was off to a promising start. High response rates for cyclophosphamide and vincristine were reported by Eagan et al.[34] and Holoye and Samuels.[35] By combining cyclophosphamide, doxorubicin, vincristine (CAV), and bleomycin, Einhorn et al.[36] produced not only high response rates in SCLC, but complete responses were also seen in 20% of cases. Bleomycin was discarded because of pulmonary toxicity, especially when combined with thoracic irradiation,[37] and the CAV regimen persists to the present as a standard regimen for SCLC.

By using principles of combination chemotherapy[38] and incorporating more and newer active agents, the search for a regimen with a high complete response rate for SCLC was intense during the 1970s. Combination chemotherapy was shown to be better than single-agent chemotherapy in three early randomized trials,[39–41] but a clearly superior regimen did not emerge. Nevertheless, in the early 1970s, a change in philosophy occurred. Because of the high response rates associated with multiagent chemotherapy, this modality became the primary therapy in LSCLC, and thoracic irradiation was relegated to an adjuvant or "consolidative" treatment.[42]

However, programs giving aggressive combination chemotherapy without thoracic irradiation[43] appeared to yield survival results similar to combined modality therapy. Median survival was in the range of 12 to 15 months, and projected long-term survival was usually in the range of 10 to 20% whether radiotherapy was given or not. Many published reports were difficult to interpret regarding long-term survival because of small trial size and inadequate follow-up. Regimens including thoracic irradiation produced a higher rate of complete remission, and an increased proportion of complete responses was felt to be essential in the evolution of therapies with curative potential.[44] However, combined modality therapy was also consistently associated with more acute and chronic toxicity, and selection of patients fit enough to receive this more demanding treatment in nonrandomized reports may have biased results against chemotherapy alone. Many investigators began to speculate that radiotherapy might not be necessary at all in LSCLC.

This debate persisted throughout the 1980s,[45,46] and many randomized trials were performed attempting to settle this vexing issue.[47–58] It was not until 1992 that metaanalyses[7,8] were published concluding that combined modality therapy moderately improves survival in patients with LSCLC.

Paradigm 5: Integrated Chemotherapy and Thoracic Irradiation

In 1976, investigators from the National Cancer Institute (NCI) in Bethesda, Maryland, performed an exploratory study that boldly went where no oncologist had gone before.[59–62] Although the protocol was influenced by the successful model of combined modality therapy for childhood lymphocytic leukemia,[63] the vigor of therapy was unprecedented in SCLC protocols. It involved initial simultaneous irradiation to the brain, primary tumor, and mediastinum and aggressive concurrent chemotherapy (cyclophosphamide 1.5 g/m^2, doxorubicin 40 mg/m^2, and vincristine 2 mg). The drugs were repeated as soon as the leukocytes increased to 3.5 × 10^9/L. All therapy was complete in 3 to 4 months.

The toxicity of this regimen was truly formidable. Radiation pneumonitis occurred in 38%, and a combination of pneumonitis and neutropenic sepsis was fatal in 24%. Severe esophagitis requiring nasogastric or parenteral nutrition occurred in 14%, and permanent strictures were observed.[64] Additionally, a previously undescribed neurologic syndrome of somnolence, poor attention span, recent memory loss, and action tremor was seen. The symptoms became evident within 2 to 4 months of starting treatment and were reversible within 4 months of onset.

The first reported survival results for LSCLC treated in this manner were spectacular, with 100% complete remissions and projected 80% long-term survival.[59] With longer follow-up, the survival curves dwindled and this trial was criticized for generation of false optimism by preliminary data reporting and unacceptably severe toxicity. Nevertheless, mature results demonstrating an 80% complete remission rate and 25% survival at 4 years in LSCLC were provocative and unprecedented.[62] Thirteen percent died without evidence of tumor at autopsy; it is speculative whether the cure rate could have been higher had modern supportive care been available. In an analysis of treatment factors contributing to long-term survival, it was concluded that concurrent chemotherapy and radiotherapy achieved better local tumor control than sequential therapy.[62] The data also suggested that if the duration of concurrent therapy is prolonged beyond three weeks, then the enhanced local tumor effect can be lost in a flood of treatment-induced toxicity.

This body of work is important because it clearly recognized the deleterious consequences of tumor repopulation permitted by sequential therapies as predicted by experimental models.[65] A generation of lung cancer investigators was both intrigued by the possibilities of early concurrent chemoradiation and troubled by a foreboding concern about the toxicity their patients would face in the quest for improved therapy.

It was evident that the combined chemoradiation model could not progress unless chemotherapy and radiotherapy could be integrated with less dire normal tissue interactions that did not compromise delivery of either modality. Sequential regimens giving thoracic irradiation during a gap in chemotherapy[66] (the "sandwich" technique) were less toxic, but efficacy was not improved, possibly because the interruption of the cadence of chemotherapy allowed tumor regrowth in unirradiated sites. Phase II results of a less aggressive CAV regimen[67] with concurrent thoracic irradia-

tion led to a large randomized trial comparing simultaneous chemoradiation to CAV chemotherapy alone, but a significant survival benefit was not observed.[68] This may have been because toxicity impaired drug delivery. Another controlled trial of CAV alone versus a tripartite split course of thoracic irradiation between CAV pulses demonstrated a survival benefit for combined modality therapy.[49] However, gastrointestinal and hematologic toxicity continued to be problematic. The severity of morbidity to normal tissue from the interaction of doxorubicin and radiotherapy has limited the utility of these approaches. Concurrent thoracic irradiation with chemotherapy containing cyclophosphamide, methotrexate, and lomustine was superior to chemotherapy given alone[47] in inducing remission and prolonging survival in patients with LSCLC, but the benefit was offset by unacceptable pulmonary toxicity. Similarly, concurrent cyclophosphamide, etoposide, and vincristine and radiotherapy have demonstrated superiority to chemotherapy alone,[48] but unacceptable chemotherapy attenuation from myelosuppression was associated with combined therapy.

The development of cisplatin and etoposide[68] as a potent combination for SCLC allowed the next step forward. Cisplatin produces no esophagitis or stomatitis and little myelosuppression at normal doses. Etoposide at standard doses has myelosuppression as its only serious side effect. More important, although cisplatin has some weak radiosensitizing properties,[69] normal tissue toxicity from concurrent chemotherapy and irradiation is not nearly so severe as with doxorubicin, nitrosoureas, or cyclophosphamide. Additionally, neither cisplatin nor etoposide have been implicated in "radiation recall"[64] toxicity. An important development in the evolution of therapy occurred when cisplatin and etoposide were integrated with thoracic irradiation. Pilot studies were independently performed at the British Columbia Cancer Agency[70,71] and by investigators associated with the Southwest Oncology Group (SWOG).[72,73] From the first report[70] in 1984, it was clear that etoposide-cisplatin chemotherapy and thoracic irradiation could be administered concurrently with manageable toxicity and little compromise in drug or radiation delivery.

The National Cancer Institute of Canada (NCIC) further improved the integration of chemotherapy and thoracic irradiation by demonstrating in a controlled trial that early concurrent cisplatin-etoposide and thoracic irradiation was superior to delayed thoracic irradiation given concurrently with cisplatin-etoposide.[74] A delay of as little as 12 weeks in the administration of thoracic irradiation for LSCLC patients resulted in an approximate 50% decline in the probability of five-year survival from 22% to 13%. The benchmark five-year survival rate for LSCLC shifted from about 10% to about 20%. Other randomized trials[48,75–77] of thoracic irradiation timing have been reported, and although not all support the superiority of early chemoradiation, the negative trials[48,74] consistently have long-term survival rates of only 10%, and the early chemoradiation arms of the positive studies[74,76,77] report long-term survival rates of 20% to 30%.

The search for improved treatment for LSCLC continues within the integrated chemotherapy and thoracic irradiation paradigm. The foci of research are the generation of more potent chemotherapy regimens and improvement in design and delivery of radiotherapy programs. Turrisi et al.[78] reported the first phase III study demonstrating a statistically significant survival advantage for more intensive twice-daily thoracic irradiation delivered early and concurrent with cisplatin-etoposide. Delayed twice-daily thoracic irradiation concurrent with EP failed to produce any evidence of survival benefit when compared to conventional radiation.[79]

Effective innovations of thoracic irradiation or chemotherapy should be more easily demonstrated in patient populations with a higher proportion of curable cases as determined by more accurate staging technology. New drugs with novel molecular targets are being explored intending to increase tumor destruction with induction therapy or prevent relapse for those in remission.

CHEMOTHERAPY FOR LSCLC

Multiagent chemotherapy is superior to single-agent therapy in most cancers for which treatment is sufficiently effective that it is given with curative intent.[38] The aggregate experience indicates that drug combinations alone in LSCLC yield a total response rate of 60% to 80% and complete response rates of 35% to 50%. Monotherapy with etoposide has been demonstrated inferior to combination chemotherapy in the palliative setting and is inappropriate for patients receiving therapy with curative intent.[80,81] There is no evidence that monotherapy with any other agent (new or old) is acceptable systemic therapy for LSCLC; multiagent chemotherapy is a necessity for patients fit enough for treatment where the goal is long-term survival.[82,83]

It is a common opinion that improvements in chemotherapy should be demonstrated in extensive-stage patients before they are adapted to LSCLC protocols. Such clear-cut evidence of increased treatment power is highly desirable, but this guideline cannot be interpreted to mean that a treatment strategy that does not improve results for incurable ESCLC patients must necessarily fail in the curable LSCLC population. Because LSCLC has a lower likelihood of drug resistance than ESCLC, the tumor burdens of SCLC patients based on stage are fundamentally different with respect to the impact of changes in both systemic and local therapy.

Median survival and rates of complete remission may not be adequate measures to judge differences between chemotherapy protocols for LSCLC.[84] When a large proportion of the patient population achieves complete remission, a therapy that produces more cures may have unimpressive differences in response rates and median survival when compared to a less efficacious treatment. Only long-term survival as shown on the "tail" of the curve may be different. Although this parameter is the outcome of greatest interest, many reports are difficult to interpret because of short follow-up and insufficient patient numbers. For these reasons, this review of chemotherapy is restricted mainly to LSCLC patient populations randomized in studies including at least 50 LSCLC patients per arm. Chemotherapy innovations include the choice of drugs, the number of drugs, and the amount to be administered.

Standard Regimens

The most commonly used programs include cyclophosphamide, doxorubicin, and vincristine (CAV), etoposide and cisplatin (EP), alternating CAV and EP, and CAV with etoposide (CAE or CAVE).[82] Chemotherapy cycles are typically given every 3 weeks for six to eight cycles. Major areas of clinical research include duration of chemotherapy, diversity of drugs within chemotherapy regimens, dose and dose-intensity escalation, and introduction of new agents.

Duration of Chemotherapy Administration

The studies by the Radiation Oncology Branch of the NCI[59–62] were provocative for several reasons, including brief duration of chemotherapy. Although toxicity may have precluded a more lengthy period of chemotherapy, durable unmaintained remissions were nevertheless demonstrated after chemotherapy duration of only 3 months.

A Cancer Research Campaign trial[85] from the United Kingdom randomized 610 patients, including 190 LSCLC patients, to receive either four or eight courses of cyclophosphamide, vincristine, and etoposide. A second randomization compared second-line chemotherapy (methotrexate and doxorubicin) on progression with symptomatic treatment only. Thoracic irradiation was used for palliative purposes only. When the effects of the treatment policies were separated according to disease extent, survival was adversely affected in patients with extensive disease who were treated with four cycles of initial chemotherapy only (no salvage chemotherapy). A similar trend was observed for LSCLC patients, but the effect was not statistically significant.

The Medical Research Council Lung Cancer Working Party[86] compared six versus twelve courses of chemotherapy (etoposide, cyclophosphamide, methotrexate, and vincristine in 497 patients, 74% with LSCLC). Limited-disease patients received thoracic irradiation between the second and third course of chemotherapy (sandwich technique). No worthwhile clinical advantage was achieved by the policy of continuing chemotherapy beyond six courses.

The European Organization for Research and Treatment of Lung Cancer (EORTC) Cooperative Group investigated 5 cycles of cyclophosphamide, doxorubicin, and vincristine versus 12 cycles in a large study[87] including 341 LSCLC patients. Chest irradiation was not routinely given. Progression-free survival (PFS) was significantly longer for patients receiving prolonged versus short chemotherapy (p = 0.01). However, PFS at 5 years was the same at approximately 8% in both arms, and overall survival was not increased by prolonged chemotherapy.

The experience from cooperative group studies with six cycles of chemotherapy is large.[74,88,89] It is improbable that useful incremental benefit can by demonstrated by administering more than six cycles of chemotherapy. In any case, compliance with additional cycles becomes increasingly problematic. Excellent phase II and III study results have been generated with as few as four cycles of cisplatin-etoposide combined with thoracic irradiation.[78,90] A comparison of four versus six courses may not be a research priority. It may be more useful to examine treatment duration on the basis of total cumulative drug doses rather than time alone.

Drug Diversity

The somatic mutation theory for drug resistance[91] suggested that drug combinations could improve the probability of overcoming resistant tumor clones by early introduction of therapeutic diversity into the treatment program. Because overlapping toxicity precludes administration of more than a few active agents at full dose at one time, the alternation of equivalent non–cross-resistant combinations was recommended. Current opinion of alternating chemotherapy in SCLC is based mainly on the outcome of large randomized studies in ESCLC.[92–94] The ESCLC experience was disappointing, showing a small or no survival advantage. The probability of resistance to all alternations tried to date is almost universal for ESCLC as revealed by the absence of a consistent proportion of long-term survivors. However, a review restricted to large LSCLC trials of alternating versus sequential chemotherapy combinations does not reach conclusions as clear-cut as ESCLC.

A randomized German multicenter trial[95] showed significant benefits for alternating chemotherapy when 306 patients (104 LSCLC) were randomized to eight cycles of CAV versus three cycles of ifosfamide, vindesine, and etoposide (weeks 1, 3, 5); three cycles of cisplatin, doxorubicin, and vincristine (weeks 2, 4, 6); and two cycles of cyclophosphamide, methotrexate, and lomustine (weeks 7, 8). Responding patients received chest radiotherapy after eight cycles of chemotherapy. In limited disease, the complete response (CR) rate was 33% in the sequential arm versus 52% in the alternating arm; median survival was 11.1 months for sequential therapy versus 13.4 months for patients receiving the more diverse regimen.

Another German multicenter study[96] compared a fixed alternation of ifosfamide/etoposide (IE) and CAV chemotherapy and response-oriented treatment with IE to maximal response and subsequently an immediate switch to

CAV. After six cycles of chemotherapy, limited-stage patients (n = 140) received thoracic irradiation. The CR rate for LSCLC was slightly higher in the alternating arm (40 versus 35%). Survival in the arms was similar, with median survival at 12.5 months versus 12.3 months and two-year survival at 21% versus 18%. However, because only a few patients achieved CR with IE, the response-oriented approach used in this trial exposed most patients in this trial to diverse chemotherapy.

The NCIC Clinical Trials Group studied 300 limited-stage patients, comparing an immediate versus a delayed alternation of CAV and EP.[88] Thoracic irradiation was given to responders after six cycles of chemotherapy in a consolidative fashion. Neither complete responses (52% versus 44%) nor median survival (14.2 versus 13.7 months) was different. The five-year survival rates for immediate and delayed alternating arms were 10% and 6%, respectively. Chemotherapy diversity between arms was similar with respect to the number of agents used.

In another large study that primarily focused on the value of thoracic irradiation in LSCLC,[58] The Southeastern Cancer Study Group (SECSG) assessed the value of the addition of two cycles of EP in responding patients after completion of six cycles of CAV (with or without thoracic irradiation). Patients randomized to receive more heterogeneous chemotherapy with "consolidative" EP experienced superior median (21.1 versus 13.2 months; p = 0.08) and two-year survival rates (44% versus 26%; p = 0.028). This result could be interpreted as an advantage for more diverse chemotherapy or simply attributed to the superiority of the EP regimen. The administration of CAV after induction with EP (first described in 1984)[97] was reexamined in an often cited but unpublished trial from Australia.[98] No advantage for the addition of CAV could be demonstrated in the total patient population, but too few limited-disease patients were included for analysis of this subgroup.

The largest randomized study (388 patients) comparing sequential and alternating chemotherapy for LSCLC was performed by the SWOG.[89] The alternating regimen was CAV and EP. The sequential regimen was CAV plus etoposide (EVAC). After six courses of chemotherapy, consolidative thoracic irradiation was given to responders. There were no significant differences in complete response (CAV/EP 51%; EVAC 48%). The survival curves overlap with median survival of 16.5 versus 15.1 months and identical long-term survival (about 10%). This study does not support the value of alternating chemotherapy, but it may not be interpreted as evidence against potential value of chemotherapy diversity. The chemotherapy in the EVAC sequential arm was not the same as either regimen used in the alternation. The drug diversity supplied by the alternating chemotherapy amounts to the addition of one agent (cisplatin) at intervals of 6 weeks on three occasions over the entire treatment program. Moreover, the dose intensity of the other drugs in the alternating regimen (cyclophosphamide, doxorubicin, etoposide, and vincristine) were reduced substantially compared to the sequential arm by the longer cycle time of the alternation.

The addition of etoposide to CAV has been examined in a controlled trial for LSCLC patients by the North Central Cancer Treatment Group (NCCTG).[99] Thoracic irradiation was given with the fourth cycle of chemotherapy (doxorubicin deleted from this cycle) in a trial in which 118 patients were randomized to CAVE and 113 to CAV. Measures of outcome for CAVE versus CAV were median survival 15 versus 13.3 months, three-year survival 17.2 versus 9.7%, and five-year survival 12.1% versus 7.0% (p = 0.13). The difficulty in interpreting studies in which the sample size is modest can be seen here because if the true effect of the addition of etoposide was to double the five-year survival, then the probability that would be declared significant in a trial of this size is only 0.32.

Only the Japanese Lung Cancer Chemotherapy Group has directly compared CAV, EP, and CAV alternating with EP in a study including LSCLC as well as ESCLC.[100] Unfortunately, the arms were not stratified by stage, so examination of LSCLC outcomes is a subgroup analysis. Each arm included about 50 LSCLC patients. Consolidative thoracic irradiation was given after four cycles of chemotherapy. The complete response rates for initial chemotherapy were similar (CAV 16%, EP 18%, and CAV/EP 22%). The median survival of the alternating regimen (16.8 months) was superior (p = 0.014) to either CAV (12.4 months) or EP (11.7 months). Mature results for the proportions of long-term survivors have not been published, but the actuarial projections appear better in the alternating chemotherapy subgroup.

Overall, the data suggest that drug diversity may be more important in LSCLC than ESCLC. However, the efficacy of EP and the ease with which it can be administered with thoracic irradiation without serious toxicity from interaction between radiation and chemotherapy on normal tissue has led several cooperative groups (Table 54.1) to simplify chemotherapy to this two-drug combination in phase III trials. It is unclear whether the loss of "therapeutic diversity" by using EP alone rather than EP plus other agents will result in negative consequences. The fact that these trials were conducted using EP chemotherapy is a powerful statement that many lung cancer experts consider this regimen to be state-of-the-art. This may be true; however, it is a poignant curiosity that, to date, EP has never demonstrated superior survival compared to any other chemotherapy regimen in a published phase III randomized trial of LSCLC or ESCLC. A standard regimen for a curable disease should have better credentials.

Dose and Dose-Intensity Escalation

The evidence that more intensive drug treatment can increase complete responses and long-term survival in animal

TABLE 54.1. PHASE III LSCLC TRIALS USING ETOPOSIDE PLUS CISPLATIN/CARBOPLATIN CHEMOTHERAPY

Group	Questions
1. SWOG[147]	Supportive Care/Maintenance —GM-CSF and Interferon
2. JCOG[77]	Radiotherapy Timing —Early Concurrent versus Sequential
3. Intergroup[78]	Radiotherapy —Standard versus Accelerated Fractionation
4. NCCTG[79]	Radiotherapy —Standard versus Hyperfractionated
5. CALGB	Resistance Modification —Tamoxifen versus Control
6. ELCWP	Cisplatin Fractionation —Standard versus Daily Cisplatin
7. Australia	Supportive Care —G-CSF versus Control

1. Southwest Oncology Group; 2. Japanese Clinical Oncology Group; 3. Intergroup; 4. North Central Cancer Treatment Group; 5. Cancer and Leukemia Group B; 6. European Lung Cancer Working Party.

models with curative potential is compelling.[101] However, the SCLC group most often studied with controlled trials of more intense therapy has been incurable extensive-stage patients.[102–105] A metaanalysis of the outcome in LSCLC patients treated with dose and dose-intensity variations of CAV, EP, and CAVE showed no consistent evidence for better response rates or median survival for more intense regimens.[106] However, the range of dose intensities was narrow and many studies included small patient numbers. Only two randomized trials[107,108] of chemotherapy intensity in LSCLC involving more than 50 patients per arm have been reported. Both demonstrate significant survival benefits for more intensive chemotherapy.

The Eastern Cooperative Oncology Group (ECOG)[107] randomized 349 patients with SCLC (38% limited stage) to induction chemotherapy with cyclophosphamide 1,500 mg/m² days 1 and 22, lomustine (70 mg/m²) day 1, and methotrexate 15 mg/m² twice per week on weeks 2, 3, 5, and 6 (without dose modification for hematologic toxicity) or to the same drugs with cyclophosphamide 700 mg/m². The abstract does not mention use of thoracic irradiation. Median survival for all intensively treated patients was 41 weeks versus 36 weeks (p = 0.04). The effect was most pronounced for limited-stage patients with median survival of 56 weeks for the intensive arm versus 42 weeks for the standard arm (p = 0.02). Long-term outcomes are not reported.

After retrospective review of treatment data on alternating chemotherapy and radiotherapy regimens for LSCLC, investigators at the Institut Gustave-Roussy concluded that the impact of the size of the initial dose of cyclophosphamide and cisplatin should be assessed in a controlled trial.[108]

Patients were randomly assigned to receive a different dose of cisplatin and cyclophosphamide (100 mg/m^2 day 2 and 300 mg/m^2 days 2–5) versus (80 mg/m^2 day 2 and 225 mg/m^2 days 2–5). The doses of doxorubicin (40 mg/m^2 day 1) and etoposide (75 mg/m^2 days 1–3) were held identical. The higher doses of cisplatin and cyclophosphamide were given for the first cycle only. Subsequently, all patients received the same schedule of alternating chemotherapy and radiotherapy with the lower cisplatin and cyclophosphamide doses. The complete remission rate for the 55 patients in the high-dose group (67%) was not significantly better than the 50 patients in the lower initial-dose group (54%). However, a significant difference in overall survival (p = 0.01) was observed in favor of the patients who received the single escalated dose of cisplatin and cyclophosphamide. Survival rates at 18 months were 52% and 32%, respectively. Although mathematical models[109] predict a disproportionately large contribution from early treatment events, the effect of escalation of the dose size for only two drugs given on one occasion is so provocative that this finding requires confirmation in trials that include more patients.

An extension of the dose-escalation rationale is that tumor resistance can be overcome by large dose size. High-dose chemotherapy with special support during severe myelosuppression, such as autologous bone marrow transplantation, peripheral blood stem cell transfusion, and hemopoietic growth factors, is commonly tested in malignancies that resist conventional strategies. This approach is an assessment of the dose-response (mg/m^2) effect rather than an investigation of dose intensity (mg/m^2 per week); the difference is not semantic. In LSCLC, high-dose chemotherapy is usually given after induction with standard-dose chemotherapy.[110–114] Trials that report the number of patients potentially eligible for such therapy[110–113] indicate that less than 40% respond well enough, remain fit enough, and consent to the high-dose treatment. Results of these investigations make it difficult to separate "late intensification" from the patient selection process. Prospective trials testing this concept must include a complete account of the overall patient population from which the randomized patients were drawn. Even if positive studies emerge, the characteristics of the overall LSCLC population restrict applications of ablative chemotherapy doses to a small subgroup.

New Cytotoxic Agents

Because analogues of existing drugs have not demonstrated convincing advantages over the parent compounds in controlled trials, chemotherapeutic agents with different structure and novel mechanisms of action are imperative to improve outcome for this systemic disease. Several new drugs with activity against SCLC have been recently described, including the taxanes,[115] gemcitabine,[116] and the topoisomerase I inhibitors.[117,118] The characteristics that new agents should have to join or displace standard therapies such as

the combination of etoposide/cisplatin are demanding. Not only must the new drug be highly active in previously untreated patients with high response rates and a proportion of complete responses, but demonstration of at least partial non–cross-resistance with existing agents is mandatory. Improved survival will not be associated with new drugs that kill the same cancer cells as the old ones. Moreover, in accordance with the theme of this chapter, it should be possible to give the new agent either concurrently with or adjacent to thoracic irradiation for LSCLC without radiotherapy-chemotherapy interactions that cause serious normal tissue toxicity; a preferential radiosensitizing effect on the tumor would be a great advantage. Activity should be present over a range of schedules so that dose-response and dose-intensity characteristics can be defined. Because it is already obvious that the new drugs are not conspicuously superior to older agents, the useful newcomer must combine with older agents with additive or preferably synergistic effects. An obvious corollary is that the new drug must have a toxicity profile that does not preclude its administration at full therapeutic doses when combined with the best standard agents or thoracic irradiation. Moreover, cumulative toxicity should not decrease the likelihood of completing the entire treatment program at full doses on time. The well-being of long-term survivors must not be endangered by chronic toxicity. The ultimate criteria will be the demonstration that the program incorporating the new drug is unequivocally superior to the best standard therapy in reproducible randomized comparisons. At this time, no phase III trials of new cytotoxic agents for LSCLC have been reported.

THORACIC IRRADIATION FOR LSCLC

Thoracic irradiation for LSCLC has long offered an attractive approach for several reasons beyond its ability to produce early responses. Because its mechanism of action is different from chemotherapeutic agents, the potential exists for additive or even synergistic damage to tumor cells. Toxicity to normal tissues is somewhat different from that produced by drugs. More important, because of its physical nature, "dose" can be administered in a focused fashion to regions containing or at high risk of tumor involvement. Most organs are thus excluded from the radiation beams, and tolerance is limited only by relatively modest volumes of normal tissue. The tumor may receive doses, which exceed by 10- to 20-fold what can be tolerated by the whole body, and the dose concentration greatly exceeds the dose concentration achievable by chemotherapy. Radiation dose is expressed in units of energy absorbed per gram of irradiated tissue (Gray), a unit of concentration or density, rather than units expressing a total body dose calculated without reference to tumor size. This capacity to strike hardest at the most populous and hence most dangerous concentration of tumor improves the probability of controlling local disease that may evolve more resistant progeny and metastasize systemically. It is intuitively reasonable that combined modality approaches including radiotherapy should improve results in the clinic.

Metaanalysis of Randomized Trials of Chemotherapy With or Without Thoracic Radiotherapy

There have been many published studies[42–58,119–122] in which this study design has been implemented (Table 54.2). There are several differences in detail between them. For example, the precise definition of "limited" stage disease varied with respect to inclusion of patients with pleural effusions. Other selection factors such as tumor size or pulmonary function were sometimes introduced. Some studies specified a requirement that patients show a complete response to chemotherapy, perhaps in the belief that thoracic irradiation could not be withheld from partial responders. The chemotherapy regimens varied widely. Most studies were initiated before 1981 when cisplatin-containing regimens were not prevalent; none of the trials included this agent. The thoracic radiotherapy protocols were also diverse because four trials employed split-course treatment, fraction sizes ranged from 1.8 to 4.0 Gy, and total dose ranged from 40 to 55 Gy. The treatment volumes all encompassed the

primary tumor with a margin of 1 to 2 centimeters. Most included the mediastinum and some treated the supraclavicular fossae electively. Most studies were designed to permit a chemotherapy response evaluation, which allows the possibility of a reduction in the radiotherapy field size. The timing of thoracic irradiation was most often after three to six cycles of chemotherapy but was concurrent with the first cycle of chemotherapy in four studies. Prophylactic brain irradiation was part of most protocols, usually at the end of induction therapy.

Nevertheless, all of these studies were designed to treat patients with regional disease in order to determine whether regional therapy would improve survival. The study populations were less than 75 in three studies, but three others included more than 290 patients. Consequently, the statistical power to detect differences varied widely and it is not surprising that many trials were negative.

The method of metaanalysis is used to study a collection of trials of similar design where each generates an estimate of treatment effect. This set of treatment effects is then subjected to statistical analysis to determine whether the average therapeutic effect can be attributed to chance alone.[123] The treatment effect can be represented by the difference between the number of events observed and the number expected if the treatment had no impact (method of Peto). The "log odds-ratio" has an approximate normal distribution and permits an estimate of the probability that

TABLE 54.2. RANDOMIZED TRIALS OF CHEMOTHERAPY ALONE VERSUS COMBINED MODALITY THERAPY IN LIMITED-STAGE SMALL CELL LUNG CANCER

Reference	Drugs	Chest Radiotherapy Start Time	Chest Radiotherapy Dose	No. of Patients	Survival Median (mos) CT	CMT	2 Yr (%) CT	CMT	p. Value
1. Perry et al.[48,174]	CAEV	I: Week 1	50Gy/25F		13.6	13.1	8	15	
				399 (All)					0.009
		II: Week 9	50Gy/25F			14.6		25	
2. Bunn et al.[47]	CML/VAP	Week 1	40Gy/15F	96 (All)	11.6	15.0	12	28	0.035
3. Greco et al.[51,58]	CAV ± PtE	Weeks 1, 2, 7	45Gy/15F split-course	369 (All)	12.8	14.4	23	33	0.077
4. Ohnoshi et al[122]	COMP-VAN	Week 2	40Gy/20F	56 (All)	13.5	15.5	7	19	NS
5. Perez et al.[49,103]	CAV	Weeks 5, 8, 11	40Gy/14F split-course	291 (All)	10.5	12.5	16	24	0.04
6. Osterlind et al.[54]	CMVL	Weeks 6, 10	40Gy/20F	145 (All)	11.5	10.5	12	5	NS
7. Creech et al.[56]	CML	Week 8	50Gy/25F	310 (CR,PR)	14.0	17.0	13	19	0.003
8. Kraft et al.[121]	CAV	I: Week 9	30Gy/15F		9.7	13.5	5	25	
				91 (All)					p=0.02
		II: Week 9	50Gy/25F			12.4		13	
9. Fox et al.[50,119]	CAV	Week 10	40Gy/20F	73 (CR + PR)	15	16.5	NA	NA	NS
10. Nou et al.[57]	CAVML	Week 12	40Gy/20F	56 (All)	14.8	15.4	17	24	NS
11. Kies et al.[52]	VMEAC	Weeks 12, 17	48Gy/22F	93 (CR)	16.0	16.0	25	35	NS
12. Souhami et al.[53]	AV/CM	Week 13	40Gy/20F	130 (CR + PR + SD)	12	13	12	14	NS
13. Carlson et al.[55]	POCC/VAM	Weeks 25 or 40	55Gy/30F	48 (CR + PR + SD)	20.3	18.9	40	40	NS

C, Cyclophosphamide; M, Methotrexate; L, Lomustine; V, Vincristine; A, Doxorubicin; P, Procarbazine; Pt, Cisplatin; E, Etoposide; N, Nimustine; CT, Chemotherapy alone; CMT, Combined modality therapy; CR, Complete response; PR, Partial response; SD, Stable disease; NS, Not significant; NA, Not available; p, Fractions.

an observed treatment effect could have been found by chance alone.[124] By a different calculation,[125] each study yields an estimate of the absolute magnitude of the effect observed, termed the *event rate difference*. One may then judge on clinical grounds whether observed effects are of practical value.

Two metaanalyses that examine the role of thoracic radiotherapy in LSCLC have been published.[7,8] One was based on published data (1,911 patients) and looked at two-year survival rates, local control, and toxicity.[7] The other included 2,140 patients and examined only survival at 3 years and prognostic factors for survival.[8] The study by Pignon et al.[8] assembled updated individual patient outcomes from the trial investigators, which yielded comprehensive reporting and more mature results than could be derived from the literature alone.

Because the majority of data in each metaanalysis was derived from the same studies, the conclusions are consistent and complementary despite differences in the methods used in the metaanalyses. Both show a modest improvement in survival rates in those patients given thoracic radiotherapy (Figure 54.1). The survival benefit becomes evident at about 15 months following start of treatment and persists beyond 5 years. At 3 years about 9% of the chemotherapy-only group are alive compared to about 14% of the combined modality group. The relative rate of death in the combined modality group as compared to the chemotherapy group was 0.86 (95% confidence interval, 0.78 to 0.94; P = 0.001), corresponding to a 14% reduction in the mortality rate. The analysis of local control was based on 1,521 patients for whom data were reported and showed marked reduction in the absolute two-year local failure rate from 23% in irradiated patients compared to 48% in nonirradiated patients (p = 0.0001). These benefits were obtained at the cost of an increase in treatment-related deaths of 1%.

The relative rate of death between the two groups was not influenced by gender or performance status. However, the improved survival of irradiated patients was largely confined to patients less than age 55; survival benefit for older patients in this data set could not be demonstrated. Similarly, treatment factors such as radiotherapy timing or chemoradiation integration (sequential, concurrent, or alternating) were not significant in the metaanalyses. An explanation for not demonstrating a benefit for older patients or the importance of timing of integration of thoracic irradiation may be found in the shape of the survival curve and the statistic methodology used in this analysis. Initially, the overall survival graph begins in favor of chemotherapy, but the curves cross at about 1 year and later demonstrate a long-term survival advantage for chemoradiation. The initial separation of the curves is not large, but many events occur on this steep portion of the curves (Figure 54.1). Because early concurrent thoracic irradiation with regimens other than EP adds excessive toxicity and may diminish chemotherapy delivery, the relative risk of death is not constant over time. The short-term mortality increase from toxicity or poor chemotherapy delivery may cancel out the long-term survival gain as measured by relative risk. Reexamination of this data set for an effect of thoracic irradiation timing on long-term survival rather than relative risk of death may be useful.

Most studies in the metanalyses began before 1981, and none delivered cisplatin and etoposide concurrently with thoracic irradiation. The safety and efficacy of early concurrent chemoradiation has been markedly improved with the administration of etoposide/cisplatin chemotherapy rather than cyclophosphamide, nitrosourea, or doxorubicin-based regimens. From the first report,[70] etoposide and cisplatin clearly could be delivered concurrently with thoracic irradiation without dire normal tissue toxicity or the need to compromise the dose of either modality. Concurrent etoposide plus cisplatin or carboplatin with thoracic irradiation has become a prevalent theme in current LSCLC regimens (Table 54.1). Lack of data of this type in the metaanalyses[7,8] reduces the capacity of these reports to provide guidance on optimal integration of chemoradiation or management of LSCLC patients that is relevant to the modern era.

Volume of Radiation

The usefulness of radiotherapy comes from its ability to be directed to target tissues of interest, sparing areas beyond

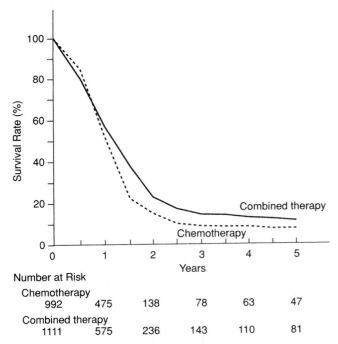

FIGURE 54.1. Survival curves for the Combined Therapy Group and the Chemotherapy Group. The three-year survival rates were 14.3% ± 1.1% in the combined-therapy group and 8.9% ± 0.9% in the chemotherapy group (for a difference of 5.4% ± 1.4%: p = 0.001 by stratified log rank test).

the treated volume, which might otherwise limit the dose delivered to the tumor. One must "see" the tumor to target it. We "see" through the use of imaging technology, knowledge of lymphatic anatomy, and experience with patterns of spread and treatment failure, but these methods have limitations.

LSCLC usually involves the mediastinal lymph nodes. Consequently, radiotherapy volumes almost always must encompass the primary node and most of the mediastinum. However, it is not clear where to draw the line. Most protocols treat the primary and clinically involved nodes; these definitions depend on imaging technology. Margins of 1.5 to 2 centimeters are commonly recommended to account for uncertainties in imaging, patient motion, and microscopic extension. Large volumes are limited as higher cumulative doses reach neighboring structures (lung, esophagus, and spinal cord). Retrospective radiation therapy quality control analysis, including dosimetric reconstruction and port film review, demonstrate lower response rates, higher chest failure rate, and statistically worse survival for patients who were considered major protocol violations.[126] Analyses suggesting that local control deteriorates with violation of thoracic irradiation protocol guidelines may be confounded by the difficulty associated with encompassing large tumor burdens.

The extension of prescribed fields to cover bilateral hila, mediastinal, and supraclavicular nodes with curative aims suggests that the disease spreads in an orderly fashion. The behavior of SCLC is characterized by disorder. The attempt to increase treatment volume may lead to two adverse consequences: Toxicity to normal tissues will increase and the dose delivered to bulk disease will be compromised. An alternative tactic is to protect normal tissue by focusing on gross disease only using radiotherapy techniques that ensure full dose to all of the target volume, leaving chemotherapy to deal with subclinical tumor.

The simulation process for trials of early integration of chemoradiation[48,74] have targeted the prechemotherapy extent of disease. When tumor has responded to chemotherapy, an opportunity exists to "trim" the volume. The SWOG performed a randomized trial of induction combination chemotherapy with or without thoracic irradiation in complete responders and with wide-field versus reduced-field radiation in partial responders.[62] Late administration of thoracic irradiation did not change survival for complete responders, but local control was better for irradiated patients. Field size of consolidative radiotherapy for partial responders influenced neither survival or local control.

Even if thoracic irradiation is given after only one cycle of chemotherapy, tumor reduction is usually evident at simulation. No scientific rationale exists for the presumption that chemotherapy-resistant elements are confined to the diminished volume.

Wide-Field Irradiation

An extension of larger radiotherapy volumes is the investigation of "systemic" radiotherapy by either whole-body or sequential half-body irradiation. This approach has been demonstrated to be feasible by Powell[127] and Urtasun.[128] In a German study, 91 LSCLC patients were randomized to receive 6 Gy sequential half-body fields alternating with chemotherapy or chemotherapy alone.[129] Outcome differences were not significantly different, but trends in time to progression and survival favored the chemotherapy-alone group.

Dose and Fractionation of Irradiation

These two parameters of radiotherapy are best considered together for radiobiologic reasons. The linear-quadratic method will not be discussed here, but the principle that dose not be considered in isolation from fractionation will be respected.[130] Major issues of thoracic irradiation dose and fractionation include the existence of a dose-response effect on outcome using conventionally fractionated treatment and the utility of unconventional fractionation schemas such as multiple fractions per day and split-course treatment (alternating with chemotherapy).

Local control is an alternative end point to survival in trials of thoracic irradiation dose. Several methodologic problems are associated with measurement of local control. Thoracic diagnostic imaging initially normalizes for complete responders, but patients receiving thoracic irradiation develop radiation fibrosis, which renders it more difficult to recognize relapse until it is moderately large. The method of locoregional failure reporting also varies. An absolute percentage of local relapse is the only information provided in many reports. A shortcoming of using the percentage with local control as an end point is that patients with brief survival and those with systemic failure may be censored from local control analysis, creating an illusory improvement in local control. The actuarial method is preferred because it shows cumulative local relapse rates as a function of time and considers the duration of exposure in the risk period.

Conventional fractionation (1.8 to 3.0 Gy/fraction) administers a dose 5 days a week, usually with no treatment on Saturday and Sunday. Because of the toxicity of combined modality therapy, the range of conventional fractionation doses employed in large studies has been narrow (Table 54.2). Thoracic irradiation dose was examined in a Canadian multicenter trial[131] that initially randomized patients to either immediate or delayed alternation of CAV/EP. After six courses of chemotherapy, responders were randomized to either 25 Gy in 10 fractions or 37.5 Gy in 10 fractions of consolidative radiotherapy. The prechemotherapy disease was treated with a 2 cm margin around the primary tumor. The spinal cord was shielded after 32 Gy. Of 333 patients enrolled in the study, 168 were randomized (88 to 25 Gy, 77 to 37.5 Gy). The complete remission rates for combined modality therapy were 65% and 69%, respectively. The actuarial incidence of local progression by 2 years was not significantly different (80% for 25 Gy and 69% for 37.5 Gy).

A retrospective analysis[132] of a broader range and larger doses of consolidative thoracic irradiation from a single institution suggest a dose-response effect for cumulative risk of locoregional failure. However, the nonrandomized nature of the data and small numbers in each subgroup allow only tentative conclusions. A relatively poor survival outcome from late thoracic irradiation (median 12 months, 5-year 8%) indicate that few LSCLC patients in this data set were at risk of local relapse by 3 years.

Altered fractionation has attracted much interest in recent years because of two biologic observations, one general and one specific. Fractionation studies have shown that late-responding normal tissues (microvasculature, neurons, etc.) are sensitive to the dose per fraction used in radiotherapy regimens with an equivalent total dose. This finding leads to the general principle that regimens with smaller doses per fraction may permit an increased dose to tumor while continuing to respect the tolerance of critical normal tissues.[133] In the specific case of SCLC, its rapid growth and responsiveness to therapy are associated with the lack of a "shoulder" on its *in vitro* cell survival curve in response to irradiation.[134] This pattern implies an inability to repair low levels of radiation damage and cell kill at exponential rates even with small doses per fraction. Multiple fractions per day potentially achieve greater kill at the expense of less late toxicity. Because these tumors exhibit high growth fractions *in vivo*, the compensatory repopulation response must be avoided by delivering multiple fractions per day to limit overall treatment time to 3 to 4 weeks. Most normal tissues are able to repair the damage of low doses in an interval of 4 to 6 hours, at least *in vitro*. As a practical matter, only two or three fractions per day are possible, two being the usual. Further therapeutic potential may arise from the tendency of surviving cells in a rapidly dividing tumor to redistribute themselves into more radiosensitive phases of the cell cycle prior to the subsequent treatment.

An influential pilot study of accelerated fractionation for LSCLC was performed by investigators at the University of Pennsylvania.[135,136] Cisplatin/etoposide chemotherapy was integrated with concurrent thoracic irradiation (1.5 Gy twice daily, total dose: 45 Gy in 3 weeks). After thoracic irradiation, patients received six further cycles of chemotherapy alternating CAV with EP. Mature results[136] from the phase II study of 32 patients show a median survival of 23 months and long-term survival of about 30%. Local failure occurred in less than 10% and occurred mainly in patients with "variant" histologic subtype, which have a shoulder on the *in vitro* cell survival curve.[137]

An intergroup phase III study,[78] including more than 400 patients has now been completed comparing accelerated fractionation to conventional fractionation while holding total dose constant. The conventional fractionation irradiation arm was 1.8 Gy once per day, five fractions per week for 5 weeks (total dose 45 Gy). The investigational arm included 1.5 Gy twice per day, 10 fractions per week for 3 weeks (total dose, 45 Gy). Both schedules of thoracic irradiation were given with initial concurrent cisplatin/etoposide. Four cycles of chemotherapy were administered. Response rates were not significantly different, but survival was significantly improved (p = 0.04) on the twice-daily treatment arm. Median survival was 23 months for twice daily versus 19 months for once daily; actual five-year survival rates were 26% versus 16%, respectively. Grade 3 esophagitis induced by twice-daily thoracic radiotherapy was significantly worse: twice-daily patients, 26% versus 11% (p = 0.001). Intrathoracic failure was 52% in the once-daily group and 36% in the twice-daily group (p = 0.06). This important trial was the first in SCLC to demonstrate an improvement in survival and local control by the sole stratagem of altering the fractionation. Improved effectiveness with approximately equal toxicity was expected on the basis of biologic considerations; the clinical result is encouraging, particularly in a disease so dominated by metastatic events. A logical next step would be to increase the total delivered dose using a similar fractionation.

Notably, twice-daily thoracic irradiation had no impact on median or long-term survival when compared to once-daily radiation in a randomized trial by Bonner et al.[79] that delivered radiotherapy in a delayed fashion (beginning concurrently with the fourth etoposide-cisplatin chemotherapy cycle).

Technical Factors

Potentially important technical radiotherapy factors include (a) the nature of imaging procedures used to specify target volumes, (b) the therapy equipment parameters, and (c) quality assurance procedures. Careful imaging and computed tomography (CT) based planning generate greater confidence in the volume definitions and tend to lead to tighter volumes and less toxicity. Recent studies using concurrent therapies have relied heavily on information provided in this way.[138] Newer planning technologies employ CT simulations (beam's-eye view) to facilitate the shielding of critical normal structures, and even dynamic methods with collimators, couch, and other equipment moving during the actual treatment exposure.[138] It is not known to what extent these technical advances will translate into clinical improvements; they do seem to improve the ability to safely deliver high doses to tumor and minimize normal tissue exposure.

Megavoltage machines are invariably used, usually linear accelerators. Pulmonary tissue is of low density compared to normal tissue, particularly in patients with chronic obstructive changes. The resultant inhomogeneities produce considerable variations in absorbed dose at high energies.[139] The importance of corrections for the distribution of lung density is unknown, but variations can produce substantial differences in the dose absorbed in the tumor.[140] This inhomogeneity is reduced with the use of higher energy photons, but another problem arises at energies above 10 MV. At the reduced tissue densities found in lung, electronic equilibrium (the condition required for "well-behaved" dose calculations), is not present.[141] Computation and image-intensive algorithms exist to perform these calculations, but they are not widely available. Dose inhomogeneities are accounted for by standard algorithms, but this remains a source of uncertainty in interpreting clinical results.

More traditional concerns have focused on issues of quality assurance of radiotherapy such as appropriate treatment of intended target volumes and shielding. Retrospective studies suggest that failure patterns can be influenced by these factors.[126,142] With the emergence of CT-directed treatment planning, it is relatively easy to apply a tumor dose to the primary tumor site and the mediastinum while avoiding excessive dose to the spinal cord through the use of oblique fields, lateral fields, or rotational techniques. When portals are delivered anteroposteriorly and posteroanteriorly (AP/PA), it is necessary to limit the spinal cord dose by a spinal cord block. Spinal cord blocks may shield centrally located SCLC. A Canadian study[131] of radiotherapy timing used anterior and posterior opposed fields to deliver 40 Gy in 15 fractions over 3 weeks. Posterior cord shielding limited the spinal cord dose to 35 Gy. A CALGB study[48] administered 40 Gy in 20 fractions during a four-week period, and a further boost of 10 Gy was given over 5 days to a "coned-down" volume. The AP/PA parallel opposed portals were used for the initial 36 to 38 Gy, then oblique portals were used for the final 12 to 14 Gy. Despite the more sophisticated treatment planning and higher total dose in the CALGB study, the cumulative risk of local relapse was about 50% at three years in both studies. The superior dose distribution and theoretical benefits of complex beam arrangements are self evident, but large trials will be needed to demonstrate a survival benefit.

Radiotherapy-Chemotherapy Interactions

Compression of combined modality therapies in time and increase in their intensity has taken them to the limits of patients' tolerance. To achieve greater antitumor effect in this way, benefits of temporal and spatial independence, which have traditionally been exploited to minimize toxicity, are partially disregarded. Additive interactions will not accrue meaningful benefits unless normal tissues are spared toxicity relative to the antitumor effect. Various mechanisms of interactions have been reviewed.[143] Comments here are restricted to those relevant to LSCLC therapy.

Radiation damage to lung is well known, and typical doses to tumor exceed the tolerance of any included lung. Oblique fields irradiate more pulmonary tissue than parallel opposed fields. When chemotherapeutic agents such as doxorubicin are given close to AP/PA thoracic irradiation, risk of pneumonitis is low.[74] Pulmonary toxicity can be severe when doxorubicin is given after three-field thoracic irradiation.[144] Lung injury from chemoradiation interaction exists for other drugs as well such as nitrosoureas and cyclophosphamide.[145] Reactions can be diminished if chemotherapy is limited to drugs that have little sensitizing effect on normal tissue, such as cisplatin and etoposide. Whether new cytotoxic agents such as the taxanes, topoisomerase I inhibitors, or gemcitabine can be incorporated into LSCLC concurrent chemoradiation protocols with an acceptable therapeutic index is unclear.

Thoracic irradiation techniques that irradiate large volumes of bone marrow increase hematologic toxicity and may reduce the intensity of ongoing chemotherapy. Larger fractions of cardiac output contained in the treatment volume may worsen myelosuppression disproportionately by irradiating hematopoietic progenitor cells.[146] Use of colony-stimulating factors during radiotherapy has been associated with an increase in the severity of thrombocytopenia,[147,148] and an increase in circulating hematologic stem cells has been proposed as the cause.[149] Marrow and blood stem cell irradiation may contribute to the documented worsening of hematologic toxicity from chemotherapy given after cranial irradiation.[150] Unless it can be convincingly demonstrated that there are advantages to giving prophylactic cranial irradiation early in the treatment program, chemotherapy attenuation from myelosuppression and risk of neurologic damage[151] should be less when elective brain irradiation is delayed until the chemotherapy is complete. Colony-stimulating factors as a supportive technique during radiotherapy requires further research because enhanced killing of circulating progenitor cells and depletion of myelopoeitic reserve may not be temporary.

Esophageal toxicity may be dose limiting. Acute esophagitis is common. Concomitant doxorubicin greatly exacerbates the reaction, and some radiation-recall esophagitis is commonly observed with doxorubicin-containing chemotherapy cycles given after thoracic irradiation.[54] Radiation-recall esophagitis is a manageable cause of morbidity, but a therapeutic effect from such a reaction on the tumor is difficult to investigate. Late strictures appear to be uncommon with standard treatment programs.

OPTIMAL INTEGRATION OF CHEMOTHERAPY AND THORACIC IRRADIATION

The rational development of the optimal integration of chemotherapy and thoracic irradiation for LSCLC requires an understanding of the causes of treatment failure and factors associated with long-term survival. In the absence of such insight, oncologists are vulnerable to either conservatively persisting with a logistically simple treatment plan or shifting with the fads and fashions of the latest new drug or appealing innovation. Even when a therapeutic approach seems logical, it must still be proven effective—not by high-profile pilot studies in prominent journals, or the force of persuasive personalities, but by the scientific method and the performance of controlled clinical trials. The intended outcome is to improve survival through reduction of both local failure and distant metastases.

Conceptual Model of LSCLC

LSCLC patients can be conceptually divided into three patient groups according to the presence or absence of chemotherapy-resistant stem cells and their location (Figure 54.2). A small proportion of patients (about 9%[7,8]) have no drug-resistant variants, and cure can be accomplished with chemotherapy alone provided that treatment is adequate with respect to dose intensity and total dose (Figure 54.2A). Thoracic irradiation for these patients would not make any contribution to cure unless chemotherapy treatment was inadequate and the only persistent disease was within the thoracic irradiation volume. The second group (Figure 54.2B) includes patients in whom drug-resistant disease is present, but the entire resistant clone of cells continues to reside within the principal repository of tumor stem cells at the primary site. Thoracic irradiation may eradicate these clones if it is delivered before they spread outside a reasonable treatment volume. Even if the local tumor mass was not eradicated by radiation, unless the proportion of chemotherapy-resistant cells was high, the effect of the radiation would be to "dilute out" the drug-resistant subpopulation. An ap-

propriate program of chemotherapy could then control the remaining local and distant chemosensitive disease. The event that leads to treatment failure in LSCLC is a very succinct one. It occurs when the first fully chemoresistant stem cell establishes itself where it cannot be destroyed by radiotherapy. Although they cannot be identified *a priori*, the majority of LSCLC patients are in this group (Figure 54.2C). Thoracic irradiation may improve local control, but it cannot change the fatal outcome for these patients.

Thoracic irradiation is acknowledged to be indicated in LSCLC, and no additional trials are underway to further examine this issue. This situation will not change unless dramatic advances are made in systemic therapy. The systemic nature of cancer implies that regional therapy can only influence the long-term outcome in those patients who will have their distant disease cured. Thoracic irradiation improves the long-term prognosis of LSCLC only in those cases where the systemic therapy is successful at treating distant disease (where present) but fails to eliminate regional disease. Thus the effect of radiation on improving long-term outcome is mathematically bounded by the effectiveness of chemotherapy. The contribution of thoracic irradiation to the cure of LSCLC depends on chemotherapy being only moderately effective. If chemotherapy is absent or weak, thoracic irradiation has trivial curative potential. If chemotherapy had the power to cure most patients, it could be difficult to demonstrate efficacy of local therapy.

Strategic Considerations for Assembly of Chemotherapy and Thoracic Irradiation

Arbitrary assembly of chemotherapy and thoracic irradiation is unlikely to yield the best results. Before review of

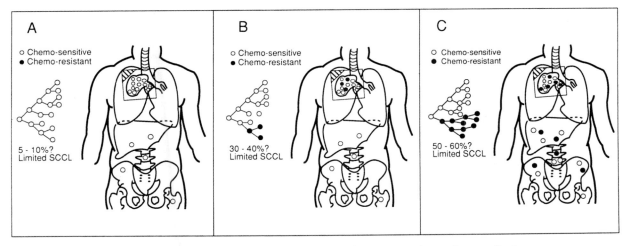

FIGURE 54.2. Conceptual model of limited small cell lung cancer shows three patient groups according to the presence or absence of chemoresistant tumor stem cells and their location. Disease depicted outside the chest is undetectable by staging procedures. Chemotherapy-resistant disease is absent in **(A)**, localized in **(B)**, and disseminated in **(C)**.

clinical investigations of chemoradiation integration, it would be useful to examine the scientific basis for various sequences of systemic and local therapeutic modalities. The goal of optimal treatment modality assembly is to maximize the probability of elimination of the last cancer stem cell, thereby attaining a durable complete remission.

A simplified overview of strategic considerations for combined modality therapy would identify two distinct plans for combining chemotherapy and thoracic irradiation (Table 54.3). The strategy of the first plan must attempt to destroy as many cancer cells as possible in the shortest period. Such front-end loaded therapy would involve using the most effective modalities early in the treatment program. Four concepts support early chemoradiation, including (a) decreased probability of metastatic events, (b) lower probability of development of chemotherapy resistance, (c) lower probability of development of resistance to radiotherapy, and (d) diminished accelerated repopulation.

The alternative model requires rationalization of the strategic superiority of deploying modalities in a sequential fashion (Table 54.3). Sequential rather than concurrent use of modalities in oncology has been prevalent for the obvious reasons of simplicity and lower toxicity. However, simplicity and low toxicity do not provide a scientific rationale for optimal tumor eradication. Existence of reversible resistance is a concept that could support sequential therapy. Additionally, if a definitive local therapy was originally impossible but was rendered feasible by neoadjuvant therapy, this concept would also support the sequential therapy model.

Concepts that Favor Early Integration of Thoracic Irradiation with Chemotherapy

The concepts that scientifically favor early integration of effective therapeutic modalities have clear-cut characteristics. The probability of treatment failure events associated with these concepts must increase fairly quickly with the elapse of time (weeks). Therefore, the chance of avoiding treatment failure should be minimized by eliminating as many tumor cells as possible in the shortest period. Rapid eradication of tumor cells requires the early integration of definitive local treatment(s) with systemic chemotherapy.

Decreased Probability of Metastatic Events

Experimental work by Hill[152,153] indicates that tumor cells mutate spontaneously and randomly to acquire metastatic potential. Moreover, once tumors reach a critical size or volume, metastatic phenotypes are generated "explosively." The cumulative probability of the existence of metastases and the number of metastases increases in proportion to elapsed time. The best way to decrease metastatic events is to quickly eliminate as much tumor as possible.

Lower Probability of Chemotherapy Resistance

A large body of experimental and clinical data exists that support the observation that variability exists for chemosensitivity within tumor cell populations.[154,155] Moreover, tumor cells display a capacity to resist many drugs concurrently.[156] The biologic basis of this evolution of resistance originates during tumor growth from mutations in the cancer genome.[157] The development of resistant mutants is a random process, and the probability of their appearance increases with time in proportion to the total number of cell divisions the neoplastic burden has undergone. The somatic mutation theory of drug resistance[109] predicts that once a tumor has reached a critical size, the probability of cure is lost over a small additional size increase in a short time period. The best way to minimize the probability of chemotherapy resistance is to eliminate as many cancer cells as possible in the shortest time.

Lower Probability of Resistance to Radiotherapy

Local control rates with radiotherapy are inversely related to tumor size.[158,159] Although microenvironmental effects such as hypoxia[160] may be relevant, increasing evidence indicates that tumor cell populations are heterogeneous with respect to inherent radiosensitivity and similar to chemo-

TABLE 54.3. CONCEPTUAL BASIS FOR EARLY INTEGRATION VERSUS SEQUENTIAL DELIVERY OF THERAPEUTIC MODALITIES IN THE ASSEMBLY OF MULTIMODALITY CANCER TREATMENT PROGRAMS

A) *Early Integration of Modalities*
   Characteristics
   — Eliminate as many cancer cells as possible in the shortest period of time.
   — Deploy multiple modalities quickly.
   — More complex logistically: requires early multidisciplinary involvement.
   — More toxic.
   Scientific Rationale
   1) Decreased probability of metastatic events.
   2) Lower probability of chemotherapy resistance.
   3) Lower probability of resistance to radiotherapy.
   4) Minimize accelerated repopulation.
B) *Sequential Assembly of Therapy*
   Characteristics
   — Modalities deployed with temporal separation.
   — Tumor burden destroyed in phases.
   — Logistically less complex: disciplines involved sequentially.
   — Chemotherapy nonresponders spared toxicity of radical local therapy.
   — Less toxic.
   Scientific Rationale
   1. Originally impossible local therapy made feasible in subset with good response to neoadjuvant chemotherapy.
   2. Requires treatment modality (chemotherapy or radiotherapy) resistance to reverse at time of planned modality deployment.

therapy resistance, resistance to ionizing radiation may be genetically determined and a stochastic process.[161] Epigenetic mechanisms for radiotherapy resistance also exist, including upregulation of DNA repair enzymes.[161] Induction of DNA repair enzymes by chemotherapy is a plausible reason why thoracic irradiation delivered after chemotherapy may be less effective. Cells that are resistant to specific chemotherapeutic agents can be very resistant[162] (a factor of several hundred compared to sensitive cells), whereas radioresistant cells are likely to be only moderately resistant (dose increase of only a factor of two or three over what is necessary for sensitive cells).[163] SCLC is less responsive to irradiation when recurrent after chemotherapy, and mechanisms of resistance may overlap; however, cross-resistance is not complete.[164] The probability of mutation to radiotherapy resistance or radioresistance as a consequence of enhanced DNA repair efficiency secondary to previous chemotherapy should be minimized by the early deployment of both modalities.

Diminished Accelerated Repopulation

"Outbursts" of cancer progression after perturbation of a tumor are not a novel observation.[165] Accelerated proliferation of tumors undergoing radiotherapy has been proposed[166,167] to explain the clinical observation that extended therapy regimens often require increased radiation dosages to achieve an isoeffective result.[168,169] Accelerated tumor growth has been reported after surgery[170] and chemotherapy[171] in animal models. Accelerated repopulation decreases local control, but additionally increased mitotic activity with larger burden of residual tumor may also hasten the tempo of metastatic events and increase the probability of developing drug and radiation resistance. Noncurative perturbation of the primary tumor may have detrimental effects (possibly mediated by cytokines) on existing metastatic lesions.[172] Accelerated repopulation is independent of modalities and an obvious form of cross-resistance. This phenomenon has not been mathematically modeled, but it appears to be well established within a few weeks after initiation of therapy.[166]

The original rationale of consolidative radiotherapy included the opinion that the smaller quantity of local disease remaining after chemotherapy would enhance the feasibility and effectiveness of local therapy. The phenomenon of repopulation imposes a different reality. Because the quantity of tumor repopulation between chemotherapy treatments depends on the size of the residual stem cell population, rapid destruction of as much cancer as possible by early integration of chemoradiation minimizes the amount of tumor capable of repopulation.

Concepts that Favor Sequential Application of Radiotherapy and Chemotherapy

Simplicity has great appeal. The model of a medical oncologist administering a series of chemotherapy treatments, assessing response, and subsequently referring the LSCLC patient for consolidative thoracic irradiation when toxicity has subsided is undoubtedly simple. This approach is also associated with fewer side effects. However, is sequential or delayed administration of thoracic irradiation after chemotherapy scientifically sound?

The strategic concepts favoring *early* combined modality have a simple rule for the timing of effective modalities; any delay is potentially detrimental because the probability of treatment failure increases as a function of time. The rules are more arcane for concepts that favor sequential modalities because an additional element of information is required. It is necessary to know the most advantageous amount of delay required for the optimum sequence of modalities. This crucial knowledge must be supplied by the concept itself or learned by the conduct of controlled clinical trials. Two strategic concepts may favor sequential therapy.

Originally Impossible Local Therapy Rendered Feasible by Neoadjuvant Therapy

An unambiguous scenario where sequential therapy would offer an advantage would be when a locally advanced tumor was originally untreatable by a definitive local therapy but such therapy was rendered feasible by downstaging. This rationale is classic for neoadjuvant chemotherapy before surgery. However, LSCLC is rarely considered for surgery, and the definition of this stage indicates that all original tumor should be encompassable within a reasonable radiotherapy treatment volume at the outset. No obvious scientific reason indicates that chemotherapy-resistant residual tumor should be confined to the postchemotherapy tumor volume.

Reversible Resistance

Sequential application of modalities could be strategically superior if resistance to a particular therapy (chemotherapy or radiotherapy) was present at one point in the treatment program but the resistance reversed later, allowing successful use of that modality. Once genetically determined resistance to chemotherapy has been acquired by a tumor, it is improbable that such elements would disappear by spontaneous mutation.[109] However, resistance to chemotherapy with an epigenetic basis could occur and would be a possible form of reversible resistance. Kinetic resistance is another type of reversible resistance. The potential superiority of sequential therapies as predicted by the Norton-Simon hypothesis[173] is based on the possible existence of kinetic resistance.

The arguments supporting either early integration of chemoradiation or sequential utilization of chemotherapy and thoracic irradiation are hypothetical and must be supported by clinical data. The most important clinical data for optimal chemoradiation integration are from randomized trials of thoracic irradiation timing.

Randomized Trials of the Timing of Thoracic Irradiation

To date, five trials[48,74–77] of thoracic irradiation timing have been performed; four trials are published in peer-reviewed journals[48,74–76] and one is currently available as an abstract.[77] Because of the importance of these trials, each study is discussed separately and summarized in Table 54.4.

The Cancer and Leukemia Group B Trial

This large trial[48,174] performed from 1981 to 1984 included 399 evaluable LSCLC patients distributed between three arms, including chemotherapy alone (cyclophosphamide, etoposide, vincristine, and doxorubicin), initial chemoradiation (50 Gy thoracic irradiation and whole-brain irradiation concurrently with the initial cycle of chemotherapy), and delayed chemoradiation (chest and brain irradiation concurrently with the fourth cycle of chemotherapy at week 9). Both arms that included thoracic irradiation had significantly superior response rates, time to progression, and overall survival rates compared to chemotherapy alone. However, no significant differences were found between the initial and delayed thoracic irradiation arms; the insignificant trend that existed favors the delayed thoracic irradiation arm. The rationale of a randomized trial is to hold all variables constant except the experimental one. Unfortunately, the interpretation of the Cancer and Leukemia Group B (CALGB) study is confounded because potential differences in outcome from thoracic irradiation timing may be obscured by unequal chemotherapy delivery. Myelosuppression from initial thoracic irradiation, brain irradiation, and concurrent CEV chemotherapy resulted in an unplanned attenuation (50% reduction) in doses of cyclophosphamide, etoposide, and doxorubicin after the first cycle. This trial clearly supports the addition of thoracic irradiation to chemotherapy in LSCLC, but the utility of the study to provide guidance for optimal integration of chemoradia-

tion is doubtful.[174] The long-term survival rates for chemoradiation in the CALGB study are low (<13%).[174]

The Aarhus Lung Cancer Group Trial

In this Danish trial[75] performed between 1981 and 1989, 199 patients with LSCLC were randomly allocated to initial chest irradiation or late chest irradiation delayed by 18 weeks. Both groups received nine cycles of combination chemotherapy: three cycles of EP and six cycles of CAV. Initial thoracic irradiation was delivered sequentially rather than concurrently with EP. The timing of radiotherapy (40–45 Gy) had no significant effect on the median survival (about 1 year) or long-term survival (about 10%).

The doses cited for the etoposide/cisplatin regimen in this study were cisplatin 60 mg/m^2 and etoposide 120 mg/m^2 on 1 day only. Conventional etoposide-cisplatin regimens deliver etoposide on at least 3 sequential days. The published doses of etoposide and cisplatin in the Aarhus study[75] do not respect the well-documented schedule dependency of this agent[175] and diminish the etoposide dose intensity to about one-third of standard levels. This trial also had an irregular randomization to prophylactic cranial irradiation.

The National Cancer Institute of Canada Trial

In 1993, the NCIC published results of a randomized trial[74] (accrual period 1985–1988) comparing early versus late thoracic irradiation that demonstrated a significant improvement in survival for early thoracic irradiation in the combined modality therapy of LSCLC. All 308 eligible patients received CAV alternating with EP for three cycles of each regimen. Patients randomized to early thoracic irradiation received 40 Gy/15F to the primary site concurrent with the first cycle of EP (week 3), and the late thoracic irradiation arm received the same radiation concurrent with the

TABLE 54.4. RANDOMIZED TRIALS OF THORACIC IRRADIATION TIMING IN LIMITED-STAGE SMALL CELL LUNG CANCER

		Thoracic Irradiation			Number of Patients		Survival Median (mo.)		Survival 5-Year (%)		
Study	Drugs	Dose	Early (Start Time)	Late	Early	Late	Early	Late	Early	Late	P-Value
1. CALGB[48,174]	CEVA	50Gy/25F/5 wk	Week 1	Week 9	125	145	13.04	14.54	6.6	12.8	NS
2. Aarhus[75]	CAV/EP	40–45Gy/22F/6 wk*	Week 1	Week 18	99	100	10.7	12.9	10.0	10.0	NS
3. NCIC[74]	CAV/EP	40/15F/3 wk	Week 3	Week 15	155	153	21.2	16.0	22.0	13.0	0.013
4. Yugoslavian[76]	Carbo/EP	54Gy/36F/3 1/2 wk	Week 1	Week 6	52	51	34	26	30	15	0.027
5. JCOG[77]	EP	45Gy/30F/3 wk	Week 1	Week 15	114	114	31.3	20.8	30	15	<0.05

* Split course
CALGB, Cancer and Leukemia Group B; NCIC, National Cancer Institute of Canada; JCOG, Japan Clinical Oncology Group; C, Cyclophosphamide; E, Etoposide; V, Vincristine; A, Doxorubicin; P, Cisplatin; Carbo, Carboplatin.

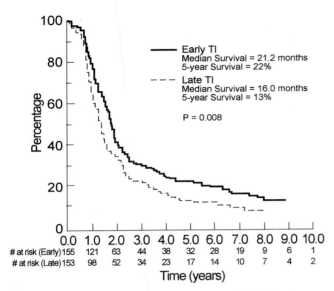

FIGURE 54.3. Updated analysis of overall survival for the National Cancer Institute (NCIC) in Canada BR6 study. (From Murray N, Coy P, Pater J, et al. Importance of timing for thoracic irradiation in the combined modality treatment of limited-stage small-cell lung cancer. *J Clin Oncol* 1993;11:336, with permission.)

last cycle of EP (week 15). Dose intensity and total dose of chemotherapy was uniform in both arms (85 to 90% delivery according to protocol).

Although complete response rates were not significantly different (CR early arm 64%, CR late arm 56%, P = 0.14), the overall survival was significantly superior (P = 0.013) in the early thoracic irradiation arm (Figure 54.3). Median survival was 21.2 months in the early arm and 16.0 months in the late arm; actual survival at 5 years was 22% in the early arm and 13% in the late arm. A delay of thoracic irradiation by 12 weeks was associated with a 50% decrease in the probability of long-term survival. This trial was the first phase III study to demonstrate that actual five-year survival rates of more than 20% were achievable using early integrated chemoradiation in LSCLC.

The Yugoslavian Trial

This extraordinary phase III study[76] performed between 1988 and 1992 achieved outcomes in LSCLC that were not only superior to any other phase III study, but survival was also better than any published phase II trial. All patients received accelerated hyperfractionated thoracic irradiation with 1.5 Gy twice daily to 54 Gy plus concurrent daily carboplatin/etoposide and four sequential cycles of EP. Early thoracic irradiation was delivered between weeks 1 to 4, and late thoracic irradiation patients received concurrent chemoradiation between weeks 6 to 9. The difference in timing of the initiation of thoracic irradiation between the two arms was only 6 weeks.

The median survival was 34 months for initial chemoradiation versus 26 months for delayed chemoradiation; five-year survival was 30% and 15%, respectively. The difference was significant on multivariate analysis (P = 0.027). This study by Jeremic and colleagues[76] shows that early integration of chemotherapy with intensive radiation for LSCLC may generate median survival times of almost 3 years, and long-term survival rates may approach 30%.

The Japan Clinical Oncology Group Trial

This study[77] by the Japan Clinical Oncology Group (JCOG) also examined the optimal sequence of chemoradiation for LSCLC by randomizing patients to initial concurrent versus sequential chemoradiation. The chemotherapy prescription was EP (four cycles), and thoracic irradiation consisted of 45 Gy over 3 weeks (two daily fractions of 1.5 Gy). Two hundred twenty-eight patients were entered between 1991 and 1995.

Initial concurrent chemoradiation was significantly superior (P < 0.05) to sequential therapy, with median survivals of 31.3 months and 20.8 months and projected five-year survival rates of 30% and 15%, respectively. These results strengthen the conclusion that long-term survival rates of more than 20% for LSCLC are obtainable with early chemoradiation.

Why Are the Randomized Trials of Thoracic Irradiation Timing Discordant?

Of the five controlled trials of thoracic irradiation timing performed, three (NCIC,[74] Yugoslavian,[76] JCOG[77]) support the concept that the optimal integration of chemotherapy and thoracic irradiation is early concurrent chemoradiation; the CALGB[174] and the Aarhus[75] studies suggest that the timing of thoracic irradiation does not influence outcome. Why are the results discordant? Three possible reasons are as follows:

1. The timing of thoracic irradiation is unimportant and the discordant results are caused by the play of chance.
2. Delivery of chemotherapy or thoracic irradiation was inadequate in the negative trials.
3. The patient populations differ.

The influence of chance cannot be discounted, but other explanations may be more plausible. Both the CALGB study[174] and the Aarhus trial[75] were associated with compromised chemotherapy delivery. Thoracic irradiation can improve the long-term prognosis of LSCLC only in those cases in which the systemic therapy successfully controls distant subclinical disease. Suboptimal systemic therapy unavoidably decreases the impact of a change in the timing of local therapy for a systemic disease. However, the most important reason for discordance of results probably is associated with differences in the trial patient populations. The prevalence of metastatic drug-resistant tumor outside the thoracic irradiation volume in the study population (Figure 54.2C) strongly affects the likelihood that thoracic irradiation or an innovation of it (timing or dose) will result in a survival advantage. If a poor prognosis LSCLC population (as evidenced by short median survival) is studied, then the proportion of cases that can have their prognosis improved by better integration of chemoradiation will be low and the benefit of early thoracic irradiation timing will be diluted out by most incurable cases. That the study populations in the CALGB[174] and Aarhus[75] trials, which fail to show superiority of early chemoradiation, were a poor prognostic group is strongly suggested by the short median survivals reported (Table 54.4). Long-term survival in these reports is also low. Adverse prognostic factors in these patients accrued to studies beginning in 1981 may have been caused by staging procedures that were less accurate than more recently reported trials. Median survival in the early chemoradiation arms of the NCIC,[74] Yugoslavian,[76] and JCOG[77] trials ranges from 21.2 to 34 months, which is two to three times longer than the median survival times in the CALGB[174] and Aarhus[75] studies. Median survival in the delayed chemoradiation arms of the trials that support early chemoradiation[74,76,77] ranges from 16 to 21 months, which indicates that *all* patients in these trials had better prognostic factors than the negative trials.[174,75] More important, long-term survival for early chemoradiation consistently exceeds 20% at 5 years.[74,76,77] Delayed chemoradiation has never approached the 20% long-term survival milestone, which should be considered minimum standard for LSCLC at this time. Delayed chemoradiation usually is associated with a long-term survival rate of approximately 10% (Table 54.4), which is not much different from the 9% rate expected from chemotherapy alone, as reported in the metaanalysis[8] of randomized trials performed in a similar era.

Ongoing or accelerated metastatic behavior of tumors that are responding to chemotherapy is counterintuitive. The data from randomized trials of thoracic irradiation timing in LSCLC suggests that the satisfaction medical oncologists experience when reviewing radiographs showing an LSCLC patient responding to drug treatment should be replaced with a sense of urgency that definitive local treatment must begin as soon as possible.

Alternating Chemotherapy and Thoracic Irradiation

Sequential and concurrent chemoradiation have previously been discussed in relation to the temporal arrangement of therapies. If interruptions in the radiotherapy sequence are permitted (split-course), then strategies of alternating chemotherapy and radiotherapy become possible, in which short courses of radiotherapy are interposed between cycles of chemotherapy without disrupting the schedule of drug treatment. Alternating chemoradiation was developed to reconcile the needs for early administration of both agents and for sequential delivery of each modality without a long break.[176] Although split-course radiotherapy in the absence of chemotherapy is believed to be detrimental, experimental evidence suggests that an alternating approach may be effective. Alternating chemotherapy and radiotherapy in the rat hepatoma model produced cures in a proportion of animals that could not be achieved by either modality administered sequentially.[177] Similar results were predicted by computer simulation studies.[178]

Clinical investigation of alternating chemoradiation for LSCLC was performed independently of the animal model and computer studies. This approach was used in one of the largest controlled studies, demonstrating superiority of combined modality therapy over chemotherapy alone.[49] The group at the Institut Gustave-Roussy[179] has performed a sequence of pilot studies pursuing an improved schedule. The alternating plan consisted of six courses of chemotherapy (doxorubicin, cyclophosphamide, etoposide, and cisplatin) and three courses of thoracic irradiation, delivering a total dose of 45, 55, and 65 Gy in consecutive protocols. Radiotherapy was started after the second cycle of chemotherapy with a gap of 1 week between modalities. Seventy percent of patients achieved complete remission. The actuarial five-year local control rate was 60% and five-year overall survival was 18%. No apparent improvement in local control or survival was achieved with higher total thoracic irradiation doses.

Lebeau et al.[180] randomized 156 eligible patients to either concurrent thoracic irradiation initiated immediately after the second cycle of chemotherapy (cyclophosphamide, doxorubicin, etoposide) versus alternating thoracic irradiation in three courses between the 2–3, 3–4, 4–5 chemotherapy cycles. Unfortunately, the conduct of the trial was frustrated by the occurrence of pulmonary toxicity that resulted in termination of the trial with less than one-half of the planned sample size. Moreover, the median survival (13 to 14 months) and three-year survival (4% to 7%) was poor and similar in both arms. Comparison of concurrent versus alternating chemotherapy may be worthwhile in a trial using more compatible chemotherapy (EP).

The concept of alternating chemotherapy was put to a direct test in a study[181] by the EORTC using the three-drug CDE (cyclophosphamide, doxorubicin, etoposide) regimen. Thoracic radiotherapy was given as 2.5 Gy daily, 5 days per week. A continuous four-week consolidation regimen given after five cycles of CDE was compared to an "alternating" regimen in which one week (12.5 Gy/5 fractions) of radiotherapy was associated with each of four chemotherapy cycles after the first. In this randomized study of 335 patients, the alternating regimen was associated with hematologic toxicity severe enough to compromise delivery of both radiation and chemotherapy. No differences in outcome were noted.

LSCLC in the Infirm and Elderly

The experience of elderly patients in two large randomized trials performed by the NCIC has been reviewed, and also discussed in Chapter 64.[182,183] The two trials included 88 patients aged 70 to 80 years in the total group of 608. The elderly subset was found to have received significantly less total drug than the younger patients, largely because of dose omissions rather than dose reductions. Dose omissions were not clearly associated with an increased rate of grade 3–4 toxicity events. Thoracic irradiation (most received 35–40 Gy), even when administered with concurrent chemotherapy, was also well tolerated by the elderly. No increased rate of treatment interruptions occurred, although when irradiation was performed late in the regimen, the elderly were slightly less likely to complete it. The overall rates of response, local relapse, and survival were similar, and age was not a significant prognostic factor. However, the elderly patients represented in these randomized trials may not be representative of elderly patients with LSCLC in general.

Elderly patients with cancer are just as likely to agree to treatment given with curative intent as younger patients, but they are more conservative with respect to trading toxicity with survival.[184] Fit elderly patients should not be denied treatment with standard regimens or access to clinical trials simply on the basis of their age. However, standard protocols are difficult for frail elderly patients or patients of any age with serious co-morbid illness. Rather than abandoning hope for long-term survival in such patients, evidence suggests that abbreviated chemotherapy (two cycles) plus thoracic irradiation has the potential to achieve the therapeutic goals of symptom palliation, prolongation of median survival, and chance of long-term survival.

In a pilot study with mature results, Murray et al.[185] reported on 55 patients with a median age of 73 years who received only two chemotherapy cycles (one CAV, one EP) plus thoracic irradiation concurrently with the EP cycle. The median survival was 54 weeks and actual five-year survival was 18%. Jeremic et al.[186] reported a median survival of 15 months and five-year survival of 13% for a regimen consisting of two cycles of carboplatin and oral etoposide concurrent with hyperfractionated thoracic irradiation. These observations provide some data that may allow realistic reassurance for LSCLC patients who are unable to complete all planned chemotherapy that a large portion of chemotherapy benefit is conferred by the first two cycles and thoracic irradiation. Abbreviated regimens should be compared to standard duration regimes in the large and increasing LSCLC patient population.

TREATMENT RECOMMENDATIONS

After the diagnosis of SCLC, accurate staging should be completed as expediently as possible. Patients with LSCLC should have consultation from both medical and radiation oncologists prior to commencing treatment. If an appropriate clinical trial is available, it should be offered to the patient. Noninvestigational therapy should be given according to a published protocol rather than assembled in an arbitrary fashion. The treatment plan should be commenced without unnecessary delay.

Integration of Chemotherapy and Radiotherapy

Theoretical and clinical data suggest that the best results are obtained with a combination of multiagent chemotherapy and radiotherapy. Thoracic irradiation should be integrated concurrently with chemotherapy early in the program in a way that allows reliable delivery of both modalities.

Chemotherapy Prescription

Standard regimens include EP and alternating CAV/EP. The standard interval between cycles is 3 weeks. The EP combination should be administered concurrently with thoracic irradiation. Chemotherapy doses should not cause more than moderately severe myelotoxicity, and no more than four to six chemotherapy cycles are necessary. Elderly, frail, or noncompliant LSCLC patients who are unable to receive standard-duration chemotherapy may have useful palliation and potential for long-term survival with abbreviated chemotherapy (two cycles) and thoracic irradiation.

Thoracic Irradiation

Evidence suggests that irradiation is best administered concurrently to (or in close association with) one of the early chemotherapy cycles (first or second). The radiotherapy volumes should encompass all areas of gross primary and mediastinal disease, based on CT planning. Through tight initial definitions or the use of volume reductions, normal tissues may be spared; it is not possible to administer full dose to all sites of potential mediastinal spread. Application of newer imaging and conformal radiotherapy planning techniques offers the possibility of improved sparing of normal tissue and of escalating the dose to known tumor. Dose-fractionation regimens may range from 40 Gy in 15 fractions to 50 Gy in 25 fractions (based on evidence from randomized trials). Twice-daily fractionation (1.5 Gy to 45 Gy) is also an appropriate standard of care. Standard regimens should start on Monday to minimize weekend interruptions. Unnecessary treatment breaks should be avoided. In the absence of evidence of infection, thoracic irradiation should not be interrupted for neutropenia, regardless of its severity.

Supportive Care

Until lung cancer symptoms are controlled by antineoplastic therapy, appropriate symptomatic treatment is essential not only for patient comfort but also because these measures may enhance the fidelity of the combined modality program. Similarly, prevention and treatment of side effects and complications minimizes protocol violations.

Standard chemotherapy regimens can be given with a good margin of safety without colony-stimulating factors. Administration of granulocyte colony-stimulating factor (G-CSF) to patients who have treatment delays or reductions because of neutropenia is reasonable when treatment is potentially curative. Because increased thrombocytopenia has been observed when CSFs are given with concurrent chemoradiation,[147] cytokine supportive care in this setting should be avoided.

Clinicians must assess the psychosocial needs of lung cancer patients and use the expertise of their health care colleagues specializing in this area. Inadequate psychological support of the patient can undermine the best treatment plan. Smoking cessation after successful treatment of SCLC is associated with fewer smoking-related second primary cancers.[187] These patients must be actively encouraged and assisted to stop smoking.

Restaging of Responding Patients

LSCLC patients who achieve a satisfactory radiographic response of thoracic disease from combined modality therapy do not require restaging.[188] Repeat bronchoscopy may identify a small proportion of complete radiographic responders with residual disease, which may be of academic interest. However, in the absence of a proven therapy that can convert partial responders who have already received both chemotherapy and thoracic irradiation into complete responders with potential for long-term survival, the patient discomfort and additional costs mitigate against restaging bronchoscopy.

RESEARCH PRIORITIES

Unlike breast and bowel cancer, no large trials (more than 1,000 patients) have set out to definitively answer important questions in the treatment of LSCLC. To a limited extent, the lack of large trials can be augmented by the metaanalysis of smaller trials, which have used similar protocols. However, heterogeneity of trial design, drug usage, and radiotherapy application among trials reduces the likelihood that differences will be seen when study patients are distributed across several studies compared to their consolidation within larger studies. The potential increase in plausibility obtained by the demonstration of a therapeutic effect in various trials is offset by the likelihood that a small but meaningful thera-

peutic advance will go unproven. A second concern with the results of metaanalyses of multimodality therapy is that multiple protocol differences may permit several interpretations of the reason(s) for any observed differences. The rationale for the creation of large intergroup trials is particularly strong in LSCLC, where modest therapeutic advance seems possible.

Lung cancer investigators must decide how much of change in long-term survival is important enough to warrant a clinical trial large enough to prove it. Most would probably agree that an increase in the cure rate of 10% is worthwhile. What about 5%? Many would reply affirmatively. For a disease this common, a true increase in the cure rate of 5% would save many patients. What about less than 5%? Probably not. Table 54.5 gives the sample sizes for trials where clinical parameters are in the range of those likely to be seen in LSCLC trials in the future. Examination of this table shows that only a few of the trials conducted to date have sample sizes that exceed the smallest of those in the table. Although most trials are small, metaanalyses have been able to demonstrate value in the use and timing of radiation. However, it will never be apparent what improvements will be missed because of the lack of large meaningful clinical trials. A substantial improvement from a succession of small advances is realistic.

Research priorities for LSCLC may include (a) further studies confirming the importance of timing of thoracic irradiation in combined modality therapy, (b) evaluation of more effective thoracic irradiation, (c) and modification of drug resistance. Investigation of chemotherapy regimens including a new drug should consider whether the combination regimen can be given concurrently or adjacent to thoracic irradiation. A large array of drugs with novel molecular targets provides welcome relief from an increasingly tedious cytotoxic drug agenda.

The clinical work performed to date appears to allay one important and serious concern. With dosage adjustments and modern methods of supportive care, it is possible to

TABLE 54.5. TOTAL SAMPLE SIZE REQUIRED FOR TWO-ARM PHASE III TRIALS AS A FUNCTION OF OVERALL SURVIVAL RATE AND IMPROVEMENT IN OVERALL SURVIVAL RATE

Control Arm Survival Rate (%)	Total Sample Size Required for Improvement in Survival Rate		
	5%	10%	15%
10	1,290	394	134
15	1,894	544	208
20	2,444	676	328
25	2,926	788	374

α, 0.05; power, 0.90
Allow for ineligibility, loss to follow-up, and late events.

put patients through fairly rigorous combined modality treatment programs without unacceptable morbidity. Thus ethical concerns that might otherwise have impeded the clinical testing of these concepts appear satisfied. The ethics of phase II and III studies for LSCLC patients must consider that standard combined modality therapy may achieve a five-year survival rate of 20% or more.

CONCLUSION

The opportunity for demonstrating treatment improvements for LSCLC would appear to be greater for systemic chemotherapy, where a large array of drug permutations and dosing variations is used. Additionally, the entire LSCLC population is a potential beneficiary of bona fide improvements in chemotherapy. For radiotherapy, the entire group is eligible for better local control, but only patients without drug-resistant metastases outside the radiotherapy volume are eligible for a contribution of thoracic irradiation to cure. It is disappointing that an advance in the efficacy of chemotherapy for SCLC has not been convincingly shown for more than 20 years. On the other hand, several radiotherapy interventions have shown significant contributions to LSCLC median and long-term survival in phase III randomized trials or metaanalyses, including (a) addition of thoracic irradiation to chemotherapy, (b) importance of early timing of thoracic irradiation, (c) increase in thoracic irradiation intensity, and (d) addition of prophylactic cranial irradiation to complete responders. Progress in the integration of modalities for LSCLC probes fundamental aspects of tumor biology. The LSCLC treatment model of early integration of local and systemic therapy should be considered for other rapidly growing cancers for which local and systemic therapy are combined with curative intent despite a high probability of the presence of metastases and chemotherapy resistance.

REFERENCES

1. Green RA, Humphrey E, Close H, et al. Alkylating agents in bronchogenic carcinoma. *Am J Med* 1969;46:516.
2. Albain KS, Crowley JJ, LeBlanc M, et al. Determinants of improved outcome in small cell lung cancer: an analysis of the 2,580-patient Southwest Oncology Group database. *J Clin Oncol* 1990;8:1563.
3. Rawson NSB, Peto J. An overview of prognostic factors in small cell lung cancer: a report from the Subcommittee for the Management of Lung Cancer of the United Kingdom Coordinating Committee on Cancer Research. *Br J Cancer* 1990;61:597.
4. Sagman U, Maki E, Evans WK, et al. Small-cell carcinoma of the lung: derivation of a prognostic staging system. *J Clin Oncol* 1991;9:1339.
5. Spiegelman D, Maurer LH, Ware JH, et al. Prognostic factors in small-cell carcinoma of the lung: an analysis of 1,521 patients. *J Clin Oncol* 1989;7:344.
6. Dearing MP, Steinberg SM, Phelps R, et al. Outcome of pa-

7. tients with small cell lung cancer: effects of changes in staging procedures and imaging technology on prognostic factors over 14 years. *J Clin Oncol* 1990;8:1042.
7. Warde P, Payne D. Does thoracic irradiation improve survival and local control in limited-stage small-cell carcinoma of the lung? A meta-analysis. *J Clin Oncol* 1992;10:890.
8. Pignon JP, Arriagada R, Ihde DC, et al. A meta-analysis of thoracic radiotherapy for small cell lung cancer. *N Engl J Med* 1992;327:1618.
9. Shepherd F, Ginsberg RJ, Haddad R, et al. Importance of clinical staging in limited small-cell lung cancer: a valuable system to separate prognostic subgroups. *J Clin Oncol* 1993;11:1592.
10. Richardson GE, Venzon DJ, Phelps R, et al. Application of an algorithm for staging small-cell lung cancer can save one third of the initial evaluation costs. *Arch Intern Med* 1993;153:329.
11. Kuhn TS. *The structure of scientific revolutions,* 2nd ed. Chicago: University of Chicago Press, 1970.
12. Shields TW, Humphrey EW, Eastridge CE, et al. Adjuvant cancer chemotherapy after resection of carcinoma of the lung. *Cancer* 1977;40:2057.
13. Higgins GA, Shields TW. Experience of the Veterans Administration Surgical Adjuvant Group. In: Muggia FM, Rozencweig M, eds. *Lung cancer progress in therapeutic research.* New York: Raven Press, 1979:433.
14. Higgins GA, Shields TW, Keehn RJ. The solitary pulmonary nodule: ten-year follow-up of Veterans Administration–Armed Forces cooperative study. *Arch Surg* 1975;110:570.
15. Barnard WG. The nature of the "oat-celled sarcoma" of the mediastinum. *J Pathol* 1926;29:241.
16. Azzopardi JG. Oat cell carcinoma of the bronchus. *J Pathol Bacteriol* 1959;78:513.
17. Watson WL, Berg JW. Oat cell lung cancer. *Cancer* 1962;15:759.
18. Zelen M. Keynote address on biostatistics and data retrieval. *Cancer Chemother Rep* (Part 3) 1973;4:31.
19. Miller AB, Fox W, Tall R. Five-year follow-up of the Medical Research Council's comparative trial of surgery and radiotherapy for the primary treatment of small celled carcinoma or oat celled carcinoma of the bronchus. *Lancet* 1969;12:501.
20. Fox W, Scadding JG. Medical Research Council comparative trial of surgery and radiotherapy for primary treatment of small celled or oat celled carcinoma of the bronchus. Ten year follow-up. *Lancet* 1973;2:63.
21. Matthews MJ, Kanhouwa S, Pickren J, et al. Frequency of residual and metastatic tumor in patients undergoing curative surgical resection for lung cancer. *Cancer Chemother Rep* (Part 3) 1973;4:63.
22. Wingfield HV. Combined surgery and chemotherapy for carcinoma of the bronchus. *Lancet* 1970;1:470.
23. Wolf J, Spear P, Yesner R, et al. Nitrogen mustard and the steroid hormones in the treatment of inoperable bronchogenic carcinoma. *Am J Med* 1960;29:1008.
24. Davis HL, Ramirez G, Korbitz BC, et al. Advanced lung cancer treated with cyclophosphamide. *Dis Chest* 1969;56:494.
25. Cameron SJ, Grant IWB, Crompton GK. Cyclophosphamide in disseminated bronchial carcinoma. *Scott Med J* 1974;19:81.
26. Brunner KW, Marthaler T, Muller W. Adjuvant chemotherapy with cyclophosphamide (NSC-26271) for radically resected bronchogenic carcinoma: nine-year follow-up. *Prog Cancer Res Ther* 1979;11:411.
27. Stott H, Stephens WF, Roy DC. Five year follow-up of cytotoxic as an adjuvant to surgery in carcinomas of the bronchus. *Br J Cancer* 1976;34:167.
28. Bergsagel DE, Jenkin RDT, Pringle JF, et al. Lung cancer: clinical trial of radiotherapy alone vs. radiotherapy plus cyclophosphamide. *Cancer* 1972;30:621.

29. Medical Research Council Lung Cancer Working Party. Radiotherapy alone or with chemotherapy in the treatment of small-cell carcinoma of the lung. *Br J Cancer* 1979;40:1.

30. Petrovich Z, Ohanian M, Cox J. Clinical research on the treatment of locally advanced lung cancer: final report of VALG protocol 13 limited. *Cancer* 1978;42:1129.

31. Perez CA, Krauss S, Bartolucci A, et al. Thoracic and elective brain irradiation with concomitant or delayed multiagent chemotherapy in the treatment of localized small cell carcinoma of the lung. *Cancer* 1981;47:2407.

32. Seydel HG, Creech R, Pagano M, et al. Small cell carcinoma: combined modality treatment of regional small cell undifferentiated carcinoma of the lung. *Int J Radiat Oncol Biol Phys* 1983; 9:113.

33. Hansen HH, Muggia FM, Andrews R, et al. Intensive combined chemotherapy and radiotherapy in patients with non-resectable bronchogenic carcinoma. *Cancer* 1972;30:315.

34. Eagan RT, Maurer LH, Forcier RJ, et al. Combination chemotherapy and radiation therapy in small cell carcinoma of the lung. *Cancer* 1973;32:371.

35. Holoye PY, Samuels ML. Cyclophosphamide, vincristine and sequential split-course radiotherapy in the treatment of small cell lung cancer. *Chest* 1975;67:675.

36. Einhorn LH, Fee WH, Farber MO, et al. Improved chemotherapy for small-cell undifferentiated lung cancer. *JAMA* 1976; 235:1225.

37. Einhorn L, Krause M, Hornback N, et al. Enhanced pulmonary toxicity with bleomycin and radiotherapy in oat cell lung cancer. *Cancer* 1976;37:2414.

38. DeVita VT, Young RC, Canellos GP. Combination versus single agent chemotherapy: a review of the basis for selection of drug treatment for cancer. *Cancer* 1975;35:98.

39. Lowenbraun S, Bartolucci A, Smalley RV, et al. The superiority of combination chemotherapy over single agent chemotherapy in small cell lung carcinoma. *Cancer* 1979;44:406.

40. Edmonson JH, Lagakos SW, Selawry OS, et al. Cyclophosphamide and CCNU in the treatment of inoperable small cell carcinoma and adenocarcinoma of the lung. *Cancer Treat Rep* 1976; 60:925.

41. Alberto P, Brunner KW, Martz G, et al. Treatment of bronchogenic carcinoma with simultaneous or sequential combination chemotherapy, including methotrexate, cyclophosphamide, procarbazine and vincristine. *Cancer* 1976;38:2208.

42. Byhardt RW, Cox JD, Holoye PY, et al. The role of consolidation irradiation in combined modality therapy of small cell carcinoma of the lung. *Int J Radiat Oncol Biol Phys* 1982;8:1271.

43. Cohen MH, Ihde DC, Bunn PA Jr, et al. Cyclic alternating combination chemotherapy for small cell bronchogenic carcinoma. *Cancer Treat Rep* 1979;63:163.

44. Greco FA, Einhorn LH, Richardson RL, et al. Small cell lung cancer: progress and perspectives. *Semin Oncol* 1978;5:323.

45. Byhardt RW, Cox JD. Is chest radiotherapy necessary in any or all patients with small cell carcinoma of the lung? Yes. *Cancer Treat Rep* 1983;67:290.

46. Cohen MH. Is thoracic radiation necessary for patients with limited-stage small cell lung cancer? No. *Cancer Treat Rep* 1983; 67:217.

47. Bunn PA, Lichter AS, Makuch RW, et al. Chemotherapy alone or chemotherapy with chest radiation therapy in limited stage small cell lung cancer: a prospective randomized trial. *Ann Intern Med* 1987;106:655.

48. Perry MC, Eaton WL, Propert KJ, et al. Chemotherapy with or without radiation therapy in limited small-cell carcinoma of the lung. *N Engl J Med* 1987;316:912.

49. Perez CA, Einhorn L, Oldham RK, et al. Randomized trial or radiotherapy to the thorax in limited small-cell carcinoma of the lung treated with multiagent chemotherapy and elective brain irradiation: a preliminary report. *J Clin Oncol* 1984;2: 1200.

50. Fox RM, Woods RL, Brodie GN, et al. A randomized study: small cell anaplastic lung cancer treated by combination chemotherapy and adjuvant radiotherapy. *Int J Radiat Oncol Biol Phys* 1980;6:1083.

51. Greco FA, Perez C, Einhorn LH, et al. Combination chemotherapy with or without concurrent thoracic radiotherapy in limited stage small cell lung cancer: a phase III trial of the Southeastern Cancer Study Group. *Proc Am Soc Clin Oncol* 1988;7:196.

52. Kies MS, Mira JG, Crowley JJ, et al. Multimodal therapy for limited small cell lung cancer: a randomized study of induction combination chemotherapy with or without thoracic radiation in complete responders; and with wide-field versus reduced-field radiation in partial responders: a Southwest Oncology Group study. *J Clin Oncol* 1987;5:592.

53. Souhami RL, Geddes DM, Spiro SG, et al. Radiotherapy in small cell cancer of the lung treated with combination chemotherapy: a controlled trial. *Br Med J* 1984;288:1643.

54. Osterlind K, Hansen HH, Hansen HS, et al. Chemotherapy versus chemotherapy plus irradiation in limited small cell lung cancer: results of a controlled trial with 5 years follow-up. *Br J Cancer* 1986;54:7.

55. Carlson RW, Sikic BI, Gandara DR, et al. Late consolidative radiation therapy in the treatment of limited-stage small cell lung cancer. *Cancer* 1991;68:948.

56. Creech R, Richter M, Finkelstein D. Combination chemotherapy with or without consolidation radiation therapy for regional small cell carcinoma of the lung. *Proc Am Soc Clin Oncol* 1988; 7:196.

57. Nou E, Brodin O, Bergh J. A randomized study of radiation treatment in small cell bronchial carcinoma treated with two types of four-drug chemotherapy regimens. *Cancer* 1988;62: 1079.

58. Johnson DH, Bass D, Einhorn LH, et al. Combination chemotherapy with or without thoracic radiotherapy in limited-stage small-cell lung cancer: a randomized trial of the Southeastern Cancer Study Group. *J Clin Oncol* 1993;11:1223.

59. Johnson RE, Brereton HD, Kent CH. Small cell carcinoma of the lung: attempt to remedy causes of past therapeutic failure. *Lancet* 1976;2:289.

60. Kent CH, Brereton HD, Johnson RE. "Total" therapy for oat cell carcinoma of the lung. *Int J Radiat Oncol Biol Phys* 1977; 2:427.

61. Johnson RE, Brereton HD, Kent CH. "Total" therapy for small cell carcinoma of the lung. *Ann Thorac Surg* 1978;25:510.

62. Catane R, Lichter A, Lee YJ, et al. Small cell lung cancer: analysis of treatment factors contributing to long term survival. *Cancer* 1981;48:1936.

63. Pinkel D. Five-year follow-up of "total therapy" of childhood lymphocytic leukemia. *JAMA* 1971;216:648.

64. Greco FA, Brereton HD, Kent CH, et al. Adriamycin and enhanced radiation reaction in normal esophagus and skin. *Ann Int Med* 1976;85:294.

65. Skipper HE. Historic milestones in cancer biology: a few that are important in cancer treatment (revisited). *Sem Oncol* 1979; 6:506.

66. Livingston RB, Moore TN, Heilbrun L, et al. Small-cell carcinoma of the lung: combined chemotherapy and radiation. A Southwest Oncology Group study. *Ann Intern Med* 1978;88: 194.

67. Greco FA, Richardson RL, Snell JD, et al. Small cell lung cancer, complete remission and improved survival. *Am J Med* 1979;66: 625.

68. Sierocki JS, Hilaris BS, Hopfan S, et al. Cis-dichlorodiammi-neplatinum (II) and VP-16-213: an active induction regimen for small cell carcinoma of the lung. *Cancer Treat Rep* 1979; 63:1593.

69. Douple FB, Richmond RC. A review of platinum complex biochemistry suggests a rationale for combined platinum-radiotherapy. *Int J Radiat Oncol Biol Phys* 1979;5:1335.

70. Murray N, Hadzic E, Shah A, et al. Alternating chemotherapy and thoracic irradiation with concurrent cisplatin-etoposide for limited stage small cell lung cancer. *Proc Am Soc Clin Oncol* 1984;3:214.

71. Murray N, Shah A, Brown E, et al. Alternating chemotherapy and thoracic radiotherapy with concurrent cisplatin-etoposide for limited-stage small-cell carcinoma of the lung. *Semin Oncol* 1986;13(suppl 3):24.

72. McCracken JD, Janaki LM, Taylor PG, et al. Concurrent chemotherapy and radiotherapy for limited small-cell carcinoma of the lung: a Southwest Oncology Group Study. *Semin Oncol* 1986;13(suppl 3):31.

73. McCracken JD, Janaki LM, Crowley JJ, et al. Concurrent chemotherapy/radiotherapy for limited small-cell lung carcinoma: a Southwest Oncology Group study. *J Clin Oncol* 1990; 8:892.

74. Murray N, Coy P, Pater J, et al. Importance of timing for thoracic irradiation in the combined modality treatment of limited-stage small-cell lung cancer. *J Clin Oncol* 1993;11:336.

75. Work E, Nielsen O, Bentzen S, et al. Randomized study of initial versus late chest irradiation combined with chemotherapy in limited-stage small cell lung cancer. *J Clin Oncol* 1997;15: 3030.

76. Jeremic B, Shibamato Y, Acimovic L, et al. Initial versus delayed accelerated hyperfractionated radiation therapy and concurrent chemotherapy in limited small-cell lung cancer: a randomized study. *J Clin Oncol* 1997;15:893.

77. Takada M, Fukuoka M, Furuse K, et al. Phase III study of concurrent versus sequential thoracic radiotherapy in combination with cisplatin and etoposide for limited-stage small cell lung cancer: preliminary results of the Japan Clinical Oncology Group (JCOG). *Proc Am Soc Clin Oncol* 1996;15:372.

78. Turrisi AT, Kim K, Blum R, et al. Twice daily thoracic radiotherapy versus once daily radiotherapy in limited small-cell lung cancer treated concurrently with cisplatin-etoposide chemotherapy. *N Engl J Med* 1999;340:265.

79. Bonner JA, Shanahan TG, Brooks BJ, et al. Phase III comparison of once-daily thoracic radiation versus twice-daily thoracic irradiation in patients with limited stage small cell lung cancer. *Proc Am Soc Clin Oncol* 1998;17:456.

80. Medical Research Council Lung Cancer Working Party. Comparison of oral etoposide and standard intravenous multidrug chemotherapy for small-cell lung cancer: a stopped multicentre randomised trial. *Lancet* 1996;348:563.

81. Souhami RL, Spiro SG, Rudd RM, et al. Five day oral etoposide treatment for advanced small-cell lung cancer: randomized comparison with intravenous chemotherapy. *J Natl Cancer Inst* 1997;89,577.

82. Ihde DH. Chemotherapy of lung cancer. *N Engl J Med* 1992; 327:1434.

83. Evans WK, Slevin ML. Multi-agent chemotherapy for small cell lung cancer: a basic necessity or basically unnecessary? *Can J Oncol* 1992;2:73.

84. Glatstein E, Makuch RW. Illusion and reality; practical pitfalls in interpreting clinical trials. *J Clin Oncol* 1984;2:488.

85. Spiro SG, Souhami RL, Geddes DM, et al. Duration of chemotherapy in small cell lung cancer: a Cancer Research Campaign trial. *Br J Cancer* 1989;59:578.

86. Medical Council Research Lung Working Party: controlled trial of twelve versus six courses of chemotherapy in the treatment of small-cell lung cancer. *Br J Cancer* 1989;59:584.

87. Giaccone G, Dalesio O, McVie G, et al. Maintenance chemotherapy in small-cell lung cancer: long-term results of a randomized trial. *J Clin Oncol* 1993;11:1230.

88. Feld R, Evans WK, Coy P, et al. Canadian multicenter randomized trial comparing sequential and alternating administration of two non-cross resistant chemotherapy combinations in patients with limited small cell carcinoma of the lung. *J Clin Oncol* 1987; 5:1401.

89. Goodman GE, Crowley JJ, Blasko JC, et al. Treatment of limited small cell lung cancer with etoposide and cisplatin alternating with vincristine, doxorubicin and cyclophosphamide versus concurrent etoposide, vincristine, doxorubicin, and cyclophosphamide and chest radiotherapy: a Southwest Oncology Group Study. *J Clin Oncol* 1990;8:39.

90. Johnson DH, Turrisi AT, Chang AY, et al. Alternating chemotherapy and twice-daily thoracic radiotherapy in limited-stage small-cell lung cancer: a pilot study of the Eastern Cooperative Oncology Group. *J Clin Oncol* 1993;11:879.

91. Goldie JH, Coldman AJ, Gudauskas GA. Rationale for the use of alternating non-cross resistant chemotherapy. *Cancer Treat Rep* 1982;66:439.

92. Evans WK, Feld R, Murray N, et al. Superiority of alternating non-cross-resistant chemotherapy in extensive stage small cell lung cancer. *Ann Intern Med* 1987;107:451.

93. Ettinger DS, Finkelstein DM, Abeloff MD, et al. A randomized comparison of standard chemotherapy versus alternating chemotherapy and maintenance versus no maintenance for extensive stage small-cell lung cancer: a phase III study of the Eastern Cooperative Oncology Group. *J Clin Oncol* 1990;8: 230.

94. Roth BJ, Johnson DH, Einhorn LH, et al. Randomized study of cyclophosphamide plus doxorubicin plus vincristine versus etoposide plus cisplatin versus alternation of these two regimens in extensive small cell lung cancer: a phase III study of the Southeastern Cancer Study Group. *J Clin Oncol* 1992;10:282.

95. Havemann K, Wolf M, Holle R, et al. Alternating versus sequential chemotherapy in small cell lung cancer: a randomized German multicenter trial. *Cancer* 1987;59:1072.

96. Wolf M, Pritsch P, Drings P, et al. Cyclic-alternating versus response-oriented chemotherapy in small-cell lung cancer: a German multicenter randomized trial of 321 patients. *J Clin Oncol* 1991;9:614.

97. Woods RL, Levi JL. Chemotherapy for small cell lung cancer: a randomized study of maintenance chemotherapy with cyclophosphamide, adriamycin, and vincristine after remission induction with cis-platinum, VP-16-213 and radiotherapy. *Proc Am Soc Clin Oncol* 1984;3:214.

98. Clarke SJ, Bell DR, Woods RL, et al. Maintenance chemotherapy for small cell carcinoma of the lung: long term follow-up. *Proc Am Soc Clin Oncol* 1989;8:248.

99. Jett JR, Everson L, Therneau TM, et al. Treatment of limited-stage small-cell lung cancer with cyclophosphamide, doxorubicin and vincristine with or without etoposide: a randomized trial of the North Central Cancer Treatment Group. *J Clin Oncol* 1990;8:33.

100. Fukuoka M, Furuse K, Saijo N, et al. Randomized trial of cyclophosphamide, doxorubicin, and vincristine versus cisplatin and etoposide versus alternation of these regimens in small cell lung cancer. *J Natl Canc Inst* 1991;83:855.

101. Skipper HE, Schabel FM Jr, Mellet LB, et al. Implications of biochemical, cytokinetic, pharmacologic and toxicologic relationships in the design of optimal therapeutic schedules. *Cancer Chemother Rep* 1970;54:431.

102. Hande KR, Oldham RK, Fer MF, et al. Randomized study

of high-dose versus low-dose methotrexate in the treatment of extensive small cell lung cancer. *Am J Med* 1982;73:413.

103. Johnson DH, Einhorn LH, Birch R, et al. A randomized comparison of high-dose versus conventional-dose cyclophosphamide, doxorubicin and vincristine for extensive-stage small-cell lung cancer: a phase III trial for the Southeastern Cancer Study Group. *J Clin Oncol* 1987;5:1731.

104. Ihde DH, Mulshine JL, Kramer BS, et al. Randomized trial of high vs. standard dose etoposide (VP-16) and cisplatin in extensive stage small cell lung cancer. *Proc Am Soc Clin Oncol* 1991; 10:240.

105. Figueredo AT, Hryniuk WM, Strautmanis I, et al. Cotrimoxazole prophylaxis during high-dose chemotherapy of small-cell lung cancer. *J Clin Oncol* 1985;3:54.

106. Klasa RJ, Murray N, Coldman AJ. Dose-intensity meta-analysis of chemotherapy regimens in small-cell carcinoma of the lung. *J Clin Oncol* 1991;9:499.

107. Mehta C, Vogl SE. High-dose cyclophosphamide in the induction therapy of small cell lung cancer: minor improvements in rate of remission and survival. *Proc Am Assoc Cancer Res* 1982; 23:155.

108. LeChevalier, Arrigada R, Pignon JP, et al. Initial chemotherapy doses have a significant impact on survival in limited small cell lung cancer—results of a multicentric prospective randomized study in 105 patients. *N Engl J Med* 1993;329:1848.

109. Goldie JG, Coldman AJ. A mathematical model for relating the drug sensitivity of tumors to their spontaneous mutation rate. *Cancer Treat Rep* 1979;63:1727.

110. Spitzer G, Farha P, Valdivieso M, et al. High dose intensification therapy with autologous bone marrow transplantation in selected small cell carcinoma of the lung: a randomized study. *J Clin Oncol* 1986;4:4.

111. Humblet Y, Symann M, Bosly A, et al. Late intensification chemotherapy with autologous bone marrow transplantation in selected small cell carcinoma of the lung: a randomized study. *J Clin Oncol* 1987;5:1864.

112. Smith IE, Evans BD, Harland SJ, et al. High dose cyclophosphamide with autologous bone marrow rescue after conventional chemotherapy in the treatment of small cell lung carcinoma. *Cancer Chemother Pharmacol* 1985;14:120.

113. Goodman GE, Crowley J, Livingston RB, et al. Treatment of limited small cell lung cancer with concurrent etoposide/cisplatin and radiotherapy followed by intensification with the high dose cyclophosphamide: a Southwest Oncology Group Study. *J Clin Oncol* 1991;9:453.

114. Elias AD, Ayash L, Frei E, et al. Intensive combined modality therapy for limited-stage small-cell lung cancer. *J Natl Canc Inst* 1993;85:559.

115. Ettinger D, Finklestein D, Sarma R, et al. Phase II study of taxol in patients with extensive-stage small cell lung cancer: an Eastern Cooperative Oncology Group study. 1993;12:329.

116. Cormier Y, Eisenhauer E, Gregg R, et al. Gemcitabine: an active new agent in patients with previously untreated small cell lung cancer: a phase II trial of the NCI Canada Clinical Trials Group. *Ann Oncol* 1994;5:283.

117. Masuda N, Fukuoka M, Kusunoki Y, et al. CPT 11: A new derivitive of camptothecin for the treatment of refractory or relapsed small-cell lung cancer. *J Clin Oncol* 1992;10:1225.

118. Schiller JH, KyungMann K, Hutson P, et al. Phase II study of topotecan in patients with extensive stage small cell carcinoma of the lung: an Eastern Cooperative Oncology Group Trial. *J Clin Oncol* 1996;14:2345.

119. Rosenthal MA, Tattersall MHN, Fox RM, et al. Adjuvant thoracic radiotherapy in small cell lung cancer. Ten-year follow-up of a randomized study. *Lung Cancer* 1991;7:235.

120. Birch R, Omura GA, Greco A, et al. Patterns of failure in combined chemotherapy and radiotherapy for limited small cell lung cancer: Southeastern Cancer Study Group experience. *Natl Canc Inst Monogr* 1988;6:265.

121. Kraft A, Arnold H, Zwingers Z, et al. Role of thoracic radiotherapy combined with chemotherapy in limited stage small cell lung cancer (SCLC). *Onkologie* 1990;13:253.

122. Ohnoshi T, Hiraki S, Kimura I. Randomized trial of chemotherapy alone or with chest irradiation in limited stage small cell lung cancer. In: Kimura K, Ota K, Herberman RB, et al., eds. *Cancer chemotherapy: challenges for the future,* Vol. 2. Proceedings of the Second Nagoya International Symposium on Cancer Treatment, Nagoya, Japan, October 16–18, 1986. Amsterdam: Excerpta Medica, 1987:186.

123. Sacks H, Berrier J, Reitman D, et al. Meta-analyses of randomized controlled trials. *N Engl J Med* 1987;316:450.

124. Chalmers T, Buyse M. *Meta-analysis. Data analysis for clinical medicine.* Rome: International University Press, 1988;75.

125. DerSimonian R, Laird N. Meta-analysis in clinical trials. *Controlled Clin Trials* 1986;7:177.

126. White J, Chen T, McCracken J. The influence of radiation therapy quality control on survival, response, and sites of relapse in oat cell carcinoma of the lung. *Cancer* 1982;50:1084.

127. Powell B, Jackson D, Scarantino C, et al. Sequential hemibody and local irradiation with combination chemotherapy for small cell lung carcinoma: a preliminary analysis. *Int J Radiat Oncol Biol Phys* 1985;11:457.

128. Urtasun RC, Belch A, Bodnar D, et al. Radiation as a non-cross-resistant systemic agent: experience with hemibody and total-body irradiation on patients with small cell lung cancer. *Cancer Treatment Symposia* 1985;2:41.

129. Brinker H, Hindberg J, Hansen P. Cyclic alternating polychemotherapy with or without upper and lower half-body irradiation in small cell anaplastic lung cancer: a randomized study. *Eur J Cancer Clin Oncol* 1987;23:205.

130. Fowler J. The linear-quadratic formula and progress in fractionated radiotherapy. *Br J Radiol* 1989;62(740):679.

131. Coy P, Hodson I, Payne D, et al. The effect of dose of thoracic irradiation on recurrence in patients with limited stage small cell lung cancer. Initial results of a Canadian multicenter randomized trial. *Int J Radiat Oncol Biol Phys* 1988;14:219.

132. Choi NC, Carey RW. Importance of radiation dose in achieving improved loco-regional tumor control in limited stage small-cell lung carcinoma: an update. *Int J Radiat Oncol Biol Phys* 1989;17:307.

133. Peters L, Ang K. *Unconventional fractionation schemas in radiotherapy. Important advances in oncology 1986.* Philadelphia: JB Lippincott, 1986;269.

134. Morstyn G, Russo A, Carney D, et al. Heterogeneity in the radiation survival curves and biochemical properties of human lung cancer cell lines. *J Natl Cancer Inst* 1984;73:801.

135. Turrisi AT, Glover DJ, Mason BA. A preliminary report: concurrent twice-daily radiotherapy plus platinum-etoposide chemotherapy for limited stage small cell lung cancer. *Int J Radiat Oncol Biol Phys* 1988;15:183.

136. Turrisi AT, Glover DJ. Thoracic radiotherapy variables: influence on local control in small cell lung cancer limited disease. *Int J Radial Biol Phys* 1990;19:1473.

137. Carney D, Mitchell J, Kinsella T. In vitro radiation and chemotherapy sensitivity of established cell lines of human small cell lung cancer and its large cell morphological variants. *Cancer Res* 1983;43:2806.

138. Emami B, Purdy J, Mandlis J, et al. Three dimensional treatment planning for lung cancer. *Int J Radiat Oncol Biol Phys* 1991;21:217.

139. Young M, Kornelson R. Dose corrections for low-density tissue

139. inhomogeneities and air channels for 10 MV x-rays. *Med Phys* 1983;10:450.
140. McKenna W, Yeakel K, Klink A, et al. Is correction for lung density in radiotherapy treatment planning necessary? *Int J Radiat Oncol Biol Phys* 1987;13(2):273.
141. Kornelson R, Young M. Changes in dose-profile of a 10 MV x-ray beam within and beyond low density material. *Med Phys* 1982;9:114.
142. Glickman AS, Reinstein LE, Laurie F. Quality assurance of radiotherapy in clinical trials. *Cancer Treat Rep* 1985;69(10):1199.
143. Vokes EE. Interactions of chemotherapy and radiation. *Semin Oncol* 1993;20:70.
144. Maurer H, Modeas C, Goutsou M, et al. Adult respiratory distress syndrome after combined modality chemotherapy and radiation therapy in limited-disease small-cell lung cancer. *Proc Am Soc Clin Oncol* 1990;9:229.
145. Maasilta P. Radiation-induced lung injury. From the chest physician's point of view. *Lung Cancer* 1991;7:367.
146. Abrams R, Lichter A, Bromer R, et al. The haematopoietic toxicity of regional radiation therapy: correlations for combined modality therapy with systemic chemotherapy. *Cancer* 1985;55:1429.
147. Bunn PA, Crowley J, Hazuka R, et al. The role of GM-CSF in limited stage SCLC: a randomized phase III study of the Southwest Oncology Group (SWOG). *Proc Am Soc Clin Oncol* 1992;11:292.
148. Momin F, Kraut M, Lattin P, et al. Thrombocytopenia in patients receiving chemoradiotherapy and G-CSF for locally advanced non-small cell lung cancer (NSCLC). *Proc Am Soc Clin Oncol* 1992;11:294.
149. Miller L. Current status of G-CSF in support of chemotherapy and radiotherapy. *Oncology* 1993;7:67.
150. Lee J, Umsawasdi T, Dhingra H, et al. Effects of brain irradiation and chemotherapy on myelosuppression in small-cell lung cancer. *J Clin Oncol* 1986;4:1615.
151. Turrisi AT. Brain irradiation and systemic chemotherapy for small-cell lung cancer: dangerous liaisons? *J Clin Oncol* 1990;8:196.
152. Hill RP, Chambers AF, Ling V. Dynamic heterogeneity: rapid generation of metastatic variants in mouse B 16 melanoma cells. *Science* 1984;224:998.
153. Hill RP, Young SD, Ling V, et al. Metastatic cell phenotypes: quantitative studies using the experimental metastasis assay. *Cancer Rev* 1986;5:118.
154. Claes Trope. Different susceptibilities of tumor cell subpopulations to cytotoxic agents and therapeutic consequences. In: Owens AH, Coffey DS, Baylin SB, eds. *Tumor cell heterogeneity: origins and implications.* New York: Academic Press, 1982;147.
155. Young RC. Drug resistance: the clinical problem. In: Ozols RF, ed. *Drug resistance in cancer therapy.* Norwell, Massachusetts: Kluwer Academic Publishers, 1989;1.
156. Cole SP, Bhardwaj G, Gerlach JH, et al. Overexpression of a transporter gene in a multidrug-resistant human lung cancer cell line. *Science* 1992;258,1650.
157. Goldie JH, Coldman AJ. Genetic origin of drug resistance in neoplasms. *Cancer Res* 1984;44:3643.
158. Tubiana M. The role of local treatment in the cure of cancer. *Eur J Cancer* 1992;28:2061.
159. Suit H. Local control and patient survival. *Int J Radiat Oncol Biol Phys* 1992;23:653.
160. Tomlinson RH, Gray LH. The histological structure of some human lung cancers and the possible implications for radiotherapy. *Br J Cancer* 1955;9:539.
161. Yaes RJ. Tumor heterogeneity, tumor size, and radioresistance. *Int J Radiat Oncol Biol Phys* 1989;17:993.

162. Skipper HE, Simpson-Herren L. The relationship between tumor stem cell heterogeneity and responsiveness to chemotherapy. In: DeVita V, Hellman S, Rosenberg S eds. *Important advances in oncology.* Philadelphia: JB Lippincott, 1985.
163. Fertil B, Malaise EP. Inherent cellular radiosensitivity as a basic concept for human tumor radiotherapy. *Int J Radiat Biol Phys* 1981;7:621.
164. Ochs JJ, Tester WJ, Cohen MH, et al. "Salvage" radiation therapy for intrathoracic small cell carcinoma of the lung progressing on combination chemotherapy. *Cancer Treat Rep* 1983;67:1123.
165. Dunphy JE. Some observations on the natural behaviour of cancer in man. *N Engl J Med* 1950;242:167.
166. Withers HR, Taylor JMG, Maciejewski B. The hazard of accelerated tumor clonogen repopulation during radiotherapy. *Acta Oncol* 1988;27:131.
167. Trott KR. Cell repopulation and overall treatment time. *Int J Radiat Oncol Phys* 1990;19:1071.
168. Maciejewski B, Preuss-Bayer G, Trott KR. The influence of the number of fractions and of overall treatment time on local control and late complication rate in squamous cell carcinoma of the larynx. *Int J Radiat Oncol Biol Phys* 1983;9:321.
169. Holsti LR, Mantyla M. Split-course versus continuous radiotherapy analysis of a randomized trial from 1964 to 1967. *Acta Oncol* 1988;27:153.
170. Simpson-Herren L, Sanford AH, Holmquist JP. Effects of surgery on the cell kinetics of residual tumor. *Cancer Treat Rep* 1976;60:1749.
171. Stephens TC, Steel GG. Regeneration of tumors after cytotoxic treatment. In: Meyn RE, Withers HR, eds. *Radiation biology in cancer research.* New York: Raven, 1980:385.
172. Fisher B, Gunduz N, Coyle J, et al. Presence of a growth stimulating factor in serum following primary tumor removal in mice. *Cancer Res* 1989;49:1996.
173. Norton L, Simon R. Tumor size, sensitivity to therapy and design of treatment schedules. *Cancer Treat Rep* 1977;61:1307.
174. Perry MC, Herndon JE, Eaton WL, et al. Thoracic radiation therapy added to chemotherapy modality treatment of limited-stage small-cell lung cancer: an update of cancer and leukemia group B study 8083. *J Clin Oncol* 1998;16:2466.
175. Slevin ML, Clark PI, Joel SP, et al. A randomized trial to evaluate the effect of schedule on the activity of etoposide in small cell lung cancer. *J Clin Oncol* 1989;7:1333.
176. Tubiana M, Arriagada R, Correct JM. Sequencing of drugs and radiation: the integrated alternating regimen. *Cancer* 1985;50:2131.
177. Looney WB, Hopkins HA. Rationale for different chemotherapeutic and radiation therapy strategies in cancer management. *Cancer* 1991;67:1471.
178. Goldie JH, Coldman AJ, Ng V, et al. A mathematical and computer based model of alternating chemotherapy and radiation therapy in experimental neoplasms. In: Arriagada R, ed. *Treatment modalities in lung cancer: antibiotics and chemotherapy.* Basel: Darger, 1988:11.
179. Arriagada R, Le Chevalier T, Ruffie P, et al. Alternating radiotherapy and chemotherapy in 173 patients with limited small cell lung carcinoma. *Int J Radiat Oncol Biol Phys* 1990;19:1135.
180. LeBeau B, Chasting C, Urban T, et al. A randomized clinical trial comparing concurrent versus alternating thoracic irradiation in limited small-cell lung cancer. *Proc Am Soc Clin Oncol* 1996;15:383.
181. Gregor A, Drings P, Burghouts J, et al. Randomized trial of alternating versus sequential radiotherapy/chemotherapy in limited-disease patients with small-cell lung cancer: a European

organization for research and treatment of cancer lung cancer cooperative group study. *J Clin Oncol* 1997;15:2840.

182. Quon H, Payne DG, Coy P, et al. The influence of age on the delivery, tolerance and efficacy of thoracic irradiation in the combined modality treatment of limited stage small cell lung cancer. *Int J Radiation Oncol Biol Phy* 1999;43:39.

183. Siu LL, Shepherd FA, Murray N, et al. The influence of age on the treatment of limited-stage small-cell lung cancer. *J Clin Oncol* 1996;14:821.

184. Yellen SB, Cella DR, Leslie WT. Age and clinical decision making in oncology patients. *J Natl Cancer Inst* 1994;86:1766.

185. Murray N, Grafton C, Shah A, et al. Abbreviated treatment for elderly, infirm, or non-compliant patients with limited-stage small-cell lung cancer. *J Clin Oncol* 1998;16:3323.

186. Jeremic B, Shibamoto Y, Acimovic L, et al. Carboplatin, etoposide and accelerated hyperfractionated radiotherapy for elderly patients with limited small cell lung carcinoma. *Cancer* 1998; 82:836.

187. Tucker MA, Murray N, Shaw EG, et al. Second primary cancers related to smoking and treatment of small-cell lung cancer. *J Natl Cancer Inst* 1997;89:1782.

188. Feld R, Pater J, Goodwin PJ, et al. The restaging of responding patients with limited small cell lung cancer; is it really useful? *Chest* 1993;103:1010.

55

SURGICAL MANAGEMENT OF SMALL CELL LUNG CANCER

FRANCES A. SHEPHERD

HISTORICAL BACKGROUND

Although small cell lung cancer (SCLC) accounts for 20% to 25% of all primary bronchogenic carcinomas, this tumor represents less than 5% of cases in most surgical series. The discrepancy can be explained by the biologic behavior of SCLC, which results in dissemination to regional lymph nodes and/or distant metastatic sites in more than 90% of patients at the time of initial presentation.[1] Even patients with apparently "limited"-stage tumors probably have micrometastic disease at distant sites, which has the potential to proliferate if only local therapeutic modalities, such as surgery or radiotherapy, are employed. This explains why almost all surgical series from the prechemotherapy era reported five-year survival rates approaching zero for patients with small cell carcinoma.[2]

Mountain reviewed the experience of the M.D. Anderson Hospital and Tumor Institute in the surgical management of 368 patients with pathologically proven SCLC[3] and found that only one patient survived longer than 5 years compared to 15% to 25% of non–small cell lung cancer (NSCLC) patients (Figure 55.1). Less than 15% of the tumors presented with a peripheral tumor mass, but no survival advantage could be identified even for this favorable subgroup. Surprisingly, the survival of the SCLC patients without lymph node involvement was not superior to those with bronchopulmonary and/or hilar nodes, or even to those with mediastinal nodal involvement (Figure 55.2). The size of the primary tumor did not seem to be prognostic, nor was the presence of atelectasis and/or pneumonitis associated with a significantly poorer outcome.

To determine whether it was ever appropriate to undertake surgery as the primary treatment for SCLC, a prospective randomized trial was mounted by the Medical Research Council of Great Britain.[4,5] In this study, 71 patients were randomized prospectively to undergo surgical resection, and 73 to receive a course of "radical radiotherapy" (30 Gy or more over 20–40 days). The median survival was 199 days for patients in the surgical arm and 300 days for patients who received radiotherapy (Figure 55.3). At 5 years, one

and three patients were alive in the surgery and radiotherapy arms, respectively (p = 0.04). At 10 years, only the three patients in the radiotherapy arm remained alive. It was concluded from this study that radical radiotherapy was preferable to surgery, but that neither of the treatment policies was really effective. The investigators concluded that other therapeutic approaches (e.g. immunotherapy, chemotherapy, or various combinations) might be more successful, and they also suggested that it would be improbable that any advance in therapy could significantly reduce the overall death rate from this disease in the absence of successful smoking prevention programs. Is it not chastening to realize that 20 years later we could draw exactly the same conclusions from many of our lung cancer clinical research trials?

The marginally superior long-term survival rate for patients treated with radiotherapy in the British Medical Research Council trial led some investigators to recommend a policy of preoperative radiotherapy followed by surgery for patients with SCLC. In a prospective phase II trial from the North Middlesex Hospital in London, 49 patients received low-dose preoperative radiotherapy (17.5 Gy) and 24 received higher dose radiotherapy (25 Gy).[6,7] Of the 90 patients who entered the study, 9 were inoperable and did not undergo surgery, and 73 eventually had resection. NSCLC was identified in nine patients. Eight patients survived 5 years, and two remained alive and disease-free more than 10 years postoperatively.

In a similar North American trial of preoperative radiotherapy that included both SCLC and NSCLC patients received higher dose radiotherapy, 30–40 Gy in 2 weeks followed by thoracotomy.[8] No long-term survivors were seen for the small population of patients with oat cell carcinoma in this trial.

It was evident to investigators in the 1960s and 1970s that patients with SCLC were dying from systemic metastases, and that no manipulation of local treatment modalities would result in significant long-term survival in the absence of effective systemic treatment. Bergsagel et al. from the Princess Margaret Hospital were among the first to test the hypothesis that chemotherapy might add to the effects of

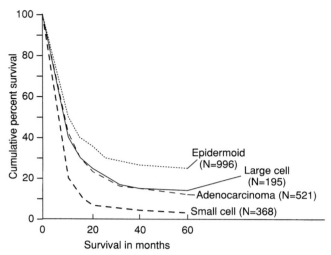

FIGURE 55.1. Bronchogenic carcinoma. Cumulative percentage of patients surviving according to morphology. (From Mountain C. Clinical biology of small cell carcinoma: relationship to surgical therapy. *Semin Oncol* 1978;5:272, with permission.)

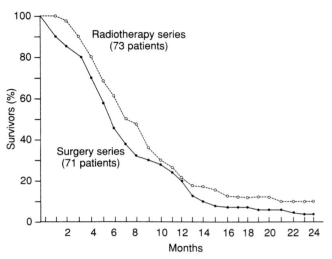

FIGURE 55.3. Survival in the two treatment series (all patients). (Working Party on the Evaluation of Different. Methods of Therapy in Carcinoma of the Bronchus. Comparative trial of surgery and radiotherapy for the primary treatment of small-celled or oat-celled carcinoma of the bronchus. *Lancet* 1966;2:979, with permission.)

local radiotherapy, and they showed a modest survival advantage for patients treated with single-agent low-dose cyclophosphamide.[9] The British Medical Research Council Lung Cancer Working Party undertook a similar trial in which 125 patients were randomized prospectively to receive 30 Gy radiotherapy delivered in 15 fractions, or the same radiotherapy with systemic chemotherapy consisting of cyclophosphamide 500 mg/m² given every 3 weeks and CCNU (1-(2-chloroethyl)-3 cyclohexyl-1-nitrosourea) 50

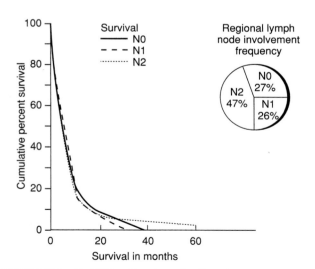

FIGURE 55.2. Undifferentiated small cell carcinoma. Percentage frequency and cumulative percentage of patients surviving according to presence and extent of regional lymph node involvement. (From Mountain C. Clinical biology of small cell carcinoma: relationship to surgical therapy. *Semin Oncol* 1978;5:272, with permission.)

mg/m² orally every 6 weeks. A significant prolongation of progression-free survival was seen for patients in the chemotherapy arm, although a long-term survival benefit was not demonstrated.[10]

Simultaneously, other investigators were applying the same adjuvant chemotherapy principles to surgical patients. In the United States, large adjuvant chemotherapy trials were conducted by the Veteran's Administration Surgical Adjuvant Group (VASOG). In a trial of 417 patients with all cell types of lung cancer, no survival benefit was identified for patients who received postoperative adjuvant cyclophosphamide alone or cyclophosphamide and methotrexate compared to a no-treatment control group.[11] Eighteen patients with SCLC were included in that trial. Of those, one of six patients in the cyclophosphamide-alone arm and three of nine patients in the cyclophosphamide and methotrexate arm were alive at 3 years compared to no patients in the control group. This was the first report to suggest that adjuvant chemotherapy might prolong survival for patients with SCLC who had undergone complete surgical resection.

In 1982, Shields reviewed the results of four VASOG adjuvant chemotherapy studies, and undertook a separate analysis of the 148 patients (47%) in those trials who had SCLC.[12] In the first trial, 28 patients were randomly assigned to receive nitrogen mustard and 27 to control, and in the second trial 26 patients were randomly assigned to receive cyclophosphamide and 20 to control. No survival advantage was seen for the patients in the chemotherapy arms of either trial. A small survival advantage was seen for patients in the chemotherapy arm of the three-arm trial, in which patients were randomized to receive prolonged

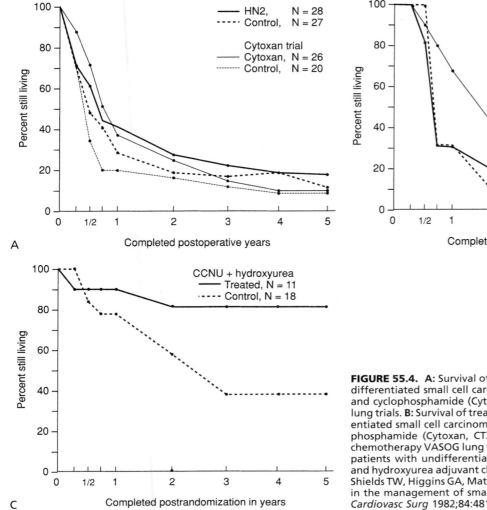

FIGURE 55.4. A: Survival of treated and control patients with undifferentiated small cell carcinoma in the nitrogen mustard (HN$_2$) and cyclophosphamide (Cytoxan) adjuvant chemotherapy VASOG lung trials. **B:** Survival of treated and control patients with undifferentiated small cell carcinoma in the prolonged intermittent cyclophosphamide (Cytoxan, CTX) and mathotrexate (MTX) adjuvant chemotherapy VASOG lung trials. **C:** Survival of treated and control patients with undifferentiated small cell carcinoma in the CCNU and hydroxyurea adjuvant chemotherapy VASOG lung trials. (From Shields TW, Higgins GA, Matthews MG, Keehn RJ. Surgical resection in the management of small cell carcinoma of the lung. *J Thorac Cardiovasc Surg* 1982;84:481, with permission.)

intermittent courses of CCNU and hydroxyurea or no further therapy (Figure 55.4).

Shields and his co-workers also made other important observations from their analysis of the SCLC patients in the VASOG trials. They demonstrated the importance of TNM (tumor, note, metastasis) staging, which has long been recognized to have prognostic significance for NSCLC. Sixty percent of patients with T1 N0 M0 tumors were alive at 5 years, whereas there were almost no five-year survivors among the patients who presented either with T2-3 tumors or with mediastinal lymph node involvement (Figure 55.5). Patients with small primary tumors with only first-level hilar nodes involved had an intermediate survival of approximately 30%.

Although it had become accepted by the 1970s that surgical resection was not appropriate for most patients with SCLC, the observations of Shields and his colleagues suggested that a subpopulation of SCLC patients might benefit

from a surgical approach. In a retrospective review of 40 patients with SCLC who underwent potentially curative resection between 1959 and 1972, Shore and Paneth reported an overall five-year survival rate of 25%. Four of ten patients (40%) without nodal involvement achieved long-term survival compared to nine of twenty-six patients (25%) who had hilar or mediastinal nodal involvement.[13] In a retrospective analysis of 106 resected patients from Japan, 87 cases were of the intermediate cell type and 19 of the oat cell type.[14] The five-year survival for the intermediate cell type was 10.3%, whereas only one of the oat cell type achieved long-term survival. Other investigators have not identified a significant survival advantage for patients with the intermediate cell type,[15] and this designation has largely been abandoned today.

SCLC usually presents with a central mass with associated hilar and mediastinal adenopathy. Lennox et al. observed that patients who had larger or more proximal tumors

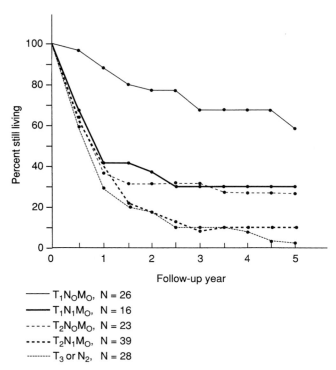

FIGURE 55.5. Survival, computed by the life-table method, from post-operative day 30 (early trials) or from randomization (recent trials) by TNM classification for patients with undifferentiated small cell carcinoma who had undergone a "curative" resection in the VASOG lung trials. (From Shields TW. Higgins GA, Matthews MG, Keehn RJ. Surgical Resection in the management of small cell carcinoma of the lung. *J Thorac Cardiovasc Surg* 1982;84:481, with permission.)

and who required a pneumonectomy were less likely to achieve long-term survival. Their two- and five-year survival rates for patients who required only a lobectomy were 32% and 18%, respectively, compared to 14.4% and 7.2%, respectively, for pneumonectomy patients.[16] Occasionally, SCLC can present as a solitary pulmonary nodule. Between 1958 and 1963, 1,134 patients with asymptomatic solitary pulmonary nodules were assessed by VASOG members.[17] Only 15 patients (4%) were found to have small cell pathology, and of those, 11 were able to undergo a curative surgical procedure. One-, five-, and ten-year survival rates for those 11 patients were 63.6%, 36.4%, and 18.2%, respectively. Because most of these patients underwent surgery before the chemotherapy era, it may be assumed that approximately one-third of patients were cured by their surgery alone as measured by survival at the five-year mark.

From this historical review it is clear that any local treatment modality alone, whether surgery or radiation, is inadequate therapy for SCLC. If surgery is to have any role to play, it must be in the context of a combined modality treatment program with systemic combination chemotherapy and perhaps radiotherapy as well.

RATIONALE FOR SURGERY IN THE MANAGEMENT OF SMALL CELL LUNG CANCER

Improved Control at the Primary Site

SCLC is a highly chemosensitive tumor (Table 55.1). Response rates of 80% or more are achieved with current chemotherapy combinations, and complete clinical response is achieved in approximately 50% of patients with limited-stage disease.[18,19] Despite this high initial response rate, most patients experience relapse shortly after discontinuing treatment, and the two-year survival rate is 20% or less in most series. For patients with limited disease, the most common site of failure is the area of the primary tumor and its hilar and/or mediastinal draining lymph nodes. Overall, 50% of patients fail at the primary site, and for one-half of those patients, the primary site may be the *only* area of failure. Similar results have been found at autopsy. In a review by Elliott, residual tumor was identified at autopsy in the primary site in 64% of patients and in the hilar and mediastinal lymph nodes in 53% of patients with limited disease who had achieved complete clinical response.[20]

Initial attempts to improve control at the primary site focused on the addition of thoracic irradiation. Two meta-analyses of thoracic radiotherapy have been published for SCLC.[21,22] The survival data for almost 2,000 patients in 16 trials were available, and data on local control rates were available for nine studies. Both metaanalyses showed that

TABLE 55.1. RATIONALE FOR SURGERY FOR LIMITED SMALL CELL LUNG CANCER

Small cell lung cancer is highly chemosensitive:

- Chemotherapy has the potential, therefore, to eradicate micrometastatic disease.

The most common site of relapse is the area of the primary tumor and/or its regional lymph nodes:

- Radiotherapy reduces local recurrence by 50%, but isolated local failure rates are still approximately 25% to 30% in most series.
- Surgery may improve control at the local site.

Mixed histology tumors respond less well to chemotherapy:

- Surgery may be necessary to treat the non–small cell component.
- Late recurrences may be of non–small cell type (a new primary) and may be treated surgically if they meet standard criteria for operability.

Retrospective reviews suggest that combined modality therapy with surgery and chemotherapy results in survival that is similar to that of patients with non–small cell tumors of similar TNM stage:

- Surgery alone may be curative for some patients with pathologic stage I tumors.

thoracic irradiation resulted in a reduction in local relapse rate from 47.9% to 23.3% (p < 0.0001).[21] They also demonstrated a small but significant survival benefit for patients who received radiotherapy.[21,22] Indirect comparisons of early to late radiotherapy and of sequential to nonsequential radiotherapy did not reveal any optimal time for the administration of this local treatment.[22]

Based on the results of these metaanalyses, the standard therapy for patients with limited SCLC now consists of combination chemotherapy and thoracic irradiation with or without prophylactic cranial irradiation. Median survival longer than 20 months and five-year survival rates of approximately 20% have been reported.[23] However, even the most successful combined modality treatment programs report isolated relapse at the primary site in 20% to 25% of patients, and a cumulative risk of recurring locally of 50%. This high local failure led several investigators to question whether surgical resection would result in improved local control. They postulated that control of bulk disease in the chest by surgery and eradication of low-volume micrometastatic disease by systemic chemotherapy would result in an increased cure rate. Small studies from several centers suggested that this might, indeed, be the case. The University of Toronto Lung Oncology Group reported only two local recurrences in 35 patients treated with combined modality therapy, which included surgical resection.[24] Similar results were reported by Comis et al., who observed no local recurrences in 16 patients who underwent adjuvant surgical resection after induction chemotherapy.[25]

Mixed Histology Tumors

In approximately 5% to 10% of cases, SCLC is found in combination with other lung cancer histologies such as adenocarcinoma or squamous cell carcinoma.[26] Investigators for the Eastern Cooperative Oncology Group (ECOG) reported that mixed histology tumors were more likely to present as peripheral lesions on chest x-ray, although they found that all other clinical characteristics were similar to those of the pure SCLC patients. When surgical series of SCLC are examined, it would appear that a higher percentage of patients have mixed small cell and non–small cell tumors. The University of Toronto Lung Oncology Group reported mixed histology in 14 of 79 patients (17.7%) who underwent initial surgery followed by adjuvant chemotherapy, and in 3 of 40 patients (7.5%) who had surgical resections after induction chemotherapy.[28]

It may be appropriate to consider a combined modality treatment program for patients with mixed histology tumors if they meet standard surgical criteria and have no evidence of extra thoracic spread. Because NSCLCs are relatively insensitive to chemotherapy, they are not likely to be controlled by systemic treatment. After initial treatment with chemotherapy for the small cell component, the addition of surgery to remove the non–small cell component might

contribute to the potential for cure of this small subgroup of patients.

Late Recurrence After Successful Treatment of Small Cell Lung Cancer

Several reviews have now suggested that long-term survivors of SCLC are at high risk of developing second primary tumors, particularly second primary lung cancers.[29–32] A review of 47 patients who survived longer than 2 years after treatment at the M.D. Anderson Cancer Center identified 14 patients who had second malignancies, and of those, 7 had second primary lung cancers.[29] In fact, their review suggested that a long-term survivor is more likely to have a second primary tumor than a relapse of SCLC. Although the patient population at risk for these second tumors is low because of the low cure rate for SCLC, clinicians seeing patients in follow-up must be aware that a new lesion on chest x-ray may not represent relapse but may be a new primary tumor. Such patients should be investigated similar to any other patient who is presenting with a lung mass for the first time. Histologic or cytologic confirmation of malignancy should be obtained, and if NSCLC pathology is found, then further workup should be directed at determining operability because surgical resection has the potential to be curative for some patients.

ADJUVANT CHEMOTHERAPY FOLLOWING SURGICAL RESECTION OF SMALL CELL LUNG CANCER

The first suggestion that adjuvant chemotherapy after surgery might prolong survival arose from Shields' review of the VASOG trials.[12] There were inadequate numbers of patients in any of these trials for the results to be statistically significant, and the chemotherapy administered would be considered inadequate by today's standards of systemic chemotherapy for SCLC. Nonetheless, the data suggested that, following complete resection of bulk disease at the primary site, systemic chemotherapy had the potential to eradicate micrometastatic tumor deposits.

These favorable results led several investigators to administer combination chemotherapy to all patients following complete resection of SCLC. A summary of 10 such trials is shown in Table 55.2.[12,33–44] All of the studies were retrospective reviews, so they suffer from the inherent weaknesses of any retrospective assessment of a treatment policy.

For many of the patients in these series, surgery was undertaken because a preoperative diagnosis of SCLC had not been made. For some, it had not been possible to obtain adequate tissue for any malignant diagnosis, and for others a preoperative diagnosis of NSCLC had been made. Some of those patients were subsequently found to have mixed histology tumors with both small cell and non–small cell

TABLE 55.2. SURVIVAL ACCORDING TO PATHOLOGIC STAGE FOR PATIENTS TREATED WITH ADJUVANT CHEMOTHERAPY AFTER SURGERY FOR SMALL CELL LUNG CANCER

Author	Number	Stage			
		I	II	III	Total
Shields, 1982[12]	No. of patients	49	55	28	132
	5-yr survival	51%	20%	3%	28%
Hayata, 1978[33]	No. of patients	27	6	39	72
	5-yr survival	26%	17%	0%	11%
Meyer, 1983, 1984[34,35]	No. of patients	6	4	10	30
	5-yr survival	>50%	50%	0	?
Osterlind, 1986[36]	No. of patients	18	8	10	36
	3 1/2-yr survival	22%	?	?	25%
Massen, 1986[37]	No. of patients	41	19	64	124
	3-yr survival	34%	21%	11%	20%
Shepherd, 1988[38]	No. of patients	19	24	20	63
	5-yr survival	48%	24%	24%	31%
Karrer, 1990, 1991[39,40]	No. of patients	63	54	40	157
	4-yr survival	61%	35%	35%	?
Macchiarini, 1991[41]	No. of patients	26	–	15 (T3N0)	42
	5-yr survival	52%	–	13%	36%
Hara, 1991[42]	No. of patients	13	10	14	37
	5-yr survival	64%	42%	10.7%	?
Davis, 1993[43]	No. of patients	11	16	5	32
	5-yr survival	50%	35%	21%	36%
Wada, 1985[44]	No. of patients	5	5	7	17
	5-yr survival	37%*	–	33%	32%

* Stages I and II combined

components whereas others had pure small cell tumors that had been incorrectly diagnosed preoperatively. Maassen[37] reported that only 18 of 24 patients had a correct histologic diagnosis of SCLC preoperatively. In a series of 63 patients reported by the University of Toronto Lung Oncology Group,[38] only 18 had a correct preoperative diagnosis of SCLC. Postoperatively, SCLC was seen in 54 patients and mixed histology tumors in 9.

For most of the studies, chemotherapy was not standardized, and because most of the reviews included patients seen over a 10 or more year period, multiple chemotherapy protocols were often employed. With the exception of the early trials reported by Shields[12] and Hayata,[33] all patients were treated with combinations of drugs that would be considered adequate even today. The duration of chemotherapy treatment was also variable and ranged from a single course of postoperative therapy to multiple courses for 18 months. Most groups administered approximately six cycles of treatment.

In addition to postoperative chemotherapy, some centers also administered local radiotherapy to the primary tumor bed and mediastinum as well as prophylactic cranial irradiation. Considering the variability in radiation treatment and incomplete reporting in several series, no conclusions can be drawn concerning the advisability of trimodality therapy.

Because so few patients with SCLC are surgical candidates, the TNM staging system is not generally applied to

this subtype of lung cancer; instead, patients are classified simply as limited or extensive disease. The patients in the reviews summarized in Table 55.2 differ from limited-stage SCLC patients overall in that they all underwent pretreatment surgical resection, and therefore detailed pathologic staging is available. From the results shown, it is clear that the TNM staging system that provides such important prognostic and therapeutic information for patients with NSCLC may also be prognostic for patients with limited SCLC. In every study, the best survival was achieved by patients who had *pathologic* stage I tumors, and the poorest survival was seen for patients with *pathologic* stage III tumors. For stage I patients, survival ranged from 22% at 3½ years in the Danish series[33] to 61% at 4 years in the International Society of Chemotherapy Lung Cancer Study Group [Figure 55.6].[39,40] On average, it would appear that approximately 50% of patients with stage I SCLC may be cured with a combined modality approach that includes surgical resection and adjuvant combination chemotherapy. In the early trials, virtually no patients with stage III tumors achieved long-term survival. In the after reviews in which more aggressive combination chemotherapy regimens were employed, long-term survival ranged from 11%[37,42] to 35%.[39,40] (See Figure 55.7). In all series, the survival of stage II patients was intermediate between that of patients at stages I and III. In fact, these survival rates are similar

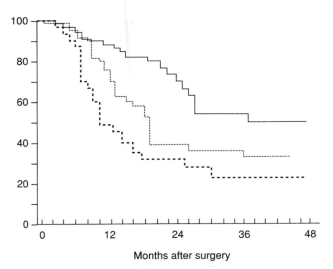

FIGURE 55.6. Life table survival curves for small cell lung cancer patients according to lymph node involvement. Patients with stage p^T, N0, MO disease (*solid line*). n, 63; pT, N1, MO (*dotted line*). (From Ulsperger E, Karrer K, Denck H, ISC-Lung Cancer Study Group. Multi-modality treatment for small-cell bronchial carcinoma. *Eur J Cardiothorac Surg* 1991;5:306, with permission.)

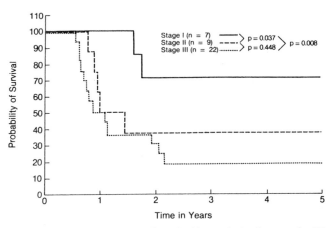

FIGURE 55.8. Comparison of survival by pathologic stage for 38 patients with small cell lung cancer treated with adjuvant surgical therapy after chemotherapy. (From Shepherd FA, Ginsberg RJ, Patterson GA, et al. A prospective study of adjuvant surgical resection after chemotherapy for limited small cell lung cancer. *J Thorac Cardiovasc Surg* 1989;97:177, with permission.)

to those seen after surgical resection for similar stage patients with NSCLC (See Figure 55.8).

What may be concluded from these series? All of the studies that employed intensive combination chemotherapy reported survival that appears to be superior to the survival seen in patients following surgery without adjuvant chemotherapy. Although these comparisons are retrospective, it

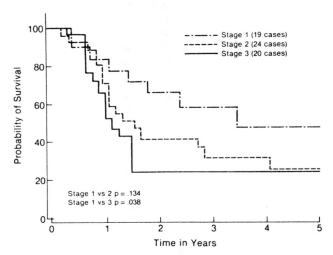

FIGURE 55.7. A comparison of survival by stage for patients treated with adjuvant chemotherapy after surgical resection for small cell lung cancer. (From Shepherd FA, Evans WK, Feld R, et al. Adjuvant chemotherapy following surgical resection for small cell carcinoma of the lung. *J Clin Oncol* 1988;6:832, with permission.)

is likely that the improved survival is attributable to the postoperative chemotherapy treatment and not to improvements in surgical techniques or supportive care. It seems appropriate, therefore, to recommend that combination chemotherapy be administered to patients who have undergone resection for limited SCLC because the short-term toxicity of such treatment is usually manageable, and the long-term toxicity is probably minimal. The University of Toronto Lung Oncology Group recommends no more than six treatment cycles[38] because survival does not seem to be superior for patients who receive 12–18 months of postoperative treatment.[36,44] Whether fewer than six cycles may also be adequate is unknown. In the study reported by Hara et al.[42] 11 patients treated between 1972 and 1981 received only one postoperative course of combination chemotherapy, and 26 patients treated from 1982 to 1989 received only two courses of chemotherapy followed by consolidation radiotherapy.

Although the five-year survival rates for patients with stage I and II tumors were excellent, only 10.7% of patients with stage III tumors were alive at 5 years. These results appear to be somewhat poorer than those achieved by other groups that administered a more prolonged course of adjuvant chemotherapy, although firm conclusions cannot be drawn from these retrospective analyses. Littlewood et al.[46] treated two young patients by pneumonectomy followed by a single course of very high-dose chemotherapy and autologus bone marrow transplantation. Both patients relapsed, 118 and 80 weeks after treatment. It would appear, therefore, that a brief course (maximum six treatment cycles) of standard-dose combination chemotherapy should be the treatment of choice for patients at this time.

Although these retrospective trials support the recommendation for adjuvant chemotherapy after surgical resection, it is not possible to state with certainty which patients have the potential to derive most benefit from adjuvant chemotherapy and whether it is necessary to administer such treatment to all patients. Shah et al.[47] reported 43.3% *actual* five-year survival for 28 patients who underwent complete surgical resection without postoperative chemotherapy. The actual five-year survival for patients with stage I disease was 51.1%, and surprisingly, was 55.5% for stage III patients. No patient with stage II disease survived 5 years. More than one-half the patients in this study had peripheral tumors, and their survival was better than that of the patients who had central tumors. Peripheral stage I NSCLC is uncommon. In the VASOG cooperative study of solitary pulmonary nodules, only 11 of 309 patients who underwent curative resection were found to have small cell tumors.[17] Their median five-year survival was 36.4% and their median ten-year survival was 18.2%. The details of postoperative therapy, if any, for these patients were not provided, but it is likely that they did not receive aggressive combination chemotherapy. It is interesting to note that their five-year survival rates were very similar to those of the other lung cancer cell types in the review. The five-year survival rate is less than that reported by Shah et al., and one can only speculate whether superior survival might have been achieved with the addition of combination chemotherapy.

On the other hand, it is not possible to draw firm conclusions concerning the contribution of the *surgery* to the overall survival of these patients. The survival of patients who undergo surgery should not be compared directly to the survival seen in trials of standard chemotherapy and radiotherapy for limited-disease SCLC. It must be remembered that surgical series include only a select subgroup within limited disease from which patients with adverse prognostic factors, such as supraclavicular adenopathy, bulky primary tumors with superior vena caval obstruction, and/or pleural effusions, have been specifically excluded.

Surgery, if it does play a role in the treatment of SCLC

will do so by improving control at the primary site. Relapse patterns were reported in only seven of the trials reviewed,[34,38,41–43,45,46] but the results from those studies suggest that surgery did contribute to local control because isolated local relapse was seen in only 8 of the 201 patients in those studies (Table 55.3). It must be remembered, though, that these patients represent only a select subgroup of the entire group of limited SCLCs in that they were considered "operable" at the time of diagnosis. It is quite possible, therefore, that this high rate of local control was attributable only to the fact that the patients in these series has less locally advanced tumors and that the local control rate might have been equivalent with a combination of systemic chemotherapy and thoracic irradiation.

PROSPECTIVE TRIALS OF INDUCTION CHEMOTHERAPY FOLLOWED BY SURGICAL RESECTION FOR SMALL CELL LUNG CANCER

Phase II Trials

The encouraging results achieved with initial surgical resection followed by adjuvant chemotherapy led several groups to undertake prospective studies of systemic chemotherapy *followed by* surgery for certain patients with limited SCLC. The results of nine such prospective phase II trials are summarized in Table 55.4.[48–56]

All of the studies administered multiple courses of combination chemotherapy, which included most of the agents that are active against SCLC (i.e., cyclophosphamide, doxorubicin, vincristine, etoposide, and cisplatin). The number of preoperative chemotherapy courses ranged from two to six, and the overall response rate was greater than 88% in all studies except that of Baker et al.[51] In that study, patients received only two preoperative courses of chemotherapy, which may explain the low complete response rate of 3% and overall response rate of only 54%. This finding might suggest that a longer course of induction chemotherapy would be advisable, although in the small study reported by Benfield et al.,[52] 88% of patients responded to treatment and 100% were able to undergo complete surgical resection after only two courses of chemotherapy. Not all responding patients underwent thoracotomy. On average, approximately 60% of patients were considered to have responded adequately enough for surgical exploration, and of those, more than 80% could be resected completely. When calculated from the total number of patients who entered the studies, the overall complete surgical resection rate was approximately 50%. Not all studies reported surgical toxicity, but it does not appear that the postoperative death rate or complication rate was significantly increased by the preoperative chemotherapy administered to these patients. Only three postoperative deaths were reported,[51,54,55] all in patients who had required a complete pneumonectomy. Other postoperative complications included infection, bronchopleural fistula formation, and reversible supraventricular

TABLE 55.3. PATTERN OF RELAPSE FOR PATIENTS WITH SMALL CELL LUNG CANCER TREATED WITH SURGERY FOLLOWED BY ADJUVANT CHEMOTHERAPY

Investigators	No. of Patients	No. of Patients with Relapse		
		Local Only	Distant Only	Both
Meyer, 1983[34]	10	—	1	—
Shepherd, 1988[38]	63	2	26	5
Macciarini, 1991[41]	42	2	24	—
Hara, 1991[42]	37	2	?	—
Davis, 1993[40]	32	—	15	2
Friess, 1985[45]	15	1	5	1
Littlewood, 1987[46]	2	1	1	—
TOTAL	201	8	72	8

TABLE 55.4. PROSPECTIVE PHASE II TRIALS OF INDUCTION CHEMOTHERAPY FOLLOWED BY SURGERY FOR LIMITED SMALL CELL LUNG CANCER

| Investigators | No. of Patients | Clinical Stage | | | Chemotherapy | Responses CR/PR (ORR%) | Surgery: Thoracotomy/CSR (%) | Complete Pathologic Responses (%) |
		I	II	III				
Prager, 1984[48]	39	2	12	25	CAVE × 2–4	13/21 (88)	11/8 (21)	2 (5)
Williams, 1987[49]	38	—	—	—	CAE × 3	5/26 (82)	25/21 (55)	4 (11)
Johnson, 1987[50]	24	3	7	14	CAV × 6 ± EP	? (100)	23/15 (62)	9 (37)
Baker, 1987[51]	37	—	—	—	CAE × 2	1/19 (54)	20/20 (54)	2 (5)
Benfield, 1989[52]	8	—	5	3	CAEV × 2	5/2 (88)	8/8 (100)	0
Shepherd, 1987[53]	72	21	16	35	CAV × 6 ± EP	27/30 (80)	38/33 (36)	3 (4)
Zatopek, 1991[54]	25	10	1	24	COPE × 3	10/14 (96)	14/10 (40)	5 (20)
Hara, 1991[55]	17	4	6	7	Various	4/10 (82)	17/17 (100)	?
Eberhardt, 1997[56]	46	6	2	38	EP	15/28 (94)	32/23 (50)	11 (24)

CR, complete response; PR, partial responses; ORR, overall response rate; CSR, complete surgical resection; V, vincristine; E, etoposide.

tachycardias, but it does not seem that the surgical complication rate was greater than that observed after similar procedures in patients who have not received chemotherapy.

Not unexpectedly, the complete pathologic response rate was considerably lower than the clinical response rate. With the exception of Benfield et al.,[52] all authors reported complete pathologic response in a few patients. The rate ranged from 4%[53] to 37%[54] and on average was approximately 10%. It is of interest that this complete pathologic response rate is similar to that which has been reported in studies of induction chemotherapy followed by surgery for patients with locally advanced (stage IIIA or IIIB) NSCLC.[58]

All investigators found that survival strongly depended on TNM stage. Patients with stage I (T1–2 N0) tumors had the best prognosis, with five-year survival rates that approached 70% for completely resected patients. Stage II and III patients fared less well, but all series reported a few patients with stage IIIA tumors (N2) who achieved long-term survival and appeared to be cured by their combined modality treatment program. The median survival for the entire group of patients who entered the trials (including those who did not procede to thoracotomy) was reported for only six studies and ranged from 13 to 33 months.[49,50,52–56] Several authors reported the highest cure rate for patients who required only a lobectomy,[49,56] although this finding was not confirmed by all authors.[48,50] Almost no long-term survival was seen in patients who were found to have unresectable tumors at the time of thoracotomy.

Patients who achieved a complete pathologic response and who had no viable tumor identified at thoracotomy had the best survival. Williams et al.[49] reported that all five patients with a pathologic complete response were cured of their tumors, compared to only 20% of patients who were operable but had viable SCLC present on pathologic review. None of their patients who had inoperable tumors at the time of thoracotomy was cured.[49]

The objective of most of these trials was to assess the feasibility of combined modality therapy, which included

chemotherapy and surgical resection, and to determine whether surgery could contribute to long-term survival and cure by reducing the local recurrence rate. Local relapse rates ranged from 0%[48] to 40% of completely resected patients.[51] Most series reported local failure rates ranging from 10% to 20% for patients who were able to undergo successful resection (Table 55.5).[48,50,52–56,59] Not surprisingly, local control was found to correlate with the degree of response to chemotherapy and the completeness of the surgical resection. Of the patients who responded to chemotherapy and proceeded to surgery, approximately 15% of patients had unresectable tumors. When these patients are added to those who relapsed locally, the local failure rate rises to more than 25% of the surgical patients.

These phase II trials led to observations that were important in the design of subsequent randomized trials of surgery

TABLE 55.5. PATTERN OF RELAPSE FOR PATIENTS WITH SMALL CELL LUNG CANCER TREATED WITH INDUCTION CHEMOTHERAPY FOLLOWED BY SURGERY*

| Investigators | No. of Patients** | No. of Patients with Relapse | | |
		Local Only	Distant Only	Both
Prager, 1984[47]	11	—	4	—
Williams, 1987[48]	25	3	6	—
Johnson, 1987[49]	23	3	7	3
Benfield, 1989[51]	8	—	6	0
Shepherd, 1987[52]	38	3	20	—
Zatopek, 1991[53]	14	—	5	—
Hara, 1991[54]	17	3	7	—
Muller, 1992[55]	45	4	15	—
Yamada, 1991[57]	20	3	7	—
TOTAL	201	19	70	6

* Excluding patients who were not resectable at time of thoracotomy
** Number of patients who underwent thoracotomy

for limited SCLC. They showed that combined modality treatment was feasible and that the preoperative administration of chemotherapy did not result in excessive postoperative morbidity or mortality. All investigators recognized that the favorable survival achieved in these trials might be caused by patient selection. The Toronto group emphasized the importance of selection bias after their review of limited-stage SCLC treated at their institutions over a ten-year period.[50] They reported a significant survival advantage for patients who had no clinical evidence of mediastinal node involvement. This group, which would include the type of patients who might be considered for surgery protocols, had a 20% cure rate with standard chemotherapy and radiation alone, compared to no long-term survival for patients with more advanced tumors. Prospective randomized trials clearly were needed to determine the true role or surgery for patients with limited SCLC.

Randomized Trials

In an attempt to determine whether the addition of surgery to combination chemotherapy and radiotherapy could prolong survival and improve the cure rate for patients with limited SCLC, the Lung Cancer Study Group initiated a prospective randomized trial of adjuvant surgical resection in 1983.[61] Most patients with limited-stage tumors were eligible for this trial, and it is important to note that patients with clinically evident mediastinal lymphadenopathy were not excluded from the study. Induction chemotherapy consisted of cyclophosphamide, doxorubicin, vincristine, and etoposide in the early phase of the trial, and cyclophosphamide, doxorubicin, and vincristine alone in the later phase. In the absence of toxicity or progressive disease, patients received five preoperative cycles of chemotherapy. They were then restaged and underwent medical assessment to determine their suitability for thoracotomy and pulmonary resection. Eligible patients were randomized to receive either surgical resection followed by radiotherapy to the chest and prophylactic cranial irradiation or to the same radiotherapy alone. Three hundred and forty patients entered the trial. The clinical response rate to chemotherapy was 68% (28% CR, 37% PR), but at the completion of induction chemotherapy, only 144 (42%) patients were randomized, 68 to receive surgery and radiotherapy and 76 to receive radiotherapy alone. Of the 68 patients who were randomized to surgery, six did not undergo thoracotomy, but eight patients had off-study surgery, so a total of 70 thoracotomies were performed. Fifty eight patients were able to undergo resection of tumor (83%), and after pathologic review, 54 were thought to have had a complete resection (77%). A complete pathologic response was documented for 18% of patients who underwent surgery. Non–small cell pathology was found in 11% of patients. All randomized patients received radiotherapy to the chest,

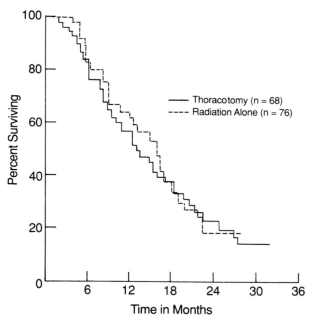

FIGURE 55.9. A comparison of survival for patients randomized to thoracotomy and radiation or radiation alone. (From Shields TW, ed. General Thoracic Surgery, ed 4. Baltimore: Williams & Wilkins, 1994, with permission.)

50 Gy delivered over 5 weeks, and prophylactic cranial irradiation, 30 Gy over 3 weeks.

The median survival from enrollment for all patients was 14 months, and for the randomized patients was 18 months, with no difference seen between the groups in either median survival or long-term survival (Figure 55.9). Because only one-half of the randomized patients in this study underwent surgical resection, it is not possible to compare survival based on pathologic stage or TNM subgroup. The Toronto Group was the first to draw attention to the discrepancy between clinical staging and pathologic staging for patients with SCLC;[53] they showed that clinical staging could not identify subgroups of patients with different prognoses (Figure 55.10).[29] Similar results were found in this study in which patients were staged carefully at the time of surgery. For all patients, it was a protocol requirement to submit multiple lymph node samples, and a mean of 10 lymph nodes were submitted for each of the 70 patients who underwent thoracotomy. Clinical and surgical TNM stages after chemotherapy were the same in only 20 patients (29%), and patients most often moved into a more advanced stage.[62] For the surgical group, no difference in *resectability* was identified for patients in any T or N subgroup, although there seemed to be a trend toward unresectability for patients with T3 tumors (p = 0.08). All pathologic T and N subsets in the surgical patients had similar survival.

Why was survival not improved by surgery, and how should we interpret the results of this Lung Cancer Study

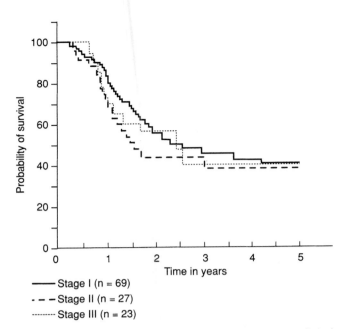

FIGURE 55.10. A comparison of survival by pretreatment clinical stage for 119 patients who underwent surgery for limited small cell lung cancer. (From Shepherd FA, Ginsberg RJ, Feld R, et al. Surgical treatment for limited small cell lung cancer. *J Thorac Cardiovasc Surg* 1991;101:385, with permission.)

Group trial? The survival curves shown in Figure 55.9 were generated on an "intent-to-treat" basis, which is, of course, proper for any prospective randomized trial. It should be noted, though, that 10% of the patients did not receive protocol-specified therapy. Six patients randomized to surgery declined operation, and of perhaps even greater significance, eight patients in the nonsurgical arm underwent thoracotomy and surgical resection. In a small study of this size, a 10% protocol violation of this nature may have masked a small but significant survival advantage in one of the treatment arms.

The next question to be asked is why complete surgical resection was possible for only three-quarters of the patients subjected to thoracotomy. Although the combination of cyclophosphamide, doxorubicin, and vincristine was considered standard therapy at the time, a disappointingly low response rate of only 65% was seen in this study. With newer regimens that incorporate etoposide and cisplatin and concurrent radiotherapy administered early in the course of the disease, response rates of 90% or more are standard.[23,50,52,55,56] Might it have been possible that a more complete response to chemotherapy could have resulted in a higher complete surgical resection rate? The answer, of course, must remain speculative.

Seventeen percent of patients underwent "open-and-closed" procedures with no attempt at surgical resection. For some patients, the residual tumor was clearly unresectable at the time of thoracotomy. For other patients, though,

the decision not to proceed to resection was based on scar tissue formation at the area of the primary tumor and in the mediastinum. Response to chemotherapy is often accompanied by an intense local schirrous reaction, which makes surgical resection more difficult. Tumors that may appear initially to be unresectable because of fibrosis may, in fact, be resected safely with careful dissection of the tumor bed and mediastinum. Because of the multi-institution, and indeed multinational nature of this large study, any individual surgeon operated on only a few patients. It is possible that had this study continued longer, the overall resectability rate might have been higher. This possibility is suggested by the observation that the resectability rate was higher for the Lung Cancer Study Group surgeons than it was in other centers that joined the trial at a later date. This difference may have resulted from their greater experience in operating on both small cell and non–small cell patients after induction chemotherapy.

Finally, patient selection undoubtedly played a large role in the ultimate results of this trial. All patients with limited disease were eligible to enter this study, with the exception of those who had supraclavicular lymph node involvement or pleural or pericardial effusions. This criteria meant that most patients had stage III (N2 and/or T3) tumors. It has long been recognized that surgery has very little role to play in the management of stage III patients with NSCLC, and this trial suggests that the same is true for patients with SCLC. Because many if not most patients with limited SCLC have mediastinal node involvement (often bulky) at the time of initial presentation, it is clear that surgical resection will have very little role to play for most patients with this disease. Nonetheless, it still remains possible that patients with early-stage disease (T1–2 N0, and perhaps nonbulky stage II) may benefit from a combined modality approach that includes surgery. Because so few patients fall into this subgroup (likely less than 10%), it will probably never be possible to undertake a prospective randomized trial to prove or disprove that surgery is appropriate in this setting.

SALVAGE OPERATIONS FOR PATIENTS WITH SMALL CELL LUNG CANCER

Treatment for patients who fail to respond to initial therapy, or who relapse after a primary response, remains unsatisfactory, and only brief periods of palliation and prolongation of survival are achieved with second-line chemotherapy and/or radiotherapy. This result has led several groups to evaluate whether surgery might be useful as salvage therapy for certain patients with limited SCLC.

Yamada et al.[59] offered surgery as salvage therapy to nine patients after chemotherapy for limited SCLC. Two patients had failed to respond to chemotherapy, six had achieved partial response, and one had experienced a complete response. Four of the nine patients achieved long-term disease-free survival, which ranged from 3 to more than 11 years. Surgery was undertaken 1 ½ to 2 ½ years after the initial diagnosis, and no details were provided to suggest why it was felt that surgery might be appropriate for this patient population. Three of the long-term survivors had stage I tumors. These results were very similar to another cohort of 11 patients reported in the same article, for whom surgery was offered as consolidation of the primary chemotherapy. Once again, long-term survival was limited almost exclusively to patients with stage I tumors.

The Toronto Group reported their experience with salvage operations for 28 patients with limited SCLC.[67] Eighteen patients in their series had pure small cell tumors. Their overall median survival was 100 weeks, but only two patients survived 5 or more years (Figure 55.11).

In view of these small numbers, surgery cannot be recommended for patients with pure small cell tumors that fail to respond or who relapse after initial standard therapy. The only possible exception to this recommendation might be the rare patient with a true stage I tumor. If surgery is contemplated for these patients, mediastinoscopy should be undertaken preoperatively because it is unlikely that any benefit will be derived if the tumor has spread to the mediastinal lymph nodes.

In a few patients, NSCLC may be found in combination with SCLC. In a review of 429 patients seen at Vanderbilt University, mixed histology tumors were identified in only nine (2%) cases.[63] Mixed histology tumors may be seen somewhat more often in patients who have been submitted to surgery, and some reviews have suggested that mixed histology tumors may be seen in more than 10% of cases.[28] In the series of salvage operations reported by the University of Toronto Group,[62] eight patients had mixed histology

tumors. The median survival for that group was 108 weeks, and four of the eight patients achieved long-term survival after operation. Three of those four patients had pathologic stage I tumors. Because a few patients with tumors of mixed histologic type may be cured by surgical treatment, consideration should be given to a second biopsy for patients who have *localized* resistant SCLC. Although few patients fall into this favorable subgroup, it is important to take the necessary steps to identify them because curative therapy may be available.

Several authors have now reported that long-term survivors of SCLC are at increased risk of developing second primary malignancies.[29–32] In fact, a long-term survivor is more likely to have a second primary malignancy than a relapse of SCLC, and many of these tumors arise in the upper aerodigestive tract, in particular the lung. In the University of Toronto series, eight patients underwent surgical resection at the time of "relapse" following a long disease-free interval after initial treatment for SCLC. Two were found to have NSCLC, and both achieved long-term survival after surgery.

It is recommended, therefore, that cytologic or histologic identification should be undertaken for long-term survivors of SCLC who develop a new lung lesion. If NSCLC pathology is documented, then the patient should be staged completely. Surgery should be considered if the standard medical and surgical criteria for resection that would be applied to all patients with NSCLCs are met. Once again, it must be recognized that any individual oncologist will see few of these patients. Nonetheless, it is the responsibility of the medical oncologist to undertake the appropriate diagnostic tests and arrange for a surgical consultation because potentially curative therapy may be available.

SUMMARY

Many lessons have been learned from the retrospective, prospective phase II and randomized trials of surgery for patients with SCLC. It is clear that patient selection is the most important determinant in the results obtained. Almost all authors have emphasized the importance of stage and have shown that, similar to NSCLC the chance of long-term survival and cure is strongly correlated to pathologic TNM subgroup. In fact, any consideration of surgery for patients with SCLC should probably be limited to those with stage I and perhaps a subgroup of stage II patients. Therefore, before surgery is ever contemplated, patients should undergo extensive staging of the mediastinum, including mediastinoscopy. Many groups have now shown that combined modality therapy with surgery either before or after chemotherapy is feasible, the toxicity is manageable, and the postoperative morbidity and mortality rates are acceptable.

The results of the Lung Cancer Study Group trial indi-

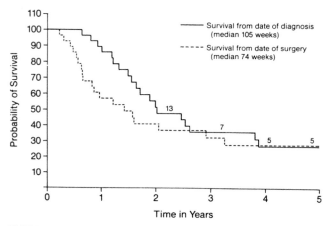

FIGURE 55.11. Survival of twenty-eight patients who underwent salvage operations for small cell lung cancer. (From Shepherd FA, Ginsberg RJ, Patterson GA, et al. Is there ever a role for salvage operations in limited small cell lung cancer? *J Thorac Cardiovasc Surg* 1991;101:196, with permission.)

cate that surgical resection will not benefit the majority of patients with limited SCLC. In general, the phase II studies suggest that the criteria of operability that are applied to NSCLC are equally valid for SCLC patients. Surgery could be considered, therefore, for all patients with T1–2 N0 small cell tumors. Whether surgery is offered as the initial treatment or after induction chemotherapy does not seem to be important. Similar results were reported by Wada et al.[44] If a small cell tumor is identified unexpectedly at the time of thoracotomy, complete resection and mediastinal lymph node resection should be undertaken if possible. Chemotherapy should be administered postoperatively to all patients, even those with pathologic stage I tumors.

With respect to stage II disease, it is not possible to make generalized recommendations regarding surgery, and treatment decisions must be individualized. If surgery is to be part of the treatment approach, it should probably be offered as adjuvant treatment only to patients who have demonstrated response to initial systemic chemotherapy. As was recommended for patients with stage I tumors, complete resection should be undertaken if SCLC is identified unexpectedly at thoracotomy, even if hilar or intrapulmonary lymph nodes are found to be positive. These patients should then receive a full course of adjuvant chemotherapy when they have recovered sufficiently from surgery.

Surgery has little role to play for patients with stage III tumors. Even though chemotherapy can result in dramatic shrinkage of bulky mediastinal tumors, the addition of surgical resection does not contribute significantly to long-term survival for most patients, as shown conclusively by the Lung Cancer Study Group trial.

The final group of patients who may benefit from surgical resection are those with combined small cell and non–small cell tumors. If a mixed histology cancer is identified at diagnosis, then the initial treatment should be with chemotherapy to control the small cell component of the disease, and surgery should be considered for the non–small cell component. For patients who demonstrate an unexpectedly poor response to chemotherapy, and for patients who experience localized late relapse after treatment for pure small cell tumors, a repeat biopsy should be performed to rule out non-small cell pathology. Complete staging should be undertaken and surgery considered for stage I and II patients who are medically fit.

REFERENCES

1. Hansen HH, Dombernowsky P, Hirsch FR. Staging procedures and prognostic features in small cell anaplastic bronchogenic carcinoma. *Semin Oncol* 1978;5:280.
2. Martini N, Wittes RE, Hilaris BS, et al. Oat cell carcinoma of the lung. *Clin Boll* 1975;5:144.
3. Mountain C. Clinical biology of small cell carcinoma: relationship to surgical therapy. *Semin Oncol* 1978;5:272.
4. Working-party on the evaluation of different methods of therapy in carcinoma of the bronchus. Comparative trial of surgery and radiotherapy for the primary treatment of small-celled, or oat-celled carcinoma of the bronchus. *Lancet* 1966;2:979.
5. Fox W, Scadding JG. Medical Research Council comparative trial of surgery and radiotherapy for primary treatment of small-celled or oat-celled carcinoma of the bronchus. Ten-year follow-up. *Lancet* 1973;2:63.
6. Bates M, Levison V, Hurt R, et al. Treatment of oat-cell carcinoma of bronchus by pre-operative radiotherapy and surgery. *Lancet* 1975;1:1134.
7. Levison V. Pre-operative radiotherapy and surgery in the treatment of oat-cell carcinoma of the bronchus. *Clin Radiol* 1980;31:345.
8. Sherman DM, Neptune W, Weichselbaum R, et al. An aggressive approach to marginally resectable lung cancer. *Cancer* 1978;41:2040.
9. Bergsagel DE, Jenkin RDT, Pringle JF. Lung cancer: clinical trial of radiotherapy alone *versus* radiotherapy plus cyclophosphamide. *Cancer* 1972;30:321.
10. Medical Research Council Lung Working Party. Radiotherapy alone or with chemotherapy in the treatment of small-cell carcinoma of the lung. *Br J Cancer* 1979;40:1.
11. Shields TW, Humphrey EW, Eastridge CE, et al. Adjuvant cancer chemotherapy after resection of carcinoma of the lung. *Cancer* 1977;40:2057.
12. Shields TW, Higgins GA, Matthews MG, et al. Surgical resection in the management of small cell carcinoma of the lung. *J Thorac Cardiovasc Surg* 1982;84:481.
13. Lennox SC, Flavell G, Pollock DJ, et al. Results of resection for oat-cell carcinoma of the lung. *Lancet* 1968;2:925.
14. Shore DF, Paneth M. Survival after resection of small cell carcinoma of the bronchus. *Thorax* 1987;35:819.
15. Hayata Y, Funatsu H, Suemasu K, et al. Surgical indications in small cell carcinoma of the lung. *Jap J Clin Oncol* 1978;8:93.
16. Shepherd FA, Ginsberg RJ, Evans WK, et al. Reduction in local recurrence and improved survival in surgically treated patients with small cell lung cancer. *J Thorac Cardiovasc Surg* 1983;86:498.
17. Higgins GS, Shields TW, Keehn RJ. The solitary pulmonary nodule. Ten-year follow-up of Veteran's Administration-Armed Forces Co-operative study. *Arch Surg* 1975;110:570.
18. Aisner J, Alberto P, Bitran J, et al. Role of chemotherapy in small cell lung cancer: a concensus report of the International Association for the Study of Lung Cancer Workshop. *Cancer Treat Rep.* 1983;67:37.
19. Livingstone RB. Current chemotherapy of small cell lung cancer. *Chest* 1986;89:2585.
20. Elliott JA, Osterlind K, Hirsch FR, et al. Metastatic patterns in small-cell lung cancer: correlation of autopsy findings with clinical parameters in 537 patients. *J Clin Oncol* 1987;5:246.
21. Warde P, Payne D. Does thoracic irradiation improve survival and local control in limited-stage small-cell carcinoma of the lung? A META-analysis. *J Clin Oncol* 1992;10:890.
22. Pingnon J-P, Arriagada R, Ihde D, et al. A META-analysis of thoracic radiotherapy for small-cell lung cancer. *N Engl J Med* 1992;327:1618.
23. Murray N, Coy P, Pater J, et al. Importance of timing for thoracic irradiation in the combined modality treatment of limited-stage small-cell lung cancer. *J Clin Oncol* 1993;11:336.
24. Shepherd FA, Ginsberg RJ, Evans WK, et al. Reduction in local recurrence and improved survival in surgically treated patients with small-cell lung cancer. *J Thorac Cardiovasc Surg* 1983;86:498.
25. Comis R, Meyer J, Ginsberg S, et al. The impact of TNM stage on results with chemotherapy and adjuvant surgery in small cell lung cancer. *Proc Am Soc Clin Oncol* 1984;3:226.
26. Hirsch FR, Osterlind K, Hansen H. The prognostic significance

of histopathologic subtyping of small-cell carcinoma of the lung according to the classification of the World Health Organization. *Cancer* 1983;52:2144.

27. Magnum MD, Greco FA, Hainsworth JD, et al. Combined small-cell and non-small cell lung cancer. *J Clin Oncol* 1989;7:607.

28. Shepherd FA, Ginsberg RJ, Feld R, et al. Surgical treatment for limited small-cell lung cancer. *J Thorac Cardiovasc Surg* 1991;101:385.

29. Heyne KH, Lippman SM, Lee JJ, et al. The incidence of second primary tumors in long-term survivors of small-cell lung cancer. *J Clin Oncol* 1992;10:1519.

30. Sagman U, Lishner M, Maki E, et al. Second primary malignancies following diagnosis of small-cell lung cancer. *J Clin Oncol* 1992;10:1525.

31. Ihde DC, Tucker MA. Second primary malignancies in small-cell lung cancer: a major consequence of modest success. *J Clin Oncol* 1992;10:1511.

32. Osterlind K, Hansen HH, Hansen M, et al. Mortality and morbidity in long-term surviving patients treated with chemotherapy with or without irradiation for small-cell lung cancer. *J Clin Oncol* 1986;4:1044.

33. Hayata Y, Funatsu H, Suemasu K, et al. Surgical indications for small cell carcinoma of the lung. *Jap J Clin Oncol* 1978;8:93.

34. Meyer J, Comis RL, Ginsberg SJ, et al. The prospect of disease control by surgery combined with chemotherapy in stage I and stage II small-cell carcinoma of the lung. *Ann Thorac Surg* 1983;36:37.

35. Meyer JA, Gullo JJ, Ikins PM, et al. Adverse prognostic effect of N2 disease in treated small-cell carcinoma of the lung. *J Thorac Cardiovasc Surg* 1984;88:495.

36. Osterlind K, Hansen M, Hansen HH, et al. Influence of surgical resection prior to chemotherapy on the long-term results in small-cell lung cancer. A study of 150 operable patients. *Eur J Cancer Clin Oncol* 1986;22:589.

37. Maassen W, Greschuchna D. Small-cell carcinoma of the lung—to operate or not? Surgical experience and results. *J Thorac Cardiovasc Surg* 1986;34:71.

38. Shepherd FA, Evans WK, Feld R, et al. Adjuvant chemotherapy following surgical resection for small-cell carcinoma of the lung. *J Clin Oncol* 1988;6:832.

39. Karrer K, Denck H, Karnicka-Mlodkowska H, et al. The importance of surgery as the first step in multi-modality treatment of small-cell bronchial carcinoma. *Int J Clin Pharm Res* 1990;10:257.

40. Ulsperger E, Karrer K, Denck H, ISC-Lung Cancer Study Group. Multi-modality treatment for small-cell bronchial carcinoma. *Eur J Cardiothorac Surg* 1991;5:306.

41. Macchiarini P, Hardin M, Basolo F, et al. Surgery plus adjuvant chemotherapy for T1-3N0M0 small-cell lung cancer. *Am J Clin Oncol* 1991;14:218.

42. Hara N, Ichinose Y, Kuda T, et al. Long-term survivors in resected and non-resected small-cell lung cancer. *Oncology* 1991;48:441.

43. Davis S, Crino L, Tonato M, et al. A prospective analysis of chemotherapy following surgical resection of clinical Stage I–II small-cell lung cancer. *Am J Clin Oncol* 1993;16:93.

44. Wada H, Yokomise H, Tanaka E, et al. Surgical treatment of small cell carcinoma of the lung: advantage of preoperative chemotherapy. *Lung Cancer* 1995;13:45.

45. Friess GG, McCracken JD, Troxell ML, et al. Effects of initial resection of small-cell carcinoma of the lung: a review of Southwest Oncology Group study 7628. *J Clin Oncol* 1985;3:964.

46. Littlewood TH, Smith AP, Bentley DP. Treatment of small-cell lung cancer by pneumonectomy and single course high dose chemotherapy. *Thorax* 1987;42:315.

47. Shah SS, Thompson J, Goldstraw P. Results of operation without adjuvant therapy in the treatment of small-cell lung cancer. *Ann Thorac Surg* 1992;54:498.

48. Prager RL, Foster JM, Hainsworth JD, et al. The feasibility of adjuvant surgery in limited-stage small cell carcinoma: a prospective evaluation. *Ann Thorac Surg* 1984;38:622.

49. Williams CJ, McMillan I, Lea R, et al. Surgery after initial chemotherapy for localized small cell carcinoma of the lung. *J Clin Oncol* 1987;5:1579.

50. Johnson DH, Einhorn LH, Mandelbaum I, et al. Post chemotherapy resection of residual tumor in limited stage small cell lung cancer. *Chest* 1987;92:241.

51. Baker RR, Ettinger DS, Ruckdeschel JD, et al. The role of surgery in the management of selected patients with small-cell carcinoma of the lung. *J Clin Oncol* 1987;5:697.

52. Benfield GFA, Matthews HR, Watson DCT, et al. Chemotherapy plus adjuvant surgery for local small cell lung cancer. *Eur J Surg Oncol* 1989;15:341.

53. Shepherd FA, Ginsberg RJ, Patterson GA, et al. A prospective study of adjuvant surgical resection after chemotherapy for limited small cell lung cancer. *J Thorac Cardiovasc Surg* 1989;97:177.

54. Zatopek N, Holoye P, Ellerbroek NA, et al. Resectability of small-cell lung cancer following induction chemotherapy in patients with limited disease (stage II–IIIb). *Am J Clin Oncol* 1991;14:427.

55. Hara N, Ohta M, Ichinose Y, et al. Influence of surgical resection before and after chemotherapy on survival in small cell lung cancer. *J Surg Oncol* 1991;47:53.

56. Eberhardt W, Wilke H, Stamatis G, et al. Preliminary results of a stage oriented multimodality treatment including surgery for selected subgroups of limited disease small cell lung cancer. *Lung Cancer* 1997;18(Suppl 1):61.

57. Muller LC, Salzer GM, Huber H, et al. Multi modal therapy of small cell lung cancer in TNM stages I–IIIa. *Ann Thorac Surg* 1992;54:493.

58. Shepherd FA. Induction chemotherapy for locally advanced non-small cell lung cancer. *Ann Thorac Surg* 1993;55:1585.

59. Yamada K, Saijo N, Kojima A, et al. A retrospective analysis of patients receiving surgery after chemotherapy for small cell lung cancer. *Jpn J Clin Oncol* 1991;21:39.

60. Shepherd FA, Ginsberg RJ, Haddad R, et al. Importance of clinical staging in limited small-cell lung cancer: a valuable system to separate prognostic subgroups. *J Clin Oncol* 1993;8:1592.

61. Lad T, Piantadosi S, Thomas P, et al. A prospective randomized trial to determine the benefit of surgical resection of residual disease following response of small cell lung cancer to combination chemotherapy. *Chest* 1994;7(Suppl 6):3205.

62. Shepherd FA, Ginsberg RJ, Patterson GA, et al. Is there ever a role for salvage operations in limited small-cell lung cancer? *J Thorac Cardiovasc Surg* 1991;101:196.

63. Mangum MD, Greco FA, Hainsworth JD, et al. Combined small-cell and non-small-cell lung cancer. *J Clin Oncol* 1989;7:607.

56

PROPHYLACTIC CRANIAL IRRADIATION IN SMALL CELL LUNG CANCER

DAVID L. BALL

The hypothesis is simple. Small cell lung cancer (SCLC) is a disseminated disease at diagnosis, best treated by systemic chemotherapy; subclinical disease in the central nervous system (CNS) is, however, in a sanctuary site protected by the blood–brain barrier; relatively low doses of prophylactic irradiation of the CNS may be able to eradicate this disease and so cure some patients who, having achieved a complete response (CR), would have relapsed in the CNS as the sole site of failure. Yet it has taken over 25 years since prophylactic cranial irradiation (PCI) was first tested in a clinical trial by the CALGB[1] before the expected survival advantage in patients with SCLC in CR could be detected by metaanalysis.[2] Even so, the role of PCI remains controversial, mainly because of concerns about late neurologic toxicity in long-term survivors.[3] Other unresolved issues include questions about the optimum dose and fractionation of the radiotherapy prescription, the timing of PCI and the net quality-of-life benefit for treated patients. It is the purpose of this review critically to examine the available randomized and nonrandomized evidence in relation to the role of PCI in SCLC and to make recommendations about its use in practice.

HISTORY

In 1971, Aur and colleagues published a paper which demonstrated that the problem of CNS relapse in children with acute lymphocytic leukaemia could be partly overcome by the administration of cranial irradiation and intrathecal methotrexate early in complete remission.[4] That the success of this approach might be reproducible in the treatment of SCLC in adults was first suggested by Hansen in 1973.[5] In the same article he reported a 40% crude incidence of cerebral metastases in 20 patients following treatment with chemotherapy and thoracic irradiation, with an apparent increase in incidence with greater elapsed time from diagnosis. However, he did not report how many patients had active disease at other sites, although it was mentioned that neurologic manifestations became the major symptomatic feature in eight of the patients with cerebral metastases. Hence, although CNS disease was a major problem for these patients, no evidence was provided to suggest that the CNS was a sanctuary site. At the time Hansen's paper appeared, the first randomized trial comparing PCI with no CNS prophylaxis had already been initiated by the CALGB in December 1972, but the results were not published until 1980.[1] By 1993, 10 randomized trials comparing PCI with no prophylaxis had been published.[1,6–14] Although PCI appeared to reduce the incidence of cerebral metastases in all studies, none revealed an associated statistically significant survival advantage. In retrospect this is not surprising—most of the studies were small: seven had fewer than 100 patients randomized and therefore had low statistical power. In only two small studies[11,14] was CR an eligibility criterion for randomization. As we shall see, patients in CR are those likely to obtain the greatest survival benefit if prevention of isolated CNS relapse can be achieved. It is now obvious that the early PCI trials suffered from a lack of sound statistical input at the study design stage, and, rather than contributing to a resolution of the controversy, the first generation of trials may have only delayed recognition of the value of PCI. The second generation of trials were, however, based on a knowledge of the magnitude of the problem of isolated CNS relapse as a cause of treatment failure and were, in statistical terms, powered accordingly. This forms the subject of the next section.

CENTRAL NERVOUS SYSTEM INVOLVEMENT AS A CAUSE OF TREATMENT FAILURE IN SCLC

The high frequency with which CNS involvement complicates the course of SCLC is well recognized.[15,16] The incidence will vary depending on the method of detection, according to the following ascending scale of sensitivity: clinical, nuclear brain scan, CT, MRI, and postmortem histopathology. High-quality CT and MRI have become readily available for staging purposes only over the last ten years, and it is conceivable that many of the patients randomized in the trials mentioned in the previous section may have already had brain metastases by current staging criteria. In theory, these patients are least likely to benefit from the relatively low doses of radiotherapy used for PCI, and their inclusion in trials may have tended to obscure the benefits of PCI for those patients whose disease was truly microscopic.

Three main sites of CNS involvement are recognized: brain, leptomeninges, and spinal cord. A review of the postmortem documented incidence of CNS metastases revealed that the brain was most commonly involved (42%) followed by the leptomeninges (14%) and spinal cord (12%).[15] In a large study of 641 patients with SCLC, 210 developed neurologic disorders during the course of their illness, including 178 cases with CNS involvement.[16] The frequency of involvement, as a percentage of the total population, was brain 24.8%, meninges 2.2%, and spinal cord 0.8%. In a nonrandomized study, PCI had no influence on the development of leptomeningeal or spinal cord metastases, although it did reduce the incidence of brain relapse.[17] Since a reduction of the incidence of meningeal or intramedullary disease is not the primary goal of PCI, the remaining discussion will concentrate on brain involvement as a cause of treatment failure.

The development of cerebral metastasis in the course of any malignancy is a catastrophic event because of the associated disabling morbidity and high mortality. The clinical features of brain involvement are likely to overshadow symptoms related to disease at other sites, even though that disease may be of greater bulk. Further, once cerebral relapse has been detected, it is unlikely that the patients will be subjected to a rigorous restaging, leading to an underestimate of the extent of extra-CNS disease. As a consequence, the frequency of the brain as a sole site of relapse may be overestimated.

In a recent review of 17 studies involving 1,202 patients with SCLC who did not receive PCI, the crude incidence of cerebral metastases was 25%.[18] The incidence was even higher (33%) in patients who had achieved a CR, possibly because of the longer survival of these patients and hence increased opportunity to develop brain metastasis. However many patients relapsed at multiple sites simultaneously, and in those studies in which first site of relapse was reported, the brain was the only site in 14%. In theory this is the proportion of patients who are most likely to benefit from eradication of subclinical disease by PCI—either curing those patients who have no disease elsewhere, or delaying death in those patients who do have extracerebral disease but who are more likely, in terms of competing risks, to die of their cerebral metastases. But as we have already seen, additional factors other than PCI—such as duration of survival—can influence the incidence of cerebral metastasis, and these need to be taken into account in any evaluation of the effect of PCI. We shall now consider these independent influences one by one.

Influence of Duration of Survival on the Risk of Cerebral Metastasis

In his original report, Hansen[5] noted an apparent increase in the risk of cerebral metastasis with lengthening survival. This observation was subsequently confirmed by others.[19,20] In the study of Nugent and colleagues,[19] the overall incidence of CNS metastasis was 49%, but for patients surviving two years, the cumulative probability rose to 80%. In the Komaki study,[20] 32 patients not receiving PCI had a 58% calculated rate of clinical failure in the brain at two years. Arrigada and colleagues[21] using a competing risk approach, reported an overall rate of 67% of patients with brain metastases at two years after achieving CR and 45% with brain metastases as a first site of failure.

The crude incidence of CNS metastases will continue to increase with increasing duration of survival unless there is a time at which the cumulative actuarial incidence reaches a plateau. For example, if the median time to CNS relapse were three years and the median overall survival duration were six months, then, assuming exponential distributions, the expected crude incidence of CNS relapse would be 14% if all patients were followed to death. If the median survival were one, two, or three years, then the expected crude incidence of CNS relapse would increase to 25%, 40%, or 50% respectively. Thus, as systemic treatment improves, CNS relapse will be an increasing cause of treatment failure in the future.

Influence of Systemic Chemotherapy on the Risk of Cerebral Metastasis

On theoretical grounds, the CNS should be impervious to the effects of systemically administered chemotherapy because of the blood–brain barrier. Recent clinical observations suggest, however, that this may not be so, since chemotherapy has been reported to induce responses in cerebral metastases in untreated and previously treated patients.[22] Twelves and colleagues[23] assessed the response in 19 patients with symptomatic cerebral metastases who were treated with chemotherapy (cyclophosphamide, vincristine, and etoposide) and in whom cranial irradiation was withheld. Of 14 patients who had postchemotherapy scans, eight had a partial response and one a complete response; of the others, one had clinical neurological improvement, giving an overall response rate of 53%. The response rate of the intrathoracic tumor in these patients was 79%, suggesting either a partial "sanctuary site" effect or, alternatively, differences in chemosensitivity between primary and metastatic disease. In a study of similar design by Kristjansen and associates[24] in which the chemotherapy consisted initially of cisplatin, teniposide, and vincristine, the CT documented response rate of the cerebral metastases was almost identical at 52%.

In an autopsy study of 85 patients with SCLC, de la

Monte and colleagues observed differences in the patterns of failure according to the type of treatment received.[25] No patient had been given PCI. The incidence of CNS involvement in patients treated with chemotherapy with or without irradiation was 50% to 55%; in patients treated exclusively with thoracic irradiation, it was 75%. Since this last group had a shorter survival than the patients treated with chemotherapy, it would have been expected that the incidence of CNS involvement would have been lower rather than higher. One possible explanation for this observation is that the chemotherapy acted directly on subclinical CNS disease to reduce the autopsy incidence. If subclinical CNS disease is as sensitive to chemotherapy as are clinically evident cerebral metastases, the development of CNS involvement in spite of chemotherapy may be at least in part a manifestation of generalized chemoresistance, and not purely a "sanctuary site" phenomenon.

Influence of Thoracic Irradiation on the Risk of Cerebral Metastasis

That thoracic irradiation may have an effect on the subsequent incidence of CNS metastases was suggested by the results of a Canadian trial designed to investigate the importance of timing of thoracic irradiation in patients with limited SCLC.[26] Patients were randomized to receive thoracic irradiation either early (week 3) with chemotherapy, or later (week 15). Complete responders were given PCI when they had finished chemotherapy. Cerebral metastases developed more frequently in patients who were randomized to late thoracic irradiation, even though they had a significantly shorter survival. The authors postulated that this result may have been due, in the early radiotherapy group, to eradication of chemoresistant clones of cells at the primary site before they had the opportunity to metastasize. If radiotherapy is delayed, these cells can disseminate and proliferate outside the radiotherapy target volume, unaffected by chemotherapy. The lower incidence of brain disease contributed to but did not entirely account for the superior survival of patients randomized to early irradiation.

Two other randomized trials have been published addressing the issue of timing of thoracic irradiation and in which the incidence of CNS relapse was reported.[27,28] In contrast to the Canadian result, neither showed an influence of timing of thoracic irradiation on the incidence of cerebral metastasis. It is not possible directly to compare the three trials because of differences in the timing of both thoracic irradiation and PCI, with the result that the contrasting results cannot be easily explained and so the effect of thoracic irradiation on the probability of CNS relapse must be regarded as an open question.

Reseeding of the CNS as a Cause of Cerebral Relapse

The discussion thus far has treated the CNS as a primary site of treatment failure, but it is conceivable that the CNS could be a site of secondary relapse, even after PCI, as a result of reseeding from uncontrolled extra-CNS disease. If this were so, it would have implications for the timing of PCI, in particular whether it is appropriate to administer PCI before complete response is achieved. This issue has been considered by Hoskin and colleagues in a study of 30 patients who had achieved a complete response and who then had PCI (20 Gy in five fractions).[29] Seven patients then relapsed in the brain after first relapsing elsewhere: six initially in the thorax, and the seventh in bone. Cerebral relapse occurred at a mean interval of 4 (range one to six) months after first relapse. Basing their arguments on clinically observed doubling times of SCLC, the authors claimed that a period of 15 months would be required from the time of reseeding until clinical relapse occurred. They therefore concluded that CNS relapse in their study was more likely to be due to inadequate PCI dose rather than secondary failure.

Summary

When patients with SCLC develop progressive disease, they usually do so at multiple sites. In one autopsy study, the mean number of metastatic sites ranged from 9.1 to 11.6, depending on the type of treatment administered[25]; in another, it was 4.2.[30] Cerebral metastasis as a sole site of first treatment failure may occur in fewer than 14% of patients; it is in this subgroup of patients that PCI has the potential to increase the probability of cure (in which case extracranial CR is a prerequisite) or at least to extend survival. Overall some 25% of SCLC patients may fail in the brain. Some survival benefit could be expected from PCI in these patients if more effective treatments of noncerebral metastases were available. Finally, it is now clear that factors other than PCI can influence the risk of CNS relapse, and unless these components of the treatment program are standardized in any comparative study evaluating PCI, their independent influence on the development of CNS metastases may be mistakenly interpreted as an effect of the PCI.

TREATMENT OF ESTABLISHED CEREBRAL METASTASES

If treatment could eradicate cerebral metastases at the time they become clinically or radiologically apparent, there would be less justification for PCI, although the relative morbidity of the two treatment approaches would need to be considered carefully. Of the treatments available, only surgery, radiotherapy, and chemotherapy are theoretically capable of inducing complete response, while corticosteroids are valuable for short-term symptom control. Because brain metastases are usually multiple,[19] surgical resection or stereotactic radiotherapy are seldom options, although they

TABLE 56.1. RESPONSE TO THERAPEUTIC CRANIAL IRRADIATION IN SCLC

First Author	Total No. of Patients	Population	No. Assessed for Symptomatic Response	Symptomatic Response	
				Overall No. (%)	Complete No. (%)
Nugent 1979[19]	58	All	51	47 (92%)	NR
Cox 1980[34]	40	All	35	30 (75%)	15 (38%)
Baglan 1981[35]	47	All	39	33 (85%)	25 (85%)
Hirsch 1983[34]	24	All	24	11 (46%)	NR
Lucas 1986[35]	38†	All	39	18 (46%)	8 (21%)
Sculier 1987[16]	144	All	85	54 (64%)	NR
Giannone 1987[36]	41	All	41	18 (100%)	NR
Mira 1988[37]	64	All	31	28 (90%)	14 (45%)
Carmichael 1988[38]	61	All	59	37 (63%)	19 (32%)
Ichinose 1989[39]	17	LD in CR	17	12 (71%)	NR
Nieder 1997[32]	94	All	94*	76 (81%)*	34 (37%)*
Postmus 1998[33]	22	CR	20	12 (60%)	6 (30%)*

NR, not reported; LD, limited disease; CR, complete response.
† includes 7 patients treated with dexamethasone alone.
* measurable response assessed by CT.

can be useful for solitary metastasis resulting from other histologic types of lung cancer.[31]

Radiotherapy

This is the most frequently used treatment modality. Table 56.1 is a compilation of reports in which the response of cerebral metastases to radiotherapy was reported in patients with SCLC. The overall symptomatic response rate was 68% in 441 patients assessed for response. This represents an overall rate of 57% in the 527 patients treated, many patients dying before an assessment could be made. Complete symptomatic responses were reported in 40% of 203 patients assessed or 32% of 251 patients treated. Response as measured by follow-up CT scanning was available in only two of the studies[32,33]: only 35% of 114 assessable patients were judged to have had a complete response.

Most studies[34,35,36–38] included patients whose cerebral metastases were detected at diagnosis, a group for whom PCI could never have been possible and who may have had a better result because they benefit from chemotherapy as well as radiotherapy.[39,40] In one report[38] the complete response rate in patients treated for delayed metastases was only 28%, compared with 39% for patients with metastases at initial presentation. Hence the complete response rate in patients who develop delayed cerebral metastases may actually be 30% or less, taking into account those patients who may never be well enough to have radiotherapy.

Table 56.2 provides a representative list of some recently reported survival data following the diagnosis of cerebral metastases in SCLC. It is important to remember that not all patients actually received or completed radiotherapy, some being too unwell to have treatment, but they cannot be excluded in any evaluation of the impact of radiotherapy on survival. The results are uniformly poor, with most series

reporting median survivals of approximately three months following the diagnosis of brain metastases. In the study by Ryan and colleagues,[41] only 8% of patients survived 12 months. The longer median survival of 5.5 months observed by Mira et al[37] can be explained by the selection of their patients, all of whom had their cerebral metastases detected at diagnosis, before chemotherapy. Absence of extracranial disease may also favor improved survival, as observed by Postmus and associates[33] although not observed by others.[42]

Perhaps the clearest picture of what is achievable when patients relapse in the brain is provided by the results of a prospective study (not listed in Table 56.1) in which 127 patients underwent three-monthly brain CT surveillance after the diagnosis of SCLC; PCI was not used, but radiotherapy was begun as soon as cerebral metastases were detected, whether symptomatic or not.[43] Brain metastases were detected in 56 patients: 16 at presentation, nine of whom were asymptomatic, and 40 on follow-up, 27 of whom were asymptomatic (i.e., detected by surveillance).

TABLE 56.2. SURVIVAL FOLLOWING DIAGNOSIS OF BRAIN METASTASES IN SCLC

First Author	Total No. of Patients	Patient Population	Median Survival (months)
Mira 1988[37]	64	P	5.5
Ryan 1995[41]	122	All	3.3
Bach 1996[42]	101	X	3.6
Nussbaum 1996[46]	110	All	3
Priestman 1996[47]	103	X	2.6
Postmus 1998[33]	22	CR	4.7

P, includes only patients whose brain metastases were discovered at diagnosis; X, includes only patients given whole brain radiotherapy; CR, includes only patients with no evidence of extracranial disease.

When cerebral relapse was detected, the policy was to give 40 Gy in 20 fractions to the whole brain. Seven patients were never well enough to receive radiotherapy, and of the remainder, 26 died with active CNS disease or within a month of completing radiotherapy; hence 33 of 56 (59%) died because of or with active CNS disease. The patients whose disease was detected by surveillance showed no survival advantage in comparison with the symptomatic group; the authors concluded, therefore, that this approach was not an effective substitute for PCI.

Baglan and Marks[35] and Kristjansen and Kristensen[44] have each undertaken an exercise designed to measure the net benefit of PCI compared with delayed therapeutic irradiation. In both instances the authors concluded that the results of therapeutic radiation were such that the proportions of patients who will be left with neurologic symptoms at the end of their illness is the same whether PCI is given or not. However Baglan's and Marks's symptomatic response rates were estimated from a series including patients whose brain metastases were detected at diagnosis, thus biasing the conclusion in favor of therapeutic irradiation. Further, 17% of patients with brain metastases who either died, were lost to follow-up, or had a craniotomy with subtotal removal of metastasis were excluded from the symptomatic response calculations. The exercise took account of only symptomatic response and did not consider the poor survival (median three months) of patients following treatment of delayed metastases. Similarly, Kristjansen and Kristensen in their calculations used a rather high figure of 40% CR rate following therapeutic irradiation—30% may be more realistic; also they have not allowed for the fact that a percentage of patients who develop CNS metastases despite PCI may obtain a symptomatic CR as a result of subsequent therapeutic irradiation.

To make a realistic assessment of the value of PCI, both duration and quality of life need to be considered. Felletti and associates[45] attempted to assess the morbidity of cerebral relapse by measuring the time spent in hospital by patients who first relapsed in the brain and comparing it with the time spent by those who relapsed in the liver. Both groups had a similar survival from the time of relapse, but the brain group spent significantly more time in hospital; thus the authors concluded that brain relapse was associated with a greater morbidity. They commented that radiotherapy was relatively ineffective in producing an improvement in performance status in their patients, and that even if PCI did not influence survival, it might be justified because of its social and economic benefits.

Chemotherapy

In comparison with radiotherapy, there is much less information available on the efficacy of chemotherapy for cerebral metastases which have developed after previous treatment. In a phase II study of the EORTC Lung Cancer Cooperative Group, response and survival following treatment with teniposide were measured in 80 patients with cerebral metastases from SCLC.[46] The overall response rate was 33%, including 8% complete responses, but there were eight treatment-related deaths. These results appear inferior to those achieved with whole-brain irradiation, which the authors recommend is still the standard treatment.

Summary

The treatment of cerebral metastases which have developed following chemotherapy is unsatisfactory, resulting in short survivals and most patients dying of their cerebral cancer. Thus there appears to be ample justification for exploring ways of reducing the risk of patients' developing cerebral metastases.

RANDOMIZED TRIALS OF PCI IN PATIENTS IN COMPLETE REMISSION

From what has been said previously, it is clear that unless competing risks for death resulting from disease *outside* the CNS can be eliminated, the eradication of disease *inside* the CNS by PCI cannot be expected to increase the probability of cure in SCLC. Effectively this means that the population of patients who stand to gain from PCI, purely in survival terms, are the 14% of patients who, in the absence of PCI, relapse in the brain as the first and only site of relapse. Accordingly, if PCI is to be given "late," only those patients who are in CR should be selected. Yet only two of the early randomized trials specified CR as a criterion for randomization.[11,14] Both studies were too small to detect an influence of PCI on survival, although significant reductions in the incidence of cerebral metastases were seen in patients randomized to PCI. Several nonrandomized studies have suggested a survival advantage for patients in CR having PCI,[17,47,48] but this has not been a universal finding.[49]

Table 56.3 a compilation of randomized trials of PCI in which only those patients who had achieved a CR were eligible. Only three of these studies were large enough to have some prospect of detecting a survival advantage.[21,50,51] Two of the trials were coordinated by the Institut Gustav-Roussy: the first trial (IPC85) had a more elaborate design and included a mandatory neuropsychological assessment,[21] but the second trial (IPC88) focused on overall survival and allowed for some variation in PCI dose.[50] IPC88 was closed prematurely when the results of IPC85 became available. All studies reported a reduction in CNS metastases in patients randomized to PCI, and this was highly significant in the IPC85 and European trials.[21,51] In the studies in which it was reported, survival was consistently better in the PCI arms, although this did not achieve statistical significance in any individual trial. However, when the results of seven separate randomized trials of PCI in CR were grouped to-

TABLE 56.3. RANDOMIZED TRIALS OF PCI VERSUS NO PCI IN PATIENTS IN COMPLETE REMISSION

First Author	No. of Patients	Radiotherapy Dose/Fractionation	CNS Metastases at 2 Yrs		Survival at 2 Yrs	
			PCI	No PCI	PCI	No PCI
Aroney 1985[11]	32	30Gy/10Fx	0%*	27%*	NR	NR
Ohonoshi 1993[14]	46	40Gy/10fx	20%	50%	22%†	15%†
Arriagada 1995[21]	294	24Gy/8fx	40%	69%	29%	21.5%
Laplanche 1998[50]	211	Various	44%#	51%#	22%#	16%#
Wagner 1996[56]	31	25Gy/10fx	18%*	53%*	15.3‡	8.8‡
Gregor 1997[51]	314	Various	30%	54%	25%	19%

* crude relapse rates.
\# four-year event rates.
† five-year survival.
‡ median survival (months).

gether in a metaanalysis of individual data on 987 patients, there was a statistically significant 16% reduction in mortality in favor of PCI.[2] The survival benefit was consistent across the subgroups defined according to age, performance status, initial disease extent, and type of induction treatment. In terms of survival, however, PCI appeared to be less effective in women than in men. There was a trend for patients having higher doses or earlier PCI to have a greater reduction in risk of brain metastasis, but without an effect on survival. Thus the elusive survival benefit for PCI which had been predicted on the basis of first principles now appears to be supported by the available evidence. Interestingly the magnitude of the effect appears to be similar to what might have been expected based on what is known of the frequency of brain as the site of first failure.

THE RADIOTHERAPY PRESCRIPTION: DOSE, FRACTIONATION, TIMING, AND TARGET VOLUME CONSIDERATIONS

The objective of PCI is to eradicate subclinical disease while minimizing the risk of producing injury to normal brain. To achieve the former requires sufficient dose and an adequate target volume. However, the risk of injury is dependent not only on total dose, but also on dose per fraction, especially for late effects. In this section we will consider one by one the individual parameters of the PCI prescription and their relevance to disease control and late toxicity.

Dose

A major advance in our understanding of the dose-response relationship for subclinical disease occurred with the publication in 1995 of an analysis by Withers and colleagues of the rates of reduction of metastatic disease according to dose of elective irradiation for various tumor sites.[52] In essence they were able to demonstrate that the percentage decrease in metastases bore a linear relationship to the dose of radia-

tion administered, and that even very low doses of radiotherapy could be associated with a small reduction in the number of metastases. These observations fitted with a model in which the logarithm of the number of subclinical metastatic clonogens is distributed evenly in any series of patients between log 1 and log M, where M is the maximum number of cells that can remain clinically undetectable. Applying these principles to PCI, one would expect a greater reduction in CNS metastases in patients receiving higher doses, and in the only published study in which patients were randomized to two different dose levels of PCI (24 Gy in 12 daily fractions versus 36 Gy in 18 daily fractions), there was in fact a significantly greater reduction in cerebral metastases in the patients randomized to the higher dose.[51] The lower dose of 24 Gy was not associated with a statistically significant reduction in cerebral metastases, but the numbers in this study were small, with only 68 patients in the comparison. In the much larger French trials involving 505 patients in which the same dose of 24 Gy (given in eight fractions) was used, a highly significant reduction in metastases was detected.[50] The association between higher doses and reduced rates of cerebral metastases was confirmed in the metaanalysis, but there was no influence of dose on overall survival.[2]

Suwinski and colleagues have performed an exhaustive analysis of the published literature on the dose-response relationship for PCI, using both randomized and unrandomized data[53] and the methodology originally described by Withers and colleagues.[52] Their results are shown in Figure 56.1, in which the reduction in metastasis rate has been plotted against dose normalized to equivalent 2 Gy fractions (LQED$_{2Gy}$), using an α/β value of 10 Gy for tumors. Using a fitted regression curve, there appears to be a shallow dose-response relationship, with doses of 35 Gy or greater being required to achieve a 70% reduction in brain metastasis rate. The authors then divided the data into two subsets: an "early" group, in which PCI was initiated less than 60 days after the start of treatment for the primary, and a "late" group, in which PCI was given after 60 days.

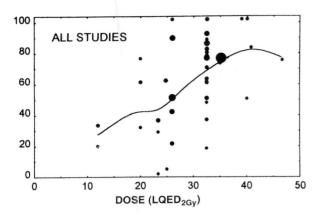

FIGURE 56.1. Percentage reduction in metastases rate as a function of dose equivalents given in 2 Gy fractions (LQED$_{2Gy}$). (From Suwinski R, Lee SP, Withers HR. Dose-response relationship for radiation therapy of subclinical disease. *Int J Radiat Oncol Biol Phys* 1995;31:353, with permission.)

The dose of radiation to achieve a 50% reduction in cerebral metastases was approximately 7 Gy greater for the "late" compared with the "early" subset. Further, it appeared that there was a 15 to 20 Gy threshold before any reduction in metastases could occur in the "late" group, unlike the "early" group, in which there appeared to be no dose threshold. The explanation advanced is that the longer PCI is delayed, the greater the increase in subclinical metastatic burden, thus requiring a higher dose to achieve the same effect. When the analysis was restricted to patients who received PCI after achieving CR, a reduction in metastasis rate was again apparent, but there was no clear dose response. The authors suggested that among other things the explanation for this observation may have been the variety of time delays between treatment of the primary and initiation of PCI among the different studies. Although the methodology of Suwinski et al. is open to criticism—particularly the inclusion of data from nonrandomized studies and the use of an assumed standard figure for brain relapse rates in the absence of PCI—their results do fit nicely with radiobiologic theory, and their study represents the best available information on the dose-response relationship of PCI in SCLC.

Dose per Fraction

One of the major disadvantages of higher-dose PCI is the greater duration and cost of treatment. In order to keep treatment times short, it has been common practice to hypofractionate PCI so that there is little or no reduction in total dose. For example, in the aforementioned paper of Suwinski and colleagues, 42 separate studies of PCI were included in their analysis, and in only six of these were fraction sizes of 2 Gy or less used.[53] But the brain is a late-reacting tissue particularly sensitive to size of dose per fraction, and if the

risk of neurotoxicity is to be minimized, treatment should be limited to 2 Gy per fraction.[54]

It is important to remember that dose per fraction can be significantly influenced by the number of fields treated at each session. For example, for a typical skull separation of 14.5 cm, the peak dose (one field per day) for cobalt-60 photons will be approximately 40% higher than the mid-separation dose; for 4 MV photons, it will be approximately 25%. Hence, for a prescribed midplane dose of 2 Gy with cobalt-60, the dose in the peak region will be 2.8 Gy. The effect of fraction size will be amplified even further if the prescribed midplane dose exceeds 2 Gy. If the dose limit of 2 Gy per fraction is to be adhered to, all fields should be treated daily.

One approach to keeping overall treatment time short without increasing fraction size is to use accelerated hyperfractionation. Although this approach has shown promise in the treatment of intrathoracic disease,[55] there are no reports of the use of multiple fractions per day for PCI.

Target Volume

Figure 56.2 is a simulation film of the skull demonstrating the field limits for a typical PCI treatment. The cross wire AB represents a line drawn from the supraorbital margin (by palpation) to the external auditory meatus, which is commonly taken to represent the base of skull, but it can be seen that this provides no margin on the middle or posterior

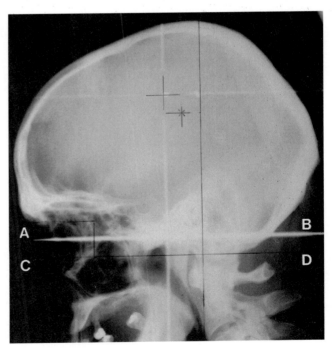

FIGURE 56.2. Simulation film for prophylactic cranial irradiation.

cranial fossae. The lower-level CD is more appropriate, and this example highlights the need to simulate all patients. The value of including a cervical extension to C2 is unknown. In the French trial[21] testing the value of PCI, a cervical extension to C2–3 was specified, but was not required in another European trial.[51]

Timing of PCI

Since the incidence of cerebral metastasis increases with lengthening survival, it could be reasoned that PCI might benefit the greatest number of patients if given at the earliest opportunity after chemotherapy. The analysis of Suwinski and colleagues suggests that the same dose of PCI has a greater effect if given early rather than later.[53] Patients in early PCI groups who achieve CR at the time of irradiation had a significantly longer brain-metastasis-free survival compared with those who had failed to achieve CR. There are two possible explanations for this observation, which has also been made by others.[17] One is that chemotherapy acts on subclinical cerebral micrometastases as well as disease at the primary site. It follows that patients achieving CR may obtain greater benefit from the effect of chemotherapy (over and above any effect of PCI) on any subclinical brain disease compared with patients not achieving CR, whose micrometastases are, like the primary site, partly chemoresistant. The second explanation is that patients not achieving CR have residual disease at the primary site which reseeds the brain *after* the subclinical metastases have been eradicated by PCI.[57] However this seems unlikely, since it has been calculated that it would require 30 months for a single clonogenic cell to become a clinically detectable metastasis.[29]

The most logical argument in favour of delaying PCI until a complete response has occurred recognizes that complete responders are the only patients for whom long-term survival is possible, while incomplete responders and nonresponders will die from uncontrolled extra-CNS disease. If PCI is given at the outset of systemic therapy, there will be additional patients treated who will never achieve CR—approximately 50%—for whom PCI is likely to be of little or no benefit. Further, there are dangers if chemotherapy and radiotherapy are given simultaneously,[58] and it may be safer to delay PCI until at least the first course of chemotherapy has been delivered. Although present indications are that PCI should be administered at the earliest possible opportunity after a CR has been achieved, a 1996 consensus report of a workshop of the International Association for the Study of Lung Cancer conceded that the optimal timing and dose of PCI are not known, and that further studies of these issues are required.[59]

TOXICITY

The acute toxicities of PCI include temporary hair loss, nausea and vomiting, and headache.[21] The risk of headache may be reduced by prophylactic administration of corticosteroids.

Late Neurotoxicity

Therapeutic radiation is a well-established cause of CNS injury.[60] The likelihood and severity of CNS injury are dependent on total dose and also on dose per fraction.[54] Since total doses in the vicinity of 60 Gy given in 2 Gy fractions have been used with comparative safety in the treatment of cerebral tumors,[61] it could not have been anticipated that lower doses in the range of 30 to 40 Gy, as used for PCI, might later be associated with irreversible long-term injury, even allowing for differences in dose per fraction. Of course, patients with brain tumors mostly have neurologic deficits prior to radiotherapy, and any late damage resulting from treatment may be obscured by preexisting deficits or features of recurrent disease. In contrast, patients for whom PCI is prescribed, are neurologically intact—or are they? Van Oosterhout and associates performed pretreatment neuropsychologic tests on 14 patients known not to have cerebral metastases and compared their performance with that of 14 matched controls.[62] The performance of the patients before they received any treatment was significantly inferior to the controls, but there was no deterioration in the performance of the patients when they were retested during and after chemotherapy and one and five months after PCI. Komaki and colleagues performed neuropsychologic tests on 30 patients with SCLC *before* going on to PCI after they had responded to chemotherapy and thoracic radiotherapy.[63] Twenty-nine of the patients had evidence of cognitive dysfunction. Excluding nine patients with a prior neurologic history, 84% had impaired verbal memory, 39% had frontal lobe dysfunction, and 21% had fine motor incoordination. It is not clear if the patients had CT or MRI of the brain at the time of testing to exclude cerebral metastases as a cause for these findings, but further studies on patients with limited disease who had not received any treatment revealed similar levels of impairment.[64] The authors concluded that the disease, rather than the treatment, somehow accounted for the cognitive deficits. However, in a study involving patients with breast cancer, some of whom had received adjuvant chemotherapy, there did appear to be an effect of chemotherapy on cognitive function, particularly in patients having high-dose therapy.[65] Thus the available evidence suggests that both the underlying disease itself *and* chemotherapy may be associated with neurologic complications independent of and preceding the administration of any PCI.

The first report of neurologic toxicity following PCI appeared in 1976 when a syndrome of poor attention span, recent-memory loss, and action tremor was described in 13 patients who had received PCI (20 to 30 Gy in 2 Gy fractions) concurrently with a doxorubicin-containing three-drug regimen.[66] The symptoms appeared within two to four months of commencing treatment and were reversible in all patients within four months of onset. An update published two years later confirmed the original observations in a larger number of patients; the symptoms were particularly severe in patients receiving 30 Gy, but the effects were not permanent.[67] That this syndrome had not been reported previously was probably due to the fact that this was one of the first reports of combined chemotherapy/radiotherapy involving doxorubicin, now recognized as a potent enhancer of radiation toxicity. Follow up of 13 long-term survivors (18 to 48 months) revealed no permanent clinical effects other than mild impairment of mental function in six patients, two of whom had not received PCI.[68] Subsequent reports of neurotoxicity following PCI confirmed the character of the syndrome—memory loss and ataxia—but also documented irreversibility of the symptoms and even fatalities. A review of 16 studies involving 691 patients revealed an overall crude incidence of significant neurologic toxicity in 19%.[18] A puzzling feature of the data was the wide variation in the reported incidence of toxicity—from under 10% in some reports[47,69] to 75% in another.[70] All studies were retrospective and most lacked information on pretreatment neurologic status. Only a small minority of studies included for comparison a cohort of patients who had not received PCI. In two nonrandomized studies there was a greater incidence of neurotoxicity in patients who had received PCI compared with those who had not.[71,72] Although it is tempting to conclude that PCI was responsible for the syndromes observed, factors such as large fraction size and concurrent chemotherapy may have been contributory. For example, in one of these studies, from the Mayo Clinic, which reported a crude incidence of neurotoxicity of 18%, the majority of patients were given 36 Gy using 3.6 Gy fractions.[71] The incidence of neurotoxicity in the other study (of the SWOG database) was 23%, which was confined to the group that had received PCI, some of whom had received concurrent chemotherapy.[72] Combining all the studies in the review, the use of concurrent chemotherapy was associated with a 26% incidence of neurotoxicity, which was significantly greater than 12% (p = 0.001) in those studies in which it was known not to be given.[18]

The lack of consistency in the reported frequency of neurotoxicity following PCI thus raises questions about a cause-and-effect relationship even though some of the differences might be explained by details of the various PCI prescriptions, some of which would now be regarded as hazardous. The issues raised by the historical data clearly required resolution by carefully conducted prospective studies. One of the French randomized trials[21] and the European trial[51] incorporated a pre- and posttreatment neuropsychologic assessment into the study design. Not all patients underwent evaluation—78% in the French study and 43% in the European study—and so the results must be interpreted with caution. Both studies found high levels of impairment (59% and up to 41% respectively) in patients tested at randomiza-

tion prior to receiving PCI. Retesting of survivors at two years in the French study and one year in the European study showed no significant differences in the cumulative incidence of neuropsychologic changes between treated and untreated groups. Furthermore, there were no significant differences in the incidence of cortical atrophy and ventricular dilatation on computed tomography scans of the brain between groups at randomization and two years later.[21] These reassuring findings in relation to the safety of PCI have now been supported by the results of recently published nonrandomized studies from the Netherlands,[73] Denmark,[74] and France.[75] Surprisingly, a large single dose of 8 Gy used as PCI in Manchester was not associated with any neurologic problems when assessment was performed at least 24 months after PCI, although 75% of patients were impaired on at least one of the four formal neuropsychometric tests used.[76] Indeed, when, in a collaborative study from the United Kingdom, the performance of the single-fraction patients was compared with that of individuals who had received a more conventional PCI regimen, they did better.[77] While there was a high frequency of impaired performance on formal neuropsychometric testing in the UK study, the majority of patients were well, with 95% having a performance status of one or less. There were insufficient patients who did not receive PCI for comparative analysis; however, the study demonstrated that the tests used were able to detect deficits of cognitive function that would have otherwise gone unnoticed.

It seems reasonable to conclude that late neurotoxicity in patients with SCLC who have received PCI may be multifactorial, and that injudicious choice of fraction size or the use of concurrent chemotherapy may be contributory. However, there is little evidence from randomized studies that PCI alone, delivered up to a dose of 36 Gy with classical fractionation, is a cause of late neurotoxicity. Nevertheless longer follow-up of the French[21] and European[51] studies will be required to confirm these preliminary findings. Since future studies of PCI are likely to focus on dose optimization,[78] the effects of treatment on cognitive and neurologic function will be critical end points. Careful pre- and posttreatment evaluation, including the use of tests capable of detecting subtle decrements in performance,[77] should continue to be part of the study design.

Finally, it should be remembered that neurologic complications of SCLC are common, occurring in 65% of patients in one large prospective study,[79] and that the vast majority of these were due to CNS metastases, which should therefore be carefully excluded before attributing the problem to treatment-related toxicity.

Quality of Life

The ideal evaluation of PCI would be a trial which takes into account not only survival but also the morbidities of treatment and cerebral relapse in both treatment arms. An example of this kind of evaluation is "TWiST" analysis, which measures the total time without disease-related symptoms *and* treatment-related toxicity.[80] None of the randomized trials of PCI has included such an analysis, but the European trial[51] did measure quality of life using the Rotterdam Symptom Checklist in a minority of the patients randomized. For all of the six commonest symptoms reported, deterioration was worse in the "no PCI" than in the "PCI" group, but the numbers were too small to draw firm conclusions.

As it seems likely that future studies of PCI will focus on fine-tuning the details of the PCI prescription, quality-of-life assessment and TWiST-type analysis will be essential components of trial design.

CONCLUSIONS

There is now incontrovertible evidence that PCI reduces the incidence of cerebral metastases in SCLC. There appears to be a shallow dose-response relationship for this effect without a detectable threshold below which some effect does not occur, especially if PCI is given early in the course of the disease. Lower doses may be required to achieve equivalent effects if PCI is given earlier rather than later. However, the only patients who can benefit in terms of cure are those who will achieve or have achieved CR, and so giving PCI early (before CR) increases the number of individuals who will be irradiated without benefit.

Although several randomized trials of PCI in patients who have achieved CR have shown that a reduction in the rate of cerebral metastasis is associated with improved survival, none has shown a statistically significant survival advantage. But when the data from all studies were combined in a metaanalysis, there was a 16% reduction in mortality in favor of PCI which was significant at the level of p = 0.01. Prospective studies of cognitive function using formal neuropsychometric tests in two of the randomized studies has not supported anecdotal observations which suggested that PCI might be a cause of serious delayed neurotoxicity, but further follow-up is required to confirm these early results.

In light of all the preceding considerations, it would seem obligatory for clinicians to inform their patients of the known benefits and potential toxicities of PCI, particularly those individuals who have achieved CR. Then it should be a case of the question being "not who needs PCI but who wants PCI?" as in the title of a recent editorial.[81] Those individuals who then wish to proceed with PCI should be offered a dose in the range of 30 to 36 Gy given in conventional 2 Gy fractions, but only at a time when chemotherapy is not being administered.

REFERENCES

1. Maurer LH, Tulloh M, Weiss RB, et al. A randomised combined modality trial in small cell carcinoma of the lung. *Cancer* 1980; 45:30.
2. Auperin A, Arriagada, R, Pignon J-P, et al. Prophylactic cranial irradiation for patients with small cell lung cancer in complete remission *N Engl J Med* 1999;341:476.
3. Einhorn LH. The case against prophylactic cranial irradiation in limited small cell lung cancer. *Semin Radiat Oncol* 1995;5:57.
4. Aur JA, Simone J, Hustu HO, et al. Central nervous system therapy and combination chemotherapy of childhood lymphocytic leukemia. *Blood* 1971;37:272.
5. Hansen HH. Should initial treatment of small cell carcinoma include systemic chemotherapy and brain irradiation? *Cancer Chemother Rep* 1973;4:239.
6. Jackson DV, Richards F, Cooper MR, et al. Prophylactic cranial irradiation in small cell carcinoma of the lung. *JAMA* 1977;237: 2730.
7. Beiler DD, Kane RC, Bernath AM, et al. Low dose elective brain irradiation in small cell carcinoma of the lung. *Int J Radiat Oncol Biol Phys* 1979;5:941.
8. Hansen HH, Dombernowsky P, Hirsch FR, et al. Prophylactic irradiation in bronchogenic small cell anaplastic carcinoma. A comparative trial of localized versus extensive radiotherapy including prophylactic brain irradiation in patients receiving combination chemotherapy. *Cancer* 1980;46:279.
9. Cox JD, Stanley K, Petrovich Z, et al. Cranial irradiation in cancer of the lung of all cell types. *JAMA* 1981;245:469.
10. Eagan RT, Creagan ET, Frytak S, et al. A case for preplanned thoracic and prophylactic whole brain irradiation therapy in limited small-cell lung cancer. *Cancer Clin Trials* 1981;4:261.
11. Aroney RS, Aisner J, Wesley MN, et al. Value of prophylactic cranial irradiation given at complete remission in small cell lung carcinoma. *Cancer Treat Rep* 1983;67:675.
12. Seydel HG, Concannon J, Creech R, et al. Prophylactic versus no brain irradiation in regional small cell lung carcinoma. *Am J Clin Oncol* 1985;8:218.
13. Niiranen A, Holsti P, Salmo M. Treatment of small cell lung cancer. Two-drug versus four-drug chemotherapy and loco-regional irradiation with or without prophylactic cranial irradiation. *Acta Oncologica* 1989;28:501.
14. Ohonoshi T, Ueoka H, Kawahara S, et al. Comparative study of prophylactic cranial irradiation in patients with small cell lung cancer achieving a complete response: a long-term follow-up result. *Lung Cancer* 1993;10:47.
15. Bunn PA, Nugent JL, Matthews MJ. Central nervous system metastases in small cell bronchogenic carcinoma. *Semin Oncol* 1978;5:314.
16. Sculier JP, Feld R, Evans WK, et al. Neurologic disorders in patients with small cell lung cancer. *Cancer* 1987;60:2275.
17. Rosen ST, Makuch RW, Lichter AS, et al. Role of prophylactic cranial irradiation in prevention of central nervous system metastases in small cell lung cancer. *Am J Med* 1983;74:615.
18. Ball DL, Matthews JP. Prophylactic cranial irradiation: more questions than answers. *Semin Radiat Oncol* 1995;5:61.
19. Nugent JL, Bunn PA, Matthews MJ, et al. CNS Metastases in small cell bronchogenic carcinoma. Increasing frequency and changing pattern with lengthening survival. *Cancer* 1979;44: 1885.
20. Komaki R, Cox JD, Whitson W. Risk of brain metastasis from small cell carcinoma of the lung related to length of survival and prophylactic irradiation. *Cancer Treat Rep* 1981;65:811.
21. Arriagada R, Le Chevalier T, Borie F, et al. Prophylactic cranial irradiation for patients with small-cell lung cancer in complete remission. *J Natl Cancer Inst* 1995;87:183.

22. Kristensen CA, Kristjansen PEG, Hansen HH. Systemic chemotherapy of brain metastases from small-cell lung cancer: a review. *J Clin Oncol* 1992;10:1498.

23. Twelves CJ, Souhami RL, Harper PG, et al. The response of cerebral metastases in small cell lung cancer to systemic chemotherapy. *Br J Cancer* 1990;61:147.

24. Kristjansen PEG, Sorensen PS, Hansen MS, et al. Prospective evaluation of the effect on initial brain metastases from small cell lung cancer of platinum-etoposide based induction chemotherapy followed by an alternating multidrug regimen. *Ann Oncol* 1993;4:579.

25. de la Monte SM, Hutchins GM, Moore GW. Altered metastatic behavior of small cell carcinoma of the lung after chemotherapy and radiation. *Cancer* 1988;61:2176.

26. Murray N, Coy P, Pater JL, et al. Importance of timing for thoracic irradiation in the combined modality treatment of limited-stage small-cell cancer. *J Clin Oncol* 1993;11:334.

27. Work E, Nielsen OS, Bentzen SM, et al., for the Aarhus Lung Cancer Group. Randomised study of initial versus chest irradiation combined with chemotherapy in limited-stage small-cell lung cancer. *J Clin Oncol* 1997;15:3030.

28. Jeremic B, Shibamoto Y, Acimovic L, et al. Initial versus delayed accelerated hyperfractionated radiation therapy and concurrent chemotherapy in limited small-cell lung cancer: a randomised study. *J Clin Oncol* 1997;15:893.

29. Hoskin PJ, Yarnold JR, Smith IE, et al. CNS relapse despite prophylactic cranial irradiation (PCI) in small cell lung cancer (SCLC). *Int J Radiat Oncol Biol Phys* 1986;12:2025.

30. Elliot JA, Osterlind K, Hirsch FR, et al. Metastatic patterns in small-cell lung cancer: correlation of autopsy findings with clinical parameters in 537 patients. *J Clin Oncol* 1987;5:246.

31. Ellis R, Gregor A. The treatment of brain metastases from lung cancer. *Lung Cancer* 1998;20:81.

32. Nieder C, Berberich W, Schnabel K. Tumor-related prognostic factors for remission of brain metastases after radiotherapy. *Int J Radiat Oncol Biol Phys* 1997;39:25.

33. Postmus PE, Haaxma-Reiche H, Gregor A, et al. Brain-only metastases of small cell lung cancer; efficacy of whole brain radiotherapy. An EORTC phase II study. *Radiother Oncol* 1998;46:29.

34. Hirsch FR, Paulson OB, Hansen HH, et al. Intracranial metastases in small cell carcinoma of the lung. Prognostic aspects. *Cancer* 1983;51:529.

35. Lucas CF, Robinson B, Hoskin PJ, et al. Morbidity of cranial relapse in small cell lung cancer and the impact of radiation therapy. *Cancer Treat Rep* 1986;70:565.

36. Giannone L, Johnson DH, Hande KR, et al. Favourable prognosis of brain metastases in small cell lung cancer. *Ann Intern Med* 1987;106:386.

37. Mira JG, Chen TT, Livingston RB, et al. Outcome of prophylactic and therapeutic cranial irradiation in disseminated small cell lung carcinoma: a Southwest Oncology Group study. *Int J Radiat Oncol Biol Phys* 1988;14:861.

38. Carmichael J, Crane JM, Bunn PA, et al. Results of therapeutic cranial irradiation in small cell lung cancer. *Int J Radiat Oncol Biol Phys* 1988;14:455.

39. Ichinose Y, Hara N, Ohta M, et al. Brain metastases in patients with limited small cell lung cancer achieving complete remission. Correlation with TNM staging. *Chest* 1989;96:1332.

40. Kochhar R, Frytak S, Shaw E. Survival of patients with extensive small-cell lung cancer who have only brain metastases at initial diagnosis. *Am J Clin Oncol* 1997;20:125.

41. Ryan GF, Ball DL, Smith JG. Treatment of brain metastases from primary lung cancer. *Int J Radiat Oncol Biol Phys* 1995;31:273.

42. Bach F, Sorensen JB, Adrian L, et al. Brain relapses in chemotherapy-treated small cell lung cancer: a retrospective review of two

43. Hardy J, Smith I, Cherryman G, et al. The value of computed tomographic (CT) scan surveillance in the detection and management of brain metastases in patients with small cell lung cancer. *Br J Cancer* 1990;62:684.

44. Kristjansen PE, Kristensen CA. The role of prophylactic cranial irradiation in the management of small cell lung cancer. *Cancer Treat Rev* 1993;19:3.

45. Felletti R, Souhami RL, Spiro SG, et al. Social consequences of brain or liver relapse in small cell carcinoma of the bronchus. *Radiother Oncol* 1985;4:335.

46. Nussbaum E, Djalilian HR, Cho KH, et al. Brain metastases. Histology, multiplicity, surgery and survival. *Cancer* 1996;78:1781.

47. Priestman TJ, Dunn J, Brada M, et al. Final results of the Royal College of Radiologists' trial comparing two different radiotherapy schedules in the treatment of cerebral metastases. *Clin Oncol* 1996;8:308.

48. Liengswangwong V, Bonner JA, Shaw EG, et al. Prophylactic cranial irradiation in limited-stage small cell lung cancer. *Cancer* 1995;75:1302.

49. Shaw EG, Su JQ, Eagan RT, et al. Prophylactic cranial irradiation in complete responders with small-cell lung cancer: Analysis of the Mayo Clinic and North Central Cancer Treatment Group data base. *J Clin Oncol* 1994;12:2327.

50. Laplanche A, Monnet I, Santos-Miranda JA, et al. Controlled clinical trial of prophylactic cranial irradiation for patients with small cell lung cancer in complete remission. *Lung Cancer* 1998;21:193.

51. Gregor A, Cull A, Stephens RJ, et al. Prophylactic cranial irradiation is indicated following complete response to induction therapy in small cell lung cancer: results of a multicentre randomised trial. *Euro J Cancer* 1997;33:1752.

52. Withers HR, Peters LJ, Taylor JMG. Dose-response relationship for radiation therapy of subclinical disease. *Int J Radiat Oncol Biol Phys* 1995;31:353.

53. Suwinski R, Lee SP, Withers HR. Dose-response relationship for prophylactic cranial irradiation in small cell lung cancer. *Int J Radiat Oncol Biol Phys* 1998;40:797.

54. Herskovic AM, Orton CG. Elective brain irradiation for small cell anaplastic lung cancer. *Int J Radiat Oncol Biol Phys* 1986;12:427.

55. Turrisi A, Kim K, Blum R, et al. Twice-daily compared with once-daily thoracic radiotherapy in limited small cell lung cancer treated concurrently with cisplatin and etoposide. *N Engl J Med* 1999;340:265.

56. Wagner J, Kin K, Turrisi A, et al. A randomised Phase III study of prophylactic cranial irradiation vs. observation in patient with small cell lung cancer achieving a complete response: final report of an incomplete trial by the Eastern cooperative Oncology Group and Radiation Therapy Oncology Group (E3589/R92–01) [Abstract]. *Proc ASCO* 1996;15:376.

57. Le Chevalier T, Arriagada R, Dewar J, et al. Prophylactic cranial irradiation in small cell lung cancer, [Letter]. *Lancet* 1985;1:692.

58. Turrisi AT. Brian irradiation and systemic chemotherapy for small-cell lung cancer: dangerous liaisons? *J Clin Oncol* 1990;8:196.

59. Ihde D, Souhami B, Comis R, et al. Consensus report: Small cell lung cancer. *Lung Cancer* 1997;17[Suppl 1]:S19.

60. Gutin PH, Leibel SA, Shelise GE, eds. *Radiation injury to the central nervous system.* New York: Raven Press, 1991.

61. Mornex F, Nayel H, Taillandier L. Radiation therapy for malignant astrocytomas in adults. *Radiother Oncol* 1993;27:181.

62. Van Oosterhout AG, Boon PJ, Houx PJ, et al. Follow-up of

time-dose regimens of therapeutic brain irradiation. *Lung Cancer* 1996;15:171.

cognitive functioning in patients with small cell lung cancer. *Int J Radiat Oncol Biol Phys* 1995;31:911.

63. Komaki R, Meyers CA, Shin DM, et al. Evaluation of cognitive function in patients with limited small cell lung cancer prior to and shortly following prophylactic cranial irradiation. *Int J Radiat Oncol Biol Phys* 1995;33:179.

64. Meyers CA, Byrne KS, Komaki R. Cognitive deficits in patients with small cell lung cancer before and after chemotherapy. *Lung Cancer* 1995;12:231.

65. van Dam FSAM, Schagen SB, Muller MJ, et al. Impairment of cognitive function in women receiving adjuvant treatment for high-risk breast cancer: high-dose versus standard-dose chemotherapy. *J Natl Cancer Inst* 1998;90:210.

66. Johnson RE, Brereton HD, Kent CH. Small-cell carcinoma of the lung: attempt to remedy causes of past therapeutic failure. *Lancet* 1976;2:289.

67. Johnson RE, Brereton HD, Kent CH. "Total" therapy for small cell carcinoma of the lung. *Ann Thorac Surg* 1978;25:510.

68. Catane R, Schwade JG, Yarr I, et al. Follow-up neurological evaluation in patients with small cell lung carcinoma treated with prophylactic cranial irradiation and chemotherapy. *Int J Radiat Oncol Biol Phys* 1981;7:105.

69. Lishner M, Fled R, Payne DG, et al. Late neurological complications after prophylactic cranial irradiation in patients with small-cell lung cancer: the Toronto experience. *J Clin Oncol* 1990;8:215.

70. Johnson BE, Becker B, Goff WB, et al. Neurologic, neuropsychologic and computed cranial tomography scan abnormalities in 2- to 10-year survivors of small-cell lung cancer. *J Clin Oncol* 1985;3:1659.

71. Frytak S, Shaw JN, O'Neill BP, et al. Leukoencephalopathy in small cell lung cancer patients receiving prophylactic cranial irradiation. *Am J Clin Oncol* 1989;12:27.

72. Albain KS, Crowley JJ, Livingston RB. Long-term survival and toxicity in small cell lung cancer. Expanded Southwest Oncology Group Experience. *Chest* 1991;99:1425.

73. Van Oosterhout AGM, Ganzevles PGL, Wilmink JT, et al. Sequelae in long-term survivors of small cell lung cancer. *Int J Radiat Oncol Biol Phys* 1996;34:1037.

74. Work E, Bentzen SM, Nielson OS, et al. Prophylactic cranial irradiation in limited stage small cell lung cancer: survival benefit in patients with favourable characteristics. *Euro J Cancer* 1996; 32:772.

75. Jacoulet P, Depierre A, Moro D, et al. Long-term survivors of small-cell lung cancer (SCLC): A French multicenter study. *Ann Oncol* 1997;8:1009.

76. Brewster AE, Hopwood P, Stout R, et al. Single fraction prophylactic cranial irradiation for small cell carcinoma of the lung. *Radiother Oncol* 1995;34:132.

77. Cull A, Gregor A, Hopwood P, et al. Neurological and cognitive impairment in long-term survivors of small cell lung cancer. *Eur J Cancer* 1994;30A:1067.

78. Gregor A. Prophylactic cranial irradiation in small cell lung cancer (SCLC) makes a comeback. *Clin Oncol* 1997;9:148.

79. van Oosterhout AGM, van de Pol M, ten Velde GP, et al. Neurologic disorders in 203 consecutive patients with small cell lung cancer. Results of a longitudinal study. *Cancer* 1996;77:1434.

80. Glasziou PP, Simes RJ, Gelber RD. Quality adjusted survival analysis. *Stat Med* 1990;9:1259.

81. Le Chevalier T, Arriagada R. Small cell lung cancer and prophylactic cranial irradiation (PCI): perhaps the question is not who needs PCI but who wants PCI? *Eur J Cancer* 1997;33:1717.

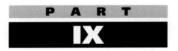

PALLIATION AND SPECIAL CONSIDERATIONS

57

PALLIATIVE CHEMOTHERAPY

MARK R. MIDDLETON
NICHOLAS THATCHER
PENELOPE HOPWOOD

The majority of patients with small cell lung cancer (SCLC) or advanced non-small cell lung cancer (NSCLC) will die of their disease. In the United States around 178,000 patients are diagnosed with lung cancer annually, and of these the disease kills 160,000.[1] Thus most treatment is delivered with palliation rather than cure in mind. In NSCLC this has been used as an argument against the use of chemotherapy, which is perceived as providing little survival benefit at the expense of unacceptable toxicity. However, modern chemotherapy has an important role to play in improving quality of life, besides offering modest but important improvements in survival. The recognition of this has required a shift away from solely traditional measures of efficacy in evaluating new drugs. Many studies now incorporate assessments of symptom relief and quality of life, as well as the usual endpoints of response, toxicity, and survival.

In SCLC the benefits of chemotherapy are more clearcut. Improvements in median survival, even in extensive-stage disease between eight and ten months against an anticipated six to eight weeks untreated, have made chemotherapy the accepted standard for this group of patients. The lung cancer population is largely elderly and often frail as a result of other illnesses. There is therefore a need to improve upon existing treatments, in particular increasing their tolerability so that more patients can benefit from them.

Choosing the optimal palliative therapy is complex. A balance must be struck between the benefits and risks of treatment that is not skewed in favor of the former, as it often is where cure is unrealistically attempted. Patients who often have considerable symptoms from their disease as well as intercurrent illnesses cannot be expected to tolerate the side effects inherent in more aggressive approaches. This is not to promote the selection of the most suitable regimen on subjective criteria. Rather, there is as great a need for objective measures in selecting patients for palliative treatments as there is in the curative scenario.

There are also several new agents available to improve the treatment of lung cancer patients, but further progress will depend upon changes in the nihilistic attitude of non-oncology physicians and funding organizations towards chemotherapy. The acceptance of enhanced quality of life as a sufficient criterion for licensing a drug and the continued evaluation and promotion of the cost-effectiveness of the approach are also important.

ASSESSING THE OUTCOME OF PALLIATIVE CHEMOTHERAPY

Response Rate and Survival

These have traditionally been the criteria by which the efficacy of new treatments has been assessed. Although they continue to play a role in the evaluation of palliative therapies, they can no longer be considered in isolation, for palliation of symptoms can occur in the absence of a conventionally defined response to treatment. Objective response to chemotherapy in NSCLC, as measured by WHO criteria, occurs in only 30% to 40% of patients, and survival benefits are modest.[2] However, there are now several studies showing that, with this objective response rate, up to 70% of patients report relief of symptoms with modern chemotherapy.[3-5]

Toxicity and Disease-Related Symptoms

The assessment of treatment-related toxicity has been codified so that side effects are recorded systematically and different therapies can be compared from trial to trial. Although a powerful tool, the Common Toxicity Criteria scheme ignores the impact of a particular side effect or symptom upon the individual; neither does it measure the combined effect of symptoms. Thus the traditional means of evaluating chemotherapy use end points that bear little relation to patients' experience of treatment. This is not to decry the use of these measures in the evaluation of new therapies, but there is a need to take into account their impact on the patient as well.

Quality of Life

The criteria that define tumor response are straightforward, as are those related to treatment toxicity, and the concepts of time to progression and overall survival are readily understood. Health-related quality of life is a more abstract entity that is much harder to define. It comprises several elements, including physical, psychological, social, emotional, and economic well-being. There are now several instruments that allow systematic collection of quality of life data so that disease-related symptoms, the side effects of treatment and their significance to the patient can be evaluated.

Although observers can readily assess some aspects of quality of life, such as physical functioning and some symptoms, there is evidence to suggest that health professionals' and other carers' interpretation of quality of life differs from that of the patient.[6,7] Since the data collected are largely subjective, it would seem best that the patients provide the information themselves. Initially studies used simple diaries to gather data. This proved very effective, for example, highlighting the (previously unsuspected) differences of dysphagia between radiotherapy regimens providing similar palliation in NSCLC.[8] However, this method is time-consuming to interpret and difficult to generalize between treatments because it does not provide systematic data. The usual method of evaluating quality of life now is by multidimensional self-report questionnaire. Depending on the design used, patients either select one of a limited number of answers to questions on their health or indicate the severity of a symptom on a visual analog scale. Several such instruments are available (Table 57.1) many of which have been validated against other indices of quality of life such as performance status, weight loss, and toxicity of treatment. This approach is acceptable to patients; indeed, many react positively to the chance to become involved in the assessment of their treatment.

The European Organisation for the Research and Treatment of Cancer (EORTC) QLQ-C30 is a well-developed example of such a questionnaire.[9] This examines quality of life across five functional scales (physical, role, cognitive, emotional, and social), three symptom scales (nausea and

vomiting, fatigue, and pain), and a global scale. There are also several other measures, and these core questions are supplemented by disease-specific modules (in the case of lung cancer, designated LC13).[10] This instrument represents only one of a number of valid scales, but the QLQ-C30 has the advantage that it has been tested successfully across several languages and cultures.[11]

There are several problems with quality-of-life assessments, not least the abysmal rate at which they have been incorporated into clinical trials. A review of four oncology journals in the period 1980 to 1995 found only 13 studies out of 871 incorporating quality-of-life assessments—and only four of the 13 were considered adequate in terms of the quality-of-life data gathered.[12] Data collection is often patchy, particularly in the palliative setting, because of limited compliance, patient attrition, and inadequate infrastructure to support studies.[13] Acute toxicities may be missed because assessments are usually made prior to each cycle of treatment, when the toxicity of the last cycle is up to three weeks past. Few trials gather data once interventions have ceased, so there is even less information about the duration of changes in quality of life. Finally, the profusion of instruments for assessing quality of life (over 50 have been used in lung cancer studies published to date) makes it difficult to draw comparisons between studies, and this is further hindered by a lack of agreed criteria for reporting results.[9] Nevertheless, quality-of-life research is critical in the evaluation of the impact of new treatments, particularly in the palliative setting where a limited improvement in survival may not be the patient's sole consideration.[14,15]

Economic Analysis

Part of the resistance to the use of palliative chemotherapy in lung cancer stems from the perception that it is expensive and, by implication, not cost-effective. However, the costs of chemotherapy are small in comparison with those of making the diagnosis and of terminal care. Chemotherapy accounted for less than 10% of the costs of care over one year in the Canadian model of lung cancer management.[16] There is also trial evidence that chemotherapy results in fewer days in hospital or hospice and less need for radiotherapy, saving costs even in NSCLC.[17,18] The need to demonstrate that palliative chemotherapy is worth it to funding bodies will persist, particularly where newer, more expensive, agents with perhaps less toxicity replace established drugs.

PALLIATION OF ADVANCED NON–SMALL CELL LUNG CANCER WITH CHEMOTHERAPY

Patient Selection

Multivariate analyses have identified a number of independent factors that predict the outcome of treatment. The presence of extrathoracic disease, some locations of metasta-

TABLE 57.1. SELECTED EXAMPLES OF QUALITY-OF-LIFE INSTRUMENTS

General
Karnofsky Performance Status
ECOG Performance Status Scale
Symptom Checklist 90
Hospital Anxiety and Depression Scale

Cancer-Specific
Functional Assessment of Cancer Therapy—General Scale
Rotterdam Symptom Checklist
Functional Living Index—Cancer
EORTC QLQ-C30

Lung-Cancer-Specific
Functional Assessment of Cancer Therapy—Lung
Lung Cancer Symptom Scale
EORTC LC-13

ses (e.g., brain), and weight loss are associated with a poor prognosis. However, neither age nor histological subtype has been shown consistently to affect outcome.[19–23] Patients suitable for palliative chemotherapy are those with stage IIIB or IV disease and fair performance status (ECOG 0 and 1, and possibly 2). Clearly, some patients with localized disease are not fit for surgery and so will be candidates for radical radiotherapy with or without chemotherapy. Patients with even moderately impaired performance status fare less well with chemotherapy: survival is reduced and the toxicity of treatment increased compared with unimpaired patients.[24] Thus chemotherapy should be offered only to patients in relatively good condition. This may change as new drugs with proven activity and fewer side effects, such as gemcitabine, become available.

Effect on Survival

The first studies, in the 1960s and 1970s, showed no benefit from chemotherapy and, as a result, radiotherapy became the standard treatment for palliating NSCLC. However, these trials used drugs that are now considered inactive.[25,26] More modern regimens have since been tested against best supportive care, with better results (Table 57.2). Supportive care was not consistently defined but was usually taken to mean any palliative therapy offered to the patient, excluding cytotoxic chemotherapy but including radiotherapy and noncytotoxic medication. The trials are difficult to interpret, as the case mix of patients was very variable, with survival times varying between 4.2 and 8.7 months in the supportive-care arms. The duration of chemotherapy also varied considerably, as did the criteria for the discontinuation of treatment. However, large metaanalyses have confirmed that platinum-based combination chemotherapy re-

duces mortality in advanced NSCLC, with an improvement in survival of around two to three months and an absolute increase of 10% (from 16% to 26%) in the proportion of patients surviving one year.[27,28]

Effect on Symptoms and Quality of Life

Although there have been few trials that measured patient-generated quality of life on chemotherapy and none as yet published with it as the primary end point, there is evidence that most patients either improve or preserve their performance status during treatment. In one report on the MIC (mitomycin C, ifosfamide, cisplatin) regimen, only 9% of patients experienced deterioration in quality of life on treatment, and 30% improved.[4] Similar results have been observed for other platinum-based regimens and with single-agent therapy.[39–41] It is also well documented that improvements in symptoms are not confined to patients with an objective response.[3,41–43] Symptoms relief with chemotherapy is comparable with that achieved by radiotherapy (Table 57.3) and decreases the need for palliative irradiation by around one third.[16,18] Trials are now being performed that examine symptom relief over time, improving on the data that are currently available.[18]

Combination Therapy

Although there are studies showing significant differences in survival in favor of combination treatment, there is as yet no consistent trial evidence that this is superior to single-agent therapy, other than with vinorelbine.[44] Despite this, most investigators use combination regimens as controls in randomized trials: usually MIC or MVP (mitomycin C, vinblastine/vindesine, cisplatin) in the U.K. and platinum

TABLE 57.2. CHEMOTHERAPY VERSUS BEST SUPPORTIVE CARE IN LOCALLY ADVANCED OR METASTATIC NSCLC IN OVER 100 PATIENTS

Reference	Regimen	Patients†	Responses (%)	Median Survival (months)		1-Year Survival (%)		p Value
				CTX	BSC	CTX	BSC	
Rapp[27]	CAP	150	15	6.1	4.2	21	10	0.01
	PV		25	8.1		22		
Woods[28]	PV	201	28	6.8	4.3	NR	NR	NS
Buccheri[29]	MACC	175	8	8.0	5.0	27	17	0.01
Cellerino[30]	CEP/MEC	128	21	8.5	5.0	32	23	NS
Leung[31]	PE	119	21	12.4	8.7	53	30	0.05
Cartei[32]	PCM	102	25	8.5	4.0	39	12	0.0001
Cullen[33]	MIC	359	31	6.9	4.8	28	18	0.009
Perrone[34]	Vin	161	20	6.2	4.8	27	5	0.04
Thatcher[35,36]	Pac	157	15	6.8	4.8	31	28	0.045

† treated and control patients; CTX, chemotherapy; BSC, best supportive care.
Chemotherapy regimens: CAP, cyclophosphamide, doxorubicin, cislatin; PV, cisplatin, vindesine; MACC, methotrexate, doxorubicin, cyclophosphamide, CCNU; CEP, cyclophosphamide, epirubicin, cisplatin alternating with MEC, methotrexate, etoposide; CCNU, cisplatin, etoposide; PCM, cisplatin, cyclophosphamide, mitomycin C; MIC, mitomycin C, Ifosfamide, cisplatin; Vin, vinorelbine; Pac, paclitaxel.

TABLE 57.3. SYMPTOMATIC RELIEF IN ADVANCED NSCLC: STUDIES OF OVER 100 PATIENTS

Reference	Treatment	Patients	OR (%)	MS (months)	Cough	Symptomatic Improvement (%) Haemoptysis	Dyspnoea	Pain	Anorexia
MRC-LCWP[8]	Radiotherapy	369	30	6.4	60	84	61	78	67
Cullen[4]	MIC	272	56	9.8	70	92	46	77	58
Ellis[5]	MVP	120	32	5.0	66	NR	59	60	NR
Anderson[18]	Gemcitabine	332	20	8.1–9.2	44	63	26	32	29

OR, overall response; MS, median survival; NR, not recorded; MIC, mitomycin C, ifosfamide, cisplatin; MVP, mitomycin C, vinblastine, cisplatin.

with paclitaxel or vinorelbine in the United States and mainland Europe. Attempts to improve outcome with dose intensification have yielded enhanced response rates but no clear survival advantage. Alternating combinations of chemotherapy have shown no advantage over their sequential administration—with a single exception.[22] Nor has any benefit been shown with increased treatment duration. Indeed, three cycles of the MVP regimen produce the same symptom relief and survival as six, but with considerably less toxicity.[45]

Attitudes to Chemotherapy

There remains a belief among physicians and other health professionals that chemotherapy inevitably causes deterioration in quality of life and performance status. Early trials in NSCLC did not show the improvements in survival seen with SCLC. Indeed, the earliest regimens, based upon alkylating agents rather than cisplatin, appeared detrimental.[25,26,38] Physicians' attitudes to chemotherapy for NSCLC were therefore profoundly negative, and have tended to remain so.[46] Subsequent combination chemotherapies have yielded some improvements in survival, as well as symptom relief as described above. Unfortunately, attitudes have not changed despite the now-abundant evidence that chemotherapy is superior to supportive care: in 1995, 79% of Canadian oncologists felt that there was no specific treatment for advanced NSCLC, a figure little changed from 1986.[47] Furthermore, this study showed that there was a tendency for physicians to overestimate the value of radiotherapy, the main plank of supportive care, and undervalue the potential contribution of chemotherapy. Patients, on the other hand, are prepared to tolerate toxic treatments for even short extensions in survival times, for symptom relief, or for an improvement in quality of life.[14,15,48]

Thus trials comparing chemotherapy with best supportive care have been, and continue to be, essential in promoting the case for palliation of advanced NSCLC with chemotherapy, particularly with reference to poorer-performance-status patients. In the fitter patient, where the benefits of chemotherapy are more clearly defined, research concen-

trates on the incorporation of new agents into combination regimens to improve outcomes. In either scenario it is vital that future studies assess the quality of life of patients during and after treatment in order to understand and decide upon the best possible palliation.

PALLIATION OF SMALL CELL LUNG CANCER WITH CHEMOTHERAPY

SCLC is exquisitely sensitive to chemotherapy, and this is the treatment modality of choice both for palliative or curative therapy, although radiotherapy too has an important role. Three quarters of patients respond to treatment, but relapse usually occurs within a few months, so that fewer than 10% of patients overall are alive two years after diagnosis.[49,50] Thus chemotherapy for SCLC is largely palliative. Chemotherapy is also effective in improving localized complications such as superior vena cava obstruction and pleural effusion.[50]

Patient Selection

As with NSCLC, the stage of disease and patient performance status are important predictors of prognosis and treatment outcome.[51] However, in SCLC the precise tumor stage is less important than the distinction between extensive and limited-stage disease. Limited-stage disease is defined as tumor confined to one hemithorax, including the mediastinum and/or supraclavicular nodes bilaterally, that is, contained within a single radiation field. This remains a useful distinction, despite evidence that SCLC disseminates early and that systemic metastases are often present in cases where screening for these is negative.[52] There are also several independent biochemical prognostic factors that predict prognosis, including lactate dehydrogenase, alkaline phosphatase, sodium, and bicarbonate.[53,54] These biochemical parameters, the disease stage, and patient performance status have been incorporated in scoring systems in selecting candidates for different therapeutic approaches (Table 57.4).[54,55] Again, age is not a predictive factor[56] but, as in NSCLC, the patient population is often frail: a consequence

TABLE 57.4. SMALL CELL LUNG CANCER: EXAMPLES OF PROGNOSTIC SCORING SYSTEMS

Manchester Score[51,4] Criteria	Ontario Cancer Institute[55]
+1 if LDH greater than ULN	Algorithm following
+1 if extensive stage	Stage (very limited/limited/extensive)
+1 if sodium is under 132 mmol/L	Gender (male/female)
+1 if KP is under 60	LDH (normal/elevated)
+1 Alk phos over 1.5×ULN	WBC (if limited stage)
+1 If bicarbonate is under 24 mmol/L	Alk phos, liver metastases (if extensive)
Groups (median survival in weeks)	
1: score 0,1[51]	A: limited-stage patients only[59]
2: score 2,3[37]	B: limited- or extensive-stage[49]
3: score 4+[26]	C: limited- or extensive-stage[35]
	D: extensive-stage only[24]

both of the aggressive nature of SCLC and the frequency of comorbid nonmalignant disease. Thus similar problems of balancing potentially toxic treatments against symptom palliation in a relatively unfit population persist. In general, prognostic factors are taken into account in determining whether treatment will be aimed at long-term survival, at cure, or at palliation, and the patient's performance status will then guide the chemotherapy regimen to be used.

Single-Agent versus Combination Chemotherapy

Combination chemotherapy has proved superior to single-agent treatment in most trials addressing this question.[57,58] Response rates, particularly complete response rates, are higher and median survival is longer. Combinations of the drugs that have shown single-agent activity are used.[59–62] Vincristine excepted, their dose-limiting toxicity is myelosuppression, and therefore combinations of up to four agents have been used (Table 57.5). The success in extend-

TABLE 57.5. STANDARD COMBINATION CHEMOTHERAPIES IN EXTENSVE SMALL CELL LUNG CANCER

Regimen	Patient Number	OR (%)	CR (%)	MS (months)
CAV[59]	140	51	7	8.3
ACE[60]	73	59	13	6.4
	89	45	10	5.8
CAVE[61,73]	110	66	26	11.9
PE[59,62]	140	61	10	8.6
	156	57	15	9.5
	150	61	14	9.9

CAV, cyclophosphamide, doxorubicin, vincristine; ACE, doxorubicin, cyclophosphamide, etoposide; CAVE, cyclophosphamide, doxorubicin, vincristine, etoposide; PE, cisplatin, etoposide; OR, objective response; CR, complete response; MS, median survival.

ing median overall survival with these regimens has meant that, until now, this and response rate have been the criteria in assessing efficacy. Although toxicity has also been well documented with these regimens, there are few studies reporting quality-of-life outcomes with combination treatments.

If combination chemotherapy is used, there remains the question of how many drugs are needed to give the best palliation. Most trials that have sought to compare four-drug regimens with three- or two-drug treatment have not addressed palliation specifically, although there are three that have. In a 310-patient randomized trial, the Medical Research Council (MRC) Lung Cancer Working Party compared ECMV (etoposide, cyclophosphamide, methotrexate, vincristine) with EV (etoposide, vincristine) in poor-prognosis SCLC.[63] No differences were seen in median survival (141 versus 137 days) or one-year survival (12% versus 10%), but toxicity was greater with the four-drug treatment, the main differences being in the rates of mucositis and of myelosuppression. Despite this, ECMV provided better symptom palliation and better relief of psychological distress, although patients reported more lethargy. The same group also compared ECMV with EI (Ifosfamide, etoposide) over six cycles, as part of a study that also assessed the effect of three cycles of ECMV.[64] Quality of life was measured by daily diary card and physician report. Survival and symptom palliation were similar in all the arms, but patients on EI reported less dysphagia and better overall condition between cycles of treatment. The third study, conducted in Switzerland, sought to compare weekly carboplatin/teniposide with standard chemotherapy (cyclophosphamide, doxorubicin, vincristine [CAV] alternating with cyclophosphamide, lomustine, methotrexate, and vincristine). This closed early when inferior survival in the less-intensive two-drug arm became apparent.[65] For now, too few data exist to indicate a preferred combination treatment for the palliation of SCLC. CAV and PE (cisplatin, etoposide) are the most widely used and are often included as control treatments in randomized trials.

Since response to treatment relates to dose intensity, it

would seem worthwhile to investigate means of attenuating the toxicity of combination treatments while maintaining the latter. In a London study of largely poor-performance-status patients, low-dose/high-frequency ACE (doxorubicin, cyclophosphamide, etoposide) was shown to be as effective as the standard three-weekly schedule in terms of response rate and overall and one-year survival.[60] Although toxicity was unaffected by schedule, quality of life (measured by daily diary card) was better in the low-dose/high-frequency arm. This demonstrates once again the added value of quality-of-life measures in evaluating palliative therapies, for the conventional outcome measures suggested that the schedules were equivalent.

Dose Intensity in Extensive SCLC

Preclinical models show a clear relationship between cure rate and dose intensity in SCLC.[66] Early clinical trials failed to establish this in clinical practice, but although dose intensification was intended, actual dose delivery often differed little between study arms.[67,68] Evidence is now emerging that growth-factor-supported dose intensification can have a significant impact upon survival,[69,70] but this approach to treatment demands a fit patient, usually with limited disease. Indeed, in extensive-stage disease, investigators have been thwarted by their inability to intensify dose owing to excessive toxicity.[71] Where intensification has been achieved in extensive-stage patients, this has had no impact upon survival, as shown in two recent trials comparing CODE (cisplatin, vincristine, doxorubicin, and etoposide) with alternating CAV and PE.[72,73] On the other hand, patients with extensive disease but good performance status benefited from dose intensification of the V-ICE regimen (vincristine, ifosfamide, carboplatin, etoposide).[74] Thus intensified therapy cannot be justified where cure is not sought.

Another approach has been to use alternating non-cross-resistant chemotherapies to enhance response rate, according to the Goldie-Coldman hypothesis.[75] Trials of PE alternating with CAV compared with one and/or other regimen alone have suggested a survival benefit for alternating treatment.[76,77] However, in the Japanese study this was confined to patients with limited-stage disease, and it failed to achieve significance in the Canadian trial of patients with extensive SCLC when those with locoregional disease were taken into account. A large United States study in extensive-stage patients found no difference in response rate or survival between six cycles of CAV, four cycles of PE, or three cycles of CAV alternating with three of PE.[59] Similarly, a German study of alternating CAV and IE (ifosfamide, etoposide) versus sequential IE then CAV found no difference in survival.[78] At present, alternating chemotherapy has no clear role in SCLC.

Duration of Treatment

There have been several studies examining the optimum number of chemotherapy cycles in SCLC, but all have used

survival rather than symptom palliation or quality of life as their yardstick. A study by Cullen and others[79] showed a survival advantage for extensive-stage patients who responded to six cycles of CAV chemotherapy if they went on to receive a further eight treatments (372 versus 259 days; p = 0.006). However, this is the only randomized trial in which prolonged chemotherapy has shown an advantage in the palliative setting. Several other studies involving extensive-stage SCLC have shown no advantage either to more cycles of chemotherapy at induction[64,80–83] or to maintenance chemotherapy for responding patients.[84–87] Prolonged chemotherapy is associated with increased toxicity, therefore the weight of evidence favors a short induction treatment (of four to six cycles) with further therapy held back for the treatment of symptomatic disease at relapse (see below).

Treatment of Poor-Prognosis, Poor-Performance-Status Patients

Although intravenous combination chemotherapy is accepted as the optimal approach in SCLC, the assumption that its use inevitably causes quality of life and performance status to deteriorate has led to some reluctance to use it on frail patients. The convenience, tolerability, and activity of single-agent oral etoposide have made this the preferred treatment for the purely palliative setting. Etoposide is schedule-dependent, with an overall response rate of 50% to 70%, depending on the regimen used and the population treated, and median survival is extended to nine or 10 months.[88–90] There are now three randomized trials comparing single-agent etoposide with intravenous combination chemotherapy, two of which examined symptom palliation or quality of life as well as conventional end points (Table 57.6). The Medical Research Council study was ended early as a result of interim analysis by an independent data-monitoring board. The study recruited patients with poor performance status. Symptom palliation, the primary end point, favored combination treatment (50% versus 39%), as did response rate and median survival.[91,92] Similar results were obtained in the London group's study of patients with extensive-stage SCLC and a poor prognosis or age of over 75 years. Quality of life was assessed using the Rotterdam Symptom Checklist and diary cards, and was shown to favor the combination regimen—with the exception of nausea and vomiting.[93] A smaller Danish study confirmed these findings in patients with extensive disease under the age of 71.[94] Together these studies show that combination chemotherapy is the treatment of choice, even for the less fit SCLC patient.

Salvage Chemotherapy

Patients who respond to induction chemotherapy generally relapse within a few months of completing treatment. There

TABLE 57.6. SINGLE-AGENT ETOPOSSIDE VERSUS COMBINATION CHEMOTHERAPY FOR POOR-PROGNOSIS SMALL CELL LUNG CANCER

Reference	Total No. Patients	Therapy	OR (%)	MS (months)	1-Year Survival (%)	p value
MRC[91,92]	370	E	61	4.0	9	0.03
		EV or CAV	77	5.4	14	
London LCG[93]	155	E	33	4.8	10	<0.05
		PE/CAV	47	5.9	19	
West Danish[94]	65	E	25	5.1	NR	NR
		EC	49	6.9	NR	

OR, objective response; MS, median survival; E, etoposide; EV, etoposide, vincristine; CAV, cyclophosphamide, doxorubicin, vincristine; PE, cisplatin, etoposide; EC, etoposide, carboplatin.

is evidence that chemotherapy can offer useful palliation in these circumstances, and this includes (unusually for SCLC) information on symptom relief and quality of life. Radiotherapy offers useful palliation, better than that achievable with chemotherapy in an early 1980s study,[95] but the increasing use of combined-modality first-line treatments means that this is not always an option. Response to second-line chemotherapy is better the longer the progression-free interval after induction therapy.[96] Normal blood parameters (specifically hemoglobin and lactate dehydrogenase) and good performance status are also associated with better response.[97]

PE can salvage patients treated with CAV chemotherapy—around half will respond.[98] Indeed, this finding is the basis for the alternating chemotherapy approach discussed above. However, with platinum-based regimens taking over from CAV as first-line treatment for limited-stage SCLC, the latter is coming into common use as a salvage therapy—to the extent that it provides the control arm in trials of treatments for relapsed SCLC.[99] The results with CAV are not particularly promising: around 20% of patients have an objective response, although more achieve symptom relief. Thus many of the newer agents discussed below are being tested as single-agent second-line treatment, and have shown activity in this setting. Topotecan, for example, has

recently been shown to have similar efficacy, both in terms of symptom control and survival, and tolerability to CAV in the treatment of recurrent SCLC.[99] The taxanes, vinorelbine and irinotecan, have also been studied (Table 56.7).

NEW DRUGS IN THE PALLIATION OF LUNG CANCER

There is a pressing need for new drugs to treat lung cancer, and there are six major new agents under evaluation: paclitaxel, docetaxel, topotecan, irinotecan, gemcitabine, and navelbine (Table 57.7). Their activity in NSCLC and extensive or relapsed SCLC has been tested in phase II studies as single agents, and they are now being incorporated into combination regimens and subject to phase II trials. The aim of the latter is to improve cure rates, but even so, the majority of patients with lung cancer will continue to die of the disease for the foreseeable future. It is therefore imperative that studies include assessments of quality of life and that palliation is adequately evaluated in order to select the best of the new regimens.

CONCLUSION

Chemotherapy is accepted as standard treatment for patients with SCLC who are fit enough to receive it. Patients with limited-stage disease are likely to be treated with multimodality regimens aimed at cure, but those with poor prognostic features and/or extensive-stage disease can gain substantial benefits, in terms of both symptom relief and longer survival, from less-intensive treatments. In NSCLC there is now ample evidence that, in selected patients, chemotherapy offers better quality of life and symptom control than supportive care, with some improvement in survival. The incorporation of new agents into current treatment schedules is likely to improve on results to date. However, their utility in palliating lung cancer can be properly evaluated

TABLE 57.7. ACTIVITY OF NEW AGENTS IN LUNG CANCER

Agent	NSCLC		ED-SCLC		Relapsed SCLC	
	RR	n	RR	n	RR	n
Gemcitabine[18,100]	20	332	27	29	–	
Topotecan[99,101]	14	153	39	48	19	301
Irinotecan[102–104]	27	138	50	8	33	38
Paclitaxel[102,105–107]	84	317	38	79	29	24
Docetaxel[102,108–111]	25	330	22	60	25	34
Navelbine[44,112–114]	24	1146	5	22	14	50

NSCLC, non small cell lung cancer: SCLC, small cell lung cancer; RR, response rate; ED, extensive disease; n, number of patients.

only if data regarding the impact of treatment on the patient is captured along with traditional outcome measures.

REFERENCES

1. Parker SL, Tong T, Bolden S, et al. Cancer statistics, 1997. *CA Cancer J Clin* 1997;43:5.
2. Ginsberg RJ, Vokes EE, Raben A. Non small cell lung cancer. In: De Vita VT Jr, Hellon S, Rosenberg SA, eds. *Cancer: principles and practice of oncology* 5th ed. New York: Lippincott-Raven, 1997:858.
3. Hardy JR, Noble T, Smith IE. Symptom relief with moderate dose chemotherapy (mitomycin-C, vinblastine, cisplatin) in advanced non–small cell lung cancer. *Br J Cancer* 1989;60:764.
4. Cullen MH. The MIC regimen in non–small cell lung cancer. *Lung Cancer* 1993;9:S81.
5. Ellis PA, Smith IE, Hardy JR, et al. Symptom relief with MVP (mitomycin-C, vinblastine, cisplatin) chemotherapy in advanced non–small cell lung cancer. *Br J Cancer* 1995;71:366.
6. Jachuck SJ, Brierly H, Jachuck S, et al. The effects of hypotensive drugs on the quality of life. *J R Coll Gen Pract* 1982;32:103.
7. Hopwood P, Thatcher N. Preliminary experience with quality of life evaluation in patients with lung cancer. *Oncology* 1990;4:158.
8. Medical Research Council, Lung Cancer Working Party. Inoperable non–small cell lung cancer (NSCLC): a Medical Research Council randomised trial of palliative radiotherapy with two fractions or ten fractions. *Br J Cancer* 1991;63:265.
9. Montazeri A, Gillis CR, McEwen J. Quality of life in patients with lung cancer. *Chest* 1998;113:467.
10. Bergman B, Aaronson NK, Ahmedzai S, et al. The EORTC QLQ-C30-LC13: a modular supplement to the EORTC score quality of life questionnaire (QLQ-C30) for use in lung cancer clinical trials. *Eur J Cancer* 1994;30A:635.
11. Aaronson NK, Ahmedzai S, Bergman B, et al. The European Organisation for the Research and Treatment of Cancer QLQ-C30: a quality-of-life instrument for use in international clinical trials in oncology. *J Natl Cancer Inst* 1993;85:365.
12. Batel-Cooper LM, Kornblith AB, Batel PC, et al. Do oncologists have an increasing interest in the quality of life of their patients? A literature review of the last 15 years. *Eur J Cancer* 1997;33:29.
13. Thatcher N, Hopwood P, Anderson H. Improving quality of life in patients with non–small cell lung cancer: research experience with gemcitabine. *Eur J Cancer* 1997;33:S8.
14. Silvestri G, Pritchard R, Welch HG. Preferences for chemotherapy in patients with advanced non–small cell lung cancer: descriptive study based on scripted interviews. *Br Med J* 1998;317:771.
15. Brundage MD, Davidson JR, Mackillop WJ. Trading treatment toxicity for survival in locally advanced non–small cell lung cancer. *J Clin Oncol* 1997;15:330.
16. Evans WK, Will BP, Berthelot J-M, et al. The cost of managing lung cancer in Canada. *Oncology* 1995;9:147.
17. Jaakkimainen L, Goodwin PJ, Pater J. Counting the costs of chemotherapy in a National Cancer Institute of Canada randomised trial in non–small cell lung cancer. *J Clin Oncol* 1990;8:1301.
18. Anderson H, Thatcher N, Walling J, et al. Gemcitabine and palliation of symptoms in non–small cell lung cancer. *Proc Am Soc Clin Oncol* 1994;13:367.
19. Stanley KE. Prognostic factors for survival in patients with inoperable lung cancer. *J Natl Cancer Inst* 1980;65:25.
20. Albain KS, Crowley JJ, LeBlanc M, et al. Survival determinants in extensive-stage non-small cell lung cancer: the Southwest Oncology Group experience. *J Clin Oncol* 1991;9:1618.
21. Lanzotti VJ, Thomas DR, Boyle LE, et al. Survival with inoperable lung cancer. An integration of prognostic variables based on simple clinical criteria. *Cancer* 1977;39:303.
22. Miller TP, Chen TT, Coltman CA, et al. Effect of alternating combination chemotherapy on survival of ambulatory patients with metastatic large cell and adenocarcinoma of the lung. A Southwest Oncology Group study. *J Clin Oncol* 1986;4:502.
23. Finkelstein DM, Ettinger DS, Ruckdeschel JC. Long term survivors in metastatic non–small cell lung cancer: An Eastern Cooperative Oncology Group study. *J Clin Oncol* 1986;4:702.
24. Ruckdeschel JC, Finkelstein DM, Ettinger DS, et al. A randomised trial of the four most active regimens for metastatic non–small cell lung cancer. *J Clin Oncol* 1986;4:702.
25. Wolf J, Spear P, Yesner R, et al. Nitrogen mustard and the steroid hormones in the treatment of inoperable bronchogenic carcinoma. *Am J Med* 1960;29:1008.
26. Green RA, Humphrey E, Close H, et al. Alkylating agents in bronchogenic carcinoma. *Am J Med* 1969;46:516.
27. Rapp E, Pater JL, Willan A, et al. Chemotherapy can prolong survival in patients with advanced non–small cell lung cancer—report of a Canadian multicenter randomised trial. *J Clin Oncol* 1990;8:1301.
28. Woods RL, Williams CJ, Levi J, et al. A randomised trial of cisplatin and vindesine versus supportive care only in advanced non–small cell lung cancer. *Br J Cancer* 1990;61:608.
29. Buccheri G, Ferrigno D, Rosso A, et al. Further evidence in favour of chemotherapy for inoperable non–small cell lung cancer. *Lung Cancer* 1990;6:87.
30. Cellerino R, Tummarello D, Guidi F, et al. A randomised trial of alternating chemotherapy versus best supportive care in advanced non–small cell lung cancer. *J Clin Oncol* 1991;9:1453.
31. Leung WT, Shiu WCT, Pang JCK, et al. Combined chemotherapy and radiotherapy versus best supportive care in the treatment of inoperable non–small cell lung cancer. *Oncology* 1992;49:321.
32. Cartei G, Cartei F, Cantone A, et al. Cisplatin-cyclophosphamide-mitomycin combination chemotherapy with supportive care versus supportive care alone for treatment of metastatic non–small cell lung cancer. *J Natl Cancer Inst* 1993;85:794.
33. Cullen MH, Woodroffe CM, Billingham LJ, et al. Mitomycin C, ifosfamide and cisplatin (MIC) in non–small cell lung cancer: 2. Results of a randomised trial in patients with extensive disease. *Lung Cancer* 1997;18(S1):5.
34. Perrone F, Rossi A, Ianniello GP, et al. Vinorelbine plus best supportive care versus best supportive care in the treatment of advanced non–small cell lung cancer elderly patients. Results of a phase III randomised trial. *Proc Am Soc Clin Oncol* 1998;17:455a.
35. Thatcher N, Ranson M, Anderson H, et al. Phase III study of paclitaxel versus best supportive care in inoperable non–small cell lung cancer. *Ann Oncol* 1998;9(S4):1.
36. Ranson M. (*Personal communication*).
37. Souquet PJ, Chauvin F, Boissel JP, et al. Polychemotherapy in advanced non–small cell lung cancer: a meta-analysis. *Lancet* 1993;342:19.
38. Non–Small Cell Lung Cancer Collaborative Group. Chemotherapy in non–small cell lung cancer: a meta-analysis using updated data on individual patients from 52 randomised clinical trials. *Br Med J* 1995;311:899.
39. Rosell R, Cardenal F, Montes A, et al. Quality of life in non–small cell lung cancer patients receiving gemcitabine plus cisplatin or etoposide plus cisplatin. *Ann Oncol* 1998;9(S4):84.
40. Billingham LJ, Cullun MH, Woods J, et al. Mitomycin, ifos-

famide and cisplatin (MIC) in non–small cell lung cancer (NSCLC): 3. Results of a randomised trial evaluating palliation & quality of life. *Lung Cancer* 1997;18(S1):9.

41. Anderson H, Lund B, Bach F, et al. Single agent activity of weekly gemcitabine in advanced non–small cell lung cancer: a phase II study. *J Clin Oncol* 1994;12:1821.

42. Fernandez C, Rosell R, Abad-Esteve A, et al. Quality of life during chemotherapy in non–small cell lung cancer patients. *Acta Oncol* 1989;28:29.

43. Hopwood P. Evidence for the impact of quality of life. *Lung Cancer* 1997;18(S2)66.

44. Gil Deza E, Balblani L, Coppola F, et al. Phase III study of navelbine vs navelbine plus cisplatin in non small cell lung cancer stage IIIB or IV. *Proc Am Soc Clin Oncol* 1996;15:394.

45. Smith IE, O'Brien MER, Norton A, et al. Duration of chemotherapy for advanced non–small cell lung cancer (NSCLC): a phase III randomised trial of 3 versus 6 cycles of mitomycin C, vinblastine, cisplatin (MVP). *Proc Am Soc Clin Oncol* 1998;17:457a.

46. Mackillop WJ, O'Sullivan B, Ward GK. Non–small cell lung cancer: how oncologists want to be treated. *Int J Radiat Oncol Biol* 1987;13:929.

47. Raby B, Pater J, Mackillop W. Does knowledge guide practice? Another look at the management of non–small cell lung cancer. *J Clin Oncol* 1995;13:1904.

48. Slevin ML, Stubbs L, Plant HJ, et al. Attitudes to chemotherapy: comparing views of patients with cancer with those of doctors, nurses and the general public. *Br Med J* 1990;300:1458.

49. Souhami RL, Law K. Longevity in small cell lung cancer. *Br J Cancer* 1990;61:584.

50. Ihde DC. Chemotherapy of lung cancer. *N Engl J Med* 1992;327:1434.

51. Rawson NSB, Peto J. An overview of prognostic factors in small cell lung cancer. *Br J Cancer* 1990;61:597.

52. Matthews MJ, Kanhouwa S, Pickren J, et al. Frequency of residual and metastatic tumour in patients undergoing curative resection for lung cancer. *Cancer Chemother Rep* 1973;4:63.

53. Albain KS, Crowley JJ, LeBlanc M, et al. Determinants of improved outcome in small cell lung cancer: an analysis of the 2580-patient South West Oncology Group data base. *J Clin Oncol* 1990;8:563.

54. Cerny T, Blair V, Anderson H, et al. Pre-treatment prognostic factors and scoring system in 407 small cell lung cancer patients. *Int J Cancer* 1987;39:146.

55. Sagman U, Maki E, Evans WK, et al. Small cell carcinoma of the lung: derivation of a prognostic staging system. *J Clin Oncol* 1991;9:1639.

56. Siu LL, Shepherd FA, Murray N, et al. Influence of age on the treatment of limited stage small cell lung cancer. *J Clin Oncol* 1996;14:821.

57. Alberto P, Brunner KW, Martz G, et al. Treatment of bronchogenic carcinoma with simultaneous or sequential combination chemotherapy, including methotrexate, cyclophosphamide, procarbazine and vincristine. *Cancer* 1976;38:2208.

58. Lowenbraun S, Bartolucci A, Smalley RV, et al. The superiority of combination chemotherapy over single agent chemotherapy in small cell lung cancer. *Cancer* 1979;44:406.

59. Roth BJ, Johnson DH, Einhorn LH, et al. Randomised study of cyclophosphamide, doxorubicin and vincristine versus etoposide and cisplatin versus alternation of these two regimens in extensive small cell lung cancer: a phase III trial of the Southeastern Cancer Study Group. *J Clin Oncol* 1992;10:282.

60. James LE, Gower NH, Rudd RM, et al. A randomised trial of low dose/high frequency chemotherapy as palliative treatment of poor prognosis small cell lung cancer: a Cancer Research Campaign trial. *Br J Cancer* 1996;73:1563.

61. Murray N, Shah A, Osoba D, et al. Intensive weekly chemotherapy for the treatment of stage extensive small cell lung cancer. *J Clin Oncol* 1991;9:1632.

62. Miller AA, Herndon JE II, Hollis DR, et al. Schedule dependency of 21-day oral versus 3-day intravenous etoposide in combination with intravenous cisplatin in extensive stage small cell lung cancer: a randomised phase III study of the Cancer and Leukaemia Group B. *J Clin Oncol* 1995;13:1871.

63. Medical Research Council Lung Cancer Working Party. Randomised trial of four-drug versus less intensive two-drug chemotherapy in the palliative treatment of patients with small cell lung cancer and poor prognosis. *Br J Cancer* 1996;73:406.

64. Bleehen NM, Girling DJ, Machin D, et al. A randomised trial of three or six courses of etoposide, cyclophosphamide, methotrexate and vincristine or six courses of etoposide and ifosfamide in small cell lung cancer. II Quality of life. *Br J Cancer* 1993;68:1157.

65. Joss RA, Alberto P, Hurny C, et al. Quality versus quantity of life in the treatment of patients with advanced small cell cancer? A randomised comparison of weekly carboplatin and teniposide versus cisplatin, adriamycin, etoposide alternating with cyclophophamide, methotrexate, vincristine and lomustine. Swiss Group for Clinical Cancer Research. *Ann Oncol* 1995;6:41.

66. Skipper HE, Schabel FM Jr, Mellett LB, et al. Implications of the biochemical, cytokinetic, pharmacologic and toxicologic relationships in the design of optimal therapeutic schedules. *Cancer Chemother Rep* 1970;54:431.

67. Sculier JP, Rudd R, Ruiz de Elvira MC, et al. Multiple drug weekly chemotherapy versus standard combination regimen in small cell lung cancer: a Phase III randomised study conducted by the European Lung Cancer Working Party. *J Clin Oncol* 1993;11:1858.

68. Souhami RL, Rudd R, Ruiz de Elvira MC, et al. Randomised trial comparing weekly versus 3-weekly chemotherapy in small cell lung cancer: a Cancer Research Campaign trial. *J Clin Oncol* 1994;12:1806.

69. Thatcher N, Sambrook RJ, Stephens RJ, et al. Dose intensification with G-CSF improves survival in small cell lung cancer: results of a randomised trial. *Proc Am Soc Clin Oncol* 1998;17:456a.

70. Steward WP, Von Pawel J, Gatzmeier U, et al. Effects of GM-CSF and dose intensification of V-ICE chemotherapy in small cell lung cancer: a prospective randomised study of 300 patients. *J Clin Oncol* 1998;16:642.

71. Pujol JL, Douillard JY, Riviere A, et al. Dose-intensity of a four-drug chemotherapy regimen with or without recombinant human granulocyte-macrophage colony-stimulating factor in extensive-stage small cell lung cancer: a multicentre randomised phase III study. *J Clin Oncol* 1997;15:2082.

72. Furuse K, Fukuoka M, Nishiwaki Y, et al. Phase III study of intensive weekly chemotherapy with recombinant human granulocyte colony-stimulating factor versus standard chemotherapy in extensive-stage small cell lung cancer. The Japan Clinical Oncology Group. *J Clin Oncol* 1998;16:2126.

73. Murray N, Livingstone RB, Shepherd FA, et al. A randomised study of CODE plus thoracic irradiation versus alternating CAV/EP for extensive stage small cell lung cancer: an intergroup study of the National Cancer Institute of Canada and the Southwest Oncology Group. *Lung Cancer* 1997;18(S1):6.

74. Steward WP, Von Pawel J, Gatzmeier U, et al. Effects of GM-CSF and dose intensification of V-ICE chemotherapy in small cell lung cancer: a prospective randomised study of 300 patients. *J Clin Oncol* 1998;16:642.

75. Goldie JH, Coldman AJ, Gudauskas GA. Rationale for the use of alternating non-cross-resistant chemotherapy. *Cancer Treat Rep* 1982;66:439.

76. Evans WK, Feld R, Murray N, et al. Superiority of alternating non-cross-resistant chemotherapy in extensive small cell lung cancer. *Ann Intern Med* 1987;107:451.

77. Fukuoka M, Furuse K, Saijo N, et al. Randomised trial of cyclophosphamide, doxorubicin and vincristine versus cisplatin and etoposide versus alternation of these regimens in small cell lung cancer. *J Natl Cancer Inst* 1991;83:855.

78. Wolf M, Pritsch M, Drings P, et al. Cyclic alternating versus response oriented chemotherapy in small cell lung cancer: a German multi-centre randomised trial of 321 patients. *J Clin Oncol* 1991;9:614.

79. Cullen MH, Morgan D, Gregory W, et al. Maintenance chemotherapy for anaplastic small cell carcinoma of the bronchus: a randomised controlled trial. *Cancer Chemother Pharmacol* 1986; 17:156.

80. Bleehen NM, Fayers PM, Girling DJ, et al. Controlled trial of twelve versus six courses of chemotherapy in the treatment of small cell lung cancer. *Br J Cancer* 1989;59:584.

81. Lebeau B, Chastang CL, Allard P, et al. Six vs. twelve cycles for complete responders to chemotherapy in small cell lung cancer: definitive results of a randomised clinical trial. *Eur Respir J* 1992;5:286.

82. Jarry O, Fournel P. A randomised trial of four versus eight courses of chemotherapy with ifosfamide, epirubicin and etoposide (EVI) in extensive small cell lung cancer. Denver, CO: IASLC-SCLC, 1994.

83. Veslemes M, Polyzos A, Latsi P, et al. Optimal duration of chemotherapy in small cell lung cancer: a randomised study of 4 versus 6 cycles of cisplatin-etoposide. *J Chemother* 1998;10: 136.

84. Giaccone G, Dalesio O, McVie GJ, et al. Maintenance chemotherapy in small cell lung cancer: long-term results of a randomised trial. *J Clin Oncol* 1993;11:1230.

85. Ettinger DS, Finkelstein DM, Abeloff MD, et al. A randomised comparison of standard chemotherapy versus alternating chemotherapy and maintenance versus no maintenance therapy for extensive stage small cell lung cancer: a phase III study of the Eastern Co-Operative Oncology Group. *J Clin Oncol* 1990; 8:230.

86. Beith JM, Clarke SJ, Woods RL, et al. Long-term follow-up of a randomised trial of combined chemoradiotherapy induction treatment, with and without maintenance chemotherapy in patients with small cell carcinoma of the lung. *Eur J Cancer* 1996; 32A:438.

87. Sculier JP, Paesmans M, Bureau G, et al. Randomised trial comparing induction chemotherapy versus induction chemotherapy followed by maintenance chemotherapy in small cell lung cancer. *J Clin Oncol* 1996;14:2337.

88. Slevin ML, Clark PI, Joel SP, et al. A randomised trial to evaluate the effect of scheduling on the activity of etoposide in small cell lung cancer. *J Clin Oncol* 1989;7:1333.

89. Clark PI, Cottier B. The activity of 10-, 14-, and 21-day schedules of single agent etoposide in previously untreated patients with extensive small cell lung cancer. *Semin Oncol* 1992;19:36.

90. Smit EF, Postmus PE. A phase II study of oral etoposide 100mg/day for 21 days every 4 weeks in untreated elderly and poor performance status small cell lung cancer patients. *Cancer Treat Res* 1991;7:136.

91. Thatcher N, Girling DJ, Clark PI, et al. Comparison of oral etoposide and standard intravenous multidrug chemotherapy for small cell lung cancer: a stopped multicentre randomised trial. *Lancet* 1996;348:563.

92. Clark PI, Thatcher N, Lallemand G, et al. Updated results of a randomised trial confirm that oral etoposide alone is inadequate palliative chemotherapy for small cell lung cancer. *Lung Cancer* 1997;18(S1):14.

93. Souhami RL, Spiro SG, Rudd RM, et al. Five-day oral etoposide treatment for advanced small cell lung cancer: a randomised comparison with intravenous chemotherapy. *J Natl Cancer Inst* 1997;89:577.

94. Pfeiffer P, Rytter C, Madsen EL, et al. Prolonged oral low-dose etoposide in SCLC. Results from randomized controlled trials. *Proc Am Soc Clin Oncol* 1998;17:498a.

95. Ochs JJ, Tester WJ, Cohen MH, et al. "Salvage" radiation therapy for intra-thoracic small cell carcinoma of the lung progressing on combination chemotherapy. *Cancer Treat Rep* 1983; 67:1123.

96. Giaccone G, Donadio M, Bonardi G, et al. Teniposide in the treatment of small cell lung cancer: the influence of prior chemotherapy. *J Clin Oncol* 1988;6:1264.

97. Albain KS, Crowley JJ, Hutchins L, et al. Predictors of survival following relapse or progression of small cell lung cancer: Southwest Oncology Group study 8605 report and analysis of recurrent disease database. *Cancer* 1993;72:1184.

98. Evans WK, Osoba D, Feld R, et al. Etoposide (VP-16) and cisplatin: an effective treatment for relapse in small cell lung cancer. *J Clin Oncol* 1985;3:65.

99. Schiller J, von Pawel J, Shepherd F, et al. Topotecan versus cyclophosphamide, doxorubicin and vincristine for the treatment of patients with recurrent small cell lung cancer: a phase III study. *Proc Am Soc Clin Oncol* 1998;17:456a.

100. Cormier Y, Eisenhauer E, Muldal A, et al. Gemcitabine is an active agent in previously untreated extensive small cell lung cancer. A study of the National Cancer Institute of Canada Clinical Trials Group. *Ann Oncol* 1994;5:283.

101. Krollmannsberger C, Mross K, Jakob A, et al. Topotecan—a novel topoisomerase I inhibitor pharmacology and clinical experience. *Oncology* 1999;56:1.

102. Bunn PA Jr, Kelly K. New chemotherapeutic agents prolong survival and improve quality of life in non–small cell lung cancer: a review of the literature and future directions. *Clin Cancer Res* 1998;5:1087.

103. Negoro S, Fukuoka M, Niitani H, et al. Phase II study of CPT-11, new camptothecin derivative, in small cell lung cancer. *Proc Am Soc Clin Oncol* 1991;10:241.

104. Masuda N, Fukuoka M, Kusunoki Y, et al. CPT-11: a new derivative of camptothecin for the treatment of refractory or relapsed small cell lung cancer. *J Clin Oncol* 1992;10:1225.

105. Ettinger D, Finkelstein D, Sarma RP, et al. Phase II study of paclitaxel in patients with extensive disease small cell lung cancer: an eastern cooperative oncology group trial. *J Clin Oncol* 1995;13:1430.

106. Kirschling RJ, Jung SH, Jett JR, et al. A phase II trial of taxol and G-CSF in previously untreated patients with extensive stage small cell lung cancer. *Proc Am Soc Clin Oncol* 1994;13:326.

107. Smit EF, Fokkema E, Biesma B, et al. A phase II study of paclitaxel in heavily pre-treated patients with small cell lung cancer. *Br J Cancer* 1998;77:347.

108. Kim NK, Park K, Park CH, et al. Phase II trial of docetaxel for advanced non–small cell lung cancer. *Proc Am Soc Clin Oncol* 1998;17:490a.

109. Burris HA, Crowley JJ, Williamson SK, et al. Docetaxel (taxotere) in extensive stage small cell lung cancer: a trial of the Southwest Oncology Group. *Proc Am Soc Clin Oncol* 1998;17:451a.

110. Latreille J, Cormier Y, Martins H, et al. Phase II study of docetaxel (taxotere) in patients with previously untreated extensive small cell lung cancer. *Invest New Drugs* 1996;13:342.

111. Smyth JF, Smith IE, Sessa C, et al. Activity of docetaxel (taxotere) in small cell lung cancer. Early Clinical Trials Group of the EORTC. *Eur J Cancer* 1994;30A:1058.

112. Le Chevalier T, Brisgand D, Douiliard JY, et al. Randomized study of vinorelbine and cisplatin versus vindesine and cisplatin

versus vinorelbine alone in advanced non small cell lung cancer: results of a European multi-centre trial including 612 patients. *J Clin Oncol* 1994;12:360.

113. Higano CS, Crowley JJ, Veith RV, et al. A phase II study of intravenous vinorelbine in previously untreated patients with extensive small cell lung cancer. *Invest New Drugs* 1997;15:153.

114. Furuse K, Kubota K, Kawahara M, et al. Phase II study of vinorelbine in heavily previously treated small cell lung cancer. Japan Lung Cancer Vinorelbine Study Group. *Oncology* 1996; 53:169.

115. Jassem J, Karnicka-Miodkowska H, van Pottelsberghe C, et al. Phase II study of vinorelbine (navelbine) in previously treated small cell lung cancer patients. EORTC Lung Cancer Co-Operative Group. *Eur J Cancer* 1993;29A:1720.

58

PALLIATIVE RADIOTHERAPY

FRANCIS J. SULLIVAN

One of the first and most fundamental principles we are taught when learning the art of radiation medicine is the distinction between radical and palliative care of the cancer patient. In defining the goals of our treatment, we clarify for ourselves and for our patients and their families realistic expectations for the (often all too short) time remaining to them. A thorough knowledge of the natural history of the disease is a prerequisite for this decision. Not infrequently we are surprised when the patient's course runs differently from the expected. Nonetheless, the inadequacies of our current treatments routinely place us in a clinical situation where cure is impossible, and improvement in the quality of life is all that we have left to offer. Some 25% to 50% of all cancer patients will require palliative radiation at some point during their illness. In no disease is this more important than in the care of the patient with lung cancer. In 1993 it was estimated that 170,000 patients would develop cancer of the lung in the United States, and 149,000 (87.6%) will die of their disease.[1] With cure rates so low that the mortality from this disease approaches the incidence, palliative care is more significant an issue in lung cancer than in almost any other single malignancy. For example, the five-year survival rates for patients presenting with locally advanced, inoperable, non–small cell lung cancer (NSCLC) (by far the majority of NSCLC patients) treated with radiation therapy with "curative" intent are 5% to 7%.[2] These figures are low enough to cause intense debate as to whether these patients are best served by aggressive therapies rather than a "palliative" approach.[3-6] Thus in lung cancer, even when the patient has locally confined disease, we are faced with a difficult decision which centers around the question of "palliation" and quality of life.

It seems generally true that management decisions for the patient requiring palliative radiotherapy may be more complex and demanding than those involving definitive or "curative" care. The patient is generally more debilitated, often has multiple coincident medical and psychosocial problems, and frequently requires complex treatment planning and support. In this context, radiation therapy is generally acknowledged as one of the most effective weapons in the armamentarium of the physician attempting to treat patients with advanced or metastatic lung cancer.[7] Radia-

tion is capable of improving symptoms in the majority of patients, and can even improve survival in selected cases. However, a wide variety of time dose and fractionation schedules are employed, with relatively little available information to guide the clinician in deciding optimal management strategies.[8-14] The final choice of dose and fractionation is often more influenced by the physician's perception of the patient's prognosis and survival, as well as by availability of resources and cultural differences in the approach to the terminal care of the cancer patient, than by clear clinical guidelines.[15] This chapter will outline the general approach to the patient with lung cancer requiring palliation of a symptom or a clinical syndrome and will thereafter focus on selected site-specific problems frequently encountered in the care of such patients.

GENERAL APPROACH TO PALLIATIVE THERAPY IN LUNG CANCER

Given the natural history of the disease, a wide spectrum of clinical conditions may confront the physician dealing with the palliative care of the patient with lung cancer.[16-18] It cannot be overemphasized that the treatment of such patients must be individualized. The tendency to categorize patients with metastatic disease as a single group, for example, is not helpful and perhaps should be avoided. For instance, there is a clear difference between the patient with a solitary brain metastasis occurring more than a year after being rendered disease-free[19] and the patient in whom multiple brain metastases occur in conjunction with other sites of extrathoracic disease.[20] A multimodality approach may be required, and physicians subspecializing in oncology should interact with one another in the management of these problems for these patients. No treatise on this topic can be all-encompassing; the following is intended as a general guideline only.

Firm Diagnosis

In the selection of the patient who might be expected to benefit from palliative irradiation, the following factors are

TABLE 58.1. GENERAL APPROACH TO PALLIATIVE CARE

- Firm diagnosis of malignancy
- Adequate life expectancy
- Performance status and coexistent medical conditions
- Clinical/radiographic correlation
- Balance of radiation-induced morbidity and expected outcome
- Technical considerations (prior therapy, treatment planning issues)
- Identification and communication of treatment goals

TABLE 58.2. THE SOLITARY METASTASIS

- Status of primary
- Patient age and performance status
- Interval from primary to development of the metastasis
- Morbidity of biopsy/resection
- Radiosensitivity of the lesion

critical (Table 58.1). In general the histologic subdivisions of lung cancer[21] are less important in the palliative management of these patients. When the patient with lung cancer requires palliative irradiation, it is often less important to know if the patient has SC versus NSC histology than it is to know that the patient has a malignant cause for the symptom. Tissue diagnosis is usually not a significant problem. The patient will commonly have a firm histologic diagnosis, so histologic reconfirmation prior to a course of palliative irradiation will not always be required. However, two clinical situations deserve mention.

Histologic Confirmation

The first involves the patient who presents with a single or multiple sites of disease in a distribution highly suggestive of a metastatic process but with no prior history of malignancy. Lung cancers not infrequently have as their initial presentation parenchymal brain lesions, spinal cord compression, or superior vena cava syndrome, requiring immediate intervention.[2,22] In the current management of these patients, it is mandatory to obtain tissue prior to instituting any anticancer therapies, including radiation.[23]

The second situation involves the patient with a known history of lung cancer who presents with a solitary lesion suggestive of metastatic disease. Table 58.2 summarizes the important issues with regard to management in this situation. Here an important issue may be whether a biopsy is required prior to palliative therapy. Although each patient must be individually evaluated, the following points may be helpful. The commonest clinical problems relating to distant metastatic disease in lung cancer are those relating to brain and skeletal metastasis.[2,16–18] Solitary lesions may account for 30% to 50% of all cases of brain metastases.[24] In selected patients, surgical resection with postoperative whole-brain radiotherapy offers a group survival benefit. So, prior to a course of palliative irradiation, selected patients may benefit from surgical intervention for both diagnostic and therapeutic reasons.

Solitary bone lesions occur in only 6% to 8% of all patients undergoing screening isotope bone scanning for metastases.[25] Not all bone scan lesions represent metastases.

Nonmalignant causes (osteoporosis, Paget's disease, prior trauma, and infection, for example) as well as other malignant entities (lymphoma, myeloma, primary bone tumors) may be characterized as metastatic lesions. The anatomic site of the lesion within the skeleton may be helpful in the differential. Although advances in diagnostic imaging have aided in the evaluation of such lesions,[26] as a rule solitary lesions should be biopsied prior to therapy. In the practical management of these problems, it is recognized that a biopsy may not be safely and easily accomplished (poor performance status or inaccessibility of the lesion). The clinician must judge each situation individually. Clearly, the assumption that a single lesion suggestive of a metastasis may be treated empirically with radiation is to be discouraged. This practice will on occasion lead to the inappropriate use of ionizing radiation for an unrelated (and possibly benign) condition or may lessen the potential for an optimal result from a curative approach (Table 58.2).

Life Expectancy and Performance Status

It need hardly be stressed that the patient's life expectancy must be factored into any decision regarding palliative irradiation. Desperately ill patients in the final stages of refractory malignancy rarely benefit from intervention. Appropriate dose fractionation, including large single fractions, may be appropriate.[11] For example, the patient with significant hemoptysis at the late stages of the disease may benefit from such an approach. The patient performance status continues to be an important prognostic factor predicting response to radiation therapy.[8,12,27] Patients with poor performance status (PS) tend to respond less well to anticancer therapies than those with good to excellent PS.[28] Coexistent medical conditions or pathophysiologic processes (related to the cancer or its treatment) may significantly impact on the patient's ability to tolerate or respond to a course of irradiation (Table 58.3).

TABLE 58.3. COEXISTENT CONDITIONS

- Anemia
- Chronic obstructive pulmonary disease
- Myocardial dysfunction
- Significant bone marrow dysfunction

Clinical/Radiographic Correlation and Target Volume Selection

A critical step in the decision to offer a course of palliative irradiation is the accurate anatomic localization of the cause of the patient's symptom or syndrome. A combination of clinical and radiographic information helps to localize a radiation portal for maximal therapeutic gain. A directed clinical history and thorough physical examination remain the best start. The practice of relying solely on radiographic studies in the selection of a treatment strategy is to be discouraged. The patient cannot always accurately localize the cause of a symptom which may vary depending upon the problem. For example, localized pain is the hallmark of skeletal metastases,[29] and a patient may accurately localize bone in many instances, whereas the ability to accurately localize the site of esophageal obstruction in the cause of dysphagia is less accurate. Clinical presentations with radiculopathy, such as brachial plexopathy from a Pancoast tumor or sciatic nerve pain from a lumbar metastasis, need to be recognized. Not infrequently, physical examinations will uncover previously unrecognized coexistent. For example, a patient with neurologic symptoms from known brain metastases may present with coexistent spinal cord compression from bony metastases. It should further be stressed that repeated clinical assessment, including physical examination, may be required during palliative therapy to ensure that the goals of treatment are being met and that such treatment remains the appropriate course, that is, is not unnecessarily protracted.

However, seldom if ever will a course of palliative radiation be instituted without some radiographic correlation (Table 58.4). The target volume irradiated must include but not necessarily be confined to the demonstrated radiographic abnormality. Knowledge of the pathophysiology and natural history of the symptom or syndrome being palliated is essential. For example, palliation of a brachial plexopathy from a Pancoast tumor requires coverage not only of the visible lesion but also of the vertebral bodies and nerve routes to the plexus. In treating multiple vertebral body metastases, the physician must remember the potential need to treat an adjacent field at a later time.

In the era of modern imaging, there is a tendency to use MRI or CT imaging techniques as initial screening evaluations prior to or instead of a plain radiograph. While there are certainly clinical situations in which this is clearly appropriate (spinal cord compression, brain metastases, etc.), plain radiographs are very useful screening evaluations in this patient population. They may be very accurate in differentiating metastatic carcinomatous lesions of bone from benign lesions as well as other bone malignancies.[29] Bone metastases from lung primaries tend to be lytic or occasionally blastic lesions localized to the spine, ribs, or metaphyseal regions of the long bones.[30] Plain radiographs of the spine can frequently complement an MRI scan and aid in the accurate localization of a vertebral body collapse or spinal cord compression. Not all bone metastases are painful. Skeletal surveys and bone scintigraphy are a powerful tool in screening for such lesions.[25,31] Scintigraphy is also useful for following responses to treatment.[25] Bone scans do not provide detail of the structural lesion in the bone; for this reason, plain radiographs should be obtained of abnormal areas of tracer accumulation detected on bone scan. In particular, painful areas and those in weight-bearing bones should be radiographed. Computerized tomography (CT) has gained an important role in the radiation management of the cancer patient, including the patient requiring palliative care.[32–34] CT can greatly aid in the delineation of soft tissue masses, which are often associated with bone metastases and are not easily seen on plain radiographs. Furthermore, the increasing use of ultrasound (US) and CT-guided biopsy to obtain tissue from previously inaccessible locations has made tissue confirmation prior to therapy a much more attainable goal.[35–37] Lastly, the incorporation of CT dosimetry into treatment planning systems[37] has enhanced the delivery of effective radiation doses with less normal-tissue morbidity.

Recent advances in magnetic resonance imaging (MRI) have greatly aided the palliative care in the cancer patient. MRI, coupled with radionuclide bone scanning, detected occult metastatic disease to the brain or skeleton in 28% of a small series of patients with operable NSCLC.[38] MRI has been shown to be effective in the early detection of vertebral body metastases[39] and is now considered to be the procedure of choice in assessing patients with medullary symptoms and cancer.[40,41] Prospective as well as retrospective studies have shown a high degree of sensitivity and specificity (90% or more) in evaluating patients with suspected metastatic spinal compression syndromes.[42,43] In situations where isotope bone scintigraphy is equivocal or negative, MRI has been shown to be a complementary noninvasive test.[44–46] With appropriate technique, differentiation between osteoporotic fractures and metastases is possible with MRI alone, and this test is now becoming increasingly useful in obviating the need for biopsy confirmation in this situation.[26] In evaluating patients with suspected spinal cord compression, the MRI has demonstrated ability in precisely characterizing the mass and its relationship to the spinal cord. It allows simultaneous demonstration of multiple sites of involvement and thus can obviate the need

TABLE 58.4. RADIOGRAPHIC EVALUATION IN PALLIATIVE IRRADIATION

- Plain radiography
- Bone scintigraphy
- Computerized tomography
- Magnetic resonance imaging
- Other: angiography, myelography

for invasive and less sensitive tests such as myelography.[47] MR has also been found superior to CT in the detection of cerebral metastases.[48] Coupled with an increasing role in radiation treatment planning,[49] it has therefore become invaluable in the staging and palliative management of the patient with lung cancer.[50]

The combined use of some or all of the aforementioned techniques, allied to the less frequently used sonography and angiography, generally compliment the history and physical examination in planning a course of palliative irradiation.

Time Dose and Fractionation in Palliative Care

There is perhaps no more important aspect to planning and administering palliative irradiation than choosing an appropriate time dose and fractionation (TDF) schedule (Table 58.5). The generally held assumption is that hypofractionated irradiation, utilizing fewer but larger doses of irradiation, is the appropriate course. Radiobiologically, these fractionation schedules are predicted to be associated with a greater long-term radiation morbidity (see Chapter 12). This approach is considered acceptable because the majority of patients will not survive long enough to experience these toxities. However it has been estimated that some 10% of all cancer patients treated palliatively will survive longer than one year. Therefore, the indiscriminate use of such schedules may cause long-term toxicity in surviving patients. Where possible, patients with a longer life expectancy should be identified because they are at greater risk for long-term morbidity related to their treatment. Because there is relatively little available literature critically analyzing the outcome when various TDF schedules are compared, good studies are needed to address this important question. Reliable and reproducible outcomes allowing comparison of various treatments must be agreed upon (see Table 58.6).

In this context, the work of patterns of care studies (PCS) and cooperative study groups such as the Radiation Therapy Oncology Group (RTOG) should be acknowledged. Recent physician-targeted studies have identified important international differences in the approach to these patients.[15,51–53] Such studies highlight as significant the availability of resources (government-funded versus private), physician and patient expectations, as well as a lack of relia-

TABLE 58.5. FACTORS IN CHOOSING PALLIATIVE RADIATION SCHEDULES

- Natural history of the disease
- Resources for treatment
- Recognizing cultural differences in palliative care
- Identifying meaningful goals for evaluating various treatments
- Communicating with patient and family
- Individualizing treatment approaches

TABLE 58.6. POSSIBLE PALLIATIVE CARE STUDY END POINTS

- Median survival
- Failure-free survival
- Percent symptom response
- Time to symptom response
- Duration of response
- Change in performance status
- Tumor volume changes
- Functional independence
- Quality of life

ble patient prognostic factors. For example, physicians who are funded privately tend to choose longer treatment courses with higher total radiation doses, as opposed to government-funded doctors, when they (the physicians) believe their treatment will prolong life or prevent the occurrence of future symptoms ("prophylactic" palliation). Further differences are seen depending on which physician has the responsibility for the terminal care of the patient.[54] These choices are often made in the absence of any demonstrable benefit in terms of survival or quality of life. As a final point, it is worth remembering that the palliative care of the patient with cancer is not necessarily synonymous with cytotoxic therapy. It is often appropriate to care for the patient with general medical treatments (analgesics etc.), allowing them to *live with* their cancer in a way that preserves their comfort, independence, and dignity for as long as possible.

SPECIFIC PROBLEMS IN PALLIATING LUNG CANCER WITH RADIATION

Brain and Central Nervous System Metastasis

Incidence

Metastasis to the central nervous system (CNS) occurs in 25% to 35% of all cancer patients.[55,56] It presents in three distinct temporal patterns relative to the primary lesion: precocious (occult primary), synchronous (simultaneous primary), and metachronous (antecedent primary). It has been estimated that lung cancer is the most common cause, accounting for 40% to 60% of all parenchymal metastases, translating to almost 45,000 cases in the U.S. in 1992.[57] In addition to being a frequent occurrence in newly diagnosed lung cancer, brain metastases constitute more than 25% of all recurrences in patients with resected NSCLC.[58] Brain metastases are present at the time of diagnosis in approximately 10% of patients with SCLC and occur at some point during the illness of a further 25% to 35%.[59] In fact, the incidence in SCLC increases with length of survival, so that 50% to 80% of patients surviving two years will develop brain metastases if no therapy is directed at their prevention.[60] The use of prophylactic cranial irradiation (PCI) in lung cancer is dealt with in Chapter 56. Brain metastases are often dramatically symptomatic and distressing to the patient and family. It is thought that as many as 50% of patients will die of progressive CNS metastases.[61,62] Thus parenchymal brain metastases represent a significant cause of morbidity and mortality in the patient with lung cancer and require careful evaluation and therapy. However, the prognosis of patients with brain metastases varies widely, once again emphasizing the need for individualized management depending on the clinical setting.

Natural History and Prognostic Factors

CNS metastases arise either from hematogenous dissemination or from direct extension from adjacent sites (skull, soft tissues of head and neck, vertebral column, etc.). This section will deal only with parenchymal brain metastases. Clinical series estimate that 53% of brain metastases are multiple, though autopsy examination would suggest an even higher frequency.[55,63,64] Lung cancer more typically presents with multiple rather than single brain metastases. Although synchronous presentations are not uncommon, the usual occurrence in lung cancer is that of metachronous presentation. In contrast to other histologies (breast, colorectal), the time interval to the development of brain metastases is relatively short in lung cancer.[56] Without treatment, the median survival for all patients is four to eight weeks.[65] With active therapy, the median survival is increased to three to six months, with measurable if modest one- and two-year survival rates. For example, of 1,292 patients with CT-documented brain metastases, the survival rates at six months, one year, and two years were 36%, 12%, and 4%, respectively. The authors identified performance status, response to steroids, systemic tumor activity, and serum LDH as independent prognostic factors with the strongest impact on survival, second only to treatment modality. Patients treated with steroids only had a 1.3-month median survival, while those receiving radiation had a 3.6-month median survival.[66] The presence of symptoms related to the primary lung tumor has also been associated with a poorer outcome.[67] The RTOG has identified a series of prognostic factors for patients with brain metastases from all causes (Table 58.7).[68] The presence of four favorable prognostic factors is associated with a 52% predicted probability of surviving six months (10% of patients), while the absence of any of these factors is associated with a dismal prognosis—less than 10% chance of six-month survival. Approximately 10% to 15% of patients will live more than one year, emphasizing the need for careful patient selection and appropriate choice of therapy so as to minimize long-term morbidities in such patients.

Presentation

The diagnosis of brain metastases in cancer patients is based upon patient history, neurologic examination, and diagnos-

TABLE 58.7. PROGNOSTIC FACTORS IN BRAIN METASTASES

- Karnofsky Performance Status (70–100)
- Status of primary (absent or controlled)
- Patient age (under 60 years)
- Histology (breast better than other)
- RTOG Neurologic function (class I = 6.6 months versus class IV = 1.2 months)
- Brain only site of metastasis (4.8 months versus 3.4 months)
- Number of metastases (single versus multiple and under 4 versus 4 or more)

tic radiologic procedures. Patients may describe headaches (over 50%), focal weakness (40%), seizures (15%), loss of sensation, or difficulties with gait or balance.[56] Often, however, patients are brought by family members or friends who have noticed the patient's lethargy, emotional lability, or personality change. Physical examination may demonstrate objective neurologic signs, but often only minor cognitive signs are present. The definitive diagnosis cannot be based solely on clinical examination alone, because the presenting symptoms and signs are not distinct from those of other intracranial space–occupying lesions. In addition, metabolic disturbance, carcinomatous meningitis, and paraneoplastic conditions may also present with CNS symptomatology, and these must be distinguished. CT and MRI scanning are the most sensitive and specific diagnostic tests.[69] They are useful not only for diagnosis but also for treatment planning (surgery as well as radiation), to follow response, and to detect recurrence or complications of therapy.

Management

Prompt and often urgent intervention is required in the management of brain metastases to avoid or minimize progressive neurologic injury. It is far more effective to prevent neurologic deterioration than to regain deficits already lost. The quality of survival is greatly improved if clinical control of intracranial metastases is achieved. Initial management is generally directed at controlling raised intracranial pressure (ICP) if present. Steroid preparations (dexamethasone, methylprednisone, prednisone) are rapidly effective (six to 48 hours) and have long been the cornerstone of initial management.[70,71] The use of steroids alone is associated with a modest survival benefit (2.5 months median) when compared with no treatment. A common regimen is dexamethasone 4 to 6 mg q.i.d. (per oram [po] or intravenously) with or without a loading dose of 10 mg. Equivalent dosages of other steroids may be used. Higher doses are sometimes effective where lower doses have failed. This is especially true in the treatment of chronically raised ICP in patients with end-stage disease.[72,73] After radiation, steroids are tapered to the lowest dose necessary to suppress neurologic symptoms, and can often be discontinued. No specific tapering schedule is preferred, and the clinician must judge on an individual basis. Other maneuvers to reduce ICP, including diuretics (furosemide, mannitol) and hyperventilation, are far less frequently required in general oncologic practice and will not be further discussed here.[56] Not all patients will show clinical evidence of raised ICP, and therefore many patients may be safely managed with radiation therapy without the use of steroids. Anticonvulsant therapy (phenytoin, carbamazepine) is recommended only if seizures occur, and is not required on a generalized basis.

Radiation Therapy of Brain Metastases

Therapeutic irradiation is used in virtually all referred patients with brain metastases, either as primary therapy or as an adjunct to surgical excision of a single lesion. The basis for the use of radiation is outlined in Table 58.8.

The commonest technique is the use of whole-brain external-beam irradiation, generally administered using 4 to 6 MV photons from a linear accelerator. [60]Co teletherapy is also appropriate. Opposed lateral technique with customized shielding of the ocular lens and soft tissues of the oropharynx and anterior neck is preferred by some. The inferior margin may be placed at the base of brain, but for ease of possible future field matching this border may also be placed to include the second cervical vertebra. The optimal time dose and fractionation schedule has been studied by the RTOG in a series of randomized prospective clinical trials.[74,75] All schedules studied were comparable in terms of frequency of improvement of symptoms and time to progression, but the duration of response and rate of complete disappearance of neurologic symptoms were not as good for ultrarapid schedules using one or two large fractions. Even where more favorable prognostic patients were evaluated using more protracted radiation courses (50 Gy in four weeks) no advantage was seen over the shorter treatment schedules.[68,76] Relatively little data exists on the long-term toxicity of these treatment regimens for obvious reasons. One report suggests a 10% to 15% dementia rate amongst long-term survivors treated with 30 Gy in two weeks.[77] More recently the RTOG has evaluated accelerated fraction-ated radiation schedules at 1.6 Gy b.i.d. to doses up to 54.4 Gy, and found improvements in survival (not reaching statistical significance) at the higher dose levels, with acceptable toxicity rates.[13] This higher dose will now be the subject of a randomized comparison versus standard therapy. Until the results of this and similar studies are available, the standard recommended time dose fraction schedule for palliative whole-brain radiotherapy in the United States continues to be 20 to 30 Gy in five to 10 fractions over one to two weeks. These are cost-effective regimens offering maximal palliative benefit with acceptable long-term morbidity rates.

The Solitary Brain Metastasis

Solitary lesions account for 30% to 50% of all cases of brain metastases.[24,63] There is emerging evidence in selected patients that surgical resection with postoperative whole-brain radiotherapy offers a potential survival benefit.[8,78–84] Patients with cancer and single metastases to the brain who receive treatment with surgical resection and postoperative radiotherapy have fewer recurrences of cancer in the brain and are less likely to die of neurologic causes than similar patients treated with surgical resection alone.[85] While the argument for resection is less strong in patients with highly radiosensitive histologies and those with other sites of disease systemically, those patients with a good performance status presenting with metachronous brain metastasis and control of the primary tumor gained maximal benefit from the combined approach. Advances in neuroanaesthesia, surgical technique, and perioperative care have broadened the availability of neurosurgical intervention in this patient population. However, even with such improvements, less than half of the patients with solitary metastases will be able to undergo such an aggressive approach.[86] Factors associated with the best short-term results from the combined approach are listed in Table 58.9.[87] One of the more influential recent studies has been that of Patchell and colleagues[80] which suggested a modest survival benefit with combined surgery and postoperative irradiation versus radiation therapy alone in a selected population with biopsy-confirmed single brain metastases. Of note was that as many as 11% of the patients entered were ineligible because they were found to have other than metastatic lesions (glioma, abscess, etc.), reinforcing the need for biopsy confirmation in the setting. A prolonged median survival (40 versus 15 weeks) and improved local control rate (80% versus 48%) was ini-

---

TABLE 58.8. BASIS FOR RADIATION THERAPY IN BRAIN METASTASES

- Median survival modestly improved to 4 to 6 months
- Selected patients with long-term (1- and 2-year) survival
- Improves symptoms 69% to 90% (RTOG)
- Improvement in KPS of 10 to 20 points
- 2 of 3 of patients with serious neurologic dysfunction improve
- 1 of 3 of patients with moderate neurologic dysfunction improve

---

TABLE 58.9. PROGNOSTIC FACTORS IN SINGLE BRAIN METASTASES

- Preoperative neurologic status
- Presence or absence of systemic disease
- Patient age
- Time interval from primary to metastasis

tially observed in the combined arm. However, by 90 weeks the overall survival in both arms was less than 10%, confirming the still-poor prognosis in these patients irrespective of treatment. Patchell and associates extended these observations in a multicenter randomized trial,[85] noting that recurrence of tumor anywhere in the brain was less frequent in the radiotherapy group than in the observation group (nine [18%] of 49 versus 32 [70%] of 46; p = less than 0.001). Postoperative radiotherapy prevented brain recurrence at the site of the original metastasis (five [10%] of 49 versus 21 [46%] of 46; p = less than 0.001) and at other sites in the brain (seven [14%] of 49 versus 17 [37%] of 46; p = less than 0.01). Patients in the radiotherapy group were less likely to die of neurologic causes than patients in the observation group (six [14%] of 43 who died versus 17 [44%] of 39; p = 0.003). Again, there was no significant difference between the two groups in overall length of survival or the length of time that patients remained functionally independent.

The optimal postoperative radiation technique has not been defined. The initial study by Patchell and associates used whole-brain radiotherapy, 3 Gy per day to 36 Gy. The dose was delivered via opposed laterals using a ^{60}Co machine. One large retrospective review suggested a radiation dose response, with improved results in patients receiving 39 Gy or more (89% local control) versus less than 39 Gy (69% local control) in the adjuvant setting.[79] Another reported treatment schedule with similar results was 2.5 Gy per day to 40 Gy whole-brain, followed by a 10 Gy boost to the metastatic lesion.[8] There is increasing acceptance for the use of combined surgery and postoperative radiation therapy in the management of selected lung cancer patients with isolated intracranial metastases.

Specialized Radiation Techniques in Brain Metastases

Retreatment

Since 30% to 50% of patients with brain metastases will develop progressive or recurrent intracerebral disease, selected patients will be considered for reirradiation. Limited data exist on the use of external beam radiation in retreating patients who have received prior whole-brain therapy.[82] Cooper and colleagues have shown that if patients are carefully selected (Table 58.10), they can benefit from reirradiation, either partial or whole-brain, in dosages up to 25 Gy in 10 fractions.[88] Patients so chosen had a mean survival

TABLE 58.10. SELECTION OF PATIENTS FOR REIRRADIATION

- At least 4 months from initial irradiation
- Neurolgic deterioration as their primary clinical problem

time of 5.6 months posttreatment and demonstrated improved average neurologic function. Less favorable reports show median duration of survival of only two to 3.5 months after retreatment and little improvement in neurologic status, illustrating that the margin of benefit is probably slim and careful patient selection is likely the key factor.[89,90]

Focal Irradiation Including Stereotactic and Brachytherapy Techniques

The ability of these techniques to limit the dose of radiation to surrounding tissues has led to their evaluation in the setting of retreatment of cerebral metastases. Stereotactic "radiosurgery" uses sophisticated computerized techniques to identify targets and to focus multiple nonplanar radiation beams on these targets, allowing the delivery of large (usually single) doses while minimizing irradiation of surrounding tissue. Therapeutic gain is maximal when the ratio of the tumor volume to that of the surrounding normal tissue is large. In practice, small (3.5 cm or less), single, favorably located lesions are suitable for this approach. Therefore the impact of this technique on cerebral metastases, frequently large, and usually multiple, will be limited. However, selected patients with single recurrent lesions appear to benefit.[91,92] A similar rationale, and therefore limitation, holds for the use of brachytherapy in this setting. This approach has been used as a boost technique in selected cases and as retreatment in patients with recurrent disease.[93,94]

Radiation Sensitizers and Chemotherapy

The high response rates of SCLC to chemotherapy has led to the observation of regression of intracerebral metastases in patients responding to primary therapy.[95–97] The response of cerebral metastases to "salvage" chemotherapy is less impressive. The fact that patients presenting with brain metastases as their only site of "extensive"-stage disease fare as well as patients with limited-stage disease is a testament to this phenomenon.[20] The response rates for brain metastases from NSCLC is obviously less striking. No studies address the role of combined chemotherapy or neoadjuvant chemotherapy with radiation.[56] Although responses may occur, this approach cannot yet be endorsed outside of a study setting. Lastly, the use of radiation sensitizers has been evaluated but shown to be of no benefit in the management of the patient with brain metastases.[9,98] There is much need for the investigation and development of novel effective approaches in the management of this important clinical problem.

Bone Metastases and Related Clinical Problems

Incidence

Annually more than 100,000 people in the U.S. suffer with painful bone metastases.[99] Bone metastases occur in 20% to

40% of patients with lung cancer,[100] amounting to almost 70,000 cases in the U.S. in 1993. Lung cancer accounted for one third of the bone metastases in one large autopsy series of patients dying of epithelial neoplasms.[101] The commonest sites are the vertebrae, pelvis, and femora, with the skull and distal extremities being less frequently involved.[101,102] When long bones are involved, it is most usually the metaphyseal and less often the mid-diaphyseal regions which are affected. Pathologic fractures requiring surgical intervention occur in less than 10% of patients with metastatic disease but are an important cause of morbidity in the cancer patient.[103] Interestingly, lung cancer less frequently accounts for such fractures than other histologies, possibly relating to the short life expectancy in this disease.[29]

Pathophysiology and Presentation

Normal bone remodelling is a coupled process balancing resorption by osteoclasts and regrowth by osteoblasts.[104] Bone metastases are either osteolytic, osteoblastic, or mixed. The osteoblastic variety is uncommon in lung cancer and will not be further discussed here. The typical bone metastasis from lung cancer is osteolytic. The mechanism of bone destruction is not completely understood and is the subject of intense research.[29] Evidence is emerging that both tumor cells and bone itself are capable of secreting factors that can stimulate osteoclastic activity. Several of the factors (TGF, OAF, IL-1, IL-6 etc.) are being evaluated as target molecules in the systemic treatment of bone metastases.[104] Skeletal metastases occur via hematogenous spread possibly through a low-pressure venous plexus described by Batson in 1940.[105] The important clinical consequences of bone metastases are pain and bony destruction. The pain is generally well localized, initially intermittent, but eventually constant and unremitting. Depending on the location of the lesion, the pain may be referred to a nearby joint (e.g., "frozen shoulder"), the anterior chest or abdominal wall, or extremity. Bone destruction may compromise the biomechanical strength of the bone and lead to pathologic fracture. The strength of normal bone depends on an intact cortex and underlying medullary system.[29] Typical metastatic lesions destroy a segment of both the cortex and medulla. Cortical defects weaken the bone, especially to torsion or rotational forces. It has been estimated that such a defect whose length is greater than the diameter of the bone may weaken the bone by as much as 90%.[106]

The consequences of pathologic fracture may be severe and debilitating. This is especially true of fractures involving weight-bearing bones, humerus, and the spine, where epidural compression of the spinal cord may be a paralyzing and even a preterminal event. Pathologic fractures from metastases will not heal without anticancer therapy. The rate of subsequent union has been shown to vary with histology (poor in lung metastases), as well as type of intervention (orthopedic, radiotherapy, or chemotherapy) employed.[107]

The following sections will deal with the use of radiation for clinical syndromes common in patients with lung cancer metastatic to bone. Unlike other histologies such as breast and prostate cancer, where systemic treatment with hormonal therapies and novel agents such as bisphosphonates[108,109] and pamidronate[110,111] can bring about valuable responses and palliation, radiation therapy (with or without surgery) is often the only therapeutic option available to lung cancer patients. The aims of such treatment are pain relief, maintenance of normal function including ambulation, and prevention or management of complications of bone destruction such as pathologic fracture or cord compression. At present the role of radiation in preventing the progression of subclinical disease is being explored.

The Radiation Management of Painful Bone Metastasis

Localized Radiotherapy

Focal external-beam radiotherapy is the commonest technique used to treat bone metastases. Factors associated with optimal radiotherapy treatment planning are listed in Table 58.11. It need hardly be stressed that any prior radiation treatments must be accounted for and the portals and techniques used should be reviewed prior to initiating therapy. It is useful practice at simulation to localize any prior portals with reference to skin tattoos and prior documentation, and delineate such portals with a wire placed on skin, to minimize the likelihood for unexpected overlap of radiation fields. The choice of the most appropriate TDF schedule for the palliation of bone metastases is a complex topic. Physician bias influences therapy selection in palliative care.[15,51] Although patients with lung cancer metastatic to bone have a median survival of less than six months and a good outcome is thought less likely with lung than other histologies,[112,113] there is sufficient heterogeneity even in this patient population to warrant careful selection in the choice of technique.

Several retrospective reviews[114–116] and a number of prospective randomized controlled trials, including those of the RTOG and others[112,117–123] are available to document the

TABLE 58.11. RADIATION TREATMENT PLANNING FOR BONE METASTASES

- History and physical examination
- Imaging studies (plain radiography, bone scanning, CT and MR imaging, myelogram, etc.)
- Radiation tolerance of normal structures (bone marrow, spinal cord, brachial plexus, etc.)
- Extent of prior therapy (radiation as well as chemotherapy)
- Target volume based on pathophysiology, prior, and possible future radiation therapy
- Appropriate choice of TDF
- Performance status, availability of resources, etc.

rough equivalence of single-dose to fractionated radiotherapy, as well as a number of multifraction schedules (10 Gy in 2 to 2.7 Gy in 15 fractions). A prospective nonrandomized study has also compared various TDF schemes in this context.[113] A number of general statements may be made. Some 80% to 90% of patients can anticipate at least partial pain relief, irrespective of the schedule used.[29,119] As many as 50% to 62% of patients experience complete pain relief.[112,113] The majority of patients will respond within two to 12 weeks from start of therapy. Some authors have argued for more protracted treatment courses and higher radiation doses, on the basis that they are more likely to produce complete responses with full withdrawal of narcotic medications than shorter courses,[118] a greater likelihood of complete pain relief, and a longer time to progression.[113] A second argument for more protracted treatment points to the increased frequency of reirradiation among patients treated with single doses, inferring less therapeutic effect. However, as has been pointed out by Malawar and Delaney,[29] this may simply reflect the reluctance of radiation oncologists to retreat areas that have received prior high-dose (tolerance dose) schedules. It has been our practice to avoid the use of large single doses of radiation in anatomic locations where potential toxicity to surrounding structures may limit the effectiveness of the therapy. Thus, for bone metastases to the skull and spine, fractionated doses are preferred, minimizing the risk of injury to the brain, spinal cord, and major organs. In the United States, 30 Gy in 10 fractions is probably the commonest schedule used. When very large spinal column fields are required, we have found 30 to 35 Gy in 12 to 14 fractions a useful alternative with acceptable acute gastrointestinal morbidity. Careful individualization is required.

Single or Limited-Number Bone Metastases

As described above, histologic confirmation is frequently required prior to irradiation. Although uncommon in lung cancer, such patients may enjoy relatively long disease-free and overall survival periods.[29] Although no clear evidence of dose response exists in palliating bone metastases, there are suggestions that doses in excess of 40 Gy may be beneficial[124] and may therefore be considered in this circumstance.

Spinal Cord Compression (SCC)

Incidence

After brain metastasis, SCC is the second most common neurologic complication of malignancy and the most common malignant lesion to affect the spinal cord. Lung cancer is its most frequent cause.[125,126] SCC is the commonest radiation emergency in the cancer patient. Although it may be the presenting feature of malignancy in lung cancer, it more typically occurs at an interval following the diagno-

sis.[127] The main determinant of neurological outcome after treatment is the pretreatment neurological status, whereas the prognosis for survival is related more to the underlying disease.[128,129] The relationship between functional outcome and pretreatment neurologic status deserves emphasis. Even with modern approaches, it has been reported that zero to 16% of paraplegic patients will regain ambulatory status with treatment.[130–132] Additionally, in a retrospective analysis of patients with lung cancer and SCC, all ambulatory small cell lung cancer patients retained function with therapy, while only 15% of the nonambulatory small cell patients regained walking ability. Similarly, 95% of patients with non–small cell lung cancers retained ambulatory function, while only 22% of nonambulatory patients were able to walk posttreatment.[133] Early recognition of the problem is essential so that therapy may be initiated and neurologic deterioration avoided.[134,135] Despite increasing awareness of the presenting features of this syndrome among oncologists as well as general physicians, 75% to 80% of patients still present with significant neurologic compromise, and these patients uncommonly recover function even with aggressive multimodal therapy.[129,136] However, it should be borne in mind that with appropriate recognition and treatment, 40% to 60% of patients will remain ambulatory.[126] Posttreatment physical therapy is also important. Functional improvements in mobility and self-care can be obtained and maintained in appropriate patients.[137]

Pathophysiology and Presentation

Although metastases to the cord itself or the epidural space can occur, by far the commonest mode of compression is that due to expansion or collapse of the vertebral body (85%) or neural arch.[126] Lung cancer may also directly invade the spinal column and epidural space, producing SCC.[138,139] With the advent of high-resolution tomography and MRI, cord compression with associated paravertebral mass is being recognized with increasing frequency.[132] The anatomic distribution of SCC reflects the number of vertebral bodies at risk (70% thoracic, 20% lumbosacral, and 10% cervical).[126] Increasing use of MRI in the diagnosis of SCC has highlighted the fact that multiple levels may be involved.[47] The clinical syndrome is summarized in Table 58.12. Pain usually precedes other symptoms and must never be ignored in the cancer patient. Sensory changes may follow or accompany motor loss. Findlay proposed a motor grading system that is useful in categorizing patients pretreatment and predicting outcome (Table 58.13).[131,134]

The evaluation of the patient with SCC must be speedy and decisive. Delay may allow the development of irreversible neurologic deficit. Although 80% of patients will show abnormalities on plain spinal radiography, normal spine films do not exclude epidural metastases. MRI with gadolinium enhancement is now being increasingly recognized as the diagnostic method of choice in SCC (see Table

TABLE 58.12. SPINAL CORD COMPRESSION

- Back pain (90%)
  Localized, aggravated by stooping, coughing, sneezing
  Radicular pain referred to extremities or anterior torso
  New onset or acute worsening
- Spinal tenderness
- Motor weakness
  Flaccid or spastic paresis
  Extensor plantar responses
- Sensory loss
  May begin distally and ascend
  Sensory level to pain and light touch
  Loss of proprioception
- Autonomic dysfunction (late and ominous signs)
  Incontinence of bladder and or bowel
  Loss of rectal tone

TABLE 58.14. MRI ADVANTAGES IN DIAGNOSING/MANAGING SCC

- Excellent sensitivity and specificity rates (over 95%)
- Selected patients may be spared the need for biopsy confirmation
- Noninvasive, avoiding need for lumbar puncture
- Rapid (usually less than 90 minutes)
- Entire spine may be imaged, detecting multiple-level involvement
- Accurate anatomic localization
  intramedullary versus subdural or epidural
  paravertebral masses
- Vital treatment planning information (radiation therapy and surgery)
- Progress and response to treatment

58.14.[126] Figure 58.1 illustrates an algorithm which allows for the practical evaluation of the patient with suspected SCC.

Management of Spinal Cord Compression

Appropriate assessment and management requires close cooperation among subspecializing physicians. Primary physicians and medical oncologists, neurologists, neurosurgeons, orthopedists, and radiation oncologists may all contribute to a successful outcome. It is incumbent on each, however, to be aware of the indications and limitations of the techniques available. Absolute management recommendations cannot be made. However, most patients will require radiation with or without surgical intervention. Selected patients with chemosensitive tumors may also require chemotherapy. Initial therapy generally consists of corticosteroid administration. Steroids can reduce pain and limit neurologic progression prior to definitive therapy. The presumed mechanism of action is reduction of edema. The optimal dose has not been established. Typically 10 mg of dexamethasone given intravenously at diagnosis is followed by 4 mg t.i.d. or q.i.d. (either intravenously or by mouth). There is no clearly established benefit to exceeding these doses, although doses up to 100 mg have been evaluated.[140]

Although a full discussion of the neurosurgical aspects of managing SCC is beyond the scope of this chapter, certain points should be made. The optimal timing of neurosurgical intervention has yet to be defined, but it would

seem logical that, if surgery is contemplated at all, the sooner the better. At least one retrospective review of 84 cases showed improved functional outcome (61.5% versus 25%) if the surgery was performed within 24 hours. Improvement was even seen in patients incontinent and immobile prior to intervention.[141] There has been a reevaluation of the role of posterior laminectomy in the surgical approach to these

TABLE 58.13. FINDLAY MOTOR GRADING SYSTEM IN SCC[134]

Grade I: ambulant with or without use of walking aid
Grade II: paraparetic and nonambulant
Grade III: complete paraplegia

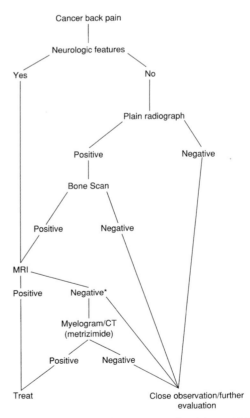

FIGURE 58.1. This figure illustrates an algorithm which allows for the practical evaluation of the patient with suspected SCC.

TABLE 58.15. INDICATIONS TO CONSIDER NEUROSURGERY IN SCC

- Appropriate surgical candidate
- Pathologic fracture of the vertebral body
- Spinal instability
- Compression of the cord by bone fragments in the canal
- Requirement for tissue diagnosis
- Radioresistant primary (progressive deterioration on or following radiation)

patients, and the radiation oncologist must be aware of the indications and contraindications for this procedure. Formerly, when the combined approach was used, laminectomy was the preferred neurosurgical intervention. Some series report good results with this technique.[142] Recent neurosurgical literature, however, emphasizes the importance of a selective operative approach based on the anatomic location of the tumor. Since 85% of epidural compressions are anteriorly located, the focus of the surgery should be the vertebral body.[126] There is evidence that posterior laminectomy may fail to deal adequately with this problem and may in fact worsen the neurologic outcome.[130,134] It has been reported that less than 10% of patients with anteriorly based lesions benefit from laminectomy.[126,143] Removal of the spinal arches in a patient with vertebral body involvement or collapse can greatly increase spinal instability and worsen neurologic function. Anterior approaches can allow stabilization of the spine. Using optimal neurosurgical approaches, as many as 94% of patients retain ambulation after treatment.[126] The indications for neurosurgery in SCC are listed in Table 58.15.

Radiation Management of Spinal Cord Compression

The role of radiation therapy alone in the management of SCC is well established. Retrospective reviews comparing radiation alone versus radiation and surgery combined are fraught with selection bias, precluding meaningful statements regarding the benefit of one versus the other. However, there is evidence of comparability in selected series.[144] Only one small randomized trial of radiation alone versus surgery and radiation has been published, and shows no significant difference between the two.[145] It is hardly surprising that radiation therapy alone is associated with better results in the more radiosensitive malignancies.[144,146] Although SCLC might be expected to exhibit a somewhat better response to radiation than NSCLC, when analyzed, histologic subtype has not proven to be important.[129] A tendency for patients with NSCLC in this study to do better with the combined approach is probably the result of patient selection. In general, response rates to radiation alone in this situation are in the 40% to 60% range. As is true in surgical and combined series, the pretreatment neurologic status is the principle prognostic marker of response to ra-

diation.[126,129] The radiation portal should be based on all available clinical and radiographic information. Paravertebral extension should be included in the portal. Since lung cancer is commonly associated with paravertebral masses, imaging must assess for such problems.[132] By time-honored practice, the typical radiation portal includes the affected vertebral body, including two vertebral bodies above and below. Cervical spine fields are generally arranged laterally and opposed. A single posterior (PA) is used for upper- and mid-thoracic levels, while lower thoracic and lumbosacral lesions may be optimally dosed via the anteroposterior (APPA) approach.

Energy and prescription depths must be individualized. The optimal radiation TDF schedule for spinal cord compression has not been clearly established. Spinal cord tolerance to radiation must be respected, and there is no objective evidence that this tolerance varies from cervical to thoracic levels.[147,148] There appears to be no clear dose response relationship in lung cancer patients irradiated for SCC.[126] Attempts to treat lung cancer patients with associated paravertebral masses to doses of 40 Gy in 16 fractions have yielded no improvement.[132] Limited experimental data in a rat model suggesting a benefit to using large initial fractions (300 to 500 cGy) has no human clinical evidence in support but is a frequently utilized regimen. The standard TDF schedule for radiation therapy alone in lung cancer SCC is 30 Gy in 10 fractions. No clear consensus on the optimal postoperative radiation TDF schedule exists. When the SCC lesion represents the only site of metastatic disease, it has been our practice to employ doses in the 40 to 50 Gy range at standard fractionation, in view of the somewhat better prognosis expected in such cases.

Prevention and Management of Pathologic Fracture

Radiation therapy is capable of halting osteolytic bone destruction and even of promoting reossification in up to 80% of lesions.[149,150] Although pathologic fracture has been thought less commonly a problem in the patient with lung cancer than in osteolytic metastases from other histologies, this clinical issue is frequently presented to the radiation oncologist for consideration. The commonest anatomic locations are the femur and humerus. Both are extremely important clinical issues, since fracture in these locations can bring about major functional impairment. Prognostic factors predicting patients at high risk for subsequent fracture have been published and used as a guide for prophylactic management,[29] both surgical and radiotherapeutic. The question as to whether the patient at high risk for pathologic fracture should be managed surgically or with radiation is a difficult one. Since radiation will take time to bring about reossification, any patient considered at imminent risk for fracture should be considered for surgery. The criteria used for operative repair of lesions of the hip and femur at Memo-

TABLE 58.16. CRITERIA FOR PROPHYLACTIC SURGERY TO PREVENT FRACTURE (MSK)

- Painful intramedullary lytic lesion 50% or more of the cross-sectional diameter of the bone
- Painful lytic lesion involving a length of cortex equal to or greater than the cross-sectional diameter of the bone
- Painful lytic lesion involving a length of cortex 2.5 cm or more in length
- Lesion of bone in which pain is unrelieved after radiation

rial Sloan-Kettering (MSK) have been published (Table 58.16).[151]

Radiographic criteria alone may be insufficient, and Mirels has described a clinico-radiographic scoring system based on four clinical factors (Table 58.17).[152] The author suggests that lesions of the long bones with scores of 7 or less could be irradiated, while those of 8 or more should be fixed surgically with postoperative irradiation.

The principles and techniques for irradiation, be it prophylactic palliation or definitive therapy, do not differ form those relating to bone metastases described above. The entire bone should be evaluated radiographically and with scintigraphy so that coexistant lesions do not go unrecognized. All patients treated with surgical intervention should be irradiated postoperatively to aid in bone healing. Postoperative irradiation is usually commenced two to three weeks after surgery to allow wound healing. Doses of 20 to 30 Gy in 5 to 10 fractions are customary, with boost doses of 600 to 900 cGy where appropriate. As before, the isolated bone lesion may be considered for a more protracted TDF course.

SPECIALIZED RADIOTHERAPEUTIC TECHNIQUES IN BONE METASTASES

Wide-Field and Systemic Irradiation

The ability to deliver tumoricidal doses of ionizing radiation systemically or at least to wider "fields" requiring treatment is an extremely appealing concept in the management of patients with or at high risk of developing overt metastatic

TABLE 58.17. SCORING SYSTEM FOR PATHOLOGIC FRACTURES

	Score (Range 3–12)		
Factor	1	2	3
Site	Upper limb	Lower limb	Peritrochanteric
Pain	Mild	Moderate	Functional
Lesion	Blastic	Mixed	Lytic
Size*	<1/3	1/3–2/3	>2/3

* Relative to the diameter of the bone.

disease. Radiation remains the most effective single anticancer agent in solid malignancies. However, the toxicities of such approaches have traditionally rendered them less desirable in this context in the opinion of most clinicians. The use of "hemibody" irradiation (HBI) or sequential double-hemibody irradiation (DHBI), either in single or multiple fractions, is not new.[153–156] With the advent of radioprotectors such as interleukin-1 and nitroxides,[157,158] along with recombinant growth factors allowing a degree of bone marrow protection, the use of HBI/DHBI with these agents is enjoying a revival in the investigative management of systemic malignancies. Included are those cancers affecting bone marrow (multiple myeloma and non-Hodgkin's lymphoma) as well as bone metastases from solid malignancies (primarily prostate and breast).

Although response rates are less than those usually expected from fractionated local-field irradiation (complete responses 20% and partial responses 50%), the pain relief may be rapid (24 to 48 hours). The use of fractionated (30 Gy in 10 fractions) versus single-dose (600 to 800 cGy in 1 fraction) may be more effective in terms of time to and duration of response, as well as toxicity, but offered no survival benefit where evaluated.[155] The optimal fractionation scheme for HBI has not yet been defined but has been evaluated by the RTOG in a phase I-II trial.[156] The dose-limiting toxicity appeared to be hematological, but gastrointestinal toxicities were also significant.

The RTOG also assessed the role of wide-field irradiation in delaying the progression of subclinical disease. A randomized prospective study found that the addition of wide-field to local irradiation delayed the onset of new disease in the targeted hemibody field, with a doubling of time to progression (6.3 to 12.6 months).[10] The same investigative approach was used in the evaluation of radionuclides in the therapy of bone metastases. Injectable radionuclides such as phosphorus-32, strontium-89, iodine-131-diphosphonates, rhenium-186, and samarium-153 are bone-seeking compounds which have been shown to be effective in relieving pain from bone metastases.[159] Much attention has been recently focussed on strontium-89 (^{89}Sr). Randomized comparisons of local field irradiation and local field plus ^{89}Sr have shown a benefit in terms of improvements in quality of life and reduction in analgesic requirements, as well as delaying the requirement for further radiotherapy in prostate cancer.[160,161] Current trials are evaluating the combination of HBI/DHBI with radionuclides and may bring about improvements applicable to treatment of bone metastases from lung cancer.

PALLIATING LOCOREGIONAL PROBLEMS IN LUNG CANCER

Superior Vena Cava Syndrome (SVCS)

Modern reports show that obstruction to the flow of blood through the superior vena cava is due to intrathoracic malig-

TABLE 58.18. COMMON SYMPTOMS AND SIGNS IN SVCS

- Dyspnea aggravated by lying flat
- Facial swelling/fullness
- Cough
- Sensation of fullness in chest
- Orthopnea
- Venous distension of neck and chest wall
- Facial swelling and plethora

nancy in almost 90% of cases.[162] Lung cancer (usually the right lung) is the commonest malignant cause, accounting for 70% of all cases.[163,164] Although SVCS occurs in less than 5% of all patients with lung cancer,[165,166] it is an important syndrome requiring recognition and relatively urgent management. Small cell (40%) and squamous cell (25%) are the commonest histologic culprits.[163,167] The SVC is a large, thin-walled vessel in the middle mediastinum and is intimately related to the right bronchus, hilum, and paratracheal lymph nodes, draining the entire right and left lower thoracic contents. It is not surprising, therefore, that it is vulnerable to compression in lung and other intrathoracic malignancies. The rapidity of onset of the obstruction is an important determinant of the type of clinical syndrome produced. Rapid occlusion of the vessel produces acute and at times dramatic clinical signs. Gradual occlusion allows time for the development of collateral vessels. This syndrome has been modeled in animals.[168] The commonest presenting symptoms and signs are listed in Table 58.18. It is important to bear in mind that the syndrome varies from an acute and dramatic presentation to a more insidious and indolent picture. Frequently, the facial and neck swelling may be apparent only on comparing appearances with an old photograph or driver's license. Although SVC has long been considered a "medical emergency," it should be emphasized that in general the only threat to the patient's life is when the patient's airway is impeded, either from the mass itself, from laryngeal edema secondary to venous hypertension, or from raised intracranial pressure.

Diagnosis and Management of SVCS

The practice of irradiating the patient with SVCS without a tissue diagnosis is inappropriate.[23,163,169] The presence of SVCS itself does not preclude a curative therapeutic strategy. The prognosis of this syndrome is strongly correlated with that of its underlying cause. On assessing the patient clinically, particular attention should be paid to the presence of airway compromise, since this will guide the diagnostic approach and therapy. The chest radiograph is usually although not invariably abnormal.[170] CT and MRI scanning provide valuable anatomic detail and staging information as well as vital detail for treatment planning. The majority

of patients with SVCS present prior to an established tissue diagnosis.[169] Some tissue diagnoses may be obtained by sputum cytology, thoracentesis, and bone marrow and lymph node biopsy, with positivity rates of 23% to 67%.[163] However, bronchoscopy, mediastinoscopy, and even thoracotomy may be required. Recent series point to acceptable complication rates where these tests have been employed.[171–173] Although radiation is frequently employed in the management of this syndrome, other therapeutic options are often appropriate. Chemotherapy may be the preferred initial option in patients with SCLC (see below), and has been used successfully in patients with recurrent disease.[174] Stenting has been used successfully in selected cases.[175–178] Even long-standing lesions can be successfully recanalized.[179] Extended surgical resections in cases of NSCLC with direct invasion on the SVC can also be effective.[180]

The optimal initial management for the patient with small cell lung cancer and SVCS is generally combination chemotherapy, although radiation has been used in selected series. There is no difference in outcome or time to resolution between the two,[163,167] but chemotherapy offers the advantage of simultaneous management of systemic disease and avoidance of large-field irradiation to the heart and lung. Resolution of the syndrome is prompt (seven to 10 days) and is achieved in 43% to 100% of cases.[181,182] One randomized study in small cell patients with SVCS assessed the value of radiation versus chemotherapy in patients initially managed with chemotherapy and found no benefit to the radiation in this circumstance.[183]

Radiation Management of SVCS in Lung Cancer

Radiation is generally central to the management of the patient with NSCLC and SVCS. Initial treatment with 2 to 4 fractions of 300 to 400 cGy has been advocated,[163] based on limited evidence suggesting a more prompt response with this schedule.[166] The choice of higher initial radiation fractions has also been advocated in patients with poor performance status.[184] However, the optimal TDF schedule in SVCS has not been established, and there is no clinical data to suggest a dose response in terms of the final dose required. Where possible, all locoregional disease, including involved hilar and supraclavicular regions, with appropriate margins should be treated. Failure of resolution of SVCS despite optimal management should prompt the search for ancillary problems such as intravascular coagulation within the SVC itself. Refractory or recurrent SVCS, especially in the patient who has received prior radiation, may require the placement of an expandable or rigid stent to reestablish patency.[175–178,185] Sharp recanalization might also be effective in these circumstances.[179] Neoadjuvant chemotherapy is of uncertain and untested value in this circumstance; however, it is not without potential merit.

Locoregional Problems in Lung Cancer

Up to 70% of patients with lung cancer present with problems related to locoregional disease. Both at presentation and relapse, locoregional symptoms are of major importance in this tumor. Radiation represents the most active agent available in the management of these problems. The use of brachytherapy techniques, both low- and high-dose rate, are increasingly popular in this context. A detailed discussion of these is seen in Chapter 49. As with other palliative issues, radiation response rates are available from a variety of studies (mostly retrospective) within a heterogeneous patient population. Therefore individualization is required, and the results quoted should be used as a rough guide only. The major symptoms and response rates are presented in Table 58.19. Randomized studies of a variety of TDF schedules in the palliative management of locally advanced NSCLC have shown equivalent survivals on the whole, irrespective of the technique used.[186-188] Typically, approximately 25% of patients experience complete relief of symptoms, while almost 50% obtain partial but measurable improvements. The duration of this palliation is generally meaningful, and persists for more than half of the expected life of the patient.[188,189] Selected retrospective reviews have shown symptom response rates equivalent to those quoted from these larger randomized studies.[189,190] As discussed in above, the final choice of TDF schedules in the palliatve care of the patient with lung cancer varies significantly from physician to physician and country to country.[15] Since these patients have limited median survivals (generally six months) and there is no evidence of improvement in survival, response rates, time to, and duration of response, shorter TDF schedules are generally preferred. Doses of 30 to 35 Gy at 250 to 300 cGy per fraction are generally considered standard in the United States, while 17 Gy in two fractions (one week apart) is gaining favor in Britain. The significant rates of local relapse have made the issue of re-treatment of locoregional disease a recently addressed issue. In general, 20 to 30 Gy using 200 cGy fractions may be safely administered to mediastinal and lung fields, with selected patient benefit.

TABLE 58.19. PALLIATING LOCOREGIONAL PROBLEMS IN LUNG CANCER

Symptom	Frequency	Improved	Complete Relief
▪ Cough	61%–93%	56%–65%	30%–54%
▪ Hemoptysis	31%–47%	81%–86%	74%–82%
▪ Dyspnoea	54%	—	37%
▪ Pain	42%–57%	74%	50%–52%
▪ Atelectasis/infection	26%	—	62%
▪ Hoarseness/TVC	25%	—	49%
▪ Dysphagia	11%	—	—

Results from randomized RTOG and MRC trials. From Bleehan N. Inoperable non–small cell lung cancer (NSCLC): a Medical Research Council randomized trial of palliative radiotherapy with two fractions or ten fractions. *Br J Cancer* 1991;63:265; and Majid OA, Lee S, Khushalani S, et al. The response of atelectasis from lung cancer to radiation therapy. *Int J Radiat Oncol Biol Phys* 1986;12:231, with permission.

REFERENCES

1. Boring CC, Squires TS, Tong T. Cancer statistics 1993. *CA Cancer J Clin* 1993;43:7.
2. Minna JD, Pass HI, Glatstein E, et al. Cancer of the lung. In: *Cancer, principles and practice of oncology.* Devita V, Hollman S, and Rosenberg S, eds. 3rd ed. Philadelphia, JB Lippincott 1989;1:591.
3. Smart J. Can cancer of the lung be cured by radiation alone? *JAMA* 1966;195:1034.
4. Cox JD, Komaki R, Byhardt RW. Is immediate chest radiotherapy obligatory for any or all patients with limited-stage non–small cell carcinoma of the lung? Yes. *Cancer Treat Rep* 1983;67:327.
5. Cohen M. Is immediate radiation therapy indicated for patients with unresectable non–small cell lung cancer? No. *Cancer Treat Rep* 1983;67:333.
6. Haffty BG. Can lung cancer be cured with irradiation alone? *Int J Radiation Biol Phys* 1992;24:181.
7. Mulshine JL, Glatstein E, Ruckdeschel JC. Treatment of non–small cell lung cancer. *J Clin Oncol* 1986;4:1704.
8. Sause WT, Crowley JJ, Morantz R, et al. Solitary brain metastases: results of an RTOG/SWOG protocol evaluation surgery + RT versus RT alone. *Am J Clin Oncol* 1990;13:427.
9. Komarnicky LT, Phillips TL, Martz K, et al. A randomized phase III protocol for the evaluation of misonidazole combined with radiation in the treatment of patients with brain metastases (RTOG-7916). *Int J Radiat Oncol Biol Phys* 1991;20:53.
10. Poulter CA, Cosmatos D, Rubin P, et al. A report of RTOG 8206: a phase III study of whether the addition of single dose hemibody irradiation to standard fractionated local field irradiation is more effective than local field irradiation alone in the treatment of symptomatic osseous metastases. *Int J Radiat Oncol Biol Phys* 1992;23:207.
11. MRC. A Medical Research Council (MRC) randomised trial of palliative radiotherapy with two fractions or a single fraction in patients with inoperable non-small-cell lung cancer (NSCLC) and poor performance status. Medical Research Council Lung Cancer Working Party. *Br J Cancer* 1992;65:934.
12. Spanos WJJ, Perez CA, Marcus S, et al. Effect of rest interval on tumor and normal tissue response—a report of phase III study of accelerated split course palliative radiation for advanced pelvic malignancies (RTOG-8502). *Int J Radiat Oncol Biol Phys* 1993;25:399.
13. Sause WT, Scott C, Krisch R, et al. Phase I/II trial of accelerated fractionation in brain metastases RTOG-8528. *Int J Radiat Oncol Biol Phys* 1993;26:653.
14. Russell AH, Clyde C, Wasserman TH, et al. Accelerated hyperfractionated hepatic irradiation in the management of patients with liver metastases: results of the RTOG dose escalating protocol. *Int J Radiat Oncol Biol Phys* 1993;27:117.
15. Maher EJ. The influence of national attitudes on the use of radiotherapy in advanced and metastatic cancer, with particular reference to differences between the United Kingdom and the United States of America: implications for future studies. *Int J Radiat Oncol Biol Phys* 1991;20:1369.
16. Line DH, Deeley TJ. The necropsy findings in carcinoma of the bronchus. *Br J Dis Chest* 1971;64:238.
17. Matthews MJ, Kanhouwa S, Pickren J, et al. Frequency of resid-

ual and metastatic tumor in patients undergoing curative surgical resection for lung cancer. *Cancer Chemother Rep* 1973;4:63.

18. Matthews MJ. Problems in morphology and behavior of bronchopulmonary malignant disease. In: *Lung cancer: natural history, prognosis and therapy.* New York, Academic Press 1976;23.

19. Fadul C, Misulis KE, Wiley RG. Cerebellar metastases: diagnostic and management considerations. *J Clin Oncol* 1987;5:1107.

20. Carmichael J, Crane JM, Bunn PA, et al. Results of therapeutic cranial irradiation in small cell lung cancer. *Int J Radiat Oncol Biol Phys* 1987;14:455.

21. Matthews MJ, Gazdar AF. Pathology of small cell carcinoma of the lung and its subtypes. A clinico-pathologic correlation. *Lung Cancer* 1981;1:283.

22. Escalante CP. Causes and management of superior vena cava syndrome. *Oncology* 1993;7:61.

23. Sullivan FJ. Causes and management of superior vena cava syndrome. The Escalente article reviewed. *Oncology* 1993;7:71.

24. Delattre JY, Krol G, Thaler HT, et al. Distribution of brain metastases. *Arch Neurol* 1988;45:741.

25. McNeil BJ. Value of bone scanning in neoplastic disease. *Semin Nuc Med* 1984;14:277.

26. Stabler A, Krimmel K, Seiderer M, et al. The nuclear magnetic resonance tomographic differentiation of osteoporotic and tumor related vertebral fractures. The value of subtractive TR gradient-echo sequences, STIR sequences and Gd-DTPA. *Rofo Fortschr Geb Rontgenstr Neuen Bildgeb Verfahr* 1992;157:215.

27. Leibel SA, Guse C, Order SE, et al. Accelerated fractionation radiation therapy for liver metastases: selection of an optimal patient population for the evaluation of late hepatic injury in RTOG studies. *Int J Radiat Oncol Biol Phys* 1990;18:523.

28. Finkelstein DM, Ettinger DS, Ruckdeschel JC. Long term survivors in metastatic non small cell lung cancer: An Eastern Cooperative Group Study. *J Clin Oncol* 1986;4:702.

29. Malawar MM, Delaney TF. Treatment of metastatic cancer to bone. In: *Cancer, principles and practice of oncology,* 4th ed. 1993; 2:2225.

30. Wilner D. Cancer metastasis to bone. In: *Radiology of bone tumors and allied disorders.* Philadelphia, WB Saunders 1982; 3641.

31. Goris ML, Bretille J. Skeletal scintigraphy for the diagnosis of malignant metastatic diseases of bone. *Radiother Oncol* 1985;4: 319.

32. Smith RE, Berg D, Hansen RM. Computerized tomography in metastatic evaluation. *Wis Med J* 1989;88:25.

33. Hirsch FR, Osterlind K, Jensen LI, et al. The impact of abdominal computerized tomography on the pretreatment staging and prognosis of small cell lung cancer. *Ann Oncol* 1992;3:469.

34. Dragani M, Ciccotosto C, Storto ML, et al. Bronchogenic carcinoma staging: comparison of magnetic resonance/computerized tomography. *Radiol Med (Torino)* 1992;84:372.

35. Levin AB. Experience in the first 100 patients undergoing computerized tomography-guided stereotactic procedures utilizing the Brown-Roberts-Wells guidance system. *Appl Neurophysiol* 1985;48:45.

36. Beutel EW, Frank SJ, Loren A, et al. A useful technique for computerized tomography directed needle biopsy. *Surg Gynecol Obstet* 1986;162:491.

37. Hitchcock E. Stereotactic-computerized tomography interface device. *Appl Neurophysiol* 1987;50:63.

38. Earnest FT, Ryu JH, Miller GM, et al. Suspected non–small cell lung cancer: incidence of occult brain and skeletal metastases and effectiveness of imaging for detection—pilot study. *Radiology* 1999;211:137.

39. Verger E, Conill C, Vila A, et al. Contribution of magnetic resonance imaging in the early diagnosis of epidural metastasis. *Med Clin (Barc)* 1992;99:329.

40. Greco A. The role of magnetic resonance imaging in an oncology centre. *Radiol Med (Torino)* 1990;79:593.

41. Offenbacher H. The diagnostic impact of magnetic resonance imaging on the evaluation of suspected spinal cord disease. *Wien Klin Wochenschr* 1992;104:589.

42. Carmody RF, Yang PJ, Seeley GW, et al. Spinal cord compression due to metastatic disease: Diagnosis with MR imaging versus myelography. *Radiology* 1989;173:225.

43. Li KC, Poon PY. Sensitivity and specificity of MRI in detecting malignant spinal cord compression and in distinguishing malignant from benign compression fractures of vertebrae. *Magn Reson Imaging* 1988;6:547.

44. Kattapuram SV, Khurna JS, Scott JA, et al. Negative scintigriphy with positive magnetic resonance imaging in bone metastases. *Skeletal Radiol* 1990;19:113.

45. Chadwick DJ, Gillatt DA, Mukerjee A, et al. Magnetic resonance imaging of spinal metastases. *J R Soc Med* 1991;84:196.

46. Aitchison FA, Poon FW, Hadley MD, et al. Vertebral metastases and an equivocal bone scan: value of magnetic resonance imaging. *Nucl Med Commun* 1992;13:429.

47. Lien HH, Blomlie V, Heimdal K. Magnetic resonance imaging of extradural tumors with acute spinal cord compression. *Acta Radiol* 1990;31:187.

48. Golfieri R, Cherryman GR, Olliff JF, et al. Comparative evaluation of computerized tomography/magnetic resonance (1.5 T) in the detection of brain metastasis. *Radiol Med (Torino)* 1991; 82:27.

49. Flentje M, Zierhut D, Schraube P, et al. Integration of coronal magnetic resonance imaging (MRI) into radiation treatment planning of mediastinal tumors. *Strahlenther Onkol* 1993;169: 351.

50. Layer G, Jarosch K. Magnetic resonance tomography of the bone marrow for the detection of metastases of solid tumors. *Radiologe* 1992;32:502.

51. Coia LR, Owen JB, Maher EJ, et al. Factors affecting treatment patterns of radiation oncologists in the United States in the palliative treatment of cancer. *Clin Oncol (R Coll Radiol)* 1992; 4:6.

52. Maher EJ. The use of palliative radiotherapy in the management of breast cancer. *Eur J Cancer* 1992;28:706.

53. Lawton PA, Maher EJ. Treatment strategies for advanced and metastatic cancer in Europe. *Radiother Oncol* 1991;22:1.

54. Duncan G, Duncan W, Maher EJ. Patterns of palliative radiotherapy in Canada. Division of Radiation Oncology, BCCA, Vancouver, Canada. *Clin Oncol (R Coll Radiol)* 1993;5:92.

55. Posner JB. Brain metastases: A clinicians view. *Brain metastases* 1980;2.

56. Wright DC, Delaney TF, Buckner JC. Treatment of metastatic cancer to the brain. In: *Cancer, principles and practice of oncology,* 4th ed. Philadelphia, JB Lippincott 1993;2:2170.

57. Boring CC, Squires TS, Tong T. Cancer statistics, 1992. *CA Cancer J Clin* 1992;42:19.

58. Ginsberg RJ, Kris MG, Armstrong JG. Non–small cell lung cancer. In: *Cancer, principles and practice of oncology,* 4th ed. 1993;1:673.

59. Nugent JL, Bunn PAJ, Matthews MJ, et al. CNS metastases in small cell bronchogenic carcinoma: increasing frequency and changing pattern with lengthening survival. *Cancer* 1979;44: 1885.

60. Komaki R, Cox JD, Whitson W. Risk of brain metastases from small cell carcinoma of the lung related to length of survival and prophylactic irradiation. *Cancer Treat Rep* 1981;65:811.

61. Order SE, Hellman S, VonEssen CF, et al. Improvement in quality of survival following whole brain irradiation for brain metastases. *Radiology* 1968;91:149.

62. Hendrickson F. The optimum schedule for palliative radiother-

apy for metastatic brain cancer. *Int J Radiat Biol Phys* 1977;2: 165.

63. Posner JB, Chernik NL. Intracranial metastases from systemic cancer. *Adv Neurol* 1978;19:575.

64. Hildebrand J. Lesions of the nervous system in cancer patients. Monograph series of the European Organization for the Research and Treatment of Cancer 1978;5,1.

65. Lang EFJ, Slater J. Metastatic brain tumors. results of surgical and non-surgical treatment. *Surg Clin North Am* 1964;44:865.

66. Lagerwaard FJ, Levendag PC, Nowak PJ, et al. Identification of prognostic factors in patients with brain metastases: a review of 1292 patients. *Int J Radiat Oncol Biol Phys* 1999;43:795.

67. Sen M, Demiral AS, Cetingoz R, et al. Prognostic factors in lung cancer with brain metastasis. *Radiother Oncol* 1998;46(1): 33.

68. Diener-West M, Dobbins TW, Phillips TL, et al. Identification of an optimal subgroup for treatment evaluation of patients with brain metastases using RTOG study 7916. *Int J Radiat Oncol Biol Phys* 1989;16:669.

69. Sze G, Milano E, Johnson C, et al. Detection of brain metastases: Comparison of contrast-enhanced MR with unenhanced MR and enhanced CT. *Am J Neuroradiol* 1990;11:785.

70. Galicich JH, French LA, Ueki K, et al. Use of dexamethasone in the treatment of cerebral edema associated with brain tumors. *Lancet* 1961;81:46.

71. French LA. The use of steroids in the treatment of cerebral edema. *Bull N Y Acad Med* 1966;42:301.

72. Ehrenkranz JRL, Posner JB. Adrenocorticosteroid hormones. In: *Brain metastases.* 1980;340.

73. Samuals MA. *Manual of neurologic therapeutics: with essentials of diagnosis,* 3rd ed. 1986;1.

74. Borgelt B, Gelber R, Kramer S, et al. The palliation of brain metastases: Final results of the first two studies by the Radiation Therapy Oncology Group. *Int J Radiat Oncol Biol Phys* 1980; 6:1.

75. Borgelt B, Gelber R, Larson M, et al. Ultra rapid high dose irradiation schedules for the palliation of brain metastases: final results of the first two studies by the Radiation Therapy Oncology Group. *Int J Radiat Biol Phys* 1981;7:1633.

76. Kurtz JM, Gelber R, Brady LW, et al. The palliation of brain metastases in a favorable patient population: a randomized clinical trial by the Radiation Therapy Oncology Group. *Int J Radiat Oncol Biol Phys* 1981;7:891.

77. Posner JB. Management of central nervous system metastases. *Semin Oncol* 1977;4:81.

78. Mandell L, Hilaris B, Sullivan M, et al. The treatment of single brain metastasis from non–oat cell lung carcinoma. *Cancer* 1986;58:641.

79. Smalley SR, Schray MF, Laws ER, et al. Adjuvant radiation therapy after surgical resection of brain metastasis: Association with patterns of failure and survival. *Int J Radiat Oncol Biol Phys* 1987;13:1611.

80. Patchell RA, Tibbs PA, Walsh JW, et al. A randomized trial of surgery in the treatment of single metastases to the brain. *N Eng J Med* 1990;322:494.

81. Amornmarn R, Prempree T, Ostrowski ML, et al. Long term survival of lung cancer with brain metastasis. *J Fla Med Assoc* 1990;77:659.

82. Buckner J. Surgery, radiation therapy, and chemotherapy for metastatic tumors to the brain. *Curr Opin Oncol* 1992;4:518.

83. Mussi A, Pistolesi M, Lucchi M, et al. Resection of single brain metastasis in non-small-cell lung cancer: prognostic factors. *J Thorac Cardiovasc Surg* 1996;112:146.

84. Hwang SL, Howng SL. Prognostic analysis in patients of lung cancer with brain metastasis under surgical removal. *Kao Hsiung I Hsueh Ko Hsueh Tsa Chih* 1998;14:126.

85. Patchell RA, Tibbs PA, Regine WF, et al. Postoperative radiotherapy in the treatment of single metastases to the brain: a randomized trial. *JAMA* 1998;280(17):1485.

86. Patchell RA, Cirrincone C, Thaler HT, et al. Single brain metastasis: surgery plus radiation or radiation alone. *Neurology* 1986; 36:447.

87. Galicich JG, Sundaresan N, Arbit E, et al. Surgical treatment of single brain metastasis: Factors associated with survival. *Cancer* 1980;45:381.

88. Cooper JS, Steinfeld AD, Lerch IA. Cerebral metastases: value of reirradiation in selected patients. *Radiology* 1990;174:883.

89. Kurup P, Reddy S, Hendrickson FR. Results of re-irradiation for cerebral metastases. *Cancer* 1980;46:2587.

90. Hazuka MB, Kinzie JJ. Brain metastases: results and effects of re-irradiation. *Int J Radiat Oncol Biol Phys* 1988;15:433.

91. Loeffler JS, Kooy HM, Wen PY, et al. The treatment of recurrent brain metastases with stereotactic radiosurgery. *J Clin Oncol* 1990;8:576.

92. Coffey RJ, Flickenger JC, Bissonette DJ, et al. Radiosurgery for solitary brain metastases using the cobalt 60 gamma unit: methods and results in 24 patients. *Int J Radiat Oncol Biol Phys* 1991;20:1287.

93. Heros DO, Kasdon DL, Chun M. Brachytherapy in the treatment of recurrent solitary brain metastases. *Neurosurgery* 1988; 23:733.

94. Prados M, Leibel S, Barnett CM, et al. Interstitial brachytherapy for metastatic brain tumors. *Cancer* 1989;63:657.

95. Lee JS, Murphy WK, Glisson BS, et al. Primary chemotherapy of brain metastasis in small-cell lung cancer. *J Clin Oncol* 1987; 7:916.

96. Twelves CJ, Souhami RL, Harper PG, et al. The response of cerebral metastases in small cell lung cancer to systemic chemotherapy. *Br J Cancer* 1989;61:147.

97. Postmus PE, Haaxma-Reiche H, Sleijfer DT, et al. High dose etoposide for brain metastases of small cell lung cancer. A phase II study. *Br J Cancer* 1989;59:254.

98. DeAngelis LM, Mandell LR, Thaler HT, et al. The role of postoperative radiotherapy after resection of single brain metastases. *Neurosurgery* 1989;24:798.

99. American Cancer Society. *Cancer facts and figures—1992.* Atlanta, American Cancer Society 1992;1.

100. Napoli LD, Hansen HH, Muggia FM, et al. The incidence of osseous involvement in lung cancer, with special reference to the development of osteoblastic changes. *Radiology* 1973;108: 17.

101. Abrams HL, Spiro R, Goldstein N. Metastases in carcinoma. Analysis of 1000 autopsied cases. *Cancer* 1950;23:74.

102. Clain A. Secondary malignant disease of bone. *Br J Cancer* 1965; 19:15.

103. Higinbotham NL, Marcove RC. The management of pathologic fractures. *J Trauma* 1965;5:792.

104. Garrett IR. Bone destruction in cancer. *Semin Oncol* 1993;20: 4.

105. Batson OV. The function of the vertebral veins and their role in the spread of metastases. *Ann Surg* 1940;112:138.

106. Pugh J, Sherry H, Futterman B, et al. Biomechanics of pathologic fractures. *Clin Orthop* 1982;169:109.

107. Gainor BJ, Buchert P. Fracture healing in metastatic bone disease. *Clin Orthop* 1983;178:297.

108. Lipton A. Bisphosphonates and breast carcinoma. *Cancer* 1997; 80:1668.

109. Coleman RE. How can we improve the treatment of bone metastases further? *Curr Opin Oncol* 1998;10:S7.

110. Hortobagyi GN, Theriault RL, Porter L, et al. Efficacy of pamidronate in reducing skeletal complications in patients with

breast cancer and lytic bone metastases. Protocol 19 Aredia Breast Cancer Study Group. *N Engl J Med* 1996;335:1785.

111. Coukell AJ, Markham A. Pamidronate. A review of its use in the management of osteolytic bone metastases, tumour-induced hypercalcaemia and Paget's disease of bone. *Drugs Aging* 1998; 12:149.

112. Tong D, Gillick L, Hendrickson FR. The palliation of symptomatic osseus metastases: Final results of the Radiation Therapy Oncology Group. *Cancer* 1982;50:893.

113. Arcangeli G, Giovinazzo G, Saracino B, et al. Radiation therapy in the management of symptomatic bone metastases: the effect of total dose and histology on pain relief and response duration. *Int J Radiat Oncol Biol Phys* 1998;42:1119.

114. Vargha ZO, Glicksman AS, Boland J. Single-dose radiation therapy in the palliation of metastatic disease. *Radiology* 1969; 93:1181.

115. Penn CRH. Single dose and fractionated palliative irradiation for osseus metastases. *Clin Radiol* 1976;27:405.

116. Qasim MM. Single dose palliative irradiation for bony metastases. *Strahlentherapie* 1977;153:531.

117. Madsen EL. Painful bony metastases: efficacy of radiotherapy assessed by the patients: a randomized trial comparing 4 Gy × 6 versus 10 Gy × 2. *Int J Radiat Oncol Biol Phys* 1983;9:1775.

118. Blitzer PH. Reanalysis of the RTOG study of the palliation of symptomatic osseus metastases. *Cancer* 1985;55:1468.

119. Price P, Hoskin PJ, Easton D, et al. Prospective randomized trial of single and multifraction radiotherapy schedules in the treatment of painful bony metastases. *Radiother Oncol* 1986;6: 247.

120. Cole DJ. A randomized trial of single treatment versus conventional fractionation in the palliative radiotherapy of painful bone metastases. *Clin Oncol* 1989;1:59.

121. Niewald M, Tkocz HJ, Abel U, et al. Rapid course radiation therapy vs. more standard treatment: a randomized trial for bone metastases. *Int J Radiat Oncol Biol Phys* 1996;36:1085.

122. Gaze MN, Kelly CG, Kerr GR, et al. Pain relief and quality of life following radiotherapy for bone metastases: a randomised trial of two fractionation schedules. *Radiother Oncol* 1997;45: 109.

123. Nielsen OS, Bentzen SM, Sandberg E, et al. Randomized trial of single dose versus fractionated palliative radiotherapy of bone metastases. *Radiother Oncol* 1998;47:233.

124. Arcangeli G, Micheli A, Arcangeli G, et al. The responsiveness of bone metastases to radiotherapy: the effect of site, histology, and radiation dose on pain relief. *Radiother Oncol* 1989;14:95.

125. Bruckman JE, Bloomer WD. Management of spinal cord compression. *Semin Oncol* 1978;5:135.

126. Delaney TF, Oldfield EH. Spinal cord compression. In: DeVita VT, Hellman S, Rosenberg SA. *Cancer: principles and practice of oncology,* 4th ed. Philadelphia, JB Lippincott 1993;2:2118.

127. Stark RJ, Henson RA, Evans SJW. Spinal metastases: a retrospective survey from a general hospital. *Brain* 1982;105:189.

128. Bach F, Larsen BH, Rohde K, et al. Metastatic spinal cord compression. Occurrence, symptoms, clinical presentations and prognosis in 398 patients with spinal cord compression. *Acta Neurochir* 1990;107:37.

129. Bach F, Agerlin N, Sorensen JB, et al. Metastatic spinal cord compression secondary to lung cancer. *J Clin Oncol* 1992;10: 1781.

130. Findlay GF. Adverse effects of the management of spinal cord compression. *J Neurol Neurosurg Psychiatry* 1984;47:761.

131. Leviov M, Dale J, Stein M, et al. The management of spinal cord compression: a radiotherapeutic success ceiling. *Int J Radiat Oncol Biol Phys* 1993;27:231.

132. Kim RY, Smith JW, Spencer SA, et al. Malignant epidural spinal cord compression associated with a paravertebral mass: its radio-

133. Bach F, Agerlin N, Sorensen JB, et al. Metastatic spinal cord compression in patients with lung cancer. *Ugeskr Laeger* 1996; 158:5606.

134. Findlay GF. The role of vertebral body collapse in the management of spinal cord compression. *J Neurol Neurosurg Psychiatry* 1987;50:151.

135. Sorensen PS, Borgeson SE, Rohde K, et al. Metastatic spinal cord compression. Results of treatment and survival. *Cancer* 1990;65:1502.

136. Kim RY, Spencer SA, Meredith RF, et al. Extradural spinal cord compression: analysis of factors determining functional prognosis—prospective study. *Radiology* 1990;176:279.

137. McKinley WO, Conti-Wyneken AR, Vokac CW, et al. Rehabilitative functional outcome of patients with neoplastic spinal cord compressions. *Arch Phys Med Rehabil* 1996;77:892.

138. Nori D, Sundaresan N, Bains M, et al. Bronchogenic carcinoma with invasion of the spine. Treatment with combined surgery and perioperative brachytherapy. *JAMA* 1982;248:2491.

139. Armstrong JG, Fass DE, Bains M, et al. Paraspinal tumors: techniques and results of brachytherapy. *Int J Radiat Oncol Biol Phys* 1991;20:787.

140. Vecht CJ, Haaxma-Reiche H, VanPutten WLJ, et al. Initial bolus of conventional versus high-dose dexamethasone in metastatic spinal cord compression. *Neurology* 1989;39:1255.

141. Harris JK, Sutcliff JC, Robinson NE. The role of emergency surgery in malignant spinal extradural compression: assessment of functional outcome. *Br J Neurosurg* 1996;10:27.

142. Landmann C, Hunig R, Gratzl O. The role of laminectomy in the combined treatment of metastatic spinal cord compression. *Int J Radiat Oncol Biol Phys* 1992;24:627.

143. Hall AJ, MacKay NNS. The results of laminectomy for compression of the cord and cauda equina by extradural malignant tumor. *J Bone Joint Surg Br* 1973;55:497.

144. Gilbert RW, Kim JH, Posner JB. Epidural spinal cord compression from metastatic tumor: diagnosis and treatment. *Ann Neurol* 1978;3:40.

145. Young RF, Post EM, King GA. Treatment of epidural metastases. Randomized prospective comparison of laminectomy and radiotherapy. *J Neurosurg* 1980;53:741.

146. Mones RJ, Dozier D, Berrett A. Analysis of medical treatment of malignant extradural spinal cord tumors. *Cancer* 1966;19: 1842.

147. Marcus RB, Million RR. The incidence of myelitis after irradiation of the cervical spinal cord. *Int J Radiat Oncol Biol Phys* 1990;19:3.

148. Schultheiss TE. Spinal cord radiation "tolerance": Doctrine versus data. *Int J Radiat Oncol Biol Phys* 1990;19:219.

149. Greenberg EJ, Chu FCH, Dwyer AJ, et al. Effects of radiotherapy on bone lesions as measured by 47-Ca and 85-Sr local kinetics. *J Nucl Med* 1972;13:747.

150. Unger JD, Chiang FC, Unger GF. Apparent reformation of the base of the skull following radiotherapy for nasopharyngeal carcinoma. *Radiology* 1978;126:779.

151. Lane JM, Sculco TP, Zolen S. Treatment of pathologic fractures of the hip by endoprosthetic replacement. *J Bone Joint Surg Am* 1980;62:954.

152. Mirels H. Metastatic disease in long bones. A proposed scoring system. *Clin Orthop* 1989;249:256.

153. Fitzpatrick PJ, Rider WD. Half-body radiotherapy. *Int J Radiat Oncol Biol Phys* 1976;1:197.

154. Salazar OM, Rubin P, Hendrickson FR, et al. Single-dose halfbody irradiation for palliation of multiple bone metastases from solid tumors: Final Radiation Therapy Oncology Group report. *Cancer* 1986;58:29.

155. Zelefsky MJ, Scher HI, Forman JD, et al. Palliative hemiskeletal irradiation for widespread metastatic prostate cancer: A comparison of single dose and fractionated regimens. *Int J Radiat Oncol Biol Phys* 1989;17:1281.

156. Scarantino CW, Caplan R, Rotman M, et al. A phase I/II study to evaluate the effect of fractionated hemibody irradiation in the treatment of osseous metastases—RTOG-8822. *Int J Radiat Oncol Biol Phys* 1996;36:37.

157. Mitchell JB, DeGraff W, Kaufman D, et al. Inhibition of oxygen-dependent radiation-induced damage by the nitroxide superoxide dismutase mimic, Tempol. *Arch Biochem Biophys* 1991;289:62.

158. Hahn SM, Tochner Z, Krishna MC, et al. Tempol, a stable free radical, is a novel murine radiation protector. *Cancer Res* 1992;52:1750.

159. Porter AT, Chisholm GD. Palliation of pain in bony metastases. *Semin Oncol* 1993;20:1.

160. Porter AT, McEwan AJB, Powe JE, et al. Results of a randomized phase III trial to evaluate the efficacy of strontium-89 adjuvant to local field external irradiation in the management of endocrine resistant metastatic prostate cancer. *Int J Radiat Oncol Biol Phys* 1993;25:805.

161. Porter AT, McEwan AJB. Strontium-89 as an adjuvant to external beam radiation improves pain relief and delays disease progression in advanced prostate cancer: results of a randomized controlled trial. *Semin Oncol* 1993;20:38.

162. Fincher RE. Superior vena cava syndrome: experience in a teaching hospital. *South Med J* 1987;80:1243.

163. Yahalom J. Superior vena cava syndrome. In: *Cancer, principles and practice of oncology,* 4th ed. Philadelphia, JB Lippincott 1993;2:2111.

164. Markman M. Diagnosis and management of superior vena cava syndrome. *Cleve Clin J Med* 1999;66:59.

165. Salsali M, Cliffton EE. Superior vena caval obstruction in carcinoma of the lung. *N Y State J Med* 1969;69:2875.

166. Armstrong BA, Perez CA, Simpson JR, et al. Role of radiation in the management of superior vena cava syndrome. *Int J Radiat Oncol Biol Phys* 1987;13:531.

167. Chan RH, Dar AR, Yu E, et al. Superior vena cava obstruction in small-cell lung cancer. *Int J Radiat Oncol Biol Phys* 1997;38:513.

168. Carlson HA. Obstruction of the superior vena cava: an experimental study. *Arch Surg* 1969;29:669.

169. Schraufnagel DE, Hill R, Leech JA, et al. Superior vena caval obstruction. Is it an emergency? *Am J Med* 1981;70:1169.

170. Parish JM, Marschke RF, Dines DE, et al. Etiologic considerations insuperior vena cava syndrome. *Mayo Clin Proc* 1981;56:407.

171. Lewis RJ, Sisler GE, Mackenzie JW. Mediastinoscopy in advanced superior cava obstruction. *Ann Thorac Surg* 1981;32:458.

172. Ahmann FR. A reassessment of the clinical implications of the superior vena cava syndrome. *J Clin Oncol* 1984;2:961.

173. Cosmos L, Haponek EF, Dariak JJ, et al. Neoplastic superior vena caval obstruction: diagnosis with percutaneous needle aspiration. *Am J Med Sci* 1987;293:99.

174. Taira N, Shinozaki Y, Kawai T, et al. Palliation for a recurrent lung cancer patient with superior vena cava syndrome by arterial infusion of CDDP through the implantable port system—a case report. *Gan To Kagaku Ryoho* 1999;26:531.

175. Wilkinson P, MacMahon J, Johnston L. Stenting and superior vena caval syndrome. *Ir J Med Sci* 1995;164:128.

176. Michel-Behnke I, Hagel KJ, Bauer J, et al. Superior caval venous syndrome after atrial switch procedure: relief of complete venous obstruction by gradual angioplasty and placement of stents. *Cardiol Young* 1998;8:443.

177. Laing AD, Thomson KR, Vrazas JI. Stenting in malignant and benign vena caval obstruction. *Australas Radiol* 1998;42:313.

178. Hochrein J, Bashore TM, O'Laughlin MP, et al. Percutaneous stenting of superior vena cava syndrome: a case report and review of the literature. *Am J Med* 1998;104:78.

179. Farrell T, Lang EV, Barnhart W. Sharp recanalization of central venous occlusions. *J Vasc Interv Radiol* 1999;10:149.

180. Fukuse T, Wada H, Hitomi S. Extended operation for non–small cell lung cancer invading great vessels and left atrium. *Eur J Cardiothorac Surg* 1997;11:664.

181. Dombernowsky P, Hansen HH. Combination chemotherapy in the management of superior vena caval obstruction in small cell anaplastic of the lung. *Acta Med Scand* 1978;204:513.

182. Maddox AM, Valdivieso M, Lukeman J, et al. Superior vena cava obstruction in small cell bronchogenic carcinoma. *Cancer* 1983;52:2165.

183. Spiro SG, Shah S, Harper PG, et al. Treatment of obstruction of the superior vena cava by combination chemotherapy with and without irradiation in small cell carcinoma of the bronchus. *Thorax* 1983;38:501.

184. Egelmeers A, Goor C, van Meerbeeck J, et al. Palliative effectiveness of radiation therapy in the treatment of superior vena cava syndrome. *Bull Cancer Radiother* 1996;83:153.

185. Putnam JS, Uchida BT, Antonovic R, et al. Superior vena cava syndrome associated with massive thrombosis: treatment with expandible wire stents. *Radiology* 1988;167:727.

186. Simpson J, Francis M, Perez-Tamayo R, et al. Palliative radiotherapy for inoperable carcinoma of the lung: Final report of the RTOG multi-institutional trial. *Int J Radiat Oncol Biol Phys* 1988;11:751.

187. Teo P, Tai T, Choy D, et al. A randomized study on palliative radiation therapy for inoperable non–small cell carcinoma of the lung. *Int J Radiat Oncol Biol Phys* 1988;14:867.

188. Bleehan N. Inoperable non–small cell lung cancer (NSCLC): a Medical Research Council randomized trial of palliative radiotherapy with two fractions or ten fractions. *Br J Cancer* 1991;63:265.

189. Collins TM, Ash DV, Close HJ, et al. An evaluation of the palliative role of radiotherapy in inoperable carcinoma of the bronchus. *Clin Radiol* 1988;39:284.

190. Majid OA, Lee S, Khushalani S, et al. The response of atelectasis from lung cancer to radiation therapy. *Int J Radiat Oncol Biol Phys* 1986;12:231.

SPECIAL CONSIDERATIONS

59

MALIGNANT PLEURAL EFFUSION

FRANK A. BACIEWICZ, JR

The discovery of a pleural effusion is a common clinical problem. The most frequent cause for a pleural effusion is an underlying malignancy.[1] Lung cancer is the most common cause of malignant effusion, followed by breast cancer and lymphoma.[2] Pleural effusions have been reported to occur in up to 50% of patients with breast cancer,[2] in about 25% of patients with lung cancer[3] and a third of patients with lymphoma.[4] These tumors are responsible for nearly 75% of all malignant pleural effusions. The remaining malignancies include the gastrointestinal tract, genitourinary tract, melanoma, mesothelioma, sarcoma, thyroid, and leukemia. Adenocarcinoma of the lung is the most frequent pulmonary malignancy-causing effusion. The primary tumor is unknown in 15% of patients.

Pleural effusions may be the presenting sign or symptom of the carcinoma or they may occur near the terminal period of the illness. Survival following presentation is related to the primary tumor. Survival is usually limited to months with lung carcinoma but in patients with breast cancer, survival can be much longer.

Since the patient presents with dyspnea and pleuritic pain, treatment of malignant pleural effusion is an important component of therapy. In addition, the respiratory distress may compound the anxiety the patient has due to the malignancy. Even if the patient's disease process cannot be cured, treatment of malignant pleural effusion will not only improve his or her symptoms but alter his or her emotional state. Prompt and efficacious treatment of malignant pleural effusion will not only contribute to patient well-being but decrease time of hospitalization and cost to the health care system.

PATHOPHYSIOLOGY OF MALIGNANT PLEURAL FLUID FORMATION

Anatomy of the Pleura

The parietal pleural receives its blood supply from the intercostal arteries and is drained by systemic intercostal and bronchial veins. The visceral pleural receives its blood supply from the bronchial (systemic) circulation.[5] Its venous drainage is via the subvisceral pleural capillaries into the pulmonary veins.

Lymphatic drainage[6] of the parietal pleura drains into both internal mammary nodes anteriorly and intercostal nodes posteriorly. The anterior and posterior mediastinal nodes also receive drainage from the diaphragmatic pleural lymphatics. The lymph from the visceral pleura flows centripetally toward the hilum. The lymph eventually reaches the right lymphatic trunk or the thoracic duct, which empties into the junction of the left internal jugular and subclavian veins.

Mesothelial cells form the lining of the parietal and visceral pleura. In addition stomata, 2 to 12 mm, form openings between the mesothelial cells. They are centered over the lymphatic channels. Stomata are the entry point of pleural fluid, particulate matter and protein from the parietal pleural space. Through the stomata there is a direct communication to the lymphatic channels. No communication exists between the lymphatics and the visceral pleura and the pleural space.

Normal Pleural Fluid Formation

Pleural fluid formation had been thought to be dependent on the visceral and parietal pleural hydrostatic and colloid oncotic pressures. Following Starling's law,[7] the pleural fluid formation was the result of the mean capillary hydrostatic pressure minus the capillary colloid oncotic pressure which favored the movement of fluid from the parietal pleura into the pleural space (Figure 59.1). These forces also favored the reabsorption of fluid from the pleural space to the visceral pleura. Based on these calculations, there was a net movement of pleural fluid from the parietal pleura to the visceral pleura. The protein within the pleural space was cleared by the lymphatic system. Given this application of Starling's law, the rate of pleural fluid and protein production was thought to be as high as 7 L per day.[8]

These concepts have been updated recently.[6,9] The parietal pleura has assumed the major role in movement of pleural fluid. The parietal pleura, which is only 10 to 20 microns from the visceral pleura, produces 100 to 200 mL of fluid per 24 hours. Since the visceral pleural microcapil-

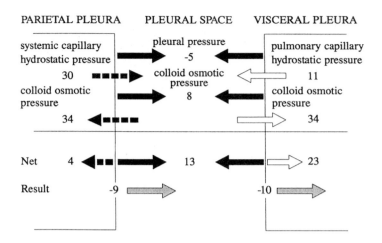

FIGURE 59.1. Net flow of protein-free fluid in accordance with Starling's law and assuming that the visceral pleura is supplied by pulmonary circulation. Pressures are provided in cm H_2O.

laries are removed from the visceral surface, they play only a minimal role in reabsorption of pleural fluid. Conceptually the pleural fluid can be thought of as being in continuity with the parietal pleura interstitium.

The current concept is that the parietal systemic capillaries produce a low-protein filtrate which enters the parietal pleura interstitium and then passes through the mesothelial cells into the pleural space. The protein content of the fluid in the pleural space is about 1.5 grams per dl.[10] The stomata lining of the parietal pleura allow the exit of pleura fluid, particulate matter, and protein from the pleural space. This passes into the lymphatic channels. Lymphatic fluid in the pleural space has a large reserve of up to 500 mL. With the equal entry and exit of fluid from the pleural space there is no accumulation of fluid (Figure 59.2).

Mechanisms of Abnormal Pleural Fluid Formation

Abnormal pleural fluid formation can be due to single or multiple etiologies. Changes in the hydrostatic or colloid oncotic pressure can result in transudative effusions.[11,12] Clinical scenarios including hypoalbuminemia, atelectasis, or congestive heart failure produce transudative effusions.

The usual cause of malignant pleural effusion is changes in the lymphatic drainage from the pleural space.[3,13] The etiology may be tumor obstruction of the parietal pleura stomata, mediastinal node involvement with impaired lymphatic drainage, or increased parietal capillary permeability due to lymphangitic tumor spread. The extent of metastatic pleural involvement does not correlate with the development of pleural effusion.[14] Pleural implants can alter capillary permeability by their production of vasoactive peptides.

Malignant pleural effusions are usually secondary to pulmonary artery invasion[12] by lung cancer and embolization of tumor cells to the visceral pleura with subsequent seeding of the pleural space. More peripheral lesions may have direct involvement of the pleural space. Direct extension from breast carcinoma involving the chest wall can cause malignant pleural effusion.

Pleural effusions can also be caused by factors that do not directly involve the pleural space.[15] Changes in the hydrostatic pressure from cardiac or pericardial disease or superior vena cava syndrome can be the underlying reason for pleural effusion. Mediastinal and chest radiation can impair lymphatic drainage and be the cause of pleural effusion. Pneumonic processes such as lung atelectasis can alter the pleural pressure. Communication from malignant ascites through diaphragmatic lymphatic channels can also cause secondary malignant pleural effusion. Conditions such as cirrhosis, connective tissue diseases, and hypoalbuminemia may also affect the rate of pleural fluid production and need to be considered when therapeutic interventions are made.

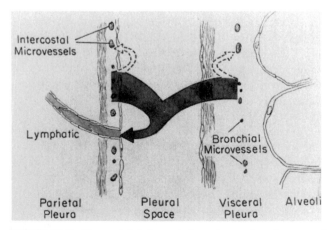

FIGURE 59.2. The parietal pleura is the primary site of entry and exit of fluid and protein. (From Broaddus C, Staub NC. Pleura liquid and protein turnover in health and disease. *Semin Respir Med* 1987;9:7, with permission.)

CLINICAL MANIFESTATIONS

Characteristics of Malignant Pleural Effusions

At the time of presentation, 77% of patients with malignant pleural effusions have symptoms. A malignant pleural effusion is the initial presentation in up to 90% of patients with primary or metastatic pleural malignancy.[16,17]

The most common respiratory symptom is shortness of breath. Dry cough and pleuritic chest pain are other commonly voiced complaints. The cough is a result of the underlying lung atelectasis and chest pain is due to the inflammation of the parietal pleura. Ipisilateral shoulder discomfort may be present when there is diaphragmatic parietal pleura involvement.

On physical examination there is dullness to percussion in the lower aspect of the thorax and with a larger pleural effusion there is dullness over the entire thorax. Breath sounds in the area of the effusion will be decreased. The effusion may also elicit a change in the character of the transmitted sound. Atelectasis of the compressed lung may result in hyperresonance above the fluid level due to distended alveolar air space. Below the fluid there may be loud bronchial breathing.

With significant tumor involvement of the chest wall there may be restricted expansion or intercostal fullness. The trachea may deviate to or away from the side of the effusion. The trachea is shifted away from the side of the pleural fluid when the malignant effusion is secondary to breast or ovarian carcinoma. When the trachea shifts toward the pleural effusion, the most likely etiology is carcinoma of the lung with either complete or partial bronchial obstruction.

The patients with an advanced stage of the malignant disease will have weight loss, appear cachetic, and feel chronically tired.

DIAGNOSIS

Radiologic Assessment

A chest radiograph is usually the initial test in a patient who presents with respiratory symptoms or physical examination suggestive of pleural effusion. The chest x-ray can demonstrate a varied appearance, with blunting of the costophrenic angle, a concave meniscus, disappearance of the diaphragmatic shadow, an apical cap, or fluid in the intralobar fissure. An upright chest film can demonstrate blunting of the costophrenic angle with as little as 175 mL of fluid.[18] A lateral chest x-ray can detect as little as 100 mL of fluid, and decubitus films can demonstrate free from loculated fluid collection. Decubitus films can also assist in diagnosis of some pulmonic effusions. Subpulmonic effusions are suggested when there is increased space between the inferior

surface of the left lower lobe and the gastric air bubble on an upright chest film.[19]

Pulmonic effusion can sometimes be confused with atelectasis. Pulmonic effusion can cause mediastinal shift to the contralateral side, while atelectasis produces a shift in the mediastinum toward the same side. When the mediastinum is fixed in the case of a mesothelium or a patient with significant mediastinal adenopathy, this radiologic finding may not be helpful.

Computerized tomography (CT) can help distinguish between effusion, atelectasis, or pleural-based tumor. The Housefield units may distinguish between pleural effusions which have a density of 20 units compared with tumors or solid lesions which have higher Housefield units.[20] The Housefield units cannot differentiate between different causes of the pleural fluid. CT can distinguish or actively define loculated fluid collections and assess mediastinal adenopathy, which is important in determining treatment.

Characteristics of Malignant Pleural Effusion

A typical malignant pleural effusion is grossly bloody and exudative in nature. However, only 30% to 60% of bloody effusions are malignant.[21] Other possible diagnoses include infection (tuberculosis) and pulmonary infarction. The effusions are bloody because of tumor involvement of blood vessels, tumor occlusion of systemic or pulmonary veins, or parietal pleural capillary dilation secondary to the release of vasoactive substances from the primary tumor.

The effusion usually has a leukocyte count of 1,000 to 10,000. The cells are usually lymphocytes.[22] If neutrophils are the dominant cells, the pleural effusion is most likely inflammatory.

Eight-five percent of malignant effusions are exudates. Exudates characteristically have a pleural-to-serum-protein ratio greater than 0.5, pleural lactic dehydrogenase (LDH)-to-serum LDH ratio greater than 0.6, and a pleural fluid LDH level of greater than 200 international units.[23,24] Exudative effusions can also have a low pH (less than 7.30) and a pleural glucose serum glucose ratio less than 0.5. Patients who are found to have a malignant effusion with a pH of less than 7.3 and a low pleural-to-serum-glucose ratio (less than 0.5) usually have a shortened survival and do not respond well to therapeutic intervention for the malignant effusion.[25]

Adenocarcinoma of the lung or ovary may have an elevated amylase detected in the pleural fluid.[26] If the malignant pleural effusion is a transudate, it is usually early in the course of the malignant process. The transudates are usually related to mediastinal lymphatic involvement with impaired lymphatic drainage.

If thoracic duct flow is decreased either due to direct tumor invasion, obstruction, or from tumor emboli, chylothorax can occur. The malignancies most frequently associated with a chylothorax include lymphoma, lymphosarcoma, and bronchogenic carcinoma.

The pleural fluid has a characteristic milky appearance. The chylothorax has specific gravity between 1.012 and 1.025, lymphocytes of 400 to 7,000 per mL, fat of 4 to 5 grams per dL, cholesterol/triglyceride ratio of less than 1, a total protein of 2 to 6 grams per dL, albumin of 1 to 4 grams per dL, glucose of 50 to 100 mg per dL, and electrolytes identical to that in serum.

Cytology

The most straightforward way of making a diagnosis of a malignant pleural effusion is with thoracentesis. The procedure is usually done at the bedside after placing 1% lidocaine in the skin and intercostal space through which the thoracentesis will be performed. If the effusion is loculated or the patient has had a previous thoracotomy requiring precise localization of the fluid, the thoracentesis may be performed under CT scan or echographic direction. The patient's prothrombin, coagulation studies, and platelet count should be normal prior to doing thoracentesis.

A minimal sample of 250 mL should be removed and sent to the laboratory for examination. The samples may be cytocentrifuged and air dried or prepared as wet mounts with toluidine blue or 95% alcohol. Any cell blocks should undergo paraffin imbedding and sectioning. Malignant cells are recognized by clusters or single malignant cells. These cells will characteristically be pleomorphic, large, have a prominent nucleus with large nucleolus, and have a high nuclear-to-cytoplasmic ratio.[27] Adenocarcinoma of the lung is most commonly responsible for a positive malignant pleural effusion.[13,28]

The thoracentesis fluid may also be subjected to immunochemical testing using monoclonal antibodies, polyclonal antisera to epithelial membrane antigen, carcinoembryonic antigen (CEA), and IGG 1 antibody B72-3. There is a positive reaction to the CEA antisera in 50% and to the polyclonal antisera in 54% of malignant effusions.[29] Adenocarcinoma of the lung, breast, and ovary have a positive reaction to the IGG 1 antibody B72-3 in 100% of malignant effusions.[30,31] Other monoclonal antibodies that demonstrate a positive reaction with malignant cells include HMFG-2, AUA-1, Mbr, and Mov 2.

The laboratory is able to establish a diagnosis from 50% of patients with malignant effusion on initial thoracentesis. With a second thoracentesis, diagnosis is obtained in up to 65% of patients, and with a third thoracentesis, diagnosis is made in slightly more than 70% of patients.[32,33] Thoracentesis carries a 3% false-positive diagnosis rate. A pleural biopsy in conjunction with thoracentesis can raise the expected diagnosis of malignant pleural effusion to 80%. By itself, a pleural biopsy has only a 45% successful diagnosis

which may be explained by localized pleural involvement with the malignant process.[34]

When thoracentesis or closed pleural biopsy have not established a diagnosis, thoracoscopy is the next diagnostic alternative. Thoracoscopy allows the direct biopsy of involved areas of the pleura or lung and is nearly 100% sensitive. This procedure requires that the patient have a good performance status, as a general anesthetic is usually administered. Video-assisted thoracoscopy (VATS) will be necessary in only 15% to 20% of patients for diagnosis.[35,36] Thoracoscopy may also allow insertion of a chest tube and sclerosis at the conclusion of the procedure. Localized pleurectomy may also be done at the time of diagnosis. Thoracoscopy is not indicated in patients who have had previous thoracic operations or previous chest radiation or may have loculated fluid collection due to previous thoracentesis or pleural biopsy. These patients may require an open biopsy for diagnosis.

Evaluation of tumor markers in the pleural fluid may became another adjunct to diagnosing malignant pleural effusion. Pleural fluid levels of CEA, creatinine kinase BB, galactosyl transferase, and adenosine deaminase[21,37,38] have been investigated in the pleural fluid. Markers have been neither sensitive or specific enough to establish a diagnosis.[39,40] When thoracentesis is not able to establish a diagnosis, cytogenic testing and chromosome analysis may be useful. Pleural effusion diagnosis using cytogenics has been reported in the range of 65% to 90%.[41-43] These changes have been most frequently abnormal in patients with lymphoma or leukemia.

TREATMENT
Approach

If pleural effusion is noted in a patient with a non–small cell lung cancer, the prognosis is poor. A complete diagnostic evaluation will usually demonstrate that the patient has advanced stage III B to stage IV lung carcinoma. All patients should undergo diagnostic evaluation, as the pleural effusions may be the result of lung atelectasis, congestive heart failure, cirrhosis, hypoalbuminemia, or pulmonary embolus. If even one of these etiologies is present, only 5.5% of patients with lung malignancy and negative pleural effusion are candidates for surgical resection.[44]

Malignant pleural effusion related to lymphoma, small cell carcinoma, or breast carcinoma and treated with systemic therapy may result in resolution of the effusion.[45] If the patient should be symptomatic with one of these diseases that are amenable to systemic therapy, thoracentesis can be performed for relief of symptoms while awaiting the effect of the systemic therapy.

Asymptomatic patients with a malignant effusion (25% to 30% of the patient population) do not need immediate treatment. Seventy-five percent of patients who will be symptomatic need treatment. The treatment must be effective in a short period, not lead to other complications, and have a low recurrence rate, as patients with malignant pleural effusions secondary to lung cancer have an average survival of only 2.2 months.[16] Since the patient's expected overall survival time is low, minimizing hospitalization or avoiding it by keeping the patient mobile and causing minimal distress are important factors when determining treatment.

Thoracentesis

Thoracentesis, in addition to being diagnostic, can also provide the patient with significant therapeutic improvement. Usually no more than 1,000 mL is removed with thoracentesis. Reexpansion pulmonary edema may occur with removal of a greater volume. Thoracentesis may cause vasovagal reaction from irritating the parietal pleura. The physician must have atropine and volume infusion available.[46,47]

After thoracentesis, the effusion will usually recur in 4.2 days[48] and consequently this treatment option is recommended only if the patient has a very short expected life span or is waiting the effect of systemic therapy.

Repeated thoracentesis can result in loculated fluid accumulation, empyema, or pneumothorax. Chemical pleurodesis can be performed through thoracentesis needle but is less effective than pleurodesis via a tube thoracostomy, as there is residual pleural fluid and the lung is not completely reexpanded.

Tube Thoracostomy Alone

The placement of a 28–32 French chest tube will be effective in relieving respiratory symptoms. As with thoracentesis, no more than 1,000 mL should be drained initially and then the tube clamped to avoid pulmonary reexpansion edema. Recurrence rates of 60% to 100% have been reported with tube thoracostomy alone.[49,50]

Tube Thoracostomy and Pleurodesis

Tube thoracostomy with subsequent pleurodesis is the most successful strategy to prevent the recurrence of malignant effusion. The chest tube, a 28–32 French, is inserted through the fifth intercostal space anterior axillary line and directed posteriorly and toward the diaphragm. If the pleural effusion is large, 1,000 mL of fluid is removed and then 500 mL amounts every four hours to prevent reexpansion pulmonary edema. The chest tube is placed to water seal and 20 cm of water suction. This allows for the lung to reexpand completely and the visceral and parietal pleura to come into contact. If the pleura are apposed, adhesion formation can begin.

For the pleurodesis to be successful, the lung needs to

be completely reexpanded with visceral and parietal pleural in contact. There should be no loculated fluid collection in the pleural space which would prevent the sclerosing agent from bathing the pleural space. The sclerosing agent is introduced when there is less than 150 mL of drainage for 24 hours.[22] In addition, the chest x-ray must show absence of the pleural effusion and reexpansion of the lung. In addition to the mechanical pleuritis induced by reexpansion of the lung and the chest tube irritating the pleura, pleurodesis is thought to be successful because of cytoreduction and chemical pleuritis from the sclerosing agent.

When the drainage has met criteria, the sclerosing agent is delivered after premedicating the patient with a narcotic analgesic; 20 mL of 1% lidocaine should be added to the sclerosant for local anesthetic effect. The sclerosing agent is usually instilled in 50 mL of 0.9% normal saline. After instilling the sclerosing agent, the chest tube is clamped and the patient is rotated in the supine position, prone, left and right decubitis positions every fifteen minutes to improve distribution of the sclerosing agent. A publication studying the movement of radiolabeled tetracycline demonstrated that the rotation of the patient did not influence distribution of the sclerosing agent.[51] After the chest tube has been clamped for four hours, the clamp on the chest tube is removed. It is important to leave the chest tube in place for several days after instilling sclerosing agent to further adhesion formation. Usually the chest tube is discontinued when there is less than 150 cc of drainage for 24 hours.[52]

Recently a small pigtail catheter (up to 24 French) has been inserted under CT or echo guidance.[53–55] The catheters have been placed to a drainage bag and the patient's pleural effusion has been drained on an outpatient basis. Prior to removing the pigtail catheter, the sclerosing agent has been inserted. This approach allows the patient to be managed on an outpatient basis with a smaller tube which is more comfortable. In a preliminary trial from Duke University Medical Center, 19 consecutive patients with symptomatic malignant pleural effusions were enrolled. A fluoroscopically placed 10.3 French catheter was connected to a closed gravity drainage bag system. Sclerotherapy was performed when daily drainage was less than 100 mL. The tubes remained in place for two to 11 days (mean, 5.1 days). At 30 days, 10 (53%) patients had a complete response, five (26%) had a partial response, and four (21%) had progressive disease. Problems with this approach have included pneumothoraces requiring regular-sized chest tube insertion, inadequate drainage, and inability to use talc, which is the most effective sclerosing agent, through the small-bore catheter. When the chest tube has been discontinued, a suture is usually placed in the wound to prevent drainage of pleural contents through the chest tube site.

A unique but small, prospective, randomized study has compared pleurodesis using a small percutaneous catheter (10 French) inserted at bedside in patients with recurrent malignant pleural effusion with a conventional large-bore chest tube (24 French) placed in connection with diagnostic thoracoscopy. After drainage, pleurodesis was performed, with tetracycline as sclerosing agent. Of 18 evaluable consecutive patients (mean age 67.8 years), nine were randomized for pleurodesis with the small, and nine with the large catheter. The authors concluded that pleurodesis in patients with recurrent malignant pleural effusion using a small percutaneous catheter had similar efficacy to that obtained with a large-bore chest tube and with less discomfort for the patient. Trials with larger numbers of patients will certainly be necessary to evaluate whether small-bore catheters are as effective and cheaper for the patient during his or her care than the more standard techniques of drainage and sclerosis.[56]

Talc Pleurodesis

A highly effective treatment for recurrent malignant pleural effusions is thoracoscopic talc poudrage. Using either local anesthetic technique with intravenous sedation in a nonintubated patient or general anesthesia with a double lumen endotracheal tube, the 5 gm of talc is instilled over the entire pleural space and lung surface, usually with a simple bulb aspirating syringe. The response rate to thoracoscopic talc insertion is 90% to 96%.[35,57–59] Since this technique has such a high success rate, some physicians recommend it as an initial treatment.

A talc slurry of 5 grams in 250 mL of saline with lidocaine added has been successful in 93% of patients.[60] Complications including pneumonitis and respiratory distress syndrome have been reported.[59–64]

Other Sclerosing Agents

Many agents besides talc have been used as sclerosing agents. Successful response is defined as no reaccumulation on chest x-ray for at least one month after the removal of the chest tube and no need for additional thoracentesis. One of the initial agents, nitrogen mustard, was administered at a dose of 0.4 mg per kg. The response rate was 52% with this agent.[2] The side effects included pain, fever, nausea, vomiting, and bone marrow depression.[65]

Tetracycline had been the agent of choice until 1991 when it was withdrawn from the market as it did not meet the U.S. Food and Drug Administration purity standards. Tetracycline was instilled in a dose of 500 to 1,000 mg, usually diluted in 50 mL of NaCl 0.9% solution with 20 mL of 1% lidocaine. Significant complications included pain in 20% to 70% and fever in up to 33% of the patients.[66–72] Since tetracycline has been withdrawn, doxycycline has been used as a replacement agent in doses of 500 to 1,000 mg. When doxycycline has been instilled, there is a 90% success rate. Doxycycline is a relatively inexpensive sclerosing agent.[73–76]

Bleomycin 60 units dissolved in 100 mL of normal saline has given a response rate of 84%.[2,77,78] Bleomycin was responsible for two deaths and has not been used extensively since it is an expensive sclerosing agent.

Quinacrine has had multiple toxicities including hallucinations, hypotension, and fever.[79] Pain is not a complication with this drug. The usual dose was 800 mg, and instillation through thoracostomy tube gave a 70% to 90% response rate.[80,81]

Other agents include *Corynebacterium parvum*, which elicits an inflammatory response when used as a sclerosing agent. Four mg of *C. parvum* has been used after thoracentesis, as the agent usually requires multiple injections, with 30% of patients needing two injections, 60% three injections, and 10% four injections.[82–86]

Other agents that have been used for pleurodesis include methylprednisolone, doxorubicin,[87,88] cisplatin, cytarabine,[89] etoposide,[90] mitomycin-C,[91] radioisotopes including gold and phosphorus,[49] interferon,[92–94] and interleukin-2.[95–97]

Randomized Trials Comparing the Most Frequently Used Agents

There are few randomized trials comparing treatment for pleural malignancies for a number of reasons. Because life expectancy is limited, a large number of patients must be entered into a trial to have statistically meaningful numbers to analyze response rates. Pleurodesis is seldom an isolated variable, because many patients are simultaneously undergoing chemotherapy or radiotherapy. Moreover, there is no standard method of measuring response, and interpretation of radiologic response may be hindered by underlying lung disease. Because the goal of pleurodesis is palliation, quality-of-life issues, cost, and toxicity must be uniformly assessed.

A review of randomized trials reveals that most consist of small numbers of patients, dosages and administration vary, long-term follow-up is often lacking, and there is no central review of radiologic response. These trials are summarized in Table 59.1.

In the trial by Bayly and colleagues comparing tetracycline (500 mg) to quinacrine (100 mg initially, followed by four daily doses of 200 mg), the agents were equally effective in controlling the pleural effusions (complete response equaled 66%).[98] However, the toxicity of quinacrine was higher.

Gupta and colleagues[99] and Kessinger and Wigton[100] reported that there was no difference between patient responses to bleomycin or tetracycline. Small numbers of patients were evaluable in these studies. However, in the multiinstitutional trial reported by Ruckdeschel and colleagues,[72] 30-day recurrences were significantly less for bleomycin versus tetracycline (36% versus 67%; p = 0.023) and remained less at 90 days (30% versus 53%; p = 0.047). The median time to recurrence was significantly longer for the bleomycin group than for tetracycline. The

TABLE 59.1. RANDOMIZED TRIALS COMPARING SCLEROSING AGENTS

Investigators	Agents	Total Number of Patients	Result
Bayly[98]	TCN Quinacrine	20	Equal
Gupta[99]	Bleo TCN	25	Equal
Fentiman[119]	Nitrogen mustard Talc	46	Talc superior
Leahy[83]	CP TCN	32	Equal
Fentiman[101]	TCN Talc	41	Talc superior
Kessinger[100]	Bleo TCN	34	Equal
Hamed[102]	Bleo Talc	29	Talc superior
Masuno[120]	Doxorubicin Doixorubicin and LC 9018	95	Doxorubicin and LC 9018 superior
Ruckdeschel[72]	Bleo TCN	85	Bleo superior
Hartman[103]	Bleo TCN Talc	99	Talc superior
Patz[121]	Bleo DCN	106	Equal

Bleo, bleomycin; CP, Corynebacterium parvum; TCN, tetracycline, DCN, doxycycline. From Keller SM. Current and future therapy for malignant pleural effusion. *Chest* 1993;103:63S, with permission.

toxicities were low and equal between the two agents. Lung cancer accounted for 34% of the effusions in each group.

The trials reported by Fentiman and associates[101] and Hamed and colleagues[102] are instructive but included only patients with pleural effusions secondary to breast cancer. Leahy and colleagues[83] randomized patients to tetracycline (500 mg) versus *C. parvum* (7 mg) and found no significant difference between prevention of recurrence at one month. However, pain and pyrexia were significantly greater in patients receiving *C. parvum*.

Hartman and colleagues[103] reported a prospective phase II study that evaluated 39 patients undergoing talc insufflation under thoracoscopic guidance, as compared to patients enrolled in a multicenter study evaluating tube drainage followed by administration of either tetracycline (41 patients) or bleomycin (44 patients). Mean time of chest tube drainage was significantly less for the talc group than for patients randomized to bleomycin or tetracycline. Thirty-day success rates were 97% for the talc, 64% for bleomycin, and 32% for tetracycline. The 90-day success rates were 95% for talc, 70% for bleomycin, and 47% for tetracycline.

One of the more recent randomized trials compared the efficacy of bleomycin with doxycycline sclerotherapy using small-bore catheters. In this study, a 14 F self-retaining catheter was inserted into the pleural space and connected to continuous wall suction. When drainage fell below 200 mL per day, patients were randomized to 60 U of bleomycin or 500 mg of doxycycline sclerotherapy. Response at 30 days was determined. Of 106 patients enrolled in the study, 15 men (29%) and 37 women (71%) with a mean age of 57 years received bleomycin sclerotherapy; 21 of the 29 patients (72%) alive and evaluable at 30 days had successful sclerotherapy. Twenty-three men (43%) and 31 women (57%) with a mean age of 61 years received doxycycline sclerotherapy. Twenty-three of the 29 patients (79%) alive and evaluable at 30 days had successful sclerotherapy. There was no significant difference in response rates between doxycycline and bleomycin (p = 0.760).

Other Treatment Modalities

Biologic Response Modifiers

Use of standard treatment for malignant pleural effusions is occasionally not successful, necessiatating novel approaches. Other avenues have been tried, such as intrapleural installation of recombinant interleukin-2 (rIL-2). A response has been recorded in 22% to 50% of the patients.[95,97] Installation of beta-interferon was responsible for a 28% complete response rate in patients with non–small cell malignant effusion.[104] OK-432,[91,105] which is prepared from a substrain of *Streptococcus pyogenes* A3, and LC 9018, prepared from the *Lactobacillus casei* YIT9018,[106] have been able to effect complete responses in up to 70% of patients with protocols requiring more than one injection spaced over several weeks.

Management of the Recurrent or Refractory Malignant Pleural Effusion

When faced with the failure to control a malignant pleural effusion or reaccumulation of fluid after initial success, the need for retreatment should first be reassessed. If life expectancy is short (i.e., a few weeks or less), thoracentesis alone may be appropriate. The clinician must also decide whether the patient's predominant symptoms relate to the presence of pleural fluid and therefore whether expectation of relief warrants reintervention.

Failure of pleurodesis may result from a lung encased in scar or tumor (i.e., trapped lung), loculation of the pleural space by fibrin or adhesions, loss of pulmonary elasticity, high liquid output, or extensive pleural metastases. If the lung is fully expandable, the clinician's first inclination is to repeat the pleurodesis with the same or a different agent. For patients with lungs that do not expand completely, pleural peritoneal shunting or thoracoscopy could be considered.

Pleural Peritoneal Shunting

The first option to consider for patients with recurrent or newly diagnosed pleural effusions *with lung nonexpansion* is pleuroperitoneal shunting.[107–110] The shunt can be placed under general or local anesthetic. It is a unidirectional pumping chamber with connected arms, usually inserted with the pleural arm being in the most inferior aspect of the pleural space. The pumping chamber is placed over a rib or costal margin, and then the peritoneal arm placed through a pursestring suture through a muscle-splitting incision in the abdomen. The Denver or pleuroperitoneal shunt requires a cooperative patient to press the pump consecutively for 10 minutes on four to six occasions during the day. Each compression will propel 1.5 mL of fluid. A cooperative patient is required for its successful use.

There are a number of studies which document the utility of pleuroperitoneal shunting in recurrent effusions.[111–113] Tsang and colleagues[114] achieved good palliation without recurrence of symptoms in 15 of 16 patients. Mean duration of shunt function was 8.6 months. Ponn and colleagues[115] achieved similar results in a group of patients who did not benefit from chemical pleurodesis or who had a trapped lung. This group constituted 4% of patients undergoing treatment for pleural effusion.

Contraindications for placing the Denver pleuroperitoneal shunt include lack of patient cooperation, loculated pleural effusion, peritoneal space which is not free secondary to previous surgery, peritoneal dialysis, pleural infection, or a short life expectancy for the patient. The shunt can become occluded in 10% to 15% of patients with fibrinous material. Shunt occlusion requires revision, usually in the form of total replacement.[116]

Thoracoscopy

When pleurodesis has not been successful or a malignant effusion recurs, thoracoscopy under local or general anesthesia can be used to install talc under direct vision, but only after there is release of a trapped lung from adhesions, or loculated pockets have been obliterated which caused the pleurodesis failure. Since the procedure usually requires general anesthesia, the patient will need to have a high performance status and an acceptable expected long-term survival.[117]

Pleurectomy

Stripping of the parietal pleura has close to a 100% success rate in obliterating malignant effusions. This is a procedure which requires general anesthetic, and consequently the patients must have a high performance status and good prognosis. Few patients with malignant pleural effusion will have a survival rate which rate justifies the 30-day mortality of over 10% and a significant morbidity.[17,48]

Malignant Effusion Discovered at Thoracotomy

When new effusions are recognized at thoracotomy, chest tube placement effectively obliterates the pleural space. Thoracic surgeons have performed localized pleural resection to aid in the obliteration of the pleural space. A study of the infusion of hyperthermic cisplatinum in this setting with an extra corporeal circuit has 100% control of malignant pleural effusions, with patients having a mean survival time of 20 months.[118]

SUMMARY

Treatment of patients with malignant pleural effusions depends on the etiology of the malignancy and the patient's expected survival. Patients with non–small cell lung cancer have an expected survival of only several months, whereas patients with breast cancer have a much longer survival.

The first step is to perform a thoracentesis to establish the diagnosis, if not already known. In patients with short expected survival, thoracentesis alone can provide significant relief. In patients with a better prognosis, drainage of the pleural space with a CT-guided drainage catheter or a standard chest tube is the preferred treatment. After the chest tube drainage is less than 150 mL per day and the lung is in contact with the pleural surface, a sclerosing agent, most often talc 5 grams, can be instilled through a chest tube or drainage catheter. It can be repeated on several occasions if necessary.

If chest tube drainage and pleurodesis are not successful, other treatment options are available. Thoracoscopy can be used to free a trapped lung and break up loculated effusions prior to installation of talc. This treatment modality would require the patient to have an expected lengthy survival. If thoracoscopy is not an option, a pleuroperitoneal shunt can be considered, although our experience has been that these often become occluded.

Under special circumstances pleurectomy can be considered to obliterate the pleural space.

In patients with breast cancer or lymphoma, treatment of the malignancy with chemotherapy and radiation itself may result in resolution of the malignant effusion.

The treatment protocols outlined above are dedicated to improving the patient's symptoms and making them comfortable. The length of the treatment and the time the patient is in the hospital for that treatment figure prominently in the prescribed therapy. For this reason the experience of the clinician is important.

Future trials using small-bore catheters for treatment of malignant effusions, new biological modifiers, and new sclerosing agents may well affect the treatment of malignant effusions. The clinician must keep up to date with these trials and advances in the therapeutic management of the malignant pleural effusion.

REFERENCES

1. Vladutiu A. *Pleural effusion.* Mount Kisco, NY: Futura, 1999.
2. Hausheer FH, Yarbro JW. Diagnosis and treatment of malignant pleural effusion. *Semin Oncol* 1985;12:54.
3. Sahn SA. Malignant pleural effusions. *Clin Chest Med* 1985;6:113.
4. Bruneau R, Rubin P. The management of pleural effusions and chylothorax in lymphoma. *Radiology* 1965;85:1085.
5. Sahn SA. The pathophysiology of pleural effusions. *Annu Rev Med* 1990;41:7.
6. Henschke CI, Davis SD, Romano PM, et al. Pleural effusions: pathogenesis, radiologic evaluation, and therapy. *J Thorac Imaging* 1989;4:49.
7. Kinasewitz GT, Fishman AP. Influence of alterations in Starling forces on visceral pleural fluid movement. *J Appl Physiol* 1981;51:671.
8. Black LF. The pleural space and pleural fluid. *Mayo Clin Proc* 1972;47:493.
9. Wiener-Kronish JP, Goldstein R, Matthay RA, et al. Lack of association of pleural effusion with chronic pulmonary arterial and right atrial hypertension. *Chest* 1987;92:967.
10. Agostoni E Mechanics of the pleural space. *Physiol Rev* 1972;52:57.
11. Leff A, Honeywell PC, Costello J. Pleural effusion from malignancy. *Ann Intern Med* 1978;88:532.
12. Meyer PL. Metastatic carcinoma of the pleura. *Thorax* 1966;21:437.
13. Lynch TE. Management of malignant pleural effusions. *Chest* 1993;103:385S.
14. Sahn SA. Malignant pleural effusions. *Clin Chest Med* 1998;6:113.
15. Rusch V, Harper GR. *Pleural effusion in patients with malignancy.* Philadelphia: W.B. Saunders, 1989.
16. Chernow B, Sahn SA. Carcinomatous involvement of the pleura. *Am J Med* 1977;37:291.
17. Martini N, Bains MS, Beattie EJ Jr. Indications for pleurectomy in malignant effusion. *Cancer* 1975;35:734.
18. Woodring JH. Recognition of pleural effusion on supine radiographs: how much fluid is required? *AJR* 1984;142:59.
19. Peterson JA. Recognition of intrapulmonary pleural effusions. *Radiology* 1960;74:34.
20. Flower CDR, Williams MP. The pleural space. In: Husband JES, ed. *CT review.* London: Churchill Livingstone, 1989:23.
21. Dhillon DP, Spiro SG. Pleural disease: malignant pleural effusion. *Br J Hosp Med* 1983;23:506.
22. Sahn SA. Pleural effusions in lung cancer. *Clin Chest Med* 1993;14:189.
23. Ruckdeschel JC. Management of malignant pleural effusion: an overview. *Semin Oncol* 1988;15:24.
24. Light RW. Pleural effusion. *Med Clin North Am* 1977;61:1339.
25. Sahn SA, Good JT Jr. Pleural fluid pH in malignant effusions. Diagnostic, prognostic, and therapeutic implications. *Ann Intern Med* 1988;108:345.
26. Krener MR, Saldana MJ, Cepero RJ, et al. High amylase levels in neoplasm related pleural effusion. *Ann Intern Med* 1989;110:567.
27. Bottles K, Reznicek MJ, Holly EA, et al. Cytologic criteria used to diagnose adenocarcinoma in pleural effusions [see comments]. *Mod Pathol* 1991;4:677.
28. DiBonito L, Falconieri G, Colautti I, et al. The positive pleural effusion. A retrospective study of cytopathologic diagnoses with autopsy confirmation. *Acta Cytol* 1992;36:329.
29. Estaban JM, Yukuta S, Husain S, et al. Immunocytochemical profile of benign and carcinomatous effusions. A practical approach to difficult diagnosis. *Am J Clin Pathol* 1990;94:608.
30. Martin SE, Moshiri S, Thor A, et al. Identification of adenocarcinoma in cytologic preparation of effusion using monoclonal antibody B72.3. *Am J Clin Pathol* 1986;86:10.
31. Johnston WW, Szpalc CA, Lottich SC, et al. Use of a monoclonal antibody (B72.3) as an immunological adjunct to diagnosis of adenocarcinoma in tumor effusions. *Cancer Res* 1985;45:1894.
32. Salyer WR, Eggleston JC, Erozan YS. Efficiency of pleural needle biopsy and pleural fluid cytopathology in the diagnosis of malignant neoplasm involving the pleura. *Chest* 1975;67:536.
33. Winkleman, J. Intracellular localization of hematoporphyrin in a transplanted tumor. *J Natl Cancer Inst* 1961;27:1369.
34. Nance KV, Shermer RW, Askin FB. Diagnostic efficacy of pleural biopsy as compared with that of pleural fluid examination. *Mod Pathol* 1991;4:320.
35. Daniel TM. Diagnostic thoracoscopy for pleural disease. *Ann Thorac Surg* 1993;56:639.
36. Colt HG. Thoracoscopic management of malignant pleural effusions. *Clin Chest Med* 1995;16:505.
37. Kim JW, Yang IA, Oh EA, et al. C-reactive protein, sialic acid and adenosine deaminase levels in serum and pleural fluid from patients with pleural effusion. *Korean J Intern Med* 1988;3:122.
38. Petersson T, Ojala K, Weber R. Adenosine deaminase in the diagnosis of pleural effusions. *Acta Med Scand* 1984;215:299.
39. Tamura S, Nishigaki T, Moriwaki Y, et al. Tumor markers in pleural effusion diagnosis. *Cancer* 1988;61:298.
40. Pavesi F, Lotzniker M, Cremaschi P, et al. Detection of malignant pleural effusions by tumor marker evaluation [published erratum appears in *Eur J Cancer Clin Oncol* 1988;24(9):1559]. *Eur J Cancer Clin Oncol* 1988;24:1005.
41. Dewald G, Dines DE, Weiland LH, et al. Usefulness of chromosome examination in the diagnosis of malignant pleural effusion. *N Engl J Med* 1976;295:1494.
42. Unger KM, Raber M, Bedrossian CW, et al. Analysis of pleural effusions using automated flow cytometry. *Cancer* 1983;52:873.
43. Fraisse J, Brizard CO, Emonot A, et al. Diagnosis of malignancy by cytogenetic means in effusions. *Clin Genet* 1978;14:288.
44. Decker DA, Dines DE, Payne WS, et al. The significance of a cytologically negative pleural effusion in bronchogenic carcinoma. *Chest* 1978;74:640.
45. Livingston RB, McCracken JD, Trauth CJ, et al. Isolated pleural effusion in small cell lung carcinoma: favorable prognosis. A review of the Southwest Oncology Group experience. *Chest* 1982;81:208.
46. Mahfood S, Hix WR, Aaron BL, et al. Reexpansion pulmonary edema. *Ann Thorac Surg* 1988;45:340.
47. Trachiotis GD, Vricella LA, Aaron BL, et al. Reexpansion pulmonary edema. *Ann Thorac Surg* 1992;63:1205.
48. Anderson CB, Philpott GW, Ferguson TB. The treatment of malignant pleural effusions. *Cancer* 1974;33:916.
49. Izbicki R. Pleural effusion in cancer patients. A prospective randomized study of pleural drainage with the addition of radioactive phsophorous to the pleural space vs. pleural drainage alone. *Cancer* 1975;36:1511.
50. O'Neill W, Spurr C, Muss H, et al. A prospective study of chest tube drainage and tetracycline sclerosis versus chest tube drainage in the treatment of malignant pleural effusion. *Proc Am Soc Clin Oncol* 1879;21:349.
51. Lorch DG, Gordon I, Wooten J, et al. Effect of patient positioning on distribution of tetracycline in the pleural space during pleurodesis. *Chest* 1988;93:527.
52. Fentiman IS. Effective treatment of malignant pleural effusions. *Br J Hosp Med* 1987;37:421.
53. Morrison MC, Mueller PR, Lee MJ, et al. Sclerotherapy of

malignant pleural effusion through sonographically placed small-bore catheters. *AJR* 1992;158:41.

54. Parker LA, Charnock GC, Delany DJ. Small bore catheter drainage and sclerotherapy for malignant pleural effusions. *Cancer* 1989;64:1218.

55. Goff BA, Mueller PR, Muntz HG, et al. Small chest-tube drainage followed by bleomycin sclerosis for malignant pleural effusion. *Obstet Gynecol* 1993;81:993.

56. Clementsen P, Evald T, Grode G, et al. Treatment of malignant pleural effusion: pleurodesis using a small percutaneous catheter. A prospective randomized study. *Respir Med* 1998;92:593.

57. Boutin C, Loddenkemper R, Astoul P. Diagnostic and therapeutic thoracoscopy: techniques and indications in pulmonary medicine. *Tuber Lung Dis* 1993;74:225.

58. Kohri K, Kataoka K, Yachiku S, et al. Changes in cyclic AMP and electrolytes after parathyroidectomy in primary hyperparathyroidism. *Clin Endocrinol* 1983;18:371.

59. Aelony Y, King R, Boutin C. Thoracoscopic talc poudrage pleurodesis for chronic recurrent pleural effusions. *Ann Intern Med* 1991;115:778.

60. Adler RH, Sayek I. Treatment of malignant pleural effusion: a method using tube thoracostomy and talc. *Ann Thor Surg* 1976; 22:8.

61. Pearson FG. Talc poudrage for malignant pleural effusion. *J Thorac Cardiovasc Surg* 1966;51:732.

62. Aelony Y, Boutin C. Local anesthesia with thoracoscopic talc poudrage pleurodesis [Letter; Comment]. *Chest* 1996;110: 1126.

63. Rinaldo JE, Owens GR, Rogers RM. Adult respiratory distress syndrome following intrapleural instillation of talc. *J Thorac Cardiovasc Surg* 1983;85:523.

64. Rehse DH, Aye RW, Florence MG. Respiratory failure following talc pleurodesis. *Am J Surg* 1999;177:437.

65. Greenwald DW. Management of malignant pleural effusion. *J Surg Oncol* 1978;10:361.

66. Oszko MA. Pleural effusions: pathophysiology and management with intrapleural tetracycline. *Drug Intell Clin Pharm* 1988;22:15.

67. Wallach HW. Intrapleural tetracycline for malignant pleural effusions. *Chest* 1975;68:510.

68. Zaloznik AJ, Oswald SG, Langin M. Intrapleural tetracycline in malignant pleural effusions. *Cancer* 1983;51:752.

69. Gravelyn TR, Michelson MK, Gross BH, et al. Tetracycline pleurodesis for malignant pleural effusions. *Cancer* 1987;59: 1973.

70. Landvater L, Hix WR, Mills M, et al. Malignant pleural effusions treated by tetracycline sclerotherapy. *Chest* 1988;93:1196.

71. Sherman S, Grady KJ, Seidman JC. Clinical experience with tetracycline pleurodesis of malignant pleural effusions. *South Med J* 1987;80:716.

72. Ruckdeschel JC, Moores D, Lee JY, et al. Intrapleural therapy for malignant pleural effusions. A randomized comparison of bleomycin and tetracycline. *Chest* 1991;100:1528.

73. Mansson T. Treatment of malignant pleural effusions with deoxycycline. *Scand J Infect Dis* 1988;53:29.

74. Robinson LA, Fleming WH, Galbraith TA. Intrapleural doxycycline control of malignant pleural effusions [see comments]. *Ann Thorac Surg* 1993;55:1115.

75. Muir JF, Defouilloy C, Ndaruinze S, et al. [Use of intrapleural doxycycline via lavage-drainage in recurrent effusions of neoplastic origin]. [French]. *Rev Mal Respir* 1987;4:29.

76. Kitzmura S, Sugiyama Y, Izumi T, et al. Intrapleural deoxycycline for control of malignant pleural effusions. *Curr Ther Res* 1981;30:515.

77. Ostrowski MJ. Intracavitary therapy with bleomycin for the treatment of malignant pleural effusions [Review]. *J Surg Oncol* 1989;1[Suppl.]:7.

78. Bitran JD, Brown C, Desser RK, et al. Intracavitary bleomycin for the control of malignant effusions. *J Surg Oncol* 1981;16: 273.

79. Borja ER, Pugh RP. Single-dose quinacrine (atabrine) and thoracostomy in the control of pleural effusions in patients with neoplastic diseases. *Cancer* 1973;31:899.

80. Taylor SA, Hooton NS, Macarthur AM. Quinacrine in the management of malignant pleural effusion. *Br J Surg* 1977;64: 52.

81. Borda I. Convulsions following intrapleural administration of quinacrine hydrochloride. *JAMA* 1967;201:1049.

82. Casali A. Treatment of malignant pleural effusions with intracavitary Corynebacterium parvum. *Cancer* 1988;62:806.

83. Leahy BC. Treatment of malignant pleural effusions with intrapleural Corynebacterium parvum or tetracycline. *Eur J Respir Dis* 1985;66:50.

84. Hillerdal G. Corynebacterium parvum in malignant pleural effusion. A randomized prospective study. *Eur J Respir Dis* 1986; 69:204.

85. Rossi GA. Symptomatic treatment of recurrent malignant pleural effusions with intrapleurally administered Corynebacterium parvum. Clinical response is not associated with evidence of enhancement of local cellular-mediated immunity. *Am Rev Respir Dis* 1987;135:885.

86. Felletti R. Intrapleural Corynebacterium parvum for malignant pleural effusions. *Thorax* 1983;38:22.

87. Ike O. Treatment of malignant pleural effusions with doxorubicin hydrochloride-containing poly(L-lactic acid) microspheres. *Chest* 1991;99:911.

88. Desai SD. Intracavitary doxorubicin in malignant effusions. *Lancet* 1979;1:872.

89. Figlin R, Mendoza E, Piantadosi S, et al. Intrapleural chemotherapy without pleurodesis for malignant pleural effusions. LCSG Trial 861. *Chest* 1994;106:363S.

90. Holoye PY, Jeffries DG, Dhingra HM, et al. Intrapleural etoposide for malignant effusion. *Cancer Chemother Pharmacol* 1990; 26:147.

91. Luh KT. Comparison of OK-432 and mitomycin C pleurodesis for malignant pleural effusion caused by lung cancer. A randomized trial. *Cancer* 1992;69:674.

92. Gebbia V. Intracavitary beta-interferon for the management of pleural and/or abdominal effusions in patients with advanced cancer refractory to chemotherapy. *In Vivo* 1991;5:579.

93. Davis M. A phase I-II study of recombinant intrapleural alpha interferon in malignant pleural effusions. *Am J Clin Oncol* 1992; 15:328.

94. Goldman CA. Interferon instillation for malignant pleural effusions. *Ann Oncol* 1993;4:141.

95. Viallat JR. Intrapleural immunotherapy with escalating doses of interleukin-2 in metastatic pleural effusions. *Cancer* 1993; 71:4067.

96. Astoul P. Intrapleural recombinant IL-2 in passive immunotherapy for malignant pleural effusion. *Chest* 1993;103:209.

97. Yasumoto K. Intrapleural application of recombinant interleukin-2 in patients with malignant pleurisy due to lung cancer. A multi-institutional cooperative study. *Biotherapy* 1991;3:345.

98. Bayly TC, Kisner DL, Sybert A, et al. Tetracycline and qinacrine in the control of malignant pleural effusions: a randomized trial. *Cancer* 1978;41:1188.

99. Gupta N, Opfell RW, Padova C, et al. Intrapleural bleomycin vs tetracycline for control of malignant pleural effusions. A randomized study. *Am Soc Clin Oncol Abstr* 1980;C-189:366.

100. Kessinger A, Wigton RS. Intracavitary bleomycin and tetracy-

cline in the management of malignant pleural effusions: a randomized study. *J Surg Oncol* 1987;36:81.

101. Fentiman IS, Rubens RD, Haward JL. A comparison of intracavitary talc and tetracycline for the control of pleural effusions secondary to breast cancer. *Eur J Cancer Clin Oncol* 1986;22:1079.

102. Hamed H, Fentiman IS, Chaudary MA, et al. Comparison of intracavitary bleomycin and talc for control of pleural effusions secondary to carcinoma of the breast. *Br J Surg* 1989;76:1266.

103. Hartman DI, Gaither JM, Kesler KA, et al. Comparison of insufflated talc under theracoscopic guidance with standard tetracycline and bleomycin pleurodesis for control of malignant pleural effusions. *J Thorac Cardiovasc Surg* 1993;105:743.

104. Rosso R. Intrapleural natural beta interferon in the treatment of malignant pleural effusions. *Oncology* 1988;45:253.

105. Uchida A. Intrapleural administration of OK432 in cancer patients: augmentation of autologous tumor killing activity of tumor-associated large granular lymphocytes. *Cancer Immunol Immunother* 1984;18:5.

106. Boutin C, Viallat JR, Van Zandwijk N, et al. Activity of intrapleural recombinant gamma-interferon in malignant mesothelioma. *Cancer* 1991;67:2033.

107. Little AG. Pleuroperitoneal shunting for malignant pleural effusions. *Cancer* 1986;58:2740.

108. Little AG, Ferguson MK, Golomb HM, et al. Pleuroperitoneal shunting for malignant pleural effusions. *Cancer* 1986;58:2740.

109. Weese JL. Pleural peritoneal shunts for the treatment of malignant pleural effusions. *Surg Gynecol Obstet* 1982;154:391.

110. Reich H. Pleuroperitoneal shunt for malignant pleural effusions: a one-year experience. *Semin Surg Oncol* 1993;9:160.

111. Sahn SA. Malignancy metastatic to the pleura. *Clin Chest Med* 1998;19:351.

112. Petrou M, Kaplan D, Goldstraw P. Management of recurrent malignant pleural effusions. *Cancer* 1995;75:801.

113. McCall E. The use of the pleuro-peritoneal shunt. *Nurs Times* 1997;93:62.

114. Tsang V, Fernando HC, Goldstraw P. Pleuroperitoneal shunt for recurrent malignant pleural effusions. *Thorax* 1990;45:369.

115. Ponn RB, Blancaflor J, D'Agostino RS, et al. Pleuroperitoneal shunting for intractable pleural effusions. *Ann Thorac Surg* 1991;51:605.

116. al Kattan KM, Kaplan DK, Goldstraw P. The non-functioning pleuro-peritoneal shunt: revise or replace? *Thorac Cardiovasc Surg* 1994;42:310.

117. Keller SM. Current and future therapy for malignant pleural effusion. *Chest* 1993;103:63S.

118. Matsuzaki Y. Intrapleural perfusion hyperthermo-chemotherapy for malignant pleural dissemination and effusion. *Ann Thorac Surg* 1995;59:127.

119. Fentiman S, Rubens RD, Hayward JL. Control of pleural effusions in patients with breast cancer: a randomized trial. *Cancer* 1983;52:737.

120. Masuno TA. Comparative trial of LC9018 plus doxorubicin and doxorubicin alone for the treatment of malignant pleural effusion secondary to lung cancer. *Cancer* 1991;68:1495.

121. Patz EF Jr, McAdams HP, Erasmus JJ, et al. Sclerotherapy for malignant pleural effusions: a prospective randomized trial of bleomycin vs doxycycline with small-bore catheter drainage. *Chest* 1998;113:1305.

60

MALIGNANT PERICARDIAL EFFUSION

JOSEPH B. ZWISCHENBERGER
ARAVIND B. SANKAR
RAYMAN LEE

Pericardial effusion is the most common manifestation of malignant pericardial involvement. In a series of 3,327 autopsies for cancer-related deaths, cardiac-related malignancy was detected in 5.1%.[1] Of these, the pericardium alone was involved in 45% of cases, the myocardium in 32%, and both in 22%.[2–4] Primary malignancies with a propensity for cardiac involvement, in decreasing order of frequency, include lung, breast, lymphoma (including Hodgkin's), leukemia, melanoma, gastrointestinal malignancies, and sarcomas. Malignant pericardial effusion (MPE) presents a clinical spectrum that ranges from totally asymptomatic to acute cardiac tamponade. Fortunately, clinically significant MPE is uncommon. Neoplastic cardiac tamponade is a clinical oncologic emergency, which may appear suddenly and precipitate death in a patient who would otherwise have a good short-term life expectancy. Patients presenting with cardiac tamponade usually have a known pulmonary primary.[5–7]

PATHOGENESIS

The pericardium is a strong, inelastic sac composed of two layers surrounding the heart. The outer fibrous parietal pericardium is commonly referred to as the pericardium. The thin, inner, serosal layer is the visceral pericardium, also known as the epicardium. These two layers form a thin, lubricated space which usually contains between 15 and 50 mL of fluid. Pericardial fluid is a clear ultrafiltrate of blood with a protein concentration one third that of plasma. Microscopically the pericardium has microvilli that decrease friction and increase the surface area of reabsorption. A fundamental knowledge of the lymphatic drainage patterns of the heart and pericardium is important in understanding the pathogenesis of MPE (Figure 60.1). The parietal lymphatics drain preferentially to the anterior and posterior mediastinal nodes, while the visceral lymphatics drain to the tracheal and bronchial mediastinal lymph nodes.[8] The pericardium itself is deficient in lymphatics, so most of the drainage occurs through the cardiac lymphatics. Flow begins in the extensive subendocardial plexus, which drains through an interconnecting system of myocardial channels into a subepicardial plexus. Efferent branches of the subepicardial plexus give rise to the cardiac lymphatic trunk, which runs with the coronary arteries to the root of the aorta. The cardiac lymphatic trunk then travels between the innominate artery and the superior vena cava directly to the cardiac node. The cardiac node then drains into the mediastinal nodes.[5] Tamura and colleagues reviewed 74 autopsies of primary lung cancer patients.[9] Metastases to the heart, or pericardium, were documented in 23 cases. MPE was present in 15 of the 23 cases. The metastatic pathway was lymphatic in 14 of 15 cases, utilizing hilar lymphatics in 10, and mediastinal lymphatics in four. Early development of MPE in lung cancer is primarily by hilar lymphatic spread.[9]

Venous and lymphatic drainage obstructed by neoplastic invasion leads to a disruption in the usual osmotic and hydrostatic forces, causing an accumulation of pericardial fluid. If the fluid accumulation is slow, the pericardial volume can expand to remarkable amounts (up to 3 to 4 L) and be clinically silent. The onset of tamponade can be rapid if the pericardium is fibrosed or thickened from previous radiation or inflammation or the fluid accumulation is rapid.

CLINICAL PRESENTATION

The clinical presentation of MPE varies dramatically from a complete lack of symptoms to acute cardiogenic shock. Fluid accumulation from lymphatic obstruction with a noncompliant pericardium results in acute restriction of atrial and ventricular filling, an increase in systemic venous pressure, and then an acute decrease in cardiac output. Since decreased cardiac filling decreases stroke volume, the initial cardiovascular response is increased sympathetic tone with compensatory vasoconstriction and tachycardia. Patients presenting with acute cardiac tamponade are typically in extremis with marked agitation or confusion, tachycardia, and tachypnea. In this setting, the classic clinical syndrome

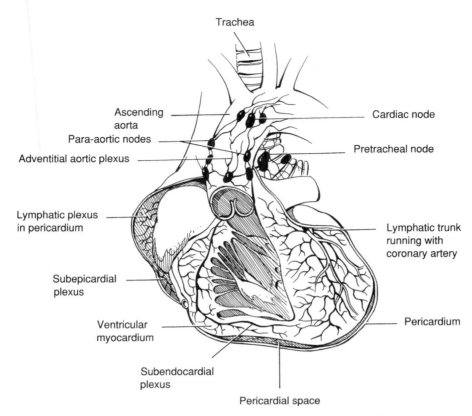

FIGURE 60.1. Lymphatic drainage of the heart and pericardium.

of Beck's triad can be seen with elevation of systemic venous pressures, systemic arterial hypotension, and a small quiet heart. When tamponade develops slowly, symptoms resemble heart failure, with orthopnea, tachycardia, and hepatic engorgement. The main complaint is usually dyspnea on exertion, accompanied by anorexia, lethargy, edema, or weight loss. In these patients there is almost always jugular venous distention and a parodoxical pulse. Table 60.1 describes the relative frequency of symptoms, signs, and laboratory findings in MPE.[10]

DIAGNOSTIC EVALUATION

Physical Examination

Acute cardiac tamponade associated with MPE often requires immediate diagnosis and treatment. Pulsus paradoxus, an important finding in cardiac tamponade, was first described as the disappearance of the radial pulse despite a palpable heartbeat. Pulsus is not really parodoxical, but an exaggeration of the normal inspiratory drop in systolic pressure. It can be measured with a sphygmomanometer by inflating the cuff above the arterial pressure and very slowly deflating the cuff until the first Korotokoff sound is heard. At this point, the Korotokoff sound will disappear with inspiration. With further slow deflation of the cuff, a continuous pulsation will be heard. The difference in the systolic pressure of these two points is the amount of pulsus. A greater than 10 mm Hg fall in the systolic pressure with inspiration signifies a pulsus parodoxus.[10] In tachypneic patients, pulsus may be difficult to measure, but with invasive arterial monitoring, the inspiratory blood pressure drop can be visualized graphically. Upon palpation of the precordium the cardiac impulse is diminished or absent. Percussion of the anterior thorax may reveal dullness in the left lung base secondary to compression from a large effusion, called Ewert's sign. On auscultation, heart sounds may be distant and weak, with tachycardia or supraventricular arrhythmias. Surprising, only occasionally will a pericardial rub or splash be heard.

Radiographs

Chest radiographs show nonspecific but often supportive evidence for the diagnosis of MPE. Enlargement of the cardiac silhouette on chest radiograph does not occur until approximately 250 cc of fluid is present in the pericardial space. The classic "water bottle" cardiac silhouette may be seen on PA chest x-ray with long-standing MPE. In one third of cases a coexisting pleural effusion is seen. Press

TABLE 60.1. RELATIVE FREQUENCY OF SYMPTOMS, SIGNS, AND LABORATORY FINDINGS IN MALIGNANT PERICARDIAL EFFUSION

Findings	Frequency (%)
Symptoms	
1. Dyspnea	79
2. Cough	47
3. Chest pain	27
4. Orthopnea	26
5. Weakness	20
6. Dysphagia	18
7. Syncope	4
8. Palpitations	3
Signs	
1. Pleural effusion	51
2. Tachycardia	50
3. Jugular venous distention	45
4. Hepatomegaly	37
5. Peripheral edema	35
6. Pulsus paradoxus	31
7. Hypotension	31
8. Distant heart sounds	17
9. Rales	15
10. Pericardial rub	12
Laboratory Findings	
1. Echocardiographic fluid	100
2. Abnormal electrocardiogram	91
a. Nonspecific ST-T segment changes	63
b. Low voltage	59
c. Sinus tachycardia	25
d. Atrial flutter or fibrillation	20
e. Premature ventricular beats	14
f. Heart block	8
g. Electrical alternans	6
3. Abnormal chest radiograph	87
a. Signs of pericardial disease on chest radiograph	46
4. Positive pericardial fluid cytology	80
5. Positive pericardial biopsy	55

From Press OW, Livingston R. Management of malignant pericardial effusion. *JAMA* 1987;257:1088, with permission.

and Livingston showed that 90% of patients had abnormal radiographs and about 45% had signs of pericardial disease.[11] Unfortunately, an enlarged cardiac silhouette is suggestive, but not specific for pericardial fluid, and other conditions, especially congestive heart failure, have a similar appearance.[12] Computed tomography (CT) defines the size of the effusion, location of intracardiac or extracardiac masses, and often the origin of the primary cancer (usually of pulmonary origin). Johnson and colleagues have proposed several CT criteria for the diagnosis of MPE: (a) pericardial effusion of high CT density, (b) localized or irregular pericardial thickening, (c) masses arising from or continuous with the pericardium, and (d) obliteration of normal tissue planes between a paracardiac mass and the heart or pericar-

dium.[13] Once the diagnosis of MPE is established, CT or echocardiography can be used to guide insertion of drainage catheters for diagnosis or treatment.

Electrocardiograms

About 90% of patients with symptomatic MPE have abnormal EKG findings, including nonspecific ST segment changes (63%), low voltage (59%), sinus tachycardia (25%), atrial flutter or fibrillation (21%), premature ventricular beats, and heart block.[11] With large effusions, the heart may develop a swinging motion within the pericardial sac, which is thought to cause electrical alternans seen in 5% of patients. Usually electrical alternans involve only the QRS complex in a two-to-one or three-to-one pattern, but when the P, QRS, and T wave are all involved, it is pathognomonic for a severe tamponade.[14–16]

Echocardiography

Echocardiography is the most specific and sensitive noninvasive test for the evaluation of MPE. Transthoracic echocardiography is initially used to evaluate the anatomy and physiologic consequences of the pericardial fluid. Transesophageal and Doppler ultrasonography are complementary in patients who do not manifest characteristic transthoracic echocardiographic findings.[17] By using parasternal, subxiphoid, and transesophageal views, the entire pericardium can be inspected. Echocardiographic changes are best seen in the posterior cardiac wall, where normally a single echo is seen moving synchronously with the heartbeat. When a pericardial effusion is present separating the pericardium and epicardium, two distinct echoes are seen: one from the pericardium and one from the epicardium.[18] The quality of the pericardial fluid (homogenous versus heterogeneous), pericardial masses, or loculations, right and left ventricular function, and right and left ventricular diastolic collapse are imaged by echocardiography. Equalization of diastolic pressures across all cardiac chambers is the hallmark of symptomatic cardiac tamponade. Diastolic collapse of the right ventricle and atrium has been proposed as an echocardiographic indicator of cardiac tamponade.[19] Patients with this finding should undergo immediate drainage of the pericardium. If the echo is indeterminate, CT and MRI may be helpful, especially with loculated effusions, pericardial thickening, calcifications, blood, fat, or chyle.

TREATMENT

Management decisions in the treatment of MPE should include consideration of age, symptoms, general condition, origin, and prognosis of the tumor (Figure 60.2). The risks versus benefits of intervention for MPE may not be favorable in patients with end-stage metastatic cancer. The median

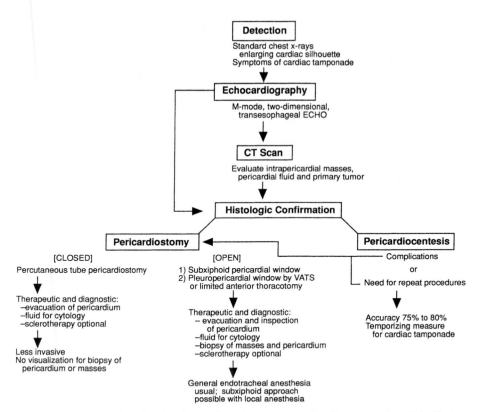

FIGURE 60.2. Algorithm for the diagnosis and treatment of malignant pericardial effusion.

survival for all malignant pericardial effusions is two to four months, with a 25% one-year survival.[20] In patients with known metastatic cancer, MPE and tamponade should always be considered when signs and symptoms of hemodynamic compromise present. Acute pericardial tamponade with cyanosis, dyspnea, impaired consciousness, shock, pulsus paradoxus greater than 50% of pulse pressure, or a decrease of more than 20 mm Hg in pulse pressure are indications for emergent drainage. If the patient is hemodynamically stable then a more definite procedure can be performed, including percutaneous insertion of a pericardial drain by Seldinger technique under radiographic guidance, open pericardiostomy by the subxiphoid approach, video-assisted thoracoscopic surgery (VATS), or limited anterior thoracotomy (see Table 60.2).[21-29] In a review of different malignant pericardial effusion treatments, no modality was clearly superior to another (Figure 60.3).

Needle- or catheter-based procedures are best image-directed by transthoracic or transesophageal echocardiography or by computed tomography. In all instances the basic technique is the same and has been well described.[23,27,29,30] Imaging by any of the mentioned modalities is used to identify the largest collection of pericardial fluid in close proximity to the skin, to identify the safest needle entry site. After local infiltration with 1% lidocaine, a sheathed needle (16

to 18 gauge) is used for the initial pericardial entry. Upon aspirating pericardial fluid, the needle is removed, leaving only the sheath in the pericardial space. A small amount of saline can be used for echocardiographic confirmation of the sheath position. If prolonged drainage is desired, a guide wire is introduced through the sheath, the sheath withdrawn, and a dilator (6–7 F) advanced over the guide wire. A multisidehole pigtail angiographic catheter (6–7 F) is placed in the pericardial space. The catheter typically re-

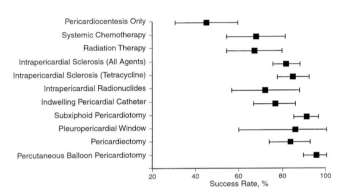

FIGURE 60.3. Success rates for treatment of malignant pericardial effusion.

TABLE 60.2. COMPARISON OF PERICARDIAL PROCEDURES

Procedure	Position	Anesthesia	Incision	Biopsy/Window/Resection Size	Pain	Advantages	Disadvantages
Pericardiocentesis	supine	local	percutaneous	none	minimal	Can be done emergently at bedside Fluid drainage/analysis Catheter for prolonged drainage or sclerosis	Drainage may be inadequate Blind approach associated with higher risk Higher recurrence rate
Balloon Pericardiotomy	supine	local	percutaneous	small window, no biopsy	minimal	Low morbidity Can be done in the cath lab	Limited availability
Subxiphoid Pericardiotomy	supine	local or single-lumen	small incision	small window, 4×4 cm anterior sample	mild	Good drainage Low morbidity	Limited access
VATS Pericardiotomy	lateral decubitus	double-lumen single-lung anesthesia	3 port video equipment	larger	mild	Good drainage Low morbidity Access to pleura and lung	Surgeon unable to feel tissue
Anterolateral Pericardiotomy or Pericardiectomy	lateral decubitus	double-lumen single-lung anesthesia	anterolateral thoracotomy	larger	most	Limited pericardiectomy Surgeon able to feel tissue Access to pleura and lung	Higher morbidity than with subxiphoid pericardiotomy
Radical Pericardiotomy	supine	single-lumen	median sternotomy	larger	moderate	Complete pericardial resection Access for cardiopulmonary bypass	Pain/morbidity Operative risk

mains in place until the fluid return is less than 50 cc every 24 hours and follow-up imaging shows insignificant residual effusion.

General endotracheal anesthesia in the setting of acute tamponade increases the risk of any intervention and should be avoided if possible. Patients in cardiac tamponade have markedly increased endogenous catecholamines for circulatory support. Induction of anesthesia inhibits these compensatory autonomic responses and may lead to circulatory collapse before drainage can be effected. Positive pressure ventilation can further impede venous return in these compromised patients. Inotropes and intravenous fluids to improve contractility and maintain preload to the heart may be temporarily necessary to allow the induction of anesthesia. Because of the risk of anesthesia, percutaneous drainage of MPE using local anesthesia only has become the procedure of choice.

Pericardiocentesis

Controversy exists regarding the roles of pericardiocentesis, pigtail catheter drainage, and pericardiotomy. Pericardiocentesis is both a diagnostic and therapeutic tool in the management of MPE. In the setting of acute hemodynamic compromise, the procedure of choice is urgent pericardiocentesis (see Figure 60.4). An 18-gauge spinal needle with an ECG lead is inserted into the pericardial sac by aiming

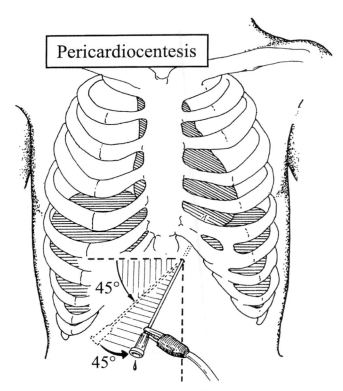

FIGURE 60.4. Pericardiocentesis.

the needle toward the patient's left shoulder at a 45 degree angle, while constantly maintaining negative pressure. If an ECG injury pattern or arrhythmia is seen, the needle is repositioned. Occasionally the pressure is so great that the plunger is pushed out. Two thirds of these patients will develop recurrence and require repeat drainage.[26]

The use of M-mode echocardiography to guide pericardiocentesis was first reported by Goldberg and Pollack in 1973 and quickly replaced ECG for directing needle placement.[31] Two-dimensional echocardiography has currently replaced M-mode. The transducer is placed at the cardiac apex while pericardiocentesis is performed from the subcostal position. The interpericardial position of the needle is confirmed by the appearance of microbubbles in the pericardial sac. If the needle has penetrated the cardiac chamber then intracardiac bubbles may be seen.[30] Once the needle is in the pericardial space, the fluid can be evacuated and a guidewire inserted for pigtail catheter drainage. Wiener and colleagues reviewed 95 cases of pericardial effusion treated initially with pericardiocentesis.[32] Pericardial fluid collected from known cancer patients revealed neoplastic cells in 66% of these patients. When the pericardial fluid was correlated with the known primary, it was 100% specific. Similar results by Press and Livingston confirm that cytology of pericardial fluid remains valuable in the diagnosis of MPE.[11] The fluid is generally hemorrhagic with a high LDH level. Pericardial fluid analysis includes cell count, glucose, protein, lactate dehydrogenase, bacterial culture, and cytology.[33]

With drainage, the crisis of acute cardiac tamponade is averted. A single pericardiocentesis is unlikely to prevent recurrence of the tamponade unless the underlying malignancy is addressed. Recurrence rates as high as 90% within 90 days are reported.[7] MPE indicates advanced systemic disease; therefore a multidisciplinary approach with oncology, radiation therapy, and thoracic surgery is necessary for appropriate palliative management.

Complications of pericardiocentesis are uncommon but can be catastrophic. In a review of medical patients requiring pericardiocentesis, 40 of 46 (87%) experienced symptomatic relief after therapeutic pericardiocentesis, but 3 (7%) had major complications including right ventricular laceration, cardiac arrest with hypoxic brain damage, and emergency ventricular repair.[34] Other potential complications include laceration of the coronary arteries, internal mammary artery, or lung, contamination of the pericardial or pleural space, and injuries to intra-abdominal organs.

Open Pericardiotomy

Open pericardiotomy, or "pericardial window," is usually performed in the operating room under general endotracheal anesthesia, although it can also be performed with local anesthesia. The procedure can be performed quickly (15 to 20 minutes), especially if hemodynamic compromise

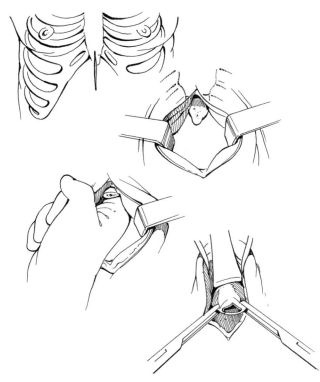

FIGURE 60.5. Subxiphoid pericardiotomy.

develops. The subxiphoid approach requires a midline incision from the xiphoid/sternal junction extending caudad 6 cm (Figure 60.5). The xiphoid is resected and the linea alba is divided without entering the peritoneum or diaphragm. The sternum is firmly retracted anteriorly, and the fatty tissue overlying the pericardium is incised and retracted laterally to allow the pericardium to be identified. The pericardium is elevated and incised. One should be ready for a sudden gush of blood under pressure if any tamponade is present. An immediate improvement of pulse pressure should be noted. The serosanguinous pericardial fluid is then sent for a cell count, cytology, gram stain, and culture if the diagnosis is uncertain. The pericardium is then digitally explored, and loculations, nodules, and masses are noted. A generous anterior portion of the pericardium is excised and sent for pathology. One should strive to excise the largest extent of pericardium possible. Large drainage tubes are placed anteriorly and posteriorly, and placed to -20 cm H_2O suction. The drains are removed when the drainage is less than 50 cc per day. Some evidence indicates that the pericardiotomy remains open long after the effusive process ends. Sugimoto and colleagues believe that obliteration of the space is the goal, and maintain drainage for as long as four weeks.[35] These observations have prompted the use of sclerosing agents similar to those used to treat malignant pleural effusions.

VATS is a minimally invasive technique that provides excellent visualization of the pericardium (Figure 60.6) and perhaps decreased morbidity when compared with a thoracotomy.[40] VATS allows complete visualization of the hemithorax, during which the pericardium hemithorax can be inspected and drained.[36] One disadvantage is that VATS requires a double lumen endotracheal tube with lung collapse for visualization of the pericardium, therefore the subxiphiod approach is still preferred by most.

Pericardial Biopsy

Pericardial biopsy can be obtained by several approaches, including subxiphoid or subcostal pericardiostomy, limited anterior thoracotomy, or VATS.[20,37] A new technique of pericardioscopy with guided biopsies increased the diagnostic yield an additional 20% in patients with malignancy when cytology and conventional biopsy were negative.[38]

Pharmacologic Agents

The recurrence rate of catheter-drained pericardial effusions has been reported at 3% to 20%. If the effusion recurs, the pericardium is again drained, followed by sclerotherapy. We initially use bleomycin, 30 to 120 mg in 30 cc of 1% lidocaine for sclerotherapy. For refractory MPE we use sterile talc, 10 g in 50 cc of normal saline. Shepherd recommends the instillation of tetracycline for persistent effusions.[6] They report 74% success in control of effusions longer than 30 days with a median survival of 168 days. Recommended agents include oxytetracycline, OK-432, a penicillin-treated and heat-treated lyophilized powder of the substrain of *Streptococcus pyogenes* A3, cisplatin, bleomycin, vinblastine, interferon, and sterile talc.[39–45] Piehler and colleagues have reported that the amount of pericardium left in the patient is directly related to the rate of recurrence, postoperative pericardial constriction, and the need for repeated therapy.[46] Since most patients with MPE have an end-stage malignancy, long-term survival is rarely affected, emphasizing the desirability of a quick, less-invasive, and short-term effective treatment approach. Complications of sclerotherapy include transient atrial arrhythmia, pain after injection, and fever. When constrictive pericarditis or extensive involvement of tumor exists, pericardiectomy is a rare option. Although this is a highly morbid procedure, it has been reported in carefully considered circumstances.[47]

Radiotherapy is generally reserved for pericardial effusions associated with lymphoma. The recommended dosage is 2 to 3 Gy, which is given over a two to three week course. Pericardial inflammation is a complication of radiotherapy. Stewart and colleagues describe giving 40 Gy for fractionated radiotherapy of the heart and adjacent structures.[48] Acute pericarditis is a complication of radiation but is usually self-limited.

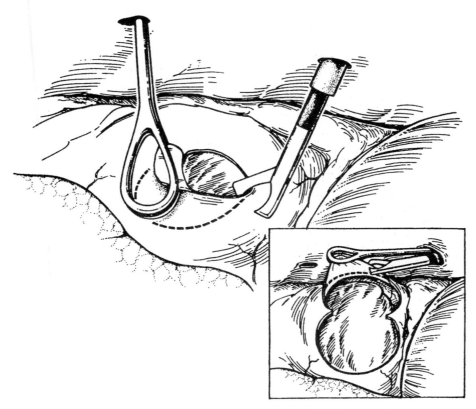

FIGURE 60.6. Video-assisted thoracoscopic surgery (VATS) pericardiotomy.

SUMMARY

The treatment of MPE should proceed in a stepwise fashion. We use CT- or echocardiography-guided percutaneous tube pericardiostomy to accomplish both diagnosis and therapy. Once the pericardium is drained, we use bleomycin or talc for sclerotherapy. If sclerotherapy fails, we proceed with subxiphoid pericardiotomy for evacuation of effusion, resection of pericardium, biopsy, and placement of drains. If the effusion recurs, this is again followed by sclerotherapy. Patients responding to treatment should have a mean life expectancy of nine to 13 months if tamponade does not recur. Even with cardiac tamponade, short-term palliation is possible.

REFERENCES

1. Shkvatsabaja LV. Secondary malignant lesions of the heart and pericardium in malignant disease. *Oncology* 1986;43:103.
2. Scott RW, Garvin CF. Tumors of the heart and pericardium. *Am Heart J* 1939;17:431.
3. Goudie RB. Secondary tumors of the heart and pericardium. *Br Heart J* 1955;17:183.
4. Theologides A. Neoplastic cardiac tamponade. *Semin Oncol* 1978;5:181.
5. Fraser RS, Viloria JB, Wang N. Cardiac tamponade as a presentation of extracardiac malignancy. *Cancer* 1980;45:1697.
6. Shepherd FA, Morgan C, Evans WK, et al. Medical management of malignant pericardial effusion by tetracycline sclerosis. *Am J Cardiol* 1987;60:1161.
7. Celermajer DS, Boyer MJ, Bailey BP, et al. Pericardiocentesis for symptomatic malignant pericardial effusion. *Med J Aust* 1991; 154:69.
8. Eliskova M, Eliska O, Miller AJ. The lymphatic drainage of the parietal pericardium in man. *Lymphology* 1995;28:208.
9. Tamura A, Masubara O, Yoshimura N, et al. Cardiac metastasis of lung cancer. A study of metastatic pathway and clinical manifestations. *Cancer* 1992;70:437.
10. McGregor M. Current concepts: pulsus paradoxus. *N Engl J Med* 1979;301:480.
11. Press OW, Livingston R. Management of malignant pericardial effusion and tamponade. *JAMA* 1987;257:1088.
12. Eisenberg MJ, Dunn MM, Kanth N, et al. Diagnostic value of chest radiography for pericardial effusion. *J Am Coll Cardiol* 1993;22:588.
13. Johnson FE, Wolverson MK, Sundaram M, et al. Unsuspected malignant pericardial effusion causing cardiac tamponade: rapid diagnosis by computed tomography. *Chest* 1982;82:501.
14. Lorell BH, Braunwald E. Pericardial disease. In: Braunwald E, ed. *Heart disease: a textbook of cardiovascular medicine.* Philadelphia: WB Saunders, 1984:1470.
15. Eisenberg MJ, de Romeral LM, Heidenreich PA et al. The diagnosis of pericardial effusion and cardiac tamponade by 12-lead ECG. A technology assessment. *Chest* 1996;11:318.
16. Meyers DG, Bagin RG, Levene JF. Electrocardiographic changes in pericardial effusion. *Chest* 1993;104:1422.
17. Chandraratna PAN. Echocardiography and Doppler ultrasound in the evaluation of pericardial disease. *Circulation* 1991;84:I302.

18. Schutzman JJ, Obarski TP, Pearce GL, et al. Comparison of Doppler and two dimensional echocardiography for assessment of pericardial effusion. *Am J Cardiol* 1992;70:1353.

19. Shina S, Yaginuma T, Kondo K, et al. Echocardiographic evaluation of impending cardiac tamponade. *J Cardiol* 1979;9:555.

20. Posner MR, Cohen GI, Skarkin AT. Pericardial disease in patients with cancer. *Am J Med* 1981;71:407.

21. Devlin GP, Smyth D, Charleston HA. Balloon pericardiostomy: a new therapeutic option for malignant pericardial effusion. *Aust N Z J Med* 1996;26:556.

22. Longo JM, Bilbao JL, Laurea JA. Malignant pericardial effusion: percutaneous creation of a pericardial window. *Am J Roetgenol* 1995;165:1305.

23. Bellon RJ, et al. CT guided pericardial drainage catheter placement with subsequent pericardial sclerosis. *J Comput Assist Tomogr* 1995;19:672.

24. Yim AP, et al. Video assisted subxiphoid pericardiectomy. *J Laparoendosc Surg* 1995;5:193.

25. Moores DW, Allen KB, Faber LP, et al. Subxiphoid pericardial drainage for pericardial tamponade. *J Thorac Cardiovasc Surg* 1995;109:546.

26. Laham RJ, Cohen DJ, Kuntz RE, et al. Pericardial effusion in patients with cancer: outcome with contemporary management strategies. *Heart* 1996;75:67.

27. Lee LN, Yang PC, Chang DB, et al. Ultrasound guided pericardial drainage and intrapericardial instillation of mitomycin C for malignant pericardial effusion. *Thorax* 1994;49:594.

28. Linder A, Friedel A, Toomes H. Prerequisites, indications, and techniques of video assisted thorascopic surgery. *J Thorac Cardiovasc Surg* 1993;41:140.

29. Gatenby RA, Harty WH, Kessler HB. Percutaneous catheter drainage for malignant pericardial effusion. *J Vasc Interv Radiol* 1991;2:151.

30. Callahan JA, Seward JB, Tajik AJ, et al. Pericardiocentesis assisted by two dimensional echocardiography. *J Thorac Cardiovasc Surg* 1983;85:877.

31. Goldberg BB, Pollack HM, Ultrasonically guided pericardiocentesis. *Am J Cardiol* 1973;85:877.

32. Wiener HG, Kristensen IB, Haubek A, et al. The diagnostic value of pericardial cytology: an analysis of 95 cases. *Acta Cytol* 1991;35:149.

33. Meyers DG, Meyers RE, Prendergast TW. The usefulness of diagnostic tests on pericardial fluid. *Chest* 1997;111:1213.

34. Guberman BA, Fowler NO, Engel PJ. Cardiac tamponade in medical patients. *Circulation* 1981;64:633.

35. Sugimoto J, Little A, Ferguson M, et al. Pericardial window mechanisms of efficacy. *Ann Thorac Surg* 1990;50:442.

36. Canto, Guýarro R, Amav A, et al. Thorascopic pericardial fenestration: diagnostic and therapeutic aspects. *Thorax* 1993;48:1178.

37. Mueller XM, Tevaearai HT, Hurni M, et al. Etiologic diagnosis of pericardial disease: the value of routine tests during surgical procedures. *J Am Coll Surgeons* 1997;184:645.

38. Nugue O, Millaire A, Porte H, et al. Pericardioscopy in the etiologic diagnosis of pericardial effusion in 141 consecutive patients. *Circulation* 1996;94:1635.

39. Norum J, Lunde P, Aasbo U, et al. Mitoxantrone in malignant pericardial effusion. *J Chemother* 1998;10:399.

40. Wilkins HE, Cacioppo S, Connolly MM, et al. Intrapericardial interferon in the management of malignant pericardial effusion. *Chest* 1998;114:330.

41. Colleoni M, Martinelli G, Beretta F, et al. Intracavitary chemotherapy with thiopeta in malignant pericardial effusions: an active and well-tolerated regimen. *J Clin Oncol* 1998;16:2371.

42. Tomkowski WZ, Filipecki S. Intrapericardial cisplatin for the management of patients with large malignant pericardial effusion in the course of lung cancer. *Lung Cancer* 1997;16:215.

43. Lerner-Tung MB, Chang AY, Ony LS, et al. Pharmokinetics of intrapericardial administration of 5-fluorouracil. *Cancer Chemother Pharmacol* 1997;40:318.

44. Liu G, Crump M, Goss PE, et al. Prospective comparison of the sclerosing agents doxycycline and bleomycin for the primary management of malignant pericardial effusion and cardiac tamponade. *J Clin Oncol* 1996;14:3141.

45. Imamura T, Tamura K, Takenga M, et al. Intrapericardial OK-432 instillation for the management of malignant pericardial effusion. *Cancer* 1991;68:259.

46. Piehler JM, Pluth JR, Schaff HV, et al. Surgical management of effusive pericardial disease: influence of extent of pericardial resection on clinical course. *J Thorac Cardiovasc Surg* 1985;90:506.

47. Caccavale RJ, Newman J, Sisler GE, et al. Pericardial disease. In: Kaiser LR, Daniel TM, eds. *Thoracoscopic surgery*. Boston: Little Brown, 1983:177.

48. Cohn KE, Stewart JR, Fajardo LF, et al. Heart disease following radiation. *Medicine* 1967;46:281.

61

MANAGEMENT OF MALIGNANT AIRWAY OBSTRUCTION

RALPH DE LA TORRE
MARK MOSTOVYCH
CHRISTOPHER MUTRIE
ATA ERDOGAN
DOUGLAS MATHISEN

BACKGROUND INFORMATION/INTRODUCTION

Lung cancer, with more than 150,000 cases every year, represents a major oncologic challenge.[1] There are more than 120,000 deaths annually, and most therapeutic approaches result in a high incidence of local failure that frequently manifests as malignant airway occlusion.[2,3] According to one estimate, 20% to 30% of newly diagnosed malignant neoplasms will present with atelectasis and pneumonia due to endobronchial disease.[3] Death from airway occlusion is often a painful process of slow asphyxiation, frequently complicated by obstructive pneumonia and hemoptysis. The management of patients with malignant airway obstruction represents a therapeutic challenge for physicians engaged in their care. With either unresectable disease at presentation, recurrence after attempted curative resection, or metastatic disease, the surgical alternatives are limited, and chemotherapy is, for most patients, ineffective or response is brief.

The ability to manage acute airway obstruction can be lifesaving. Airway relief should be expeditious and immediate, with low morbidity and mortality. It should not interfere with future definitive therapy. In patients with terminal malignancy, it should be economical in costs and should minimize hospitalization.

Acute respiratory distress, stridor, and obstructive pneumonia may be the presenting signs of advanced airway neoplasms.[4] Reduction of the tracheal lumen by 80% (3 to 5 mm) may occur before symptoms become severe. However, inflammatory swelling or poststenotic retention of mucus or blood may lead to acute obstruction and severe hypoxia.[5]

Symptoms depend on location and extent of the tumor. Neoplasms of the trachea and carina may cause obstructive airway symptoms, as opposed to neoplasms of the distal airway, which are more likely to show initial symptoms of postobstructive pneumonia. Dyspnea may initially be present only with exertion, but may progress as the tumor enlarges to dyspnea at rest, stridor, and acute respiratory distress. In patients with pedunculated tumors, symptoms may vary with body position.

Management of patients with malignant airway obstruction depends on the urgency of presentation, etiology, localization, extent of obstruction, and prognosis of the disease. Complications from the obstruction, therapeutic measures available, and the experience of the physician influence the management of such patients.[5] Many methods of relieving airway obstruction are available. Palliation of symptoms and establishment of an airway in an expeditious manner are the goal.[4]

When patients present with respiratory distress, efforts are aimed at relief of symptoms rather than extensive evaluation of the patient. Functional assessment of the patient and evaluation of the extent of disease can be performed after the airway obstruction has been relieved. For those patients who present in a less acute fashion, functional assessment of the patient and radiologic evaluation of the extent of disease are appropriate. Above all else, one should consider the possibility of curative resection even in patients with obstructing airway neoplasms. Bronchoplastic techniques are available to allow resection and reconstruction of the trachea, carina, main bronchi, and lobar orifices.[6] Opening an obstructed airway in patients who have acute respiratory distress with potentially resectable tumors will allow time for a thorough workup, correction of underlying medical problems, or tapering of steroid administration if the patients have been incorrectly treated for "asthma."[4]

RADIOLOGIC EVALUATION

If time permits, careful radiologic evaluation is a valuable asset to operative management. Frequently the site of tracheal obstruction may be seen on chest x-ray in two planes. Tomography of the trachea and carina provides information about the extent of involvement, configuration, axis of the airway, and patency of the distal airway.[7] A lateral neck with oblique tracheal views along with AP views of the larynx and trachea may show stenoses, intraluminal densities, or luminal narrowing and displacement. Computerized tomography with axial 4 mm. sections may be used to assess intraluminal and extraluminal malignant tumors, including lymph node metastases. Magnetic resonance imaging with axial coronal and sagittal T1 and T2-CW images delineates tumors in the coronal, axial, and lateral projections; it is helpful in the evaluation of extraluminal tumor extension, vascular invasion, and lymph node metastases.[8,9,10]

ANESTHESIA

When there is a significant degree of airway obstruction, it is desirable to induce anesthesia with a controlled inhalation technique, as described by Wilson.[11] Ethrane is our agent of choice. When adequate alveolar ventilation exists and there is no need for an extremely high (99%) inspired oxygen concentration, nitrous oxide is often used to hasten and smooth induction of anesthesia. Muscle relaxants should not be used, because ventilation provided with mask and positive pressure through an obstructed airway is generally less satisfactory than the degree of gas exchange produced with spontaneous ventilation using assisted positive-pressure breathing. Anesthesia administration is continued until the patient is at a suitable depth to withstand bronchoscopy. This technique allows a patient to maintain spontaneous ventilation throughout the procedure. It can be time-consuming and requires patience on the part of the anesthesiologist and surgeon, but the disadvantage this imposes is greatly outweighed by the tremendous advantage of having the patient spontaneously ventilating throughout the procedure. This is especially important because the exact nature of the obstruction may not be known. During the course of tumor removal, maintaining the airway may be difficult and the patient's ability to breath is often the only thing that sustains him or her through this period.[4] When spontaneous ventilation is preserved, the surgeon will have more time to establish an airway than in the paralyzed, apneic patient. For this reason, we have avoided the use of narcotics, barbiturates, and paralyzing agents.

TECHNIQUES

Coring Out

The combination of biopsy forceps and the tip of the rigid bronchoscope to "core out" the tumor is very effective and satisfies many of the requirements for opening an obstructed airway. The authors find this to be the procedure of choice

for management of malignant airway obstruction. This technique demands that the surgeon and assistants be in attendance during induction of anesthesia and have all necessary instruments available to establish an emergency airway. Rigid bronchoscopes of graded sizes should be available (3.59 mm). The small pediatric bronchoscope may be the only bronchoscope that can be inserted through a very proximal, tight stricture. This allows immediate control of the airway subsequent to further manipulations. The bronchoscope is introduced and insinuated with gentle pressure past the malignant stricture. It is almost always possible to pass a rigid bronchoscope beyond an obstructing tumor. If the tumor is not based circumferentially, the rigid bronchoscope may be insinuated along the wall of the trachea that is not involved. Once the patient has an airway and is well ventilated, the bronchoscope may be withdrawn above the tumor and the bulk of the tumor removed. The tumor is first biopsied to determine its consistency and vascularity. The tip of the bronchoscope is then used as a coring device to shave larger pieces of tumor. Once a piece is dislodged, suction or biopsy forceps are used to extract it. This is repeated until an adequate airway is achieved. It is vitally important to perform this in the axis of the airway to avoid penetration through the wall and injury to vascular structures or creation of a pneumothorax. The procedure usually takes 15 to 30 minutes[12] (Figure 61.1).

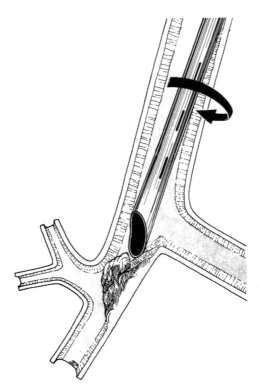

FIGURE 61.1. Technique of "coring out" utilizing the rigid bronchoscope.

For more distal tumors, insertion of a larger broncho-scope in the proximal airway allows careful inspection and suctioning of any secretions. The distal airway can be evaluated by inserting a flexible bronchoscope through the rigid bronchoscope. It is important to establish an airway, clear retained secretions, and stabilize the patient before proceeding with tumor removal. Using standard rigid bronchoscopy techniques, even lobar obstructions can often be managed with this technique.

Mathisen and Grillo reported our results of treating malignant obstruction with this technique in 1989.[4] The location of the obstruction was trachea in 16 patients, carina in 24, main bronchi in eight and distal airway in eight. Improvement in the airway was accomplished in 90% of patients. A single bronchoscopy was sufficient in 96%. There were numerous histologic types of tumors amenable to this approach (Table 61.1). An improved airway was achieved in 51 of the 56 patients after endoscopic removal of tumor, with no intraoperative deaths in the series. Only two patients required repeat bronchoscopy within two months of initial successful core-out. Nineteen complications occurred in 11 patients, including pneumonia, bleeding, pneumothorax, hypoxia, hypocarbia, arrhythmias, and laryngeal edema. Four patients died within two weeks of endoscopy of causes unrelated to the procedure. All patients had received no benefit from previous radiation therapy and were in desperate condition with postobstructive pneumonia.

Major hemorrhage rarely occurs with this technique and did not occur in this series of patients. Only three out of 56 patients had more than minor bleeding (500 mL).[4] Minor bleeding is easily controlled with simple measures such as irrigation with saline or tamponade with epinephrine (0.1 mg per mL) soaked pledgets on long applicators. Use of the rigid bronchoscope to tamponade the raw surface of the tumor is also effective. Tamponade with Fogarty venous occlusion catheters or an inflated endotracheal tube balloon against the raw surface is also effective for persistent oozing from a raw surface.

Short-term survival depends on the success of the endoscopic core-out of the tumor and long-term survival depends on the effectiveness of proposed treatments. The survival of inoperable patients after radiation or chemotherapy in the series presented by Mathisen ranged from two months to 82 months, with a median of six months. Histology, location, and extent of disease determine success of treatment. For patients with failed previous therapies, endoscopic removal of the tumor is a temporary measure that allows a patent airway. Use of tracheotomy tubes, T-tubes, or other stents may be effective in maintaining an airway in this group of patients who have no other options.

Cryotherapy

Cryotherapy is of limited usefulness, especially in the acute setting. Treatment requires application of probes that are cooled to $-60°$ C to $-80°$ C with liquid nitrogen. Tumors may be frozen and removed mechanically. The stated advantage of endoscopic cryosurgery is the capacity to extend it to extramural parts of tumors up to 1.5 to 2 cm. With this technique, only tumors of 1 to 2 cm. on half the circumference of the trachea can be removed in one session. Reepithelization after removal is reportedly very good.[5] The obvious disadvantages in its application for severe tracheal obstruction are in the actual mechanics of its application. The probes are clumsy and make exact endoscopic placement difficult. Acute manipulation of the airway is limited, because the probe cannot be removed immediately but remains stuck to the tissues for about one minute. If the diameter of the probe is reduced, then the speed of cooling may be diminished. With a slower rate of cooling, tumor cells are preserved rather than destroyed. Coring out and laser surgery, along with endobronchial brachytherapy, have supplanted the role of cryotherapy in malignant airway obstruction.

Expandable Metallic Stents

The last several years have seen a substantial growth in the availability and use of endolumenal stents. Available expandable stents basically break down into covered and uncovered metallic stents. The first stent commonly used, the Gianturco stent, is a self-expandable, stainless steel stent made of a thin-diameter stainless steel wire laced into a zigzag cylinder that expands on placement. Use of the Gianturco self-expandable stent was initially intended for treatment of stenoses within the vascular system and biliary tree.[13,14,15] Similarly, the covered Wallstent was first used

TABLE 61.1. HISTOLOGY OF OBSTRUCTING NEOPLASMS

Histology	Location of Tumor*		
	Trachea	Carina	Bronchus
Squamous carcinoma	8	11	6
Adenoidcystic	2	7	0
Adenocarcinoma	0	3	4
Thyroid	3	0	0
Sarcoma	1	1	2
Carcinoid	1	0	1
Mucoepidermoid	1	0	0
Lymphoma	0	1	0
Small cell carcinoma	0	1	1
Metastatic melanoma	0	0	1
Metastatic acinar carcinoma	0	0	1

* In numbers of patients
From the Society of Thoracic Surgeons. Mathisen DJ, Grillo HC. Endoscopic relief of malignant airway obstruction. *Ann Thorac Surg* 1989;48:469, with permission.

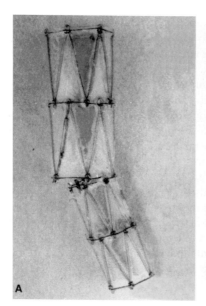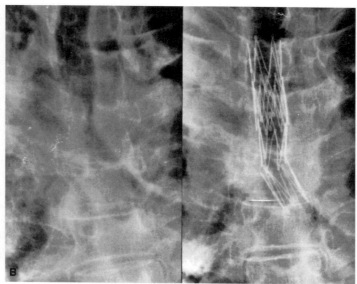

FIGURE 61.2. A: Gianturco stent for endobronchial stenting. (Photo, courtesy of Dr. Rosch, Professor of Radiology, Oregon Health Sciences University.) **B:** Chest x-ray of endobronchial stent in place. (Photo, courtesy of Dr. Rosch, Professor of Radiology, Oregon Health Sciences University.)

in the vascular tree and has recently gained popularity within the tracheobronchial tree.

Different lengths and widths are available, and commonly, two Gianturco stents are joined together with lateral barbs affixed to the stent to minimize migration (Figure 61.2). Varela and colleagues, Wilson and colleagues, and others have described a technique for stent placement.[16,17] A guidewire is passed through a flexible bronchoscope through the obstruction. The bronchoscope is then reinserted so that the deployment of the stent can be observed. The stents are inserted in a compressed form, loaded in a 12 French Teflon sheath over the guidewire. The stent is advanced through the Teflon sheath until it reaches the distal aspect of the sheath. The pusher is held with one hand while the Teflon sheath is removed, allowing the distal aspect of the stent to expand. Two or more stents may be required, and the stents should always be longer than the obstructing lesion. Correct placement is confirmed with the fiber-optic bronchoscope.[15,16,17,18,19]

The deployment of the covered Wallstent was well described by Monnier and associates in a prospective multicenter study. Two methods for deployment currently exist. The Rigistep device consists of a rigid bronchoscope through which the stent is deployed after the lesion has been crossed. If the lesion cannot be crossed with a rigid bronchoscope or the resources for rigid bronchoscopy do not exist, the telestep device can be used to deploy the stent while observing with a flexible bronchoscope or under fluoroscopy. This proceeds in a manner similar to that described above.[20]

Multiple studies have now looked at the efficacy of expandable stents. Wilson and colleagues looked at 56 patients with inoperable malignancy and significant airway compromise. These patients underwent stenting with the Gianturco expandable stent. Of the patients treated, 77% showed significant symptomatic improvement and 67% showed improvement in pulmonary function tests. Four patients died perioperatively, two of respiratory causes and two of myocardial infarction. One patient suffered a pneumothorax and one suffered a hemopneumothorax. Mean survival of all patients was 77 days (1 to 477 days).[17] Another study by Monnier and associates looked at the efficacy of covered Wallstents in 40 patients presenting with inoperable tracheobronchial cancer. Except in cases of pure extrinsic compression, an initial lumen was created using the Neodymium-Ytrium-Garnet (Nd:YAG) laser. The tumor was situated in the trachea in 11 patients, in the carina in six, right main or intermediate in 12, and the left main in 11. Following stent deployment, the lumen was returned to within 92% of normal (plus or minus 6.3%). Patients were evaluated post procedure and at 30 and 90 days. At 30 days, 22 patients were alive and 19 underwent bronchoscopy. Eleven showed partial obstruction and three showed minor stent migration. There was no significant progression of dyspnea. At 90 days, 13 were still alive and 10 underwent bronchoscopy. All patients showed incomplete tumor coverage but once again, there was no significant difference in dyspnea.[20] Tojo and associates sought to compare these stents. They used Gianturco stents to treat 11 patients with extrinsic compression; the airway remained open in 10 of these patients. Sixteen patients with intraluminal tumor were treated as follows: Nine with bare metal stents, four with covered metal stents, three with Dumon stents. Four of the patients treated with a covered stent suffered tumor ingrowth necessitating laser therapy. None of the covered stent or Dumon stent patients needed further therapy.[21] None of the patients treated with bare stents for extrinsic compression required further therapy.

In conclusion, expandable stents represent a viable option in the treatment of obstructing malignant airway disease. While hard data are lacking, several inferences can be made. It appears that bare metal stents are more secure and tend to migrate less. On the other hand, tumor ingrowth through the metal lattice appears a real phenomena. At present these properties suggest that bare metal stents are more suitable for extrinsic airway compression and covered stents are more suitable for intraluminal tumor growth. Both stents become intensely incorporated after about two weeks. It also appears that deployable metallic stents induce a granulation response at their anchoring points. These properties make them contraindicated in the treatment of benign disease.[20,22] As with all devices, innovations and revisions are surely underway.

Silastic Stents

The T-tube that is presently in clinical use was developed in 1965 by Montgomery[23] and has been most widely used by otolaryngologists and thoracic surgeons[24,25] as a stent in subglottic and tracheal obstructions.

The T-tube is made of a light and pliable silicone rubber and comes with a silicone plug secured in place by friction from a slight twisting motion. The intratracheal edges of the tube are trimmed and smoothed to avoid trauma to the tracheal mucosa. Tissue reaction to silicone is usually minimal, and the stent can remain in place for extended periods of time. The flexibility of the cannula allows easy insertion and removal via tracheostomy. If the laryngeal airway is adequate, normal phonation and humidification through the nasopharynx are preserved. The Montgomery T-tube endoprosthesis comes in a variety of sizes and shapes (Figure 61.3). Sizes range from 4 to 16 mm in outside diameter. A variety of tubes are available with long inferior limbs for intrathoracic tracheal obstructions. There are also available either single-armed or Y-shaped cannulas with the lower ends acting as stents for the carina and main bronchi when the lesion involves that area.[26,27]

In cases where malignant obstruction of the airway cannot be operated on because of extent of disease, the T-tube can be inserted to relieve asphyxia and allow a relatively good quality of life. Insertion of the T-tube requires careful preoperative assessment of the airway. Measurements are obtained with a rigid bronchoscope to determine proximal and distal extent of the tumor, carina, stoma, and vocal cords. The T-tube is inserted through a preexisting tracheal stoma or a newly created stoma.[28] After the proper diameter T-tube is selected and the ends trimmed to the desired length, the upper limb of the intratracheal tube is grasped with a Kelley clamp and the lower end is introduced into the stoma. With the tube inserted, the lower limb is advanced toward the distal trachea until the entire endotracheal portion is within the lumen. A second Kelley grasps the outside horizontal branch, pulling it to seat the cannula in the proper position. This is all done with the aid of

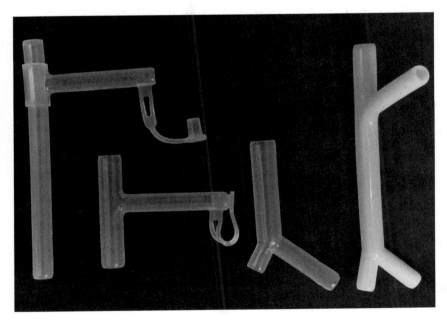

FIGURE 61.3. Variety of available Montgomery T-tubes with modifications shown.

the rigid bronchoscope under direct vision to minimize any iatrogenic injury to the trachea and provide an airway. The upper limb of the tube should be positioned, unless contraindicated by involvement of the subglottic and glottic region, about 1 cm below the vocal cords. If the upper limb is too long, irritation of the subglottic region and vocal cords will lead to laryngeal edema or predispose to aspiration. In rare cases, however, the proximal extent of the T-tube has been placed through the vocal cords, with some patients even developing pharyngeal speech. The side arm should be plugged as soon as possible to allow speech and natural humidification. Failure to plug the side arm will quickly lead to crusting and obstruction of the tube. Humidification should be provided and the tube suctioned frequently. Acetylcysteine can be instilled with normal saline to prevent formation of mucous plugs. The skin around the stoma should be cleaned regularly to minimize contamination. Patients can be easily trained to perform routine care of the tube at home.

Similar to the T-tube, the Dumon tube is a silastic stent placed directly into the airway. Unlike the T-tube, there is no stomal connection. Instead, the tube is held in place by a series of silastic studs that line the outside of the stent (see Fig. 61.3). The Dumon tube requires rigid bronchoscopy for placement and comes in a Y shape for stenting of the mainstems or carina. The Dumon tube has both advantages and disadvantages compared to the T-tube. Its advantages include cosmesis and placement without the need for a stoma. Its disadvantages include the lack of a stoma through which suctioning of secretions is facilitated and, despite the silastic studs, a greater tendency to migrate.

In general, the authors favor the use of a T-tube over the Dumon tube. We find dealing with inspisated secretions considerably easier with a stomal component in place. Patients with an end tracheal stoma who develop an intratracheal recurrence, however, pose a specific problem. In these patients, a Dumon tube is preferable to an amputated T-tube, primarily due to its anchoring capabilities. A special situation that requires close monitoring is the patient with a Y stent in place and a severe forceful cough. On occasion these patients have dislodged an arm of the Y stent causing the stent to buckle and occlude the airway.

Lasers

Laser is an acronym for light amplification by the stimulated emission of radiation. The principle upon which lasers are based was expounded by Einstein in 1917[29] but was not put into practical use until 1958, when groups at Bell Laboratories and Hughes began using a doped ruby crystal.[30] Endoscopic application of laser technology began in 1973 with the use of carbon dioxide CO_2 laser therapy to ablate benign neoplasms such as papillomas and later to palliate malignant obstruction of the major airways.[31] Laser mediated ablation of tissue proceeds from the rapid deposition

of energy into a small area. Following absorption of this energy, a primarily thermal process ensues, culminating in a phase change and vaporization of tissue. The absolute quantity of energy deposited, the wavelength of light used, and the pulse duration all significantly impact the process. The wavelength of the emitted light determines the molecule within the tissue that will act as the absorber. The pulse duration affects thermal dissipation and hence lateral thermal injury.

The carbon dioxide laser emits an invisible beam of light with a wavelength of 10,600 nm. The beam has a very high water-absorption coefficient and is absorbed by all tissues with little or no scatter or penetration. This produces a precisely localized vaporizing instrument with very little surrounding edema or trauma adjacent to the focal point of the beam. CO_2 laser light cannot at present be transmitted through fiber-optic bundles but must be reflected in transit off prisms and articulation, and therefore requires a cumbersome delivery system of articulated arms. Because of these mechanics of delivery, only tracheal and proximal bronchial lesions are accessible. The CO_2 laser is a precise cutting instrument and affords hemostasis only to the microcirculation. Vessels greater than 0.5 mm. are ineffectively coagulated. However, because of minimal edema next to the focal point of the beam, there is excellent healing ability in the adjacent tissues. With the advent of the Nd: YAG laser for similar lesions, the CO_2 laser has become less important. Ablation and resection of tumor mass in major airways is much more effectively and safely performed with the Nd: YAG laser.[32]

The Nd:YAG laser can be delivered through an optical fiber and produces excellent vaporization. The high thermal energy can produce vaporization, coagulative necrosis, and coagulative hemostasis. The energy output of this laser far exceeds that of the CO_2 laser. This laser system can be used through flexible optical fibers and allows for resection of tumor by vaporization and for effective coagulation and hemostasis of larger vessels (1 mm).[33-35]

Contraindications to Nd:YAG laser therapy include the following: obstruction due to extrinsic compression; obstruction due to lack of cartilaginous support; tracheoesophageal fistula; lobar or more distal occlusion; total obstruction over 4 to 6 cm with no probable distal airway, and bleeding diathesis.[32]

Use of a No. 9 Wolf ventilating bronchoscope with a Sanders injector for ventilation is recommended. The FI02 should be less than 40% to prevent combustion and/or fire. The tumor is assessed through the rigid scope, and any large bulky portions are dislodged by manipulations of the tip of the bronchoscope as previously described in the coring-out technique. Hemorrhage from the tumor is usually only mild to moderate. Indeed, most of the tumor bulk can be removed through this simple method of debridement. A flexible bronchoscope can then be passed through an occluding grommet at the open end of the scope, and a laser fiber can be passed through the channel of the fiberoptic scope and positioned under direct vision of the operator. Smoke is aspirated with the use of a vinyl suction catheter in the rigid scope. The power output is between 45 and 55 watts in half-second pulses.

If during laser therapy there is need for suctioning of secretions, purulent material, or blood, or removal of large portions of necrotic debris, the flexible scope can be removed, the ventilation converted to a jet system with the Sanders injector, and a large-bore suction catheter and biopsy forceps inserted directly into the open end of the bronchoscope. This particular technique allows for simple and rapid conversion from one delivery system to another. Repetitive treatments may be necessary to obtain an adequate airway. A dilute solution of epinephrine is occasionally injected into the scope to arrest bleeding from the raw tumor bed. The patient can either be extubated in the operating room, or reintubated with an endotracheal tube after the rigid bronchoscope has been removed and extubated in the recovery room.

The major advantages of the Nd:YAG laser over other lasers are the superior vaporization, excellent coagulative necrosis, and deeper penetration achieved. Safe and effective ablation can be performed much more quickly with this laser. The procedure may be done either through a flexible bronchoscope, as described, or through a rigid bronchoscope exclusively, as described by Dumon.[34] Complications include hypoxemia, hemorrhage, perforation, fire, pneumothorax, and endobronchial spillage of distal obstructive purulent material.

McDougall and Cortese[33] defined the selection criteria for laser therapy. They stated that these patients should have malignant airway obstruction which has failed all other reasonable therapy, and the lesion should be protruding into the bronchial wall without obvious extension beyond the cartilage. They further stated that the actual length of the endobronchial component of the tumor should be less than 4 cm, and that the bronchoscopist should be able to see the bronchial lumen at all times. There should be functioning lung tissue beyond the obstruction. Their initial series included 22 patients who received 28 treatments during a five-month period. After the initial treatment, immediate improvement in airway diameter and symptomatic relief was achieved in 20 of 22 patients.

The efficacy of the Nd:YAG laser in endobronchial tracheal obstructive lesions has been shown by several series.[35–38] Perhaps the largest is from France, where Dumon and colleagues reported 1,503 endoscopic YAG laser treatments on 839 patients.[34] Brutinel and associates, from the Mayo Clinic,[38] reported that airway caliber improvement was achieved in up to 83.4% of treatments. Obstructions at the level of the trachea, mainstem bronchi, and bronchus intermedius were improved more often than those at the lobar bronchi. At follow-up, 36% of patients in his series were alive at one year. The median time to retreatment or

death was 130 days. In Parr's and colleagues' series of 40 patients,[36] patients had primary lung malignancies. Of those treated with the Nd:YAG laser, results were reported as excellent in 22 patients. Kvale and associates at Henry Ford Hospital reported a series of 55 patients treated a total of 82 times. Satisfactory results (doubling of airway size with relief of dyspnea or drainage of obstructive pneumonitis) were obtained in 12 of 13 patients with bronchogenic carcinoma initially managed with laser and in 22 of 32 patients with recurrent malignancies.[37]

The major cause of death during or after laser resection is hypoxemia and perforation (less than 40%).[32] Hemorrhage is rare in the series listed (1% to 3%).[31,33–38] Dumon and colleagues[34] state that experimental data suggests a continuous radiation at a power setting of 40 watts or more creates massive tissue coagulation and uncontrolled penetration. Consequently, to preclude perforation and exsanguinating hemorrhage, the endoscopists must use the laser sparingly over intermittent exposures (0.5 to 1 second) at power settings not higher than 45 watts. For coagulation, long low-powered shots are used; for resection, short high-powered shots are needed. Another rule of safety consists in firing parallel to the airway wall and strictly avoiding perpendicular shots. Further economy in laser firing can be had by photocoagulation and mechanical removal of the tumor mass using the tip of the bronchoscope to shave off fragments and the suction tubing to evacuate them. Oxygen concentration should not exceed 50% during laser resection to avoid fire at the fiber-optic tip. Kvale and associates[37] utilized computer axial tomography (CAT) with contrast infusion and rapid sequence imaging to display the relationships between the involved bronchus and the surrounding structures, particularly the large intrathoracic blood vessels. The image provided by the CAT scan may be useful, particularly when the lesion is obstructing the distal trachea or more peripherally.

In summary, exophytic lesions of the trachea and mainstem bronchi are most amenable to therapy by laser, and improvement in symptoms correlate best with improved patency of large airways. In most patients the major portion of the endobronchial debulking procedure can be performed quickly and safely by physically coring out the exophytic tumor mass with the rigid end of the bronchoscope. The laser can then be used to remove any remaining tumor and produce hemostasis by coagulation of the tumor bed.[32]

Bronchoscopic Balloon Dilatation

Bronchoscopic balloon dilatation is a well-known technique in the management of children and infants with tracheobronchial stenosis. Its usefulness, however, in the management of malignant airway obstruction has been quite limited. For now, its use is primarily as an adjunct to laser photoresection or stenting. It serves to create an adequate lumen for the deployment of more definitive modalities.[39]

Intratumoral Injections

When other modalities have been unavailable, some physicians have turned to direct intratumoral injection of chemotherapeutic agents. Celikoglu and associates recently looked at 93 patients who presented with over 50% obstruction of at least one major airway. All patients were treated with 5-fluorouracil, mitomycin, methotrexate, bleomycin, and mitoxantrone, injected directly into the tumor. Thirty-five patients presented with complete obstruction of one lung; of these, 18 saw complete reexpansion, six had partial reexpansion, and 11 had no effect. Overall, 39 of the 93 patients showed an increase in the lumenal diameter to over 50%, and 42 showed a 25% to 50% increase.[40]

While direct intratumoral injection does not appear as efficacious as other modalities, it clearly holds promise. Its role as an adjunct to other techniques, for example, has not been investigated. Furthermore, the development of other chemotherapeutic regimens and/or selective activation (as with esophageal PDT) may greatly extend its efficacy.

CONCLUSION

Short-term survival is directly dependent on the ability to open the obstructed airway; long-term survival depends on the effectiveness of proposed treatments of the underlying cancer. For patients who have failed previous therapy, endoscopic removal of tumor is a temporary measure to relieve airway obstruction. Use of tracheotomy tubes and T-tubes may ultimately be effective in maintaining an airway in this group of patients who have no other options. The use of the Nd:YAG laser is an acceptable alternative to core-out, but more costly. Endoluminal stenting, although more costly than silastic stents or core-out, has the advantage of not requiring rigid bronchoscopy or general anesthesia. Endobronchial brachytherapy, although very labor-intensive, has also shown good success. It is important to note that all these modalities are acute therapy for airway occlusion and do not treat the underlying problem. Since no modality has proven clearly superior, the choice of therapy should depend on the expertise and resources of the staff and institution. Also, these therapies should not deter definitive therapy—tracheal resections, carinal resections, and sleeve resections of the tracheobronchial tree are accepted methods of treatment and can be curative.[6] These should always be considered on patients with obstructed airways so as not to deny patients the opportunity for cure.

REFERENCES

1. Silverberg E, Lubera JA. Cancer statistics. *Cancer* 1989;39:3.
2. Perez CA, Bauer M, Edelstein S, et al. Impact of tumor control on survival in carcinoma of the lung treated with irradiation. *Int J Radiat Oncol Biol Phys* 1986;12:539.
3. Minna JD, Higgins GA, Glatstein EJ. Cancer of the lung. In: VT Devita, S Hellman, SA Rosenberg, eds. *Cancer: principles and practice of oncology,* 2nd ed. Philadelphia: JB Lippincott; 1985:518.
4. Mathisen DJ, Grillo HC. Endoscopic relief of malignant airway obstruction. *Ann Thorac Surg* 1989;48:469.
5. Becker HD, Blersch E, Vogt-Moykopf I. Urgent treatment of tracheal obstruction. In: *International trends in general thoracic surgery,* vol. II. Grillo H and Eschapasse H, eds. Philadelphia: W.B. Saunders, 1987:13.
6. Grillo HC. Tracheal tumors: surgical management. *Ann Thorac Surg* 1978;26:112.
7. Felson B. Neoplasms of trachea and mainstem bronchi. *Semin Roentgenol* 1983;18(1):13.
8. Gamsu G, Webb WR. Computed tomography of the trachea and mainstem bronchi. *Semin Roentgenol* 1983;18(1):51.
9. Gamsu G, Webb WR. Computed tomography of the trachea: normal and abnormal. AJR *Am J Roentgenol* 1982;129:321.
10. Weber AL. Symposium on the larynx and trachea. *Radio Clin North Am* 1978;16(2).
11. Wilson RS. Anesthetic management for tracheal reconstruction. In: *International trends in general thoracic surgery,* vol. II. Grillo H and Eschapasse H, eds. Philadelphia: W.B. Saunders, 1987: 3;261.
12. Grillo HC. Urgent treatment of tracheal obstruction—discussion. In: *International trends in general thoracic surgery,* vol. II. Grillo H and Eschapasse H, eds. Philadelphia: W.B. Saunders, 1987:19.
13. Wright KC, Wallace S, Charnsangavey C, et al. Percutaneous endovascular stents: an experimental evaluation. *Radiology* 1985; 156:69.
14. Carrasco CH, Wallace S, Charnsangavey C, et al. Expandable biliary endoprosthesis: an experimental study. AJR *Am J Roentgenol* 1985;145:1279.
15. Wallace MJ, Charnsangavey C, Ogawa K, et al. Tracheobronchial tree: expandable metallic stents used in experimental and clinical application. *Radiology* 1986;158:309.
16. Varela A, Maynar M, Irving D, et al. Use of Gianturco self-expandable stents in the tracheobronchial tree. *Ann Thorac Surg* 1990;49:806.
17. Wilson GE, Walshaw MJ, Hind CRK. Treatment of large airway obstruction in lung cancer using expandable metal stents inserted under direct vision via the fibreoptic bronchoscope. *Thorax* 1996; 51:248.
18. Simonds AK, Irving JD, Clarke SW, et al. Use of expandable metal stents in the treatment of bronchial obstruction. *Thorax* 1989;44:680.
19. Coolen D, Slabbynck H, Galdermans D, et al. Insertion of a self-expandable endotracheal metal stent using topical anaesthesia and a fibreoptic bronchoscope: a comfortable way to offer palliation. *Thorax* 1994;49:87.
20. Monnier P, Mudry A, Stanzel F, et al. The use of the covered Wallstent for the palliative treatment of inoperable tracheobronchial cancers. *Chest* 1996;110:1161.
21. Tojo T, Iioka S, Kitamura S, et al. Management of malignant tracheobronchial stenosis with metal stents and Dumon stents. *Ann Thorac Surg* 1998;61:1074.
22. Fraga JC, Filler RM, Forte V, et al. Experimental trial of balloon-expandable, metallic palmaz stent in the trachea. *Arch Otolaryngol Head Neck Surg* 1997;123:522.
23. Montgomery WW. T-tube tracheal stent. *Arch Otolaryngol* 1965; 82:320.
24. Gaissert HA, Grillo HC, Mathisen DJ, et al. Temporary and permanent restoration of airway continuity with the tracheal T-tube. *J Thorac Cardiovasc Surg* 1994;107:600.
25. Cooper JD, Pearson FG, Patterson GA, et al. Use of silicone stents in the management of airway problems. *Ann Thorac Surg* 1989;47:371.

26. Westaby S, Jackson JW, Pearson FG. A bifurcated silicone rubber stent for relief of tracheobronchial obstruction. *J Thorac Cardiovasc Surg* 1982;83:414.

27. Westaby S, Sheperd MP. Palliation of intrathoracic tracheal compression with a silastic tracheobronchial stent. *Thorax* 1983;38:314.

28. Landa L. The tracheal T tube. In: *Tracheal surgery. International trends in general thoracic surgery,* vol. II. Grillo H and Eschapasse H, eds. Philadelphia: W.B. Saunders, 1987:124.

29. Einstein A. On the quantum theory of radiation. *Physikal* 1917;18:121.

30. Maiman TH. Stimulated optical radiation in ruby. *Nature* 1960;187:493.

31. Shapshay SM, Davis RK, Vaughan CW, et al. Palliation of airway obstruction from tracheobronchial malignancy: Use of the CO_2 laser bronchoscope. *Otolaryngol Head Neck Surg* 1983;91:615.

32. Goldberg M. Endoscopic laser treatment for bronchogenic carcinoma. *Surg Clin North Am* 1988;68:635.

33. McDougall JC, Cortese DA. Neodymium-YAG laser, therapy of malignant airway obstruction: a preliminary report. *Mayo Clin Proc* 1983;58:35.

34. Dumon JF, Shapshay S, Bourareau J, et al. Principles for safety in application of neodymium-YAG laser in bronchology. *Chest* 1984;86:163.

35. Toty L, Personne CL, Colchen A, et al. Bronchoscopic management of tracheal lesions by laser photoresection. *Chest* 1982;81:278.

36. Parr GVS, Unger M, Trout RG, et al. One hundred ND-YAG laser ablations of obstructing tracheal neoplasms. *Ann Thorac Surg* 1984;38:374.

37. Kvale PA, Eichenhorn MC, Radke JR, et al. YAG laser photoresection of lesions obstruction the central airways. *Chest* 1985;87:283.

38. Brutinel WM, Cortese DA, McDougall JC, et al. A two-year experience with neodymium YAG laser in endobronchial obstruction. *Chest* 1987;91:159.

39. Noppen M, Schlesser M, Meysman M, et al. Bronchoscopic balloon dilatation in the combined management of postintubation stenosis of the trachea in adults. *Chest* 1997;112:1136.

40. Celikoglu S. Karayel T, Demirci S, et al. Direct injection of anticancer drugs into endobronchial tumours for palliation of major airway obstruction. *Postgrad Med J* 1997;73:159.

62

SUPERIOR VENA CAVA SYNDROME: SURGERY AND STENTS

JONATHAN C. NESBITT

INTRODUCTION AND HISTORY

Obstruction of the superior vena cava (SVC) is well recognized as a complication of lung cancer. The degree of clinical manifestation varies among patients, but recognition and prompt management are essential. Although the usual treatment is nonsurgical, selected patients can benefit significantly from operative or interventional measures.

Superior vena cava syndrome (SVCS) was originally described by William Hunter in 1757 in a patient with a saccular aneurysm of the ascending aorta.[1] At autopsy, he noted that the SVC and innominate vein were "both so much compressed by the dilated artery, as hardly to have any thing left of their natural capacity and appearance." William Stokes in 1837 reported SVCS secondary to a right-lung malignancy, noting that the progressive physical findings were a consequence of the compressive effects of tumors on the SVC and the development of collateral circulation.[2] He described a patient whose "face was bloated, pale, and slightly edematous, which, with an appearance of the eyes as if the balls were protruded from the sockets, and a marked dilatation of the nostrils during breathing, gave his countenance an expression of distress and suffering. . . . The right jugular vein was much distended, as were the veins in the right axilla; but this symptom was chiefly remarkable on the surface of the belly, where two veins . . . pursued a remarkably tortuous course . . . being turgid and dilated to the size of swan quills." In his comprehensive review of lung cancer in the nineteenth century, Rosenblatt refers to several reports from Ireland and Germany that describe SVCS secondary to bronchogenic carcinoma.[3]

Prior to the mid twentieth century, malignancy accounted for roughly one-third of all cases of SVCS. Most cases occurred secondary to infectious conditions such as luetic aortic aneurysms, tuberculosis, and fibrotic mediastinitis.[4] Today, however, intrathoracic malignancy has far surpassed benign disease as the primary cause of SVC obstruction. The increased incidence of bronchogenic carcinoma over the past several decades and improved treatment for granulomatous and infectious diseases have accounted for these etiologic changes.

ANATOMY AND PATHOGENESIS

The normal SVC measures 6 to 8 cm in length and 1 to 2 cm in diameter. It is formed by a union of the left and right innominate veins and is positioned in the middle mediastinum to the right of the aorta and anterior to the trachea. The inferior aspect of the SVC resides within the pericardial cavity for a length of 2 to 3 cm. For most of its length, the azygos vein is located posteriorly and adjacent to the vertebral column. As it approaches the SVC, it courses anteriorly over the right mainstem bronchus and enters the posterior wall of the SVC above the level of the pericardial reflection, several centimeters cephalad to the right atrium.

There are eight principal collateral pathways for drainage of the venous system in the chest: the paravertebral, azygos-hemiazygos, internal mammary, lateral thoracic, anterior jugular, thyroidal, thymic, and pericardiophrenic veins. The five major venous collateral networks are depicted in Figure 62.1. Each system is elaborately interconnected to provide innumerable possibilities for variations and directions in flow, depending on the situation. The presence of SVCS depends on individual anatomic patterns and compensatory changes during the evolution of the pathologic process. The location of the obstruction, the extent of the process, the presence of access pathways, and the capability of the pathways to adapt to excess blood flow determine the severity of the syndrome.

By using contrast venography, Stanford and Doty have described four patterns of associated venous flow determined by the degree of SVC obstruction[5] (Figures 62.2 to 62.5). Obstruction of the SVC below the insertion of the azygos vein may result in use of the azygos arch as the major collateral pathway, with reversal of flow and drainage into the inferior vena cava. Obstruction of the SVC above the level of insertion of the azygos vein results in flow through alternative pathways, primarily the cervical and paravertebral plexuses. The collateral vessels, in turn, drain into the azygos system, which flows retrograde into the inferior vena cava. A sparse number of central venous collaterals appear when the SVC and the major venous channels undergo

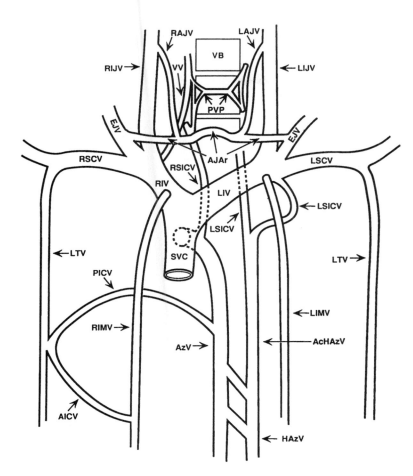

FIGURE 62.1. The five major collateral venous networks of the thorax. The thyroidal, thymic, and pericardiophrenic veins are not depicted. AcHAzV, accessory hemiazygos vein; AICV, anterior intercostal vein; AJAr, anterior jugular arch; AzV, azygos vein; EJV, external jugular vein; HAzV, hemiazygos vein; LAJV, left anterior jugular vein; LIJV, left internal jugular vein; LIMV, left internal mammary vein; LIV, left innominate vein; LSCV, left subclavian vein; LSICV, left superior intercostal vein; LSCV, left subclavian vein; LTV, lateral thoracic vein; PICV, posterior intercostal vein; PVP, paravertebral plexus; RAJV, right anterior jugular vein; RIJV, right internal jugular vein; RIMV, right internal mammary vein; RIV, right innominate vein; RSCV, right subclavian vein; RSICV, right superior intercostal vein; SVC, superior vena cava; VB, vertebral body; VV, vertebral vein. (From Chasen MH, Charnsangavej C. Venous chest anatomy: clinical implications. In: Greene R, Muhm JR, eds. *Syllabus: a categorical course in diagnostic radiology.* Presented at the 78th Scientific Assembly and Annual Meeting of the Radiological Society of North America. 1992:121, with permission.)

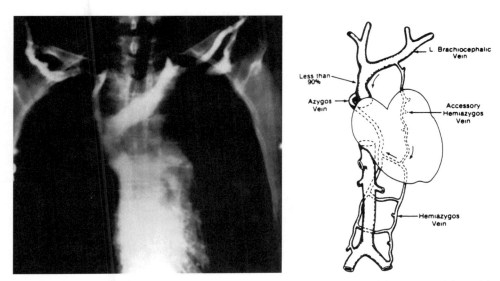

FIGURE 62.2. Partial obstruction of the superior vena cava with patency of the azygos; right atrial pathway. (From Stanford W, Doty DB. The role of venography and surgery in the management of patients with superior vena cava obstruction. *Ann Thorac Surg* 1986;41:158, with permission.)

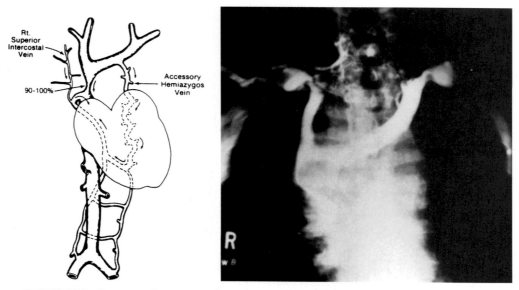

FIGURE 62.3. Near-complete to complete obstruction of the superior vena cava with pathway and antegrade flow in the azygos; right atrial pathway. (From Stanford W, Doty DB. The role of venography and surgery in the management of patients with superior vena cava obstruction. *Ann Thorac Surg* 1986;41:158, with permission.)

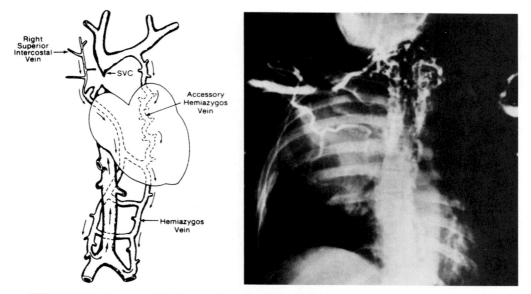

FIGURE 62.4. Near-complete to complete obstruction of the superior vena cava with reversal of azygos blood flow to the inferior vena cava. (From Stanford W, Doty DB. The role of venography and surgery in the management of patients with superior vena cava obstruction. *Ann Thorac Surg* 1986;41:158, with permission.)

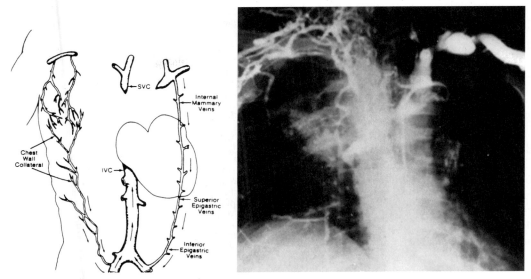

FIGURE 62.5. Complete obstruction of the superior vena cava and one or more of the major vena caval accessory pathways, including the azygos systems. (From Stanford W, Doty DB. The role of venography and surgery in the management of patients with superior vena cava obstruction. *Ann Thorac Surg* 1986;41:158, with permission.)

extensive thrombosis. In such circumstances, collateralization occurs through a network of extrathoracic pathways within the chest wall musculature and skin.

The progress of the vena caval obstructive process determines the severity of the syndrome and the changes associated with alterations of venous flow. Gradual strangulation of a major venous pathway (i.e., vena cava, innominate vein, or azygos vein) induces compensatory rerouting of flow into smaller systems. The process usually evolves as a subacute or chronic phenomenon which develops more quickly than the body's ability to create collateral vessels to circumvent the resulting congestion. The high venous circulatory pressure above the obstruction causes shunting into the adjacent lower pressure plexuses and venules. As time passes over weeks or months, the sustained pressure imposed upon the collateral pathways invokes their gradual distension and dilation. Eventually, small veins become major channels for flow.

When cutaneous veins are recruited to unload back pressure, increased venous blood in the skin is manifested clinically by a ruborous hue which gives the impression of cyanosis. Swelling and edema from the increase in capillary hydrostatic pressure are common; the extent of these conditions is determined primarily by the degree of collateral flow to reduce venous hypertension. If obstruction is insidious, the circulatory system has the ability to adapt to flow changes, often with only subtle clinical signs. In a few instances no clinical signs are expressed. Typical anatomic and physiologic changes which reflect congestion of flow include facial plethora, mild edema and rubor of the face and upper extremities, and dilated cutaneous veins. When the obstruc-

tive process is acute or subacute, physiologic changes of venous collateralization cannot occur quickly enough to compensate: compensatory collaterals for pressure unloading are nonexistent and pronounced venous hypertension results. In this situation, clinical signs and symptoms are more evident and are manifested more overtly by more severe facial, neck, and arm edema; headache; dyspnea; periorbital swelling; and facial erythema.

ETIOLOGY

Obstruction of the vena cava is due to extrinsic pressure, tumor invasion, thrombosis, or impedance of venous return from intra-atrial or intraluminal pathology. Approximately 73% to 97% of cases of SVCS occur secondary to malignancy.[6–11] Malignant encroachment on the SVC occurs either by direct extension or compression by the primary tumor or by invasion of superior mediastinal lymph nodes that contain malignancy. In addition, progressive tumor growth may violate the vascular intima and serve as a nidus for thrombus formation, which can evolve to extensive thrombosis of the SVC, branch vessels, and collateral tributaries. The malignancy that most frequently causes SVCS is lung cancer. Approximately 3% to 5% of patients with lung cancer develop the syndrome,[11–15] and approximately 10% to 15% of patients with right-sided chest malignancies will develop SVCS.[6,14] Of 337 patients with malignancies and SVCS registered at the University of Texas M.D. Anderson Cancer Center Department of Patient Studies through 1992, 218 (64.7%) had lung cancer. The histologic type varied: 77 (35%) had small cell carcinoma, 46 (21%) adenocarcinoma, 44 (20%) squamous cell, 8 (4%) large cell, and 63 (29%) nonspecified carcinomas. Other reviews have noted that lung cancer constituted 65% to 95% of all malignant causes of SVCS.[8,11,16–20]

CLINICAL PRESENTATION

The signs and symptoms of mature SVCS are usually easily recognized. Common symptoms and physical findings are noted in Tables 62.1 and 62.2. Early in the course, the presenting changes are subtle with minimal physical changes and no symptoms. On rare occasions, the SVC can be completely occluded without the development of physiologic or anatomic changes. At the other extreme, acute SVCS can result in the abrupt onset of symptoms with pronounced clinical manifestations reflective of the rapidly obstructive process. The average duration of symptoms is approximately 45 days,[21] with 90% of patients noting the duration of symptoms as less than eight weeks.[17]

The typical presentation reflects venous hypertension above the level of the obstruction. At a certain point in the process, venous collaterals will develop, including small, tortuous, vertically oriented cutaneous tributaries above the level of the rib cage margin. Features include upper body venous engorgement with dilated primary venous tributaries of the trunk, upper extremities, and neck. Facial plethora

TABLE 62.1. COMMON SYMPTOMS OF SUPERIOR VENA CAVA SYNDROME

	%
Facial swelling	71.9
Dyspnea	60
Cough	37.7
Arm swelling	27.6
Orthopnea	23.5
Pain	15.3
Dysphagia	10.6
Syncope	7.9
Headache	6.3
Stridor	4.2

Compiled from data on 571 patients from the following series; Fincher RE. Superior vena cava syndrome: experience in teaching hospital. *South Med J* 1987;80:1243. Parish JM, Marschke RF, Dines DE, et al. Etiologic considerations in superior vena cava syndrome. *Mayo Clin Proc* 1981;56:407. Lockridge SK, Knibbe WP, Doty DB. Obstruction of the superior vena cava. *Surgery* 1979;85:14. Armstrong BA, Perez CA, Simpson JR, et al. Role of irradiation in the management of superior vena cava syndrome. *Int J Radiat Oncol Biol Phys* 1987;3:531. Chen JC, Bongard F, Klein SR. A contemporary perspective on superior vena cava syndrome. *Am J Surg* 1990;160:207. Yellin A, Rosen A, Reichert N, et al. Superior vena cava syndrome: the myth—the facts. *Am Rev Resp Dis* 1990; 141:1114. Schraufnagel DE, Hill R, Leech JA, et al. Superior vena cava obstruction. *Am J Med* 1981;70:1169. Maddox AM, Valdivieso M, Lukeman J, et al. Superior vena cava obstruction in small cell bronchogenic carcinoma. *Cancer* 1983;52:2165, all with permission.

TABLE 62.2. COMMON PHYSICAL SIGNS OF SUPERIOR VENA CAVA SYNDROME

	%
Dilated neck veins	70.1
Facial plethora	68.1
Prominent cutaneous veins	60.1
Arm swelling	41.3
Edema	30.5
Cyanosis	22.7
Vocal cord paralysis	4.7
Obtundation	1.8

Compiled from data on 592 patients from the following series Fincher RE. Superior vena cava syndrome: experience in teaching hospital. *South Med J* 1987;80:1243. Parish JM, Marschke RF, Dines DE, et al. Etiologic considerations in superior vena cava syndrome. *Mayo Clin Proc* 1981;56:407. Lockridge SK, Knibbe WP, Doty DB. Obstruction of the superior vena cava. *Surgery* 1979;85:14. Armstrong BA, Perez CA, Simpson JR, et al. Role of irradiation in the management of superior vena cava syndrome. *Int J Radiat Oncol Biol Phys* 1987;3:531. Chen JC, Bongard F, Klein SR. A contemporary perspective on superior vena cava syndrome. *Am J Surg* 1990;160:207. Yellin A, Rosen A, Reichert N, et al. Superior vena cava syndrome: the myth—the facts. *Am Rev Resp Dis* 1990; 141:1114. Schraufnagel DE, Hill R, Leech JA, et al. Superior vena cava obstruction. *Am J Med* 1981;70:1169. Maddox AM, Valdivieso M, Lukeman J, et al. Superior vena cava obstruction in small cell bronchogenic carcinoma. *Cancer* 1983;52:2165, all with permission.

is most common, and unrecognized facial swelling is a frequent manifestation. The skin may appear ruddy or with a slight violet hue, giving the impression of cyanosis or flushing. Mild edema of the neck, face, and periorbital region with proptosis and conjunctival suffusion may be present. Assuming a recumbent position, bending over, and coughing exacerbate symptoms from transient elevations in venous pressure that is already hypertensive. Headache, nausea, dizziness, and visual disturbances are not uncommon. Lethargy, obtundation, syncope, stupor and/or coma occur in fewer than 2% of cases and appear more commonly in patients with rapidly progressive and severe SVCS. Such neurologic symptoms may be secondary to metastatic disease, not cerebral edema from venous occlusion. Laryngeal edema and glottic swelling can occur, but it is unusual for respiratory decompensation to occur from laryngeal edema alone. Significant compromise of the airway is uncommon, but when it does occur, it may be caused by the SVCS or by other factors that include glottic swelling, vocal cord paralysis, and extrinsic tracheal compression.

EVALUATION AND DIAGNOSIS

The superior vena cava syndrome is a clinical diagnosis; the signs and symptoms usually permit easy recognition. Confirmation by radiologic studies is not necessary, but histologic diagnosis is essential prior to the initiation of treatment.

Ultrasonography

Ultrasonography is valuable in evaluating the patency of the jugular, subclavian, and axillary veins. It is a safe, quick, and noninvasive bedside procedure. As a screening study to evaluate the presence of obstructive pathology, Doppler flow measurements are easy and accurate but are limited by their inability to view the intrathoracic veins adequately.[22,23] Further assessment of the intrathoracic venous system can be accomplished by transesophageal echocardiography (TEE), which has been shown to be an excellent method for evaluating the SVC and surrounding structures.[24,25]

Radionuclide Venography

Nuclear scintigraphy is an accurate and relatively noninvasive method of imaging the venous system. The images are not as precise as contrast venography in clearly defining the venous anatomy, but technetium-99m DPTA studies can readily confirm the presence of SVCS, allow visualization of the site of obstruction, demonstrate regions of collateral flow, assess the general quantity of accessory circulatory patterns, and identify areas of pulmonary emboli.[26–28] When evaluation of the venous system is desired in anticipation of surgery, nuclear scintigraphy is not the study of choice; contrast venography should be performed.

Computed Tomography and Magnetic Resonance Imaging

Computed tomography (CT) provides much information about SVCS. CT shows details of the thoracic anatomy, including tumor proximity to the SVC, heart, trachea, and other major structures; visualizes the extent of vena caval occlusion, including thrombi; permits visualization of collateral venous pathways, including the "collateral loop" of interconnecting intrathoracic veins[29]; and assists in directing diagnostic and therapeutic maneuvers. Using chest CT, Raptopoulos[30] has identified five categories of SVC compression that correspond to the severity of symptoms.

Type Ia is moderate narrowing of the SVC without collateral flow or increase in the size of the azygos vein.

Type Ib is severe narrowing of the SVC with retrograde flow into the azygos vein.

Type II is obstruction of the SVC above the azygos arch with retrograde flow into the thoracic, vertebral, and other peripheral veins.

Type III is obstruction of the SVC below the azygos arch with retrograde flow through the azygos arch into the inferior vena cava.

Type IV is obstruction of the SVC at the azygos arch with multiple peripheral collaterals and nonvisualization of the azygos vein.

Opacification of thoracic venous collaterals by CT often is suggestive of SVCS, but opacification of the anterior thoracic subcutaneous channels is the best indicator of SVC occlusion, with a specificity of 96%.[31] Moncada and colleagues noted the specific advantages of combining CT scans with CT digital phlebography for patients with SVCS to highlight detailed resolution of the thoracic and venous anatomy.[32] Magnetic resonance imaging (MRI) allows images in multiple planes and does not require iodinated contrast material. The ability of MRI to diagnose thoracic venous obstruction is high, with sensitivity and specificity rates of 94% and 100%, respectively.[33] Disadvantages of MRI include increased scanning time and cost.

Contrast Venography

Venacavography is an essential procedure when operative intervention is being considered and is a fundamental aspect of evaluation in anticipation of endovascular stent placement. The exact location and severity of caval obstruction, the sites of major vascular patency, the degree of associated thrombosis, and the extent of collateralization—key information in formulating an operative plan—can be precisely identified by contrast venography. Venography can be performed by bilateral antecubital venous injections or by conventional single-catheter injection, depending on the extent and location of the obstruction.

In a series of 36 patients, Stanford and Doty used venography to identify those patients whom they felt would most likely benefit from surgical bypass procedures[5] (Figures 62.2 to 62.5). Each radiographic pattern appeared to have a uniquely similar clinical presentation. As expected, the worst obstructive patterns and most severe symptoms were seen in patients with complete or near-complete obstruction of the SVC along with reversal or occlusion of flow in the azygous vein. The severity of the symptoms was the basis for selecting patients for palliative bypass grafting. Their results suggested that the patients who benefitted the most from surgical bypass were those with severe symptoms and with the worst obstructive patterns on venography.

Sputum Cytology, Fine-Needle Aspiration, and Lymph Node Biopsy

The simplest method of obtaining a histologic diagnosis is sputum cytologic analysis, which can yield a diagnosis in two thirds of patients.[17] Fine-needle aspiration or lymph node biopsy are important diagnostic methods that also yield a diagnosis in most cases. For lesions that are amenable to these procedures, they should be employed before proceeding to other more invasive methods, because hemorrhage or hematoma formation at the biopsy site is a concern. Prudent attention to the potential for associated coagulopathy and the reduction in venous hypertension while maintaining head and shoulder elevation is important. In most cases these procedures can be performed readily without complications.[34]

Transluminal Radiographic Biopsy

Another method for obtaining a histologic diagnosis is transluminal biopsy under fluoroscopic guidance. This combined procedure allows evaluation of the venous system as well as pathologic diagnosis,[35,36] but only rarely is it indicated. It is best used in circumstances of diagnostic difficulty when surgical intervention is being considered. If contrast venography is performed and identifies an intraluminal tumor, fluoroscopic transluminal biopsy can be performed.

Mediastinoscopy

The safety of mediastinoscopy in patients with SVCS has been questioned; in fact, some clinicians feel that it is contraindicated. Fears of hemorrhage, hematoma formation, perioperative respiratory distress, and infection have served as the principle factors discouraging many physicians from recommending or performing the procedure, but such fears are unjustified. SVCS has been the direct cause of very few complications in patients who have undergone mediastinoscopy. Kirschner performed mediastinoscopy in 16 patients with SVCS without a complication.[37] Callejas and colleagues, noting that mediastinoscopy is useful and reliable in the diagnosis of tumors that cause SVCS, reported one wound infection and one carotid artery injury in eight such cases.[38] Little and colleagues had no complications in eight patients who underwent cervical mediastinoscopy.[34] Jahangiri and colleagues performed mediastinoscopy in 14 patients with SVCS and had only one complication, an innominate artery injury.[39] They concluded that the procedure is safe and effective for establishing a diagnosis when other less invasive techniques have been unsuccessful. In two series of 53 patients with SVCS who underwent mediastinoscopy, one patient had excessive bleeding[40] and another had respiratory compromise requiring intubation for three days.[41]

When considering mediastinoscopy in patients with SVCS, the surgeon should be cognizant of SVCS physiology and take appropriate measures to reduce the potential for bleeding. Assuring adequate coagulation parameters is fundamental. Placing the patient in the reverse Trendelenburg position will help to reduce some of the upper-body venous hypertension, which in turn alleviates capillary oozing during the procedure. Enlarged subcutaneous venous collaterals should be avoided and pushed to the side. Heightened attention to hemostasis is key to the prevention of postoperative hemorrhage. When these usual precautionary measures are taken, mediastinoscopy is a safe procedure to perform in patients with SVCS.

MANAGEMENT

SVCS is an alarming phenomenon with seemingly dire consequences. Although it is often characterized as a medical emergency,[42–44] this is rarely the case. In a review of 90 publications that described 1986 cases of SVCS, there was only one death, of aspiration of epistaxis, that was directly attributable to SVC obstruction.[10] Frequently mentioned severe complications of SVCS include cerebral edema and laryngeal edema with associated respiratory distress,[5,12,42] but actual experiences of these types have been reported infrequently.[7,11,45] In fact, cerebral edema and seizures may be secondary to associated metastatic disease, and respiratory compromise may be caused by tracheal compression from a tumor that is also causing SVC compression. Therefore, by recognizing that SVCS is very rarely a true oncologic emergency, clinicians should be able to identify the etiology prior to embarking on a therapeutic course. Treatment can be and should be delayed until appropriate evaluation is undertaken to determine the cause.

The management of SVCS depends on the severity of the patient's symptoms, the cause of the obstruction, and the histologic type of the tumor. Conservative measures such as head elevation, rest, judicious administration of fluids, and supplemental oxygen are important primary maneuvers until a diagnosis is made and more definitive treatment can begin. The roles of diuretics and corticosteroids in the treatment of SVCS are unclear. After a diagnosis is made, therapy should be initiated promptly. Treatment should not be initiated until a diagnosis is made.

Most patients with SVCS secondary to malignancy have traditionally been treated nonoperatively, with radiotherapy, chemotherapy, or both. More recently, endovascular stents have been successfully used to alleviate symptoms; a prompt and durable resolution of symptoms is achieved in 75% to 95% of patients.[46–56] Such success occurs from direct thrombolysis of SVC clot and mechanical enlargement of the SVC to reestablish normal flow. With radiotherapy, diminished venous distension and subjective improvement usually do not occur until three to seven days after beginning therapy. Approximately 46% to 70% of patients with bronchogenic carcinoma will demonstrate a symptomatic response to radiotherapy or combined radiotherapy and chemotherapy within the first two weeks.[17,41] This improvement reflects either reestablishment of vena caval patency through recanalization or the further development of venous collaterals. Imaging studies performed after improvement of SVCS often show persistent SVC occlusion by stenosis, thrombosis, or residual tumor; the improvement in the syndrome in such instances is usually due to the recruitment of collateral flow.

Surgery has a very limited role in the management of SVCS. Some authors believe that surgery with bypass grafting has no role in the treatment of patients with SVCS secondary to malignant disease because of the morbidity

TABLE 62.3. RELATIVE INDICATIONS FOR OPERATIVE INTERVENTION IN SUPERIOR VENA CAVA SYNDROME

Chronic occlusion with moderate to severe refractory symptoms
Acute occlusion with severe symptoms
Recurrent occlusion with severe symptoms

Venography shows superior vena cava occlusion with absence or thrombosis of collaterals.

associated with a major operation,[7,57] but others believe that surgery has a role in treating selected patients such as those with acute SVC occlusion and severe symptoms or those with complete occlusion of the SVC, severe refractory symptoms, and thrombosis of venous collaterals (Table 62.3). An operation can provide almost immediate, sustained relief of symptoms in most patients. The decision for any invasive procedure must be made with regard to the acuity of the syndrome, severity of the underlying disease, the patient's overall health, the risk of surgical intervention, the patient's life expectancy, and the anatomy of the receptive vein. In the current setting of improved anesthesia and perioperative monitoring, surgical procedures can be performed safely and effectively in selected patients.

Surgical Procedures

A number of surgical procedures have been described for the treatment of SVCS secondary to both benign and malignant conditions (Table 62.4). The objective is to decompress safely the venous system above the level of the obstruction. Two techniques of operative management exist: bypass and resection. Bypass procedures reroute the venous blood of the upper compartment around the obstructed segment to the right atrium. The tumor itself is not handled. A single major vein (i.e., jugular, innominate, or subclavian) is used for the bypass; unilateral decompression relies on the normal venous flow patterns that readily cross the midline within

TABLE 62.4. SURGICAL PROCEDURES FOR SUPERIOR VENA CAVA SYNDROME

SVC to right atrial appendage[58,60]
Innominate vein to right atrium[20,58–60,72,103,104,118]
Jugular vein to intrapericardial SVC[72]
Jugular vein to right atrium[59,60,72]
Right subclavian vein to SVC[105]
Left subclavian vein to right atrium[105]
Azygos vein to right atrium[59–61]
Azygos vein to intrapericardial SVC[62]
Azygos vein to inferior vena cava[63]
Extra-anatomic bypass to femoral vein[59,60,64–67]
Resection with interposition graft[69,93,94,106–114]
Endarterectomy with patch[115,116]

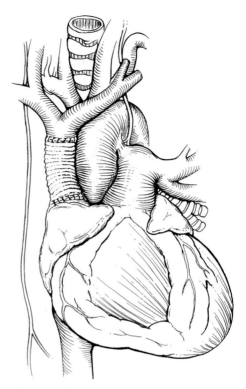

FIGURE 62.6. Superior vena cava resection and reconstruction with a synthetic graft.

the head and neck to decompress the contralateral side. The other operative technique, surgical resection (Figure 62.6), involves *en bloc* removal of the SVC and the tumor, followed by reconstruction of the SVC with an interposition graft.

As previously mentioned, venacavography is essential prior to operative intervention for SVCS. Contrast venography accurately delineates the major venous structures to be used for the bypass procedure. The degree of collateralization, the proximity of SVC occlusion, and the presence of intraluminal thrombosis should be noted for operative planning. Some thrombus exists in approximately 20% of cases[20]; thrombectomy can be accomplished at the time of surgery in most circumstances. Extensive thrombotic occlusion of the innominate, subclavian, or jugular veins may preclude bypass.

Surgical Bypass

Median sternotomy provides the best exposure to the heart and innominate vein for bypass procedures. If no diagnosis has been obtained, biopsy should be performed to confirm the histology prior to proceeding with surgical treatment of the SVCS. In a few patients, tissue diagnosis requires an open procedure when other methods have failed. In such circumstances, simultaneous biopsy and bypass grafting have been performed with satisfactory results.[58] The innominate vein is the vein most amenable for bypass, though other major veins can be used. The innominate vein is usually easily identified and can be encircled with tapes proximally and distally to expose an adequate length that is free from thrombosis or tumor involvement. With tourniquet pressure to the tapes, a 1 cm incision is made along the inferior aspect to permit a Fogarty catheter. The catheter should be passed proximally and distally to remove potential thrombi. A side-biting vascular clamp is applied, and the venotomy is extended for 2.5 to 3 cm. Autologous vein or synthetic graft is used for the bypass; both are discussed in the following section. If a synthetic graft is used, a 10 to 14 mm graft is most favorable. The graft is sutured to the vein in an end-to-side fashion using 5–0 monofilament suture. Alternatively, an end-to-end anastomosis can be performed after ligation and division of the innominate vein (Figure 62.7). After the anastomosis is complete, the graft should be flushed with heparinized saline, clamped, and measured for length to the right atrium. A comfortable length should be determined with the graft coursing to the side of the aorta. The graft may be sutured to the atrial appendage or the atrium proper, taking care to divide intra-atrial bands before performing the anastomosis.

Other types of bypass procedures have been described for the treatment of SVCS. Several reports have noted use of the azygos vein for bypass.[59–63] Such approaches can be performed through a right thoracotomy, which provides satisfactory exposure to both the vein and the right atrium. Extra-anatomic bypasses have been successfully used and are appealing because they are less invasive,[59,60,64–67] but they have suffered from poor patency rates caused by inherent low flow rates.

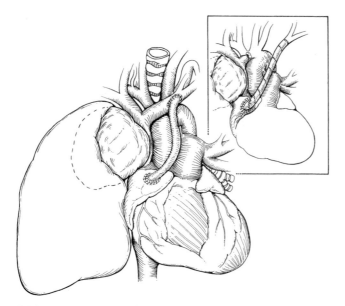

FIGURE 62.7. Innominate vein to right atrial bypass can be performed using autologous vein, synthetic graft, or spiral vein.

TABLE 62.5. GRAFTS

Polytetrafluoroethylene (PTFE)[58,64,69,93–95,103,106,107,109–113,117]
Spiral vein[69,72,93,108]
Saphenous vein[95,104]
Femoral vein[118]
Dacron[20,94,109]
Pericardial tube[94,95,119]
Umbilical vein[95]

Grafts

Bypass procedures use a variety of conduits to reroute the venous return to the right atrium (Table 62.5). The autogenous vein has the obvious advantage of providing a conduit of native tissue, which historically has allowed the highest patency rates of all conduits. One disadvantage, however, is the easy compressibility of the conduit, which can lead to occlusion. With connection of a bypass graft from peripheral to central veins, surrounding mediastinal tissues have the propensity to apply pressure along the course of the conduit. Lack of rigidity of the graft may lead to compression with consequent restrictive flow and graft occlusion. Another disadvantage of autogenous veins exists with the size discrepancy: a larger vein is more desirable. Doty[23] has championed the use of the composite spiral, autogenous vein graft that was originally described by Chiu in 1974.[68] Other authors also prefer the spiral vein to other graft types.[69,70] In several articles, Doty describes his technique for preparation of the vein and for bypass procedures from the jugular or innominate veins to the right atrium for both benign and malignant disease.[23,71] In 1990 he reported his experience with nine patients with benign disease and noted success in seven of 10 grafts placed.[72] In a separate report, he noted 100% success in six patients with lung malignancies.[5] Certainly the advantages of a spiral vein are its autogenicity and its larger size, which theoretically permits greater volumes of flow. The disadvantage is its compressibility which subjects it to occlusion. Alimi and colleagues have noted success with the placement of endovascular stents in grafts that develop stenoses or occlusions.[70]

Expanded or ringed polytetrafluoroethylene (PTFE) seems to be the most popular synthetic graft for bypass and for interposition. It is preferred for several reasons, including its excellent immediate and long-term patency rates, and noncompressibility.[73] With its inherent skeleton, ringed PTFE prevents the problem of extrinsic compression leading to occlusion.

Other conduits have been used with less uniform success, although only scattered reports exist. Dacron, pericardial tubes, and umbilical vein are not considered desirable options because of their marginal patency rates; these conduits are not recommended unless others are unavailable.

Endovascular Stents

Over the past 15 years, expanding (self-expanding and balloon-expandable) endovascular stents have been effectively used for treatment of stenoses of the arterial system[74] venous system,[56,75,76] esophagus,[77,78] biliary tree,[79–82] urologic tract,[83,84] and airway.[85–89] Stents mechanically expand and support structures that are obstructed by either an intrinsic or extrinsic process. They provide immediate palliation of symptoms and often render a long-term effect.

The advantages of expanding stents include the simplicity of insertion, dynamic expansiveness, and low profile. While stents open the stenoses and obstructions, their thin meshwork slowly sinks into the inner lining of the adjacent tissue, where it is incorporated. The stent, in essence, becomes a part of the wall of the structure into which it is inserted. Several types of expanding stents are available. Each has a different fundamental design, though they were developed with the same goal of low-profile expandability.

Self-Expanding Stents

Symphony Stent

The Symphony stent (Medi-Tech, Boston Scientific Corporation, Quincy, Massachusetts) is made of a nickel-titanium alloy called nitinol and is constructed from a single strand using an open knitted loop mesh design. The ends of the stent are looped and atraumatic, and the unique design allows the stent to bend easily to conform to angled lumen and to maintain a uniformly fixed open radius in all twisting positions. It can be deployed through a 7–10 French vascular introducer. Its low-profile release mechanism allows controlled incremental deployment to permit proximal readjustment of the position during deployment. Whereas most other deployment systems require protective introducer sheaths, this stent requires only an exchange guidewire over which the delivery catheter is placed.

Wallstent

The Wallstent (Medi-Tech, Boston Scientific Corporation, Quincy, Massachusetts) is composed of stainless steel monofilaments braided into a cylindrical tube. The stent is longitudinally stretched to fit within a delivery catheter that can be compressed into a 7–9 French introducer. The Wallstent has a larger surface area in contact with the wall of the vessel to provide position stability and to reduce the potential for erosion. A quality of the Wallstent is its excellent flexibility and conformance, which allows it to adapt particularly well to angulated, tortuous lesions. It requires a protective sheath for insertion and deployment.

Gianturco Stent

The Gianturco stent (William Cook Inc.) is constructed from 0.018 inch (460 μm in diameter) stainless steel monofilament wire fashioned in a zigzag pattern with five to ten bends. The two ends are joined to create a cylinder. Compressed, a stent will fit within an 8 French introducer sheath. Several modifications have been made since the stent was first designed to reduce migration and to facilitate precision in placement. The current stent is a tandem stent of two individual stents connected in multiple locations with monofilament sutures, which allows much better control of positioning, insertion, and deployment. The stent has very little longitudinal elasticity, which makes it less effective in a tortuous or highly angulated vascular stenosis. But it tends to have a slightly greater dynamic pressure of outward expandability than the other self-expanding stents.

Balloon-Expandable Stents

Palmaz Stent and Strecker Stent

In 1985, Palmaz and associates introduced the balloon-expandable stent (Johnson & Johnson Interventional Systems, Warren, NJ) that has been used extensively as an intravascular stent.[90] The stent consists of a slotted, seamless, stainless steel tube with a wall thickness of 0.15 mm. An angioplasty balloon catheter is used to inflate the malleable framework into staggered rows of diamond-shaped slots which are resistant to collapse. The Strecker stent (Medi-Tech, Boston Scientific Corporation, Quincy, Massachusetts) is comprised of a knitted meshwork of tantalum wire 0.1 mm in diameter. The design provides greater flexibility when inserted into narrow, tortuous vessels. As opposed to the Palmaz stent, the Strecker stent is compressible in a longitudinal and radial fashion. Both types of stents are crimp-mounted on a folded angioplasty balloon catheter. The Palmaz stent is inserted through a protective introducer sheath. The Strecker stent requires no protective sheath and is inserted into the vascular system with a slightly smaller introducer.

Covered Expanding Stents

The meshwork of metal alloy is a fundamental design of all expanding stents. Unfortunately, this property has a downside because tissue, or tumor, can grow through the interstices of the stent and lumenal occlusion can subsequently recur. In recognition of this potential problem for patients who have disease within the vascular lumen, covered stents have been developed using a thin membrane of silastic or dacron to surround the stent cylinder.[91] Each type of expanding stent has a covered version, most of which remain in developmental stages and are not commercially available.

Insertion of Expanding Prostheses

Endovascular stents are inserted with fluoroscopic guidance. Initially, the anatomy of the SVC system is evaluated with venography. The extent of endovascular thrombus, the degree of SVC narrowing, and the length of lumenal stricture are ascertained. Thrombolytic agents are often locally delivered to enhance visualization of the anatomy and to provide access to the target site. Balloon dilation of the SVC is performed as an initial step, depending on the degree of obstruction. The size and length of stent are determined, as well as type, covered or uncovered. Standard sizes range from 10 to 14 mm in diameter and 4 to 10 cm in length. Following insertion of the stent, confirmation of SVC patency is established by repeat venography. A second stent is inserted if residual stenosis is present proximal or distal to the initial stent.

RESULTS

For patients with SVCS secondary to malignancy, survival varies significantly depending on the tumor histologic type. The prognosis correlates with that implied by the natural history of the underlying disease. Patients with SVCS from lung cancer have a very poor prognosis, as shown by the five-year survival rates of 337 patients registered at M.D. Anderson Cancer Center with the diagnosis of SVC obstruction (Figure 62.8): lung 2%, breast 10%, lymphoma 40%, and all other 7%. None of these patients underwent surgical bypass. The response to therapy in patients with lung cancer and SVCS may have an impact on survival. In one series, those who did not respond to nonoperative therapy within 30 days had a significantly lower rate of one-year survival (7%) than those who did respond to therapy (17% to 24%).[17] Patients who receive no therapy or who develop mentation changes and airway compromise have a median survival of only six weeks.[5,92]

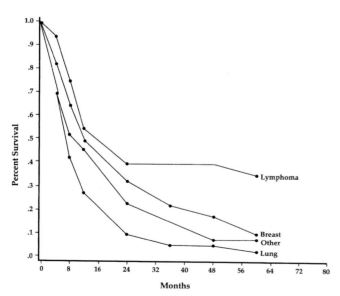

FIGURE 62.8. Survival by histology of 337 patients with malignancy and superior vena cava syndrome at the M.D. Anderson Cancer Center.

Surgery

Because of the infrequency of bypass procedures, large collections of patients from single centers do not exist. Moghissi and colleagues reported a series of 43 patients with bronchogenic carcinoma who underwent bypass procedures for malignant SVCS.[20] This group experienced an operative mortality rate of 4.4% and an average survival of 32 weeks. Stanford and Doty, reviewing their series of six patients with SVCS from lung cancer, noted no operative mortality and a mean survival of 10.8 months.[5] The mean survival for those who did not undergo bypass was 8.2 months. In each of the series, immediate graft occlusion rates were low and long-term patency rates were unknown. In the few patients with lung carcinoma who have undergone SVC resection, one, from the six-patient series of Dartevelle and colleagues[106-107], died of pneumonia after surgery, whereas no operative mortality was noted in three other small series.[93-95] In none of these series did surgery have a significant impact on long term survival rates.

The purpose of bypass procedures is to provide immediate relief of the SVCS prior to the patient's undergoing more definitive treatment for the underlying disorder. The objective is not to provide sustained rechanneling for blood flow but to palliate the patient by promptly alleviating symptoms before administering more definitive therapy directed at the tumor. It is believed that most bypass grafts placed in patients with malignant obstructions become occluded within five to six months. Usually, by the time the graft becomes occluded, the vena caval obstruction has been adequately relieved by the development of collateral vessels, recanalization of the SVC, or reduction of the tumor compressive effects. In most patients the SVCS will not return, and if it does, it usually will do so without significant symptoms.

Endovascular Stents

The Wallstent and Gianturco stent have been the most common endovascular devices used for treatment of SVCS (Figures 62.9 and 62.10), though the Palmaz stent has also been used with success.[51] Clinical experiences are limited, because this technique for management of SVCS has truly evolved during this decade, but the uniformly successful results suggest that stent placement should be considered the optimal form of management. Several clinical groups comprising the largest experiences have established that the procedure for insertion is straightforward and can be performed with a low complication rate. Kee and colleagues[54] performed catheter-directed thrombolysis and/or endovascular stent placement to treat SVCS. They achieved technical success in 56 of 59 patients (95%) with mortality and morbidity rates of 3% and 10%, respectively. Mathias and colleagues[96] had a success rate of 96% using Gianturco and Wallstents in 176 patients with SVCS. Overall success rates

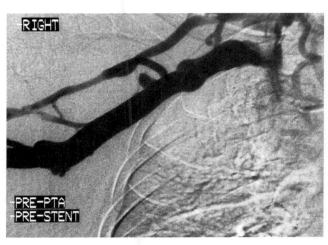

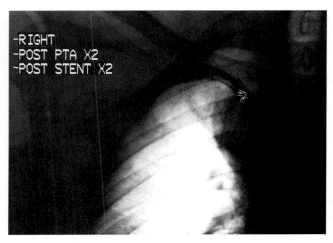

FIGURE 62.9. A: A right-arm venogram shows occlusion of the SVC with adjacent collateral vessels. **B:** Two Wallstents have been placed after transluminal dilation. A repeat venogram shows excellent patency of the SVC.

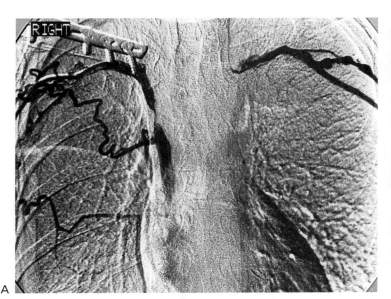

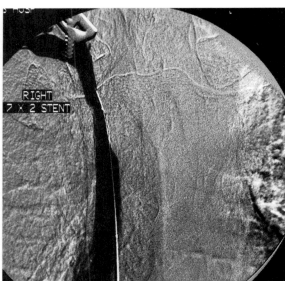

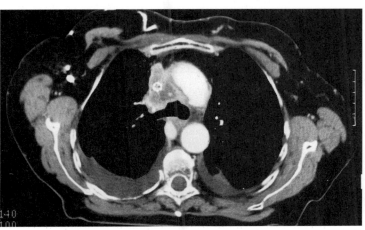

FIGURE 62.10. A: Bilateral upper extremity venography shows significant stenosis of the upper SVC with collateral flow and reconstitution of the lower SVC. **B:** Repeat venography following SVC dilation and placement of two Wallstents demonstrates near-normal flow into the right atrium. **C:** Computed tomography of the same patient shows tumor surrounding the SVC that contains the stent.

have ranged from 85% to 96%.[54–56,96–98] Mortality has ranged from 0% to 4%.[47,55,56] The most common complication is early stent thrombosis 8% to 20%.[100] Late thrombosis (more than a month postprocedure) is manifested by recurrence of symptoms (5% to 45%) and has been successfully treated with further thrombolysis or further stent insertion.[47,53–56,97,99,100] It is significantly reduced when chronic anticoagulants (warfarin, platelet inhibitors) are administered following the procedure.[101]

Stent placement for SVCS provides rapid relief of symptoms within six to 48 hours in most patients, as opposed to the relief associated with radiotherapy, which gradually evolves, beginning three to seven days after the initiation of treatment. Nicholson and colleagues[98] prospectively compared radiation therapy to stent placement for patients with SVCS. They concluded that stent placement was a more effective palliative therapy and recommended that stent placement should be the procedure of choice.

CONCLUSIONS

SVCS is commonly caused by lung cancer and requires prompt recognition and management. In the absence of tracheal compression and airway compromise, however, the syndrome is rarely an oncologic emergency. Management depends on the etiology of the obstructive process and should not be undertaken until a diagnosis is obtained. Traditionally, patients with SVCS secondary to lung cancer have been treated with nonsurgical methods, which include appropriately directed chemotherapy and radiotherapy. Operative decompressive measures are rarely necessary, though they can be accomplished with good palliation and low morbidity. Over this decade, percutaneous implantation of endovascular stents has proven to be an excellent and safe palliative measure for the relief of SVCS. It provides prompt and sustained resolution of symptoms with minimal morbidity. In the setting of SVCS secondary to lung cancer, endovascular stent placement not only should be considered the optimal method of treatment but also should be considered early in the course of management.

REFERENCES

1. Hunter W. History of aneurysm of the aorta with some remarks on aneurysms in general. *Med Obs Inq* 1757;323.
2. Stokes W. *A treatise on the diagnosis and treatment of diseases of the chest.* Dublin: Hodges Smith 1837;370.
3. Rosenblatt MB. Lung cancer in the 19th century. *Bull Hist Med* 1964;38:395.
4. McIntyre FT, Sykes EM. Obstruction of the superior vena cava: a review of the literature and report of two personal cases. *Ann Intern Med* 1949;925.
5. Stanford W, Doty DB. The role of venography and surgery in the management of patients with superior vena cava obstruction. *Ann Thorac Surg* 1986;41:158.
6. Fincher RE. Superior vena cava syndrome: experience in teaching hospital. *South Med J* 1987;80:1243.
7. Parish JM, Marschke RF, Dines DE, et al. Etiologic considerations in superior vena cava syndrome. *Mayo Clin Proc* 1981; 56:407.
8. Banker VP, Maddison FE. Superior vena cava syndrome secondary to aortic disease: a report of two cases and review of the literature. *Dis Chest* 1967;51:656.
9. Kamiya K, Nahata Y, Naiki K, et al. Superior vena cava syndrome. *Vasc Dis* 1967;4:59.
10. Ahmann FR. A reassessment of the clinical implications of the superior vena caval syndrome. *J Clin Oncol* 1984;2:961.
11. Lockridge SK, Knibbe WP, Doty DB. Obstruction of the superior vena cava. *Surgery* 1979;85:14.
12. Perez CA, Presant CA, Van Amburg AL. Management of superior vena cava syndrome. *Semin Oncol* 1978;5:123.
13. Salsali M, Clifton EE. Superior vena caval obstruction with carcinoma of the lung. *Surg Gynecol Obstet* 1965;121:783.
14. Escalante CP. Causes and management of superior vena cava syndrome. *Oncology* 1993;7:61.
15. Nogeire C, Mincer F, Botstein C. Long survival in patients with bronchogenic carcinoma complicated by superior vena cava obstruction. *Chest* 1979;75:325.
16. Cofield RH, Dozois RR, Gerich JE, et al. Etiologic considerations in superior vena cava syndrome. *Mayo Clin Proc* 1981; 56:407.
17. Armstrong BA, Perez CA, Simpson JR, et al. Role of irradiation in the management of superior vena cava syndrome. *Int J Radiat Oncol Biol Phys* 1987;3:531.
18. Chen JC, Bongard F, Klein SR. A contemporary perspective on superior vena cava syndrome. *Am J Surg* 1990;160:207.
19. Lokich JJ, Goodman F. Superior vena cava syndrome. *JAMA* 1975;231:58.
20. Moghissi K, Dhumale R, Sench M. Innominate to right atrium bypass graft for malignant superior vena caval obstruction. Paper presented to the Society of Thoracic Cardiovascular Surgeons of Great Britain and Ireland, 1983.
21. Yellin A, Rosen A, Reichert N, et al. Superior vena cava syndrome: the myth—the facts. *Am Rev Resp Dis* 1990;141:1114.
22. Khimji T, Zeiss J. MRI versus CT and US in the evaluation of a patient presenting with superior vena cava syndrome. *Clin Imaging* 1992;16:269.
23. Doty DB. Bypass of superior vena cava: six years experience with spiral vein graft for obstruction of the superior vena cava due to benign and malignant disease. *J Thorac Cardiovasc Surg* 1982;83:326.
24. Ayala K, Chandrasekaran K, Karalis DG, et al. Diagnosis of superior vena caval obstruction by transesophageal echocardiography. *Chest* 1992;101:874.
25. Dawkins PR, Stoddard MF, Lindell NE, et al. Utility of transesophageal echocardiography in the assessment of mediastinal masses and superior vena cava obstruction. *Am Heart J* 1991; 122:1469.
26. Muramatsu T, Miyamae T, Dohi Y. Collateral pathways observed by radionuclide superior vena caval obstruction. *Clin Nucl Med* 1991;16:609.
27. Podoloff DA, Kim EE. Evaluation of sensitivity and specificity of upper extremity radionuclide venography in cancer patients with indwelling central venous catheters. *Clin Nucl Med* 1992; 17:457.
28. Savolaine ER, Schlembach PJ. Scintigraphy compared to other imaging modalities in benign superior vena caval obstruction accompanying fibrosing mediastinitis. *Clin Imaging* 1989;13: 234.
29. Chasen MH, Charnsangavej C. Venous chest anatomy: clinical

implications. In: Green R, Muhm JR, eds. *Chest Radiology.* 1992:121.

30. Raptopoulos V. Computed tomography of the superior vena cava. *Crit Rev Diagn Imaging* 1986;25:373.

31. Trigaux JP, Van-Beers B. Thoracic collateral venous channels: normal and pathologic CT findings. *J Comput Assist Tomogr* 1990;14:769.

32. Moncada R, Cardella R, Demos TC, et al. Evaluation of superior vena cava syndrome by axial CT AND CT phlebography. *AJR Am J Roentgenol* 1984;143:731.

33. Hansen ME, Spritzer CE, Sostman HD. Assessing the patency of mediastinal and thoracic inlet veins: value of MR imaging. *Am J Radiol* 1990;155:1177.

34. Little AG, Golomb HM, Ferguson MK, et al. Malignant superior vena cava obstruction reconsidered: the role of diagnostic surgical intervention. *Ann Thorac Surg* 1985;40:285.

35. Kumar PP, Good RR. Need for invasive diagnostic procedures in the management of superior vena cava syndrome. *J Natl Med Assoc* 1989;81:41.

36. Nataf P, Regnard JF, Solvignon F, et al. Epithelioid hemangio-endothelioma of the azygos vein. *Arch Mal Coeur Vaiss* 1989; 82:1919.

37. Kirschner PA. Mediastinoscopy in superior vena cava obstruction. In: Jepssen O, Ruhbek-Sorenson H, eds. *Mediastinoscopy: proceedings of an international symposium.* Odense, Denmark: Odense University Press, 1971:40.

38. Callejas MA, Rami R, Catalan M, et al. Mediastinoscopy as an emergency diagnostic procedure in superior vena cava syndrome. *Scand J Thorac Cardiovasc Surg* 1991;25:137.

39. Jahangiri M, Taggart DP, Goldstraw P. Role of mediastinoscopy in superior vena cava obstruction. *Cancer* 1993;71:3006.

40. Schraufnagel DE, Hill R, Leech JA, et al. Superior vena cava obstruction. *Am J Med* 1981;70:1169.

41. Davenport D, Ferree C, Blake D, et al. Response of superior vena cava syndrome to radiation therapy. *Cancer* 1976;38:1577.

42. Baker GL, Barnes JH. Superior vena cava syndrome: etiology, diagnosis, and treatment. *Am J Crit Care* 1992;1:54.

43. Helms SR, Carlson MD. Cardiovascular emergencies. *Semin Oncol* 1989;16:463.

44. Adelstein DJ. Managing three common oncologic emergencies. *Cleve Clin J Med* 1991;58:457.

45. Hussey JJ, Katz S, Yayer WM. The superior vena caval syndrome: report of thirty-five cases. *Am Heart J* 1946;31:1.

46. Eng J, Sabanathan S. Management of superior vena cava obstruction with self-expanding intraluminal stents. Two case reports. *Scand J Thorac Cardiovasc Surg* 1993;27:53.

47. Oudkerk M, Heystraten FM, Stoter G. Stenting in malignant vena caval obstruction. *Cancer* 1993;71:142.

48. Irving JD, Dondelinger RF, Reidy JF, et al. Gianturco self-expanding stents: clinical experience in the vena cava and large veins. *Cardiovasc Intervent Radiol* 1992;15:328.

49. Rosch J, Uchida BT, Hall LD, et al. Gianturco-Rosch expandable Z-stents in the treatment of superior vena cava syndrome. *Cardiovasc Intervent Radiol* 1992;15:319.

50. Edwards RD, Cassidy J, Taylor A. Case report: supervisor vena cava obstruction complicated by central venous thrombosis—treatment with thrombolysis and Gianturco-Z stents. *Clin Radiol* 1992;45:278.

51. Solomon N, Wholey MH, Jarmolowski CR. Intravascular stents in the management of superior vena cava syndrome. *Cathet Cardiovasc Diagn* 1991;23:245.

52. Morita R, Akaogi E, Mitsui K, et al. Gianturco expandable metallic stents in the treatment of superior vena cava syndrome caused by lung cancer. *Nippon Kyobu Shikkan Gakkai Zasshi* 1992;30:1110.

53. Hochrein J, Bashore TM, O'Laughlin MP, et al. Percutaneous stenting of superior vena cava syndrome: a case report and review of the literature. *Am J Med* 1998;104:78.

54. Kee ST, Kinoshitda L, Razavi MK, et al. Superior vena cava syndrome: treatment with catheter-directed dthrombolysis and endovascular stent placement. *Radiology* 1998;206:187.

55. Hennequin LM, Fade O, Fays JG, et al. Superior vena cava stent placement: results with the Wallstent endoprosthesis. *Radiology* 1995;196:353.

56. Shah R, Sabanathan S, Lowe RA, et al. Stenting in malignant obstruction of superior vena cava. *J Thorac Cardiovasc Surg* 1996;112:335.

57. Effler DB, Groves LK. Superior vena caval obstruction. *J Thorac Cardiovasc Surg* 1962;43:574.

58. Majid AA. Simultaneous bypass grafting of the SVC and intrathoracic biopsy in fulminant SVC syndrome. *J R Coll Surg Edinb* 1991;36:406.

59. Li YZ. Surgical treatment of obstructed superior vena cava. *Chung Hua Wai Ko Tsa Chih* 1992;30:142.

60. Wang ZG. Surgical treatment of superior vena cava syndrome. *Chung Hua Wai Ko Tsa Chin* 1992;30:218.

61. Gerbode F, Yee J, Rundle F. Experimental anastomosis of vessels to the heart. *Surgery* 1949;25:556.

62. Klassen KP, Andrews NC, Curtis GM. Diagnosis and treatment of superior vena cava obstruction. *Arch Surg* 1951;63:311.

63. Cooley DA, Hallman GL. Superior vena cava syndrome treated by azygos vein to inferior vena cava anastomosis. *J Thorac Cardiovasc Surg* 1962;43:574.

64. Yamashita C, Nakamura K, Okada M, et al. Surgical treatment of superior vena cava syndrome (SVCS). *Kyobu Geka* 1989;42: 129.

65. Gutowicz MA, Quinones-Baldrich WJ, Lieber CP, et al. Operative treatment of refactory superior vena cava syndrome. *Am Surg* 1984;50:399.

66. Taylor GA, Miller HA, Standen JR, et al. Bypassing the obstructed superior vena cava with a subcutaneous long saphaneous vein graft. *J Thorac Cardiovasc Surg* 1974;68:237.

67. Berman IR, Mergenthaler FW, Clauss RH. An extracorporeal venous shunting procedure for the symptomatic relief of superior vena cava obstruction and report of a case. *Ann Surg* 1968; 167:269.

68. Chiu CJ, Terzis J, MacRae ML. Replacement of superior vena cava with the spiral composite vein graft. *Ann Thorac Surg* 1974; 17:555.

69. Gloviczki P, Pairoler PC, Cherry KJ, et al. Reconstruction of the vena cava and of its primary tributaries: a preliminary report. *J Vasc Surg* 1990;11:373.

70. Alimi YS, Gloviczki P, Vrtiska TJ, et al. Reconstruction of the superior vena cava: benefits of postoperative surveillance and secondary endovascular interventions. *J Vasc Surg* 1998;27:287.

71. Doty DB, Baker WH. Bypass of the superior vena cava with spiral vein graft. *Ann Thorac Surg* 1976;22:490.

72. Doty DB, Doty JR, Jones KW. Bypass of superior vena cava. Fifteen years' experience with spiral vein graft for obstruction of superior vena cava caused by benign disease. *J Thorac Cardiov Surg* 1990;99:889.

73. Masuda H, Ogata T, Kikuchi K, et al. Longevity of expanded polytetrafluoroethylene grafts for superior vena cava. *Ann Thorac Surg* 1989;48:376.

74. Katzen BT, Becker GJ. Intravascular stents. Status of development and clinical application. *Surg Clin North Am* 1992;72: 941.

75. Watkinson AF, Hansell DM. Expandable Wallstent for the treatment of obstruction of the superior vena cava. *Thorax* 1993; 48:915.

76. Zollikofer CL, Antonucci F, Stuckmann G, et al. Use of the

Wallstent in the venous system including hemodialysis-related stenoses. *Cardiovasc Intervent Radiol* 1992;15:334.

77. Schaer J, Katon RM, Ivancev K, et al. Treatment of malignant esophageal obstruction with silicone-coated metallic self-expanding stents. *Gastrointest Endosc* 1992;38:7.

78. Kozarek RA, Ball TJ, Patterson DJ. Metallic self-expanding stent application in the upper gastrointestinal tract: caveats and concerns. *Gastrointest Endosc* 1992;38:1.

79. Hoepffner N, Foerster EC, Hogemann B, et al. Long-term experience in Wallstent therapy for malignant choledochal stenosis. *Endoscopy* 1994;26:597.

80. Rossi P, Bezzi M, Rossi M, et al. Metallic stents in malignant biliary obstruction: results of a multicenter European study of 240 patients. *J Vasc Interv Radiol* 1994;5:279.

81. Stoker J, Lam'eris JS, Jeekel J. Percutaneously placed Wallstent endoprosthesis in patients with malignant distal biliary obstruction. *Br J Surg* 1993;80:1185.

82. Stoker J, Lam'eris JS, van Blankenstein M. Percutaneous metallic self-expandable endoprostheses in malignant hilar biliary obstruction. *Gastrointest Endosc* 1993;39:43.

83. Baert L, Verhamme L, Van Poppel H, et al. Long-term consequences of urethral stents. *J Urol* 1993;150:853.

84. Lugmayr H, Pauer W. Self-expanding metal stents for palliative treatment of malignant ureteral obstruction. *AJR Am J Roentgenol* 1992;159:1091.

85. Carrasco CH, Nesbitt JC, Charnsangavej C, et al. Management of tracheal and bronchial stenosis with the Gianturco stent. *Ann Thorac Surg* 1994;58:1012.

86. Nashef SAM, Dromer C, Velly FJ, et al. Expanding wire stents in benign tracheobronchial disease: indications and complications. *Ann Thorac Surg* 1992;54:937.

87. Nomori H, Kobayashi R, Kodera K, et al. Indications for an expandable metallic stent for tracheobronchial stenosis. *Ann Thorac Surg* 1993;56:1324.

88. Sawada S, Tanigawa N, Cobayashi M, et al. Malignant tracheobronchial obstructive lesions: treatment with Gianturco expandable metallic stents. *J Radiol* 1993;188:205.

89. Tsang V, Goldstraw P. Self-expanding metal stent for tracheobronchial strictures. *Eur J Cardiothorac Surg* 1992;6:555.

90. Palmaz JC. Intravascular stenting: from basic research to clinical application. *Cardiovasc Intervent Radiol* 1992;15:279.

91. Chin DH, Peterson BD, Timmermans H, et al. Stent-graft in the management of superior vena cava syndrome. *Cardiovasc Intervent Radiol* 1996;19:302.

92. Rosenbloom SE. Superior vena cava obstruction in primary cancer of the lung. *Ann Intern Med* 1949;31:470.

93. Nakahara K, Ohno K, Mastumura A, et al. Extended operation for lung cancer invading the aortic arch and superior vena cava. *J Thorac Cardiovasc Surg* 1989;97:428.

94. Lai WW, Wu MH, Chou NS, et al. Surgery for malignant involvement of the superior vena cava. *J Formos Med Assoc* 1992; 91:991.

95. Larsson S, Lepore V. Technical options in reconstruction of large mediastinal veins. *Surgery* 1992;111:311.

96. Mathias K, Jager H, Willaschek J, et al. Interventional radiology in central venous obstructions. Dilation—stent implantation—thrombolysis. *Radiologe* 1998;38:606.

97. Crowe MT, Cavies CH, et al. Percutaneous management of superior vena cava occlusions. *Cardiovasc Intervent Radiol* 1995; 18:367.

98. Nicholson AA, Ettles DF, Arnold A, et al. Treatment of malignant superior vena cava obstruction: metal stents or radiation therapy. *J Vasc Interv Radiol* 1997;8:781.

99. Oudkerk M, Kuijpers TJ, Schmitz PI, et al. Self-expanding metal stents for palliative treatment of superior vena caval syndrome. *Cardiovasc Intervent Radiol* 1996;19:146.

100. Stock KW, Jacob AL, Proske M, et al. Treatment of malignant obstruction of the superior vena cava with the self-expanding Wallstent. *Thorax* 1995;50:1151.

101. Gross CM, Kramer J, Waigand J, et al. Stent implantation in patients with superior vena cava syndrome. *Am J Roentgenol* 1997;169:429.

102. Maddox AM, Valdivieso M, Lukeman J, et al. Superior vena cava obstruction in small cell bronchogenic carcinoma. *Cancer* 1983;52:2165.

103. Minami H, Kubota F, Kawafuchi T, et al. A case of idiopathic fibrous mediastinitis with superior vena caval obstruction. *Kyobu Geka* 1990;43:245.

104. Bordigoni L, Blin D, Magnan PE, et al. Ectatic tumoral thrombobis of the superior vena cava revealing thyroid cancer. *Ann Radiol* 1992;35:5595.

105. Baker GL, Barnes JH. Etiology, diagnosis, and treatment. *Am J Crit Care* 1992;1:54.

106. Dartevelle PG, Chapelier A, Navajas M, et al. Replacement of the superior vena cava with polytetrafluoroethylene grafts combined with resection of mediastinal-pulmonary malignant tumors. *J Thorac Cardiovasc Surg* 1987;94:361.

107. Dartevelle PG, Chapelier AR, Pastorino U, et al. Long-term follow-up after prosthetic replacement of the superior vena cava combined with resection of mediastinal-pulmonary malignant tumors. *J Thorac Cardiovasc Surg* 1991;102:259.

108. Rutegard J, Granstrand M, Aberg T. Intracaval paraganglioma causing superior vena cava syndrome. *Eur J Cardiothorac Surg* 1992;6:337.

109. Shimizu N, Date H, Moriyama S, et al. Reconstruction of the superior vena cava in patients with mediastinal malignancies. *Eur J Cardiothorac Surg* 1992;5:575.

110. Fujisawa T, Yamaguchi Y, Iwai N, et al. A case of mediastinal germ cell tumor radically operated on after neoadjuvant chemotherapy-combined resection of the superior vena cava and reconstruction with expanded-PTFE graft. *Jpn J Surg* 1988;18:336.

111. Ikeuchi K, Nagata Y, Kobayashi S, et al. Replacement of superior vena cava with resection of Hodgkin's disease of the thymus: a case report. *Kyobu Geka* 1990;43:305.

112. Yamaguchi T, Hasegawa T, Fukushima K, et al. A case of superior vena cava syndrome caused by adenocarcinoma of the mediastinum: the significance of pulsed Doppler echocardiography in the SVC reconstruction. *Nippon Kyobu Geka Gakai Zasshi* 1992;41:780.

113. Brachet A, Thevenet F, Gilly FN, et al. Inflammatory pseudotumor of the superior vena cava: rare etiology of mediastinal tumor. *Ann Chir* 1993;47:170.

114. Oka M, Kusano M, Miyasaka T, et al. A case of adenosquamous carcinoma with unknown origin and with superior vena cava syndrome as the first symptom. *Kekkaku* 1992;67:457.

115. Gomes MN, Hufnagel CA. Superior vena cava obstruction. *Ann Thorac Surg* 1975;20:344.

116. Templeton JY. Endovenectomy for relief of obstruction of the superior vena cava. *Am J Surg* 1962;104:70.

117. Nomori H, Nara S, Kobayashki R, et al. A case of malignant lymphoma of anterior mediastinum requiring superior vena cava reconstruction. *Kyobu Geka* 1992;45:446.

118. Gladstone DJ, Pillai R, Paneth M, et al. Relief of superior vena caval syndrome with autologous femoral vein used as a bypass graft. *J Thorac Cardiovasc Surg* 1985;89:750.

119. Lemmer JH, Behrendt DM, Beekman RH, et al. Pedicled right atrial pericardial tissue conduit for bypass of the obstructed superior vena cava in children. *J Thorac Cardiovasc Surg* 1989; 98:417.

63

TREATMENT OF NON-SMALL CELL LUNG CANCER IN THE ELDERLY PATIENT

SUSAN BLACKWELL
JEFFREY CRAWFORD

EPIDEMIOLOGY OF LUNG CANCER IN THE ELDERLY

Cancer is a major concern for people age 65 and older, with 58% of all cancers occurring in this segment of the population. Incidence data from the National Cancer Institute's (NCI) surveillance epidemiology and results (SEER) have shown that older persons have a 10 times greater risk of developing cancer than those individuals under age 65. In the United States, the leading cause of cancer deaths in men and women is lung cancer. When incidence rates are calculated for age specificity, lung cancer rates escalate to more than 500 per 100,000 persons for those 70 to 84 years of age, with a peak of 567 per 100,000 in the 80–84-year-old group. In women, lung cancer incidence rates peak in the 70–79-year-old group, with more than 200 per 100,000. The number of older people who will develop lung cancer is expected to increase as the smoking exposure time effects on birth cohorts become more apparent.[1]

An American Cancer Society study provides further insight into the risk of lung cancer mortality as a function of age and smoking history.[2] In a prospective cohort study of more than 900,000 people, with 6 years of follow-up, the absolute risk of lung cancer mortality was compared in individuals who had never smoked, those currently smoking, and former smokers. As expected, those individuals who quit smoking early in life had a lower lung cancer death risk, and the risk for those who were former smokers was significantly lower than those who continued to smoke. However, the influence of age was remarkable (Figure 63.1). The lung cancer death risk for those who stopped smoking between the ages of 30 and 49 rose gradually with age at a rate slightly greater than for those persons who had never smoked. For a person who quit smoking between the age of 50 and 64, the lung cancer death risk leveled off at the risk attained at the time of quitting until around the age of 75 when it significantly increased. The annual lung cancer mortality for current smokers at age 75 was estimated at 1 per 100 for men and 1 per 200 for women (Table 63.1).

Nonsmokers have a relative risk of lung cancer death of 0.05 or less compared to current smokers. However, former smokers had a relative risk of lung cancer death of approximately .45 if they quit smoking in their early 60s, 0.20 if they stopped smoking in their early 50s, and 0.10 for those who had stopped smoking in their 30s.

In terms of reducing risk of lung cancer mortality, stopping smoking at any age is beneficial, but it is much more beneficial for those quitting at a younger age. It was also shown that even though absolute lung cancer risks can plateau following smoking cessation, the lung cancer risk for former smokers is still consistently greater than for those who have never smoked.[2]

In addition to age effects, a dose-response relationship exists for smoking and lung cancer. The risk for lung cancer increases with longer smoking duration and greater number of cigarettes smoked, early age of onset of smoking, greater use of unfiltered cigarettes, high tar and nicotine content, and greater degree of inhalation.[3,4] A survey of tobacco use found that older smokers smoked cigarettes with a higher nicotine content than younger smokers, although the number of cigarettes smoked per day was similar.[5] In this analysis, it was estimated that 50% of Americans age 21 to 49 years were ever smokers, including 31% current smokers and 22% former smokers. In the older population, age 50 to 74, 58% were ever smokers, including 23% current smokers and 35% former smokers. Even though the older smokers had smoked for more than twice as many years as the younger group, the AUTS survey showed very little difference between older and younger smokers, either in smoking habits or quitting history. Although the older smokers had smoked longer, they did not report an increased number of quitting attempts.[6]

CLINICAL PRESENTATION AND EARLY DETECTION

Most patients with lung cancer are symptomatic at the time of diagnosis. Unfortunately, the symptoms they present

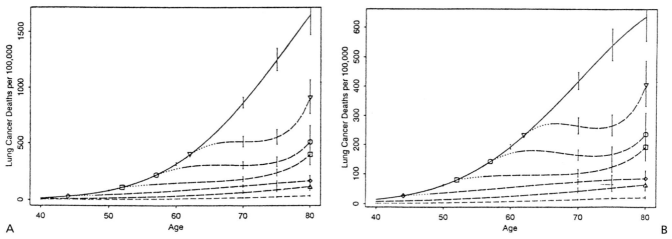

FIGURE 63.1. **A:** Model estimates of lung cancer death rates by age for male current, former, and never smokers, based on smokers who started at age 17.5 and smoked 26 cigarettes per day. Estimates are plotted for current smokers (*solid line*), never smokers (*dotted line*), and former smokers (*dashed lines*). The five age-at-quitting cohorts are distinguished by the following symbols on the graph at the age of quitting and also at age 80: △ 30–39, ◇ 40–49, □ 50–54, ○ 55–59, ▽ 60–64. **B:** Model estimates of lung cancer death rates by age for female current, former, and never smokers, based on smokers who started at age 18.5 and smoked 22 cigarettes per day. Estimates are plotted for current smokers (*solid line*), never smokers (*dotted line*), and former smokers (*dashed lines*). The five age-at-quitting cohorts are distinguished by the following symbols on the graph at the age of quitting and also at age 80: △ 30–39, ◇ 40–49, □ 50–54, ○ 55–59, ▽ 60–64.

with are often caused by locally advanced or distant disease. Depending on the location of the tumor, patients can present with a variety of signs or symptoms. Unfortunately, many of the symptoms of lung cancer are nonspecific, and in elderly patients these symptoms may be attributed to comorbid disease. This often can result in a delay in diagnos-

TABLE 63.1. ESTIMATED RR OF LUNG CANCER DEATH FOLLOWING SMOKING CESSATION: NEVER AND FORMER SMOKERS COMPARED WITH CURRENT SMOKERS

	RR		
	Age 55	Age 65	Age 75
Men			
Never smokers	0.05	0.03	0.03
Quit 30–39	0.14	0.09	0.07
Quit 40–49	0.36	0.18	0.12
Quit 50–54	—	0.29	0.19
Quit 55–59	—	0.56	0.27
Quit 60–64	—	—	0.45
Current smokers	1.0	1.0	1.0
Women			
Never smokers	0.07	0.05	0.04
Quit 30–39	0.17	0.11	0.10
Quit 40–49	0.40	0.22	0.15
Quit 50–54	—	0.33	0.23
Quit 55–59	—	0.60	0.31
Quit 60–64	—	—	0.49
Current smokers	1.0	1.0	1.0

tic testing for the older patient. In a study by DeMaria and Cohen, it was shown that patients of all ages had similar presentation of cough, hoarseness, dysphagia, and weight loss. However, patients greater than 70 years of age presented more often with dyspnea but less often with chest pain than did younger patients.[7]

Although routine screening for lung cancer has not been recommended, this is currently being reevaluated. High-risk patients (smokers/former smokers) over age 65 might benefit from screening because of the high incidence of lung cancer in this population. The prospective randomized studies using serial chest x-rays complemented by sputum cytology did not demonstrate that intensive screening led to a lower death rate, but these studies focused on a younger population, largely 45–55, where the incidence is substantially lower. In addition to the high frequency of lung cancer in the elderly, data suggest that lung cancer may present at a less advanced stage with increasing age.[8] Twenty-two thousand, eight hundred seventy-four cases from the centralized cancer patient data system information were analyzed. The percentage of lung cancer patients with local disease increased from 15.3% for patients age 54 years of younger to 25.4% for those 75 years or older. In addition, 6,332 cases were analyzed after undergoing surgical staging, and there was a greater likelihood of local stage disease as age increased. Screening trials targeted at the elderly with current techniques are warranted. In the interim, the clinician should now have a high index of suspicion for lung cancer in the older smoker or former smoker and have a low threshold for obtaining a chest x-ray in this population when symptoms arise.

TREATMENT APPROACHES IN THE ELDERLY

Even though cancer is a disease of the elderly, older patients are often treated less aggressively. This may be due, in some cases, to the presence of comorbid conditions in the elderly. Whether young or old, the patient's ability to tolerate treatment is of great importance, whether the planned treatment is surgery, radiation therapy, chemotherapy, or multimodality. Older patients have the same right as younger patients to take part in the decision-making process about their treatment. Cancer is no less a devastating illness to an elderly person than to a younger person. For most older patients, quality of life is equally important, and they often prefer improved quality over quantity of life.[9]

Non–small cell lung cancer (NSCLC) represents 80% of all lung cancers. Treatment recommendations for patients with NSCLC have clearly been affected by the age of the patient at presentation. Younger patients, despite presenting with more advanced disease, are more likely to be offered surgical resection than older patients. In older populations, the option of surgery may be more limited because of associated comorbidity or because of beliefs within the medical community that chronological age automatically excludes an aggressive surgical approach.[10] By contrast, age seems to have less influence on whether patients are offered radiation therapy.[11] Lung cancer is one of the most common tumors treated with primary radiation therapy in the over 65 age group. Despite this, studies evaluating the benefits and toxicities in the elderly are limited.

The therapeutic nihilism that has surrounded the role of chemotherapy in NSCLC is even more pronounced in treatment decisions regarding the elderly. Many physicians are hesitant to subject older patients to aggressive chemotherapy. However, studies over the last decade have shown that elderly patients may be able to cope with the impact of chemotherapy as well as younger patients.[12] Older patients do not report any greater frequency of toxic side effects, and when compared to younger patients, often experience lower levels of emotional distress and life disruption.

Lastly, the "quantity of life" available to the elderly is often underappreciated by health care providers and needs to be factored into any treatment decision. An 80-year-old American man has a current life expectancy of 6.7 years and an 80-year-old woman has a life expectancy of 8.8 years. At age 85 a man can expect to live 5.3 years and a woman 6.7 years.[13] In addition, a 75-year-old can expect 75% of his or her remaining years to be spent active as opposed to dependent. At age 85, about 50% of one's life is independent.[14] With this in mind, the degree of potential for quality

longevity far exceeds the expected survival of untreated or treated lung cancer patients at any stage.[15]

As the population ages, the number of older patients presenting with lung cancer will indeed increase. In the past, this older age group has been under-represented in clinical studies, resulting in a general decreased knowledge and, therefore, uncertainty about the best management of the older lung cancer patient. Fortunately, recently studies have begun to clarify the treatment options for this population and are reviewed here.

SURGERY IN THE ELDERLY LUNG CANCER PATIENT

Surgical treatment of lung cancer in the elderly patient is still a controversial area because of concern about the increased morbidity and mortality from pulmonary resection in the older patient. However, as the life expectancy rises and numbers of elderly people increase, surgeons and oncologists will be faced with increasing numbers of patients in their 70s and 80s who present at a resectable stage. The observation from cancer center databases that the older patient may actually present with an earlier stage lung cancer,[8] is supported in surgical series.[16] In the report by Gebitekan from the *European Journal of Cardiothoracic Surgery*, 58% of patients above the age of 70 presented with stage I disease versus 40% in younger patients, whereas 13% of older patients had stage III disease versus 22% in the younger population.

In the 1970s, Thompson-Evans reported the outcomes of surgical treatment in the elderly.[17] He showed that patients aged 65 years or more were resectable in a range comparable to that of younger patients. Twenty-three percent were operable and 15% were suitable for curative resection. However, the operative mortality exceeded 15%, making the benefits debatable. Over the last two decades with refined staging approaches and improved surgical techniques and postoperative support, considerably lower mortality rates have been reported.

Massard et al. reviewed 1,616 patients who underwent thoracotomy for lung cancer from January 1983 to December 1992 with 233 patients age 70 years or more, at the University Hospital in Strasbourg, France.[18] Twenty-nine percent of these patients had no medical history, 26% had a history of cardiovascular disease, and 19% had a previous history of malignancy that was in complete remission; 48% of patients were stage I, 17% stage II, and 30% stage III. Two hundred ten patients were able to undergo resection, with 60 receiving pneumonectomies and 150 lobectomies. A total of 16 patients died postoperatively—7.2% for the whole series, 10% after pneumonectomy, and 6.6% after lobectomy. The mortality was similar below and above 75 years. The five-year survival for stage I was 45%, 36.3% for stage II, and 13.8% for stage III, with an overall five-year survival of 39.9%. Survival was not influenced by age.

In a series from St. Rafael and Yale New Haven Hospital, Pagni et al. reviewed the short-term and long-term results of pulmonary resection with the intention of cure from lung cancer in patients 80 years and older.[19] There were 54 octogenarians, which represented 4% of 1,328 operations for lung cancer between 1980–1995. There were 28 men and 26 women, with the mean age of 82 years in the range of 80 to 88 years. Thirty-one percent of these patients had chronic obstructive pulmonary disease, 24% had a history of angina pectoris, myocardial infarction, or cardiac arrhythmia requiring treatment, and 19% had previous treatment for malignant disease or were free of evidence of recurrence at the time of their lung cancer operation. None of these patients received induction chemotherapy or chemotherapy/radiotherapy with the exception of two patients who were treated with preoperative radiation for clinical nodal stage III-A disease. The types of surgery performed were 43 standard lobectomies, 2 extended lobectomies, 2 bilobectomies, 3 lower lobe superior segmentectomies, 3 wedge resections, and 1 left pneumonectomy. There were two perioperative deaths for a 3.7% operative mortality rate. Twenty-three patients had nonlethal complications, with cardiac problems making up the majority of these complications. There were six nonfatal problems, which were considered major complications because they extended the hospital stay and required unusual intervention. These problems were air leaks, congestive heart failure, pneumonia, recurrent laryngeal nerve injury, and reoperation for evacuation of hemothorax. Minor complications occurred in 17 patients, including atrial arrhythmia, urinary retention, depression, or confusion. Forty-nine of the 52 patients were discharged to home after their operation; however, three patients required temporary care at a convalescent facility. The actuarial survival of the 52 discharged patients was 86% at 1 year, 62% at 3 years, and 43% at 5 years. For stage I patients, survival was 97% at 1 year, 78% at 3 years, and 57% at 5 years. Those patients with more advanced lung cancer did poorly. There were 13 patients in this group and only two were alive at 8 and 27 months after the operation. The remainder died between 4 and 40 months postoperatively. The median survival for the combined stage II and III cohort was only 15 months. The authors concluded that age in the 80s was neither a contraindication to operative treatment nor routine indication for lesser resection.

In a second study evaluating the surgical treatment of lung cancer in octogenarians, Hanagiri et al. reviewed 20 patients aged 80 or older who underwent surgery for lung cancer in Japan.[20] In this review, the authors found that the postoperative complication rate was 50% in patients over 80; however, there were no fatal complications. The most common postoperative complication seen in these patients was transient cardiorespiratory complications such as difficulty in expectoration and arrhythmia. A five-year sur-vival rate was 42.6%, which was similar to that obtained in younger patients.

From the University of Milan, Italy, Santambrogio et al. compared the short- and long-term results of treatment of patients age 70 and older with a group of younger patients undergoing surgical treatment for lung cancer.[21] From March 1986 to March 1997, 424 consecutive patients were evaluated. These patients had documented NSCLC stage I or II. Of 519 evaluable cases, 54 were age 70 or over and 465 were between the ages of 40 and 69 with a mean age of 58. Although the composition of the two groups was homogeneous, for the most part, there was noted a reduced forced vital capacity and FEV1 in the patients over 70 as well as significantly higher incidence of risk factors, including heart disease, hypertension, diabetes, chronic obstructive pulmonary disease (COPD), and peripheral vascular disease. For both groups, the most frequent operation undertaken was lobectomy; however, pneumonectomy was performed significantly less in the older patient group. The operative mortality as occurring within 30 days of surgery was 5.5% in the older group and 1.3% in the younger group. The total complications were 7.4% and 6.9%, respectively. At 5 years, patients with stage I disease, the older group had a 52% survival and the younger patients had a 57.8% survival. In stage II disease, five-year survival was 50% and 30.6% in the older and younger groups, respectively. In another study from Milan, Italy, Cicraco et al. determined that the postoperative outcome and survival at 12 months in patients 70 years or older, who underwent surgical resection for stage I, II, or III-A disease, was determined not by stage or histology but by the postoperative complications and concomitant cardiopulmonary disease.[22] Seventy-six patients underwent surgical resection between January 1992 and June 1996. There were 15 cases of postoperative complications and a 30-day operative mortality of 1.3%. Overall actual survival at 54 months was 53%. Mortality at 12 months was found not to relate to the stage of disease, histology, or whether patients underwent lobectomy versus wedge resection. Specifically, compromised preoperative pulmonary function and spirometry and concomitant cardiac disease were predictive of postoperative complications.

From these series of lung cancer patients undergoing surgery,[18–22] it appears clear that the operative mortality and postoperative complication rate has substantially decreased in the 1990s compared to the 1970s. In addition to better preoperative staging of these patients, significant improvements have been made in pre- and postoperative care. Furthermore, because all of these studies are retrospective, patient selection continues to be a critical factor in achieving comparable surgical outcomes in the elderly compared to younger patients. Even in this setting, it is clear that the comorbid cardiac and pulmonary disease does lead to a somewhat higher, although fortunately manageable, complication rate in these series of patients. Thus age alone should not be a factor in determining the best operative procedure for lung cancer patients with adequate physiologic status and functional reserve.

For patients who do have significant pulmonary compromise that might otherwise preclude standard surgical approaches, newer minimally invasive techniques have been developed that may be particularly useful in the elderly population. Preliminary reports have suggested that video-assisted lobectomy can be performed in the elderly[23] with less morbidity. Secondly, thoroscopic surgery[24] is a useful diagnostic and potential therapeutic tool in this population. One report of video-assisted thoroscopic surgery for partial pulmonary resection for lung cancer in elderly patients with severe emphysema demonstrated not only successful removal of the tumor but actual improvement in the pulmonary function.[25] Thus in appropriate candidates such pulmonary resection may not only remove the cancer but also improve underlying pulmonary function. These small series of patients require larger prospective surgical trials to better define both the short-term complications of this procedure as well as long-term benefits compared to more standard surgical approaches. In the interim, however, the standard surgical staging of mediastinoscopy takes on an even more important role in the elderly lung cancer patients to be as certain as possible about the nodal status of the patient before undertaking definitive surgical resection.

RADIATION

Radiation is an important treatment modality in the management of lung cancer. The acute side effects of radiation may result in physicians altering or interrupting a course of treatment in elderly patients. This action may compromise the efficacy of treatment even though most of these side effects are reversible. In contrast, the late side effects of radiation therapy may be neglected in older patients but can significantly impact on quality of life. Pignon et al. reviewed radiation data from patients treated on European Research Organization for Treatment of Cancer, (EORTC) trials to determine the influence of age on the frequency and severity of acute and late side effects of radiation therapy and if the prognosis of tumors sufficiently differed between patients of six age groups.[26] One-thousand three-hundred seventy-seven patients with lung cancer or esophageal cancer enrolled from 1976 to 1987 in six trials initiated by the lung cooperative group or by the gastrointestinal cooperative group of the EORTC were examined. Survival and toxicities according to age were analyzed in six age groups: less than 50, 50–54, 55–59, 60–64, 65–70 and more than 70 years. Data regarding age and acute toxicity were available for 1,208 patients who experienced 640 greater than 1 World Health Organization (WHO) toxicities. Of the patients evaluated for nausea, 30% had toxicity. The difference in distribution of the occurrence of nausea between

age groups was not significant, but there was a trend toward more nausea in the younger age groups. Only two cases of grade IV nausea were seen in the 55–59 and 60–64-year-old age groups. Weight loss during the treatment affected 228 of 470 patients evaluated. By contrast to nausea, there was a statistical difference in the distribution of weight loss with regard to age with a trend toward more weight loss in the older patients (p = .0002). Common symptoms included 16% of patients experiencing dyspnea, 30% esophagitis, and 23% weakness. There was no difference in the distribution of these complications according to age.

There was also no significant difference in the distribution of WHO performance status in relation to age; change in performance status was evaluated in 112 patients during radiation therapy, and they did not show an age effect. Regarding late side effects, 1,082 grade more than 1 late toxicities were recorded in 935 of 1,106 patients available for analysis, after 90 days. Approximately 40% of patients were free of late toxicity at 4 years in each age group. The comparison of late toxicity for all complications and all grades in each age group showed no significant difference in the actuarial incidence of late effects among age groups. When the analysis was restricted to grade more than 2 toxicities, there was a trend for more severe complications in older groups. However, only esophagitis demonstrated a significant difference with a higher frequency in the older patient (p = .01). Importantly, overall survival was related to stage and no differences were reported between the various age groups. These results, similar to the surgical data, suggest that age alone is not a reason to withhold another standard radiation treatment in the elderly patient with adequate physiologic reserve. Lastly, the addition of chemotherapy to radiation therapy had no influence on late complications as a function of age. Specifically, posttreatment weakness was noted to be equally distributed in all age groups. This finding is important because a common reason for applying a shortened course of radiation, or less aggressive treatment, in older patients is to reduce the duration to decrease the risk of fatigue.

In a study from Japan conducted between 1976 and 1992, 32 patients age 75 and older with a mean age of 79 years and 11 patients over 80 years with stage I and II NSCLC were given definitive radiation therapy.[27] Four patients were T_1N_0, 9 patients were T_2N_0, and 19 patients were T_2N_1. Twenty-six patients had a performance status of 0 to 1 and six patients had a $\geq$ 2 performance status. A total dose more than 60 Gy radiation was given to each patient, and all 32 patients completed treatment without treatment-related complications. The two-year survival rate was 40% and the five-year overall survival rate was 16%. There were 11 intercurrent deaths with 7 patients dying with heart disease. The two- and five-year cause-specific survival rates were 57% and 36%, respectively. In Japan most patients receive radiation treatment as inpatients, and all but three patients on this study were treated on an inpatient basis. None of the patients developed pneumonitis requiring hospitalization.

Another retrospective study of radiotherapy for lung cancer patients age 75 years and over by Patterson et al. from the United Kingdom concluded that radiation therapy for elderly patients with lung cancer is well tolerated with similar responses as seen in younger patients;[28] however, patient selection was deemed important. There were 149 patients over 75 years of age referred for radiation therapy. Eighty-three percent of these patients were ambulatory and independent in self-care but 12% were dependent. These patients had non–small cell and small cell carcinoma of the lung, 24% had known metastatic disease, and 91% had received previous treatment either with surgery or chemotherapy. No patients received chemotherapy during radiation. One hundred forty-two patients received radiation therapy, 8 received aggressive treatment with curative intent because they were either unfit or refused surgery, and 134 patients received palliative radiotherapy, 25 receiving a single fraction, 104 receiving two to five fractions over 1 week, and 5 patients were treated 9 to 14 days. One patient died before completing the treatment. The most common pretreatment symptoms reported by about 50% of the patients were cough and breathlessness. Hemoptysis and chest pain were seen in one-third of the patients and one-quarter of patients experienced weight loss. A complete or moderate response was reported in 80% of patients with hemoptysis (34/44), 56% with chest pain (25/45), 44% with dyspnea (32/73), 25% with cough (14/57), and 18% with dysphagia (2/11). Twenty-five patients reported side effects, 12 with dysphagia, 7 with lethargy, and 5 with pain. These reported side effects were for the most part graded as mild (61%), 50% (4/8) patients who received aggressive radiotherapy were alive after 21 to 25 months, the mean survival being 12 months. Only 4 (3%) of the 133 patients who completed palliative radiotherapy were alive 15 to 24 months later with the mean survival being 5 months. Thus these institutional experiences suggest that radiation treatment can be delivered in the lung cancer patient over 75 years of age with curative[27] or palliative[28] intent, with results comparable to younger patients.

Combined modality treatment with radiation therapy and chemotherapy in patients with unresectable stage III NSCLC is becoming standard of care in good performance status patients, as discussed elsewhere in this book. Older patients have been included in many of these trials, but studies evaluating combined modality aproaches in NSCLC as a function of age are limited. By contrast, radiation therapy and chemotherapy as a combined modality has been a standard of care for limited-stage small cell lung cancer (SCLC) for many years, and trials evaluating this approach in the elderly have been reported. A treatment regimen consisting of carboplatin and etoposide with accelerated hypertractionated radiation therapy achieved encouraging results in elderly patients with limited-stage SCLC.[29] Seventy-five

patients who were 70 years of age or older with Karnofsky performance status greater than or equal to 60 and no other major medical problems were treated on this protocol. The patients received carboplatin at 400 mg/m² on days 1 and 29, oral etoposide 50 mg/m² on days 1 through 21 and days 29 through 49, with accelerated hyperfractionated radiation at a dose of 1.5 Gy twice daily for a total dose of 45 Gy beginning on day 1 of treatment. There was a median follow-up of 61 months with a response rate of 75% complete response in 57% of patients and a median survival time of 15 months. The two-year survival rate was 32% and the five-year survival rate 13%. Grade III toxicities included leukopenia in 8.3% of patients, thrombocytopenia in 11% of patients, and esophagitis in 2.8% of patients. Only one patient experienced grade IV thrombocytopenia. There was no grade III or higher late toxicity seen. Fifty-two of the 61 patients who began treatment with a Karnofsky performance status of less than or equal to 90% had an improvement in their performance status.

In a retrospective review of two studies from the NCI Canada in which patients with limited-stage SCLC were randomized to received combined modality therapy, 88 of 608 patients were 70 years or older.[30,31] The conclusion of this study was that potentially curative combined modality therapy for limited-stage SCLC should not be withheld from patients because of their age. In this trial there were two arms: patients could, on arm A, receive CAV chemotherapy for three cycles alternating with etoposide/platinum chemotherapy for three cycles or CAV chemotherapy followed by etoposide/platinum chemotherapy for three cycles. In this arm, patients received radiation at week 18 for 25 Gy in 10 fractions or 37.5 Gy in 15 fractions. In the second arm, patients received CAV for three cycles alternating with etoposide/platinum for three cycles and then were randomized to receive either early thoracic radiation beginning at week 4 for 40 Gy at 15 fractions or late thoracic radiation beginning at week 16 for 40 Gy at 15 fractions. There was no significant difference in the tolerance between the two age groups; however, there was a trend toward a greater number of days required to complete treatment in patients receiving the late thoracic radiation with a greater variation seen in the older population. There were similar incidence of both acute and late grade III or IV toxicities between the two age groups. Incidence of esophagitis was not noted to be increased for the elderly group, although it was increased for all patients with increasing doses of radiation. There was no significant difference in response rates, local relapse rate, or overall survival in the two groups. The authors concluded that it is possible to administer combined modality therapy with chemotherapy and thoracic radiation safely in older patients presenting with limited-stage SCLC.

Although these results may differ in NSCLC patients, at a minimum it suggests that combined modality approaches should be evaluated in physiologically fit elderly patients with inoperable stage III NSCLC in an attempt to offer curative therapy.

Chemotherapy In the Elderly Patient

Of all the treatment modalities, the use of chemotherapy in the elderly has remained the most controversial. This relates to a variety of factors, including the perception of limited benefit of chemotherapy in NSCLC in general, as well as the potential for increased toxicity in the elderly. Over the last decade (as discussed elsewhere in this book), the benefit of chemotherapy has been well recognized in patients with advanced-stage cancer, as well as in patients with locally advanced disease in combination with either radiation treatment, surgery, or both. Unfortunately, most of the clinical trials that have documented this benefit have focused on patients in general younger than 70. In addition, most of the trials that have documented the benefit of chemotherapy have been combination chemotherapy regimens including cisplatin. Therefore, because of the relatively small database with regard to the benefit of combination chemotherapy in the elderly as well as the presumed increased toxicity in this population, there has been a reluctance to treat elderly patients with advanced NSCLC in the same way that younger patients have been treated. Fortunately, in the last few years several trials specific to the elderly have been conducted that clarify the benefits of treatment in this population.

In treatment of patients with advanced NSCLC, the most consistent factor predicting for survival has been performance status.[32] Of interest in this review published by Dr. Albain from the Southwest Oncology Group (SWOG) experience, increasing age in fact had a positive influence on survival. This may reflect a somewhat different biology of lung cancer in the elderly or simply that physician selection of elderly patients might be even more rigorous than in younger patients enrolling on chemotherapy trials. A more recent report reviewed the outcome of chemotherapy in patients with advanced NSCLC treated at the Royal Marsden Hospital from 1990–1995.[33] Of the 290 patients enrolled, 44% were over the age of 60 and 12% were over the age of 70. A variety of combination chemotherapy regimens were administered. In a multivaried analysis of the overall population, poor performance status elevated alkaline phosphatase more than 2 times normal, extensive-stage disease, and hypoalbumenia were all predictors of poor survival. However, in this study, age had no influence either positive or negative on survival or symptom relief because equivalent benefit was seen across all populations.

Although these trials suggest that elderly patients with comparable performance status to younger patients may receive the same benefit of chemotherapy without added toxicity, preselection remains a major problem in interpreting the data of such retrospective reviews. Fortunately, several prospective trials targeting elderly patients have now been

performed and reported. It is instructive to review the work of Gridelli[34] as an initial attempt to develop a less toxic regimen. Carboplatin at a dose of 300 mg/m^2 intravenously on day 1 was combined with oral etoposide 100 mg per day for 7 days, with the treatment to be cycled every 4 weeks. Of the first 14 patients treated, no objective response was observed and remarkable hematologic toxicity was recorded.[34] This regimen was developed to be "kinder and gentler" treatment, but declining renal function in the elderly was likely a significant factor in the toxicity of carboplatin dosed on body surface area. By contrast, Dr. Frasci performed another trial with carboplatin and oral etoposide, but in this study initiated carboplatin and an area under the curve (AUC) of 4, which allows correction for the decreased renal function in the elderly, and combined this with etoposide 50 mg twice daily orally for 14 days.[35] If no excess toxicity was noted, then the carboplatin dose was increased to an AUC of 5 on the second course and the etoposide course was extended to 21 days of administration on the third course. A total of 38 NSCLC patients over the age of 70 were enrolled in this trial. The overall response to treatment was 22%, with a median survival time of 11 months in the elderly patients. Of significance was that the quality of life improved in 41% of patients. Thus these phase II trials not nicely document that by adjusting chemotherapy for differences in organ function in the elderly, both improvement in clinical benefit and reduction in toxicity may be seen.

The new agents have had a major impact in the treatment of NSCLC with a potential to have an even greater impact in the elderly. The new agents (discussed elsewhere in this textbook) have significant advantages in terms of less fatigue and less effect on appetite and weight loss, which may be particularly important to the elderly. Also, because these agents have been largely tested with contemporary populations, more detailed toxicity data is available. Lastly, in order to establish the activity of these agents, single-agent studies have been conducted, and it appears that monotherapy may be a very appropriate alternative for elderly patients with advanced NSCLC.

Vinorelbine was the first new agent approved for treatment for NSCLC.[36,37] In the U.S. trial,[36] single-agent vinorelbine at 30 mg/m^2 intravenously weekly was compared to a five-day 5FU leucovorin regimen administered monthly. This trial documented a survival advantage for a single-agent vinorelbine compared to 5FU leucovorin with 25% of patients with stage IV NSCLC alive at 1 year compared to 16% on the control arm. Similar results were seen in the European trial.[37] In this study, both stage IIIb and IV patients were included, and the one-year survival for vinorelbine was 30% with a combination of vinorelbine and cisplatin superior at 35%. In both of these trials, elderly patients were included, but the median age of the patients was 61. Therefore, limited conclusions can be made from these two trials about the absolute benefit of either single-agent vinorelbine or vinorelbine and cisplatin in elderly patients over 70. Of interest, in a subsequent analysis of the European trials,[38] the benefit of cisplatin/vinorelbine in combination over single-agent vinorelbine was limited to patients with a performance status of 0 and 1. No additional benefit of the combination chemotherapy was seen in the performance status 2 patients.

In light of these data, it is interesting that Vernisi evaluated the role of single-agent vinorelbine in an elderly population of patients felt to be "unfit" for cisplatin-based chemotherapy. There were 23 patients over the age of 70 out of 83 patients treated.[39] In this study, the overall response was 30% and toxicities were mild with a median survival of 9 months. No effect of age on outcome was detected, and it was suggested that single-agent vinorelbine was a reasonable option for patients with advanced NSCLC, particularly in the elderly.

With this background, the most significant trial of chemotherapy in the elderly to date is the study performed by Dr. Gridelli and the Elderly Lung Cancer Vinorelbine Italian Study Group, also known as the ELVIS trial.[40] Elderly patients over the age of 70 with stage IIIb or IV NSCLC ineligible for radiotherapy with a performance status of 0 to 2 were enrolled in a trial that compared vinorelbine to supportive care alone. The vinorelbine dose was 30 mg/m^2 intravenously on days 1 and 8 with no planned dose on day 15. This three-week cycle was repeated for a maximum of 6 cycles of treatment. In addition to standard follow-up studies, a quality-of-life assessment was performed using the EORTC core questionnaire as well as the lung cancer specific module. A statistically significant survival advantage was seen in patients receiving vinorelbine (p = .03). The median survival was 28 weeks in the vinorelbine arm versus 21 weeks in the control arm, and survival of 1 year was 32% in the vinorelbine group and 14% in the control arm (Figure 63.2). These survival outcomes are similar to, if not superior to, the U.S. trials of single-agent vinorelbine versus 5FU leucovorin in younger patients. Of the 71 patients assessed for toxicity of vinorelbine, treatment was stopped in five patients because of severe toxic events. Four of the five patients developed constipation after multiple cycles of treatment. Other milder toxicities, as the vinorelbine were seen, but despite the treatment-related side effects, there was an overall improvement in quality-of-life scores for patients receiving vinorelbine versus supportive care alone. This trial clearly establishes the potential benefit of single-agent therapy in the elderly population across the range of performance status categories. These results confirm the earlier work of Dr. Gridelli and colleagues in the phase II study that preceded the ELVIS trial.[41] This large phase II and phase III experience with vinorelbine in the elderly provides an excellent database against which other new agents or combinations may be tested.

A second agent that also has a favorable side effect profile has been gemcitabine.[42] Like vinorelbine, extensive studies

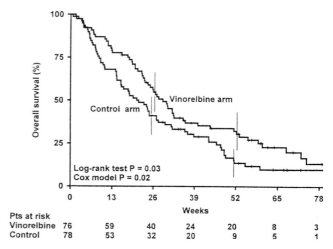

FIGURE 63.2. Estimated survival according to treatment arm as calculated by the Kaplan-Meier method. Number of patients at risk by treatment arm is shown at the bottom. Pts, patients; vertical bars, representative of 955 confidence intervals.

have been performed with gemcitabine as a single agent in advanced NSCLC across a range of ages. Specific review of gemcitabine experience in patients over age 65 enrolled in phase II trials has also been reported.[43] In these trials, gemcitabine dose ranged from 800 to 1,250 mg/m^2 weekly for 3 weeks out of 4 with repeated monthly cycles of treatment. In these studies 255 patients were under the age of 65 and 105 patients were over the age of 65. Of interest was the fact that the group under 65 had a median survival of 8.1 months and a one-year survival of 27%. By contrast, the older population had a median survival of 9.1 months and a 36% one-year survival. Several cycles associated with dose reduction or dose omissions in the mean number of treatment cycles administered were similar between the two groups. Although this trial has the same limitations as other retrospective reviews with regard to patient selection, it supports the conclusion that gemcitabine is active and well tolerated in elderly patients with NSCLC and may also be a potential consideration for monotherapy in the elderly. To help explore the relative benefits of vinorelbine versus gemcitabine, the Multiagent Italian Lung Cancer Elderly Trial (MILES) is ongoing, which is randomizing patients to single-agent vinorelbine versus single-agent gemcitabine versus the combination of the two agents. These trials will be invaluable in determining the relative benefits of chemotherapy in general and the new agents specifically in elderly patients with NSCLC.

Although monotherapy is certainly an appropriate alternative to combination chemotherapy in the elderly patients and those with lower performance status, for the higher performance status, physiologically fit, elderly lung cancer patients with potential curable NSCLC, a much larger prospective database is needed to establish the benefits of combination chemotherapy in stage III patients and in the adjuvant setting. Until such trials are performed, we must look to ongoing cooperative group trials that cross the age groups to determine relative benefits of combination chemotherapy in this population. Specifically, the taxanes, paclitaxel and docetaxel, have demonstrated substantial clinical activity as single agents and in combination treatment. Because of the increased toxicities associated with cisplatin in association with paclitaxel and docetaxel, there has also been a shift from cisplatin use to carboplatin use in combination with these agents. The relative benefits of these newer combinations are the subject of ongoing trials.

The initial report by the SWOG has suggested that cisplatin and vinorelbine and carboplatin and paclitaxel have a similar impact on survival in advanced NSCLC patients across the range of ages.[44] Although detailed quality-of-life data and economic analyses are pending, there was a higher dropout rate noted for patients on the cisplatin arm of the study, supporting the better tolerability of carboplatin-based therapy. A second trial of major importance in this area is an ongoing trial performed by the Eastern Cooperative Oncology Group (ECOG) also comparing carboplatin and paclitaxel to three cisplatin-based regimens, including cisplatin and paclitaxel, cisplatin and docetaxel, and cisplatin and gemcitabine. Full analysis of this study awaits completion of the trial, but a preliminary analysis has suggested that the carboplatin arm of the trial had an improved toxicity profile compared to all three of the cisplatin-based therapies.[45] Because of the increased toxicity in the performance status to patients compared to historical controls in the ECOG database, the trial was closed to performance 2 patients. Analysis of the data, however, reflected statistical differences favoring carboplatin and paclitaxel over the other three arms of the study in terms of grade 3–5 toxicities. Survival data and other outcomes await completion of the trial and its subsequent analysis, but it appears from the safety data that carboplatin is the preferred platinum agent.

Lastly, a third trial of importance by the Cancer and Leukemia Group B (CALGB) is evaluating the role of single-agent paclitaxel versus carboplatin and paclitaxel. This trial is open to enrollment of performance status 0 to 2 patients, and a monitoring committee is in place to review potential toxicities seen in the performance 2 patients. However, in view of the lower toxicity profile of this combination regimen in the ECOG trial, it is hoped that this trial will reach its completion. Because elderly patients are eligible for this trial and are being actively enrolled, it is hoped that this study will help address the relative benefit of monotherapy versus combination chemotherapy in elderly patients with NSCLC.

SUMMARY

Because of the demographics of lung cancer, the elderly population has become an increasingly important group for evaluation of the relative benefits of both curative and palliative approaches to this disease. In addition to the specific trials of surgery, radiation therapy, and chemotherapy that have recently been performed in this population, increasing experience is being gained in the supportive care of all cancer patients, and the elderly may particularly benefit from the improvements in pain management, reduction in hematologic toxicity, and in improving our understanding of fatigue as well as other supportive care approaches. The growing database and number of clinical trials specifically targeted to the elderly is encouraging and should be useful to the clinician and the patient in making informed decisions about treatment options in this disease.

REFERENCES

1. Yancik R, Reis LA. Cancer in older persons—magnitude of the problem. How do we apply what we know? *Cancer* 1994;74(suppl 1):1995.
2. Halpem M, Gillespie B, Warner K. Patterns of absolute risk of lung cancer: mortality in former smokers. *J Natl Cancer Inst* 1993;85:457.
3. Doll R, Hill AB. Lung cancer and other causes of death related to smoking: a second report on the mortality of British doctors. *Br Med J* 1956;2:1071.
4. Pathak DR, Samet JM, Humble CG, et al. Determinants of lung cancer risk in cigarette smokers in New Mexico. *J Natl Cancer Inst* 1986;76:597.
5. Halpern M, Gillespie B, Warner K. Patterns of absolute risk of lung cancer: mortality in former smokers. *J Natl Cancer Inst* 1993;85:457.
6. Orleans TC, Jepson C, Resch N, et al. Quitting motives and barriers among older smokers: the 1987 Adult Use of Tobacco Survey revisited. *Cancer* 1994;74(suppl):2055.
7. DeMaria LC, Cohen JH. Characteristics of lung cancer in the elderly patient. *J Gerontol* 1987;42:540.
8. O'Rourke MA, Feussner JR, Ferge P, et al. Age trends of lung cancer at diagnosis. *JAMA* 1987;258:921.
9. McKenna RJ. Clinical aspects of cancer in the elderly. Treatment decision, treatment choices and follow up. *Cancer* 1994;74:2107.
10. Sherman S, Geudot C. The feasibility of thoracotomy for lung cancer in the elderly. *JAMA* 1987;258:927.
11. Crocker I, Prosnitz L. Radiation therapy of the elderly. In: *Clinics in geriatric medicine*, vol. 3. Philadelphia: WB Saunders, 1987:473.
12. Walsh SJ, Begg CB, Carbone PP. Cancer chemotherapy in the elderly. *Semin Oncol* 1989;16:66.
13. United States National Center for Health Statistics. Changing mortality patterns, health services utilization and health care expenditures 1978–1003. Publication no. 83-1047, Bethesda Maryland: NCHS Analytical & Epidemiological Studies, Vital and Health Statistics, 1983.
14. Katz S, Branch LG, Branson MH, et al. Active life expectancy. *N Engl J Med* 1983;309:1218.
15. Kirsh MM, Rotman H, Bove E, et al. Major pulmonary resection for bronchogenic carcinoma in the elderly. *Ann Thorac Surg* 1976;22:369.
16. Gebitekin C, Gupta NK, Martin PG, et al. Long term results in the elderly following pulmonary resection for non-small cell; lung cancer. *Eur J Cardiothorac Surg* 1993;7:653.
17. Thompson-Evans EW. Resection for bronchial carcinoma in the elderly. *Thorax* 1973;28:86.

18. Massard G, Moog R, Wihlm JM, et al. Bronchogenic cancer in the elderly: operative risk and long-term prognosis. *Thorac Cardiovasc Surg* 1996;44:40.

19. Pagni S, Federico JA, Ponn RB. Pulmonary resection for lung cancer in octogenarians. *Ann Thorac Surg* 1997;63:785.

20. Hanagiri T, Muranaka H, Hashimoto M, et al. Results of surgical treatment of lung cancer in octogenarians. *Lung Cancer* 1999; 23:129.

21. Santambrogio L, Nosotti M, Bellaviti N, et al. Journal of Gerontology: Prospective study of surgical treatment of lung cancer in the elderly patient. *Medical Sciences* 1996;51A(6):M267.

22. Ciriaco P, Zannini P, Carretta A, et al. Surgical treatment of non-small cell lung cancer in patients 70 years of age or older. *Int Surg* 1998;83:4.

23. Asamura H, Nakayama H, Kondo H, et al. Video-assisted lobectomy in the elderly. *Chest* 1997;111:1101.

24. Yim, APC. Thoracoscopic surgery in the elderly population. *Surg Endosc* 1996;10:880.

25. Ohtsuka T, Kohno T, Nakajima J, et al. Thoracoscopic surgery for lung cancer complicated by emphysema in elderly patients. Report of three cases. *Int Surg* 1996;81:245.

26. Pignon T, Gregor A, Koning CS, et al. Age has no impact on acute and late toxicity of curative thoracic radiotherapy. *Radiother Oncol* 1996;46:239.

27. Furuta M, Hayakawa K, Katano S, et al. Radiation therapy for stage I-II non-small cell lung cancer in patients aged 75 years and older. *Jpn J Clin Oncol* 1996;26:95.

28. Patterson CJ, Hocking M, Bond M, et al. Retrospective study of radiotherapy for lung cancer in patients aged 75 years and over. *Age and aging* 1998;27:515.

29. Jeremic B, Shibamoto Y, Acimovic L, et al. Carboplatin, etoposide and accelerated hyperfractionated radiotherapy for elderly patients with limited small cell lung carcinoma. A phase II study. *Cancer* 1998;82:836.

30. Siu LL, Shepherd FA, Murray N, et al. Influence of age on the treatment of limited-stage small-cell lung cancer. *J Clin Oncol* 1996;14(3):821.

31. Quon H, Shepherd FA, Payne DG, et al. The influence of age on the delivery, tolerance and efficacy of thoracic irradiation in the combined modality treatment of limited stage small cell lung cancer. *Int J Radiation Oncology Biol Phys* 1999;43(1):39.

32. Albain KS, Crowley JJ, Leblanc M, et al. Survival determinants in extensive-stage non-small–cell lung cancer: the Southwest Oncology Group Experience. *J Clin Oncol* 1997;9:1618.

33. Hickish TF, Smith IE, O'Brien ME, et al. Clinical benefit from palliative chemotherapy in non-small-cell lung cancer extends to the elderly and those with poor prognostic factors. *Br J Cancer* 1998;78(1):28.

34. Gridelli C, Rossi A, Scognamiglio F, et al. Carboplatin plus oral etoposide in elderly patients with advanced non small cell lung cancer. A phase II study. *Anticancer Res* 1997;17:4755.

35. Frasci G, Comella P, Panza N, et al. *Eur J Cancer* 1998;34(11): 1710.

36. Crawford J, O'Rourke M, Schiller JH, et al. Randomized trial of vinorelbine compared with fluorouracil plus leucovorin in patients with stage IV non-small-cell lung cancer. *J Clin Oncol* 1996;14(10):2774.

37. Le Chevalier T, Brisgand D, Douillard J, et al. Randomized study of vinorelbine and cisplatin versus vindesine and cisplatin versus vinorelbine alone in advanced non-small cell lung cancer. *Proc Am Soc Clin Oncol* 1992;11:287.

38. Soria JC, Douillard JY, Pujol JL, et al. Gustave Roussy, Villejuif, France. Proceedings of ASCO, Volume 18, 1999. #1893.

39. Veronesi A, Crivellari D, Magri MD, et al. Vinorelbine treatment of advanced non-small cell lung cancer with special emphasis on elderly patients. *Eur J Cancer* 1996;32(10):1809.

40. The Elderly Lung Cancer Vinorelbine Italian Study Group. Effects of vinorelbine on quality of life and survival of elderly patients with advanced non-small-cell lung cancer. *J Nat Canc Inst* 1999;91(1):66.

41. Gridelli C, Perrone F, Gallo C, et al. Vinorelbine is well tolerated and active in the treatment of elderly patients with advanced non-small cell lung cancer. A two-stage phase II study. *Eur J Cancer* 1997;33(3):392.

42. Le Chevalier T. Single-agent activity of gemcitabine in advanced non-small cell lung cancer. *Semin Oncol* 1996;23(5):36.

43. Shepherd FA, Abratt RP, Anderson H, et al. Gemcitabine in the treatment of elderly patients with advanced non-small cell lung cancer. *Semin Oncol* 1997;24(2):S7-50.

44. Kelly K, Crowley J, Bunn PA, et al. A randomized phase III trial of paclitaxel plus carboplatin (PC) versus vinorelbine plus cisplatin (VC) in untreated advanced non-small cell lung cancer (NSCLC): a Southwest Oncology Group (SWOG) trial. Proceedings of ASCO, Volume 18, 1999. Abs #1777.

45. Johnson DH, Zhu J, Schiller J, et al. E1594—A randomized phase III trial in metastatic non-small cell lung cancer (NSCLS)—outcome of PS 2 patients (Pts): an Eastern Cooperative Group trial (ECOG). Proceedings of ASCO, Volume 18, 1999. Abs #1779.

64

TREATMENT OF SMALL CELL LUNG CANCER IN THE ELDERLY PATIENT

FRANCES A. SHEPHERD
ANDREA BEZJAK

The global incidence of lung cancer is increasing at a rate of 0.5% per year, and is the leading cause of cancer mortality for both men and women in most countries.[1] Although in North America the age-adjusted incidence rates for men began to decline in the 1980s, they continued to increase for women and are still increasing to this day. The average age of patients with lung cancer is also rising such that the age-specific incidence for men peaks at 75–79 years and for women at age 70–74. Incidence rates decline thereafter in both genders, likely due to the lower prevalence of smoking in the population at the beginning of the century. In some areas of the world, all-cancer mortality rates in the elderly have increased substantially over the past two decades, due almost exclusively to an increase in lung cancer and other tobacco-related cancers in both men and women.[2,3]

Small cell lung cancer (SCLC) accounts for approximately 20% of all pulmonary neoplsms, and unlike squamous cell lung cancer, which tends to increase in incidence with increasing age, SCLC appears to be equally distributed over all age groups.[4,5] Some investigators have shown an inverse relationship between age and stage of disease.[5,6] This trend has been shown most clearly for patients with non–small cell lung cancer (NSCLC), but has also been reported in several series of small cell patients.[5–7]

It is clear that large numbers of elderly patients have lung cancer, including SCLC, for whom treatment decisions must be made. However, there are few data on how treatment for this group of patients differs or should differ from that of younger patients. Until recently, elderly patients were often excluded from clinical research trials, and few studies have been designed specifically for the elderly population. Goodwin et al. reported that although 31% of all adult patients with cancer were over 70 years of age, only 7% of patients enrolled in the Southwest Oncology Group (SWOG) trials were in that age group.[8] Specifically, in the SWOG lung cancer trials, only 18% of the patients were over age 65, and 9% were over age 70. Dajczman et al. reported that only 1 of 81 elderly patients was enrolled on an experimental protocol for SCLC compared to 19% of

patients age 60–69 and 28% of patients less than 60 years of age.[9] Furthermore, several investigators have shown that treatment *of any kind* may be withheld from elderly patients with SCLC despite a high expectation of benefit and even a chance of cure for patients with limited-stage disease.[7–10] The University of Toronto group reported that over the 12-year period 1976–1988, only 78 of 123 patients (63%) age 70 years or greater were treated with chemotherapy (only one-third over age 80), and 25 patients received no treatment at all.[7] The most important determinant in the decision to treat or not to treat was performance status: only 38% of patients with performance status 3 or 4 received treatment, compared to 66% of patients with performance status 0, 1, or 2. Similar statistics were reported by de Rijke et al. from the Netherlands, where 52% of patients over age 70 were offered no treatment at all compared to 14% and 22% for patients age 50–59 and 60–69, respectively.[10]

It would appear that the reasons for not referring older patients for investigation and treatment of SCLC are based on widely held beliefs and perceptions rather than on well-documented scientific data. It is possible that many primary care physicians assume that elderly patients have a limited life expectancy and, therefore, do not warrant treatment of malignant disease in general and lung cancer in particular. In fact, the life expectancy of a woman who reaches age 70 is 15 years, and 8–10 years for a man that age.[11] It is also a commonly held belief that elderly patients have a poorer prognosis and tolerate therapy less well than younger patients, perhaps due to the presence of other comorbid illnesses that commonly occur in this population. These issues will be addressed in the sections that follow. Finally, some physicians view the elderly as emotionally as well as physically frail, which may lead to the extreme of withholding not just treatment but even the diagnosis from older patients. However, this view does not seem to be justified, as shown by Nerenz et al.[12] and Ginsburg et al.[13]

In view of these attitudes, it is clear that the treatment of elderly patients with SCLC requires critical evaluation. Should all elderly patients be offered the same therapy as younger patients, and if not, what guidelines are available to help determine which patients are most likely to benefit from treatment? Should treatment be attenuated in dose or duration, and is combined modality therapy appropriate in the older population? Should specific protocols be designed to meet the needs of the elderly patient? Because elderly patients were excluded from most clinical research trials until recently, it is difficult to address these questions with data that are not heavily influenced by referral bias and physician treatment bias. Furthermore, even in the overviews of large cooperative group databases, the extremely elderly population of over 75 or over 80 years of age is under-represented. Clearly, clinical trials for older patients are desperately needed.[14]

AGE AS A PROGNOSTIC FACTOR

Several of the cooperative groups have analyzed their databases to determine the relative prognostic importance of various baseline clinical and laboratory factors in SCLC.[15–18] There is universal agreement that stage is the most important determinant of prognosis, with median survival times of 12 to 16 months reported for limited-stage compared to only 7 to 11 months for extensive-disease patients. Other important clinical parameters include performance status, gender, and baseline level of lactate dehydrogenase (LDH).[15,16]

A summary of the findings related specifically to age is shown in Table 64.1. The largest study was that of the SWOG database reported by Albain et al.[15] They found that age under 70 years was significantly favorable in both limited- and extensive-stage patients. Furthermore, age was significant even when entered into the Cox regression model of multiple prognostic indices. In a retrospective review of 1,521 patients, the Cancer and Leukemia Group B (CALGB) identified female gender and performance status as important predictors of survival in both limited- and

extensive-stage disease.[17] Limited-stage patients older than 60 years had a higher mortality rate than younger patients ($p < 0.008$), but age was not predictive of survival duration among patients with extensive disease.

Sagman et al. analyzed 614 patients from the University of Toronto database and reported a modest survival advantage for patients less than 70 years (RR 1.32, $p = 0.023$);[16] however, using recursive partitioning and amalgamation modeling (RECPAM) techniques, age was not significant and did not appear in any of the terminal pods of the four prognostic groups identified by the model. Albain et al.[15] also applied the RECPAM technique to the SWOG data set and identified four separate prognostic groups. Age was of importance only in the two limited-stage subgroups. This observation is similar to that reported by Spiegelman et al. for the CALGB.[17]

Siu et al. analyzed the National Cancer Institute of Canada, Clinical Trials Group (NCIC-CTG) BR.3 and BR.6 trials in limited-stage SCLC to determine the influence of age on both outcome and chemotherapy delivery.[18] This analysis is particularly important because all 618 patients received the same chemotherapy. They showed that, when analyzed as a continuous variable, age was of modest prognostic significance ($p = 0.02$), but when the survival of patients less than 70 years was compared to that of the older patients, there was no significant difference ($p = 0.14$). In fact, survival was similar for patients of all age groups, with the exception of the 13 patients age 75–80 who had significantly poorer survival than the rest of the group (Figure 64.1).

Pignon et al. reported the results of a metaanalysis of 2,140 patients who participated in 13 randomized trials designed to assess the importance of thoracic radiotherapy in limited-stage SCLC.[19] The relative risk of death in the combined therapy group compared to the chemotherapy-alone group was 0.86 (CI 0.78–0.94, $p = 0.001$), and the benefit in terms of overall survival at 3 years was 5.4%. There was a trend toward a larger reduction in mortality

TABLE 64.1. THE IMPORTANCE OF AGE AS A PROGNOSTIC FACTOR IN SMALL CELL LUNG CANCER

Author	Age Break	Limited Stage		Extensive Stage	
		Univariate	Multivariate	Univariate	Multivariate
Albain et al.[15] n = 2,580	70	Hazards ratio 1.4 (p = <0.0001)	Hazards ratio 1.5 (p = <0.00005)	Hazards ratio 1.3 (p = 0.002)	Hazards ratio 1.3 (p = 0.006)
Sagman et al.[16] n = 614	70	Relative risk 1.32 (p = 0.023)*	Not significant	—	Not significant
Spiegelman et al.[17] n = 1,521	60	—	Relative hazard 1.23 (p = 0.008)	—	Relative hazard 1.03 (p = 0.74)
Siu et al.[18] n = 608	70	Age as a continuous variable p = 0.02 Age 0–69 vs. ≥70, p = 0.14	Not significant	—	—

* The effect of age was examined together for limited and extensive disease

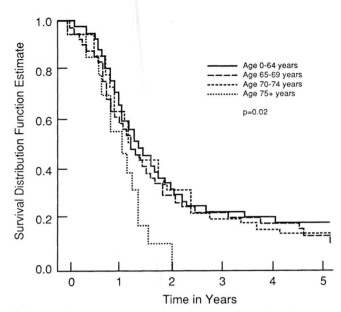

FIGURE 64.1. Comparison of survival by age group: 0–64, 65–69, 70–74, and 75+. (From Siu L, Shepherd FA, Murray N, et al. Influence of age on the treatment of limited-stage small-cell lung cancer. *J Clin Oncol* 1996;14:821, with permission.)

in younger patients, with a relative risk of death in the radiation group being 0.72 for patients less than 55 years of age. In contrast, the relative risk of death was actually *increased* at 1.07 (CI 0.70–1.64) with radiotherapy in patients over 70. Three-year survival rates estimated using the Kaplan-Meier method were 9.2% for chemotherapy alone compared to 17.4% for chemotherapy and radiotherapy in patients less than 55 years. For patients over 70, the rates were 10.2% and 8.75%, respectively.

CHEMOTHERAPY

With the exception of two studies that included elderly patients among other poor-prognosis populations,[20,21] there have been no randomized clinical trials of chemotherapy for SCLC in the elderly. For that reason, it is necessary to rely on retrospective reviews of large data sets that have compared the results achieved by elderly patients to those of younger patients in the same cohort, or to small prospective trials designed specifically for the elderly population. The definition of elderly has not been standard in these studies and has even been as low as 55 years or greater.[23] Most reports dealing with SCLC, however, have used age 70 years or greater to distinguish between the young and the elderly.

Retrospective Reviews

The results of nine retrospective reviews have been summarized in Table 64.2.[7,9,18,22–27] Several authors reported that

many patients with SCLC were not offered treatment of any kind.[7,9,22,24] In the Toronto Hospital review,[7] 25 of 123 patients received no therapy and 20 were offered palliative radiation only. Survival correlated significantly with treatment received, ranging from 1.1 months for those not treated to 10.7 months for those who completed four to six cycles of combination chemotherapy (p = 0.0001). Dajczman et al.[9] also reported that suboptimal treatment was given to 57% of patients age 60–69 and 77% of patients over 70. Furthermore, the administration of suboptimal treatment was associated with significantly poorer survival, although this was true across all age groups studied. Shepherd et al.[7] and Dajczman et al.[9] examined the possible reasons for withholding or delivering less than standard treatment to elderly patients, and both investigators reported that performance status was the most important determinant in decision making. In the Toronto study,[7] only 38% of patients with Eastern Cooperative Oncology Group (ECOG) performance status 3 or 4 were treated with chemotherapy. In fact, performance status played a greater role than age itself, stage of the tumor, or the presence of other comorbid diseases. Several investigators have reported that the elderly population have more comorbid illnesses than their younger counterparts;[7,9,22] however, even serious illnesses such as chronic obstructive pulmonary disease, atherosclerotic heart disease, hypertension, diabetes, and so on do not seem to influence the decision to treat the elderly patient, nor do they affect the ability to deliver therapy.

Once a decision has been made to treat with chemotherapy, elderly patients often receive lower doses than younger patients. Shepherd et al.[9] showed, once again, that the decision to reduce initial doses was based most often on performance status. Physician decision to reduce doses for the elderly is based largely on the perception of poorer bone marrow reserve in the elderly and poorer tolerance for other toxicities. Although there are theoretical reasons why physiological changes in the elderly might lead to higher area under the curve (AUC) drug concentrations, and hence increased toxicity, this does not always seem to be the case in clinical practice.[28] Begg et al.[29,30] reported that with the exception of methyl-CCNU and methotrexate, agents that are seldom used in the treatment of SCLC any longer, neither the frequency nor the severity of toxicity was increased in the elderly.

More recent studies have also shown that elderly patients, if they meet the criteria for entry into SCLC clinical trials, do not experience increased rates of toxicity.[18,31] Siu et al. reported that grade 3 and 4 toxicity was not increased in elderly patients treated in two NCIC-CTG trials of limited SCLC in which patients received three cycles of cyclophosphamide, doxorubicin, and vincristine, and three cycles of etoposide and cisplatin. However, in an older study that used the more myelosuppressive regimen doxorubicin, cyclophosphamide, and etoposide, Poplin et al.[23] found that the incidence of fever and infection increased with age. Nou

TABLE 64.2. RETROSPECTIVE ANALYSES OF CHEMOTHERAPY IN ELDERLY PATIENTS WITH SMALL CELL LUNG CANCER*

Author	Number Young/Old	Drugs	Response		Median Survival		Toxic Death	
			Young	Old	Young	Old	Young	Old
Clamon et al.[22]	0/20	Various	NA	50%	NA	10 mos	NA	1
Poplin et al.[23]	164/49	CAE	LD	LD	—	~12 mos	19	10
			60%**	75%**				
			ED	ED				
			44%**	40%**				
Kelly et al.[24]	62/34	Various	NR	NR	27 wks	25 wks	0	3
Findlay et al.[25]	0/64	Various	NA	67%	NA	25 wks	NA	3
Shepherd et al.[7]	0/78	CAV or EP	NA	62%	NA	LD	NA	0
						11.9 mos		
						ED		
						5.2 mos		
Nou.[26]	235/110	CAV or CME	NR	NR	10.9 mos	7.4 mos	15	9
Dajczman et al.[9]	231/81	CAV or EP	50%	51%	~9 mos	6 mos	12	4
Siu et al.[18]	520/70	CAV and EP	78%	82%	15 mos	13 mos	9	4
					11% 5-yr	8% 5-yr		
Tebbutt et al.[27]	73/29	CAV or EC	LD	LD	LD	LD	0	3
			71%	68%	45 wks	36 wks		
			ED	ED	ED	ED		
			65%	38%	39 wks	23.5 wks		

* Results summarized only for patients treated with chemotherapy in each series
** Only complete remission rates reported.
CAE, cyclophosphamide, doxorubicin, etoposide; CAV, cyclophosphamide, doxorubicin, vincristine; EP, etoposide, cisplatin; EC, etoposide carboplatin; CME, CCNU, methotrexate, etoposide; LD, limited disease; ED, extensive disease; NA, not applicable; NR, not reported.

et al.[26] also reported that although nadir blood counts were similar in patients less than or greater than 70 years of age, the rates of septicemia per course and lethal septicemia were significantly higher in the older patients. However, this group also used highly myelosuppressive combinations that included both methotrexate and CCNU. With the possible exception of peripheral neuropathy,[24] significantly increased nonhematologic toxicity has not been reported in any series to date. It would appear, therefore, that elderly patients of good performance status tolerate chemotherapy well, and that when regimens associated with modest degrees of myelosuppression are used, the risk of severe or fatal infectious complications is not increased.

Even though toxicity rates in elderly patients do not appear to be higher than those seen in younger patients, several authors have reported that elderly patients receive significantly fewer chemotherapy cycles than younger patients, and this situation appears to occur even in the stricter setting of a clinical research trial.[7,9,18,27] Siu et al.[18] reported that only 69% of elderly patients completed six chemotherapy cycles compared to 82% of younger patients (p = 0.01) in two NCIC-CTG trials. They did not find that the elderly patients had higher rates of dose reduction, although this finding has been reported by other authors.[9,27] When initial dose reductions, subsequent dose reductions for toxicity, and dose omissions are considered, the elderly population

may actually received only one-half to two-thirds the treatment given to younger patients.

Clearly, the most important question to be asked is whether this attenuation of treatment in the elderly has a significant effect on survival. The results for the patients who received chemotherapy in several reported series are summarized in Table 64.2. All studies were retrospective reviews and some looked only at an elderly population, whereas others compared the results in elderly and young patients using variable age cutoffs. Siu et al.[18] showed that for patients with limited disease, response rates and median and five-year survival rates were similar for elderly and young patients. These observations are important because all patients were treated on a clinical trial and received the same chemotherapy. Poplin et al.[23] showed wider variations among four age subgroups of patients with limited disease (Figure 64.2), but it is interesting to note that the patients with the poorest survival were those in the *youngest* age group less than 55 years. Less difference was seen for patients with extensive-stage tumors (Figure 64.3). Other investigators who treated the elderly and the young with relatively uniform chemotherapy combinations reported similar response rates in both age groups, particularly for limited-stage disease patients,[9,26,27] and the Montreal group showed that median and two-year survival rates were similar for patients in three age groups if they were of good perfor-

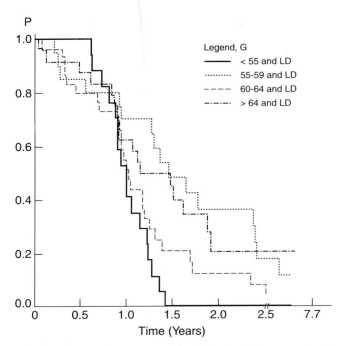

FIGURE 64.2. Kaplan-Meier survival plots for different ages; all patients had LD. (From Poplin E, Thompson B, Whitacre M, et al. Small cell carcinoma of the lung; influence of age on treatment outcome. *Cancer Treat Rep* 1987;71:291, with permission.)

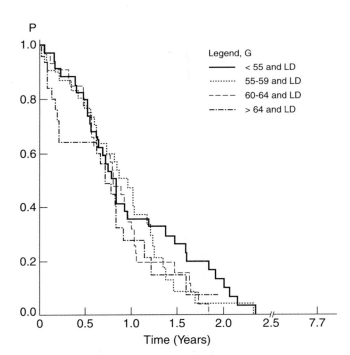

FIGURE 64.3. Kaplan-Meier survival plots for different ages; all patients had ED. (From Poplin E, Thompson B, Whitacre M, et al. Small cell carcinoma of the lung; influence of age on treatment outcome. *Cancer Treat Rep* 1987;71:291, with permission.)

mance staus and received chemotherapy.[9] However, both Nou[26] and Tebbutt et al.[27] reported shorter survival for elderly patients, although the difference was statistically significant only in the Nou study[26] when examined in a multivariate analysis.

A closer examination of Table 64.2 shows that for each report that compares young to elderly patients, survival in the older group is less. Frequently, the differences were not statistically different in the individual studies, and further deductions should probably not be drawn in view of the variability in treatment delivered and the differing definitions of elderly. However, these data suggest that the true impact of age on treatment outcome still requires further examination. Furthermore, little can be said about chemotherapy for the extremely elderly. Siu et al.[18] reported that the patients with the worst survival in the NCIC trials were those in the 75–80 age group. Only 46% of patients completed all six courses of chemotherapy, and no patient survived beyond 2 years (Figure 64.1). Patients over age 80 were excluded from all research trials until recently, and some authors have reported that patients in this age group are seldom offered chemotherapy of any kind, even that which is considered to be "gentle."[7] As the likelihood of surviving past 80 years of age increases, more attention will have to be paid to determining appropriate treatment for this group.

Prospective Trials for the Elderly

It is clear that some elderly patients can derive significant benefit from combination chemotherapy for SCLC. However, many investigators continue to question whether such treatment is appropriate for the elderly, and some have suggested that less aggressive treatment might be more appropriate even if this results in some compromise in overall response or survival rates.[25] Findlay et al.[25] reviewed their results for 72 elderly patients treated with either intensive combination chemotherapy or less rigorous treatment using either single agents or reduced doses of combination chemotherapy. In the intensive group, there were three treatment-related deaths, but despite this, median survival was longer (36 weeks versus 16 weeks), particularly for patients with limited disease (43 versus 26 weeks). Although other investigators might have reached a different conclusion from these results, these authors summarized by saying that intensive chemotherapy for elderly patients results in higher response rates and higher toxicity but not a major survival benefit.

In an attempt to avoid the toxicity of combination chemotherapy without compromising efficacy, several groups have developed treatment strategies specifically for elderly patients with SCLC. The results of several prospective trials are summarized in Table 64.3.[32–41] The epipodophyllotoxins, etoposide and teniposide, are among the most active agents for the treatment of SCLC, and as single agents produce response rates of 70% or more. Three trials of sin-

TABLE 64.3. PROSPECTIVE SINGLE-ARM TRIALS OF CHEMOTHERAPY FOR ELDERLY PATIENTS WITH SMALL CELL LUNG CANCER

Author	Drugs	Number of Patients	Response	Median Survival	Toxic Deaths
Smit et al.[32]	Etoposide 160 mg/m² PO daily × 5	35	ORR 71%	LD 16 mos ED 9 mos	
Gatzemeier et al.[33]	Etoposide 500 mg/m² over 3 days every 8–10 days	55	ORR 57%	LD 7.5 mos ED 6.6 mos	
Keane et al.[34]	Etoposide 200 mg P.O. daily × 5	63	CR 20% PR 56%	38 wks	0
Bork et al.[35]	Teniposide 60 mg/m² daily × 5	33	90%	8+ mos	0
Cerny et al.[36]	Teniposide 100 mg/m² daily × 5	30	33%	5.6 mos	5
Byrne et al.[37]	Etoposide 200 mg P.O. daily × 5 Carboplatin 300 mg/m² day 1	70	CR 28% PR 51%	40 wks	1
Michel et al.[38]	Teniposide 80 mg/m² weekly Carboplatin 80 mg/m² weekly	24	CR 21% PR 46%	33 wks	1
Evans et al.[39]	Etoposide 100 mg/m² P.O. daily × 7 Carboplatin 150 mg/m² day 1	47	CR 23% PR 37%	46 wks	4
Cascinu et al.[40]	Teniposide 60 mg/m² daily × 5	22	CR 5% PR 18%	not reported	0
Westeel et al.[41]	PAVE	66	CR 44% PR 18%	LD 70 wks ED 46 wks	1

CR, complete response; PR, partial response; ORR, overall response rate; LD, limited disease; ED, extensive disease.
PAVE: cisplatin 30 mg/m² day 1, doxorubicin 40 mg/m² day 1, vincristine 1 mg/m² day 1, etoposide 100 mg/m² intravenously day 1 and orally days 3 and 5.

gle-agent teniposide in the elderly produced conflicting results. Borke et al.[35] treated 33 patients (27 over age 70) and reported 90% response, median survival exceeding 8 months, and virtually no toxicity. In contrast, Cerny et al.[36] reported only 48% response and an unacceptably high toxic death rate of five patients in the first cycle despite using the same dose and schedule of teniposide. This may have been due to the inclusion of seven patients of poor ECOG performance status 3. However, Cascinu et al.[40] also reported a low response rate of only 23% without toxic deaths.

Etoposide may be administered orally and is associated with only modest toxicity when used this way.[42] The Dublin group were among the first to use single-agent oral etoposide in the treatment of elderly SCLC patients.[32] Keane et al.[34] treated 63 elderly patients with etoposide, 200 mg orally daily for 5 days, and reported an overall response rate of 76% and median survival of 38 weeks. Using slightly different doses and schedules of etoposide, other investigators have also found similar response and survival rates as shown in Table 64.3.

These favorable results led to two randomized trials of single-agent oral etoposide in the United Kingdom, one by the Medical Research Council (MRC) Lung Cancer Working Party,[21] and the other by the London Lung Cancer Group.[20] The schemata and results of these two studies

are summarized in Table 64.4. The MRC compared oral etoposide, 50 mg twice daily for 10 days to two standard combinations of chemotherapy. The survival of the patients treated with single-agent etoposide was significantly shorter than that of patients treated with combination chemotherapy (130 versus 183 days, p = 0.03). Furthermore, quite unexpectedly, the etoposide group experienced more life-threatening side effects (19% versus 10%, p = 0.05). The London group compared etoposide, 100 mg twice daily for 5 days to alternating combination chemotherapy. It should be noted that this trial was limited to the extremely elderly over age 75, or to younger patients with extensive disease and poor performance status. Overall response rates (39% versus 61%, p = 0.01), median survival (146 days versus 189 dates), and one-year survival rates (6.5% versus 17%) all favored the combination chemotherapy arm. Although toxicity was greater in the combination arm, severe grade 3 and 4 toxicities were uncommon in either arm.

Although the aforementioned studies have shown that elderly patients of good performance status may tolerate combination chemotherapy, several investigators have attempted to modify current regimens to improve the therapeutic index for this patient population. The most common maneuver has been to substitute carboplatin for cisplatin and to combine it with either etoposide or teniposide. The results of three trials are shown in Table 64.3.[37–39] All inves-

TABLE 64.4. PROSPECTIVE-RANDOMIZED TRIALS FOR ELDERLY PATIENTS WITH SMALL CELL LUNG CANCER

Author	Drugs	Number of Patients	Response	Median Survival	Toxic Deaths
London Lung Cancer Group[20]	Etoposide 100 mg, BID × 5 days *versus*	75	ORR 33%	146 days 6.5% 1-yr	2
	CAV alternating with EP	80	ORR 46%	189 days 17% 1-yr	1
Medical Research Council[21]	Etoposide 50 mg P.O. BID × 10 days *versus*	171	ORR 61%	130 days 11% 1-yr	17
	EV or CAV[2]	168	ORR 73%	183 days 13% 1-yr	10

ORR, overall response rate; CAV[1], cyclophosphamide 600 mg/m^2, doxorubicin 50 mg/m^2, vincristine 2 mg; EP, etoposide 120 mg/m^2 IV day 1 and 100 mg P.O. twice daily days 2, 3; cisplatin 60 mg/m^2; EV, Etoposide 120 mg/m^2 IV day 1 and 240 mg/m^2 P.O. days 2, 3; vincristine 1.3 mg/m^2; CAV[2], cyclophosphamide 750 mg/m^2, doxorubicin 40 mg/m^2, vincristine 1.3 mg/m^2.

tigators reported response rates that ranged from 60%[39] to 89%,[37] and median survival that ranged from 33 weeks[38] to 40 weeks.[39] In general, the regimens were well tolerated, although Evans et al. reported that 4 of 40 patients suffered toxic deaths due to treatment.[39]

Westeel et al.[41] elected to use the standard chemotherapy agents cisplatin, doxorubicin, vincristine, and etoposide given in smaller doses in their PAVE regimen. For patients with limited-stage tumors, thoracic irradiation was administered concurrently with chemotherapy in cycle 2, but only cisplatin and etoposide were administered during that cycle. They reported a favorable overall response rate of 895, and median survival times of 70 and 46 weeks for limited and extensive stages, respectively.

RADIOTHERAPY

Radiation therapy plays several important roles in the treatment of patients with SCLC. Thoracic irradiation has been shown to improve response rates, and two large metaanalyses found significant improvements in two- and three-year survival rates in patients with limited-stage tumors.[19,43] All studies of prophylactic cranial irradiation reported a decreased risk of isolated cranial metastases for treated patients, and a metaanalysis has shown that this treatment is accompanied by a modest survival benefit in patients achieving a complete clinical response.[44] Radiation also has an important role in symptom palliation in patients who have relapsed or who are not candidates for aggressive treatment.

Given the essential role of thoracic irradiation in the treatment of limited-stage SCLC and the relatively modest side effects seen with conventional doses and fractionation schemes, many studies of combined modality chemotherapy and radiotherapy have included elderly patients. Despite the limitations of lack of uniformity in the dose and timing of radiation among studies, some conclusions may be drawn

from analyses of the small populations of elderly patients in these trials.

Retrospective Reviews

There have been only a few analyses of the efficacy and tolerability of thoracic radiation in older patients with SCLC. Quon et al.[45] undertook a retrospective review of two NCIC-CTG studies of combined modality treatment for limited-stage SCLC, BR.3 and BR.6. Of 608 patients, 520 were less than age 70 and 88 were older (254 younger and 46 older patients in BR.3, and 266 younger and 42 older patients in BR.6). In the BR.3 study, patients were randomized to receive thoracic irradiation with either 25 Gy in 10 fractions or 37.5 Gy in 15 fractions, after completing six courses of chemotherapy consisting of cyclophosphamide, doxorubicin, vincristine (CAV), and etoposide and cisplatin (EP) administered in either sequential or alternating fashion. In BR.6, all patients received CAV alternating with EP, and randomization was to early (with cycle 2) or late (with cycle 6) thoracic irradiation (40 Gy in 15 fractions), administered concurrently with EP. In BR.3, 179 patients (60%) participated in radiotherapy randomization (61% of the young, 52% of the elderly), and 176 actually received radiation. In BR.6, randomization occurred at study entry for all patients, and 282 patients (91.6%) received radiation (92% young, 88% elderly). More patients of both age groups randomized to late radiation did not receive treatment, but this did not differ by age. The authors could identify no tendency to reduce field size in the elderly, even at the higher radiation doses. Once radiation started, there was no significant difference between the age groups with respect to the proportion of patients who completed treatment, and no differences were seen in time to complete radiation therapy dose delivered, or incidence of acute and late radiation toxicity. Some trends were noted, with elderly patients being somewhat less likely to complete late radiation in the BR.6 study. Elderly patients also tended to have lower rates of complete response in the BR.3 trial, although this was not the case in the BR.6 trial in which chemotherapy and radiotherapy were delivered concurrently. Local control rates were similar for both age groups in both trials.

Pignon et al.[46] analyzed the effect of age on acute and late toxicity of curative thoracic irradiation given to 1,208 patients who participated in six randomized trials of lung and esophageal cancer conducted by the European Organization Research for the Treatment of Cancer (EORTC). The largest of these trials compared sequential to alternating radiochemotherapy in 389 patients with limited-stage SCLC.[46] Patients received either 50 Gy in 20 fractions after chemotherapy (sequential design), or four courses of 12.5 Gy in 5 fractions (alternating with chemotherapy). Of 389 patients, 95 (24%) were 65–70 years of age, and 29 (7%) were older than 70. This study contributed to the analysis of the effect of age on the pulmonary and esophageal toxicity, although results were reported collectively for all of the six EORTC trials. There was no difference in the distribution of either acute or late pneumonitis or esophagitis with increasing age. The analysis of other toxicities revealed no difference with age in the severity or incidence of nausea, weakness, or late side effects. The only difference related to age was significantly greater weight loss seen in older patients, which suggests that the clinical impact of esophagitis may have been greater in this population. This outcome however, was not accompanied by a greater decline in performance status in the elderly compared to the younger patients. The authors concluded that good general condition and performance status, rather than age alone, are the best predictors of tolerance of curative thoracic radiotherapy.

Other reports of radiation side effects in older patients treated for a variety of tumors document that radiation is well tolerated by patients 80 and older[47] and even patients over 90.[49] The high degree of tolerability of radiation in the elderly population with SCLC may be due to the relatively modest doses of radiation traditionally employed to treat this type of cancer. The standard dose is 40–50 Gy delivered in 15–25 fractions, although an increasing number of studies of dose escalation and hyperfractionation have been conducted,[50–52] which may affect future practice.

Despite the good overall tolerance of thoracic irradiation, one cannot ignore the physiological decline in organ function, including a decline in pulmonary reserve, that occurs with increasing age. Studies of radiologic changes of radiation pneumonitis have documented a lower tissue density of lung with increasing age,[53] which would lead to a greater dose transmission through the lung in an older patient. This response is even more pronounced in patients with emphysema or other lung disease. The impact of radiation damage is also clinically more apparent in patients whose lung reserve is reduced due to chronic obstructive pulmonary emphysema (COPD) or other factors. The radiation portals

for SCLC that traditionally include the initial tumor volume (prior to any treatment), although whether or not uninvolved nodes need to be included is controversial. If a large volume needs to be irradiated, then the potential for radiation toxicity is greater. For this reason, some investigators have suggested that there might be merit in giving a higher radiation dose to a smaller volume by treating areas of residual disease only.[54] However, the review by Quon et al.[45] did not suggest that practicing radiation oncologists felt that it was necessary to reduce field size in the elderly, and there was no evidence of increased pulmonary toxicity in the older patients, even when radiation was administered concurrently with chemotherapy.

Side effects may also be influenced by the type of chemotherapy used. This is especially true when doxorubicin is employed because the incidence of esophagitis increases greatly when it is administered concurrently or soon after radiation. In the NCIC-CTG trials reviewed by Quon et al,[45] all patients received chemotherapy with a doxorubicin-containing regimen, and no differences in the rates of esophagitis were seen.

Prospective Trials of Combined Modality Treatment for the in Elderly

Several studies described in the chemotherapy section of this chapter included radiation; however, these studies, although they included elderly patients, were not designed specifically for this population. Recently, though, some investigators have undertaken combined modality therapy trials of abbreviated chemotherapy and radiation for elderly patients, and their results are summarized in Table 64.5.[41,55,56]

Westeel et al.[41] treated 66 elderly patients with PAVE chemotherapy given every 3 weeks for five cycles. The 25 patients with limited-stage tumors also received concurrent thoracic irradiation (dose and schedule was variable) administered with etoposide and cisplatin in cycle 2. The overall response rate for the limited patients was 92%, and 76% achieved complete remission. Their median survival was 70 weeks, and 25% remained alive at 5 years. There were no toxic deaths in this group, although one patient with extensive disease died from neutropenic sepsis, and the febrile neutropenia rate for patients treated with combined modality therapy was 18%.

Jeremic et al.[55] administered accelerated hyperfractioned radiotherapy, giving 1.5 Gy twice a day to a total dose of 45 Gy over 3 weeks administered concurrently with carboplatin intravenously days 1 and 29, and oral etoposide days 1–21 and 29–49. No further chemotherapy was given. They treated 77 patients aged 70–77 years. All patients had limited-stage disease, but 12 patients had a Karnofsky performance status of only 60% or 70%, and 18 patients had weight loss of more than 5% of body weight. The patients tolerated treatment remarkably well with only 2.8% grade 3 esophagitis, 8.3% grade 3 leukopenia, and 4.2%

TABLE 64.5. PROSPECTIVE TRIALS OF COMBINED MODALITY THERAPY FOR ELDERLY PATIENTS WITH LIMITED SMALL CELL LUNG CANCER

Author	Treatment	Number of Patients	Response	Median Survival	Toxic Deaths
Westeel et al.[41]	PAVE × 5	25	ORR 92% CR 76%	70 weeks 25% 5-yr	0
Murray et al.[56]	Thoracic XRT (Variable doses and fractionation) CAV × 1	55	ORR 89% CR 51%	12.5 months 28% 2-yr 18% 5-yr	3
Jeremic et al.[55]	EP × 1 Thoracic XRT 20–30 Gy with EP EC × 2	75	ORR 75% CR 57%	15 months 32% 2-yr 13% 5-yr	0
	Accelerated hyperfractionated XRT 1.5 Gy BID × 15 days starting day 1				

ORR, overall response rate; CR, complete response; CAV, cyclophosphamide 1,000 mg/m^2, doxorubicin 50 mg/m^2, vincristine 2 mg;
EP, etoposide 100 mg/m^2 IV days 1–3, cisplatin 25 mg/m^2 IV days 1–3;
EC, etoposide 50 mg/m^2 P.O. days 1–21 and 29–49 and carboplatin 400 mg/m^2 IV days 1 and 29;
PAVE, cisplatin 30 mg/m^2 day 1, doxorubicin 40 mg/m^2 day 1, vincristine 1 mg/m^2 day 1, etoposide 100 mg/m^2 intravenously day 1 and orally days 3 and 5.

grade 3 infection. Despite the abbreviated chemotherapy treatment, the overall response rate was 75%, and survival rates were promising (74% 1-year, 32% 2-year, 19% 3-year).

In a trial of similar design, Murray et al.[55] gave only two cycles of chemotherapy (CAV followed by EP) and radiation consisting of either 20 Gy in 5 fractions or 30 Gy in 10 fractions concurrently with EP to the frail elderly (more than 70 years) as well as to younger patients who had significant comorbidity or who refused standard chemotherapy. Although 14 of the 55 patients were less than 70 years of age, the remainder were elderly, with 22 older than 75, and four were above age 80. Three patients died of treatment-related complications, although two of these deaths were acute cardiac events that may have had other causes in this elderly or infirm patient cohort. Other toxicities were no different than expected. The overall response rate was 89%, and median survival was 12.5 months with 28% and 18% of patients alive at 2 and 5 years, respectively.

The results of these phase II studies are compelling, and they raise interesting questions for the treatment of both elderly and younger patients. As shown from the analyses in the chemotherapy section, elderly patients complete fewer cycles of chemotherapy than younger patients even when participating in clinical research protocols. However, their overall outcome does not seem to be significantly worse because of this regimen. The results of the Murray and Jeremic pilot studies suggest that when combined with early concurrent thoracic irradiation, chemotherapy may be further abbreviated to as few as two cycles without compromising efficacy. This approach deserves further study in a randomized clinical trial of elderly or infirm patients.

Radiation Alone

If a patient is not only elderly but also frail and not suitable or interested in standard chemotherapy or combined modality treatment, radiation alone may be considered with the intent of improving symptoms and palliating the disease. Given the radiosensitive nature of SCLC, symptom improvement is likely, especially in patients with thoracic symptoms, painful bone lesion, or symptomatic soft tissue, nodal, or brain metastases.

In this clinical setting, shorter fractionation courses are appropriate because symptom improvement does not necessarily depend on complete eradication of the local tumor. This is especially true for patients with extensive-stage disease, who may require and benefit from palliative radiotherapy to several symptomatic disease sites.

Although the intent of such treatment is largely palliative, some patients with localized thoracic disease may achieve prolonged symptom-free survival with radiation alone. In the Toronto Hospital review,[7] 20 of 123 patients over the age of 70 received radiation only. Their median survival was 7.8 months, which was superior to the 1.1 month survival of the 25 patients who had no treatment, and 3.9 month survival of the 27 patients who had fewer than three courses of chemotherapy without radiation. This is shown graphically in Figure 64.4.

This degree of potential benefit from radiation alone, especially given its high degree of tolerance by most elderly patients, emphasizes the need for informing patients of this therapeutic option should they decline to have chemotherapy. However, that is not to say that it should be recommended as an equal alternative to all elderly patients. Yellen

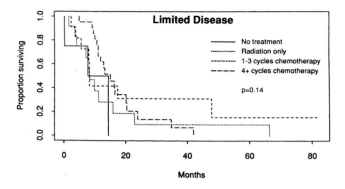

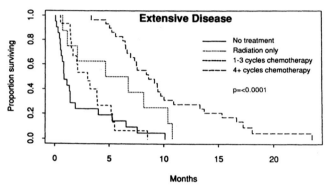

FIGURE 64.4. A comparison of survival by treatment modality for patients with limited (*above*) or extensive disease (*below*). (From Shepherd FA, Amdemichael E, Evans WK, et al. Treatment of small cell lung cancer in the elderly. *J Am Geriatr Soc* 1994;42: 64, with permission.)

et al.[57] in a survey of cancer patients given hypothetical vignettes of different disease stage and treatment toxicity showed that older patients are as likely as younger ones to accept both curative and palliative chemotherapy. They were, however, less willing to accept higher degrees of treatment toxicity for a given treatment benefit. Thus all treatment options need to be presented to elderly patients and discussed in the framework of their values and goals of therapy to determine the optimal treatment plan for each patient.

SUMMARY

To summarize, it appears that elderly patients can derive benefit from treatment for SCLC that is similar to that achieved by younger patients. However, this can only be stated with a word of caution because of the limitations of the studies of elderly patients performed to date. To tolerate therapy, older patients must be of good performance status, and this should be the major determinant in reaching a decision to treat and how to treat. Firm recommendations cannot be made for the extremely elderly population of 75

years or more, and further studies of this subgroup and all elderly patients must be encouraged in the future.

REFERENCES

1. Schottenfeld D. Epidemiology of lung cancer. In: Pass HI, Mitchell JB, Johnson DH, et al. eds. *Lung cancer: principles and practice*. Philadelphia: Lippincott-Raven, 1996:305.
2. Grulich AE, Swerdlow AJ, dos Santos Silva I, et al. Is the apparent rise in cancer mortality in the elderly real? Analysis of changes in certification and coding of cause of death in England and Wales 1970–1990. *Int J Cancer* 1995;63:164.
3. Levi F, La Veccia C, Luccini F, et al. World-wide trends in cancer mortality in the elderly, 1955–1992. *Eur J Cancer* 1996;32A: 569.
4. O'Rourke MA, Crawford J. Lung cancer in the elderly. *Clin Geriatr Med* 1987;3:595.
5. Di Maria LC, Cohen HJ. Characteristics of lung cancer in elderly patients. *J Gerentol* 1965;42:540.
6. Teeter SM, Holmes SF, McFarlane MJ. Lung carcinoma in the elderly population. Influence of histology on the inverse relationship of stage to age. *Cancer* 1987;60:1331.
7. Shepherd FA, Amdemichael E, Evans WK, et al. Treatment of small cell lung cancer in the elderly. *J Am Geriatr Soc* 1994;42: 64.
8. Goodwin JS, Hunt WG, Humble CG, et al. Cancer treatment protocols. Who gets chosen? *Arch Int Med* 1998;148:2258.
9. Dajczman E, Fu LY, Small D, et al. Treatment of small cell lung carcinoma in the elderly. *Cancer* 1996;77:2032.
10. de Rijke JM, Schouten LJ, Schouten HC, et al. Age-specific differences in the diagnostics and treatment of cancer patients aged 50 years and older in the province of Limburg, the Netherlands. *Ann Oncol* 1996;7:677.
11. Festen J. Lung cancer in the elderly. *Eur J Cancer* 1991;27:1544.
12. Nerenz DR, Love RR, Leventhal H, et al. Psychological consequences of cancer chemotherapy for elderly patients. *Health Serv Rev* 1986;20:961.
13. Ginsburg ML, Quirt C, Ginsburg AD, et al. Psychiatric illness and psychosocial concerns of patients with newly diagnosed lung cancer. *Can Med Assoc J* 1995;152:701.
14. Kennedy BJ. Needed: clinical trials for older patients. *J Clin Oncol* 1991;9:718.
15. Albain K, Crowley J, LeBlanc M, et al. Determinants of improved outcome in small-cell lung cancer: an analysis of the 2580-patient Southwest Oncology Group data base. *J Clin Oncol* 1990;8:1563.
16. Sagman U, Maki E, Evans WK, et al. Small-cell carcinoma of the lung: derivation of a prognostic staging system. *J Clin Oncol* 1991;9:1639.
17. Spiegelman D, Maurer H, Ware JH, et al. Prognostic factors in small-cell carcinoma of the lung. *J Clin Oncol* 1989;7:344.
18. Siu L, Shepherd FA, Murray N, et al. Influence of age on the treatment of limited-stage small-cell lung cancer. *J Clin Oncol* 1996;14:821.
19. Pignon J-P, Arriagada R, Ihde D, et al. A meta-analysis of thoracic radiotherapy for small-cell lung cancer. *N Engl J Med* 1992;327: 1618.
20. Harper P, Underhill C, Ruiz de Elvira MC, et al. A randomized study of oral etoposide versus combination chemotherapy in poor prognosis small cell lung cancer. *Proc Am Soc Clin Oncol* 1996; 15:27(abst).
21. Medical Research Council Lung Cancer Working Party. Comparison of oral etoposide and standard intravenous multi-drug chemotherapy for small cell lung cancer: a stopped multicentre trial. *Lancet* 1996;348:563.

22. Clamon GH, Audeh MW, Pinnick S. Small cell lung carcinoma in the elderly. *J Amer Geriatr Soc* 1982;30:299.
23. Poplin E, Thompson B, Whitacre M, et al. Small cell carcinoma of the lung: influence of age on treatment outcome. *Cancer Treat Rep* 1987;71:291.
24. Kelly P, O'Brien AAJ, Daly P, et al. Small-cell lung cancer in elderly patients: the case for chemotherapy. *Age and Aging* 1991; 20:19.
25. Findlay MPN, Griffin A-M, Raghaven D, et al. Retrospective review of chemotherapy for small cell lung cancer in the elderly: does the end justify the means? *Eur J Cancer* 1991;27: 1597.
26. Nou E. Full chemotherapy in elderly patients with small cell bronchial carcinoma. *Acta Oncol* 1996;35:399.
27. Tebbutt NC, Snyder RD, Burns WI. An analysis of the outcome of treatment of small cell lung cancer in the elderly. *Aus NZ J Med* 1997;27:160.
28. Smit EF, Postmus PE, Sleijfer DTH. Small cell lung cancer in the elderly. Factors influencing the results of chemotherapy: a review. *Lung Cancer* 1989;5:82.
29. Begg CB, Chohe JL, Ellerton J. Are the elderly predisposed to toxicity from cancer chemotherapy? An investigation using data from the Eastern Cooperative Oncology Group. *Cancer Clin Trials* 1980;3:369.
30. Begg CB, Carbone PP. Clinical trials and drug toxicity in the elderly. The experience of the Eastern Cooperative Oncology Group. *Cancer* 1983;52:1986.
31. Giovanazzi-Bannon S, Rademaker A, Lai G, et al. Treatment tolerance of elderly cancer patients entered onto phase II clinical trials: an Illinois Cancer Center study. *J Clin Oncol* 1994;12: 2447.
32. Smit EF, Carney DN, Harford P. A phase II study of oral etoposide in elderly patients with small cell lung cancer. *Thorax* 1989; 44:631.
33. Gatzemeier U, Neuhauss R, Heckmayr M. Single agent oral etoposide in advanced non-small cell lung cancer, and in elderly patients with small cell lung cancer. *Lung Cancer* 1991;7(suppl): 102(abst).
34. Keane M, Carney DM. Treatment for elderly patients with small cell lung cancer. *Lung Cancer* 1993;9(suppl 1):S91.
35. Bork E, Hansen M, Dombernowsky P, et al. Teniposide (VM-26), an overlooked highly active agent in small cell lung cancer. Results of a phase II trial in untreated patients. *J Clin Oncol* 1986;4:524.
36. Cerny T, Pedrazzini A, Joss RA, et al. Unexpected high toxicity in a phase II study of teniposide (VM-26) in elderly patients with unresected small cell lung cancer. *Eur J Cancer Clin Oncol* 1988;24:1791.
37. Byrne A, Carney D. Small cell lung cancer in the elderly. *Semin Oncol* 1994;3(suppl 6):43.
38. Michel G, Leyvraz S, Bauer J, et al. Weekly carboplatin and VM-26 for elderly patients with small cell lung cancer. *Ann Oncol* 1994;5:369.
39. Evans WK, Radwi A, Tomiak E, et al. Oral etoposide and carboplatin. Effective therapy for elderly patients with small cell lung cancer. *Am J Clin Oncol* 1995;18:149.
40. Cascinu S, Del Ferro E, Ligi M, et al. The clinical impact of teniposide in the treatment of elderly patients with small cell lung cancer. *Am J Clin Oncol* 1997;10:477.
41. Westeel V, Murray N, Gelmon K, et al. New combination of the old drugs for elderly patients with small-cell lung cancer: a

42. phase II study of the PAVE regimen. *J Clin Oncol* 1998;16: 1940.
43. Carney D, Grogan L, Smit EF. Single-agent oral etoposide for elderly small cell lung cancer patients. *Semin Oncol* 1990; 17(suppl 2):29.
44. Warde P, Payne D. Does thoracic irradiation improve survival and local control in limited-stage small-cell carcinoma of the lung? A meta-analysis *J Clin Oncol* 1992;10:890.
45. Arriagada R, Auperin A, Pignon JP, et al. Prophylactic cranial irradiation overview (PCIO) in patients with small cell lung cancer (SCLC) in complete remission (CR). *Proc Am Soc Clin Oncol* 1998;17:457a.
46. Quon H, Shepherd FA, Payne DG, et al. The influence of age on the delivery, tolerance and efficacy of thoracic irradiation in the combined modality treatment of limited stage small cell lung cancer. *Int J Radiat Oncol Biol Phys* 1999;43:39.
47. Pignon T, Gregor A, Koning CS, et al. Age has no impact on acute and late toxicity of curative thoracic radiotherapy. *Radiother Oncol* 1998;46:239.
48. Gregor A, Drings P, Schuster L, et al. Acute toxicity of alternating schedule of chemotherapy and irradiation in limited small-cell lung cancer in a pilot study (08877) of the EORTC Lung Cancer Cooperative Group. *Ann Oncol* 1995;6:403.
49. Zachariah B, Balducci L, Venkattaramanbalaji GV, et al. Radiotherapy for cancer patients aged 80 and older: a study of effectiveness and side effects. *Int J Radiat Oncol Biol Phys* 1997;39:1125.
50. Oguchi M, Ikeda H, Watanabe T, et al. Experience of 23 patients >90 years of age treated with radiation therapy. *Int J Radiat Oncol Biol Phys* 1998;41:407.
51. Choi NC, Hemdon J, Rosenman J, et al. Phase I study to determine the maximum tolerated dose (MTD) of radiation in standard daily (QD) and accelerated twice daily (bid) radiation schedules with concurrent chemotherapy (CT) for limited stage small cell lung cancer: CALGB 8837. *Proc Am Soc Clin Oncol* 1995; 14:363.
52. Johnson DH, Kim K, Sause W, et al. for the Eastern Cooperative Oncology Group. Cisplatin (P) & Etoposide (E) + thoracic radiotherapy (TRT) administered once or twice daily (bid) in limited stage (LS) small cell lung cancer (SCLC): final report of intergroup trial 0096. *Proc Am Soc Clin Oncol* 1996;15:374.
53. Takada M, Fukuoka M, Furuse K, et al. for the JCOG-Lung Cancer Study Group. Phase III study of concurrent versus sequential thoracic radiotherapy (TRT) in combination with cisplatin (C) and etoposide (E) for limited-stage (LS) small cell lung cancer (SCLC): preliminary results of the Japan Clinical Oncology Group (JCOG). *Proc Am Soc Clin Oncol* 1996;15: 372.
54. Mah K, Keane TJ, Van dyk J, et al. Quantitative effect of combined chemotherapy and fractionated radiotherapy on the incidence of radiation-induced lung damage: a prospective clinical study. *Int J Radiat Oncol Biol Phys* 1994;28:563.
55. Lichter AS, Turrisi AT III. Small cell lung cancer: the influence of dose and treatment volume on outcome. *Sem Rad Onc* 1995; 5:44.
56. Jeremic B, Shibamoto Y, Acimovic L, et al. Carboplatin, etoposide, accelerated hyperfractionated radiotherapy for elderly patients with limited small cell lung cancer. A phase II study. *Cancer* 1998;82:836.
57. Murray N, Grafton C, Shah A, et al. Abbreviated treatment for elderly, infirm or non-compliant paatients with limited small cell lung cancer. *J Clin Oncol* 1998;16:3323.
58. Yellen SB, Cella DF, Leslie WT. Age and clinical decision making in oncology patients. *J Natl Cancer Inst* 1994;86:1766.

65

COST EFFECTIVENESS AND LUNG CANCER

CRAIG C. EARLE
DOUGLAS COYLE
WILLIAM K. EVANS

There have been many recent advances in lung cancer treatment, particularly for patients with locally advanced or metastatic tumors; however, lung cancer is a common disease, and these interventions can be costly. Health care systems around the world are feeling economic pressures from multiple sources. Western countries have an aging population that is developing age-related infirmities such as cancer and heart disease. At the same time, new technologies have increased the complexity and expense of medical care. Patients are also generally more informed about treatment options and often demand access to the latest interventions. As a result, the health economic literature is growing rapidly. In this chapter, we present an overview of the methodological components of an economic analysis, review the current literature of economic studies in lung cancer, and discuss how these result relate to policy issues.

METHODOLOGICAL COMPONENTS OF AN ECONOMIC STUDY

Research Question

The first step in doing an economic study is to clearly identify the research question. The essential elements of the question are (a) the alternatives being compared, (b) the perspective of the analysis, and (c) the analytic technique. The analytic technique is largely determined by the outcome being measured. From an assessment of these components, readers should quickly be able to determine whether a particular study is relevant to their practice.

Treatment Alternatives

A full economic evaluation is a systematic comparison of at least two alternative healthcare strategies. The reader should be able to easily identify the alternatives being compared and find them fully described; however, there can be different comparators in different situations. If appropriate, a "do nothing" alternative should be included to determine whether there should be any intervention at all for the con-

dition. In addition, guidelines have proposed that the cheapest[1] and the most commonly used options[2] should be considered. The reader must decide whether any appropriate alternative has been excluded.

Perspective

The perspective of an analysis affects the range of costs and benefits considered, and ultimately the conclusions of the evaluation. Ideally, a full economic evaluation should include the costs and benefits to all sectors of society affected by the interventions. However, evaluations often are carried out from one relevant perspective, such as that of the providers or purchasers of health care. The most economic management strategy from the perspective of a hospital may not be the same as that from the perspective of the entire healthcare system. For example, a program of early discharge after a lung resection might save a hospital money, but increased costs for home care services may offset these savings. On the other hand, the perspective of healthcare institutions or the healthcare system may ignore important costs to social service agencies or to family members who may lose wages staying home to provide care.[3] One solution to this problem is to take a broader perspective and to present the costs and benefits broken down into the component parts of that broader perspective.[4] In this way, various stakeholders can examine the results from their own perspective.

Analytic Technique

There are four types of commonly used economic evaluations (Table 65.1). Each involves a comparison of both the costs and consequences of alternative interventions. The main differences among them are the methods used to measure the consequences.

Cost-Minimization Analysis

Also called a "cost-analysis," cost-minimization analysis is the simplest form of economic evaluation. This type of study assumes that the outcomes or effectiveness of the in-

TABLE 65.1. TYPES OF ECONOMIC ANALYSES

Cost-minimization analysis	Compares strategies of equal effectiveness to determine which is least expensive.
Cost-effectiveness analysis	Compares ratios of the incremental cost over the incremental effectiveness of alternative strategies.
Cost-utility analysis	Compares ratios of the incremental cost over the incremental utility. The utility is a measure of the value attributed to a health state, usually measured in quality-adjusted life-years (QALY).
Cost-benefit analysis	Assigns monetary value to the health benefits of an intervention. If the cost/benefit ratio is <1, then the intervention is attractive.

terventions are equal. Resource utilization is the only significant difference between the options. The direct costs associated with each intervention are compared, and the least costly strategy is the preferred choice. No assessment of the consequences of treatment is required. Although some examples in the oncology literature address staging procedures,[5,6] radiotherapy techniques,[7–9] and systemic therapy,[10] cost-minimization studies are not common because cancer treatments rarely produce equivalent survival or quality of life.

Cost-Effectiveness Analysis

If the interventions being assessed are not of equal effectiveness, thus a more sophisticated analysis is required. Cost-effectiveness analysis includes a comparison of outcomes as well as costs. In this form of analysis, the effectiveness of alternatives is measured in natural units, such as life-years gained, cases successfully treated, or cases averted. These outcomes are then related to the direct costs of the procedure by calculating ratios of cost per unit of effectiveness, such as cost per life-year gained.

Cost-effectiveness analysis has the advantage of being easily understandable. As a result, it is the most common approach to economic evaluation in healthcare.[11] However, only one measure of effectiveness can be related to the cost of the interventions. A cost per life-year gained looks only at survival, but not at toxicity, inconvenience, or effects on quality of life, which are also important considerations in cancer treatment. For example, surgery versus radiation for the primary treatment of a specific cancer can be compared in terms of their costs per life-year gained, but this comparison may lead to an invalid conclusion if the treatments effects on quality of life are different. Therefore, cost-effectiveness analysis can help choose between similar treatments for a specific disease but not for choices across dissimilar treatments and conditions.

Cost-Utility Analysis

A cost-utility analysis is similar to a cost-effectiveness analysis. The main difference is that cost utility combines mortal-

ity and morbidity data into a single multidimensional measure, usually a quality-adjusted life-year (QALY).[12] The QALY is a measure of the *quantity* of life gained by a treatment, weighted by the *quality* of that life. This measure is relevant in oncology because many anticancer treatments are inconvenient and have substantial toxicities that impair quality of life. Because the QALY is not disease-specific, it allows comparison of the relative efficiency of healthcare interventions for different conditions.

Quality of life is approximated by a *utility*, which is a measure of preference for a given health state rated on a scale where 0 equals death and 1 equals perfect health. Theoretically, a utility is most accurately determined using a "standard gamble" exercise, where a subject in a particular health state finds the balance between a chance of returning to perfect health and a risk of possibly dying in the process. Other techniques such as time trade off and direct rating on visual analogue scales have also been employed.[13] Alternatively, instruments such as the Health Utilities Index[14] and the EuroQoL[15] have been administered alongside standard gamble exercises in order to relate their scores to utilities; however, most quality-of-life instruments have not undergone such testing. An approach often used to integrate quality and quantity of life calculates the quality-adjusted time with and without symptoms or toxicity (Q-TWiST).[16] It is particularly useful when looking at interventions that have health effects persisting beyond the duration of treatment (e.g., adjuvant chemotherapy).

Controversy exists regarding whether utilities should be derived from patients, their families, healthcare workers, or lay societal "jurors" given detailed scenarios describing the health state. Recent guidelines favor the latter approach as being most consistent with a societal perspective.[17] However, there is concern that people without relevant disease experience may not properly understand the health (disease) state. Any of these approaches to defining utilities is defensible, as long as it is stated clearly in the methods section of the publication.

Cost-Benefit Analysis

Cost-benefit analysis takes cost-utility analysis one step further. It tries to determine whether the benefits of an intervention outweigh its cost. As a result, cost-benefit analysis is in theory the gold standard of the different forms of economic evaluation. The quality-adjusted life-years in the denominator are valued in monetary terms to arrive at the absolute benefit of the intervention. An intervention is "cost-beneficial" if the benefits (measured in currency) are greater than the costs. Because these analyses always produce a monetary outcome, it is relatively easy to compare different potential uses of resources. However, placing a monetary value on the often intangible outcomes of health care, in particular the value of a life, is problematic. As a result, true cost-benefit analyses are rare.

Each of these analytic techniques has its place. Cost-utility analysis is ideal for comparing toxic treatment options, whereas a cost-effectiveness analysis may be adequate when deciding between two diagnostic strategies.

Assessing Costs

Identification and Assessment of Costs and Benefits

Depending on the perspective taken, the resource costs (inputs) in an economic analysis can include:

- *Direct treatment costs:* the resources used by the health sector to provide treatment (e.g., healthcare provider time, drugs, equipment, diagnostic tests, overhead).
- *Direct nontreatment costs:* the resources used by patients and family to gain access to and participate in treatment, such as travel, parking, and accommodations near a cancer treatment center. These costs are often measured by having patients complete diaries of their out-of-pocket expenses.
- *Indirect costs:* costs such as lost work time for the patient or caregiver, or the time of volunteers assisting with treatment. In accounting practice, the term "indirect cost" refers to overhead, but in health economics, overhead is considered a direct cost.
- *Intangible costs:* the costs of anxiety, uncertainty, or pain caused by the treatment itself. These costs have proved difficult to measure. Techniques, such as "willingness to pay" have been developed, but can be affected by each subject's own economic circumstance.

The choice of *time horizon* is important to ensure that the analysis has considered all relevant resources. If a new treatment intervention has an impact on the natural history of a disease, it could affect "downstream" costs. For example, when analyzing the cost of treating lung cancer, upfront costs include the costs of physician visits, diagnostic tests and procedures, hospitalization, as well as drugs and dispensing fees. Downstream costs include those for treatment of long-term complications and terminal care. One of these downstream costs, hospitalization for terminal care, has been found in the Canadian health care system to be the largest single component of management over the entire course of illness.[18] Interventions that affect terminal care can have large impacts on the lifetime costs of the disease[19,20] that might be missed if the time horizon only included the active phase of disease treatment.

If satisfied that all relevant resources have been considered, then it is important to assess whether they have been quantified accurately and valued credibly. It is important to consider whether the analysis is based on costs or charges. Charges for health care are influenced by market forces, government regulations, and taxation laws[21] and often bear little resemblance to actual incremental resource costs.[22] Medicare providers are required to provide cost-to-charge ratios that can be used to estimate costs; however, the accuracy of these ratios is undetermined.

Another issue is whether resource consumption data have been collected prospectively or retrospectively. Prospectively collected data, such as those gathered as part of a clinical trial, are more likely to be complete. This process also allows for the timely availability of economic data to help decision-makers after an important clinical result is found; however, prospective data is more expensive to collect. Furthermore, care in clinical trials is often more resource intensive than routine practice. For example, trials usually take place in expensive tertiary care teaching hospital settings and involve more frequent monitoring with blood tests and imaging studies. As a result, retrospective data or prospective data collected outside a clinical trial can each be effectively used in many circumstances.

It is often necessary to determine costs in several steps and to use a combination of empirical data and modeling in the analysis. Resource consumption data such as hospital days could first be gathered from a clinical trial. Then, this data could be adjusted to reflect anticipated usual care. For example, the frequency of imaging studies might be greater in a study situation than in routine practice. Lastly, the costs can be allocated to the resources consumed to calculate the cost of delivering the intervention. By separating resource consumption from cost, local variations in costs or charges can be assessed.

Discounting

Costs and benefits that occur in the future should be adjusted, or discounted, to their present value because of "time preference." We generally prefer to incur benefits sooner rather than later and costs later rather than sooner. Thus future costs and benefits have less weight than current costs and benefits, and are usually accounted for by multiplying them by a constant discount rate with the formula:

$$\frac{1}{(1 + r)^n}$$

where r is the discount rate, and n is the number of years.[23] Such adjustment favors therapeutic procedures that provide immediate benefit, while rendering preventive and screening programs, which require immediate expenditure for future benefits, less attractive.

There is a lack of consensus over what the appropriate discount rate should be. Recent American guidelines suggest 3%,[12] whereas Canadian guidelines have recommended 5%[24] and British recommendations have been 6%.[25] The choice of discount rate can seriously affect the results of evaluations[26] and should be subject to sensitivity analysis. Also of debate is whether benefits and costs should be discounted at the same rate because empirical studies have demonstrated that people do not have the same preferences for future health benefits as for future costs.[27-30]

Assessing Effectiveness

Healthcare benefits (outputs) can be measured as:

- *Direct benefits:* monetary savings in treatment-related resource consumption
- *Indirect benefits:* from increased productivity
- *Intangible benefits:* such as prolonged survival, or alleviation of pain and suffering associated with health improvements

As described previously, the type of study (cost-effectiveness, cost-utility, etc.) determines the type of benefit considered.

Large, randomized controlled trials or metaanalyses provide good measures of clinical effectiveness; however, extrapolation of economic and clinical data to routine practice is not always straightforward. Controlled clinical trials usually test the *efficacy* of a procedure under strictly defined "ideal world" conditions. Differences in the demographic characteristics of the population, variations in clinical practice, and availability of resources may mean that the procedure is less *effective* in routine clinical management.[31] For example, we might expect an elderly patient with multiple comorbidities to have a different experience with chemotherapy for advanced lung cancer than the highly selected patients studied in a clinical trial. Clinicians must decide whether patients are likely to derive the same benefits as the patients included in the study.

Similarly, toxicity of therapy may differ between the experimental and normal practice settings. The complication rate reported in a trial of complex therapy given to highly selected patients in a tertiary care setting might not be the same as that seen when the treatment is moved into general practice. As a result of the costs associated with these complications, the treatment might prove to be more expensive than predicted by the economic model.

When survival is the outcome of interest, it is important to accurately quantify the benefit. Because survival distributions are skewed, the median survival is most often reported in cancer trials; however, this measure may disregard important information when trying to determine the average benefit a patient can expect from a therapy. For example, an intervention that results in some cures creates a long tail on the survival curve that contributes to the number of life-years gained. Such an intervention can be highly cost-effective, even if there is little or no increase in the median survival time (Figure 65.1). As a result, economic evaluations should use the area between two survival curves to determine the average benefit from treatment.

Assessing cost-effectiveness

The cost-effectiveness ratio (CE) is the *incremental* cost of an intervention divided by its *incremental* benefits, as given by the formula:

$$CE = \frac{C_1 - C_2}{E_1 - E_2} \quad \frac{(\$)}{(\text{e.g., time})}$$

where C represents the cost of each intervention and E represents their effectiveness.

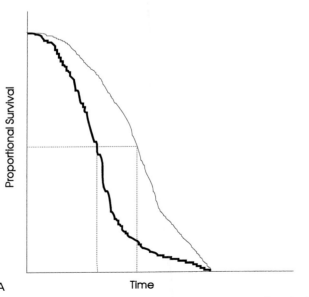
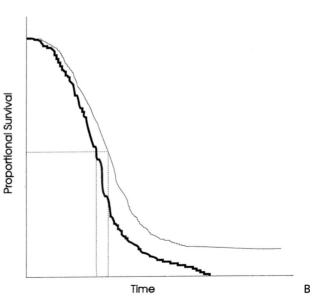

FIGURE 65.1. The effect of the shape of survival curves on life years gained from an intervention. **A:** This treatment results in a relatively large increase in medium survival time, but there are no cures. **B:** This treatment causes a small increase in median survival time; however, because some patients are cured, there is a plateau on the tail of the curve that may eventually produce a larger increase in the area between the two.

TABLE 65.2. AN EXAMPLE OF A LEAGUE TABLE

Medical Intervention	Cost Per Life-Year Gained*
Liver transplantation	251,000
Screening mammography, <50 years old	245,000
Zidovudine for HIV infection	87,000
Renal dialysis, in-center benefit, men	53,000
Screening mammography, >50 years old	37,000
Smoking cessation counselling, men	1,400

* 1994 U.S. dollars
From Desch CE, Hillner BE, Smith TJ. Economic considerations in the care of lung cancer patients. *Curr Opin Oncol* 1996;8:126, with permission.

Many people use thresholds to decide whether an intervention is cost-effective. Canadian authors have proposed that interventions costing less than $20,000 per QALY be considered cost-effective.[32] Americans tend to set the threshold at approximately $50,000 per QALY.[21] However, these cutoff points are arbitrary.

Another type of decision rule is a "league table." Economic evaluations assume that resources are limited and have alternative uses if not applied to the intervention in question. Policymakers must make decisions that will maximize health by getting the highest value for the resources consumed. Their decisions often reflect a utilitarian philosophy of doing the greatest good for the greatest number of people. In order to achieve this goal, a technology must be assessed for its efficiency relative to all other potential uses of the same resources. Cost-effectiveness league tables such as Table 65.2 rank interventions by cost per life-year or cost per QALY gained.

There are two major attractions to league tables: (a) they place results in the context of the cost-effectiveness of other technologies, and (b) they offer an easy mechanism to inform or justify resource allocation decisions. Resources can then be spent on the most cost-effective programs until the resources are exhausted. Numerous examples of league tables have been published across specialties,[33–35] and in oncology in particular.[36]

There are many methodological difficulties in creating league tables, necessitating caution when using them for resource allocation.[37] One major problem is that they often group studies that were undertaken at different points in time. Cost-effectiveness figures can be adjusted to a base year, but this method requires assumptions of constancy of relative costs, resource use, disease management, and treatment efficacy over time.

There may also be differences in study methodology, including the choice of treatment comparisons, the length of follow-up of patients, the quality-of-life or utility instrument adopted, the assumptions made, and the range and sources of costs included.[37] Such differences may affect the ranking of various technologies within a league table, leading to erroneous conclusions.

Both the threshold and league table approaches assume that QALYs have the same value in all situations; however, empirical evidence tells us otherwise. Society generally adheres to the "rule of rescue": we value interventions that actually save a patient from dying from a disease more than one that may make many patients live a little longer. We are also more willing to pay for an intervention that saves an identifiable life, such as an individual who requires a heart transplant, than one for which a "statistical" life may be saved, as in preventive programs.

Because of these problems, neither league tables nor thresholds should be seen as providing accurate answers to difficult resource allocation decision; rather, they should be seen only as an aid to inform decision-makers.

Deciding Whether to Believe the Results

Knowledge of the key methodological principles that well-conducted studies should follow[23,38,39] is important in order to avoid inappropriately applying the results of a poor study or using data that are not applicable in a certain setting. Because of this need, American guidelines have recently been published for reporting economic studies,[17] and useful strategies have been proposed for critically appraising economic analyses.[40,41] Table 65.3 summarizes some important considerations when appraising economic studies.

Sensitivity Analysis

Sensitivity analyses assess the effect of varying the estimates of resource use (such as the number of treatments of a new drug, the number of hospital days for treatment administra-

TABLE 65.3. KEY CONSIDERATIONS IN THE EVALUATION OF ECONOMIC STUDIES

1. The study question, perspective, and design must be clearly stated. Are they relevant and appropriate?
2. The study should involve a comparison of at least two alternative interventions. Are they the most relevant ones? The "do nothing," the least costly, and the most used options should be considered. Are any other important alternatives missing?
3. All relevant costs and benefits of the alternatives should be identified. Were they measured accurately and valued credibly? Are they likely to be transferable to your setting?
4. Future costs and benefits should be discounted. Is the discount rate appropriate?
5. The setting and type of patients analyzed should be clear to allow inference about the likelihood of similar costs, benefits, and toxicity in your particular patient or practice.
6. Detailed sensitivity analyses should be conducted. Did they include all relevant parameters across an adequate range of values?
7. Data should be presented in a transparent fashion.

tion or for palliative care), and effectiveness (e.g., the amount of survival gained, utility estimates) over a range of plausible possibilities. No matter how accurately costs and benefits have been quantified and valued, it is likely that certain assumptions have been required. Skeptics often attack these assumptions to dismiss a study. If altering the value of key parameters significantly changes the outcome of the study, then the analysis is said to be "sensitive" to that variable. If not, it is "robust." The question becomes not whether all estimates of resource use and survival were accurate, but whether any errors would have a meaningful impact on the results.

Setting

Economic evaluations are relatively specific to the healthcare system in which they are performed. Countries such as Canada have single-payer universal healthcare systems in which the government funds virtually the entire system. In contrast, health care in the United States is funded by multiple payers, primarily private insurers, and providers compete for contracts to manage the care of groups of individuals. A third type of system, common in European countries, provides universal health care with patients responsible for a copayment.

Extrapolating the results of a study from one healthcare environment to another involves more than simply adjusting the figures by the exchange rate. Costs for a health care intervention may be affected by differences in (a) demographics and disease incidence, (b) clinical practice patterns, and (c) relative prices. Practice patterns may be influenced by the availability of alternative treatments and diagnostic tests, as well as incentives to professionals and institutions (e.g., salary versus fee for service).[42] There have been few studies reported to date addressing this issue. Drummond et al. assessed misoprostal for the prevention of nonsteroidal antiinflammatory drug (NSAID) induced ulcers simultaneously in four countries (i.e., Belgium, France, United Kingdom, and the United States) using identical methodology. They found misoprostol to be more cost-effective in the United States despite the drug being 36% more expensive because it averted surgical procedures that were relatively more costly in America.[43] Recently, Copley-Merriman et al.[44] made similar observations when they found that gemcitabine monotherapy in advance non–small cell, cancer (NSCLC) compared to standard etoposide/cisplatin (excluding chemotherapy drug costs) saved more money in the United States than in Germany or Spain because it averted more costly hospitalization and antiemetic use.

Transparency

A concern with many economic papers is a lack of *transparency* in the description of methods and assumptions. Transparency refers to how easy it is to see exactly what the au-

thors of a study have done. After reading the results of an economic analysis, the reader should not be left with the impression that the study was done in a "black box." It is best to report disaggregated data on costs, resource use, and quality of life.[4] Ideally, the numerator and denominator of cost-effectiveness ratios should be reported separately. Costs should be shown in the format:

$$quantity \times unit\ price = cost$$

while effectiveness measures should be separated from their utility weightings. Obviously, it is important to know the currency and year of the costs; however, reports should also identify instances of price adjustment, such as use of the consumer price index to inflate prices from another time period, or the date and exchange rate used to translate costs from other countries.

PUBLISHED ECONOMIC STUDIES RELATED TO LUNG CANCER

Prevention

Smokers accrue significant lifetime medical costs[45] as well as costs due to passive smoking, accidental fires, and lost productivity due to illness.[46] However, studies have generally found that smoking is not an economic burden on society. Savings in other medical costs due to early mortality offset the treatment of smoking-related diseases.[47–49] Furthermore, costs to society are offset by tobacco taxation and unclaimed pensions.[50] These conclusions tend to be sensitive to the discount rate used because the costs from smoking occur in the present, whereas the savings occur in the future.

Smoking cessation is the main form of lung cancer prevention. Intervention studies focus on restrictions on smoking and smoking advertisement,[45] and taxation,[51] which are modestly effective and appear to be cost-effective.[52] For example, a mass media campaign costing $759,436 over 4 years was estimated to cost $754 per smoker averted, with a cost per life-year gained of $696.[53] Although the effectiveness of screening programs for lung cancer has not been established, an economic model has indicated that screening programs involving detection of genetic aberrations in the sputum would likely be cost-effective if shown to be clinically effective.[54]

Diagnosis and Staging

Economic studies have also tried to define an optimal diagnostic strategy for NSCLC. For example, Govert et al. determined that the addition of either brushings or washings to bronchoscopic biopsy increased the sensitivity of the test at relatively low cost; however, addition of both procedures was unnecessary and not cost-effective.[55] Several groups have shown that computed tomography (CT) chest with

TABLE 65.4. SUMMARY OF DIRECT CARE COSTS PER CASE FOR NSCLC IN CANADA BY STAGE*

Stage	Primary Treatment	Lifetime
I	$14,110	$21,400
II	$14,110	$23,881
IIIa	$12,474	$22,131
IIIb	$11,714	$19,366
IV	$6,333	$16,501

* 1988 Canadian dollars.

selective mediastinoscopy is more cost-effective than routine mediastinoscopy.[56,57] Furthermore, positron emission tomography (PET) scanning may eventually be a cost-effective addition to CT scanning in this setting.[58] However, routine CT of the head in patients without clinical evidence of metastases has been shown not to be a cost-effective staging procedure.[59]

Similar techniques allowed Richardson et al. to develop an optimal protocol for staging small cell lung cancer (SCLC) patients.[60] Clinical exam and biochemistry followed by bone scan, abdominal CT, head CT, bone marrow aspirate and biopsy, CT chest, and finally pulmonary function testing were able to avert one-third of the overall cost of staging as long as the workup was discontinued as soon as a metastasis was identified.

Cost of NSCLC

It has been estimated that lung cancer management accounts for approximately 20% of cancer care costs and 2% of all healthcare costs in the United States.[61] Several studies have examined the costs associated with lung cancer.[62] Evans et al. calculated the average direct care costs for diagnosis and treatment of NSCLC in Canada to be $19,778 in 1988 Canadian dollars over 5 years. The first-year costs ranged from $6,333 for supportive care for stage IV disease, to $17,889 for surgery and radiotherapy in earlier stage lung cancer (Table 65.4). Hospital costs were found to dominate, accounting for 36.8% of all costs (Figure 65.2). About one-third of the total cost is for hospitalization during the initial diagnostic workup. Terminal care accounts for about one-half of the total cost whether a patient receives chemotherapy or not. The five-year costs ranged from $16,501 to $23,881.

In the United States, Riley et al. compared the Medicare payments for patients aged 65 and over with common cancers.[63] They found that lung cancer was the most expensive cancer site for initial treatment at $17,518 (1990 US$) due to high costs for hospitalization ($10,782, or 62%); however, because of the relatively short survival of lung cancer patients, it was among the least expensive in terms of total payments from diagnosis to death at $29,184.

Recently, Hillner et al. looked at the cost of lung cancer for a commercially insured cohort in Virginia.[64] These patients were younger and fees generally were higher than those for the Medicare population studied by Riley et al. They found that the total cost of treatment from diagnosis to death was $47,941 (in 1992 US$), with inpatient hospital facility costs accounting for up to 65% of the total cost. Patients receiving no active treatment still incurred significant costs ($26,597 in the first year after diagnosis). On

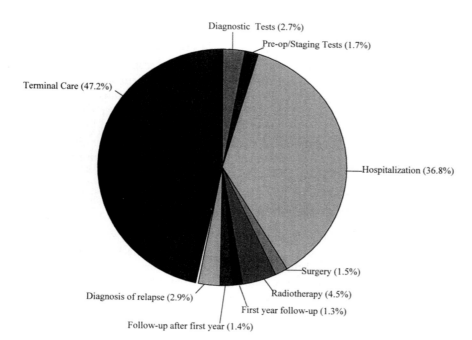

FIGURE 65.2. The cost component of lung cancer management.

TABLE 65.5. ECONOMIC EVALUATIONS OF TREATMENT ALTERNATIVES IN LUNG CANCER

Reference	Country	Form of Analysis	Disease and Stage	Comparators	Main Results
Coyle et al.[72] (1997)	UK	CEA	Stage III NSCLC	CHART RT	CHART more costly than conventional treatment but cost-effective given survival benefits.
Evans et al.[73] (1997)	Canada	CEA	Stage III NSCLC	Chemo + RT Chemo + RT +/− surgery	Multimodality treatment cost-effective at $3,348–$14,958/LYG relative to standard surgery or radiation.
Earle et al.[74] (1997)	Canada	CEA	Stage IV NSCLC	TAX BSC	TAX cost-effective at $4,778/LYG relative to BSC.
Evans[75] (1996)	Canada	CEA	Stage IV NSCLC	GEM BSC	GEM is more costly, but cost-effective relative to BSC.
Palmer et al.[76] (1996)	Italy	CEA	Stage IIIB & IV NSCLC	GEM-P MIP VP-P NVB-P	GEM-P had the lowest cost per response at 85,700,000 lira.
Evans et al.[77] (1996)	Canada	CEA	Stage IV NSCLC	NVB NVB-P VP-P VLB-P BSC	VLB-P was most cost-effective relative to BSC, however, NVB-P yielded the best survival at $5,551/LYG.
Doyle et al.[78] (1996)	USA	CMA	Limited & extensive SCLC	VP-P P + Etoposide phosphate	Etoposide phosphate, a prodrug with shorter administration time, consumes fewer resources than standard etoposide.
Copley Merriman et al.[44] (1996)	USA, Germany, Spain	CMA	Stage III/IV NSCLC	GEM VP-P VP-I	GEM was cost saving compared to the other regimens when the drug costs for chemotherapy were excluded.
Copley Merriman et al.[79] (1996)	USA	CMA	Stage III/IV NSCLC	GEM VP-P	If the cost of the drugs is ignored, GEM uses fewer resources than VP-P.
Vergnenegre et al.[83] (1996)	France	CEA	Stage III/IV NSCLC	M-NVP-P M-VDS-P	Calculated that MNP cost 12,339.40 francs less per response than MVP.
Koch et al.[80] (1995)	USA	CMA	Stage III/IV NSCLC	GEM VP-I	GEM uses fewer resources than VP-I.
Smith et al.[81] (1995)	USA	CEA	Stage III/IV NSCLC	NVB NVB-P VDS-P	If NVB's toxicity profile is acceptable, then NVB-P is cost-effective at $17,700/LYG relative to NVB, and $15,500 compared to VDS-P.
Kennedy et al.[82] (1995)	Canada	CEA	Stage III/IV NSCLC	CAP VDS-P BSC	Redid the Jaakkimainen et al. study incorporating health professional–derived utilities: CAP $42,833 and VDS-P $43,496/QALY.
Jaakkimainen et al.[20] (1990)	Canada	CEA	Stage III/IV NSCLC	CAP VDS-P BSC	Both chemotherapy regimens cost-effective compared to BSC. CAP actually led to cost savings compared to BSC.
Goodwin et al.[84] (1988)	Canada	CEA/CUA	Extensive SCLC	CAV CAV alternating with VP	Alternating chemotherapy cost $3,370/LYG and $4,495/QALY.

A, doxorubicin
BSC, best supportive care
C, cyclophosphamide
CEA, cost-effectiveness analysis
CHART, continuous hyperfractionated accelerated radiotherapy
Chemo, chemotherapy
CMA, cost-minimization analysis
CUA, cost-utility analysis
GEM, gemcitabine
I, ifosfamide
LYG, life year gained

M, mitomycin
NSCLC, non–small cell lung cancer
NVB, vinorelbine
P, cisplatin
QALY, quality-adjusted life-year
RT, conventional radiotherapy
SCLC, small cell lung cancer
TAX, paclitaxel
V, vincristine
VDS, vindesine
VP, etoposide

average, patients spent 27.6 days in the hospital in the last 6 months of life.

Methodological differences and different time frames make these studies not completely comparable; however, hospitalization consistently stands out as the dominant cost in all of them. Similar findings have been seen in other tumor sites.[65–67] This sort of research has led to the shift in recent years of treatment in the ambulatory setting, development of care maps and algorithms to expedite diagnosis,[68] and increased use of hospices for terminal care.[69]

Cost of SCLC

Less work has been published on the costs associated with SCLC treatment. Evans et al. found that direct care costs for the diagnosis and initial treatment of SCLC ranged from $18,691 (1988 Canadian dollars) for management of limited-stage disease, to $4,739 for the supportive care of patients with extensive disease who were not candidates for chemotherapy. The average total cost for treating SCLC was $25,988.[18,70] This figure is comparable to the $18,234 (1990 Australian dollars) for limited and $13,177 for extensive disease calculated by Rosenthal.[71] Again, hospitalization was the dominant cost.

Cost-Effectiveness of Treatment

Through a MEDLINE search to identify studies whose principal objective was to examine the cost-effectiveness of lung cancer treatment options, and by searching the references of relevant articles, we identified 15 economic evaluations[20,44,72–84] (Table 65.5). All but one study included an evaluation of the cost-effectiveness of chemotherapeutic alternatives in lung cancer treatment.[72] The one exception involved a comparison of two different radiotherapy regimens for NSCLC: conventional radiotherapy treatment *versus* continuous hyperfractionated accelerated radiotherapy. Despite the recognition of the importance of quality-of-life effects on treatment choice, only two studies incorporated estimates of patient's quality of life into QALYs.[82,84]

All studies used effectiveness data derived from clinical trials, although not all were based on randomized evidence. Several studies examined resource consumption from those same trials,[20,72,78,82–84] whereas others adopted an approach whereby resource use estimates were obtained from other sources (e.g., institutional databases) and were combined with effectiveness data within a modeling framework.[44,73–75,77,79–81]

In most cases, costly but effective treatment options were found to be cost-effective due to savings in the consumption of other resources. For example, a cost analysis performed by the National Cancer Institute of Canada (NCIC) on a multicenter randomized trial comparing chemotherapy with best supportive care (BSC) found chemotherapy to be not only cost-effective but also cost-saving by reducing the

need for palliative radiotherapy and the length of terminal care hospitalization.[20] A record linkage study of more than 600 patients in the province of Manitoba recently corroborated this finding (Statistics Canada, personal communication, 1999). Although another analysis of the same trial failed to confirm this result,[82] in general, effective interventions tend to be cost-effective.

Supportive interventions have also been evaluated. Ondansetron has been shown to be cost-effective for prophylaxis against cisplatin-induced emesis.[85] On the other hand, granulocyte colony-stimulating factor (G-CSF) was not found to be a cost-effective adjunct to SCLC treatment.[86]

LUNG CANCER ECONOMICS AND HEALTH CARE POLICY

The expenditures associated with medical practice are coming under increased scrutiny. Both public and private payers are demanding increased efficiency and "value for money" in the provision of healthcare services. As a result, policymakers in both Australia and the province of Ontario (Canada) have developed formal guidelines for economic analyses that are to be part of drug reimbursement submissions.[1,2]

Recent practice guidelines[87,88] have recommended that it is "reasonable to offer cisplatin-based chemotherapy to medically suitable patients as a treatment option" for survival, symptom control, and quality-of-life outcomes in metastatic NSCLC patients.[87] As Evans et al. reported,[89] the average cost (all stages) of managing a lung cancer patient from diagnosis to death without palliative chemotherapy is just under $20,000. Therefore, for all 17,128 cases diagnosed in Canada in 1992, the total cost was approximately $350 million (and about 10 times as much in the United States). Even though palliative chemotherapy is considered cost-effective,[90] by virtue of lung cancer's high incidence, the cost of treating all advanced-stage patients with chemotherapy would add significantly to healthcare budgets and labor requirements.

Oncologists are still fairly conservative in their management of advanced lung cancer.[91] Additionally, many patients are not candidates for systemic therapy because of biologic age, performance status, or comorbid conditions; therefore, the actual impact of a new treatment for lung cancer on national health budgets is likely to be less than projected.

CONCLUSION

Because of its high incidence, lung cancer is a significant burden on healthcare systems. Studies indicate that strategies to minimize hospitalization are likely to have the greatest impact on these expenditures.[74] Despite common perceptions to the contrary, supportive care for advanced lung cancer is associated with significant cost, and many chemotherapeutic treatments are cost-effective relative to other commonly accepted medical interventions; however, decision-makers sometimes have trouble seeing past the price of these interventions. Therefore, it is important to understand how to assess these technologies in the broader context of the costs and consequences associated with their use. Providing decision-makers with useful information from methodologically sound studies will help optimize use of health care resources and ensure continuing access to care for lung cancer patients in the future.

REFERENCES

1. Ontario Ministry of Health. Guidelines for preparation of economic analysis in submission to drug programs branch for listing in the Ontario Benefit Formulary/Comparative Drug Index. Toronto: Ontario Ministry of Health, 1991.
2. Commonwealth of Australia. Guidelines for the pharmaceutical industry on preparation of submissions to the Pharmaceutical Benefits Advisory Committee: including submissions involving economic analyses. Canberra: Department of Health, Housing and Community Services, 1992.
3. Grunfeld E, Glossop R, McDowell I, et al. Caring for elderly people at home: the consequences to caregivers. *Can Med Assoc J* 1997;157:1101.
4. Drummond MF, Jefferson TO. Guidelines for authors and peer reviewers of economic submissions to the BMJ. *Br Med J* 1996;313:275.
5. Eddy RJ. Cost effectiveness of CT scanning compared with mediastinoscopy in the preoperative staging of lung cancer. *J Can Assoc Radiol* 1989;40:189.
6. Houston BA, Griffith JE, Sanders JA, et al. Staging of lung cancer. A cost-effectiveness analysis. *Am J Clin Oncol* (CCT) 1985;8:224.
7. Kesteloot K, Dutreix A, Scheuren Evd. Quality assurance in radiotherapy-economic criteria to support decision making. *Intl J Tech Assess Health Care* 1993;9:274.
8. Kesteloot K, Dutreix A, van der Scheuren E. A model for calculating the costs of in vivo dosimetry and portal imaging in radiotherapy departments. *Radiother Oncol* 1993;28:108.
9. Weltens C, Desteloot G, Vandevelde R, et al. Comparison of plastic and orfit masks for patient head fixation during radiotherapy; precision and costs. *Int J Radiat Oncol Biol Phys* 1995;33:499.
10. Evans WK, Burpee C, Skinn B, et al. An evaluation of the costs of outpatient chemotherapy administration for small cell lung cancer. *Can J Oncol* 1993;3:225.
11. Williams C, Coyle D, Gray A, et al. European School of Oncology advisory report to the Commission of the European Communities for the "Europe Against Cancer Programme" cost-effectiveness in cancer care. *Eur J Cancer* 1995;31A:1410.
12. Gudex C, Kind P. The QALY Toolkit. Centre for Health Economics Discussion Paper 38. University of York, York, England, 1988.
13. Torrance GW, Feeny D. Utilities and quality-adjusted life years. *Intl J Tech Assess Health Care* 1989;5:559.
14. Torrance GW, Furlong W, Feeny D, et al. Multi-attribute preference functions. Health Utilities Index. *Pharmacoeconomics* 1995;7:503.
15. Euroqol Group. Euroqol—A new facility for the measurement of health related quality of life. *Health Policy* 1990;16:199.
16. Goldhirsch A, Gelber RD, Simes RJ, et al. Costs and benefits of adjuvant therapy in breast cancer: a quality-adjusted survival analysis. *J Clin Oncol* 1989;7:36.
17. Siegel JE, Weinstein MC, Russell LB, et al. Recommendations for reporting cost-effectiveness analyses. *JAMA* 1996;276:1339.
18. Evans WK, Will BP, Berthelot J-M, et al. Estimating the cost of lung cancer diagnosis and treatment in Canada: the POHEM model. *Can J Oncol* 1995;5:408.
19. Rapp E, Pater JL, Willan A, et al. Chemotherapy can prolong survival in patients with advanced non-small-cell lung cancer—report of a Canadian multicenter randomized trial. *J Clin Oncol* 1988;6:633.
20. Jaakkimainen L, Goodwin PJ, Pater J. Counting the costs of chemotherapy in a National Cancer Institute of Canada randomized trial in non-small cell lung cancer. *J Clin Oncol* 1990;8:1301.
21. Hayman J, Weeks J, Mauch P. Economic analyses in health care: an introduction to the methodology with an emphasis on radiation therapy. *Int J Rad Oncol Biol Phys* 1996;35:827.
22. Finkler SA. The distinction between costs and charges. *Ann Intern Med* 1982;96:102.
23. Drummond MF, Stoddart GL, Torrance GW. *Methods for the economic evaluation of health care programmes.* Oxford: Oxford University Press, 1987.
24. Torrance GW, Blaker D, Detsky A, et al. Canadian guidelines for economic evaluation of pharmaceuticals. *Pharmacoeconomics* 1996;9:535.
25. Gold MR, Siegel JE, Russell LB, et al. *Cost-effectiveness in health and medicine.* New York: Oxford University Press, 1996.
26. Drummond MF, Coyle D. Assessing the economic value of antihypertensive medicines. *J Hum Hypertension* 1992;6:495.
27. Parsonage M, Neuberger H. Discounting and health benefits. *Health Econ* 1992;1:71.
28. Coyle D, Tolley K. Discounting of health benefits in the pharmacoeconomic analysis of drug therapies: an issue for debate? *Pharmacoeconomics* 1992;2:153.
29. Cairns J. Discounting and health benefits: another perspective. *Health Econ* 1992;1:76.
30. Sheldon TA. Discounting in health-care decision-making—time for a change. *J Pub Health Med* 1992;14:250.
31. Fayers PM, Hand DJ. Generalisation from phase III clinical trials: survival, quality of life, and health economics. *Lancet* 1997;350:1025.
32. Laupacis A, Feeny D, Detsky A, et al. How attractive does a new technology have to be to warrant adoption and utilization? Tentative guidelines for using clinical and economic evaluations. *Can Med Assoc J* 1992;146:473.
33. Williams AH. Economics of coronary artery bypass grafting. *Br Med J* 1985;291:326.
34. Maynard A. Developing the health care market. *Econ J* 1990;101:1277.
35. Schulman KA, Lynn LA, Glick HA, et al. Cost-effectiveness of low-dose zidovudine therapy for asymptomatic patients with human deficiency virus (HIV) infection. *Ann Int Med* 1991;114:798.
36. Smith TJ, Hillner BE, Desch CE. Efficacy and cost-effectiveness of cancer treatment: rational allocation of resources based on decision analysis. *J Natl Cancer Inst* 1993;85:1460.
37. Drummond MF, Torrance GW, Mason J. Cost-effectiveness league tables: more harm than good? *Soc Sci Med* 1993;37:33.
38. Williams A. The cost benefit approach. *Br Med Bull* 1974;249:326.
39. Maynard A. The design of future cost-benefit studies. *Am Heart J* 1990;119:761.
40. Drummond MF, Richardson WS, O'Brien BJ. Users' guides to the medical literature XIII. How to use an article on economic

analysis of clinical practice A. Are the results of the study valid? *JAMA* 1997;277:1552.

41. O'Brien BJ, Heyland D, Richardson WS, et al. Users' guides to the medical literature XIII. How to use an article on economic analysis of clinical practice B. What are the results and will they help me in caring for my patients? *JAMA* 1997;277:1802.

42. Drummond MF. Comparing cost-effectiveness across countries. The model of acid-related disease. *Pharmacoeconomics* 1994;5:60.

43. Drummond MF, Bloom BS, Carrin G, et al. Issues in the cross-national assessment of health technology. *Intl J Tech Assess Health Care* 1992;8:671.

44. Copley-Merriman C, Martin C, Johnson N, et al. Economic value of gemcitabine in non-small cell lung cancer. *Semin Oncol* 1996;23,Suppl 10:90.

45. MacKenzie TD, Bartecchi CE, Schrier RW. The human costs of tobacco use. *N Engl J Med* 1994;330:975.

46. Lesmes GR, Donofrio KH. Passive smoking: the medical and economic issues. *Am J Med* 1992;93(suppl. 1A):38S.

47. Leu RE, Schaub T. Does smoking increase medical care expenditure? *Soc Sci Med* 1983;17:1907.

48. Lippiatt BC. Measuring medical cost and life expectancy impacts of changes in cigarette sales. *Prev Med* 1990;19:532.

49. Barendregt JJ, Bonneux L, van der Maas PJ. The health care costs of smoking. *N Engl J Med* 1997;337:1052.

50. Manning WG, Keeler EB, Newhouse JP, et al. The taxes of sin. Do smokers and drinkers pay their way? *JAMA* 1989;261:1604.

51. Peterson DE, Zeger SL, Remington PL, et al. The effect of state cigarette tax increases on cigarette sales, 1955 to 1988. *Am J Pub Health* 1992;82:94.

52. Phillips CJ, Prowle MJ. Economics of a reduction in smoking: case study from Heartbeat Wales. *J Epidemiol Comm Health* 1993;47:215.

53. Secker-Walker RH, Worden JK, Holland RR, et al. A mass media programme to prevent smoking among adolescents: costs and cost-effectiveness. *Tobacco Control* 1997;6:207.

54. Berthelot J-M, Earle CC, Will BP, et al. Sputum dual antibody testing (SDAT) and chemoprevention for lung cancer: a decision analytic model. *Proc Am Soc Clin Oncol* 1998;17:[abstr.]2173.

55. Govert JA, Kopita JM, Matchar D, et al. Cost-effectiveness of collecting routine cytologic specimens during fiberoptic bronchoscopy for endoscopically visible lung tumor. *Chest* 1996;109:451.

56. Black WC, Armstrong P, Daniel TM. Cost effectiveness of chest CT in T1N0M0 lung cancer. *Radiology* 1988;167:373.

57. The Canadian Lung Oncology Group. Investigation for mediastinal disease in patients with apparently operable lung cancer. *Ann Thorac Surg* 1995;60:1382.

58. Gambhir SS, Hoh CK, Phelps ME, et al. Decision tree sensitivity analysis for cost-effectiveness of FDG-PET in the staging and management of non-small cell lung carcinoma. *J Nuc Med* 1996;37:1428.

59. Colice GL, Birkmeyer JD, Black WC, et al. Cost-effectiveness of head CT in patients with lung cancer without clinical evidence of metastases. *Chest* 1995;108:1264.

60. Richardson GE, Venzon DJ, Phelps R, et al. Application of an algorithm for staging small-cell lung cancer can save one third of the initial evaluation costs. *Arch Intern Med* 1993;153:329.

61. Desch CE, Hillner BE, Smith TJ. Economic considerations in the care of lung cancer patients. *Curr Opin Oncol* 1996;8:126.

62. Coy P, Schaafsma J, Schofield JA, et al. Comparative costs of lung cancer management. *Clin Invest Med* 1994;17:577.

63. Riley GF, Potosky AL, Lubitz JD, et al. Medicare payments from diagnosis to death for elderly cancer patients by stage at diagnosis. *Med Care* 1995;33:828.

64. Hillner BE, McDonald MK, Desch CE, et al. Costs of care associated with non-small cell lung cancer in a commercially insured cohort. *J Clin Oncol* 1998;16:1420.

65. Hurley SF, Huggins RM, Snyder RD, et al. The cost of breast cancer recurrences. *Br J Cancer* 1992;65:449.

66. Barr R, Furlong W, Henwook J, et al. Economic evaluation of allogeneic bone marrow transplantation: a rudimentary model to generate estimates for the timely formulation of clinical policy. *J Clin Oncol* 1996;14:1413.

67. Covens A, Boucher S, Roche K, et al. Is paclitaxel and cisplatin a cost-effective first-line therapy for advanced ovarian carcinoma. *Cancer* 1996;77:2086.

68. Smith TJ, Desch CE, Hillner BE. Ways to reduce the cost of oncology care without compromising the quality. *Cancer Inves* 1994;12:257.

69. Emanuel EJ, Emanuel LL. The economics of dying. The illusion of cost savings at the end of life. *N Engl J Med* 1994;330:540.

70. Evans WK, Earle CC, Berthelot J-M, et al. The cost and cost-effectiveness of small cell lung cancer treatment in Canada. *Proc Am Soc Clin Oncol* 1997;16[abstr.]1503.

71. Rosenthal MA, Webster PJ, Gebski VJ, et al. The cost of treating small cell lung cancer. *Med J Aust* 1992;156:605.

72. Coyle D, Drummond MF. Costs of conventional radical radiotherapy versus continuous hyperfractionated accelerated radiotherapy (CHART) in the treatment of patients with head and neck cancer or carcinoma of the bronchus. *Clin Oncol* 1997;9:313.

73. Evans WK, Will BP, Berthelot J-M, et al. The cost of combined modality interventions for stage III non-small cell lung cancer. *J Clin Oncol* 1997;15:3038.

74. Earle CC, Evans WK. A comparison of the cost of paclitaxel versus best supportive care in stage IV non-small cell lung cancer. *Cancer Prev Control* 1997;1:282.

75. Evans WK. Cost-effectiveness of gemcitabine in stage IV non-small cell lung cancer: an estimate using the POpulation HEalth Model lung cancer module. *Semin Oncol* 1997;24(2 suppl 7):S7-56.

76. Palmer AJ, Brandt A. The cost-effectiveness of four cisplatin-containing chemotherapy regimens in the treatment of stages IIIB and IV non-small cell lung cancer: an Italian perspective. *Monaldi Arch Chest Dis* 1996;51:279.

77. Evans WK, Chevalier T. The cost-effectiveness of Navelbine alone or in combination with cisplatin in comparison to standard therapies in stage IV non-small cell lung cancer. *Eur J Cancer* 1996;32A:2249.

78. Doyle JJ, Dezii CM, Sadana S. A pharmacoeconomic evaluation of cisplatin in combination with either etoposide or etoposide phosphate in small cell lung cancer. *Semin Oncol* 1996;23(suppl 13):51.

79. Copley-Merriman C, Corral J, King K, et al. Economic value of gemcitabine compared to cisplatin and etoposide in non-small cell lung cancer. *Lung Cancer* 1996;14:45.

80. Koch P, Johnson N, van Schaik J, et al. Gemcitabine: clinical and economic impact in inoperable non-small cell lung cancer. *Anti-Cancer Drugs* 1995;6(suppl 6):49.

81. Smith TJ, Hillner BE, Neighbors DM, et al. An economic evaluation of a randomized clinical trial comparing vinorelbine, vinorelbine plus cisplatin, and vindesine plus cisplatin for non-small cell lung cancer. *J Clin Oncol* 1995;13:2166.

82. Kennedy W, Reinharz D, Tessier G, et al. Cost utility of chemotherapy and best supportive care in non-small cell lung cancer. *Pharmacoeconomics* 1995;8:316.

83. Vergnenegre A, Perol M, Pham E. Cost analysis of hospital treatment—two chemotherapic (sic) regimens for non-surgical non-small cell lung cancer. *Lung Cancer* 1996;14:31.

84. Goodwin PJ, Feld R, Evans WK, et al. Cost-effectiveness of cancer chemotherapy: an economic evaluation of a randomized trial in small-cell lung cancer. *J Clin Oncol* 1988;6:1537.

85. Stewart DJ, Dahrouge S, Coyle D, et al. Impact of ondansetron on costs of preventing and treating nausea and vomiting. *Proc Am Soc Clin Oncol* 1998;17:[abstr.]270.

86. Nichols CR, Fox EP, Roth BJ, et al. Incidence of neutropenic fever in patients treated with standard-dose combination chemotherapy for small-cell lung cancer and the cost impact of treatment with granulocyte colony-stimulating factor. *J Clin Oncol* 1994;12:1245.

87. Lopez PG, Stewart DJ, Newman TE, et al. Chemotherapy in stage IV (metastatic) non-small-cell lung cancer. *Cancer Prev Control* 1997;1:18.

88. American Society of Clinical Oncology. Clinical practice guidelines for the treatment of unresectable non-small-cell lung cancer. *J Clin Ocol* 1997;15:2996.

89. Evans WK, Will BP, Berthelot J-M, et al. The economics of lung cancer management in Canada. *Lung Cancer* 1996;14:19.

90. Evans WK, Will BP, Berthelot JM, et al. The cost of managing lung cancer in Canada. *Oncology* 1995;9:147.

91. Raby B, Pater J, Mackillop W. Does knowledge guide practice? Another look at the management of non-small-cell lung cancer. *J Clin Oncol* 1995;13:1904.

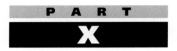

STATISTICS AND TRIAL DESIGN

66

STATISTICS AND TRIAL DESIGN

SETH M. STEINBERG

The purpose of this chapter is to provide a brief description of the types of clinical trials that are currently used to evaluate treatments for cancer and to discuss statistical techniques involved in analyzing such trials. These techniques include such methods as Kaplan-Meier survival curves, Cox proportional hazards models, and metaanalysis, all of which are common in the literature today. Before beginning any discussion of specific types of clinical trials, it is useful to define a clinical trial: a clinical trial is a carefully planned study used to determine the effect and value of interventions in human subjects. In order to conduct a trial, there must be a primary question of interest, a detailed study protocol, and availability of resources. These needed resources include patients for the study, clinicians, any study drugs, and any other types of equipment or supplies that would be needed for the trial.

In oncology, three types of clinical trials are generally conducted, known as phase I, phase II, and phase III. A phase I trial is typically the first trial that is conducted in humans. It is used to determine the maximum tolerated dose of therapy and may indicate whether or not there is some degree of benefit from the drug or drugs. A phase II trial usually measures the disease response to a single therapy or combination of therapies, whereas a phase III trial compares the effectiveness of two or more therapies in a randomized, prospective fashion. In addition to these three main types, other variations exist such as phase I/II trials, phase II/III trials, and trials that are known as *pilot,* or *feasibility,* studies. A pilot, or feasibility, study is a trial of limited numbers of patients intended to determine whether a new procedure may be safely carried out using human subjects. Such trials rarely have efficacy end points and are typically limited to no more than 10 patients. The next few sections discuss some of the statistical issues in each type of trial.

PHASE I TRIALS

The objective of a phase I trial is to determine dose levels of a single agent or combination of agents that balance toxicity with efficacy. Patients enrolled in a phase I trial may come from a wide variety of disease types. In general, the starting dose of drug for a phase I trial is one-tenth of the mouse LD_{10}, which has been determined previously in preclinical studies. A common procedure that can be used for determining the rate of dose escalation for a phase I trial is called a *modified Fibonacci approach.* Table 66.1 provides a hypothetical example of a modified Fibonacci procedure for selecting dose levels for a Phase I clinical trial. As can be seen in this table, the initial dose would be one-tenth of the mouse LD_{10}. In step 2 this amount would be doubled. The third step would be 67% above step 2; the fourth step would be 50% above that of step 3; and finally the smallest increment that is normally used for escalating doses is 33%. As shown in this table, with a hypothetical starting dose of some drug of 100 mg/m^2, by the sixth step the dose is approximately nine times the initial starting dose.

The standard procedure for enrolling patients in a phase I trial is as follows: at the lowest starting dose, three patients are entered. Those three patients would be treated and followed for toxicity. If none of those three patients have unacceptable toxicity as defined by the protocol, then the next dose to be evaluated would be that of the second dose level. However; if one patient of the three experiences dose-limiting toxicity, then up to three additional patients would be treated on that same dose level. If none of those additional three patients experiences dose-limiting toxicity, then the next three patients would be entered at the next higher dose level. If, however, a dose level is identified at which two or more patients have dose-limiting toxicity, then that dose would be the highest dose level examined. The next patients to enter the study would be placed at the preceding dose; that is, the dose below the one in which toxicity was noted, in order to verify safety at that level. This dose, if found to be acceptable, would be called the *maximum tolerated dose* (MTD). Escalation continues in this fashion until the MTD is reached.

Because of the nature of the standard accrual scheme of phase I clinical trials, three times the number of dose levels, plus six, would be an estimate of the maximum number of patients that would be needed to evaluate an agent during phase I using a standard accrual approach. For example, if a clinical trial were to be conducted with six dose levels,

TABLE 66.1. EXAMPLE OF MODIFIED FIBONACCI PROCEDURE FOR SELECTING DOSE LEVELS FOR A PHASE I CLINICAL TRIAL

Step Number	Relative Dose	Example
1	1/10 Mouse LD_{10}	100 mg/m^2
2	Double Step 1	200 mg/m^2
3	67% Above Step 2	333 mg/m^2
4	50% Above Step 3	500 mg/m^2
5	33% Greater Than Step 4	667 mg/m^2
6	33% Greater Than Step 5	890 mg/m^2

then it would be expected that up to 24 patients might be required on this trial. This information can be useful for planning accrual to the study.

Recently, Simon and co-workers developed an alternative design approach, based on rapidly escalating doses treating one patient per dose level until evidence of any toxicity is encountered, followed by a standard dose-escalation until an MTD is reached.[1] Under appropriate assumptions, this design can attain the identical MTD as a conventional escalation scheme but may require far fewer patients. In another report, Ahn compares a variety of novel phase I escalation methods and makes recommendations for selecting one of these newer designs.[2]

It is commonly believed that a phase I trial is not designed for evaluating efficacy of a therapy. That is generally true, especially with conventional phase I trials, because most patients are treated at doses that are below the one that would most likely produce a response; however, it may be possible to see responses in patients, even at the lowest doses of therapy. In general, no more than 5% of patients would be expected to respond to a phase I study; thus, although phase I studies are conducted with therapeutic intent, clear efficacy from phase I trials is believed to not be readily determinable.

Data from phase I trials are typically analyzed using descriptive methods. A wide range of toxicity results by dose level are often tabulated to demonstrate the degree to which patients treated at the various doses are effected adversely by the treatment. Any responses identified may also be noted.

A specific type of phase I trial, known as a *biologic response modifier trial,* is often conducted in two phases. In phase IA, the objective is to find the maximum tolerated dose much as one would do customarily in a standard phase I trial. In phase IB, one would try to find the optimal biologic response modifying dose. This dose may not be the same as the maximum tolerated dose. The MTD is used to define the upper limit of therapy that is safe to evaluate in patients, whereas the OBRMB is the dose that is believed to have the most potential benefit for patients. For additional, more detailed discussion on phase I clinical trials, consult a reference book on this topic.[3]

PHASE II TRIALS

The objectives of a phase II trial are to screen the drug or drugs evaluated for any antitumor activity in a specific disease, and to try to increase knowledge of pharmacology and toxicology of drugs that are being evaluated. In general, success or failure from a phase II study is determined according to whether or not an observed response proportion in patients with measurable disease (i.e., the fraction of patients who successfully receive treatment and are able to experience a well-defined clinical response) is consistent with, greater than, or less than a hypothesized response proportion. One needs to have strictly stated objective criteria for response prior to initiation of the study to ensure correct evaluation of efficacy.

Phase II trials normally treat patients using approximately 75% to 90% of the MTD as found in a phase I trial. This dosage ensures that the study can be conducted safely. It should be noted that in the absence of severe toxicity found in a phase I trial, there are no scientific grounds for terminating a drug's clinical development without conducting a phase II trial because only a phase II trial has sufficient patients enrolled at potentially therapeutic doses in order to make an evaluation of whether the drug has benefit.

Phase II trials are not generally comparative. They are used to indicate whether a new treatment should be pursued further, and to determine its priority relative to other agents being evaluated for treatment of the same disease. A randomized phase II trial provides a means of making a comparison between two or more agents. In this type of trial, two or more agents are randomized against one another so that patient characteristics are similar for each of the agents being evaluated; no formal statistical comparison is undertaken between the groups. It is expected, though, that the agent that produces the greatest response rate from among those compared is the one that is most likely to be useful for advancement into the larger phase III trials.

Several factors should be considered when designing a phase II trial. First, it is important to plan to accrue a homogeneous group of patients with respect to disease type and estimated prognosis. Homogeneity enhances the interpretability and meaningfulness of the findings from this study. It is also important to try to estimate the potential response rate to this agent or combination of agents. This estimation can be determined to some extent from literature results of trials in patients treated for this disease. Careful consideration of the possible differences in prognosis between the historical group and the present group of patients should be taken into consideration. Furthermore, with tumor shrinkage as the end point in most phase II trials, it is important that potentially measurable changes in size of tumor be used. Also, if a trial is to evaluate efficacy in subgroups of patients, it is important to allow adequate numbers of patients in each subgroup.

Determination of sample size for a phase II trial can range from being simple to somewhat complex depending on the assumptions one is willing to make. One of the earliest types of designs commonly used was developed by Gehan[4] and is a straightforward two-stage design. In the first stage, 14 patients are accrued, treated, and evaluated. If no responses occur in the first stage, then accrual is terminated because there is less than a 5% probability that the true response rate is at least 20%. If at least one of the initial 14 patients has an objective response to therapy, then a second stage would be conducted with accrual of at least 11 additional patients. The more patients entered on the second stage, the more precise the estimate of the response. However, with this particular example, if the true response probability was 5%, then there is a 51% chance of observing one or more responses in 14 patients. Thus if an agent had a true response probability that was very low, this design would not likely result in an appropriate early termination with high probability.

Lee and Wesley[5] describe another relatively simple approach to determining the number of patients to enter as a function of acceptable or unacceptable response proportions. With their method, if one was interested in stopping a study if the results are inconsistent with 30% response, then accruing nine patients and observing no responses would allow accrual to end. Or, to quickly rule out consistency with a 50% response proportion, entering five patients and observing no responses could result in termination at this point.

An improved design was developed by Simon.[6] His design is called an *optimal two-stage design* for a phase II clinical trial and is optimal in the sense that the expected sample size required for evaluation is minimized if the agent has a low activity level. Potentially, one could stop accrual to a study evaluating a poor agent with fewer patients on average than with a standard two-stage design because many poor agents would end up being evaluated in both stages using the standard Gehan approach. To design a study of this type, one first needs to decide on two error probabilities (the probability of accepting an uninteresting drug and the probability of rejecting a desirable drug), the response probability which is uninterestingly low, P_0, and that worthy of further exploration, P_1. After deciding on these parameters, one can determine a two-stage design that specifies the number of patients to accrue and corresponding maximum number of responses consistent with an insufficiently active agent. Table 66.2 provides a few examples (with 10% as each error probability) of numbers of patients to be accrued at an interim point and the highest number of responses observed that would cause termination of the study at that point. This table also indicates the highest final response proportion that is inconsistent with a desirable drug. For example, if it were considered uninteresting in a particular disease to have a response proportion of 20% and of more interest to have a response proportion of 40%, if 17 patients

TABLE 66.2. EXAMPLES OF RESPONSE PROPORTIONS CAUSING REJECTION OF DRUG, USING OPTIMAL TWO-STAGE DESIGN

Reject Drug if Observed Response Rate is Below:

P_0*	P_1**	Interim Point	Final Evaluation
0.20	0.40	3/17	10/37
0.30	0.50	7/22	17/46
0.40	0.60	7/18	22/46
0.20	0.35	5/22	19/72
0.30	0.45	9/30	29/82

* Response probability if drug is uninteresting.
** Response probability if drug is desirable.
From Simon RM. Optimal two-stage designs for Phase II Clinical Trials. *Controlled Clinical Trials* 1989;10:1, with permission.

were initially entered into the trial, and if no more than 3 experienced objective clinical responses, then accrual would be terminated and the drug would be declared unsatisfactory. However, if in the initial 17 patients there were 4 or more responses, then accrual would continue until 37 patients were entered into the trial. In that event, if there were 10 or fewer total responses, the agent would be considered unsatisfactory. Otherwise, with 11 or more responses, the agent would be considered worthy of further investigation. Other examples are presented in this table as well as in the original article.

Analysis of the main results of the phase II study typically includes a summary of the demographic and clinical characteristics of the patients accrued, the toxicities observed, and categorization of the responses observed according to how complete the responses are. In addition, confidence intervals about the observed response proportions are often presented to assess the precision of the results obtained and to indicate the approximate degree of consistency with other studies. Confidence intervals that are appropriate to the two-stage nature of many designs may be employed.

Finally, it is important to realize that in a Phase II study there are many sources of variability that can affect the responses observed and the interpretation of study results.[3] First, the doses and schedules of drugs administered can vary, and the eligibility criteria for patients to be entered into the studies may also vary considerably. Such things to consider in assessing comparability of studies include the extent of disease, performance status, and any prior treatments the patients may have received. The response criteria may also differ. It is important that these criteria be consistently defined. There could be inter-observer variability because individuals do not necessarily agree on every aspect of evaluation of a patient's response. Dosage modifications and protocol compliance issues could also vary from institution to institution. Differences in reporting procedures, primarily regarding which patients are to be included in the analyses, may be identified. For example, every patient who has entered into the study that was initially found eligible or only those who successfully completed the treatment may ultimately be included in analysis. Finally, the sample size of an individual study can effect the interpretation. Tighter confidence limits are obtained with more patients, and results based on larger numbers of patients could therefore be more likely to be better estimates of the responses that would be observed in a population of similar patients. These considerations may suggest that, in phase II trials designed to test agents or combinations in diseases for which active agents already exist, an appropriate randomized concurrent active control group may be useful to help estimate the clinical importance of the new agent or combination prior to attempting to evaluate a phase II agent or combination in a larger, more definitive trial.

PHASE III TRIALS

Phase III clinical trials require the largest number of patients. These trials are designed to compare the ability of two or more therapies, or combinations of therapies, to treat patients with a particular disease. Three or more treatments can be randomized against one another; however, the remainder of this section focuses on studies comparing two treatments. Although these studies can be accomplished at single institutions, randomized phase III trials often involve groups of institutions that combine their resources to accrue larger numbers of patients in order to answer study questions within a reasonable period.

Phase III trials are randomized to ensure unbiased placement of patients into the study arms and to allow probability to provide approximately equivalent patients on the arms. Ideally, differences noted between two arms of a randomized study should be due to the treatment, not to imbalances in patient characteristics. In order to randomize, a computer program that creates random sequences of treatment group identifiers is typically employed. A procedure known as *blocking* is often employed to ensure even numbers of patients on each arm throughout the trial. For every fixed number of patients (e.g., 4, 6, 8), equal numbers of patients receive both treatments by the end of the block. For example, with a block size of six, three patients would each receive treatment A and three would receive treatment B in some random order in the first block. In the next block, three patients would each receive treatment A and treatment B but in a (probably) different random order from the prior block. The objective is to provide balance in the study after fixed periods and to create a pattern of treatment assignment that is difficult to discern by investigators in order to prevent bias in entering patients in the study.

Conducting randomized studies is sometimes difficult when the treatments administered might have different long-term physical effects or changes in patients being entered into the trial. For example, in early-stage breast cancer,

it can be difficult to enroll patients into a study randomizing between lumpectomy plus radiation versus mastectomy. Other designs can be used if randomization is overly problematic to accomplish; however, these other approaches have potentially serious drawbacks. Consultation with a statistician about alternatives to standard randomization schemes may be worthwhile in those situations.

Patients are typically randomized in equal proportions between the two arms; that is, in a 1:1 ratio. However, a 2:1 randomization is sometimes employed. In such cases, typically two patients would receive the newer treatment to every one patient who receives the more conventional therapy. The best rationale for this method would be to gain more information about the new treatment. For example, in some studies it may be considered more of an inducement for investigators to put patients in a trial if they believed that their patients will have a better than 50% chance of receiving the new or experimental therapy. On the other hand, 50% allocation is more consistent with the belief of equipoise, or genuine unbiased indifference toward the placement of patients in trials, which in theory is required for physicians before entering patients into randomized studies. In a 2:1 randomization trial, only 10% to 15% additional patients would be required than a corresponding 1:1 allocation, so the numbers of additional patients needed are small. On the other hand, by using this design, it may be a clue to the subject and to the physician that one intervention is preferred over the other. Thus potential for unintended bias may result.

Stratification

In order to balance prognostic characteristics among patients on the two or more treatment arms in a randomized phase III trial, stratification is often employed. Stratification refers to placing patients into relatively homogeneous groups before performing the randomization. With this approach, patients are randomized within one stratum independently of patients who have characteristics of another stratum. Stratification is more helpful in trials with relatively few patients where probability might not permit patients to balance out with respect to important characteristics over the course of accrual. Stratification at time of randomization is not necessary to perform stratified or subgroup analysis at the end of the trial. One should try to limit the number of strata. Overstratification, defined as placing patients into an excessive number of strata, is not useful and may result in situations in which there will be so few patients in any given stratum that the final trial may end up with a greatly imbalanced number of patients between the two arms.

As an example of stratification in a phase III trial, consider the following: the two treatment arms are designated as A and B, and it is assumed that there were two important prognostic factors for patients with the particular disease: (a) size of tumor and (b) nodal involvement, each with two categories. Size may be classified as being less than 2 cm or more than 2 cm and patients may either have or not have nodal involvement. Thus four possible categories result from these two factors: (a) less than 2 cm with nodal involvement, less than 2 cm without nodal involvement, more than 2 cm with nodal involvements, and more than 2 cm without nodal involvement. Patients are randomized separately to treatment A or B within each of these four categories to ensure an approximately equal number of patients receiving both treatments within each category.

Sample Size Determination

Determination of sample size for a phase III trial is a multi-step process. The first step is to decide the primary end point of interest. For example, a simple end point would be a comparison of the proportions of patients responding to therapy; for example, does the proportion responding to one therapy equal the proportion responding to the other therapy or do the response proportions differ? Another end point could be disease-free survival; for example, for patients who have their disease eliminated at or before the start of therapy, how long does it take for the disease to return with either therapy, and are these intervals different? Survival is a common end point that is measured from date of randomization until the date of death or last follow up. Progression-free survival can also be determined from the date of randomization until the date progression is first noted.

The next step is to decide whether a one-tailed or two-tailed hypothesis test should be used. A one-tailed test would indicate that the difference between the two groups is of interest in only one direction; for example, to test whether therapy A would be better than therapy B. A two-tailed test is used to determine whether the two therapies are different and allows for the possibility that either one could be better. The reason for making this decision is that the significance level, known as *alpha (α)*, is affected by it. A two-tailed test would require somewhat greater numbers of patients than a one-tailed test, all else being equal. A two-tailed test is generally preferred unless there is strong justification for expecting a difference in only one direction.[7]

Once the decision has been made about whether to use a one-tailed or two-tailed test, the next step is to estimate the magnitude of results to be obtained and the minimum difference of interest between study arms. In order to do so, it is best to use estimates based on the literature in the same patient population, if such data exist. It is most important to try not to assume that the two arms would result in extreme differences in outcome because the study will end up with too few patients to identify a significant difference if an effect is noted. Therefore, it is useful to be conservative.

The next step is to estimate the approximate accrual rate of the particular types of patients to be treated. Again, it is useful to be conservative. If the trial is unable to accrue patients at the expected rate, this deficiency could lead to termination of the trial without useful results. The fifth step is to decide the magnitude of errors that would be acceptable to make. Table 66.3 presents definitions of alpha and beta, known as the type I and type II error in the context of a comparative trial. As shown in this table, type I and type II errors are made when clinical trial results differ from the real relationship between the two arms.

Based on the preceding steps, a preliminary sample size estimate can be made. In order to do so, a variety of methods are possible depending on the outcome of interest. In Table 66.4, an example of the number of patients required to detect a difference between two proportions is presented for a two-tailed alpha level of 0.05. Based on hypothetical values of response proportions in two arms on a trial, the number of patients required per arm is tabled according to the specified power, where power is defined as $(1 - beta \times 100\%$. As can be seen by examining Table 66.4, the number of patients required per arm for this type of study varies greatly depending on the anticipated or clinically meaningful difference between the two arms. For a study with 80% power, a comparison of 20% versus 50% responses requires only 45 patients per arm, whereas a trial seeking a difference between 20% and 30% would require 313 patients per arm.

This method of determining the sample size is simple. Other more complex methods are available for determining sample size with survival-type end points, such as overall survival, disease-free survival, or progression-free survival. These techniques consider factors such as the relative ratios of median survival, disease-free survival, or progression-free survival between the two groups, the amount of follow-up time per patient, and the accrual rate. These methods can be more complex to implement, but they can result in a requirement for fewer patients than using the method based

TABLE 66.3. DEFINITIONS OF TYPE I AND TYPE II ERRORS IN CONTEXT OF COMPARATIVE CLINICAL TRIAL

		Decision	
		Two Treatments Equal	One Treatment Better Than the Other
Actual Relationship	Two Treatments are Equal	OK	α-Type 1 Error
	One Treatment Better	β-Type II Error Power-$(1-\beta) \times 100\%$	OK

TABLE 66.4. NUMBER OF PATIENTS REQUIRED TO DETECT DIFFERENCE BETWEEN TWO PROPORTIONS (TWO-TAILED $\alpha = 0.05$)

Hypothetical Values		Patients Per Arm According to Power		
		70%	80%	90%
P_2	P_2			
0.2	0.25	900	1,134	1,504
0.2	0.30	250	313	412
0.2	0.35	122	151	197
0.2	0.40	74	91	118
0.2	0.45	50	62	79
0.2	0.50	37	45	57

From Fleiss JL. *Statistical methods for rates and proportions,* 2nd ed. New York: John Wiley and Sons, 1981:266, with permission.

on comparing proportions of patients alive or disease-free by a fixed point in time. It is important to realize that the sample size estimate is just a guess of the number of patients needed to find a significant difference. The final end point results may be different from those projected. Thus it may be sufficient to use a sample size estimate based on something as simple as a proportion alive at a given point in time because the assumptions that were employed with the more complex approaches may not turn out to be correct.

Once this preliminary sample size estimate has been determined, the length of the accrual period required can be calculated. If this accrual period is likely to be too lengthy, then it may be necessary to reevaluate the parameters used for calculating the sample size. For example, if there is willingness to tolerate greater errors in the study, or there are ways to increase the accrual by including additional institutions in the study, or a difference of a larger magnitude would be acceptable to try to detect with the trial, then these decisions can be used to address the feasibility of conducting the trial. It is important to realize that, for a specific number of patients accrued, only a difference of a given magnitude can be detected. Thus if not enough patients can be accrued for the study in order to detect a difference of a reasonable magnitude, then whether the study can be conducted in the framework that has been selected must be evaluated. For example, it is not a good practice to reevaluate study design parameters and then decide that it is acceptable to detect only an unrealistically large difference. Failure to conclude that an observed difference is statistically significant may be due to either a correct finding of no (or little) difference or a type II error; that is, the lack of power to correctly identify the difference. Freiman et al.[8] determined that of 71 randomized studies with conclusions of no difference between therapies, 50 of these studies were too small to have 90% power to identify a 50% difference in outcome. Thus trials with insufficient patients were found to be prevalent but should be avoided because of the lack of certainty about the interpretations of results.

Analysis

The type of analysis used in phase III trials largely depends on the type of end point being considered in the trial. When the proportions of patients responding to treatment are the primary end point, a test for differences of binomial proportions is sufficient. For example, depending on the numbers of patients being evaluated in these trials, a Chi-squared statistic or Fisher's exact test might be appropriate.

Many trials in oncology focus on end points such as survival, disease-free survival, or progression-free survival. When the main end point in a trial is time to an event, in order to describe the data, the most common approach used is the Kaplan-Meier method.[9] An example of a pair of Kaplan-Meier curves is presented in Figure 66.1. As can be seen, the curves have the following characteristics: initially, all of the patients were alive or in remission and thus the proportion surviving, or remaining disease-free, was 100%. As time progressed, events were noted by drops in the curve at the times at which the events took place. Patients who did not have the event in question occur during the period of observation were considered to have censored observations and had their follow-up times denoted by small, vertical tick marks on the curves. Thus Kaplan-Meier curves incorporate all follow-up data on all patients. They only reach 0% if the patient with the longest follow-up has the event in question. In the example in Figure 66.1, the patient with the longest follow-up in the arm (denoted by open squares) dies shortly after 36 months, whereas in the other arm, a patient with approximately 39 months of follow-up remains alive. These curves are constructed such that the magnitude of the drop is proportional to the number of patients who remain at risk for the event at the time at which the event occurs. Thus, early in time, any drops are small because a large number of patients are potentially at risk, whereas at later time points, few patients are at risk

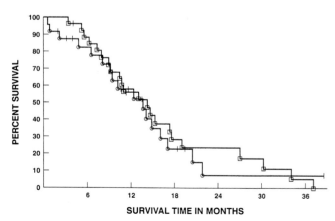

FIGURE 66.1. Example of Kaplan-Meier survival curves. Treatment A denoted by circles (○) and treatment B denoted by squares (□). The two curves are not statistically significantly different from one another ($P_6 = 0.73$).

and the drops are larger. As would be expected, because the drops in the curve are larger later on, greater variability is introduced at this point in the curve. In studies with large numbers of patients, it may be difficult to graphically display the follow-up time of every patient entered into the study, whether a failure or a censored observation. In those cases, it is useful to provide a count of the number of patients remaining at risk along the time axis.

Evaluation of the difference between two survival curves, such as those shown in Figure 66.1, may be done through a variety of methods. The most commonly used technique is known as the Mantel-Haenszel method[10] which considers the actual times of events and provides a generally accepted test for the difference between two curves. This type of test is not always the most appropriate, especially if curves cross one another. In those cases, other methods of analysis can be used. However, in general, it is important to decide in advance of seeing the results of the study which method to use in order to avoid selecting the test that results in the most significant result. For example, in Figure 66.1, the two treatments have approximately the same results. Using a Mantel-Haenszel statistic, the p-value is 0.73. Thus it is easy to see that neither treatment is preferred. In Figure 66.2, however, a difference could be interpreted as being of borderline statistical significance, $p_2 = 0.06$, between the two groups.

Kaplan-Meier survival curves and Mantel-Haenszel statistics can be useful to help identify potential prognostic factors in patients on randomized studies. In Figure 66.3A, all six patients with a low value of a potential prognostic marker survive, whereas the 27 patients with a higher value of the prognostic marker experience significantly greater mortality ($p_2 = .05$). In Figure 66.3B, the patients are further divided according to whether they have metastatic or localized disease. All patients with a low value of the marker had localized disease. As shown in this figure, when

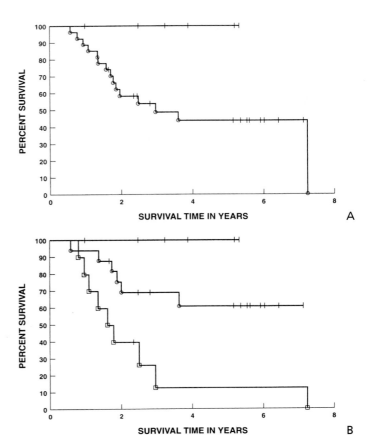

FIGURE 66.3 A: Use of Kaplan-Meier curves to help elucidate prognostic effects. In the top curve (no symbols), all six patients with a low value of a potential prognostic marker survive, whereas those with a higher value experience significantly greater mortality ($p_2 = 0.05$). **B:** Same data as Figure 66.3A, but now examining effect of metastatic disease as well. Top curve (no symbols): localized disease with low levels of the marker; middle curve ($\bigcirc$), localized disease with high levels of the marker; bottom curve ($\square$), metastatic disease with high levels of the marker. Statistical comparisons are as follows: local/low vs. local/high: $p_2 = 0.14$; local/high vs. metastatic/high: $p_2 = 0.012$.

one divides the patients according to whether the disease is metastatic or localized, it becomes less clear whether the marker has the beneficial effect or whether the effect is more an attribute of having localized or metastatic disease. The top and middle curves present a comparison of patients with localized disease according to low versus high values of the marker, and in this group of patients, the p-value for the difference between the two curves is 0.14. Patients with metastatic disease all had high marker values, and their survival curve drops rapidly. The comparison between patients with a high marker value for the localized versus metastatic disease is significant ($p_2 = 0.012$). This example illustrates how Kaplan-Meier curves can help explain the effects of more than one prognostic factor on a time-to-event (e.g., survival) end point.

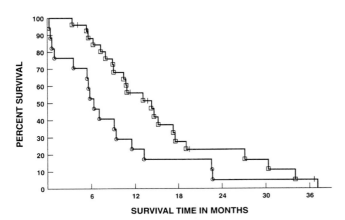

FIGURE 66.2. Example of two Kaplan-Meier survival curves in which two treatments have virtually significantly different effects on outcome ($p_2 = 0.060$).

COX PROPORTIONAL HAZARDS REGRESSION MODELS

In 1972, Professor D. R. Cox published a method for analyzing multiple prognostic factors from clinical trials with time-to-event end points.[11] The method, known as the *Cox proportional hazards model,* is widely used today and is generally considered an acceptable method for determining the relative importance of potentially prognostic factors in a group of patients under investigation in a clinical trial with a time-to-event end point. An excellent discussion of the Cox proportional hazards model can be found in a book intended to be read by clinicians.[12]

The Cox proportional hazards model assumes that the risks of failure on two or more Kaplan-Meier survival curves are proportional. That is, the death rates for individuals with nonbaseline values of some factor under evaluation are constant multiples of the death rates of patients who have baseline values of the factors. Specifically, this assumption means that the Cox proportional hazards model is not suitable when the Kaplan-Meier survival curves crossed at some point in time. Because this is a regression technique, some of the general guidelines that apply to linear regression analysis apply to proportional hazards regression analysis as well. For example, it is not good practice to include more parameters in a model than the square root of the number of failures in the data set. For example, in a study of 100 patients with a total of 30 patients dying, it might be reasonable to develop a model with up to five parameters, provided that such a large number of factors could be suitably interpreted.

An important outcome measure from the Cox proportional hazards model is an estimate of the relative risk of death for patients having one level of a potentially prognostic variable compared to patients who have the baseline level of the potentially prognostic variable. For example, Table 66.5 shows that three parameters (i.e., stage, gender, and metastases) were simultaneously identified to be associated with survival in a group of patients. According to the results shown in the table, each of these parameters is statistically significant in the presence of one another. Stage, which has a p-value of .031, is shown to have a relative risk of 3.74. If only patients with either stage 3 or stage 4 disease are entered into the study, then patients with stage 4 disease have approximately 3.74 times the risk of dying at any given point than patients who have stage 3 disease. Similarly with gender, if the baseline group were males, then females would have approximately 50% more risk (e.g., 1.5 times the relative risk) of dying during any small interval of time. Patients with metastatic disease would have 15 times the relative risk of dying compared to patients with localized disease only. These statistics are the results of all three of these characteristics taken simultaneously. In the Kaplan-Meier survival curve, typically only one factor is portrayed at a time. In the Cox proportional hazards model results, the effects can be identified simultaneously and are adjusted for the effects of the other parameters. Because patients have a constellation of traits that could be important in prognosis, the Cox proportional hazards model results, if based on appropriate factors, are considered preferable to results obtained only in a univariate fashion. The univariate results, however, are useful for illustrative purposes and for leading one to identify factors for consideration in proportional hazards models. Also shown in Table 66.5 is the 95% confidence interval for the relative risk for each of the three factors in the model. This figure is important because it provides an indication of the preciseness of the estimated relative risk. For example, although stage has a relative risk of 3.74, the 95% confidence interval ranges from 1.26 to 11.1, meaning that it is likely that the true relative risk is between 1.25 and 11.00. For gender, there is a tighter interval from approximately 1 to approximately 2, whereas the interval for metastases ranges from 4 roughly to 53.

GROUP SEQUENTIAL DESIGNS

Some small clinical trials are designed to accrue the total number of patients originally intended without any interim evaluations for efficacy; however, in many phase III studies, particularly those of moderate to large size, the design must allow for the possibility of early termination of the trial if results appear to be statistically significant early on. Trials that allow for formal evaluations that could result in termination after fixed prespecified points are called *group sequential designs.* A whole body of literature exists on these designs. Two specific, easily described designs permit examination of the data at prespecified time points and adjust the p-values required for termination so that highly significant findings may lead to termination of the trial depending on proximity to the planned end of the trial. These two methods were developed in the late 1970s. The first, by Pocock,[13] allows one to terminate the trial when a p-value of less than some small fixed value, which remains constant for each potential evaluation, is reached. For example, in a study with plans for up to five equally spaced looks at the data prior to termination of accrual, if at any of the five looks the significance of the difference between the two

TABLE 66.5. EXAMPLE OF COX PROPORTIONAL HAZARDS MODEL RESULTS

Variable	Parameter Estimate	p-Value	Relative Risk (RR)	95% Confidence Interval for RR
Stage	1.32	0.031	3.74	(1.26, 11.10)
Gender	0.74	0.027	1.49	(1.07, 2.08)
Metastases	2.71	0.0037	15.03	(4.25, 53.15)

groups was such that p_2 was less than 0.008, then accrual to the study could be terminated because this result could be shown to be consistent with a final p-value of less than 0.05. Another approach, developed by O'Brien and Fleming,[14] allows for decreasingly stringent p-values to be used in the evaluation at successive interim looks. For example, in this same example with five interim evaluations, if at the first evaluation the p-value were less than approximately 3×10^{-6}, then accrual would terminate. The p-value required for termination would increase gradually, so that at the second evaluation the required p-value would be 7×10^{-4}; 4×10^{-3} would be the threshold for the third evaluation, .011 for the fourth, and .021 for the fifth interim evaluation. Many other possible designs have been studied and can be considered for use in clinical trials. The important point is that stopping a trial early because of an interim significant finding requires great care. It is insufficient to stop accrual with an early p-value of .05 because it can be shown that it is likely, if the study were to progress to the intended accrual target, that the ultimate p-value could be much greater than .05 and thus one would have erred in making this early decision.

METAANALYSIS

Conducting a randomized clinical trial can be a time-consuming and expensive process, and sometimes the answer to a major clinical question might be obtained by examining and synthesizing the results of other research that has been previously conducted. *Metaanalysis* is a term that was first used in the mid 1970s by an educational researcher, and is a discipline that critically reviews and systematically statistically combines the results of previously conducted research studies. An article by Sacks et al.[15] provides a description of the subject. The purposes of metaanalysis are to increase the statistical power of primary end points and within subgroups, to resolve uncertainty when reports disagree, to understand interstudy differences and results, to improve estimates of effect size, and to answer questions not posed at the start of individual trials.[15] When studies that are pooled are similar with respect to the treatment, the patient population, and data quality, then averaging results makes sense.[16] However, in practice, the doses of drugs actually delivered differ, the patient population may differ, and there may be different degrees of protocol compliance, adequacy of follow-up, and reliability of data. Perhaps well-designed and well-conducted clinical trials are still the best means of answering questions concerning what treatments are effective and how effective they are.

Sacks et al. published a careful evaluation of metaanalyses in the English language medical literature.[15] In order to be included in their report, data from more than one study had to be combined, and at least one of the studies pooled had to be a randomized controlled trial. This study determined that the number of articles that can be included in their metaanalysis increased rapidly through the mid-1980s, from a starting point in the 1950s, when few such articles existed. These authors identified six major areas for determining the quality of a metaanalysis: study design, combinability, control and measurement of potential bias, statistical analysis and methodology used, sensitivity analysis, and the application of the results. These six major areas were further subdivided into 23 individual items. Their study determined that 28% of the metaanalyses addressed all six of these major areas, 36% addressed five, 29% addressed four, and 7% addressed either two or three of these areas. When the individual items, and thus the quality of the metaanalyses, were examined, out of 23 possible items, not a single paper received more than 14 adequate ratings, and in most articles, 5 to 8 of the 23 points were addressed. Thus it was believed that many metaanalyses that were reported were not adequate on several grounds.

A properly performed metaanalysis can be useful in a setting where one wants to obtain a global answer to an important question incorporating the results from a large number of properly done and reported studies. Metaanalyses should be reported with sufficient information in order for the readers to draw conclusions about the validity of the results reported. A metaanalysis should be conducted like a scientific experiment with a clear study design, evaluation methods, and results presented. Because metaanalyses typically use results of published clinical trials, there is a potential bias in the articles that can be included in a metaanalysis. It is well known that clinical trials with positive results are more likely to be published than ones with negative results. Unpublished trials might be less reliable and might not be conducted with the same care as published studies. Nonetheless, this is a bias because not all studies may be included in the metaanalysis.

There are instances, however, of metaanalyses that are conducted on large numbers of trials that can produce interesting results, which could not necessarily have been found from the examination of any single trial. As an example, the Early Breast Cancer Trialist's Collaborative Group performed a metaanalysis based on 133 randomized trials from around the world involving 24,000 deaths among 75,000 women.[17] This metaanalysis was able to demonstrate highly significant reductions in the annual rates of recurrence and of death by use of Tamoxifen, although the results varied. Because this metaanalysis was performed on an extensive group of randomized clinical trials run by centers and consortiums from around the world and conducted with great care by the organizing committee in Oxford, England, this metaanalysis may be valuable because complex questions were able to be answered without the need to resort to additional randomized clinical trials.

As a second example, the Non-small Cell Lung Cancer Collaborative Group performed a metaanalysis based on 52 randomized clinical trials from around the world, which included 9,387 patients, of whom 7,151 died.[18] The objective of the metaanalysis was to determine the impact of cytotoxic chemotherapy on survival in patients with non–small cell lung cancer. This study demonstrated that modern chemotherapy regimens containing cisplatin were favored in all comparisons performed, and that the benefit attained conventional levels of statistical significance when combined with radical radiotherapy and supportive care. This metaanalysis was carefully performed, involved a large worldwide set of all available trials, including unpublished studies, and was done under the auspices of a group with substantial expertise in conducting such studies. Thus the conclusions of this metaanalysis are likely to be reliable and would obviate the need for additional randomized trials to address the specific questions being posed in this study, which had remained controversial and uncertain until this metaanalysis was performed.

REFERENCES

1. Simon R, Freidlin B, Rubinstein L, et al. Accelerated titration designs for Phase I clinical trials in oncology. *J Natl Cancer Inst* 1997;89:1138.
2. Ahn C. An evaluation of phase I cancer clinical trial designs. *Stat Med* 1998;17:1537.
3. Leventhal BG, Wittes RE. *Research methods in clinical oncology.* New York: Raven Press, 1988:41.
4. Gehan EA. The determination of the number of patients required in a follow-up trial of a new chemotherapeutic agent. *J Chronic Diseases* 1961;13:346.
5. Lee YJ, Wesley RA. Statistical contributions to phase II trials in cancer: interpretation, analysis and design. *Semin Oncol* 1981;8:403.
6. Simon RM. Optimal two-stage designs for phase II clinical trials. *Controlled Clinical Trials* 1989;10:1.
7. Friedman LM, Furburg CD, DeMets DL. *Fundamentals of clinical trials,* 3rd ed. New York: Springer, 1998.
8. Freiman JA, Chalmers TC, Smith H Jr, et al. The importance of Beta, the type II error, and sample size in the design and interpretation of the randomized control trial. *N Engl J Med* 1978;299:690.
9. Kaplan E, Meier P. Non-parametric estimation from incomplete observations. *J Am Stat Assoc* 1958;53:457.
10. Mantel N. Evaluation of survival data and two new rank order statistics arising in its consideration. *Cancer Chemo Rep* 1966;50:163.
11. Cox DR. Regression models and life tables. *J Royal Statistical Society* 1972;34:187.
12. Matthews DE, Farewell VT. *Using and understanding medical statistics.* Basel: Karger, 1985:148.
13. Pocock SJ. Group sequential methods in the design and analysis of clinical trials. *Biometrika* 1977;64:191.
14. O'Brien PC, Fleming TR. A multiple testing procedure for clinical trials. *Biometrics* 1979;35:549.
15. Sacks BS, Berrier J, Reitman D, et al. Meta-analyses of randomized controlled trials. *N Engl J Med* 1987;316:450.
16. Simon R. Overviews of randomized clinical trials (editorial). *Cancer Treat Rep* 1987;71:3.
17. Early Breast Cancer Trialists' Collaborative Group. Systemic treatment of early breast cancer by hormonal, cytotoxic, or immune therapy. *Lancet* 1992;339:1.
18. Non-small Cell Lung Cancer Collaborative Group. Chemotherapy in non-small cell lung cancer: a meta-analysis using updated data on individual patients from 52 randomized clinical trials. *Br Med J* 1995;311:899.

SUBJECT INDEX

Page numbers followed by f indicate figures; those followed by t indicate tables.